DAVID A. MORROW, D.V.M., Ph.D

Professor of Large Animal Clinical Sciences
Michigan State University
College of Veterinary Medicine
East Lansing, Michigan

CURRENT THERAPY IN
Theriogenology

2

DIAGNOSIS, TREATMENT
AND PREVENTION OF
REPRODUCTIVE DISEASES
IN SMALL AND
LARGE ANIMALS

W. B. Saunders Company   1986
Philadelphia London Toronto Mexico City
Rio de Janeiro Sydney Tokyo Hong Kong

W. B. Saunders Company: West Washington Square
                         Philadelphia, PA 19105

Library of Congress Cataloging in Publication Data

Main entry under title:

Current therapy in theriogenology.

  Includes bibliographies and index.
1. Theriogenology.   I. Morrow, David A. [DNLM:
  1. Genital Diseases, Female—veterinary.   2. Obstetrics—
  veterinary.   3. Reproduction.   4. Veterinary Medicine.
  SF 871 C976]

SF871.C84 1986   636.089'8   85-11937

ISBN 0-7216-6580-2

Designer: Karen O'Keefe
Production Managers: Laura Tarves and Frank Polizzano
Manuscript Editor: Roger Wall
Illustration Coordinator: Walter Verbitski

Cover Illustration: Courtesy of Margaret Muns, B.A., who is a veterinary student at Michigan State University.

Current Therapy in Theriogenology   ISBN   0–7216–6580–2

Last digit is the print number: 9   8   7   6   5   4   3   2   1

Contributors

GEORGE P. ALLEN, Ph.D., Associate Professor, Department of Veterinary Science, College of Agriculture, University of Kentucky, Lexington, Kentucky.

RUPERT P. AMANN, Ph.D., Professor, Animal Reproduction Laboratory, Colorado State University, Ft. Collins, Colorado.

KEVIN L. ANDERSON, D.V.M., M.S., Ph.D., Assistant Professor, Department of Food Animal and Equine Medicine, School of Veterinary Medicine, North Carolina State University, Raleigh, North Carolina.

JOAN M. ARNOLDI, D.V.M., M.S., Director, Bureau of Technical Services, State Humane Agent, Wisconsin Department of Agriculture, Madison, Wisconsin.

A. C. ASBURY, D.V.M., Professor, College of Veterinary Medicine, University of Florida, and Clinician, Veterinary Medical Teaching Hospital, University of Florida, Gainesville, Florida.

MARIANNE ASH, D.V.M., Staff Veterinarian, Yeager & Sullivan, Inc., Camden, Indiana.

MELVIN W. BALK, D.V.M., M.S., Charles River Breeding Laboratories, Inc., Wilmington, Massachusetts.

LESLIE BALL, D.V.M., M.S., Diplomate, American College of Theriogenologists, Professor, Department of Clinical Science, College of Veterinary Medicine and Biomedical Science, and Clinician, Veterinary Teaching Hospital, Colorado State University, Ft. Collins, Colorado.

DONELLE R. BANKS, Ph.D., Lecturer, Department of Biological Sciences, California State University, Sacramento, California.

JEANNE A. BARSANTI, D.V.M., M.S., Diplomate, American College of Veterinary Internal Medicine, Associate Professor of Internal Medicine, College of Veterinary Medicine, and Clinician, University Teaching Hospital, University of Georgia, Athens, Georgia.

ALBERT D. BARTH, D.V.M., M.V.Sc., Associate Professor, Theriogenology, Western College of Veterinary Medicine, University of Saskatchewan, Saskatoon, Saskatchewan, Canada.

PAUL C. BARTLETT, D.V.M., M.P.H., Assistant Professor, Department of Large Animal Clinical Sciences, College of Veterinary Medicine, Michigan State University, East Lansing, Michigan.

PARVATHI K. BASRUR, B.Sc., M.Sc., Ph.D., Professor, Department of Biomedical Sciences, and Consultant, Medical Genetics, Teaching Hospital, Ontario Veterinary College, University of Guelph, Guelph, Ontario, Canada.

H. NEIL BECKER, D.V.M., M.S., Associate Professor, College of Veterinary Medicine and Service Chief, Rural Animal Medicine Service, Veterinary Medical Teaching Hospital, College of Veterinary Medicine, University of Florida, Gainesville, Florida.

ANNE-CHARLOTTE BENGTSSON, M.Sc., Research Assistant, Swedish University of Agricultural Sciences, Department of Farm Buildings, Lund, Sweden.

EZRA BERMAN, D.V.M., Chief, Physiology Section, Experimental Biology Division, Health Effects Research Laboratory, Environmental Protection Agency, Research Triangle Park, North Carolina.

GREGG W. BEVIER, D.V.M., M.S., Visiting Assistant Professor, University of Illinois, Champaign, Illinois; Pig Improvement Co., Franklin, Kentucky.

W. SHELDON BIVIN, D.V.M., Ph.D., Professor, Veterinary Clinical Sciences, Director, Laboratory Animal Medicine, and Clinician, Exotic Animal Medicine and Surgery, Veterinary Teaching Hospital and Clinic, Louisiana State University, Baton Rouge, Louisiana.

ROBERT H. BONDURANT, D.V.M., Associate Professor of Veterinary Reproduction, School of Veterinary Medicine, and Service Chief, Food Animal Reproduction and Herd Health, Veterinary Medical Teaching Hospital, University of California, Davis, California.

J. M. BOWEN, F.R.C.V.S., Associate Professor, College of Veterinary Medicine, Texas A&M University, College Station, Texas.

MONICA J. BOWEN, B.V.Sc., M.R.C.V.S., Research Associate, Veterinary Physiology and Pharmacology, College of Veterinary Medicine, Texas A&M University, College Station, Texas.

R. KENNETH BRAUN, D.V.M., M.S., Specialty Board, American College of Theriogenologists, Professor and Chairman, Department of Preventive Medicine, College of Veterinary Medicine, Clinician, Food Animal Herd Health, Veterinary Medical Teaching Hospital, University of Florida, Gainesville, Florida.

WILLIAM F. BRAUN, JR., D.V.M., Diplomate, American College of Theriogenologists, Associate Professor of Veterinary Medicine and Surgery, Theriogenology Section, College of Veterinary Medicine, University of Missouri, Columbia, Missouri.

KATHERINE N. BRETZLAFF, D.V.M., M.S., Research Associate, College of Veterinary Medicine, University of Illinois, Urbana, Illinois.

F. BRISTOL, B.V.Sc., M.Sc., Professor, Department of Herd Medicine and Theriogenology, Western College of Veterinary Medicine, and Clinician, Large Animal Clinic, University of Saskatchewan, Saskatoon, Saskatchewan, Canada.

JACK H. BRITT, Ph.D., Professor of Reproductive Physiology, Department of Animal Science, North Carolina State University, Raleigh, North Carolina.

A. NEIL BRUERE, B.V.Sc., Ph.D., D.V.Sc., F.A.C.V.Sc., Professor of Veterinary Medicine and Head, Department of Veterinary Clinical Sciences, Massey University, Palmerston North, New Zealand.

DAVID B. BRUNSON, D.V.M., M.S., Assistant Professor of Anesthesiology, Department of Surgical Sciences, School of Veterinary Medicine, University of Wisconsin, Madison, Wisconsin.

JOHN T. BRYANS, Ph.D., Professor and Chairman, Department of Veterinary Science, College of Agriculture University of Kentucky, Lexington, Kentucky.

J. ROSS BUDDLE, B.Sc., B.V.Sc., D.V.P.H., M.A.C.V.Sc., Senior Lecturer in Pig Medicine and Production, School of Veterinary Studies, Murdoch University, Western Australia.

MARIE S. BULGIN, D.V.M., Diplomate, American College of Veterinary Medicine, Associate Professor, WOI Interstate Veterinary Program, University of Idaho, Moscow, Idaho, Food Animal Medicine Clinic, Caldwell Veterinary Teaching Center, Caldwell, Idaho.

STUART J. BURNS, D.V.M., M.S., Associate Professor of Veterinary Medicine, College of Veterinary Medicine Large Animal Clinic, Texas A&M University, College Station, Texas.

THOMAS J. BURKE, D.V.M., M.S., Associate Professor of Medicine, College of Veterinary Medicine, University of Illinois, Urbana, Illinois; Consultant, Capitol Illini Veterinary Hospital, Springfield, Illinois.

MITCHELL BUSH, D.V.M., National Zoological Park, Smithsonian Institution, Washington, D.C.

JERRY CALDWELL, Ph.D., President, ImmGen Inc., College Station, Texas.

CARLA L. CARLETON, D.V.M., M.S., Diplomate, American College of Theriogenologists, Assistant Professor, Equine Theriogenology, College of Veterinary Medicine, and Clinician, Michigan State University Veterinary Clinical Center, Department of Large Animal Clinical Sciences, Michigan State University, East Lansing, Michigan.

TERRY D. CARRUTHERS, D.V.M., Ph.D., Associate Professor, Department of Veterinary Physiological Sciences, University of Saskatchewan, Saskatoon, Saskatchewan, Canada.

PETER J. CHENOWETH, B.V.Sc., Ph.D., Diplomate, American College of Theriogenologists, Senior Lecturer, Department of Veterinary Medicine, School of Veterinary Science, University of Queensland, St. Lucia, Queensland, Australia.

CHARLES J. CHRISTIANS, B.S., M.S., Ph.D., Professor of Animal Science, University of Minnesota, St. Paul, Minnesota.

L. KIRK CLARK, D.V.M., Ph.D., Associate Professor of Veterinary Medicine, College of Veterinary Medicine, Department of Large Animal Clinics, Purdue University, West Lafayette, Indiana.

EMERSON D. COLBY, D.V.M., M.S., Director, Animal Research Facilities, Associate Professor in Physiology, Dartmouth Medical School, Hanover, New Hampshire.

ROBERT J. COLLIER, Ph.D., Monsanto, St. Louis, Missouri.

PATRICK W. CONCANNON, Ph.D., Senior Research Associate, Department of Physiology, New York State College of Veterinary Medicine, Cornell University, Ithaca, New York.

M. D. COPLAND, B.V.Sc., M.A.C.V.S., M.R.C.V.S., Central Veterinary Laboratories, Adelaide, South Australia.

GLENN H. COULTER, B.Sc., (Agr.), Ph.D., Research Scientist (Reproductive Physiology), Agriculture Canada Research Station, Lethbridge, Alberta, Canada.

VICTOR S. COX, D.V.M., Ph.D., Associate Professor of Anatomy, Veterinary Biology Department, College of Veterinary Medicine, University of Minnesota, St. Paul, Minnesota.

BO G. CRABO, D.V.M., Ph.D., Professor of Reproductive Physiology, Department of Animal Science, University of Minnesota, St. Paul, Minnesota.

TERRIE L. CUNLIFFE-BEAMER, D.V.M., M.S., Head, Clinical Laboratory Animal Medicine, Assistant Director, Research Animal Facility, The Jackson Laboratory, Bar Harbor, Maine.

STANLEY E. CURTIS, Ph.D., Professor of Animal Sciences, University of Illinois, Urbana, Illinois.

ROSS CUTLER, B.V.Sc., Ph.D., Department of Food Animal and Equine Medicine, College of Veterinary Medicine, North Carolina State University, Raleigh, North Carolina.

N. M. CZEKALA, B.S., Zoological Society of San Diego, San Diego, California.

ANNA M. DAVIS, B.S., M.S., University of Idaho, Moscow, Idaho.

LLOYD E. DAVIS, D.V.M., Ph.D., Professor of Veterinary Clinical Medicine and Pharmacology, College of Veterinary Medicine, and Director, Clinical Pharmacology Studies Unit, Veterinary Medical Teaching Hospital, University of Illinois, Urbana, Illinois.

S. R. DAVIS, Ph.D., Ruakura Animal Research Station, Ministry of Agriculture and Fisheries, Hamilton, New Zealand.

C. H. W. DE BOIS, Professor of Veterinary Medicine (EM), Veterinary Faculty, Clinic for Veterinary Obstetrics, A.I. and Reproduction, State University of Utrecht, Utrecht, The Netherlands.

PAUL J. DEKEYSER, D.V.M., Head, Department Large Animal Pathology, National Institute of Veterinary Research, Brussels, Belgium.

STANLEY M. DENNIS, B.V.Sc., Ph.D., F.R.C.V.S., F.R.C.Path., Diplomate, American College of Theriogenologists, Professor of Pathology, College of Veterinary Medicine, Kansas State University, Manhattan, Kansas.

GARY D. DIAL, D.V.M., Ph.D., Assistant Professor, School of Veterinary Medicine and Veterinary Teaching Hospital, North Carolina State University, Raleigh, North Carolina.

PAUL A. DOIG, D.V.M., M.Sc., Manager, New Product Development and Technical Services, Syntex Agribusiness, Mississauga, Ontario, Canada.

ROBERT H. DOUGLAS, Ph.D., President, BET Farms and BET Reproductive Laboratories, Lexington, Kentucky.

MAARTEN DROST, D.V.M., Professor of Veterinary Medicine, Department of Reproduction, College of Veterinary Medicine, University of Florida, Gainesville, Florida.

J. P. DUBEY, M.V.Sc., Ph.D., Animal Parasitology Institute, United States Department of Agriculture, Beltsville, Maryland.

BARBARA S. DURRANT, Ph.D., Reproductive Physiologist, Zoological Society of San Diego, San Diego, California.

NANCY E. EAST, D.V.M., M.S., M.P.V.M., Department of Medicine, School of Veterinary Medicine, Veterinary Medicine Teaching Hospital, University of California, Davis, California.

STIG EINARSSON, D.V.M., Ph.D., Professor, Department of Obstetrics and Gynaecology, College of Veterinary Medicine, Swedish University of Agricultural Sciences, Uppsala, Sweden.

WILLIAM A. ELLIS, Ph.D., B.V.M.S., F.R.C.V.S., Senior Veterinary Research Officer, Department of Agriculture, Belfast, Northern Ireland, United Kingdom.

KENNTH L. ESBENSHADE, Ph.D., Associate Professor, Department of Animal Science, School of Veterinary Medicine, North Carolina State University, Raleigh, North Carolina.

L. E. EVANS, D.V.M., Ph.D., Chairman, Department of Veterinary Clinical Sciences, College of Veterinary Medicine, and Director, Veterinary Teaching Hospital, Iowa State University, Ames, Iowa.

E. C. FELDMAN, D.V.M., Associate Professor, School of Veterinary Medicine, and Internist, Veterinary Medical Teaching Hospital, University of California, Davis, California.

E. D. FIELDEN, B.Agr.Sc., B.V.Sc., F.A.C.V.Sc., F.R.C.V.S., Professor of Veterinary Clinical Sciences, Massey University, Palmerston North, New Zealand.

DELMAR R. FINCO, D.V.M., Department of Physiology, College of Veterinary Medicine, University of Georgia, Athens, Georgia.

REG. J. FITZPATRICK, Ph.D., M.R.C.V.S., Professor of Animal Reproduction, Faculty of Veterinary Science, University of Liverpool, and Professor of Animal Reproduction, Division of Farm Animal Medicine, Department of Veterinary Clinical Science, University of Liverpool Veterinary Field Station, Leahurst, Neston, South Wirral, United Kingdom.

JESSICA S. FRANKLIN, D.V.M., Associate Veterinarian, Dundee Veterinary Clinic, Dundee, Michigan.

BRIAN J. GERLOFF, D.V.M., Ph.D., Seneca Bovine Services, Marengo, Illinois.

CHARLES D. GIBSON, D.V.M., Ph.D., Professor of Large Animal Clinical Sciences, College of Veterinary Medicine, Michigan State University, East Lansing, Michigan.

EBERHARD GRUNERT, D.V.M., Ph.D., Professor of Veterinary Obstetrics and Gynecology, Veterinary College of Hanover; Director of the Bovine Clinic of Obstetrics and Gynecology, Hanover, Germany (FRG).

BORJE K. GUSTAFSSON, D.V.M., Ph.D, Professor and Head, Department of Veterinary Clinical Medicine, College of Veterinary Medicine, University of Illinois, Urbana, Illinois.

GEORGE K. HAIBEL, D.V.M., Diplomate, American College of Theriogenologists, Assistant Professor, Department of Veterinary Clinical Sciences, The Ohio State University, Columbus, Ohio.

W. C. D. HARE, M.A.(h.c.), B.Sc., Ph.D., D.V.M.&S., F.R.C.V.S, Head, Reproduction Section, Animal Diseases Research Institute, Animal Pathology Division, Food Production and Inspection Branch, Agriculture Canada, Nepean, Ontario, Canada.

JOHN E. HARKNESS, D.V.M., M.S., M.Ed., Professor of Veterinary Medicine, College of Veterinary Medicine, Mississippi State University, Mississippi State, Mississippi.

AKIRA HASHIMOTO, D.V.M., Ph.D., Assistant Professor, Veterinary Hospital, Faculty of Agriculture, Gifu University, Gifu, Japan.

K. G. HAUGHEY, B.V.Sc., M.A.C.V. Sc., Senior Lecturer in Veterinary Medicine (Sheep), Faculty of Veterinary Science, University of Sydney, Camden, New South Wales, Australia.

NABIL A. HEMEIDA, D.V.M., Ph.D., Professor of Theriogenology and Attending Clinician, Division of Theriogenology, Veterinary Medical Teaching Hospital, Artificial Insemination Center, Faculty of Veterinary Medicine, Cairo University, Giza, Egypt.

P. H. HEMSWORTH, B.Ag.Sci. (Hon), Ph.D., Animal Research Institute, Department of Agriculture, Werribee, Victoria, Australia.

S. C. HENRY, B.S., D.V.M., Clinician, Abilene Animal Hospital, Abilene, Kansas.

MARY A. HERRON, D.V.M., Ph.D., Professor, Department of Veterinary Anatomy, College of Veterinary Medicine, Texas A&M University, College Station, Texas.

HARVEY D. HILLEY, D.V.M., Ph.D., Associate Professor, Leader, Swine Section, Department of Food Animal and Equine Medicine, School of Veterinary Medicine, North Carolina State University, Raleigh, North Carolina.

KATSUYA HIRAI, D.V.M., Ph.D., Assistant Professor, Department of Veterinary Microbiology, Faculty of Agriculture, Gifu University, Gifu, Japan.

R. J. HOLMES, B.V.M.&S., Ph.D., M.R.C.V.S., Senior Lecturer in Animal Behavior, Department of Veterinary Clinical Sciences, Massey University, Palmerston North, New Zealand.

PHYLLIS A. HOLST, D.V.M., M.S., Animal Medical Clinic, Longmont, Colorado.

PETER G. HONEY, B.V.Sc., M.S., Diplomate, American College of Theriogenologists, Practitioner, Snowy River Veterinary Clinic, Orbost, Victoria, Australia.

STEVEN M. HOPKINS, D.V.M., Diplomate, American College of Theriogenologists, Associate Professor, Veterinary Clinical Sciences, College of Veterinary Medicine, Iowa State University, Ames, Iowa.

JOGAYLE HOWARD, D.V.M., National Zoological Park, Smithsonian Institution, Washington, D.C.

THOMAS H. HOWARD, D.V.M., Ph.D., Veterinarian, American Breeders Service, DeForest, Wisconsin.

ROBERT S. HUDSON, D.V.M., M.S., Diplomate, American College of Theriogenologists, Professor, Large Animal Surgery and Medicine, Auburn University, Alabama.

WILLIAM D. HUESTON, D.V.M., M.S., Ph.D., Assistant Professor, Department of Veterinary Preventive Medicine, and Clinical Epidemiologist, Field Services, College of Veterinary Medicine, The Ohio State University, Columbus, Ohio.

JOHN P. HURTGEN, D.V.M., M.S., Ph.D., Private Practitioner, New Freedom, Pennsylvania.

PAUL W. HUSTED, V.M.D., M.S., Assistant Professor, Section Chief, Small Animal Medicine, College of Veterinary Medicine, Colorado State University, Ft. Collins, Colorado.

M. R. JAINUDEEN, B.V.Sc., M.S., Ph.D., Professor of Animal Reproduction, School of Veterinary Medicine, and Director, University Veterinary Hospital, University Pertanian Malaysia, Serdang, Selangor, Malaysia.

CHERI A. JOHNSON, D.V.M., M.S., Diplomate, American College of Veterinary Internal Medicine, Assistant Professor, Small Animal Clinical Sciences, College of Veterinary Medicine, Michigan State University; Head of Internal Medicine, Veterinary Clinical Center, East Lansing, Michigan.

WALTER H. JOHNSON, D.V.M., M.V.Sc., Associate Professor, Ontario Veterinary College, University of Guelph, Guelph, Ontario, Canada.

SHIRLEY D. JOHNSTON, D.V.M., Ph.D., Diplomate, American College of Theriogenologists, Associate Professor, Internal Medicine, College of Veterinary Medicine, University of Minnesota, St. Paul, Minnesota.

ROBERT L. JONES, D.V.M., Ph.D., Assistant Professor, Department of Microbiology, and Head, Bacteriology Section, Diagnostic Laboratory, Colorado State University, Ft. Collins, Colorado.

ROBERT F. KAHRS, D.V.M., Ph.D., Dean, College of Veterinary Medicine, University of Missouri-Columbia, Columbia, Missouri

L. H. KASMAN, Oklahoma City Zoo, Oklahoma City, Oklahoma.

JOHANNA KAUFMAN, D.V.M., M.S. Bulger Animal Hospital, N. Andover, Massachusetts.

KEITH W. KELLY, Ph.D., Professor of Animal Sciences, College of Veterinary Medicine, University of Illinois, Urbana, Illinois.

ROBERT M. KENNEY, D.V.M., Ph.D., Professor of Reproduction, School of Veterinary Medicine, University of Pennsylvania, Philadelphia, Pennsylvania.

M. KIERSTAD, R.T., A.R.T. (Microbiology), Veterinary Laboratory Services, Ontario Ministry of Agriculture and Food, Guelph, Ontario, Canada.

PAUL B. KIMSEY, Ph.D., Research Virologist, Division of Comparative Medicine, Massachusetts Institute of Technology, Cambridge, Massachusetts.

JOHN H. KIRK, D.V.M., Associate Professor, Department of Large Animal Clinical Science, and Head, Field Service Section, College of Veterinary Medicine, Michigan State University, East Lansing, Michigan.

JEFFREY J. KNICKERBOCKER, Ph.D., NIH Postdoctoral Trainee, Department of Physiology and Biophysics, Colorado State University, Ft. Collins, Colorado.

DUANE C. KRAEMER, D.V.M., Ph.D., Professor of Veterinary Physiology and Pharmacology, Animal Science, and Genetics, College of Veterinary Medicine, Texas A&M University, College Station, Texas.

LOUISE LALIBERTÉ, D.M.V., M.Sc., Consultant, Hôpital Vétérinaire Vimont, Auteuil-Laval, Québec, Canada.

K. R. LAPWOOD, B.V.Sc., Ph.D., Reader in Physiology, Faculty of Veterinary Science, Massey University, Palmerston North, New Zealand.

ROLF E. LARSEN, D.V.M., Ph.D., Associate Professor, Department of Reproduction, College of Veterinary Medicine, University of Florida, Gainesville, Florida.

LESTER L. LARSON, D.V.M., Ph.D., Head, Veterinary Department, American Breeders Service Division, W. R. Grace & Co., DeForest, Wisconsin.

KJELL LARSSON, D.V.M., Ph.D., Professor of Artificial Insemination, College of Veterinary Medicine, Swedish University of Agricultural Sciences, Uppsala, Sweden.

WILLIAM L. LASLEY, Ph.D., Department of Reproduction, School of Veterinary Medicine, University of California, Davis, California.

GORDON E. LAYTON, D.V.M., Private Equine Practice, Paris, Kentucky.

MICHELLE M. LEBLANC, D.V.M., Diplomate, American College of Theriogenologists, Assistant Professor of Reproduction, College of Veterinary Medicine, and Clinician, Large and Small Animal Clinic, Veterinary Medical Teaching Hospital, University of Florida, Gainesville, Florida.

DONALD H. LEIN, D.V.M., Ph.D., Associate Professor of Pathology and Theriogenology, New York College of Veterinary Medicine, and Consulting Clinician, Small Animal Clinic, Cornell University, Ithaca, New York.

HORST W. LEIPOLD, Dr. Med. Vet., M.S., Ph.D., Professor of Pathology, College of Veterinary Medicine, Kansas State University, Manhattan, Kansas.

ALLEN D. LEMAN, D.V.M., Ph.D., Professor, Large Animal Clinical Science, College of Veterinary Medicine, University of Minnesota, St. Paul, Minnesota.

TED F. LOCK, D.V.M., M.S., Associate Professor, College of Veterinary Medicine, and Clinician, Large Animal Clinic, University of Illinois, Urbana, Illinois.

R. M. LÖFSTEDT, B.V.Sc., M.C., Diplomate, American College of Theriogenologists, Assistant Professor, School of Veterinary Medicine, and Head, Section of Theriogenology, Large and Small Animal Hospitals, Tufts University, North Grafton, Massachusetts.

N. M. LOSKUTOFF, M.S., Department of Veterinary Physiology, College of Veterinary Medicine, Texas A&M University, College Station, Texas.

JOHN W. LUDDERS, D.V.M., Assistant Professor of Anesthesiology, Department of Surgical Sciences, School of Veterinary Medicine, University of Wisconsin, Madison, Wisconsin.

MAURICE F. McDONALD, M.Agr.Sc., Ph.D., Reader in Animal Science, Massey University, Palmerston North, New Zealand.

DONALD J. MCKENNA, D.V.M., M.S., Assistant Professor of Veterinary Clinical Medicine, College of Veterinary Medicine, University of Illinois, Urbana, Illinois.

ANGUS O. McKINNON, B.V.Sc., M.Sc., Diplomate, American Board of Veterinary Practitioners, Assistant Professor, Veterinary Teaching Hospital, College of Veterinary Medicine, Colorado State University, Ft. Collins, Colorado.

MICHAEL L. MAGNE, D.V.M., M.S, Diplomate, American College Veterinary Internal Medicine, Staff Internist, Santa Cruz Veterinary Hospital, Santa Cruz, California.

JOE E. MANSPEAKER, V.M.D., Associate Professor, VA-MD Regional College of Veterinary Medicine, University of Maryland, College Park, Maryland.

REUBEN J. MAPLETOFT, D.V.M., M.S., Ph.D., Professor of Theriogenology, Department of Herd Medicine and Theriogenology, Western College of Veterinary Medicine, University of Saskatchewan, Saskatoon, Saskatchewan, Canada.

I. C. A. MARTIN, B.V.Sc., Ph.D., F.R.C.V.S., Reader, Department of Veterinary Physiology, University of Sydney, Sydney, Australia.

PAUL A. MARTIN, D.V.M., Ph.D., Associate Professor, Veterinary Medical Research Institute, Iowa State University, Ames, Iowa.

EDWARD C. MATHER, D.V.M., Ph.D., Professor and Chairman, Department of Large Animal Clinical Sciences, College of Veterinary Medicine, Michigan State University, East Lansing, Michigan.

PETER MAZUR, Ph.D., Professor, University of Tennessee–Oak Ridge Graduate School of Biomedical Sciences, and Senior Research Staff, Biology Division, Oak Ridge National Laboratory, Oak Ridge, Tennessee.

WILLIAM L. MENGELING, D.V.M., Ph.D., Chief, Virological Research Laboratory, National Animal Disease Center, Ames, Iowa.

MICHAEL J. MEREDITH, B.Sc., B. Vet. Med., Ph.D., M.R.C.V.S, Lecturer in Animal Health, Department of Clinical Veterinary Medicine, University of Cambridge, England.

VICKI N. MEYERS-WALLEN, V.M.D., Postdoctoral Fellow, School of Veterinary Medicine, University of Pennsylvania, Philadelphia, Pennsylvania.

R. B. MILLER, B.Sc., D.V.M., Ph.D, Professor and Chairman, Department of Pathology, Ontario Veterinary College, University of Guelph, Guelph, Ontario, Canada.

S. J. MILLER, M.V.Sc., F.A.C.V.Sc., Veterinary Practitioner, Warwick, Australia.

DAVID A. MORROW, D.V.M., Ph.D., Professor of Large Animal Clinical Sciences, College of Veterinary Medicine, Michigan State University, East Lansing, Michigan.

ROBERT G. MORTIMER, D.V.M., M.S., Diplomate, American College of Theriogenologists, Assistant Professor, Department of Clinical Science, College of Veterinary Medicine and Biomedical Science, and Clinician, Veterinary Teaching Hospital, Colorado State University, Ft. Collins, Colorado.

RAY F. NACHREINER, D.V.M., Ph.D., Professor, Departments of Physiology and Large Animal Clinical Sciences, College of Veterinary Medicine, and Section Chief, Endocrine Diagnostic Section,

Animal Health Diagnostic Laboratory, Michigan State University, East Lansing, Michigan.

R. W. NELSON, D.V.M., Assistant Professor, School of Veterinary Medicine, Purdue University; Internist, Small Animal Clinic, W. Lafayette, Indiana.

TERRY M. NETT, Ph.D., Department of Physiology and Biophysics, College of Veterinary Medicine and Biomedical Sciences, Colorado State University, Ft. Collins, Colorado.

PAUL NICOLETTI, D.V.M., M.S., Professor, College of Veterinary Medicine, University of Florida, Gainesville, Florida.

JERRY D. OLSON, D.V.M., M.S., Diplomate, American College of Theriogenologists, Associate Professor, Department of Clinical Science, College of Veterinary Medicine and Biomedical Science, and Clinician, Veterinary Teaching Hospital, Colorado State University, Ft. Collins, Colorado.

PATRICIA N. OLSON, D.V.M., Ph.D., Associate Professor, Departments of Clinical Sciences and Physiology and Biophysics, College of Veterinary Medicine and Biomedical Sciences, Colorado State University, Ft. Collins, Colorado.

BENNIE I. OSBURN, D.V.M., Ph.D., Professor of Pathology, School of Veterinary Medicine, University of California, Davis, California.

RANDALL S. OTT, D.V.M., M.S., Diplomate, American College of Theriogenologists, Department of Veterinary Clinical Medicine, College of Veterinary Medicine, University of Illinois, Urbana, Illinois.

N. C. PALMER, D.V.M., M.Sc., Ph.D., Veterinary Laboratory Services, Ontario Ministry of Agriculture and Food, Guelph, Ontario, Canada.

DONALD F. PATTERSON, D.V.M., D.Sc., Professor of Medicine, Chief, Section of Medical Genetics, School of Veterinary Medicine, University of Pennsylvania, Philadelphia, Pennsylvania

JOHN W. PAUL, D.V.M., M.S., Manager, Professional Services, Hoechst-Roussel Agri-Vet Co., Somerville, New Jersey.

JAMES E. PETTIGREW, JR., Ph.D., Associate Professor of Animal Science, University of Minnesota, St. Paul, Minnesota.

MAURICIO H. PINEDA, D.V.M., Ph.D., Professor of Physiology, Department of Veterinary Physiology and Pharmacology, College of Veterinary Medicine, Iowa State University, Ames, Iowa.

L. E. L. PINHEIRO, D.V.M., M.Sc., Ph.D., Associate Professor, Faculty of Veterinary Medicine, UNESP, and Clinics Veterinary Hospital, DCCV-FCAV-UNESP, Jaboticabal, Brazil.

DAVID G. POWELL, B.V.Sc., F.R.C.V.S., Assistant Extension Professor, Department of Veterinary Science, University of Kentucky, Lexington, Kentucky.

A. L. RAE, M.Agr.Sc., Ph.D., Professor of Animal Science, Massey University, Palmerston North, New Zealand.

GEOFFREY C. B. RANDALL, Ph.D., B.V.Sc, M.R.C.V.S., Research Scientist, Animal Diseases Research Institute, Agriculture Canada. Nepean, Ontario, Canada.

CHESTER L. RAWSON, D.V.M., Practitioner, Hazel Green, Wisconsin.

KENT R. REFSAL, D.V.M., M.S., Assistant Professor, Department of Small Animal Clinical Science, College of Veterinary Medicine, Michigan State University, East Lansing, Michigan.

LAWRENCE E. RICE, D.V.M., M.S., Professor, Department of Medicine and Surgery, College of Veterinary Medicine, and Section Head, Food Animal Section, Veterinary Teaching Hospital, Oklahoma State University, Stillwater, Oklahoma.

S. J. ROBERTS, D.V.M., M.S., Professor (Emeritus), Large Animal Medicine, Obstetrics and Surgery, New York State College of Veterinary Medicine, Cornell University, Ithaca, New York; Practitioner, Woodstock Veterinary Clinic, Woodstock, Vermont.

DONALD G. ROBINSON, JR., B.S., Tumblebrook Farm, Inc., West Brookfield, Massachusetts.

JAMES F. ROCHE, M.Agr.Sc., Ph.D., D.Sc., Professor of Animal Husbandry and Production, Faculty of Veterinary Medicine, University College Dublin, Dublin, Ireland.

ROBERT F. ROWE, D.V.M., Ph.D., Veterinary Reproductive Specialties, Inc., Middleton, Wisconsin.

H. LOUISE RUHNKE, B.S.A., M.Sc., Microbiologist, Veterinary Laboratory Services, Ontario, Ministry of Agriculture and Food, and Associated Graduate Faculty, University of Guelph, Guelph, Ontario, Canada.

ULRICH SCHNEIDER, Dr. Med. Vet., Research Associate, Biology Division, Oak Ridge National Laboratory, Oak Ridge, Tennessee.

GERRIT SCHUIJT, D.V.M., Senior Lecturer and Clinician in Veterinary Obstetrics, State University of Utrecht, Utrecht, The Netherlands.

STEPHEN W. J. SEAGER, D.V.M., Department of Physiology, College of Veterinary Medicine, Texas A&M University, College Station, Texas.

BRADLEY E. SEGUIN, D.V.M., Ph.D., Professor, College of Veterinary Medicine, and Clinician, Large Animal Clinic, University of Minnesota, St. Paul, Minnesota.

GEORGE E. SEIDEL, JR., Ph.D., Professor of Physiology, College of Veterinary Medicine and Biomedical Sciences, Colorado State University, Ft. Collins, Colorado.

PHILIP L. SENGER, B.S., M.S., Ph.D., Professor, Department of Animal Sciences, Washington State University, Pullman, Washington.

DAN C. SHARP, Ph.D., Professor of Physiology, Animal Science Department, College of Veterinary Medicine, University of Florida, Gainesville, Florida.

MAURICE SHELTON, Ph.D., Professor, Texas A&M University, Texas Agricultural Experiment Station, San Angelo, Texas.

PATRICIA E. SHEWEN, B.Sc., D.V.M., M.Sc., Ph.D., Assistant Professor of Immunology, Department of Veterinary Microbiology and Immunology, Ontario Veterinary College, University of Guelph, Guelph, Ontario, Canada.

SUSAN E. SHIDELER, Ph.D., Zoological Society of San Diego, San Diego, California.

VICTOR M. SHILLE, D.V.M., Ph.D., Associate Professor of Theriogenology, College of Veterinary Medicine, University of Florida, Gainesville, Florida.

ELIZABETH L. SINGH, B.Sc., M.Sc., Animal Diseases Research Institute, Animal Pathology Division, Food Production and Inspection Branch, Agriculture Canada, Nepean, Ontario, Canada.

WAYNE L. SINGLETON, Ph.D., Professor of Animal Science, Animal Science Department, Purdue University, West Lafayette, Indiana.

GILBERT M. SLATER, Charles River Breeding Laboratories, Inc., Wilmington, Massachusetts.

FRANCES O. SMITH, D.V.M., Ph.D., Clinical Assistant Professor, College of Veterinary Medicine, University of Minnesota, St. Paul, Minnesota.

MARY C. SMITH, D.V.M., Associate Professor of Veterinary Medicine, Ambulatory Clinician, De-

partment of Clinical Sciences, New York State College of Veterinary Medicine, Cornell University, Ithaca, New York.

R. DAVID SMITH, Ph.D., Associate Professor of Animal Science (Reproductive Physiology), Department of Animal Science, Cornell University, Ithaca, New York.

SUSAN F. SODERBERG, D.V.M., Northeast Veterinary Hospital, Detroit, Michigan.

NICKOLAS J. SOJKA, D.V.M., M.S., Professor and Chairman, Department of Comparative Medicine, Charlottsville, Virginia.

JOHN C. SPITZER, B.S., M.S., Ph.D., Associate Professor of Reproductive Physiology, Animal Science Department, Clemson University, Clemson, South Carolina.

THOMAS E. STEIN, D.V.M., M.S., Ph.D., Assistant Professor, College of Veterinary Medicine, University of Minnesota, St. Paul, Minnesota.

BARBARA E. STRAW, D.V.M., Ph.D., Associate Professor, New York State College of Veterinary Medicine, and Clinician, Swine Extension, College of Veterinary Medicine, Cornell University, Ithaca, New York.

STEVEN J. SUSANECK, D.V.M., M.S., Resident in Oncology, Comparative Oncology Unit, Colorado State University, Ft. Collins, Colorado.

JØRGEN SVENDSEN, D.V.M., M.Sc., Ph.D., Research Leader, Department of Farm Buildings, Swedish University of Agricultural Sciences, Lund, Sweden.

LORRAINE STEEN SVENDSEN, M.Sc., Ph.D., Research Assistant, Department of Farm Buildings, Swedish University of Agricultural Sciences, Lund, Sweden.

T. W. SWERCZEK, D.V.M., Ph.D., Professor, Department of Veterinary Science, University of Kentucky, Lexington, Kentucky.

BRAD J. THACKER, D.V.M., Ph.D., Assistant Professor, Department of Large Animal Clinical Sciences, College of Veterinary Medicine, Michigan State University, East Lansing, Michigan.

WILLIAM W. THATCHER, Ph.D., Professor of Dairy Science, College of Veterinary Sciences, University of Florida, Gainesville, Florida.

WALTER R. THRELFALL, D.V.M., M.S., Ph.D., Diplomate, American College of Theriogenologists, Professor of Veterinary Medicine, College of Veterinary Medicine, and Clinician, Theriogenology Area, Veterinary Hospital, The Ohio State University, Columbus, Ohio.

GREGORY C. TROY, D.V.M., M.S., Diplomate, American College of Veterinary Internal Medicine, Associate Professor, Department of Small Animal Medicine and Surgery, College of Veterinary Medicine, and Clinician, Small Animal Clinic, Veterinary Teaching Hospital, Texas A&M University, College Station, Texas.

V. R. VALE-FILHO, Federal University of Minas Geraio, Belo-horizonte, Brazil.

STEVEN D. VAN CAMP, D.V.M., School of Veterinary Medicine, North Carolina State University, Raleigh, North Carolina.

MARCEL M. VANDEPLASSCHE, D.V.M., Professor of Veterinary Reproduction and Obstetrics, Faculty of Veterinary Medicine, State University, Gent, Belgium.

J. T. VAUGHAN, D.V.M., M.S., Diplomate, College of Veterinary Surgeons, Dean of the College and Professor of Large Animal Surgery and Medicine, School of Veterinary Medicine, Auburn University, Auburn, Alabama.

SALLY VIVRETTE, D.V.M., Resident, Large Animal Medicine, School of Veterinary Medicine, University of California, Davis, California.

W. C. WAGNER, D.V.M., Ph.D., Professor and Head, Department of Veterinary Biosciences, College of Veterinary Medicine, University of Illinois, Urbana, Illinois.

W. R. WARD, Ph.D., B.V.Sc., M.R.C.V.S., Senior Lecturer, Faculty of Veterinary Science, Liverpool University, South Wiral, United Kingdom.

LEON D. WEAVER, V.M.D., Senior Lecturer, School of Veterinary Medicine, University of California, Davis; Veterinary Medicine Teaching and Research Center, Tulare, California.

MARTIN S. WENKOFF, D.V.M., M.V.Sc., Diplomate, American College of Theriogenologists, Theriogenologist, Advanced Genetic Research Ltd., Calgary, Alberta, Canada.

DAVID M. WEST, B.V.Sc., Ph.D., F.A.C.V.Sc., Senior Lecturer, Department of Veterinary Clinical Sciences, Massey University, Palmerston North, New Zealand.

STEVEN L. WHEELER, D.V.M., M.S., Fellow in Oncology, College of Veterinary Medicine and Biomedical Sciences, Colorado State University, Ft. Collins, Colorado.

HOWARD L. WHITMORE, D.V.M., Ph.D., Professor of Veterinary Clinical Medicine, College of

Veterinary Medicine, University of Illinois, Urbana, Illinois.

DAVID E. WILDT, Ph.D., Head, Reproductive Biology Section, Department of Animal Health, National Zoological Park, Smithsonian Institution, Washington, D.C.

CHRISTINE S. F. WILLIAMS, B.V.Sc., M.R.C.V.S., Director, Laboratory Animal Care Service, College of Veterinary Medicine, Michigan State University, East Lansing, Michigan.

NORMAN BRUCE WILLIAMSON, M.V.Sc., Professor, College of Veterinary Medicine, University of Minnesota, St. Paul, Miinesota.

GARY L. WILSON, D.V.M., M.S., Director, Equine Reproductive Clinic, Lexington, Kentucky.

MICHAEL R. WILSON, B.V.Sc., Ph.D., Professor, Clinical Sciences, University of Guelph, Ontario Veterinary College, Guelph, Ontario, Canada.

C. G. WINFIELD, B.Sc. (Agr.), M.Sc., Animal Research Institute, Department of Agriculture, Werribee, Victoria, Australia.

AMELIA E. WING, B.S., Zoological Society of San Diego, San Diego, California.

STEPHEN J. WITHROW, D.V.M., Professor of Surgery, Chief, Clinical Oncology Service, Comparative Oncology Unit, Colorado State University, Ft. Collins, Colorado.

DWIGHT F. WOLFE, D.V.M., M.S., Assistant Professor, Large Animal Surgery and Medicine, College of Veterinary Medicine, Auburn University, Auburn University, Alabama.

DONALD S. WOOD, D.V.M., Staff Surgeon, Coast Pet Clinic, Hermosa Beach, California.

MOLLIE WRIGHT, D.V.M., M.S., Diplomate, American College of Veterinary Anesthesiologists, Small Animal Associate, River Valley Veterinary Clinic, Plain, Wisconsin.

RAYMOND W. WRIGHT, JR., Ph.D., Professor, Department of Animal Science, Washington State University, Pullman, Washington; Director, Human in Vitro Fertilization Program, Deaconess Hospital, Spokane, Washington.

PEGGY M. WYKES, D.V.M., M.S., Reference Surgical Veterinary Practice, Englewood, Colorado.

ROBERT S. YOUNGQUIST, D.V.M., Diplomate, American College of Theriogenologists, Associate Professor of Veterinary Medicine and Surgery, and Clinician, Veterinary Teaching Hospital, University of Missouri-Columbia, Columbia, Missouri.

Preface

The objective of this second edition of *Current Therapy in Theriogenology* is to provide the practicing veterinarian and veterinary student with a concise source of current information documented by controlled research on the diagnosis, treatment and prevention of reproductive conditions in large and small animals. This book is designed to supplement existing publications on theriogenology.

The information is presented in a problem-oriented manner in an effort to help the reader solve the reproductive problem and also to provide rational, scientific reasons for the solution. The first part of the book includes information on principles of hormone and antibiotic therapy and embryo transfer. In subsequent sections reproductive problems are discussed by animal species. The role of computers in theriogenology is discussed in the final section before the Appendix of tables summarizing various reproductive parameters.

While the authors have tried to present information documented by controlled research, the reader is referred to existing publications in theriogenology for additional information. The references at the end of each chapter are designed to provide the reader with access to the literature. They have been limited to conserve space except in situations in which reviews are limited or unavailable.

Members of the American College of Theriogenologists and Society for Theriogenology indicated strong support for the project, and many subsequently served as consulting editors, authors and reviewers.

The editor would like to express his appreciation for the cooperation and support provided by the consulting editors, authors, reviewers and colleagues in completing this book, and especially for Dr. Brad Thacker's commentary on the swine section. The editorial assistance provided by Helene E. Pazak is gratefully acknowledged. The help provided by Robert Reinhardt and staff at the WB Saunders Company is also gratefully acknowledged. Suggestions for improving the content and presentation of information for the next edition are welcome.

The editor would like to thank his wife, Linda, and children, David Austin, Laurie and Melanie, for being understanding and for providing support during the preparation of *Current Therapy in Theriogenology*.

DAVID MORROW

NOTICE

Each country may at a specific time approve or disapprove usage of an individual drug and define withdrawal times for milk and meat in food-producing animals. Therefore, the clinician is responsible for knowing current regulations and observing the manufacturer's instructions on the label with regard to approved animals, recommended dosage and withdrawal times for the specific drug.

The authors, editors and publishers have made every effort possible to assure the accuracy of information provided in this book; however, they cannot assume responsibility for changing local regulations.

THE EDITORS

Contents

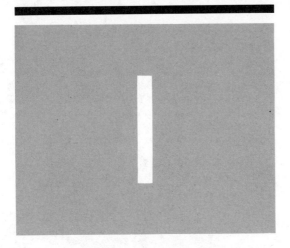

SECTION

I

PRINCIPLES OF HORMONE THERAPY

Terry Carruthers, D.V.M., Ph.D.

Consulting Editor

Principles of Hormone Therapy in Theriogenology

Terry D. Carruthers, D.V.M., Ph.D.
University of Saskatchewan
Saskatoon, Saskatchewan

The use of hormones is a major component of theriogenology. Hormone preparations are utilized as reproductive management tools, diagnostic aids and therapeutic agents. The intention of this chapter is to provide a general introduction to the physiological and pharmacologic bases for this extensive use of hormones in animal reproduction. For an in-depth review of the physiology and endocrinology of reproduction in domestic animals, the reader is referred to the numerous textbooks and related research and clinical publications in this field. When applicable, this text will also contain additional discussions of the secretion patterns and actions of specific hormones for individual species. Furthermore, specific diagnostic and therapeutic applications of hormones constitute a major portion of the remainder of this text and, therefore, will be discussed in the first part of this article only to illustrate general principles or concepts in hormonal therapy.

PRINCIPLES OF REPRODUCTIVE ENDOCRINOLOGY

Overview of Reproductive Hormones

A *hormone* can be defined as a chemical substance synthesized and secreted by specialized ductless glands and transported by the blood stream to other parts of the body, where it influences the activities of target tissues in such a way as to coordinate or integrate bodily functions. Although fundamentally valid, this definition has been expanded in recent years to include numerous local hormones or *parahormones*, which have their regulatory effects within the tissue or organ of origin. A number of parahormones are found in the ovaries and testes, but at present their functions are poorly understood, and they do not yet play a role in clinical theriogenology. Many of the diverse functions of the prostaglandins are of a local nature (e.g., their involvement in ovulation), yet their commonly exploited role as a luteolytic agent better fits the classical definition of a hormone.

The sources and principle actions of the major reproductive hormones are summarized in Table 1. Although much of the remaining discussion will concern these hormones and their clinically important derivatives, it is important to recall that reproductive function tends to be secondary to general health. This, in turn, is influenced by a multitude of factors, including hormones not normally considered to be involved in reproduction. Thyroid dysfunction, for example, can result in reproductive failure or infertility even when the thyroid condition itself is subclinical in nature.

Chemically, the hormones of reproduction can be grouped as peptides, glycoproteins and steroids, plus a miscellaneous group. Although varying considerably in terms of origin and biologic functions, the members of a specific chemical group have many similarities in terms of synthesis, metabolism and mechanisms of action. Also, they tend to share clinically important attributes, such as routes of administration, possible side effects and suitability for chemical synthesis or derivatization.

Peptide Hormones

The small peptide hormones of reproduction, gonadotropin-releasing hormone (GnRH) and oxytocin, are both synthesized by neurons located in the hypothalamus. Once identified, the simple structure of these peptides allowed them to be readily synthesized, and extensive research, particularly with GnRH, has resulted in the production of potent agonistic and antagonistic analogs of the natural peptides.

Gonadotropin-releasing hormone is synthesized primarily in the arcuate nucleus of the hypothalamus. It is transported axonally to the median eminence, where it is stored until appropriate stimulation causes its release into the hypothalamo-hypophyseal portal vessels. These vessels carry the releasing hormone to the anterior pituitary gland, where it stimulates synthesis and secretion of the gonadotropic hormones, luteinizing hormone (LH) and follicle-stimulating hormone (FSH). Very little GnRH appears to escape the pituitary, and meaningful concentrations are not detectable in the peripheral circulation.

The applications of GnRH and its analogs in theriogenology are mainly based on their ability to stimulate a surgelike release of LH and FSH from the anterior pituitary when administered as a single bolus injection. This induced LH surge has been used successfully to cause ovulation in ewes and cows, in which the normal preovulatory LH surge is quite short. GnRH-induced LH release does not result in ovulation in estrus mares, in which the normal preovulatory gonadotropin surge occurs over a period of days not hours. This example illustrates the importance of knowing the normal endocrine patterns in a given species when designing

Table 1. Principal Reproductive Hormones

Hormones	Major Sources	Function
Gonadotropin-releasing hormone (GnRH)	Hypothalamus	Stimulation of LH and FSH synthesis and secretion
Oxytocin	Neurohypophysis	Milk let-down, parturition and gamete transport
Luteinizing hormone (LH)	Adenohypophysis	Stimulation of ovulation, corpus luteum function and secretion of steroids
Follicle-stimulating hormone (FSH)	Adenohypophysis	Stimulation of follicle growth, spermatogenesis and estrogen secretion
Prolactin	Adenohypophysis	Lactogenic and luteotropic in some species
Chorionic gonadotropin	Placenta	Gonadotropin-like activity
hCG	women	LH activity
eCG	mares	FSH and LH activity (maintenance of luteal function?)
Placental lactogen	Placenta	Mammary development and fetal growth and metabolism
Progestogens	Corpus luteum and placenta	Establishment and maintanance of pregnancy, mammary growth, regulation of LH and FSH secretion
Estrogens	Follicles and placenta	Sexual behavior, female sex characteristics, growth of mammary gland and reproductive tract, regulation of LH and FSH secretion
Androgens	Testes	Male sexual differentiation and behavior, spermatogenesis

treatments or evaluating responses to hormonal therapy. The therapeutic use of GnRH to induce luteinization of ovarian cysts in dairy cows is again a reflection of its ability to induce pituitary LH secretion. However, in this example, the lower cost and lack of antigenicity of GnRH as compared with that of human chorionic gonadotropin (HCG) or pituitary LH preparations are primary considerations in its use.

A "GnRH-like" *gonadocrinin* has been reported to be present in the gonads of some species, and potent GnRH analogs have been reported to exert direct effects on ovarian and testicular function. Although potentially of clinical importance, the significance of these findings is at present unclear.

Oxytocin is synthesized by neurons of the supraoptic nucleus and transported axonally to storage sites in the posterior pituitary. Stimulation of the appropriate neural reflex results in release of oxytocin into the general circulation, where it stimulates the smooth muscle of the genital and mammary system. Oxytocin has well-defined functions in milk let-down, parturition and transportation of both egg and sperm in the tubular genitalia. In addition, oxytocin has been reported to be produced by luteal tissue and implicated in control of luteal regression

in sheep. A corresponding testicular production of oxytocin activity has not been reported.

Oxytocin has a number of clinical uses, including stimulation of milk let-down, parturition, uterine involution and expulsion of retained placenta. The response of a given tissue to a hormonal treatment is frequently influenced by its concurrent or prior exposure to other hormones. Adrenaline will block oxytocin's contractile effects on the mammary myoepithelial cells; therefore, a wildly excited heifer would not be likely to give a good milk let-down response to oxytocin. As well, the myometrium responds best to oxytocin when in an estrogen-dominated condition; therefore, use of oxytocin to induce uterine involution will be considerably more effective shortly after parturition than several days later.

Glycoprotein Hormones

This class of reproductive hormones are gonadotropic in function; Table 2 summarizes their principal features. All species produce the pituitary gonadotropins (LH and FSH), but the placental gonadotropins are apparently produced by only a few species. Pregnant mare serum gonadotropin

Table 2. Characteristics of Gonadotropic Hormones

Hormone	Molecular Weight	Carbohydrate	Sialic Acid	Half-Life
Luteinizing hormone (LH)	28–34,000	12–24%	1–2%	<30 min
Follicle-stimulating hormone (FSH)	32–37,000	25%	5%	2 hr
Human chorionic gonadotropin (hCG)	38,000	32%	8.5%	11 hr
Equine chorionic gonadotropin (eCG)	68,000	48%	10.4%	26 hr

(PMSG), or equine chorionic gonadotropin (eCG) as it has been called more recently, and human chorionic gonadotropin (hCG) are two major examples of placental gonadotropins.

The glycoprotein hormones are relatively large carbohydrate-containing proteins, each consisting of two nonidentical subunits (α and β), which are held together by noncovalent forces. Within a species, the structure of the α subunit is identical among hormones, and there is also considerable similarity among different species. It is the β subunit that provides the functional specificity of each gonadotropin. Significant biologic activity is only present when both subunits are combined, and individual subunits are not normally secreted or present in the circulation.

Carbohydrate content varies among gonadotropins and by species for a particular gonadotropin. The carbohydrates are covalently linked to the protein structure, primarily in the form of oligosaccharide chains, some of which terminate in sialic acid residues. Both pituitary and placental gonadotropins require their carbohydrate component for in vivo biologic activity. The number of sialic acid residues in particular has a direct relationship to the circulatory half-life of each gonadotropin.

Although the amino acid structure of a number of gonadotropins is known, the size of the molecules alone precludes their economical synthesis. Fortunately, the biologic activity of the gonadotropins tends not to be species specific, and a relatively diverse range of activities are available from various pituitary, serum and urine extracts.

Luteinizing hormone is secreted by the basophilic gonadotrophs of the anterior pituitary and stimulates both the testes and ovaries. The primary gonadal response is steroidogenic, as LH stimulates androgen secretion from both ovarian thecal cells and testicular Leydig cells as well as progesterone secretion from luteal cells in the ovary. Ovulation of mature follicles, oocyte maturation and corpus luteum formation and maintenance are also major effects of LH in the female.

Generally, pituitary LH preparations receive relatively little use in theriogenology because there are more appropriate hormones available. Endogenous LH secretion of short duration can be readily induced with GnRH, and more prolonged LH action is more easily achieved by using hCG, which has a significantly longer biologic half-life.

Follicle-stimulating hormone is secreted by the same population of anterior pituitary cells that produce LH. It acts to stimulate follicular growth, spermatogenesis and estrogen production. Estrogens are produced primarily by aromatization of androgen precursors in follicular granulosa cells and testicular Sertoli's cells. Until recently, assay methodology for FSH in domestic species lagged behind that for LH, and the longer half-life and more stable circulating concentrations of FSH have frequently led to its being dismissed as having a permissive role. Now that sensitive and specific assays are

available and with the increasing understanding of the control of FSH secretion, this relatively naive view may change.

Induction of follicular growth for the purposes of superovulation and out-of-season breeding has been the principal use of pituitary FSH preparations. Repeated injections are required owing to the relatively short half-life, but this inconvenience is offset by the ability to readily control the duration of the stimulation. It should be remembered that commercial FSH preparations contain large amounts of "contaminating" LH, which may explain the success of superovulatory regimens that feature decreasing doses of FSH. Excessive LH during the later stages of follicle growth is probably detrimental to normal maturation and ovulation. This points out a problem inherent in most hormones derived from natural sources, that is, they are seldom pure in either the chemical or biologic sense. This "impurity" is also reflected in the lot-to-lot variations in biologic activity that occur with these products.

Equine chorionic gonadotropin is secreted by the fetal trophoblastic cells of the endometrial cups between approximately the fortieth and one hundred fiftieth days of pregnancy in the mare. Its function in the mare was believed to be formation and maintenance of the secondary or accessory corpora lutea of pregnancy. Recent research, including intraspecies embryo transfer between donkeys and horses, has demonstrated that accessory corpora lutea can form and function normally in the absence of eCG production. Also, death or surgical removal of the fetus after the endometrial cups have formed will result in regression of the corpora lutea, even though eCG production will continue normally until regression of the endometrial cups. It has been suggested that the massive quantities of eCG produced may be involved in immunoprotection of the developing fetus, but at present the true function of eCG in the mare is not clear. The mare is relatively insensitive to the gonadotropic, follicle-stimulating activity of eCG, and this appears due to a failure of eCG to bind to the FSH receptors in the mare ovary. In other species, eCG exhibits both FSH and LH bioactivity.

As with pituitary FSH, the principle use of eCG is induction of follicular growth either for superovulation or for out-of-season breeding. The long half-life of eCG is a major advantage, as only a single injection is required. However, poor success with this preparation has frequently been attributed to an inappropriately prolonged period of stimulation. Immunoneutralization with anti-eCG serum has been used to terminate the biologic effects of eCG and to improve the superovulatory response.

Human chorionic gonadotropin and related hormones in nonhuman primates are produced during the period from implantation to near parturition by syncytial trophoblast cells of the placenta. In primates, these hormones are involved in recognition of pregnancy and act to maintain luteal steroid secretion until maturation of the placenta's steroidogenic capability. In most species, hCG has potent LH-bioactivity, with little or no FSH effects. In the bitch, hCG induces estrogen secretion, as indicated by vaginal cytology, but whether this is an FSH-like property or due to LH-like activity increasing the androgenic precursors for estrogen synthesis is unknown. Certainly, the in vitro binding of hCG is highly specific for the LH receptors, with very little binding to FSH receptors.

The major clinical advantage of hCG over pituitary LH (exogenous or GnRH-induced) is its long half-life, which increases its effectiveness for inducing ovulation in species like the mare, in which the normal LH surge is prolonged.

Steroid Hormones

These hormones consist of a family of four-ringed organic compounds that are synthetically related. The reproductive steroid hormones can be separated into four groups: progestogens, androgens, estrogens and corticosteroids (Fig. 1). The primary steroid-producing tissues of the body are the testes, ovaries, adrenals, placenta and fetal gonads; the steroid products of a tissue are the result of its intrinsic enzymatic pathways and the metabolic precursors available to it at a given time. It is also possible for otherwise nonendocrine tissues to possess the enzymes required to convert a precursor steroid to another more or less active steroid. The aromatization of androgens to estrogens by the central nervous system or the conversion of testosterone to dihydrotestosterone by accessory sex organs in the male are two examples.

Steroid hormones differ from the previously discussed peptide and glycoprotein hormones in that they are small, lipophilic compounds, which have relatively low solubilities in the aqueous fluids of the body but can pass readily through the predominately lipid cell membranes. The majority of steroids circulating in the blood are bound to large carrier proteins. A principal protein carrier for many steroids is albumin, although most species also possess a sex steroid–binding globulin. The steroid carrier proteins function to increase the solubility of the steroids, extend their biologic half-life by reducing renal filtration and modify their bioavailability, since only the free, unbound steroid can enter a cell to exert its effects or to be metabolized.

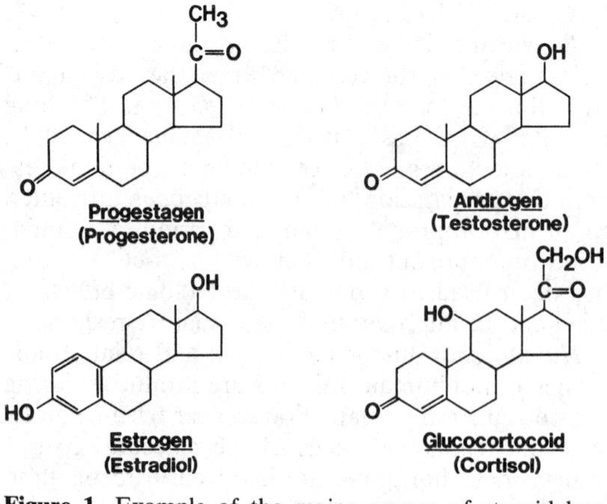

Because steroids are small and relatively simple molecules, they can be readily synthesized, and therefore, naturally occurring steroids are available as chemically pure preparations. In addition, extensive research has resulted in numerous synthetic steroids and steroid derivatives that exhibit clinically important attributes such as increased potency, prolonged action, increased specificity of effect, reduced side effects and easier administration. Most steroid hormones used routinely in animal reproduction are either wholly synthetic or altered in some fashion from the naturally occurring compounds. Research in developing competitive and noncompetitive blockers of steroid hormone action has yielded several promising therapeutic approaches in human medicine. Little clinical or research use has been made of these agents in domestic animal reproduction, although antiandrogens have been used to treat behavioral problems and prostatic disease in dogs.

Sex steroids and their derivatives have been used extensively in food animal production as growth promotants. Androgens and estrogens have nitrogen-sparing anabolic effects, which increase the rate and efficiency of gain in castrated animals. Progestogens are used in intact heifers to suppress the behavioral disruption and inefficiencies resulting from estrus activity.

Progestogens, the most common being progesterone, are important regulators of reproductive function in the female. Their primary sites of secretion are the ovarian luteal tissue and the placenta. They function in coordinating the estrous cycle through their negative feedback effects on LH secretion and act as the "hormone of pregnancy." They suppress myometrial activity, promote endometrial secretion, block estrous behavior and, in general, support the establishment of a viable conceptus within the uterus. They act synergistically with estrogens to promote uterine and mammary growth.

There is widespread use of progestogens, both synthetic and natural, as management aids in veterinary medicine. They are used to block estrus in feedlot heifers, mares and bitches. In a related use, their short-term administration and timed withdrawal can be used to synchronize estrus and ovulation in most species. Forms of administration for these purposes include feed additives, oral tablets, injections, and slow-release vaginal sponges or subcutaneous Silastic implants. The duration of progestogen administration prior to the synchronized withdrawal is important. An insufficient interval

Figure 1. Example of the major groups of steroid hormones with reproductive functions.

will not allow time for regression of an existing CL; therefore, synchrony will be poor. Prolonged administration may result in good synchrony but impaired fertility due to changes induced in the tubular genitalia. The concept that hormonally induced effects are dynamic and time dependent is important to the correct application of hormones as management and therapeutic agents.

Androgens, testosterone being a major example, are the principal circulating reproductive steroids in the male. Leydig or interstitial cells of the testes are the main source of secretion. Androgens are responsible for maintenance of spermatogenesis, accessory sex gland function and secondary sex characteristics, including sex drive.

Androgens are the precursors for estrogen production in both sexes, and alterations in androgen levels can influence reproductive function in females (e.g., ovulation rate) as well as in males. Also, many of the actions of androgens in males appear to require conversion of a circulating form (e.g., testosterone) to an active form in the target tissues (e.g., dihydrotestosterone in the accessory sex glands or estradiol in the brain).

Androgens have been used relatively little in the reproductive management of domestic animals. They are utilized to increase sexual behavior in males with poor libido, and in heifers they are used as estrus detectors in artificial insemination (AI) programs. Problems with masculinization can be seen in fillies that receive anabolic steroid treatment as part of competitive training, since these steroids also have androgenic activity. Prolonged administration of androgens in either sex results in feedback inhibition of the hypothalamopituitary axis, thereby, reducing gonadotropin secretion and resulting in atrophy of the gonads.

Estrogens, for example 17β-estradiol, have wide-ranging functions most obvious in the female but no less important in the male. Estrogen is primarily responsible for behavioral estrus, although small amounts of progesterone or a progesterone pre-exposure will enhance this effect. Estrogens induce the changes in the tubular genitalia required for successful mating and gamete transport. They act with progestogens to stimulate growth of the uterus and mammary gland. When not blocked by progestogens, they stimulate myometrial activity and sensitize it to the effects of oxytocin and prostaglandins during estrus and parturition. Their actions are required for maturation of the graafian follicle and stimulation of the ovulatory surge of gonadotropins. As mentioned previously, in the male many of the androgen effects on spermatogenesis and sexual behavior are mediated by a conversion of androgens to estrogens in the target cells.

Induction of behavioral estrus is a frequent use of estrogens, primarily to produce mount animals for semen collection or libido-testing programs. Although estrogen administration can induce a preovulatory-like LH surge, it does not reliably result in ovulation, since the critical follicular maturation

that normally accompanies the proestrus estrogen increase will not be stimulated. In a number of species, estrogens are used to increase uterine tone and motility in order to aid in expelling unwanted contents as in the case of pyometra.

Corticosteroids are produced by the adrenal cortex in response to pituitary corticotropin stimulation. Glucocorticoids play an important role as a fetal signal for induction of parturition in a number of species. By their actions on placental enzymes, they induce a fall in progesterone and an increase in estrogen, which is accompanied by an increase in prostaglandins and the initiation of labor.

Potent synthetic glucocorticoids are used to induce parturition in a number of species. Viability of near-term offspring does not appear to be impaired, and although the incidence of retained placentae may increase, postpartum fertility does not appear to be reduced.

Glucocorticoid release in response to "stressful" stimuli has also been linked to various reproductive dysfunctions, including postpartum anestrus and cystic ovarian disease; however, the degree and mechanism of involvement are uncertain.

Other Hormones

Prostaglandins are highly modified 20-carbon fatty acids produced by many tissues and with a multitude of forms and functions. Of primary concern to reproduction is prostaglandin $F_{2\alpha}$ ($PGF_{2\alpha}$), which has been demonstrated to play a role in luteolysis, ovulation, parturition and gamete transport in both the male and the female. Again, because prostaglandins have a relatively simple structure, potent synthetic analogs have been produced and are in commercial use (Fig. 2).

The capacity of $PGF_{2\alpha}$ to induce luteolysis has been extensively exploited in recent years as a tool for manipulating the estrous cycle of domestic animals, and this will be discussed in detail in later chapters. An area that may see increased activity in the future is the use of prostaglandin inhibitors or antagonists to block luteolysis or inhibit uterine motility.

Prolactin is a large polypeptide hormone secreted by the anterior pituitary. It is required for the initiation and maintenance of lactation in most species. This hormone is luteotropic in some species and appears to play a role in the mediation of seasonal and lactational effects on reproduction in others.

There are a large number of additional hormones and putative hormones with reproductive functions that are not yet of practical use. Among these are relaxin, inhibin, various early pregnancy factors, intragonadal regulators and a growing number of neurotransmitters. Some or all of these may one day become tools for reproductive management or treatment, but at this time even their potential uses are unclear.

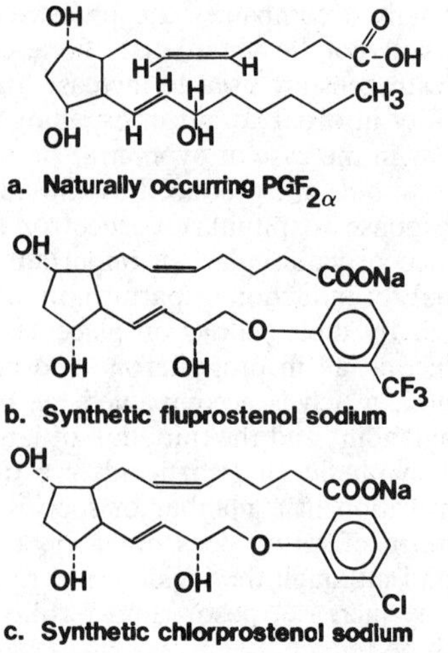

a. Naturally occurring PGF$_{2\alpha}$

b. Synthetic fluprostenol sodium

c. Synthetic chlorprostenol sodium

Figure 2. Structure of a reproductively important prostaglandin (PGF$_{2\alpha}$) and two clinically important derivatives.

Control of Hormone Synthesis and Secretion

The control of synthesis and secretion of a particular hormone is primarily a consequence of the effects exerted by other hormones on the cells of origin. These hormonal effects consist of direct stimulatory or trophic inputs such as stimulation of LH and FSH secretion by GnRH and synthesis and secretion of testosterone by LH-stimulated Leydig cells in the testis.

There is also a feedback component to control of hormone secretion, whereby a hormone influences either positively or negatively the secretion of the trophic stimuli that have caused its own release. For example, LH is required for normal progesterone secretion by the corpus luteum, and progesterone will, in turn, inhibit the secretion of pituitary LH by actions on both the pituitary gonadotrophs and the GnRH-secreting hypothalamic neurons. This type of negative feedback control is common and essential to maintenance of controlled hormone secretory patterns. The ability of estradiol to cause a progressive increase in the secretion of pituitary gonadotropins, culminating in a preovulatory surge of LH and FSH, is an example of positive feedback. This type of feedback is much less common and more specialized; it relies on some form of self-terminating mechanism for control. In the example of the preovulatory surge induced by estrogen, at least two such brakes exist. First, although some LH is required to drive estradiol production, the high levels reached during the surge result in changes to the follicular theca and granulosa cells. These cells cease to secrete estrogen and convert to secreting progesterone, which is an inhibitor of LH secretion. Secondly, the pituitary exhausts its supply of readily releasable gonadotropin and becomes

refractory to further stimulation by the hypothalamus. The clinical significance of these feedback systems is that prolonged administration of any hormonal product not only will cause effects in target organs but also may disrupt the normal mechanisms controlling endogenous secretion. The use of androgenically active anabolic steroids in race horses has already been mentioned.

In the case of peptide and protein hormones, the control of synthesis and secretion can be somewhat independent, since these hormones are stored within the cells of origin as membrane-bound granules. A large and rapid release of hormone can therefore occur in advance of any de novo synthesis. Steroid hormones and prostaglandins are not stored in any appreciable quantity by their cells of origin; therefore, secretion is essentially synonymous with synthesis. However, since the synthesis of these small molecules often involves relatively minor changes in an abundant precursor, the response to stimulation can be very rapid.

The major endocrine interactions of the *hypothalamo-hypophyseal-testicular axis*, shown in Figure 3, illustrate the degree and complexity of the interrelationships involved in the control of hormone secretion. This is probably one of the more straightforward systems and, as yet, is still only partially understood. For example, most studies have concentrated on the major androgens such as testosterone, but various other androgen metabo-

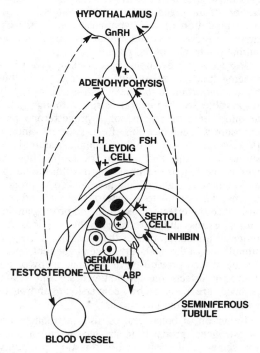

Figure 3. The *hypothalamo-hypophyseal-testicular axis,* an example of the complex endocrine interrelationships that regulate reproductive function.

lites may be just as important in controlling testicular function and secondary sex characteristics. Also, the role of various intragonadal parahormones is only beginning to be elucidated.

Another central aspect of the control of secretion is the temporal pattern of hormone secretion. First, there is the distinction to be made between basal and stimulated secretion. Hormone secretion is seldom an on-off proposition; rather there is a state of minimal or basal secretion that may function to maintain a target organ's status. For example, the low levels of LH secreted during the luteal phase of the estrous cycle are required for normal maintenance and progesterone secretion by the corpus luteum. On the other hand, stimulated secretion such as the preovulatory LH surge tends to have more dynamic effects such as ovulation of a follicle and formation of a corpus luteum.

It has become increasingly evident that normal secretion is not simply a matter of serum or tissue concentration of hormone; it is also the result of the duration and frequency of exposure to these concentrations. It appears that most, if not all, peptide and protein hormones are secreted in an episodic or pulsatile pattern, with the amplitude of each pulse and the frequency of pulses being critical to the biologic effects of the hormone. As an example, constant infusion of GnRH will result in an initial release of LH and FSH but, after a period of some minutes or hours, secretion will fall to baseline levels in spite of continued GnRH infusion. Repeated injection of low doses of GnRH will result in continued secretion of gonadotropins in response to each injection, and the nature and level of secretion can be regulated by changes in injection frequency, without changing the amount injected. Although it appears that steroid hormones are also released in pulses or bursts in response to pulses of their trophic hormones, the fact that they are largely carrier bound once in the circulation tends to result in the stabilization of their biologic effect; relatively constant levels of steroids appear to be quite adequate in terms of biologic efficacy.

The half-life of a hormone is also an important determinant of its secretory profile and biologic effects. Hormones with very short half-lives will reach sustained high concentrations only if secreted or administered continuously or in massive quantities, which overload the metabolic or excretory pathways that normally clear them from the circulation. Conversely, the hourly release of a hormone with a half-life of several hours will eventually give rise to relatively high serum concentrations, even if the individual pulses of hormone are quite small. Another important concept is that for many hormones, most notably steroids, the duration of biologic effects may be significantly longer than the hormone's chemical half-life in the blood or tissue. This concept is important not only when selecting treatment intervals in maintenance therapy but also when attempting to relate circulating hormone patterns to the physiological events they control.

Mechanisms of Hormone Action

There are two basic paradigms for how hormones exert their effects—one for peptide and protein hormones and a second for steroids. The following is an example of the first (Fig. 4). LH binds to specific receptors located on the Leydig cell of the testis. The receptor itself is a large protein embedded in the cell membrane and possesses both a high degree of specificity and a strong affinity for the LH hormone. Therefore, the presence of these receptors enables the Leydig cell to respond to LH at very low blood concentrations, whereas nontarget tissues for LH do not possess these receptors and are unable to respond to even very high LH concentrations. Binding of LH to its receptor results in conformational changes in the receptor, which in turn activates the membrane-bound enzyme, adenylate cyclase. This enzyme catalyzes the conversion of adenosine triphosphate (ATP) to cyclic adenosine monophosphate (cAMP), which has been referred to as the "second messenger" of hormone action. One of the known actions of cAMP is the activation of protein kinase systems, which in turn phosphorylate other enzymes, thereby causing their activation. By binding to an external receptor, a hormone such as LH is thus able to induce a cascade of events, resulting in activation (or deactivation) of one or more enzymes and thus increasing (or decreasing) the production of various cellular products such as testosterone. It is the particular internal architecture and enzyme complement of individual cells or tissues that allows one hormone to exert different effects on different tissues or a number of hormones each to act independently on one cell and exert specific effects, even though each acts through the mediation of common internal second messengers.

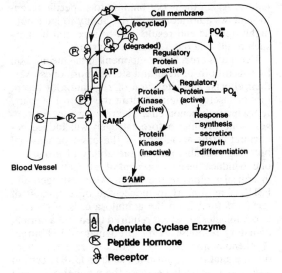

Figure 4. Mechanism of action of protein and peptide hormones such as the gonadotropins.

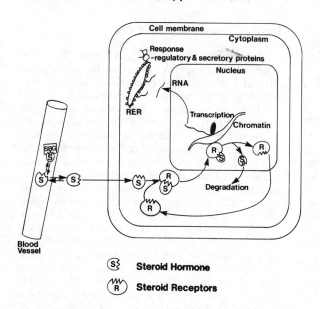

Figure 5. Mechanism of action of steroid hormones.

The model for the action of steroid hormones on a target cell is shown in Figure 5. Steroids, being lipid soluble, are thought to diffuse passively into the cytoplasm of cells; however, there is some evidence for protein-mediated transport. Target tissues for a particular steroid possess specific, high-affinity cytoplasmic receptors that bind to the hormone after it enters the cell. Binding results in transformation or activation of the receptor-hormone complex, allowing it to move (translocate) into the cell nucleus. At the nuclear site, the receptor-hormone complex binds to specific acceptor sites on the nuclear material and causes synthesis of specific messenger ribonucleic acid (mRNA) molecules. The resulting mRNA is moved to the cytoplasm, where it directs synthesis of specific proteins, which may be structural, enzymatic or secretory in nature. Again the act of binding to a specific receptor endows a hormone with the ability to have both highly specific end results and to accomplish many such results via one recognition system.

Receptors are a key component in the mechanism by which both protein and steroid hormones exert their effects, and alteration or regulation of receptors themselves is important in the control of many reproductive phenomena. The requirement for progesterone priming before estrogen will induce behavioral estrus at puberty or the onset of seasonal breeding probably reflects the ability of progesterone to induce the development of estrogen receptors in critical regions of the brain. Also, estrogen and FSH act in concert to induce the development of receptors for LH on the granulosa cells of preovulatory follicles, an event required to enable a normal ovulatory response to the preovulatory LH surge. A phenomenon also exists that is referred to as downregulation. A hormone such as GnRH can, in large doses, actually decrease the number of its own receptors on the pituitary gonadotrophs and thereby induce a period of refractoriness to further GnRH

stimulation of those cells. As the factors controlling receptor regulations are clarified, hormonal treatments that induce receptor populations or avoid events such as downregulation will be developed.

Once having bound to a hormone, membrane-bound receptors appear to be internalized, after which the hormone may be degraded and the receptor itself recycled back to the membrane surface.

Hormone Metabolism

Hormones are metabolized or cleared from the body by a number of mechanisms, and it should be noted that removal of biologic activity may precede actual physical clearance. Peptide and protein hormones are generally catabolized and broken down to their constituent amino acids. This occurs to a large degree in the liver but also in the kidneys and to some extent within the target tissues. For example, hypothalamic GnRH is metabolized by peptidases found in both the hypothalamus and anterior pituitary. In addition, any endogenous GnRH that escapes the pituitary is diluted to ineffective concentrations once it enters the general circulation.

Steroid hormones are inactivated primarily by conversion via reduction reactions to inactive or less active forms by the liver, kidney and other tissues. Both active and inactive steroids are hydroxylated and conjugated with glucuronic or sulfuric acid. This occurs primarily in the liver and results in water soluble compounds that have little biologic activity, reduced binding to carrier proteins and increased rates of urinary and fecal excretion. It is important to recall that metabolism of steroids not only is a means for their removal but also is required for many of their biologic actions. Carrier protein binding of steroids may act to reduce their biologic activity by preventing access to target cells, but it also prolongs their duration of action by reducing clearance rates.

Prostaglandins are very rapidly inactivated both at their sites of local action or when released into the general circulation, where they are removed and metabolized by the lungs and liver.

PRINCIPLES OF THERAPEUTICS

The therapeutic principles of modern pharmacology appear to have received little study relative to the use of reproductive hormones in veterinary medicine. The purpose of this section is to highlight some therapeutic principles and, it is hoped, encourage at least their consideration when planning and conducting hormonal therapy in domestic animals.

The first prerequisite of rational hormonal therapy is to gain as complete an understanding of the normal physiological functions of the hormonal product as is feasible. This includes consideration of not only the desired therapeutic effects but also the multitude of side effects both coincidental and detrimental that may occur. It is also important to recognize that both normal physiological processes and disease states are heterogeneous and dynamic; therefore, the use of uniform, static treatment regimens may often be inappropriate.

Therapeutic Goal

The goal of hormone administration should be well defined; it can fall into one or more categories. It may be management related, such as the manipulation of the estrous cycle using progestational compounds or luteolytic prostaglandins. Such goals are usually achieved using well-defined treatments. As a result, the choice of a particular approach is often based on readily definable criteria such as age of animals, stage of cycle and cost. Also, most management-related uses of hormones depend on extensively tested regimens based on relatively large bodies of basic research.

The goal may also be diagnostic. For example, an injection of hCG or LH can be used to determine if low serum testosterone concentrations in a male with poor libido are a result of gonadotropin insufficiency or testicular dysfunction. The administration of hormones for diagnostic purposes has received relatively little attention in theriogenology as compared with other areas of medicine. Many diagnostic applications of hormones utilize serum concentrations of a responding hormone as an end point. Only recently has hormone measurement begun to be available and cost effective for many practitioners. The diagnostic use of hormones must be well planned and carefully executed, otherwise the diagnostic validity is seriously weakened.

Medical use of hormones, such as in the treatment of a reproductive dysfunction (e.g., anestrus) or organic disease (e.g., endometritis), has been the area in which the principles of therapeutics are most important and have been most neglected. Too often this clinical use of a hormone concentrates on one desired effect, with too little attention given to the following points.

Diagnostic Accuracy

Obviously, an accurate diagnosis is essential to selecting the correct therapeutic hormone. It would be unwise, to say the least, to induce CL regression with prostaglandins in a cow that a dairyman has presented as anestrus without first insuring that she is not in fact pregnant.

Choice of Hormonal Product

Although often constrained by availability or affordability, choice of a particular product should be based on factors others than just "what I've always used." Stability, potency, ease of administration, duration of effects, withdrawal times for meat and milk, and known side effects should be evaluated and considered whenever possible. Informal clinical trials by individual practitioners can be very useful in determining the most effective and efficient treatments for use in each case. They also help increase confidence in the treatments ultimately selected and stimulate increased efforts at observation, which frequently yield beneficial results in terms of treatment monitoring and success.

Dose-Level–Response

Once a hormone preparation has been selected it becomes necessary to select the most appropriate dosage. A dose can be arrived at by means of personal trials, published data (including manufacturer's recommended doses), empirical calculation based on body size, volume of distribution and half-life of the material or by the use of graded doses and the monitoring of the response by measuring achieved blood concentrations or treatment response.

It is also important to distinguish between the goal of achieving a physiological response versus pharmacologic response. Attaining a physiological response may require not only much more precise dosages but also refined methods of administration and monitoring in order to mimic normal secretory patterns as well as concentrations. Pharmacologic effects, on the other hand, are often achieved using massive excesses of the hormone, with little or no concern for normal endogenous concentrations and secretion patterns. As a consequence, pharmacologic doses of hormones are much more likely to have pronounced side effects.

Some of the variables that influence the relationship among dose, achieved concentration and effect are presented in Figure 6. Most are self-explanatory; however, a few warrant additional comment. First, it should be pointed out that much of the data required to actually take many of these factors into account are not available even for commonly used hormones in the major species of domestic animals.

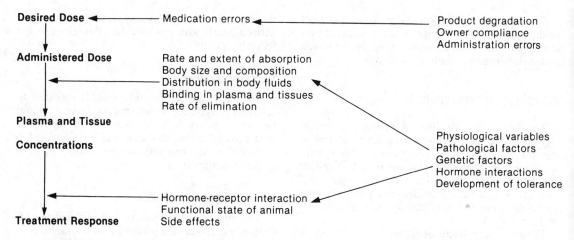

Figure 6. Factors influencing the relationship between dose, concentration and response to hormonal therapy.

Therefore, many of the concepts that can be used are based on simple common sense.

In terms of route of administration, it is obvious that peptide and protein hormones cannot be given orally, and even most naturally occurring steroids are inefficient when administered by this route. However, numerous synthetic steroids are effective when administered orally, and these receive extensive use, especially as management tools. Most other hormones are administered parenterally by injection, infusion or implantation. Various depot or slow-release methods are also used to administer steroid hormones, including specially formulated "repositol" injections and steroid impregnated Silastic implants or vaginal sponges.

The distribution and half-life of a hormone once it has entered the circulation may be altered by chemical modifications. These may delay its enzymatic degradation; reduce its binding to carrier proteins, thereby increasing its availability to target cells; or increase its affinity to target cell receptors. Many advances have been made in this field with small hormones such as steroids, prostaglandins and releasing hormones. The larger gonadotropic hormones must essentially be used "as is," but fortunately there is considerable diversity in the half-lives of the various preparations available.

The possibility of developing antibodies against large molecular weight hormones such as the gonadotropins must be recognized both in terms of developing tolerance and the possibility of anaphylatic reactions. Practical experience has indicated that this is not a major constraint, although repeated use of hCG for induction of ovulation in mares and treatment of cystic ovaries in cows has been associated with reduced efficiency.

Intentional immunization against reproductive hormones is an area of intense research. Passive and active immunization against GnRH is being investigated as a nonsurgical, potentially reversible method of sterilizing both companion and food-producing animals. Active immunization against the steroid androstenedione is being commercially used to increase lambing rates in ewes.

Hormone Residues

Hormone residues in food animals and their products are of major concern. The extensive use of reproductive-based hormones as growth promotants in ruminants has resulted in at least one major controversy, that of diethylstilbestrol. This, in turn, has drastically slowed the rate at which new reproductive hormone products have been developed for use in food animals. The prescribed withdrawal times for hormonal products should be as carefully observed as those provided for other drugs. Since route of administration, product formulation, species, sex, age, body condition and physiological status will all influence the rate at which a hormone will be cleared, it is important to be cautious in advising on withdrawal times even when using "natural" hormone products.

SUMMARY

Effective use of hormones in theriogenology requires knowledge of both normal reproductive endocrinology and the therapeutic characteristics of available hormonal preparations. The more extensive this knowledge, the more likely that hormonal treatments will be effectively designed and administered so as to manipulate and control the reproductive system with minimal unwanted side effects.

This chapter has attempted to highlight the major hormones utilized in theriogenology and characterize key concepts in their actions and uses. No attempt has been made to discuss details of the various reproductive systems and events in the different species. There is a rapidly expanding body of knowledge on the reproductive biology of domestic animals, and only a dedicated effort to read current texts and journals will enable the theriogenologist to remain up-to-date on even a few species.

The principles of therapeutics have received little serious consideration as they apply to the use of reproductive hormones in domestic animals. Most management-related uses are based on a relatively solid footing of basic research as are the limited diagnostic uses. However, to a large extent the therapeutic uses of reproductive hormones have been developed by trial-and-error, often with little apparent consideration of the underlying physiological factors. When possible, the factors influencing choice of hormonal product and method, dose and frequency of administration should be evaluated in light of both the endogenous endocrine patterns and the chemical and biologic characteristics of the product itself.

References

1. Arthur GH, Noakes DE, Pearson H: Veterinary Reproduction and Obstetrics. 5th Ed. London, Bailliere-Tindall, 1982.

2. Asbury AC (consulting ed): Reproduction. *In* Robinson NE (ed): Current Therapy in Equine Medicine. Philadelphia, WB Saunders Co., 1983, pp. 399–460.

3. Booth NH, McDonald LE (ed): Veterinary Pharmacology and Therapeutics. 5th Ed. Ames, Iowa State University Press, 1982.

4. Brander GC, Pugh DM, Bywater RJ: Veterinary Applied Pharmacology and Therapeutics. 4th Ed. London, Bailliere-Tindall, 1982.

5. Edquist LE, Stabenfeldt GH: Reproductive hormones. *In* Kaneko JJ (ed): Clinical Biochemistry of Domestic Animals. 3rd Ed. New York, Academic Press, 1980, pp. 513–544.

6. Gorbman A, Dickoff WW, Vigna SR, et al.: Comparative Endocrinology. New York, John Wiley and Sons, 1983.

7. Hafez ESE (ed): Reproduction in Farm Animals. 4th Ed. Philadelphia, Lea & Febiger, 1980.

8. Lein CK (consulting ed): Reproductive disorders. *In* Kirk RW (ed): Current Veterinary Therapy VIII. Philadelphia, WB Saunders Co., 1983, pp. 885–964.

9. Neely DP, Liu IKM, Hillman RB: Equine Reproduction: A Review for Equine Practitioners. New Jersey, Veterinary Learning Systems Co, Hoffman-La Roche, 1983.

10. Thomas JA, Mawhinney MG: Synopsis of Endocrine Pharmacology. Baltimore, University Park Press, 1973.

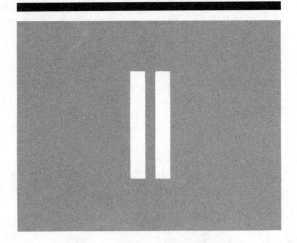

SECTION

II

DIAGNOSTIC ENDOCRINOLOGY

Ray F. Nachreiner, D.V.M., Ph.D.

Consulting Editor

Laboratory Endocrine Diagnostic Procedures in Theriogenology

Ray F. Nachreiner, D.V.M., Ph.D.
Michigan State University, East Lansing, Michigan

Since the advent of the radioimmunoassay (RIA), many hormone assay procedures have been developed. Commercial RIA kits are available for quantitating many hormones, but few are designed and developed for animal procedures. Some laboratories have diligently striven to modify these procedures so that they may be applied to animal specimens. Practitioners often utilize referral laboratories for analysis of progesterone, 17β-estradiol, testosterone and other clinically useful hormone determinations. Fortunately, research continues using procedures such as the enzyme-linked immunosorbent assay (ELISA), enzyme immunoassay (EIA), fluorescence immunoassays (FIA) and others to make hormone determinations more practical in the practitioner's office. A number of procedures are presently practical, including a recent ELISA procedure for pregnant mare serum gonadotropin (PMSG) determination, which has been marketed for veterinary use. Veterinary-oriented laboratories should be identified and utilized for technically difficult hormone quantitation.

TESTOSTERONE

The assay of testosterone usually involves an extraction procedure to remove the hormone from the serum. Hence, there are less problems with species idiosyncrasies. The assay is useful in determining male maturity (puberty), cryptorchid conditions, ovarian tumors, excess androgen production and other procedures in which testosterone quantitation is clinically relevant.

Puberty. At puberty gonadotropins stimulate changes in the interstitial cells of the testicle so that testosterone is produced. Prior to puberty in males, females and castrates, the testosterone concentration in serum is quite low. Therefore, in males the significant increase may be used to indicate onset of puberty.

Cryptorchids. In some species cryptorchid conditions occur frequently. Horses with cryptorchidism are a problem, since they continue to demonstrate the behavior of an intact male. Iden-

tification of this condition may be difficult in many animals owing to a vague clinical history. In addition, episodic surges of testosterone release in normal stallions can cause considerable variation in the "basal" testosterone concentration. In one study it was found to vary from 0.5 to 1.4 ng/ml over an 8-hour period. As a result, a provocative procedure has been established to help determine cryptorchid tissue. Human chorionic gonadotropin (hCG) and gonadotropin-releasing hormone (GnRH) response tests are quite predictable in their release of testosterone in castrate, cryptorchid and normal stallions. In the hCG response test, a basal serum sample is obtained. An injection of 10,000 IU hCG is administered intravenously (IV) and 30-, 60- and 120-minute serum samples are obtained. Normal stallions give the following response: preinjection, 0.20 to 0.98 ng/ml; 30 minutes, 1.09 to 1.77 ng/ml; 60 minutes, 1.47 to 2.35 ng/ml; and 120 minutes, 1.47 to 2.35 ng/ml. Castrates start at less than 0.10 ng/ml and show no significant response at any of the time intervals. Cryptorchid horses start between 0.10 and 1.50 ng/ml and show marked responses to the hCG, similar to normal stallions. The most common basal values in cryptorchids are 0.25 to 0.45 ng/ml and a response to 0.50 to 1.45 ng/ml in one of the postinjection samples.

A response test has also been established for differentiation of castrates and cryptorchids using GnRH. This may be more practical for smaller species, since the cost is prohibitive at this time in horses. When economically feasible, 1000 μg of GnRH can be injected IV, and samples can be obtained prior to injection and at 30-, 60- and 120-minutes postinjection, similar to the hCG response test. Testosterone release in normal stallions has been found to be as follows: preinjection, 0.40 to 1.60 ng/ml; 30 minutes, 0.35 to 1.62 ng/ml; 60 minutes, 1.25 to 2.60 ng/ml; and 120 minutes, 2.00 to 3.50 ng/ml. Cryptorchids had 0.14 to 0.75 ng/ml prior to GnRH administration and doubled these concentrations on one or more post-GnRH samples. Complete castrates, of course, will not show testosterone release after GnRH.

A GnRH response test has also been developed for the dog. A preinjection sample is obtained, and an IV injection of 0.22 μg/kg GnRH is administered. Samples are obtained at 30 and 60 minutes after injection. Average values for testosterone were the following: preinjection, 2.09 ng/ml; 30 minutes, 3.36 ng/ml; and 60 minutes, 4.28 ng/ml. 17β-estradiol was not released in response to hCG or GnRH in dogs. This procedure may be used to evaluate normal testicular function as well as to differentiate between cryptorchids and complete castrates; no testosterone response identifies the castrate.

Pituitary Function. GnRH may also be useful in the evaluation of normal gonadotropin release and testicular response in stallions used for breeding purposes, since it indicates that both the pituitary gland and testicles are capable of normal hormone release. In addition, the test may be useful for locating the site of disease in infertile animals. Release of testosterone after GnRH stimulus indicates that both pituitary and gonadal endocrine functions are normal. Release of luteinizing hormone (LH) (assuming an assay is available) without testosterone release would indicate a normal pituitary gland but an abnormal testicle. Neither testosterone nor LH release would indicate pituitary gland disease. In this final case, an hCG response test could be used to determine whether testicular function is normal or whether there is also pathologic function in the testicle.

Granulosa Cell Tumor. Palpable ovarian masses are often of concern in mares. The testosterone assay of mare serum has been useful in determining abnormal androgen production from this tissue. Concentrations greater than 100 pg/ml are common in mares with granulosa cell tumors. The results from these assays can give the practitioner additional evidence for the existence of disease and the need for surgical intervention.

ESTROGENS

Pregnancy Diagnosis and Fetal Monitoring. Numerous reports are beginning to appear outlining the usefulness of estrone sulfate (E_1S) in the diagnosis of pregnancy and as a monitor of fetal viability. Since the hormone is of fetoplacental origin, it is a useful tool for both. In goats, E_1S is produced in high concentrations beginning near day 45 of gestation. In cattle, E_1S is found in the serum or milk and may be detected near day 120 for monitoring fetal viability. Also E_1S is found in high concentrations in horses' serum and urine beginning near day 100. It is found in sows' serum early in gestation (days 26 to 32) but drops rapidly to low levels. In this early time period, a positive correlation has been reported between E_1S concentration and fetal number. Therefore, it may be practical for identifying and culling sows with small litters.

Cryptorchid Horse. Total serum estrogens have been used to determine cryptorchidism in horses. Since estrone is one of the major testicular estrogens produced by stallions, the estrone sulfate assay is also useful for determining cryptorchidism.

Monitoring Estrous Cycles. 17β-estradiol (E_2) is the major estrogen produced by the ovarian follicle in many species. Hence, the assay is available for diagnostic use in many laboratories. Some animals, such as the cow, have very low concentrations of estrogens (1 to 15 pg/ml). The concentration increases to 5 to 15 pg/ml during the follicular phase of the cycle and estrus. During the luteal phase E_2 tends to drop to about 2 to 5 pg/ml. These low concentrations are very close to the "sensitivity" of many assays. As a result, most laboratories request 2 ml of serum or more for extraction and analysis.

Milk or serum progesterone assays can also be helpful in monitoring estrous cycles.

Sertoli's Cell Tumor. Sertoli's cell tumors in older cryptorchid dogs may be difficult to diagnose, since the condition may mimic many other nonspecific dermatoses, especially in their early stages. Total estrogen assays and assays specific for individual estrogens, such as E_2, may be helpful in establishing a diagnosis. Male dogs with Sertoli's cell tumors usually have serum E_2 concentrations greater than 10 pg/ml. In our laboratory normal males have 2.0 to 6.2 pg/ml. When high E_2 is found, it is suggestive of the presence of a Sertoli's cell tumor. Unfortunately, a normal concentration does not rule out the condition, since some of these tumors may produce other estrogens in excess or none at all.

PROGESTERONE

Estrous Cycles. One of the most accurate methods of determining ovarian cyclicity in suspected anestrous animals is to take serial samples and to assay the progesterone concentration. The interval for sampling is species dependent. Samples should be obtained monthly for anestrous dogs and weekly for anestrous horses, cows, pigs, sheep and goats. "High" concentrations will be found during the luteal phase, and "low" concentrations will be found at estrus. Low concentrations will persist in anestrous females that have ovarian inactivity. Progesterone has been shown to adhere to red blood cells, so the serum must be removed from the clot within one-half hour of sample collection.

Cystic Ovarian Disease. Cows with luteinized ovarian cysts will have elevated progesterone in their serum. These cows respond poorly to attempts to induce ovulation but respond more favorably to a therapeutic regimen that includes luteolytic substances such as prostaglandin $F_{2\alpha}$. Cows with ovarian cysts that are producing low concentrations of progesterone respond favorably to GnRH, hCG or LH.

Early Embryonic Death. A poorly functioning corpus luteum (CL) may result from a lack of luteotropic substances as well as from excess luteolytic substances. Each species appears to have a progesterone threshold that is necessary for maintenance of pregnancy. When progesterone concentrations drop below this threshold, abortion may occur. In some species, however, the low progesterone can be the result of the condition rather than a cause of the abortion. One should strive to eliminate other causes of abortion before attempting to use progesterone assays in the clinical work-up. By obtaining frequent samples from animals that chronically abort, especially near the time the abortions have occurred in the past, it may be possible to detect the poor CL function prior to the abortion. Some practitioners have supplemented these animals with exogenous long-acting or slow-release progestins that may have helped to maintain the pregnancies. Progesterone's biologic half-life is less than 1 hour in most species, so depot preparations are important for therapeutic success.

Pregnancy Diagnosis. In many species the absence of progesterone is a very good indication of the absence of pregnancy. However, the presence of progesterone in serum is not unique to pregnancy, since it is also present during the luteal phase of the estrous cycle. In our laboratory, serum progesterone during the midluteal phase of the cycle is 4 to 20 ng/ml in cows, 4 to 15 ng/ml in horses and 20 to 30 ng/ml in dogs. By obtaining samples at the next expected estrus, the presence of progesterone is suggestive of pregnancy, but accuracy is poor. Accuracy can be increased by obtaining a sample low in progesterone at estrus followed by a sample at the next expected estrus that is elevated. This procedure is more practical when milk can be used for the progesterone determinations, since the farmer can readily obtain the sample.

Milk Progesterone. Milk progesterone determinations have the potential to become a good management tool in theriogenology. Progesterone in milk closely correlates with the concentrations found in serum. The progesterone is more concentrated in the fat fraction than in skim milk. Many new assays have adequate sensitivity to quantitate skim milk or whole milk. A number of practical applications have been studied in dairy cattle.

1. Pregnancy Diagnosis. By obtaining samples 22 to 25 days after estrus, a presumptive diagnosis of pregnancy can be made. The accuracy, however, ranges from 60 to 90 per cent. By obtaining a sample at breeding or insemination that has low progesterone and then finding a high progesterone at days 22 to 25, the accuracy may be increased to over 90 per cent. Early embryonic death will prevent this from becoming more accurate.

2. Estrus Check. Cows showing signs of estrus can be checked for progesterone concentration prior to insemination. If in estrus, the levels should be very low. When finding significantly high concentrations of progesterone with a "rapid turn around" assay, insemination can be withheld and valuable semen saved. In addition, this may be a useful management and educational tool in teaching the herdsman the signs of estrus. Studies have shown that 13 to 30 per cent of cattle are inseminated during nonestrous stages of the estrous cycle. This could be prevented with a rapid assay. Herdsmen have improved their techniques of estrus detection when faced with "hard" data indicating that the cow would not be in estrus.

3. Lactational Anestrous Period. Some heavy producing cows show a prolonged lactational anestrous period. Because of the value of these cows, the herdsman may become concerned about reproductive status. Weekly samples from these cows may be used to follow their ovarian activity. When luteal activity is detected, the next estrus can be approximated. Some of these cattle may have short cycles and unexpected falls in milk progesterone.

This is often a result of heavy lactation, and the cow will usually begin to cycle normally at a later date. When these short cycles are detected, the farmer can be reassured that the cow is not abnormal.

4. Silent "Heat." Some valuable high-producing cows may not exhibit strong signs of estrus. By assaying milk progesterone every 2 days on these cows, the estrous cycle can be determined quite accurately. High progesterone indicates luteal activity. Falling progesterone indicates CL regression. The cow can be inseminated on the second and third days of baseline progesterone (estrus concentrations). These days correlate highly with the days of estrus in normal cycles.

5. Early Embryonic Death. In some cows the milk progesterone concentrations are borderline on the 21- to 23-day assay. These cows should be checked again, perhaps daily, to determine their status. Some of these will remain in the borderline range for 1 week or more (cycle length 28 to 30 days) until falling to estrus levels with the cow returning to estrus. One potential cause of the borderline low progesterone is impending abortion due to early embryonic death.

HYPOTHYROIDISM

Common clinical features in hypothyroid humans include females with amenorrhea and reduced libido and fertility in both sexes. The normal ranges for thyroxine (T_4) and triiodothyronine (T_3) for dogs in our laboratory vary somewhat with season, being slightly higher in winter. Generally, they are 0.75 to 2.0 ng/ml for T_3 and 10 to 40 ng/ml for T_4. In a retrospective study only 0.1 per cent of our samples were received primarily for detection of reproductive problems. Some samples were received from bitches with irregular estrous cycles, and 7 of 19 had low thyroid function. Eighteen male dogs with breeding problems were examined, and eight of these animals had evidence of low thyroid function. Practitioners reported that some of these dogs began cycling or had improved fertility after therapy was begun, but an objective study was not performed. In a subsequent objective study of the effects of thyroidectomy on estrous cycles in 10 bitches, all cycled normally within 3 months of thyroidectomy. Serum hormone concentrations were indicative of classic primary hypothyroidism during this entire period. In a study of stallions reported at Cornell University, thyroidectomy at 18 months of age decreased sexual desire and resulted in lethargy. However, semen characteristics, testicular histologic findings and fertility were not affected. Apparently, most animals can continue to reproduce even though they are hypothyroid. However, animals with abnormal reproductive function may have low thyroid function, and therapy may help these individuals. Although a cause and effect relationship has not been scientifically established, clinical evidence indicates that the thyroid should be considered as a cause of infertility in dogs and other species if other causes have been ruled out.

SAMPLE HANDLING AND SHIPMENT

Procedures for handling and shipment of samples and hormone levels expected from different types of samples vary from laboratory to laboratory. It is imperative that practitioners utilizing an endocrine diagnostic service check with the laboratory to find out what types of samples to obtain and how these should be shipped. For instance, thyroid hormone concentrations are slightly different in serum than in plasma. Also, refrigeration of samples for thyroid hormones is not necessary, but rapid deterioration of cortisol and insulin occurs if shipments are not kept cool. For progesterone analyses of milk, some laboratories use preservatives during shipment. As a rule, check with the laboratory prior to sample collection and shipment for specific instructions.

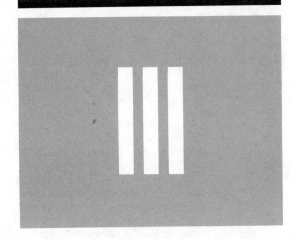

SECTION

III

PRINCIPLES OF
ANTIBIOTIC
THERAPY

Borje K. Gustafsson, D.V.M., Ph.D.

Consulting Editor

Rational Use of Antimicrobial Drugs

Lloyd E. Davis, D.V.M., Ph.D.
University of Illinois, Urbana, Illinois

Antimicrobial agents are among the most frequently used and misused drugs in veterinary practice. Overuse of antibiotics occurs because of factors such as operant conditioning, advertising, client pressure, and therapy by the laity. In response to this demand the annual production of antibiotics in the United States exceeded 26,000 tons in 1971. This quantity far exceeds any rational medical need.

Inappropriate use of drugs may result in (1) a delay in diagnosis, (2) a lack of effective therapy for a life-threatening but curable disease, (3) the production of toxicity, (4) the prolongation of a disease state, and (5) the development of a disorder to which a patient would otherwise not be subject.[4] All of these situations have been observed in veterinary practice. Inappropriate antimicrobial therapy instituted by the veterinarian or producer will lead to a subsequent delay in diagnosis by interfering with laboratory procedures for the identification of the etiologic agent. The fact that one has committed himself to inappropriate therapy tends to remove the motivation to delve deeper into other possible causes for an animal's illness. In addition, the veterinarian may induce severe toxic reactions in animals through drug interactions or direct adverse effects of drug therapy. An example of this is sudden death of cattle given intravenous antibiotics that are contained in a propylene glycol vehicle. Antibacterial drugs can prolong the course of diarrhea by inducing suprainfections within the intestinal tract. Examples of drug-induced disorders that have been observed in cattle by the author are acute anaphylactoid reactions to penicillin, drug fevers and eosinophilia associated with cephalosporins, paralysis leading to death caused by the parenteral administration of neomycin and deafness induced by dihydrostreptomycin.

A rational approach to antimicrobial therapy entails choosing the proper drug to be administered through a dosage regimen appropriate to the particular patient after consideration of potential benefits and risks. Prerequisites to rational therapy include a diagnosis, understanding of the pathophysiology of the disease and pharmacology of the drug and the establishment of therapeutic objectives. It is the purpose of this article to describe an approach to rational treatment of infections in the patient. It is the more concise definition of benefit and risk factors in drug therapy in animal patients that constitutes the principal efforts of the Clinical Pharmacology Studies Unit of the University of Illinois College of Veterinary Medicine.

DOCUMENTATION OF INFECTION

Establishment of an etiologic diagnosis is essential to the selection of the most effective drug with which to treat the infection. Ideally, this should be done for each incident of infection, but this is not often practical in most field situations. Fortunately, many infections are self-limiting in nature, and precise therapy is not essential for success in these cases. The veterinarian must make an effort to obtain additional information when he encounters the severely ill animal, the relapsed case or the patient showing no response to initial treatment. Samples of exudates, urine, cerebrospinal fluid, transtracheal aspirates and synovial fluid should be submitted to the laboratory for culture and sensitivity tests. The usual Kirby-Bauer technique for determining antimicrobial sensitivity of the isolate is helpful in the selection of an antibiotic, but the determination of minimal inhibitory concentration (MIC) of the antimicrobial is the more useful procedure. This was shown in the study of *Pasteurella* species isolated by Hjerpe from feedlot cattle.[3] He found a bimodal distribution in which some isolates were sensitive to various antimicrobics at concentrations attainable in vivo, whereas others would be resistant.

At the time of collection, it is wise to stain a smear of exudate, milk or sediment (following centrifugation) with Gram's stain and examine it microscopically. This can provide immediate information concerning the presence of bacteria and the general nature of the pathogen (gram-positive or negative, bacilli or cocci). This is a simple procedure that can be done on the farm and is inexpensive and rapidly performed. Such information will greatly improve the ability to select an effective drug for a particular case. If the Gram's stain is not used routinely, a convenient control for the staining procedure is to scrape human teeth and place this specimen on the edge of the slide prior to staining (the human mouth contains an abundance of both gram-positive and gram-negative bacteria).

In dealing with herd outbreaks of infectious disease, I advocate that the veterinarian approach the situation by doing a complete clinical evaluation of a few of the most severely affected animals. Therapy for the herd can then be predicated on the etiologic diagnosis made from this sample of the population. While there are still risks of error, this approach is more rational than institution of therapy in the absence of any information concerning the organism to be treated.

The importance of documenting the existence of a bacterial infection cannot be overemphasized. The most common treatment error I have observed in a referral practice setting is that veterinarians treat patients having viral, mycotic, neoplastic, metabolic or parasitic diseases with several antimicrobial drugs prior to referral. These patients frequently have adverse reactions to the drugs and have a multiple-resistant microbial flora. The only pathogens susceptible to antimicrobial therapy are bacteria, yeasts, chlamydia, rickettsia and certain protozoa.

The presence of fever or changes in the differential blood cell count are not in themselves adequate evidence that a patient has a bacterial infection requiring chemotherapy. Fever can be caused by immunologic disorders, neoplasia, drug reactions, excitement, exercise, increased environmental temperature, tissue damage following surgery or injury and dehydration. Neutrophilia can be produced by causes other than a suppurative process.

DRUG SELECTION

Once the clinician has documented the presence of an infection by a susceptible pathogen, he is in a position to select the most appropriate drug for therapy. Drugs approved by the Food and Drug administration for use in cattle are listed in Table 1. In addition to susceptibility of the organism to the drug, one must consider various pharmacologic, toxic and economical factors of the drugs.

To be effective, the drug must reach the site of infection at concentrations high enough to destroy or inhibit the infecting organism. Consideration should be given to drug absorption from the route of administration. Many drugs are poorly absorbed from the gut (aminoglycosides, acid-labile penicillins, some nitrofurans and cephalosporins, polymyxins and tetracyclines under certain circumstances). Chloramphenicol and trimethoprim are destroyed in the rumen, which would obviate this route for the treatment of systemic diseases. Absorption from muscle or subcutaneous sites may be poor in animals that are in shock or severely debilitated. In general, severe infections should be treated with parenterally administered drugs followed by oral administration if appropriate, during the convalescent phase.

Another factor to be considered in selecting a drug is its distribution in the body. For most body tissues, the permeation of various drugs is not a limiting factor in selecting a drug for therapy. Several of the commonly used antibacterial drugs will not enter freely into the brain, aqueous humor, prostate gland, bone, synovial fluid or serosal fluids. In such circumstances it would be appropriate to consider an alternative drug, shown to be active against the pathogen, or to increase the dosage of the drug initially selected.

Knowledge of routes of elimination of antimicrobial drugs is essential to selection of drugs for therapy. Drugs that are excreted unchanged by the kidneys—such as penicillins, aminoglycosides and certain tetracyclines or sulfonamides—must be used with caution and with dosage modification in patients with impaired renal function, e.g., pyelonephritis. Conversely, those compounds metabolized or eliminated by the liver (chlortetracycline and chloramphenicol) should be avoided in patients with hepatic dysfunction, e.g., "fat cow syndrome." In treating urinary tract or biliary infections, it is desirable to use an effective drug that is eliminated unchanged by these routes.

If everything else is equal, the least toxic and the lowest priced drug should be used to accomplish therapeutic objectives. Very seldom are combinations of antibacterial drugs needed in practice. The fewer drugs employed in a given patient, the less likelihood there will be of producing adverse reactions in the animal as a result of drug interactions or other untoward effects. In some circumstances the simultaneous use of two antimicrobial drugs can be advantageous because of their synergistic effects. Some examples are (1) penicillin and streptomycin in endocarditis caused by *Escherichia coli*, (2) polymyxin and sulfonamides in urinary tract infections caused by certain strains of *Proteus*, (3) carbenicillin and gentamicin for gentamicin-resistant *Pseudomonas* infections, (4) cephalothin and gentamicin for infections caused by resistant *E. coli, Klebsiella* or *Proteus* species, and (5) a sulfonamide with trimethoprim for nocardiosis.[1] These drugs should be employed separately and administered according to the usual dosage regimens for each drug. The only fixed dosage combination products that I advocate are the combination of a sulfonamide with trimethoprim and amoxicillin confined with clavulanic acid.

DRUG DOSAGE

The dosage of antimicrobial drugs is not a fixed entity, as suggested by Tables 1 to 5 but should be adjusted to the organism being treated. This is part of the art of veterinary practice. During drug development, the manufacturer is required to prove safety and efficacy of the drug. Efficacy will generally be established against an infection caused by an organism that is highly sensitive to the drug. Thus, the recommended dose appearing on the label or package insert will frequently be lower than the dose required for effective therapy against more resistant but still suceptible organisms. If the veterinarian has made an intelligent selection of a therapeutic agent based on a specific diagnosis, and the patient does not respond, he should increase the dose of the same drug rather than change drugs. We have had much better clinical results against several organisms susceptible to oxytetracycline at a dosage of 22 mg/kg repeated every 12 hours instead of the usual dose of 11 mg/kg given once daily. It was shown by studies conducted in our hospital that 11 mg/kg would maintain therapeutic concentrations of oxytetracycline in the uterus of

Table 1. Conventional Regimens for Some Antimicrobial Drugs in Ruminant Animals (Approved Drugs)

Drug	Dosage	Route	Repeat	Withhold Meat/Milk (days)
Ampicillin	11 mg/kg	IM	Daily	6/2
Cephapirin	200 mg/quarter	Intramammary	12 hr, lactating	0/4
Cloxacillin	500 mg/quarter	Intramammary	Dry cow	—
Dihydrostreptomycin	11 mg/kg	IM	12 hr	30/2
Erythromycin	4.4 mg/kg	IM	Daily	14/3
	216 mg/quarter	Intramammary	12 hr	—
Neomycin	11 mg/kg	Oral	Daily	30/0
	1–2 gm	Intrauterine	Daily	—
Oxytetracycline	11 mg/kg	IV, IM	Daily	5/2.5
	426 mg/quarter	Intramammary	12–24 hr	0/4
Penicillin G procaine	6600 U/kg	IM	Daily	5/3
	1,000,000 U/quarter	Intramammary	Dry cow	—
Sodium sulfamethazine	206 mg/kg initial, 103 mg/kg maintenance	IV, IM	Daily	15/4
	220 & 110 mg/kg	Oral	Daily	10/0
Sodium sulfapyridine	66 mg/kg	IV	Daily	
Sulfadimethoxine	55 mg/kg initial, 27.5 mg/kg maintenance	IV, oral	Daily	7/2.5
Sulfaethoxypyridazine	55 mg/kg	Oral	Daily	16/3
Triple sulfonamides	198 mg/kg initial, 132 mg/kg maintenance	IV, intraperitoneal, oral	12 hr	15/4
Tylosin	4.4 mg/kg	IM	Daily	8/4

Table 2. Extralabel Regimens for Some Antimicrobial Drugs in Ruminant Animals*

Drug	Dose	Route	Repeat
Cephalothin	30 mg/kg	IM	8 hr
Clotrimazole	100 mg/quarter	Intramammary	12 hr
Cloxacillin	10 mg/kg	IM	8 hr
Dihydrostreptomycin	11 mg/kg	IM	6 hr
Gentamicin	4 mg/kg	IM, IV	12 hr
Kanamycin	5 mg/kg	IM	8 hr
Oxytetracycline	22 mg/kg	IM, IV	12 hr
Penicillin G procaine	22,000 U/kg	IM	12 or 24 hr
Polymyxin B	55 mg/kg	IM	12 hr
	200 mg/quarter	Intramammary	12 hr
Trimethoprim + sulfapyridine	30 mg/kg	IM	12 hr

*Either the drug or the dosage suggested is not approved by the FDA for use in food-producing animals. The practitioner would assume liability associated with such usage.

Table 3. Conventional Regimens for Antimicrobial Drugs Approved for Use in Swine

Drug	Dose	Route	Repeat (Hours)	Withhold (Days)
Amoxicillin	40 mg/animal	Oral	12	15
Ampicillin	11 mg/kg	Oral	12	1
	6 mg/kg	IM	12	15
Chlortetracycline	22 mg/kg	Oral	24	5
Dihydrostreptomycin	11 mg/kg	IM	12	30
Erythromycin	6 mg/kg	IM	24	7
Furazolidone	100 mg/piglet	Oral	24	5
Lincomycin	11 mg/kg	IM	24	2
Neomycin	11 mg/kg	Oral	24	20
Oxytetracycline	6 mg/kg, 8 hrs before farrowing	IM	—	22
Penicillin G procaine	22,000 U/kg	IM	24	5
Sodium sulfachloropyridazine	35 mg/kg	Oral	12	4
Spectinomycin	22 mg/kg	Oral	12	21
Sulfaethoxypyridazine	110 mg/kg	Oral	24	10
Sulfamethazine	220 mg/kg	Oral	24	15
Tetracycline	11 mg/kg	Oral	12	4
Tylosin	9 mg/kg	IM	24	4

(From Lewis BP, Wilken LO: Veterinary Drug Index. Philadelphia, WB Saunders Co, 1982.)

Table 4. Dosage of Antimicrobial Drugs in Horses

Drug	Dose Range	Route	Dose Interval
Amphotericin B	0.5 mg/kg	IV	48 hrs
Ampicillin sodium	6.6–22 mg/kg	IM, IV	8 hrs
Benzyl penicillins:			
Sodium or potassium	20,000–60,000 U/kg	IM, SC, IV	6 hrs
Procaine	20,000–50,000 U/kg	IM	12–24 hrs
Benzathine	10,000 U/kg	IM	48 hrs
Carbenicillin	12.5–50 mg/kg	IM, IV	6 hrs
Cephalothin	10–25 mg/kg	IV	6 hrs
Chloramphenicol succinate	25–50 mg/kg	IM, SC, IV	2 hrs IV, 8 hrs SC or IM
Chloramphenicol base	25–50 mg/kg	Oral	8 hrs
Clindamycin	Contraindicated in horse		
Erythromycin	2.5 mg/kg	IV	6 hrs
Gentamicin	2–4 mg/kg	IM	8 hrs
Griseofulvin	10 mg/kg	Oral	24 hrs
Kanamycin	5–10 mg/kg	IM	8 hrs
Oxacillin	12.5–25 mg/kg	IM, IV	6 hrs
Oxytetracycline	8–15 mg/kg	IV	12 hrs
Polymyxin B sulfate	2 mg/kg	IM	12 hrs
Streptomycin	10–20 mg/kg	IM	6 hrs
Sulfamethazine	66–132 mg/kg	IV	12 hrs
Sulfadimethoxine	27.5–55 mg/kg	IV	24 hrs
Trimethoprim-Sulfapyridine	30 mg/kg (sulfa)	Oral	12 hrs

SC = subcutaneous

Table 5. Conventional Regimens for Some Antimicrobial Drugs in Dogs and Cats

Drug	Dose	Route	Repeat Dose
Amphotericin B	0.5–1.0 mg/kg	IV	2 or 3 days
Ampicillin	10–20 mg/kg	PO	6 hrs
	5–10 mg/kg	IV, IM, SC	6 hrs
Amoxicillin	11 mg/kg	PO, IM	12 hrs
Carbenicillin	15 mg/kg	IV	8 hrs
Cephalexin	30 mg/kg	PO	12 hrs
Cephaloridine	10 mg/kg	IM, SC	8–12 hrs
Cephalothin	35 mg/kg	IM, SC	8 hrs
Chloramphenicol	50 mg/kg	PO, IV, IM, SC	8 hrs (dog), 12 hrs (cat)
Chlortetracycline	20 mg/kg	PO	8 hrs
Cloxacillin	10 mg/kg	PO, IV, IM	6 hrs
Colistin	1 mg/kg	IM	6 hrs
Dihydrostreptomycin	20 mg/kg	PO	6 hrs (not absorbed)
	10 mg/kg	IM, SC	8 hrs
Erythromycin	10 mg/kg	PO	8 hrs
Framycetin	20 mg/kg	PO	6 hrs (not absorbed)
Gentamicin	4 mg/kg	IM, SC	12 hrs first day, then 24 hrs
Griseofulvin	20 mg/kg	PO	24 hrs, with fat
	140 mg/kg	PO	1 wk, with fat
Hetacillin	10–20 mg/kg	PO	8 hrs
Kanamycin	10 mg/kg	PO	6 hrs (not absorbed)
	7 mg/kg	IM, SC	6 hrs
Lincomycin	15 mg/kg	PO	8 hrs
	10 mg/kg	IV, IM	12 hrs
Methicillin	20 mg/kg	IV, IM	6 hrs
Metronidazole	60 mg/kg	PO	24 hrs
Nafcillin	10 mg/kg	PO, IM	6 hrs
Neomycin	20 mg/kg	PO	6 hrs (not absorbed)
	10 mg/kg	IM, SC	12 hrs
Nitrofurantoin	4 mg/kg	PO	8 hrs
	3 mg/kg	IM	12 hrs
Nystatin	100,000 U	PO	6 hrs (not absorbed)
Oxacillin	10 mg/kg	PO, IV, IM	6 hrs
Oxytetracycline	20 mg/kg	PO	8 hrs
	7 mg/kg	IV, IM	12 hrs
Penicillin G sodium or potassium	40,000 U/kg	PO	6 hrs (not with food)
	20,000 U/kg	IV, IM, SC	4 hrs
Penicillin G benzathine	40,000 U/kg	IM	5 days
Penicillin G procaine	20,000 U/kg	IM, SC	12–24 hrs
Penicillin V	10 mg/kg	PO	8 hrs
Phenethicillin	10 mg/kg	PO	8 hrs
Phthalylsulfathiazole	50 mg/kg	PO	6 hrs (not absorbed)
Polymyxin B	2 mg (20,000 U)/kg	IM	12 hrs
Pyrimethamine (initial)	1 mg/kg	PO	24 hrs for 3 days
(subsequent)	0.5 mg/kg	PO	24 hrs
Streptomycin	20 mg/kg	PO	6 hrs (not absorbed)
	10 mg/kg	IM, SC	8 hrs
Sulfadiazine, sulfamerazine, sulfamethazine	50 mg/kg	PO, IV	12 hrs
Sulfadimethoxine	25 mg/kg	PO, IV, IM	24 hrs
Sulfamethizole, sulfisoxazole	50 mg/kg	PO	8 hrs
Sulfasalazine	15 mg/kg	PO	6 hrs (dog only)
Tetracycline	20 mg/kg	PO	8 hrs
	7 mg/kg	IV, IM	12 hrs
Trimethoprim + sulfadiazine	30 mg/kg	PO	12 hrs
Trimethoprim + sulfadoxine	15 mg (combined)/kg	IV, IM	24 hrs
Tylosin	10 mg/kg	PO	8 hrs
	5 mg/kg	IV, IM	12 hrs

(From Davis LE: Antimicrobial therapy. In Kirk RW (ed) Current Veterinary Therapy VII. Philadelphia, WB Saunders Co, 1980, p 9.)

the cow for 12 hours but not for 24 hours.[2] Regimens for drugs not approved in the United States for use in food-producing animals and for approved drugs whose recommended doses are inadequate are listed in Table 2.

PITFALLS IN ANTIMICROBIAL THERAPY

The other half of the benefit-risk equation for antimicrobial chemotherapy involves hazards associated with the use of the various members of this class of drugs in patients. For discussion purposes risks can be divided into therapeutic failures and direct pharmacologic hazards caused by the presence of the drug in the patient.

Frequently Encountered Causes of Therapeutic Failure

Failure of a patient to respond to drug therapy can be of considerable importance to the patient and its owner when therapy is urgently needed. Some common causes of failure are listed in Table 6. These various possibilities should be considered and investigated in patients with documented infections not responding properly to chosen drug therapy.

Pharmacologic Hazards of Antimicrobial Therapy

Three principal mechanisms of toxicity produced by antimicrobial drugs are (1) dose-related toxicity, which can generally be predicted and which is related to overdosage or impaired pathways of drug elimination, (2) idiosyncratic or allergic reactions, which are not dose related and cannot often be predicted, and (3) drug interactions, which can be anticipated and prevented.

Dose-related toxicity will vary depending on the chemical class of drugs involved, and it will be manifested by organ toxicity. Neurotoxic antibiotics include the aminoglycosides, which will selectively damage either the vestibular or auditory nucleus of the eighth cranial nerve, and the penicillins, which will cause convulsions if directly applied to nervous tissue. Nephrotoxic drugs can (1) decrease the glomerular filtration rate (GFR) and damage renal tubules (aminoglycosides, polymyxins, amphotericin B, cephaloridine), (2) cause lower nephron nephrosis secondary to crystalluria (sulfonamides), or (3) produce renal tubular acidosis (amphotericin B or outdated tetracycline preparations). Hepatotoxic drugs include isoniazid, oxacillin, and erythromycin estolate. Tetracyclines can produce fulminant fatty metamorphosis of the liver late in pregnancy. Hematologic disorders include dose-related neutropenia with chloramphenicol, thrombocytopenia produced by isoniazid or chloramphenicol and hemolytic anemia associated with nitrofurantoin and sulfonamides.

Table 6. Frequent Causes of Failure of Antimicrobial Therapy*

1. Pharmacologic factors
   Drug interactions
   Inactivation due to incompatibilities
2. Presence of nondraining, deep-seated abscess
3. Obstruction of natural drainage of an infected area
4. Presence of a foreign body
   Soft tissues
   Bronchus
   Cystic calculi
5. Emergence of drug resistance
6. Antagonism from simultaneously administered antibiotics
7. Protection of a penicillin-susceptible pathogen on mucosal surfaces by a penicillinase-producing member of the normal host flora
8. Elimination of competing normal bacterial flora
9. Diseases impairing normal host defenses
10. Incorrect diagnoses
    Underlying noninfectious disease
    Drug reactions that may mimic signs of infectious disease
11. Incorrect dosage or route of administration
12. Presence of nontreatable diseases
    Viral, neoplastic, immune-mediated

*Adapted from Davis LE: Rational Therapy with Newer Antibacterial Drugs. Proc 45th Ann Meet Am Anim Hosp Assoc, 1978, p 72.

Chloramphenicol can suppress antibody production and may interfere with the development of active immunity. Until this situation is clarified, it would be wise not to immunize animals during a period of treatment with chloramphenicol.

Some antibiotics can be enterocolotoxic, and these include the broad-spectrum antibiotics, lincomycin, clindamycin and ampicillin. These effects are mediated, in part, by their alteration of the flora of the gut. The pathogenesis of hemorrhagic diarrhea associated with ampicillin has not been clarified. It has been demonstrated in experiments with hamsters that lincomycin produces pseudomembranous colitis by suppression of normal competing flora, which permits overgrowth by a fastidious, exotoxin-producing *Clostridium*. It is this exotoxin that induces the characteristic lesions. Pulmonary infiltrates may occur in animals treated with nitrofurantoin.

Tetracyclines administered during pregnancy or the neonatal period may cause enamel hypoplasia of the developing teeth and interfere with long bone growth. This group of antibiotics exerts an antianabolic effect by inhibiting protein synthesis. By virtue of this action, they can exacerbate uremia in patients with impaired renal function, and when employed in combination with high doses of corticosteroids, they can produce rapid development of general ill health and malnutrition.

Allergic reactions to antimicrobial drugs can manifest themselves in a variety of ways, including anaphylaxis, urticaria, angioneurotic edema, serum sickness, purpura, eosinophilia or drug fever. This type of drug reaction sometimes can be very misleading to the clinician. Fever caused by the drug might be interpreted as a worsening of the infectious process under treatment. Observation of eosinophilia might cause the veterinarian to question the original diagnosis of a bacterial infection, which was correct, and lead to suspicion of a parasitic or primary immune-mediated disease. The key diagnostic features of an allergic drug reaction are the following: (1) it is not dose related, (2) the clinical signs abate upon withdrawal of the drug, (3) some allergic manifestation will occur upon challenge with the same or similar drug, and (4) the fever is out of proportion to the clinical well-being of the animal. In a patient with no prior history of allergy, allergic reactions will be entirely unpredictable. The author is aware of healthy animals that were given antibiotics prophylactically and that died of anaphylactic reactions. In case of an acute allergic reaction such as anaphylaxis, urticaria, laryngeal edema or angioneurotic edema, one should *immediately administer epinephrine* intravenously or intramuscularly. Corticosteroids or antihistaminics are not effective in this situation. Administration of an antihistaminic is of value after the reaction has been controlled with epinephrine, in order to prevent a relapse.

A variety of drug interactions can occur between various antibiotics and other drugs. A complete discussion of drug interactions is beyond the scope of this article (see Veterinary Values, listed in the references). Some of the more common interactions with which the veterinarian should be familiar will be discussed here.

Chloramphenicol and the tetracyclines inhibit microsomal enzymes in the liver that metabolize a variety of drugs. If a second, pharmacologically active drug were administered to a patient receiving one of these drugs, the pharmacokinetics of the second drug would be modified, thus leading to accumulation or prolongation of its effect. Sleeping time with barbiturates is increased with the result that recovery from anesthesia will be prolonged.

Interactions can occur that will influence renal excretion of antimicrobial drugs. Probenecid and thiazide diuretics can compete with the penicillins for active transport by the proximal tubules and prolong the elimination rate of the penicillins leading to possible drug sensitization or elevated milk- and meat-drug residues. On the other hand, drugs with a high affinity for binding with albumin (e.g., phenylbutazone) can displace highly protein-bound antimicrobial drugs, such as sulfadimethoxine, which are excreted by glomerular filtration. This will cause more *rapid* excretion of the antimicrobial drug with resultant lower plasma concentrations and therapeutic values. Furthermore, displacement of drugs from protein will increase the concentration of unbound drug in the plasma, which is free to diffuse into tissues. Furosemide is normally about 98 per cent bound to serum albumin and is potentially ototoxic. If this drug were displaced by an aminoglycoside, the two drugs may have additive effects and cause loss of hearing.

A serious and not uncommon interaction occurs among anesthetic agents, and some other drugs, and aminoglycoside antibiotics that blocks the myoneural junction and inhibits the release of acetylcholine from motor nerve endings. This curariform effect results in paralysis of skeletal muscle with apnea. It is most commonly observed with administration of neomycin or polymyxin to animals during surgery. The use of aminoglycosides in patients receiving anesthetic agents, muscle relaxants, quinidine, promethazine or sodium citrate (blood transfusions) should be avoided. Should paralysis occur under these circumstances, the cause should be recognized as a drug interaction because it is reversible, and prompt action can be lifesaving. Paralysis may be corrected by administration of calcium gluconate solution or neostigmine.

Another common interaction can occur in the gastrointestinal tract to impair the absorption of certain antibiotics. Antacids, dairy products and iron salts will impair absorption of tetracyclines. Antidiarrheal preparations containing kaolin, pectin or bismuth will decrease the absorption of lincomycin and erythromycin from the gut. Slow absorption due to interactions of antimicrobial drugs with other drugs or foods will result in inadequate blood concentrations, slow onset of action and sustained release with possible prolonged undesirable effects. Some suggestions for minimizing the chance of an interaction are the following:

1. Whenever possible, avoid multiple drug therapy.

2. Avoid combination products.

3. With oral dosage forms, adjust the regimen relative to feeding times; i.e., tetracyclines are better given between meals.

4. Avoid simultaneous use of drugs that might be antagonistic; e.g., tetracyclines and penicillins.

5. Try to minimize the personal formulary to a point at which you are thoroughly familiar with each drug.

6. When in doubt, consult a pharmacist.

The use of chloramphenicol in food-producing animals has been absolutely prohibited by the U.S. Food and Drug Administration since this article was written. The author no longer advocates the use of chloramphenicol in the treatment of cattle and swine.

References

1. Anderson KL, Wilcke JR: Potentiated sulfonamides in the treatment of bovine pulmonary nocardiosis. J Vet Pharmacol Therap 3:217, 1980.
2. Bretzlaff KN, Ott RS, Koritz GD, et al.: Distribution of oxytetracycline in the genital tract of cows. Am J Vet Res 43:12, 1982.
3. Hjerpe CA, Routen TA: Practical and theoretical considerations concerning treatment of bacterial pneumonia in feedlot cattle, with special reference to antimicrobic therapy. Proc. 9th Ann Conven Am Assoc Bovine Pract 1976, pp 97–140.
4. Melmon KL, Morrelli HF: Clinical Pharmacology: Basic Principles in Therapeutics. 2nd ed. New York, Macmillan, 1978.
5. Veterinary Values '81. Available from Ag Resources, 15 West 44th St, New York, NY 10036.

Drug Interactions and Incompatibilities

John W. Paul, D.V.M., M.S.
Hoechst-Roussel Agri-Vet Company, Somerville,
New Jersey

The objective of this chapter is to describe interactions and incompatibilities of drugs used to treat reproductive diseases or to regulate reproductive functions. Some other drugs will also be discussed that can affect reproductive performance although administered for other purposes; namely, antiparasitic agents. Incompatibility of two or more drugs, usually in vitro, leads to an undesirable event. The outcome may be manifest by inactivation of the drugs or accumulation of toxic byproducts. Adverse reactions may occur as a result of an imcompatibility of a drug with an organ system. Drug interactions, on the other hand, are considered as events that occur resulting from two or more drugs reacting in vivo. The outcome of such interactions is often adverse or antagonistic; however, an enhanced or synergistic effect may occur. Finally, the interaction of certain drugs with laboratory tests is an important consideration for the interpretation of test results.

DRUG INTERACTIONS AND INCOMPATIBILITIES IN VIVO

Antimicrobials

Antimicrobials are the most commonly used drugs in animal health and have a prominent role with the theriogenologist. Use of combinations of antimicrobial drugs can affect their efficacy or safety. An example of enhanced efficacy or synergism can be found in the combined use of penicillin and streptomycin against some bacteria, especially streptococci. This may be due to the effect of penicillin on the cell wall of the bacterium, allowing streptomycin to enter the organism more readily.[8]

The interaction of edetate trisodium (EDTA-tris) and various antibiotics has been shown to be strongly synergistic.[19] Body cavities such as the uterus, bladder or external ear canal are lavaged with EDTA-tris and then infused with an antibiotic solution. The degree of edetate trisodium potentiation varies according to both the antibiotic selected and the infecting bacteria.

The combination of sulfadiazine and trimethoprim provides another example of a synergistic drug interaction by sequential inhibition of bacterial metabolism of para-aminobenzoic acid (PABA) and folic acid. This results in a bactericidal action of the combination.[3]

A classic example of drug antagonism is the concomitant use of bacteriostatic drugs (e.g., tetracyclines, chloramphenicol, sulfonamides) with bactericidal drugs (e.g., penicillins, cephalosporins, aminoglycosides). The reason is that bacteriostatic drugs inhibit bacterial multiplication, while bactericidal drugs kill multiplying bacteria.[8] In effect, bactericidal and bacteriostatic agents work against each other in terms of the growth phase during which organisms are susceptible. It must be emphasized that the foregoing example may be affected by drug concentrations and/or metabolic characteristics of various bacteria. Recent reports indicate that aminoglycosides can be inactivated by carbenicillin and ticarcillin. This has been observed more extensively in vitro; however, limited observations of an in vivo interaction suggest that these drugs should be used together only with strict monitoring.[13]

Interactions of antimicrobial drugs also affect safety. The aminoglycosides (streptomycin, dihydrostreptomycin, neomycin, kanamycin, gentamicin, amikacin, tobramycin) possess a potential for ototoxicity, nephrotoxicity and neuromuscular blockade. These toxic effects are additive with combinations of aminoglycosides.[11] Concurrent use of aminoglycosides with known neuromuscular blockers, including various anesthetics and depolarizing muscle relaxants, can result in respiratory distress and even failure, as well as reduced cardiac output.[1] The neuromuscular blocking effects of aminoglycosides are attributed to an inhibition of calcium.[1] Caution is advised in use of these drugs in postpartum cows, especially in those with a history of milk fever.[6]

Tetracyclines exert an antianabolic effect by virtue of their inhibition of protein synthesis. This action may also interfere with antibody production; however, this has not been well documented. Because of their antianabolic action and associated build-up of nitrogenous waste products, tetracyclines should not be used in animals with renal failure.[10] Tetracyclines are chelated by bivalent and trivalent cations such as calcium, magnesium, aluminum, and iron. Concurrent administration of milk products, antacids, calcium gluconate and other compounds containing these cations will reduce the antimicrobial action of tetracyclines.[8]

Administration of oxytetracycline to horses has been reported to result in severe diarrhea and occasionally death. This reaction may be associated with predisposing stress, such as hospitalization or surgery, and a latent *Salmonella* infection.[2] Tetracyclines also have neuromuscular blocking properties and can interact with anesthetics and muscle relaxants as already described.[1] Tetracyclines as well as chloramphenicol inhibit hepatic microsomal enzymes. The consequence is an interaction with barbiturates, phenytoin and analgesic-antipyretic drugs, resulting in prolonged effects of the latter drugs.[1]

Chloramphenicol can cause various toxic syndromes, including depression, anorexia, and bone marrow depression with dose-related anemia or non–dose-related aplastic anemia. Because chloramphenicol inhibits protein synthesis, antibody formation may also be impaired; however, this has been demonstrated only in animals given very large doses.[5]

Penicillin and its semisynthetic derivatives or impurities in their formulations can produce anaphylactoid reactions in sensitive individuals. Occasionally, a single treatment may appear to serve as the sensitizing as well as the shock dose; however, previous exposures may not be apparent if the veterinarian does not or cannot obtain an adequate history. Owing to the longer duration of blood levels of penicillin when administered as the benzathine salt, the duration of shock potential is proportionately longer.[11]

Cephalosporins are chemically related to penicillin. Evidence exists of partial cross sensitivity with penicillin. Chronic use in cats depresses the red blood cell count, packed cell volume and hemoglobin level. Large doses can be nephrotoxic. Cephaloridine can cause pain at the site of IM injection.[17]

Reactions to sulfonamides vary according to the specific drug. The older sulfas are less soluble compared with more recent derivatives. Insoluble sulfas are more likely to cause crystalluria and associated renal problems. This condition is more likely to occur in animals with low water intake and a low urine pH. Some individuals are hypersensitive to sulfonamides. Prolonged therapy in cattle can alter the rumen flora and interfere with rumen function.[17]

Sulfonamides represent an interesting example of improved safety resulting from the interaction of combined sulfas. Sulfamethazine, sulfamerazine and sulfathiazole (triple sulfa) are additive in respect to antimicrobial action; however, the solubility of each sulfa is independent—not additive—resulting in greater safety of the combination with reference to crystalluria.[17]

Hormones

Hormones offer an exquisite example of naturally occurring interactions; for instance, estrogens sensitize the uterus to respond to oxytocin, stimulate the hypothalamus to secrete gonadotropin-releasing hormone (GnRH) and prime the pituitary to release follicle stimulating hormone (FSH) and luteinizing hormone (LH) in response to GnRH. These are positive actions that are involved with "turning on" reproductive functions. Progestins, on the other hand, "turn off" the cycle by suppressing secretion of GnRH by the pituitary. Progestins also interact with the events of pregnancy to prepare the uterus

for pregnancy and to sustain pregnancy. It must be emphasized that estrogens and progestins do not act independent of one another, but these two hormones interact either synergistically or antagonistically in all respects.[7]

A thorough understanding of functions and interactions of naturally occurring hormones provides the veterinarian with an opportunity to improve reproductive efficiency. Synchronization or regulation of estrus is an important reproductive management tool. This can be achieved in a wide variety of ways, all of which utilize strategic administration of hormones, including progestins, estradiol, GnRH, human chorionic gonadotropin (hCG) and $PGF_{2\alpha}$.

Other potential effects, some favorable and some adverse, must be considered. Estrogens have a beneficial effect on the uterus in respect to infectious processes[18] but can cause aplastic anemia with prolonged treatment; the bitch is especially sensitive to this adverse effect.[14] Progesterone can increase the susceptibility to uterine infection[18]; again, the bitch with cystic hyperplasia-pyometra complex is a prime example of an adverse effect of progestin on the uterus.[9]

Anabolic steroids are often used in horses to improve performance and accelerate growth. Detrimental effects of these drugs have been shown in both males and females. In a study with stallions, LH concentration was reduced, as was sperm concentration, motility and total sperm per ejaculate; size of the testes was also reduced.[16] Mares treated with anabolic steroids had abnormal heat periods, smaller ovaries and fewer follicles. These mares also demonstrated signs of masculinity.[15]

Antiparasitics

Breeding animals are often treated for parasitism in an effort to improve the condition of the parents and to reduce parasitic infective stages in the environment to which the newborn is exposed. Most of the newer antiparasitic drugs enjoy wide margins of safety, including their use in breeding animals. The following warnings are taken from product labeling:

1. Bunamidine should not be given to male dogs within 28 days of breeding.

2. Butamisole should not be given to bitches during the first three weeks of pregnancy.

3. Cyothiate should not be given to pregnant bitches for flea control.

4. Cambendazole should not be given to mares during the first 3 months of pregnancy.

5. The effects of ivermectin on pregnant mares have not been determined.

6. The safety of oxibendazole has not been investigated in stallions; therefore, do not use in stallions at stud.

· 7. Products containing phenothiazine should not be given to mares during the last month of pregnancy.

DRUG INCOMPATIBILITIES IN VITRO

Veterinarians are often tempted to mix two or more drugs in vitro, either in the same vial or in the same syringe, to reduce the number of injection sites and to save time. In some situations this practice can be justified; however, the possibility of drugs being physically or chemically incompatible in admixtures must be considered. Drug incompatibilities in admixtures often become apparent, as evidenced by precipitation, color change, or gas formation. The real danger lies with those incompatibilities that do not show visible signs, but nevertheless an ingredient may be rendered inactive. For example, the high pH of sulfonamides inactivates penicillin, without visible signs to the user when mixed in vitro.[11] Extreme storage temperature, specifically freezing, can inactivate drugs. One must closely examine drugs that have been frozen.[4] If doubt exists about the integrity of a drug that has been frozen or exposed to high temperatures or if there are questions about the compatibility of drugs, one should consult a pharmacist or the drug manufacturer. Table 1 lists in vitro incompatibilities of some commonly used drugs.

Table 1. In Vitro Drug Incompatibilities

Drug	Incompatibility
Ampicillin	Do not mix with other drugs
Acepromazine	Chloramphenicol, phenylbutazone, sulfonamides
Calcium gluconate	Sodium bicarbonate, tetracyclines, phenylbutazone, sulfonamides
Chloral hydrate	Alkaline solutions
Chloramphenicol	Erythromycin, hydrocortisone, tetracyclines, procaine, vitamin B complex
Diazepam	Do not mix with other drugs
Erythromycin	Hydrocortisone, penicillin G, streptomycin, chloramphenicol
Furosemide	Ringer's solution
Gentamicin	Do not mix with other drugs
Hydrocortisone	Chloramphenicol, erythromycin, kanamycin, promazine, tylosin, tetracyclines
Kanamycin	Do not mix with other drugs
Levamisole	Neomycin, phenylbutazone, sulfonamides, tetracyclines
Lincomycin	Do not mix with other drugs
Penicillin G	Sulfonamides, erythromycin, tetracyclines
Sulfonamides	Acepromazine, calcium gluconate, dextrose, kanamycin, penicillin G, procaine, tylosin
Tetracyclines	Many solutions, including calcium
Tylosin	Hydrocortisone, tetracyclines, streptomycin, sulfonamides
Vitamin B complex	Many solutions, especially antibiotics
Xylazine	Thiamylal

Table 2. Potential Effects of Drugs on Laboratory Test Results

Drug	Laboratory Test Results
Acetylpromazine	Increased: glucose, bilirubin, alkaline phosphatase Decreased: cholinesterase, RBC count, WBC count, platelet count, hemoglobin, PCV
Ampicillin	Increased: alkaline phosphatase, eosinophils, SGOT, SGPT Decreased: none
Anabolic Steroids	Increased: calcium, phosphorus, BUN, total protein, total bilirubin, SGOT, SGPT Decreased: glucose, T_4
Corticosteroids	Increased: bilirubin, glucose, sodium, chloride Decreased: coagulation time, prothrombin time, WBC count, potassium
Erythromycin	Increased: alkaline phosphatase, SGOT, SGPT Decreased: cholesterol
Furosemide	Increased: BUN, glucose Decreased: sodium, potassium, calcium
Gentamicin	Increased: BUN, SGOT, SGPT Decreased: none
Nitrofurantoin	Increased: brownish urine, bilirubin, eosinophils, SGOT, SGPT Decreased: none
Penicillin	Increased: alkaline phosphatase, protein, Coombs' test Decreased: RBC count, WBC count
Phenothiazine	Increased: red-brown urine, bilirubin, glucose, SGOT, SGPT Decreased: none
Phenylbutazone	Increased: BUN, creatinine, glucose, bilirubin, SGOT, SGPT, sodium, chloride Decreased: RBC count, hemoglobin, PCV
Phenytoin	Increased: red-brown urine, glucose, bilirubin, alkaline phosphatase Decreased: none
Sulfonamides	Increased: amino acids, bilirubin, BUN, SGOT, WBC count, prothrombin time, urine crystals, brownish urine, urine glucose Decreased: protein-bound iodine, RBC count
Tetracycline	Increased: BUN, coagulation time, WBC count, urine glucose, urine protein Decreased: calcium, potassium
Thiabendazole	Increased: chloride, glucose, SGOT Decreased: WBC count
Xylazine	Increased: blood glucose, urine glucose, BUN Decreased: RBC count, hemoglobin, PCV, blood insulin

INTERACTION OF DRUGS WITH LABORATORY TESTS

Deviation from normal laboratory test values may be caused by the influence of drugs on enzyme systems or directly on the chemistry of a test procedure. The presence of a drug may also cause pathologic changes in organs, which may be reflected in laboratory test results. This is a very important aspect of drug interactions and one that is often overlooked. Table 2 lists potential effects of various drugs on laboratory test results.

Sound clinical judgment must be used in the interpretation of laboratory test results when the patient is under medication or has recently been medicated. When considering laboratory test values, one might pose the following questions: Am I aware of the patient's complete medication history? Am I sufficiently familiar with the laboratory procedure to be able to rule out the possibility of drug interference? Am I making a diagnostic or therapeutic decision based upon the most specific laboratory determination?[12]

The concept of drug interactions and incompatibilities is worthy of consideration when one evaluates laboratory test results or observes changes in the appearance of a drug, especially in an admixture. The same concept may be valid when adverse reactions are encountered or when expected efficacy is not achieved. The clinical significance of many drug interactions in animals is often minor, while in some cases an interaction may be fatal. The temptation to use multiple drug therapy and/or high doses of drugs in the critically ill patient increases the chances for severe drug interactions, which could mean the difference between recovery or death.

References

1. Adams HR: Acute adverse effects of antibiotics. JAVMA 166:983, 1975.
2. Baker JR, Leyland A: Diarrhea in the horse associated with stress and tetracycline therapy. Vet Rec 93:583, 1973.
3. Bushby S: Biochemical basis of chemotherapy and bacteriology concepts of trimethoprim-sulfonamide combinations. Proc Symp Trimethoprim/sulfadiazine. Burroughs-Wellcome Co, 1978, pp 4–13.
4. Cutie MR: Effects of cold and freezing on pharmaceuticals. US Pharmacist 4:38, 1979.
5. Clark CH: Metabolic effects and toxicities of chloramphenicol. MVP 59:663, 1978.
6. Crawford LM, et al.: Hypocalcemic effect of aminoglycoside antibiotics in the dairy cow. Can J Comp Med 41:251, 1977.
7. Dickson WM: Endocrinology, reproduction, and lactation. In Swenson MJ (ed): Dukes' Physiology of Domestic Animals. 9th ed, Ithaca, Comstock Publishing Assoc, 1977, pp 763–764.
8. Glaser U: Drug interaction with antimicrobial substances. Dtsche Tierarztl Wschr 86:274, 1979.
9. Hardy RM: Cystic endometrial hyperplasia-pyometra complex. In Morrow DA (ed): Current Therapy in Theriogenology. Philadelphia, WB Saunders Co, 1980, pp 624–630.
10. Osborne CA, Klausner JS: In Veterinarian Medicine Reproduction. University of Minnesota, Minneapolis, 1977, p 103.
11. Paul JW: Drug interactions. In Howard JL (ed): Current Veterinary Therapy: Food Animal Practice. Philadelphia, WB Saunders Co, 1981, pp 38–41.
12. Reiss BS: Interactions of drugs and laboratory tests. J Clin Pharmacol 15:135, 1975.
13. Rich DS: Recent information about inactivation of aminoglycosides by carbenicillin and ticarcillin: Clinical implications. Hosp Pharm 18:41, 1983.
14. Schalm OW: Exogenous estrogen toxicity in the dog. Canine Pract 5:57, 1978.
15. Squires EL, et al: Effect of anabolic steroids on reproductive function of young mares. Proc. 8th Equine Nutr Physiol Symp, 1983, p 279.
16. Squires EL, et al.: Effect of anabolic steroids on reproductive function of young stallions. J Anim Sci 54:576, 1982.
17. Upson DW: Upson's Handbook of Clinical Veterinary Pharmacology. Bonner Springs, VM Publishing Co, 1980, p 230.
18. Washburn SM, et al.: Effect of estrogen and progesterone on the phagocytic response of ovariectomized mares infected in utero with β-hemolytic streptococci. Am J Vet Res 43:1367, 1982.
19. Wooley RE: EDTA-tris potentiation of antimicrobial agents. MVP 64:113, 1983.

Factors of Importance for the Disposition of Antibiotics in the Female Genital Tract

Katherine N. Bretzlaff, D.V.M., M.S.
University of Illinois, Urbana, Illinois

Infections of the genital tract have been treated over the years with a wide variety of antibiotics. Although much remains to be learned about proper dosage regimens for effective antimicrobial therapy of the reproductive system, current knowledge permits recognition of some of the factors influencing drug disposition in genital tissues.

ROUTE OF ADMINISTRATION

Primarily, two methods of antimicrobial administration are used for treatment of genital tract infections: (1) systemic (intravenous, intramuscular, subcutaneous) and (2) intrauterine.

Following systemic administration of an antimicrobial, plasma concentrations will be achieved depending on the drug's absorptive, distributive, metabolic and excretive properties. Blood plasma concentrations will then be related to genital tissue concentrations depending on numerous factors, including plasma protein and tissue binding, blood flow to the genital tract, diffusion characteristics of the drug, concentration gradients between blood and genital tissues, lipid solubility of the drug and the differential between blood and tissue fluid pH.

Following local, or intrauterine (IU), administration of an antimicrobial, genital tissue concentrations will be related to factors such as physical distribution of the drug in the genital tract, genital tissue or other binding of the drug within the tract, diffusion from the lumen into genital tissues and absorption into the blood.

Many studies have considered serum or plasma concentrations of the drugs following intrauterine application. This information allows determinations of rate and efficiency of absorption from the uterus. It does not reveal concentrations of antimicrobials that exist in the genital tissues. More recently, studies have included assessment of genital tract tissue concentrations of antibiotics following transcervical biopsies, surgical removal or post-mortem collection of uterine tissue specimens after both

systemic (single IV or IM injections or continuous IV infusions) and IU administration. Such data permit the determination of actual tissue concentrations of these compounds.

A number of antimicrobials have been determined to be absorbed from the genital tract of cows and mares following IU administration. Sulfonamides, tetracyclines, dihydrostreptomycin, penicillin G sodium and procaine, ampicillin, ticarcillin, gentamicin, amikacin and chloramphenicol have been among the antibiotics investigated.

In cows, a number of sulfonamides have been shown to be absorbed from the uterus, with peak blood concentrations occurring 2 hours after infusion, with detectable levels remaining in the blood for 12 to 24 hours.[1, 2, 3, 4] Penicillin was absorbed rapidly after an IU infusion, reaching peak plasma concentrations 1 hour after administration and declining to less than 1 IU per ml by 4 hours.[2, 5, 6] Endometrial concentrations were detectable for 24 hours after IU infusion.[4] Following IM injections of sodium penicillin G, peak blood concentrations were higher, occurred more quickly and lasted longer than those after IU infusions. Endometrial concentrations were present for 8 hours but were considerably less than those achieved following IU administration.[5]

Peak concentrations of dihydrostreptomycin in serum occurred 1 to 2 hours following IU administration to cows.[2] Detectable concentrations were present in serum 24 hours after infusion.

Chlortetracycline has been shown to be absorbed from the bovine uterus, with peak blood concentrations occurring approximately 2 hours after infusion.[7] Serum concentrations following IU infusion were noticeably less than those following IV administration.

Oxytetracycline has been shown to reach peak blood concentration levels 2 to 4 hours after IU administration to cows, with detectable concentrations remaining at 24 hours.[2, 8, 9, 10] Intramuscular administration resulted in more rapid and complete absorption of the drug into the blood than after IU administration. Detectable concentrations of the drug were present in all tissues of the reproductive tract 24 hours after IM injection. Oxytetracycline concentrations were extremely high in the lumen and endometrium 24 hours after IU infusion, but very low, or nondetectable, in the ovaries, oviducts, myometrium, serosa, cervix and vagina.[9, 10]

Recent studies with gentamicin in the cow demonstrated that the drug was poorly absorbed from the uterus of diestrous cows, suggesting that concentrations in the lumen would remain high but that the drug would not reach subendometrial tissues.[11] Following IM administration of 4 mg/kg of gentamicin, therapeutic concentrations were achieved in the uterine lumen 6 hours after injection. Tissue concentrations were not determined, but plasma concentrations remained above therapeutic concentrations for 6 hours after administration.

Chloramphenicol was rapidly absorbed from the bovine uterus, with peak serum concentrations appearing 30 minutes after infusion.[12] Approximately 50 per cent of an IU dose was absorbed into the blood.

Studies conducted in mares have demonstrated that penicillin G sodium is rapidly absorbed from the uterus, with peak blood concentrations occurring 15 minutes after IU infusion and decreasing to very low concentrations after 5 hours.[13] One study showed that in general endometrial tissues contained only 50 to 75 per cent of blood concentrations after IM or IV administration of penicillin G sodium, while tissue concentrations after IV dosages of sodium ampicillin were equal to, or greater than, serum concentrations.[14] With either drug, serum concentrations declined rapidly, so that systemic administration every 4 to 5 hours was recommended for treatment of genital infections. Absorption of penicillin G sodium from the uterus was incomplete in one study in which plasma concentrations after IU infusion peaked at only 10 to 50 per cent of the peak concentrations after IM administration.[15] Therefore, it is possible that uterine tissue concentrations might remain elevated after blood concentrations have declined, as has been demonstrated in the cow.

Chloramphenicol is rapidly absorbed from the equine uterus,[16] with peak serum concentrations occurring 45 minutes after infusion. Approximately 50 per cent of an IU dose was found to be absorbed from the uterus, similar to findings in the cow.

Oxytetracycline has been studied in the mare,[17, 18] showing that absorption from the uterus following IU administration is slow and prolonged, with detectable serum concentrations still present 24 hours after infusion. Uterine and ovarian tissue concentrations greater than or equal to serum concentrations were observed at 12 and 24 hours after IV administration. Very high concentrations remained in uterine tissue 24 hours after IU administration.

Ticarcillin, a synthetic penicillin, was shown to be poorly absorbed from the equine uterus, with plasma concentrations disappearing 2 hours after IU infusion. Both IM and IU administration resulted in therapeutic uterine tissue concentration 2 hours after administration.[18]

Amikacin, a semisynthetic aminoglycoside, was not detected in serum following IU infusion in mares.[37] A dose of 2 gm administered IU resulted in peak concentrations of the drug in the endometrium 1 hour after infusion. Endometrial tissue concentrations were still detectable 24 hours after infusion.

A potentially complicating factor in the evaluation of IU application of antibiotics is the escape of the drug through the oviducts into the peritoneal cavity, where rapid and complete absorption might be expected. Occlusion of the oviducts in both cows and mares has resulted in lesser absorption of penicillin G sodium following IU administration.[19]

Although direct comparisons among experiments are not always possible, because different doses of the drugs are used and different analytical methods are employed, general conclusions can be drawn. Following intrauterine administration of antimicrobials, the drugs are absorbed into the general circulation, although not as rapidly, or as completely, as when systemic administration is employed. Concentrations of the drug in uterine contents and in tissues lining the uterine lumen are significantly higher and last longer following IU rather than systemic administration. However, other genital tract tissues achieve much lower drug concentrations after IU administration. Following systemic administration, significant concentrations of the drug occur in all genital tissues, as well as in the uterine lumen. After peak blood concentrations have been reached, concentrations in genital tissues may exceed those found in the blood, probably because elimination from genital tissues lags behind owing to the time required for equilibration.

When deciding between systemic and intrauterine routes of administration, it is important to assess the goal of therapy, i.e., to produce therapeutic concentrations of the drug at the appropriate site in order to produce the desired result. The precise anatomic location of the "appropriate site" may be debatable. There is little doubt that a primary focus of microbial growth is within the lumen of the tubular genital tract, suggesting that sufficient antibiotic concentrations in the uterine contents are of major concern. Likewise, it is logical that in animals with a septic metritis, there is an invasion of microorganisms into deeper layers of the uterine wall. This would imply that effective concentrations of the antimicrobial would be desired in all regions of the genital tract. Less certainty exists about desired distributions of drugs in animals with mild localized postpartum metritis or moderate postpartum metritis accompanied by some degree of systemic involvement or chronic purulent endometritis or pyometra. Distinguishing between "metritis" and "endometritis," which inherently suggests inflammations of differing involvements, may be of major importance when devising optimal treatment regimens. Additional considerations are the concentrations achieved in the often neglected portions of the reproductive tract: the oviducts, ovaries, cervix and vagina.

PHYSIOLOGIC STATE OF THE GENITAL TRACT

Studies with sulfonamides revealed that the proestrual or estrual bovine uterus absorbed a greater amount of the drug than the postestrual or anestrual uterus.[3] Benzyl penicillin sodium administered IU to estrous cows resulted in peak concentrations in plasma that were three times those following administration to diestrous cows.[20] Although another study suggested that absorption of sulfadimidine was decreased from the estrous bovine uterus, reflux through the cervix was a complicating factor.[21] Experimentally, IM or IU administration of estradiol benzoate to cycling cows resulted in absorption of enhanced penicillin benzyl sodium from the uterus, confirming the positive effect of estrogen on antibiotic absorption from this organ.[22] This effect was considered to be due to the increased uterine blood supply or the increased endometrial capillary permeability attributable to estrogen.

It is not clear whether progesterone has a negative effect on antibiotic concentrations achieved in the uterus. In rabbits that received IM injections of four different penicillins, uterine tubal fluid collected from doses in early pregnancy contained drug concentrations that were only 50 per cent of those collected from estrous doses.[23] It was considered that this result was possibly associated with the effects of progesterone on secretion of uterine tubal fluids.

Contrary to findings in cows, absorption of penicillin G sodium and ticarcillin from the equine uterus has been reported not to be affected by stage of the estrous cycle.[13, 18]

Decreased absorption of antimicrobials from the postpartum bovine uterus has been observed following IU administration. The rate and efficiency of absorption of sulfamethazine, oxytetracycline, penicillin G procaine and dihydrostreptomycin have all been demonstrated to be reduced and of less magnitude during the first 2 to 3 days postpartum than after 12 days.[2] Absorption of chloramphenicol from the bovine uterus was decreased during the first 60 days postpartum, although individual variation was considerable.[12]

Recent studies conducted with oxytetracycline have confirmed the differences between the early postpartum and the cycling bovine uterus.[25, 26] Using continuous IV infusions of the drug, a steady state equilibrium was approached between plasma and genital tissues. Plasma to uterine tissue ratios of oxytetracyclines at equilibrium approached 1.00 in cycling cows. In 3- to 4-day postpartum cows, however, significantly higher ratios were obtained. When uterine tissues were separated into caruncles, endometrium and uterine wall, mean plasma-to-tissue ratios were found to be 0.95, 1.33 and 1.88, respectively. The mean plasma-to-ovarian tissue ratio was 1.04. This suggested that significantly lower concentrations of the antibiotic were achieved in the endometrium, and especially the subendometrial uterine tissues, than were achieved in the blood. Preliminary results from studies with chloramphenicol indicate a similar trend.[27]

Potential reasons for decreased absorption of antibiotics from the early postpartum uterus include the involutional processes of denudation of epithelium, necrosis of caruncles, production of lochia and vascular regression. However, the decreased tissue concentrations resulting from systemic administration suggest that extraluminal factors are also involved, such as decreased blood flow to these tissues.

Although studies on the disposition of antimicrobials in the genital tract of postpartum mares are limited, no significant difference was reported in the absorption of penicillin G sodium from the uterus of postpartum and cycling mares.[13] Possibly, the more rapid involution of the equine uterus compared with that of the bovine uterus is involved.

The irritating effect of several substances commonly infused into the bovine uterus has been documented. Commercial preparations of oxytetracycline in propylene glycol, aqueous solutions of oxytetracycline hydrochloride and Lugol's (dilute iodine) solution have all been shown to cause endometrial necrosis.[28, 29] It would be logical to assume that the increased vascularity coincident with the irritation would result in increased absorption of these antimicrobials. However, in one study in which cows were infused with 10 per cent Lugol's iodine solution 30 minutes prior to IU administration of benzyl penicillin sodium, absorption of the drug from the uteri was not enhanced over that from uteri of cows receiving penicillin only.[20]

Contrary to findings in cows, infusion of Lugol's solution into the equine uterus 13 to 50 minutes prior to IU administration of benzyl penicillin sodium markedly increased absorption.[15] Swabbing of the uterus prior to antibiotic administration also increased antibiotic absorption in this species.[13]

PRESENCE OF PATHOLOGY

Many studies of antibiotic distribution in the genital tract have involved healthy cycling animals. Information derived from such studies may not be relevant to the treatment of animals with genital infections. The presence of inflammation and its byproducts could potentially influence the distribution and activity of antimicrobials.

A few studies have included comparative aspects of genital disease on antibiotic distribution. When oxytetracycline was administered IU to cows with chronic endometritis, absorption from the uterus into the bloodstream was less than that in healthy cycling animals. After IM administration, endometrial concentrations in diseased uteri were lower than those in the uteri of healthy counterparts 12 through 72 hours after administration.[9]

After continuous IV infusions of oxytetracycline to early postpartum cows with and without acute endometritis, no significant differences were found in plasma-to-genital tissue ratios.[26] However, following IU infusions into early postpartum cows with or without acute endometritis, uterine disease was associated with decreased drug absorption. This was reflected in reduced plasma concentrations and, therefore, lower tissue concentrations of oxytetracycline in subendometrial tissues.[10]

When acute endometritis was induced in healthy diestrous cows by infusion of *Corynebacterium pyogenes* and traumatization of the uterine wall, absorption of benzyl penicillin sodium, infused 11 to 18 hours after inoculation, was increased over that of control diestrous uteri.[22] Increased blood flow to the acutely inflamed involuted uterus may have been responsible.

The presence of retained fetal membranes (RFM) might prevent uniform drug distribution and absorption following IU administration. Controlled studies of this phenomenon are lacking. Following IU administration of penicillin, penicillin plus dihydrostreptomycin or penicillin plus dihydrostreptomycin plus nitrofurazone to 3-day postpartum cows with or without retained fetal membranes, no significant differences in required milk withholding times were observed.[30]

CHARACTERISTICS OF THE ANTIMICROBIALS

The binding of antimicrobials to blood plasma proteins is widely recognized as a phenomenon that could affect therapeutic efficacy because only the unbound drug is active and free to undergo equilibration with tissues.[31]

Binding of antimicrobials to tissues and body secretions may also occur, but the significance of this phenomenon in the treatment of genital tract disease is largely unknown. It would be of interest to know if the reduced absorption of antibiotics in the uteri of cows with endometritis is due to binding of the drugs to uterine secretions or to endometrial surfaces.

Physiochemical characteristics of the individual antimicrobial compounds influence their distribution in the genital tract. Diffusion of compounds in general, whether from blood to genital tissues (following systemic administration) or from the uterine lumen into blood (following IU administration) will be dictated by the nature of the drug (weak acid or weak base), pK_a values, pH of the local environment, molecular size and lipid solubility. The pH of the healthy bovine uterus has been reported to range from 5.5 to 7.0, which is less than the value of 7.4 reported for plasma.[32] The pH of uterine contents in cows with endometritis has been determined to be slightly more alkaline (7.5 to 8.5) than that of plasma. In other studies of bovine endometritis a less pronounced increase of uterine pH was observed.[22] When a differential pH occurs across biologic membranes, a corresponding differential in the degree of ionization of certain drugs occurs at equilibrium. Ionized drug is then trapped on one side of the membrane. In the case in which uterine contents are more acidic than plasma, an antimicrobial drug acting as a weak acid (e.g., penicillins, cephalosporins, and sulfonamides) would be ionized to a greater degree in plasma, resulting in a uterine contents-to-plasma drug ratio of less than one. An antimicrobial drug acting as a weak base (e.g., aminoglycosides, erythromycin, tylosin, lincomycin, trimethoprim) would be less ionized in plasma than in the uterus, resulting in a uterine contents-to-plasma drug ratio of greater than one. If uterine pH were more alkaline than plasma pH, the relationships would be reversed. In theory, then, the uterine concentration of a drug acting as a weak acid would be greater in a cow with endometritis than in a healthy cow. The reverse would be true

for a drug acting as a weak base. The actual significance of pH partitioning with respect to uterine infections is unknown. Other factors such as protein binding, ionization in serum, lipid solubility, molecular size and polarity also influence the movement of drugs across biologic membranes. In addition, equilibrium between uterine contents and plasma may not be achieved because of the larger volume of plasma and because of elimination of the drug from plasma.

The movement of a number of sulfonamides across the uterine membrane of guinea pigs has been determined to occur by passive diffusion.[34] More studies evaluating the uterine mucosa as a biologic membrane with respect to movement of antimicrobials need to be done.

A chelated formulation of oxytetracycline was demonstrated to be less absorbed from the bovine uterus than a nonchelated form, illustrating the importance of molecular structure.[8]

The pharmacokinetic properties of each drug influence its distribution in the genital tract. Following systemic administration, blood and, therefore, tissue concentrations will depend on the absorption, distribution, metabolism and excretion of each compound. Water soluble compounds are often more rapidly and completely absorbed than compounds solubilized in organic solvents such as propylene glycol. Therefore, an equivalent dose of an aqueous drug solution may result in higher tissue concentrations but may need to be administered more frequently to maintain these concentrations.

The *appropriate volume* of a drug solution to infuse for IU treatment is a much discussed topic, with little concrete data to support conclusions. It would be desirable to achieve a complete and uniform distribution of an antimicrobial agent throughout the uterine lumen. Of course, volumes should not be so large as to rupture the endometrium. Small volumes, especially in the early postpartum uterus, would not seem likely to be well distributed, particularly if RFM are present. However, large volumes of irritating solutions such as those containing organic solvents cannot be recommended. Large volumes also increase the chance of reflux through a relaxed cervix. One must also consider the existing volume of uterine contents. Infusion of large volumes of a dilute antimicrobial solution into an already fluid-filled uterus might result in an intraluminal concentration that is below the minimal inhibitory concentration of the drug.

Formulation of the antimicrobial is another important consideration. Antimicrobials have been placed intrauterinely in the form of pills, boluses, powders in gelatin capsules, powders wiped around the surface of the endometrium and aqueous and saline solutions. They are also often combined with estrogens, foaming preparations and other compounds designed, in theory, to disinfect and empty the uterine cavity. The efficacy of the various formulations is poorly documented.

The distribution of antibiotics in pressed, concentrated formulations such as boluses cannot be the same as that of an aqueous solution. Because of the requirement for dissolution, boluses result in lower, more prolonged blood concentrations. The distribution of such antimicrobials within the uterine lumen must be inconsistent at best. Critical studies evaluating the efficacy of such formulations are sorely needed.

A remarkable effect of *vehicle* on intrauterine absorption of gentamicin was recently described in cows.[35] Over 80 per cent of a dose of gentamicin dissolved in water, and when administered intrauterinely, disappeared from the uterine lumen within 6 hours after infusion; less than 20 per cent disappeared following IU application of the drug dissolved in saline. Therefore, it appears that tonicity of an infused solution can influence absorption of the dissolved drug.

The fate of a compound infused in the uterus deserves consideration. Although penicillin has been very popular for IU therapy in the past, it is known that some organisms commonly residing in the uterus produce penicillinase. Little is known about the metabolic or other inactivation of antibiotics in the uterine environment.

SPECIFIC RECOMMENDATIONS

The selection of an antimicrobial drug for treatment of a genital tract infection should be based upon a knowledge of the microorganisms present and the prospects for achieving an effective drug concentration in the uterine environment. Factors governing drug behavior in various environments have been reviewed.[36] As more information concerning the uterine environment becomes available, more specific recommendations concerning selection of appropriate drugs for the treatment of genital tract infections will be forthcoming.

Prior to the initiation of antimicrobial treatment of a genital tract infection, a thorough physical examination should be performed, in order to evaluate the extent and severity of the infection. If antimicrobial therapy is deemed necessary, mild, localized infections might be effectively and most economically treated by the IU route. Use of slow-release, long-acting or poorly absorbed formulations such as boluses or chelated compounds should be restricted to such infections. For more extensive or chronic infections, including those accompanied by systemic signs of illness, systemic administration should be considered.

Rigorous attempts to maintain inhibitory blood concentrations of antibiotics must be made in early postpartum cows if effective genital tissue concentrations of the drugs are to be realized. Because of high plasma-uterine-tissue drug concentration ratios in early postpartum cows, more intensive dosage regimens may be required than are typically used for infections of other organs. Based on limited information, a similar concern would not seem to be necessary in the mare.

The volumes of diluent chosen for IU administration of antimicrobials should be sufficiently large to achieve distribution throughout the uterine lumen without causing trauma. The size and potential luminal capacity of the uterus, as well as the volume of any uterine contents present, should be estimated during the physical examination. Removal of uterine contents prior to IU infusions would reduce dilutional effects. However, excessive manipulations of the genital tract should be avoided. In general, infusion volumes (IU) in the cow or mare should not exceed 50 to 150 ml in an involuted uterus, or 1 to 2 liters in an early postpartum uterus.

Because drugs administered by IU infusion are absorbed into the general circulation, milk-withholding times should be observed in dairy animals. Reducing the doses of antimicrobials used for IU administration in order to circumvent proper withholding times should be avoided in order to reduce the possibility of treatment failures.

References

1. Bierschwal CJ, Dale HE, Uren AW: The absorption of sulfamethazine by the bovine uterus. JAVMA 126:398, 1955.
2. Righter HF, Mercer HD, Cline DA, Carter GC: Absorption of antibacterial agents by the bovine involuting uterus. Can Vet J 16:10, 1975.
3. Miller GE, Rouse G: Passage of drugs from the bovine uterus into blood, milk, and urine. J Dairy Sci 53:652, 1970.
4. Huang J, Hawkinson D, Miller GE: Passage of sulfadimethoxine from the bovine uterus into blood, milk, and urine. J Dairy Sci 55:705, 1972.
5. Masera J, Gustafsson BK, Afiefy MM: Blood plasma and uterine tissue concentrations of sodium penicillin G in cows at intramuscular vs. intrauterine administration. 9th Int Cong Anim Reprod AI (Madrid), 1980.
6. Ayliffe TF, Noakes DE: Some preliminary studies on the uptake of sodium benzylpenicillin by the endometrium of the cow. Vet Rec 102:215, 1978.
7. Bierschwal CJ, Uren AW: The absorption of chlortetracycline (Aureomycin) by the bovine uterus. JAVMA 129:373, 1956.
8. Miller GE, Bergt GP: Oxytetracycline in bovine plasma, milk, and urine after intrauterine administration. J Dairy Sci 59:315, 1976.
9. Masera J, Gustafsson BK, Afiefy MM, et al.: Disposition of oxytetracycline in the bovine genital tract at systematic vs. intrauterine administration. JAVMA 176:1099, 1980.
10. Bretzlaff KN, Ott RS, Koritz GD, et al.: Distribution of oxytetracycline in genital tract tissues of postpartum cows given the drug by intravenous and intrauterine routes. AJVR 44:764, 1983.
11. Al-Guedawy S, Neff-Davis CA, Davis LE, et al.: Disposition of gentamicin in the genital tract of cows. 63rd Ann Meet Conf Res Workers in Anim Dis, Chicago, 1982, p 41.
12. Niedweske I, Threlfall WR: The influence of days postpartum on chloramphenicol absorption from the bovine uterus. Theriogenology 14:319, 1980.
13. Allen WE: Plasma concentrations of sodium benzylpenicillin after intrauterine infusion in pony mares. Equine Vet J 10:171, 1978.
14. Arbeiter VK, Awad-Maselmeh M, Kopschitz MM, et al: Uterusgewebespiegel und Blutserumspiegelbestimmungen bei der Stute nach parenteraler Verabreichung von Penicillin (Penicillin Novo gepuffert) und Ampicillin (Binotal). Wien tierarztl Mschr 63:298–304, 1976.
15. Allen WE, Clarke AR: Absorption of sodium benzylpenicillin from the equine uterus after local Lugol's iodine treatment, compared with absorption after intramuscular injection. Equine Vet J 10:174, 1978.
16. Threlfall WR: Antibiotic infusion of the uterus of the mare. Proc Soc Theriogenology, Mobile, 1979, p 45–47.
17. Lock T, Bevill R, Memon M, et al.: Absorption of oxytetracycline following intrauterine treatment in mares. 9th Int Congr Anim Reprod AI, Madrid, 1980.

18. Lock TF: Distribution of antibiotics in the mare reproductive tract after various routes of administration. Proc 3rd Int Symp Equine Reprod 1982, pp 640–641.
19. Ayliffe TR, Allen WE: Effect of experimental uterine tube occlusion on plasma penicillin concentrations following intrauterine instillation in pony mares. Equine Vet J 14:336, 1982.
20. Ayliffe TR, Noakes DE: Intrauterine absorption of sodium benzylpenicillin in the cow. J Vet Pharmacol Therap 1:267, 1978.
21. Bu J: Studies on local treatment of the uterus in oestrual and luteal phase of the cycle. Nord Vet Med 7:917, 1955.
22. Ayliffe TR: Effects of exogenous oestrogen and experimentally induced endometritis on absorption of sodium benzylpenicillin from the cow's uterus. Vet Rec 110:96, 1982.
23. Sander PD, Foley CW, Goetsch DD: Passage of certain penicillins into the uterine tubal fluid of estrous and pregnant rabbits. Theriogenology 8:3, 1977.
24. Bretzlaff KN: Unpublished data.
25. Bretzlaff KN, Ott RS, Koritz GD, et al.: Distribution of oxytetracycline in the genital tract of cows. AJVR 43:12, 1982.
26. Bretzlaff KN, Ott RS, Koritz GD, et al.: Distribution of oxytetracycline in the healthy and diseased postpartum genital tract of cows. AJVR 44:759, 1983.
27. Bretzlaff KN, Ott RS, Koritz GD, et al.: Disposition of chloramphenicol in the genital tract of postpartum cows. 63rd Ann Meet Conf Res Workers in Anim Dis, Chicago, 1982, p 41.
28. Oxender WD, Seguin BE: Bovine intrauterine therapy. JAVMA 168:217, 1976.
29. Bretzlaff KN, Ott RS, Weston PG, McEntee K: Luteolysis in cows after the intrauterine administration of oxytetracycline. 63rd Ann Meet Conf Res Workers in Anim Dis, Chicago, 1982, p 41.
30. Abdurahman E, Parsons JG: Duration of antibiotics in milk from cows treated via intrauterine infusion. J Dairy Sci 63(Suppl 1):39, 1980.
31. Baggot JD: Drug Distribution. In: Principles of Drug Disposition in Domestic Animals: The Basis of Veterinary Clinical Pharmacology. Philadelphia, WB Saunders Co, 1977, pp 48–72.
32. Boiter I, Muntean M, Mates N, et al.: Laboratory and therapeutic studies of puerperal endometritis and repeat breeding in the cow. Vet Bull 53:755, 1982.
33. Miller GE, Banerjee NC, Stowe CM: Drug movement between bovine milk and plasma as affected by milk pH. J Dairy Sci 50:1395, 1967.
34. Huang J, Miller GE: Mechanism of movement of sulfanilamide, sulfaethoxypyridazine, sulfamethazine, sulfadimethoxine, sulfacetamide, and salicylic acid across the uterine membrane of the guinea pig. J Dairy Sci 55:705, 1972.
35. Al-Guedawy SA, Vasquez LA, Neff-Davis CA, et al.: Effect of vehicle on intrauterine absorption of gentamicin in cattle. Theriogenology 19:771, 1983.
36. Hjerpe CA: Systemic antimicrobial therapy in beef cattle: Pharmacologic and therapeutic considerations. Proc Am Assoc Bovine Pract 15:92, 1982.
37. Caudle AB, Purswell BJ, Williams DJ, et al.: Endometrial levels of amikacin in the mare after intrauterine infusion of amikacin sulfate. Theriogenology 19:433, 1983.

The Efficacy of Uterine Treatment with Antimicrobial Drugs

Randall S. Ott, D.V.M., M.S.
University of Illinois, Urbana, Illinois

Husbandry and sanitation practices commonly employed with some species at parturition expose the uterus to a broad range of bacterial contamination and provide an increased opportunity for postpartum uterine infections. For example, bacteria are present in the uterus of up to 90 per cent of dairy cows during the first 10 days postpartum, whereas beef cows are known to have a much lower infection rate at this time. This higher incidence of postpartum uterine infections in dairy cows as compared with beef cows is partly due to sanitation and environmental influences. Many dairy cows calve in continually occupied maternity stalls, whereas most beef cows calve on relatively clean and uncontaminated pastures.

Most information available about the etiology and significance of postpartum uterine infection concerns the cow. The composition of uterine flora in the postpartum cow has been demonstrated to fluctuate constantly throughout the first 7 weeks after calving, as a result of spontaneous contamination, clearance and recontamination. However, the 50-day interval between calving and rebreeding usually allows sufficient time for the elimination of pyogenic uterine infection and the resolution of associated endometritis from the majority of animals. Leukocytic infiltration and phagocytosis eliminate invading organisms from the uterus. *Corynebacterium pyogenes* appears to be the pathogen most often causing a persistent infection and the development of a purulent discharge.

Uterine infections have generally been treated with either antibiotics or disinfectants, such as iodine solutions, sodium hypochlorite or chlorhexidine. Various disinfectants have been proposed as uterine treatments in the dairy cow in an attempt to circumvent problems caused by antibiotic residues in the milk of treated cows; however, broad spectrum antibiotics have become generally accepted as the products of choice for intrauterine therapy.

INDICATIONS

Uterine therapy with antimicrobials has been aimed at ameliorating the effects of acute puerperal metritis, pyometra and endometritis. Prophylactic uterine treatments have been used in animals that have experienced dystocia, fetal membrane retention or repeat breeding.

Pneumovagina, dystocia, unsanitary breeding practices, excessive multiple breedings and insertion of unsanitary equipment into the genital tract have been implicated as conditions leading to uterine infections in the mare. Uterine infection is a common sequela to dystocia and/or retained fetal membranes in the cow. Uterine involution and ovarian activity progress more slowly in these cows. The metritis that often develops in dairy cows retaining fetal membranes causes a significant increase in the interval from calving to first estrus and services per conception. Recent data have failed to implicate nonspecific infections as a cause of endometritis in repeat-breeder cows. Therefore, the use of antimicrobial therapy would not be indicated for these cows.

The occurrence of favorable results from antimicrobial therapy varies because of many factors, including the sensitivity of the offending organisms to the antimicrobial selected, dosage and length of treatment, route of administration, the time at which treatment was initiated during the course of the infection, presence of concurrent maladies, age, nutritional status and stress resulting from environmental or management factors. The mere presence of microorganisms in the uterus after parturition should not be viewed as a detriment to reproductive function. Evidence has accumulated that little significance can be attributed to a single sample from the uterus containing nonspecific bacteria. Routine use of antimicrobials may not be economically feasible and may result in development of resistant strains of microorganisms.

ROUTE OF ADMINISTRATION

Intrauterine administration of antimicrobials has been most commonly chosen for treatment of uterine infections in the cow, sow and mare. Recent studies have suggested that concentrations of certain antibiotics are greatest throughout the genital organs when the systemic route of administration is used.[6] The local route of administration offers a high concentration of the drug superficially adjacent to the endometrium. However, infections may involve the myometrium and other parts of the genital tract (cervix, oviducts). In small ruminants and dogs and cats, systemic routes are usually chosen.

Infusion of certain substances into the uterus may alter the length of the estrous cycle. The estrous cycle of cows can be shortened when iodine solution, oxytetracycline or nitrofurazone is infused into the uterus. Mares are reported to exhibit estrus 2 to 4 days after intrauterine infusion of isotonic saline solution. In addition, infusion of antimicrobials into the uterus may result in irritation of the endometrium and reduction of subsequent fertility. For example, breedings required per conception and days from treatment to conception were recently reported to be higher in cows infused with 5 per cent Lugol's solution compared with chlorhexidine, propylene glycol, 0.2 per cent nitrofurozone or oxytetracycline for therapy of mild postpartum endometritis.[8]

EFFICACY OF TREATMENTS

It is likely that most, if not all, antibiotics and disinfectants that are available to veterinarians have been placed into the uterine cavities of a cow or mare, singly or in various combinations. Unfortunately, there is a paucity of information regarding the efficacy of uterine treatments in these two species, and even less information is available concerning other species. Most of the information available concerning the efficacy of uterine therapy involves the cow. Some examples are reviewed below.

A recent study at the University of Illinois evaluated two antimicrobial treatments as a prophylactic measure in cows with assisted births and as therapy for uterine infections.[2] The treatments were tetracycline intrauterinely (IU) plus penicillin IM for 3 days or sulfaurea boluses given IU. Neither treatment appeared effective as a prophylactic measure, as 26 of 34 cows (76 per cent) having either assisted birth or retained fetal membranes developed metritis. Neither treatment regimen was superior to the other. These results were very different from those reported in a California study, in which cows retaining fetal membranes received an intrauterine tetracycline bolus every other day until 1 day after membranes were expelled. These cows experienced fertility rates similar to nonaffected cows.[9] Negative results were obtained in a study in which routine treatment of all cows, consisting of intrauterine boluses containing a total of 1000 mg neomycin sulfate given 24 hours postpartum, was compared with controls.[5] The treated cows required more services per conception (1.7 versus 1.4) and were open more days before conception (100.5 versus 88.5) than controls.

Treatment failure in some studies may be attributed to either ineffective drugs or inadequate dosage regimens. Despite the fact that chloramphenicol is not FDA approved for use in food animals, it has received attention by practitioners because bacterial isolates from cows with postpartum uterine infections show resistance to the more commonly used antimicrobials. Sensitivity testing of cows with postpartum reproductive problems in the Illinois study revealed that chloramphenicol was the most effective antimicrobial tested (96 per cent of all isolates were sensitive). A study was subsequently undertaken in this same herd,[1] in which a very intensive treatment regimen of 5 gm chloramphenicol (oral solution) was infused in the uterus every 12 hours for six treatments in an attempt to prevent metritis and detrimental effects on milk production and subsequent fertility of the cow. Untreated cows served as controls in this study; removal or nonremoval of retained fetal membranes was also tested. Chloramphenicol did not prevent metritis even with this intensive treatment regimen, and only transient ameliorating effects were observed (decreased temperature and decreased prevalence of purulent discharges during the treatment). Most importantly, milk production remained depressed in treated cows, and there was no improvement in reproductive performance of the treated cows compared with

Table 1. Fertility of Cows in the Various Uterine Groups

Uterine Group	Total Cows Examined	Total Cows Used for Analysis*	Conceived First Service	Per Cent†	Cows in Analysis for Days Open	Cows Open 150 Days Postpartum	Per Cent†	Mean Days Open
A	1450	1140	498	44[a]	937	184	16[a]	94
B	1568	1206	550	46[a]	1008	192	16[a]	96
B$_c$	631	465	219	47[a]	398	63	14[a]	96
B$_t$	937	741	331	45[a]	610	124	17[a]	97
C	564	345	111	32[b]	246	104	30[b]	105

B = All cows in group B
B$_c$ = Group B controls
B$_t$ = Group B treated
*Total cows examined less those culled during the project
†Statistical comparisons within columns
a to b = p<.001

the untreated controls. In this study the cost of treatment was very high; however, no significant benefit could be demonstrated.

Intrauterine infusion of antimicrobial drugs shortly after breeding has been used in an attempt to rid the uterus of organisms that might be detrimental to the survival of the conceptus. However, there appear to be no convincing data that would encourage this method. In one study, intrauterine infusion of gentamicin sulfate at the rate of 200 mg 10 minutes following first-service insemination did not enhance fertility. Pregnancy rates combined for both first and second services were 68.7 per cent for treated cows and 71.1 per cent for controls.[3]

In one of the most extensive studies reported concerning endometritis in cattle, 3582 dairy cows in California were examined between 21 and 35 days postpartum.[7] The cows were divided into three groups; A, normal uterus; B, moderately affected with endometritis; and C, severely affected. Group B was subdivided into a control and a treatment group that received a single intrauterine infusion of tetracycline and nitrofurazone (Furacin) or penicillin and dihydrostreptomycin. All cows in group C were treated with several intrauterine infusions (Table 1).

There were no differences in fertility in group B cows, whether or not they were treated. Cows in group C had lower fertility rates, and since all were treated, it was not known whether the treatments had any effect. In this study, endometritis was diagnosed in some cows by rectal examination, while examination with a vaginal speculum was used in others. A comparison of the percentage of uterine samples yielding bacterial isolates between these two techniques revealed that the vaginal method was more accurate than the rectal examination, 59 per cent versus 22 per cent, respectively. The authors speculated that inclusion of nonaffected cows in the moderately affected group, because of inaccurate diagnosis and the spontaneous recovery of some affected cows, may have accounted for the similar results in groups A and B. Concerning group C, it was felt that repeated treatments every 24

hours might have improved results, and the authors encouraged further investigations.

Poor results from uterine infusion were obtained in another recent study, in which 152 pyometritic cows were utilized to study cloprostenol and estradiol cypionate with or without nitrofurazone solution infusions. These infusions failed to prevent relapses and increased the number of services required for conception.[4]

Concerning efficacy of uterine treatments in the cow, the following conclusions have been made:

1. More effort is needed to improve sanitation and management practices to prevent postpartum uterine infections in individual herds.

2. Cows that are not severely affected will most likely resolve these infections with their own inherent defense mechanisms. Antimicrobial therapy may not offer any advantage.

3. Cows severely affected by uterine infection may suffer some degree of impairment of fertility, whether or not treated. Few definitive studies are available to guide the veterinarian in the choice of therapy to ameliorate the degree of fertility impairment.

Most investigators agree that while commonly used treatments may not be beneficial, more intensive treatments *may* prove helpful and deserve investigation. However, more intensive treatments can greatly increase costs because of the greater expense of a more effective antimicrobial or the increased dosage used, the increased number of treatments used in an attempt to achieve and maintain therapeutic concentrations during an appropriate treatment interval and the loss of income from discarding milk following treatments to ensure that milk is free of drug residues. Therefore, research is also needed to determine whether the cost of treatment might result in a satisfactory economic return to the producer who bears these costs.

The literature presents a similar but smaller picture concerning antimicrobial therapy for uterine infections in mares. In one study, five different antibiotics were used to treat problem and normal mares by intrauterine infusion 24 to 48 hours after breeding.[10] No treatment advantage was demonstrated in the percentage of live foals. No statistically significant difference in the percentage of live foals was observed between the mares given penicillin G procaine, nitrofurazone solution or chloramphenicol and the untreated controls. However, there was a decrease in live foal percentage in those mares treated with polymyxin B and Daribiotic Improved.

Studies involving the use of ampicillin, gentamicin or amikacin given IU once daily for 3 to 5 days to mares with endometritis and metritis have been published; however, no data from contemporary control mares were available.

SUMMARY AND CONCLUSIONS

Uterine infections are commonly diagnosed and treated in cows and mares. Results from recent studies that have attempted objectively to measure the efficacy of uterine therapy with antimicrobial agents have been varied. It is not known whether more intensive treatment regimens might be either more efficacious or economically feasible. There is an *urgent need* for controlled clinical studies involving both the *efficacy* and the *economic benefit* of uterine treatment regimens in domestic animals.

References

1. Bretzlaff KN: Results of a clinical trial using chloramphenicol for treatment of retained fetal membranes in dairy cows. Proc Theriogenology 1982, p 72.
2. Bretzlaff KN, Whitmore HL, Spahr SL, Ott RS: Incidence, cause and treatment of postpartum metritis in dairy cattle. Theriogenology 17:527, 1982.
3. Daniels WH, Morrow DA, Pickett BW, Ball L: Effects of intrauterine infusion of gentamicin sulfate on bovine fertility. Theriogenology. 6:61, 1976.
4. Fazeli MA: A comparison of treatments for bovine pyometra: Cloprostenol vs. estradiol cypionate, with or without nitrofurazone. Proc Soc Theriogenology, 1979, p 75.
5. Fuquay JW, Harris RA, McGee WH, Beatty JF, Arnold BL: Routine postpartum treatment of dairy cattle with intrauterine neomycin sulfate boluses. J Dairy Sci 58:1367, 1974.
6. Gustafsson BK, Ott RS: Current trends in the treatment of genital infections in large animals. Comp Cont Ed 3:5147, 1981.
7. Miller HV, Kimsey PB, Kendrick JW, et al.: Endometritis of dairy cattle: Diagnosis, treatment and fertility. Bovine Pract 15:13, 1980.
8. Oxenreider SL: Evaluation of various treatments for chronic uterine infection in dairy cattle. Proc Soc Theriogenology 1982, p 64.
9. Squire AG: Therapy for retained placenta. In Morrow DA (ed): Current Therapy for Theriogenology. Philadelphia WB Saunders Co, 1980, pp 186–189.
10. Wearly WK, Murdick PW, Hensel JD: Five year study of the use of post-breeding treatment in mares in a Standardbred stud. Proc Am Assoc Equine Pract 1971, p 89.

Possible Adverse Effects of Antimicrobial Treatment of Uterine Infections

Howard L. Whitmore, D.V.M., Ph.D.
Kevin L. Anderson, D.V.M., Ph.D.
University of Illinois, Urbana, Illinois

A significant and highly variable percentage of dairy and beef cows are treated for metritis or endometritis by intrauterine infusion of antibiotics,[1,2] with published reports indicating that approximately 20 per cent of all cows on a reproductive herd-health program are treated for endometritis in this manner. In these reports diagnosis of endometritis was based on either rectal palpation or vaginal examination plus a history of vaginal discharge in some cases.

ANTIMICROBIAL TREATMENT IN THE UTERUS FOLLOWING PARTURITION

Intrauterine antimicrobial therapy is routinely administered to cows with retained fetal membranes, with or without careful sanitary manual removal of the membranes. The most common antimicrobial used may be 1 to 5 gm of tetracycline (Polyotic, tetracycline hydrochloride soluble powder, American Cyanamid Co., Berdan Avenue, Wayne, NJ 07470) administered in the uterus. Adverse side effects are normally limited to accidents occurring during intrauterine therapy such as penetration of the uterus by the pipette. However, vehicles like propylene glycol and disinfectants like iodine may, if they are inadvertently placed in the vagina or expelled from the uterus into the vagina, cause apparent irritation. Cows will strain, switch their tails and in some cases lay down for a period of 1 to 2 hours. On the other hand, propylene glycol and iodine do not cause a painful response when administered in the uterus.

Dairymen experiencing a relatively high incidence of postpartum metritis often want some form of routine postpartum treatment for all cows following calving. This has resulted in the owner routinely placing various types of antibiotic boluses or powders directly into the uterus using a plastic sleeve. Tetracycline powder in gelatine capsules or sulfaurea boluses are most commonly used. The authors have seen this practice result in a 50 to 100 per cent incidence of acute metritis and subsequent pyometra in several herds of dairy cattle. Bacteriology revealed that the acute metritis and pyometra were due to *Corynebacterium pyogenes*. Failure to maintain satisfactory sanitary conditions and trauma appeared to be factors leading to establishment of this type of herd problem. This practice should be strongly discouraged.

Another risky procedure is the practice of "flushing" the postpartum uterus with rather large volumes (1 to 10 liters) of antibiotic or antiseptic solutions. Veterinary practitioners sometimes judge it necessary to pump antibiotic solutions into the uterus to help "flush out" or remove toxic uterine contents. This procedure has resulted in some beneficial effects but also has risks associated with it. The greatest risk in flushing the uterus comes from pumping too large a volume of antimicrobial solution into the postpartum uterus. This may force fluid from the uterus into the uterine tubes or rupture the uterus wall. Careful siphoning of fluid from the uterus is safe, but pumping fluids into the uterus should be discouraged. In most cases, solutions pumped into the uterus cannot be removed, and thus potential damage may result. There is also some risk of penetrating the wall of the uterus if hard plastic hoses are used.

Veterinarians are well aware of the absorption of antibiotics from the uterus and their subsequent presence in meat and milk; therefore, nonantibiotic treatments have been attempted in order to avoid the required withholding of milk from the market. Hydrogen peroxide has been used as a substitute therapy for antibiotics; however, this has risk involved owing to hydrogen peroxide gas plus purulent exudate being forced out through the uterine tubes. Personal communications with practicing veterinarians and dairymen have revealed that intrauterine treatment with hydrogen peroxide has resulted in peritonitis and death of some cows. Small amounts of hydrogen peroxide (25 to 50 ml) infused into the uterus seldom cause problems, but large amounts (100 to 500 ml) are very risky. Therefore, use of hydrogen peroxide in the uterus should be strongly discouraged.

Another possible adverse effect of antimicrobial treatment of the uterus may be inhibition of phagocytosis. Several reports have shown that some antibiotics, their vehicles, antiseptics and preservatives present in injectable antibiotics may inhibit phagocytosis or migration of leukocytes.[3] Leukocytes (polymorphonuclear and macrophages) are the principal phagocytic cells in the body and constitute one of the essential defenses against microbial infection.

One study dealing specifically with treatments for retained placenta compared the effects of various antibiotics on in vivo phagocytosis in the uterus.[4] The results indicate that some intrauterine medications and manipulations, e.g., manual removal of the placenta, adversely affect uterine phagocytosis.

Much more work needs to be done on this topic before specific recommendations can be given.

ANTIMICROBIAL TREATMENT IN THE UTERUS OF CYCLING ANIMALS

Intrauterine antimicrobial treatments are often given to cycling animals that have mild endometritis and to "repeat-breeder" cows. Again, owners place rather strong demands on the veterinarian to infuse antibiotics into the uterus of problem-breeder cows to improve herd reproductive performance. However, the value of intrauterine antibiotics in cycling and repeat-breeder cows is questionable. Antibiotics are certainly beneficial in some cases of obvious uterus infection but should be restricted to a small percentage of the herd.

Decreased conception rates following postbreeding infusion of neomycin and oxytetracycline have been reported. In one trial,[5] 48 repeat breeders were randomized into two groups. Twenty-four cows were treated with antibiotics, and 24 were untreated controls. All 48 cows were slaughtered 34 days after insemination and examined for embryos. The conception rate was 35 per cent for treated cows and 56 per cent for untreated cows; thus, antibiotics can reduce conception rates but may have some value in selected problem breeders. In general, the authors do not recommend pre- or postinfusion of antimicrobials in the uterus. We believe they should be used only in selected cases after vaginal and genital examination for endometritis.

The effect of postbreeding intrauterine infusions of antibiotics in mares has been summarized. The antibiotics used were usually selected on the basis of culture and sensitivity tests. One study showed no difference in conception rates or percentage of live foals born as a result of treatment with penicillin, nitrofurazone or chloramphenicol.[6] However, there was a significant decrease in live foals born when polymyxin B and a proprietary mixture of polymyxin and neomycin were infused into the uterus.

It has been shown that irritating substances infused into the uterus will alter the length of the estrous cycle in cows. Dilute iodine solution (5 ml of Lugol's solution diluted in 250 ml of saline) was infused into the uteri of cows on days 4 and 15 of the estrous cycle.[7] The mean cycle length was 10.6 and 25.1 days, respectively. Mean cycle length of control cows was 21.3 days. Thus, the dilute iodine solution resulted in significant shortening or lengthening of the cycle, depending on the stage of the cycle when iodine was given. Necrotizing endometritis was diagnosed by biopsy 24 hours after infusion of dilute iodine solution. Surface epithelium had been regenerated by the subsequent estrus. The mechanism of action was thought to be caused by endometrial irritation rather than distention of the uterus. Intrauterine infusion of saline in the cow did not alter the cycle; however, in mares, this caused a shortening of the cycle. When cows were given intrauterine infusions of iodine solution on day 15 and a luteolytic dose of prostaglandin on day 16, estrus occurred in 3.1 days. These results indicate that intrauterine infusion of dilute iodine solution may have destroyed the source of the luteolytic factor in the endometrium. Synthesis of luteolysin probably resumed during endometrial repair. Other irritating substances such as oxytetracycline in propylene glycol have been shown to alter the estrous cycle following intrauterine infusion. It has not been determined whether this irritation is beneficial or harmful in cows with metritis. Until results are available, iodine infusions in early postpartum cows should probably not be used.

Although dilute iodine solutions are thought to cause only temporary irritation of the endometrium in cycling cows, this is not the case in mares. Several reports provide rather convincing evidence that intrauterine infusions of dilute iodine solution in mares result in severe transluminal, cervical and uterine adhesions.[8] Therefore, intrauterine iodine therapy in mares should not be used.

Overuse of antibiotics in the bovine and equine uterus could lead to a shift in the nature of pathogenic bacteria or to the development of antibiotic-resistant strains. Many pathogens isolated from the equine uterus are resistant to most antibiotics except the lesser-used ones such as chloramphenicol or gentamicin. This will probably change with time. Organisms once considered to be facultative saprophytes (e.g., *Pseudomonas aeruginosa* and *Candida albicans*) are now seen more regularly as pathogens in the equine uterus. Fungal and yeast infections have become slightly more prevalent, probably owing to excessive use of intrauterine therapy with broad spectrum antibiotics. Veterinarians must continuously assume responsibility for governing the use of antibiotics in the management of reproductive problems. Antibiotics are usually of secondary importance in the prevention and management of reproductive problems in farm animals.

PUBLIC HEALTH SIGNIFICANCE OF ANTIBIOTICS IN THE UTERUS

There are numerous reports showing that antibiotics are rapidly absorbed from the uterus. It should probably be assumed that all antibiotics and antiseptics are absorbed from the uterus and thus appear in serum, milk and tissues. There are differences among antibiotics in absorption and disappearance rates in the uterus. For example, some antibiotics, such as ampicillin, in mares may precipitate and remain in the lumen of the uterus for extended periods. Recently, a closed system was developed to monitor absorption of antibiotics from the lumen of the uterus.[9] This technique involves insertion of a Foley catheter into one horn of the uterus, inflation of the cuff and infusion of a known concentration of antibiotic solution plus a marker dye. The Foley catheter is clamped shut and left in the uterine horn. Samples are withdrawn from the Foley catheter every hour for 6 hours. Initial trials using this technique revealed that significantly more antibiotic was absorbed from the uterus when gentamicin was diluted in sterile water when compared with gentamicin diluted with saline. Therefore, the diluent used for intrauterine antibiotics is another important factor affecting the absorption rate from the uterus.

The presence of antibiotics and antiseptics in milk and tissues of food-producing animals causes concern for human health, thus proper withholding time on the sale of milk and slaughter of treated animals must be adhered to. More programs are being developed to monitor antibiotic residues in milk and meat. These surveillance programs are designed to assist livestock owners and veterinarians with the safe use of antibiotics and, thus, ensure protection of human health.

References

1. Miller HV, Kimsey PP, Kendrick JW, et al.: Endometritis of dairy cattle: Diagnosis, treatment and fertility. Bovine Pract 15:13, 1980.
2. Whitmore HL, Mather EC, Hurtgen JP, Zemjanis R: Evaluation of reproductive efficiency in dairy herds on a fertility program. Proc Soc Theriogenology, pp 160–162, 1977.
3. Frank T, Anderson KL, Smith AR, et al.: Phagocytosis in the uterus: A review. Theriogenology 20:103, 1983.
4. Bouters R, Vandeplassche M: Postpartum infection in cattle: Diagnosis and prevention and curative treatment. J S Afr Vet Assoc 46:237, 1977.
5. Ulberg LC, Black WG, Kidder HE, et al.: The use of antibiotics in the treatment of low fertility cows. JAVMA 121:436, 1952.
6. Davis LE, Abbitt B: Clinical pharmacology of antibacterial drugs in the uterus of the mare. JAVMA 170:204, 1977.
7. Seguin BE, Morrow DA, Louis TM: Luteolysis, luteostasis and the effect of prostaglandins in cows after endometrial irritation. Am J Vet Res 35:57, 1974.
8. Mather EC, Refsal KR, Gustafsson BK, Seguin BE, Whitmore HL: The use of fiberoptic techniques in clinical diagnosis and visual assessment of experimental intrauterine therapy in mares. J Reprod Fertil Suppl 27:293, 1979.
9. Al-Guedawy SA, Vasquez L, Neff-Davis CA, et al.: Effect of vehicle on intrauterine absorption of gentamicin in cattle. Theriogenology 19:771, 1983.

Therapy of Uterine Infections: Alternatives to Antibiotics

Nabil A. Hemeida, D.V.M., Ph.D.
Borje K. Gustafsson, D.V.M., Ph.D.
Howard L. Whitmore, D.V.M., Ph.D.
University of Illinois, Urbana, Illinois

Antibiotics have prevailed for many years as the treatment of choice for genital infections. Increasing awareness of treatment failures, the risk for bacterial resistance, the risk for residues in tissues and milk and the possibility of undesirable effects on the natural defense mechanisms have increased the interest in alternative (nonantibiotic) treatment methods. The need for nonantibiotic methods is obviously greatest in food producing animals, particularly cattle. Therefore, for the most part this article focuses on cattle.

THE EARLY POSTPARTUM PERIOD

Nonantibiotic drugs of interest in this period are those that are capable of stimulating uterine contractility (e.g., oxytocin, prostaglandin, ergonovine, estrogens) and/or the uterine defense mechanisms (e.g., estrogens, gonadotropin releasing hormone). These drugs are almost exclusively administered systemically. Local use of disinfectants, which is another possible nonantibiotic approach (e.g., iodine, chlorhexidine and other similar disinfectants), may adversely influence the local defense mechanisms,[5] and restricted use is therefore recommended.

Oxytocin. There are conflicting reports about the effectiveness of oxytocin in prevention of retained placenta and postpartum infections. One of the reasons for frequent failures in response may be an incorrect timing of the treatment or an inappropriate dose. Recent research indicates that oxytocin given in a dose of 20 IU intramuscularly immediately following calving and preferably repeated 2 to 4 hours later reduces the incidence of retained placenta in cows, especially after difficult calvings.[13] The results indicate that uterine atony due to blockage of oxytocin release may be of greater importance as a cause of retained placenta than previously thought. The blockage of oxytocin release is thought to be provoked by an increased synthesis of endorphins due to stress and pain.[13] The uterotonic effect

of an endorphin antagonist (10 mg naltrexone—an analogue of naloxone) given IM to cows with postpartum uterine atony supports the theory. Additional tests are needed to determine the therapeutic and practical values of these drugs.

The therapeutic effect of exogenous oxytocin on a fully manifested postpartum metritis as an alternative to antibiotics is not well established. Undoubtedly, stimulation of uterine contractions is beneficial by draining the uterus of pathologic secretions. Recent experimental evidence indicates that oxytocin is uterotonic in the postpartum cow.[1, 3] The effect is more pronounced on a uterus sensitized by estrogens, which might explain the beneficial effects seen very early postpartum while the effect of the high prepartum estrogen levels still remains. The best way to administer oxytocin would be in intravenous drip infusion (60 to 100 IU oxytocin over 6 to 10 hours). Since this is not practical in most cases, the best alternative is to administer relatively small doses (20 IU to cow and mare and 5 to 10 IU to small ruminants and swine) IM 3 to 4 times a day over a period of 2 to 3 days. In mild to moderate cases of acute postpartum metritis this may be used as the only treatment, especially if estrogens have been used to sensitize the uterus.

Ergonovine. Most of the usage of this drug in large animals is based on empirical results rather than controlled experiments. Ergonovine is thought to produce a prolonged series of uterine contractions, which would make it valuable in uterine atony. The usually recommended doses for cattle are 2 to 5 mg IM. However, in the postpartum cow Zerobin failed to demonstrate any increased uterine activity after administration of 5 to 20 mg of ergometrine maleate. No consistent improvement of reproductive parameters has been found in controlled clinical trials.

Prostaglandin. The effect of prostaglandin $F_{2\alpha}$ ($PGF_{2\alpha}$) and its analogues on chronic endometritis, especially the classical pyometra, is well established and will be described in other sections of this book. It is generally believed that the effect requires the presence of a corpus luteum. However, in early postpartum metritis or early in subinvolution syndrome there is no corpus luteum present. It is therefore questionable whether prostaglandin $F_{2\alpha}$ would have any effect. If it has effect, it would likely be through increased uterine contractions, but other mechanisms of action cannot be ruled out. There is some evidence that retained placenta and delayed involution in the postpartum cow are related to subnormal levels of prostaglandins.[8, 9] Furthermore, preliminary results indicate that twice daily treatments with $PGF_{2\alpha}$ during the first 10 days postpartum may enhance uterine involution. Successful one-time treatment of the early postpartum cow with no functional corpus luteum has also been reported. The result might be related to a beneficial effect on uterine contractions but might also be due to factors involved in the uterine natural defense. At present, prostaglandin treatment (25 mg $PGF_{2\alpha}$

or 0.5 mg of a prostaglandin $F_{2\alpha}$ analogue) one or several times during the first 2 weeks postpartum is frequently used by practitioners in cases of delayed involution and metritis. More controlled field trials are needed to evaluate the effects.

Estrogens. The importance of resumption of normal cyclicity for the spontaneous recovery from uterine infections in the cow is well known. The mechanism of the beneficial effects is thought to be the exposure of the genital tract to estrogens, which increases the natural defense, i.e., uterine phagocytosis.[5] The protective action of estrogens has been confirmed in experimental studies. Other beneficial effects of estrogen are associated with its uterotonic effect.[3] The early postpartum cow has just been deprived of estrogen production, which will not resume until the cow comes into estrus in about 2 to 3 weeks. It seems logical to assume that administration of small amounts of estrogen during this period would be useful to protect the cow from uterine infections and to enhance the uterine involution. Estrogens are therefore frequently used as the only treatment for cows with mild to moderate postpartum infections with or without retained placenta. The recommended doses are 3 to 10 mg of estradiol benzoate, estradiol valerate or estradiol cypionate given intramuscularly. The treatment can be repeated twice at an interval of 3 days. Recent studies show that in mild and moderate cases of postpartum endometritis, treatment with estrogen alone was as effective as treatments with estrogens followed by various antibacterial and antimicrobial agents.[12] In cases of uterine atony with accumulation of exudate in the uterus it is sometimes beneficial to administer low doses (10 to 20 IU) of oxytocin within 4 to 6 hours of the estrogen injection.

Intrauterine Infusion of Disinfectants. Intrauterine infusion with various disinfectants is a relatively common nonantibiotic alternative for treatment of postpartum infections. Although some positive results have been reported, very few controlled evaluations of this form of treatment have been made. One recent trial[10] evaluated the effect of routine intrauterine treatment of 360 ml of dilute Lugol's solution (2 per cent solution made from a 7 per cent iodine stock solution) at 3 days postpartum. There was no effect on the rate of progression or recovery from metritis, involution of the uterus, days to first estrus or cystic ovarian disease. There is increasing evidence that intrauterine use of disinfectants—as well as antibiotics—suppress the natural defense mechanisms such as the uterine phagocytosis.[5] Given the present state of knowledge, a general use of intrauterine infusions in the postpartum cow is therefore not recommended.

Gonadotropin-Releasing Hormone (GnRH). Early resumption of cyclicity after calving promotes spontaneous recovery of uterine infections probably through beneficial effects of endogenous estrogens. Administration of GnRH is one of the methods to reduce the interval from calving to first ovulation and to increase the number of ovulations during the first 3 months after calving.[4] Recent field trials[2]

demonstrated that IM administration of 20 µg of a GnRH analogue on days 10 to 12 postpartum improved uterine involution in cows with retained placenta, significantly shortened the interval from calving to conception and increased the conception rate compared with untreated controls. This indicates that GnRH may become a viable alternative to antibiotics to improve the fertility of cows with retained placenta. In this context, it seems appropriate to refer to a recent experiment that evaluated the effect of GnRH (100 µg IM) given to postpartum cows (day 14) and to repeat breeder cows at the time of the third insemination.[7] The postpartum treatment resulted in a significantly improved conception rate. In repeat breeders the conception rate for treated cows was 25 per cent higher than in the controls.

ENDOMETRITIS IN CYCLING ANIMALS

Postpartum infections (acute metritis, endometritis) in the cow often results in a chronic endometritis characterized by a slightly to moderately enlarged uterus caused by a thickening of the uterine wall. These animals, which often have a mucopurulent discharge from the vulva, demonstrate a form of purulent endometritis with little, if any, accumulation of fluid in the uterus. Such cows are usually cycling, although the cycle length may be irregular. Empirically, it is quite clear that spontaneous recovery in many cases is good after the cow has gone through several estrous cycles. This is probably because of the positive effect of estrogens on the natural defense mechanisms. Therefore, methods that increase the number of estrous periods occurring in a short time interval have become a valuable alternative to antibiotics to enhance the recovery from endometritis. In principle, two methods are used today for that purpose: (1) prostaglandin treatment with prostaglandin $F_{2\alpha}$ or its analogues and (2) shortening of the estrous cycle by intrauterine infusion of iodine.

Prostaglandin Treatment. This method is based upon the luteolytic effect of prostaglandins which brings the cow into estrus within 2 to 4 days of the injection. The doses used are those generally recommended for induction of estrus. The number of treatments needed varies with the severity of the cases. In a mild to moderate case of endometritis it appears that one or two treatments would be adequate. If two treatments are performed, they should be done 10 to 14 days apart. The treatment appears to hasten recovery and reduce the interval from calving to breeding.

Intrauterine Infusions. It has been known since the late 1960's that irritating solutions infused during the early part of the estrous cycle (day 4 or 5 of the cycle, with the day of previous estrus equaling day 1) induce estrus within 4 to 7 days of the treatment. Seguin and colleagues[14] demonstrated that a necrotizing endometritis occurred as early as 24 hours after intrauterine infusion of a dilute Lugol's solution. The dilute iodine solution was prepared by mixing 5 ml of a strong iodine solution (Lugol's solution, Humco Laboratory, Texarkana, TX) with 250 ml of saline solution. The 255 ml of dilute iodine solution that was infused into the uterus contained 3.3 gm of iodine and 6.6 gm of potassium iodide. When this mixture was infused into the uterus on day 5 (day of estrus was day 1) the cows had short cycles and returned to estrus on day 11. The endometrium had regenerated by day 11. They postulated that the premature estrus was induced by endogenous release of $PGF_{2\alpha}$ during endometrial repair. Later, Kindahl and colleagues[6] confirmed that the infusion of Lugol's solution was followed by a $PFG_{2\alpha}$ release preceding the luteal regression and estrus in a similar pattern to that of a spontaneous estrus. No alteration of the estrous cycle occurs after infusions during midcycle or estrus. Infusions in late cycle (days 16 to 19), on the other hand, prolong cycle length 4 to 5 days.[6, 14] Can the induction of premature estrus by intrauterine infusions be useful for therapy purposes in cows with endometritis? Although few data are available from controlled experiments, it appears empirically that this might be an alternative to prostaglandins in lactating animals or in countries in which prostaglandin is not available or too expensive. Furthermore this treatment may be more valuable than prostaglandin treatment in cases of repeat breeding in which no or very mild symptoms of endometritis exist. The treatment of true repeat breeders with this method is, in our view, more attractive than other regimens, local or systemic, that commonly are used in such cases. The effect in repeat breeders may be caused by a change in the uterine environment, making the endometrium more suitable for implantation, or the effect could be related to a normalization of hormonal events that affect the gamete transport or fertilization (compare with the old practice of corpus luteum enucleation in repeat breeders). Further experimental and controlled clinical studies are needed to confirm the positive effects that have been found empirically and to elucidate the mechanisms involved. The regimen that we suggest consists of an intrauterine infusion of 4 per cent Lugol's solution (4 ml of commercial Lugol's solution per 100 ml of saline) on day 4 or 5 of the cycle (day 1 equals day of previous estrus). The volume of the infused solution is not critical, since volumes as low as 5 ml of Lugol's solution have proved effective in inducing estrus. We infuse 25 to 50 ml of this mixture into each horn. This frequently results in estrus within 5 to 7 days of treatment.

Breeding on the induced estrus might improve conception rates in repeat breeders without any signs of endometritis. If the method is used in clear cases of mild to moderate endometritis, it is recommended not to breed the animal on the induced estrus but to wait until the next spontaneous estrus at an appropriate time postpartum.

References

1. Armstrong-Backus CS, Hopkins FM, Eiler H: The uterotonic effect of prostaglandin $F_{2\alpha}$ and oxytocin on the postpartum cow. Proc 64th Ann Meet Conf Res Workers, Chicago, 1983, Abstract 93.
2. Bostedt H, Maurer G: The reproduction performance of cows after an injection of a GnRH-analogue in the early puerperium. In Karg, Schallenberger (eds): Factors Influencing Fertility in the Postpartum Cow. Boston, Martinus-Nijhoff Publishers, 1982, pp 562–565.
3. Bretzlaff KN, Ott RS: Postpartum reproductive problems in a large dairy herd. Bovine Clin Vol. 1, no. 4, 1981.
4. Britt JH, Koftock RJ, Harrison DS: Ovulation estrus and endocrine response after GnRH in early postpartum cows. J Anim Sci 39:915, 1974.
5. Frank T, Anderson KL, Smith AR, Whitmore HL, Gustafsson BK: Phagocytosis in the uterus: A Review. Theriogenology 20:103, 1983.
6. Kindahl H, Granstrom E, Edquist LE, Gustafsson B, Astrom G, Stabenfeldt GH: Progesterone and 15-keto-13,14-dihydro-prostaglandin $F_{2\alpha}$ levels in peripheral circulation after intrauterine infusions in cows. Acta Vet Scand 18:274, 1977.
7. Lee CN, Maurice E, Ax RL et al: Efficacy of gonadotropin-releasing hormone administered at the time of artificial insemination of heifers and postpartum and repeat breeder dairy cows. Am J Vet Res 44:2160, 1983.
8. Leidl W, Hegner D, Rockel P: Investigations on the $PGF_{2\alpha}$ concentration in maternal and foetal cotyledons of cows with and without retained foetal membranes. Zentralblatt fur Vet Med 27A:691, 1980.
9. Lindell JO, Kindahl H, Jansson L, Edquist LE: Postpartum release of prostaglandin $F_{2\alpha}$ and uterine involution in the cow. Theriogenology 17:237, 1982.
10. Neuhardt VA, Hancock DD, Harrison JH: Effect of routine postpartum intrauterine infusion of Lugol's solution on uterine involution, rate of metritis and other reproductive parameters. Proc 64th Ann Meet Conf Res Workers, Chicago, 1983 Abstract 94.
11. Ott RS, Gustafsson BK: Use of prostaglandins for the treatment of bovine pyometra and postpartum infections: A Review. Comp Cont Ed 3:184, 1981.
12. Oxenreider SL: Evaluation of various treatments for chronic uterine infections in dairy cattle. Proc Ann Meet Soc Theriogenology, 1982, pp 64–72.
13. Russe M: Myometrial activity postpartum. In Karg, Schallenberger (eds): Factors Influencing Fertility in the Postpartum Cow. Boston, Martinus-Nijhoff Publishers, 1982, pp 55–60.
14. Seguin BE, Morrow DA, Louis TM: Luteolysis, luteostasis, and the effect of prostaglandin $F_{2\alpha}$ in cows after endometrial irritation. Am J Vet Res 35:57, 1974.
15. Zerobin K: Die Uterusmotorischen Ablaufe Waehrend Geburt und Puerperium beim Rind und deren Beeninflussbarkeit Proc 11th Int Congr Dis Cattle 2:1157, 1980.

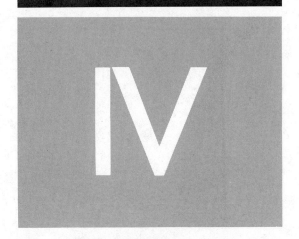

SECTION IV

EMBRYO TRANSFER AND GENETIC ENGINEERING

Reuben J. Mapletoft

Consulting Editor

Introduction

Reuben J. Mapletoft, D.V.M., M.S., Ph.D.
University of Saskatchewan,
Saskatoon, Saskatchewan, Canada

Embryo transfer is a technique by which fertilized embryos are collected from a donor female and transferred to a recipient female that serves as a surrogate mother for the remainder of pregnancy. Embryo transfer techniques have now been applied to nearly every species of domestic animal and to many species of wildlife and exotic animals, including humans and nonhuman primates.

It must be appreciated that the embryo transfer procedures as presently practiced are highly sophisticated, requiring knowledge, practice and dexterity. The veterinary practitioner must recognize the time commitment that successful embryo transfer requires. If the practitioner is unable to make this commitment, then a greater service can be provided by advising the client and supervising the program with a specialized group providing the technical service. (Researchers and those requiring additional information are referred to the first edition of *Current Therapy in Theriogenology*. In addition, the proceedings of the annual meeting of the International Embryo Transfer Society (IETS, 3101 Arrowhead Road, LaPorte, CO 80535) are published annually in the January issue of Theriogenology. The IETS also publishes a quarterly bibliography that thoroughly reviews current literature in the area.

HISTORY

The successful transfer of rabbit embryos was first performed in 1890, and bovine embryos were first collected in the 1930's. However, it was not until the early 1970's that great commercial interest in bovine embryo transfer occurred. In North America there were 20 registered embryo transfer units by 1976, and in 1982 it was estimated that approximately 35,000 pregnancies resulted from bovine embryo transfer. Further, in 1974 the IETS membership was 82, representing seven countries, whereas in 1983 it boasted 832 members, representing 35 countries.

APPLICATION

Genetic Improvement. Most geneticists agree that genetic progress will be slower through the use of embryo transfer than it will be using conventional artificial insemination (AI). This is particularly true on a national herd basis. However, with increased selection intensity and shortened generation intervals, i.e., transferring female offspring, very definite genetic gain can be made on a within-herd basis. It has been shown that the production of about six offspring per donor could double selection intensity and the rate of response to genetic selection for traits such as growth, which can be measured in both sexes. This would be especially worthwhile in improving elite herds, the genetics of which could be spread over a large population through the use of AI. The same principle applies to selection for sex-limited traits, such as milk production.

Planned Matings. By far the most common use of embryo transfer in animal production programs is the proliferation of so-called desirable genotypes. AI has permitted the widespread dissemination of a male's genetics. Embryo transfer provides the opportunity of disseminating the genetics of highly proven elite females. Many AI sires today are produced through the use of embryo transfer. Embryo transfer has also been used to rapidly expand a limited gene pool. The rapid development of the embryo transfer industry in North America is a direct result of the introduction of so-called "exotic" breeds of cattle from Europe, which were then in short supply in North America.

Genetic Testings. A common use of embryo transfer procedures is to genetically test AI sires for deleterious hereditary traits. Some AI organizations keep known carriers of certain genetic defects on hand to serve as donors in testing new sires. Embryos are transferred into unrelated recipients, and depending upon the defect, pregnancy may be terminated at various stages to examine fetuses for presence or absence of the defect. Depending upon the heritability of the defect, generally eight to ten nonaffected fetuses are sufficient to declare a bull free of that trait. Another alternative is to mate the bull in question to seven or eight of his superovulated daughters. Offspring will then represent all recessive traits that a bull may carry. A less attractive alternative would be to mate the bull in question to 40 to 50 of his single ovulating daughters.

Twinning in Cattle. Genetic selection for twinning in cattle has been largely unsuccessful. Similarly, gonadotropin treatments to induce twinning have been unreliable. However, it has been estimated that unit beef production can be increased by 60 per cent through twinning in intensively managed herds. Embryo transfer does provide a very real alternative in the production of twins. The most limiting factor at this time is the cost of transfer. It must be remembered that recipients carrying twins will require extra nutrition and management, especially around the time of calving. Furthermore, recipients must be sufficiently large to carry twins and to produce enough milk to feed twins. Freemartins make twinning less attractive for purebreeding purposes. However, the incidence is relatively low, and sexing of embryos would eliminate the problem entirely. Similarly, the production of identical twins would make twinning very feasible for embryo transfer programs in purebred herds.

Import and Export. The international movement of livestock has become extremely costly. Whereas the intercontinental transport of a live animal may cost $1000 or more, an entire herd can be transported, frozen in the form of embryos, for less than the price of a single plane fare. This may be the single most important potential benefit of embryo transfer. Additional benefits of the export of embryos over that of live animals include a wider genetic base from which to select, the retention of genetics within the exporting country and resolution of the problems. This is particularly true of countries with tropical and subtropical climates, where the fetus would have the opportunity to adapt both within the country and then on a recipient dam indigenous to the area.

There are several potential problems that must be overcome in order to make the international movement of embryos commonplace. First, successful freezing of embryos is imperative. Another problem is the inadvertent introduction of disease into a herd and/or country with or within the embryo. This presents some very difficult regulatory problems. Finally, the international movement of embryos is very dependent on technology transfer. The task of training personnel in the importing countries is one of the greater challenges for the exporting countries.

Salvage of Reproductive Function. Embryo transfer procedures have proved to be extremely useful in the diagnosis, treatment and, finally, the salvage of reproductive function in so-called infertile cows. There has been great benefit demonstrated in the mare as well. It is recommended that the cause of the infertility not be of genetic origin; however, this is difficult to determine. Furthermore, the marketplace is likely to sort out a problem if it is inadvertently propagated through embryo transfer.

Another very important use of embryo transfer is to salvage the genetics of terminally ill animals. It is often possible to produce an additional two or three offspring through embryo transfer before the animal dies.

Disease Control. The embryo is most unlikely to transmit infectious disease. Consequently, it has been suggested that embryo transfer be used to salvage genetics in the face of a disease outbreak. This is a very useful alternative in the establishment of dairy herds that are free of bovine leukosis virus. Similarly, embryo transfer has proved to be a safe way of introducing new bloodlines into specific pathogen-free pig herds. This is one of the most common uses of swine embryo transfer.

Research. Over the years, embryo transfer techniques have proved to be a very useful research tool. In fact, many technical developments in embryo transfer prior to 1970 were directed toward research purposes rather than toward the propagation of superior livestock. Much of the research utilizing embryo transfer involves the physiology, pathology and endocrinology of embryo-utero-ovarian relationships.

DONOR SELECTION

Every breeder will have his own reasons, which are more often economic than genetic, for wanting to perform embryo transfer on a given animal. Certainly, economics will always be the most important factor in determining the utilization of embryo transfer. As optimal results will in turn reduce costs, donor selection may involve using an animal with a previous history of success in embryo transfer. In addition, it has been suggested that the following criteria be used in selecting a cow for embryo transfer:

1. Regular estrous cycles beginning at a young age.
2. No more than two breeding services per conception.
3. First three calves born within two calendar years.
4. Superior individual performance for traits of economic importance.
5. Above average productive performance of offspring from previous matings of the same sire and dam.
6. No parturition difficulties or reproductive irregularities.
7. No conformational or detectable genetic defects.
8. From 3 to 10 years of age.

Selection criteria of this nature will not only ensure genetic superiority but should also ensure a high level of success. It is imperative that the practicing veterinarian be prepared to advise and to assist his clients in the selection of donors and recipients, in the selection of AI bulls and in the overall operation of an embryo transfer program. This is true whether the veterinarian is conducting the embryo transfer service or simply supervising the program. A herd-health service includes genetic consultation in addition to attention to health needs.

REGISTRATION OF OFFSPRING

It is imperative for the veterinarian to become familiar with the breed association requirements for embryo transfer. Generally, confirmation of parentage by blood typing and certification of transfer by the veterinarian doing the work is all that is required for registration. However, individual breed organizations occasionally have unique requirements. This is particularly true of the equine industry. Before a client embarks on an embryo transfer program, he must be advised to consult breed association regulations.

The freezing of embryos has added new problems to documentation and identification. Presently, the IETS is registering firms performing embryo freezing and provides guidelines for identification, documentation and registration of offspring. However, every country and every breed organization again, may have unique requirements. The practitioner must be able to advise his clients in this regard and then be able to complete the necessary paperwork so that offspring may be registered.

COSTS AND SUCCESS RATES

Costs and success rates in embryo transfer are interdependent. Certainly, embryo transfer will be used in animal production programs if it is cost effective. At the same time there are many intangible factors from both the breeder's and the veterinarian's point of view, which are difficult to quantify and may not show up on a balance sheet. Further, inherent fertility, management, weather, semen quality and recipient quality are factors that affect results and costs and are difficult to predict.

It is generally assumed that sex ratios will be 50:50; however, sex ratios may vary a great deal. Results also tend to be extremely good or extremely poor. Data from Colorado State University indicate that approximately one third of donor cows will not produce transferable embryos, and clients must be warned of these possibilities.

With existing technology, the average for each donor cow superovulated would be eight to ten ova collected, six to seven embryos transferred and three to four resulting pregnancies. It must be emphasized that very few donor cows are average. Pregnancy rates are generally around 60 per cent with fresh embryos and range from 30 to 40 per cent with frozen embryos. One can anticipate a fetal death loss of 10 per cent between pregnancy diagnosis and when the calf is 6 months old.

Generally, veterinarians are charging two to four times regular hourly fees for embryo transfer work. Furthermore, many fee schedules are on a per pregnancy basis, which means that successes must cover the costs of failures. As a client becomes more confident of a veterinarian's ability, he may prefer to work by the hour, which will be beneficial to both the veterinarian and the breeder. Fee schedules for bovine embryo transfer in North America at the present time range from $200 to $600 per pregnancy or $100 to $300 per hour. Usually, drug costs and travel costs are extra. As techniques are streamlined, and as results improve, fees will be less, and embryo transfer should be available to most breeders. This would also mean embryo transfer would become a very important part of all herd-health programs.

Costs can be broken down into direct and indirect costs. Direct costs include embryo transfer services (e.g., entrance fees, drugs, board and pregnancy fees) and those costs related to recipient and calf (e.g., transportation, net recipient costs, feed, blood typing). Indirect costs include interest on investment and losses. One must also consider what it would cost to produce a purebred calf by conventional means, which is in excess of $1000 by 1983 standards. With these points in mind, it can be estimated that calves must be worth from $2000 to $3000 at weaning for embryo transfer to be profitable.

Work done on-farm will tend to cost less, whereas calves produced at an embryo transfer center will cost slightly more. This is because labor that is considered essentially free on-farm is taken into consideration. In addition, work on-farm provides many of the so-called intangible benefits for both the breeder and the veterinarian. On-farm embryo transfer can be most economical if three to four donors are superovulated at a time and scheduled to utilize animals of lesser genetic merit as recipients just prior to the beginning of the normal breeding season. A successful embryo transfer program must complement, rather than detract from, a regular breeding program.

References

1. Adams CE (ed): Mammalian Egg Transfer. Boca Raton, CRC Press Inc, 1982.
2. Betteridge KJ: A commemoration of the fiftieth anniversary of the first recovery of a bovine embryo. Bovine Pract 15:4, 1980.
3. Betteridge KJ: A historical look at embryo transfer. J Reprod Fert 62:1, 1981.
4. Brackett BG, Seidel GE, Seidel SM (eds): New Technologies in Animal Breeding. New York, Academic Press Inc, 1981.
5. Church RB, Shea BF: The role of embryo transfer in cattle improvement programs. Can J Anim Sci 57:33, 1977.
6. Elsden RP: Bovine embryo transfer. Proc Soc Theriogenology. Omaha, 1980, p 101.
7. Mapletoft RJ: Embryo transfer for the practitioner. Bovine Pract 13:154, 1980.
8. Betteridge KJ (ed): Embryo Transfer in Farm Animals. Monograph No. 16. Ottawa, Agriculture Canada, 1977.
9. Rowson LEA (ed): Egg Transfer in Cattle. Publications No. EUR 5491, Luxembourg, Commission of the European Communities, 1976.
10. Seidel GE Jr: Costs and success rates of embryo transfer with beef cattle. Proc Ann Conf on AI and Embryo Trans in Beef Cattle. Denver, NAAB, IETS, 1982.

Bovine Embryo Transfer

Reuben J. Mapletoft, D.V.M., M.S., Ph.D.
University of Saskatchewan,
Saskatoon, Saskatchewan, Canada

Embryo transfer in the cow consists of several steps, each of which is critical. Failure in any portion of the procedure will probably result in overall failure. Therefore, success depends on knowledge, practice and constant attention to detail.

The superovulation procedure is an area that requires strict attention to detail. Research over the past decade has not provided the information required to reduce variability in superovulatory response, to increase fertilization rate or to improve embryo quality. In contrast, the technology associated with embryo collection and transfer has been well studied and has been developed to a fairly efficient art. However, there may be no other step in the procedure requiring greater dexterity and more practice.

SUPEROVULATION

General. The majority of donor cows will respond most predictably and optimally if superovulation treatments are instituted between days 8 and 14 of the cycle. We have initiated treatments as early as day 6 of the cycle (estrus = day 0) with success but will not begin treatment after day 14 of the cycle because of the variability in estrous cycle length.

Treatments. Traditionally, a single injection of 1500 to 3000 IU of pregnant mare's serum gonadotropin (PMSG) has been used to superovulate cows. However, more ovulations, embryos recovered and pregnancies have been reported after a superovulatory regimen with follicle-stimulating hormone (FSH) and luteinizing hormone (LH) in a 5:1 ratio, administered twice daily in decreasing doses for 5 days. We have recently demonstrated an improved response when LH was not added to a decreasing dose of FSH. However, certain cows do seem to require 20 per cent LH in order to superovulate successfully. Furthermore, there may be cows that will only superovulate with PMSG. Another treatment that is commonly used, especially because of its simplicity for on-farm work, is 5 mg of FSH twice daily for 5 days. Care must be taken not to induce an overdose, as this will result in a marked reduction in embryo quality. FSH and PMSG may be given either subcutaneously or intramuscularly. Three methods of superovulation are outlined in Table 1.

Synchronization. Normally, a luteolytic dose of prostaglandin $F_{2\alpha}$ ($PGF_{2\alpha}$) is administered 48 to 72 hours after initiation of treatment. Estrus is expected to occur around 48 hours after the administration of $PGF_{2\alpha}$. Cows that are late coming into heat by one or more days usually yield poor results. Occasionally, estrus will occur 12 to 24 hours early. These cows usually have a good superovulatory response with good embryo quality. Once heat is expressed, treatments cease and inseminations begin. If ovulation problems are suspected in a given donor cow (based on previous experience), 2500 IU of human chorionic gonadotropin (hCG) or 200 µg of gonadotropin-releasing hormone (GnRH) may be administered at the onset of heat. Donor cows can be superovulated every 50 to 60 days rather indefinitely. However, it is often useful to allow a

Table 1. Superovulation Treatments in the Cow

Day	Time	Treatment 1	Treatment 2	Treatment 3
10	AM	2500 IU PMSG	5 mg FSH	5 mg FSH
	PM		5 mg FSH	5 mg FSH
11	AM		4 mg FSH	5 mg FSH
	PM	Recipients receive $PGF_{2\alpha}$	4 mg FSH	5 mg FSH
12	AM	Donors receive $PGF_{2\alpha}$	3 mg FSH	5 mg FSH
	PM		3 mg FSH	5 mg FSH
13	AM		2 mg FSH	5 mg FSH
	PM		2 mg FSH	5 mg FSH
14	AM			
	PM	AI	AI	AI
15	AM	AI	AI	AI
	PM	AI	AI	AI

donor cow to have a calf to rejuvenate the system and to milk some fat off her back.

Recipients are normally injected with a luteolytic dose of $PGF_{2\alpha}$ 12 to 18 hours earlier than the donor cow. Recipients should be in heat slightly before or exactly at the same time as the donor cow. Recipient quality is one of the most important factors contributing to transfer success rates.

The superovulation schedule for donor cows and synchronization of recipients require meticulous attention to detail. The donor cow must always be examined prior to treatment to determine any abnormalities and to determine the presence of a normal, functional corpus luteum (CL). Both the breeder and the practitioner must have a complete set of instructions. Furthermore, the local practitioner must serve a very important role in the selection, health, and nutrition and synchronization of recipients. Good communications are essential so that simple things, such as checking and recording onset of heat for recipients or checking donor cows for heat prior to expected estrus, are not overlooked.

Breeding/Insemination. Ovulation in superovulated cows has been shown to be spread over as much as 24 hours; however, the time from onset of estrus to first ovulation is essentially unchanged. Therefore, superovulated cows are inseminated three or four times at 12-hour intervals, beginning 8 to 12 hours after the onset of heat. Some breeders use two doses of semen at each insemination time. Fresh semen or natural service also provides good fertilization rates. The insemination schedule and the inherent fertility of the bull used have been shown to be one of the most limiting factors in numbers of fertilized ova recovered. If at all possible, semen should be evaluated prior to use, paying particular attention to morphology and the per cent of intact acrosomes. Finally, meticulous attention to cleanliness and to good insemination techniques must be emphasized.

EMBRYO COLLECTION

Until 1975, most ova were recovered by surgical methods. However, surgical techniques often resulted in adhesions of the reproductive tract, which in turn reduced the fertility of valuable donor cows. In addition, elaborate facilities were required and on-farm recoveries were impossible. Nonsurgical techniques are preferred, as they are not damaging to the reproductive tract, are repeatable and can be performed on the farm. Nonsurgical techniques can only be performed when embryos enter the uterus and on cows in which the cervix can be penetrated during diestrum.

Nonsurgical Methods. Normally, embryos are collected on days 6 to 8 after the onset of estrus. Prior to this time embryos may still be in the oviduct, and after this time ova begin to hatch from the zona pellucida and are extremely difficult to find. Older dairy cows in particular do not have good muscle tone in the perineal region and tend to "suck" air into the uterus and rectum when an epidural anesthetic is administered. This is overcome in part by making sure that the rumen is full. It is also useful to elevate the front feet or provide a "belly band" to lift abdominal structures to the level of the pelvis and to produce a positive, rather than a negative, pressure in the abdomen.

Preparation. The donor is placed in a squeeze chute and the rectum is evacuated of feces and air. The number of CL is estimated either at this time or at the beginning of collection. Collection is not attempted until a satisfactory epidural anesthesia is attained. Then the perineal region and vulvar lips are thoroughly washed, and the tail is tied out of the way. It is important to avoid ballooning of the rectum with air. In difficult cases, a stomach tube and pump may be used to remove air.

Catheters. There are three basic types of catheters used in nonsurgical embryo collection. Original reports described the use of two-way and three-way Foley catheters. Many groups still use the Foley catheter, as it is inexpensive and readily available. However, the rubber is soft and the catheter is difficult to thread into the uterine horn. Furthermore, the Foley catheter is rather short for large cows, and the distance from the cuff to the catheter tip is short. The "Modell Neustadt/Aisch" two-way Rusch catheter is preferred by many. It is 67 cm long and has an 18-gauge outside diameter and Luer-Lok fittings. The tip in front of the cuff measures 5.5 cm and has four holes. The catheter is stiffened for passage through the cervix by a stainless steel stilette, which locks into the Luer-Lok fitting. It is long enough for large cows and is stiff enough that it can be easily threaded down the uterine lumen. Newcomb has developed an embryo collection catheter that is also very long (115 cm), with an extension of 42.5 cm from cuff to the fluid outlet. Fluid is passed into the uterus through an inlet hole at the leading extremity of the catheter and recovered through an outlet hole immediately before the inflated cuff. In Newcomb's experience with heifers, this catheter has resulted in higher embryo recovery rates than conventional catheters.

Techniques. There are two methods of collection: the continuous-flow, closed-circuit system and the interrupted-syringe method. Any combination of those described is possible. Each system has advantages and disadvantages relative to the other system. Each operator must develop a technique that results in the best personal success. With the closed system, it is easier to maintain sterility, and there is less chance of losing medium and, consequently, embryos. However, the closed system is cumbersome, and the extra tubing provides extra potential for contamination from either bacteria or chemicals. The interrupted syringe method allows for the use of completely disposable equipment, with the exception of catheters. This also permits the searching for embryos during the collection.

Interrupted Syringe Technique. A brief review of the use of the "Modell Neustadt/Aisch" two-way

Rusch catheter and the interrupted-syringe collection technique is presented as follows. The catheter with the stilette in place is coated with a sterile lubricant and is passed through the vagina and the cervix. If vaginitis exists, it is often advisable to use a double-catheter threading technique to prevent contamination of the uterus. Furthermore, every attempt must be made to be sure that the catheter itself will not contribute to bacterial contamination. Catheters may be sterilized with either ethylene oxide or a cold sterilizing solution. It is absolutely necessary to make sure that catheters are dry prior to sterilization with ethylene oxide and to allow "airing out" for 1 week after sterilization; as ethylene oxide can kill embryos. Similarly, most cold sterilizing solutions are embryo-toxic and must be rinsed from the catheter with saline.

It is very seldom that it takes more than a few seconds to thread the catheter into the cervix. Occasionally, it is necessary to use a "cervical dilator" to enlarge the cervical canal before a catheter can be passed. The catheter is directed into the right uterine horn, and the stilette is gradually removed as the catheter is threaded down the horn. The catheter is placed so that the inflated cuff is located approximately half-way between the uterine body and the uterine tip. The cuff is inflated initially with 5 ml of sterile saline, then palpated, with additional saline added until the cuff completely fills the uterine lumen. Over-inflation or too rapid inflation of the cuff may split the endometrium, causing hemorrhage and loss of flushing medium into the broad ligament. The stilette is then removed and a clamp is placed on the catheter at its exteriorized end.

Collection is normally done with disposable syringes using 25 to 35 ml of medium per flush. This is particularly useful when one is collecting a single embryo, as flushes are placed singly into sterile, disposable petri dishes and examined microscopically by an assistant to locate embryos. The embryo is usually found in one of the first four flushes. In the superovulated donor, each uterine horn is flushed with eight individual flushes, which are placed in a 500-ml graduated cylinder. Normally, 85 per cent of the embryos will be found in the first four flushes of each horn.

The technique for collection of embryos is one of the most difficult steps to master. One must be gentle and yet ensure that the medium mixes and reaches all areas of the endometrium. Two or more flushes are often placed in the horn together before agitation and aspiration. It is important to ensure that medium is not forced into the uterus under too much pressure, as the endometrium may split, resulting in hemorrhage and loss of fluid and embryos into the broad ligament. It is also important to prevent kinking of the uterine horn, as a small portion may become over-inflated, again causing a split in the endometrium. It is necessary to achieve some distention of the horn to wash embryos from folds in the endometrium.

When the collection of the right horn is completed, the stilette is reinserted without withdrawing the catheter from the uterus. The catheter with the stilette in place is then inserted into the left horn, and the cuff is positioned as previously described. When the flush is completed, each uterine horn is infused with 30 to 40 ml of an antibacterial or antibiotic solution using a syringe and a uterine infusion catheter. $PGF_{2\alpha}$ may be given at this time or approximately 1 week later to induce luteolysis. However, return to estrus cannot be expected for 1 to 2 weeks. Conception on the first estrus is not as high as it will be on subsequent heats.

Continuous-Flow Technique. Embryo collection by way of a three-way Foley catheter and a continuous-flow, closed-circuit system has been described by Elsden. A sterile 18- or 24-gauge three-way Foley catheter with a stiffening rod of stainless steel inside it is gently inserted through the vagina and into the cervix. It is then manipulated into the selected horn so that the inflatable cuff is situated at the palpable bifurcation of the uterus. Some operators situate the cuff just beyond the internal os of the cervix; however, it is difficult to flush each horn separately with this positioning. The cuff may be inflated with 15 ml of air or fluid, more being added if necessary, to hold the cuff in place. Approximately 500 to 800 ml of medium heated to 37°C is placed in an Erlenmeyer flask fitted for infusion with a 1.0-m length of Tygon tubing with an inside diameter of 6 to 8 mm. The tubing from the flask is attached to the inflow tube of the Foley catheter with a glass connector. Another piece of Tygon tubing, 1.0 m in length, is connected to the outflow tube of the Foley catheter with a glass connector, and the other free end is held at the top of a 1000-ml graduated cylinder. Should a two-way Foley catheter be used, a glass "T" is connected to the inflow and outflow tubing and to the lumen of the Foley catheter.

The first 20 to 30 ml of medium are allowed to flow in and out of the uterus freely to ensure that there are no blockages in the system and to clear any mucus or blood clots. The outflow tube is then clamped, and the horn is filled with medium by way of the inflow tube. Usually, the uterine horn of a heifer is distended to the size of a 35-day pregnancy and that of a cow to a 45-day pregnancy. The uterus is gently massaged and fluid is agitated to dislodge ova from the endometrial folds. The outflow clamp is released, the inflow is clamped off and the fluid is allowed to drain from the uterus into the cylinder. Once the initial rush of fluid is over, the remaining medium is "milked" out of the uterus. This process is repeated until approximately 800 ml of medium pass through the uterine lumen.

The relatively gentle gravity flow allows tissues to expand gradually to their greatest capacity without damage. The uterus of multiparous cows will gradually expand more and more with each flush, thus resulting in greater penetration of the endometrial folds and release of trapped ova. The endometrium should be thoroughly expanded and washed at least three times before the Foley catheter is removed and inserted into the other uterine horn, where the process is repeated. Experience will indicate how much manipulation and how much medium are necessary to collect most, if not all, ova. One should normally collect approximately 80 to 90 per cent of ova based on palpable CL counts.

Searching for Embryos. Regardless of the method of collection, medium is allowed to settle for a minimum of 35 minutes in a straight-sided cylinder. A siphon of sterile silastic tubing may then be set up to remove all but the bottom 50 ml of medium. The remaining medium is then swirled, aspirated into a syringe with a uterine infusion pipette and placed in sterile, disposable petri dishes (100 × 15 mm in size) for searching. Occasionally, an embryo will be siphoned off. It is imperative that the medium not be agitated, as currents may develop while siphoning is occurring. Alternatively, one may simply aspirate 35 ml from the bottom of the cylinder after the medium settles. This is repeated again 10 to 15 minutes later. This has resulted in as high a recovery rate as siphoning. It is also possible to use a 50-μm plankton filter with good success. Medium is passed through the filter and then rinsed off into a petri dish for embryo searching.

There is no question that one of the most difficult tasks facing a practitioner who is learning embryo transfer techniques is searching for, identifying and evaluating embryos. Select the stereoscopic microscope you intend to work with, use it and establish confidence with it. A grid is placed on the base of the microscope, and the petri dish is searched at 10 × magnification. Once the dish is searched, it is swirled to move the embryo away from the perimeter and searched again. Each dish should be searched at least twice after the last embryo is found, with the swirling motion repeated in each case.

Media. Flushing medium is prepared prior to preparation of the cow. Dulbecco's phosphate-buffered saline (PBS) is commonly used and is refrigerated in 500-ml bottles ready for use. In addition, 10-ml quantities of heat-inactivated fetal calf serum (FCS) and 5 ml of an antibiotic/antimycotic solution are kept frozen so that a single quantity is available for each 500 ml of PBS. Medium then contains 100 IU of penicillin, 100 μg of streptomycin and 25 μg of amphotericin B (Fungizone). Glucose and pyruvate can also be added so that the medium contains 1 mg/ml glucose and 0.33 mM sodium pyruvate. Eight ml of FCS are added to the flushing medium to produce a 2 per cent solution, while 8 ml of the flushing medium are added in turn to the remaining 2 ml of FCS to produce 10 ml of culture medium, which is a 20 per cent FCS solution for culture prior to transfer. Culture medium is passed through a 0.22 μm Millipore filter prior to use. It would seem that glucose and pyruvate are only necessary for longer periods of embryo culture. Therefore, medium for on-farm work need only contain PBS, antibiotics and 2 per cent FCS for collection and 10 to 20 per cent FCS for culture prior to transfer.

The culture medium containing 10 to 20 per cent FCS is deposited in a smaller sterile disposable petri dish (35 × 15 mm), which in turn is placed in one of the large petri dishes to provide stability. Embryos, when they are located, are picked up with a sterile disposable 20-gauge plastic intravenous catheter, attached to a 1-ml syringe and deposited in the culture dish. Once searching ceases, embryos are placed in fresh medium, evaluated at 50 × magnification, illustrated or described. Washing of embryos should take place three or four times before transfer. The culture dishes are then placed at room temperature on the counter top between two layers of terry towels or at 35 to 37°C on a warm stage or in an incubator. Just prior to transfer, embryos may be again placed in fresh culture medium.

Temperature and Sterility. Temperature does not seem to be critical. Room temperature is satisfactory, provided chills and drafts are avoided. Similarly, sterility is not possible but every attempt should be made to be as clean as possible. Sterilization with chemicals is as likely to kill embryos as bacterial contaminants. Although embryos may be cultured in PBS over the course of a day, culture medium should be changed from time to time, as contamination and evaporation will occur.

EVALUATION OF EMBRYOS

General. Evaluation of bovine embryos is normally done at 50 to 100 × magnification, with the embryo in the small culture dish. It is important to be able to recognize the various stages of development and to compare these with the developmental stage that the embryo should be at based on the occurrence of heat (Fig. 1). Embryos that are of doubtful quality can be cultured for a few hours. An improvement in appearance will indicate that the embryo is of transferable quality. Often a decision as to whether an embryo is worthy of transfer will depend on the availability of a recipient. Embryos classified as good or excellent result in high pregnancy rates. However, fair and poor quality embryos may also result in pregnancies, and consideration should be given to their use if recipients are available.

Classification. The overall diameter of the bovine embryo is 150 to 190 μm, including a zona pellucida thickness of approximately 12 to 15 μm. The overall diameter of the embryo remains virtually unchanged from the one-cell stage until blastocyst expansion. Early cleavage stage embryos are commonly referred to by the number of cells present, such as one-cell and two-cell, up to the 16-cell stage. In embryos developed beyond the 16-cell stage other morphologic criteria must be used. Generally, the embryo is described in terms of its stage of development and its quality or health as follows:

Stage

MORULA. A mass of at least 16 cells. Individual blastomeres are difficult to discern from one another. The cellular mass of the embryo occupies most of the perivitelline space.

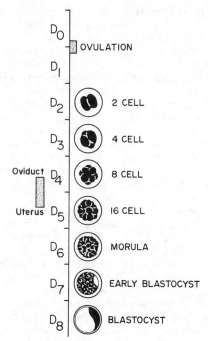

Figure 1. Ovulation and embryo development in the superovulated cow. Ovulation takes place 24 to 48 hours after the onset of estrus. Embryos enter the uterus between days 4 and 5. On days 6 to 8, during which nonsurgical embryo collections are done, embryo development should range from early morula to expanded blastocyst.

COMPACT MORULA. Individual blastomeres have coalesced, forming a compact mass. The embryo mass occupies 60 to 70 per cent of the perivitelline space.

EARLY BLASTOCYST. An embryo that has formed a fluid-filled cavity or blastocoele and gives a general appearance of a signet ring. The embryo occupies 70 to 80 per cent of the perivitelline space. Early in this stage the embryo may appear of very questionable quality.

BLASTOCYST. Pronounced differentiation of the outer trophoblast layer and of the darker, more compact inner cell mass is evident. The blastocoele is highly prominent, with the embryo occupying most of the perivitelline space. Visual differentiation between the trophoblast and the inner cell mass is possible at this stage of development.

EXPANDED BLASTOCYST. The overall diameter of the embryo dramatically increases, with a concurrent thinning of the zona pellucida to approximately one third of its original thickness.

HATCHED BLASTOCYST. Embryos recovered at this developmental stage can be undergoing the process of hatching or may have completely shed the zona pellucida. Hatched blastocysts may be spherical with a well-defined blastocoele or may be collapsed. Identification of embryos at this stage can be difficult for the inexperienced operator.

Quality

EXCELLENT. An ideal embryo, spherical, symmetrical and with cells of uniform size, color and texture.

GOOD. Small imperfections such as a few extruded blastomeres, irregular shape and few vesicles.

FAIR. More definite problems including presence of extruded blastomeres, vesiculation and a few degenerated cells.

POOR. Severe problems, numerous extruded blastomeres, degenerated cells, cells of varying sizes, large numerous vesicles but an apparently viable embryo mass. These are generally not of transferable quality.

Results. In the superovulated cow, there is likely to be a considerable range of stages on any given day during development. On day 7 after estrus, there may be morulae and hatching blastocysts within the same flush. At the same time, there may be embryos of excellent quality and also unfertilized ova and degenerate embryos. The reasons for these variations is not known, but they may be due to differences in ovulation time and in endocrine environments. Generally, wide variations in embryo quality and stages of development are signals that existing embryos are not entirely normal and that pregnancy rates may be disappointing. Embryos of good and excellent quality at the developmental stages of late morula to blastocyst yield the best pregnancy rates. It may be advisable to select the stage of the embryo for the synchrony of t ecipient. It would also seem that fair and poor quality embryos are most likely to survive in the most synchronous recipients.

References

1. Betteridge KJ (ed): Embryo Transfer in Farm Animals. Monograph No. 16. Ottawa, Agriculture Canada, 1977.
2. Drost M, Brand A, Aarts MH: A device for non-surgical recovery of bovine embryos. Theriogenology 6:503, 1976.
3. Elsden RP, Hasler JF, Seidel GE Jr: Non-surgical recovery of bovine eggs. Theriogenology 6:523, 1976.
4. Elsden RP, Nelson LD, Seidel GE Jr: Superovulation of cows with follicle stimulating hormone and pregnant mare's serum gonadotrophin. Theriogenology 9:17, 1978.
5. Eldsen RP: Bovine embryo transfer. Proc Ann Meet Soc Theriogenology. Omaha, 1980, p 101.
6. Lindner GM, Wright RW Jr: Bovine embryo morphology and evaluation. Proc Workshop, IX Ann Meet IETS. Denver, 1983, p 21.
7. Mapletoft RJ: Embryo transfer for the practitioner. Bovine Pract 13:154, 1980.
8. Newcomb R, Christie WB, Rowson LEA: Non-surgical recovery of bovine embryos. Vet Rec 102:414, 1978.
9. Rowe RF, Del Campo MR, Eilts CL, et al.: A single cannula technique for non-surgical collection of ova from cattle. Theriogenology 6:471, 1976.
10. Schneider U, Hahn JF: Bovine embryo transfer in Germany. Theriogenology 11:63, 1979.

Transfer of Bovine Embryos

Robert F. Rowe, D.V.M., Ph.D.
Veterinary Reproductive Specialties, Inc.,
Middleton, Wisconsin

Since the inception of the idea of embryo transfer in cattle, the goal has been successful nonsurgical processes to collect and to transfer embryos. Much of the progress in the development of these techniques can be traced to commercial firms whose continued existence depended on success (pregnant recipient animals). Advancement toward the goal of successful nonsurgical transfers was often put aside in favor of the more successful, surgical technique.

The chronological development of embryo transfer techniques has paralleled embryo collection techniques. When donors were surgically flushed under general anesthesia at 3 to 5 days after heat, recipients were also placed under general anesthesia in the dorsal recumbent position to allow surgical replacement of the embryo into the approximate area of the reproductive tract from where it had been recovered.

In an effort to eliminate the problems associated with general anesthesia and yet maintain good surgical collection rates, some firms resorted to local anesthesia and flank collections. Similarly, locally anesthetized recipients became the next logical step for surgical transfers. Indeed, this process continues to be used by a great number of embryo transfer firms.

When nonsurgical collection procedures became as successful as surgical techniques, while eliminating many of the problems associated with surgery, they were rapidly adopted by the industry. As pregnancy rates achieved by nonsurgical procedures continue to improve and approximate those achieved with surgical techniques, while eliminating problems associated with surgery, more firms will transfer all embryos using nonsurgical techniques.

SURGICAL TRANSFER TECHNIQUES

Although most commercial firms that transfer embryos surgically use the flank approach, some still utilize the midventral technique. This involves general anesthesia of the recipient, placing her in dorsal recumbency, surgical preparation of the midline just anterior to the mammary gland and surgical invasion of the abdominal cavity. Once the uterus has been located and a suitable corpus luteum (CL) has been confirmed in one of the ovaries, a small puncture is made into the lumen of the uterine horn ipsilateral to the CL. The pipette loaded with the embryo is introduced through the puncture and the embryo is deposited. Routine closure, extubation and postoperative recovery follow. To facilitate the procedure, most firms withhold feed (24 to 48 hours) and water (12 to 24 hours) from recipients prior to midventral surgery.

Most commercial firms have adopted the flank approach for surgical transfers. Preliminary preparations include palpation of the recipients to identify the site of the CL, which must correspond with the side of the flank incision. Paravertebral and/or local (L-block) anesthesia is accomplished with a local anesthetic, and the flank area is surgically prepared. Routine opening is accomplished, and the site of the CL is confirmed. The uterine horn is grasped and gently retracted to the incision. Transfer is similar to that in the midventral approach, and closure is again routine. Some of the advantages of flank transfer over the midventral technique include the need for less equipment (anesthesia machines and equipment to handle cows under general anesthesia), fewer facilities (holding pens, recovery facilities and surgical suites) and the option to perform the transfers on-farm into the client's own recipients.

NONSURGICAL TECHNIQUES

Several variations of nonsurgical techniques have appeared in the literature. These include sets of telescoping stainless steel rods with flexible polyethylene tubing, to deposit the embryo ultimately to a cranial position in the uterine horn, transvaginal techniques using stainless steel needles to circumvent the cervix and polyethylene tubes for embryo deposition. However, the most commonly used equipment for nonsurgical embryo transfers in the cow is the Cassou AI gun and either 0.5- or 0.25-ml French straws.

When using the Cassou equipment, each embryo is loaded into a straw with an air bubble on either side of the fluid containing the embryo itself. The air bubbles act as barriers to prevent the indiscriminate movement of the embryos.

The recipient is examined for the presence of an appropriate CL and a normal uterus, and an epidural anesthetic is given to eliminate rectal contractions. The straw is loaded into the Cassou syringe, and the sheath is placed over it. The vulvar area is cleaned and wiped dry. Some practitioners use a "soda straw" or other protective double sheath to reduce contamination from the recipient's vagina. The Cassou gun is inserted to the external cervical os, punched through the protective sheath and threaded through the cervix into the uterine horn ipsilateral to the CL.

Most practitioners attempt to place the embryo cranial to the external uterine bifurcation, and all agree that a rapid atraumatic placement more caudal in the horn is preferable to a prolonged, difficult placement extremely cranial into the horn. The actual deposition of the fluid and embryo is accomplished with a slow, steady motion similar to that of depositing semen.

Advantages of nonsurgical techniques include the reduced amount of time required, the need for little or no special facilities and the reduced cost to the cattle breeders. The biggest disadvantages are the extensive practice required to become and to remain proficient in the techniques and the occasional recipient whose cervix is difficult or impossible to penetrate.

RECIPIENT CONSIDERATIONS

The two requirements for a successful embryo transfer are a good embryo and a good recipient. Recipients must be healthy, cycling and on an increasing plane of nutrition; they must also be sufficiently well grown to produce a live, healthy calf. Recipients that are too thin or too fat will have suboptimal pregnancy rates with embryo transfer, just as they would in an artificial insemination program. In well-managed herds cows can be as good recipients as heifers, or better, because of the equal transfer success rates and lower occurrence of perinatal mortality.

Most practitioners agree that a high degree of estrous synchronization of donors and recipients is essential for high pregnancy rates. However, variation does occur. The most important factor would appear to be the embryo quality. An embryo that is of high quality (compacted morula or blastocyst) can adjust to asynchrony, whereas an embryo graded lower in quality has a smaller range of acceptable uterine environment. The best recipients are usually those in heat the day before and the same day as the donor.

SUPPORTIVE TREATMENTS

Over the years commercial embryo transfer firms have attempted to increase pregnancy rates with the use of exogenous hormone products. Treatments with these agents have been shown to increase pregnancy rates in certain animals. None has shown to be consistently effective in increasing overall pregnancy rates in controlled studies. In the final analysis, a good quality embryo and a high quality recipient with less than ± 24-hour asynchrony will yield optimal pregnancy rates, providing transfer techniques are also of a high quality.

Suggested Readings

1. Rowe RF, Del Campo MR, Critser JK, Ginther OJ: Embryo transfer in cattle: Nonsurgical transfer. Am J Vet Res 41:1024, 1980.
2. Wright JM: Nonsurgical embryo transfer in cattle. Theriogenology 15:43, 1981.

Embryo Transfer in Repeat-Breeder Cows

Walter H. Johnson, D.V.M., M.V.Sc.
University of Guelph,
Guelph, Ontario, Canada

There are many factors that impair conception, ranging from those that are impossible to detect clinically to those that are very easily diagnosed. Factors that render an animal infertile but are difficult to detect clinically include oviductal obstructions, minor periovarian adhesions, inhospitable uterine environment and functional deficiencies. Other conditions, such as chronic, purulent metritis, advanced adhesions, hydrosalpinx and cervical tears, may be easily detected on clinical examination.

FACTORS IMPAIRING CONCEPTION

Adhesions. Adhesions of the genital tract of cows may have many causes, including surgery, such as caesarian section or surgical embryo collection; poor AI technique, with puncture of the uterus; rape of young heifers by a large bull, with penetration of the dorsal vaginal wall; ascending infection as a result of pyometra; and descending infections as a result of peritonitis. Many of these causes also result in blockage of the oviducts. Occluded oviducts often show evidence of fibrosis, with constriction of the lumen and localized dilations. It has been estimated that 10 per cent of oviducts on post-mortem specimens were occluded. Bursal adhesions may result in malfunction of the fimbria, causing improper recovery of the oocytes and their loss into the abdomen.

Embryonic Death. It is often felt that the main factor in infertility is early embryonic death, rather than fertilization failure. If early embryonic death is occurring, early removal of these embryos from this environment, with transplantation into suitable recipient animals may result in an acceptable pregnancy rate. The longer the embryo is allowed to remain in the infertile host, the greater are the chances of degeneration.

Fertilization Failure. Information obtained through embryo transfer suggests that fertilization failure may be the most important factor in repeat breeding animals. The cause of this is not clear. However, one must again consider an environment that is inhospitable to sperm survival and transport. Certain morphologic and biologic defects in the production of oocytes may also make them unfertilizable or cause them to degenerate early.

DIAGNOSIS

The diagnosis of the cause of infertility must begin with a good history. The clinical examination of the genital tract should include careful rectal palpation of the cervix, uterine horns, ovaries, bursae and oviducts, along with palpation of the surrounding tissues plus endoscopic examination and palpation of the vagina and cervix. A uterine culture should be taken for identification of pathogenic organisms, and possibly a uterine biopsy should be taken in order to identify the quality of the endometrium. Specialized diagnostic techniques include a hormone profile to assess gonadotropin and sex steroid levels, a cytologic study to detect chromosomal abnormalities, oviduct patency tests to detect occluded oviducts, laparotomy to visualize the extent of pathologic abnormalities and an embryo collection. The procedure of superovulation and embryo collection has proved to be a useful diagnostic procedure, as it will indicate whether oviducts are patent and functional, whether fertilization has occurred and whether normal embryonic development is proceeding.

TREATMENT

The appropriate treatment will, of course, vary with the diagnosis. In many cases it is entirely possible that conception will occur following simple procedures. Uterine lavage associated with embryo collection has been shown to have excellent therapeutic value in infertile cows. Appropriate antibiotic treatments should also be instituted in conjunction with lavage to treat inflammation or infection of the vagina, uterus or cervix.

Appropriate surgery may also be performed to aid in the restoration of fertility. This may include urethral extension to prevent urovagina, ovariectomy of a severely diseased ovary and forcing fluid through occluded oviducts to remove the blockage. However, in our experience oviductal occlusions generally recur. It must be remembered that any reproductive surgery, unless done with extreme care, may result in the formation of extensive adhesions in the delicate tissues of the reproductive tract.

EMBRYO COLLECTION

Embryo transfer procedures, as applied to subinfertile or repeat-breeder cows, are very practical ways of salvaging the genetics of these often valuable animals. However, the success rate with repeat-breeder cows is reduced from that of normal animals. Embryo transfer may also be viewed as a multifaceted procedure because it is a sound diagnostic procedure and, at the same time, provides excellent uterine therapy.

Superovulation. The induction of superovulation may increase the possibility of oocytes being picked up by the fimbria, thus enabling fertilization and collection of embryos to occur. Superovulation in cows that have normal estrous cycles is done in the routine manner using follicle-stimulating hormone (FSH) or pregnant mare serum gonadotropin (PMSG) in conjunction with prostaglandin $F_{2\alpha}$ ($PGF_{2\alpha}$). Animals that have abnormal estrous cycles or animals that do not cycle may be superovulated using progesterone injections or a progestogen implant (Synchro-Mate B) to control the estrous cycle. Daily injection of 100 mg of aqueous progesterone for 7 days and 50 mg for 2 days will prevent estrus. Superovulation should be instituted on day 7 and $PGF_{2\alpha}$ should be administered on day 9. Synchro-Mate B treatment consists of an ear implant containing norgestomet, a synthetic progestogen, plus an injection of norgestomet and estradiol on day 1. Superovulation is begun on day 7, and the ear implant is removed on day 9. Estrus is expressed 24 to 48 hours following implant removal or last progesterone injection. With either method, breeding and embryo collection can be done in the routine manner.

Embryo Collection. The embryo collection procedure is also an excellent diagnostic tool, whether or not animals have obvious disease. Provided a good superovulatory response has occurred and a good collection procedure followed, many questions may be answered. The flush from each horn should be kept separate. If no embryos are recovered from one or either uterine horn, it strongly suggests that they were not in the uterine lumen, the reasons being that oocytes were either not captured by the fimbria or that blockage of the oviducts prevented oocyte passage into the uterus. Diseases of the fimbria, such as adhesions, can be detected per rectum, as can advanced cases of salpingitis. However, occluded oviducts are often not palpable per rectum.

The collection of unfertilized oocytes in the flush may indicate a fertilization problem, and confirms that ovulation has occurred and that the oviduct on that side is patent. Fertilization failure may be due to an inhospitable uterine environment so that the semen is destroyed, poor quality semen or improper time and technique of insemination. Certain morphologic and biologic defects may also occur in the production of oocytes that make them unfertilizable or cause them to degenerate early. Because superovulation creates such an artificial environment, single egg collections after a normal estrus may more specifically solve the riddle of fertilization failure.

THERAPEUTIC FLUSH

The flushing procedure used to attempt recovery of embryos from infertile animals is extremely beneficial as a therapeutic technique, and in many cases it may be performed by itself in the absence of superovulation and insemination. The therapeutic uterine lavage should be performed during diestrus to ensure that the uterotubal junction is tightly closed and that contaminated fluid will not be forced into the oviducts. The entire uterus should be washed, with particular care taken to reach the tips of each uterine horn to ensure that there is not a nidus of infection remaining in that location.

A wide variety of fluids may be used to lavage the uterus, but physiological saline is probably adequate. In the mare it produces a short-term superficial inflammatory reaction in the endometrium, which is probably adequate to induce a chemical curettage effect. Twenty per cent nitrofurazone also produces a superficial inflammatory reaction with longer duration, while 20 per cent povidone-iodine (Betadine) or 10 per cent oxytetracycline (Liquamycin 100) produces a more severe and long-lasting reaction.

The majority of cases require only a single lavage treatment plus a luteolytic dose of $PGF_{2\alpha}$ to induce estrus, at which time breeding can occur. More severe endometritis or pyometra may require more aggressive therapy, with lavage treatments every second day for several days until all purulent material is removed and the endometrium has returned to normal. It may also be advantageous to lavage the uterus with physiological saline 24 hours after insemination.

It is important to use large volumes of fluid in the lavage procedure and to remove as much of the fluid as possible. Lavage should continue until clear fluid is recovered. Antibiotics may be infused into the uterus after lavage; however, greater concentrations of some antibiotics may be achieved in uterine tissue by systemic administration rather than by intrauterine infusion.

The endometrium of animals with a chronic endometritis may have such severe damage that the maintenance of a pregnancy to term is impossible. Embryo transfer certainly can be considered in these cases. Aggressive treatment and lavage can improve the endometrial environment to the point at which viable embryos can be obtained and pregnancies can result through the use of embryo transfer.

CONCLUSION

Infertility in the cattle population is an economically significant problem. If the animal is not genetically valuable, slaughter must be considered. However, in the valuable animal, embryo transfer must be considered as a practical method for propagating the genetics of that animal. One must be cognizant of possible heritability factors of infertility and of the possibility of propagating a line of subfertile animals. Embryo transfer techniques have proved useful not only in the salvage of valuable genetics but also in the diagnosis and treatment of infertility. Uterine lavage has been shown to be an excellent therapeutic technique to be employed in the treatment of repeat-breeder animals and should be used by practitioners performing fertility work.

Suggested Readings

1. Bowen RA, Elsden RP, Seidel GE Jr: Embryo transfer for cows with reproductive problems. JAVMA 172:1303, 1978.
2. Greve T: Embryo transplant in cattle: Non-surgical recovery of embryos from repeat breeders. Acta Vet Scand 21:26, 1980.
3. Linares T, King WA, Ploen L: Observations on the early development of embryos from repeat breeder heifers. Nord Vet Med 32:433, 1980.
4. Mapletoft RJ, Johnson WH, Adams WM: Effects of a progestagen ear implant on superovulatory response in the cow. Theriogenology 13:102, 1980.
5. Mapletoft RJ, Johnson WH, Miller DM: Embryo transfer techniques in repeat breeding cows. Theriogenology 13:103, 1980.

Embryo Transfer in Sheep and Goats

R. H. Bondurant, D.V.M.
University of California,
Davis, California

INDICATIONS

The low unit-value of most sheep and goats restricts widespread use of embryo transfer technology as it is presently practiced, but specific applications have included the following:

1. The introduction of new breeds or bloodlines, especially when international transport of live animals is otherwise impractical or restricted by law.

2. Rapid multiplication of exceptional females, with acceleration of genetic intervals.

3. Increasing the benefit of "out of season" breeding.

4. Research.

The procedures for superovulation, collection and transfer of embryos from sheep and goats are essentially identical and will be described together, except in the few cases in which major differences exist. Several breeds of sheep have been successfully superovulated and their embryos transferred; however, most data on caprine embryo transfer have been collected from Angora goats.

SELECTION OF DONORS AND RECIPIENTS

The essential prerequisite for both donor and recipient animals is that they exhibit normal estrous cycles. For this reason, embryo transfer in small ruminants is usually done during the normal breeding season, when cyclic behavior can be expected.

It is possible, however, to induce estrus and superovulation during the anestrous period by a variety of means. In addition, recipients should have proven fertility (i.e., offspring at expected intervals), good mothering ability and milk production and sound feet and legs and should be available at a reasonable price.

Superovulation. Both sheep and goats can be superovulated during the breeding and anestrous seasons. Some reports suggest a slightly lower response in the anestrous period, particularly for those breeds with strict seasonal limitations on cyclic behavior. In the cyclic donor gonadotropins are administered near the end of the luteal phase of the cycle (day 12 in the ewe and days 17 to 18 in the doe) so that follicles are recruited immediately prior to lysis of the existing corpus luteum. Commonly, the precise stage of the cycle is not known so that the donor's estrous cycle must be artificially controlled.

Several gonadotropins have proved successful, among them pregnant mare serum gonadotropin (PMSG), porcine follicle-stimulating hormone (FSH) and equine pituitary extract (EPE) or horse anterior pituitary (HAP) hormone. Table 1 lists the doses and timing for each of these drugs in sheep and goats.

It should be understood from the outset that wide variation in response of donor animals to *any* superovulating drug is the rule rather than the exception. This variation arises from several factors, among them the sensitivity of the ovary to stimulation by gonadotropins, a trait that is almost certainly determined genetically. Breeds noted for fecundity, e.g., Finnish Landrace, will generally show a greater response to gonadotropins than breeds of lower fecundity. Other factors involved include the age of the donor (ewe lambs and yearling does show diminished responses), the nutritional status of the donor, the particular drug used and perhaps even the particular lot or batch of that drug.

In several trials with Angora goats (Fig. 1), and in limited experiments with sheep, FSH has provided a greater ovulatory response and embryo recovery rate than PMSG, probably because of more specific FSH activity. Greater numbers of

Table 1. Superovulation in Sheep and Goats

Drug	Dose/Route	Days of Estrous Cycle* Sheep	Days of Estrous Cycle* Goat	Comments
PMSG	1000 to 2000 IU IM	11 or 12	14 to 18	Single injection
FSH	18 to 24 mg IM or SC (begin at 5 mg)	Begin days 11 to 13	Begin days 13 to 16	Twice daily decreasing dose for 3 to 4 days
HAP EPE‡	40 to 45 mg/day SC 600 to 1000 FHRU† IM or SC	Begin days 10 to 12	Begin days 13 to 17	Crude extract once daily for 3 days

*When PGF$_{2\alpha}$ is used, it is given 1 to 2 days after initiation of gonadotropin treatment.
†Fevold-Hisaw rat units.
‡Not tested in sheep and goats.

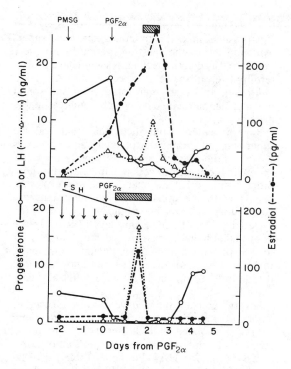

Figure 1. Estradiol, progesterone and luteinizing hormone (LH) profiles in Angora does superovulated with a combination of gonadotropin (PMSG or FSH) and prostaglandin. Stipled area indicates duration of estrus. Note the rise in progesterone immediately following PMSG injection. (Adapted from Armstrong et al.: J Reprod Fert 67:395, 1983.)

unovulated follicles have been associated with superovulation induced by PMSG than by FSH or HAP, apparently because of the long half-life of PMSG. The periestrous endocrine patterns of estradiol, progesterone and luteinizing hormone (LH) in caprine donors superovulated with FSH more closely resembled "normal" patterns than those treated with PMSG. In both sheep and goats superovulation with PMSG has been associated with premature regression of the induced corpora lutea, resulting in short cycles and risk of embryo death and/or expulsion. All of these factors notwithstanding, PMSG is still a useful drug because of its

availability in many countries and its convenient dosage.

It is often necessary to control the time of estrus and ovulation in donors so that gonadotropin treatment can be administered properly timed to the recruitment of follicles and subsequent estrus. When information is available about the stage of the donor's estrous cycle, a single injection of prostaglandin $F_{2\alpha}$ ($PGF_{2\alpha}$), given 2 days after initiation of gonadotropin treatment (middle to late cycle), will induce estrus in 1 to 4 days. In animals for which no such information is available, two injections of $PGF_{2\alpha}$ may be given 8 to 10 days apart (sheep) or 10 to 12 days apart (goat). Gonadotropin treatment is begun 2 days before the second injection of $PGF_{2\alpha}$.

In either cyclic or anestrous donors, estrus and ovulation may be controlled with progesterone or synthetic progestins (Table 2). When progesterone is used, it is administered as daily injections of 10 to 12 mg for 12 days in the ewe and 14 to 18 days in the doe. A more convenient method of control employs the use of vaginal sponges or pessaries containing either flurogestone acetate (Cronolone) or methyl-acetoxyprogesterone. Sponges are inserted intravaginally and are removed 12 to 14 days later (sheep) or 16 to 20 days later (goat). Gonadotropin treatment begins 1 to 2 days before sponge removal, and estrus commences 1 to 2 days after removal.

It is possible to combine progestin and $PGF_{2\alpha}$ treatment in goats by inserting progestins for 9 days, beginning on day 3 of the cycle, and administering $PGF_{2\alpha}$ at sponge withdrawal. While this system shortens the duration of progestin treatment, it is limited to use during the breeding season and requires detection of estrus.

Synchronization of Recipients. If large numbers of potential recipients are available, estrous animals may be identified by a teaser male and may be scheduled for transfer accordingly. When numbers are limited, recipients may be synchronized with a single or double $PGF_{2\alpha}$ regimen or by insertion of intravaginal progestins. Because the donors have been stimulated with gonadotropins, sponges or pessaries should be removed from recipients 1 day earlier than from donors. Some advocate treatment of recipients with low doses of gonadotropins, spe-

Table 2. Estrous Control in Sheep and Goats

Drug	Dose	Route	Duration (Days)	Comments
Progesterone	10 to 12 mg	IM	12–14*	In oil
Cronolone	30 to 45 mg	Vaginal pessaries	12–14*	Immature animals may require higher dose
Methyl-acetoxyprogesterone	60 mg	Vaginal pessaries	12–14*	
$PGF_{2\alpha}$	8 to 15 mg†	IM	1	At midcycle
Cloprostenol	150 to 250 μg‡	IM	1	At midcycle

*Goats—14 to 18 days.
†Goats—4 to 10 mg $PGF_{2\alpha}$.
‡Goats—100 to 250 μg cloprostenol.

cifically 300 to 500 IU of PMSG, at the time of sponge withdrawal to ensure ovulation. This would be especially important for synchronizing anestrous recipients. Goat embryos tolerate as much as 24 hours of asynchrony between donor and recipient, while sheep embryos, especially early in development, are apparently less tolerant.

Breeding of Donors. In the superovulated ewe, fertilization failure, caused by apparently inhibited sperm transport through the cervix, seems to be a problem. This occurs whether the ewes are naturally bred or artificially inseminated intracervically. This may be due to the influence of progestin or to the gonadotropin. It has recently been demonstrated that PMSG treatment raises plasma progesterone concentration almost immediately. Thus, the gonadotropin's negative effects may be mediated through endogenous progesterone. In any case, the recovery of fertilized ova rarely exceeds 40 to 70 per cent, based on corpora lutea counts, with more unfertilized ova encountered as the ovulation rate increases.

When high fertilization rates for ovine donors are essential, 0.02 ml of raw semen may be surgically inseminated into the lumen of the uterine horn, near the uterotubal junction. This is done under local anesthesia through a small ventral abdominal incision. Ewes should be inseminated while in estrus, or at the time of expected estrus, 24 to 48 hours after progestin sponge removal.

Goats, on the other hand, have fairly high fertilization rates after superovulation. While some studies have indicated a lower fertilization rate for PMSG-treated does than for FSH-treated does, the general rate of ovum fertilization for the species tends to be higher than for sheep, and natural mating of superovulated does is generally successful. Fertilization rates after artificial insemination of superovulated does have not been as high.

Collection of Embryos

Timing. Embryos may be recovered from very shortly after fertilization until hatching from the zona pellucida. In general, recovery rates tend to decrease with increasing estrus-to-collection intervals. This may result from the early death of genetically nonviable embryos, the increased difficulty in removing a microscopic embryo from a relatively voluminous uterus or the premature luteal regression and expulsion of the embryo.

Because very early embryos may be more susceptible to manipulation, embryo collection is usually done on days 3 or 4 (estrus = day 0). At this time the embryo is in the 8- to 16-cell stage, at which time normal development can be readily distinguished from retarded development or unfertilized ova. Collection at this early stage may also allow for "rescue" of viable embryos from donors, who may otherwise undergo premature luteal regression on days 4 to 6.

Methods. Surgical collection is performed under either general or local anesthesia. A midline incision is made as near to the udder as possible, and the uterus and ovaries are exteriorized. Corpora lutea may be counted and evaluated for developmental stage. The infundibulum of the oviduct is cannulated with a small-bore smooth catheter, which is secured in place by clips or ligatures. After a pediatric Foley catheter is introduced through the uterine wall into the lumen near the bifurcation, oviductal embryos may be flushed into the uterus. A small amount of flushing medium (3 to 6 ml) is used to force the embryos into the uterus, and then 10 to 25 ml is introduced via a blunt needle near the tip of the uterine horn. Embryos are expelled through the Foley catheter into a collecting dish.

A simpler method involves cannulation of the oviduct with as large a catheter as possible (usually 2 mm outside diameter) and flushing of the uterus and oviducts in a retrograde fashion with 25 to 35 ml of medium. A blunt needle is inserted through the uterine wall a few centimeters from the tip on day 3 or earlier. The caudal segment of the uterine horn is held off with intestinal forceps or with the fingers and thumb, while the portion of the horn cranial to the blunt needle is gently "milked" toward the oviduct. Caution is advised, as too much pressure can rupture the endometrium. Potential postsurgical adhesions can be minimized by careful handling and by the irrigation of manipulated tissues with heparinized saline or high-molecular weight dextran.

Flushing Media. Several flushing media have been used successfully. All contain a balanced salt solution enriched with a protein source, which may be either homologous serum (10 to 20 per cent v/v) or bovine serum albumin (BSA, 3 mg/ml). The most commonly used medium is Dulbecco's phosphate-buffered saline (PBS), supplemented with a protein source and antimicrobials. Potassium penicillin (100 U/ml) and streptomycin sulfate (50 μg/ml) are commonly used, as are commercial preparations containing both antibiotics and antimycotics. If serum is used as the protein source, it should be heat treated at 56°C for 30 minutes to inactivate complement and should be filtered through a 0.45 μm Millipore filter before adding it to the PBS. Likewise, PBS should be filter sterilized (0.3 μ filter) before adding the antimicrobials and protein source.

Evaluation of Embryos. Morphologic assessment is still the most practical criterion for evaluating sheep and goat embryos. Table 3 shows the expected cell number and developmental stage for embryos of a given age. In general, an early embryo should be within one "cleavage" of its expected stage to be considered normal. Those embryos that are retarded by more than one cleavage, relative to the majority of embryos in a collection, should be considered suspect. Blastomeres should be reasonably symmetrical and spherical, with a minimum of extruded cytoplasm. A great many exceptions to these guidelines occur, and considerable experience is required to classify embryos into the various categories of viability.

Handling and Storage. Ovine and caprine embryos can be cultured for 1 to 2 days at 37°C in bicarbonate- or phosphate-buffered media, and they

Table 3. Embryo Development in the Ewe

Day†	"Expected" Stage
1	1 to 2 cells
2	2 to 4 cells*
3	4 to 16 cells*
4	16 to 32 cells*
5	>32 cells (morula)
6	Late morula/early blastocyst

*The relative development of goat embryos is similar; however, it may be delayed by as much as one cleavage per day.
†Estrus = day 0.

can be slowly cooled to −4°C for up to 2 or 3 days. This may allow asynchronous recipients to "catch up" with the temporarily arrested embryo. Ovine and caprine embryos can also be deep-frozen in liquid nitrogen, by procedures very similar to those used for bovine embryos.

Transfer of Embryos. Most transfers in small ruminants are performed surgically, although there are a very few reports of successful nonsurgical transfer in the goat. For surgical transfer, the reproductive tract is approached through a ventral midline incision and elevated far enough to allow for visual confirmation of at least one corpus luteum. Embryos of less than eight cells are generally transferred into the oviducts in 0.01 to 0.02 ml of medium. This is accomplished by placing a fire-polished glass pipette or 1.0 mm tom cat catheter well into the infundibulum (2 to 4 cm) and gently expelling the embryos. Embryos of more than eight cells are transferred to the lumen of the uterine horn, about 2 to 3 cm from the uterotubal junction. A blunt needle (e.g., the eye-end of a small suture needle) is used to puncture the wall of the uterus, and a polished pipette is inserted through the hole to expel the embryo into the lumen 2 to 5 cm beyond the hole.

Pregnancy Diagnosis. Recipients should be observed for signs of estrus at the expected interval. Plasma or milk progesterone concentrations can also be assayed at this time. This is especially helpful when transfers are done during the anestrous season, since recipients that fail to retain their embryos will revert to an anestrous (minimal progesterone) status, making a diagnosis of "not pregnant" obvious.

If real-time ultrasound diagnostic equipment is available, sheep and goats can be accurately examined for pregnancy at about 35 days gestation. The number of fetuses present cannot be determined with great accuracy by this method. By 75 to 85 days, fetuses can be enumerated by radiography.

Suggested Readings

1. Armstrong DT, Evans G: Factors influencing success of embryo transfer in sheep and goats. Theriogenology 19:31, 1983.
2. Armstrong DT, Pfitzner AP, Warnes GM, et al.: Endocrine responses of goats after induction of superovulation with PMSG and FSH. J Reprod Fert 67:395, 1983.
3. Bondioli, KR, Allen RL, Wright RW, Jr: Induction of estrus and superovulation in seasonally anestrous ewes. Theriogenology 18:209, 1982.

Embryo Transfer in Swine

Paul A. Martin, D.V.M., Ph.D.
Iowa State University,
Ames, Iowa

SELECTION OF DONORS

The choice of donors for commercial embryo transfer in swine is dictated largely by the needs of the owner of the donor and/or the owner of the recipient herd. However, only animals that have the genetic potential to improve the breed or that

Note: The FDA has not approved PMSG, Pg, E, P and hCG for the uses discussed in this article.

have terminal crosses in commercial herds should be selected as donors. Moreover, they should be in sound health not only because embryos must be recovered surgically but also because embryos may be collected on two or more consecutive estrous cycles. Although sows and gilts can be used as donors, sows are the usual source of embryos.

SPECIFIC USES OF EMBRYO TRANSFER

The major reason for performing commercial embryo transfer in swine is to prevent and/or control disease. Although swine producers invariably exploit superior females, this is seldom the primary reason given for doing embryo transfer in swine, because even the most valuable donors and embryos are inexpensive compared with costs incurred when some of the common diseases of swine are introduced into a susceptible herd. Table 1 shows the primary reasons why swine embryos entered recipient herds in the United States in 1981. Export of swine embryos will likely become another important reason for doing embryo transfer once long-term storage of swine embryos becomes possible.

SYNCHRONIZATION OF ESTRUS

There are two methods commonly used to synchronize estrus for embryo transfer purposes. The first method involves weaning a group of sows on the same day, with estrus occurring 4 to 10 days later. However, if the sows are injected subcutaneously with 500 to 750 IU of pregnant mare serum gonadotropin (PMSG) at weaning, a high proportion of sows will come into estrus 4 to 5 days later. Another method frequently used to synchronize sows is breeding and then aborting sows when they are between days 16 and 45 of pregnancy. Sows are aborted with one injection followed 12 hours later by a second injection of prostaglandin $F_{2\alpha}$ ($PGF_{2\alpha}$) or one of its analogs. A high proportion of sows come into estrus 4 to 7 days after treatment, and conception rates are high. Better synchrony can be achieved by injecting 500 to 750 IU of PMSG 12 hours after the second injection of $PGF_{2\alpha}$. With this regimen, nearly all sows come into estrus 4 to 5 days after the first injection of $PGF_{2\alpha}$. Often, a group of sows will be synchronized by using both the weaning and the abortion methods.

Two other methods are sometimes used to synchronize estrus in swine. Pseudopregnancy may be induced with daily injections of estrogen preparations on days 11 through 15 of the estrous cycle. The corpora lutea of pseudopregnancy, which can be maintained for as long as 90 to 120 days, can be induced to regress with $PGF_{2\alpha}$. Most sows return to estrus 4 to 7 days later. Another synchronization method is to inject or to feed progestogens for about 14 to 16 days. However, most of these progestogens induce ovarian cysts and are seldom used.

SUPEROVULATION AND INSEMINATION

Superovulation. Sows are usually superovulated with one injection of 1200 to 1500 IU of PMSG at weaning or 24 hours after the first injection of $PGF_{2\alpha}$ in sows that were synchronized by first being made

pregnant or pseudopregnant. For gilts and sows in which embryos are collected on more than two consecutive estrous cycles, the time of estrus is not controlled, and the animals are not usually superovulated. If these sows are superovulated, PMSG is given on alternate estrous cycles 4 to 5 days before the expected onset of estrus.

As with other species, the superovulatory response is quite variable within and among breeds. However, the average response for small groups of sows to 1200 to 1500 IU of PMSG ranges from 30 to 45 ovulations. Ovulation rates of 45 or more are not desirable because of the increase in the proportion of abnormal embryos and the proportion of unfertilized eggs. Human chorionic gonadotropin (hCG), which can be used to control the time of ovulation, is seldom used by embryo transfer specialists. If hCG is used, 500 IU is given 3 to 4 days after administration of PMSG. Ovulation occurs about 40 to 42 hours after hCG injection.

Insemination. For optimum conception and fertilization rates, donors should be mated or inseminated every 12 hours throughout estrus. If hCG is used to control the time of ovulation, the most important inseminations of fresh and frozen semen are those done at 24 and 36 hours, respectively, after hCG injection. The volume of the inseminate should be 50 to 100 ml and contain at least 4 to 5 billion live spermatozoa.

DAY OF EMBRYO COLLECTION

Timing. Swine embryos are usually collected 4 to 6 days after the onset of estrus. Four days after the onset of estrus most embryos are at the four- to eight-cell stage, whereas on the sixth day after the onset of estrus, most are in the expanded unhatched blastocyst stage. Most collections of swine embryos are done 4 days after the onset of estrus because four- to eight-cell embryos are easily identified and evaluated. In contrast, morulae and the early blastocysts, which are most frequently collected on day

Table 1. Primary Reasons for Performing Commercial Embryo Transfer in Swine in the United States in 1981 and the Number of Transfers and Recipient Herds Involved

Group No.	Reason	No. of Recipients (%)	No. of Herds
1	Establish new herds from herds with pseudorabies	113 (43)	4
2	Make additions to specific-pathogen free (SPF) herds	67 (26)	13
3	Obtain boars for closed commercial herd	61 (23)	11
4	Obtain more offspring from superior gilts and sows	19 (7)	8
		260	36*

*One herd in group 2 is also represented in group 4. (Adapted from Martin PA: Theriogenology 19:43, 1983.)

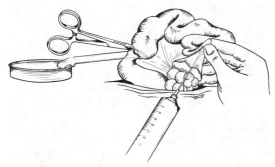

Figure 1. Collection of embryos from donor sow.

5, are more difficult to identify and to distinguish from unfertilized eggs.

Collection and transfer are seldom done before day 4, not only because embryos, which are usually located in the oviduct of the donor, must be transferred to the oviduct of the recipient, but also because it is more difficult to deposit embryos in the oviduct than in the uterus. The collection of embryos on day 7 or later is not usually done because sows that receive hatched blastocysts may be less likely to farrow than sows that receive unhatched embryos.

Surgical Collection. Embryos are collected surgically in a clinic or laboratory. Anesthesia is induced by injecting a barbiturate into the marginal ear vein and is maintained with halothane using a closed-circuit anesthesia machine. A small midventral incision is made to expose one ovary along with the adjacent oviduct and about 30 cm of the uterine horn. A small incision is made for insertion of a glass cannula on the antimesometrial side of the uterine horn at about 20 to 25 cm from the uterotubal junction. To avoid contaminating the cannula with blood when it is introduced into the uterine horn, it is important (1) to squeeze the blood vessels on the mesometrial side with thumb and forefinger while forcing the blunt end of a scalpel handle through the wall of the uterus on the opposite side and (2) to insert the cannula into the uterine lumen as soon as pressure on the blood vessels is removed.

The glass cannula should be about 12 to 15 cm long and 9 to 11 mm in diameter. The end that goes into the uterine horn should be cut at a 45° angle and flared. The opposite end of the cannula should have a bend of about 45° located 1 to 2 cm from the end. The glass cannula is inserted about 2 to 3 cm into the uterine horn and is held in place with a towel clamp.

To collect the embryos (Fig. 1), about 40 to 50 ml of the medium warmed to 37°C is placed in a syringe fitted with a blunt 12- to 14-gauge needle. The needle is inserted into the oviduct, and all of the medium is flushed into the oviduct, through the uterine horn, out the cannula and into a petri dish. After removing all of the flushing medium from the uterine horn, the incision is closed before repeating the entire procedure in the second uterine horn.

Following the surgical collection of embryos, swine are especially prone to form adhesions of the reproductive organs. Therefore, to reduce the possibility of adhesions forming, it is essential to (1) maintain asepsis throughout the procedure, (2) handle the reproductive organs gently and only when necessary and (3) keep the exposed reproductive organs moist at all times with saline or another physiological solution.

HANDLING EMBRYOS

Searching for and Handling Embryos. The flushings are examined for embryos with a stereomicroscope. Searches are done at 10- to 12-× magnification and the evaluation of embryos at 50 to 70 ×. Good optics and high magnification are particularly important for distinguishing morulae and early blastocysts from unfertilized eggs. As embryos are located, they are transferred to culture plates or other dishes that contain fresh medium warmed to 37°C. After several rinses in fresh medium, the embryos are stored until transferred to the recipient. Tuberculin syringes fitted with a tom cat catheter or a glass pipette are frequently used to handle embryos.

Short-term Storage. The medium for the flushing procedure can also be used to store embryos in vitro for several hours. Some of the media used for flushing and storing embryos include Brinster's solution, Ham's F-10 and TCM-199 with bicarbonate. Embryos should be stored in fresh medium at 37°C. Although not recommended, it is possible to obtain acceptable conception rates with embryos stored at room temperature for 2 hours. Swine embryos have been cultured for 24 hours without a decrease in embryonic survival rates after transfer to recipients. However, high survival rates were not obtained after using similar conditions for the long-distance shipment of swine embryos.

Evaluation of Embryos. Evaluation of the quality of embryos is done by examining the general morphologic appearance of the embryos at the time of collection. In general, the cleavage rate of embryos collected from a donor is quite uniform. On days 4, 5 or 6 the stage of development for most normally developing embryos ranges from four to eight cells, eight cells to morulae and blastocysts, respectively. Once embryos pass the eight-cell stage, cells fuse, making it difficult to identify and to count individual cells. Therefore, considerable experience is required to distinguish 8- to 16-cell embryos, morulae and early blastocysts from degenerating unfertilized eggs. Because four- to eight-cell embryos are easily identified and evaluated, most embryo transfer specialists prefer to collect embryos from donors when the embryos are expected to be at the four- to eight-cell stage. However, in a recent study it was shown that sows that received morulae were more likely to farrow than sows that received four- to eight-cell embryos.

TRANSFER OF EMBRYOS

Practical methods for the nonsurgical transfer of swine embryos have not been developed. Surgical

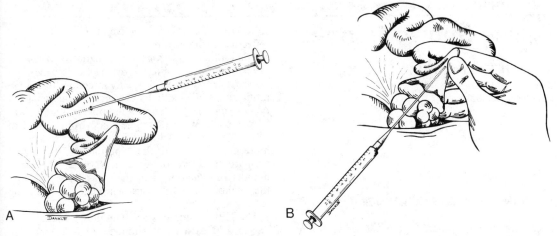

Figure 2. *A, B,* Transfer of embryos to recipient sow.

transfers are usually done on the farm rather than in a clinic or a laboratory to reduce the risk of introducing disease. Anesthesia is induced and maintained by injecting a barbiturate into the marginal ear vein. The reproductive tract is reached through a midventral incision. Corpora lutea should be examined for appropriate stage of development before embryos are transferred to the recipient. The uterine horns should also be examined for abnormalities, especially if gilts are used as recipients.

Embryos are usually transferred to the anterior one fourth of one uterine horn. However, it is likely that other sites are equally suitable. It is not necessary to transfer embryos to each uterine horn because embryos migrate from one horn to the other and become equally distributed throughout both horns.

Embryos are transferred to the recipient by one of two methods (Fig. 2). In one method a fine catheter or pipette that contains the embryos is passed through a small puncture wound into the lumen of the uterus. The embryos are deposited about 3 to 5 cm from the puncture wound, and the wound does not require sutures. Inexperienced individuals should be especially careful not to deposit the embryos into the endometrium or the myometrium. Depositing embryos into the wall of the uterus is more easily done in swine than in bovine or in ovine. However, this complication and hemorrhaging of the puncture wound, which sometimes occur, can be avoided. This is accomplished by introducing a tom cat catheter or a piece of rubber tubing, which contains the embryos, into the oviduct. The distal end of the tubing is held firmly in place while the embryos are flushed into the uterus with a syringe that is attached to the other end of the tubing.

FACTORS AFFECTING RESULTS

Best results are obtained when the donor comes into estrus from 2 days before to 1 day after the recipient. Little information is available concerning the possible effect of duration of estrus of the donor and recipient on the success rate of embryo transfer. Perhaps results could be improved if donors and recipients were matched according to the day of onset as well as duration of estrus. The day of collection and transfer of embryos may influence results.

Higher rates of farrowing may be possible when embryos are collected and transferred within 6 days after the onset of estrus.

For optimum results, at least 12 embryos of high quality should be transferred to each recipient. Pregnancy fails to occur if there are too few embryos between days 12 and 17 or if embryos are not distributed throughout most of the uterine horns. In recipient sows that farrow about 30 per cent of the embryos do not survive to farrowing. This loss, which is similar to losses in normally bred sows, and the loss of all embryos in about 30 per cent of recipients that fail to farrow represent a substantial loss of embryos after transfer.

As in other species, the time and conditions of in vitro storage also influence results. Until culture methods improve, swine embryos should be transferred to the recipient as soon as possible after collection. If embryos must be stored for 4 hours or more before transfer, better results may be obtained by collecting embryos that are past the eight-cell stage.

Lastly, considerable experience with surgical collection of embryos is required to minimize the possibility of donors forming adhesions of the reproductive tract, which can cause infertility. Sows are more likely than ewes and cows to form adhesions following the surgical collection of embryos.

Suggested Readings

1. James JE, James DM, Martin PA, et al.: Embryo transfer for salvaging valuable genetic material from swine herds with pseudorabies. JAVMA (in press).
2. Martin PA: Commercial embryo transfer in swine: Who is interested in it and why. Theriogenology 19:1, 1983.

Equine Embryo Transfer

Robert H. Douglas, Ph.D.
University of Kentucky,
Lexington, Kentucky

POTENTIAL USE OF EMBRYO TRANSFER

From a purely academic point of view, equine embryo transfer can be used for the following: (1) to obtain foals from subfertile mares; (2) to better manage older, valuable broodmares; (3) to circumvent problems with neonatal isoerythrolysis (jaundice); (4) to obtain foals from mares engaged in competition; (5) to manage mares that chronically abort twins; (6) to further the knowledge of the mechanisms of the maternal recognition of pregnancy; (7) to produce multiple offspring and (8) to advance genetic progress.

The first successful equine embryo transfers were reported in England a little more than 10 years ago.[1] Acceptance of the technique as an approved method for producing foals by a major American breed association occurred less than 5 years ago. The procedure was initially adopted to produce a single foal per year from barren mares that could not carry a pregnancy to term; however, more recently, embryo transfer is also being used to produce pregnancies from maiden fillies that are in show competition. This is probably most often done in the Arabian breed.

Irrespective of the reason for performing embryo transfer, the efficacy of the procedure in horses is confounded by the inability to produce multiple viable embryos via superovulation, a relatively short in vitro survival of the equine embryo, difficulty in synchronizing ovulation among donors and recipients and the high incidence of uterine infections in barren donor mares. Moreover, in the United States and in virtually all other countries, the two major racing breeds, Standardbreds and Thoroughbreds, do not accept foals produced by embryo transfer in their registries.

SPECIAL PROBLEMS

Superovulation. The first published reports of superovulation in the mare appeared in 1940. Pregnant mare serum gonadotropin (PMSG) and human chorionic gonadotropin (hCG) alone or in combination were used unsuccessfully in this initial attempt to induce follicular growth in the mare. Both PMSG and porcine follicle stimulating hormone (FSH) are relatively ineffective in the mare. This is reflective of the apparent insensitivity of the mare's ovarian follicles to exogenous gonadotropins.

The first encouraging report regarding superovulation appeared in 1974.[1] Daily injections of equine pituitary extract (EPE) were given to anovulatory ponies, and the incidence of multiple ovulations was 54 per cent. Since that time, data from a total of 112 mares treated with EPE have appeared in the literature.[6] Out of all the experiments 70 per cent of mares had two or more ovulations. The mean number of ovulations per mare was 3.0 ± 0.2, and the number of ovulations per multiple ovulating mare was 4.0 ± 0.2.

The EPE treatments are generally initiated after day 11 of diestrus and continued for 7 days or until a 35-mm follicle is detected. The minimum effective dose of EPE appears to be 750 Fevold-Hisaw rat units (FHRU) per day in seasonally ovulatory mares. On the first day of estrus or on the last day of EPE treatment, 3000 to 4000 IU of hCG are administered intramuscularly to synchronize the occurrence of ovulation. For example, multiple ovulations occurred on the same day in 10 out of 10 hCG-injected mares but in only 3 of 12 non–hCG-injected mares.

Without superovulation, one expects an embryo recovery rate of approximately 70 per cent in reproductively sound donor mares. The expected pregnancy rate in properly synchronized recipient mares is 50 per cent. Therefore, the probability of obtaining a pregnancy on a single attempt is 35 per cent (70 × 50 per cent). With an expected ovulation rate of 3.0 by EPE treatment, one would anticipate a possible increase in this probability to 105 per cent (35 per cent × 3 ovulations). In practice this has not been the case. When 21 day 7 embryos were recovered and transferred from eight EPE-treated donor mares that had multiple ovulations, the pregnancy rate at 21 days was significantly lower (47 per cent) than when embryos from single, natural-ovulating donors were transferred (88 per cent). Pregnancy rates at 49 days were 33 and 50 per cent for embryos originating from EPE-treated and non–EPE-treated donor mares, respectively.[6]

The eight EPE-treated donors produced 21 embryos (260 per cent collection rate), resulting in a 33 per cent pregnancy rate; therefore, the probability for a pregnancy using EPE in donor mares would be 87 per cent. This is more than double that expected in non–EPE-treated donor mares. The extra cost and management of having more recipients available per collection attempt plus the fact that EPE is not commercially available may make this nothing more than an academic exercise, although a very interesting one. Further, repeated treatments with EPE during a single breeding season may not be possible, since some mares apparently have prolonged luteal phases following EPE treatments. The effectiveness of repeated EPE treatments over a season has not been studied.

A very exciting research area has evolved from work with EPE. It appears that the lower pregnancy rate with embryos from EPE-treated donors may be due to a biologic embryo-reduction mechanism that seems to occur between days 7 and 11 after ovulation. That is, one embryo can eliminate another embryo. This is supported both by experimental models in which mares with induced multiple ovulations developed only one fetus and by the significant reduction in twin pregnancies in spontaneously double-ovulating mares in which ovulations are synchronous (occur within 24 hours) compared with asynchronous ovulations. However, the viability of multiple embryos collected on day 6, presumably before the embryo reduction mechanism occurs, has not been determined.

Synchronization. Ovulation is difficult to synchronize in the mare in comparison to other farm species. This is likely because of the longer follicular phase and the difficulty of adequately controlling follicle growth. This aspect of equine embryo transfer is further complicated by the recent realization that pregnancy rates are significantly higher in recipients that ovulate 24 to 48 hours after the donor. The more effective the synchronization treatment, the fewer the number of recipients required. Single or complex regimens using prostaglandin $F_{2\alpha}$ ($PGF_{2\alpha}$), progestogens, gonadotropin-releasing hormone (GnRH) and hCG have been used. Even when the above hormone treatments are combined, only approximately 75 per cent of mares will ovulate over a 4-day period.

An important concept to remember when evaluating a synchronizing regimen is that $PGF_{2\alpha}$ chemically lyses the corpus luteum, whereas progestogens, when given, block ovulation while the corpus luteum is allowed to regress. When progestogens are given alone, relatively long treatment periods are required (15 days); however, the treatment period can be shortened to 10 days if a luteolytic dose of $PGF_{2\alpha}$ is administered on the last day of progestogen treatment. Either oral (altrenogest—Regumate, 20 mg/day) or injectable progesterone in oil (200 mg/day) may be used. With any progestogen treatment, the effects on follicular growth are not uniform. Upon withdrawal of the progestogen, mares with more mature follicles will ovulate sooner than mares with immature follicles. Injection of hCG (3000 IU) can be used to reduce this variation, although only moderately.

A more effective synchronization regimen has recently been published that utilizes a combined intramuscular treatment of progesterone (150 mg/day) and 17-β estradiol (10 mg/day) for a 10-day period. $PGF_{2\alpha}$ is given on the tenth day of treatment.[4] In one study 18 of 20 mares ovulated 10 to 12 days after the last injection. This is probably the optimum synchronization that one could obtain and appears to be due primarily to the inhibitory effects of 17-β estradiol on follicular growth. When this hormone combination is withdrawn, a more uniform population of follicles is present, so the interval to ovulation is correspondingly more uniform.

Typically, a donor mare is started on progesterone/estradiol treatment on one day, one recipient is started on the next day and a second recipient is started the following day. This increases the likelihood of a recipient ovulating 24 to 48 hours after the donor. Injections of hCG are given on an individual basis to advance ovulation in the donor or recipients, as indicated. This treatment can be initiated on any day of the estrous cycle, but it is necessary to inject $PGF_{2\alpha}$ on the last day of treatment. Mares beginning treatment during estrus will often not respond unless $PGF_{2\alpha}$ is given at the end of treatment. This is owning to the inability of ovarian steroids to inhibit ovulation in about 40 per cent of mares treated during estrus. The treatment period may also be extended if management factors require it.

As a general guideline, when synchronization regimens without 17-β estradiol are used, approximately four to five recipients should be synchronized per donor mare. Regardless of the regimen, treatment of the recipients should be initiated 1 to 2 days after initiation in donors. Obviously, batching of donors greatly reduces the costs of the embryo transfer program. Ideally, three donors can be started on the same day and five to six recipients on the following day.

Uterine Infections. The embryo recovery rate in 74 experimental mares with no history of breeding problems was higher (56 per cent) than that in 20 barren mares (34.3 per cent).[2] The major factor responsible for this decrease in barren mares is the presence of uterine infection. In these and other barren mares presented for embryo transfer, the author has found pathogenic organisms in the uterine effluent from 30 per cent of these mares. The typical mare in this category has been barren 2 or more years and has not been detectably pregnant during this period. This mare, without intense management, is a poor candidate for embryo transfer.

In the field a cloudy uterine effluent upon collection of the embryo recovery medium is strongly suggestive of the presence of uterine infection. Invariably, no embryo is found in this collection, and if one is present, it is most often degenerate. In over 50 collections in which the collection effluent was cloudy, only three embryos were found. None of the three resulted in a pregnancy. Culture of every collection effluent is strongly indicated.

Prior to placing a barren donor mare in an embryo transfer program, a thorough inspection of the reproductive tract is warranted. The first evaluation the author makes is by hysteroscopy, followed by culture of the cervicouterine area and clitoral fossa. In addition, a uterine lavage with physiological saline is performed when the donor mare is in diestrus. The lavage effluent is graded for clarity and cellular debris and is cultured.

If infection is present, treatment would include, in order of priority of application, uterine lavages, curettage and antibiotics, with the latter treatment indicated by sensitivity of the organisms. Treatment regimens of short duration are usually ineffective in such chronically infected mares. Treatments are performed during diestrus to maximize time and management more efficiently. Efforts are also made to collect embryos on day 6 after ovulation, which may reduce the exposure of the embryo to pathogens. Uterine lavages may also be performed every day from day 2 after ovulation to day 6, at which time the embryo can be collected.

Even if chronically infected mares respond to treatment, they appear to be easily reinfected after the embryo collection procedure. Close monitoring of these mares immediately following embryo collection is essential. A uterine lavage using 1 liter of 0.02 per cent tamed-iodine solution on the day of collection appears to be beneficial.

PROCEDURES

Medium Preparation. Dulbecco's phosphate-buffered saline (PBS) supplemented with 1 per cent heat-inactivated fetal bovine serum appears to be the most suitable medium for field use. It should be noted that currently there does not seem to be an optimal medium for equine embryos, as in vitro survival in all media investigated seems to be much shorter than that for other species. Dulbecco's PBS is supplemented with 1 per cent fetal bovine serum and 100 IU penicillin plus 100 μg streptomycin/ml to prepare the embryo recovery medium. This is done by adding powdered Dulbecco's PBS and antibiotics to autoclaved, deionized, distilled water. Fetal bovine serum is kept frozen before use. Other investigators have used heat-inactivated steer or mare serum with seemingly equal results. Embryo culture and transfer medium is prepared by adding 20 per cent heat-inactivated fetal bovine serum to a volume of recovery medium. This is then Millipore-filtered through a 0.22 μm disposable Falcon filter.

Collection of Embryos. Embryo collections are performed nonsurgically on days 6 to 9 after ovulation (day of ovulation = day 0). The equine embryo does not enter the uterus until day 6 after ovulation, precluding earlier collection nonsurgically. After day 9, equine embryos are generally too large to transfer without breakage. The diameter of equine embryos over days 6 to 9 after ovulation will range from 0.1 to 4.5 mm. By day 8 the equine embryo is generally 10-fold larger than a bovine embryo of the same age.

The nonsurgical collection procedure is a modification of the one developed for cattle. An extended 30-French Foley or an 18-French Rusch catheter with a 30-ml inflatable cuff is inserted through the cervix into the uterine body and is secured in position by inflating the cuff with 15 to 30 ml of sterile water or recovery medium. Once the catheter is properly positioned, both uterine horns and the uterine body are filled simultaneously with 1 liter of medium by gravity flow. The medium is then collected by gravity flow into sterile, 1 liter Erlenmeyer flasks or graduated cylinders. This procedure is repeated three additional times. Uterine

palpation is used to facilitate recovery of medium from the uterus during the last three flushes.

Embryo Handling. Embryos are of greater density than the medium and therefore settle to the bottom of the collection vessel within approximately 20 to 30 minutes following collection. The upper 850 to 900 ml of medium is removed by pouring or siphoning into another sterile container. The bottom portion of the medium is then poured into a gridded sterile plastic Petri dish. Attempts are first made to identify the embryo macroscopically, and then the dish is searched with a dissecting microscope under low magnification (10 ×). Once identified, the embryo is aspirated into a 14-gauge catheter (Sovereign) attached to a 1-ml syringe and is then deposited into a sterile plastic Petri dish containing transfer medium. The embryo is then gently agitated (washed) for approximately 1 to 2 minutes and then placed in a second Petri dish containing transfer medium. The embryo is stored in this dish until transfer.

Results have indicated that equine embryos do not remain viable for more than approximately 3 hours in Dulbecco's PBS. Therefore, transport of fresh equine embryos over long distances would seem impossible. Embryo freezing would be an obvious solution to this problem. Although limited, research to date suggests that the optimal age of equine embryos for freezing is day 6 after ovulation and that protocols for freezing bovine embryos can be used for equine embryos. The first known foal birth resulting from transfer of a frozen-thawed equine embryo occurred in 1983.

Embryo Transfer
Nonsurgical. Embryos are aspirated into a Luer-Flex 22-inch sterile large animal pipette or similar pipette, which contains 10,000 IU penicillin plus 10,000 μg streptomycin. The aspiration procedure has the following sequence: 1 ml antibiotics, 0.25 ml air, 0.5 ml transfer medium, 0.25 air, 0.5 ml transfer medium containing the embryo, 0.25 air and 0.5 ml transfer medium.

The perineal area of the recipient is scrubbed with a dilute Betadine solution and water before transfer. The infusion pipette containing the embryo is passed through the vagina and into the cervix following manual dilation of the external cervical os. The operator's hand is covered by a plastic palpation sleeve and a sterile surgical glove. Before passing the pipette into the uterine body, the operator's hand is transferred from the vagina into the rectum to grasp the uterus. The uterus is elevated, and the pipette is then passed into the lumen of the uterine body. Precaution is taken to keep physical trauma to the endometrium to a minimum. The contents of the pipette are deposited at a point approximately equally distant from the internal cervical os and uterine bifurcation.

Surgical. The most practical method for field use is via a flank incision.[3] This method is similar to that used in cattle. Mares are given 250 mg xylazine IV and 25 mg of acepromazine IM. The paralumbar fossa is prepared for aseptic surgery, and the incision site is infiltrated with 30 to 50 ml of lidocaine. A 15- to 20-cm vertical incision is made beginning approximately 10 cm ventral to the lumbar processes. After the skin is incised, the muscle layers and peritoneum are bluntly dissected. The tip of the uterine horn adjacent to the corpus luteum is exteriorized, and a small puncture is made into the lumen of the uterine horn with the blunt end of a cutting needle. The embryo is loaded into a 14-gauge large animal Sovereign catheter or glass pipette in a total volume of approximately 0.5 ml of transfer medium. The embryo is usually positioned between two air spaces in the catheter to stabilize its position. The catheter is passed through the uterine puncture, and its contents are deposited into the uterine lumen. The abdominal wall is then closed in a routine manner.

Results. Embryo recovery rates can be expected to be from 50 to 80 per cent in reproductively sound mares with no history of breeding problems and bred to highly fertile stallions. An often-ignored component of the embryo transfer program is stallion fertility. When chronically barren mares are used as donors, transferable embryos can be expected to be recovered in only 30 per cent of collection attempts.

Probably the most important factor in determining nonsurgical pregnancy rates is operator experience. Pregnancy rates of 50 per cent have been achieved with nonsurgical transfers of equine embryos. However, published data indicate that pregnancy rates approaching or exceeding 50 per cent are more rapidly attained using surgical transfer methods.[5] Thus, at the onset of an equine embryo transfer program more rapid success will likely be achieved by transferring embryos surgically. Irrespective of the method used or the skill of the operator, the success of the embryo transfer program is directly related to the quality of donors, recipients and management.

References

1. Douglas RH: Review of induction of superovulation and embryo transfer in the equine. Theriogenology 11:33, 1979.
2. Douglas RH: Some aspects of equine embryo transfer. J Reprod Fert Suppl 32:405, 1982.
3. Imel KJ, Squires EL, Elsden RP, Shideler RK: Collection and transfer of equine embryos. JAVMA 179:987, 1981.
4. Loy RG, Penstein R, O'Canna D, Douglas RH: Control of ovulation in mares with ovarian steroids and prostaglandin. Theriogenology 15:191, 1981.
5. Squires EL, Imel KS, Iuliano MF, Shideler RK: Factors affecting reproductive efficiency in an equine embryo transfer programme. J Reprod Fert Suppl 32:409, 1982.
6. Woods GL, Ginther OJ: Recent studies relating to the collection of multiple embryos in mares. Theriogenology 19:101, 1983.

Embryo Transfer in Laboratory Animals

Duane C. Kraemer, D.V.M., Ph.D.
Monica J. Bowen, B.V.Sc., M.R.C.V.S.
Texas A&M University,
College Station, Texas

The reasons for undertaking embryo transfer in laboratory animals include the following: development of embryo transfer techniques, studies of fertilization and gestation, oocyte and embryo preservation, developmental genetics, cell differentiation, disease transmission, oncogenesis, maternal environmental physiology, contraceptive development and gene transfer.

MOUSE

In general, prepubertal mice that are maintained on a photoperiod of 10 hours in dark, 14 hours in light can be superovulated by administering 2 to 10 IU pregnant mare serum gonadotropin (PMSG) at approximately 4 PM on day 0. Following that, 2 to 10 IU of human chorionic gonadotropin (hCG) is generally given 44 to 48 hours later (noon of day 2). These gonadotropins may be administered by either intraperitoneal (IP) or subcutaneous (SC) injection; however, the former is usually most convenient. The females may be placed with males at the time of injection of hCG and checked for vaginal plugs the following morning. Mature mice can be superovulated using the same regimen. However, improved results can be obtained using vaginal smears and administering the PMSG approximately 2 days before the expected mating. In the most productive strains, immature and mature superovulated mice can be expected to yield around 60 and 20 ovulations, respectively.[4]

Tubal stage mouse embryos are collected from the excised oviducts during the first 3 days of pregnancy (day 1 = day of confirmed mating). During the morning of day 1, the embryos in cumulus may be recovered by cutting or dissecting the ampulla of the oviduct longitudinally. An alternate procedure consists of cutting the oviduct in half and flushing the ampullary end by inserting a blunted 30-gauge hypodermic needle into the uterine end of this segment of the oviduct. Later stage tubal embryos are usually free of cumulus and corona cells and can be collected by flushing collection medium from the ampullary end of the oviduct to the uterine end.

From days 3½ to 4 embryos may be in the area of the uterotubal junction (UTJ) or in the tip of the uterus. A portion of the uterus may be removed with the oviduct, and the entire unit is flushed as previously described. If difficulty is encountered in forcing fluid through the UTJ, the ampullary portion of the oviduct can be removed so that only the isthmic portion is flushed, allowing pressure to be applied.

Uterine-stage embryos may be collected from the excised uterus either by a surgical in situ method or by a nonsurgical procedure. The excised uterus is flushed by inserting a blunted 23-gauge needle into the tubal end and holding it in place with a forceps. For the in situ surgical flush, a 4- to 5-mm diameter speculum is placed into the vagina and held firmly around the cervical os. Fluid is injected surgically, simultaneously into the tips of the uterine horns and out through the cervix, where it is conducted to a collection vessel via the vaginal cannula. Uterine stage embryos can also be collected from adult mice nonsurgically.[7] A vaginal speculum (4 to 5 mm in diameter) is used to visualize the cervix, and a stainless steel catheter with a length, 4 cm length, 1.2 mm outside diameter (OD) and 0.9 mm internal diameter (ID) is inserted into the cervix. Collection fluid is introduced into the uterine horn via a plastic catheter and collected via the stainless steel catheter. The major problem with this technique is puncture of the uterine wall by the plastic catheter.

Recipient females may be prepared either by a fertile mating, if mixed litters are desired or by mating with a vasectomized male. Stimulation of the cervix with an artificial insemination pipette and sterile saline may also be used to induce pseudopregnancy in naturally ovulating females or in adult females stimulated with 1.5 to 3.0 IU of both PMSG and hCG.

Surgical procedures are necessary for transfer of tubal stage embryos. At least four different anesthetics have been successfully used for surgical transfer of mouse embryos; (1) ether to effect, (2) pentobarbital (35 mg/kg IV or 60 mg/kg IP), (3) droperidol and fentanyl citrate (Innovar) (10 per cent solution, 0.3 ml/100gm IM) and (4) acepromazine maleate and ketamine hydrochloride (1:4 combination, 0.3 ml/20gm IM or IP).

Incisions through the paralumbar fossae are used to expose the ovaries and oviducts, which are observed using a dissecting microscope. Embryos in cumulus may be transferred into the ovarian bursa through the bursal foramen. Cumulus-free embryos must be transferred into the oviduct. A small incision is made in an avascular region of the bursa, and the transfer pipette is inserted through this opening into the fimbriated end of the oviduct. Although several types of transfer pipettes have been used, the most convenient type utilizes a glass capillary tube and a metal plunger so that the embryos can be delivered in less than 1 μl of medium without the introduction of air.

Uterine-stage embryos may be transferred either surgically or nonsurgically. Surgical transfer is achieved by exposing the uterine horns via a mid-ventral laparotomy; the embryos are then deposited via a puncture wound in the ovarian end of the uterus using a transfer pipette similar to that used for tubal transfer. Nonsurgical transfer can be accomplished without anesthesia. The mouse is placed on a grasping surface, and the buttocks are elevated by grasping the tail. A speculum is placed in the vagina and a transfer pipette (wire-trol, Drummond Scientific Co., Broomal PA) is inserted through the cervix and directed into the appropriate horn.

Pregnancy rates are highly variable; however with practice, using strains that are well adapted to embryo transfer, one might expect an 85 per cent pregnancy rate, with 60 per cent survival of embryos.

RAT

Embryo collection and transfer procedures for the rat are very similar to those described for the mouse.[4] There are, however, two major differences. First, the dosage of PMSG for superovulation of the mature rat is 30 IU, given on the morning of estrus, followed 52 to 58 hours later by 30 IU hCG. Immature (21- to 30-day old) rats can be superovulated with 20 IU of PMSG, followed by 20 IU of hCG 52 to 58 hours later. Second, the ovarian bursa of the rat is more vascular than that of the mouse. Therefore, it is helpful to use electrocautery to open the ovarian bursa for transfer of tubal stage embryos in the rat.

MONGOLIAN GERBIL

Gerbils[1] are spontaneous ovulators, with ovulation starting approximately 21 hours after mating (day 0) and lasting for a period of 6 to 10 hours. Egg transport through the oviducts is slow in the gerbil. Embryos are not found in the uterus until days 5 to 6 when most are blastocysts. Both mature and immature female gerbils can be superovulated with 10 IU PMSG in the immature and 20 IU PMSG in the adult female followed by 20 IU hCG 50 or 54 hours later, respectively. This treatment will yield an average response of 30 to 33 eggs/female. Blastocysts can be surgically flushed from the uterus between days 7 and 10 using approximately 0.5 ml of phosphate buffered saline (PBS). This can be done either by a midline exposure of the uterus after sacrificing the gerbil or by anesthetizing the gerbil with methoxyflurane and exposing the uterine horn via a flank incision. Transfer is also done via the flank approach using a 25-gauge hypodermic needle to facilitate entry of the micropipette into the uterine horn. The embryos should be transferred in the smallest volume of fluid possible.[1]

GOLDEN HAMSTER

Embryo transfer in the hamster was first reported in 1964. Adult hamsters (2- to 3-months old, 80- to

120-gm live weight) kept on a 12-hour light/dark cycle can be superovulated by treatment with 30 IU of PMSG on the day of ovulation followed by 25 IU of hCG 76 hours later; estrus occurs within 5 hours after the hCG injection. Normally, 40 to 45 embryos can be collected 2 to 3 days after mating. Immature hamsters (5- to 6-weeks old, 60- to 80-gm live weight) can also be induced to superovulate by IP injection of 25 IU of PMSG and 25 IU of hCG 48 to 56 hours later.

Hamster embryos enter the uterus on days 3 to 4 (day 1 = day of spermatozoa in the vaginal smear). On day 3½, recovery is difficult, as the blastocyst may be already attached to the uterine wall. The blastocyst is zona pellucida-free at 2¾ days after ovulation. For embryo collection the oviducts and uteri are taken from sacrificed hamsters and flushed with 0.2 ml of sterile TCM-199. As hamster embryos are very sensitive to the type of medium used, they must be rinsed twice and transferred within 20 minutes. Embryos are transferred via a lateral approach to the uterine lumen or ampulla through the infundibulum, depending on the developmental stage of the embryo. As hamsters are induced ovulators, potential recipients must be given hCG at the same time as the donors or must have mechanical stimulation to the vagina and cervix to induce pseudopregnancy late on the fourth day.

FERRET

Embryo transfer in the ferret was first reported in 1968.[3] Ovulation in the ferret normally occurs approximately 30 hours after coitus. However, it can also be induced by giving 90 IU of hCG IP to the estrous female, in which case ovulation occurs 30 to 36 hours later. The majority of the eggs (average 8 to 13) enter the uterus between days 4½ and 7 after hCG administration and can be collected on days 5, 6, 7 or 8 by flushing the uterine horns with a small amount of medium.

Embryos can be transferred to the recipient under general anesthesia via a midline or flank approach into the uterine horn. It is of the utmost importance to have donors and recipients closely synchronized. In order to achieve this, the same dose of hCG must be given to both at the same time.

MINK

Embryo transfer is an uncommon procedure in the mink, and the conception rate is not very high.[1] Mink are induced ovulators, with ovulation occurring from 33 to 72 hours after coitus; there is considerable variation both among animals and among cycles. Ovulation can also be induced with 50 IU of hCG SC or 90 IU of hCG IP, with ovulation occurring 35 to 40 hours later. Embryos enter the uterus approximately 8 days after coitus (5 to 6 days after ovulation), usually at the expanded blastocyst stage of development. Mink have facultative de-

layed implantation for 5 to 25 days, depending on the season. Therefore, it should be possible to collect viable embryos for transfer over an extended period of time. The oviducts of the mink are rather small and require the use of a stereomicroscope for flushing. After sacrifice, each oviduct is dissected from the ovary that it surrounds and straightened out, and a blunt-ended 25-gauge needle is introduced into the fimbria and held in place by forceps. Each oviduct is flushed with approximately 0.5 ml of medium. On days 7 or 8 after coitus the oviducts can be flushed into the uterus. However, on days 5 or 6 fluid cannot be forced through the oviducts unless the UTJ is first removed. The uterine horns may be flushed by inserting a regular 25-gauge hypodermic needle into the uterine lumen just posterior to the UTJ and flushing with approximately 1 ml of medium for each horn.

Transfer is done surgically under general anesthesia, usually via a midventral approach. It is necessary to pierce the wall of the uterus with a hypodermic needle before introducing the egg-carrying pipette.

RABBIT

Embryo transfer was first performed successfully in the rabbit on April 24, 1980, by Heape, and ever since that time it has remained a popular choice for gamete research. Most embryo transfer work is done in mature does, that is, female rabbits over 5 to 6 months of age.

Does are easy to superovulate by different regimens, which have been used with varying degrees of success. A single dose of 150 to 200 IU of PMSG (SC or IM) followed by 50 IU of hCG at the time of mating, 66 to 72 hours (up to 80 hours) later, is commonly used. Hafez[6] reported that best results were obtained from three SC injections of 50 IU of PMSG given once daily starting on day 1 at 4 PM, day 2 at 4 PM and day 3 at 8 AM, with 50 IU of hCG IV on day 4 at 4 PM. Follicle stimulating hormone (FSH) can also be used. Twice daily injections of 0.5 mg of FSH for 3 days with 1.5 mg of luteinizing hormone (LH)/kg IV or 30 to 50 IU of hCG 12 to 24 hours after the last FSH injection consistently produce 40 to 60 ovulations. Horse anterior pituitary extract (HAP), 2 mg/day for 5 days, also gives very good results. The average number of embryos recovered from superovulated rabbits is 50 (range of 6 to 135). Fertilization rates are normally high, i.e., 90 per cent or greater.

As the rabbit is an induced ovulator, it is necessary to give the proposed recipient doe either hCG or gonadotropin-releasing hormone (GnRH) to stimulate ovulation. Unfortunately, does become refractory to repeated hCG treatments. However, GnRH does not appear to cause refractoriness and is, therefore, to be recommended. It is also possible to induce the recipient to ovulate by mating her with a vasectomized male. In the rabbit, the fertilized eggs enter the uterus 72 to 84 hours after coitus, i.e., 60 to 72 hours after ovulation. When ovulation is induced with hCG, this time period is shortened slightly. On the way through the oviduct, each egg receives a thick coating of mucin, which is peculiar to the rabbit.

Embryos normally enter the uterus as early blastocysts, remaining near the UTJ for some time, and are easy to collect. After the embryos have entered the uterus, blastocysts may be flushed from the uterus until at least 5½ days after coitus. Attachment occurs at about 6¾ days.

Embryos may be collected surgically or by sacrificing the donor doe. For collection of tubal stage ova the oviducts can be flushed in either direction using a blunt-ended 26-gauge hypodermic needle. Retrograde flushing (flushing from the uterine end) appears to require less pressure. Two ml of medium is usually adequate to flush the oviduct.

In surgical collection strict aseptic procedures must be followed, using either the flank or midventral approach. For collection of early embryos from the oviduct, a small curved glass cannula (ID of 0.3 to 0.5 mm) is inserted into the fimbriated end of the oviduct and held in place manually or with a small clamp. Next, a blunted 18-gauge hypodermic needle is inserted into the UTJ, and 2 to 3 ml of medium is used to flush the oviduct in a retrograde direction. This is repeated for the other oviduct. The procedure for surgical collection of uterine stage embryos is very similar except that the glass cannula is introduced through a puncture wound at the cervical end of the uterine horn. The blunted 18-gauge hypodermic needle is inserted at the UTJ, and 5 to 8 ml of medium is used to flush the blastocysts down the horn and through the cannula. Both horns must be cannulated separately, as the rabbit has two cervices.

Several safe methods of administering anesthesia are available. One reliable and simple method is the use of ketamine hydrochloride IM at a dose of 60 to 75 mg/kg body weight, with 2 mg of acepromazine maleate added to each 10 ml of ketamine (100 mg/ml). This results in better relaxation than when ketamine is used alone. Both surgical collection and transfer can be done by midventral laparotomy. A flank approach can be used when a surgical transfer into an oviduct is carried out; however, for manipulation of the uterus the midventral approach is most convenient.

Embryos are transferred surgically to the oviducts or the uterus depending on the stage of development. Zygotes and embryos up to the 32-cell stage are best transferred to the oviducts, while morulae and older embryos are best transferred to the uterus. Those embryos transferred to the oviduct (using a fire-polished 2-mm glass pipette) are inserted 5 to 10 mm into the infundibulum via the fimbria, taking care not to use more than 0.2 ml of fluid. Transfer to the uterus is similar except that in many cases it is necessary first to puncture the wall of the uterus with a 25-gauge hypodermic needle or with the blunt end of a suture needle before introducing the pipette.

Better results are obtained in transferring morulae or early blastocysts than in transferring late stage blastocysts. Zygotes will rupture if collection is attempted later than 5½ to 6 days after coitus, and it has been found that zygotes transferred without a zona pellucida do not develop, as the blastocyst does not "hatch" in the rabbit. The zona pellucida is normally retained up to implantation. Pregnancy can be diagnosed by palpation as early as days 9 to 10.

The rabbit egg and embryo are quite tolerant to a wide variety of transfer media. However, best collection results were obtained using Dulbecco's phosphate-buffered saline, although physiological saline solution (0.9 per cent w/v sodium chloride) has also been widely used. If the zygotes are to be held in culture for more than a few hours, a more sophisticated medium containing either bovine serum albumin (BSA) or homologous plasma should be used. As bacterial contamination is probably the most important cause of embryo transfer failure, antibiotics should also be added.

It is important for the donor and recipient to be synchronized, and if the recipient has ovulated in advance of the donor by 2 or more days, few, if any, pregnancies will result. The embryos have a better chance of survival if the recipient ovulates slightly later than the donor. In addition, an optimal number of embryos (around 15) should be transferred to each horn. There is no transuterine migration of zygotes in the rabbit, and at least two implanted embryos are required for fetal survival.

FELINE

There have been only two reported studies of successful embryo transfer in cats.[5, 8] Synchronization of donors and recipients is easily achieved with domestic cats, since they ovulate in response to mating or hCG injection during estrus. Anestrous queens can be induced to ovulate by administration of 2.0 mg of FSH-P IM daily (for up to 5 days) until estrus is observed. This is followed by 250 IU of hCG on the first and second day of estrus. Increasing the FSH dosage to 3.0 mg/day and extending the duration of administration to 7 days appear to result in a reduced ovulation rate and more unovulated follicles.

The embryos are collected from the uterus on day 6 rather than from the oviducts at an earlier time to minimize the formation of adhesions involving the ovary and oviduct. Ovulation should be confirmed by laparoscopy to avoid unnecessary surgery. If ovulations have occurred, the uterus is exposed via midventral laparotomy. The donor is anesthetized with an IM injection of a combination of ketamine hydrochloride and acepromazine maleate and maintained with supplemental injections of ketamine. A ball-tipped metal catheter (14- to 18-gauge) is inserted through a puncture wound in the uterine horn just anterior to the uterine bifurcation and is held in place by digital pressure.

Collection medium is introduced at the tip of the uterine horn using a 20-gauge plastic indwelling catheter, and the fluid is collected in glass bowls as it flows from the metal catheter. This procedure is repeated on the remaining uterine horn, and the puncture wounds at the base of the horns are closed with 4–0 absorbable surgical suture. Recovery rates of around 90 per cent of the ova can be anticipated with this procedure.

Recipient queens may be prepared either by mating to a vasectomized male or by two daily injections of 250 IU of hCG. Anesthesia and the surgical exposure of the recipient reproductive tract are similar to those described for the donor. A puncture wound is made approximately 4 cm from the tip of the uterine horn using an 18-gauge indwelling catheter, and the embryos are deposited toward the tip of the horn in 1 to 5 μl of medium. Ham's F-10 medium with 25 mM HEPES buffer and L-glutamine plus 10 per cent heat-treated fetal bovine serum and antibiotics (50 U/ml of penicillin and 50 μg/ml of streptomycin) have been used successfully. Improved results would probably be obtained with the use of bicarbonate-CO_2 buffer rather than HEPES buffer.

CANINE

The few canine embryos that have been successfully transferred were obtained from naturally ovulating donors and were transferred to naturally ovulating recipients.[8] The most promising approach to superovulating the bitch consists of intramuscular administration of 44 IU of PMSG/kg body weight daily for 9 days during the anestrous period of the cycle, followed by 500 IU of hCG on day 10.[2] Current research on pulsatile administration of GnRH may yield clinically useful information for induction of synchronized ovulation in donor and recipient canidae.

The methods for collecting canine embryos involve surgery. However, with an appropriately designed vaginal speculum, it would seem to be possible to pass a balloon-tipped catheter through the cervix for nonsurgical collection of embryos. A Foley catheter can be introduced through the cervix during surgery, and embryos can be recovered by introducing collection medium into the tips of the uterine horns and out of the Foley catheter.[2]

For surgical collections animals are fasted for 12 hours, anesthetized using ketamine hydrochloride (11 mg/kg) and xylazine (2.2 mg/kg) and maintained on halothane (Fluothane). The uterus is exposed via midventral laparotomy, and a ball-tipped metal or a fluted glass catheter is inserted into the uterine lumen anterior to the uterine bifurcation and held in place manually. Collection fluid is introduced into the uterine lumen near the tip of the horn using an indwelling catheter and collected via the previously placed catheters. Ham's F-10 with 25 mM HEPES buffer and L-glutamine plus 10 per cent heat-treated fetal bovine serum and penicillin (50 U/ml) and streptomycin (50 mg/ml) have been used as the medium. On the basis of experience with bovine embryos, the use of bicarbonate-CO_2 buffer may yield better results.

The degree of synchrony that is essential for successful embryo transfer in the canine has not been determined. Canine embryos may be transferred surgically using anesthesia and procedures similar to those described for the donors. A puncture wound is made through the uterine wall into the lumen around 4 cm from the UTJ, and the embryos are deposited into the lumen using a 1- to 5-μl glass pipette. To date, only four live offspring have been produced by embryo transfer, and these were from three pregnancies in seven recipients.

Determining the appropriate time for embryo collection from the canine is more difficult than in many other species. Cannulation of the canine oviduct is difficult because of the ovarian bursa. Therefore, uterine-stage embryos are the most easily obtained. Uterine stage preimplantation embryos have been obtained on days 13 to 18 (day 1 = first day of standing estrus).

NONHUMAN PRIMATES

The strategy for performing embryo transfer in nonhuman primates, as with other laboratory animals, depends upon several factors, such as the objectives of the experiment, the relative value of the donor and recipient, the anatomic and physiological limitations of the reproductive system and the status of procedure development. For example, in attempting to develop a procedure that can be used to induce and to maintain pregnancy in the ovariectomized female using rhesus and cynomolgus monkeys as the animal model, it is appropriate to use surgical collection and transfer of tubal stage embryos. In this case the recipients are more valuable than the donors, and adhesions that develop following surgical collection of tubal embryos can be tolerated. Also, in the macaques the cervix is difficult to cannulate so that nonsurgical collection procedures have not yet been developed.

Attempts to superovulate nonhuman primates have generally been unrewarding. Although multiple follicles can be rescued using exogenous gonadotropins, very few of them ovulate, and when they do, the fertilization rate and embryo quality are usually low. It is possible, however, to obtain oocytes from such follicles, which are useful for in vitro fertilization. Various regimens used to induce follicle development and superovulation in nonhuman primates have been previously reviewed.[8]

Uterine-stage embryos can be collected nonsurgically from baboons using a modified endometrial cell sampler.[9] The tip of the sampler is passed through the cervix into the uterine lumen. Collection fluid is infused slowly into the uterus via a fine plastic tube that is inserted through the sampler; the fluid is collected as it returns via the sampler. If fluid is introduced too rapidly, the embryo may be forced back through the oviduct and into the peritoneal cavity. With practice, about a 50 per cent recovery rate of ova or embryos can be obtained from parous baboons by this method. Nonsurgical embryo collection methods have not been developed for any other species of nonhuman primates. Nevertheless, the method described for the baboon would very likely be useful for any of the larger nonhuman primate species in which the cervix can be cannulated.

Uterine-stage embryos may be collected surgically by a variety of procedures that have been discussed previously.[1] The procedures that do the least damage to the reproductive tract involve introduction of fluid into the uterine fundus either via laparoscopy or midventral laparotomy. The embryos are collected via a vaginal speculum as they are forced through the cervix or via a second needle puncture into either the fundus or base of the uterus, with the cervix clamped. Care must be taken to avoid forcing the embryos out through the oviducts. Higher recovery rates are possible by cannulation of the oviducts, clamping of the cervix and forcing the fluid through the UTJ and out the cannulated oviduct. However, adhesion formation between the oviduct and the ovary will usually limit the number of collections to three per animal.

Tubal-stage embryos may be obtained by cannulation of the oviduct with a fluted plastic catheter on the side ipsilateral to the ovulation. The collection fluid is introduced into the oviduct lumen a few millimeters above the UTJ with a 25- to 30-gauge hypodermic needle. Since only one oviduct is cannulated per collection, the number of collections per animal before adhesion formation becomes a limitation is approximately twice that for surgical collection of uterine stage embryos via the cannulated oviduct.

Selection of collection and culture media for nonhuman primate embryos is difficult because few controlled comparisons of various media have been conducted. Baboon embryos were cultured from the 12- to 16-cell stage to the hatched blastocyst stage of development.[9] These embryos were collected in a bicarbonate-buffered salt solution containing bovine serum albumin, glucose, lactate, pyruvate, penicillin and streptomycin (Biggers,

Whitten and Whittingham medium). The embryos were then cultured in CMRL-1066 medium supplemented with glutamine (1 mM), pyruvate (0.37 mM), penicillin (100 U/ml), streptomycin (50 g/ml) and 20 per cent of heat-inactivated human placental cord serum or fetal calf serum. The embryos were cultured at 37°C in an atmosphere of 100 per cent humidity and 5 per cent CO_2, 5 per cent O_2 and 90 per cent N_2. Around 50 per cent of embryos at the 12-cell stage or greater can be expected to hatch from the zona pellucida, but only approximately 10 per cent of earlier stage embryos are likely to hatch in this system.

Tubal-stage nonhuman primate embryos are usually transferred to the oviducts; however, it has been shown that tubal-stage embryos can be successfully autotransferred to the uterus. The highest conception rate achieved with the transfer of embryos in nonhuman primates was four of seven (57 per cent). Macaque embryos were transferred surgically to the oviducts of ovariectomized recipients that had been prepared by exogenous administration of estrogen and progesterone.

References

1. Adams CE (ed): Mammalian Egg Transfer. Boca Raton, CRC Press, 1982, p 53.
2. Archbald LF, Baker BA, Clooney LL, Godke RA: A surgical method for collecting canine embryos after induction of estrus and ovulation with exogenous gonadotropins. Vet Med/Sm Anim Clin, February 1980, pp 228–238.
3. Chang MC: Reciprocal insemination and egg transfer between ferrets and mink. J Exp Zool 168:49, 1968.
4. Dickmann Z: Egg transfer in the mouse and rat. In Adams CE (ed): Mammalian Egg Transfer. Boca Raton, CRE Press, 1982.
5. Gruffydd-Jones TJ, David JSE: Embryo collection and transfer in cats. In Proceedings of the 2nd World Conference on Embryo Transfer and In Vitro Fertilization. Annecy, France, 1982, p 93.
6. Hafez ESE: Reproduction and Breeding Techniques for Laboratory Animals. Philadelphia, Lea & Febiger, 1970.
7. Kraemer DC: Intra- and interspecific embryo transfer. J Exp Zool 228:363, 1983.
8. Kraemer DC, Flow BL, Schriver MD, et al.: Embryo transfer in the non-human primate, feline and canine. Theriogenology 11:51, 1979.
9. Pope CE, Pope JZ, Beck LR: Development of baboon preimplantation embryos to post-implantation stages in vitro. Biol Reprod 27:915, 1982.

Culture and Short-term Storage of Embryos

Raymond W. Wright, Ph.D.
Washington State University,
Pullman, Washington

Culture systems for embryos of major farm species were designed to meet one of two objectives. The first was for long-term culture (days), in which various media, gaseous atmospheres and embryo handling methods could be studied. The second was a short-term culture system (hours), in which embryos could be held for brief periods of time before transfer to recipient females.

MEDIA COMPONENTS

Embryos from farm animals have been cultured in a wide variety of defined and undefined media. Defined media, rather than undefined media (in which the composition is unknown and the components can vary considerably), are the media of choice when the objective is to study embryo development. However, when the objective is to provide a system that supports in vitro embryo survival, the appropriate medium is the one that is effective.

The ions required for successful embryo development include K^+, Ca^{+2}, Na^+, Mg^{+2}, Cl^-, PO_4^{-3} and HCO_3^-. Optimum levels of these ions in media are similar to serum values except for K^+, which is sometimes found in higher concentration in synthetic oviduct fluid (SOF) and Menezo's medium. The role of individual ions in embryonic development is not well understood; however, Ca^{+2} is known to be important in membrane stability and permeability and also at the time of morula compaction. It is generally agreed that the role of sodium chloride is primarily for osmotic balance of the medium. The osmolarity of commonly used media is in the range of 250 to 300 millosmoles (mOsm). Studies in the mouse suggest that hypoosmotic medium may be more effective when culturing very early-stage embryos. However, using a variety of media with different osmolarities suggests that the effect of osmolarity on embryo development is limited.

It is often difficult when working under field conditions to maintain embryos under a controlled gaseous atmosphere. This has led to the use of phosphate-buffered medium, which eliminates the need for CO_2 incubators or alternative gassing systems. This is of some concern because it has been found that mouse embryo development decreased following incubation in phosphate- rather than bicarbonate-buffered medium. Further, it has been established that the mouse embryo utilizes CO_2 as a carbon source during development. However, phosphate-buffered medium is preferred owing to the radical change in pH that can occur with bicarbonate-buffered medium when care is not taken to maintain a 5 per cent CO_2 in air atmosphere under field conditions.

The most commonly used gas atmosphere for embryo culture is 5 per cent CO_2 in air. Some investigators have found that reducing the oxygen concentration from 20 to 5 per cent (a total gas phase of 5 per cent CO_2, 5 per cent O_2 and 90 per cent N_2), was beneficial for embryo development. No development occurs in the absence of O_2, and the lower O_2 tensions are probably closer to physiological states. No role for N_2 in this mixture has been found, and it is generally considered to be inert.

The role of the bicarbonate ion in the medium is to control the pH, but it also functions in equilibrium with CO_2 as a carbon source during embryo development. For this reason, long-term storage of embryos in phosphate- compared with bicarbonate-buffered medium is not recommended.

Pyruvate and lactate are preferred energy sources for early preimplantation embryos, while glucose is incorporated into the embryo at all stages of development in much greater amounts than either pyruvate or lactate. There seems to be little benefit in including pyruvate or lactate in media for the culture of embryos of eight cells or greater in development. Glucose should be a component of phosphate- as well as bicarbonate-buffered medium at a concentration of 0.5 to 1.0 gm/l. Research on the mouse suggests that in vitro processes such as hatching, attachment and trophoblast outgrowth are glucose-dependent events.

Little benefit is gained by using a concentration of serum greater than 10 per cent in complete culture medium. However, when using a phosphate-buffered medium, serum concentrations of 20 per cent are recommended for holding embryos up to several hours. Considerably less serum, from 1 to 10 per cent, can be used for flushing. All serum should be heat treated to remove complement activity and should be sterilized before being used in any medium. Recent results suggest that newborn calf serum and steer serum can be used in place of the more expensive and difficult to obtain fetal calf serum for embryo flushing and transfer. Bovine serum albumin (BSA) can be an effective media supplement for long-term culture. However, care should be taken to adjust the pH of the medium, particularly when concentrations of BSA are greater than 1 per cent. As a matter of convenience, serum is used more frequently than BSA, which is generally supplied in a powdered form.

EMBRYO CULTURE AS A TOOL IN EVALUATING EMBRYO QUALITY

Several studies have attempted to use embryo culture as a means of predicting viability following freezing and/or direct transfer. Results suggest that there is little advantage in culturing embryos as a means of predicting subsequent viability, although the results are probably as much a reflection of the culture system employed as embryo quality. However, grading embryos by categories of good, fair and poor clearly shows that pregnancy rates following direct transfer and/or freezing are lower when using embryos of poor quality. In summary, embryos should be graded at collection, with the realization that transfer of embryos of poor quality will result in lower pregnancy rates. Further, unless embryo cultures are conducted in an extremely controlled system, embryo viability will be reduced.

METHODS FOR SHORT-TERM EMBRYO CULTURE IN THE FIELD

Embryos should be stored in the same medium that was used for flushing. It is not desirable to move embryos, for example, from a phosphate- to a bicarbonate-buffered medium because of the possible changes in osmolarity, pH and energy substrates. Precautions should be taken if a bicarbonate-buffered medium is used, to prevent changes in pH due to CO_2 escape into the atmosphere. This can be accomplished by using capped tubes, which have been previously gassed, or by placing embryo vessels in an incubator in which the atmosphere can be controlled. No precautions are necessary with phosphate-buffered medium, and it is recommended that a 20 per cent serum concentration be used if less than this amount was employed for the flush.

Flushing and holding medium should contain antibiotics to prevent bacterial contamination. Also, embryo vessels should be sterilized before use and kept in a dust-free environment. No particular precautions need to be taken to maintain embryos at 37°C, but extremes in temperature should be avoided.

Results from our laboratory indicate that bovine and ovine embryo viability begins to decline following 12 hours of storage in phosphate-buffered medium supplemented with serum. Thus, embryos that need to be stored longer than this period of time before transfer should be frozen. If freezing is not possible, sheep and cattle embryos should be placed in a bicarbonate-buffered medium with 1 gm/l glucose and 10 per cent heat-treated serum or BSA 1.5 per cent w/v and held at 37°C in a 5 per cent CO_2 in air gaseous atmosphere.

Recently, evidence has indicated that bovine embryos will survive for 2 to 3 days at 4°C. Basically, embryos in culture medium were placed in a stoppered tube in a water bath in a refrigerator. Survival was very good up to 48 hours. This does provide an alternative for transporting embryos or retarding the development of embryos while recipients are allowed to "catch up."

Attempts to freeze porcine embryos or even cool them to temperatures below 5°C have proved unsuccessful. Long-term storage systems for porcine embryos should include a bicarbonate-buffered medium supplemented with glucose and BSA at a concentration of 1.5 per cent w/v. Porcine embryos should be held at 37°C in a gaseous atmosphere of 5 per cent CO_2 in air for optimal results.

In order to maintain a temperature of 37°C for long periods of time, our experience has shown that a Trans-Temp Container holds a temperature of 37°C for 48 hours and still offers enough space for an embryo container. In addition, this system is well padded and secure enough for shipment under most conditions. We prefer to ship embryos in plastic tubes with tight caps that have been previously gassed with a 5 per cent CO_2 in air mixture. It should be remembered that the gas will leak from the tube and that the atmosphere will not be maintained indefinitely. For this reason, we place plastic tubes in a stainless steel anerobic chamber, which can then be gassed directly by 5 per cent CO_2 in air source. Next, the anerobic chamber is placed in the Trans-Temp Container. This system controls both temperature and gas atmosphere and places the embryos in a secure environment.

TECHNIQUES AND METHODS FOR QUALITY CONTROL OF EMBRYO CULTURE

The use of high quality water, equivalent to at least twice glass-distilled water, has been shown to be an important factor in successful culture of embryos from laboratory animals. Several reports exist concerning the use of deionized water prepared for common household application in preparing flushing medium. Pregnancy rates using this water appear to be satisfactory, but the direct effect on embryo survival has not been evaluated.

Media for flushing can be purchased completely formulated in a liquid form or purchased as a powder that requires the addition of water. Completely formulated media eliminate the necessity of providing a high-quality water but are also much more expensive than preparations from powder. Results in our laboratory suggest that commercially prepared media can vary considerably in osmolarity and pH. In order to ensure quality control, routine measurements of these parameters should be performed.

References

1. Betteridge KJ (ed): Embryo Transfer in Farm Animals. Monograph No. 16. Ottawa, Agriculture Canada, 1977.
2. Lindner GM, Anderson GB, BonDurant RH, Cupps PT: Survival of bovine embryos stored at 4°C. Theriogenology 20:311, 1983.
3. Wright RW Jr, Bondioli KR: Various aspects of in vitro fertilization and embryo culture in farm animals. J Anim Sci 53:702, 1981.

Implications and Applications of the Long-term Preservation of Embryos by Freezing

Ulrich Schneider, Dr. Vet. Med.
Peter Mazur, Ph.D.
Oak Ridge National Laboratory,
Oak Ridge, Tennessee

Modern agriculture and biology increasingly involve the manipulation of germ plasm in procedures such as artificial insemination (AI) and embryo transfer. The efficacy of these procedures depends on maintaining the viability of the germ cells from the time of collection to the time of transfer, and freezing offers a practical solution for long-term storage.

Since its first success in 1972, low-temperature preservation of mammalian embryos has developed from a scientific feat to a routine technique in two areas of animal breeding: (1) banking of the embryos of mutant strains of mice and (2) the use of frozen embryos in bovine embryo transfer programs. Additionally, mammalian embryos have proved to be excellent models for research in basic cryobiology because of their comparatively large size and because of the existence of in vitro and in vivo survival assays. Thus, as further knowledge is gained from basic research on embryos, it has had and will continue to have an immediate impact on the methodology of freezing.

Numerous implications in the use of frozen embryos have been discussed. Those relevant to embryo transfer in farm animals include the following:

1. Recipients do not have to be synchronized for the day of embryo collection. Transfer can be done whenever recipients come into the proper stage of the cycle. As a consequence large recipient herds do not have to be kept.

2. Parturition can be timed to achieve optimum herd management and the best utilization of food resources.

3. Frozen embryos can be shipped far more easily and inexpensively than live animals. So far, disease control regulations have limited the export and import of embryos. Frozen embryos, however, will help lessen the problems, for collected embryos can be stored in the frozen state while the parents are being tested for diseases, including those with longer incubation periods.

4. Progeny and performance tests of full siblings can be carried out more rapidly and efficiently.

5. Germ plasm of rare breeds can be preserved.

BASIC PRINCIPLES

The freezing of a living cell constitutes a complex physicochemical process of heat and water transport between the cell and its surrounding medium. There usually exists an optimum cooling rate. It is dependent on the size of a cell, its surface-to-volume ratio, its permeability to water and the temperature coefficient of that permeability.

Cooling. The medium, including the embryos, initially cools below the freezing point without ice crystal formation, a phenomenon referred to as supercooling. Then, at some lower temperature, ice nucleation occurs, followed by a rapid rise in temperature due to the release of latent heat of fusion. To avoid extensive supercooling and thereby to avoid ice nucleation of the embryos, crystallization is induced in the extracellular medium some 2°C below the freezing point of the solution by seeding the medium with an ice crystal. During further cooling the solute concentration rises with decreasing temperature. The embryo responds osmotically to this increase in solute concentration by losing water.

At slow cooling rates, the compositional changes in the intracellular solution follow very closely those in the extracellular solution. At higher cooling rates, however, the dehydration of the cell falls behind that of the solution. The extent of dehydration depends also on the subzero temperature to which the embryo is exposed and on the molar ratio of salt to cryoprotectant in the freezing medium. As long as the temperature is above the eutectic point (the temperature below which no liquid remains—about $-45°C$ for glycerol solutions), the embryos will be surrounded by at least some unfrozen solution.

Freezing Injury. Cells are injured during freezing and thawing primarily by two mechanisms: solution effects and intracellular ice formation. At high cooling rates heat transport dominates over water transport so that water cannot leave the cells fast enough to maintain equilibrium. Consequently, the cells supercool. Equilibrium is eventually restored by the formation of intracellular ice, a generally lethal event. Intracellular ice is especially detrimental when relatively large amounts of large crystals are formed. To avoid intracellular freezing, embryos must be cooled at 1°C/minute or slower. However, too slow a rate of cooling can also damage cells by what has been referred to as "solution effect damage."

Until recently, injury from solution effects has been thought to result from damage to cell membranes and cell organelles by the high concentrations of electrolytes generated during slow cooling.

However, the increase in the concentration of electrolytes can be reduced by the presence of a cryoprotectant in a suitable concentration. This reduction, a colligative effect, has been thought to be the basis of the protective effects of these solutes. However, this view of solution effect injury and its prevention has recently been challenged by Mazur and his colleagues. They have shown, using human erythrocytes as a model, that the decrease in the fraction of unfrozen water is more responsible for slow freezing injury than is the rise in solute concentration. We have evidence that this mechanism also applies to embryos.

Storage. Any temperature below $-120°C$ will provide long-term viability because no ordinary, thermally driven reactions can occur. A storage temperature of $-196°C$ is commonly used because it is the boiling point of liquid nitrogen, a relatively cheap cold source. The only reactions that occur at $-196°C$ are direct ionizations from background radiation. Consequently, storage times of about 200 years are unlikely to produce any detectable reduction in the survival of frozen embryos or any detectable genetic change. A pragmatic advantage of liquid nitrogen storage is that it can make use of the reliable equipment that has been used for frozen semen under field conditions for two decades.

Thawing. The required thawing rate depends on the freezing regimen used. When embryos are cooled slowly to temperatures between -30 and $-40°C$ and then rapidly to $-196°C$ (the so-called modified two-step procedure), then thawing has to be rapid (about $200°C/minute$). Cells treated in this way may contain some intracellular ice, and thawing has to be rapid to prevent injury from the recrystallization of that ice. On the other hand, if embryos are cooled slowly to temperatures below $-60°C$ before transfer to liquid nitrogen, then thawing is normally done slowly at about $20°C/minute$.

Cryoprotectant. Embryos survive cryopreservation only in the presence of the cryoprotectants glycerol or dimethylsulfoxide (DMSO) in concentrations ranging from 1.0 to 2.0 M. Other cryoprotectants might work but have rarely been tested. Criteria for a cryoprotectant are high solubility, low toxicity at high concentrations and a low molecular weight both for easier permeation and for exertion of a maximum colligative effect.

Permeability of Cryoprotectants. During the addition and dilution of a permeating cryoprotectant, the cell undergoes osmotic changes in size. As a consequence, if the addition or particularly the dilution of the cryoprotectant is carried out inappropriately, the viability of cells can be affected. In general, when the embryo is exposed to a cryoprotectant it will initially shrink by losing water both because of the initial hyperosmoticity of the extracellular solution and because the embryo is much more permeable to water than to the cryoprotectant. Shrinkage will continue until the efflux of water is balanced by the influx of cryoprotectant. The cryoprotectant will then enter the embryo at a rate dependent on the permeability coefficient and

the temperature. Concomitantly, water will reenter the cell, causing it to gradually increase its volume. Equilibration is complete when the water volume of the embryo regains its isotonic volume.

The opposite reaction occurs when the cryoprotectant is removed from the cell. When the extracellular cryoprotectant concentration is first lowered, water will enter the embryo abruptly. If the dilution is not carried out carefully, the cells can swell to a damaging size.

Equations that model the influx and efflux of cryoprotectants in cells can be used to calculate the optimum procedure and to design the most practical addition and removal method. However, the equations require the permeability coefficient of the cryoprotectant, and this has not been experimentally determined for most of the developmental stages of embryos of different species. For this reason we have recently determined the permeability coefficient for DMSO and glycerol in day 7 bovine embryos. At room temperature the values are 1.4×10^{-3} cm/minute for DMSO and 2.2×10^{-3} cm/minute for glycerol.

Addition of Cryoprotectant. To date, most investigators have not used these permeability equations to compute optimum addition and dilution protocols but have derived them empirically. There is debate, in fact, whether the rate of addition of cryoprotectant is critical. Still, most investigators add the cryoprotectant step-wise, typically in 0.25 M increments.

Removal of Cryoprotectants. In contrast, there is clear evidence that the rate of removal of cryoprotectants is critical. The standard, empirical method is to dilute it by step-wise addition of culture medium or to pipette the embryos into decreasing concentrations of cryoprotectant solution.

Leibo and Mazur suggested a modification in the procedure of cryoprotectant removal by including nonpermeable solutes like sucrose into the dilution medium to control the amount of swelling. The sucrose acts as an osmotic counterforce to restrict water movement across the membranes. In fact, as the cryoprotectant is leaving the embryo, it will shrink in response to the extracellular hypertonic dilution medium. It regains its normal volume when at the end of the process the sucrose is removed from the dilution medium, thereby returning the medium to isotonic conditions. The observed shrinkage and swelling of embryos during a sucrose dilution treatment are preliminary indications that they have survived freezing because they demonstrate that the cell membranes are functioning normally.

Biologic Freezers. The current embryo freezing techniques require slow cooling at 0.3 to $0.8°C/minute$ from the seeding temperature to between -30 and $-40°C$. Various devices have been used for cooling the samples. All freezers follow the principle that the temperature in a chamber is lowered at a controlled rate, thus removing heat from the samples. Some systems cool an air-filled chamber by the injection and the mixing of liquid nitrogen vapor. Others use a compressor and cooling coils to cool a large volume of a well-stirred fluid (usually alcohol), in which the samples are immersed.

The temperature is measured either in the chamber or preferably in a reference sample. The rate of decrease in temperature is controlled by a mechanical or electronic programmer. Some control units contain microprocessors with memory to allow the preprogramming of the various steps of a cooling protocol. Finally, some freezers permit the automatic seeding of samples at a predetermined temperature.

The exact equipment is not critical to successful freezing. Far more important is an understanding of the cryobiologic events that are especially critical to survival.

Methodology. The following protocol is representative of those used for the cryopreservation of day 7 bovine embryos. Dulbecco's phosphate-buffered saline (PBS) supplemented with sodium pyruvate, glucose, protein and glycerol (1.0 to 1.5 M) is used as the freezing medium. Embryos are pipetted into the freezing medium at room temperature (20°C) and are kept for 8 to 10 minutes at that temperature to permit the glycerol to equilibrate. During this equilibration period the embryos are transferred in volumes of 0.2 to 0.5 ml of freezing medium into vials or French straws. The container is then securely sealed. Labeling should follow the standards of the International Embryo Transfer Society. Since the cooling rate to the seeding temperature (-5 to $-7°C$) is unimportant, the samples can be immediately transferred into the seeding bath. Crystallization (seeding) of the extracellular medium is initiated by touching the outside wall of the straw or vial with cold forceps at a location distant from the embryos. The forceps are usually precooled in liquid nitrogen. The samples are kept at the seeding temperature for 5 to 10 minutes to allow for the crystallization of the medium to progress to equilibrium. Next, they are cooled at 0.3 to 0.8°C/minute to between -30 and $-40°C$, and then immersed in liquid nitrogen and stored.

Thawing is carried out by placing the straw or vial into a water bath at 20 or 37°C, respectively. The rate of thawing is critical to success and must be consistent from sample to sample. Different temperatures are used for French straws and vials to compensate for the differences in the sample surface-to-volume ratio. The rate of thawing can also be significantly affected by the vigor with which the water bath is stirred or with which the sample is agitated. Therefore, any thawing procedure should be carefully tested before it is used with valuable embryos.

Next, the cryoprotectant must be removed without causing osmotic damage. The method of choice is dilution in a sucrose-PBS medium. Sucrose in a concentration that is isosmolal or lower, with the glycerol solution, is either added to the freezing medium at a volume ratio of 10:1, or the embryos are pipetted into a suitable volume of sucrose-PBS medium. The embryos are allowed to remain in contact with the dilution medium for about 5 to 10 minutes at room temperature. Thereafter, the embryos are pipetted into isotonic PBS medium.

Survival can be assayed by morphologic criteria (membrane appearance, presence of a blastocoele) or by vital staining with fluorescent compounds such as fluorescein-diacetate (FDA) or 6-carboxylfluoresceindiacetate (CFDA). A more functional test of viability is whether the embryos are capable of development in vitro, and the ultimate test is whether the embryos result in pregnancies after transfer to recipients.

Differences between Developmental Stages and Species. Procedures similar to those described have resulted in the successful freezing (i.e., live-born offspring) of morulae and blastocysts from cattle, goats, sheep and horses. Freezing of earlier embryonic stages of farm animals, unlike that of laboratory animals, has been unsuccessful. For example, pig zygotes do not even survive cooling to temperatures below $+10°C$. Temperature sensitivity of the early developmental stages of embryos may be associated with the presence of large amounts of lipids in the cells. The sensitivity of the early stages as well as differences among species could also be related to differences in permeability to water or to the cryoprotectant. Mouse oocytes for example, have lower permeabilities to glycerol than do later stages. Embryos with ruptured zonae pellucidae or those without zonae pellucidae, as well as retarded or degenerating embryos, survive present freezing techniques very poorly.

RESULTS

Survival rates of cryopreserved embryos are steadily improving. Only a few years ago the number of live offspring from transferred frozen-thawed bovine embryos was about half of that obtained from transferred nonfrozen embryos. Now that difference has almost disappeared, and overall pregnancy rates of close to 50 per cent are reported for frozen-thawed cattle embryos. However, unless all steps are controlled closely, the pregnancy rates from day 7 bovine embryos may vary considerably among different donors. The extent of variation can be a significant factor in the cost-effectiveness of an embryo transfer program.

References

1. Leibo SP, Mazur P: Methods for the preservation of mammalian embryos by freezing. In Daniel JC (ed): Methods in Mammalian Reproduction. New York, Academic Press, 1978, pp 179–201.
2. Mazur P: Freezing of living cells: Mechanisms and implications. Am J Physiol (Cell Physiol, 16) 247:C125, 1984.
3. Schneider U, Maurer RR: Factors affecting survival of frozen-thawed mouse embryos. Biol Reprod 29:121, 1983.
4. Schneider U, Mazur P: Osmotic influence of cryoprotectant permeability and its relation to survival of frozen-thawed embryos. Theriogenology 21:68, 1984.

Embryo-Pathogen Interactions in Relation to Disease Transmission

Elizabeth L. Singh, M.Sc.
W. C. D. Hare, D.V.M., Ph.D., F.R.C.V.S.
Agriculture Canada, Animal Diseases Research
Institute, Nepean, Ontario, Canada

Theoretically, the potential of embryos to transmit infectious disease is considerably less than that of semen or live animals. Embryos can only be infected in two ways: (1) The pathogenic organism may be carried in/on the gametes so that infection occurs at fertilization, or (2) the developing embryo may be infected with the organism present in the reproductive tract of its mother. Thus, the success of embryo transfer for disease control depends on the pathogenic organism in question not being transmitted via the gametes and not infecting the embryo prior to or during collection.

There has been a limited amount of work on the mode of transmission of prenatal infections in domestic animals. However, few pathogens have been implicated in the infection of the oocyte, and pathogens found in semen are usually present in the seminal fluid rather than within the sperm cell. Thus, it is likely that most infections found in early embryos originate from their environment and not directly via the gametes.

DISEASES OF CONCERN

At present, few countries have regulations in place for the exchange of embryos. For those countries that do, certification differs in regard to diseases included and requirements to be met. Generally, developed countries are concerned about diseases, depending on the health status of the national herd/flock and on the significance of breeding stock and meat exports to their agricultural economies. In all cases, however, existing regulations relate to the donor and sire and to the herd of origin rather than to the embryo itself. This is because information regarding the potential for disease transmission by embryos is either incomplete or not available, and the technology for testing embryos has not yet been developed.

It should be recognized that the disease transmission potential of embryos is quite different from that of the live animal. The zona pellucida of embryos has been shown to be an effective barrier against certain viruses,[8] and thus, on a strictly physical basis, it is unlikely that the zona pellucida would allow the passage of bacterial and fungal agents. For these latter agents, there is also the added deterrent in the uterine flush fluid of antibiotics, which are generally bacteriostatic and in some cases bacteriocidal. Thus, transmissible disease agents of concern in embryo transfer are likely to be viral rather than bacterial in nature.

SUMMARY OF RESEARCH

Research on the disease transmission potential of livestock embryos is costly and time consuming; however, it is probably the interpretation of research results that presents the greatest difficulty. Much of the work has involved in vitro experimentation, and caution must always be taken in extending these results to in vivo situations.

Generally, embryos being tested are subjected to higher levels of virus in vitro than they would be under the most extreme in vivo situation. The rationale for doing this is that if a virus cannot be transmitted under these extreme conditions, it is unlikely to be transmitted in embryos collected from healthy seropositive donors. However, if transmission of the virus does occur under extreme conditions, it is not proof that this would occur under natural circumstances.

The method for determining embryonic "infection" must also be critically studied. Demonstration of viruslike particles in embryos is often accepted as proof of embryonic "infection." However, in some cases, embryos with viruslike particles in their cells have been found to be noninfective when assayed and capable of producing normal uninfected fetuses.[11] Thus, it would seem that some viruslike particles observed in embryos are incomplete and incapable of producing infectious virus. Before this conclusion can be reached, however, it is essential to demonstrate that "negative" infectivity results are due to the absence of virus and not to a lack of sensitivity of the assay system.

The embryo-pathogen interaction may also change because of in vitro conditions. For instance, low pH has been used to remove the zona pellucida from embryos prior to viral exposure. However, it has not been established whether this low pH might also result in temporary membrane permeability, which could then allow viruses to enter the cells.

The greatest difficulty with in vivo research is in obtaining significant numbers on which to base a conclusion. Transferring embryos from viremic donors is both time consuming and costly, and it will be some time before sufficient numbers of transfers have been carried out to fully assess the transmissibility of each virus via embryo transfer.

Thus, before any conclusions can be reached about the disease transmission potential of embryos, it is essential to evaluate critically both the methodology and data of the experiments involved.

CATTLE

Most research efforts to date have been directed toward those diseases of specific concern to the bovine species. The following is a brief review of the research that has been carried out and an assessment of the probability of disease spread by way of the embryo for each of the pathogens.

Bovine Leukemia Virus (BLV). The evidence for the use of embryo transfer in the control of BLV is most encouraging. There have been 480 transfers carried out with embryos from BLV-seropositive donors to BLV-seronegative recipients.[9] All of the recipients and all of the 143 calves produced from these transfers have remained BLV-seronegative. Since BLV was found in 16 per cent of the flush fluids examined, it is essential that embryos derived from BLV-seropositive animals be washed prior to transfer.

Blue Tongue Virus (BTV). BTV did not infect 120 zona pellucida-intact embryos exposed in vitro to 10^{-2} to 10^{-7} pfu/ml of BTV.[6, 12] Similarly, the virus could not be isolated from 63 zona pellucida-intact embryos recovered from BTV-infected donors.[7] In three studies involving the transfer of zona pellucida-intact embryos from viremic donors to seronegative recipients, all of the calves (n = 37) and recipients remained BTV-seronegative.[7, 12, 15]

The data indicate that BTV is unlikely to be spread by the zona pellucida-intact embryo. When the zona pellucida is removed, BTV will enter embryonic cells, killing the embryo (n = 18).[6] Therefore, these embryos and those infected at fertilization would not be candidates for transfer, and the disease cycle would be broken.

Infectious Bovine Rhinotracheitis (IBRV). Attempts to isolate IBRV from 31 zona pellucida-intact embryos derived from IBRV-seropositive donors have proved unsuccessful. However, when embryos were exposed to 10^6 to 10^8 tissue culture infective dose $(TCID)_{50}$/ml of IBRV and then washed, approximately 65 per cent of the embryos retained infectious virus, although their development was not affected. Both trypsin and IBRV-antiserum were effective in removing the infectious IBRV from the embryos (n = 32).[12]

Embryos derived from donors shedding IBRV have also been transferred, after trypsin treatment, to IBRV-seronegative recipients. To date, 20 seronegative calves have been produced, 14 of which were derived from donors that had IBRV in their uterus and/or oviducts at the time of collection. All of the recipients have also remained IBRV-seronegative.[12]

As IBRV has been isolated from semen, it will also be necessary to show that IBRV does not enter or attach to the spermatozoa infecting the egg during fertilization.

Bovine Viral Diarrhea Virus (BVDV). In one study zona pellucida-intact embryos (n = 96) exposed to 10^4 to 10^5 TCID$_{50}$/ml BVDV for 24 hours did not become infected, and their development proceeded normally.[12] Twenty-nine eggs/embryos collected from BVDV-seropositive donors were also found to be negative for BVDV.[12] However, in another study[1] there was evidence that BVDV penetrated the zona pellucida and interfered with normal embryonic development. Structures resembling BVDV were also seen beneath the zona pellucida of the degenerating embryos.

More experiments must be conducted before the feasibility of controlling BVDV with embryo transfer can be assessed. It is possible that BVDV causes embryonic degeneration and retardation by infection of the endometrium, resulting in a change in uterine environment. However, the relationship between the viruslike particles found in the embryonic cells and the lack of infection of embryos exposed to BVDV must be further established. It must be determined whether the particles would be capable of replication in a recipient's reproductive tract. In addition, as BVDV has been isolated from semen, studies must determine whether there may be a male contribution to embryonic infection.

Foot and Mouth Disease Virus (FMDV). Based on infectivity assays and animal inoculations, preliminary results show that FMDV does not penetrate or attach to the zona pellucida.[13a] Zona pellucida-intact embryos (n = 169) exposed to 10^6 pfu/ml of FMDV for 4 to 18 hours did not become infected and developed normally. Similarly, FMDV was not found to be associated with 48 embryos collected from cattle during the acute stages of the disease.[13a] However, when hatched bovine embryos were exposed to 10^6 pfu/ml of FMDV (n = 42) for 2 hours, 35 per cent of the embryos carried infectious virus after washing. Transfers of zona pellucida-intact embryos from FMDV-viremic donors to uninfected recipients must be conducted, and since FMDV has been isolated from semen, the possibility of a male contribution to embryonic infection must be studied.

Bovine Parvovirus (BPV). Zona pellucida-free morula stage embryos continued to develop normally after exposure to BPV and showed no evidence of embryonic infection when they were examined by electron microscopy.[5] However, since it has been shown that porcine parvovirus does not infect pig embryos but does bind to the zona pellucida,[16] it is essential to determine whether BPV sticks to the zona pellucida of bovine embryos.

Akabane Virus (AV). Zona pellucida-intact bovine embryos (n = 80) exposed to 10^4 to 10^6 pfu/ml of AV for 1 to 24 hours were negative when assayed for infection. AV also had no effect on embryonic development compared with controls.[12]

Brucella Abortus. *Brucella abortus* has been isolated from uterine flush fluid up to 41 days after abortion. Evidence tends to indicate, however, that provided embryos are washed, this agent is unlikely to be transmitted during embryo transfer procedures.[14]

Mycobacterium Paratuberculosis. M. paratuberculosis was not isolated from embryos (n = 7) or flush fluids from three experimentally infected donors.[10a]

SWINE

Embryo transfer has been used in swine for the control of infectious disease. Some of the diseases that have been studied are included here.

African Swine Fever Virus (ASFV). Infectious ASFV was detected on or in 95 per cent of 80 zona pellucida-intact porcine embryos that had been exposed to 10^6 to 10^7 HAdD$_{50}$/ml of ASFV for 18 hours, washed and then cultured. Papain, versene or ficin treatment of 24 embryos had no effect on the retained virus, whereas trypsin-edetic acid (EDTA) and pronase treatment of 141 embryos were found to be effective in reducing the number of embryos carrying virus (30 versus 95 per cent) and the amount of virus on the embryos.[13] It has not been determined whether ASFV enters the embryonic cells, but evidence suggests that most, if not all, of the virus retained is bound to the zona pellucida. Although these experiments indicate that ASFV could be transmitted via embryo transfer, it remains to be established whether ASFV is ever shed into the reproductive tract. If it is, then chances are that the virus would bind to the zona pellucida of any embryos present in the tract.

Porcine Parvovirus (PPV). Although infectious virus did bind to the zona pellucida, 38 zona pellucida-intact embryos did not become infected when exposed to 10^4 CCID$_{50}$/ml of PPV.[16] When 76 PPV-exposed embryos were washed and transferred to four recipients, the recipients became PPV-seropositive, and PPV-specific fluorescent material was observed in embryonic cells.[17] In addition, PPV has been found on or immediately below the outer surface of the zona pellucida of 25 porcine embryos exposed to PPV.[4] If PPV is shed into the reproductive tract of an infected animal, it would seem that the potential for the transmission of PPV by embryo transfer does exist.

Pseudorabies Virus (PrV). In one study 72 zona pellucida-intact porcine embryos were exposed to 10^6 pfu/ml of PrV for 24 hours, washed, cultured and assayed for PrV. Although all embryos developed normally, approximately 45 per cent were found to be positive for PrV.[13b] In another research study 155 zona pellucida-intact and 48 zona pellucida-free embryos were assayed and found to be negative after exposure to 10^4 or 10^8 TCID$_{50}$/ml of PrV for 1 hour.[2] When the embryos were exposed to 10^8 TCID$_{50}$/ml in vitro, washed and then transferred to five seronegative recipients, all of the recipients developed antibodies to PrV. Similarly, seroconversion occurred in two of five recipients receiving embryos from donors infected both intranasally and intrauterinely.[3] Electron micrographs also have demonstrated PrV adsorbed to the outer surface of the zona pellucida and buried in the sperm tracts of 20 embryos exposed to PrV. Washing failed to remove this adsorbed virus.[4]

However, 805 embryos derived from 38 PrV-seropositive sows have been transferred to 34 uninfected recipients. All recipients remained PrV-seronegative, and 22 of the recipients farrowed 208 piglets that were also PrV-seronegative.[10] Therefore, it would seem that in order for transmission of PrV to occur, embryos must be exposed to a threshold level of virus that does not appear to be present in the oviducts and uteri of seropositive pigs in a PrV-infected herd.

Swine Vesicular Disease Virus (SVDV). When zona pellucida-intact embryos (n = 186) were exposed to 10^6 pfu/ml of SVDV, washed and cultured, infectious virus could still be isolated from most of the embryos. Replication of the virus did not take place in the embryos, and it appeared that most, if not all, of the virus was attached to the zona pellucida. Treatment with trypsin-EDTA or pronase after washing resulted in a reduction both in the number of positive embryos and in the amount of virus on the embryos. However, no treatment was found to be effective in rendering all of the embryos "clean."[13b] Therefore, if SVDV is excreted into the reproductive tract, it could stick to the zona pellucida of embryos present there.

Enteroviruses (ECOP-3 and ECOP-6). Porcine embryos (n = 48) that had been cocultivated with cultures infected with ECOP-3 or ECOP-6 were found to have virions in pores of the zona pellucida and were associated with sperm that were at or near the outer surface of the zona pellucida.[4]

Foot and Mouth Disease Virus (FMDV). When 196 zona pellucida-intact porcine embryos were exposed to 10^6 pfu/ml for 4 to 18 hours, approximately 3 per cent retained infectious virus after washing.[13b] These results are in contrast with those found with bovine embryos in which no embryos carried infectious virus. The difference may be due to the presence of sperm tracts that are usually found in the zona pellucida of porcine embryos. These sperm tracts may trap FMDV, making it inaccessible to washing procedures. To fully assess the potential for the transmission of FMDV via embryos, it must now be determined whether the virus is excreted into the reproductive tract.

SHEEP AND GOATS

The least amount of research has been done on those diseases specific to sheep and goats. Experiments are now underway that will examine the potential of embryo transfer for the spread of blue tongue virus, maedi-visna virus and the scrapie agent.

RECOMMENDED PROCESSING FOR EMBRYOS

Collection and Transfer. It is essential that no disease be introduced during embryo collection and transfer. All equipment and solutions should be sterile, and the perineum and vulva of the animal should be cleaned and disinfected for the nonsurgical procedure. Any serum added to the flush medium should be mycoplasma and virus free. The addition of antibiotics to the flush medium is a desirable precaution but should not be used in lieu of aseptic technique.

Washing. Since a number of viruses and bacteria have been isolated from uterine flush fluids, it is essential to wash embryos prior to transfer to reduce the possibility of disease transmission. Embryos should be washed by transferring them through 10 changes of medium. Each wash should constitute a hundredfold dilution of the previous one. The embryos should be gently agitated in each wash and the pipette used to transfer the embryos should be changed after each of the 10 transfers. Under these conditions, it is consistently possible to remove 10^6 to 10^7 of virus, if the virus does not bind to the embryo.[12]

Treatments. To date, antiserum, trypsin, pronase, papain and ficin have been used to treat embryos in an attempt to remove virus bound to the zona pellucida.[12] The advantage of cleaning embryos enzymatically is that if it is effective, it is irreversible. This has not always been found to be true with antiserum. Embryos carrying SVDV and treated with SVDV-antiserum were negative for virus immediately after treatment. However, if the embryos were cultured and then assayed, an increasing number of embryos become SVDV positive. Presumably, the antibody-antigen complexes disassociated over time.

It is unlikely at this time that disinfection of embryos will be considered acceptable for the international exchange of embryos. However, within a particular country, treatment of embryos can and is being used to develop clean herds or introduce new genetic material into SPF herds. This will allow the effectiveness of the treatment to be better assessed, which may eventually allow it to be used internationally.

Freezing. The importation of frozen embryos rather than fresh embryos can be to a country's advantage. It allows the importer time to ascertain the disease status of the donor and the sire of the embryos not only before and at the time of collection but also for a period of time after collection. When the importing country is fully satisfied with the health of the donor and sire, the embryos can be released for transfer.

However, it should be recognized that in terms of the embryo itself the disease potential of frozen embryos may be greater than that of fresh embryos. This is because the zona pellucida affords the embryo protection against certain viruses, and this structure is often cracked during the freezing-thawing procedure. In addition, movement of water into the embryo during thawing may allow a virus access to embryonic cells. Thus, embryos must be thoroughly washed prior to freezing, since once the zona pellucida has cracked and a virus has entered the embryonic cells, further washing would be to no avail.

POTENTIAL OF EMBRYO TRANSFER IN TERMS OF DISEASE CONTROL

It would be enormously beneficial if embryo transfer could be used for disease control. Briefly, the reasons for this are as follows: If uninfected embryos can be obtained from infected parents or herds, then disease-free genetic material can be exported from infected areas, breeders will be able to eliminate diseases from their herds and flocks within one generation without loss of the gene pool and new blood lines can be introduced into specific pathogen-free herds.

References

1. Archbald LF, Fulton RW, Seager CL, et al.: Effect of bovine viral diarrhea (BVD) virus on preimplantation bovine embryos: A preliminary study. Theriogenology 11:81, 1979.
2. Bolin SR, Runnels LJ, Sawyer CA, et al.: Resistance of porcine preimplantation embryos to pseudorabies virus. Am J Vet Res 42:1711, 1981.
3. Bolin SR, Runnels LJ, Sawyer CA, Gustafson DP: Experimental transmission of pseudorabies virus in swine by embryo transfer. Am J Vet Res 43:278, 1982.
4. Bolin SR, Turek JJ, Runnels LJ, Gustafson DP: Pseudorabies virus, porcine parvovirus and porcine enterovirus interactions, with the zona pellucida of the porcine embryo. Am J Vet Res 44:1036, 1983.
5. Bowen RA, Storz J, Leary J: Interaction of viral pathogens with preimplantation embryos. Theriogenology 9:88, 1978.
6. Bowen RA, Howard TH, Pickett BW: Interaction of blue tongue virus with preimplantation embryos from mice and cattle. Am J Vet Res 43:1907, 1982.
7. Bowen RA, Howard TH, Elsden RP, Seidel GE: Embryo transfer from cattle infected with blue tongue virus. Am J Vet Res 44:1625, 1983.
8. Eaglesome MD, Hare WCD, Singh, EL: Embryo transfer: A discussion on its potential for infectious disease control based on a review of studies on infection of gametes and early embryos by various agents. Can Vet J 21:106, 1980.
9. Hare WCD, Mitchell D, Singh EL, et al.: Embryo transfer in relation to bovine leukemia virus control and eradication. Can Vet J Vol 26, 1985.
10. James JE, James DM, Martin PA, et al.: Embryo transfer for conserving valuable genetic material from swine herds with pseudorabies. JAVMA 183:525, 1983.
10a. Jorgenson B, Rasbech NO: Unpublished data.
11. Neighbour PA: Studies on the susceptibility of the mouse implantation embryo to infection with cytomegalovirus. J Reprod Fert 54:15, 1978.
12. Singh EL: Disease transmission: Embryo-pathogen interactions in cattle. 10th Int Cong Anim Reprod AI, Urbana-Champaign. Vol 4, No 9, pp 17–24, 1984.
13. Singh EL, Dulac GC, Hare WCD: Embryo transfer as a means of controlling the transmission of viral infections. V. The in vitro exposure of zona pellucida-intact porcine embryos to African Swine Fever. Theriogenology 22:693, 1984.
13a. Singh EL, McVicar JW: Unpublished data.
13b. Singh EL, Thomas FC: Unpublished data.
14. Stringfellow DA, Howell VL, Schnurrenberger PA: Investigations into the potential for embryo transfer from *Brucella abortus*-infected cows without transmission of infection. Theriogenology 18:733, 1982.
15. Thomas FC, Singh EL, Hare WCD: Embryo transfer as a means of controlling viral infections. VI. Blue tongue virus-free calves from infectious semen. Theriogenology (In press).
16. Wrathall AE, Mengeling WL: Effect of porcine parvovirus on development of fertilized pig eggs in vitro. Br Vet J 135:249, 1979.
17. Wrathall AE, Mengeling WL: Effect of transferring parvovirus-infected fertilized pig eggs into seronegative gilts. Br Vet J 135:255, 1979.

Genetic Engineering

George E. Seidel, Jr., Ph.D.
Colorado State University,
Fort Collins, Colorado

Genetic engineering might be narrowly defined as modification of the chemical structure of DNA or RNA. However, it seems more appropriate to broaden the definition to include any directed change in the genetic make-up of a population. Thus, a farmer who selects bulls for artificial insemination (AI) on the basis of superior milk production of their daughters would be a genetic engineer in the broad sense. Artificial insemination and embryo transfer are clearly useful tools for genetic engineering. A number of genetic engineering strategies will be considered here.

STATE OF THE ART OF IN VITRO FERTILIZATION IN MAMMALS

To date, the production of young from in vitro fertilization has been accomplished in nine mammalian species, but only in the mouse, rabbit, and human have more than a few dozen young been produced. Great strides have recently been made in obtaining sperm penetration of the oocyte in vitro. However, continued development into a normal two-cell embryo that grows into a fetus after embryo transfer does not often follow the in vitro sperm penetration. Probably the most difficult aspect of in vitro fertilization is effecting capacitation. Ejaculated sperm of mammals are incapable of fertilizing ova until they are capacitated, a process that normally takes place in the female reproductive tract over a period of 30 minutes to 10 or more hours, depending on the species. Capacitation has also been accomplished in vitro in many species.[9] The molecular basis of capacitation is not yet clear, although considerable evidence indicates that it involves removal of membrane-stabilizing proteins from the sperm surface.[3] Membrane destabilization should facilitate the acrosome reaction and fusion of sperm and oocyte membranes during fertilization.

Laboratory Rodents and Rabbits. In vitro fertilization with mouse gametes represents the most studied, most successful and best-defined model of mammalian in vitro fertilization. Epididymal sperm can be capacitated in vitro in 1 hour, and sperm penetration rates are in excess of 80 per cent.[9] Embryos from some strains of mice can be cultured in vitro fairly easily, but there is considerable diffi-

culty in getting mouse ova from other strains to develop, owing to the "two-cell block." In vitro fertilized mouse ova develop into normal fetuses after embryo transfer, provided that they are at a normal stage of development when transferred. Procedures for in vitro fertilization with rat gametes are less commonly performed but are similar to those with mice except that it is somewhat more difficult to culture rat embryos in vitro. Procedures for hamsters are more defined on a biochemical basis, but methods for culture of one-cell hamster ova are ineffective, and development of fetuses after transfer of such in vitro fertilized ova does not occur. These problems will be overcome with additional research.

In vitro fertilization with rabbit gametes is a completely different process than that for rodents. First, rabbit sperm are much more difficult to capacitate in vitro, possibly because the process takes 6 to 10 hours in vivo. Since rabbits are much more expensive than mice, ejaculated sperm collected with an artificial vagina are frequently used instead of sacrificing the males for epididymal sperm. There is circumstantial evidence that it is more difficult to capacitate ejaculated than epididymal sperm. In many cases, in vivo capacitated sperm, recovered from the rabbit uterus, are used in rabbit studies. One advantage of rabbits over most strains of rodents is the ease with which the fertilized one-cell ovum can be cultured. Many investigators have produced young from embryo transfer of in vitro fertilized rabbit ova.

Domestic Animals. In vitro fertilization procedures for farm animals have been reviewed recently.[3, 15] With a few exceptions, success rates have been poor, and criteria of fertilization have frequently been unconvincing. The most common measure of fertilization is division to the two-cell stage, but parthenogenesis and fragmentation of the ovum are difficult to distinguish from cell division of fertilized embryos. The recent birth of a genetically marked calf is the first unequivocal evidence of successful in vitro fertilization in farm animals;[4] however, much more needs to be done before routine procedures are available. Thus, it may be some years before in vitro fertilization with gametes of domestic animals becomes a routine procedure.

Primates. Procedures for in vitro fertilization of nonhuman primate gametes have been reviewed recently.[5] The situation is nearly identical to that with domestic animals, i.e., poor success rates, unconvincing evidence for fertilization and only a few successful pregnancies to date. These studies are, of course, very difficult and expensive, but progress is being made.

The situation with human in vitro fertilization is much more promising, partly because of the huge resources allocated and partly because of the ease of capacitating human sperm in vitro. The major problems in this species are obtaining normal oocytes and culturing the embryos after fertilization until they are at a suitable stage for transcervical deposition into the uterus. A common practice is to transfer two to four embryos in the hope that one will develop. Another problem is that the same woman is usually both donor of oocytes and recipient, and the hormonal manipulations to induce oocyte maturation and ovulation frequently result in an inappropriate hormonal milieu for a recipient. The most common application of in vitro fertilization in *Homo sapiens* is to circumvent female infertility. Interestingly, a second application is to circumvent some types of male infertility; i.e., with oligospermia, too few sperm may be produced for in vivo fertility, but sufficient normal sperm may be produced so that fertilization can occur when they are placed next to oocytes in a small droplet of medium.

Other Considerations. In recent years it has become popular to use the zona pellucida-free hamster oocyte for preliminary studies of in vitro fertilization because only capacitated sperm seem to fuse with the hamster oocyte, and there is no barrier to penetration because of species differences. This is an appropriate, approximate test for capacitation, but it is not necessarily a good test of fertilizing ability of sperm. In many respects intact and even dead oocytes from ovarian follicles of the same species as the sperm are a more stringent test, as the most difficult barrier to sperm penetration seems to be getting through the zona pellucida.

One other approach worth mentioning is xenogenous fertilization, placing gametes of both sexes into the reproductive tract of a different species.[6] In some cases this works well, and one can recover the embryos and transfer them to a recipient of the same species as the gametes for gestation.

CURRENT STATUS OF PRENATAL SEX SELECTION

Sperm. At a recent conference on prospects for sexing mammalian sperm, it was concluded that no reliable nondamaging methods of separating X- and Y-bearing sperm were available.[1] However, there was also a consensus that powerful tools were becoming available that would likely lead to separation of X- and Y-bearing sperm within a decade. Such techniques would have wide application, particularly in humans and cattle, if they were accurate and inexpensive and did not result in reduced fertility.

Embryos. The first approach to sexing embryos was conducted on the basis of sex chromatin in biopsied trophoblast cells. Since then, numerous investigators have successfully sexed mammalian embryos on the basis of the karyotype of biopsied cells.[3] Under ideal circumstances, about two thirds of the embryos can be karyotyped accurately for sex chromosomes; suitable metaphase chromosome preparations are not obtained from the other one third. The net result is a 1:1:1 sex ratio of males, females and unknown. The biopsy and karyotyping

procedures are tedious and time consuming, making them impractical for routine commercial use.

A second method of sexing embryos is to use an antibody to H-Y antigen, a protein found on the cell membrane of male, but not female, mammalian cells.[11] Detectable H-Y antigen is present at the eight-cell stage if the ovum was fertilized by a Y-bearing sperm, which contains the genetic information for producing this protein. For sexing, the antibodies to H-Y antigens are usually made in rodents, although monoclonal antibodies are also used. The embryos are exposed to anti–H-Y antibodies, which bind to the male embryos. Two methods are commonly used to detect the bound antibodies. The first method involves adding complement, which results in death of the male embryos. The more practical method is the second antibody method (Fig. 1). This consists of producing a fluorescent-labeled antibody to the first antibody so that the male embryos will fluoresce in the appropriate light. This procedure is about 80 per cent accurate for sexing mouse embryos[11] and is being developed by several companies for use with bovine embryos. A major concern is that the procedures might damage embryos. One way around this might be to detect sex-specific secretion products after short-term culture of embryos. Development of sexing procedures is expensive, and the commercial companies will have to charge high rates for sexing embryos to recover these costs. However, with continued research and development, costs are likely to drop quickly to less than $50 per embryo sexed, but they must be even lower for profitable application in most circumstances.

APPLICATIONS OF MICROSURGERY TO EMBRYOS

Manufacture of Identical Multiplets. One method of making identical twins is to separate cells of two-cell embryos and allow each half to develop independently. The most successful means for accomplishing this has been developed by Willadsen,[12] who embeds the half embryos in agar blocks, which are then transferred to the sheep oviduct for 3 to 5 days, where they develop to morulae or blastocysts. They are then recovered, dissected from the agar and retransferred to the appropriate species for gestation to term. Blastomeres from four- and eight-cell embryos can also be used to make half and quarter embryos. This method has been used to produce identical quadruplet sheep, triplet cattle and twin horses and pigs.[12] The method also works for later stage embryos. Success rates are fairly high for identical twins but drop off considerably when identical quadruplets are attempted (although twins or triplets frequently result). Nearly all embryos fail to develop to term when identical octuplets are attempted in this way. However, an elegant procedure can be used, which has already resulted in identical quintuplets. This involves mixture of cells of four- and eight-cell embryos such that the blas-

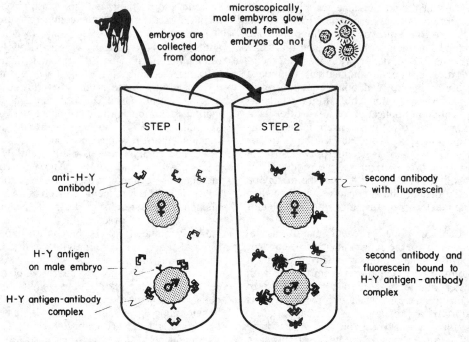

Figure 1. Sexing embryos with a fluorescent antibody technique.

tomeres of the eight-cell embryo develop into fetuses, while those of the four-cell embryos form placentas.[10, 13]

A much simpler method has been developed for producing identical twins from postcompaction morulae and early blastocysts by microsurgically dividing the embryos into two groups of cells followed by immediate embryo transfer.[14] In some cases, surrogate zonae pellucidae are used, although this may not be necessary, at least in later stages. This procedure takes approximately 10 minutes per embryo, and its simplicity cannot be overemphasized. Of course, proper equipment and appropriately trained personnel are necessary. Pregnancy rates of 50 per cent or more per half-embryo are common in cattle, which results in a net pregnancy rate in excess of 100 per cent per original embryo. Thus, about 50 per cent more calves result with half-embryos than with whole embryos. Also, half of the calves so produced are members of identical twin sets; i.e., both halves developed to term, and these are extremely valuable for experimental purposes. For example, some two-treatment experiments are as valid when about one third as many identical twin animals are used than if unrelated animals are used. However, this is not true for all kinds of experimental designs.

Methods of making identical multiplets are, in many respects, methods of cloning, as genetically identical animals are produced asexually. Sometimes cloning is defined in a narrower sense as nuclear transplantation. Illmensee and Hoppe have demonstrated that nuclear transplantation can be accomplished successfully in one-cell mouse ova if the donor nucleus comes from an embryonic cell.[7] Although very few mice have been born as a result of such procedures, one could theoretically make hundreds of genetically identical animals in this way by serial nuclear transplantation.

Strategies for Cloning Adults. To date, it has not been possible to clone adults reliably, even in fish and amphibians. However, if one combines cryopreservation of embryos with the methods just described, one can, in effect, clone adults. The simplest example is to split an embryo, transfer one of the half-embryos to a recipient and freeze the other. If the first half-embryo turns into a desirable adult animal, the copy in the liquid nitrogen tank can be thawed and transferred. This process can be amplified by using quarter embryos or by transplantation of nuclei from cells of frozen blastocysts.

Androgenesis, Gynogenesis and Parthenogenesis. Androgenesis refers to reproduction without a nuclear genetic contribution from the female and gynogenesis to reproduction without a genetic contribution from the male, although a sperm may activate the oocyte. Parthenogenesis is a special case of gynogenesis, in which males are not involved at all. The most simple example of androgenesis would be fertilization of an ovum with two sperm followed by removal of the female genetic material. This would result in a sex ratio of 1XX:2XY:1YY, the latter being a lethal condition.[10] There seems to be no theoretical reason why such a procedure would not work, although hydatidiform molar pregnancies might occur in the human, especially if both sperm were from the same male. If both haploid genetic complements come from the same animal, the process is termed "selfing" and results in 50 per cent inbreeding. An alternate method of androgenesis or gynogenesis could be accomplished by pronuclear removal and fusion.[8]

Diploid parthenogenesis can be accomplished in several ways in mammals.[10] Perhaps the most simple conceptual method is fertilization of an ovum with another ovum instead of a sperm. Another method would be suppression of second polar body formation, or fertilization of the ovum with the second polar body. A most interesting aspect of mammalian parthenogenesis is that development to term has never been observed, even with inbred strains of animals that have no deleterious recessive alleles. Under these circumstances normal animals are produced in other classes of vertebrates. There are at least two possible explanations for failure of term development of mammalian parthenotes. First, methods of activating the ovum, i.e., initiating parthenogenetic development, may damage it or be less effective than activation that occurs during normal fertilization. Second, the sperm may be complementary to the ovum in some epigenetic sense, e.g., methylation of DNA. In any case, this is an intriguing problem because when cells of parthenogenetic embryos are mixed with those of normal embryos, the resulting chimeras develop to term and contain both kinds of cells.

Chimeras. One of the most powerful embryologic techniques ever devised is aggregation of cells of two or more preimplantation embryos to produce offspring that have cells from more than one cell line. The most common procedure is to aggregate two four-cell mouse embryos by removing the zona pellucida, which would result in a tetraparental mouse. Another method is to inject cells of one embryo into the blastocoelic cavity of another. These procedures appear to work for embryos of all mammals. In some cases, cells of only one of the lines contribute to the fetus. The biggest problem with the technique is the inability to direct which portion of the resulting animal will have which genotype. By chance, some of the chimeric animals produced are very useful experimentally. An example of such animals comes from mixing *Bos taurus* and *Bos indicus* embryos and obtaining a phenotypic *Bos taurus* calf with a *Bos indicus* immune system. In cattle, animals that are chimeric in hemopoietic tissue arise simply by producing fraternal twins via embryo transfer due to anastomosis of placental circulations of twin cattle.

Direct Addition or Modification of DNA. A remarkable technique has recently been developed whereby DNA is injected into pronuclei of one-cell fertilized ova. In some instances, the injected DNA is integrated into the genome and expressed in cells and transmitted to future generations.[10] The possibility that such a procedure could work would have been ridiculed by most scientists a few years ago. This procedure permits modification of genetic material in a fundamentally different way from conventional procedures. One might add genes for disease resistance directly to embryos rather than

breeding for it by selection methods. Genes can even be transferred from one species to another. Success rates however are low, but methods are being refined at a rapid pace.

Future Considerations. It is difficult, even for basic scientists, to keep up with the rapid advances in the field of genetic engineering. For example, much can be written about the potentially very useful technique of sperm injection into the ovum. One could also discuss the possibilities of numerous other technologies, such as manipulation of individual chromosomes. One general notion worth stressing is that cloning would merely produce copies of the best animal available and that we need to be thinking of producing something better than the best available.

It is probably not possible to overrate the value of genetic engineering techniques as research tools. Our basic knowledge of life processes is increasing exponentially, partly because of these techniques. However, there is very much more to learn.

On the other hand, genetic engineering is probably greatly overrated as a short-term means of improving animal production before perhaps the year 2000. However, there are bound to be a few spectacular successes, and all phases of animal production probably will be affected by genetic engineering. Nevertheless, it is instructive to remember that fewer than 5 per cent of beef cows in North America conceive by artificial insemination, and this is a proven technology that is inexpensive and easy to apply compared with most genetic engineering techniques. Thus, because a technology is available does not mean that it will be widely applied. Nevertheless, we need to be aware of new genetic engineering tools and be prepared to develop, refine and apply them to serve the needs of mankind.

References

1. Amann RP, Seidel GE Jr (eds): Prospects for Sexing Mammalian Sperm. Boulder, Colorado Associated University Press, 1982.
2. Betteridge KJ, Hare WCD, Singh EL: Approaches to sex selection in farm animals. In Brackett BG, Seidel GE Jr, Seidel SM (eds) New Technologies in Animal Breeding. New York, Academic Press, 1981, p 109.
3. Brackett BG: A review of bovine fertilization in vitro. Theriogenology 19:1, 1983.
4. Brackett BG, Bousquet D, Boice ML, et al.: Normal development following in vitro fertilization in the cow. Biol Reprod 27:147, 1982.
5. Dukelow WR: Early development of the in vitro fertilized preimplantation primate embryo. J Exptl Zool 228:353, 1983.
6. Hirst PJ, De Mayo FJ, Dukelow WR: Xenogenous fertilization of laboratory and domestic animals in the oviduct of the pseudopregnant rabbit. Theriogenology 15:67, 1981.
7. Illmensee K, Hoppe PC: Nuclear transplantation in Mus musculus: Developmental potential of nuclei from preimplantation embryos. Cell 23:9, 1981.
8. McGrath J, Solter D: Nuclear transplantation in the mouse embryo by microsurgery and cell fusion. Science 220:1300, 1983.
9. Rogers BJ: Mammalian sperm capacitation and fertilization in vitro: A critique of methodology. Gamete Res 1:165, 1978

10. Seidel GE Jr: Mammalian oocytes and preimplantation embryos as methodological components. Biol Reprod 28:36, 1983.
11. White KL, Lindner GM, Anderson GB, BonDurant RH: Cytolytic and fluorescent detection of H-Y antigen on preimplantation mouse embryos. Theriogenology 19:701, 1983.
12. Willadsen SM: Micromanipulation of embryos of the large domestic species. In Adams CE (ed): Mammalian Egg Transfer. Boca Raton, CRC Press, 1982, p 185.
13. Willadsen SM, Fehilly DB: The developmental potential and regulatory capacity of blastomeres from 2-, 4-, and 8-cell sheep embryos. In Beier HM, Lindner HR (eds): Fertilization of the Human Egg In Vitro—Biological Basis and Clinical Applications. Berlin, Springer-Verlag, 1983, p 353.
14. Williams TJ, Elsden RP, Seidel GE Jr: Pregnancy rates with bisected bovine embryos. Theriogenology 22:521, 1984.
15. Wright RW Jr, Bondioli KR: Aspects of in vitro fertilization and embryo culture in domestic animals. J Anim Sci 53:702, 1981.

SECTION

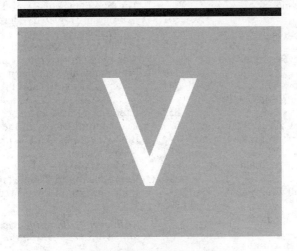

V

BOVINE

Maarten Drost, D.V.M.

Consulting Editor

***Additional Pertinent Information Found in the first
edition of Current Therapy in Theriogenology:***

Schuijt G, Ball L: Delivery by Forced Extraction and Other
Aspects of Bovine Obstetrics, p 247.

Examination of the Reproductive Tract of the Cow and Heifer

Robert H. BonDurant, D.V.M.
University of California, Davis, California

INDICATIONS

A thorough examination of the female and her reproductive tract is essential for diagnosis of pregnancy, estimation of the gestational age of the conceptus and characterization of her reproductive physiological pathologic status. A complete examination allows the astute clinician not only to assess the current status of the patient but also to predict important events to come, such as estrus, ovulation, parturition or abortion. It also allows for a rational approach to therapy and for establishing a prognosis for conditions of the uterus, uterine tubes, ovaries and supporting structures. As with any physical examination, the findings must be reconciled with information gathered in the history and perhaps with additional laboratory findings.

HISTORY

Taking a history need not be a formal process, and indeed is done by most clinicians while the animal is being examined. The important issues that need to be addressed include the following:

1. Parity (virgin heifer, pregnant heifer, uniparous or multiparous cow)
2. Age (including age at first calving)
3. Cyclic history (normal or abnormal cycle lengths, anestrus, nymphomania)
4. Calving dates and comments (dystocia, twins, retained placenta, surgical or mechanical intervention, viability of calf)
5. Breeding dates and methods (artificial insemination or natural service, estrous detection methods and personnel, semen supplier and quality, previous record of bull fertility, including examination for venereal disease)
6. Previous treatments (drugs, dosages and routes; treatment intervals; clinical outcome; drug withdrawal times)
7. Nutritional program (periparturient supplementation of beef cows, dry-period feeding of dairy cows, body conditions of cows at calving, milk production levels).

METHODS OF PHYSICAL EXAMINATION

At present, the most cost-effective and accurate method of examination of the reproductive tract is per rectum palpation of the cervix, uterus, ovaries and supporting structures. Most dairy cattle can be rectally examined with minimal restraint (stanchion or halter), while beef cattle may need to be controlled in a squeeze chute to assure the safety of both patient and examiner. A latex obstetrical sleeve, or a disposable plastic sleeve should be worn. Greater sensitivity and less rectal irritation may be obtained if the tips of the fingers of the plastic sleeve are removed, and a disposable latex exam glove is applied over the sleeve. A nonirritating water soluble lubricant is applied to a gloved arm, and the hand is inserted through the anus into the rectum. In order to complete the examination before the animal's peristaltic and abdominal efforts can interfere, one should proceed quickly to examine the reproductive tract, using the following three-step retraction method:

Cervix. The cervix will generally be located in the anterior pelvic canal, although in cases in which the uterus is enlarged the cervix may be pulled anteriorly into the abdomen. It is very firm, cylindrical, 5 to 12 cm in length and 2 to 6 cm in diameter in the healthy animal. In contrast to the mare, the palpable characteristics of the bovine cervix change very little with the stage of the estrous cycle. The cervix can be grasped, palpated and retracted into the pelvic cavity while simultaneously turning it perpendicularly. The examiner then holds the cervix to the floor of the pelvis with a thumb, while extending the fingers craniolaterally to the edge of the broad ligament.

Broad Ligament. The cervical retraction will tense this supporting structure, making its edge easier to find. The ovary may be noticed near the edge but should be ignored until the uterus has been examined. Hooking the fingers over the lateral edge of the broad ligament and retracting it will usually deliver the uterus into the pelvic cavity. By securing the retracted broad ligament with the thumb, the examiner may then complete the retraction process by locating the ventral intercornual ligament.

Ventral Intercornual Ligament. This connective tissue band is much thicker than the dorsal intercornual ligament and will better tolerate retraction. This is accomplished by hooking the ligament with the middle finger, and gently pulling the entire uterus further into the pelvis. The two uterine horns should now be reflected dorsally, such that the base of each horn is directed at the examiner. The uterus is now ready for complete examination. (Table 1 lists conditions under which the uterus may not be retractable). The size, muscular tone and contents of the uterus should be assessed. (This can be done simultaneously with the "membrane slip" for pregnancy determination, discussed later). Commonly

Table 1. Differential Findings (Per Rectum) of Various Commonly Encountered Uterine Conditions

	Pregnancy 30–65 Days	Pregnancy 65–120 Days	Pregnancy 120 + Days	Endo-metritis	Pyometra	Fetal Mummy	Metritis	Uterine Adhesions	Segmental Aplasia
Heavy, less retractable uterus	−	+	+	±	±	+	+	+	±
Thinning of uterine wall	+	+	+	−	±	−	−	−	±
Fluctuation	+	+	+	−	+	−	+	±	+
Chorioallantoic slip	+	+	+	−	−	−	−	−	−
Amniotic vesicle	+	−	−	−	−	−	−	−	−
Placentomes	−	+	+	−	−	−	−	−	−
Fetus	−	+	+	−	−	+	−	−	−
Fremitus in uterine artery	−	−	+	−	−	−	±	−	−
Presence of corpus luteum	+	+	+	±	+	+	±	±	±

used terms for characterizing uterine tone include the following:

Estrous tone—a turgid, contracted uterus that is often curled into a rather tight configuration.

Diestrous ("normal")—a relaxed muscular uterus.

Edematous—a somewhat turgid uterus but without muscular contraction; may be palpable for a few days after estrus.

Flaccid—a limp, soft, usually thin-walled uterus that does not contract in response to palpation.

Thickened ("doughy")—a pathologic description, indicating thickening of the endometrium and possibly the myometrium as well.

Fluctuant—a uterus in which there is intraluminal fluid.

PREGNANCY DIAGNOSIS

Membrane Slip. Table 1 lists the characteristic rectal examination findings for various stages of pregnancy and contrasts them with commonly encountered pathologic conditions. Pregnancies from 30 days to term can be diagnosed by the detection of a so-called membrane slip, in which the connective tissue band on the lesser curvature of the chorioallantoic membrane is noted as a palpable "blip" as it passes between the examiner's finger and thumb. This phenomenon can be felt throughout the uterine horns, from the bifurcation to the tips, so that each horn should be explored in its entirety. It is important to appreciate the fragile nature of these tissues so that one does not risk damage to the fetal membranes by pinching. The fingers and thumb should always be flatly opposed. It is also important to note that the entire diameter of each uterine horn must be palpated so that if a chorioallantoic slip is present, it will not be missed. Studies that have attempted to assess the risk to the conceptus of membrane slipping have suffered from lack of controls and have shown considerable variation among investigators (from <1 to 14 per cent fetal loss).

Amniotic Vesicle. From approximately 30 to 65 days gestation the amniotic vesicle can be detected as a moveable oval object within the uterine lumen. The vesicle is turgid early in pregnancy but becomes flaccid with advancing gestation until days 65 to 70 when it is difficult to detect at all. The width of the vesicle correlates very well with gestational age (Table 2).

Placentomes. The presence of placentomes is another positive sign of pregnancy and is detectable from about 75 days to term. Since there is great variation in size among individual placentomes (those nearest the fetus are the largest), their usefulness in aging a pregnancy is limited. In general, they can be detected as soft, thickened lumps in the uterine wall and are more easily detected as pregnancy advances.

Palpation of the Fetus. Of course, the presence

Table 2. Relationships of Palpable Parameters to Gestational Age

Parameter	Size		Gestational Age
Amnionic vesicle	1 (finger widths)	1.5 (cm)	42 (days)
	2	3.5	48
	3	5.5	52
	4	7.5	58
	4+*	9.0	62
	5	10.5	65
Fetal poll to snout distance	1 (finger widths)	1.5 (cm)	70 (days)
	2	3.5	80
	3	5.5	90
	4	7.5	100
	4+*	9.0	110
	5	10.5	120
Placentomes	—	—	75 + days
Fetus		mouse	2 (months)
		rat	3
		small cat	4
		large cat	5
		beagle dog	6
Fremitus in uterine artery (bicornual twins)	unilateral		120 + days
	bilateral, asymmetrical		210 + days
	bilateral, symmetrical		120 + days

*Width of the hand minus the thumb

of the fetus itself is a positive sign of pregnancy. Depending on the skill of the examiner and the location of the fetus, the fetus can be palpated from the time of amniotic softening (65 to 70 days) to term. Fetal growth is quite uniform up to about the sixth month, so that fetal size can be used to estimate fetal age accurately (Table 2).

Uterine Artery Fremitus. The major supply of blood for the gravid uterus arrives via the uterine arteries, which enlarge considerably as pregnancy progresses. These bilateral vessels travel in the broad ligaments, just below and anterior to the iliac shafts, reflecting in a cranioventral direction. The uterine arteries branch from the pudendal artery at the level of the iliac shaft, extending ventrally at right angles from the pudendal artery, to course in the broad ligaments. Because of their location in the broad ligaments, they are freely movable, thus differentiating them from the external iliac arteries, which are tightly applied to the medial shaft of each ilium. Enlargement of the uterine artery ipsilateral to the pregnant horn is detectable after 80 to 90 days of gestation. By approximately 120 days, the blood flow within the ipsilateral uterine artery has increased to the point at which turbulence is palpable as a buzzing sensation, also referred to as a thrill or fremitus. Initially, it may be necessary to place very slight pressure on the artery to elicit the fremitus, but as pregnancy progresses the buzzing becomes obvious without pressure. By about 7 to 8 months fremitus is often palpable in the contralateral uterine artery as well. The presence of bilateral fremitus before 7 to 8 months, especially when the two arteries are symmetrical, strongly suggests bicornual twins. Individuals in which true fremitus occurs in the absence of a pregnancy are rare, so its detection can be considered a positive sign of pregnancy in nearly all cases.

PALPATION FOR UTERINE DISORDERS

During routine postpartum examinations in cases in which pregnancy diagnosis is negative or in examinations of "problem cows," the reproductive tract should be examined for palpable abnormalities. The essential questions for the examiner to answer are the following: (1) Is the uterus completely involuted (i.e., symmetrical and approximately the size and tone of the pregravid tract); (2) is there evidence that the patient is cycling (i.e., a corpus luteum or an ovarian follicle associated with increased uterine tone); and (3) are there palpable lesions of the reproductive tract.

Uterine Inflammation. It is generally possible to diagnose moderate to severe endometritis, acute metritis or pyometra by rectal examination. The specific criteria for these diagnoses are presented with the specific conditions elsewhere in this text.

Adhesions. Additionally, the experienced clinician should be able to detect the presence of uterine or utero-ovarian adhesions, which result from inflammatory insults involving the serosal surfaces of the reproductive tract. If the three-step retraction method is employed, the presence of uterine adhesions will interfere with normal retraction of some part of the tract. Commonly, the uterus will adhere to the rumen, the omentum or the ovarian bursae. The prognosis will depend on the severity of adhesions, the degree of involvement of the oviducts and fimbriae and the presence of pathogens.

Abscesses. Uterine abscesses can occur following dystocia or as a sequela to the improper use of an intrauterine pipette. In the former case, the location and the size of the abscess will vary with the site of mechanical trauma and the degree of endometrial/myometrial insult; in the latter case, the abscess is most often in the area of the uterine body and is approximately the size of a golf ball (2 to 6 cm in diameter). In either case the abscess is firm and raised and may cause discomfort when palpated. Adhesions of the abscessed portion of the uterus to other abdominal or pelvic organs are common.

Tumors. Tumors of the bovine uterus are not common but when seen occur predominantly in older cows. Uterine lymphosarcoma, leiomyoma and rarely carcinoma have been diagnosed. Lymphosarcoma may be detectable as multiple smooth nodular enlargements of the uterine wall, often with concurrent enlargement of the deep inguinal and iliac lymph nodes.

Fetal Remnants. Other detectable uterine abnormalities include the presence of fetal remnants. Occasionally, a fragment of an autolyzed term fetus, e.g., a claw, may remain in the uterine lumen following parturition. This is generally detectable as a moveable firm mass in the lumen of an involuting uterus. A foul vaginal discharge will often be noted.

In cases in which cows or heifers do not calve at the expected time following a positive pregnancy diagnosis, one may find either a mummified or macerated fetus on rectal examination. In the former condition the fetal and placental fluids are absorbed, leaving the uterus drawn rather snugly around the fetus. On rectal examination, a heavy, nonfluctuant uterus is palpable. Careful examination will usually reveal firm fetal outlines, the presence of a thick, almost tarlike placenta and a corpus luteum (CL) on the ipsilateral ovary. A vaginal discharge is not seen. Because actual endometrial damage is usually slight or absent in cows carrying mummified fetuses, the prognosis for future fertility is favorable if the mummy can be removed.

In cases of fetal maceration, however, bacterial degradation of fetal soft tissues occurs, leaving a distended uterus with palpably crepitant fetal bones in the lumen. An ipsilateral CL may be present, as well as a fetid vaginal discharge. Because of severe damage to the endometrium during maceration of the fetus, the prognosis for future fertility of such cows is grave.

PALPATION OF THE OVARIES

In the reproductive tract of nonpregnant cows the ovaries lie at the tip of the uterine horns, which in

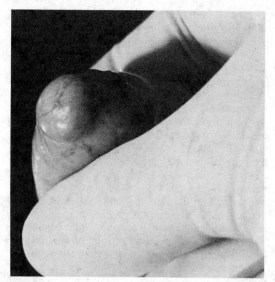

Figure 1. A corpus luteum with a prominent, palpable papilla.

turn lie just cranioventral and lateral to the bifurcation of the uterine horns. It is easier to locate the ovaries if the retracted uterus is first returned to its original location. By sliding the hand down the cervix and uterine body to the bifurcation, the examiner can identify the ovaries as the distinct oval or round masses on either side of the uterus, suspended in the edge of the broad ligament. Left-handed palpators may more easily locate the left ovary by sweeping the entire tract to the right, so that the left broad ligament is tensed, thus revealing the left ovary. Pulling the tract to the left will usually expose the right ovary. The ovary should be cradled between the middle and ring fingers so that its surface can be explored with the index finger and thumb. Significant structures can be differentiated by the following characteristics:

Follicles. These are vesicular structures; i.e., they have a smooth outline with fluctuation just below the surface. Normal antral follicles vary in diameter from 5 to 20 mm and project only slightly from the surface. The presence of follicles can be detected at almost any time throughout the estrous cycle, so by themselves follicles are not a reliable parameter for assessing the stage of the cycle. However, they are most likely to be palpated immediately prior to and during estrus and again 7 to 11 days after estrus.

Corpora Lutea. These are transient endocrine glands and as such have a consistency that changes with the stage of the cycle, from soft, crepitant blood clots in the period immediately following ovulation, to a liverlike consistency at midcycle and to firm, smooth structures near the end of the luteal phase. Variation in size, shape and consistency of CL is common, so one can rarely be entirely confident of the stage of the cycle only by palpating a CL.

Most CL have a papilla, or crownlike projection, above the surface of the ovary (Fig. 1). This papilla

and its characteristic glandular consistency generally make it easy to detect. The papilla will often be large enough so that the entire ovary is distorted from its normal almond shape.

Some CL, including those associated with pregnancies of greater than 30 days duration, do not exhibit a papilla. Instead, extensive remodelling and vascularization cause the CL to be embedded within the ovary, resulting in a large, soft ovary that may be distorted in shape. Careful deep palpation of such an ovary may allow for detection of this CL by noting within the ovary the presence of a "waist-line" that marks the boundary between the base of the CL and the remaining ovarian stroma (Fig. 2). The CL of pregnancy can sometimes resemble a cystic ovary but any confusion can be avoided by first determining the pregnancy status of the uterus.

Corpora Albicantia. These are small, very firm, inactive remnants of CL from previous cycles. It is important to differentiate them from softer, larger, active CL, and from the firm nodular area of attachment of the utero-ovarian ligament to the ovary.

"Smooth Ovaries." This term is often applied to ovaries on which no significant structures can be palpated. If smooth ovaries are repeatedly palpated on an individual cow, it can be safely assumed that she is not cycling, and systemic or local causes should be investigated. However, it should be remembered that the detection of smooth ovaries at a single examination can occur in cycling cows, especially during the first few days following ovulation when the developing CL is not palpable.

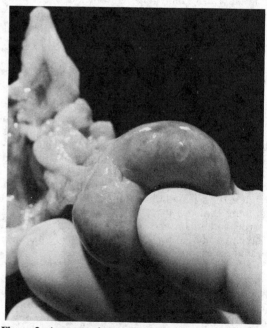

Figure 2. An ovary demonstrating a corpus luteum (CL) without a papilla. Note the "waistline" which is defined by the tip of the palpator's thumb, with the CL above and the ovarian stroma below.

Ovarian Cysts. These are discussed elsewhere in detail but generally include any fluid-filled structure greater than 25 mm in diameter found in the absence of a detectable CL. They should be differentiated from parovarian cysts, which do not involve the ovary but rather involve remnants of the mesonephric or paramesonephric duct systems.

Ovarian Bursa. These may not be routinely palpated but may warrant inspection in cases of "problem-breeder" cows. The bursa can be examined by elevating the ovary with the thumb and index finger while sliding the remaining fingers down the lateral surface of the ovary into the bursa. The thin, bandlike bursa can be lifted and spread on the fingers while the thumb explores the surface for evidence of adhesions, oviductal fluctuation or thickening.

Miscellaneous Ovarian Conditions. These include abscesses (uncommon) and tumors (rare). Both of these conditions result in a greatly enlarged, usually firm ovary and may be associated with bursal and uterine adhesions. Abscessed ovaries may have a softened area within the firm mass and may cause the cow pain when palpated. The unaffected ovary

may function normally so that cyclic structures may be palpated. In the few reported cases of ovarian tumors in cattle (particularly granulosa cell tumors), the contralateral ovary was apparently small and inactive.

VAGINAL EXAMINATION

Vaginal examination can yield supplemental information that may refine the tentative diagnosis made after rectal examinations. Indeed, in some intensive dairy practices vaginal examination of postpartum cows has virtually replaced rectal examination, since it has been shown to be a more sensitive method for the diagnosis of mild to moderate endometritis.

Manual Examination. Although not commonly indicated, manual examination of the vagina and cervix of the early postpartum cow will aid in the diagnosis of vaginal/cervical trauma, retention of fetal membranes and patency of the cervical canal. The cow's vulva and perineum should be carefully washed with a mild disinfectant soap, and a well-

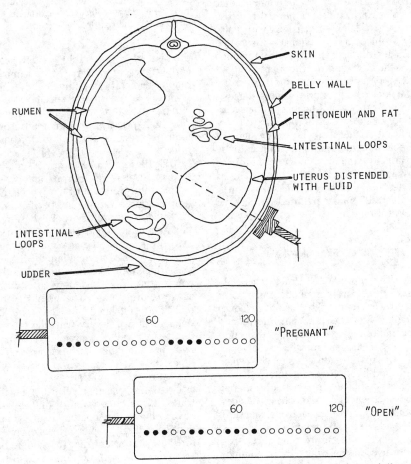

Figure 3. Diagrammatic representation of A-mode ultrasonic pregnancy diagnosis in a ruminant. A "pregnant" diagnosis depends on the detection of a fluid-filled uterus, as inferred from the large gap between "blips" on an oscilloscope screen or linear light scale. (From BonDurant RH: Calif Vet *34*:27, 1980.)

lubricated disposable plastic sleeve should be worn by the examiner.

Vaginoscopic Exam. A cylindrical glass or plastic speculum, approximately 50×5 cm, and a penlight are sufficient for vaginoscopy. If the speculum is to be used on several patients, it should be cleaned between cows and sanitized in a disinfectant that is known to be effective against potential pathogens (infectious bovine rhinotracheitis—IBR—virus, ureaplasma). The vulva and perineum are washed, and the speculum is inserted first in a dorsal-cranial direction until the ischial symphysis has been passed, then in a cranial direction. Some resistance will be noticed at the vestibulovaginal junction. This is easily overcome by gentle pressure.

With a light, the vaginal vault should be examined for the location of the cervix, cervical/vaginal color and secretions, cervical anomalies, trauma and discharges. Physiological secretions, such as cervical mucus, may rather accurately indicate the stage of the estrous cycle. The appearance of large quantities of stringy, water-clear mucus places the cow in the periestrous phase of her cycle, while the discharge of a small amount of blood through the cervix into a mucus pool in the anterior vagina places the cow in the metestrous phase of her cycle. Vaginoscopic findings during diestrus include a rather pale mucosa with scant amounts of sticky mucus. As with palpable findings, visible cervical changes associated with various stages of the estrous cycle are much more subtle for the cow than for the mare.

The presence of pus in the external os of the cervix or on the floor of the anterior vagina suggests endometritis. Small amounts of tacky opaque secretions on the floor of the posterior vagina are probably not significant if there are no other signs of cervical or vaginal inflammation and can usually be ignored. Occasionally, one may find a pool of urine mixed with mucus in the anterior vagina. This is generally a self-limiting problem, but "urovagina" may temporarily result in an irritated, hyperemic vaginal and cervical mucosa.

ALTERNATIVE METHODS OF EXAMINATION

Laparoscopy. The reproductive tract can be directly visualized by laparoscopy/endoscopy. (For details, see the article Genital Surgery of the Cow.)

Ultrasonographic Examination. The uterus and ovaries can be indirectly examined by ultrasonographic techniques. These include the use of "amplitude-depth" (A mode) sonography, in which the presence of fluid-filled viscera is inferred from sonarlike echoes displayed on a cathode ray tube/oscilloscope screen (Fig. 3). These devices, originally developed for swine back fat measurements and later adapted for pregnancy diagnosis, generally have been less accurate than rectal palpation. False-positive diagnoses are more common than false-negatives, suggesting a lack of specificity. Real-time ultrasound, in which a two-dimensional "sonic picture" is generated from echoes, offers the

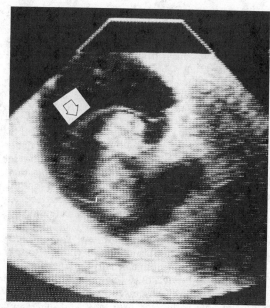

Figure 4. Real-time ultrasonogram of a 48-day bovine fetus in utero. Note the edges of the amniotic vesicle (arrow) surrounding the fetus. The fetal head is at the top, with the umbilicus appearing as a wedge-shaped structure to the right of the picture.

promise of considerably greater accuracy. In the early stages of pregnancy the amniotic vesicle is readily detectable by this method (Fig. 4); later, it is possible to visualize specific fetal anatomy, including a beating heart and major blood vessels. The high price of real-time ultrasonic equipment limits its practical applications for bovine use at this time.

Milk/Plasma Progesterone Assay. The pregnancy status of a cow can be reasonably assessed by the proper interpretation of her plasma or milk progesterone concentrations at specific times. The accuracy of this laboratory tool is based on two important assumptions: (1) The cow was in standing estrus at the time of breeding; and (2) the cow exhibits estrous cycles of normal length. If these criteria are met, then the detection of elevated progesterone concentrations 21 to 24 days after breeding strongly suggests pregnancy. The boundary between "normal" and "elevated" progesterone levels is hazily defined, and will vary with the laboratory method used, the type of sample taken (plasma or milk) and the handling of the sample after collection. Since progesterone is a fat-soluble hormone, it is concentrated in milk at levels 2 to 8 times as high as circulating plasma levels. It is specifically concentrated in the fat portion of milk, so strippings that have a higher fat content than foremilk will have correspondingly higher progesterone levels. Therefore, it is important that the sample be collected in accordance with the criteria established by the diagnostic laboratory. If the restrictions regarding timing of sample collection are observed, accuracy of progesterone determination for pregnancy diagnosis is about 80 to 85 per cent, whereas its accuracy for making a diagnosis of *nonpregnancy* approaches 100 per cent. It is important to note that progesterone concentrations will decay in improperly preserved samples, so plasma should be immediately separated from blood cells and chilled or frozen; milk should be frozen or chemically preserved with approximately 2 mg/ml potassium dichromate until it can be delivered to a laboratory.

The same progesterone assay can be employed to assess the intensity and the accuracy of estrus detection in an artificial insemination program. By periodically sampling groups of cows eligible for breeding (e.g., every other day for 2 to 3 weeks), one can determine the proportion of cows that are actually cycling and compare this number with the number of cows that are actually bred. By sampling cows at the time of breeding when progesterone concentrations should be at basal levels it is possible to detect those cows that are mistakenly bred during the luteal phase of the cycle or even to detect early pregnancy.

Examination of the Reproductive System of the Bull

Lester L. Larson
American Breeders Service, DeForest, Wisconsin

The proper examination of the bull for adequacy of reproductive function is a unique procedure for the veterinarian in that it demands a combination of proficiencies rarely required. It is necessary to employ a good amount of (1) clinical competence, (2) animal psychology, (3) patience, (4) common sense, (5) knowledge of clinical pathology and, in some cases, (6) athletic prowess coupled with raw courage.

Since standard anatomy texts generally treat anatomy of the bull's reproductive organs in a cursory manner, this article will include detailed anatomic illustrations of the genital organs of the bull.

Through the generosity of Erik Blom and N.O. Christensen,[5] their classic anatomic illustrations of the bull's genital organs have been made available for this book (see Figures 2 to 4 and 6). It is the wish of these highly respected Danish colleagues that these illustrations be superbly reproduced in the veterinary literature of North America in commemoration of Paul H. Winther, the artist, now deceased, whose skill has captured so precisely the anatomic details of these structures.

This article places major emphasis on the examination of the mature dairy bull. An effort will be made to point out differences between beef and dairy bulls from the point of view of the examiner. The underlying clinical principles, however, remain the same regardless of the kind of bull or the intended purpose of the examination.

PREPARATION

Restraint. This requirement takes on unusual significance when, as in the examination of a mature bull, one is required to perform all observations and manipulative procedures with all of the bull's faculties intact. These faculties may include an intense desire to demolish veterinarians or to be at a place different than the location at which the examination is scheduled to take place. These desires are often enforced with 2000 to 3000 pounds of a highly coordinated neuromusculoskeletal system.

It is patently obvious that application of restraint to a fractious 2500-pound bull must be on the veterinarian's, rather than a bull's, terms. There is little doubt of the outcome if bull mentality is applied to bull restraint.

In the absence of adequate facilities, competent handlers and a bull accustomed to being restrained by a nose ring, which is often the case, the principles of good restraint for mature bulls must be fully utilized.

The bull should be secured in a roomy box or tie stall by anchoring the head to a structural beam or post with a strong halter, neck chain or neck strap, preferably through a stanchion or headgate. One handler must remain at the bull's head. A light but strong rope is attached to the nose ring and half-hitched to a structure directly forward of the bull, so that the rigging that actually secures the head tightens before the nose tie as the bull pulls back. With one hand on the nose ring and one on the rope to prevent the half-hitch from slipping, the bull's attention can usually be adequately maintained. The nose ring may be quickly released to prevent tearing of the muzzle if the bull becomes excessively fractious.

The bull must be afforded the opportunity to gain confidence in the examiner. The degree of the bull's nervousness will determine the time requirement for the bull's realization that the upcoming ordeal is not painful. It is *absolutely essential* that physical contact is achieved between bull and examiner and that the bull's initial sensation to the contact is pleasurable. Approach is best made slowly, deliberately and with the hand extended toward the shoulder area while talking in tones of kindness and confidence. The move into contact is made only as the bull's cowering subsides. Essentially, all bulls react favorably to rubbing or currying over the withers and dorsal neck area if given enough time. It may take 10 to 30 minutes to reach this "end point," but it is time well spent.

With this state of restraint achieved, the examination can usually proceed uninterrupted if reinforcement is provided by continuing verbal and body-contact reassurance. Sudden moves and loud noises must be completely avoided by all participants.

Identification. The examining veterinarian has an important responsibility as a neutral party to check for agreement between the bull's permanent identifying marks and the official written record. This is particularly necessary so that blood obtained for typing can be correctly identified.

Access to the immunolo᷈ ᷈ identification of the red blood cell–associated antigens of cattle is an absolutely essential initial point of reference for determining the facts in all animal identification disputes.

THE EXAMINATION

Health History and General Physical Examination

Other than to point out factors particularly pertinent to the examination of a large bovine male and, especially, to attempt to categorize clinically the potency-impairing diseases of the neuromusculoskeletal system, it is not within the scope of this article to elaborate on the classic approach to general physical examinations. The following outline lists the components of special significance in the general examination of the bull.

History of Disease

In addition to using the bull's breeding history and physical examination findings as evidence for the presence or absence of infectious venereal disease, these must also be used to determine the presence of recessive genes in the bull, which if brought together through mating with other similar genes from a female would create lethal, semilethal or economically undesirable conditions in offspring.

Systems Review

Integument and Body Wall. Bulls with umbilical, inguinal or other hernias or with surgically repaired hernias may not be justifiably recommended for use in breeding.

Lymphatic System. During palpation of internalia (pelvic and abdominal genital organs), the iliac, mesenteric and deep inguinal lymph nodes are easily accessible for detailed examination.

Circulatory System. Typically, the thickness of the body wall in large bulls makes meaningful cardiac auscultation difficult. Characterizing the pulse by direct palpation of distal aortic, iliac or hypogastric arteries is easily accomplished. This enables one to recognize minimal pulse aberrations, which are rare.

Digestive System. Detailed examination of the oropharyngeal cavity by visual inspection or palpa-

tion or both and examination by palpation of the abdominal digestive organs within reach via the rectum are always a necessary part of a complete examination of the digestive system.

Urinary System. The examiner should give full attention to the urinary organs, either before or after conducting the detailed examination of the internalia.

Locomotor (Neuromusculoskeletal and Hooves, NMSH) System. Liberty is taken to use this systems conglomeration in order to more easily emphasize the significance that these individual body systems, in consort, play in determining a bull's potency, that is, the function of his semen delivery system. The semen delivery system can loosely be divided into two components: the penis with its complex support systems, which is a marvel of efficiency and durability, and the NMSH system, which is unsound in many ways and fails all too often.

Through genetic improvement of cattle for production, larger animals have been developed without necessarily providing a system for locomotion and coition that is proportionately stronger. Therefore, situations arise at coitus that require the pelvic limbs of a bull to support upward of 3000 pounds while engaging in highly coordinated movements. It cannot be overemphasized, therefore, that veterinarians examining bulls for adequacy of reproductive function must critically evaluate NMSH.

Conformation

The examiner must be fully aware, as an anatomist, of limb-hoof conformation traits that are functionally sound and therefore contribute to the bull's longevity and usefulness. The veterinarian will, thereby, readily recognize the significant conformation defects. Pertinent questions such as the following must be answered:

1. Are the angles of the tarsal joints proper (Fig. 1*D*), i.e., not excessively small and "sickle-hocked" (Fig. 1*E*) or excessively large and "posty" (Fig. 1*F*)?
2. Do the axes of the stifle, tarsal and fetlock joints approximately intersect single right and left sagittal planes (Fig. 1*A*) or are the pelvic limbs rotated laterally so a "cow-hocked" trait is evident (Fig. 1*C*)? Are the pelvic limbs rotated medially, resulting in a "bow-legged" attitude (Fig. 1*B*)?
3. Do the axes of the joints of the forelimbs approximately intersect single right and left sagittal planes, or is there excessive outward rotation (supination) with consequent "toeing out"?
4. Is the slope of the pasterns (angle of metatarsophalangeal, metacarpophalangeal joints) proper as in Figure 1*D* and not too "weak" as in Figure 1*F* or too straight?
5. Are the hooves of adequate size consistent with age? Are the shape and placement of the hooves upon the third phalanx such that:
   a. Adequate weight-bearing surfaces are present?

b. The medial and lateral hooves are symmetrical in size and shape?

c. The axial hoof walls are flat, parallel to and equidistant from the sagittal plane in which the limbs are located and that they are in close apposition to each other?

d. The anterior and abaxial hoof walls, together with the bulbs of the heels, form hooves of medium length with adequate width and depth of the heel, rather than hooves that are long and narrow with shallow heels? Such hooves many times are associated with weak pasterns and turning axially of the distal abaxial hoof wall, forming the so-called corkscrew or scissor hooves.

6. Is the gait that of a well-coordinated animal?

Evaluation of conformation of hooves is often complicated by gross horn overgrowth because of neglect in hoof care.

Pathology. Limb conformation defects resulting in dysfunction are by definition pathologic conditions. Defects of a lesser degree may be termed blemishes, when dysfunction is not a consequence of the lesion.

It is not the intent here to discuss the pathologic conditions of NMSH, which are so superbly handled in the book by Greenough and colleagues.[8] However, in case of the potency-impairing degenerative disease conditions of the rear limbs that are not primarily arthritic and are most frequently observed in mature bulls, there are nomenclature contradictions in the literature that need to be clarified.

A summary of extensive clinical-pathologic experiences clearly identifies three such disease entities of rear limbs: (1) progressive posterior paralysis, (2) "postiness" and sequelae and (3) spastic syndrome. A fourth, closely related condition, spastic paresis, or Elso heel, although not a disease of mature bulls, will be discussed briefly from the standpoint of differential diagnosis. Unfortunately, the terms progressive posterior paralysis, spastic syndrome and "crampy" have been applied to a combination of rear limb diseases. It is proposed that the term progressive posterior paralysis be reserved for the disease for which the description follows and for which the term itself is highly descriptive.

Progressive Posterior Paresis. This is a clinically specific paralyzing disease of older bulls. It is rarely seen in bulls under 6 years of age and is generally characterized by a slow onset with signs of ataxia. Impairment seems to be exclusively of motor and proprioceptive function. Skin esthesia usually remains intact.

Typically, the bilateral partial paralysis worsens perceptibly from week to week, as though there is progressive destruction of motor nerve fibers, or neurons, in the spinal cord. Given adequate time, the bull usually becomes fully paralyzed in the rear limbs. The disease may reach a plateau for many months at certain levels of severity. Apparent improvement, which occurs rarely, is seemingly by compensation through learning rather than by an improvement in neurologic function.

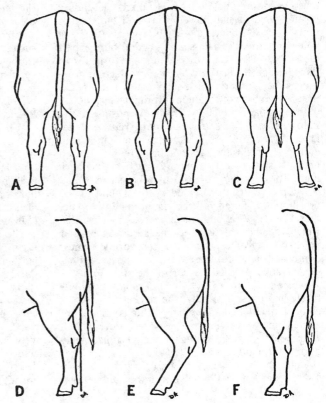

Figure 1. Normal and abnormal conformation characteristics of rear limbs of bulls. *A* and *D*, Normal. *B*, "Bow-legged," medial rotation, narrow base. *C*, "Cow-hocked," lateral rotation, wide base. *E*, "Sickle-hocked," angle of tarsus small. *F*, "Post-leg," angle of tarsus large, and "weak pastern," angle of metatarsophalangeal joint reduced. (From Ott RS: Vet Med/Small Anim Clinician, November 1976, pp 1592–1595.)

Occasionally, other structures whose nerve supply is from lumbosacral segments of spinal cord are affected. The terminal rectum and anus may become paralyzed so that fecal evacuation is by abdominal press. The urinary bladder may lose capacity to contract reflexly so that urination is by spillover. Tail muscles may become fully or partially paralyzed.

Vertebral osteophytosis/ankylosis/spondylosis as part of nutritional hypercalcitoninism may well be a contributing cause. Bone spicules encroaching upon the vertebral canal have been observed on rare occasions at necropsy in affected bulls. In most cases, however, no such specific lesions are evident. Other, more subtle, etiologies that are degenerative in nature at the central nervous system level may also cause this defect.

Progressive posterior paresis has a relatively high incidence among older bulls. The distribution among breeds, both beef and dairy, appears to be quite uniform. The average age of 66 affected bulls was 9.8 years. Only five were below 7 years of age.

"Postiness" ("Post-Leg"). This defect (Fig. 1*F*), in the severe form, is the major cause of more rear limb disease than any other abnormal conformation trait in mature bulls. In this condition the anatomic system (peroneus tertius and gastrocnemius muscles) that causes hock and stifle joints to flex or extend together is so structured that joints remain in perpetual extension. Postiness nearly always becomes evident bilaterally, often by 1 to 3 years of age.

The primary condition, a conformation defect, must be differentiated from acquired, secondary postiness, which may develop in older bulls either unilaterally or bilaterally. This appears to be a voluntary (reflex?) pain-sparing action on the part of the bull as a result of degenerative arthritis of the stifle joint. Localized hyaline cartilage destruction has been observed in association with secondary postiness but is not common in primary postiness.

In essentially all cases of primary postiness, the following sequelae occur at varying rates and degrees of severity. Pain, although not common in early primary postiness, is evidenced by the affected animal's shifting of weight bearing from limb to limb. The first signs of pain may be accompanied by or preceded by increased synovial fluid in the tarsal joints. Later, as tarsitis becomes chronic, there is often development of osseous periarthritis, which, together with local edema, results in a rather postlike limb largely devoid of the normal angles, depressions and protuberances of the tarsus. Often, degenerative processes occur in the stifle joints as sequelae to lesions of the tarsus. Primary postiness rarely improves. Typically, the degenerative processes initiated by the primary fault continue unabated but at varying rates. Rarely does a bull whose tarsus is too straight remain functionally normal throughout life.

Only 2 of 37 bulls with primary postiness cited in Table 1 were of beef breeds, even though beef bull experience constitutes 24 per cent of the total bull years cited.

As with other conformation defects, the inheritance of these tendencies is complex. In the case of primary postiness, which is usually functionally debilitating, verterinarians should maintain a strong position against employing such bulls in extensive breeding programs.

Spastic Syndrome ("Crampiness," "Stretches," Neuromuscular Spasticity). This is a disease of mature dairy and dual purpose cattle. It is characterized by intermittent bilateral tonic spasms of skeletal muscle groups in the standing animal. Early in the course of the disease or in cases in which signs are slight, the rear limb muscles may be involved either unilaterally or bilaterally. Anterior progression of muscular contractions usually occurs. Such progression may vary in rate but involves all axial and trunk muscles. In the severest form, all muscles appear to be involved in contractions, causing an appearance of opisthotonus.

Spasms do not occur during recumbency but are most prominent on rising, while the bull is adapting to weight-bearing. Pain stimuli from limbs severely aggravate the signs. These and other clinical observations strongly suggest that the primary defect in this disease involves the highly complex myotatic-postural reflex system.

The aggravation of muscle contractions by pain and adaptation to weight-bearing is more readily explained if an assumption is made that spastic syndrome is the result of impaired spinal cord connections and interpretations of the afferents of the myotatic reflex, resulting in abnormally increased efferents. That is, both pain stimuli and stimulation of muscle spindle fibers by stretching, such as in weight-bearing, increase afferent stimuli. In the case of bulls with functionally abnormal cord connections, as in spastic syndrome, increased afferent stimuli result in abnormal, highly exaggerated efferent stimuli and characteristic involuntary contractions of skeletal muscles.

It has been frequently observed that some bulls, usually younger animals, show typical signs of spastic syndrome only in the presence of severely painful hoof lesions such as traumatic or infectious laminitis. This has been interpreted to mean that such bulls have latent spastic syndrome, which may surface as frank disease with advancing age. Thus, an indicator of sorts exists for latent spastic syndrome.

The mere fact that spastic syndrome is a disease exclusively of dairy and dual-purpose cattle suggests heritability in some form. A familial occurrence of the disease has been reported.[8] In an extensive statistical study conclusions were drawn that suggested inheritance for spastic syndrome ("crampy") by a single recessive factor with incomplete penetrance. However, in this study precise diagnoses were apparently not available, and bulls were included in the survey whose afflictions were variably descriptive of progressive posterior paralysis and polyarthritis in addition to spastic syndrome ("crampy"), the disease under consideration. Accurate conclusions concerning inheritance of a tendency for a single disease simply cannot be drawn from source material that includes at least three disease entities.

Semen from the 55 bulls with spastic syndrome has been sold for use in artificial insemination (AI). Conservatively estimated, more than 100,000 female offspring have been sired by these affected bulls. In spite of a feedback system designed to ferret out and to report unusual offspring, records show no such reports for spastic syndrome in offspring of these bulls. It is apparent, therefore, that neither the incidence nor severity of spastic syndrome among daughters of afflicted bulls has warranted reporting by herd owners.

Over a 30-year period the following working hypothesis has been found very useful in confronting the question of heritability of spastic syndrome. Since the expression of the disease is variable and is modified by factors such as age, standing position and pain and since definitive evidence for inheritance following a predictable pattern is lacking, the mode of inheritance is considered to be highly complex and therefore difficult to elucidate. Consequently, bulls with spastic syndrome are handled on an individual basis. Whenever signs of the disease occur at a relatively young age, are uncomplicated by pain and are typical, severe and worsening, the problem is self-limiting in that potency impairment is or will soon be complete. All such bulls should be held out of extensive breeding programs.

In cases in which onset of spastic syndrome occurs in older bulls (often associated with pain of arthritis or other painful limb afflictions and therefore amenable to treatment with analgesic drugs), the disease is handled as though it has no ramifications beyond the specific bull involved. Potency is maintained with pain-relieving drugs such as phenylbutazone.

Spastic Paresis (Elso Heel). This disease has some clinical signs and part of its name in common with spastic syndrome. Therefore, it seems appropriate to consider spastic paresis briefly from a standpoint of differential diagnosis. Spastic paresis is most common in European Friesian cattle. It is uncommon in the United States but has been reported in Holstein, Ayrshire, Angus and Beef Shorthorn breeds. Clinical signs are most frequently unilateral. Onset is rare after 1 year of age, but it may occur within a few weeks of birth. The disease is characterized and explainable by chronic contraction of gastrocnemius and superficial digital flexor muscles. As a result, hock and stifle joints are typically maintained in near full extension, holding the fibular tarsal bone and its os calcis in close apposition to the distal tibia. Partial separation of the os calcis from the fibular tarsal bone gives an increased area of reduced radiopacity at its epiphyseal plate.

Tremulous muscle contractions are present in the affected limb, especially on arising. The limb appears shorter, may not touch the ground, often swings in a pendulous manner and usually points anterolaterally. Symptomatic surgery, in which either the achilles tendon or branches from the tibial nerve to the gastrocnemius muscle are interrupted, usually gives marked relief.

Relief has also resulted through surgical transection of dorsal roots of spinal nerves supplying gastrocnemius muscle (desafferentation). This suggests that the primary neurophysiologic defect in spastic paresis is, as suggested herein for spastic syndrome, an exaggerated efferent response in the myotatic (stretch) reflex.

Sire-daughter matings provide firm evidence that spastic paresis is not transmitted by a simple recessive mechanism.

It has been determined that calves with spastic paresis display deviations from normal of some components of cerebrospinal fluid. The most significant deviation may be a substantial reduction of homovanillic acid, the main metabolite of the neurotransmitter dopamine.

SPECIAL EXAMINATION OF THE REPRODUCTIVE ORGANS

Internalia

The pelvic and abdominal genital organs constitute the internalia (Figs. 2 to 4).

The *vesicular glands* are readily examined by palpation on the anterior floor of the pelvic cavity. They converge posteriorly along with the ampullae ductus deferentes at the anterior end of pelvic urethral muscle at the point at which the body of the prostate gland is palpable. The vesicular glands lie just lateral to the ampullae ductus deferentes (Fig. 2). Their normal consistency is yielding and meaty, and their lobulated outlines are readily discernible.

Disease of the vesicular glands is restricted nearly exclusively to hypoplasia and aplasia, which are rare, and infectious conditions, which may be acute or chronic. Acute seminal vesiculitis may show all the signs of localized pelvic peritonitis. On palpation pain may be severe, and the affected glands may be found markedly enlarged and firm. Fibrin exudate on the peritoneum with subsequent organization may occur. Purulent exudate is consistently present in semen.

Chronic seminal vesiculitis, which may or may not follow an acute phase, is associated with persistent or intermittent purulent exudate in semen. Usually localized or generalized fibrosis and enlargement with loss of lobulation are present, but pain on palpation ordinarily is absent.

In young beef bulls under ranch conditions, the incidence of seminal vesiculitis has been found to be 2.4 per cent. Under conditions of an AI stud, the annual incidence was determined to be 1.3 and 0.7 per cent for bulls more than 1½ and less than 1½ years of age, respectively. Incidence was proportionately distributed among beef and dairy bulls.

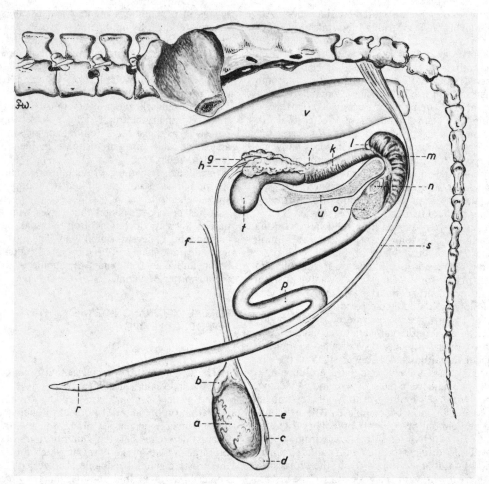

Figure 2. General view of genital organs of bull; left testis and spermatic cord have been removed. *(a)* Right testis, *(b)* head of epididymis, *(c)* body of epididymis, *(d)* tail of epididymis, *(e)* right ductus deferens, *(f)* mesorchium, *(g)* right ampulla ductus deferentes, *(h)* left vesicular gland, *(i)* body of prostate, *(k)* pelvic portion of urethra with urethralis muscle, *(l)* left bulbourethral gland, *(m)* left bulbospongiosus, *(n)* left crus penis (cut), *(o)* left ischiocavernosus (cut), *(p)* penis with sigmoid flexure, *(r)* glans penis, *(s)* retractor penis, *(t)* urinary bladder, *(u)* symphysis pelvis and *(v)* rectum. (From Blom E, Christensen NO: Skandinavisk Veterinartidskrift, 1947, pp 1–45.)

In young, group-housed bulls, seminal vesiculitis in some cases appears to be contagious. Transmission may be retrograde as a result of urethral contamination during homosexual activity. In most such cases, resolution occurs spontaneously but slowly. In older bulls, which more commonly are afflicted with chronic seminal vesiculitis, cure is rarely possible.

Etiological agents that have been reported are nonspecific opportunistic pathogens such as streptococci, staphylococci, actinobacilli, corynebacteria, mycoplasma and chlamydia or specific pathogens such as *Brucella abortus*, *Myobacterium bovis* and *Mycobacterium paratuberculosis*. Distressingly, infectious agents frequently are not isolated.

Surgical removal of offending vesicular glands has been performed with varying degrees of success, but results have mostly been poor.

The surgical principles that are violated by such a radical procedure are the following: (1) disruption

of the nerve supply to critical structures, (2) creation of a surgical field deep within the pelvic cavity such that hemorrhage is difficult to control and (3) automatic occurrence of septic inoculation upon incision of the infected gland.

The *ampullae ductus deferentes* are readily palpable in their entirety. They lie in the urogenital fold between the vesicular glands (Fig. 2). Their junction with the pelvic urethra at the body of the prostate may be dorsal to vesicular glands, as in Figure 6, or intermediate or ventral. Rarely do ampullae show hypoplasia or aplasia. If present, such anomalies are usually associated with defects of the other derivatives of the wolffian ducts. The incidence of segmental aplasia of the wolffian ducts has been reported as 0.56 per cent on necropsy specimens and 0.1 per cent on clinical specimens.

Clinically, ampullitis is not readily recognized; however, in bulls with a high incidence of seminal vesiculitis an equal or greater incidence of infection

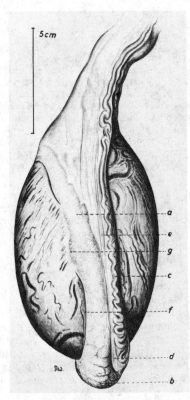

Figure 3. Left testis and epididymis from a 2-year-old bull, caudomedial view. *(a)* Body of epididymis, *(b)* tail of epididymis, *(c)* ductus deferens, *(d)* ligament of tail of epididymis (cut), *(e)* mesorchium (cut), *(f)* testicular bursa and *(g)* part of epididymis attached to testis; no testicular bursa is formed. (From Blom E, Christensen NO: Skandinavisk Veterinartidskrift, 1947, pp 1–45.)

Again, just as the sperm in semen represent the condition in the seminiferous tubules, the presence of cells other than sperm (COTS) in the fluid portion of semen indicates the condition of the tubular genital tract. Examination for COTS, therefore, is an important component of any genital examination.

The *inguinal rings* are easily palpable at a point 12 to 18 cm ventral to the deep inguinal lymph nodes. If the opening is too large, i.e., transmits three or more fingers, the animal is predisposed to inguinal hernia. Hereditary implications of enlarged inguinal rings may be of greater significance than the abnormality itself in an individual bull. Incidences of enlarged inguinal rings of 0.15 per cent and 0.11 per cent have been observed.

Externalia

Scrotum and Testes. Examination of the scrotum and testes is by visual inspection and palpation. The tunica dartos should be fully relaxed in warm

in the ampullae was found at necropsy. Müllerian cysts are rather commonly encountered in the urogenital fold of the interampullar space. Very rarely a uterus masculinus is found in the same location.

The *prostate gland* is composed of the palpable *body* and nonpalpable *pars disseminata*, which lies deep to the pelvic urethralis muscle (Fig. 2). Inflammatory processes have been identified at necropsy, but not clinically, in 43 per cent of bulls with a high incidence of seminal vesiculitis.

The *bulbourethral glands* (Fig. 2) are not palpable, being imbedded under the bulbospongiosus muscle. Thus, disease of these glands, determined clinically, has not been reported. However, at necropsy of bulls with a 49 per cent incidence of seminal vesiculitis, 15 per cent showed bulbourethral adenitis. A significant anatomic aspect of the bulbourethral glands is the urethral recess, which is formed in the dorsal wall of the urethra at the ischial arch by a fold of urethral mucosa. The excretory ducts of the bulbourethral glands enter the urethra at the free end of this mucosal fold. Because of its location and structure, the urethral recess forms an obstruction to passage of a sound or catheter into the urinary bladder via the urethra.

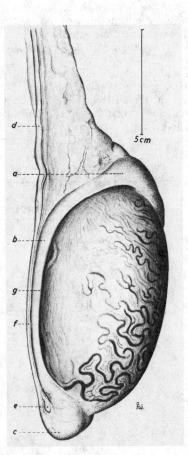

Figure 4. Right testis and epididymis from 3-year-old bull, caudolateral view. *(a)* head of epididymis, *(b)* body of epididymis, *(c)* tail of epididymis, *(d)* ductus deferens, *(e)* ligament of tail of epididymis (cut), *(f)* mesorchium (cut) and *(g)* testicular bursa. (From Blom E, Christensen NO: Skandinavisk Veterinartidskrift, 1947, pp 1–45.)

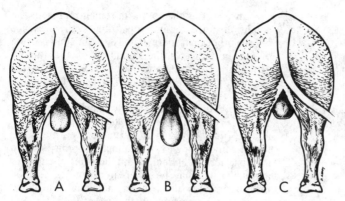

Figure 5. Scrotal configurations. *A,* Flat-sided scrotum associated with moderate-sized testes. *B,* Normal scrotum. Testes are usually large. *C,* Short, ventrally tapered scrotum, often associated with small testes. (From Cates WE: Observations on scrotal circumference and its relationship to classification of bulls. Proceedings of the Annual Meeting of the Society for Theriogenology. Cheyenne, Wyoming, September 1975.)

weather, revealing a scrotal "neck" that is trim and is free of fat and of varicoceles of the pampiniform plexus. The scrotal abaxial contour should be convex (Fig. 5), and the relaxed scrotal wall should be thin and pliable. Adhesions involving visceral and parietal layers of tunica vaginalis propria should not exist between testes and scrotum.

The normally suspended testis hangs in the scrotum so that the body of the epididymis is located caudomedially and the head of the epididymis lies on the proximoanterolateral surface. Thus, the view of the left testis in Figure 3 is from the caudomedial aspect.

Rarely, there is malformation of the scrotum by differential growth of the scrotal wall or septum. Typically, the former results in an abbreviated caudal scrotal wall so that the testes are unilaterally or bilaterally held in a near horizontal position. This condition seems mainly restricted to young beef bulls. A shortened scrotal septum results in a midventral scrotal cleft. In older bulls the scrotum, if unpigmented, seems uniquely susceptible to "blood warts," which are varicose dilatations of scrotal veins.[9]

Ventral scrotal scab formation as a sequela to scrotal frostbite is substantial evidence that supercooling of the testis has occurred and that resultant transitory (at best) testicular degeneration has taken place.

The normal left testicle with the epididymis and proximal ductus deferens is well illustrated in Figure 3. Note that testicular length is roughly 2 times its diameter.

The mean testicular size in mature bulls, both beef and dairy, when expressed as length and diameter, is approximately 14 to 16 cm × 7 to 8 cm. Expressed as scrotal circumference (SC), testicular size in such bulls is 41 to 44 cm (Table 1). The

Table 1. Changes in Testicular Size in Holstein and Angus Bulls with Age

	Scrotal Circumference			
	Holstein		Angus	
Age in Months	No. of Measurements	Measurement (cm)	No. of Measurements	Measurement (cm)
6–12	371	30.0 ± 3.3*	3	33.5 ± 3.1*
12–18	696	34.9 ± 2.4	19	36.1 ± 3.0
18–24	597	37.4 ± 2.2	19	40.1 ± 4.0
24–30	510	39.1 ± 2.9	43	40.0 ± 2.7
30–36	488	40.1 ± 2.3	37	39.5 ± 3.2
36–42	466	40.8 ± 2.7	38	40.6 ± 2.5
42–48	431	41.2 ± 2.5	18	40.5 ± 3.1
48–54	375	41.6 ± 2.5	25	40.3 ± 3.1
54–60	361	41.7 ± 2.9	8	39.7 ± 2.5
60–72	616	42.1 ± 2.7	16	40.0 ± 2.3
72–84	307	42.6 ± 2.7	21	41.0 ± 2.4
84–96	219	42.6 ± 3.9	21	41.1 ± 2.9
96–108	158	43.3 ± 2.5	23	42.1 ± 2.3
108–120	116	43.5 ± 2.6	18	42.1 ± 2.3
120–132	82	43.9 ± 2.7	12	41.6 ± 2.0
132–144	62	43.5 ± 2.8	8	40.0 ± 2.9
144–156	30	43.1 ± 2.6	6	40.3 ± 2.1
156–168	16	41.5 ± 2.7	3	41.0 ± 3.0
168–180	6	41.8 ± 3.9	1	39.0
Total	5909		339	

*Mean ± standard deviation. (From Coulter GH, Larson LL, Foote RH: J Anim Sci 41:1383, 1975.)

normal consistency of the testes is turgescent yet resilient.

Testicular hypoplasia has been determined to be heritable in Swedish Highland cattle. An association has been made between testicular hypoplasia and autosomal secondary constrictions, as determined by cytogenetic studies. By definition, testicular hypoplasia connotes both small size and spermatogenic malfunction. The latter, if slight, is often indistinguishable on histologic examination from testicular degeneration, to which bulls with slight degrees of testicular hypoplasia are particularly susceptible. The difference between these two conditions may, under some circumstances, only be in definition or underlying cause, and the diagnosis must be based upon history, clinical findings and evaluation of repeated semen samples. Incidence has been reported to be 0.2 per cent, 1.3 per cent and 0.3 per cent, depending on populations studied.

Cryptorchidism is of low frequency in bulls. Two comprehensive studies reveal a near identical incidence of 0.1 per cent. Evidence for heritability has been cited.

Testicular degeneration is the partial or complete failure of the spermatogenic epithelium to proceed normally with spermatogenesis. It may be transitory or permanent. As the degree of degeneration increases, palpable and tonometric testicular flaccidity and the numbers of spermatocytes, spermatogonia and malformed spermatozoa in ejaculated semen increase as well. In gradual testicular degeneration, such as in aging, there is concurrent fibrosis of the seminiferous tubules. The products of degeneration become calcified. With rapid but permanent degeneration, fibrosis takes place after the degenerative process, and the connective tissue itself may become calcified.[9]

Etiological factors regarded as significant in testicular degeneration are (1) elevation of testicular temperature, whether caused by local or environmental factors; (2) super-cooling, such as occurs in scrotal frostbite; (3) circulatory ischemia to the testes, whether due to trauma or to degenerative vascular lesions; (4) congenital occlusion of efferent tubules—as spermatogenesis commences at puberty, and back pressure and edema of the testes cause megalotestis and complete testicular degeneration; (5) autoimmunity; (6) toxins; (7) gonadotropin deficiencies—actual difference between testicular degeneration due to gonadotropin deficiency and testicular hypoplasia may be only a matter of degree and (8) viral infection.

Orchitis-periorchitis is usually unilateral. An incidence of 0.45 per cent has been reported in an extensive survey of young ranch beef bulls, and an annual incidence of 0.12 per cent has been recorded in bulls maintained under conditions of an AI stud. If source infection is hematogenous, a testis is infected first, but periorchitis often eventually occurs. If infection is retrograde via the ductus deferens, the corresponding epididymis is usually infected first. Often periorchitis, which also involves the peritoneum, is primary. In acute cases classic inflammatory signs are present, followed by testicular degeneration, which ordinarily is complete. In no instance is the prognosis other than poor. Unilateral castration has been used to retain function of the contralateral gland.

Brucella abortus (including Strain 19), *Corynebacterium pyogenes,* streptococci and other bacterial opportunists are among the etiological agents for orchitis-periorchitis. Figure 6 illustrates an eventual lesion in which adhesion about the distal testis and tail of the epididymis has occurred. Rarely, abscessation is a final outcome.

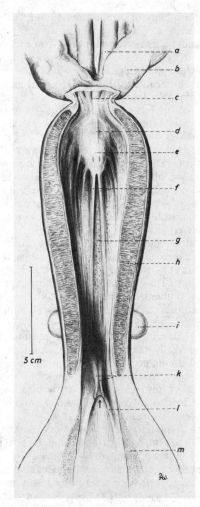

Figure 6. The proximal part of urethra opened ventrally. *(a)* Ampulla ductus deferentis, *(b)* vesicular gland, *(c)* neck of bladder, *(d)* urethral crest, *(e)* colliculus seminalis with ejaculatory orifices, *(f)* frenula of colliculus seminalis, *(g)* excretory orifices from pars disseminata of prostate, *(h)* urethralis, *(i)* bulbourethral gland loosened and moved laterally, *(k)* excretory ducts from bulbourethral glands distended by injection of plaster of Paris, *(l)* the free distal border of the mucosal fold forming urethral recess into which the arrow points and *(m)* corpus spongiosum. (From Blom E, Christensen NO: Skandinavisk Veterinartidskrift, 1947, pp 1–45.)

Testicular tumors diagnosed clinically are extremely rare. However, at necropsy a considerable incidence of primary testicular tumors in aging bulls has been reported.[9]

Hydrocele, the accumulation of transudate within the processus vaginalis, has been observed but is extremely infrequent in bulls.

Hematocele, traumatically induced by testicular rupture in group-housed bulls, is the most common traumatic disease of the scrotum and testes in bulls so maintained. Typically, there is extreme distention of the affected scrotum. Resolution is by organization of the blood clot with complete fibrosis, resulting in acquired monorchism.

The variability of fertility among bulls with normal potency, i.e., semen delivery system function, is dependent upon the number of normal sperm produced in the testes and made available to the tails of the epididymides, from which final delivery is made at ejaculation. In turn, the total number of sperm ejaculated is related to the adequacy and amount of the parenchymal mass of the testes and the functional normalcy of the efferent ducts and epididymides.

Thus, clinicians, after determining that all components of the scrotum and its contents are present and free of obvious abnormalities, have at their disposal only the characteristics of size and consistency with which to substantiate data regarding fertility/infertility derived from laboratory findings on collected semen.

Scrotal circumference (SC) is the most easily reproducible single measurement of testicular mass. Table 1 is very useful to the clinician, as it gives SC averages for Holstein and Angus bulls at age increments of 6 months between age 6 and 180 months. Other studies are in close agreement with these findings.

As a clinical guideline in interpretation of SC data, especially if obtained prior to sexual maturity, a scrotal circumference that is more than one standard deviation less than average indicates a marked deficiency in testicular mass. At two standard deviations less than average, a clinical diagnosis of "hypoplasia" is mandatory.

Slight asymmetry in testicular size is very common. If size ratio exceeds 60:40, unilateral hypoplasia may not be adequately reflected by scrotal circumference. Obviously, scrotal circumference for unusually spherical or elongated testes must be modified by an appropriate decreasing or increasing factor, respectively, to reflect testicular mass accurately.

Within limits, the degree and significance of testicular turgescence, flaccidity and fibrosis can be readily determined by palpation by experienced clinicians. However, correct diagnosis can be made with assurance in the absence of semen evaluation only in cases of testicular degeneration that are severe and acute or those that are severe and chronic with fibrosis. In cases in which degeneration is moderate and acute or is moderate and chronic with fibrosis, there must be supporting data concerning semen quality for a definitive diagnosis.

A more precise measure of testicular consistency may be obtained with a tonometer. If used properly, a highly repeatable number that characterizes the degree of turgescence will be obtained. Consistently high relationships have been found between tonometer ratio and semen quality as determined in the laboratory. Used in conjunction with palpation, this instrument provides useful points of reference for the clinician. Testicular degeneration with fibrosis will, obviously, give a false-high tonometer reading for which the correct interpretation is possible only after careful palpation.

Epididymis. An epididymis (Figs. 2, 3, 4) is palpable in its entirety. The head is easily recognized as a flattened structure, more firm than the testis, on the proximoanterolateral surface of the testis (Fig. 4). The body is readily exposed for palpation by raising the contralateral testis. The tail is composed of the terminal epididymal tubule and mostly, but not always, protrudes well beyond the ventral limits of the testis.

The epididymis is a single, tightly convoluted tube, 30 to 35 m in length, whose diameter increases as it progresses through the arbitrary segments designated head, body and tail. Most disorders of this structure, therefore, are related to nonpatency, the cause of which may be segmental aplasia, trauma or infection with cicatrix formation.

Spermatocele is often a sequela to epididymal occlusion for whatever reason. It is a cystic dilation of an epididymis, with accumulation of inspissated sperm immediately proximal to the occlusion. Since efferent ducts of the testes have the capability of resorbing noncellular products of the seminiferous tubules, back pressure and resultant testicular degeneration are delayed. Congenital occlusion of efferent ducts, however, results in rapid back pressure producing a large, markedly turgescent testis with complete testicular degeneration at the onset of spermatogenesis.

Eventually, most spermatoceles develop into spermatic granulomas as the epididymal wall degenerates and permits direct contact of sperm with epididymal stroma, whereupon a granulomatous reaction is elicited.[9] These, plus inflammatory lesions, constitute the vast majority of palpable conditions of the epididymis.

Penis and Prepuce. The penis and prepuce are best examined at the time of semen collection with an artificial vagina. Penile protrusion for examination may also be accomplished with an electroejaculator or with regional anesthesia of the pudendal nerves. When visual observation of the penis and free preputial membrane is not possible, these structures are readily palpable.

Failure of full penile development, especially in bulls with "paunchy" abdomens or in bulls that fail to properly flex vertebral joints at penile intromission, results in impotency due to inadequate penile protrusion.

Other forms of impotency caused by failure of normal penile protrusion are the following:

1. Lack of erection with normal mounting. This is extremely rare (annual rate of 0.02 per cent).

2. Congenital persistence of the penile frenulum. This is found most frequently in Beef Shorthorn and polled beef bulls.

3. Phimosis caused by adhesions as a result of (a) traumatic, physical or chemical injury; (b) non-specific balanoposthitis, e.g., caused by filth and/or trauma or (c) specific balanoposthisis, such as in infectious pustular balanoposthitis (IPB).

4. Large penile papillofibromata.

5. Penile fracture with a hematoma and its organization.

Avulsion of the free preputial membrane at the fornix during intromission into an artificial vagina, usually with copious preputial hemorrhage, is by far the most common preputial injury among bulls in AI. Successful surgical repair is readily achieved in the standing bull under pudendal nerve block, provided early closure is possible.

A deviated or corkscrew penis created by abaxial tensions at erection by the apical ligament results in impotency at coitus but usually not for service of an artificial vagina.

Patency of the tunica albuginea of the glans penis with blood loss at erection (a very difficult lesion to handle surgically) creates a situation in which ejaculated semen is consistently contaminated with blood.

In bulls of Brahman breeding, pendulous prepuce coupled with chronic eversion of free preputial membrane, predisposes such animals to paraphimosis as a result of the vicious circle of trauma, edema, increased trauma and increased edema. This conformation defect frequently requires surgical correction in order to maintain potency of the affected bull. Polled bulls, however, which tend to have chronically everted free preputial membranes with a sheath that is not pendulant, do not seem to have an increased incidence of traumatic preputial disease.

CLINICAL ASPECTS OF SEMEN COLLECTION

An attempt will be made here to discuss briefly the art of semen collection under other than ideal circumstances and to point out the unqualified usefulness of semen collection via the artificial vagina (AV) in the clinical interpretation of potency-related neuromusculoskeletal function.

The employment of the AV makes collection of a physiological semen sample as a "biopsy" for study of spermatogenic membrane an extremely simple procedure. Also, it creates a confrontation between bull and veterinarian, enabling clinical evaluation of nonspermatogenic components of bull fertility—namely, potency and libido, the interrelationships of which are depicted in the following outline:

Bull Fertility—fertility in the larger sense.*

Spermatogenesis—capacity to produce optimal numbers of sperm with high fertilizing capability.

Potency—ability to readily deliver sperm to anterior vagina, natural or artificial. This requires:

A. Physiological and physical soundness of the tubular components and accessory glands of the genital system.

B. Integrity and coordination of the neuromusculoskeletal system and hooves (NMSH).

C. Libido—sexual desire:
   1. Innate libido—genetically conferred.
   2. Environmental modifiers of innate libido:
      a. Painful disease of NMSH.
      b. Nutrition—malnutrition or obesity.
      c. Age.
      d. Poor management practices that have produced pain or anxiety at coitus or at semen collections or that have resulted in sexual exhaustion.

Freedom from infectious agents—if present in the bull may impair fertility in cows/heifers similarly infected at coitus or from AI with contaminated semen.

Semen collection with an electroejaculator reveals partial information concerning spermatogenesis and essentially no information regarding potency.

Leading, Restraint and Safety. All bulls must be considered extremely dangerous with but few individual and breed exceptions. The safest and most suitable means of leading bulls is to use two 15- to 25-foot light and flexible, yet strong, ropes of ⅝-inch braided nylon. One, for restraining, should be tied in a bowline around the horns or neck, and then passed through a strong nose ring. The other, for leading, may be tied directly to the nose ring.

It is an illusion that mature aggresive bulls can be safely handled with a bull staff. A staff requires the handler to be much too close to a bull's head. Should the bull make a fast move or lower his head so that control is lost, the staff can become a deadly instrument for impaling, entangling or flailing the handler.

---

*Effective bull fertility, obviously, is equally dependent upon normal spermatogenesis, normal potency and freedom from venereal or semen-borne pathogens. Availability for ejaculation and delivery of spermatozoa in optimal numbers and of superb fertilizing capacity has no fertility value unless the spermatozoa can readily be delivered at coitus or through AI to a site in a fertile cow/heifer at which their capacity to fertilize may be realized. Conversely, vigorous libido coupled with virile potency contributes nothing to effective bull fertility other than to insure the proper delivery of the spermatozoa. Likewise, if high quality semen is produced and properly delivered but becomes contaminated with pathogens from a diseased bull, the resultant infertility may be as complete as though fertilization had not occurred. It is important in all fertility/infertility contemplations to be able to conceptualize the interrelationships of the male and female fertility components, which together make up the actual, expressed fertility.

Under no circumstances must one get caught in a corner from which there is no escape when a bull attacks.

English beef bulls are usually not aggressive; neither are they usually accustomed to being handled by ropes. With such bulls, the practical solution may be to use no restraint, or at most a rope halter, on a bull broken to a lead.

"Mount" Animal and Semen Collection Site. A cow in estrus, obviously, is most suitable as a "mount." But an in-heat cow is seldom available when needed. Therefore, substitution with a sturdy, nonestrous cow that is easy to handle is often necessary.

Suitable breeding chutes are rarely available for confining the "mount" animal. Characteristically, chutes on farms or ranches have been built for natural mating. Some have been modified for semen collection by people unfamiliar with hazards of semen collection with an AV. Such stocks generally are constructed with maximum emphasis on bull-escape prevention. Chute side panels and approach alley walls are high, and openings for the person handling the AV are small and in the wrong location and often are perfectly designed to enhance to the ultimate degree the arm-breaking hazard for the semen collector. In most cases the procedure is safer, and opportunity for success is greater, at an improvised collection site than in an improperly constructed chute-alley.

The desirable elements of an improvised collection site are the following: (1) Sidewise and back and forth movement of the "mount" must be restricted; (2) the ground surface must not be excessively smooth, slippery, rough or muddy; (3) there must be space available for freedom of movement and escape by the collector and (4) bull handlers must be able to maintain a fence between themselves and the bull. One arrangement that provides most of these desirable elements is to halter-tie a "mount" snugly into a corner of a sturdy board fence that is readily available to the bull.

In this set-up, the fence on the far side from the collector serves to prevent the "mount" from moving excessively away from the collector and also serves as a safety rail for the bull handlers. It is often necessary to hand-hold a nose-lead in the "mount's" nares to keep attention away from what must seem to the nonestrous cow as an impending disaster.

An assistant on the "mount's" near side can be very useful in preventing excessive "mount" movement toward the collector by firmly holding the end of a blunt stick or bar into the "mount's" midthorax.

With "mount" and collection site thus arranged and the collector ready with a properly prepared AV in hand, the bull is brought in with a lead rope, while the restraining rope is being paid out from a hitch around a strong post or plank. The handlers must always maintain at least a 20-foot distance from a bulls' head unless working over a sturdy fence.

In order to obtain a physiological ejaculate, it is essential that the bull be restrained from mounting until his penis is partially erect and a flow of seminal fluid from accessory sex glands is well underway. During this period of 5 to 10 minutes of "teasing," it is well not to permit direct nuzzling of the vulva of the nonestrous "mount." This is in an effort to delay full realization by the bull that the cow is nonestrous. During this preparatory period, the veterinarian-collector must utilize every opportunity to evaluate the bull for lameness, coordination, gait, conformation and intensity of libido.

At the moment when the bull shows partial erection, i.e., the glans penis protrudes from its prepuce, or the glans penis distends the prepuce near its orifice, and there is liberal dripping of seminal fluid, along with display of willingness to mount, the handlers should, on the veterinarian's command, give the bull freedom but should keep the restraining rope anchored. They should be especially watchful for a fast move by the bull toward the collector. The attendant at the "mount's" head should, at the same time, place some tension on the nose-lead while the blunt stick or bar is being placed more snugly into the mid-seventh to eighth intercostal space by a person so assigned.

To avoid natural intromission, as the bull mounts the collector moves in quickly, but quietly, from a point lateral to and slightly behind the bull.

The penis is gently deflected laterally toward the collector with near cupped hand on the distal sheath.*

As the bull makes probing movements with his penis, the artificial vagina is placed in direct line with the diverted penis, which is permitted to probe the AV. If consistency, temperature, lubrication and pressure of the artificial vagina closely approximate the bovine vagina, the bull will typically enter his penis deeply and forcefully into the AV. Ejaculation with semen emission occurs within 1 second of the time that intromission commences. The bull should be permitted to retract his penis from the AV voluntarily. Frequently, this is not done prior to dismounting, in which instance it may be necessary to follow the bull down, with the AV remaining on the penis, as dismounting occurs. At this point also, bull handlers must be especially alert to prevent the bull from making a pass at the collector.

Evaluative observations regarding a bull's potency are best made during the act of semen collection. Was libido intense, adequate or subnormal? If apparent libido was subnormal, could this be

---

*It may be desirable not to permit the bull to find the AV at first mounting but to allow him to make repeated probings with the penis diverted away, so the "mount" is not contacted. This is termed a false-mount. Such precoital stimulation has the advantage of increasing sperm numbers in a prospective ejaculate and permitting closer scrutiny by the veterinarian of the erected penis and of the bull's mounting behavior. The obvious disadvantage of a false-mount is that if a bull is not accustomed to mounting without attaining ejaculation, the opportunity for obtaining a subsequent semen collection may be lost, especially if conditions for collection are less than optimal.

attributed to low innate libido or to normal libido, environmentally modified, as previously described?

Is the bull an athlete? Was mounting accomplished readily without the bull's partially supporting his weight by employing his head and neck in order to "slide" onto the "mount"? A bull's need for such support may be evidence of pain in vertebral, pelvic or limb joints. Was the "mount" animal firmly grasped with the bull's forelimbs? Was intromission vigorous, and was it made without hesitation? If not, could the failure be attributed to an improperly prepared AV or to the imperfect coordination by the collector of the bull's probing movements with accessibility of the AV for the bull's "finding"?

In the evaluation of properly collected semen it cannot be overemphasized that semen is at its highest quality the moment it leaves the external urethral orifice. It is, therefore, axiomatic that meaningful semen evaluation is impossible unless semen is ejaculated into, and maintained in, an environment that closely simulates that from which sperm cells were ejaculated. Semen must be handled out of direct sunlight, at body temperature and in an environment free of filth and deleterious foreign ions. Microscopic examination of the semen must not be unduly delayed.

EXAMINATION FOR SPECIFIC INFECTIOUS DISEASES OF BULLS

The subject of venereal or semen-borne diseases of bulls, as well as other (emerging?) diseases of special concern in examination of bulls, such as blue tongue, bovine leukosis, chlamydial infections and the ubiquitous pathogens, has recently been reviewed.[3] Therefore, cursory discussion only seems indicated here, with emphasis on testing methods for bulls.

Bovine Tuberculosis. Full consideration must be given to tuberculosis in the health evaluation of bulls. Not only can *Mycobacterium bovis* be transmitted from an infected bull to contact cattle via the usual respiratory-alimentary route, but in the case of urogenital tuberculosis, the infection can be transmitted at coitus and by artificial insemination.

The insidious nature of bovine tuberculosis and the inherent inaccuracy of the intradermal test when applied diagnostically to a single animal demand employment of additional testing methods in order to be certain that the animal is disease-free.

In addition to the intradermal test (preferably comparative cervical) of the bull in question, it is important to obtain a complete history about herd additions, outside contacts by the bull and recent herd test results. If recent and frequent complete herd tests have not been done, such testing often is essential in arriving at a diagnosis for the bull.

Bovine Brucellosis. A battery of effective seriologic tests are available for determining the brucellosis status of cattle. Of particular interest in bulls is the need to determine whether or not infection of the genital organs has occurred, resulting in liberation of infective organisms in semen. It has been established that the semen plasma tube agglutination test identifies genital infection with discharge of purulent material and infectious organisms in the semen earlier and with higher titer than do serologic tests. Bulls with negative serologic findings but which were shedding brucella organisms in semen have been identified.[4, 13]

The semen plasma tube test, therefore, is most critical and meaningful in determining the brucellosis disease status of bulls of semen-producing age and must be a part of every bull examination, along with appropriate serologic brucella tests, herd disease history evaluation and herd test results for the disease.

Bull calves should not be vaccinated for brucellosis with Strain 19 vaccine. Vaccination may destroy bull's fertility by infecting genital organs, and Strain 19 may be shed in semen from the infected organs.

Bovine Campylobacteriosis and Bovine Venereal Trichomoniasis. Diagnosis in the bull of these well-established, true venereal diseases of cattle depends largely upon obtaining an adequate sample from the fornix-glans penis area of the prepuce. Unless the bull has had at least 4 days without sexual activity to permit population build-up of organisms lost at coitus or semen collection, opportunity for obtaining a reliable sample is reduced. Necessary assurance that these infectious agents are not present in the genital organs of bulls may be achieved only if adequate preputial specimens are obtained and competently examined on three or more occasions during a 3- to 4-week period. ·

Of importance is the fact that it was possible to create and to maintain herds of AI semen donor bulls totally free of *Campylobacter fetus* only after instituting dihydrostreptomycin preputial (10 ml 50 per cent solution) and subcutaneous (22 mg/kg of body weight) treatments as described by Seger[11] on all bulls.

A sampling system has been developed that enables a veterinarian readily to obtain simultaneously useful samples for examination for both *Campylobacter fetus* and *Trichomonas foetus*.

The disposable sample collecting device (Fig. 7*D*) is composed of a plastic preputial sampling pipette (Fig. 7*A*) within a plastic sheath outfitted with a break-through cap (Fig. 7*B*) so that the sampling pipette is protected during preputial entry and passage to the fornix. A sanitized 1-ounce rubber bulb (Fig. 7*C*) is attached to the exposed end immediately prior to use.

In preparation for obtaining the required smegma sample the envelope is removed, and the unit is passed to within 10 cm of the glans penis. With the plastic protection sheath fixed in this position, the aspirating pipette is popped through the cap and brought to the area of the preputial fornix.

The actual technique for picking up smegma from the recesses of the convoluted skin of the glans and fornix is by aspiration. While diligently and firmly

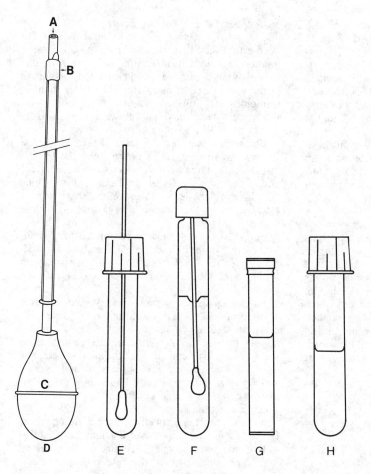

Figure 7. Apparatus and media used in preputial sample collection, transport, and culture. *A,* Plastic sampling pipette. *B,* Plastic sheath with breakthrough cap. (*A* and *B* sterilized in plastic envelope available from Continental Plastic Corp., Delavan, WI.) *C,* Rubber bulb, 1 oz capacity. *D,* Sampling device assembled. Plastic envelope not shown. *E,* Sterile plastic vial with swab. *F,* Modified Stuart's carrier medium with inoculating swab in place. *G,* Sterile physiological saline in 8 ml plastic tube for *Trichomonas foetus* sample transport. *H,* thyoglycollate or Diamond's medium in plastic vial for *T. foetus* culture.

massaging the glans with one hand, the rubber bulb is compressed and released successively with the other hand. This is done while simultaneously moving the aspiration pipette back and forth with its tip in close apposition with, and sometimes lightly scraping, the glans and fornix area. Fifteen to 30 such strokes are required to obtain a good sample.

Prior to removal from the prepuce, the aspiration pipette is withdrawn into the plastic sheath. The entire device is removed from the prepuce maintaining this configuration until transfer of the sample. It is important to place samples promptly into respective carrier/culture media.

First, a portion of the sample (approximately three drops) destined to be cultured for *C. fetus venerealis* is best expelled into the bottom of a sterile vial (Fig. 7*E*). The remainder, to be examined for *T. foetus,* is flushed into 3 to 4 ml sterile physiological saline in an 8 ml test tube (Fig. 7*G*). This smegma inoculum should be sufficient to create marked turbidity of the saline. If direct microscopic examination for *T. foetus* is not intended, the sample may be gently flushed directly into the upper layer of *T. foetus* culture medium (Fig. 7*H*). (Details for *T. foetus* examination/culture are described after those for *C. fetus venerealis.*)

The *C. fetus venerealis* sample may be transported to the laboratory in any of several suitable transport media. Stuart's,[29] Clark's[13, 35] and Selective Enrich-

ment Transport (SET)[18] are described in the footnote on the opposite page.

Inoculation into Stuart's medium should be done *immediately* after collection and is best accomplished by absorbing the sample into the sterile cotton swab (Fig. 7*E*) and then stab-inoculating it to a depth of 4 to 5 cm, where the swab should remain until removed in the laboratory (Fig. 7*F*). Stuart's medium is best stored at refrigerator temperature but should be warmed to room temperature for inoculation and transport.

Clark's medium is a bovine serum enrichment medium requiring microaerophilic conditions for full effectiveness. Properly employed, this medium maintains viability of *C. fetus venerealis* for 72 to 96 hours at room temperature. The need to maintain the medium in a microaerophilic environment renders it somewhat cumbersome to use, especially under field conditions. For example, in order for a sample, absorbed onto a sterile swab or placed in a sterile vial, to be inoculated it is necessary first to prepare a fluid suspension of the smegma suitable for air (O_2)-free injection into the sealed vial containing Clark's medium.

In SET medium, as with Stuart's, the smegma-soaked cotton swab (Fig. 7*E*) is used for inoculation by breaking it aseptically into the anaerobic culture tube. Prompt and tight restoppering is important. Inoculation and transport should be done at room temperature. Under these conditions, viability of *C. fetus venerealis* can be expected to be maintained in SET for up to 5 days while in transit. Laboratory culture procedures for *C. fetus venerealis* have been competently described by Foley and colleagues[7] and Stalheim and colleagues.[14]

The *T. foetus* sample, which has been placed into sterile saline, must be maintained at room temperature and must be permitted to settle for at least 1 hour. Centrifugation is contraindicated. For direct microscopic evaluation remove 1 or 2 drops of sediment with a sterile pipette and spread onto one-half of a microscopic slide. Do not coverslip. Examine this entire sample systematically at 100 × in reduced light. Proper examination will take more than 10 minutes. Repeat. The entire remainder of the sedimented sample is then layered onto an appropriate culture medium (Fig. 7*H*). Either modified Thioglycollate Broth Medium (TBM) or modified Diamond's Medium (DM) is suitable (see footnote).

A drop from the bottom of a culture tube is examined for the presence of *T. foetus* after 24 to 48 hours and 72- to 96-hour incubation at 37°C. If present in culture, the protozoa will be numerous. This is in contrast to directly examined samples, which require a higher degree of diligence and

technical competence in order to find and recognize *T. foetus*.

The morphologic identifying features of *T. foetus* are its size (6 to 8 × 10 to 25 microns), its spindle or pear shape and its continual motility, characterized by an undulating membrane. There are three anterior and one posterior flagella. The characteristic continual motility, size and spindle shape are recognizable under 100 × magnification in reduced light. The details of the undulating membrane and number of flagella are best recognized in an organism showing reduced motility examined at 400 ×.

Leptospirosis. The definitive immunological test in cattle for identification of species-specific antibodies is the blood serum microscopic agglutination (MA) test.[10] This method ordinarily identifies specific antibodies at 8 days following infection. The highest titer is usually reached in 3 to 4 weeks and may remain high for several months before declining.

Since the hazard for venereal transmission exits largely from urine contamination of semen in older bulls, it is imperative that bulls with significant titers be further tested for the presence of leptospires in urine[10] or be monitored by additional MA testing for stabilization or regression of titer.

One subcutaneous dose of dihydrostreptomycin

Stuart's: To a liter aspirator bottle, place 475 ml of distilled water, 5 gm of Bacto agar, 0.25 ml of thioglycollic acid, 5 gm of sodium glycerophosphate, 5 ml of 1 per cent $CaCl_2$ (in water), 0.025 gm of cysteine hydrochloride and 1 ml of 0.1 per cent methylene blue (in water). Heat to boiling to dissolve the agar. Cool to 56°C in a water bath and adjust pH to 7.2 using 1N NaOH. Dispense 10 ml medium into glass screw-cap tubes. Place caps on loosely and evacuate atmosphere four times in a dessicator jar, replacing each time with N_2 gas. Quickly screw caps on tightly and atuoclave for 20 minutes at 10 pounds pressure. These tubes can be stored upright for about 4 weeks at room temperature. Blue coloration of the media indicates the presence of oxygen. This medium permits samples to remain useful for culture for up to 48 hours.

Clark's: To each milliliter of freshly prepared bovine serum add 300 μg of 5-fluorouracil, 100 U of polymyxin B sulfate, 50 μg of brilliant green, 3 ug of nalidixic acid, and 100 μg of cycloheximide. The serum is then dispensed in 10 ml quantities into widemouth vaccine bottles (30 ml capacity), and rubber stoppers are inserted. The vials are placed into a boiling water bath for 2 minutes, which results in solidification of the serum and development of a blue-green color. After cooling, the medium is dispensed by stirring with a sterile glass rod. An 18-gauge needle is inserted through each firmly fixed stopper, the vials are placed into a dessicator, and the air in the vials is replaced by a mixture of 2.5 per cent O_2, 10 per cent CO_2 and 87.5 per cent N_2. The dessicator is opened, the needles are removed immediately and the vials incubated at 4°C for at least 1 week before use. During this period of storage the medium develops a dark green color. It should be stored at 4°C and used within 4 weeks.

SET: The medium is composed of prereduced and anaerobically sterilized chopped meat broth medium prepared according to the method outlined in the Anaerobe Laboratory Manual[2] with the addition of 300 μg per ml of 5-fluorouracil, 50 μg per ml of brilliant green and 100 μg

per ml of cycloheximide prior to autoclaving. The medium is dispensed in 10 ml volumes in 18 × 142 mm anaerobic culture tubes stoppered with black rubber stoppers. Prior to use, 0.1 ml of 10,000 U/ml solution of polymyxin B sulfate is introduced into each tube along the side of the stopper using a 1 cc syringe fitted with a 23-gauge × 1-inch needle. The final concentration of polymyxin B sulfate is then 100 U/ml. Stoppers are not removed from the tubes until the time of use in order to preserve the anaerobic condition. SET tubes displaying a uniform pink to red color, indicating oxidation, should be discarded. SET has a shelf life of 6 months.

TBM preparation[10]: For approximately 500 ml, dissolve 14.9 gm Fluid Thioglycollate Medium, dry form in 500 ml distilled water. Autoclave for 20 minutes, cool to 56°C. Aseptically, add 50 ml Fetal Bovine Serum, 2.25 ml aqueous suspension of procaine penicillin (200,000 U/2 ml) and dihydrostreptomycin sulfate (0.5 gm/2 ml). Inactivate at 56°C for 30 minutes. Finally, aseptically, add 1 mg amphotericin B (2 mcg/ml final concentration).

Dispense 5 ml, aseptically, into sterile 17 × 100 mm clear plastic tubes with cap (Fig. 7*H*). Incubate overnight to reveal contaminating bacteria. Refrigerate until used. Store no more than 30 days prior to use.

DM preparation[1]: Mix 2 gm trypticase peptone, 1 gm yeast extract, 0.5 gm maltose, 0.1 gm L-cystine hydrochloride, 0.02 gm L-ascorbic acid, 0.08 gm each of K_2HPO_4 and KH_2PO_4 in distilled water to make 90 ml. Determine pH. If not in range of 7.2 to 7.4, adjust pH with NaOH or HCl.

Add 0.5 gm agar and autoclave for 10 minutes at 121°C. Then cool to 49°C and aseptically add 10 ml of heat-inactivated (56°C for 30 minutes) bovine serum, 100,000 U penicillin G (1 ml of stock solution prepared by adding 10 ml sterile water to 10^6 units of crystallin penicillin G) and 0.1 gm of streptomycin sulfate (0.5 ml of stock solution prepared by adding 5 ml sterile water to 1 gm of streptomycin sulfate).

at the level of 25 mg/kg body weight has been shown effective in treatment of bovine renal leptospirosis.[15] It should be used as an adjunct to MA and urine culture to ascertain that leptospires do not contaminate semen.

The incidence of various *Leptospira* species varies with locality. Generally, *L. pomona, L. hardjo, L. grippotyphosa, L. canicola* and *L. icterohaemorrhagiae* are the species for which MA testing is indicated in the United States.

Infectious Bovine Rhinotracheitis/Infectious Pustular Vulvovaginitis/Infectious Pustular Balanoposthitis (IBR/IPV/IPB). Clinically, in bulls the highly characteristic pustular ulcers of the preputial-penile membrane are pathognomonic. The virus, during the clinical course of IPB, is highly contagious and readily infects the vulva-vagina on contact in susceptible females.

As is characteristic for herpes viral infections, a latent infection remains, presumably for life. Generally, thereafter, antibody titers are remarkably persistent. Substantial research evidence is accumulating that indicates in spite of persistent infectious shedding of the virus in semen rarely, if ever, occurs except under conditions of stress or as a result of repeated administration of corticosteroids. Under these conditions, recrudescence of the virus may occur without clinical signs of disease. Testing for presence of IPB virus in semen may be done with a tissue culture-serum neutralization method. Modified live virus vaccination via the nasal route at 4- to 6-month intervals apparently prevents all shedding of the virus from the genital tract of bulls.[12]

Johne's Disease (Paratuberculosis). In addition to its classic form, it has now been well established as a disease deserving of major concern among veterinarians examining bulls for genital health. *M. paratuberculosis* has been isolated from the genital organs, except the testes, and from semen of six of six bulls that showed clinical evidence of the disease.

Negative fecal culture along with a history of negative herd of origin for the disease are indicated prior to moving the bull into a new herd and into extensive service.

DIAGNOSIS AND PROGNOSIS

In undertaking the assignment of the examination of a bull for normalcy of reproductive function, the veterinarian assumes the responsibility for arriving at and communicating to his client in writing the diagnoses and prognoses for the various aspects of the examination. All determinations of unusual risks

in placing a bull in service and the options open to the client must be thoroughly explained.

The veterinarian must take an especially hard line on holding out of service those bulls with infectious genital diseases, pathologic conformation traits and conditions that are known to be heritable in a predictable manner.

References

1. Abbitt B: Trichomoniasis. Soc Theriogenology, Proc Fall Conf, Spokane, September 1981, pp 31–37.
2. Anaerobe Laboratory Manual. 4th ed. Blacksburg, Virginia Polytechnic Institute and State University.
3. Bartlett DE, Larson LL, Parker WG, Howard TH: Specific pathogen free (SPF) frozen bovine semen: A goal. Proc 6th Tech Conf Art Insemin Repro. Milwaukee, National Association of Animal Breeders, 1976, pp 11–22.
4. Bendixen HO, Blom E: Undersøgelser over forkomsten of Brucellose hos tyre specielt med henblik paa betydningen ved den Kunstige Insemination. Maanedsskr Dyrl 59:61, 1947.
5. Blom E, Christensen NO: Studies on pathological conditions in the testis, epididymis and accessory sex glands in the bull. Skand Vet 1, 1947.
6. Clark BL, Monsbourgh MJ, Dufty JH: Isolation of *Campylobacter fetus* subsp. *venerealis* and *Campylobacter fetus* subsp. *intermedius* from preputial secretions of bulls. Aust Vet J 50:324, 1974.
7. Foley JW, Bryner JH, Hughes DE, Barstard RD: Improved method for diagnosis of *Campylobacter fetus* infection in cattle using selective enrichment transport medium. Proc Am Assoc Vet Lab Diag 22:367, 1979.
8. Greenough PR, MacCallum FJ, Weaver AD: Lameness in Cattle. 2nd ed. Littleton, John Wright PSG Inc, 1981, pp 124, 353, 407.
9. Jubb KVF, Kennedy PC: Pathology of Domestic Animals. 2nd ed, Vol 1. New York, Academic Press, 1970, pp 445, 450–452, 458–463.
10. Lyle WE, Brown LN, Bryner JH, Hanson LE, Kirkbride CA, Larson AB: Recommended uniform diagnostic procedures qualifying bulls for the production of semen. Minneapolis, Proc 77th Ann Meet USAHA, 1973, pp 455–473.
11. Seger CL, Lank RB, Levy HE: Dihydrostreptomycin for treatment of genital vibriosis in the bull. JAVMA 149:1634, 1966.
12. Schultz RD, Hall CE, Sheffy BE, Bean BH: Current status of IBR-IPV infection in bulls. Miami, Proc 80th Ann Meet USAHA. Miami, 1976, pp 156–168.
13. Smith GF, Monroe JB: The testing of bulls for *Brucella abortus* infection with some reference to A.I. stud experience. England, Report Prod Div Milk Market Board, 1956, p 120.
14. Stalheim OHV, Bartlett DE, Carbrey EH, Knutson WW, Langford EV, Seigfried L: Recommended Procedures for the Microbiologic Examination of Semen. Reprinted from Proc 21st Ann Meet Am Assoc Vet Lab Diag, Madison, 1979, p 14.
15. Stalheim OHV: Chemotherapy of renal leptospirosis in cattle. Am J Vet Res 30:1317, 1969.
16. Thoen CO, Hines EM, Stumpff CD, Parks TW, Sturkie HN: Isolation of *Mycobacterium bovis* from the prepuce of a herd bull. Am J Vet Res 38:877, 1977.
17. Winter AJ, Caveney NT: Evaluation of transport medium for *Campylobacter* (Vibrio) *fetus*. JAVMA 173:472, 1978.

Endocrine Patterns During the Initiation of Puberty, the Estrous Cycle, Pregnancy and Parturition in Cattle

J. J. Knickerbocker
Colorado State University, Fort Collins, Colorado
Maarten Drost
William W. Thatcher
University of Florida. Gainesville, Florida

During the last several years our understanding of endocrine events regulating bovine reproductive processes has expanded considerably. This article will review the major endocrine events associated with puberty, the estrous cycle, pregnancy and parturition in cattle. In addition, current concepts relevant to the physiological significance of these events will be discussed.

PUBERTY

Reproductive function is normally initiated around 1 year of age in heifers. However, numerous genetic (sex and breed) and environmental (nutritional status, social interactions, temperature and photoperiod) factors influence the onset of puberty, so that age at puberty may be extremely variable, ranging from 4 months to over 2 years.

Onset of puberty in heifers (as in other species) results via a synchronized and interdependent cascade of maturational changes in the central nervous system (CNS), hypothalamus, pituitary and ovaries. Characterization of endocrine profiles and study of mechanisms controlling the prepubertal-to-pubertal transition in heifers have, at least partially, unraveled the dynamics of this maturational process.

As early as 4 months of age, the pituitary is capable of releasing luteinizing hormone (LH) in response to exogenous gonadotropin-releasing hormone (GnRH). Likewise, the ovaries respond to exogenous and endogenous (GnRH-induced) gonadotropins by increasing steroidogenic activity. Data such as these suggest that hypothalamic inactivity is responsible for the prepubertal state rather than an inability of the pituitary or ovaries to respond to GnRH and gonadotropin secretions, respectively. The mechanisms by which hypothalamic inactivity exists have not been resolved clearly in the bovine female. Maturation of the GnRH-releasing system may involve the CNS, since increased hypothalamic turnover rates and decreased sensitivity to the neurotransmitters norepinephrine (NE) and dopamine (DA) occur in rats approaching puberty. Increased hypothalamic NE turnover rates normally accompany LH pulses in this species.

Furthermore, evidence in both the ewe lamb and heifer suggest that the prepubertal GnRH-releasing system is extremely responsive to negative feedback from ovarian estrogen, such that estrogen inhibits the pulsatile mode of LH secretion. The threshold to negative feedback is elevated gradually as puberty approaches. Thus, the mechanisms modulating pulsatile LH secretion become derepressed, resulting in more frequent LH pulse patterns and ovarian activity.[28]

Endogenous spikes or episodes of LH occur at a frequency of one to four episodes per 24 hours during the prepubertal period in heifers. Amplitudes of these LH episodes range from 3 to 12 ng/ml of plasma, and baseline concentrations of LH are maintained generally below 1.5 ng/ml of plasma[20] (Fig. 1). Prior to 20 days before puberty, plasma progesterone (P_4) concentrations seldom rise above 0.5 ng/ml. Thus, it appears that the frequency of LH episodic release is insufficient to support ovarian activity during this period[11, 20] (Fig. 1).

Transition between prepuberty and puberty occurs 2 to 4 weeks prior to the first ovulation. Transition is characterized first by an increased frequency of LH episodes and then by the onset of ovarian activity, as determined by plasma P_4 concentrations[11, 26] (Fig. 1).

McLeod and colleagues[11] reported an increased frequency of LH episodic release in 1 of 12 prepubertal heifers. Detection of estrus in this animal occurred 10 days following a 24-hour sampling period. However, none of the remaining 11 heifers, which exhibited less frequent LH episodes, displayed estrus within the ensuing 6 weeks.

In nearly all cases, heifers in the transitional period exhibited one to two transient (duration of 2 to 5 days) elevations in plasma P_4. These P_4 elevations are of a lower magnitude (1 to 2 ng/ml plasma) than concentrations following corpus luteum (CL) formation during the first estrous cycle. Transitional elevations in P_4 are always preceeded by "priming" LH episodes. Palpation data suggest that this rise in P_4 results from the luteinization of ovarian follicles.[11] The first preovulatory surge of LH occurs only after the prepubertal P_4 elevation declines to baseline levels. Behavioral estrus is observed in some but not all heifers at this time.

Onset of ovarian steroidogenic activity may act to establish regulation of hypothalamic GnRH and pituitary gonadotropin release patterns, as depicted in the cyclic cow.[24] In addition, steroid-induced intraovarian regulation of ovarian follicular development may be important before the first ovulation.

Plasma 17-β estradiol (E_2) concentrations in heifers are elevated (approximately 60 pg/ml) at 2

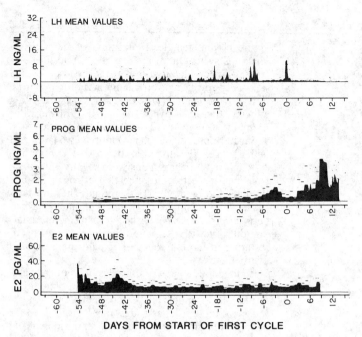

Figure 1. Average concentrations of luteinizing hormone (LH), progesterone (PROG) and estradiol-17β (E_2) in plasma samples collected at 6-hour intervals in six heifers (progesterone and estradiol-17β were analyzed in daily pools). Each dot or bar represents the standard deviation at a given period (from Gonzalez-Padilla et al., 1975).

months prior to first ovulation, then decline gradually to a baseline concentration of approximately 15 pg/ml by the first ovulation at puberty (Fig. 1). The decline in E_2 concentration is accompanied by a reduction in mean concentration of plasma follicle stimulating hormone (FSH) from approximately 52 ng/ml to 35 ng/ml. No discernible trends in pulsatile patterns or baseline concentrations of FSH or prolactin (PRL) occur throughout the prepubertal and early pubertal periods. McLeod and colleagues[20] suggest that the failure to detect clear episodic release patterns of FSH during prepuberty may be due to the higher threshold dose of GnRH required to evoke FSH release versus LH release.

THE ESTROUS CYCLE

The nature of the estrous cycle and its endocrine regulation have been extensively described in cattle. Estrous cycles in domestic cattle occur approximately every 21 days, with a range of 17 to 25 days considered normal. Cycle lengths of nulliparous heifers are, in general, slightly shorter (approximately 1 day) than those of cows. There does not appear to be a consistent season of the year (photoperiod) effect on length of estrous cycle in cattle. However, extremely high temperature does reduce expression of behavioral estrus, blood flow to the reproductive tract and reproductive efficiency and may alter normal hormonal profiles.[29]

Historically, observations regarding ovarian morphology and behavioral changes led to the division of the estrous cycle into four phases: estrus (day 0), metestrus (days 1 to 3), diestrus (days 4 to 18) and proestrus (day 19 to behavioral estrus). It should be kept in mind, however, that morphologic, functional and behavioral changes during the estrous cycle occur in response to and result in cyclical

endocrine patterns (Figs. 2, 3 and 4). Thus, cyclical alterations in tissue morphology and function, behavior and endocrine patterns are manifestations of the integrated regulation achieved between the hypothalamus, pituitary gland, ovaries and uterus during the estrous cycle.

For purposes of describing these interactions,

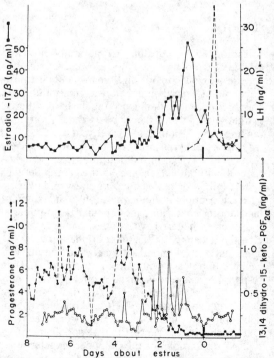

Figure 2. Two-hourly changes in peripheral plasma concentrations of estradiol-17β, progesterone, luteinizing hormone (LH) and 13,14 dihydro-15 keto-PGF$_{2\alpha}$ around estrus in one dairy cow (from Peterson et al., 1975).

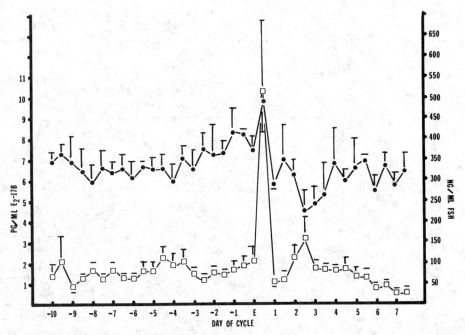

Figure 3. Concentrations of plasma follicle stimulating hormone (FSH; □———□) and estradiol-17β (E₂; ●———●) (± S.E.) in cycling dairy heifers around estrus (E) (from Kazmer, Barnes and Halman, 1981).

Hansel and Convey[12] recently reviewed the physiology and endocrinology of the estrous cycle in terms of three endocrine phases: (1) pregonadotropin surge, (2) postgonadotropin surge and (3) luteal. Such a format will be incorporated in the following discussion. Prior to the preovulatory surge of gonadotropins, E_2 begins to increase concurrently with the initiation and accelerated growth of the preovulatory follicle. Conversely, plasma P_4 concentrations decline as the CL regresses. Appreciable and sustained increases in E_2 do not occur until P_4 levels have begun to decline.[23] This observation can be explained by the fact that P_4 exerts a negative feedback effect on the hypothalamus and/or pituitary that reduces gonadotropin release. Removal of this negative influence during CL regression results in elevated LH baseline concentrations,[2] with a pulsatile release pattern characterized by high frequency and low amplitude[24] (Fig. 5). Although

follicular growth may be stimulated with FSH alone, a combination of FSH and LH has been shown to induce maximal E_2 biosynthesis in vitro. Thus, both gonadotropins probably influence follicular growth and E_2 production. Our understanding of FSH release patterns and mechanisms of control in the cow is not well established. However, it appears that E_2 is able to exert an inhibitory effect on FSH release, since exogenous E_2 administered to ovariectomized heifers reduced FSH concentrations to precastration levels. Additionally, plasma FSH concentrations appear lower just prior to the preovulatory surge of gonadotropins when E_2 levels are highest.

Peak follicular production and the resulting plasma concentrations of E_2 potentiate the onset of behavioral estrus and trigger the preovulatory surge release of both LH and FSH from the anterior pituitary. Evidence in the cow and ewe suggests that E_2 acts via increasing pulsatile GnRH secretion

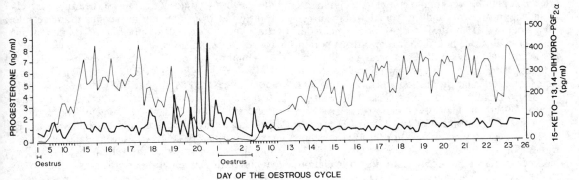

Figure 4. Peripheral plasma concentrations of progesterone (———) and 15-keto-13, 14 dihydro-PGF$_{2\alpha}$ (———) during the estrous cycle and early pregnancy in one heifer (from Kindahl et al., 1976).

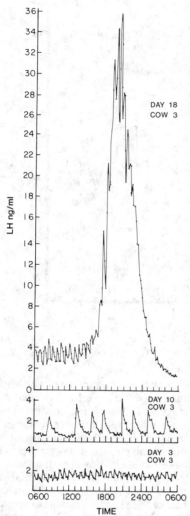

Figure 5. Patterns of plasma luteinizing hormone (LH) concentrations on days 3 (early luteal), 10 (midluteal) and 18 (preovulatory LH surge) of the estrous cycle in cow 3 (from Rahe et al., 1980).

by the hypothalamus and via enhancing pituitary responsiveness to GnRH. Both factors are essential for creating the preovulatory LH and FSH surges.[12] In addition, low basal P_4 concentrations must be maintained if E_2 is to exert its positive feedback effects. A high P_4 background completely eliminates E_2 induction of estrus and the gonadotropin surge. The surge of LH and FSH release occurs near the onset of a 12- to 22-hour behavioral estrous period in the cow and lasts for 8 to 10 hours.

During and immediately following the preovulatory surge, follicular production and circulating levels of E_2 rapidly decline as follicle luteinization occurs. During the majority of metestrus (days 1 to 3), plasma concentrations of E_2, P_4 and LH remain low. However, a second elevation in FSH concentrations of lower magnitude than the first (Fig. 3) has been reported[15] to occur just prior to ovulation in the cow, ewe and sow. This second rise in FSH may be a result of a reduction in follicular inhibin

production during the ovulatory process. The function of this rise is currently unknown; however, FSH may play a role in the recruitment of preantral follicles.[12]

Ovulation occurs on day 1 of the estrous cycle, approximately 24 to 30 hours after the preovulatory surge of LH and FSH. Following ovulation, the CL develops, and plasma P_4 concentrations rise from approximately 1 ng/ml on day 3 after estrus to a plateau of 6 to 10 ng/ml from days 7 to 18. During the luteal phase, LH secretion is again altered in response to steroid hormone concentrations. Low frequency and high amplitude LH pulses occur during the P_4-dominated phase of the cycle[24] (Fig. 5).

Follicular growth and atresia occur continuously throughout the estrous cycle, with moderate rises in plasma E_2 occurring responsively. The largest follicle present on the ovaries during the luteal phase of the cycle will, in most cases, become atretic. Only after day 18 is there an increase in the probability that the largest follicle will ovulate. Thus, the rapid growth of a small- or medium-sized antral follicle to a large antral follicle that is subsequently identified as a mature preovulatory graafian follicle probably occurs from days 15 to 18 in the cow. Elevated plasma E_2 concentrations during this period[2, 23] occur simultaneously with the development of the preovulatory graafian follicle.[3]

Estrogens, produced primarily by a developing large antral follicle, are thought to initiate the process of luteal regression during late diestrus via induction of uterine prostaglandin $F_{2\alpha}$ ($PGF_{2\alpha}$) production. Administration of exogenous estrogens initiates luteolysis in cattle[6] and has been shown to stimulate uterine $PGF_{2\alpha}$ production during late diestrus.[29] Conversely, removal of ovarian follicles results in extended luteal function in cattle.[35]

Uterine involvement in the luteolytic process is supported, since prolonged maintenance of CL function results after surgical removal of the uterus during mid-diestrus. Additionally, cattle with a congenitally absent uterine horn (uterus unicornis) adjacent to the CL-bearing ovary display prolonged luteal life spans. Such observations and surgical preparations have provided evidence for a local utero-ovarian control of CL life span. Current data suggest that $PGF_{2\alpha}$ (luteolysin) produced by the uterine horn adjacent to the CL-bearing ovary is transferred from the uterine venous drainage into the ovarian arterial supply via a countercurrent transfer mechanism.[10]

A major and more stable metabolite of $PGF_{2\alpha}$, 15-keto-13, 14-dihydro-$PGF_{2\alpha}$ (PGFM), is commonly measured as an index of uterine $PGF_{2\alpha}$ production.[29] Luteolytic pulses of uterine $PGF_{2\alpha}$ (peripheral PGFM)[16] (Fig. 4) are detected concurrently with increasing plasma E_2 and declining plasma P_4 concentrations[2, 23] (Fig. 2). Recent data on cattle[33] and sheep[8] demonstrate the release of ovarian oxytocin during luteolysis. Oxytocin is believed to augment uterine $PGF_{2\alpha}$ release, thus ensuring a rapid and complete luteal regression.[8]

PREGNANCY

Pregnancy is defined as the period from fertilization to parturition. Gestation in domestic cattle extends for approximately 280 days after mating (range 270 to 292 days). Variability in length of gestation is influenced by fetal sex, number of fetuses, breed and genotype of the sire or dam or fetus, plane of nutrition and environmental temperature.

An opportunity for establishment of pregnancy is provided with each estrous cycle. When conception occurs following insemination at estrus, the development of a CL becomes essential for establishment and maintenance of pregnancy. As a consequence of luteal P_4 production, glandular epithelium of the uterine endometrium becomes secretory in nature, providing the sole source of nutrients (histotroph) for conceptus growth and development prior to placentome formation (day 45). In addition, elevated P_4 concentrations reduce uterine tone and myometrial contractility, thus allowing for conceptus expansion and attachment and preventing constriction and expulsion of the conceptus from the uterus.

Endocrinologically, the first 15 days of the estrous cycle and of pregnancy are, generally speaking, identical, and early events contributing to an embryotrophic uterine environment occur regardless of the presence or absence of a viable conceptus within the uterine lumen. Beyond this point, however, a viable conceptus within the uterus must play an active role in the perpetuation of its embryotrophic environment. Consequently, luteal maintenance, characteristic of pregnancy, reflects responses of the uterus and ovary to physiological conditions initiated by the conceptus and its products. The process by which the periattachment conceptus signals its presence to the maternal unit, as reflected by luteal maintenance, is referred to as "maternal recognition of pregnancy."[29]

The bovine conceptus is active endocrinologically by day 13 of gestation, producing an array of steroids, prostaglandins and proteins within the uterine lumen. Noticeable conceptus-induced alterations in maternal physiology do not occur until day 16 or 17 of gestation. During this critical period, the cyclical events involved with CL regression are modified to accommodate pregnancy maintenance.

Specific conceptus signals and their mechanisms of action are currently being examined. Recent data on cyclic cows demonstrate that proteins secreted by day 16 to 18 of bovine conceptuses extend luteal function and interestrous interval when administered into the uterine lumen between days 15 and 21.[18] It appears that conceptus secretory proteins reduce the capacity of the uterus to synthesize and to secrete $PGF_{2\alpha}$, thus providing for CL and pregnancy maintenance.[17] In addition, Kindahl and colleagues[16] have reported that pulsatile episodes of prostaglandins are depressed during early pregnancy (Fig. 4).

Conceptus interactions with the maternal system during the establishment and maintenance of pregnancy also influence maternal vascular permeability, uterine blood flow, fluid movement, response of the CL to $PGF_{2\alpha}$, uterine synthetic and metabolic activity, nutrient transfer and immunosuppressive activity as well as mammary gland growth and development. All of these phenomena occur as a result of conceptus endocrine signals, acting both independently and cooperatively, to ensure that requirements of the fetoplacental unit are met by the maternal system throughout pregnancy.

As described, the CL is maintained for the duration of pregnancy and P_4 concentrations fluctuate between 6 and 15 ng/ml throughout gestation. The bovine adrenal glands also contribute to the maternal P_4 pool during gestation (1 to 4 ng/ml plasma) and are capable of maintaining pregnancy in the absence of ovaries from approximately day 200.[34] Elevated concentrations of plasma P_4 and placental estrogens during pregnancy inhibit pituitary gonadotropin production so that a preovulatory surge of LH and ovulation does not occur. Placental steroidogenic activity, as determined by plasma estrone sulfate (E_1SO_4), increases throughout pregnancy in conjunction with fetoplacental growth and development. Estrone (E_1) and 17-α estradiol (17-αE_2) are the major steroids synthesized by the fetoplacental unit. A major portion of these estrogens are conjugated immediately at the placentomes, so that conjugated estrogens exceed free estrogens by 10- to 100-fold. Local conjugation of estrogens probably reduces excessive estrogenic activity on peripheral maternal tissues. 17-α estradiol sulfate is the major estrogen in fetal plasma.[13] However, E_1SO_4 predominates in fluids of the chorioallantois and amnion and of maternal plasma.[5, 25] Maternal plasma concentrations of E_1SO_4 increase gradually from a baseline of 30 to 60 pg/ml before day 60, to approximately 500 pg/ml by day 100 of pregnancy. A rapid elevation then occurs until day 150 when E_1SO_4 concentrations approach 3000 pg/ml. Plasma E_1SO_4 concentrations are highly variable beyond day 150 but tend to increase gradually until approximately day 240 when E_1SO_4 again increases rapidly to term[25, 30] (Figs. 6 and 7). Characterization of estrone (E_1), pooled 17-α/β estradiol sulfates (E_2SO_4), androstenedione (A_2) and testosterone (T) throughout pregnancy in cattle reflects profiles similar to that of E_1SO_4[9, 25, 30] (Figs. 6 and 7). These steroids appear to be synthesized in the placenta as well, since concentrations in maternal blood are depleted immediately following birth of the calf and expulsion of the placenta.[4, 22]

In dairy cattle P_4, A_2, T, E_1 and E_1SO_4 have been measured in milk. Milk hormone patterns during pregnancy are in most cases comparable to those found in plasma. Steroid concentrations, however, may be higher (e.g., P_4, A_2 and E_1) or lower (e.g., T and E_1SO_4) than plasma values during the same sampling period.[22] Compartmentalization of biologically active steroids in milk, as well as plasma, may be important for mammary gland growth and development. The major portion of mammary gland

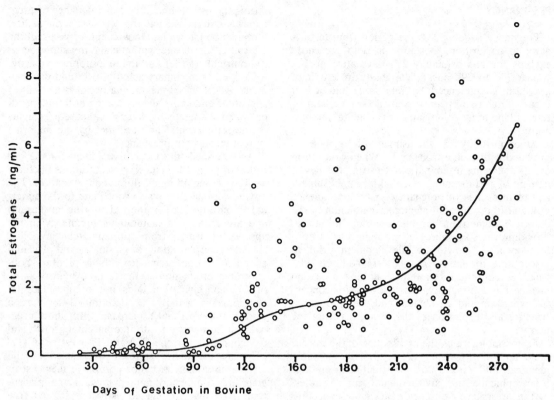

Figure 6. Patterns of peripheral estrogens throughout gestation in cattle. (From M. Terqui personal communication.)

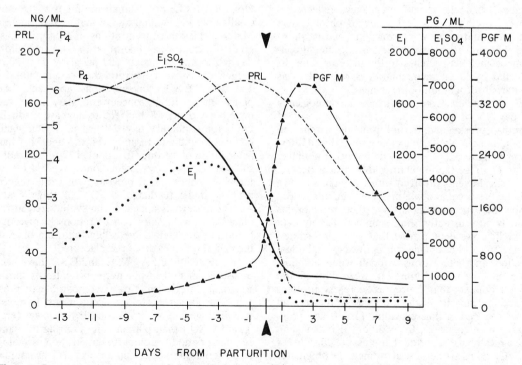

Figure 7. Least squares regressions of plasma progesterone (P_4), estrone sulfate (E_1SO_4), estrone (E_1), prolactin (PRL) and 15-keto-13, 14 dihydro-$PGF_{2\alpha}$ (PGF M) during the periparturient period in cattle (from Eley et al., 1981).

development in heifers occurs during pregnancy in response to placental hormones.

As previously mentioned, significant changes in patterns of LH (range 0.7 to 1.0 ng/ml) are not evident during gestation. This is also the case for growth hormone (range 5.0 to 10.0 ng/ml). Prolactin concentrations, on the other hand, begin to rise from a variable baseline of approximately 80 ng/ml 2 weeks prepartum and reach peak values of 200 to 400 ng/ml just prior to calving (Fig. 7). Approximately 1 week prepartum, PGFM concentrations gradually increase in maternal plasma. A final abrupt increase in PGFM is accompanied by a decline in progesterone associated with CL regression just prior to parturition (Fig. 7).

PARTURITION

The process of parturition marks the termination of pregnancy, at which time the fetus is capable of independent existence outside the uterus. Endocrine events during the periparturient period (Figs. 7 and 8) represent the final stages of fetoplacental maturation and provide the impetus for synchronous mammary gland function at birth, postpartum uterine involution, and reinitiation of postpartum ovarian cyclicity.

The initiation of parturition in cattle, as in other domestic species, centers around activation of the fetal hypothalamic-pituitary-adrenal axis. Thus, surgical removal of the fetal anterior pituitary or adrenal glands results in prolongation of gestation. Additionally, genetic abnormalities shown to reduce or to eliminate the fetal anterior pituitary gland or the adrenal cortex result in delay of onset of parturition in cattle. In cattle, sheep, goats and pigs infusions of either adrenocorticotropic hormone (ACTH) or corticosteroids into the fetus or dam during the last trimester of pregnancy result in the initiation of parturition.

As parturition approaches, the fetal adrenal cortex becomes increasingly sensitive to ACTH. Increased cortical growth in fetal adrenals during late pregnancy occurs in the absence of noticeable elevations in fetal ACTH concentrations, as does the production of adrenal corticosteroids. Fetal plasma concentrations of corticosterone rise gradually from 3 weeks (5 ng/ml) to 4 days (25 ng/ml) prepartum. Fetal plasma ACTH becomes noticeably elevated 1 to 2 days prepartum, coincident with a rapid increase in corticosterone to term (70 ng/ml).[14] There is some evidence to suggest that another pituitary hormone, α-melanocyte stimulating hormone (α-MSH) from the pars intermedia, may influence fetal adrenal function in sheep. The physiology of α-MSH in cattle is at present uncertain.

The rise in fetal corticoids during the last month of gestation may be responsible for activation of enzyme systems within the cotyledons, which increase the capacity of the bovine placenta to convert C-21 steroids (e.g., P_4 and pregnenolone) to C-19 estrogen precursors (e.g., A_2 and DHEA) and estrogens during normal parturition.[19] Such an increase in placental steroidogenic activity is evidenced by the dramatic prepartum elevations of estrogens, estrogen sulfates and estrogen precursors A_2 and T in maternal plasma from approximately day 240 of gestation to term.

Maternal plasma P_4 declines gradually from approximately 2 weeks to 3 days prepartum before falling precipitously to less than 1 ng/ml at term. The gradual decline in serum P_4 may in part be due to increased placental metabolism of P_4 to androgens and estrogens, as has been suggested in sheep. In addition, elevated placental estrogens may initiate events leading to CL demise. Estrogens are known to stimulate the production of the uterine luteolysin $PGF_{2\alpha}$ in cattle. Prostaglandin $F_{2\alpha}$ production may also be influenced by oxytocin actions on the endometrium, since oxytocin administered to cattle causes $PGF_{2\alpha}$ elevations during the cycle. Estrogen has been shown to increase uterine oxytocin receptor concentrations in a number of species. Progesterone, on the other hand, is antagonistic to this estrogen action. Increased uterine responsiveness to oxytocin as parturition approaches may therefore be regulated by the increasing estrogen-to-progesterone ratio and subsequent induction of oxytocin receptor numbers.

In cattle[27] and sheep[21] there is a transient increase in oxytocin levels as the fetus enters the birth canal and dilates the cervix (Fig. 8). Following expulsion of the fetus and placenta, oxytocin levels return to low baseline levels. In addition, milk ejection during the calving and milking processes occurs simultaneously with the elevation of oxytocin concentrations in plasma.[27]

As a result of alterations in steroid patterns, increased uterine sensitivity to oxytocin and production of $PGF_{2\alpha}$, myometrial contractility becomes more coordinated and intensifies as parturition approaches.

In conjunction with myometrial activity, a softening of the cervix, relaxation of pelvic ligaments and a generalized expansion of the birth canal become evident 1 to 2 days prior to parturition. An ovarian hormone, relaxin, has been implicated in regulating this process, as have placental estrogens and uterine $PGF_{2\alpha}$. In the pregnant pig, relaxin is produced by the CL and released into the general circulation during luteolysis. Relaxin concentrations, in this species, become elevated 2 days prepartum, peak between 1 and 0.5 days prepartum and fall to basal levels at parturition.[1] A similar relaxin profile has been reported during parturition in beef cattle.[1] The majority of relaxin data collected in the cow, however, have relied upon indirect bioassay methods for measuring relaxinlike activity. Isolation of bovine relaxinlike peptides has been reported in CL[7] and placenta.[32] Porcine relaxin has been shown to cause cervical dilation and increase the pelvic area in cattle under an estrogen-dominated endocrine environment.[1] Further studies dealing with direct relaxin measurements in blood and tissues are required to understand the importance of this hormone in bovine parturition.

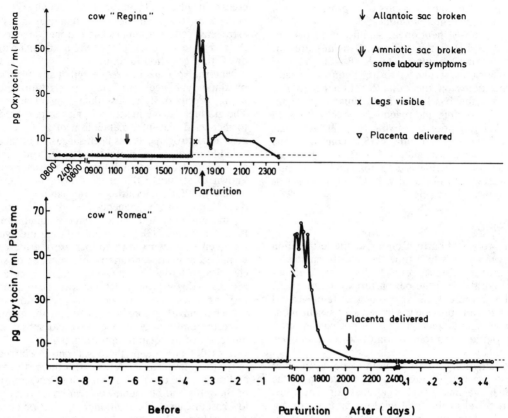

Figure 8. Plasma concentrations of oxytocin from two cows before, during and after parturition (from Schams, Schmidt-Polex and Kruse, 1979).

During the stress of labor and fetal passage through the birth canal, maternal adrenal corticoids become acutely elevated (approximately 15 ng/ml). Glucocorticoids are essential in the cow for the establishment of mammary gland lactogenesis. Likewise, prolactin serves a similar function during the periparturient period.

Following birth of the fetus and expulsion of the placenta, the uterus begins the process of involution, characterized by elevated uterine $PGF_{2\alpha}$ production. Uterine $PGF_{2\alpha}$ production, as determined by measurements of PGFM in the peripheral circulation, increases to maximal concentration 1 to 4 days postpartum and gradually declines to baseline values by 15 days postpartum[4] (Fig. 7).

Postpartum ovarian activity is reinitiated by days 11 to 13 in dairy cattle, and ovulation occurs by approximately 15 to 20 days. The luteal phase resulting from this ovulation is short lived and characterized by P_4 concentrations of a lower magnitude than those found during the luteal phase of normal estrous cycles. In addition, estrous behavior is absent prior to the first postpartum ovulation in most cases.

Initiation of behavioral estrus and cyclical endocrine events characteristic of the estrous cycle occur around 25 to 30 days postpartum.

Postpartum intervals to ovarian activity, ovulation and estrus are considerably longer in suckled beef cows. Resumption of ovarian activity and cyclicity are physiological indications that the cow is approaching a reproductive condition capable of supporting another pregnancy. This involves a restoration of hypothalamic, pituitary, ovarian and uterine components that must interact in a coordinated manner for successful reproductive function. Effects of management, nutrition, suckling and animal health influence the efficiency by which this axis functions and thereby affect reproductive competence.

References

1. Anderson LL, Perezgrovas R: Biological actions of relaxin in pigs and beef cattle. Ann NY Acad Sci 380:131, 1982.
2. Chenault JR, Thatcher WW, Kalra PS, et al.: Transitory changes in plasma progestins, estradiol, and luteinizing hormone approaching ovulation in the bovine. J Dairy Sci 58:709, 1975.
3. Dufour J, Whitmore HL, Ginther OJ, Casida LE: Identification of the ovulating follicle by its size on different days of the estrous cycle in heifers. J Anim Sci 34:85, 1972.
4. Eley DS, Thatcher WW, Head HH, et al.: Periparturient and postpartum endocrine changes of conceptus and maternal units in Jersey cows bred for milk yield. J Dairy Sci 64:312, 1981.
5. Eley RM, Thatcher WW, Bazer FW: Hormonal and physical changes associated with bovine conceptus development. J Repro Fert 55:181, 1979.

6. Eley RM, Thatcher WW, Bazer FW: Luteolytic effect of oestrone sulphate on cyclic beef heifers. J Repro Fert 55:191, 1979.

7. Fields MJ, Fields PA, Castro-Hernandez A, Larkin LH: Evidence for relaxin from corpora lutea of late pregnant cows. Endocrinology 107:869, 1980.

8. Flint APF, Scheldrick EL: Ovarian secretion of oxytocin is stimulated by prostaglandin. Nature 197:587, 1982.

9. Gaiani R, Chiesa F, Mattioli M, et al.: Androstenedione and testosterone concentrations in plasma and milk of the cow throughout pregnancy. J Repro Fert 70:55, 1984.

10. Ginther OJ: Local versus systemic uteroovarian relationships in farm animals. Acta Vet Scand Suppl 77:103, 1981.

11. Gonzalez-Padilla E, Wiltbank JN, Niswender GD: Puberty in beef heifers. 1. The interrelationship between pituitary, hypothalamic and ovarian hormones. J Anim Sci 40:1091, 1975.

12. Hansel W, Convey EM: Physiology of the estrous cycle. J Anim Sci 57 (Suppl 2):404, 1983.

13. Hoffman B, Wagner WC, Gimenez T: Free and conjugated steroids in maternal and fetal plasma in the cow near term. Biol Reprod 15:126, 1976.

14. Hunter JT, Fairclough RJ, Peterson AT, Welch RAS: Foetal and maternal hormonal changes preceding normal bovine parturition. Acta Endocrinologica 84:653, 1977.

15. Kazmer GW, Barnes MA, Halman RD: Endogenous hormone response and fertility in dairy heifers treated with norgestomet and estradiol valerate. J Anim Sci 53:1333, 1981.

16. Kindahl H, Edqvist LE, Bane A, Granstrom E: Blood levels of progesterone and 15-keto-13,14-dihydro-prostaglandin $F_{2\alpha}$ during the normal estrous cycle and early pregnancy in heifers. Acta Endocrinologica 82:134, 1976.

17. Knickerbocker JJ, Thatcher WW, Bazer FW, et al.: Inhibition of estradiol-17β-induced uterine $PGF_{2\alpha}$ production by bovine conceptus secretory proteins. J Anim Sci 59 (Suppl 1):368, abstract 543, 1984.

18. Knickerbocker JJ, Thatcher WW, Bazer FW, et al.: Proteins secreted by cultured day 17 bovine conceptuses extend luteal function in cattle. 10th Int Cong Anim Reprod Art Insemin. June 10–14, 1984, abstract and paper No. 88.

19. Larsson K, Wagner CW, Sachs M: Oestrogen synthesis by bovine foetal placenta at normal parturition. Acta Endocrinologica 98:118, 1981.

20. McLeod BJ, Haresign W, Peters AR, Lamming GE: Plasma LH and FSH concentrations in prepubertal beef heifers before and in response to repeated injections of low doses of GnRH. J Repro Fert 70:137, 1984.

21. Mitchell MD, Kraemer DL, Brennecke SP, Webb R: Pulsatile release of oxytocin during the estrous cycle, pregnancy and parturition in sheep. Biol Repro 27:1169, 1982.

22. Mostl E, Mostl K, Choi HS, et al.: Plasma levels of androstenedione, epitestosterone, testosterone and oestrogens in cows at parturition. J Endocrinology 89:251, 1981.

23. Peterson AJ, Fairclough RJ, Payne E, Smith JF: Hormonal changes around bovine luteolysis. Prostaglandins 10:675, 1975.

24. Rahe CH, Owens RE, Fleeger JL, et al.: Pattern of plasma luteinizing hormone in the cyclic cow: Dependence upon the period of the cycle. Endocrinology 107:498, 1980.

25. Robertson HA, King GJ: Conjugated and unconjugated oestrogens in fetal and maternal fluids of the cow throughout pregnancy. J Repro Fert 55:463, 1979.

26. Schams D, Schallenberger E, Gombe S, Karg H: Endocrine patterns associated with puberty in male and female cattle. J Repro Fert Suppl 30:103, 1981.

27. Schams D, Schmidt-Polex B, Kruse V: Oxytocin determination by radioimmunoassay in cattle. Acta Endocrinologica 92:258, 1979.

28. Schillo KK, Dierschke DJ, Hauser ER: Regulation of luteinizing hormone secretion in prepubertal heifers: Increased threshold to negative feedback action of estradiol. J Anim Sci 54:325, 1982.

29. Thatcher WW, Collier RJ: Effects of climate on bovine reproduction. In Morrow D (ed): Current Therapy in Theriogenology. 2nd ed. Philadelphia, WB Saunders Co, 1985.

30. Thatcher WW, Guilbault LA, Collier RJ, et al.: The impact of ante-partum physiology of postpartum performance in cows. In Karg H, Schallenberger E (eds): Current Topics in Veterinary Medicine and Animal Science. Vol 20. Factors Influencing Fertility in the Postpartum Cow. Boston, Commission of the European Communities, Martinus Nijhoff, Publ, 1982, pp 1–25.

31. Thatcher WW, Wolfenson D, Curl JS, et al.: Prostaglandin dynamics associated with development of the bovine conceptus. Anim Reprod Sci 7:149, 1984.

32. Wada H, Yuhara M: Concentration of relaxin in the blood serum of pregnant cow and cow with ovarian cyst. Proc Silver Jubilee, Kyoto University, 1961, pp 61–66.

33. Walters DL, Schams D, Bullermann B, Schallenberger E: Pulsatile secretion of gonadotropins, ovarian steroids and ovarian oxytocin during lutelysis in the cow. Biol Repro 28 (Suppl 1):142, abstract 220, 1983.

34. Wendorf GL, Lawyer MS, First NL: Role of the adrenals in the maintenance of pregnancy in cows. J Repro Fert 68:281, 1983.

35. Villa-Godoy A, Ireland JJ, Wortman JA, et al.: Luteal function in heifers following destruction of ovarian follicles at three stages of diestrus. J Anim Sci 52 (Suppl 1):372, abstract 603, 1981.

Breeding Soundness Examination of Bulls

Randall S. Ott, D.V.M., M.S.
University of Illinois, Urbana, Illinois

The concept of a breeding soundness examination was developed by members of the Society for Theriogenology to assist veterinarians who perform routine bull examinations as a service for cattle raisers.

Breeding soundness examinations in the United States are mostly performed on beef bulls used for natural service, although some dairy bulls are examined for natural service or for entry into artificial insemination organizations. Following examination, a bull is classified as a *satisfactory potential breeder, a questionable potential breeder* or *an unsatisfactory potential breeder.* The overall classification of the bull must be the lowest classification obtained on any part of the examination. A bull classified as questionable may deserve reexamination at a later date. It is recommended that the owner of a bull be given a written report containing results of the examination and a prognosis. The value of a breeding soundness examination is related to both the knowledge and the experience of the individual performing the examination; therefore, the validity of these examinations is enhanced as the practitioner learns and does more.

INDICATIONS FOR BREEDING SOUNDNESS EXAMINATIONS

Prepurchase (Sale). A prepurchase examination provides the buyer with information that may prevent future loss of income. Breeders of bulls can benefit by protecting their reputations as sellers of sound breeding animals and by eliminating the need for the standard "breeding guarantee," which usually states that if an animal is found to be an unsatisfactory breeder within 6 months after the date of sale, the buyer can return the animal to the seller. The seller then has 6 months to prove that the animal is a breeder, replace the animal with one of equal value, or refund the buyer's money. Obviously, the effects of injury, infections or nutritional status may decrease fertility of the animal once it is in the hands of the buyer, even though the animal was sound on the day of purchase.

Prebreeding Season. Breeding soundness examinations performed 30 to 60 days prior to the breeding season give the cattleman an appraisal of available bull power. Examinations performed at this time will be valid for the breeding season and the cattleman will have time to locate adequate replacements, if necessary. The consequences of turning infertile bulls into the breeding pasture include the obvious loss of gross income due to a decrease in the calf crop. Also, cows may calve late in the season in subsequent years, and it can be difficult to move their calving dates back again. In herds in which weaning age calves are marketed as a group at the same time each year, the late-born calves will weigh less.

Postbreeding Problem. In many practices the most common time for the examination of bulls is after breeding failure. The history of the bull's performance should be carefully recorded and evaluated. Breeding soundness examinations can be used as a diagnostic aid in herd fertility problems. Finding that the bulls are satisfactory potential breeders can "rule out" this parameter and suggest investigation of management factors or reproductive diseases in the cow herd. Many times breeding soundness examinations are used to confirm a suspected case of bull infertility. These cases may seem obvious to the practitioner, but the examination results may allow the owner to receive compensation or a replacement animal from the seller if the bull is under warranty.

PHYSICAL HEALTH

Evaluation of physical health should include a general physical examination of bulls, with special attention to the reproductive organs. The breeding history or results of the physical examination may indicate that specific tests for reproductive or other diseases should be conducted. Information concerning diagnosis and therapy of reproductive diseases is presented in separate articles of this text.

Examination of the eyes may detect pinkeye scars and lesions of squamous cell carcinomas. Early detection of cancerous eye lesions should be reason for slaughter of the bull because these lesions can develop rapidly and greatly reduce salvage value. An oral examination will determine whether bulls have adequate teeth to allow them to eat the available roughages while in the breeding pasture. A bull with dental lesions or a bull that has lost its teeth will lose weight rapidly during the breeding season. The *overall condition* of the bull is important. Bulls should not be fat but should carry some extra weight when entering the breeding pasture, as they can be expected to lose weight during the breeding season. Young bulls completing gain performance tests at 12 to 15 months of age are frequently used to service a small number of cows during their first breeding season. These bulls are usually fed a high concentrate ration during the test period, and they lose weight very rapidly when placed in the breeding pasture unless supplemental feed is provided. Feeding a high roughage diet during a "let down" period 1 to 2 months prior to pasture use is a good practice.

Rear Leg Structure and Feet Examination. Examination of *rear leg conformation* is often overlooked when bulls are evaluated for breeding soundness. Sound rear legs are vital to the breeding capacity of bulls. During copulation, most of the bull's weight is supported by the rear legs. While bearing this weight, extension of the bull's rear legs enables forward thrusting and ejaculation. A bull with rear leg impairment may not move around freely to find cows in estrus and may be unable to mount successfully. A more subtle problem is the bull that does mount cows in estrus, but fewer times, because of rear leg discomfort. Observations of bulls for mobility and structural soundness are best accomplished while the bulls are loose in pastures or on dirt lots prior to being restrained on artificial surfaces or in crowded alleys and chutes.

A careful examination of hooves and feet will detect interdigital fibromas, abscesses and abnormal hoof growth. In most cases the need for trimming a bull's feet results from faulty rear leg conformation. Hooves of structurally sound bulls wear evenly under normal conditions. *The prognosis for structural unsoundness is usually poor.* As a bull with faulty rear leg conformation ages, the defect becomes more apparent and tends to interfere more with the animal's breeding ability. Breeders should be warned that structural faults of the rear legs are heritable. Figures 1 and 5 illustrate desirable conformation of rear legs. Common structural faults are depicted in Figures 2 through 4 and 6 and 7.

Libido and Mating Ability. Libido is an important component of a bull's breeding ability; however, it is difficult to make an assessment of libido during a breeding soundness examination. Although young bulls must learn to identify cows in estrus properly and to mount them, this learning usually takes place in a short period of time. It has been demonstrated in a research trial that bulls graded high for libido and placed with 50 cyclic heifers impregnated more

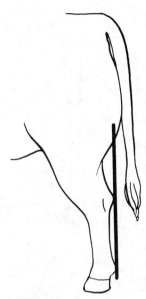

Figure 1. Desirable conformation of the rear legs as seen from the side.

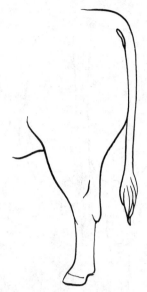

Figure 3. Postlegged. Bulls with this fault lack proper angulation of the hock and stifle joint. These animals may "stifle" (rupture cruciate ligament and meniscus). Their pasterns may be noticeably weakened.

heifers during a 20-day breeding period than bulls with low libido. Differences in libido among pasture-mated bulls with fewer cows in the breeding unit may also exist but may be difficult to document unless the bull has extremely poor libido. Older bulls tend to mount cows in estrus less frequently than young bulls, with no apparent decrease in pregnancy rate of the cows. Some bulls service cows only after dark. A more detailed discussion of libido is presented in the section on male behavior.

Mating ability can be assessed to some degree if semen is collected with an artificial vagina; however, test matings are usually required. Mating ability is impaired by problems of the musculoskeletal system, especially unsoundness of the rear legs and back. Penile deviations and loss of innervation of the penis (usually a sequelae to hematoma of the penis) may also reduce mating ability. Careful questioning of the owner can provide clues concerning mating ability and libido of bulls.

When more than one bull is present in a breeding pasture, problems concerning social dominance may come into play. Bull subfertility is magnified when

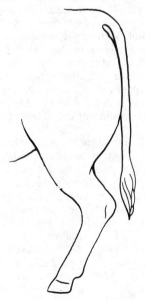

Figure 2. Sickle-hock conformation. This fault can lead to swollen hocks and lameness.

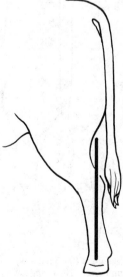

Figure 4. Camped behind. With this defect bulls shift their rear legs frequently in an effort to find a comfortable stance. They are usually swayback.

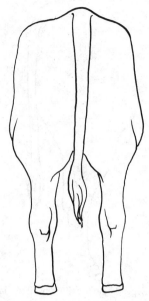

Figure 5. Desirable conformation of the hind legs as seen from the rear.

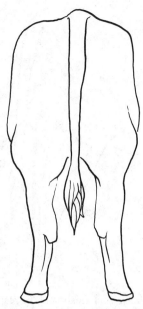

Figure 7. Toed-out stance (base wide). This fault is usually seen in conjunction with the sickle-hock conformation.

the less fertile or the impaired bull is also the dominant bull in multiple-bull mating systems.

Examination of Prepuce and Penis. The *prepuce* should be thoroughly palpated for adhesions caused by injury or penile hematomas. The prepuce of *Bos indicus* bulls or breeds utilizing Brahman, such as Santa Gertrudis, Beefmaster and Brangus, can have a very loose and pendulous development that predisposes them to preputial injury and prolapse (Fig.

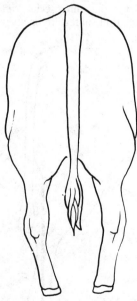

Figure 6. Bowleggedness (base narrow). The outside wall of the hoof is compressed. The outer toe may curl upward, growing over the inside toe and requiring frequent trimming. Bulls with this fault show various degrees of lameness.

8). *Eversion of the prepuce* (Fig. 9) is found to some degree in all naturally polled bulls and in *Bos indicus* bulls but not in horned animals. The extent of an eversion may range from 1 to 10 cm. Bulls with an advanced degree of preputial eversion are predisposed to preputial injury due to trauma or frostbite.

The *penis* can be manually exteriorized but is usually examined after erection and protrusion during electroejaculation. Sequelae to a penile hematoma (resulting from a rupture of the tunica albuginea) include adhesions between the penis and prepuce and sensory nerve damage to the penis. A diagnosis of lateral, ventral or corkscrew deviation of the penis should be made during a test mating and not during a forced erection with the electroejaculator. Bulls with penile deviations are usually sold for slaughter because the cost of surgical correction is seldom justified for commercial bulls used as terminal sires (all offspring slaughtered). Surgical correction of penile deviations in bulls used to sire purebred calves is not prudent because of the possibility of transmission of the defect to future generations.

Virgin bulls should be examined for normal development of the penis and for freedom from developmental anomalies such as a persistent penile frenulum (Fig. 10). Hair rings around the penis are probably the result of young bulls mounting each other. Hair rings located just posterior to the glans penis can restrict circulation, resulting in amputation of the glans. Fibropapillomas occur most often on the penis of young bulls. To prevent the spread of fibropapillomas to other bulls or cows, bulls should not be used for natural service or collection with the artificial vagina until the fibropapillomas have been surgically removed and the penis has completely healed.

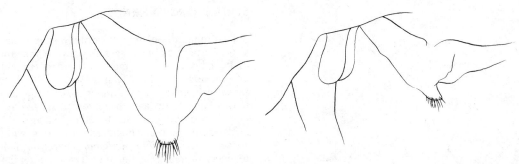

Figure 8. A very pendulous development of the prepuce, which predisposes to preputial lesions (left) compared with a more desirable conformation (right) in *Bos indicus*.

Examination of Scrotum, Testes and Epididymides. Examples of variations in scrotal conformation are depicted in Figure 11. Some bulls may have a significant cleavage between the right and the left cauda epididymis. This modification of the scrotum does not seem to interfere with testicular function. In rare cases, testes may be rotated up to 40 degrees with no apparent ill effects. The testes, epididymides and the scrotal contents should be carefully palpated and evaluated during the examination. Some examples of abnormal scrotal conformation are shown in Figure 12.

Cryptorchidism does occur in bulls, but a more commonly observed condition is a bull with one testis only partially descended into the scrotum. These bulls are commonly called "high flankers," and the partially retained testis can usually be palpated in the scrotal cord. Scrotal hernias are encountered less frequently now than in the past when bulls were customarily more highly "fitted" (fattened). Testes that are soft may be undergoing degeneration and are usually smaller than normal. The importance of determining testes size is discussed in the section on scrotal circumference.

Since normal testes and epididymides are almost always symmetrical, *any deviation in size, shape or relative position should be viewed with suspicion.* Alternately, each testis with epididymis may be displaced dorsally in the scrotum to facilitate a thorough examination of the adjacent testis and epididymis. This procedure also assesses mobility of these organs within the scrotum, indicating a lack of adhesions.

The caput (head), corpus (body) and cauda (tail) of the epididymis are readily palpable in the normal bull. Hypoplasia or aplasia of the epididymis can occur; however, the most commonly encountered epididymal lesions involve enlargement of the epididymis due to inflammation, fibrosis, tumors, abscesses and sperm granulomas. Sperm granulomas, secondary to adenomyosis in the epididymis, have recently been found to be common in bulls implanted as calves with Zeranol (Ralgro, available from International Minerals and Chemical Corp., Terre Haute, Indiana). Conditions producing gross

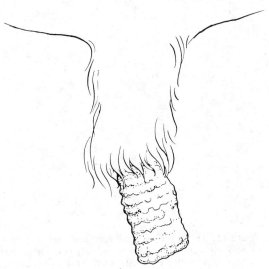

Figure 9. Eversion of the prepuce is found in all polled bulls and bulls of *Bos indicus* breeds. Bulls severe in this trait may experience more preputial damage.

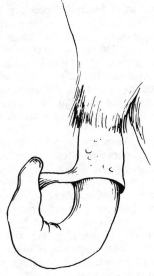

Figure 10. A persistent penile frenulum results from an abnormal development of the penis and sheath and prevents service. This condition is easily corrected by surgery. However, bulls with this genetic defect should not be used to sire purebred calves.

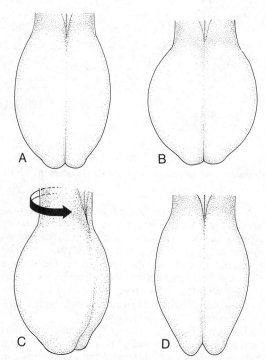

Figure 11. Variations of scrotal conformation. *A,* Normal scrotal conformation with elongated testes. *B,* Normal scrotal conformation with rounded testes. *C,* Scrotum may be rotated in some bulls with no apparent ill effects. *D,* Cleavage between caudal epididymides is sometimes very distinct.

enlargement of the epididymis can be the result of many causes; however, *the net results of most are occlusion of the epididymal duct and a poor prognosis for recovery.*

Examination of Internal Accessory Sex Organs. The ampullae of the vas deferens, the vesicular glands, the prostate gland and the pelvic urethral muscle can be palpated via rectal examination. The body of the prostate gland is palpable as an elevated band of tissue at the anterior end of the pelvic urethral muscle; however, the disseminate part of the prostate is not palpable. Abnormalities of the prostate gland are seldom detected during a rectal examination.

The most commonly encountered lesion during the rectal examination is chronic inflammation of the vesicular glands, which are lobulated paired organs. Increased firmness of the vesicular glands along with increased numbers of white blood cells in the semen help establish a diagnosis of vesiculitis. Vesiculitis is most often seen in young bulls and very old bulls. Vesicular gland disease is often accompanied by inflammation of other parts of the tubular genital tract, the vas deferens, ampullae, epididymides or the testes.

During the rectal examination, the fecal contents should be removed in preparation for the insertion of the probe of the electroejaculator.

SCROTAL CIRCUMFERENCE

Determination of scrotal circumference is an essential aspect of breeding soundness examinations of beef bulls. Measurements of scrotal circumference have great value as indicators of *puberty, total semen production, semen quality, pathologic conditions* of the testes and the potential *subfertility or infertility* of bulls in the breeding pasture. Most importantly, scrotal circumference, along with its consequences, is *highly heritable.* Therefore, failure to select properly for this trait has the potential of decreasing fertility and production for generations to come. A yearling bull with a scrotal circumference greater than 36 cm has very good testes size for its age, since most bulls range from 32 to 36 cm at this age. Excellent testes size in 2- to 3-year-old bulls can exceed 40 cm.

Methods. Measurements of scrotal circumference have been demonstrated to be highly repeatable, both among different people taking the measurements and among different measurements taken by the same person, if care is taken in obtaining the measurement. It is extremely important that veterinarians consistently utilize *similar* and *accurate* methods (Fig. 13). The measurement for scrotal circumference (in centimeters) is taken at the area of the largest diameter of the scrotum, using a special tape constructed for this purpose (Scrotal Tape, Lane Manufacturing Inc., Denver, Colo-

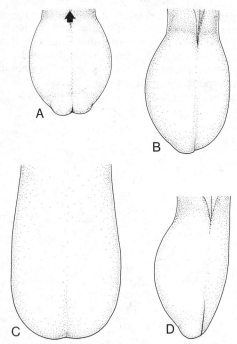

Figure 12. Any deviation from normal scrotal conformation usually leads to a poor prognosis. *A,* Testes held close to the body wall are usually small or hypoplastic. *B,* Unilateral hypoplasia. *C,* Scrotal hernia. *D,* Incomplete descent of right testis.

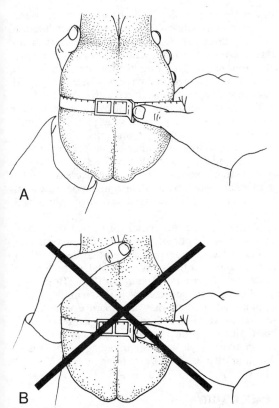

Figure 13. Correct method for measurement of scrotal circumference. The testes are pulled *firmly* into the lower part of the scrotum by encircling its base with the hand and pulling down on the testes *(A)*. The scrotal tape is formed into a loop and slipped over the scrotum and pulled up snugly around the *greatest diameter* of the scrotal contents. The thumbs and fingers should be located on the side of the scrotum rather than between the testes *(B)* to prevent separation of the testes and inaccurate measurement.

rado). Scrotal circumference is an indirect but effective method for determining the weight of the testes of a live bull. Testicular weight provides an accurate estimate of the sperm-producing parenchyma of the testes of young bulls.

Puberty. Measurements of scrotal circumference have been shown to be more accurate predictors of puberty than either age or body weight, regardless of breed or breed cross. Bulls in one study reached puberty (defined as the time when a bull first produced an ejaculate containing at least 50×10^6 spermatozoa and at least 10 per cent motility) at an average scrotal circumference of 27.9 cm. Age at puberty in heifers has been shown to be favorably correlated with scrotal circumference in their half-sib yearling brothers. Young bulls with an above average scrotal circumference should produce heifer offspring with earlier inherent ages at puberty. Conversely, use of bulls with below average scrotal circumference could delay the age at puberty in heifer offspring and impair the heifer's ability to cycle and to conceive at an early age.

Semen Production and Semen Quality Related to Testes Size. Scrotal circumference measurements are accurate predictors of sperm output in young bulls. Bulls with larger testes produce more spermatozoa. Scrotal circumference in young bulls also gives an accurate indication of future testicular characteristics. Scrotal circumference of bulls at 12 and 18 months of age has been shown to be favorably correlated with weekly sperm output of mature bulls. Other studies of beef bulls during and after weight gain trials have demonstrated that most bulls with inadequate scrotal circumference at 12 months of age and inadequate semen at 16 months of age did not correct their deficiencies by 2 years of age. Therefore, bulls with scrotal circumference measurements below that of their herdmates as early as 1 year of age are unlikely to catch up later.

Scrotal circumference in young bulls is favorably correlated with semen traits. As scrotal circumference increases, estimates of sperm motility and percentage of normal sperm increases, while percentage of abnormal sperm decreases. Increased motility of sperm and a higher percentage of normal sperm occurs earlier in bulls that reach sexual maturity earlier. In older bulls, an increase in abnormal spermatozoa associated with small testes is usually attributed to pathologic conditions in the testes.

Scrotal circumference has also been shown to be positively correlated with pregnancy rate of cows. This could be viewed as the ultimate test of semen quality in beef bulls.

Factors Affecting Scrotal Circumference. Scrotal circumference increases rapidly in young bulls, more gradually in mature bulls and may even decline in old bulls. As a bull gains weight, testicular weight also increases, especially in growing bulls. However, heavily fitted 2-year-old bulls may have a larger scrotal circumference because of fat deposition in the scrotal area.

Zeranol, an anabolic steroid, is used widely in the beef cattle industry to increase weight gain of growing cattle. Zeranol is derived from zearalenone, which interacts directly with estrogen receptors and evokes many of the same biologic and biochemical responses that are evoked by estradiol. Although Zeranol is not recommended for use in breeding animals, some breeding bulls have been implanted with it to increase feed-gain records and skeletal growth. Breeders should be warned that the use of zeranol implants in prepuberal bulls will decrease scrotal circumference and retard sexual development.

Differences in scrotal circumference among breeds have been recorded. For example, Angus and Simmental have larger scrotal circumferences than Polled Herefords, Charolais or Limousin. Brahman bulls tend to have the smallest scrotal circumferences as yearling bulls. However, there is great variation in scrotal circumference among individuals within breeds. For example, 25 Angus bulls from one herd ranged in scrotal circumference from 28 to 37.5 cm at 13 months of age at the completion of a 140-day gain test. *This variation offers cattlemen an opportunity to increase reproductive and productive traits in beef cattle by selecting individuals within breeds that have above average scrotal circumferences.*

Beef bulls are generally selected for performance traits (rate of gain, feed conversion, red meat "muscle" yield of carcass), rather than reproductive traits. It has been demonstrated that selection for increased growth rate in bulls results in later maturing lean types. Later maturing lean types tend to have smaller scrotal circumferences. Small testes have also been reported to be associated with bulls with muscular hypertrophy characteristics that produce high cutability carcasses. It is extremely important that high performance bulls be reproductively sound. *A high rate of gain or superior muscling will not compensate for inadequate scrotal circumference.* In a recent study involving over 3,000 yearling beef bulls of twelve breed groups, testicular size and body weight were found to be largely independent, regardless of breed. It should, therefore, be possible to produce bulls with both superior growth traits *and* large testicular size for age.

Testicular Lesions Associated with Small Testes. Inadequate scrotal circumference is commonly observed in bulls examined after poor performance in the breeding pasture. While lower sperm production is a characteristic of bulls with small testes, a decrease in sperm numbers alone is not sufficient to explain the subfertility or infertility that is often observed in these bulls. Bulls in pasture service usually have a large reserve capacity of sperm production in relation to the demands placed upon them. If low numbers of sperm were the major consideration, then bulls with small testes might be expected to be equally as fertile as those with large testes, if mated with fewer cows. This does not appear to hold true, however, as there are other factors involved. Infertility associated with small testes is usually attributed to testicular hypoplasia and/or testicular degeneration. Although the histopathologic lesions of both testicular hypoplasia and degeneration have been characterized, it is difficult to differentiate between the conditions clinically without an accurate history showing that infertility was an acquired trait.

Bulls with *total hypoplasia* can have a scrotal circumference of only 27 to 29 cm at 2 to 3 years of age. Essentially no germinal epithelium is present in the seminiferous tubules, and the affected bulls are azoospermic. Chromosomal abnormalities have been observed in some cases of severe bilateral testicular hypoplasia. A more commonly encountered condition is *partial hypoplasia,* in which both hypoplastic and normal seminiferous tubules are present in the same testis. Bulls with partial hypoplasia may produce sperm with fertility rates approaching those of normal bulls for 1 or more years. These animals eventually become less fertile or completely sterile because the normal seminiferous tubules tend to undergo degeneration earlier and at a more rapid rate. Clinical examinations often reveal a higher prevalence of abnormal sperm in the semen of bulls with small testes, most likely because of early testicular degeneration of the normal tubules. Hypoplasia is present in most cattle breeds. *All forms of hypoplasia are likely heritable.* Selection of bulls with large scrotal circumference for age will discriminate against bloodlines with hypoplasia.

Testicular degeneration, which is not associated with hypoplasia, can occur in young bulls as a result of extreme heat, cold, systemic infections, trauma, nutritional factors and other causes. Degeneration of the seminiferous epithelium can decrease the scrotal circumference of bulls. This decrease can be permanent or reversible, depending upon the causal factors involved, including duration of insults and age of bulls.

Because of the association of scrotal circumference with age of puberty, semen traits and testicular health, it has been recommended that beef bulls on performance test trials have a scrotal circumference of *at least 32 cm at 12 months of age.* Beef bulls usually average between 34 to 36 cm in scrotal circumference when they are mature enough for service as yearlings. Studies have suggested that bulls with a scrotal circumference of less than 30 cm should not be used for breeding even if most sperm in the ejaculate are normal.

SEMEN QUALITY

Methods of Semen Collection. Most bulls evaluated for breeding soundness in the United States are beef bulls. Because beef bulls are usually not trained to the artificial vagina and are seldom halter broken, the electroejaculator is most often used to collect a semen sample. Several types of electroejaculators are available commercially, but little improvement has been made in the design of electroejaculators since they first came into wide use. A significant improvement in probe design, however, has been available for a number of years. With the improved design, the electrodes are located ventrally on the probe and are not equally spaced around the probe. This arrangement seems to reduce excessive muscular contractions associated with electroejaculation. These types of probes* are available in three sizes (60 mm, 75 mm and 90 mm). One should always use the largest probe size that the bull will easily accommodate for best results. This will almost always be either the 75 or 90 mm size. The weakest link in the electroejaculator system is the cord-probe connection. It is advisable to always have an extra cord available as a spare. Electrojac† applies rhythmically preprogrammed alternating periods of stimulation and rest to the electrodes and automatically increases the signal strength during 32 successive stimulation periods.

It is important to collect only the semen-rich

---

*3-Electrode Probe, Lane Manufacturing, Inc., Denver, Colorado.

†Electrojac, Ideal Instruments, Inc., Chicago, Illinois.

portion of the ejaculate and not the accessory sex fluid, which may be profuse in some bulls. The collection tube should be warm and properly insulated to protect against cold shock, and the semen should be immediately moved to a waterbath maintained at 37°C. Not all bulls respond to the electroejaculator. *The most difficult aspect of collection with the electroejaculator is the determination of whether a representative sample of ejaculate has been obtained from an unresponsive bull.* Multiple attempts to obtain a satisfactory sample may be necessary in some bulls. The bull should be allowed a 10- to 15-minute rest between attempts for best results. A diagnosis of azoospermia or oligospermia determined from a sample of an ejaculate obtained with the electroejaculator needs corroborating evidence such as epididymitis, sperm granulomas or testicular hypoplasia.

Manual massage of the pelvic genitalia (vesicular glands, ampullae, and pelvic urethra) can produce a quantity of semen sufficient for examination. Success depends upon the age of the bull and the experience of clinician using this method. Younger bulls are usually more responsive.

The *artificial vagina* is an expedient method of collection of the semen sample if conditions permit its use. This method offers the advantage of simultaneous evaluation of mating ability and, to some extent, libido during the collection.

Motility of Spermatozoa. A semen sample should be evaluated for motility only if the temperature of the sample has been kept constant from the time of collection until the time of examination under the microscope. Small portable slide warmers are available for this purpose. A drop of semen is placed directly on a prewarmed slide for examination. Gross motility is judged according to the swirling movement of the semen. Individual motility of the sperm cells exhibiting progressive movement can be estimated as a percentage if the sample is diluted with either physiologic saline or sodium citrate solution.

Research indicating a positive correlation between individual motility of spermatozoa and fertility has been conducted at artificial insemination centers that have controlled environmental conditions, semen handling techniques and well-trained technicians. *However, in recent studies, motility has been found to be of limited value in predicting the potential fertility of beef bulls used in pasture-mating systems.* Numerous factors can decrease motility estimates of a semen sample that is collected with the aid of an electroejaculator under field conditions. Semen samples that are not properly fractionated during the collection process are dilute and do not give the rapidly swirling appearance of properly collected samples when gross motility is estimated. The presence of urine in the sample will greatly reduce motility. Environmental insults such as heat, cold or chemical contamination of the collection apparatus can immobilize spermatozoa. When semen samples are diluted for individual motility estimations, care must be taken that the diluent is

of the same temperature as the semen and that these diluents are freshly prepared.

Morphology of Spermatozoa. Our interest in sperm morphology concerns its influence upon fertility. Lagerlof, in 1934, was among the first to show that an increased prevalence of abnormal sperm is associated with a decrease in fertility. The appearance of an increased number of abnormal sperm in the ejaculate is a reflection of lesions of the testes and/or of the excurrent duct system and provides a convenient clinical diagnostic aid.

To some degree, phagocytosis masks the evidence of lesions in the seminiferous epithelium by eliminating some abnormal sperm during their passage through the tubular genital tract. In bulls whose fertility is impaired, a high number of head abnormalities is found in sperm leaving the rete testis. Phagocytosis occurs in the excurrent duct system of these bulls and reduces the number of abnormal heads appearing in the ejaculate. Tail abnormalities generally increase as the sperm pass through the excurrent duct system. Some tail abnormalities may originate in the testes of bulls with impaired fertility, but an increased prevalence of tail abnormalities is usually the result of epididymal dysfunction.

Methods. The prevalence of abnormal spermatozoa is usually determined by a stained semen smear examined under the light microscope or by a wet mount of spermatozoa preserved in formol saline solution and examined under a phase contrast microscope. Generally, abnormal sperm are categorized and percentages recorded while counting a total of 200 sperm cells.

An eosin-nigrosin stain is commonly used as a morphology stain. Semen smears can be prepared by placing a small drop of semen and an equivalent drop of stain at one end of a slide. With a second slide placed across both semen and stain, this slide is rotated to mix the semen with the stain. The slide is then pulled across the top of the first slide, leaving a thin smear.

The other method involves the addition of a few drops of semen to 2 ml of of a buffered formol saline solution to preserve the sperm for immediate or future examination. A wet mount is prepared by placing a drop of this mixture on a glass slide and adding a coverslip. Samples preserved in this manner can be easily shipped when additional interpretations or a second opinion is needed.

Examination of sperm morphology is best accomplished with the use of a phase contrast microscope because certain types of sperm abnormalities cannot be detected when sperm are viewed under the light microscope. In research studies, greater magnification may be required. Figure 14 shows spermatozoa with the crater defect, as viewed with phase contrast, differential interference contrast and transmission electron microscopy.

Classification of Abnormal Sperm. If a bull has a very high prevalence of a specific sperm abnormality, we expect the animal to be infertile. An example of this type of defect would be the "decapitated sperm defect" first reported in 1949. Separation of

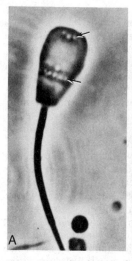
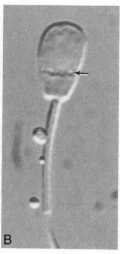
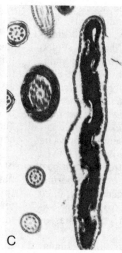

Figure 14. *A,* Phase micrograph of an affected spermatozoon. Craters appear as clear refractile bodies in the diadem position postacrosomally (arrow) as well as near the acrosomal ridge (arrow). *B,* Differential interference contrast micrograph of an affected spermatozoon. *C,* Transmission electron microscopy transverse profile of the diadem arrangement of craters in the postacrosomal region. The craters are located alternately on both faces of the nucleus.

the spermatozoa into detached heads and active tails involved nearly 100 per cent of the ejaculated sperm cells and resulted in sterility. An example of a specific abnormality associated with subfertility is the "Dag defect," in which half of the sperm had strongly coiled, folded or broken tails. Other specific sperm abnormalities that have been reported to be abundant in the spermiogram of an infertile or subfertile bull include "knobbed sperm," in which a protrusion of the acrosome occurs at the apical ridge; the "tail stump defect," in which many of the sperm have rudimentary tails; "pseudodroplets," in which a droplet with inclusion bodies is located on the middle piece and a specific middle piece abnormality descriptively named the "corkscrew defect." In addition to these, there are many nonspecific sperm abnormalities that are frequently encountered during breeding soundness examinations.

The classification of commonly observed sperm abnormalities as *primary abnormalities* or *secondary abnormalities* is not correct but is still widely used. The designation of primary abnormalities was reserved for those abnormalities of the sperm cells that occur within the seminiferous epithelium. Examples were abnormal head shapes, midpiece abnormalities and strongly coiled tails. Secondary abnormalities were thought to occur as the sperm traverse the epididymis or during ejaculation. These included proximal and distal cytoplasmic droplets, detached normal heads and simple bent tails. This classification of sperm abnormalities has become troublesome. More importantly, retention of the proximal droplet is now thought to be a result of a malfunction of the process of formation of the spermatozoa in the seminiferous epithelium, rather than the result of epididymal dysfunction. Furthermore, classification of sperm abnormalities as *primary* and *secondary* implies that secondary abnormalities are less important than primary. Proximal droplets were considered a secondary abnormality, but they have great importance as indicators of testicular degeneration.

In 1973 Blom suggested that a more appropriate designation of abnormalities might be categorization as *major* or *minor*, according to their significance as indicators of potential breeding soundness. Examples of some of the more common major and minor sperm abnormalities are shown in Figures 15 and 16. This classification should only be used as a guide, since much of the evidence linking the prevalence of morphologically abnormal sperm with infertility is circumstantial. More studies are needed to determine the significance of the presence of abnormal sperm in the ejaculate and their subsequent effect on fertility.

Interpretation of the Spermiogram. An increased prevalence of sperm with morphologic abnormalities such as head abnormalities and retained proximal droplets may be evidence of either *sexual immaturity* or *degenerative changes* in the seminiferous epithelium of the testes. A rapid decrease in the prevalence of spermatozoa with head abnormalities, retained proximal cytoplasmic droplets, kinked and coiled tails occurs in ejaculates of bulls during the first several months after puberty. Abnormal sperm will usually disappear from the ejaculate of a late maturing bull as the bull ages and, in some bulls, as the testes become larger. *A bull that does not exhibit a normal spermiogram by 18 months of age is a poor risk as a future breeding animal.*

It is difficult in many cases to determine whether testicular degeneration will be *transient* or *permanent.* Our prognostications are complicated by the fact that 49 days are required for sperm to complete the spermatogenic cycle plus an additional 2 weeks are required for passage of the sperm through the epididymis. One condition that causes a transient increase in morphologic abnormalities of sperm cells and a consequent decrease in fertility is heat stress. Approximately 2 weeks after the insult of heat stress, abnormal sperm will appear in the ejaculate and will continue to increase as long as 1 month later. After that time, improvements should be seen. If the heat stress were continued over a longer

palpable testicular or epididymal lesions or inadequate scrotal circumference, is sufficient reason to classify a bull as a questionable or, depending upon severity, as an unsatisfactory potential breeder. A bull should remain a questionable or an unsatisfactory potential breeder until a normal sample is obtained in a later examination.

Several points concerning the determination of the prevalence of abnormal spermatozoa in an ejaculate should be emphasized.

1. Accuracy of classification of sperm as normal or abnormal may vary greatly according to the *training* and *experience* of the examiner. Pitfalls include artifacts that may be classified as abnormal sperm and failure to recognize discrete but important abnormalities. Yet another variable concerns the type of microscope used to examine samples of ejaculate. Equipment used to view spermatozoa can range from the light microscope to phase contrast, differential interference contrast, scanning electron or transmission electron microscope. At one extreme, one may not always be seeing enough to be helpful, while at the other, one may be seeing too much with little hope of proper interpretation.

2. There is great danger in trying to arrive at a diagnosis and a prognosis after viewing a sample from only one ejaculate. Variations in the spermiogram among successive ejaculates taken with the electroejaculator from the same bull at 10 to 15

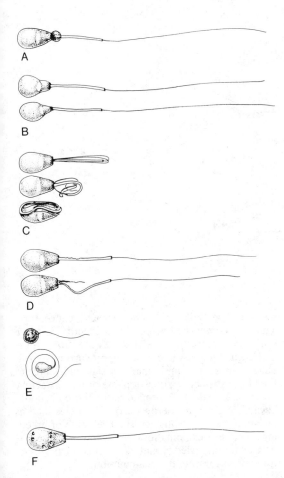

Figure 15. Major sperm abnormalities. *A,* Proximal cytoplasmic droplets. *B,* Pyriform heads. *C,* Strongly folded or coiled tails, tails coiled around the head. *D,* Middle piece defects. *E,* Maldeveloped. *F,* Craters.

period of time, improvement in semen quality and fertility would also be delayed. Figure 17 shows an actual case of heat stress in a bull and its effect on abnormal heads, abnormal acrosomes, proximal droplets and sperm motility. In general, there was an increase in these abnormalities, especially proximal droplets, reaching a maximum by mid-September after heat stress in late July to early August. At this same time, there was a corresponding decrease in motility from 70 to 20 per cent during the time of the greatest number of abnormal sperm. Proximal droplets increased from levels below 5 per cent to 90 per cent during this time period. By mid-December, the spermiogram approached normality.

Classification of a Bull with an Abnormal Spermiogram. A spermiogram exhibiting an increased percentage of sperm with major or minor abnormalities should be viewed with suspicion. The presence of more than 15 per cent major abnormalities or more than 30 per cent total abnormalities, especially when coupled with other findings such as

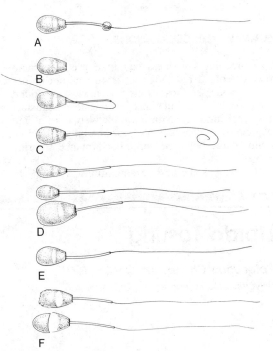

Figure 16. Minor sperm abnormalities. *A,* Distal cytoplasmic droplets. *B,* Tailless normal heads. *C,* Simple bend or terminally coiled tails. *D,* Narrow, small or giant heads. *E,* Abaxial implantation. *F,* Abnormal acrosomes (ruffled, detached).

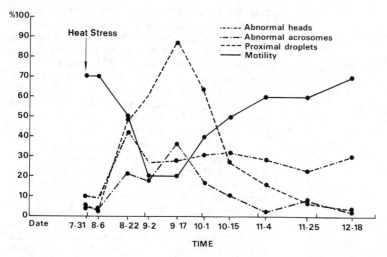

Figure 17. Effects of heat stress on a bull.

minute intervals are common. Therefore, two or *more* samples are usually required. In some cases, examination of samples collected over a period of months may be necessary to gain insight required for an accurate diagnosis and prognosis.

3. Interpretation of a spermiogram requires information concerning the bull's breeding history and the results obtained from a thorough clinical examination of the bull. This is very important.

SUMMARY AND CONCLUSIONS

A breeding soundness examination is the practitioner's considered judgment as to whether or not a bull possesses those traits that have been found common to other bulls that have achieved satisfactory conception rates in reproductively normal and eligible cows. The only *true* test of a bull's breeding ability is the bull's measured performance of siring calves.

Breeding soundness examinations attempt to measure the bull's *potential* to cause conception. This is accomplished primarily by identifying those bulls with characteristics that deviate from "normal," attaching a value based upon current knowledge to these data and, finally, assigning a status to the bull (satisfactory, questionable or unsatisfactory potential breeder). A prognosis for the bull should always be given to the owner of a bull classified as questionable or unsatisfactory. The value of breeding soundness examinations varies in direct proportion to the knowledge and experience of the practitioner performing the examination.

References

1. Ball L, Ott RS, Mortimer RG, Simons JC: Manual for Breeding Soundness Examination of Bulls. J Soc Theriogenology 12:1983.
2. McEntee K: The male genital system. In Jubb KVF, Kennedy PC (eds): Pathology of Domestic Animals. 2nd ed. vol 1. New York, Academic Press, 1970, p 443.
3. Roberts SJ: Infertility in male animals. In Veterinary Obstetrics and Genital Diseases. 2nd ed. Ann Arbor, Edwards Brothers, Inc., 1971, p 713.

Libido Testing

Peter John Chenoweth, B.V.Sc., Ph.D.
University of Queensland, St. Lucia, Australia

Libido in bulls has been defined as the willingness and eagerness to mount and attempt service, with mating ability described as the ability to complete service. Deficiencies in either can seriously compromise herd production. Such deficiencies represent significant causes of bull wastage, and they often have a genetic basis. High libido in bulls is advantageous to herd fertility and has probable beneficial effects on the fertility of subsequent female progeny.

Despite these considerations, interest in bull sexual behavior has burgeoned only recently, with the first literature reference to bull libido appearing in 1941. Even today, with breeding soundness examinations (BSE) of bulls being widely accepted, there is little routine screening of bulls for libido and mating ability, despite evidence that such omission enables a number of substandard bulls to be classed as satisfactory potential breeders. Unfortunately, there is no relationship between BSE and libido assessments, and use of the electroejaculator precludes concurrent assessment of both libido and semen quality.

THE DEVELOPMENT OF TEST PROCEDURES

Bulls Used for Artificial Insemination

Early studies on bull libido were stimulated by problems in maintaining libido in dairy bulls at artificial insemination (AI) centers. Progression from this work led to the development of procedures such as sexual preparation and stimulation to optimize sperm harvests.

Anderson[2] summarized the earliest efforts at assessing bull sexual behavior into three categories:

1. Studies in which bulls were exposed to suitable stimuli on different occasions, with the number of successful services being recorded.

2. Studies in which the number of mounts and services within a stipulated time period were counted.

3. Studies in which elapsed time was measured between exposure of bulls to a suitable stimulus and their first service ("provocative" or "reaction" time).

"Reaction" time was used quite extensively as a measure of bull libido in the 1950's, particularly in work with AI bulls. Almquist and Hale[1] obtained a high reliability with this method in 28 bulls but warned that assessment accuracy could be influenced by the presence or absence of prior stimulation. Both "exhaustion" and "depletion" tests of bulls were also developed during the 1950's; however, although they contributed greatly to our knowledge of the reproductive capacity of bulls, they were generally too demanding of time and labor for use as routine testing procedures.

Hultnas[8] described a technique for assessing libido and mating ability in AI bulls by employing a nonestrous cow restrained in a service bail as the stimulus. Three attempts were made to collect semen with an artificial vagina over a 10-minute period. The reaction of the bull to the cow, his approach to service and his behavior in completing service were scored, and libido was quantified as follows:

0 = No interest in cow, although bull was led up and invited to mount.

1 = Little interest in mounting, despite sniffing at the rear end of the cow and perhaps vague mounting attempts.

2 = Mounting after obvious repeated hesitation with weak clasping and seeking.

3 = Comparatively quick mounting without obvious eagerness. Satisfactory holding and seeking.

4 = Quick mounting with bull's attention focused upon the cow with very good holding and seeking.

5 = Eager mounting with very good holding and seeking.

6 = Uncontrolled eager mounting with very good holding and intensive seeking.

Beef Bulls

The next logical development in the refinement of testing procedures was to develop a test for untrained beef bulls. Osborne and colleagues[10] proposed a scheme in which individual bulls were exposed to an estrous female for 5 minutes. The procedures employed by these authors were as follows:

Virgin heifers were ovariectomized. Immediately prior to their use they were treated as follows:

Day 1: 6 to 7 AM, 10 mg of dexaprogesterone acetate in oil IM

Day 2: 6 to 7 AM, 10 mg of dexaprogesterone acetate in oil IM

Day 3: 6 to 7 AM, 10 mg of dexaprogesterone acetate in oil IM

Day 4: 5 to 6 PM, 5 mg of diethyl stilbestrol diproprionate in oil IM

Most heifers showed evidence of estrus 12 to 20 hours after the last injection and remained in this state for approximately 6 to 8 hours. Heifers required for use on succeeding days were given 5 mg of diethylstilbestrol diproprionate IM on the preceding evenings. With this technique, heifers were successfully used for up to 4 successive days.

The examination for libido and breeding ability was performed in a small yard where the bull and heifers could be easily observed. Bulls were admitted individually and were allowed exactly 5 minutes with one of the prepared heifers that had been selected as exhibiting behavioral estrus.

Research with this program led to separate scoring systems being used for both libido and mating ability[4] as follows:

Libido Scoring System

0 = Bull showed no sexual interest.

1 = Sexual interest shown only once (e.g., sniffing at perineal region).

2 = Positive sexual interest in female on more than one occasion.

3 = Active pursuit of female with persistent sexual interest.

4 = One mount or mounting attempt with no service.

5 = Two mounts or mounting attempts, with no service.

6 = More than two mounts or mounting attempts with no service.

7 = One service followed by no further sexual interest.

8 = One service followed by sexual interest, including mounts or mounting attempts.

9 = Two services followed by no further sexual interest.

10 = Two services followed by sexual interest, including mounts, mounting attempts or further services.

Each bull was tested twice at each testing period and the worst result of the two tests was discarded.

Mating Ability Scoring System

Group 1 = Bulls that served satisfactorily.

Group 2 = Bulls that made mounting attempts

that did not culminate in service because of inexperience, faulty mating technique or pathologic factors.

Group 3 = Bulls that mounted but did not achieve service owing to lack of cooperation by the female. This could reflect factors such as bull inexperience, low libido or use of an unsuitable female.

Group 4 = Bulls for which there was no record of mating ability because of lack of sufficient activity for an assessment to be made.

This procedure proved useful in testing young beef bulls, as it enabled a score to be given that was not dependent solely upon service. In single-sire breeding trials the libido scores obtained by 56 bulls were more highly correlated with the subsequent pregnancy rates than were seminal quality scores. However, considerable time and effort were necessary to prepare the heifers for this test (although the advent of effective estrus synchronization agents, such as the prostaglandins, has simplified procedures for heifer preparation).

A "serving capacity test" for beef bulls was developed that minimized these difficulties.[3] The procedure for this test was as follows:

1. Nonestrous cows or heifers were restrained in service crates in a pen.

2. Bulls were "prepared" prior to their exposure to the test by allowing them to observe sexual activity within the pen for 10 or more minutes.

3. Bulls were admitted to the yard containing the restrained cows at a bull-to-female ratio of 5:2 or 5:3.

4. The duration of the yard test was 40 minutes.

5. The number of services performed by each bull during that period was recorded as his serving capacity score.

This test was applied to 75 bulls (aged 2 to 5 years) that were then placed in groups with heifers at a bull-to-female ratio of 1:5. The heifers had been ovariectomized and given an intramuscular injection of 0.75 mg estradiol benzoate (in oil) 16.5 to 18.5 hours previously. It was found that the serving capacity score of groups of bulls was highly correlated with the proportion of estrous heifers the groups of bulls served (r = 0.94) and the proportion of heifers the bulls served 2+ times (r = 0.98) in a simulated breeding season. However, this test was only valid if the groups of bulls used for testing were kept intact for the breeding season, as libido and dominance were confounded.

Libido and serving capacity scores, as well as reaction times to mounts and service, were compared in 113 yearling beef bulls in Colorado.[5] The overall repeatabilities (phenotypic correlations) of the libido and serving capacity scores were similar (r = 0.67 and 0.60, respectively), while reaction times were not significantly correlated. Fifty-seven per cent of the bulls did not achieve a service in both 30-minute serving capacity tests and thus received no score.

The libido score method had the advantages that more bulls received a positive score, and the test duration (in this case, 10 minutes) was shorter than that of the serving capacity test. The shorter test (utilizing fewer bulls) reduced the opportunity for agonistic interactions among bulls, which was a source of concern in the longer serving capacity tests. Thus, it was concluded that the libido score method was most advantageous in assessing sex drive in yearling beef bulls and that a short test (e.g., 10 minutes) gave as much comparative information about bull libido as longer tests (e.g., 30 minutes). However, an assessment period longer than 10 minutes may be necessary to define certain types of breeding disabilities. The total number of services achieved by the bulls did not differ when estrous or nonestrous heifers were employed as stimuli, and it was concluded that the use of females in estrus was unnecessary to assess bull sex drive satisfactorily, provided the females acting as stimuli were properly restrained and presented. It should be noted that this last conclusion has doubtful validity for testing of *Bos indicus* type bulls.

A testing procedure employing features of several systems has now been used successfully with large numbers of beef bulls.[4] This procedure is as follows:

1. Two mildly sedated, nonestrous females are restrained in service crates in a small pen about 5 to 7 m apart.

2. Bulls to be tested are allowed to observe the testing procedure for at least 10 minutes prior to their exposure.

3. Two bulls are admitted to the pen at a time and observed for exactly 10 minutes.

4. The libido scoring system (as previously described) is applied.

5. The bulls are retested on at least one more occasion (preferably on different days).

6. The worst score obtained by an individual bull is discarded.

Work at Clay Centre[9] resulted in the development of a testing procedure employing four restrained, estrus-induced ovariectomized females as stimuli for randomized groups of five yearling bulls for 30 minutes. Each bull received six exposures to the test over a 21-day period prior to pen and hand-mating trials of selected bulls. Although this testing procedure is impractical for on-ranch testing, a significant difference was found between the pregnancy rate achieved by the low libido bulls (50 per cent) and the medium and high libido bulls (61 per cent) in the pen-mating trials. In these tests a learning process occurred in the bulls over consecutive libido tests—a trend also observed by the author in one study with 26 yearling bulls[4a] but not in another employing 113 yearling bulls.[5]

In Australia promising results have been obtained in relating bull reproductive performance to changes in peripheral blood testosterone concentrations following GnRH or hCG challenge. Such changes were highly repeatable within bulls and were significantly related to both their 24-hour testosterone profiles and to the pregnancy rates that they achieved in single-sire mating programs.[11]

PITFALLS

In general successful testing of bulls for libido and breeding ability requires careful planning, lots of patience and a modicum of luck. Pitfalls include the following:

1. Testing of bulls that are excessively apprehensive or agitated. Apart from taking precautions to handle cattle quietly and to avoid distractions, there is no easy solution to this problem that can lead to depressed scores.

2. Testing of bulls immediately following their subjection to other stressful procedures such as electroejaculation, vaccination and parasite control measures.

3. Testing under adverse weather conditions (e.g., in extreme heat or cold or during inclement weather).

4. Testing of bulls in groups in which one or more bulls are markedly dominant (e.g., with mixed-age groups of bulls). The exposure of only two bulls to the test at a time and the subsequent retesting with a different bull help to minimize this problem. It should be noted however that a dominant bull can exert an inhibitory effect on submissive bulls from a distance (e.g., from an adjacent pen).

5. Use of inadequate stimuli. Restrained females should be incapable of excessive movement of their rear ends, or some bulls will be deterred. If nonrestrained females are employed, care should be taken to ensure that they are in full estrus.

6. Spreading of venereal diseases. Every precaution should be taken to ensure that venereal diseases such as vibriosis and trichomoniasis are not transmitted via such procedures.

7. Injury or excessive stress to restrained females. Humane considerations mandate that females are closely observed for signs of stress and that they are replaced when these become evident. Mild sedation of the females for the test period is also recommended.

Causes of Low Libido Scores in Bulls

Libido in bulls has a strong genetic component. It is best assessed in young bulls as older bulls can have superimposed learning patterns, musculoskeletal problems and inhibitions that adversely affect libido scores. However, some young bulls raised in all male groups may show temporary deficiencies in libido.

Bulls that are overconditioned or that have been on high feeding levels may show decreased libido. Also, bulls in very poor condition, or those suffering from disease or pain, can show a secondary lack of libido. Bulls that are stressed (either from handling or environmental influences) will generally give poor results.

If the stimuli are inadequate (e.g., the females are poorly restrained or unrestrained females are not fully in estrus) depressed scores will be obtained. Similarly, bulls that have become satiated with particular stimuli will show decreased libido, although new stimuli will often regenerate them.

Causes of Poor Breeding Ability in Bulls

Low libido in bulls can contribute to disorientation and lack of motivation in sexual foreplay and mounting. Young bulls raised in all male groups often show delayed expression of competent mating ability, and this can lead to lowered reproductive performance early in restricted breeding seasons.

A five-part classification system for different types of breeding disabilities in bulls has been proposed[6] and is outlined here.

Serving Disability with No Other Apparent Clinical Signs. This is generally observed in younger bulls and can be due to low libido, inexperience, or spondylosis deformans. In this latter situation bulls place their hind legs too far back when mounting, leading to a concavity of the back when seeking (Fig. 1). The penis is not fully extended and seeking

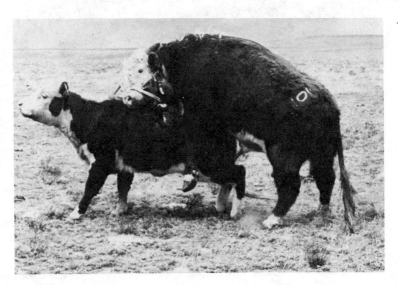

Figure 1. Mature bull exhibiting symptoms of spondylosis deformans. Note the concavity of the back and the ventral direction of the penis.

is typified by short, quick movements with the penis being directed below the level of the vulva. Lesions may be detected, especially in the lumbosacral intervertebral joints. There is possibly a genetic basis for this condition.

Serving Disability Associated with Back Problems. This is more commonly seen in older bulls (although not exclusively so) and is often due to wear and tear on articular surfaces. Pathologic conditions of the skeletal system in old bulls (9 to 16 years) with impaired fertility have been described. Degenerative changes in the articular cartilages of various joints were commonly encountered, as were vertebral exostoses. No difference was found between beef and dairy bulls in the occurrence of spinal bone lesions. Also, there was no evidence that the degree of force of the ejaculatory thrust or the ejaculation frequency influenced the development of these lesions. Other work suggests a relationship between the feeding of high dietary calcium levels to bulls and the occurrence of similar conditions.

Spondylosis deformans is not uncommon in older bulls. Affected bulls often "step short" in their hind limbs and display a hunched back. There is often unilateral or bilateral wasting of the gluteal muscles, periodic lameness and sometimes paralysis of the tail. Some individuals will use their neck muscles to "lever" themselves up onto the back of the female when mounting. These bulls mount with a stiff back and show a gradual decrease in penile protrusion and the vigor of both seeking and thrusting (Fig. 2). This condition is probably caused by prolonged attrition of the lumbar intervertebral spaces, resulting in osteophytic outgrowths and ankylosis.

Serving Disability Due to Abnormalities of Feet and Legs. Joint lesions are increasingly being detected in young bulls. Genetic, nutritional and conformational factors have been implicated. A degen-erative arthropathy of the hip has been reported in young Hereford bulls, affecting approximately one quarter of the male progeny of one sire. This condition, which primarily affects the stifle joint, can have variable effects on breeding ability. Evidence implicating both heredity and nutrition in the pathogenesis of this condition is strong.

In one report all of 223 fattened young European bulls examined showed joint lesions of varying severity in the forelimbs. The most severe lesions occurred in those bulls fed most intensively and that grew the fastest. Overweight, straight-hocked bulls were also predisposed to stifle lameness.

Conformational defects such as straight legs, "sickle hocks" and "pigeon toes" can not only lead to mating disabilities but can also contribute to associated problems such as penile hematomas. In addition, it has been shown that conformational defects of the feet and legs of young bulls can be highly heritable.

A progressive spastic syndrome affecting one or both hind legs in young calves (and occasionally older animals) has been reported. This disease is manifested by a straightening and backward extension of the affected hindlimb with certain breeds (e.g., Holstein) and conformations (e.g., "post legs") being predisposed. The disease is inherited and has been referred to as spastic paresis, spastic syndrome and "Elso heel."

Another condition has been reported in older animals. This is characterized by clonic-tonic muscular spasms, generally first evident in the hind quarters. It has been termed "crampy," "stretches" and progressive hindlimb paralysis. The condition is incurable, inherited and probably sex linked. Its development has been associated with arthritis, straight hindlimbs, and weak hocks and with lumbar spondylosis and lumbosacral disc protrusions.

Foot problems such as overgrown hooves, inter-

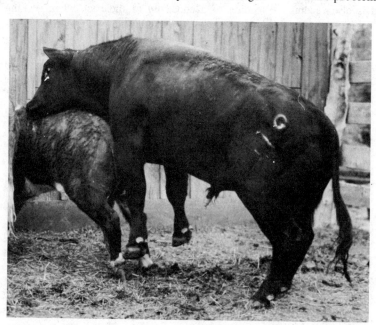

Figure 2. Mature bull exhibiting symptoms of spondylosis deformans. Note the use of head and neck muscles to lever himself onto the female, the stiff back and the poor penile protrusion.

digital necrobacillosis, bruised sole, pododermatitis, interdigital fibromas and laminitis can interfere with breeding ability. For a complete review of these and other foot and limb conditions that may affect breeding ability in bulls, readers are referred to the work of Greenough and colleagues.[7]

Serving Disability Associated with Abnormalities of the Penis and Prepuce. Inability to attain normal penile protrusion can be caused by a short retractor penis muscle or by a congenitally short penis. Both conditions may be inherited. Care must be taken to avoid premature diagnosis of the latter problem in young, overfat bulls that may be slow in penile development or penile-preputial separation.

Both decreased libido and copulative dysfunction are associated with penile phimosis. This can be caused by stenosis of the preputial passage or orifice, adhesions within the penile-preputial system, neoplasms of the penis or prepuce and balanitis or balanoposthitis.

Paraphimosis of the penis, or inability to retract the penis, occurs when there is constriction of the preputial passage or orifice. Other causes include penile paralysis and increased fluid pressure within the penile-preputial system secondary to penile hematomas.

A persistent penile frenulum was detected in 57 bulls out of 10,940 examined in one survey, with the main breeds represented being Beef Shorthorns and polled beef breeds. This was seen as a bandlike attachment from the glans penis to the prepuce along the ventral median raphe, varying from a short, cordlike structure to a continuous band of tissue. This condition represents a failure of normal prepuberal adhesions between the penis and prepuce to separate properly. Some breeds and lines of bulls are more susceptible than others, indicating a probable genetic predisposition.

Preputial prolapse in the bull is a serious condition that can adversely affect copulative ability. Breed differences in the occurrence of this condition have been reported. Two factors possibly associated with these differences are an excessive amount of parietal preputial epithelium and an absence of the retractor muscle of the prepuce (particularly in polled breeds). Those bulls of breeds commonly affected (Santa Gertrudis, Brahman, Angus and Poll Hereford) were shown to have a greater total prepuce length than other, less susceptible, beef breeds. In another report, it was shown that a significant difference existed between the mean lengths of the prepuce in Hereford bulls that everted (13.0 cm) and those that did not (11.4 cm).

Rupture of the tunica albuginea leading to a penile hematoma is a common condition in beef bulls. It generally occurs at service and is associated with the very high blood pressures within the corpus cavernosum penis (CCP) at this time. Sequelae include paraphimosis, adhesions and sensory nerve damage.

An important cause of copulative disability in beef bulls is penile deviation (or phallocampsis).

Three main types of spontaneous deviation have been described; namely, ventral, S-shaped and spiral (or corkscrew). The last is seen most commonly. Deviations may occur secondarily to trauma, such as lacerations or hematomas of the penis and, here, the presence of scar tissue readily indicates the cause. Spontaneous deviations are often seen in 3- or 4-year-old bulls following one or two successful breeding seasons. Ventral deviations may be diagnosed with the aid of a suitable electroejaculator, whereas corkscrew deviations can only be properly diagnosed at natural service. The heritability of such conditions has been reported to be low, although circumstantial evidence of a genetic basis for the corkscrew type abnormality has been collated. Because surgical correction often affords only temporary relief, it is possible that the problem is of neuromuscular origin and represents a premature occurrence or incoordination of a "normal" event. Support for this theory is furnished in one study that showed that the bull's penis often coiled during ejaculation. The penis of the bull has a natural tendency to deviate ventrally and to the right when the integument is stretched, and thus caution must be exercised in the diagnosis of penile deviations under conditions other than natural service.

A bull's inability to perform service has been associated with peripheral nerve degeneration to the penis. Damage to the sensory nerve supply to the dorsum of the penis can occur subsequently to a penile hematoma. Affected bulls often lose the ability to "seek" accurately and commonly direct the penis over the gluteal area of the mount animal. Hair rings around the penis are a common malady in bulls and can cause restricted circulation and even necrosis of areas of the penis distal to them.

Abnormalities in the degree of erection of the penis, or "filling defects," have been reported. Here, the erection may commence in an abnormal fashion from the posterior part of the prepuce and spread slowly towards the glans; or the penis may curve out of the prepuce in a semierect state and remain in this fashion for some seconds after the bull has dismounted. A consideration of the mechanisms of erection in the bull (subsequently confirmed by corpus cavernosography studies) strongly suggests that some of these problems are related to leakage or abnormal anastomoses from the CCP or blockage of the CCP by a persistent thrombus. Cavernosal venal shunts may be either congenital or traumatic in origin.

Penile papillomatosis is not uncommon in young bulls, particularly when they are reared together. It is caused by a similar papilloma virus to that which causes body warts and can be spread among bulls by homosexual behavior. The papillomas are often subepithelial on the penis, can grow quite large in size and can interfere with normal copulation.

Miscellaneous Problems Leading to Service Disability. A number of physical problems can interfere with the ability of a bull to perform natural service. These include excessive paunchiness and the presence of either scrotal or umbilical hernias. Marked disparity in size between bulls and mount animals can also lead to apparent faults in breeding ability.

CONCLUSION

Bulls vary greatly in libido and mating ability. A number of contributing factors to this variation and different methods of assessing these traits have been discussed. Such assessments improve fertility prognosis in bulls and are valuable in the detection of specific abnormalities. Different surveys indicate that between 10 and 20 per cent of bulls have unacceptably low libido, which underlines the importance of assessment for this trait.

Bulls of high libido generally get more females pregnant earlier in the breeding season than bulls of lower libido, leading to improved calving rates and weaning weights. High libido bulls are superior in the detection of females in estrus, and they tend to service estrous females more often than lesser bulls. As fertility differences among sires have been related to the interval between ovulation and fertilization, this latter consideration is important. High libido bulls tend to produce uniform calf groups as they achieve more pregnancies within limited time periods than lower libido bulls. This facilitates genetic selection programs as well as managerial tasks.

The limiting factor in the reproductive performance of high libido bulls is their capability to produce sufficient numbers of viable spermatozoa to sustain fertility through multiple ejaculations at short intervals. As libido and BSE components are not related to each other, it is advisable to assess bulls in both categories.

References

1. Almquist JO, Hale EB: An approach to the measurement of sexual behavior and semen production of dairy bulls. Proc 3rd Int Cong Anim Repro, Cambridge, Plenary papers, pp 50–39, 1956.
2. Anderson J: The semen of animals and its use for artificial insemination. Tech Comm Imp Bur Anim Breed Genetics Edinburgh, 1945.
3. Blockey MA de B: Serving capacity—a measure of the serving efficiency of bulls during pasture mating. Theriogenology 6:393, 1976.
4. Chenoweth PJ: Libido and mating ability in bulls. In Morrow DA (ed): Current Therapy in Theriogenology. Philadelphia, WB Saunders Co, 1980.
4a. Chenoweth PJ, Berndtson: Unpublished data.
5. Chenoweth PJ, Brinks JS, Nett TM: A comparison of three methods of assessing sex-drive in yearling beef bulls and relationships with testosterone and LH levels. Theriogenology 12:223, 1979.
6. Galloway DB: Factors affecting fertility in bulls. Proceeding of refresher course for veterinarians on beef production. The Postgraduate Foundation in Veterinarian Science, University of Sydney, 1970, p 36.
7. Greenough PR, MacCallum FJ, Weaver AD: Lameness in cattle. Weaver AD (ed): Bristol, John Wright & Sons, 1981.
8. Hultnas CA: Studies on variation in mating behavior and semen picture in young beef bulls of the Swedish Red and White Breed and on causes of this variation. Acta Agric Scand Suppl 6:1, 1959.
9. Lunstra DD: Evaluation of libido in beef bulls. Proc Soc Theriogenology Ann Gen Meet. Omaha, 1980, pp 169–178.
10. Osborne HC, Williams LG, Galloway DB: A test for libido and serving ability in beef bulls. Aust Vet J 47:465, 1971.
11. Post TB, Reich MM: Relationship between fertility and the testosterone response to GnRH or hCG in bulls. Proc 2nd Anim Sci Cong Asian Australasia Assoc Anim Prod Soc. Manila, 1982.

Puberty and Postpuberal Development of Beef Bulls

Glenn H. Coulter, B.Sc. (Agr.), Ph.D.
Agriculture Canada Research Station,
Lethbridge, Alberta, Canada

In recent years increased attention has been given to the reproductive development and performance of young beef bulls. However, it is the opinion of this author that emphasis by breeders on reproductive performance still ranks third, behind growth performance and conformational traits, in most beef-breeding programs. In terms of economic importance to the cow-calf producer, reproductive performance, growth performance and product quality (for example, carcass quality) have been ranked in the ratio of 10:2:1. That is, reproductive performance is five times more important than growth performance and ten times more important than quality traits. Reproductive performance is of particular importance in beef bulls that breed 90 to 95 per cent of North American beef females by natural service and are traditionally used at a bull-to-female ratio of 1:25 to 1:40. Pressure to improve growth traits of beef cattle has resulted in the selection and use of younger bulls in an effort to shorten generation interval. As beef breeders increasingly realize the important role of reproductive performance, more interest and emphasis on reproductive performance of young beef bulls can be expected. In turn, the beef breeder will demand from the veterinary practitioner more answers about the selection and management of young beef bulls.

Puberty has been defined as the period at which the sexual organs are functionally developed, the sexual instincts are prominent and reproduction is possible. In bull calves puberty is indicated by the ability to produce spermatozoa and to copulate, resulting in paternity, usually occurring at less than 1 year of age. It should be noted that attainment of puberty does not equal attainment of sexual maturity and full reproductive capacity, although the two appear to be related. Many different definitions of puberty are used in the scientific literature. One commonly associated with young bulls is that puberty occurs upon the collection of the first ejaculate having at least 50×10^6 spermatozoa/ml with at least 10 per cent progressive motility.

This article will address some of the physiological changes occurring in young beef bulls up to puberty and early postpuberal development, as well as factors that should be considered when selecting and managing young beef bulls in order to improve reproductive performance. The behavioral aspects of puberty and reproductive performance will be covered elsewhere.

ENDOCRINOLOGY

Puberty in the bull appears to result from a continuous, dynamic endocrine process that begins soon after birth. Shortly after 2 months of age, the first prominent endocrine activity begins with the frequent pulsatile discharge of luteinizing hormone (LH).[2] By 3 months of age, prepuberal LH concentrations peak and start to decline slowly. The frequency of LH peaks increases until about 4 months of age.[2] Serum LH concentrations increase linearly ($P < .01$) from 7 months of age through puberty until at least 13 months of age. No differences in LH concentration because of breed have been observed between 7 and 11 months of age.[5] Induced LH surges do not stimulate increased average serum testosterone (T) secretion until bulls are about 6 months of age, indicating that the Leydig's cells of prepuberal bulls may become more sensitive to LH stimulation as puberty approaches. Steroidogenesis begins at about 3 months of age, with androstenedione levels being greatest in 4-month-old bulls, likely as a result of LH-induced differentiation of the Leydig's cell. Further differentiation of the Leydig's cell is believed to result in high T levels at 5 months of age, about 1 month subsequent to increased frequency of LH episodic peaks. Serum testosterone also increases linearly ($P < 0.01$) from 7 months through puberty until 13 months of age. Breed differences in T ($P < 0.05$) were observed over the evaluation period. The correlation between average T and age at puberty in young beef bulls was -0.51 ($P < 0.01$), while average T was not correlated with LH concentration at puberty ($r = 0.26$).[5] The gradual increase in LH and T as puberty approaches supports the theory of sexual maturation through hypothalamic-hypophysis complex desensitization by gonadal steroids. Follicle stimulating hormone (FSH) concentrations do not appear to change appreciably with age. FSH remains relatively constant and free of episodic peaks throughout the prepuberal period.[2] Prolactin concentrations tend to increase in young bulls from 1 through 5 months of age, while the increase in frequency of prolactin peaks appears to increase through 4 months of age. The role of prolactin in sexual maturation is not yet clear.

SPERMATOGENESIS

Parallel to the endocrine changes leading to puberty in the bull are continuous quantitative and qualitative morphologic developmental changes in the seminiferous tubules of the testes. The development of spermatogenic function is dependent on endocrine activity. Abdel-Raouf has broken down the initiation of spermatogenesis into four phases.[1]

The first or infantile phase extends from birth to the beginning of the eighth week of age. During this phase the solid sex cords are composed of gonocytes and undifferentiated supporting cells. Some gonocytes degenerate; others divide mitotically while retaining relatively constant gonocyte numbers. Indifferent basal supporting cells divide actively and increase in number, and some appear in the center of the solid cords.

The second or proliferation phase begins during the eighth postnatal week and continues until 20 to 24 weeks of age, depending on the level of nutrition. Spermatogonia first appear at 8 weeks and increase in number until they are found in all tubules by 20 weeks of age. Both the basal and the central indifferent supporting cells have reached their maximal relative numbers and begin to decrease. The increase in number of indifferent supporting cells is higher than that of spermatogonia.

The third, or prepuberal, phase extends from the beginning of the twentieth postnatal week until the beginning of week 32. In bulls fed at low levels, this begins at week 24 and ends between week 32 and 40. In this phase lumen formation begins and is completed. The indifferent supporting cells decrease rapidly in relative numbers, giving rise to Sertoli's cells, which are first observed at about week 28. Primary spermatocytes make their appearance at the beginning of this phase (20 weeks). By 32 weeks of age the average number of primary spermatocytes exceeds that of spermatogonia. Primary spermatocytes will increase in number until about 60 weeks of age. Secondary spermatocytes first appear sometime between 20 and 28 weeks. At the latter age spermatids begin to appear. Spermatozoa are first seen late in the prepuberal phase.

The fourth, or puberal, phase extends from week 32 until about week 44, when spermatogonia reach adult levels. By 40 weeks all indifferent cells have matured to Sertoli's cells and have reached adult levels. By 44 weeks primary spermatocyte numbers increase, owing to the active division of the spermatogonia, and either spermatids or spermatozoa or both are present. From the time puberty occurs at about 44 weeks until senility, the main changes in spermatogenesis are quantitative.

Naturally, the ages discussed here are averages

for a particular group of bulls. Considerable variation in the time of onset of different aspects of spermatogenic activity is expected among bulls within a breed, among breeds and as a result of environmental factors such as nutrition, as mentioned previously.

The growth curve for seminiferous tubule diameter is not linear, but somewhat S-shaped. The increase in tubule diameter can be divided into three periods according to age. From birth to 20 weeks of age constitutes the first period when diameter increases twofold. The second period extends to about 36 weeks of age. At this time rapid increases in size occur followed by a slower growth rate in the third period after 36 weeks of age. Little increase in tubule diameter occurs after 60 weeks of age.

ANATOMIC CHANGES

Discussion of the early development of the epididymis is facilitated by dividing it into five regions: region I and II in the caput, region III in the corpus and regions IV and V in the cauda epididymis.[1] Variation in the epithelial lining of the epididymis is evident at birth. Region V is lined with pseudostratified epithelial cells, while the other regions are lined with simple columnar epithelial cells. The other regions acquire the pseudostratified epithelium in ascending order, with differentiation completed by 32 weeks of age. It is suggested that testicular androgens diffuse through the tunica albuginea and enhance the differentiation process, particularly in region III. Stereocilia are observed in regions I and V at birth, followed by development in the other regions. The adult height of the epididymal epithelium is attained by 52 weeks, well after puberty. Sperm are first observed in the lumen of the epididymis at 32 weeks of age. Feeding at low levels results in delayed epithelial differentiation, delayed maximum epithelial height and delayed appearance of sperm in the lumen. The first two effects are eliminated by 36 weeks and the third by 48 weeks of age.

The tubelike seminal vesicles of newborn bulls increase in length accompanied by a double bending. The first curvature develops at 4 to 8 weeks and the second at 24 weeks of age. In young bulls the lobules of the seminal vesicles are small and cover only the cranial aspect of the gland. The lobules increase in size and extend caudally over a larger area with advancing age. The consistency of the glands becomes softer and the color darker with age. Fructose and citric acid are present in the glands at birth; however, the amounts of these substances greatly increase after 20 weeks of age, presumably in response to testicular androgens. Glandular secretions begin by 24 weeks of age. Lower nutritional levels result in delayed morphologic development that is eliminated by 36 weeks of age.[1] The size of the seminal vesicles continues to increase to sexual maturity. As seminal vesiculitis is a relatively common problem in young bulls, particularly those reared in groups, the practitioner should be familiar with the size, shape and consistency of the seminal vesicles of bulls of different ages.

Penile growth is most rapid in young bulls from birth to 24 to 28 weeks of age. The sigmoid flexure begins to develop at about 12 weeks of age and becomes more prominent thereafter. Separation of the penis from the prepuce begins on the left dorsal aspect of the glans penis and progresses ventrally and caudally. Separation of the penis from the prepuce begins at 4 weeks of age, the urethral process is fully separated by 8 weeks of age, and the entire separation is completed by 32 to 40 weeks.[1] Penile separation can be retarded through inadequate nutrition or accelerated through androgen administration. A highly significant correlation of -0.48 has been reported between average serum T concentration and age of prepuce-penis detachment in young beef bulls.[5] The penis increases in length by up to 5 times by the onset of puberty and continues to increase in length until sexual maturity.

TESTICULAR DEVELOPMENT

Puberty, defined in this case as when a bull first produces an ejaculate with at least 50×10^6 spermatozoa/ml and 10 per cent progressive motility, can be accurately predicted using scrotal circumference. A scrotal circumference of 27.9 ± 0.2 cm at puberty is relatively constant among breeds differing in biologic type and among bulls differing widely in age and weight at puberty.[5] This puberal scrotal circumference measurement, obtained with the measurement technique used is equal to 26.1 ± 0.2 cm using the scrotal circumference technique recommended by the Society for Theriogenology.

Testicular growth in the young bull is very rapid from 6 months through puberty. Puberty in the bull seems to be a focal point whereby testicular growth either continues at a normal rate or slows, resulting in underdeveloped testes in breeding-age bulls. It is this author's opinion that decisions on the acceptability of testicular development of a bull cannot be made with any degree of authority until several months after puberty.

The age of the bull is the factor that has the greatest effect on testicular development from 6 through 24 months of age. Figure 1 illustrates a distribution of scrotal circumference by age in a sample of 1275 Angus bulls. The shape of the best fitting regression line shown for Angus bulls is similar for all *Bos taurus* beef breeds. An important characteristic of this growth curve is the rapid increase in testicular growth rate from 6 through 24 months of age, particularly during the last 8 to 10 months. By 24 months of age testicles of the beef bull have developed to approximately 90 per cent of mature size. Therefore, if a bull has not achieved anticipated growth by 2 years of age, there is a very low probability that appreciable additional growth will occur.

A striking aspect of the distribution shown in

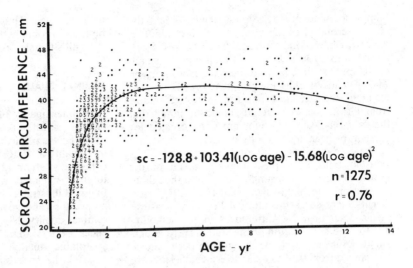

Figure 1. Distribution of scrotal circumference by age in Aberdeen Angus bulls. Note the rapid growth rate in young bulls and the large variation in testicular size at a given age ("age" in the regression equation is in days). Scrotal circumference measurements taken as per Foote. (From Coulter GH: Proc 8th Tech Conf AI Reprod, NAAB, 1980, p 106.)

$$sc = -128.8 + 103.41(\text{LOG age}) - 15.68(\text{LOG age})^2$$

$$n = 1275$$

$$r = 0.76$$

Figure 1 is the great range in testicular size for bulls of the same age within breed. Paired testes weight of bulls of the same breed may vary by as much as 550 gm. A similar pattern is observed for bulls of most breeds. This variation within a breed, coupled with the high heritability of testicular size ($h^2 = 0.44$ to 0.69), facilitates a relatively rapid response to selection.

Figure 2 illustrates differences in testicular development as related to body weight in five beef breeds. A contrast is observed between the best-fitting regression lines for the "British" (Hereford and Angus) versus "Continental" (Charolais, Maine Anjou and Simmental) breeds. Between 200 and 600 kg of body weight, the regression lines for the British breeds are curvilinear. Testicular growth rates are faster initially but slow to rates below those of the Continental breeds. Within the same weight range, testicular growth rate is linear for all three Continental breeds. These testicular growth patterns relative to body weight are not unexpected. British breed cattle tend to reach mature size at a younger age and lower body weight than Continen-

tal breeds. The relationship between body weight and scrotal circumference was examined in a 4-year study involving 1770 yearling beef bulls of several breeds as they completed 140-day growth performance tests. A highly significant correlation coefficient of 0.43 was observed between body weight and scrotal circumference.

Testicular development does not appear to be highly related to postweaning weight gain. One study reported a genetic correlation of 0.22 ± 0.34 ($n = 401$) between scrotal circumference at 365 days of age and postweaning gain, while a second study reported no significant relationship ($n = 1770$) between average daily gain over a 140-day growth performance test and scrotal circumference at 365 days of age. In the latter study a negative relationship ($P < 0.05$) was observed between weight per day of age and scrotal circumference at 365 days of age. Although significant, this relationship appears not to be of any practical importance.

Breed contributes significantly to variation in testicular development of young beef bulls. In a study on the effect of breed in 3063 1-year-old beef

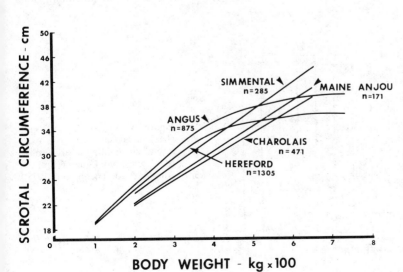

Figure 2. Regression lines illustrating the effect of body weight on scrotal circumference in five breeds of beef bulls. Scrotal circumference measurements taken as per Foote. (From Coulter GH: 8th Tech Conf AI Reprod, NAAB, 1980, p 106.)

bulls from nine breeds, Simmental bulls had the largest scrotal circumference at 365 days (35.9 ± 0.2 cm), while Blonde d'Aquitaine (30.6 ± 0.5 cm) and Limousin (30.3 ± 0.3 cm) bulls had the smallest. Unpublished data from the same laboratory on 7447 2-year-old bulls indicate that breeds tend to maintain their relative position in testicular size from 1 to 2 years of age. It should be noted that the data for 2-year-old bulls are not corrected for location or year, age or body weight.

The predictabilities of scrotal circumference in 1-year-old bulls from measurements taken during growth-performance testing reveal that although all correlations are highly significant (P <0.01), coefficients increase as the interval between measurements decreases. No differences in predictability due to breed or location of the studies were apparent. Coefficients early in the growth-performance test ranged from 0.44 to 0.68. These coefficients are too small to predict final scrotal measurements accurately. In contrast, measurements taken during the last month of the growth performance test were useful in predicting whether a bull would achieve a specified culling level. It was determined that taking scrotal circumference measurements on young bulls within a month of the end of the test would save time during the final weighing procedure. Bulls estimated to be borderline with respect to a culling level could be measured again at the end of the test.

Testicular development in young beef bulls is highly heritable. Estimates of heritability (h^2) of scrotal circumference at 365 days of age range from 0.44 ± 0.24 in 401 Hereford bulls to 0.69 ± 0.15 in 1984 bulls of eight breeds at completion of their respective performance tests. A h^2 score for scrotal circumference in 438 Hereford and 331 Angus bulls 16 to 22 months old on a within-breed basis is reported as 0.40 ± 0.15 or 0.21 ± 0.15 when corrected for body weight. The high h^2 of the scrotal circumference trait, the considerable variance in the trait in bulls of a given age and the ease and repeatability with which the measurement can be taken provide an opportunity to readily increase

testicular size. Thus, the breeding performance of bulls and probably the reproductive performance of the bull's female progeny are also improved.

SEMINAL QUALITY

Seminal quality of young beef bulls is the most difficult aspect of reproductive performance to evaluate. This is particularly true when predicting seminal quality at 16 to 18 months of age from samples collected at about 12 months of age. Scrotal circumference is related to seminal quality in beef bulls. Figure 3 illustrates the proportion of beef bulls with a given scrotal measurement having satisfactory seminal quality. No bulls having scrotal circumferences of less than 30.0 cm produced semen of acceptable quality. As scrotal circumference increased, the probability of a bull having acceptable seminal quality increased linearly until a scrotal measurement of 38.0 cm was attained. At this point 88 per cent of bulls were classified as satisfactory.

As discussed earlier, bulls reach puberty once they have a scrotal circumference of 26.1 cm. As complete spermatogenic function is just beginning at this time, continued improvement in sperm numbers and seminal quality would be expected as testicular development proceeds. Extensive variation has been noted in seminal quality traits of young beef bulls. These differences occur both within and among breeds. It has been demonstrated[4] that adjustment of seminal quality data for age at puberty negates breed differences. This suggests that for the breeds evaluated, seminal characteristics were similar at puberty. The seminal traits of spermatozoa concentration, progressive motility, seminal protein concentration, proportion of spermatozoa with normal head and tail morphology and proportion of spermatozoa with normal acrosomal morphology all increase until at least 4 months after puberty.[4] Changes in scrotal circumference and seminal quality traits relative to puberty are illustrated in Figures 4 and 5. Age at puberty varies among breeds and to a still greater extent among bulls

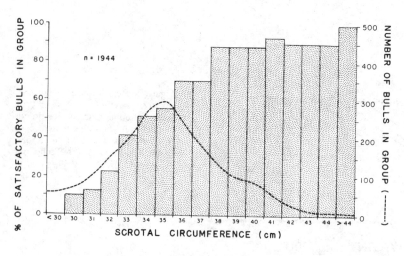

Figure 3. Proportion of bulls classified as satisfactory in each scrotal circumference size group. (Adapted from Cates WF: Proc Ann Meet Soc Theriogenol, 1975.)

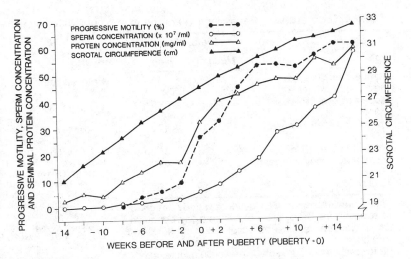

Figure 4. Patterns of change in scrotal circumference (cm), sperm concentration ($\times$ 10^7/ml), progressive motility (%) and seminal protein concentration in semen (mg/ml) of 31 beef bulls during the period from 14 weeks before through 16 weeks after onset of puberty (50×10^6 sperm/ml, 10% motile). Increases ($P < 0.01$) occurred in all four traits. Scrotal circumference measurements taken as per Foote. (From Lunstra DD, Echternkamp SE: J Anim Sci 55:638, 1982.)

within breeds. Therefore, careful evaluation of the stage of puberal development in individual bulls is highly recommended when carrying out breeding soundness examinations to determine the desirability of young bulls for breeding programs. The greater the sexual development beyond puberty, which can be estimated by testicular size, the more critical the practitioner should be in evaluating seminal quality characteristics of a bull, keeping in mind normal testicular development for the breed and age of bull.

INFLUENCE OF NUTRITION

Diets adequate in protein, vitamins, minerals and energy appear to hasten the onset of puberty in young beef bulls.[1] The early attainment of puberty improves the opportunity for early postpuberal development. This implies greater numbers and higher quality spermatozoa available when the bull is first used for breeding. However, the feeding of high energy diets beyond puberty is of no benefit and may cause substantial harm to the reproductive potential of young beef bulls. Feeding of high versus

medium energy diets from weaning through 15 months of age has been reported to result in substantial reductions in epididymal sperm reserves in Hereford and Angus bulls. Parallel studies[3] in which Hereford and Angus bulls were fed high- versus medium-energy diets from weaning through 24 months of age show reductions in total epididymal sperm reserves. Reserves were depressed by 75 per cent ($P < 0.01$) and 13 per cent ($P > 0.05$) for Hereford and Angus bulls, respectively, in the first year, and by 35 and 14 per cent ($P = 0.06$) in the second year of the study. Seminal quality in bulls fed high energy diets was also inferior. Preliminary results from subsequent experiments comparing lean and obese bulls at 2 years of age (Table 1) show that lean bulls had about twice as many total epididymal sperm reserves, twice the number of progressively motile sperm, one third as many morphologic abnormalities and 11 times more total services as did obese bulls. These data strongly suggest that the current practice of feeding high-energy diets is detrimental to the reproductive capacity of young beef bulls. Further research is needed to delineate the nutritional requirements of young beef bulls to optimize their reproductive

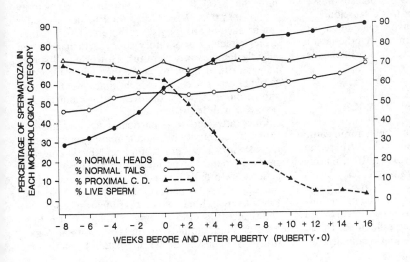

Figure 5. Patterns of change in the percentages of spermatozoa with normal head morphology (excluding acrosomes), normal tail morphology (excluding proximal cytoplasmic droplets) and proximal cytoplasmic droplets and in the percentage of spermatozoa alive (unstained) in semen of 31 bulls during the period from 8 weeks before through 16 weeks after the onset of puberty (50×10^6 sperm/ml, 10% motile). Increases ($P < 0.01$) occurred in the percentage of normal heads and tails, and a marked decrease ($P < 0.01$) occurred in the percentage of proximal droplets during the evaluation period. (From Lunstra DD, Echternkamp SE: J Anim Sci 55:638, 1982.)

Table 1. Suppression of Reproductive Potential*

Trait	Dietary Energy	
	Medium	High
Number of bulls	8	8
Mean body weight (kg)	578	796
Mean back fat thickness (mm)	5.4	39.9
Epididymal sperm reserves ($\times 10^9$)	40.6	19.8
Mean sperm motility (%)	66	35
Mean total abnormal sperm (%)	22	64
Total services†	55	5

*Preliminary results from GH Coulter on a study designed to examine the mechanism by which body condition suppresses reproductive potential in 2-year-old Hereford bulls.

†Total services accumulated in two 30-minute exposures by all bulls in group.

potential. Generally, postpuberal bulls should be maintained in lean condition.

References

1. Abdel-Raouf M: The postnatal development of the reproductive organs in bulls with special reference to puberty. Copenh Acta Endocrinology (Suppl) 49:9, 1960.
2. Amann RP, Schanbacher BD: Physiology of male reproduction. J Anim Sci 57:380 (Suppl 2), 1983.
3. Coulter GH, Kozub GC: Testicular development, epididymal sperm reserves and seminal quality in two-year-old Hereford and Angus bulls: Effects of two levels of dietary energy. J Anim Sci 59:432, 1984.
4. Lunstra DD, Echternkamp SE: Puberty in beef bulls: Acrosome morphology and semen quality in bulls of different breeds. J Anim Sci 55:638, 1982.
5. Lunstra DD, Ford JJ, Echternkamp SE: Puberty in beef bulls: Hormone concentrations, growth, testicular development, sperm production and sexual aggressiveness in bulls of different breeds. J Anim Sci 46:1054, 1978.

Reproductive Behavior of Bulls

Peter J. Chenoweth, B.V.Sc., Ph.D.
University of Queensland, St. Lucia, Australia

Cattle, like most domesticated mammals, are social animals with the unit of their "society" consisting of the herd. Similar to other societies, certain rules and procedures have developed to ensure group survival, cohesion, defense and propogation. Domestication by man, with his emphasis on production characteristics (which are not necessarily in concert with these social needs) has placed stresses upon the system. The object of this discussion is to review current knowledge of bovine male behavior, with particular reference to reproductive behavior, so that the interaction of natural and artificial demands may be better understood.

EARLY DEVELOPMENT OF SEXUAL BEHAVIOR

The basic pattern of male sexual behavior in cattle appears to be innate, as postpuberal bulls reared in complete isolation will often display normal mating behavior when exposed to estrous females. Calves of both sexes exhibit sexual behavior during play, with the most common manifestation being mounting behavior. This impulse is also seen in castrated bulls and in females under steroid influences. In the intact bull, however, such activities gradually de-

velop into coordinated mating behavior under the mediation of nervous and hormonal influences. Full puberty (or sexual maturity) occurs when the physical, spermatogenic and behavioral development of the bull are all sufficiently developed and coordinated to allow fertile service to occur. Breed differences occur in the time period required for such attainment, with dairy breeds generally requiring a shorter period than beef breeds. Within beef breeds, sexual maturity generally occurs earlier in *Bos taurus* breeds than in *Bos indicus* breeds, with a differential as great as 9 months.

NORMAL MATING BEHAVIOR

In the breeding herd, females generally play the major role in soliciting sexual partners and often from a sexually active group (SAG) that although highly mobile generally stays within eyeshot of the bull (or bull group). The bull is usually attracted into the SAG by the sight of mounting activity within its ranks. Visual cues tend to be of greater importance in arousing sexual interest in bulls than either olfactory or auditory cues, particularly when eligible females are plentiful. However, all senses may be called upon for assistance when receptive females are scarce, at which time the bull may shown more evidence of investigatory and tending behavior with individual females.

Once attracted to a particular female, the bull tests her receptivity by making real or sham mounting attempts, by chin testing and by licking and sniffing around her perineal region. These last two actions are often followed by a curling upwards of the upper lip to perform the flehmen response. Recent research has shown that this response is the end result of a series of tongue actions that help to transfer fluid samples to the vomeronasal organ, which is believed to be the site of pheromone identification. The greatest single stimulus to a bull to mount and to attempt service is a female's rear quarters or something similar. Physiological estrus is not necessary for the bull to attempt mounting and service, providing adequate immobility is displayed. A suitable stimulus need not even be female, confirming that an inverted "U" shape is the visual configuration most stimulatory to the release of mounting behavior in bulls. This phenomenon has been exploited widely in bull studs in which steers instead of females are often employed as stimulus animals. The main criteria for an ideal stimulus for a bull to carry out mounting and service are considered to be adequate strength, appropriate height and immobility. Although "dummies" can be used satisfactorily, bulls tend to prefer teaser animals, with older bulls being more discriminatory.

The process of "seeking" is the penis' movement to and fro until its tip reaches and penetrates the vulva. This process is aided by movements of the bulls' hindlimbs to align the glans penis both vertically and horizontally with the vulva. Contractions of his abdominal muscles and hind leg movements help bring the pelvic region of the bull into direct apposition with the external genitalia of the female. The detection of vulval heat and moisture by superficial nerve endings in the glans penis is the major factor leading to proper intromission. However, ejaculation following intromission is apparently dependent upon nerve impulses from the dorsum of the free portion of the penis. The ejaculatory thrust of the bull is achieved mainly by contractions of the abdominal muscles. Ejaculation coincides with the utmost lengthening of the penis, ensuring that semen is sprayed around the external cervical os. Momentary peak pressure within the corpus cavernosum penis (CCP) may exceed 14,000 mm Hg during ejaculation. Bulls often coil the penis during ejaculation, and the duration of ejaculation is approximately 1.3 seconds.

Bulls are often capable of great sexual activity, and it is not uncommon for pasture-mated bulls to service 30 or 35 times in 1 day, providing stimulus pressure is adequate. In trials in which bulls were mated with estrus-synchronized females, they averaged 55 services within a 30-hour period (range 14 to 101). Whether estrus was induced or natural, bulls tended to serve receptive females between 3 and 10 times per estrous period. Fertility (i.e., pregnancy rates) did not significantly decrease with consecutive services even when very high service rates were achieved, although optimal service rates per female estrous cycle averaged between four and six. Bulls tend to be more attracted to females at the beginning of their estrous cycles, and the presentation of new stimuli can revitalize sexual interest in apparently satiated or jaded bulls.

Obviously, workload affects the ability of bulls to achieve satisfactory pregnancy rates. The amount of work that an individual bull is called upon to perform daily depends on the bull-to-female ratio (BFR), the cyclicity of females, the nature of the terrain, the length of the breeding season and the social interactions among animals within the breeding pasture. In general, the standard recommendation of employing one bull per 20 to 25 females is relatively "safe" when groups of bulls of unknown potential are used in a variety of terrains. Such BFR represent considerable underutilization of superior bulls, as bulls of high libido and having good sperm production can adequately service 60 to 100 females within a limited breeding season. These high breeding ratios are not recommended for young (e.g., yearling) or old bulls or those with suboptimal mobility, sexual stamina or sperm production.

FACTORS AFFECTING BULL MATING BEHAVIOR

Social Interaction. Social ranking of bulls can influence their sexual activity when they are mated in groups, and this can severely compromise group libido testing. Such effects have been well illustrated in studies in which calves from multisire matings were identified by blood typing. Dominant bulls generally sired the majority of calves, with bulls at the bottom end of the social order having relatively little impact on the calf crop. The presence of competition for sexual partners can have a stimulatory effect on the dominant bull even when that competition is suppressed.

In young bulls social dominance ranking has been shown not to be favorably related to either sex drive or breeding soundness criteria. This would explain why in a number of studies pregnancy rates were lower with multisire breeding compared with single-sire breeding. In such cases the dominant bulls could act to depress herd fertility by failing to service or to impregnate all females under their influence and by preventing other bulls from compensating. This effect of social status on reproductive performance is probably most evident when young and old bulls are placed together in mating groups.

Dominance in bulls appears to be mainly a function of age and seniority within the herd or group and less a function of size and presence of horns. With dairy bulls, serious agonistic behavior did not develop until they were 3½ to 4½ years of age. Thus, dominance effects, with their attendant disadvantages, would tend to be less evident when homogenous groups of young bulls are employed in breeding programs. It is also probably more evident with lower BFR and smaller breeding pastures where competition for mating becomes more intense.

There is some interesting information available on dominance in bulls. One study has shown some indication of genetic influences upon dominance in yearling beef bulls, with differences occuring among sires within lines. Several observers have reported apparent breed effects, with *Bos taurus* bulls in particular, being dominant over *Bos indicus* bulls. However, these observations were based on phenotypes within the calf crop, and age and fertility effects among bulls were not studied.

One study has shown that dominance ranking in

yearling beef bulls that had just completed individual performance testing was not related to average daily gain or final test weight. Conversely, in another report a significant partial correlation was found between dominance and weight gain in young bulls, although this relationship only existed during a period of supplementary feeding when competition for feed occurred.

Genetic Effects. Both libido and mating ability in bulls are strongly influenced by genetic factors. Monozygous twin bulls exhibit great similarities in libido and mating ability despite separation into different managerial and nutritional regimes. Variations in libido among sire-son groups have been shown to be significantly greater than variations within such groups, and differences in libido have been reported among different lines and breeds of bulls. A within-breed heritability estimate of 0.59 ± 0.16 was reported for libido of young beef bulls. There are strong indications that some specific forms of mating disability are caused by genetic factors and that certain structural abnormalities causing mating disability are highly heritable.

An interesting possibility is that bull libido and female fertility are linked genetically in a similar fashion to scrotal circumference in bulls and age at puberty in heifers. In sheep female progeny of high-libido rams achieved significantly higher cycling and lambing rates than female progeny of rams with low libido. Ovulation rate in ewes and scrotal circumference in rams are genetically linked. It is probable that genetic relationships occur between similar and other fertility components in male and female cattle. This should be a fruitful area for investigation. If libido in bulls and fertility measures in females (such as age at puberty or ovarian activity post-partum) were genetically linked, there would be a stronger case for libido screening of sires used for artificial insemination.

Libido in bulls apparently is not related to either seminal characteristics or scrotal circumference. It is possible to obtain good semen from a bull with low libido, and high libido bulls may have poor semen quality. The use of aids such as the electro-ejaculator to obtain bull semen precludes the necessity of the subjects' having good or even adequate libido. Thus, bulls of low libido could have their genes widely disseminated with unknown deleterious effects on cattle production.

Differences in sexual behavior at semen collection have been reported for different breeds of bulls, with dairy bulls responding with greater alacrity than beef breeds. Zebu bulls have been reported to exhibit marked sexual sluggishness and a tendency to mount cows in full estrus only. One author observed considerable differences among Indo-Pakistani breeds in the alacrity with which they completed service. Comparison of libido and mating ability in young beef bulls of six different breed groups in Queensland (Brahman, Africander, Hereford, Brahman cross, Africander cross and Short-horn-Hereford cross) showed that the cross-bred bulls generally performed better than the pure-breeds. Those cross-bred bulls with an Africander component in their breeding were superior to those with a Brahman component, while the British type crossbreeds were mostly intermediate. In a Texas study Angus bulls consistently displayed higher libido than high-grade Brahman bulls, although the Brahman bulls were considered to be more efficient at detecting estrus.

Hormonal Influences. Bulls, like other animals, appear to require a threshold level of circulating androgens to initiate true sexual behavior. Once this threshold is attained, the level of sexual activity displayed is not directly linked to circulating testosterone or LH levels, although some promising results have been obtained relating bull libido and fertility to testosterone levels following gonadotropin-releasing hormone (GnRH) or human chorionic gonadotropin (HCG) challenge. Our understanding of the hormonal basis of sex drive is limited. Individual variations in libido are probably influenced by differences in target site responsiveness to androgens and/or their metabolites as well as by the stimulation value of exteroceptive factors. Relating blood levels of hormones to such traits as sex drive is further complicated by the pulsatile nature of the release of many hormones and by the suppressive effects of stress (e.g., restraint) on gonadotropin release.

Thus, it is not surprising that sporadic sampling of peripheral blood with subsequent assay for androgens has yielded disappointing relationships with traits such as sex-drive and fertility. One approach to circumventing the above difficulties is to study the function and size of androgen-dependent organs such as the accessory sex organs. In male rats the size of the accessory sex glands has been associated with intensity of sexual behavior. In one study the libido score was significantly correlated with physical measurements of the vesicular glands in young bulls. Although the correlations obtained were not of a high order, this question deserves further study.

Early Experience. Sexual inhibition in male animals has been reported to occur when management systems congregate young postpuberal males in bachelor groups. Although libido is largely genetic, mating ability has a learned component that could be influenced when bulls are so raised. It has been suggested that a loss of sex drive in bachelor groups of animals is a behavioral adaptation to suppress libido during the nonbreeding season. In one study the libido of Zebu bulls was influenced by management systems, with bulls raised in large mixed age groups on open pasture generally lacking interest in estrous females in comparison with those raised in small homogenous groups in small pastures. However, all bulls eventually displayed "adequate" sexual interest. The possibility that a learned factor is necessary before inexperienced bulls can perform to their capabilities is suggested by the abrupt development of sexual interest in some inexperienced bulls after being mounted by females. Unpublished data from the National Cattle Breeding Station in Australia indicate that young bulls reared together often show delayed reproductive activity when used in single-sire breedings with older cows. On the other hand, there is no evidence to suggest that excessive sexual usage of young bulls has a detrimental effect on subsequent libido, mating behavior or reproductive life, providing adequate growth is maintained.

Nutrition. Conflicting reports exist about the effects of nutrition on sexual behavior of bulls, especially in the peripuberal period. Gross malnutrition, specific protein deprivation and certain hypovitaminoses can adversely affect both steroid secretion and target tissue responsiveness, with the most damaging effects being on the peripuberal male. Several workers have shown that reduced food intake in bull calves may cause sexual maturity to be delayed, although affected animals often achieved normality eventually. Pronounced hypovitaminosis A, phosphorus deficiency, excessive or deficient intake of water and molybdenum poisoning have been reported to have adverse effects on the sex drive of bulls.

At the other end of the spectrum there are a number of reports linking excessive growth rate (particularly concentrate induced) in young bulls with diminished sex drive and semen quality. In one report this disparity in libido between overconditioned and "normal" young bulls was greater under conditions of high environmental temperatures.

Season. The effect of season on bull libido has been poorly documented. A review of earlier work concluded that the greatest variations occurred in tropical and subtropical areas where the libido of bulls could be greatly reduced during the hotter periods of the year. This is probably more associated with physical discomfort than with intrinsic physiological mechanisms, as Leydig cell function is relatively resistant to high temperatures. In one report it was observed that bulls in Europe displayed a less intensive libido in autumn than in spring. In Sweden it was found that libido did not vary with season in young bulls (15 to 26 months) of the Swedish Red and White breed, although a significantly greater number of bulls showed satisfactory natural mating during the summer months. In both subtropical Australia and in Texas, no seasonal effects on libido of young bulls of both *Bos indicus* and *Bos taurus* derivation were observed, although Queensland studies indicated that testosterone levels (based on 24-hour profiles) peaked in early summer and dropped significantly in autumn.

Temperament. Various attempts have been made to categorize temperament of bulls and to relate this to reproductive behavior. These have not generally yielded much valuable information, although there is no doubt that excessively apprehensive or disturbed bulls generally perform poorly in pen assessments of sex drive. Some producers believe that very aggressive bulls are better breeders under conditions of adverse terrain or environment. This relationship has not been established experimentally, and most indications are that aggression and sex drive are not synonymous.

SEXUAL BEHAVIOR AND SEMEN COLLECTION

Early interest in bull sexual behavior was derived from problems associated with libido maintenance in dairy bulls at artificial insemination (AI) centers. Studies in the 1950's and 1960's established procedures for sexual stimulation and preparation of bulls for optimal sperm harvest. Sexual stimulation of bulls is the presentation of a stimulus situation adequate to elicit mounting and ejaculation, whereas sexual preparation is defined as prolongation of the period of stimulation beyond that which is sufficient for mounting and ejaculation. The objective of sexual stimulation is to produce an ejaculate within the shortest possible time, whereas that of sexual preparation is to maximize the number of spermatozoa within the ejaculate. Although work in the past 20 years emphasized sperm harvests per collection, developments of increased periods of semen storage, lower insemination doses and increased usage of beef bulls have led to renewed emphasis on libido maintenance in AI bulls.

Two sexual preparation procedures that have an additive effect on sperm harvest per ejaculate in dairy bulls are false mounting and additional time spent in preparing for ejaculation. One false mount, 2 minutes of restraint and two additional false mounts prior to ejaculation have been recommended for optimal sperm harvest. Beef bulls have responded differently from dairy bulls, with both false mounts and restraint being less effective. Three false mounts did not increase the number of spermatozoa in the second ejaculate from Hereford and Angus bulls in contrast to dairy bulls. It was recommended that beef bulls be given three false mounts prior to the first ejaculate and no false mounts prior to the second ejaculate. Beef bulls generally exhibit lower sexual activity than dairy bulls, and, at the same frequency of ejaculation, they require more frequent changes of teaser cows and of location to maintain effective sexual stimulation.

Although techniques of sexual preparation and stimulation, such as restraint and false mounts, have positively influenced sperm harvest, there is less evidence for their effect on qualitative seminal characteristics. However, characteristics such as spermatozoal motility, spermatozoal survival rate and conception rate are positively influenced by precoital stimulation. Increased sperm numbers harvested in ejaculates following sexual preparation could be attributed to enhanced movement of sperm in the excurrent ducts. Exogenous prostaglandin $F_{2\alpha}$ can cause a similar increase in ejaculated sperm numbers, although it does not influence sperm production.

Increases in qualitative seminal characteristics following such treatment are not explained so easily, although it is possible that sexual stimulation can favorably influence the composition of seminal plasma through enhanced accessory gland function. It is not unreasonable to assume that the libido of individual bulls is a major factor in affecting their degree of response to sexual preparation and stimulation. If both quantitative and qualitative seminal characteristics are affected favorably by such procedures, then the best semen should be consistently obtained from high libido bulls in AI centers. Properly controlled studies are needed to confirm this hypothesis.

Biostimulation

There is considerable evidence in a number of species of a stimulatory male effect on estrous and ovulatory responses in females. This male effect has been termed biostimulation. Biostimulation can accelerate the onset of puberty in females, stimulate cyclic activity to resume in females undergoing seasonal or lactational anestrus and alter times associated with estrus and ovulation.

In domestic animals of economic importance, effects of biostimulation are most evident in sheep and swine, in whom management techniques are commonly employed to exploit this phenomenon. Such techniques include sudden introduction of rams to ewes during transitional periods from the "nonbreeding" to "breeding" season to stimulate group cyclic activity and the exposure of peripuberal gilts to boars to advance and synchronize puberty.

In cattle effects of biostimulation are less dramatic, although the timing of LH peaks, estrus and ovulation in cows can be influenced by various stimuli. Data suggestive of a biostimulatory effect have come from breeding programs in which AI and natural breeding were compared. Although there are grave difficulties in comparing pregnancy and calving rates from AI with natural service, a number of studies reported an advantage for the latter. This advantage (which was not discerned in all studies) could be caused by a number of factors, of which biostimulation may or may not be of greatest importance.

In those studies showing an advantage for natural service over AI, part of this advantage could be caused by genital stimulation of the female by the bull, either before or during service. Nuzzling, nudging and licking of the perineal region of the female by the bull can act to induce estrous behavior and also to prepare the female genital tract for optimal gamete transport. The act of intromission provides the female with an important source of genital stimulation, which in some species (e.g., the cat and rabbit) is necessary for ovulation and in others (e.g., the laboratory rat) is necessary for inducing the "progestational state" necessary for pregnancy. The idea that genital stimulation can favorably influence pregnancy rates in cattle has been shown in several studies on the effects of clitoral stimulation during AI. In these studies clitoral stimulation improved pregnancy rates by 6.3 to 7.5 per cent in cows, but no advantage was seen in yearling heifers. Other possible advantages for natural service include multiple services and more optimal timing of services relative to ovulation than AI.

Other reports have shown positive effects from the presence of bulls or bull-like behavior on estrous behavior and pregnancy rates in females, although not all data are universally supportive of this effect. It would appear that biostimulation is most effective when males are introduced as a novel stimulus. Both the time of the male introduction and female susceptibility are critical. Although intact males would logically be the most effective biostimulators, one experiment reports enhanced estrous and pregnancy responses in estrus-synchronized heifers exposed to androgenized females. The use of behavioral methodology to synchronize estrus and enhance fertility in females obviously has wide implications for both the beef and dairy industries; more research is warranted. For example, it remains to be determined whether bulls of high libido are more effective as biostimulators than bulls of low libido.

In conclusion, application of behavioral principles to cattle management has yielded positive dividends. Exploitation of current knowledge of bull behavior holds the key to maximum sire exploitation, whether in natural service or AI, and indicates possible fruitful areas for future research.

References

1. Amann RP, Almquist JO: Bull management to maximize sperm output. Proc 6th Tech Conf Anim Reprod AI (NAAB). Milwaukee, 1976.
2. Bane A: Studies on monozygotic cattle twins. XV. Sexual functions in bulls in relation to heredity, rearing intensity and somatic conditions. Acta Agric Scan 4:95, 1954.
3. Blockey MA de B: Observations on group mating of bulls at pasture. Appl Anim Ethol 5:15, 1979.
4. Brinks JS, McInerney MJ, Chenoweth PJ: Relationship of age at puberty in heifers to reproductive traits in young bulls. Am Soc Anim Sci (West Sect) abstract No 2, 1978.
5. Chenoweth PJ: Libido and mating behavior in bulls, boars and rams. A review. Theriogenology 16:155, 1981.
6. Hafez ESE, Boissou MF: The behavior of cattle. In Hafex ESE (ed): The Behavior of Domestic Animals. 3rd ed Baltimore, Williams & Wilkins Co., 1975.
7. Jacobs VL, Sis RF, Chenoweth PJ, et al.: Tongue manipulation of the palate assists estrous detection in the bovine. Theriogenology 13:353, 1980.
8. Land RB: Selection among males for the genetic improvement of female fertility. XII. Bienn Symp Anim Repro J Anim Sci (Suppl 11) 47:48, 1975.
9. Ologun AF, Chenoweth PJ, Brinks JS: Relationships among production traits and estimates of sex-drive and dominance value in yearling beef bulls. Theriogenology 15:379, 1981.
10. Randel RD, Short RE, Christensen DS, Bellows RA: Effects of various mating stimuli on the LH surge and ovulation time following synchronization of estrus in the bovine. J Anim Sci 37:128, 1973.
11. Wodzicka-Tomaszewska M, Kilgour R, Ryan M: "Libido" in the large farm animals. A review. Appl Anim Ethol 7:203, 1981.

Estrus Detection

R. David Smith, Ph.D.
Cornell University, Ithaca, New York

Cows in dairy and beef herds should calve at regular 12- to 13-month intervals in order to maximize the efficiency of production, genetic progress, through the use of artificial insemination (AI), and profit. To maintain a 12- to 13-month calving interval, cows must become pregnant within 85 to 115 days after calving. A waiting period of 40 to 50 days before the first postcalving breeding is usually recommended, leaving a 35- to 75-day breeding period. Thus, cows must conceive within one to three estrous cycles after breeding begins.

To help ensure that these goals are met, it is recommended that farmers establish veterinary reproductive health programs. These programs stress the early diagnosis and effective treatment of reproductive disorders that can delay the resumption of normal estrous cycle activity after calving and can lower conception rate.

Furthermore, it is obvious that effective estrus detection is the key to maximizing reproductive efficiency. Accurate identification of as many estrous periods as possible is critical if the benefits of the reproductive health program are to be realized and if its value is to be recognized by the farmer; but estrus detection continues to be cited by farmers, veterinarians and researchers as the major cause of low reproductive efficiency.

Therefore, a complete reproductive health program must include an evaluation of estrus detection procedures and recommendations for improvement when they are needed. This article discusses the economic importance of estrus detection, outlines the problems associated with this activity and describes how they might be solved through improved estrus detection practices and the proper use of estrus detection aids.

THE ECONOMIC IMPORTANCE OF EFFECTIVE ESTRUS DETECTION

Research suggests that on most farms improved estrus detection will have the greatest impact when improvements in reproductive efficiency are sought. Cornell University studies have shown that increasing the percentage of estrous periods accurately detected from 35 to 55 per cent in herds in which conception rate averages 55 per cent will reduce the average calving interval from 13.7 to 13.1 months and the percentage of the herd culled for reproductive reasons from 21 to 13 per cent. A further increase so that 75 per cent of the heat periods are detected will reduce the calving interval to 12.7 months and reproductive culls to 11 per cent.

Cornell University researchers predicted that increasing estrus detection efficiency from 35 to 55 per cent would increase income per cow by $72 and that increasing it from 55 to 75 per cent would result in an additional $28 per cow.

Costs associated with making the changes necessary to improve estrus detection efficiency were not considered in the Cornell study. There is little doubt, however, that improving heat detection will pay dividends. For instance, if increasing heat detection from 35 to 55 per cent in a 100-cow herd required an average daily investment of $5 for labor (30 minutes at $8/hour) and estrus detection aids, the net return would be $5400, or $3 for each dollar invested.

EVALUATING ESTRUS DETECTION EFFICIENCY

Complete and accurate herd records are essential for evaluating the efficiency and accuracy of estrus detection. Calving dates, heat and breeding dates and the results of prebreeding and pregnancy examinations are needed. From these data the following measures of reproductive efficiency relating to estrus detection can be determined.

1. Percentage of cows observed in estrus within 60 days after calving.

2. Interval from calving to first breeding.

3. Intervals between breedings.

4. Estrus detection index, which is defined as the average number of breedable heats per cow divided by the average number of breedings per cow. The average number of breedable heats is estimated using the following formula:

$$1 + \frac{[\text{average days open} - (\text{voluntary wait before first breeding} + 10)]}{21}$$

5. Percentage of cows found to be open when examined for pregnancy.

6. Percentage of eligible cows observed in estrus during a 3- to 4-week period.

Realistic goals for these measures of performance are shown in Table 1.

The milk progesterone assay can also be used to monitor reproductive status. The normal pattern of changes in the milk progesterone level as a cow resumes estrous cycle activity and becomes pregnant after calving is illustrated in Figure 1.

Coupling the day of breeding samples with 22- to 24-day postbreeding samples provides an accurate assessment of estrus detection accuracy and efficiency in problem herds. Heat detection *accuracy* can be determined by sampling cows on the day of

Table 1. Goals for Measures of Reproductive Performance That Reflect the Effectiveness of Estrus Detection Programs

Measure of Performance	Goal
Percentage of cows in estrus within 60 days postpartum	85 per cent or more
Average interval from calving to first breeding	70 days or less
Intervals between breedings:	
Less than 4 days	5 per cent or less
5 to 17 days	10 per cent or less
18 to 24 days	60 per cent of more
more than 24 days	25 per cent or less
Estrus detection index	0.70 or higher
Percentage of cows open at pregnancy exam	15 per cent or less
Percentage of eligible cows observed in estrus during a 3 to 4 week period	70 per cent or more

insemination. Cows with low levels of progesterone in their milk are in or near estrus. Cows with elevated progesterone levels are not in true estrus. Heat detection *efficiency* can be monitored if cows are sampled at 22 to 24 days after breeding. A low level of progesterone at this time indicates that the cow is open with an accuracy of greater than 95 per cent. If estrus was not observed, estrus detection methods are assumed to have failed.

ESTRUS DETECTION PROBLEMS AND THEIR CAUSES

Basically, there are two estrus detection problems: (1) missed or unobserved estrous periods and (2) estrus detection errors. The latter results in the insemination of cows that are not in the proper stage of the estrous cycle for conception to occur. Some are near estrus but are bred 1 to 2 days too early or too late, some are open but in the luteal phase of the cycle and some are pregnant.

Unobserved Estrus

Research using the milk progesterone assay to monitor reproductive status has demonstrated that in well-fed, healthy dairy herds 90 per cent of the cows resume normal estrous cycle activity within 50 to 60 days after calving. In a Canadian study in which TV cameras were used for 24-hour observation 90 per cent of the cows were observed in standing estrus before 60 days postpartum. Yet, only 50 to 60 per cent of the estrous periods that occurred were observed by the herdsperson.

It should be noted, however, that true anestrus should not be overlooked as a possible cause of poor reproductive performance in problem herds. In a New York field study it was found that in 2 of

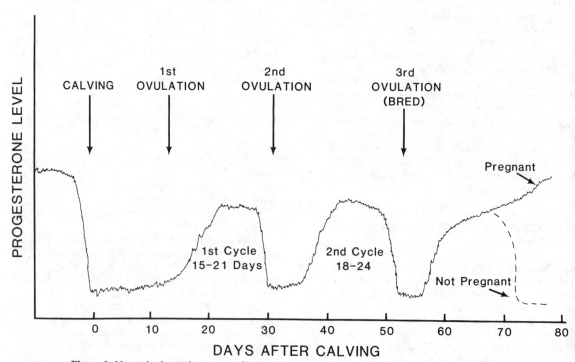

Figure 1. Normal schematic pattern of a cow's progesterone cycle during the postpartum period.

12 cooperating dairy herds up to 30 per cent of the cows had *not* resumed normal estrous cycle activity prior to 60 days postcalving. Anestrus is a more significant problem in some beef herds in which nutrition may be limiting.

A study of the farm records can provide valuable information for the evaluation of estrus detection efficiency. Herds, with poor estrus detection efficiency, are characterized by one or more of the following:

1. Prolonged calving to first service interval. The interval should be no more than 15 to 18 days longer than the farmer's goal and/or average no more than 70 days.

2. Prolonged intervals between breedings, especially when many are multiples of a normal 18- to 24-day cycle.

3. Veterinary examinations confirming that cows are cycling normally, although estrus is not observed.

4. More than 10 to 15 per cent of the cows confirmed to be open at a 35- to 50-day pregnancy check.

5. Heat detection index less than 0.50 or less than 50 per cent of the eligible cows observed in estrus within a period of 3 to 4 weeks.

If in most herds essentially all cows are cycling normally, why does the dairy farmer have difficulty "catching the cycling cow"? There are several reasons: Some represent "people problems," but there are several "cow factors" that make estrus detection difficult. The major factors contributing to poor heat detection efficiency are the following:

1. *Failure to spend sufficient time on a daily basis for estrus detection.* Only 44 per cent of 225 New York dairy farmers completing a reproductive management questionnaire set aside a specific time each day to observe cows for signs of estrous activity.

2. *Most mounting activity occurs at night in loosely-housed herds.* Research in Canada and England indicates that 70 per cent of the activity occurs between 6 PM and 6 AM.

3. *Heat periods are short.* Several studies indicate that as many as 65 per cent of the cows are in standing heat for 16 hours or less; 25 per cent for less than 8 hours.

4. *Low levels of estrous activity when few cows are in heat.* This can be a significant problem in small herds and in groups of cows in large herds in which many cows are either pregnant, not cycling or in the luteal phase of their estrous cycles. In one study of a group of 33 cows there were only 12 mounts during the entire estrous period when only one cow was in heat. The duration of standing estrus was 10 hours, resulting in an average of 1.2 mounts per hour.

5. *Mounts last 10 seconds or less.* Farmers must concentrate on estrus detection. Too many still try to combine it with other activities. Forty-six per cent of 225 New York farmers reported that they *always* combine estrus detection with other chores.

6. *Feet and leg problems, slippery floors, summer heat, winter cold and other environmental factors reduce estrous activity.* For example, North Carolina researchers compared standing and mounting activities when cows were in a dirt lot with those observed when they were in a grooved concrete free-stall alley. Both activities were twofold higher in the freestall alley than when cows were in the dirt lot.

Heat detection programs that limit the effects of these "people" and "cow" factors must be developed in order to maximize heat detection efficiency.

Estrus Detection Errors

Recent research using milk progesterone analysis on the day of insemination has shown that up to 30 per cent of the cows presented for insemination in some problem herds are not in heat. Some cows are pregnant, while others are open but just not in estrus. The effect of estrus detection errors on reproductive performance is illustrated in Table 2.

Estrus detection in dairy herds is a difficult task. The observation of standing behavior is the most definitive sign that a cow should be inseminated, but because of the factors already outlined, herd managers often rely on secondary signs of estrus (vaginal mucous discharge, mounting behavior, vocalization or failure to let down milk) and on various estrus detection aids to identify cows for insemination. In some herds, relying too heavily on secondary signs of estrus and on estrus detection aids apparently results in the poorly timed insemination of cows that are near heat. The effect of this type of error is illustrated in Table 3.

Herds in which a large number of estrus detection errors are made often are characterized by the following:

1. More than 5 to 10 per cent of the intervals between breedings are too short (3 to 17 days).

Table 2. The Effect of Heat Detection Errors on Conception Rate

Status	Milk Progesterone	Number Bred	Conception Rate*
Not in heat	High	25	0
In or near heat	Low	49	61 per cent
Total	—	74	41 per cent

*Based on rectal examination at 40 to 50 days after breeding. (From Smith RD: Proceedings National Invitational Dairy Cattle Reproduction Workshop, 1982.)

Table 3. The Relationship Between Signs of Estrus and Conception Rate

Signs of Heat	Milk Progesterone	Number Bred	Conception Rate*
Standing	Low	163	55 per cent
Not standing	Low	197	37 per cent

*Based on rectal examination at 40 to 50 days after breeding. (From Smith RD: Proceedings National Invitational Dairy Cattle Reproduction Workshop, 1982.)

2. More than 5 to 10 per cent of the cows are bred twice within 3 days.

3. More than 10 per cent of the intervals between breedings are 25 to 35 days.

4. Cows are checked pregnant and/or calve to a breeding that occurred earlier than the last one recorded.

Estrus detection errors must be avoided. Breeding pregnant cows can cause abortion. Breeding nonestrous, open cows wastes time, semen and money.

In order to reduce the number of errors, potential causes of the problem must be identified. In most herds errors result from (1) misidentification of cows, (2) misinterpretation of the signs of heat, (3) misuse or misinterpretation of heat detection aids—15 to 20 per cent of cows bred on the basis of activated mount detectors in 476 dairy herds in the northeastern United States were not in heat and (4) cows transmitting the wrong signals—up to 10 per cent of pregnant cows may stand to be mounted.

WISE USE OF ESTRUS DETECTION AIDS

Estrus detection is difficult, so estrus detection aids are needed in many herds to identify effectively all the cows that must be inseminated. The most important consideration for farmers is to remember that they are only aids. For best results aids must be used in conjunction with good visual detection programs, not as a substitute for visual detection. Some valuable estrus detection aids are described below.

Wall Charts, Breeding Wheels, Herd Monitors and Individual Cow Records. These systems are the least expensive heat detection aids. Their use is based upon anticipation of the next heat period. If the farm workers know when closely to observe individual cows for signs of estrus, more short- or weak-heat periods can be identified. Keys to successful use of these management aids are (1) the *accurate* recording of *every* heat beginning with the *first* after calving and (2) their daily use to identify those cows that are due to return to estrus.

Secondary Signs of Estrus. Secondary signs indicate that a cow is in or near heat. They should be used primarily to identify cows that need careful observation for standing estrus. A twice-daily walk behind the cows when most of them are lying down provides a good opportunity to check for the secondary signs of estrus.

Palpation of the Reproductive Organs. Routine rectal examination of all cows between 30 and 40 days after calving and of individual problem cows that have not been inseminated within 70 days after calving should be encouraged to confirm that the reproductive tract is normal and to predict when the next estrus will occur or to identify cows for prostaglandin treatment when estrous cycles are occurring, but estrus has not been detected.

Mount Detection. Two methods are widely used for mount detection: (1) pressure-sensitive devices and (2) paint stick, chalk or paint on the tail head. When animals are in estrus, mounting activity changes the color of the detector or erases the chalk or paint stick markings. With good management and proper interpretation, pressure-sensitive mount detectors provide excellent results. But care must be taken to position the detectors properly and to minimize the opportunities for false activation of the devices.

False activation of mount detectors can be reduced by removing cows that are in estrus from the herd. The disadvantage of this practice is that it removes sexually active cows that stimulate increased mounting behavior in others that may be in estrus but are less active.

Recent studies show that the accuracy of mount detectors, when used as the sole method of heat detection, may be as low as 30 to 50 per cent. These results strongly suggest that mount detectors should be used only to identify cows that require additional observation. Breeding on the basis of activated mount detectors without additional signs to confirm that cows are in estrus should be discouraged.

Chalking the tail head is a less expensive alternative for mount detection. False-positives are sometimes a problem, and animals must be restrained and marked every few days, since mud and manure may obscure the chalk or paint stick marking. Paint can be used instead of chalk or paint stick. When the paint dries, it becomes brittle and flakes off when the cow is mounted.

Heat Detector Animals. Sexually active animals can be used to identify estrous cows. They may be fitted with halters containing ink-filled reservoirs and ball point pen type devices (chin-ball markers) that will mark animals that are mounted, or they can be used without these devices to increase sexual activity and make visual detection programs more effective. Bulls, "cystic" cows, hormone-treated steers and hormone-treated cows and heifers have been used. Cows with chronic follicular cysts are inconsistent, and there appears to be variation in effectiveness among hormone-treated steers. In a Michigan study, testosterone-treated cows and heifers identified 74 to 80 per cent of the estrous cows.

The marker bull is the most effective detector animal. Copulation must be prevented even in sterilized animals to ensure against the spread of venereal diseases. Use of surgical techniques that prevent sexual contact (deviation or removal of the penis) is preferred. Mechanical devices that prevent copulation are less desirable because they sometimes fail, cause infection and tend to reduce the sex drive of the bull.

Bulls are dangerous. Injuries to cows and farm workers can and do occur. For this reason, other bulls must be available so that bulls can be replaced when they become too aggressive. Hormone-treated heifers and cows are more docile. Although they may be slightly less effective, they are the animal of choice on most farms.

When marker animals are used, cows should be removed from the herd as they come into estrus. This will stimulate the marker animal to seek out and identify additional cows that may be in heat. The ratio of cows to markers should be no greater than 40:1.

Marker animals have disadvantages. Some cows may be marked when they are not in estrus. Others that are coming into estrus may be marked before they stand to be mounted. Therefore, care must be exercised when interpreting the marks. For these reasons, the best results are obtained when marker animals are used in addition to a good visual detection program. Also, marker animals tend to become too fat if feed intake is not restricted. A possible solution to the latter problem in loose-housed herds is to put the marker with the herd only at night or other periods during the day when visual observation is limited.

Heat Check Report System. A heat check report system for herds experiencing estrus detection problems has been developed by Eastern AI Cooperative and Cornell University. It has been particularly useful in herds in which more than one person routinely reports estrous cows. In these herds the best "cow person" is given responsibility for the estrus detection and breeding programs. Workers return heat reports to the person in charge, who then makes the decision on whether or not to breed the cow. In one herd, estrus detection errors decreased from 34 per cent to less than 5 per cent after 1 month on the system.

Prostaglandin. One of the greatest potential uses of prostaglandin is as an estrus detection aid in dairy cows in which estrus has not been observed. Research has shown that prostaglandin treatment of cows with functional corpora lutea will induce a fertile estrus within 2 to 7 days. Approximately 50 per cent will be observed in estrus within 80 hours after treatment and will demonstrate normal fertility. For best results, insemination should be based on estrus observation, but insemination at 80 hours after treatment for cows that have not been observed in estrus by that time has been recommended. In these cases estrus detection efforts should continue because some cows will come into estrus after the "80-hour breeding" and will have to be inseminated again.

The Electronic Probe. When the cow is in heat, the volume and ionic composition of the cervical-vaginal mucus change. The result is a decrease in the resistance of the mucus to the passage of an electrical current. The estrus probe is designed to monitor this change in resistance. Estrus is associated with "low probe readings." The use of the probe for estrus detection is time consuming because cows must be probed once or twice daily, and cow-to-cow variation makes it necessary to develop a profile for each cow.

Pedometers. Because cows become more active when they are in estrus, activity monitoring through the use of pedometers is a potentially valuable method of identifying estrous cows. Studies at the United States Department of Agriculture (USDA) showing that cow activity measured by pedometers strapped to the cows' rear legs increased approximately 400 per cent in cows housed in free stalls and 275 per cent in cows in comfort-stall housing support this concept. Twenty-three of 108 heat periods in free-stall housed cows were identified by activity monitoring but missed by herders.

"Tricks of the Trade." In certain management situations various tricks can be used to improve estrus detection. First, cows in heat can be left with the herd to stimulate activity. Canadian studies showed that mounting activity increased 3- to 5-fold when more than one cow was in heat. However, an argument for removing estrous cows is that animals who are actively mounting sometimes choose favorites. This can reduce the chances of detecting additional cows that are in heat but less aggressive. Second, questionable cows can be placed with strange animals to stimulate activity. Third, simply moving cows as a group from one area to another, such as from concrete to a dirt lot, sometimes stimulates activity. Heat checking should always include getting all cows up and moving them if they are in free stalls or outside. These tricks will not be feasible in all operations, but for those in which they can be used more heats may be accurately detected.

The Bottom Line. Adequate visual observation and keen cow sense are the keys to successful heat detection. However, it is unrealistic to expect that every cow will be observed in standing estrus. The goal should be to develop a program that will (1) result in as many cows as possible being observed in standing estrus and (2) make optimum use of a *combination* of secondary signs of heat and heat detection aids to identify those cows in which standing behavior is not observed. Aids should only be used in conjunction with adequate visual detection programs.

References

1. Esslemont RJ, Bryant MJ: Oestrous behavior in a herd of dairy cows. Vet Rec 99:472, 1976.
2. Foote RH: Estrus detection and estrus detection aids. J Dairy Sci 58:248, 1975.
3. Hurnik JF, King GJ, Robertson HA: Estrous and related behavior in postpartum Holstein cows. Appl Anim Ethol 2:55, 1975.
4. Oltenacu PA, Rounsaville TR, Milligan RA, Foote RH: Sys-tems analysis for designing reproductive management programs to increase production and profits in dairy herds. J Dairy Sci 64:2096, 1981.
5. Williamson NB, Morris, RS, Blood DC, Cannon CM: A study of oestrus behavior and oestrus detection methods in a large commercial dairy herd. I. The relative efficiency of methods of oestrus detection. Vet Rec 91:50, 1972.
6. Williamson NB, Morris RS, Blood DC, et al.: A study of oestrus behavior and oestrus detection methods in a large commercial dairy herd. II. Oestrus signs and behavior patterns. Vet Rec 91:58, 1972.

Estrus Synchronization in Cattle

Martin Wenkoff, D.V.M., M.V.Sc.
Bova Tech Livestock Ltd., Shaughnessy, Alberta, Canada

Because effective estrus detection requires much time, labor, skill and expense, it has often been cited as a major factor limiting the widespread use of artificial insemination (AI) in cattle. Therefore, the elimination of estrus detection from artificial breeding programs was the principal stimulus that led to research in the development of prostaglandin and progestational compounds that have the ability to control estrus without affecting fertility. Although some estrus synchronization programs using these products can achieve rates of synchrony high enough to allow insemination without estrus detection, it is ironic that the best conception rates from most synchronization programs occur when breeding follows twice daily heat detection.

Synchronization of estrus, however, does offer many benefits in addition to reductions in estrus detection, such as overall improvements in herd productivity and reproductive efficiency. For example, if a herd is synchronized early in the breeding season, the breeding season and the resultant calving season will be shortened. As a result, the average length of the following postpartum interval will be increased, which has a positive effect on first service conception rates. Also, a greater percentage of the herd will have had, by the beginning of the next breeding season, the required postpartum interval to be eligible for the next synchronization program.

Estrus control offers several applications in addition to synchronized breeding programs. These include management of replacement heifers in beef and dairy herds, breeding control for controlled lactation in dairy herds and estrus synchronization in embryo transfer programs.

SYNCHRONIZATION PROGRAMS

Prostaglandins

Prostaglandin $F_{2\alpha}$ ($PGF_{2\alpha}$) has generally been accepted as the luteolytic agent that ends the lifespan of the bovine cyclic corpus luteum (CL) at the end of diestrus. Regression of the CL results in a drop in blood progesterone that in turn allows the release of gonadotropins from the anterior pituitary, and the animal returns to estrus. The administration of exogenous $PGF_{2\alpha}$ (or its synthetic analogs) in most stages of diestrus results in luteolysis, which is followed by the normal sequence of endocrinologic and physiological events that proceed estrus. This shortening of the luteal phase is the mechanism by which prostaglandins can be used to control estrus. There is no effect on the fertility of estrus following a prostaglandin-shortened diestrus.

Programs

Program A (Fig. 1 and Table 1). The basic objective of "double-injection" programs is to have a high percentage of the herd in diestrus at the time of the second injection. In a cycling herd approximately two thirds of the animals should be in diestrus at any given time, and hence the majority should respond to a single injection. In those cows that respond, luteolysis is followed by estrus in about 2 to 5 days. Eleven days after the injection the cows that responded should be on days 6 through 9 of the estrous cycle; the remainder would be on days 6 through 15. Most of the animals should now have a functional CL, and a second injection at this time should induce a synchronized estrus. One should not, however, expect the entire herd to become synchronized because both the ages of the animal and the CL at the time of the injections influence the rate of luteolysis and therefore the rate of synchrony (see the Endocrinologic Considerations section).

Program A is used most often when heat detection is impossible, limited or very inefficient. It can be an efficient program in beef herds and in replacement dairy heifer programs. In program A cyclicity of the herd is established either by limited heat detection or by rectal palpation of the ovaries. The ovaries could be palpated prior to the first injection, with all anestrous animals eliminated from the pro-

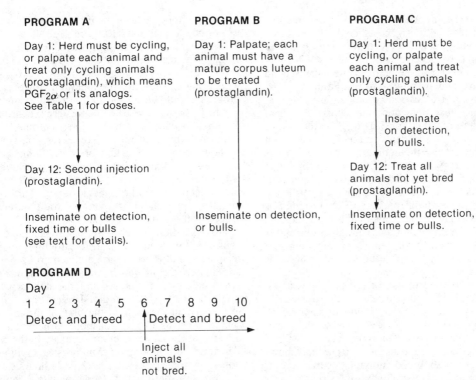

Figure 1. Suggested controlled breeding programs. Programs must be selected, modified and customized to fit individual management situations.

gram at this time. Some veterinarians have more confidence in identifying cycling animals at the time of the second injection, i.e., only animals with a mature CL are given the second injection. This procedure is probably more accurate than palpation prior to the initial injection, but it may result in higher drug costs. It does have the advantage of eliminating from the program animals with abnormal estrous cycles and animals that did not respond to the first injection.

The rate of synchrony in program A can be high enough for insemination to be done at fixed times following the second injection. Satisfactory conception rates can be achieved by performing insemination at 72 and 96 hours after the last injection, but this is probably impractical in beef herds in which calves are at foot. Generally, cows could be inseminated somewhere between 72 and 80 hours after injection, with heifers inseminated up to 10

hours earlier than cows. Insemination based on heat detection is still the best way to achieve the highest possible conception rates. A reasonable compromise might be to observe the synchronized herd and breed the entire herd relative to maximum estrous activity. This technique must be used with caution in herds that are a mixture of cows and heifers.

Program B. This is a practical and useful management tool in programs for dairy replacement heifers in which heat detection is possible and in which eligible heifers can be chosen from large numbers by age, weight and identification of a functional CL per rectum. Program B can also be used in beef herds. Insemination in this program should always be based on heat detection or by natural service because the rate of synchrony following a single dose of prostaglandin is not high enough for fixed-time inseminations.

Program C. This is a variation of program A and

Table 1. Prostaglandin and Prostaglandin Analogs

Drug	Trade Name	Manufacturer	Dose*	Route
Alfaprostol†	Alfavet	Hoffmann-La Roche	5.0 mg	IM
Cloprostenol†	Estrumate	ICI Pharma	500 μgm	IM
Dinoprost	Lutalyse	Upjohn	25 mg	IM
Fenprostalene†	Bovilene	Syntex	1.0 mg	SC

*Manufacturers' recommended doses
†Prostaglandin analog

provides for the opportunity to use varying amounts of heat detection. Drug costs could be reduced proportionately by heat detection in that a smaller number of cows receive two injections. The recommendations for insemination after the second injection are similar to those for program A.

Program D. This uses a combination of prostaglandin and heat detection and consists of heat detection and breeding for 5 days. If by the end of day 5 at least 24 per cent of the herd has been observed in estrus, the remainder of the herd is injected on day 6, and detection and breeding continue until the end of day 10. Over 80 per cent of the cows (in a cycling herd) will have had one breeding in the 10-day period. This program is economical (only 75 per cent of the herd receives an injection), requires no ovarian palpations and is a practical method of shortening the breeding season in herds in which AI is used as well as in herds in which natural service is used.

Bulls can be used in any of the programs as an alternate to AI. It is not unreasonable to expect a high capacity bull with good libido to serve 25 to 30 cows in a 48-hour period. Mature bulls will generally serve any one cow only once or twice if other estrous cows are available. Virgin bulls, however, may tend to breed individual cows several times and may not cover all cows in estrus.

Successful synchronization programs involve much more planning than simply following a chart or recipe and can rarely be achieved without considering and adjusting for several endocrinologic, product, animal and management factors. It is in these areas that competent veterinary advice is required.

Endocrinologic Considerations

The luteolytic rate is low in young (days 5 to 6) corpora lutea and does not approach 90 per cent until CL are over 7 to 9 days old. This could partially account for a less than expected response in cattle that have functional corpora lutea.

The stage of the cycle at which an injection is given has an effect on the interval to estrus. Cows and heifers injected during the first half of the functional lifespan of the CL have an interval to estrus that is 10 to 12 hours shorter than that of animals injected near the middle or end of the cycle. This factor alone can drop the degree of synchrony to the point at which a reasonable conception rate cannot be achieved with a single fixed-time insemination following a single synchronizing injection. This is why programs based on rectal identification of mature CL followed by a single injection and a single fixed-time breeding should be avoided.

The stage of diestrus at which a prostaglandin injection is given also has an influence on the variability of the interval to estrus. The interval to estrus varies from about 2½ or 3 to 5 days for cows and from 2 to 4 days for heifers. The greatest variability appears to occur if the injection is given when the CL is in days 10 through 13.

The degree of synchrony following a second injection (see program A or C) could be high enough for a satisfactory conception rate to be obtained with a single fixed-time insemination. However, this program should be approached with caution in herds in which cows and yearling heifers are synchronized together, because prostaglandin-synchronized heifers usually have an interval to estrus that is 10 to 12 hours shorter than that of cows. If the heifers are bred at the same time as the cows, the breeding will occur several hours too late in the heifers, and the conception rate will be lowered. This factor alone may be largely responsible for reputed low success rates in heifer programs.

This variation in response is also an important consideration in embryo transfer programs in which recipients and/or donors are a mixed group of cows and heifers or in which an attempt is made to synchronize the recipients and the donors with a single dose of prostaglandin. Heifers that happen to be early in the cycle at the time of the injection can be in estrus 24 hours or more earlier than cows injected at the same time but were late in the cycle. Furthermore, the interval from prostaglandin injection to the onset of estrus is 12 to 24 hours shorter in gonadotropin-treated (superovulated) animals than in single ovulating donors or recipients.

Product Differences

There may be differences in the action, duration of action or reliability of different prostaglandin products. However, to date, there are no supporting data to suggest superiority of one product over another.

Management Criteria for Successful Programs

The inclusion of anestrus cows or heifers in synchronization programs is a major factor that contributes to program failures. The following factors should be considered in the management of controlled breeding programs in cattle:

Nutrition. Cows that are fed less than the amount needed to maintain energy levels and, hence, lose weight over winter are plagued with delayed onset of postcalving estrus, resulting in anestrus at the beginning of the breeding season. The mechanism causing this state appears to be an inhibition of the release of gonadotropins from the pituitary. Also, inadequate postcalving energy intake results in low first service conception rates. Similarly, over-winter phosphorus deficiency has a negative influence on subsequent first service conception rates. The National Research Council (NRC) recommends 4.08 kg (9 lb) of total digestible nutrients (TDN) over winter and 7.26 kg (16 lb) of TDN for flushing after calving.

Cows with adequate energy levels should gain about 0.45 kg (1 lb) per day during the last 4 months of gestation and about 0.34 kg (0.75 lb) per day after calving. A simple way to monitor weight gains is to weigh a sample of the herd monthly. It is of utmost importance that cows and heifers, even if they are fit, are in a positive energy balance during the breeding season because high endometrial glycogen levels are essential for sperm cell and embryonal survival. Also, at estrus glycogen is converted to lactate in the vaginal epithelium under the influence of estrogens as part of the local defense mechanism.

Inefficient reproductive performance caused by inadequate vitamin A or protein levels can occur but usually does not become a problem unless levels are so low that clinical signs of deficiencies are first apparent. In fact, if adequate energy is being supplied in the form of forage and grains, adequate phosphorus and protein are undoubtedly also being supplied. However, phosphorus supplementation should be considered if over-winter intake is below the NRC recommendations of 15 gm per head of cattle per day.

Herd Cyclicity. The level of herd cyclicity needs to be established because the entire herd must be cycling if prostaglandin is to be used as the synchronizing drug. Herd cyclicity can be assessed by blood or milk progesterone and estrogen assays, limited estrus detection or rectal palpation of the ovaries. The latter two techniques are the most practical.

Limited heat detection involves observing the herd for 5 days. If the herd is cycling, about 4.5 per cent should be in estrus on any particular day. If less than 24 per cent has been observed in estrus over a 5-day period, either the herd is not cycling adequately for a successful synchronization program or heat detection is not efficient enough for programs that require detection.

Rectal palpation is an efficient and accurate method of identifying cycling cows and heifers and has the added advantage of eliminating from the program animals that are pregnant and animals with uterine, ovarian, cervical or tubal disorders. One disadvantage of rectal palpation is that it requires special skills.

Postpartum Interval. The length of the postpartum interval is an important consideration in planning synchronization programs. It is well known that conception rates improve as the postpartum interval increases. The endometrium, especially the caruncular areas, does not become completely histologically normal until several weeks after calving. Cows less than 50 days postpartum should be excluded from synchronization programs. This can be accomplished only if adequate records of calving dates are kept and if cows are adequately identified. First and second calf heifers usually require a postpartum interval 3 weeks longer than cows (i.e., 70 days).

Heifers. Unlike adult cows, heifers need extra energy for body growth. Inadequate nutrition could result in inadequate body weights and resultant delayed puberty in virgin heifers. The best results are obtained if heifers are 14 months of age or older and have reached at least 65 per cent of expected adult weight, i.e., about 320 kg (700 lb) for British dairy breeds. Heifers should be gaining about 0.45 kg (1 lb) per day prior to the breeding season. First and second calf heifers are lactating and growing at the same time, and return to estrus is usually delayed for up to 3 weeks. Rectal palpation of the ovaries may be necessary to cull anestrous heifers from the program.

Herd Health. The general health of the herd should be evaluated for conditions that can affect reproductive performance. For example, severe pediculosis can lead to anemia, which in turn can lower conception rates.

AI Technicians and Semen. Adequate and sufficient AI technology should be ensured, especially if large number of cows are to be bred over a short period of time. Facilities should be adequate and should include protection from wind and sun. Frozen semen should be examined prior to use; inadequate semen quality could cause an otherwise well-managed program to fail.

First Service Conception Rates. Prostaglandin is not a "fertility drug" and will not increase first service conception rates nor will it replace good management. If the previous years first service conception rates in a herd that is being considered for estrus synchronization are below 40 per cent, synchronization should not be attempted unless the factors responsible for the low rates can first be identified and corrected.

Progesterones

Progestational compounds such as 6-chloro-6-dihydro-17-acetoxyprogesterone (CAP), 6-α-methyl-17α-acetoxyprogesterone (MAP) and melengestrol acetate (MGA) were researched in the 1960's as possible synchronization compounds. The level of synchrony was adequate but conception rates were low because of delayed embryo cleavage, probably because of the long exposure times to the compounds (i.e., 20 to 25 days). The recently developed synthetic progesterone norgestomet, on the other hand, can be used to synchronize estrus without lowering fertility.

Syncro-Mate B (SMB) treatment consists of an ear implant that contains 6 mg of norgestomet and an intramuscular injection of 5 mg estradiol valerate and 3 mg norgestomet mixed together in a single 2-ml dose. The norgestomet acts as an "artificial CL" and therefore prevents luteinizing hormone (LH) surges and ovulation, CL formation and CL maintenance. The lack of CL maintenance along with the estradiol valerate induces CL regression. When the implant is removed 9 days later, the pituitary gland is released from the inhibitory effects of norgestomet, and the animal returns to estrus in 24 to 36 hours. The degree of synchrony is high, and satisfactory conception rates can be achieved with a single fixed-time insemination 48 to 54 hours after the implant is removed. Insemination based on estrus detection after removal of the implant does not appear to result in conception rates higher than those achieved by a single fixed-time insemination.

Conception rates in herds of cows can be much improved if the calves are removed during the 48-hour interval from removal of implant to breeding. This so-called "shang" treatment does not harm the calves, and at least some of its positive effects may be due to the induction of estrus in anestrous cows. It has been suggested but not clearly established that SMB treatment will induce estrus in a significant percentage of true anestrous cows. On the other hand, there is good evidence that SMB could induce a fertile estrus in prepubertal heifers that are over 14 months of age and weigh over 250 kg.

Successful SMB programs, like prostaglandin programs, are dependent on good management of nutrition, postpartum interval and breeding technology.

Results Obtainable with Controlled Breeding Programs

Conception rates of 45 to 55 per cent in cows in synchronized estrus and 75 to 85 per cent or higher in a 35-day breeding period can be achieved. Success should be measured in terms of the pregnancy rate achieved by 21 days or 35 days following the synchronization injection, rather than in terms of first service conception rate. A moderately successful program in 1 year will have a positive carry-over effect on the average postpartum interval by the beginning of the next breeding season.

Research

More research is needed to clarify the optimum insemination times for fixed-time insemination in different age groups of animals, especially heifers, following synchronization with prostaglandins. Programs using SMB and prostaglandin combinations are currently being researched and may prove to be useful in synchronization programs as well as in embryo transfer management.

References

1. Burfening PJ, Anderson DC, Kinkie RA, et al.: Synchronization of estrus with PGF$_{2\alpha}$ in beef cattle. J Anim Sci 47:999, 1978.
2. King ME, Kiracofe GA, Stevenson JS, Schalles RR: Effect of stage of the estrous cycle on interval to estrus after PGF$_{2\alpha}$ in beef cattle. Theriogenology 18:191, 1982.
3. Seguin BE: Role of prostaglandins in bovine reproduction. JAVMA 176:1178, 1980.
4. Spitzer JC, Mares SE, Peterson LA: Pregnancy rate among beef heifers from timed insemination with a progestin treatment. J Anim Sci 53:1, 1981.
5. Walters DL, Smith MF, Harms PG, Wiltbank NJ: Effect of steroids and/or 48 hour calf removal on serum luteinizing hormone concentrations in anestrous beef cows. Theriogenology 18:349, 1982.
6. Wenkoff M, Crowe-Swords PR: The management of prostaglandin-controlled breeding programs in beef cattle—a five year study. Can Vet J 24:50, 1983.
7. Wiltbank JN, Rowden WW, Ingalls JE, Zimmerman DR: Influence of postpartum energy level on reproductive performance of Hereford cows restricted in energy intake prior to calving. J Anim Sci 23:1049, 1964.

Principles and Procedures for Storing and Using Frozen Bovine Semen

Phillip L. Senger
Washington State University, Pullman, Washington

During the last 15 years there has been a significant increase in the number of dairy and beef producers that artificially inseminate their own cattle. In 1981 semen sold directly to dairy and beef producers accounted for 50 to 60 per cent of all semen sales in the United States. These producers purchase semen, manage liquid nitrogen (LN) refrigerators, thaw semen and prepare the inseminating device to inseminate the cow. Proper practice of these techniques requires a high degree of technical awareness by the producer. This was not necessary when professional AI technicians were totally responsible for artificial insemination. Producers and veterinarians must understand the proper methods and the scientific rationale for the procedures they employ if they are to maximize the fertility of AI services. Therefore, the purpose of this article is to discuss proper methods for LN refrigerator management and seminal handling. Discussions will be limited to the 0.5-ml plastic straw, since this unit is the predominant packaging unit used by the AI industry in the United States.

MANAGEMENT AND CARE OF THE LIQUID NITROGEN REFRIGERATOR

Construction of the Refrigerator. Because of its rugged external appearance and bulk, the LN refrigerator is often thought to be indestructible.

Many refrigerators are mishandled because the user lacks an understanding of its internal construction. Mishandling undoubtedly leads to premature refrigerator failure.

A cryogenic refrigerator provides an extremely cold environment for the storage of frozen semen. Liquid nitrogen at a temperature of −196°C is used as the refrigerant. A high quality refrigerator conserves the LN for the longest possible period of time by retarding evaporation of the liquid. To do this, the refrigerator must be designed so that it has maximum insulating properties.

The LN refrigerator is a double chambered vessel (Fig. 1). The inner chamber (Fig. 1A), which contains the LN, the canisters and the racks of frozen semen, is suspended from the outer chamber by a nonmetal neck tube (Fig. 1D). This structure retards conduction of heat from the outside of the refrigerator to the inner chamber containing the LN. Thus, heat cannot move easily into the inner chamber and cause rapid evaporation of LN. The neck tube is structurally weaker than the metal components of the refrigerator, and the addition of LN to the inner chamber significantly increases the weight that the neck tube must support. Sudden movements, such as skidding the refrigerator across a floor, transporting it in the back of a pickup truck

or automobile (without securing *and* cushioning) and bumping into stationary objects can vibrate the inner chamber. As the chamber swings slightly from side-to-side, a high degree of stress is placed on the neck tube, which greatly increases the likelihood of mechanical damage. Thus, the LN refrigerator should be moved infrequently and positioned where it is unlikely to be disturbed except when removing semen or refilling with liquid nitrogen.

To retard the evaporation of LN, two types of insulation are used. The wall of the inner chamber (Fig. 1A) is wrapped with a very high quality insulation, and the outer chamber (Fig. 1E) is often filled with a solid insulation material. The most important insulating component of the refrigerator, however, is the vacuum that is created in the outer chamber. Air is evacuated from the outer chamber through a port (Fig. 1F) so that a vacuum exists in the outer chamber. This is accomplished at the factory. The vacuum port should never be manipulated. If the vacuum is lost (i.e., equilibration to atmosphere) the LN boils and is rapidly lost from the inner chamber. Such loss occurs when the neck tube is cracked or the outer chamber is mechanically punctured. Generally, the loss of vacuum in the outer chamber of the refrigerator is associated with a damaged neck tube.

Rapid evaporation of the LN causes the accumulation of highly visible frost around the top portion of the refrigerator. If this frost build-up is observed, obtain an alternate working refrigerator and transfer the semen to it immediately.

Refrigerator Location. In a recent report[16] the distance from the location of the LN refrigerator to the site of LN and semen delivery was often excessive and involved moving the refrigerator around obstacles (doors, stanchions, bulk tanks, steps, chairs, buckets). Damage to the refrigerator is most likely to occur when the refrigerator is moved, particularly if it makes abrupt contact with door frames or other stationary objects. Placement of the refrigerator at a point close to the site of LN delivery in a clean, dry, ventilated area reduces the risk of mechanical damage. This placement furthermore increases the convenience to both the distributor and the owner at refilling time. Placing the refrigerator directly on concrete floors promotes corrosion and should be avoided. Placement on a wooden pallet or on a dolly with wheels is a good way to provide ventilation. Store the refrigerator in a location where routine activity occurs, so that the refrigerator will be observed at least twice daily. Such a situation greatly increases the probability of observing a faulty refrigerator and minimizes the chance of losing semen.

INVENTORIES OF SEMEN

Semen refrigerator inventory systems in 57 dairy herds were found to be poor.[16] As a result, a simple semen inventory device was developed (Fig. 2). This device enables the exact location of the semen in the refrigerator to be determined at a glance.

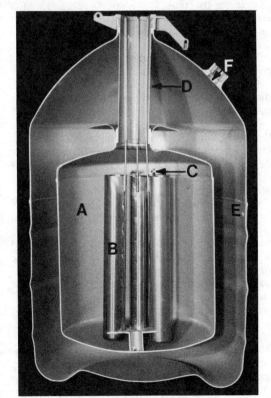

Figure 1. Cutaway view of a typical field liquid nitrogen (LN) refrigerator. *A*, Inner chamber containing LN. *B*, Canister containing racks (canes) of frozen semen. *C*, Racks holding goblets of semen. *D*, Neck tube. *E*, Outer chamber. *F*, Evacuation port.

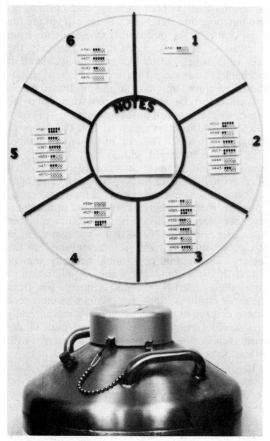

Figure 2. Inventory wheel and its relationship to liquid nitrogen refrigerator.

Furthermore, the quantity of semen remaining in the refrigerator can be determined quickly.

An inventory wheel can be accomplished as follows:

1. The wheel is made of one-quarter inch Plexiglas and is cut into a circle about 20 inches in diameter. The circle represents the cross section of the inner chamber of the refrigerator.

2. Each numbered section (1 to 6) represents a canister within the tank. The divisions are made by applying a high adhesion tape to the Plexiglas. The large canister numbers are adhesive numbers.

3. Each set of numbers within each canister section represents the bull number. The bull ID tags are made by Avery International. They can be easily removed from the Plexiglas without losing their adhesive properties. The labels can then be placed into a notebook to keep a record of semen usage. By writing the date of purchase and the date of last use on each label, records on the duration of semen storage can be kept.

4. The 10 circles after each bull ID number represent the 10 straws on a full rack. The top five circles represent the straws in the top goblet and the bottom five circles represent the straws in the bottom goblet.

5. As each straw of semen is used, the circle is filled in, indicating use. The number of open circles represents the number of unused units of semen. If four circles are filled in on the top goblet, this prompts the user to be aware that a goblet must be removed along with the next straw. By observing the number of solid versus open circles the producer and the semen distributor are clearly aware of the space available in the tank as well as future semen needs.

6. The entire wheel can be attached to the wall directly above the semen tank with mirror hangers. The cost of this wheel is about $12 to $15.

Refrigerator Holding Time and Size. Holding time refers to the length of time the LN will remain in a refrigerator and reflects the refrigerator's insulating capability. Generally, holding times range from 8 to 32 weeks, depending on the manufacturer and model. Regardless of the manufacturer's designated holding time, regular checks of the LN should be made. The checks should be made every 2 to 3 weeks. Results should be recorded so that evaporation rate can be determined. By making routine checks and recording the LN levels over time, one can develop an LN evaporation profile for the refrigerator under the specific use condition for a given setting. Deviation from expected evaporation rates is cause for alarm. Checks are made by dipping a ruler into the LN refrigerator until it strikes the bottom of the tank. The rule should remain in the tank for 5 to 10 seconds. After removal, frost will form on the rule after a short period of time. The frost line indicates the level of the LN within the refrigerator. Black is a preferred color for the measuring ruler, since it provides good contrast between the white frost and black rule.

Many dairy and beef producers own refrigerators that have a storage capacity greater than their usage needs. As a rule, the refrigerator should not hold more units at any time than the number of cows in the herd. Since semen distributors generally visit farms on a monthly basis, there is little danger of depleting the supply of semen or LN. On-farm LN refrigerators are not the place for maintaining large semen inventories.

Impact of Tank Failure. Damage to a single LN refrigerator can be very costly to the individual producer, particularly if large inventories of high-cost semen are kept. The present nationwide trend is for increasing herd sizes. As this happens, more and more producers are becoming herders-inseminators. This growth trend will probably also result in larger inventories of semen in on-farm LN refrigerators. Therefore, the total value of semen stored in LN refrigerators is likely to increase with time, particularly if semen from high demand bulls is stored by herders-inseminators in the hope of increased future values. Regardless of the value per unit of semen, as the number of units grows, the total value of semen within the refrigerator increases, thus raising the net loss should failure occur. To help protect the producer from this possibility, refrigerator insurance policies are available through AI organizations.

Figure 3. Schematic illustration of three zones that exist in a straw of frozen semen. The "ice front" zone results from rapid freezing, which occurs on the outer edge of the straw. The majority of sperm in this zone sustain damage. The "optimum" zone is a region of maximum sperm survival because the ice crystal–solute conditions are compatible with viability. The "solute" zone results from increasing concentration of salts. Spermatozoa in this area are damaged owing to dehydration. (Modified from Saacke RG: Proc Ninth NAAB Confer Artif Insemin Reprod, 1982, pp 6–12.)

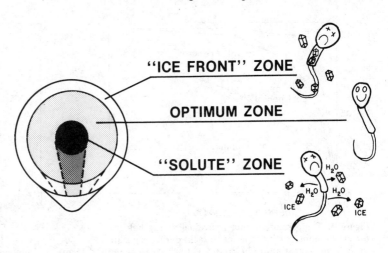

PRINCIPLES OF FREEZING SEMEN

Freezing and thawing of bull semen is necessary for widespread utilization of genetically superior sires. Artificial insemination organizations are devoted to assuring that maximum numbers of spermatozoa survive the freeze-thaw process, thus providing high numbers of viable sperm for insemination. They are also committed to providing semen from disease-free bulls and to ensuring that semen packages are properly labeled. Guidelines for these important areas are provided to member organizations by Certified Semen Services, Inc. (CSS), a subsidiary of the National Association of Animal Breeders (Box 1033, Columbia, MO 65205-1033). Participants in CSS have their health and identification procedures audited annually.

Regardless of successful research to improve cryopreservation, some spermatozoa fail to survive freezing and thawing. The reasons for cell death due to freezing and thawing are not fully understood. Two known causes of sperm injury/death are (1) formation of ice crystals within spermatozoa when fast cooling rates are used and (2) development of regions of high solute concentrations that dehydrate the cell when slow rates of cooling are employed. Regardless of the degree to which freez-

ing techniques are controlled, both sets of conditions exist in each straw of semen. Thus, a certain proportion of spermatozoa within each packaging unit are killed (Fig. 3). The objective of any freezing procedure is to optimize the cooling rate so that cell death due to formation of intracellular ice and hypertonic solutions is minimized. Under optimum sets of cooling conditions the "ice front" zone (Fig. 3) is small in width (or volume), thus damaging the fewest possible number of sperm. Likewise, the width (volume) of the "solute" zone should be small. The greater the volume of the "optimum" zone, the higher the number of spermatozoa surviving.

POSTFREEZING HANDLING OF FROZEN SEMEN

Physical Characteristics of Seminal Packaging Units. The surface-to-volume ratio of the packaging unit is the most important characteristic determining the method of handling frozen semen. The surface-to-volume ratio governs the rate at which temperature changes occur within the packaging unit. The higher the surface-to-volume ratio, the greater the temperature change per unit of time. Table 1 com-

Table 1. Surface Area and Surface-to-Volume Ratio of Various Seminal Packaging Units*

Type of Packaging Unit	Approximate Surface Area (mm²)	Approximate Volume of Semen Within Unit (ml)	Approximate Surface-to-Volume Ratio
1 ml ampule	1153	0.75	1537
0.5 ml ampule	696	0.50	1392
0.5 ml French straw	1152	0.50	2304
0.25 ml Continental straw	555	0.25	2220
0.25 ml French straw	823	0.25	3292

*Surface area values were computed by considering the top of the ampule as a cone and using the formula $\pi R \sqrt{R^2 + h^2}$. All other surface area values were computed by considering the unit as a cylinder and using the formula $2\pi Rh$ in which R = radius of the base and h = height of cone or length of straw (modified from Senger PL, 1980).

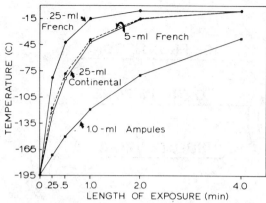

Figure 4. Temperature within individual straws held by forceps or ampules clipped to metal racks during exposure to ambient temperature (20 ± .6°C). Each curve is the mean of 5 replicates. (From Berndtson et al.: Proc Sixth NAAB Confer Artif Insemin Reprod, 1976, pp 51–60.)

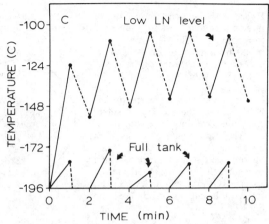

Figure 5. Influence of level of liquid nitrogen (LN) on temperature of semen packaged in 0.5 ml French straws (5 straws per goblet) during repeated exposure to the neck of a LN refrigerator. (From Berndtson et al.: Proc Sixth NAAB Confer Artif Insemin Reprod, 1976, pp 51–60.)

pares the surface-to-volume ratio for various packaging units. Because of the high surface-to-volume ratio, straws are very sensitive to changes in temperature caused by (1) transfer of the semen from LN refrigerator to LN refrigerator, (2) manipulation of the semen within the refrigerator, (3) thawing and (4) exposure to post-thaw environments of varying temperatures. The first opportunity for temperature change occurs during transfer from refrigerator to refrigerator during delivery of the semen to the farm. The length of time the semen is exposed to ambient temperature is critical and affects the viability of spermatozoa. Figure 4 compares the temperature changes that occur in various packaging units when they were exposed to ambient temperature (20°C) for varying lengths of time. Figure 4 also illustrates the extremely rapid increase in temperature that occurs in plastic straws when they are exposed to ambient temperature (20°C). This increase in temperature following exposure to ambient conditions is translated into loss of sperm viability. In all types of straws motility declined significantly after a 1-minute exposure to ambient temperatures and became dangerously low after a 2-minute exposure.[4] The cause for this loss of viability is believed to be from shifting of ice crystals and growth of ice crystals within and around the cell, thus damaging the plasma membrane. Straws packaged in goblets are more resistant to temperature changes than single straws.

Handling of Semen in the Tank. During removal of semen from the LN refrigerator for breeding, the canister containing the racks of straws must be raised into the neck of the refrigerator. Following removal of the semen, the canister must be lowered into the LN again. Such manipulation causes temperature fluctuations within the frozen straws.

Figure 5 illustrates the degree to which the temperature changes when the LN level is either high or low (approximately 14 cm). When the refrigerator was full of LN, elevation of the semen into the neck of the refrigerator for periods of approximately

1 minute resulted in a temperature increase in the semen of only 15°C (from −196° to approximately −180°C). On the other hand, in tanks with low LN levels (14 cm) the temperature increased from −196 to −124°C (approximately 72°C). In addition, the influence of raising and lowering the semen in the tank was additive in tanks containing low LN levels. When semen was raised into the neck and held for 1 minute and then lowered back into the tank, the seminal temperature increased rapidly during the first minute of exposure but did not return to the original storage temperature of −196°C when replaced. When this was repeated, the temperature increased further with successive raising and lowering of the canister.

Spermatozoal motility and percentage of intact acrosomes, both measures of sperm viability, declined significantly when semen packaged in straws was raised and lowered in the LN tank approximately 480 times during a 6-month period.[9] This averages approximately 2.5 up-down cycles per day. The study also showed that spermatozoa stored in the top goblet sustained more acrosomal damage than semen in the bottom goblet, indicating that semen in the top goblets are more susceptible to damage. More recent studies[7, 15, 16] have shown that there were no significant differences in viability of spermatozoa when top and bottom goblets were compared in on-farm refrigerators. Semen was removed from these tanks after 6, 12, 18 and 24 months of storage for evaluation of motility and acrosomal maintenance. While the extent to which the semen was raised and lowered in the farm tanks was not measured, it was doubtful whether semen stored under farm conditions was subjected to the frequent up-down manipulations as reported by Pace and Sullivan.[9] Nevertheless, extreme care should be taken when raising the semen into the neck of the LN storage refrigerator. The canister should remain in the neck for very short periods

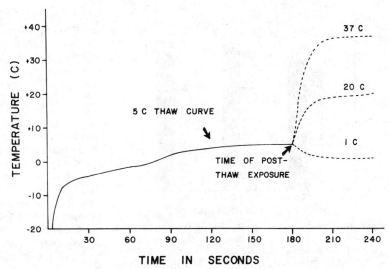

Figure 6. Temperature changes within the French straw during the 5°C thaw and during immediate post-thaw exposure to 1°C, 20°C and 37°C (10 replications). (From Senger et al.: J Anim Sci 42:932, 1976.)

and should be elevated only to the point at which the straw can be grasped with forceps.

Thawing of Semen. Because of the high surface-to-volume ratio and thus the high sensitivity to thermal change, the rate of thawing in straws is rapid regardless of the temperature. Much research has been conducted in order to describe and to refine the procedures for processing and thawing semen packaged in plastic straws. It is clear from controlled research that warm thaws result in improved recovery of viable spermatozoa.[2, 10, 11, 14, 17]

It is recommended that warm thaws (35°C) be used under field conditions. While temperatures of greater than 35°C result in greater survival,[10] it should be noted that the duration of the thaw must be shortened and carefully timed. This is particularly important at temperatures above which protein denaturation occurs. Prolonged exposure of the semen to temperatures higher than 35°C will result in death of the spermatozoa and inevitable loss of fertility.

Influence of Post-thaw Temperature. One point that continues to receive debate is the duration at which the straw should remain in the warm water

thaw bath (35°C). Straws removed from a 35°C water bath at 10 to 12 seconds have a terminal thaw temperature of −8 to 0°C,[2, 14] while straws removed after 1-minute exposure have reached 35°C (Fig. 7). Since the straw is thermally sensitive, the possibility of post-thaw cold shock injury has been of major concern. Spermatozoa packaged in straws and thawed in warm water (35°C) sustained post-thaw temperatures.[1, 14] When straws were thawed in warm water and removed before the temperature could rise above 5°C, there was no evidence of cold shock when straws were subsequently placed in iced water.[11]

Senger and colleagues[14] conducted a study to compare directly the degree of post-thaw spermatozoal damage when semen frozen in 0.25-ml Continental straws was thawed at either 5 or 35°C and subsequently plunged in water baths at 1°C, 20°C and 35°C. (Note: Continental straws are similar in diameter to the 0.5-ml French straw and thus have similar thermal behavior.) Temperature changes occurring within the straws during iced water (5°C) and warm water thaws (35°C) and during the post-thaw treatments are presented in Figures 6 and 7.

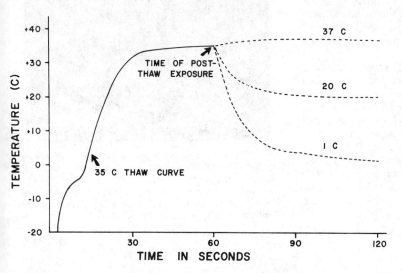

Figure 7. Temperature changes within the French straw during the 35°C thaw and during immediate post-thaw exposure to 1°C, 20°C, and 37°C (10 replications). (From Senger et al.: J Anim Sci 42:932 1976.)

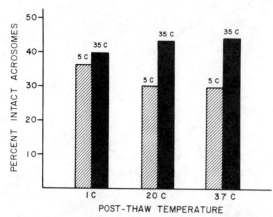

Figure 8. Influence of thawing rate (5°C or 35°C) and post-thaw temperature (1, 20, 37°C) on acrosomal maintenance. Values depicted by each bar are the overall means for 0-, 4- and 8-hour post-thaw incubations (37°C) for one ejaculate from each of 13 bulls. (Adapted from Senger et al.: J Anim Sci 42:932, 1976.)

Figure 6 illustrates that slow thaws (5°C) with a low terminal post-thaw temperature cannot be subject to a sudden decline in temperature, and therefore cold shock cannot occur. Rapid thaws (35°C), however, have a higher terminal temperature (Fig. 7) and are susceptible to a wide range of cold post-thaw temperatures. This greatly increases the probability of post-thaw cold shock.

Damage to the acrosomes occurred only under extreme cold shock conditions when semen thawed at 35°C for 1 minute was immediately plunged into iced water at 1°C (Fig. 8). Acrosomal integrity, however, was still higher than semen thawed in iced water (5°C) for 3 minutes (Fig. 8). Acrosomal damage was not observed when semen with a terminal temperature of 35°C was plunged into water baths of 20°C (Fig. 8). Such treatment resulted in a temperature decrease of 15°C. When semen was thawed in iced water (5°C) for 3 minutes and immediately plunged into water baths of 20 or 35°C, significant acrosomal damage occurred (Fig. 8).

This response is contrary to the accepted belief that a continual increase in post-thaw seminal temperature is not deleterious. More recent studies[5, 6] have confirmed the finding that post-thaw warming damages spermatozoa.

A fertility trial involving 13,543 services and nine technicians over a 10-month period was conducted to compare the fertility of semen packaged in 0.3 ml Continental straws and thawed at 35°C and held in the thaw bath for either 12 or 30 seconds.[2] Fertility resulting from the two thawing times was compared using 66-day nonreturn rates. Percentages of nonreturns (NR) were higher (P < 0.01) when semen was thawed for 30 seconds (72 per cent NR) than for semen thawed for 12 seconds (70.1 per cent NR). Semen thawed at 35°C for 12 seconds had a terminal thaw temperature of above 0°C,

while semen held at the thaw bath for 30 seconds reached approximately 32°C. Semen removed from the thaw after 12 seconds was inevitably warmed when deposited into the reproductive tract of the cow, and this warming presumably damaged spermatozoa. An additional important finding was that the improvement in fertility with longer thawing was not affected by month or season of the year. During the coldest months of December, January and February the mean temperature in the area of the experiment was −2.2, −7.9, and −0.2°C, respectively. The corresponding differences in nonreturns in favor of the 30-second thaw were 5.9, −0.9 and 0.49 per cent for the months of December, January and February, respectively. It should be pointed out that the AI technicians involved in this study were instructed to guard against cold shock by wrapping the inseminating gun in a paper towel and placing it inside the outer garment before moving to the place of insemination. Thus, it appears that if precautions against post-thaw cold shock are taken by the inseminator significant fertility advantages can be realized when warm water thaws of between 30 and 60 seconds are used.

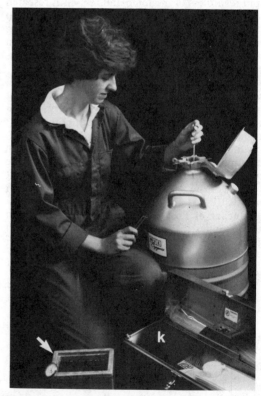

Figure 9. Be prepared. Have all necessary equipment ready and conveniently at-hand before opening the liquid nitrogen refrigerator. Thaw bath (arrow) should be 35°C and within close range of the refrigerator. The insemination kit (k) should be kept in a warm (70°C) room so that the insemination device is never cold.

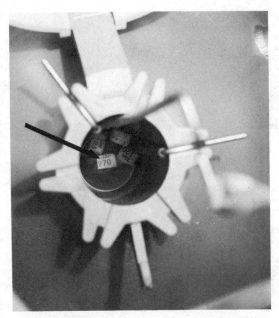

Figure 10. Identify the semen from the desired bull by the number on the top of each rack (arrow). Be sure that the canister containing the semen is well below the top of the refrigerator neck (see Fig. 11).

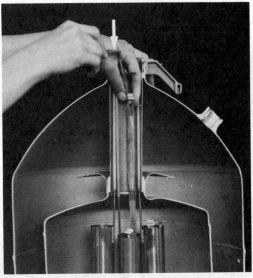

Figure 11. *This step takes practice.* Reach within the semen tank neck to grasp the top of the rack. Remove the straw using tweezers as shown (arrow). When properly elevated, the bottom end of the rack does not come out of the canister. Therefore, when the straw is removed, the rack may be released, and it will drop inside the canister. (See Fig. 23 for an additional method of straw removal.)

The data presented here strongly suggest that semen should be allowed to reach body temperature (thaws at 35°C for 30 to 60 seconds) before insemination. The physiological reasons for spermatozoal damage because of post-thaw warming are not understood, and this phenomenon needs further study.

PROPER STEPS FOR SEMEN HANDLING

The sequence of photographs presented in Figures 9 to 23 illustrates important steps in semen handling, beginning with removal of semen from the LN refrigerator and progressing through important steps required for successful semen handling.

SUMMARY

The little extra effort and time spent to manage semen refrigerators properly and handle and thaw semen will help optimize the number of viable spermatozoa inseminated. Recommendations that have been made are supported by valid research. Common sense and attention to detail should contribute to achieving optimum conception rates.

Text continued on page 174

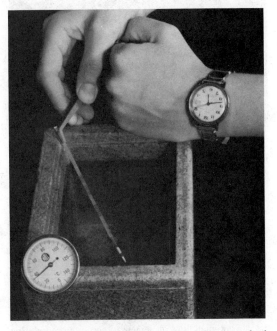

Figure 12. Immediately place the straw into the water bath at 35°C. Thaw time should be no less than 30 seconds and no longer than 1 minute.

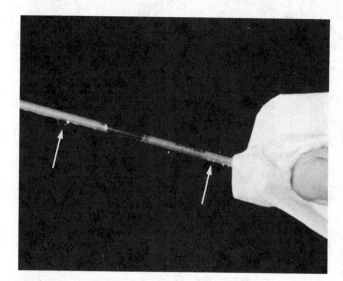

Figure 13. After the thawing period, remove the straw from the water bath. Remove all water from the external surface (arrows) of the straw with an absorbant tissue. *Water is lethal to spermatozoa.*

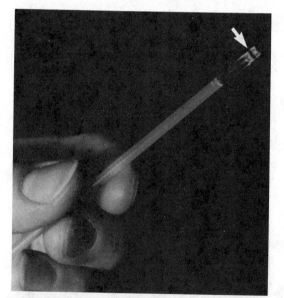

Figure 14. Shake the air bubble from the middle of the straw (seen in Fig. 13) to the end of the straw as shown here. This can be done by grasping the straw at the "factory" seal (arrow) and shaking it once or twice like a thermometer. The location of the air bubble should be at the sealed end of the straw (arrow). This location is important so that when the straw is cut no semen is lost, and a continual flow of semen is accomplished during deposition of the semen.

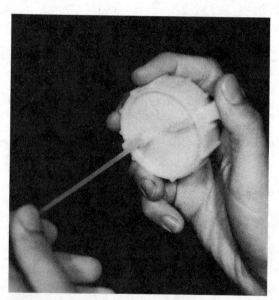

Figure 15. Cut the end of the straw with a straw cutter as shown or with a pair of scissors. If scissors are used, care must be taken so that the end of the straw is not crimped, thus preventing a secure fit into the plastic inseminating sheath (shown in Fig. 16).

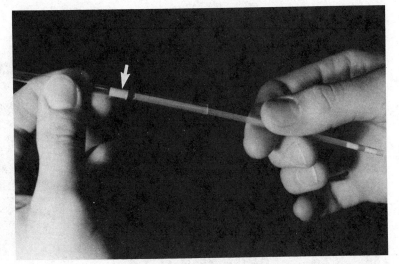

Figure 16. Carefully place the straw into the inseminating sheath. The cut end of the straw should be snugly placed in the adapter (arrow) within the plastic sheath. Grasp the adapter with the thumb and forefinger while twisting the straw into the adapter. This will insure proper seating of the straw within the adapter.

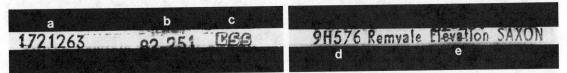

Figure 17. *Double check the sire identification.* The numbers on the straw represent: *a*, registration number of the bull; *b*, freeze code (this provides the AI organization with the date of collection and freezing); *c*, indication that the semen supplier has followed guidelines provided by Certified Semen Services (CSS); *d*, stud ID number and sire code; *e*, bull's name.

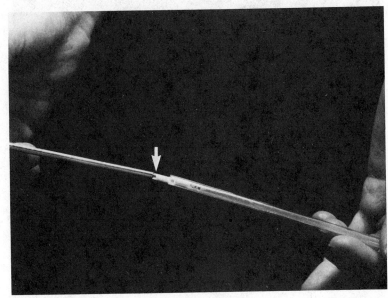

Figure 18. Place the stainless steel inseminating device over the straw (arrow) and slide the device between the plastic sheath and straw. *Do not use a cold stainless steel inseminating device.* Gently push the stainless steel device and the straw toward the end of the plastic sheath.

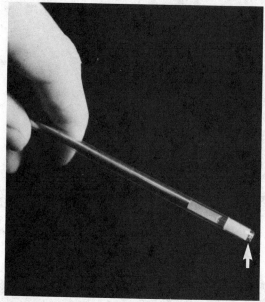

Figure 19. A properly seated 0.5-ml straw in the French inseminating device. Be sure the plastic adapter is fitted snugly against the end of the plastic sheath (arrow).

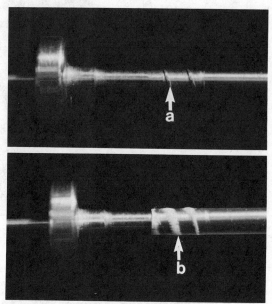

Figure 21. An alternative inseminating device for the 0.5-ml French straw contains machined screw-threads (arrow a), which serve to anchor the plastic inseminating sheath (arrow b). The O ring (Fig. 20) is not required with this device.

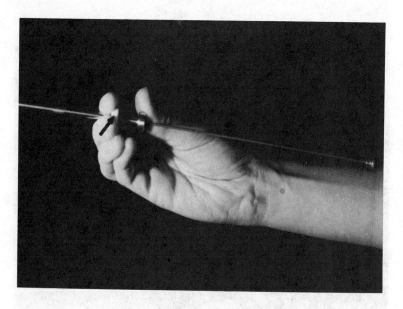

Figure 20. Securely set the O ring (arrow) by pushing it forcefully against the flanged portion of the syringe. The plastic sheath should not move during the insemination procedure.

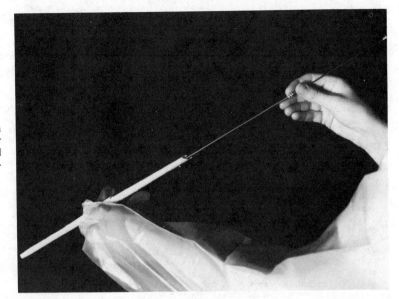

Figure 22. The tip of the sheath should be wrapped with a paper towel so that the possibility of cold shock is minimized during movement to the cow.

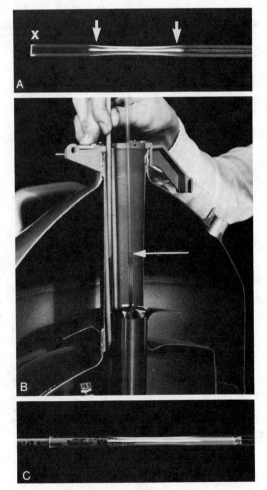

Figure 23. Straw retrieval device *(A)* made from an inseminating pipette sheath. Cut off one end *(x)* and pinch the sheath (arrows) so that it is flattened. Next, *(B)* pass sheath over end of straw (arrow) and retrieve. Straw *(C)* will remain in the sheath because of friction. An improvement over the technique shown in *A* is to cut the end of the sheath to a point. This enables the sheath to fit over the straw with greater ease. Be sure to test the sheath on a used straw to insure that it will secure the straw. When this method is used, the canister does not need to be elevated as high as in the method shown in Figure 11. (This procedure was developed by Mr. Gene Lowe, Training Coordinator, COBA/Select Sires, Tyler, Texas. See Advanced Animal Breeder, May 15, 1984, p 13.)

References

1. Almquist JO: Effect of cold shock after thawing on acrosomal maintenance and motility of bovine spermatozoa frozen in plastic straws. J Dairy Sci 59:1825, 1976.
2. Almquist JO, Rosenberger JL, Branas RJ: Effect of thawing time in warm water on fertility of bovine spermatozoa in plastic straws. J Dairy Sci 62:772, 1979.
3. Almquist JO, Grube KE, Rosenberger JL: Effect of thawing time on fertility of bovine spermatozoa in French straws. J Dairy Sci, 65:824, 1982.
4. Berndtson WE, Pickett BW, Rugg CD: Procedures for field handling of bovine semen in plastic straws. Proc 6th NAAB Tech Conf Artif Insem Reprod, 1976, pp 51–60.
5. Brown JL, Senger PL, Hillers JK: Influence of thawing time and post-thaw temperature on acrosomal maintenance and motility of bovine spermatozoa frozen in 0.5 ml French straws. J Anim Sci 54:938, 1982.
6. De Abreu RM, Berndtson WE, Smith RL, Pickett BW: Effect of post-thaw warming on viability of bovine spermatozoa thawed at different rates in French straws. J Dairy Sci 62:1449, 1979.
7. Lineweaver JA, Saacke RG, Gwazdauskas FC: Effect of double decking and storage time on semen stored in farm storage tanks. Proc 1979 ADSA Meet, 1979, p 175.
8. Mazur P: Fundamental aspects of the freezing of cells with emphasis on mammalian ova and embryos. Proc 9th Int Cong Anim Reprod AI, Madrid, 1980 Vol 1, p 99.
9. Pace MM, Sullivan JJ: A biological comparison of the 0.5-ml ampule and 0.5-ml French straw for packaging bovine spermatozoa. Proc 7th NAAB Tech Conf Artif Insemin Reprod, 1978, pp 22–25.
10. Robbins RK, Saacke RG, Chandler PT: Influence of freeze rate, thaw rate and glycerol level on acrosomal retention and survival of bovine spermatozoa frozen in French straws. J Anim Sci 42:145, 1976.
11. Rodriquez OL, Berndtson WE, Enne BD, Pickett BW: Effect of rates of freezing, thawing and level of glycerol on the survival of bovine spermatozoa in straws. J Anim Sci 41:129, 1975.
12. Saacke RG: What happens when a sperm is frozen and thawed? Proc 9th NAAB Tech Conf Artif Insemin Reprod, 1982, pp 6–12.
13. Senger PL: Handling frozen bovine semen—factors which influence viability and fertility. Theriogenology 13:51, 1980.
14. Senger PL, Becker WC, Hillers JK: Effect of thawing rate and post-thaw temperatures on motility and acrosomal maintenance in bovine semen frozen in plastic straws. J Anim Sci 42:932, 1976.
15. Senger PL, Becker WC, Hillers JK: Quality of semen stored in on-the-farm semen tanks. J Dairy Sci 63:646, 1980.
16. Senger PL, Hillers JK, Fleming WN: On-the-farm management of semen tanks. Proc 8th NAAB Tech Conf Artif Insemin Reprod, 1980, pp 25–29.
17. Wiggin HB, Almquist JO: Effect of glycerol equilibration time and thawing rate upon acrosomal maintenance and motility of bull spermatozoa frozen in plastic straws. J Anim Sci 40:302, 1975.

Recommended Review

Pickett BW, Berndtson WE, Sullivan JJ: Influence of seminal additives and packaging systems on fertility of frozen bovine spermatozoa. J Anim Sci (Suppl 2) 47:12, 1978.

Evaluating Artificial Inseminators' Placement of Semen in Cattle

Brad Seguin, D.V.M., Ph.D.
University of Minnesota, St. Paul, Minnesota

Unsatisfactory conception rates identified in a herd can stem from several possible causes, which fall into four major categories: cow fertility, bull (or semen) fertility, heat detection accuracy and insemination technique. One component of insemination technique is the accuracy of the inseminator's placement of semen. Incorrect placement of the semen dose, usually by going beyond the uterine body into one of the uterine horns, can lower the pregnancy results. In this situation normal fertility is expected when ovulation occurs on the side of semen deposition. When ovulation occurs opposite the side of deposition, pregnancy results may drop as much as 20 to 30 per cent, but a drop to near zero would not be characteristic of this problem.

A test system for cattle has been developed to evaluate pregnancy results achieved in relation to the side of the reproductive tract inseminated. This on-farm system can be used to determine if, and to what extent, differences in pregnancy rates between sides of the reproductive tract might be influencing overall pregnancy rates. To do this, ovaries of cows inseminated 7 to 18 days previously are palpated to determine which ovary contains the corpus luteum (CL), i.e., the side of last ovulation. Subsequently, results for each service are analyzed according to side of CL location, and left- and right-side pregnancy rates are calculated. The following set of trials have been conducted to validate this procedure.

The effect of the test procedure on pregnancy results was evaluated by testing (palpating) every other cow serviced (216 services on two farms). Results were similar on each location and were combined. The test did not affect pregnancy rates, as 46 per cent of 116 tested cows and 42 per cent of 110 control cows conceived. Palpation did not affect the interestrous interval in the nonpregnant cows.

In 2374 services tested in 16 locations (inseminator units or individual farms inseminating their own cows), more CL were located on the right ovary than on the left. The overall left-to-right ratio was 41.9:58.1. This ratio varied considerably among inseminator units and farms (from 37.2:62.8 to 50.4:49.6). This variation is too great to use the overall average in determining influence of semen deposition on conception rate.

Table 1. Guidelines for Numbers of Observations Needed to Show Statistically (P < 0.05) That an Individual Has a Conception Rate Difference Between Sides of the Cow's Reproductive Tract

Conception Rate Difference Between Sides of Tract (Per Cent)	No. of Services Needed to Show Side Effect at P < 0.05
40*	25–30
30	50
20	100
10	400
5	1600

*e.g., left = 30 per cent, right = 70 per cent

Pregnancy rate differences between sides of the tract for the 16 inseminators ranged from 1.0 to 18.0 percentage points and averaged 7.3 percentage points. Two individuals had differences exceeding 15 percentage points, four more exceeded a 10-point difference, three exceeded a 5-point difference and seven had differences of less than 5 percentage points. Among the nine inseminators with differences exceeding 5 points, eight used the left arm, and one used the right arm per rectum; but the arm used per rectum and the side of higher results were not consistently related. Therefore, pregnancy rate differences between sides of the tract represented insemination technique rather than physiological tendencies in the cow. Numbers of observations

(services) that must be made to establish statistically (P < 0.05) that an individual is having conception differences between sides of the reproductive tract are presented in Table 1.

In a subset of 1187 test results, ovarian findings were more thoroughly analyzed. Most (1067 or 89.9 per cent) of the cows had a normal single CL. Another 20 cows (1.7 per cent) had two CL. These findings in 91.6 per cent of the cows examined were consistent with a developing pregnancy. In the remaining 100 services (8.4 per cent of the total), a functional CL could not be detected. In 62 of these cases ovarian follicular cysts were found, and in 38 cases no functional ovarian structures of any type were detected. Thus, in these 1187 postservice examinations, findings in 8.4 per cent were inconsistent with a developing pregnancy. Therefore, this system of ovarian examination 7 to 18 days after service can provide additional information about factors such as ovulation failure that influence pregnancy results.

In summary, this method can be used to learn—on the farm during routine herd health visits—whether the inseminator's semen deposition adversely affects conception rate. Specifically, the test determines whether semen is consistently deposited beyond the uterine body in one uterine horn. Because this flaw in technique affects conception rates achieved among inseminators, this test method should be included in the list of several possible areas for investigating herds with disappointing pregnancy results.

Monitoring Trends in Pregnancy Results

Brad Seguin, D.V.M., Ph.D.
University of Minnesota, St. Paul, Minnesota

Monitoring results of a breeding program, especially evaluating trends in pregnancy rate, should be an integral part of a reproductive herd health program.[1] "Pregnancy rate" is defined here as the number of pregnancies resulting from a given number of services that when multiplied by 100 becomes a percentage. The number of services used as the denominator should include *all* services in a given period, including those used in cows that ultimately leave the herd without conceiving. Counting only those services used in cows that eventually conceive gives an artificially high result and one that is unduly affected by culling. This policy also complicates and delays pregnancy rate calculation, as no decision

can be made about the inclusion or the exclusion of unsuccessful services in cows still being bred. Although average days open is the reproductive parameter with greatest economic significance in a dairy herd, there are several reasons for using pregnancy rate as an indicator of herd performance. It is one of the three factors that determine days open, the other two being estrus detection efficiency and length of the postpartum rest interval. Pregnancy rate data, when used with early pregnancy diagnosis, can indicate reproductive performance to within 21 to 35 days. These data also are easily calculated and are accepted as a standard index for dairy cattle reproduction. The most productive way of using pregnancy rate data is to examine the time trends rather than look at one numerical figure representing an extended period, for example, 1 year.

A graph system consecutively listing service results according to service date has been developed.[2] From a list of services and service results (e.g., pregnant or nonpregnant) a graph is constructed using one input for each service. One symbol is used for each pregnancy achieved (a P is used in the sample graph in Fig. 1) and another symbol (O) is used for each unsuccessful service. The first entry starts from an arbitrary point on the left side of a sheet of graph paper; Ps are entered one row up

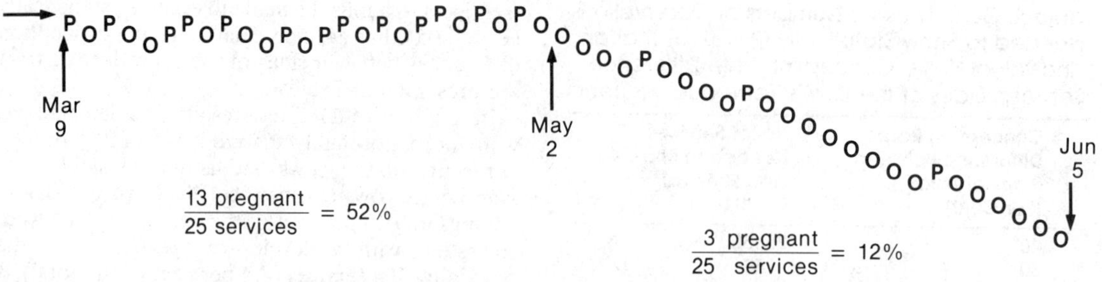

Figure 1. Graphic presentation of service results in a herd from March 9 through June 5. Services resulting in pregnancy are indicated by a P and those not producing a pregnancy are shown by an O. The pregnancy rate for each group of 25 services is presented, along with the beginning and ending dates for each of these groups.

from the last entry and Os are entered one row down. The slope of the composite line formed by these entries indicates conception rate trends in the herd. A line that goes approximately straight across the page indicates a pregnancy rate of about 50 per cent. In Figure 1 the starting date and dates at increments of 25 services are indicated, and the pregnancy rate for each 25-service group is calculated. Graph paper with 100 columns therefore will allow 100 services to be conveniently recorded per page. The service list can be maintained by the client, and the graph should be updated and inspected at the completion of reproductive examinations during each veterinary visit. This list becomes a handy checklist to see if all cows ready to be checked for pregnancy have been examined. The system can record the results of all services or only first services. Using only first-service results in small and medium herds, however, eliminates data needed to show performance trends. Another reason to use all services is that repeat service frequently costs the same as first service. In addition, results for first services and for all services are frequently so similar that distinguishing between them is not important. Therefore, using results of all services is recommended, with the possible exception of very large herds. This record system can be used with any method of pregnancy diagnosis,

but for the greatest benefit pregnancy status should be determined by an early and highly accurate method.

This graph system is an excellent method to determine pregnancy rates accurately on farms. Replacing the common but erroneous practice of equating pregnancy rate and pregnancy palpation results (i.e., number of cows pregnant of those examined for pregnancy) with a system such as this should be encouraged. Percentage of cows pregnant at palpation effectively indicates estrus detection but not pregnancy rate. The graph system also quickly indicates when pregnancy rate changes. Notice in Figure 1 that the onset of a low pregnancy rate can be pinpointed close to May 2. With this information, an investigation can be focused on this period, which may obviate a diagnosis. Similarly, this graph quickly indicates when results have improved.

References

1. Seguin BE: A reproductive herd health program for dairy herds. Comp Cont Ed Vet Pract 3:S445, 1981.
2. Meek AH, Mitchell WR, Curtis RA, et al.: A proposed information management and disease monitoring system for dairy herds. Can Vet J 16:329, 1975.

Congenital Defects Affecting Bovine Reproduction

Horst W. Leipold
Stanley M. Dennis
Kansas State University, Manhattan, Kansas

A variety of structural and functional defects have been described in newborn calves that range from variant through blemish, to imperfection and deviant and to malformation and monstrosity. Only when the defect occurs repeatedly in the same herd or geographic area is a defective neonate likely to be brought to the attention of investigators concerned with congenital defects. Most defective neonates, however, go unrecorded by veterinarians, animal scientists and geneticists.[11]

Recently, there has been a perceptible change in attitude by veterinarians, geneticists, animal scientists and livestock industries toward the importance of congenital defects or diseases. Much of the change resulted from experiences of artificial insemination and breed registry organizations as they found that they and their consulting experts required more scientific information than was available. They have now developed programs for monitoring undesirable genetic traits, controlling specific ones and sharing with herd owners the names of cattle known to transmit the defect. This has and will cause many more herd owners to seek advice from veterinary practitioners about appropriate genetic control measures. Current assessment of bovine congenital defects reveals the major problems to be inadequate information, i.e., too few case reports; inadequate anatomic and pathologic investigations or descriptions; inadequate and inappropriate genetic analyses and failure to integrate underlying embryologic, pathologic and genetic processes.[11]

IDENTIFYING CONGENITAL DEFECTS

Definition and Classification

Congenital defects, or diseases, are abnormalities of structure or function present at birth. They may affect a single anatomic structure or function, an entire system, parts of several systems or both a structure and a function. All body structures and functions may be affected. Congenital defects are usually classified by the body system primarily affected.

Nature and Effect

Defective development may be manifested by embryonic mortality, fetal death, mummification, abortion, dysmaturity, full-term stillbirth or nonviable or viable neonate. Congenitally defective calves pose a diagnostic challenge to veterinarians, act as sentinels of man's environment and are of comparative biomedical significance for other animal species.

Susceptibility to injurious environmental or genetic agents varies with the stage of development and decreases with fetal age. Before day 14 the zygote is resistant to teratogens but susceptible to genetic mutations and chromosomal aberrations. During the embryonic period (days 14 to 42), the embryo is highly susceptible to teratogens, but this decreases with embryonic age as the critical developmental periods of various organs or organ systems are passed. The fetus (day 42 plus) becomes increasingly resistant to teratogenic agents with age except for its later-differentiating structures such as cerebellum, palate and urogenital system.

Congenital defects may be lethal, semilethal or compatible with life and may impair viability, may have little effect on viability or may have an esthetic effect and thus lower economic value. The frequency with which various body parts are affected varies according to breed, geographic location, season, sex, age of parent and level of nutrition. Additional economic losses occur when congenital defects are only one manifestation of a syndrome including embryonic and fetal mortality. Herd improvement is lessened through loss of replacements and consequent reduction in culling potential. Congenital defects may be an added source of confusion in diagnosing other diseases or abortion. Control measures may require expensive adjustments of breeding programs if the defect is genetic, as they are repeated generation after generation. With increasing use of artificial insemination in cattle, defects no longer are rare; all are important. Collectively, congenital defects cause economic losses by increasing perinatal calf mortality, decreasing maternal productivity and decreasing the value of viable defective calves and their relatives.

Frequency

The frequency of congenital defects in cattle is not a fixed proportion of all births but varies because congenital defects are caused either by hereditary and environmental factors or by the interactions of these factors. The frequency of individual defects will vary among breeds, geographic locations and seasons. Frequencies of all congenital defects, as well as those of individual structures or functions,

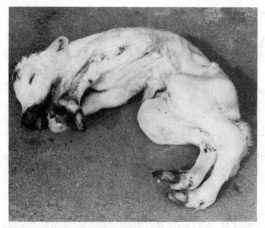

Figure 1. Arthrogryposis in a neonatal Charolais calf. Note the bilateral symmetrical contracture of the joints.

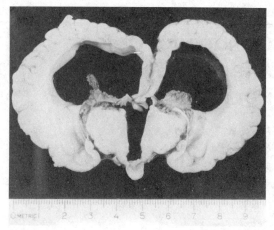

Figure 3. Cross section of internal hydrocephalus in a neonatal calf. The lateral ventricles are markedly dilated.

are difficult to obtain because many can be identified only by necropsy. Many defects go unnoticed, others are not reported for economic reasons and others occur so rarely as to defy accurate accounting. Frequent reporting of some defects may reflect high interest of the observer rather than high incidence of the defect.[3, 11]

Incidence of congenital defects among all calves seems to range from 0.2 to 3.0 per cent, with 40 to 50 per cent born dead, and only a small fraction of reported defects not being externally visible.

The most frequently encountered congenital defects in cattle involve the skeletal, central nervous and muscular systems. The most common are skeletal defects, as they are more easily recognized than internal defects. Common bovine defects include arthrogryposis, internal hydrocephalus, cleft palate, syndactyly, rectovaginal constriction (RVC) and degenerative progressive myeloencephalopathy ("weaver") (Figs. 1–10).[2, 3, 9–11]

Causes

Many congenital defects have no clearly established cause, others are caused by environmental or genetic factors or from environmental-genetic interaction.

Genetic. Hereditary defects are pathologic or pathophysiological results determined by mutant genes or chromosomal aberrations. Chromosomal aberrations have been demonstrated in cattle but as yet have not gained the diagnostic prominence as in humans. A common chromosomal defect frequently encountered in cattle is centric fusion of acrocentric chromosomes to form robertsonian translocation.[1]

Diagnosis of genetic defects is based on the rule that genetic diseases run in families in typical intergenerational and intragenerational patterns requiring enumeration of normal and abnormal offspring and identification of their familial relationships.

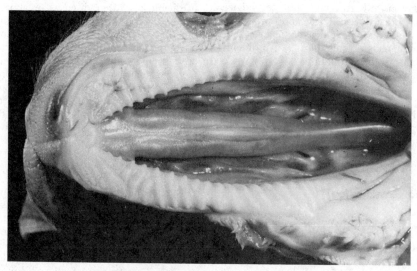

Figure 2. Cleft palate in the arthrogrypotic calf depicted in Figure 1.

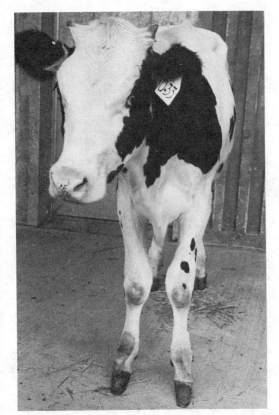

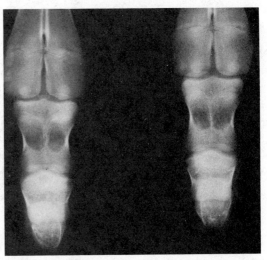

Figure 5. Radiograph of front legs of a neonatal syndactylous calf. Notice horizontal fusion of corresponding phalanges.

Figure 4. Holstein heifer affected with syndactyly of both front feet.

Various statistical methods are used to analyze such data, and breeding trials may be necessary to confirm inheritance patterns. Many congenital diseases in cattle follow the patterns of simple Mendelian inheritance, mostly simple autosomal recessive. Other monofactorial inheritance patterns described are overdominant, dominant or incompletely dominant, whereas only a few reports describe sex linkage. Congenital defects may also be inherited as polygenic traits.

Environmental. Teratogenic factors reported include toxic plants, viruses, drugs, trace elements and physical agents such as irradiation, hyperthermia and pressure during rectal examination. They are difficult to identify but often follow seasonal patterns and known stressful conditions and may be linked to maternal disease. They do not follow a familial pattern as do genetic causes. They occur in any genotype during the appropriate critical period. Maternal disease patterns vary, but neonates from primiparous dams are more frequently affected: Fetal immunoglobulin levels to infectious agents are

Figure 6. Bovine fetus, 60 days, taken by preterminal cesarean section. Notice syndactyly of both front feet.

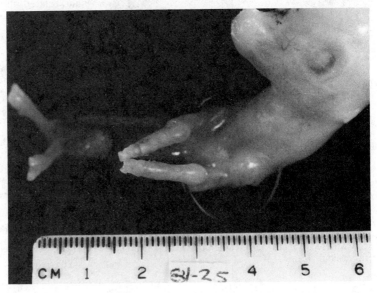

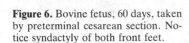

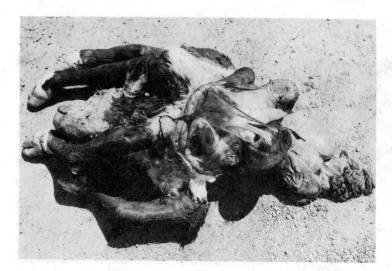

Figure 7. Schistosomus reflexus—a common cause of dystocia due to a defective calf.

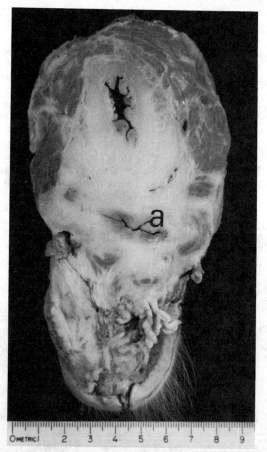

Figure 8. Cross section of vestibule and rectum of a Jersey cow with rectovaginal constriction (RVC). Note hypoplastic vestibule *(a)*.

frequently detected abortion incidence is increased and morbidity may be observed in the herd or in other animals on the farm. Field studies have usually led to observations on frequency and pattern of a defect in a herd or in a population. They have usually suggested what kind of plant was consumed or what viral infection appeared likely.

Plant Teratogens. Ingestion of lupines has resulted in crooked calves characterized by arthrogryposis and possibly torticollis, scoliosis or kyphosis, cleft palate and combinations of these defects. The alkaloid anagyrine has been identified as the teratogen. Other plants incriminated or suspected of causing defective calves include *Conium maculatum, Senecio, Indigofera spicata, Cycadales, Blighia,* locoweeds, *Papaveraceae, Colchicum, Vinca,* tobacco and related plants.[6]

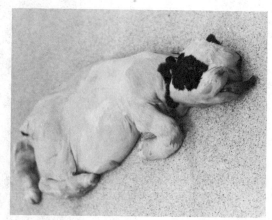

Figure 9. Holstein calf afflicted with chondrodysplasia ("bull dog").

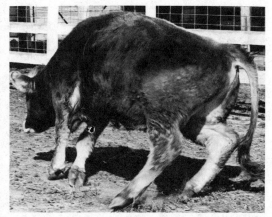

Figure 10. Brown Swiss bull afflicted with bovine progressive degenerative myeloencephalopathy.

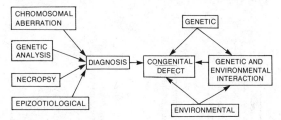

Figure 11. Factors involved in diagnosing congenitally defective calves.

Viruses. Certain prenatal viruses have been found to be teratogenic for cattle: Akabane virus causes abortion, premature births and arthrogryposis-hydranencephaly (A-H) syndrome; bovine virus diarrhea induces congenital defects such as cerebellar dysplasia, ocular defects, brachygnathia inferior, alopecia, dysmyelinogenesis, internal hydrocephalus, dysmaturity (intrauterine growth retardation) and impaired immunologic competence; blue tongue virus affects fetal calves, resulting in abortion, stillbirths and congenital defects such as arthrogryposis, campylognathia, prognathism, hydranencephaly, and "dummy calf" syndrome; Wesselsbron virus is reported in South Africa to cause porencephalia and cerebellar hypoplasia.[7, 11]

Others. The following have been incriminated or suspected of being teratogenic in cattle: rectal palpation, manganese deficiency, hyperthermia, irradiation, iodine deficiency, vitamin A deficiency, fetal hypoxia, aging of ova and spermatozoa and various drugs.

Recent work in Germany has revealed rectal palpation and pressure on the amnion between days 33 to 40 of gestation may cause atresia coli and occasionally atresia jejuni. Male calves were affected more frequently than females.[11]

SPECIFIC DEFECTS

Congenital defects reported in cattle are summarized in Table 1, which is divided into sections according to the principal body system involved.

Factors Influencing Diagnosis of Congenital Defects

Because diagnosis of bovine congenital defects is complex, various limiting factors need to be considered (Fig. 11).

Defects Not Reported. Defective calves are frequently not reported unless they are unusually bizarre or several defective births have occurred. Nonreporting is a major difficulty limiting our knowledge of congenital defects in cattle. Cooperation of breeders through reporting all defective calves to the appropriate cattle associations and artificial insemination (AI) centers is essential for controlling or for eliminating undesirable genetic traits.

Professional Knowledge. Limited knowledge and incomplete examination have led to defective calves being mistaken for premature births or abortions. Practitioners should be familiar with the more common cattle defects and if in doubt should seek specialized assistance. Practitioners are required to advise breeders about control measures, which may require altering herd management or breeding programs, depending on whether they consider the congenital defect to be environmentally or genetically induced. Veterinarians, both practitioners and laboratory diagnosticians, should always be cognizant of their role in preventive bovine teratology.

Inadequate History. Too often defective calves are submitted for diagnosis with little available history. Diagnostic judgment and documentation of congenital defects require information on the geographic region, gestation season, feeding and management practices, types of pastures, presence of poisonous or teratogenic plants, vaccinations, stresses and any sickness or medication during pregnancy.

Breeding Records. Diagnosis of genetic defects is handicapped by lack of or inadequate records. This restricts genetic analysis, requiring enumerating normal and defective calves and recording their familial relationships. Most known genetic defects in cattle follow a simple autosomal recessive pattern.

Classification and Terminology. Lack of a standardized system for classifying birth defects makes comparisons in the literature difficult. This deficiency interferes with exchange among the various disciplines and with accumulating readily retrievable data on congenital birth defects. Consequently, many reports are virtually lost in the literature. For easy reference and to facilitate interdisciplinary comparisons, it is recommended that congenital defects be classified by the body system primarily affected.

Text continued on page 196

Table 1. Congenital Defects of Cattle Classified by Body System

Defect	Description	Etiology	Frequency	Diagnosis	Associated Defects
Congenital Defects of the Entire Skeletal System					
Dwarfism	Disturbance of longitudinal epiphyseal growth; appositional bone growth normal; abnormal head	Genetic, recessive	Rare	Short stature, x-ray of lumbar vertebrae	May be affected with internal hydrocephalus
Chondrodysplasia ("Bulldog")	Craniofacial defect giving a "bulldog" appearance, legs short and stubby; several types described	Genetic, recessive, polygenic, reported	Common	X-ray, necropsy	Cleft palate, ventricular septal defect, ascites
Osteogenesis imperfecta	Fragile bones, reduced bone mass	Genetic, recessive; polygenic	Rare	X-ray, histologic examination	None
Osteopetrosis	Continuous formation of chondro-osseous matrix, lack of resorption and remodeling of bones; premature stillborn	Genetic, recessive	Common	X-ray, necropsy	Short lower jaw, dam may have hydramnios
Acroteriasis (congenital "amputated")	Involves entire skeleton, amputation of all four legs, defects of facial skeleton, cleft palate and short lower jaw	Genetic, recessive	Rare	External examination and x-ray	Vertebral column, eye defects
Porphyria (pink tooth)	Metabolic defect; teeth and bone store porphyrin, giving characteristic brown appearance	Genetic, recessive	Common	Clinical examination	Photosensitivity
Congenital Defects of the Facial Skeleton					
Cleft palate without associated defects	Median cleft due to nonclosure of hard palate	Unknown	Rare	Clinical examination	None
Cleft palate associated with arthrogryposis	Complete nonclosure of hard palate; permanent joint contractures present at birth	Recessive, other cases sporadic	Common	Necropsy examination	Hypoplasia of patella
Cleft palate associated with crooked legs	Variable degrees of cleft palate and joint contractures	Maternal ingestion of lupine between days 40 and 70 of pregnancy	Common	Clinical and necropsy examination	Variable
Short lower jaw	Shortened mandible	Unknown	Common	External examination	None
Prognathism	Shortened upper jaw and protruding lower jaw	Possibly genetic	Uncommon	External examination	None
Campylognathia	Curved jaw	Unknown	Rare	External examination	None
Agnathia	Aplasia of mandible	Possibly genetic	Uncommon	External examination, x-ray	Other mandibulofacial defects
Craniofacial dysplasia	Deficient ossification of frontal sutures, convex profile of nose, short lower jaw	Incompletely dominant with incomplete penetrance	Rare	External examination	Macroglossia, patent ductus arteriosus

Congenital Defects of the Axial Skeleton

Defect	Description	Cause	Frequency	Diagnosis	Associated Defects
Scoliosis	Lateral deviation of vertebral column	Unknown	Rare	External examination	May have arthrogryposis or no associated defects
Kyphosis	Dorsal deviation of vertebral column	Unknown	Rare	External examination	May be associated with other musculoskeletal defects
Kyphoscoliosis	Dorsal and lateral deviation of vertebral column	Genetic and environmental causes	Common	External examination	Frequently associated with arthrogryposis
Torticollis	Twisted neck (wryneck)	Genetic and environmental causes	Fairly common	External examination	None
Short spine	Reduction and fusion of vertebrae and ribs from 13 to 6 or 7	Recessive	Rare	External examination	CNS defects
Atlanto-occipital fusion	Fusion of first cervical spine to occipital bones; hypoplasia of dens of axis	Unknown	Rare	X-ray, necropsy	Spinal cord defect
Perosomus elumbis	Agenesis of lumbosacral and coccygeal vertebrae with spinal cord ending in thoracic area	Unknown	Fairly common	External examination and necropsy	CNS defects
Anury (tail absent)	Agenesis of coccygeal vertebrae	Nongenetic environmental cause unknown	Common	External examination	About 50 per cent have high ventricular septal defect and/or microphthalmia
Wrytail	Kink between coccygeal vertebrae	Recessive	Rare	External examination	None

Congenital Defects of Appendicular Skeleton

Defect	Description	Cause	Frequency	Diagnosis	Associated Defects
Polymelia	Duplication of one or more limbs	Unknown	Uncommon	External examination and x-ray	None
Polymelia, heterotopic	One or two supernumerary limbs attached to various regions, e.g., thoracomelia, if attached to thorax	Unknown	Uncommon	External examination	None
Abrachia	Agenesis of both front limbs	Unknown	Uncommon	External examination	None
Apodia	Agenesis of both hind legs	Unknown	Uncommon	External examination	None
Monobrachia	Agenesis of one front limb	Unknown	Uncommon	External examination	None
Monopodia	Agenesis of one hind limb	Unknown	Uncommon	External examination	None
Micromelia	All parts of appendicular skeleton present but hypoplastic	Unknown	Uncommon	External examination and x-ray	None
Peromelia	Agenesis of distal appendicular parts	Unknown	Uncommon	Clinical examination and x-ray	None

Table continued on following page

Table 1. Congenital Defects of Cattle Classified by Body System *Continued*

Defect	Description	Etiology	Frequency	Diagnosis	Associated Defects
Phocomelia	Agenesis of proximal appendicular parts, distal parts are developed	Unknown	Uncommon	Clinical examination and x-ray	None
Tibial hemimelia	Agenesis of both tibias	Recessive	Common	Clinical examination	Encephalocele, ventral abdominal hernia, male-cryptorchid; female nonunion of müllerian ducts
Ectrodactyly	Partial or complete absence of digits	Possibly genetic	Rare	Clinical examination and x-ray	None or arthrogryposis
Adactyly	Complete or partial lack of digits	Recessive	Rare	Clinical examination and x-ray	None
Polydactyly	Development of additional digits on one or more limbs	Polygenic	Common	Clinical examination and x-ray	None
Syndactyly	Fusion or nondivision of functional digits	Recessive with incomplete penetrance and varying degrees of expressivity	Common	Clinical examination and x-ray	Hyperthermia
Brachydactyly	Short stature caused by shortness of metacarpal and metatarsal bones	Possibly genetic	Rare	Clinical examination and x-ray	None
Congenital Defects of the Muscular System					
Arthrogryposis	Permanent joint contractures present at birth	Genetic, recessive. Sporadic cases occur. Needs careful analysis.	Common	Clinical examination, necropsy	Cleft palate, kyphoscoliosis
Double muscling	Fine neck and head, bulging muscles in back and hind quarters, deep creases between muscles, reduced fat	Recessive; other hereditary modes are currently being investigated	Common in some breeds	Inspection at slaughter	Abnormalities of bone and reproductive systems, dystocia
Congenital Defects of the Cerebrum					
Agenesis of corpus callosum	Absence of corpus callosum	Unknown	Rare	Necropsy	Absence of septum pellucidum and other CNS defects
Anencephaly	Absence of cerebral hemispheres, nonclosure of anterior portion of neural tube, brain stem and eyes present	Unknown	Rare	Necropsy	Acrania, cranioschisis, craniorachischisis, cleft palate, absence of pituitary, taillessness, atresia ani

Defect	Description	Cause	Frequency	Diagnosis	Associated defects
Cerebellar atrophy	Cerebellum reduced in size; mild to severe depletion of cortical layers and narrow, fiber-depleted streaks to large, irregular cavities in the folial white matter	BVD virus	Rare	Necropsy and histologic examination	Ocular lesions: cataract, retinal degeneration, hypoplasia and neuritis of optic nerves; also fetal mummification, mandibular brachygnathia, skin defects may occur
Cerebellar ataxia and hypomyelinogenesis congenita	CNS grossly normal; histologic changes consist of diffuse spongy appearance	Recessive	Rare	Histologic examination	None
Neuraxial edema	CNS grossly normal, sometimes brain pale and swollen; histologic examination reveals spongy vacuolation of long axis of myelinated fibers in white and gray matter	Recessive	Rare	Histologic examination	None
Arnold-Chiari malformation	Herniation of tonguelike processes of cerebellar tissue through foramen magnum dorsal to anterior cervical spinal cord, displacement of medulla oblongata, pons and fourth ventricle	Unknown	Rare	Necropsy	Spina bifida of lumbar spinal column
Cerebellar abiotrophy	Ataxia, dysmetria, rhythmic head movements, degeneration of cerebellar neurons	Possibly recessive	Rare	Clinical histologic examinations	None
Progressive ataxia	Hypermetria, incoordination, muscular weakness, rhythmic head movements	Possibly recessive	Rare	Clinical and histologic examinations	None
Progressive degenerative myeloencephalopathy ("weaver")	Hindleg weakness, dysmetria, ataxia	Possibly recessive	Common	Clinical and histologic examinations	None
Arhinencephalia	Absence of olfactory bulbs, tracts and nerves	Unknown	Rare	Necropsy	Aprosopia, nasal atresia, cleft palate, other CNS defects, aplastic pituitary (prolonged gestation)
Exencephaly	Exposure of brain in a defectively developed cranium	Unknown	Rare	Necropsy	Acrania, cervical spina bifida
Hydranencephaly	Cerebral tissue replaced by thin fluid-filled tissue	Unknown, blue tongue and Akabane viruses	Uncommon	Necropsy	Arthrogryposis
Hydrocephalus, internal	Accumulation of excessive CNS fluid within lateral and other ventricles leading to dilation	Recessive, environmental causes possible	Common	Necropsy	Cleft palate, eye defects, cerebellar and spinal cord defects, myopathy, arthrogryposis, heart defects may occur

Table continued on following page

Table 1. Congenital Defects of Cattle Classified by Body System *Continued*

Defect	Description	Etiology	Frequency	Diagnosis	Associated Defects
Meningoencephalocele	Herniation of meninges and/or cerebral tissue through a cranial defect, usually in frontal region	Unknown	Common	Necropsy	Agnathia, cleft palate, other CNS and eye defects, arthrogryposis, atresia ani
Microencephaly	Abnormally small brain, small and reduced number of gyri	Possibly genetic	Rare	Necropsy	Micrognathia, agenesis of corpus callosum, pachygyria, enlarged third cerebral ventricle, arthrogryposis
Congenital Defects of the Cerebellum					
Cerebellar hypoplasia	Cerebellum absent or small, smooth surface, cross section reveals small and narrow cortex and folia; cerebral hemispheres and brain stem normal	Possibly genetic, recessive trait	Rare	Necropsy and histologic examination	None
Genetic Spastic Diseases					
Spastic paresis	Spastic contracture of muscles and extension of stifle and tarsal joints of one or both hind limbs; progressive, varies in severity and time of onset from 3 to 6 months of age or as late as 2 years	Genetic and environmental factors	Common	Clinical examination	None
Spastic syndrome	Chronic progressive disease characterized by intermittent spastic contractures of muscles of both hind limbs; straight rear limbs and weak hocks; no CNS lesions	Recessive	Common	Clinical examination	None
Spastic lethal (neonatal) syndrome	Spasms and incoordination involving all four limbs, present at birth or developing later; sudden touch and noise will precipitate spasms; no pathologic lesions	Recessive	Rare	Clinical examination	None
Epilepsy	True epilepsy is a convulsive state without definitive CNS lesions	Dominant	Uncommon	Clinical examination	None
Congenital tremor	Tremor of forelimbs, no CNS lesions	Unknown	Uncommon	Clinical examination	None
Doddlers	Muscle spasm, convulsions, nystagmus, incoordination, calcification of small vessels and neurons of brain stem	Possibly genetic	Uncommon	Clinical and histologic examinations	None

Defect	Description	Inheritance	Incidence	Diagnosis	Associated Defects
Ataxia and stagger	Ataxia, incoordination and staggering; no CNS lesions reported	Unknown	Uncommon	Clinical examination	None
Congenital Defects of the Spinal Cord					
Spina bifida	Segmental nonclosure of arches, with or without associated spinal cord defects	Possibly genetic, recessive or dominant gene with low penetrance and variable expressivity	Uncommon	Necropsy	Arthrogryposis, kyphoscoliosis, varying internal defects, atresia ani, taillessness
Spinal dysraphism	Varying segmental lesions; hydromyelia, dilation of central spinal canal and syringomyelia and cavitation of spinal cord	Possibly genetic	Uncommon	Necropsy and histologic examination	Spina bifida, Arnold-Chiari malformation. Cerebellar agenesis, arthrogryposis, hydranencephaly, internal hydrocephalus, cleft palate, facial-digital syndrome
Hereditary Storage Diseases of the Central Nervous System					
α-Mannosidosis (pseudolipidosis)	Deficiency of mannosidase with accumulation of oligosaccharides in neurons, reticuloendothelial system and other cells. Characterized clinically by ataxia, incoordination, head tremor, failure to thrive, aggressive behavior; onset 6 to 12 months of age	Recessive	New Zealand and Australia common, recently diagnosed in United States	Clinical and histologic examination, blood biochemistry for α-mannosidase	None
GM-gangliosidosis	Deficiency of β-galactosidase resulting in accumulation of GM-gangliosides in neurons; clinical signs in calves are swaying of hind quarters, reluctance to move, stiff gait, failure to thrive	Recessive	Uncommon	Clinical and histologic examination, enzyme studies	None
Type II gluconeogenesis (generalized)	Incoordination, muscular weakness, deficiency of α-1,4 glucosidase and accumulation of PAS positive diastase soluble granules in most tissues	Recessive	Rare	Clinical and clinicopathologic examinations	None
Neuronal lipodystrophy	History of blindness, intermittent circling, periodic convulsions, coma; histologic lesions of eosinophilic granules in cytoplasm of neurons and macrophages	Familial	Uncommon	Clinical and histologic examination	None

Table continued on following page

Table 1. Congenital Defects of Cattle Classified by Body System *Continued*

Defect	Description	Etiology	Frequency	Diagnosis	Associated Defects
Congenital Defects of the Eye					
Exophthalmos	Protrusion of eyeballs; initially, impaired vision	Recessive	Rare	Clinical examination	None
Strabismus	Deviation of eyeballs from proper axis	Recessive	Rare	Clinical examination	None
Anophthalmia	Absence of one or both eyes	Unknown	Rare	Clinical examination	Some cattle have no tails
Microphthalmia	One or both eyeballs abnormally small	Unknown	Common	Clinical examination	Tailless, high ventricular septal defect
Microphthalmia associated with other ocular defects and internal hydrocephalus	Usually bilateral reduction size of eyeballs with internal hydrocephalus	Recessive	Common	Clinical examination	Myopathy, cerebellar hypoplasia
Glaucoma	Increased intraocular pressure	Dominant	Rare	Clinical examination	Cataracts, lens luxated
Entropion	One or both eyelids turned inwards; leads to conjunctivitis and corneal lesions	Possibly genetic	Rare	Clinical examination	None
Ectropion	One or both eyelids turned outwards	Possibly genetic	Rare	Clinical examination	None
Distichiasis	Double row of eyelids	Unknown	Uncommon	Clinical examination	None
Dermoid	Skinlike appendage on eyelids, conjunctive, nictitating membrane or cornea; same color as eyelid, contains hair	Polygenic	Common	Clinical examination	None
Corneal edema	Mild corneal edema and cloudinesss present at birth; condition progresses with age and may lead to blindness	Possibly genetic, recessive	Rare	Clinical examination	None
Heterochromia iridis	Multicolored iris	Genetic, recessive, others dominant	Rare	Clinical examination	Deafness, coloboma
Albinism, complete	Lack of pigment, ocular structures pink	Recessive	Rare	Clinical examination	Enzyme deficiencies
Albinism, incomplete	Gray to blue irides, skin white or may have a few pigmented spots	Dominant	Rare	Clinical examination	Deafness, coloboma of optic disc
Chédiak-Higashi syndrome	Gray iris, color reduction in skin	Recessive	Rare	Clinical examination, blood smears to demonstrate intracytoplasmic inclusions in leukocytes	Susceptible to bacterial infections
Cataract	Lens opacity or one or both eyes	Genetic	Common	Clinical examination	Calves may have multiple ocular defects

Defect	Description	Cause	Frequency	Diagnosis	Associated defects
Retinal dysplasia	Nonattached retina dysplastic	Genetic, environmental	Rare	Clinical examination	May have internal hydrocephalus, myopathy and other defects
Coloboma of optic disc	Defect occurs in ventral position of optic disc, characterized by hypoplasia of sclera, choroid, retinal thinning and gliosis	Dominant	Rare	Clinical examination	None

Congenital Defects of the Heart and Large Vessels

Defect	Description	Cause	Frequency	Diagnosis	Associated defects
Ectopia cordis cervicalis	Heart located outside thoracic cavity, usually in ventral neck area, and covered by skin	Possibly genetic	Common	External examination	Abnormalities of ribs and large vessels
Ectopia cordis sternalis	Fissure in sternum, heart located outside thorax, not covered by skin	Unknown	Uncommon	External examination	Sternum has fissure, large vessels abnormal
Ectopia cordis abdominalis	Heart located in abdominal cavity	Unknown	Uncommon	Clinical examination	Large vessels abnormal
Cor triloculare biventriculare	Three-chambered heart, one atrium and two ventricles; calves die shortly after birth	Unknown	Uncommon	Necropsy	Vascular defects, arthrogryposis
Cor triloculare biatriatum	Three-chambered heart, two atria and one ventricle; calves die shortly after birth	Unknown	Uncommon	Necropsy	Vessels abnormal
Cor biloculare	Two-chambered heart, calves usually stillborn	Unknown	Uncommon	Necropsy	Multiple defects of bones and muscles
Patent foramen ovale	Persistence of foramen ovale, opening between right and left atrium, usually partially covered by membrane	Unknown	Common	Clinical examination, necropsy	About half the calves may have patent ductus arteriosus
Ventricular septal defect	Opening between right and left ventricle; may vary in location and size in ventricular septum	Possibly genetic	Common	Clinical examination, necropsy	May be single isolated defect or associated with abnormalities of blood vessels, microphthalmia, taillessness
Tetralogy of Fallot	High ventricular septal defect, stenosis of pulmonary artery, dextroposition of aorta and dilation of right ventricle	Unknown	Rare	Clinical examination	None
Patent ductus arteriosus	Persistence of fetal vessel from pulmonary artery to aorta that shunts blood away from lung	Unknown	Common	Clinical examination	May have patent foramen ovale
Common aortic trunk	Failure of separation of common trunk of aorta and pulmonary artery	Unknown	Rare	Clinical examination, necropsy	None

Table continued on following page

Table 1. Congenital Defects of Cattle Classified by Body System *Continued*

Defect	Description	Etiology	Frequency	Diagnosis	Associated Defects
Persistence of right aortic arch	Encircling of esophagus by pulmonary artery, aorta, ligamentum arteriosum and trachea	Unknown	Uncommon	Clinical examination, necropsy	None
Left cardiac hypoplasia	Hypoplasia of aorta and left ventricle; calves die shortly after birth	Possibly genetic	Rare	Clinical examination, necropsy	Atrial septal defect and patent ductus arteriosus
Valvular hematocysts	Blood-filled cysts at margins of the atrioventricular valves, measuring up to 1.0 cm in diameter	Unknown	Common	Usually no clinical signs	None
Endocardial fibroelastosis	Abnormal diffuse thickening of endocardium in left ventricle, hypertrophy of left ventricle; death in late neonatal period	Unknown	Rare	Necropsy	May have other vessel and heart defects
Congenital Defects of the Intestinal System					
Atresia ani	Rectum ends blindly in a cul-de-sac or opens into urinary bladder, urethra or vagina; distended abdomen, no feces around anal area	Unknown	Rare	Clinical examination	May be associated with defects of urogenital system, or taillessness or spinal dysraphism of lumbar spinal cord or atresia coli
Atresia of rectum	Rectum ends blindly in cul-de-sac, more extensive than atresia ani; distended abdomen, no feces at anal area	Unknown	Rare	Clinical examination	Older calves may have urogenital or skeletal defects
Atresia coli	Rectum and anus usually patent; passage of some meconium; distended abdomen; location of atresia is variable	Unknown, amnion palpation between days 33 to 40 of gestation	Rare	Clinical examination, laparotomy, necropsy	May have atresia ani, skeletal or urogenital defects
Atresia ilei	Ileum ends blindly	Possibly genetic	Uncommon	Necropsy	None
Congenital Defects of the Skin					
Epitheliogenesis imperfecta	Discontinuity of squamous epithelium, epithelial defects of circumscribed areas (1 to 2 cm) in areas distal to carpus and tarsus, muzzle, nostrils, tongue, hard palate, cheeks, esophagus, forestomach; one or more claws may be defective, ears may lack epithelium	Recessive	Common	Clinical and histopathologic examinations	Lesions may involve jaw, anus and vagina

Defect	Description	Inheritance	Frequency	Diagnosis	
Congenital ichthyosis	Severe skin defect; characterized by large scales of horn; separated by deep fissures; lethal	Recessive	Uncommon	Clinical examination	None
Collagenous tissue dysplasia	Collagenous tissue dysplasia (dermatoparaxis, skin fragility) characterized by skin fragility, resulting in severe lacerations with nominal trauma and delayed skin healing; histologic and ultrastructural studies disclose lack of mature collagen fibers	Recessive	Rare	Clinical examination	None
Acantholysis	Shedding of epidermis, leaving ulcers in oral mucosa, skin of carpus, phalanges and coronary border, hooves may separate	Recessive	Rare	Clinical and histologic examination	None
Lethal hairlessness	Calves die shortly after birth; hair present only on muzzle, eyelids, ears, tail and perineum; otherwise naked	Recessive	Rare	Clinical examination and genetic analysis	None
Semi-hairlessness	Affected calves are viable; have fine, thin, curly hair coat; skin is patchy, wrinkled and scaly	Recessive	Rare	Clinical examination and genetic analysis	None
Hypotrichosis with anodontia	Completely hairless at birth, may develop a fine short hair coat later in life; teeth missing; calves do not thrive	Sex-linked recessive	Uncommon	Clinical examination and genetic analysis	None
Viable hypotrichosis	Completely or partially hairless at birth; may develop patches of hair later	Recessive	Rare	Clinical examination and genetic analysis	None
Hypotrichosis with missing incisors	Patches of short hair at birth on face and neck; later hair coat is normal; agenesis of four to six incisor teeth	Genetic, possibly a dominant trait	Uncommon	Clinical examination and genetic analysis	None
Streaked hairlessness	Affected calf lacks hair development; vertical streaks involving lip, lateral abdominal and leg areas; apparently lethal to males	Sex-linked dominant	Uncommon	Clinical examination and genetic analysis	None
Protoporphyria	Affected cattle presented because of dermatitis and hair loss	Recessive	Rare	Clinical, biochemical and histologic examinations	Liver fibrosis, convulsions in some calves

Table continued on following page

Table 1. Congenital Defects of Cattle Classified by Body System *Continued*

Defect	Description	Etiology	Frequency	Diagnosis	Associated Defects
Congenital Defects of the Body Cavities					
Schistosomus reflexus	Severe closure defect characterized by extreme spinal retroflexion and abdominal and thoracic viscera eventrated so the fetus appears turned inside-out	Unknown	Common	Clinical examination	Spinal column defective and twisted
Abdominal fissure	Variable degrees of opening in ventral abdominal wall with herniation of organs	Unknown	Uncommon	Clinical examination	None
Umbilical hernia	Hernia involving umbilical area and covered by skin	Polygenic	Common	Clinical examination	None
Congenital Defects of the Female Reproductive System					
Vulva and vagina: Atresia	Vulva nonpatent	Unknown	Rare	Clinical examination	Associated with atresia ani
Cloaca	Failure of vulva and vestibule to separate from the urogenital sinus	Unknown	Common	Clinical examination	Associated with majority of cases of atresia ani
Rectovaginal constriction	Stenotic vestibule and anus	Recessive	Common in Jersey cows, possibly Friesians	Rectal and vaginal examinations	Udder edema in cows and anal stenosis in bulls
Persistent hymen	Persistent hymen strands	Genetic	Relatively common	Vaginal examination	Associated with white heifer disease or freemartinism
Dysplasia of müllerian ducts Segmental aplasia (white heifer disease)	Part or all of the vagina, cervix or uterus may be missing	Recessive	Not uncommon	Rectal examination	Oviducts rarely involved and usually normal. Mucovagina, mucocervix and mucometra
Uterus unicornis	Segmental aplasia of one horn	Recessive	Rare	Rectal examination	None
Uterus didelphys	Double uterus resulting from failure of the müllerian ducts to fuse	Unknown	Rare	Rectal examination	Double cervix
Double cervix	Failure of the müllerian ducts to fuse in the cervical region	Recessive	Common	Rectal examination	None
Ovaries: Aplasia	One or both ovaries missing	Unknown	Rare	Rectal examination	Usually associated with other more extensive defects
Hypoplasia	One or both ovaries smaller than normal	Recessive	Common	Rectal examination,	Usually none;

Mammary glands					
Aplasia	One or more quarters missing.	Unknown	Rare	Clinical examination	None
Hypoplasia	One or more quarters smaller than normal	Unknown	Rare	Clinical examination	Freemartinism
Agenesis of a teat	Missing teat	Unknown	Rare	Clinical examination	None
Polythelia	Supernumerary teats, usually caudal	Unknown	Relatively common	Clinical examination	None
Synthelia	Fused teats	Recessive	Relatively common	Clinical examination	None
Intersexuality:					
Hermaphroditism	Internal genitalia and gonadal tissue of both sexes; external genitalia intermediate	Unknown	Rare	Clinical examination	None
Pseudohermaphroditism	Male variety more common	Unknown	Relatively common	Clinical examination	None
Freemartinism	Vagina nonpatent, small vulva, uterus cordlike, ovaries hypoplastic	Inconclusive	Relatively common	Clinical examination	Usually co-twin to a male
Congenital Defects Usually Resulting in Dystocia					
Asymmetrical twins: Holoacardius acephalus	Small nonviable twin with a trunk, two hind legs and no heart, neck and head	Unknown; chromosomal?	Rare	Clinical examination	Many
Amorphus globosus	Rounded, edematous structure having no general body form	Unknown; chromosomal	Rare	Clinical examination	Many
Conjoined twins: Anterior or posterior types	Various combinations	Unknown	Not uncommon	Clinical examination	Many, depending upon attachment
Hematic mummification	Usually occurs between fourth and sixth months of gestation	Recessive	Not uncommon	Clinical examination	None
Fetal dropsy	Edematous fetus, milder form may be associated with edema of the hind legs	Recessive	Not common	Clinical examination	None
Hydramnios	Slowly developing edema, viscid amniotic fluid	Recessive	Not common	Usually diagnosed at parturition by syrupy, viscid amniotic fluid and small defective calf	Defective cell
Prolonged gestation	Two types recognized, a large nonviable calf (Holstein) and a small defective fetus (Guernsey) with cranial anomalies	Recessive	Not common	Based on appearance and size of the calf, length of gestation and associated lesions	First type has hypoplastic adrenals; second is associated with adenohypophyseal aplasia

Table continued on following page

Table 1. Congenital Defects of Cattle Classified by Body System Continued

Defect	Description	Etiology	Frequency	Diagnosis	Associated Defects
Congenital Defects of the Male Reproductive System					
Scrotum:					
Aplasia	Missing scrotum	Unknown	Rare	Clinical examination	Usually associated with pseudohermaphroditism
Partially to completely divided scrotum	Partial to complete lack of fusion of the two scrotal pouches	Unknown	Rare	Clinical examination	Hypospadias
Scrotal hernia	Unilateral or bilateral displacement of small intestine	Unknown	Not common	Clinical examination	None
Testes:					
Aplasia	One or both testes missing	Unknown	Not common	Clinical examination	Commonly associated with incomplete twinning
Cryptorchidism	Incomplete descent of one or both testes	Recessive	Common	Clinical examination	None, or other defective syndromes
Polyorchidism	More than two testes	Unknown	Rare	Clinical examination	Usually part of incomplete twinning
Hypoplasia	One or both testes smaller than normal	Recessive with incomplete penetrance	Common	Palpation, semen examination, evaluation of breeding records	None
Abnormal spermatozoa	Various abnormal spermatozoa	Many are thought to be hereditary	Common	Semen examination	None, or various conditions
Epididymis:					
Segmental aplasia	Part or all of the epididymis, vas deferens or seminal vesicular glands may be missing	Recessive	Not common	Palpation, semen examination, breeding performance	Spermatic granuloma aspermia if bilateral
Spermatic granuloma	Granulomatous reaction to extravasated spermatozoa	Unknown, traumatic or infectious	Common	Palpation, histologic examination	May or may not be associated with aplasia
Paradidymis	Small gray nodule or nodules of a few convoluted tubules from the mesonephros located in the anterior part of the spermatic cord	Unknown	Common, found in 25 to 46 per cent of calves	Incidental necropsy finding	None
Uterus masculinus	Small blind pouch arising in the prostate and opening into the seminal colliculus; remnant of the distal portion of the müllerian duct	Unknown	Common, found in 24 to 44 per cent of bulls	Incidental necropsy finding	None
Seminal vesicular glands:					
Segmental aplasia	Part or all of both lobes may be missing, usually unilateral	Recessive	Not common	Palpation	Usually associated with lack of part or all of epididymis and vas

Defect	Description	Heredity	Incidence	Diagnosis	Associated defects
Hypoplasia	One or both lobes smaller than normal	Unknown	Not common	Palpation	None, or other wolffian duct defects
Duplication	Doubling of the seminal vesicles	Unknown	Not common	Palpation	None, or other wolffian duct defects
Penis:					
Short penis	Smaller than normal	Possibly recessive	Not common, seen more in Herefords and Guernseys	Palpation and service behavior	Usually none
Corkscrew penis	Penis spirals counterclockwise ventrally and to the right	Unknown	More common in younger bulls	Service observation	Usually none
Rainbow deviation	Ventral deviation	Unknown	Not common	Observation of service	Usually none
Persistent frenulum	Persistence of the fold beneath the glans penis to prepuce	Unknown, suspected to be hereditary	Not common	Examination and observation of service	Penile
Diphallia	Penile duplication.	Unknown	Rare	Examination	Usually scrotal duplication
Hypospadias	Abnormal ventral opening in the extrapelvic urethra due to incomplete closure of the urethral folds	Possibly recessive	Not common	External examination	Bifid scrotum. Regarded as a mild form of pseudohermaphroditism
Epispadias	Dorsal opening in the penile urethra	Unknown	Rare	Careful examination of penis, evaluation of breeding records	None, or other penile and scrotal defects
Pseudohermaphroditism	See Section 16				
Spastic paresis	See Section 8				
Congenital Immunodeficiency Diseases					
IgG$_2$ deficiency	Reported in Red Danish cattle; increased susceptibility to pneumonia and gangrenous mastitis	Genetic	1 to 2 per cent incidence	Clinical and immunologic examination	None
Lethal trait A-46 (Edema lethal)	European Black Pied cattle; characterized by lymphoid and thymic hypoplasia; dermal and intestinal lesions develop in second month of life; reduced immunologic responsiveness due to reduced intestinal capacity to absorb zinc	Recessive	Rare	Clinical, pathologic and immunologic examinations	None
Chédiak-Higashi syndrome	Partial albinism, photophobia, recurrent pyogenic infections	Recessive	Rare	Clinical and clinicopathologic examinations demonstrating inclusion bodies in leukocytes	None

Differentiation of Genetic Defects. Genetic defects arise from mutant genes and tend to run in families. Mutant genes become evident over two or more generations by one of four major hereditary patterns: dominant, incomplete dominant, recessive and over-dominant. These patterns involve certain characteristic ratios of normal and defective progeny that form the basis for accurate genetic diagnosis. Characteristics of recessive mutations include defective calves coming from normal-appearing parents and usually occurring in small numbers. Recessive genes are carried generation after generation by normal carriers or heterozygotes and are insidiously perpetuated. The difficulty of identifying normal-appearing carriers makes control virtually impossible. Genetic defects may also be polygenic.

Diagnosis of genetic origin for a single defective calf is impossible without an adequate breeding record. Even when several congenital defects occur in a herd, differentiation between a genetic or environmental cause may be difficult.

Differentiation of Chromosomal Aberrations. Although chromosomal aberrations have been known in cattle for some time, they have not achieved the diagnostic significance that they have in man.

Genetic-Environmental Interaction. Even though little understood, the complex interaction between genetic and environmental factors is slowly gaining prominence as knowledge of congenital defects increases.

Etiologic Agents. Identifying etiologic agents of bovine congenital defects is often difficult for several reasons. In many cases, there is no clearly established cause. The first question that must be answered is whether the defect is genetic or environmentally induced. Even when several calves have similar defects, it is not easy to incriminate or eliminate the possibility of disease, plant or drug teratogens or nutritional deficiencies as the causative agent. When defective calves are restricted to a single herd or region, environmental factors are usually investigated first.

Confirmation. Most genetic defects are due to recessive genes. Diagnosis can be confirmed by test matings, resulting in the predictable occurrence of defective and normal progeny. When the number of defective calves is small and test matings are not possible, it is difficult to determine the mode of transmission, and a tentative diagnosis is usually made on the basis of contributing evidence. Recessive inheritance can also be detected by reporting all defective animals; this is efficient and easier to organize than test matings.

Suspected plant teratogens can be tested by feeding trials with pregnant cows or laboratory animals in early pregnancy.

BASIC GENETIC PRINCIPLES

Cattle breeders use genetic recombination or mutation to improve the breed of their cattle. Unfavorable variation can result, however, causing undesirable reproductive traits as well as genetic diseases.

Genes are units of inheritance determining growth and development within environmental limits. In using genetic variation to improve their livestock, animal breeders are concerned with the action of a single gene, gene pairs or multigene inheritance. Analyzing genetic defects is based on (1) the passage of genetic diseases by genes from parents to offspring and (2) the mating of closely related animals increasing the probability of offspring receiving a copy of the same desirable or undesirable gene. To determine if a disease is caused by genetic action, offspring have to be classified as normal or abnormal, and family relationships must be established. Most genetic defects are caused by simple inheritance (one pair of genes), and for the most part the defective gene is recessive to the normal gene (normal gene dominates the effect of the defective gene).

Diagnosing genetically caused congenital defects is based on genetic diseases running in families; i.e., they occur in typical intergenerational patterns and intragenerational family frequencies. Various statistical methods are used to analyze such data. Confirming the genetic nature and pattern of a congenital defect can be done by test matings. The recessive genetic pattern is the most common and involves only two kinds of calves: normal or defective. Among the normal calves are a few that can transmit the disease, but most calves cannot do so. Although mating two defective parents produces only defective calves, most defective animals do not reproduce. Therefore, most defective calves are born to normal-appearing parents, although most normal parents cannot transmit the disease. Each normal parent producing a defective calf transmits one of the two abnormal genes necessary to produce defective offspring.

When homozygous normal cattle are mated with other homozygous normal cattle or even with normal-appearing carriers, they produce only normal calves. When normal-appearing cattle that produced a defective offspring are mated repeatedly, 25 per cent of their offspring will be defective, and 75 per cent will be normal. Moreover, two of every three normal calves from such parents also carry a hidden abnormal gene that they, too, can transmit to offspring just as their parents transmitted a recessive gene to them. Thus, recessive defects are "carried" from generation to generation by normal-appearing carriers or heterozygotes. The defects are exposed only when heterozygous cattle are mated to other heterozygotes and defective calves appear. Eliminating defective offspring usually keeps the frequency of recessive defects low.

Other simple inheritance patterns include dominance, incomplete dominance and over-dominance (dominant being the opposite of recessive.) With dominant inheritance, normal cattle breed true, but abnormal cattle may produce both normal and abnormal calves. With dominant genetic diseases, defective calves are readily recognized, and the gene can be easily eliminated.

Incomplete dominance creates three kinds of cattle: normal, slightly abnormal and severely abnormal. Normal and severely abnormal cattle breed true. Slightly abnormal cattle mated to each other produce 25 per cent normal, 50 per cent slightly abnormal and 25 per cent severely abnormal calves. The disease is easily controlled by eliminating all abnormal calves.

Over-dominance is similar to incomplete dominance in that three kinds of cattle are recognized: normal, superior and abnormal. The normal and abnormal animals breed true. Mating superior cattle produces 25 per cent normal, 50 per cent superior and 25 per cent defective calves. The superior cattle usually are selected as replacements in preference to normal animals because the person making the selection does not know that 25 per cent of the offspring from like mates will be defective. Over-dominant traits are difficult to control because all superior animals carry the undesirable gene, and owners are reluctant to choose inferior breeding animals. Few traits, however, show over-dominance.

Few characteristics are sex linked. Some reports describe chromosomal aberrations. Congenital defects may also be inherited in a polygenic manner (many genes involved).

DIAGNOSING CONGENITAL DEFECTS IN CATTLE

For accurate diagnosis of congenital defects in cattle, the following standardized procedures are recommended.

Reporting Defects. As mentioned previously, continual efforts should be made to have breeders report all defective calves. This will require constant cooperation of veterinarians, AI centers, animal scientists and cattle breed associations. The monitoring of congenital defects by cattle breed associations and AI centers will provide information on the frequency of various defects and on the changing incidences.

Recording All Defective Calves. All defective calves should be thoroughly examined and documented.

History. The following history should be obtained and carefully evaluated: breed, geographic region, time of year, type of pasture, soil type, exposure to or suspected exposure to teratogenic plants, feeding and management practices, type of breeding, previous breeding records, maternal medical and vaccination records, disease status of herd, periods of stress, drugs administered, congenital defects observed previously and any history of similar congenital defects in neighboring herds.

Necropsy. Defective calves should be subjected to a standardized necropsy, and lesions should be

photographically documented. This should be carried out by the practitioner, the regional diagnostic laboratory or a specialist. Defects should be classified by the body system primarily involved.

Serum samples should be taken whenever possible and checked for bovine diarrhea virus, blue tongue virus, and other viral antibodies. Sections of spleen, liver and brain should be taken for possible virus isolation if a viral teratogen is suspected and if the defective calf has little autolysis. Virus isolation is difficult, as most viruses are labile and have disappeared by birth. Serologic and fluorescent antibody techniques are more reliable when a viral teratogen is suspected.

Sections of brain, spinal cord, lungs, liver, kidneys and other appropriate tissues should be collected and fixed in 10 per cent buffered neutral formalin for histopathologic examination.

Chemical Teratogens. The history should be carefully evaluated for any possible exposure to chemical or plant teratogens, especially during mating and embryogenesis. If necessary, the ranch should be visited and the pastures checked for possible plant teratogens.

Chromosome Examination. With live defective calves, leukocytes and various tissues should be collected for culture and examination for possible chromosomal aberrations.

Genetic Analysis. Breeding records should be examined for characteristic intra- and intergenerational hereditary patterns of genetic disease. Analysis should proceed along several lines: segregation analysis with full-sib families and compatibility analysis of close and distant relatives. Several methods may be used to test results of segregation analysis and to search for inbreeding.

Differential Diagnosis. Congenital defects must be differentiated from embryonic mortalities, abortions, premature births, stillbirths and neonatal deaths.

Diagnosis. Etiologic diagnosis of defective calves is made after carefully considering the results of all the criteria of the standardized approach just discussed.

Confirmation. Confirmation of a genetic defect and mode of inheritance is possible by trial matings among suspected carriers or close relatives. As mentioned before, suspected plant teratogens can be tested by feeding trials with pregnant laboratory animals or cows in early pregnancy.

TESTING SUSPECTED CARRIER BULLS

The major hereditary patterns encountered in defective calves have already been discussed. There is no need to test for a dominant trait, since it is easily recognized. It may be necessary to test a bull to determine if he is heterozygous for a simple autosomal recessive gene. If the bull is of standard phenotype (not abnormal or surgically corrected for a defect), one or more of the following tests may be used.

Table 2. Sire-Testing Procedures

Procedure	Offspring Needed To Reach Probability Level		
	0.05	0.01	0.001
Homozygous abnormals*	5	7	10
Heterozygotes*	10	16	24
Father-daughters†	22	35	52

*Checks for one trait only.
†Checks for all undesirable recessive traits.

Bred to Unknown Population. The resulting offspring are carefully monitored, and any abnormal calves are recorded. If specified defects occur or if the number of specific defective calves exceeds a predetermined threshold, the bull is regarded as a heterozygote and is removed from service.

Bred to Daughters. A suspected bull may be bred to 35 of his daughters. The procedure is expensive and time consuming.

Bred to Known Heterozygotes. A bull may be tested for a specific defect by being bred to 16 cows that are heterozygous for the defect.

Bred to Homozygous Abnormals. Another method of testing suspected bulls is to breed them to seven homozygous abnormal cows, if they can be raised to breeding age.

The commonly used sire-testing procedures are summarized in Table 2. Although they all have the disadvantage of being expensive and time consuming, they are much cheaper than trying to eliminate a genetic defect after it has insidiously spread throughout a given cattle population. Remember, there are no minor defects when AI is used. A bull siring defective calves of unknown cause should immediately be removed from service. Bulls with any defect should not be used.

Embryo transfer alone or in conjunction with preterminal cesarean section is the method of choice for testing bulls for simple autosomal recessive defects. It has the additional advantage of being less expensive and time consuming.[4, 8]

Biochemical testing procedures may become more important in the future. Heterozygotes for protoporphyria and mannosidosis can be detected by enzyme tests.[5, 12]

KANSAS GENETIC DISEASE PROGRAM

The Kansas State University genetic disease program was initiated in the early 1930's and consists of gathering and recording, analyzing and interpreting information and communicating and using the results. Epizootiology of genetic defects is considered in three etiologic contexts: unknown, suspected and known causes.

Gathering and Recording. Initial reports are received in many forms from veterinarians, breed and AI organizations, extension personnel and herd owners; these are then recorded. A history of each case is taken, as previously outlined, as well as any information of similar defects in neighboring herds. Breeding records are analyzed for evidence of inbreeding and for characteristic intergenerational transmission patterns and intragenerational frequencies.

Etiologic diagnosis of defective calves is made after evaluating these various tests and the results of a central congenital defects file.

Analysis and Interpretation. Preliminary analysis and interpretations are made during the gathering and collecting phases as they proceed through the following: a check on whether a similar defect has been reported among a bull's offspring; a check of the case against similar cases recorded in central congenital defects file; a check of the literature file for reports of similar defects in cattle; a check of literature in other species (animals and man) and a check of all herd health data, necropsies and other tests as previously outlined.

For decisions on breeding programs, the following steps should be taken. Most breed associations follow similar procedures such as blood typing to establish verified parentage, especially when an AI sire is involved, obtaining a certified statement from a veterinarian or a third party witness, drawing up an extended pedigree chart, asking a pathologist to perform a laboratory examination when applicable and withholding a decision on breeding programs until all reasonable doubt has been eliminated—this usually requires two or more thoroughly documented reports for bulls.

Communicating and Using Results. The following points should be considered: Many genetic defects have not yet been clearly identified and await description and clarification; a single undesirable recessive trait can rapidly become a real problem in a breed of cattle and maintaining a recording system by breed organization, AI centers and other institutions is the most efficient and least expensive way to monitor undesirable traits.

If evidence is presented that a bull carries an undesirable recessive gene, most organizations proceed to declare the bull as heterozygote and remove him from service. If the bull is not removed, advertisement material should carry information concerning the congenital defect.[11]

WHAT SHOULD VETERINARIANS DO?

Practitioners should be familiar with the more common cattle defects, particularly those known to occur in the various breeds in their area. When consulted about defective calves, they should attempt to diagnose the defect and to determine if it is known to be hereditary. Veterinarians should ask the following questions:

1. Were the defective calves sired by the same bull?
2. Did other bulls on the ranch sire any abnormal calves?
3. Were the dams of the defective calves related?
4. Was inbreeding practiced?

If the defect is genetic, they should recommend disposal of the bull and its offspring. If inconclusive, they should also try to determine whether the dams were sick or stressed during early pregnancy or if the dams were vaccinated or exposed to possible teratogens during this period. If negative, the veterinarian should then seek specialized help.

PREVENTION OF CONGENITAL DEFECTS

Determining whether congenital defects are genetically or environmentally induced is important, as this dictates the control measures. It is essential to recognize genetic defects early in order to control their progressive insidious spread. The difficulty of identifying heterozygotes makes control of recessive defects extremely difficult.

To minimize the effects of defective calves, it is recommended that the veterinarian observe the following precautions:

1. Establish an accurate diagnosis. If not, all congenital defects should be regarded as genetic until proved otherwise.

2. Defective calves should not be bred.

3. All newborn defective calves should be disposed of.

4. If the defect is environmentally induced, the management program should be adjusted. If in doubt, the veterinarian should seek specialized assistance.

5. All defective calves should be reported to cattle breed associations or AI centers.

IMPROVING KNOWLEDGE OF CONGENITAL DEFECTS

Breed associations, AI centers and veterinarians should actively encourage cattle breeders to report rather than hide defective calves. It is unfortunate that these calves are not reported and made available for research. The more we know the better we can control congenital defects. Research and control of congenital defects depend primarily upon individual cattle breeders and their veterinarians.

With the changing demands within the cattle industry and importation of new breeds in recent years, new inherited defects will emerge. It is hoped that complete records of such defects will be kept by the breed associations and AI centers and that appropriate cases will be available for diagnosis and research.

Expanding the knowledge of congenital defects in cattle will depend on numerous, adequately described reports containing detailed clinicopathologic examinations and genetic analyses. This will require the continual cooperation and effort of cattle breeders, veterinarians, breed associations, AI centers and animal scientists. Adopting standardized classification and terminology and diagnostic procedures should improve descriptions, diagnoses and interdisciplinary exchange of information. This, in turn, should improve knowledge and diagnosis of congenitally defective calves in the future.

References

1. Biuère AN: The application of cytogenetics to domestic animals. In Grunsell CSG, Hill FWG (eds) Veterinarian Annual 20:29, 1980.
2. Cho DY, Leipold HW: Congenital defects of the bovine central nervous system. Vet Bull 47:489, 1977.
3. Greene HJ, Leipold HW, Huston K, Dennis SM: Congenital defects in cattle. Irish Vet J 27:37, 1973.
4. Johnson JL, Leipold HW, Schalles RR, et al.: Hereditary polydactyly in Simmental cattle. J Hered 72:205, 1981.
5. Jolly RD: Two model lysosomal storage diseases. In Desnick RJ, Patterson DF, Scarpelli DG (eds) Animal Models of Inherited Metabolic Diseases. New York, Alan R. Liss Inc., 1982, pp 145–164.
6. Keeler RF: Alkaloid teratogens from *Lupinus, Conium, Veratrum* and related genera. In Keeler RF, vanKampen KR, James LF (eds) Effects of Poisonous Plants on Livestock. New York, Academic Press, 1978, pp 397–408.
7. Konno S, Moriwaki M, Nakagawa M: Akabane disease in cattle: Congenital abnormalities caused by viral infection. Spontaneous disease. Vet Pathol 19:246, 1982.
8. Leipold HW, Peeples JS: Progeny testing for bovine syndactyly. J Am Vet Med Assoc 179:69, 1981.
9. Leipold HW, Dennis SM, Huston K: Syndactyly in cattle. Vet Bull 43:399, 1973.
10. Leipold HW, Watt B, Vestweber JGE, Dennis SM: Clinical observations in rectovaginal constriction in Jersey cattle. Bovine Pract 16:76, 1981.
11. Leipold HW, Huston K, Dennis SM: Bovine congenital defects. Adv Vet Sci Comp Med 27:197, 1983.
12. Ruth JR, Schwartz S, Stephenson B: Diagnostic tests for the carrier of bovine protoporphyria. Proc Am Assoc Vet Lab Diag 23:79, 1980.

Early Embryo Loss in Cattle

James F. Roche, M.Agr.Sc., Ph.D., D.Sc.
University College, Dublin, Ireland

Embryo loss in cattle has to be distinguished from failure of fertilization. There are various estimates of fertilization rates in cattle, but in general 85 to 95 per cent of recovered ova are fertilized in normal cows;[2, 4] in repeat-breeder animals fertilization rates are lower and vary between 56 and 72 per cent. Hawk[5] concluded that when cows were managed to obtain high fertility, fertilization failure still accounted for 15 per cent of reproductive wastage, a figure in agreement with more recent work.[12] Embryo loss, therefore, accounts for the major portion (25 per cent) of the remaining reproductive wastage.

TIME OF OCCURRENCE OF EMBRYO LOSS

There is disagreement on the exact time of occurrence of embryo loss in cows after breeding; this relates mainly to the problems of monitoring embryo development in utero during the first 3 weeks of pregnancy. Data from the literature show that the major portion of embryo loss occurs gradually between days 8 and 19 after breeding and that subsequent loss is much smaller. More recent data suggest that early embryonic mortality is more important than fertilization failure in parous females in their relative contributions to reduce reproductive efficiency.[8] Estimates based on maintenance of high progesterone levels and late but irregular returns to estrus indicate that late embryo/fetal loss amounts to 5 to 10 per cent of reproductive wastage in cows. However, it must be remembered that the latter estimates of late losses are indirect and factors other than the presence of an embryo can maintain the corpus luteum. Therefore, most embryo loss occurs before the critical stage of pregnancy recognition and maintenance of the corpus luteum of pregnancy. This means that when early embryo loss occurs, cows will return to estrus at the normal 18- to 26-day interval after breeding, whereas late embryo loss manifests itself in late and irregular returns to estrus, with a consequent lengthening of the calving-to-conception interval in postpartum cows.

EFFECT OF NUTRITION

Although nutritional deficiencies are often associated with infertility problems, there is very little clear-cut scientific evidence demonstrating a direct cause and effect relationship in embryo loss in cattle.[2] Beta-carotene, selenium, phosphorus and copper deficiencies have all been implicated with increased incidences of embryo loss. However, because of the problems of establishing a direct cause and effect relationship between nutrition and fertility and the difficulties of long-term carry-over effects of nutrition often being confounded with short-term dynamic effects, very few clear-cut conclusions can be made at this time. It is important to ensure that breeding cattle are fed an adequate quantity of a balanced diet, with due regard to the physiological state and age of the animal.

CYTOGENETIC ABNORMALITIES

One of the critical requirements for normal development of the embryo after fertilization is the presence of a normal complement of chromosomes, which must be properly expressed. It has been demonstrated that ewes ovulate ova and produce zygotes with abnormal karyotypes, indicating that chromosomal aberrations play some, but as yet unquantified, role in early embryo loss in domestic animals. There is very little good scientific data quantifying the extent of chromosomal aberrations in cattle, but one report suggests an incidence of 8 per cent of abnormal karyotypes in 12- to 16-day-old cattle embryos. In the Swedish Red and White breeds a high frequency (30.8 per cent) of centric fusion between one chromosome of the first pair and one chromosome of the twenty-ninth pair (1/29 translocation) was found in a cytogenetic survey of 263 repeat-breeder heifers and was associated with lowered fertility.[6] It must be borne in mind that conventional methods of chromosome staining were used, and small inversions, single gene effects, deletions and duplications may not have been identified with this relatively simple technique. However, there are extensive data from studies on humans suggesting that chromosomal aberrations account for 33 per cent of the lost conceptions that occur in early pregnancy.

The problem with these estimates in the human is the difficulty of establishing whether or not fertilization has occurred and the subsequent viability of the preimplanting embryo. Recently, Rolfe[10] has used the presence of an immunosuppressive pregnancy specific protein (EPF) to monitor the extent of early embryo death in humans and has indeed confirmed the very high incidence of early embryo loss, provided that the presence of EPF does, in fact, mean there is an embryo present.

IMMUNOLOGIC FACTORS

Immunologic mechanisms may also play a role in the extent of embryo loss. Following conception, the cow comes into contact with both sperm and embryonic antigens, and if the immunosuppressive mechanisms are not functioning properly, the antibodies produced may reduce fertility. Recent studies in pigs[1] indicate a 12.4 per cent increase in litter size by adding cellular antigens in the form of leukocytes to semen, which should enhance the immunologic response of the female. These results strengthen the idea of possible involvement of the immune system and thus afford one possible explanation for the increased conception rate following heterospermic insemination in cattle. It is not clear how leukocytes might stimulate the immune system at present.

UTERINE ENVIRONMENT AND EMBRYO LOSS

The specificity of the uterine environment necessary for normal development of the embryo is not clear. Egg transfer experiments indicate that best pregnancy rates are obtained if synchronous transfer is carried out; there is a major drop in survival of transferred embryos when transfer is done more than 2 days out of synchrony. Research on the ewe indicates that the uterus has a more critical steroid hormonal requirement than the oviduct. In the uterus there are critical time and steroid requirements, presumably for proper protein synthesis, which must be satisfied for normal development to proceed. Morphologic transformation of the endometrium occurs in order to promote the correct uterine secretions for development of the embryo. These histologic transformations are under the control of progesterone and estradiol, and result in distinct patterns of low and high molecular weight substances being continually produced in the correct chronologic sequence. In the rabbit it has been demonstrated that normal development of the blastocyst in the uterus requires a specific and favorable uterine environment. However, relatively little is known of the protein production patterns of the cow's uterus and the relationship to embryo death. Ayalon[2] has shown that total protein levels are higher in flushings from the uterus of normal cows compared with flushings from repeat-breeder cows. In addition, differences were found in phosphorus, zinc and calcium levels in uterine flushings of cows with normal or abnormal embryos. It is clear that the quantitative and qualitative aspects of uterine secretions require further study in attempts to relate these changes to early death of the embryo in utero.

HORMONE LEVELS AND EMBRYO LOSS

Once conception has taken place, it is necessary that the cyclic corpus luteum of the cow be maintained for continual progesterone production for at least 8 months in order to maintain pregnancy. Since it is known that the uterus of the nonpregnant cow secretes a luteolytic agent, prostaglandin $F_{2\alpha}$ ($PGF_{2\alpha}$), it is necessary to overcome this luteolytic influence to maintain the corpus luteum of pregnancy. Recent evidence suggests that the embryo

has a luteotrophic effect and that this effect is exerted just prior to the time at which an increase in $PGF_{2\alpha}$ production occurs in nonpregnant cows, i.e., days 15 to 17 of the estrous cycle. This is the period when the conceptus is undergoing maximum expansion and when apposition to the endometrium occurs. Although the time of production of the embryonic signal is known, its chemical nature still remains to be elucidated.

Since the major proportion of embryo loss occurs prior to day 18 of the estrous cycle, it is questionable if embryo loss prior to day 15 is from an inappropriate signal from the embryo between days 15 and 17. This raises the question of the relationship between early embryo loss and serum concentrations of progesterone and estradiol from mating to days 15 to 17. One plausible hypothesis is that the embryo loss is caused by insufficient progesterone production during the luteal phase after mating. Thus, it is important to determine if embryo loss is initiated by insufficient steroid production.

However, there are conflicting reports on differences in concentrations of progesterone in cows that did or did not conceive after breeding. Data from Bulman and Lamming[3] indicated no differences in concentrations of progesterone in animals up to 14 days after breeding, irrespective of pregnancy status, while others[7] found that progesterone concentrations were higher in pregnant heifers from days 10 to 18 after breeding. More recent evidence from Ireland[13, 14] on large numbers of heifers bled three times daily demonstrated no differences in concentrations of progesterone between pregnant and nonpregnant heifers from 7 days before to 17 days after breeding. In addition, progesterone concentrations were not different in nonpregnant heifers and in heifers that became pregnant following embryo transfer at day 10. This further suggests that the relationship between peripheral concentrations of progesterone and embryo viability are equivocal in cattle. Further substantiation of the fact that minor alterations in luteal phase concentrations of progesterone are not directly related to embryo loss comes from data of supplementation of heifers after breeding with exogenous progesterone.[11, 14] However, there would appear to be some indication that in repeat-breeder cows administration of progesterone tends to increase the pregnancy rate.[14] Part of the problem with supplementation of progesterone arises from the high dose required to increase concentrations in blood of cows, and high doses can have a negative feedback effect on LH, possibly reducing endogenous progesterone production through decreased luteal tissue weights.

Using human chorionic gonadotropin (hCG) to induce stimulation of steroidogenesis by the corpus luteum is an alternative approach to increase endogenous progesterone levels in cows. Despite some reports indicating positive effects on pregnancy, the main bulk of literature suggests no increase in pregnancy rate following hCG administration during the luteal phase, despite increases in ovulation rate, luteal weight and progesterone concentrations in the blood.[14] It is possible that there is a critical time period early in the cycle when progesterone is required, and further experimentation will determine if such a critical phase exists. It must also be borne in mind that not only is blood concentration of steroids important, but also sufficient receptors must be occupied in order for the biologic effect of the hormone to take place. The interaction between steroid hormones and their intracellular receptors leading to the development of a secretory endometrium may be a far more fruitful area of research in determining the causes of early embryo loss.

EFFECT OF TIME OF ARTIFICIAL INSEMINATION AND FERTILITY OF SIRE

It is well accepted that optimum conception rates are obtained in cows inseminated from midestrus up to about 6 hours following standing estrus. This relates to the fact that the fertile life span of the cow ovum is about 6 hours and 18 to 24 hours for spermatozoa, depending on whether they have been frozen, the nature of the diluent and the method of storage used. The fertility of the sire affects pregnancy rate, but most of this variation is due to differences in fertilization rate rather than differences in early embryo survival rate. Therefore, low fertility sires, when used outside of the recommended optimum breeding time, will reduce conception rates primarily through decreased fertilization rate. However, when aged sperm or ova are involved in the fertilization process, the resultant zygote often dies prematurely. Therefore, it is important to avoid aging of gametes in routine reproductive management programs for cattle.

CONCLUSIONS AND RECOMMENDATIONS

Early embryo loss is a major determinant of reproductive wastage in cattle breeding, and accounts for about 25 per cent of failed conceptions. The loss occurs gradually between days 8 and 19 after breeding, with the result that animals return to estrus within a normal 3-week interval. The causes of this early loss are not clear, and shedding of genetic load, immune intolerances, nutritional imbalances, improper uterine secretory pattern, hormone deficiencies and aging of gametes are among the many factors that may be involved.

At present there are no clear-cut recommendations or hormonal preparations that can reduce the extent of this early embryo loss. The best recommendation is to ensure that cows are bred at the optimum time to bulls of high fertility or with highly fertile and adequate numbers of properly preserved spermatozoa. It is important that cows are fed a sufficient amount of a properly balanced diet, are gaining body weight and are free of uterine infections and ovarian problems. Therefore, strict attention to a good reproductive breeding program should ensure that early embryo loss does not exceed the normal level discussed. Further detailed research is required to determine if embryo loss can be reduced or whether cattle breeders will have to accept as normal the present high death rate of zygotes.

References

1. Almlid T: Does enhanced antigenicity of semen increase the litter size in pigs? Sonder. Zeits. Tierzuch. Züchtung. 98:1, 1981.
2. Ayalon N: A review of embryonic mortality in cattle. J Reprod Fertil 54:483, 1978.
3. Bulman DD, Lamming GE: Milk progesterone levels in relation to conception, repeat breeding and factors influencing acyclicity in dairy cows. J Reprod Fertil 54:447, 1978.
4. Diskin MG, Sreenan JM: Fertilization and embryonic mortality rates in beef heifers after artificial insemination. J Reprod Fertil 59:463, 1980.
5. Hawk HW: Infertility in dairy cattle. In Beltsville Symposia in Agricultural Research (3). Animal Reproduction. New York, John Wiley, 1979, p 19.
6. King WA, Linares T: A cytogenic study of repeat-heifers and their embryos. Can Vet J 24:112, 1983.
7. Lukaszewska J, Hansel W: Corpus luteum maintenance during early pregnancy in the cow. J Reprod Fertil 59:485, 1980.
8. Maurer RR, Chenault JR: Fertilization failure and embryonic mortality in parous and non-parous beef cattle. J Anim Sci 56:1186, 1983.
9. McFeely RA, Rajakoski E: Proc 6th Int Cong Anim Reprod AI Paris 2:905, 1968.
10. Rolfe BE: Detection of fetal wastage. Fertil Steril 37:655, 1982.
11. Roche JF: Control of oestrus in cattle. World Rev Anim Prod 15:49, 1979.
12. Roche JF, Boland MP, McGeady TA, Ireland JJ: Reproductive wastage following artificial insemination of heifers. Vet Record 109:401, 1981.
13. Roche JF, Ireland JJ, Boland MP, McGeady TA: Concentrations of luteinizing hormone and progesterone in pregnant and non-pregnant heifers. Vet Record 116:153, 1983.
14. Sreenan JM, Diskin MG: Early embryonic mortality in the cow. Its relationship with progesterone concentration. Irish Vet News 5:31, 1983.

Ontogeny of Immunity and Its Relationship to Diagnosis of Congenital Infections

Bennie I. Osburn

University of California,
Davis, California

FETAL RESPONSE TO INFECTION

Animal fetuses are capable of responding immunologically to a wide variety of antigens associated with infectious agents. These fetal responses can be used to diagnose the cause of abortion.

The serum of fetal ruminants normally contains minute quantities (< 0.2 mg/ml) of immunoglobulins until after birth. The inability of the ruminant placenta to transport maternal immunoglobulins actively to the developing fetus leaves the fetus without passive immunity and highly susceptible to infection. The consequences of infection depend upon virulent factors associated with the infectious agent, the ontogenic development of fetal organs and the maturity of the immune system of the fetus at the time of microbial insult. Highly pathogenic agents often kill the fetus with no response; moderately pathogenic agents may result in teratogenic lesions in the immunologically immature fetus; some microbes cause no lesions and in others, no lesions are observed until the immune response becomes active.

Ontogenetic studies suggest that the ruminant fetus sequentially develops immune responses to antigens at predetermined stages of development. Although the immune system shows signs of maturation, the nonimmune effector systems, such as complement and neutrophils, are immature and somewhat deficient in functional capacity. As a consequence, these fetuses are often unable to defend against invading microbes, and the result is abortion. Control of the maturation of the immune response is not fully understood at this time.

MORPHOLOGIC EVIDENCE OF FETAL INFECTION

Evidence from the examination of lymphoid organs for antigenic stimulation can be used as an indicator of congenital infection. The more reliable lymph nodes to use as indicators are the mediastinal and/or bronchial lymph nodes. The morphologic changes indicative of antigenic stimulation include germinal centers in the cortex, increased cellularity in the lymph node, medullary cords with plasma cells and lymphoblasts and medullary channels with increased numbers of lymphoblasts and hypertrophic macrophages. In epizootic bovine abortion (EBA), these changes occur; however, after 100 days of infection, lymphoid necrosis occurs in lymph nodes and the thymus. The massive necrosis in the thymus has been used as the pathognomonic lesion for EBA.[3]

DIAGNOSTIC USE OF FETAL SERUM

The fetal immune response can be used to determine fetal infections by measuring the serum for either immunoglobulin or specific antibody content.[6, 7] Antigenic stimulation can lead to elevated amounts as high a 3.5 mg/ml. Sometimes these levels can be obtained, and no detectable antibody activity can be associated with the immunoglobulins[7] (Table 1).

Specific antibody activity is detectable once the fetus becomes immunologically mature to the specific antigens of the agent. These changes do not necessarily occur to all antigens of the microorganism at the same time. Blue tongue virus precipitating antibody activity can be detected by 145 days ges-

Table 1. Immunoglobulin Values Reported for Microbial Infection of Fetal Calves

Microorganism	Immunoglobulin Values (mg/ml)	
	IgM	IgG
Normal, nonstimulated	0.11	0.16
Bovine virus diarrhea	0.11–0.31	0.50–4.20
Campylobacter fetus	0.09–2.65	0.17–8.72
Anaplasma marginale	0.12–0.15	1.58–4.02
Chlamydia	0.54	0.74–5.91
Epizootic bovine abortion	0.17–2.22	1.48–8.11
Blue tongue virus	0.15–2.00	0.40–6.00
Parvovirus (4)	0.11–1.25	0.20–4.00
Normal, postcolostral	1.01–3.01	2.39–24.0

Table 2. Specific Antibody Activity Occurring During Ontogeny of the Immune Response to Microorganisms

Microorganism	Fetal Age (Days Gestation)	Type of Antibody
Parainfluenza 3 virus	120	Neutralizing
Parvovirus	140	Neutralizing
Anaplasma marginale	141	Complement fixing
Blue tongue virus	145	Precipitin
Leptospira saxkoebing	162	Agglutinating
Infectious bovine rhinotracheitis virus	165	Neutralizing
Bovine virus diarrhea	190	Neutralizing
Escherichia coli	231	Agglutinating (2)
Campylobacter fetus	235	Agglutinating
Chlamydia	243	Complement fixing
Reovirus	257	Neutralizing (1)
Blue tongue virus	Newborn	Neutralizing (5)
Epizootic hemorrhagic disease virus	Newborn	Neutralizing
Brucella abortus	Newborn	Agglutinating

tation in infected fetal calves; however, virus-neutralizing antibody activity is not present until after 200 days gestation.[5] Table 2 lists the fetal ages during ontogeny when the earliest specific antibody activity for microorganisms has been reported in the calf and the type of test used to detect the antibodies.

RECOMMENDATIONS

Since it is not always possible to recover the etiologic agent causing abortion, the use of serology to analyze fetal serum or fluids may assist in making a diagnosis. Fetal sera collected from late-term calves or, if present, fluids from the abdominal cavity of fetuses may be submitted to a diagnostic laboratory for (1) quantitative radial immunodiffusion and (2) serologic tests. Commercial test kits are available for quantitating immunoglobulins IgM and IgG. Values greater than 0.4 mg/ml for either immunoglobulin should be considered as an indication of antigenic stimulation. Serologic testing can be expensive; however, clinical impressions of pos-

sible causes of abortion should be submitted along with the serum samples. This will assist laboratory personnel in narrowing the panel of tests that need to be performed.

References

1. Conner GH, Carter GR: Response of the bovine fetus to reovirus. Vet Med/Small Anim Clin 70:1463, 1975.
2. Conner GH, Richardson M, Carter GR: Prenatal immunization and protection of the newborn: ovine and bovine fetuses vaccinated with *Escherichia coli* antigen by the oral route and exposed to inoculum at birth. Am J Vet Res 34:737, 1973.
3. Kennedy PC, Casaro AP, Kimsey PB, et al.: Epizootic bovine abortion: Histogenesis of the fetal lesions. Am J Vet Res 44:1040, 1983.
4. Liggit HD, DeMantini JC, Pearson LD: Immunologic responses of the bovine fetus to parvovirus infection. Am J Vet Res 43:1355, 1982.
5. MacLachlan NJ, Schore CE, Osburn BI: Antiviral responses of blue tongue virus inoculated bovine fetuses and their dams. Am J Vet Res 46:1469, 1984.
6. Osburn BI, MacLachlan NJ, Terrell TG: Ontogeny of the immune system. J Am Vet Med Assn 181:1049, 1982.
7. Sawyer MM, Osburn BI, Knight HD, Kendrick JW: A quantitative serologic assay for diagnosing congenital infections of cattle. Am J Vet Res 34:1281, 1973.

Induced Abortion in Cattle

Albert D. Barth, D.V.M., M.V.Sc.
University of Saskatchewan,
Saskatoon, Saskatchewan, Canada

INDICATIONS FOR INDUCTION OF ABORTION

For a variety of reasons it is frequently necessary to induce abortion in cattle. Sometimes heifers inadvertently become pregnant at a very early age, predisposing them to dystocia as well as retarded growth during pregnancy and the subsequent lactation. Cows or heifers may unintentionally be bred to an undesirable bull. It may be desirable in such cases to prevent or to terminate pregnancy.

Several studies have shown that up to 50 per cent of heifers and cows entering feed lots are pregnant. Pregnancy results in reduced feed efficiency and lower slaughter prices. In addition, problems associated with calving, postpartum conditions and the rearing of calves in a feed lot situation could be avoided if abortion were induced.

Pathologic pregnancies such as hydramnios, hydrallantois, fetal maceration, fetal mummification and pathologically prolonged gestations must also be terminated in order to save the life or breeding value of affected animals.

ENDOCRINOLOGIC ASPECTS

Pregnancy maintenance is dependent on continuous adequate concentrations of circulating blood progesterone, whether the pregnancy is normal or abnormal. Pregnancy will be maintained regardless of the treatment method used for the presence of fetal life if adequate concentrations of progesterone are maintained either endogenously or exogenously. Thus, all treatment methods intended to terminate pregnancy, except surgical removal of the fetus, must directly or indirectly eliminate the sources of progesterone.

The corpus luteum is the main source of progesterone in cattle throughout pregnancy. However, the placenta and, possibly to a minor extent, the adrenal glands also contribute to circulating levels of progesterone. The presence of a functional corpus luteum is essential for maintenance of pregnancy during the first 5 months and in the final month of gestation. However, from approximately days 150 to 250 of gestation, pregnancy will be maintained in the absence of a luteal source of progesterone. During this period placental progesterone production is sufficient to maintain pregnancy. Data from two experiments conducted by the author and his colleagues indicate that circulating progesterone concentrations must be maintained above 1 ng/ml of blood plasma for pregnancy to be maintained. A small gradual decline in serum progesterone normally occurs during the final month of gestation. This may be due to a decline in placental progesterone production brought about by increasing fetal cortisol secretion. Thus, the final month of gestation again becomes dependent on a luteal source of progesterone. This is supported by experimental results indicating that when corpus luteum function was removed, either by ovariectomy or prostaglandin treatment at days 200 to 210 of gestation, parturition occurred early in the final month of gestation.

Treatment of the pregnant bovine with prostaglandin $F_{2\alpha}$ ($PGF_{2\alpha}$) results in luteolysis in both normal and abnormal gestations at any stage. In rare instances luteolysis appears to be incomplete and sufficient progesterone remains to maintain the pregnancy. In such cases, the female may undergo partial cervical dilation and may experience some abdominal straining but then returns to the normal course of gestation and maintains the pregnancy to term. Ovulation with formation of a new corpus luteum may also occur in these instances.

Glucocorticoids such as dexamethasone and flumethasone appear to reduce placental secretion of progesterone as early as the fifth month of gestation. However, luteolysis does not occur as a result of glucocorticoid treatment until the final month of gestation when these steroids are able to induce parturition. In the final month of gestation glucocorticoid treatment appears to increase the production of estradiol and $PGF_{2\alpha}$ by the placentome. $PGF_{2\alpha}$ in turn results in luteolysis, and parturition is initiated. In order for glucocorticoids to play a role in initiation of parturition, the fetoplacental unit must be functional. Thus, in cases of fetal maceration or mummification, glucocorticoids will fail to induce parturition.

In summary, the luteolytic effect of prostaglandins will induce abortion during the first 5 months of pregnancy, which are corpus luteum dependent. During the sixth, seventh and eighth months of gestation, a combination treatment of $PGF_{2\alpha}$ and glucocorticoids will eliminate luteal and placental sources of progesterone and thus induce abortion. In the final month of gestation either $PGF_{2\alpha}$ or glucocorticoid treatment alone will induce parturition.

Estrogens have been used to induce abortion in both normal and abnormal gestations. Estrogens cause luteolysis, but the exact mechanism is not clear. It appears that the endometrium must be intact for estrogens to be effective abortifacients.

In one experiment diethylstilbestrol treatments failed in three of five cases of fetal maceration to induce luteolysis and fetal expulsion. Estrogens readily induce luteolysis and abortion in the majority of cases during the first half of gestation. However, in one experiment conducted by the author, 30 mg of estradiol valerate alone or in combination with dexamethasone failed to induce abortion in any of 12 cows that were 200 to 220 days pregnant. Blood serum progesterone levels did not change in any of these cows, indicating that luteolysis did not occur.

SITUATIONS REQUIRING INDUCED ABORTION

Mismating

Veterinarians are sometimes asked to prevent pregnancy in a mismated female. The treatment of choice in these cases is to cause luteolysis and an early return to estrus. Since the bovine corpus luteum cannot be lysed by prostaglandins for at least 5 days after ovulation, treatment for mismating must be delayed for 5- to 7-days postestrus. A luteolytic dose of $PGF_{2\alpha}$ (25 mg IM) or an analog such as cloprostenol (500 μg IM) will in most cases result in a return to estrus in 3 to 5 days and prevent implantation of an embryo. If the female fails to return to estrus within 5 days, she should be retreated. If desired, the female can be rebred upon the return to estrus. Alternatively, the mismated female could be observed for return to estrus 18 to 23 days after breeding to determine if conception has actually occurred. If she failed to return to estrus she could then undergo abortion with a luteolytic dose of prostaglandin. Conception rates upon return to estrus after abortions this early in pregnancy are near normal.

The establishment of pregnancy could also be prevented by intramuscular injection of an estrogen 24 to 48 hours after the undesired service. In the cow or heifer, 40 to 80 mg of diethylstilbestrol or 4 to 8 mg of estradiol intramuscularly usually prevents implantation of the embryo. The probable mechanism by which estrogens prevent pregnancy is to prolong the passage of the embryo through the oviduct or to cause expulsion of the embryo. Signs of estrus are usually prolonged for several days after this treatment.

The embryo normally passes through the oviduct and into the uterine lumen in 4 to 5 days. Infusion of the uterus with 50 ml of an irritating solution such as 0.5 per cent aqueous iodine or 2 gm of tetracycline in saline 4 days after breeding will prevent pregnancy. Cattle treated in this manner 4 to 8 days after breeding often have an early return to estrus.

Experimentally, pregnancy has been prevented by once-daily injections of 100 to 200 IU of oxytocin from days 2 to 7 after estrus. The oxytocin treatments prevent the development of the corpus luteum necessary for pregnancy maintenance. Cattle treated in this manner usually return to estrus in 8 to 10 days.

Established pregnancies can be terminated by hormonal treatments, manual per rectum enucleation of the corpus luteum or destruction of the conceptus and embryonic or fetal destruction by uterine infusion of irritating solutions.

A single luteolytic dose of $PGF_{2\alpha}$ or a prostaglandin analog will usually induce abortion within 5 days in cattle that are up to 5 months pregnant. Up to 10 or more days may be required for some animals to abort. After the fifth month of gestation, a combination of a luteolytic dose of prostaglandin and 25 mg of dexamethasone will reliably induce abortion at a mean of 5 days after treatment. Estrous behavior often precedes or accompanies the abortion. The prostaglandin or prostaglandin-dexamethasone treatment methods are the most reliable and rapid ways to induce abortion and in most cases can be recommended over other methods.

Estrogens administered intramuscularly in large and/or repeated doses will induce abortion quite reliably in the first 5 months of gestation. Repositol diethylstilbestrol, 100 to 150 mg, or 10 to 20 mg of an ester of estradiol such as estradiol 17β-cypionate (cyclopentylpropionate), estradiol valerate or estradiol benzoate is administered intramuscularly every 4 to 7 days until abortion occurs. Abortion has been reported to occur in 60 to 80 per cent of heifers 3 to 7 days after a single treatment. Additional abortions may occur up to 14 days after treatment. Estrous behavior is observed in some aborting females. Other side effects may include mammary enlargement, vulvar swelling and a mucopurulent discharge.

Manual per rectum enucleation of the corpus luteum can be performed until the ovary is drawn out of reach by the pregnant uterus after about the fourth month of gestation. Abortion invariably results in about 3 to 5 days and is accompanied by behavioral estrus. Failure of abortion to occur may be because of incomplete removal of the corpus luteum. There is danger in causing fatal hemorrhage by using this technique. In addition, bursal or uterine adhesions may occur and prevent pregnancy in subsequent breedings.

Manual per rectum destruction of the fetus by rupture of the amnion and crushing the fetus or decapitation of the fetus has been used as a cost-saving method and as an alternative to hormonally induced abortion. The disadvantages of inducing abortion by this method include a prolonged interval from treatment to abortion and a limitation of its use to the first 120 days of gestation. Abortion will occur in 10 to 54 days with a mean of about 25 days. Mummification of the fetus may also occur following fetal decapitation.

Uterine infusions with irritating solutions such as 0.5 per cent aqueous iodine, 200 ppm chlorine solution, dilute acetic acid or potassium permanganate solution may be carried out in early pregnancy while the cervix can still be manipulated per rectum. The developing embryo or fetus is usually destroyed, and abortion ensues at a variable period.

Retained placentae can be expected in over 80 per cent of cases when abortion is induced beyond the third to fourth month of pregnancy. In most cases the placenta will be shed after approximately 1 week, and no form of therapy is routinely necessary. Metritis or pyometra may follow abortion particularly when the placenta is retained. Thus, all aborting females should be carefully observed for signs of such complications and treated as necessary.

Feed Lot Heifers

All females in a feed lot should be rectally examined for pregnancy. Abortion can be induced at the time of the rectal examination. Animals induced to abort should be in good health and well adjusted to the feed lot, since induction of abortion can be sufficiently stressful to increase the incidence of common feed lot diseases, particularly those involving the respiratory system.

Growth promotants containing progestins may interfere with induction of abortion and should be withheld until after abortion occurs. Heifers that are up to 150 days pregnant can be aborted with approximately 90 per cent effectiveness by a single intramuscular injection of 375 μg of cloprostenol. After 150 days of gestation, prostaglandin treatment alone gives poor results. However, a combination of a luteolytic dose of $PGF_{2\alpha}$ and 25 mg of dexamethasone can be expected to cause abortion in approximately 95 per cent of cattle 5 to 8 months pregnant. A reduced dose of 375 μg of cloprostenol and 10 mg of dexamethasone has been shown to be equally efficacious in feed lot heifers.

Abortion occurs over a period of 2 to 10 days, with a mean of 5 days, following treatment. Behavioral estrus of 8 to 12 hours duration precedes or accompanies abortion in 75 to 80 per cent of heifers. Abortions may occur unnoticed, especially in the first trimester. Thus, all abortions should be recorded, and heifers failing to abort should be reexamined. Lack of luteolysis is the most likely cause of abortion failure, and retreatment will in most cases induce abortion. The incidence of fetal mummification is 2 to 4 per cent. This figure is approximately twice as high as that recorded in normal populations of cattle. Fetal mummies are usually promptly expelled following retreatment with prostaglandins. Some obstetric assistance may be required. Cattle that are more than 4 months pregnant when aborted will retain the placenta in more than 80 per cent of cases. The placenta is usually passed in approximately 1 week, and treatment is rarely necessary. Postpartum metritis and purulent vaginal discharges occur in a significant number of heifers but in most cases resolve spontaneously. Rarely, acute toxic metritis occurs, and death may result if prompt treatment is not undertaken.

Cost-benefit analysis of induced abortions in feed lots have not been published. However, sufficient data have been accumulated by the author and his colleagues to indicate that heifers that were aborted were more profitable than unaborted pen-mates.

PATHOLOGIC GESTATION

Hydropic Conditions of the Uterus

Hydropic conditions of the uterus occur sporadically in beef and dairy cattle. Hydrallantois, which accounts for about 90 per cent of uterine hydrops, is characterized by a rapid accumulation of fluid over a period of 5 to 20 days in late gestation. Abnormal function of the placentomes results in transudation and collection of 80 to 150 liters of watery amber fluid. The rapid accumulation of fluid produces a distended, tense, barrel-shaped abdomen. Affected animals become anorectic, dehydrated and weak and may have difficulty with respiration. On rectal examination the uterus is greatly distended and tense and fills the abdominal cavity. Placentomes and the fetus usually cannot be palpated through the tense uterine wall. The sudden increase in weight and volume of the abdominal contents predisposes the female to ventral herniation or rupture of the prepubic tendon. Retained placenta and septic metritis usually follow termination of the pregnancy. The prognosis for life or fertility is poor even with vigorous treatment and supportive care. Thus, salvage by slaughter should be a first consideration in all cases.

In contrast to hydrallantois, hydramnios is characterized by a gradual accumulation of 20 to 100 liters of fluid in the last half of gestation. The condition is frequently associated with a genetically or congenitally defective fetus. The fluid is viscid and often contains meconium. Since the abdominal wall has more time to adjust to the increased weight and volume, the abdomen is pear shaped and less tense than that of a cow with hydrallantois. In cases of hydrallantois with ventral herniation the abdominal shape may resemble that of a cow with hydramnios. The placentomes and often the fetus may be palpated per rectum, since the uterine wall is less tense than that of a cow with hydrallantois. Although placental retention commonly follows pregnancy termination, metritis is less common and less serious than during hydrallantois, and the prognosis for life and fertility is fair to good.

Treatment of Hydropic Conditions

Slaughter of animals in good condition is the best method of handling cases of hydrallantois. In certain cases of hydrallantois, and in cows with hydramnios, treatment may be undertaken.

Most severely affected cows are very dehydrated, with marked electrolyte imbalance. Large volumes of intravenous fluids are required for several days to maintain hydration. When abdominal distention is severe enough to cause respiratory difficulty, fluid should be drained from the uterus. A catheter should be aseptically placed with a surgical approach via the right flank. In rare instances in early cases, removal of 15 to 20 liters of fluid results in recovery. Removal of 30 to 50 liters or more may induce abortion; however, treatment to cause parturition should be administered to ensure pregnancy will be terminated as early as possible. Systemic antibiotic therapy may prevent uterine sepsis and must be continued until the placenta is passed and the uterus begins to involute.

Pregnancy can be reliably terminated in 24 to 48 hours with a simultaneous injection of 25 mg of dexamethasone and a luteolytic dose of prostaglandin. Parturition can also be induced with single or repeated treatments of 20 to 40 mg of dexamethasone or 10 to 20 mg of flumethasone (Flucort). Prostaglandins alone at one to two times the luteolytic dose have been reported to be effective. Daily administration of large doses of estrogens for 4 to 7 days alone or in combination with glucocorticoids have been used; however, this form of treatment is less satisfactory than the preceding treatments.

Parturition is usually abnormal. Cervical dilation is often incomplete, and primary uterine inertia and lack of a strong abdominal press are usual. However, since the fetus is usually small, removal by repositioning and traction is commonly successful. Partial fetotomy may be necessary in a few cases.

Cesarean section has been attempted with some success. Gradual removal of the fluid with a catheter over a 24-hour period prior to surgery may help to avoid shock from sudden loss of fluid at the time of surgery. The prognosis for Cesarean section is unfavorable because the uterus is atonic and friable and the fetal membranes are almost always retained. Metritis is a common sequela and frequently causes death.

Fetal Mummification and Maceration

The incidence of fetal mummification as reported from herd data and slaughterhouse surveys of very large numbers of cattle ranges from 0.13 to 1.8 per cent. In some herds the incidence may be much higher. The incidence of fetal maceration from the same reports was 0.09 per cent. Mummification occurs from the third to eighth months of gestation but is most common in the fourth through sixth months. Maceration may occur at any stage of gestation. In the early stages of pregnancy before bone calcification occurs, maceration is often undetected but may be noted in the form of fetal tissue debris in a purulent discharge.

Fetal mummification or maceration occurs when a fetus dies without concomitant luteolysis and adequate cervical dilation to allow for expulsion. A functional corpus luteum is a cardinal feature of these conditions. Mummification occurs as a result of autolysis of fetal tissue and fluid resorption in a sterile environment. When the maternal caruncle involutes, a variable amount of hemorrhage occurs between the endometrium and placenta. Hemoglobin staining imparts a reddish-brown color to the fetal membranes and the fetus. Infectious agents that caused fetal death or organisms that entered the uterus through a partly dilated cervix result in maceration of the fetus and its membranes.

The causes of fetal death are varied and often cannot be determined, since the time of fetal death is unknown, and autolysis and resorption of the fetus and fetal membranes prevent the establishment of a definitive diagnosis. Genetic and chromosomal abnormalities may contribute to the causes of fetal death. There is evidence that fetal mummification may follow infectious causes of fetal death such as *Campylobacter fetus*, molds, leptospirosis and bovine virus diarrhea (BVD) virus. Fetal mummification occurs at a relatively high incidence of 3 to 4 per cent in feed lot heifers induced to abort with prostaglandins. The cause of fetal death is probably ischemia, since uterine contractions are quite strong for several days after the abortive treatment. If regression of the corpus luteum is incomplete, the dead fetus will be retained and mummify or macerate.

Mummification may be suspected when a cow believed to be pregnant fails to show abdominal or mammary enlargement near expected term. On rectal examination the fetus may be felt; however, fluid fluctuation in the uterus and fremitus of the uterine arteries are absent. In some large cows, the fetus may be out of reach, and because of the weight of the fetus the uterus may be impossible to retract. Two assistants raising the caudal abdomen of the cow with a plank may bring the fetus within reach during rectal palpation.

When the fetus is macerated, there is usually a chronic, fetid reddish-gray watery or mucopurulent discharge from the vulva over a period of several weeks or months that soils the tail and perineum of the cow. In early stages of fetal maceration signs of a toxic metritis may be seen; however, in later stages, signs of systemic illness are usually absent, although a gradual weight loss and decline in milk production may occur. On rectal examination crepitation of the uterus is often present, and the bones of the fetus can be felt rubbing against each other.

The treatment of choice for fetal mummification is a single injection of a luteolytic dose of $PGF_{2\alpha}$ or a prostaglandin analog. A second treatment is rarely necessary. Expulsion of the mummified fetus usually occurs in 2 to 4 days. Estrogens have also been used to cause expulsion of the mummified fetus. Fifty to 80 mg of diethylstilbestrol, 100 to 150 mg of repositol diethylstilbesterol or 5 to 10 mg of estradiol given intramuscularly will result in fetal expulsion in 24 to 72 hours in most cases. A second treatment may be necessary in about 20 per cent of cases, and in rare cases three or more treatments at 48-hour intervals are required.

Whether prostaglandins or estrogens are used, expulsion of the mummy may not be complete because of poor dilation and dryness of the cervix and birth canal. Lubrication of the birth canal and traction should allow delivery of the mummified fetus in most cases.

The prognosis for rebreeding of the female is good. Most cases will conceive 1 to 3 months after expulsion of a mummified fetus.

Cattle with long-standing fetal maceration can seldom be successfully treated because damage to the endometrium is severe. Treatment with prostaglandin and/or estrogens will result in poor cervical dilation so that manual removal of bones is not generally possible. A few of the fetal bones may be passed after treatment; however, many of the bones will be retained. Surgical removal of the macerated fetus is rarely indicated because of the likelihood of severe endometrial damage. Salvage by slaughter is the best alternative.

References

1. Barth AD, Johnson WH, Mapletoft RJ, Manns, JG: Induction of abortion in feedlot heifers with dexamethasone and prostaglandin $F_{2\alpha}$. Proc Soc Theriogenology, 1981, pp 78–95.

2. Copeland DD, Schultz RH, Kemtrup ME: Induction of abortion in feedlot heifers with cloprostenol (a synthetic analogue of prostaglandin $F_{2\alpha}$): A dose response study. Can Vet J 19:29, 1978.
3. Day AM: Cloprostenol for termination of pregnancy in cattle. B. The induction of abortion. New Zealand Vet J 25:139, 1977.
4. Parigiani E, Ball L, Lefever D, et al.: Elective termination of pregnancy in cattle by manual abortion. Theriogenology 10:283, 1978.
5. Roberts SJ: Veterinary Obstetrics and Genital Diseases. 2nd ed. Ann Arbor, Edwards Brothers, Inc., 1971.
6. Thorburn GD, Challis JRC, Currie WB: Control of parturition in domestic animals. Biol Reprod 16:18, 1977.
7. Vandeplassche M, Bouters R, Spincemaille J, Bonte P: Induction of parturition in cases of pathological gestation in cattle. Theriogenology 1:115, 1974.

Induced Parturition in Cattle

Albert D. Barth, D.V.M., M.V.Sc.
University of Saskatchewan, Saskatoon,
Saskcatchewan, Canada

ENDOCRINOLOGY OF PARTURITION

The concept of the fetus controlling the time of its own delivery was postulated by Spiegelburg in 1891. The probable endocrine mechanisms of initiation of parturition were elucidated in the late 1960's by workers such as Kennedy, Liggins, Holm and Drost. Abnormalities of the fetal pituitary or adrenal glands were found to result in prolonged gestation. The importance of these endocrine glands for initiation of parturition was verified by experiments involving fetal hypophysectomy or adrenalectomy. Further studies showed that administration of adrenocorticotropic hormone (ACTH) or cortisol to fetal limbs in utero resulted in premature parturition in both normal and hypophysectomized lambs. Large doses of corticosteroids administered parenterally to cows or ewes near the end of pregnancy resulted in parturition in 2 to 3 days. The development of radioimmuneoassays allowed more complete studies of the endocrine events surrounding parturition in both hormonally induced and natural parturitions.

It is generally believed that parturition is initiated when maturation of the fetal hypothalamo-pituitary-adrenal axis occurs. In response to pituitary ACTH, the fetal adrenals secrete increasing amounts of cortisol as parturition approaches. Fetal cortisol increases particularly sharply in the last few days before parturition. It appears that fetal cortisol gradually reduces placental progesterone production in the last few weeks of gestation and finally initiates the release of prostaglandin from the placentome. Luteolysis occurs in response to the prostaglandin release, and as a result, progesterone support for the pregnancy is lost, and parturition ensues. Hormones used to induce parturition initiate the endocrine events triggered by fetal cortisol.

INDICATIONS

The shortest interval from treatment to calving that can be achieved ranges from 24 to 72 hours. Calvings are distributed fairly evenly over the dark and daylight hours unless modified by the feeding regimen. Thus, the use of parturition induction as a management tool to concentrate calvings in daylight hours and on weekdays has not been realized.

In some of the large continental European beef breeds, calves are at times carried up to 2 weeks beyond the accepted normal gestation length. The fetal calf of these breeds may gain 0.25 to 1.0 kg daily near the end of gestation. Many beef producers prefer to induce parturition in all cows that have not calved by the "due date" according to their own herd's or breed's average length of gestation. This practice to some degree prevents excessive birth weights and dystocia related to fetal oversize. However, in most experiments, when calving was induced 1 to 2 weeks prematurely, dystocia scores were not significantly reduced even though mean calf birth weights were several pounds less than in control calves. In beef cattle a major cause for failure to become pregnant within a limited breeding season is insufficient time in the postpartum period to resume cyclicity. Cows induced to calve by their due date may gain 5 to 15 days for postpartum recovery prior to rebreeding. The incidence of placental retention in cows induced to calve near term is usually lower than in cows induced to calve earlier.

In dairy herds, parturition is sometimes induced 1 to 2 weeks early to prevent excessive udder edema and distention, which predisposes the cow to mastitis and udder breakdown.

In New Zealand the dairy industry depends on a highly seasonal system of grassland agriculture. Calving is concentrated at a time of year when grazing is optimal for milk production. In the limited breeding season that follows it is inevitable that some cows will fail to become pregnant or will become pregnant too late to calve on time the following year. These cows would ordinarily be culled. Induced calving can be applied in association with an extended mating period to reduce herd wastage. Cows that are not pregnant by the end of the usual mating season can be mated and identified by bulls with a chin ball marking harness. In the following calving season these cows can be induced to calve 1 to 3 months prematurely. Calves born more than a month prematurely will be lost; however, milk yield can be expected to be near normal.

PRECAUTIONS

Accurate knowledge of breeding dates is necessary in all cases of induced parturition in which calf viability is important. Calves born up to 2 weeks prematurely have normal vigor and are able to attain normal blood levels of gamma globulins. Most calves born more than 3 weeks prematurely have low viability. Since there is the potential for large numbers of calves to be born in a short period of time, consideration should be given to the management of obstetric problems and to the needs of large numbers of newborn calves. Close confinement of newborn calves predisposes the calves to epizootics of diarrhea or pneumonia.

When parturition occurs prematurely, for whatever reason, a high incidence of retained placenta will occur. Most retained placentae are shed by 7 days postpartum, however, a few may be retained for 10 to 14 days. In most cases no form of treatment is necessary; however, all females retaining their placentae should be carefully observed for signs of illness due to metritis. Cows that show a rise in body temperature or that become inappetent should be promptly treated parenterally with a broad spectrum antibiotic. Treatments should be continued until the placenta is passed. The fertility of induced animals was not altered in a study by Wagner and colleagues.[7] The intervals from calving to conception and services per conception in induced cows that retained the placenta were similar to induced cows that did not retain the placenta. In this study and in others, subsequent pregnancy rates of induced cattle were similar to those of cattle that calved naturally.

METHODS OF INDUCTION AND RESULTS

Parturition has been induced in cattle with corticosteroids, prostaglandins, combinations of these drugs and combinations of corticosteroids and estrogens (Table 1). Corticosteroids can be considered in two categories depending on the response of the pregnant cow: (1) dexamethasone, flumethasone or betamethasone in the free alcohol or soluble ester forms that induce calving in 2 to 3 days and (2) suspensions or insoluble esters of these steroids that induce calving in about 2 weeks.

Short-Acting Corticosteroids

In North America the most common corticosteroids used for inducing parturition are dexamethasone (20 to 30 mg) or flumethasone (Flucort, 8 to 10 mg) given as a single intramuscular injection. Parturition is induced with 80 to 90 per cent efficacy when the injection is given within 2 weeks of normal term. The interval from injection to parturition is 24 to 72 hours, with an average of 48 hours. In cows that have not calved by 72 hours after treatment the induction is considered to have failed. Retreatment in such cases is often successful in inducing parturition. Relaxation of the pelvic ligament, cervical dilation and filling of the udder occur rapidly, and labor and parturition are normal. Calving difficulty scores that have been recorded for induced parturition have generally not been different from natural calvings; however, frequently a higher incidence of minor assistance is given. This is probably because personnel are readily available during induction trials and assistance is more likely to be given even when not absolutely necessary.

Calves that are born less than 2 weeks prematurely are very vigorous, and calf mortality is not increased.

The actual secretion of milk at the onset may not be plentiful in induced cows; however, colostral immunoglobulin levels and total milk production for the lactation period are very close to normal. Induced calves attain similar blood levels of immunoglobulins as calves born naturally.

The incidence of placental retention is related to the degree of prematurity of induced parturition. Cows induced 1 to 2 weeks prematurely usually retain the placenta in over 75 per cent of cases, whereas cows induced within a few days of term or at term (over due pregnancies) have a 10 to 50 per cent incidence of placental retention.

Short-Acting Corticosteroids and Estrogen Combinations

Numerous experiments have been conducted using combinations of estrogens and dexamethasone or flumethasone in attempts to reduce the incidence of retained placentae. The combined results of these experiments indicate that estrogens do not reduce the incidence of placental retention. When large doses of estrogens (10 to 20 mg of estradiol) are administered at the time of corticosteroid treatment, the average interval to parturition may be several hours shorter than when a corticosteroid is used alone. The use of estrogens in combination with a corticosteroid appears to reduce the incidence of

Table 1. List of Drugs Used to Induce Parturition in Cattle

Name of Drug	Supplier	Dose
Betamethasone Suspension	Glaxo Laboratories Toronto, Ontario M8Z 5S6	20 mg
Cloprostenol (Estrumate)	Imperical Chemical Industries (ICI) Ltd. Macclesfield, Cheshire, England	375–500 μg
	ICI United States, Inc. Wilmington, DE 19897	
	Cooper's Agropharm Inc. 402 Consumer's Rd. Willowdale, Ontario M2J 1P8	
Dexamethasone	Shering Corporation Kenilworth, NY 07033	20–30 mg
	Rogar/STB Pointe Claire Dorval, Quebec H9R 4V2	
Dexamethasone trimethylacetate (Opticortenol)	CIBA-Geigy Corp. Ardsley, NY 19502	20 mg
	CIBA-Geigy Can. Ltd. Mississauga, Ontario L5N 2W5	
Flucort	Eli Lilly & Company Indianapolis, IN 46206	10 mg
	Syntex Corp. Palo Alto, CA 94302	
	Syntex Inc. Mississauga, Ontario L5M 2B3	
Flumethasone Susp.	Syntex Inc. Mississauga, Ontario L5M 2B3	10 mg
Prostaglandin $F_{2\alpha}$	The Upjohn Company Kalamazoo, MI 49001	20–30 mg
	The Upjohn Company of Canada Ltd. Don Mills, Ontario M3B 1Y6	
Triamcinolone acetonide (Kenalog)	Squibb Canada Inc. Montreal, Quebec H4N 2M7	30 mg

induction failures and thus may be considered a useful adjunct treatment. Other aspects of induced parturition such as ease of calving, milk production and subsequent fertility are not affected by the addition of estrogens to the induction treatment.

Long-Acting Corticosteroids

The long-acting corticosteroids are not commonly used to induce parturition in North America, where calf viability is of primary importance. However, they have gained wide acceptance in New Zealand and in other parts of the world where milk production rather than calf viability is the primary consideration. Dexamethasone trimethylacetate (Opticortenol, 20 mg), triamcinolone acetonide (Kenalog, 30 mg), flumethasone suspension (10 mg) and betamethasone suspension (20 mg) may be used and give similar results. An injection is given once intramuscularly approximately 1 month prior to the due date of calving, and parturition occurs at 15 ±

8 days (x ± SD). Usually, the further a cow is from her due date the longer it takes for a response.

In spite of prolonged elevated systemic corticosteroid levels, cow health is generally good. However, pre-existing diseases, particularly subclinical infections, may be exacerbated by the treatment, and there is a potential increase in cow mortality.

The udders of treated cows are consistently engorged with milk about 1 week after the injection, though it may be another week before they actually calve. It has been suggested that these animals should be milked prepartum if the udder is obviously full enough to prevent regression of secretory tissue. Total milk production per lactation can be expected to be reduced by 4 to 7 per cent.

The incidence of retained placentae with the use of long-acting corticosteroids is quite low (9 to 22 per cent) compared with short-acting corticosteroids. The high incidence (17 to 45 per cent) of calf mortality appears to be due to premature placental separation and an increased frequency of uterine inertia. Calves often die in utero and frequently are born partially autolysed with the membranes intact. Calf mortality could be reduced somewhat by careful observations and the provision of prompt assistance. Calves surviving premature births need more shelter and more care with feeding.

Colostral immunoglobulin secretion appears to be reduced when parturition is induced with long-acting corticosteroids. The longer a cow is exposed to the steroid prior to calving, the lower the immunoglobulin concentration in her colostrum. In addition, calves are often weak and ingest inadequate amounts of colostrum.

Data from New Zealand based on many thousands of animals over several years of study indicate that the fertility of cows induced to calve with long-acting corticosteroids is similar to that of naturally calving cows. Thus, it is feasible to move back the calving dates of late calving cows by this method of induction so that they are more likely to calve with the rest of the herd in future years.

Long-Acting Corticosteroids Followed by Short-Acting Corticosteroids of Prostaglandins

Long-acting corticosteroids induce parturition over a very wide range of 4 to 26 days. The pattern of calving can be greatly improved by administering a second injection of either a short-acting corticosteroid or prostaglandin 7 to 12 days after the depot corticosteroid injection. Most cows will calve 2 to 3 days after the second injection. The interval from injection to calving tends to be shorter and more predictable after prostaglandin than after a short-acting corticosteroid. In addition, fewer repeat injections are required with prostaglandins.

Calf mortality and the incidence of retained placentae are not reduced by giving a second injection.

Induction with Prostaglandins

Induction of parturition with $PGF_{2\alpha}$ (25 to 30 mg) or cloprostenol (500 μg) intramuscularly gives very similar results to induction with short-acting corticosteroids. The later the stage of gestation at which prostaglandins are administered, the greater the efficiency with which a single injection induces calving. The interval from injection to induced calving is 24 to 72 hours.

Reports in the literature vary greatly with regard to the mean interval from injection of prostaglandins to calving when compared with the interval from injection of short-acting corticosteroids to calving. Such variation may be due to differences in the stage of gestation during which the treatment was given and to differences in breed or age of cows. The mean treatment-to-calving interval may be considered as essentially the same for both prostaglandins and short-acting corticosteroids.

Some investigators have reported that cows with prostaglandin-induced parturitions, particularly those induced more than 2 weeks prematurely, suffered a higher than normal incidence of dystocia due to uterine inertia or malpresentation of the fetus. However, others indicated no difference in the frequency of dystocia in cows induced 1 to 2 weeks prematurely with either corticosteroids or prostaglandins. Moreover, the induced parturitions had no greater frequency of dystocia than spontaneous parturitions.

It has been reported that more than 50 per cent of cows induced to calve with prostaglandins exhibited estrous behavior within 96 hours of treatment. The estrous behavior included active seeking and mounting of other cows but not standing to be mounted. In contrast, dexamethasone-treated cows were more docile and did not exhibit estrous behavior. Estrous behavior does not occur consistently after prostaglandin injection for parturition induction. In another experiment,[6] in which the induced cows were observed every 2 hours over the duration of the calving season, no estrous activity was observed in either prostaglandin- or dexamethasone-treated groups.

Corticosteroid-Prostaglandin Combination

Recently, two experiments[6] were conducted to compare parturition induced by a combination of dexamethasone and cloprostenol, dexamethasone alone and cloprostenol alone with saline-treated controls. In the first experiment 58 cross-bred Simmental cows that were pregnant recipients from embryo transfer were treated on day 280 of gestation. Cows failing to respond to treatment within 3 days were retreated with dexamethasone when the first treatment was cloprostenol, or with cloprostenol when the first treatment was dexamethasone. Control cows not calving by day 290 of gestation

Table 2. Results of Induction of Parturition with 500 μg Cloprostenol IM (PG), 25 mg of Dexamethasone IM (Dex) or a Combination of 500 μg Cloprostenol and 25 mg Dexamethasone IM (PG-Dex)

Treatment	Number Induced	n	Treatment to Calving (hours)*	Chorioallantois to Delivery (hours)*	Placental Retention (per cent)	Birth Weight (kg)
PG	10	12	44.8 ± 2.1	5.3	50.0	43.1
Dex	14	16	43.3 ± 2.4	2.4	18.8	42.9
PG-Dex	15	15	34.6 ± 1.4	3.2	53.3	41.6
C†	—	6	153 ± 21	2.6	0	45.2
C-PG-Dex‡	9	9	269 ± 2.3	2.4	44.4	45.9

*Mean ± SEM
†C = saline treated controls
‡ C-PG-Dex = cows not responding to induction treatment within 72 hours were retreated with PG or Dex, and control cows not calving by day 290 of gestation were retreated with PG-Dex on day 290.

were treated with both drugs. The results are shown in Table 2.

A second experiment (experiment two) was designed to confirm the results of experiment one and to determine whether two injections of cloprostenol 12 hours apart would improve the efficacy of induction of parturition by a prostaglandin. One hundred and fifty cross-bred cows were randomly assigned to one of four treatment regimens on day 276 ± 1 of gestation. The treatments were control (no treatment), a single injection of cloprostenol, two injections of cloprostenol 12 hours apart and a combination of cloprostenol and dexamethasone, respectively. The results are shown in Table 3.

In both experiments cows receiving the combination treatment calved earlier, and the interval from injection to calving was less variable than with the other treatments. In addition, with the combination treatment there were no induction failures, whereas the dexamethasone and cloprostenol treatments resulted in 10.5 and 12.5 per cent induction failures, respectively, in experiment one. In experiment two, single cloprostenol treatments and two cloprostenol treatments 12 hours apart resulted in 16.6 and 11.8 per cent induction failures, respectively.

In experiment one, the interval from appearance or rupture of the chorioallantois until completion of delivery was 1 to 2 hours shorter for parturitions induced by dexamethasone alone than for parturi-

tions induced by cloprostenol alone or by the combination of dexamethasone and cloprostenol. This may indicate that the dexamethasone treatment results in better relaxation of the birth canal than when cloprostenol is used. This is a matter that requires further study.

The combined results of both experiments indicate that the rate of placental retention is significantly higher with all methods of induction of parturition than in control cows. It would appear from experiment one that the use of prostaglandins alone or in combination with dexamethasone results in higher rates of placental retention than when dexamethasone is used. Further trials will be necessary to confirm this finding.

The advantage gained by using the combination of drugs instead of dexamethasone alone may be outweighed by the additional expense of including prostaglandins in the induction regimen.

References

1. Adams WM: The elective induction of labor and parturition in cattle. JAVMA 154:261, 1969.
2. Bailey LF, McLennan MW, McLean DM, et al.: The use of dexamethasone trimethylacetate to advance parturition in dairy cows. Aust Vet J 49:567, 1973.
3. Barth AD, Adams WM, Manns JG, Rawlings NC: Induction of parturition in beef cattle using estrogens in combination with dexamethasone. Can Vet J 19:175, 1978.

Table 3. Results of Induction of Parturition with 500 μg of Cloprostenol IM (PG), Two Injections of 500 μg of cloprostenol IM 12 Hours Apart (PG-PG) and a Combination of 500 μg of Cloprostenol and 25 mg of Dexamethasone IM (PG-DEX)

Treatment	Number Induced*	n	Treatment to Calving (hours)†	Placental Retention (per cent)
Control	5	34	186.8 ± 1.57	3
PG	25	30	46.1 ± 2.0	64
PG-PG	30	34	46.4 ± 1.8	57
PG-Dex	30	30	39.1 ± 1.0	50

*Number calving within 72 hours
†Mean ± SEM

4. Drost M, Holm LW: Prolonged gestation in ewes after fetal adrenalectomy. J Endocrinol 40:293, 1968.
5. Kennedy PC, Liggins GC, Holm LW: Prolonged gestation. In Benirschke K (ed): Comparative Aspects of Reproductive Failure. New York, Springer-Verlag, 1967, pp 186–193.
6. Lewing FJ, Mapletoft RJ: Induction of parturition in the cow using dexamethasone and cloprostenol in combination. Can Vet J (in press 1985).

7. Wagner WC, Willham RL, Evans LE: Controlled parturition in cattle. J Anim Sci 38:485, 1974.
8. Welch RAS, Newling P, Anderson D: Induction of parturition in cattle with corticosteroids: An analysis of field trials. NZ Vet J 21:103, 1973.
9. Welch RAS, Day AM, Duganzich DM, Featherstone P: Induced calving: A comparison of treatment regimens. NZ Vet J 27:190, 1979.

Physical Diagnosis During Dystocia in the Cow

Gerrit Schuijt
State University of Utrecht,
Utrecht, The Netherlands

Leslie Ball
Colorado State University
Fort Collins, Colorado

With dystocia in the cow, health and fertility of the dam and survival of the calf are the important objectives of treatment. Careful examination is necessary for a well-founded prognosis and for course of treatment. The chance of survival for the calf is often dependent on the obstetrical treatment. The health of the calf during parturition is dependent on the health of the cow during both gestation and parturition. Therefore, to arrive at the proper diagnosis and prognosis and to provide the correct treatment we must include assessment of the health of the dam and the course of parturition up to the point of examination.

Economic aspects may play a role in the choice of the treatment. In dairy cattle protection of health and fertility of the cow are usually more important than health of the calf because profits are determined by milk production. In beef cattle a healthy calf may be of greater importance. The economic value of a calf is determined both by its weight and its sex. Estimation of birth weight and determination of sex may affect handling of the dystocia. The intrauterine diagnosis of congenital defects may also affect selection of obstetric procedure.

DIAGNOSTIC PROCEDURES

The examination includes history, the obstetric examination and, on occasion, a supplemental examination.

Anamnesis

In most cases a calf can be delivered without the benefit of anamnesis. However, the examination can be better guided if the anamnesis is known. This may affect the prognosis and the treatment. It may be important to ask the following questions: Why was the veterinarian consulted? Has the cow been sick recently? Were there unusual signs during gestation and/or parturition such as decreased appetite, colic, straining, prolapse of the vagina or milk fever? In general, a veterinarian will be consulted when the delivery takes too long, when progress is abnormal or when there are unusual signs.

When dealing with a healthy cow, the anamnesis is primarily an obstetric one. Determination of age and parity are important because some conditions such as juvenile pelvis, milk fever or twinning are age-related and have prognostic value for the course of parturition. The breeding history is important because some bulls sire heavy calves at birth. Whether or not this will be true at term will be answered if duration is known. Other questions to ask include what was the course of previous deliveries, especially the most recent one? How long and how forceful has the cow been straining? When were the fetal fluids expelled and what was their nature? What has happened to the cow during this parturition? Stress and activity during relocation or transport of a cow to a strange environment can delay parturition for several hours. Under these conditions, release of epinephrine and norepinephrine inhibits uterine contractions. The owner should also be asked what kind of assistance has been given thus far, as this is important to consider during the vaginal examination.

General Impression

The cow's attitude, behavior, body condition and obvious clinical abnormalities frequently provide important information. Moderate body condition of a cow may indicate a heavy calf or twins, especially if judged by comparison to the rest of the herd. Abortion, premature delivery and dystocia occur more frequently in sick cattle. A cow can also be sick as a result of abnormal gestation or parturition. It is sometimes difficult to decide which is cause and which is effect.

General Examination

If indicated, pulse, respiration, temperature, mucous membranes, hydration and rumen motility should be evaluated. Apparently sick cattle should be subjected to a more extensive internal examination. Examination of the udder should never be overlooked because severe mastitis can cause dystocia and result in serious complications during the postpartum period. Lameness in crippled cows may prevent normal parturition. When the fetus is viable and strong, a more extensive general examination can be completed after the calf is delivered. Frequently, it is also better to examine a sick cow after parturition because the uterus no longer occupies so much space. After this, a specific examination is made to determine the cause of the delay in parturition or of signs that gave reason for concern.

Obstetric Examination

The obstetric examination is made to determine the condition of the genital tract and the fetus and the cause of dystocia.

External Obstetric Examination (Inspection)

During the external examination, attention should be paid to expected prodromal changes of the udder, the pelvic ligaments, the vulva and surrounding area, vulvar discharges, the flanks and the abdominal circumference. Partial or complete lack of prodromal signs may indicate abortion, or premature delivery, and may influence the course of parturition adversely. Occasionally, prodromal signs are absent during induced parturition because the normal hormonal changes do not take place or perhaps take place so rapidly that the cervix dilates slowly, and the calf may be adversely affected. Admixture of blood or meconium in the discharge may indicate life-threatening conditions for the calf but may also be observed with healthy calves. Discharges with a bad odor usually mean that the calf has died but occasionally a live, healthy calf is delivered under such circumstances. To be more certain of a correct diagnosis, it is necessary to examine the fetus itself.

Vaginal Examination

A vaginal examination should be done only under hygienic circumstances. Infection introduced during examination or assistance may disturb the normal course of the postpartum period. The hind quarters, the vulva and surrounding area and the underside of the tail should be cleaned and disinfected. The vaginal examination may be done manually or with a speculum to prevent trauma if the vagina is too constricted for manual examination. This may be the case with abortion or premature delivery or when the cow is actually not in labor. An antepartum manual examination of the vagina of the cow

frequently leads to vaginitis. A nonirritating lubricant should be used, and when the discharge is abnormal and malodorous, plastic sleeves should be worn.

During the exploration of the vagina at the time of a term delivery, sequential attention should be paid to the following:

1. Formation of possible folds, lesions, hemorrhages or other abnormalities of the genital tract and pelvic cavity.
2. Position of the gravid horn and calf and congenital defects, if any, of the calf.
3. Signs of life in the fetus.
4. Relaxation and degree of dilation of the cervix.
5. Size of calf relative to the pelvic inlet.
6. Relaxation and dilation of the vagina and the vulva and the vulvovaginal sphincter.
7. Position of the umbilical cord, particularly of a calf in posterior presentation.

It is important to check first for folds, lesions or hemorrhage, so the owner can be informed, in case he blames the veterinarian in retrospect. Congenital or acquired abnormalities of the genital tract or the pelvic cavity should be evaluated at this time as well as abdominal organs that have entered the pelvic cavity next to the vagina. Dry feces should be removed from the rectum to minimize the danger of rectal damage.

The location and position of the gravid horn can have a deciding influence on the choice of laparotomy site for cesarean section or of side of recumbency for extraction. The tone of the uterus can be evaluated, and if possible, a partial torsion should be corrected before delivery is begun. Position of the calf should be determined and corrected to normal, if necessary, before extraction is begun. When a fetotomy or a cesarean section is chosen, reposition is less important. In some cases an abnormal presentation, position or posture of a calf leads to a poor prognosis for delivery or survival of the calf. Dorsoilial positions occur more frequently in cows with uterine atony or oversized calves. Deviations of the fetal extremities also occur more frequently in oversized calves and in those that are dead in utero. If possible, congenital abnormalities of the calf should be determined because they may influence selection of method for delivery. Abnormal calves are frequently born prematurely, but calves with such conditions as arthrogryposis or infections of *Schistosoma reflexum* are usually born at term.

It is important to evaluate vital signs of the unborn calf because they also influence the choice of obstetric treatment. If the calf is dead, it is usually best to perform a fetotomy, especially on an oversized fetus if the birth canal is sufficiently dilated, or on the calf if it is no longer fresh.

Anterior Presentation. Signs of life of a calf in anterior presentation can be determined by the interdigital claw reflex, the swallowing reflex or the eye reflex or by palpation of the heartbeat or the pulsations in the umbilical cord.

The interdigital claw reflex is elicited by firmly

pinching the interdigital web. A vigorous calf usually withdraws its foot only once. When the reaction is exaggerated, or in the form of pedaling motions, it may indicate hypoxia and/or acidosis. When the head has entered the pelvic canal, the interdigital claw reflex is sometimes absent even though the calf is normal. During straining it may appear—falsely—that a live or a dead calf actively reacts because the front limb is pressed into the pelvic cavity, which then seems to retract when the press is relaxed.

The swallowing reflex is elicited by applying pressure on the base of the tongue. A vigorous calf will usually react by swallowing or by making gentle sucking motions. Exaggerated or frequent swallowing or sucking may indicate hypoxia and/or serious acidosis. It may appear that there is a positive swallowing reflex in a dead calf during straining because its tongue is extruded from the mouth by pressure.

By placing slight pressure on the eyeballs, the eye reflex can be felt as a vibration of the eyes or as a movement of the eyelids. This reflex may still be positive when the calf is already seriously acidotic.

With worsening condition, these reflexes disappear in order. The interdigital claw reflex is negative first, and the eye reflex remains positive for the longest amount of time. Checking these reflexes is of prognostic value, provided that they are interpreted correctly. A positive response indicates a calf is still alive; however, a negative response does not always mean that it is dead.

Common Causes of Fetal Death during Parturition. Hypoxia and acidosis are the most common causes of fetal death during parturition. As a result of the increasing frequency and strength of uterine contractions the fetus' blood supply diminishes, reducing the gaseous exchange in the placenta. This occurs mostly during the last phase of the expulsion when the calf is in the birth canal because contraction of the unoccupied part of the uterus can increase considerably. Other factors, such as circulatory and respiratory problems of the dam, placentitis, placental detachment, umbilical cord stenosis and circulatory problems in the calf, may also play a role. When oxygen becomes deficient, the calf reacts with anaerobic glycolysis, and metabolic products such as lactic and pyruvic acid are released as the calf attempts to provide for its energy needs. Its buffering capacity is not enough to prevent development of acidosis. In addition centralization of the circulation occurs, allowing the heart and the brain to be supplied as long as possible by oxygen-containing blood, which is at the expense of the peripheral tissues, particularly the muscles. Accumulation of lactic acid occurs first in the muscles and decreases their reactivity. This explains why reflexes of the extremities become negative first.

To check the heartbeat and pulsations in the umbilical cord, it is best to stand over the cow, bend over and pass the hand between the front legs of the calf and along the ventral side of the neck, following the sternum to the curvature of the last ribs. Usually, this is possible only when the head has not yet entered the birth canal or after the head of the calf is repelled into the uterus. Sometimes this procedure is difficult, but it is always possible when the front legs are pushed back first followed by the head. It is absolutely necessary to do this when there is no other way in which to determine whether or not the oversized calf is alive; otherwise, fetotomy might be done on a live calf. The heartbeat can best be detected by grasping the sternum from below, preferably with the fingers on the left side of the chest wall. The umbilical cord can be felt at this same level and is reached much easier than is generally believed. It can be located by searching the area between the curvature of the last ribs and the flaccid abdomen. In many cases one can also determine sex by palpating for the scrotum. Persons with short arms are sometimes not able to palpate the umbilical cord, but they can almost always feel the heartbeat. One should never pull on the umbilical cord because this results in reflex contraction of the arterial vessels, which diminishes the blood supply to the calf, compromising its oxygen supply. Pulsation and tension of the vessels can best be evaluated by slight digital pressure on the umbilical cord. The umbilical cord may be wrapped around the abdomen of the calf, increasing the likelihood of fetal death on delivery per vaginam. On rare occasions the umbilical cord is severed, probably from rotation of the calf during hypoxic distress.

Posterior Presentation. Vitality of a calf in posterior presentation can be determined by the pedal reflex, anal reflex, pulsation in the umbilical cord and sometimes the heartbeat. The sex of the calf in posterior presentation can always be determined.

The interdigital claw reflex of the rear feet is lost sooner than that of the front feet and can sometimes be negative in a live calf. The pedal reflex can be absent when a live calf is wedged in the birth canal, consequently its prognostic value is not as good as when performed on the front feet.

The anal reflex is elicited as a constriction of the anal sphincter when a finger is pushed against or into the anus, but this reflex is not very reliable because it is absent in some vigorous calves. The umbilical cord can always be easily reached in calves in posterior presentation, and its evaluation is always effective in determining vitality of the calf. The heartbeat can be felt only by persons with long arms.

Evaluation of the Heartbeat and the Umbilical Cord

Depending on the degree of muscling of the calf, the heartbeat can be felt more or less clearly on the left thoracic wall. Double-muscled calves have a broad thorax with heavy pectoral muscles and a relatively small heart, consequently the heartbeat is sometimes felt less distinctly. Evaluation of the umbilical vessels is sometimes hampered by edema of the umbilical sheath. A regular, pounding heart-beat and well-distended and tense umbilical vessels are signs of good condition in a calf.

The heart rate drops when the uterus contracts. Its normal rate should be about 120 beats/minute but may drop to nearly 80 beats/minute during uterine contraction. The depth and duration of the drop in frequency are dependent both on the strength and duration of the uterine contractions and on the condition of the calf. A calf in poor condition will experience a greater, more protracted drop.

Evaluation of the pulse is only reliable during periods between uterine contraction or abdominal press and at least 30 seconds after repulsion of the calf. An irregular pulse in which the pulse frequency fluctuates over 10-second periods is an unfavorable sign. During normal parturition, pulse frequency gradually increases from about 90 to 120/minute. When the head and especially the thorax have difficulty in passing through the birth canal, pulse frequency sometimes drops considerably. With a prolonged, heavy pull, the frequency may even drop to near zero.

The amplitude of the pulse should not vary; if it does, the prognosis is unfavorable. Totally sponta-neous movements, particularly when they are fre-quent and violent, are also an unfavorable sign and in most cases indicate imminent death caused by hypoxia and/or acidosis. In some cases a hypoxic state can correct itself very rapidly when the circum-stances change—for example, when it is the result of excessive straining, which suddenly stops.

Congestion of the head and the tongue of the calf occurs with prolonged wedging of the head in the birth canal—often due to frequent, forcible strain-ing, especially in heifers. Severe congestion may occur in either vigorous or moribund calves, so it has little prognostic value. Sometimes the calf jerks its legs back violently when traction is applied to the chains. In most cases this is probably the result of pain caused by stretching of the front legs and has no prognostic value. When the calf develops acidosis, the frequency of its pulse can increase up to 140 beats/minute and higher, then the calf's condition deteriorates further, the frequency drops and the pulse becomes irregular. At this point, the reflexes also disappear sequentially. The heartbeat is pounding at first but becomes weak and irregular. As death approaches, spontaneous fetal movements can be felt or, at times, observed externally.

In most cases intensive examination for all signs of life are unnecessary when the course of parturi-tion does not give reason for concern and normal reflexes of the calf are present.

It is important to check cervical dilation because insufficient dilation can prevent delivery per vagi-nam. The cervix in heifers can usually be felt as a ring; cervical dilation in the cow is not often a problem. An insufficiently dilated cervix will tense around the calf like a cuff.

During preparation for parturition, the cervix first actively softens as a result of decreased muscle tone and the relaxing action of hormones on the colla-genous connective tissue. Then, the cervix is pas-sively stretched and dilated by the pressure of the fetal membranes and the fetus as the uterus con-tracts. Passive dilation can take place properly only after the active phase is complete. A cervix that is poorly dilated owing to failure of active dilation feels stiff and inelastic, but the uterus is usually well contracted and feels tense upon rectal examination. Causes of failure of active dilation include insuffi-cient or abnormal hormonal preparation, scar tissue from previous trauma or infections or congenital abnormalities. Frequently, labor will be several days old, the fetal fluids will have been voided, the fetus will be impacted against or in the cervix in such cases and the cervix will not dilate. The fetus is usually in poor condition or may be already dead as a result of the prolonged labor. The signs of life are difficult to check when the hand cannot be passed through the cervix. Signs of life can some-times be palpated per rectum. In cases of delivery before 8½ months it is less important to know the condition of the calf because the prognosis for its life is poor. Early labor resulting in fetal death may be associated with abnormal cervical preparation.

If passive dilation has not been completed after normal active dilation, the cervix feels soft and elastic, and the uterus is not yet firmly contracted around the calf. Upon rectal examination the uterus feels firm but flexible. Often, the fetal fluids have not yet been discharged, and the calf is in good condition. This situation is encountered most com-monly with large calves or with uterine atony re-sulting from milk fever, in which rotation from the lateral to the dorsosacral position has been too slow or incomplete. In both cases stretching of the cervix is not difficult and the incomplete dilation of the cervix is not the primary cause of the dystocia.

Before extraction is attempted, the size of the calf must be evaluated relative to the birth canal, and it must be decided whether or not it is reason-able and possible to extract the calf. In a calf the circumference of the head and extended legs is less than that of the thorax at the level of the points of the shoulder. Even when the head has completely entered the birth canal it may be impossible to extract the calf because its shoulders are too large to pass through the pelvic inlet.

Anterior Presentation

The prognosis for extraction is unfavorable when a cow has not managed to deliver the head of the calf in normal position completely into the birth canal after protracted labor. When the calf is wedged in the birth canal at the level of the humeri because the width at the points of the shoulder is too large, the front legs are frequently crossed. If the ventral pelvic inlet is narrow, the elbows are pressed together, causing the claws to be rotated with their volar surfaces medial. Both of these cases have an unfavorable prognosis for extraction. When the claws protrude during straining then glide back when straining stops, or when a heifer vocalizes a great deal during straining, the birth canal is still in the process of stretching. Heifers may be expected to expand somewhat more during extraction if they have been in labor only a short time. The prognosis for extraction is then more favorable. First, the head and extended forelimbs must be brought completely into the pelvic cavity. With traction of one person on both front legs it must be possible to pull the fetal head into the pelvic inlet during the abdominal press in the recumbent animal with a completely dilated birth canal. During this maneuver the hand is placed behind the head, which is guided and pulled along with the legs. When a greater amount of traction than this is required to deliver the head, extraction is not the method of choice because the fetus is oversized. Once the head has completely entered the birth canal and the legs are extended, one person can pull to wedge the calf into the pelvic inlet. The hand is then passed between the calf and the iliac shaft to feel for the point of the shoulder and evaluate the space between the cranium of the calf and the sacrum of the dam. In older cows it may be difficult to displace the sacrum dorsally because the iliosacral joint lacks mobility, or it may sag after an earlier difficult delivery.

The following criteria can be used to judge whether extraction of a calf in anterior presentation is possible: In the *standing animal* with the head completely in the pelvic cavity and with the pull of one person during straining one should be able to place a hand between the cranium and sacrum; one should be able to feel both points of the shoulder 10 cm or less cranial to the pelvic inlet. In the *recumbent animal* one must be able to feel both points of the shoulder 5 cm or less cranial to the pelvic inlet. This examination requires only a few minutes.

Posterior Presentation

Spontaneous delivery of a calf in posterior presentation lasts longer, and the likelihood of perinatal death is greater because it differs in several respects from delivery in anterior presentation. Rotation is more difficult because the hind quarters are heavier than the head and the neck and are less flexible than the thorax, hence greater uterine tone is necessary.

Pain and restlessness occur because the less flexible rear legs may poke the uterine and vaginal wall, delaying parturition.

Dilation of the cervix takes longer because stimulation of receptors in the birth canal and pelvic cavity (Fergusson's reflex) is delayed because of slower rotation. The abdominal press is delayed in turn.

Passage of the hind quarters through the pelvic inlet is also more difficult. The umbilical cord is more frequently abnormal in position and even when normal it stretches and becomes pinched earlier, often leading to fetal death.

Inspiration may be stimulated as a result of hypoxia, and more amniotic fluid enters the lung. This makes breathing difficult after delivery, and the chance of death increases. At the onset of labor, the hind quarters of the fetus in posterior presentation are further from the cervix than from the head when the fetus is in anterior presentation. Therefore, the uterus must be more contracted to expel the fetus an equal distance, which may lead to delayed expulsion and increased risk of fetal hypoxia.

Posterior presentation of a calf also creates more problems during obstetric assistance, and the veterinarian is more frequently consulted than when the calf is in anterior presentation. The determination of whether or not a calf in posterior presentation can be extracted is also more difficult. Only when the calf is clearly too large can a diagnosis be made in the standing animal; otherwise, a proper determination is possible only in the recumbent animal. The same principles for delivery of the points of the shoulder in the anterior presentation are true for the greater trochanters in posterior presentation, but palpation of the greater trochanters is usually impossible because of the thickness of the hind legs. Therefore, the determination of whether or not it is possible to extract the calf can only be determined with the pull of two people on the calf while the cow is recumbent.

Criteria for Determining Whether Extraction of a Calf in Posterior Presentation is Justified. It must be possible to expose both hocks with traction applied in a slightly dorsal direction after the fetal hind quarters have been rotated 60 to 90 degrees. The hips of the fetus are widest between its greater trochanters. The maternal pelvic inlet has a wider dorsopubic than bisiliac diameter. Therefore, the fetus must be rotated 60 to 90° into the dorsoilial position so its greatest hip diameter corresponds to the greatest diameter of the maternal pelvis.

When the greater trochanters have passed the pelvic inlet, the hocks protrude about one hand's width beyond the vulva. If it is impossible to extract the hocks so they are visible, traction should be discontinued and other methods used for delivery of the calf. This diagnosis can be made in a few seconds. A hard pull, especially a prolonged hard pull, leads to severe acidosis. If the calf is in good condition before the extraction is begun, it will recover, provided no trauma occurs. If the calf is already in poor condition, with acidosis of any degree, the chance of complications developing during the recovery is much greater.

Relaxation and dilation of the vagina, vulvovaginal sphincter and vulva is necessary before extraction can be begun. It is less important with fetotomy, and for cesarean section it is unimportant. The question is whether the calf can pass without complications, and we must check the space in relation to the calf and the stretchability of the birth canal. In heifers with posterior presentations and in anterior presentations in which the head is not in the birth canal, dilation is frequently incomplete. It is better for the cow and the calf manually to stretch the soft tissue portions of the undilated birth canal before extraction. Stretching during the extraction frequently leads to tearing and delay of extraction.

The umbilical cord may be wrapped around a leg or the trunk, or occasionally, it enters the birth canal in a loop next to the calf. Early contraction or tearing of the umbilical cord may endanger the life of the calf. Abnormal location of the umbilical cord can be handled in one of three ways: (1) repulsion of the calf or of the umbilical cord without placing it under excessive tension, (2) very rapid extraction of the calf or (3) cesarean section, if both other methods are impossible. Traction on the calf for the determination of relative size can be fatal if the umbilical cord is misplaced, consequently its location should be determined during the initial examination, especially in cases of posterior presentation.

Rectal Examination

A rectal examination is done only as part of an obstetric examination when there is a specific indication for it. The direction and degree of uterine torsion can be determined by rectal palpation of the broad ligaments.

Sometimes rectal palpation is useful for determining uterine tone and contractility. In abortion the uterus frequently feels like a tense balloon, as it does at times with a poorly dilated cervix because such animals have frequently been in protracted labor. Conversely, the uterus of a cow in false labor is atonic, and parts of the fetus can be grasped through the uterine wall.

It is also sometimes possible to elicit a positive response from the calf per rectum to determine that it is alive.

Firm feces should be removed from the rectum before an extraction to minimize the chance of damaging the rectum, and when rectal trauma, rupture of the uterus or bleeding into the broad ligaments is suspected, rectal examination can often verify a diagnosis. Subserous emphysema of the uterus and peritonitis resulting from a macerating or emphysematous fetus can be diagnosed per rectum. A supplemental examination is indicated when the veterinarian needs to provide better treatment. When the pH is less than 7, and the base excess is less than 1 in the arterial umbilical blood of the calf, the prognosis, even after cesarean section, is very unfavorable.

CLINICAL SIGNS OF THE HEALTHY NEW-BORN CALF

Respiration is initiated in a normal term calf within 30 seconds after delivery. At first, respiration is irregular, but soon it becomes fairly regular, with a frequency of 45 to 60 per minute and with a visually sufficient depth. The pulse is usually higher than 120 beats/minute and can be judged very well with a stethoscope and with the calf in right lateral recumbency. The frequencies of respiration and pulse are strongly dependent on the activity of the calf; for example, they are much higher during and immediately after activities such as attempts at standing. Calves that have been extracted frequently have a lower pulse immediately after delivery than calves born by cesarean section, because a drop in the frequency of the pulse has occurred during the extraction; the pulse then slowly returns to the normal level after delivery. The drop in the frequency of the pulse is a result of decreased venous blood supply to the heart because the thorax is compressed during passage through the birth canal. It is possible that direct stimulation of the vagus nerve also plays a role in this bradycardia. In calves delivered by cesarean section, respiration sometimes is initiated somewhat later because the partial pressure of carbon dioxide immediately after delivery in such calves is lower than that of extracted calves, and therefore respiration is stimulated less quickly. The calf will raise its head after a few minutes and pull its legs underneath its body, which places it in a stable sternal recumbency. It shakes its head, and frequent attempts to stand are made within 10 minutes after delivery. Activity is dependent on the size and the degree of muscling of the calf. Small, slightly thin calves are soon active and stand sooner in general than large muscular calves. It is therefore possible to have a calf that does not breathe for the first 30 seconds after delivery or that does not show any activity, except for respiration, for 2 minutes after the delivery while it lies flat. It is understandable that this worries the owner. However, immediately postpartum it is possible to differentiate between a well-oxygenated calf that is not breathing because the partial pressure of carbon dioxide is not yet high enough and a calf whose respiration is slow in becoming established because functions are disturbed. A normal vigorous calf whose blood pH and blood gas values are not grossly abnormal immediately after delivery has palpable muscle tone in the extremities and shows a normal pedal reflex in all four legs. A normal pedal reflex means that the calf pulls the leg back once when the interdigital web is pinched. To judge this reflex properly it is necessary that the calf be in complete lateral recumbency without weight on the limbs. Only very heavy pull on the extremities or swelling because of congestion will render the reflex of the front or hind legs unreliable. The swallowing reflex and the eye reflex are normally present. The color of the tongue is pink when there has been no severe congestion. The mucous membranes of the mouth and eyes are also pink. Additional respiratory sounds in the upper airways occur frequently in otherwise normal healthy calves and are of no serious importance per se. When these signs are noted in the calf there is no reason for panic and no reason for all types of hurried measures. Under normal circumstances the calf will be able to adapt well to the new situation. The body temperature of the calf will usually not drop below 37°C. When the environmental temperature is 15°C, the hair coat will be completely dry within 6 hours after delivery.

Immediate Postpartum Care of the Dam

George K. Haibel, D.V.M.
The Ohio State University, Columbus, Ohio

The relief that accompanies the delivery of a calf following dystocia should not divert attention away from the cow, which should be the object of primary economic concern to the herdsman or rancher. Parturition is both a culmination and a beginning. The postpartum cow is in metabolic transition between the demands of late pregnancy and ensuing lactation. Mismanagement of added stress caused by regrouping, diet change or sequelae to dystocia can spell the difference between profit and loss. The veterinary obstetrician bears responsibility for evaluation of the dam and for initiation of therapy when it is needed to maximize subsequent fertility, lactation or, at least, salvage value.

TRAUMA TO THE BIRTH CANAL

Assisted delivery increases the risk of trauma to the soft tissue of the birth canal. This seems obvious in cases of fetal/maternal disproportion with normal presentation, but the mere fact that the calf is aided with traction rather than pushed out elongates and constricts the vagina (consider the principle of novelty store "Chinese handcuffs"). Assisted delivery may also deny the cervix, vagina and vulva the aid in dilation caused by the progressive pressure of the calf. All assisted deliveries, even in the absence of hemorrhage, deserve an immediate, clean, manual examination and systematic evaluation of the uterus, cervix and vagina.

The vulva and perineum should be cleaned with soap and water. The examiner should assure the cleanliness of his own arm and with adequate lubrication should examine, by progressing inward, the entire circumference of the birth canal. While knowledge of the obstetric procedures performed can guide the thoroughness of the examination, the possibility of trauma from prior assistance should be kept in mind. The presence of a remaining calf should always be ruled out. Soluble oxytetracycline powder (Vetquamycin 25, Rochelle Laboratories, Inc., Long Beach, CA 90801) in large gelatin capsules provides some measure of antibiotic protection against the contamination inherent in any manual exam. The number of boluses used should reflect the depth and duration of manipulations and the degree of sepsis. An attempt should be made to place the boluses between the membranes and the endometrium, lest they be expelled rapidly by the contracting uterus. Intramuscular oxytocin at a dose of 60 to 100 IU, depending on the size of the cow, will aid in contracting the uterus and in expelling the fetal membranes.

The management and prognosis for trauma to birth canal depends on location, severity and existence of sepsis. Thus, a small dorsal uterine laceration sustained during delivery of a fresh calf may be managed with oxytocin and systemic antibiotics and have a favorable outcome. Conversely, comparable vaginal lacerations or bruising during fetotomy of an emphysematous fetus may result in severe perivaginal cellulitis and pelvic inflammation, with death occurring in a stressed, toxic cow not receiving aftercare.

The vulva is frequently lacerated in first calf heifers even during unassisted delivery. These lacerations are generally dorsal and heal without consequence. Lateral laceration of the labia can occur and may, if severe, be sutured to restore vulvar function.

The vagina may suffer longitudinal lacerations during assisted delivery of a large or an inadequately lubricated calf. The caudal vaginal wall frequently splits when a wave of perivaginal fat preceding a large calf meets the vestibulovaginal sphincter. This fat may prolapse following delivery and needs to be differentiated from any other abdominal structure that may have prolapsed through a more cranial vaginal defect. Lacerations of the vagina are generally left unsutured, as healing by first intention is rarely achieved. Concurrent systemic antibiotic therapy may lessen perivaginal cellulitis and abscessation. Prolapsed fat can be manually removed or trimmed without serious hemorrhage.

The effaced cervix at parturition is subtly hoop-like on manual examination per vaginam. The cervical rings are reduced to ripples of mucosa at the junction of the smooth vaginal epithelium with the endometrium, which is identified by the presence of caruncles. Interfering fetal membranes should not cause confusion in the detection of myometrial defects, which may be longitudinal or circular, paralleling the dilated cervix. Simultaneous examination per vaginam and per rectum may be necessary. Defects diminish in size as the uterus contracts; therefore, examination should be performed prior to administration of oxytocin.

Uterine laceration may have resulted from mutation of limbs with inadequate uterine relaxation or lubrication or from injudicious use of fetotomy instruments. Cows with long-standing dystocia with a dry fetus and contracted uterus or fetal emphysema with metritis and severe uterine distention are at increased risk of uterine rupture.

Uterine body and cervical lacerations may be sutured per vaginam with a hand-held Loopuyt's needle and catgut. Any enhancement of apposition will aid the fibrin seal, which, with systemic broad spectrum antibiotics, is the real salvation of the cow. Lacerations in the uterine horn may require an abdominal approach via an inguinal or caudal midline incision. Alternately, the uterus may be manually prolapsed during the 12 hours immediately postpartum following slow intravenous administration of 10 ml of 1:1000 USP epinephrine, which causes temporary complete myometrial relaxation. Caruncles at the tip of the horn of pregnancy are grasped per vaginam and gently withdrawn, producing inversion. Prolapse is aided by the cow's straining as the uterine mass enters the vagina. This procedure should not be attempted following epidural anesthesia or oxytocin administration.

HEMORRHAGE

Vaginal lacerations are a frequent source of acute hemorrhage. Some fresh blood is always present at the vulva owing to rupture of the calf's umbilicus. Bleeding can also be caused by laceration of the cervix or uterus, forcible separation of membranes or laceration of a caruncle during fetotomy. Hemorrhage from the deeper structures may not be evident at the vulva but noticed only after manual examination. Bleeding from a ruptured broad ligament may be intra-abdominal and therefore occult unless a peritoneal tap is performed. The source of serious hemorrhage should be determined. Large vaginal bleeders may be ligated, or a hemostatic forceps may be left in place for 24 to 48 hours. Bleeding of uterine origin may be decreased by administration of oxytocin. The cow's membrane color and respiratory and heart rates should be noted to follow the progress of hypovolemic shock. Whole blood transfusion may be indicated.

EVALUATION OF OTHER BODY SYSTEMS

A rapid but systematic appraisal of the dam following obstetric intervention will often reveal problems in other body systems, which can seriously alter the outcome of the case. At the very least some appraisal needs to be made of the musculoskeletal system and, particularly in dairy cows, the udder, for evidence of mastitis.

Within a half-hour postpartum the cow should be encouraged to rise. Footing should be good and assistance available at the tail, if needed. The cow should be assessed for strength and proprioception in the hind limbs. Weak animals may have some degree of paralysis due to nerve damage. Hypocalcemia could be a concurrent problem and should be suspected if the cow is unable to rise, especially if the dystocia was caused by ineffective labor. Cows with weakness are at an increased risk for further injury, such as hip luxation or rupture of the gastrocnemius.

Cows unable to rise need nursing care. Crush syndrome of the down side rear limb ensues rapidly if the animal is not well bedded and turned side-to-side at several hour intervals. Food, water and shelter should be provided. Dairy cattle must be milked. Affected cattle need frequent reevaluation, as injury such as hip dislocation often occurs following paresis. The hind legs may be hobbled to prevent spreading beyond 1 meter. If considerable improvement has not occurred after parturition, recovery is unlikely in the first 2 weeks.

Reference

1. Greenough PR, MacCallum FJ, Weaver AD: Lameness in Cattle. 2nd ed. Philadelphia, JB Lippincott Co, 1981.

Resuscitation and Intensive Care of the Newborn Calf

David B. Brunson, D.V.M., M.S.
John W. Ludders, D.V.M.
University of Wisconsin,
Madison, Wisconsin

In dairy practices the death of a calf within minutes of birth is a well-known occurrence. Data collected on Michigan dairy herds has indicated that approximately 6 per cent of calf losses occur at the time of birth.[4]

Large animal practitioners often work hard to correct a complicated dystocia only to have the calf die before establishing adequate ventilation. When delivered, these calves are usually fully developed, have normal reflex responses and have strongly beating hearts. Typically, attempts to clear the airway and stimulate breathing are not successful in saving the calf. Some of the calves that die at birth can be saved if proper resuscitation procedures are followed. The techniques are simple and easily performed without expensive equipment. Although many factors may prevent success, there are several reasons for always making an attempt at resuscitation.

First, many calves asphyxiate because of a failure to establish adequate ventilation. Since endotracheal intubation is an easily learned skill, no animal should ever die of primary ventilatory failure without an attempt by the veterinarian to perform intubation and to assist in ventilation.

Second, attempting to intubate and to ventilate all dying newborn calves will improve the skills of the practitioner and will increase the frequency of successful resuscitation. The few minutes required to prepare and administer emergency procedures will be many times repaid by the positive professional image created by the attempted and successful resuscitations.

This article will discuss the physiology of the near-term fetus, the changes that occur during parturition and the steps that can be taken to support weak and dying calves. These physiological principles and the resuscitation techniques can be applied to all mammalian species.

INTRAUTERINE PHYSIOLOGY

In order to help a newborn calf establish respiratory and circulatory independence it is essential to understand fetal and neonatal physiology and anatomy. Tremendous changes occur in both of these organ systems at the moment of birth. The events that occur are a carefully developed cascade of steps. Each event must occur in order to allow the next step to proceed.

During intrauterine development the nutrients required by the fetus are provided by the maternal circulation through the placenta. Nutrients, including oxygen, are carried from the placenta via the umbilical veins. The umbilical veins deliver the oxygenated blood into the posterior vena cava by means of the ductus venosus. The blood from the postcava is primarily diverted through the foramen ovale and into the left atrium. Blood from the fetal head and right atrium enter the right ventricle. Blood leaving the right ventricle flows into the pulmonary artery, but because of the high pulmonary vascular tone, the majority of the blood does not perfuse the lungs. Instead, the blood passes into the aortic arch via the ductus arteriosus.

This circulatory pathway effectively delivers blood that is high in oxygen and nutrients to the fetal heart and brain. The lungs that are unable to oxygenate the blood are perfused with only enough blood to meet the needs of the pulmonary tissue. At parturition this circulatory pattern must change if the calf is to survive in the extrauterine environment.

The partial pressure of oxygen in the fetal blood is lower than that required by adult animals. This relative hypoxic condition is compensated for by an increased affinity for oxygen by fetal hemoglobin and by an increased ability to release oxygen to the tissues.

In the lungs the lower oxygen tensions cause a constriction of the vasculature. This contracture produces high pulmonary vascular resistance and prevents blood flow through the nonventilated lungs. This phenomenon is called hypoxic vasoconstriction and remains as a characteristic of the pulmonary vasculature throughout adult life.

Although the fetal lungs are not involved in the elimination of carbon dioxide and the absorption of oxygen, they serve several special functions. The lungs produce amniotic fluid to cushion the fetus, and they act as an important glycogen reservoir during late pregnancy. As the end of fetal development approaches, the lungs begin to produce the surface-active substance that will be required to stabilize the air-inflated lungs. This substance is called surfactant and is an essential requirement for alveolar stability in the newly inflated lungs of the newborn.[3]

The bovine lung is highly lobulated and lacks collateral channels for ventilation. The calf must inflate each lobule of its lungs independently of the adjacent lobule. This lack of interdependence may predispose the calf to greater problems with atelectasis if small airways are occluded.

Near parturition, the fetal lung becomes primed for the initiation of breathing. The muscles used for respiration contract and relax as the functional development of the respiratory center reaches maturity. The ventilatory efforts are weak because of the mild stimuli that reach the calf through the intrauterine environment. Another indication of fetal lung maturity is the lung size. The fetal lung becomes filled with surfactant-rich fluid to a volume comparable to the functional residual capacity of the inflated neonatal lung. This ensures that the lungs will have sufficient size to sustain the newborn immediately following birth.

PARTURITION-INDUCED CHANGES IN THE NEONATE

The birth of the fetus causes the separation of the fetal life line and initiates the sequence of events necessary for the independent life of the neonate. During the birth process the calf is forced through the birth canal. Umbilical blood flow may become reduced, resulting in lower oxygen tension and higher carbon dioxide tension in the fetal blood. Central and peripheral chemoreceptors become activated, with changes in the gas tension and blood pH resulting in secondary stimulation of the respiratory center of the brain. Additionally, ventilation is stimulated by the change in ambient temperature and by the tactile stimulation caused by the new environment. All of these factors are normal respiratory center stimuli.

The first breath marks the end of fetal life and the beginning of the postnatal period. Lung inflation, in response to the numerous strong stimuli, must occur within a few minutes of placental separation. Measurements of the effort needed initially to inflate the fluid-filled fetal lung have shown that intrathoracic negative pressures in the range of -60 to -80 cm H_2O are required. Once air is retained within the lung and the fluid is absorbed, the effort of breathing is reduced to the range of -8 to -12 cm H_2O pressure.[3]

The inflation of the lungs is the first and the most important step of the cascade. If ventilation occurs spontaneously, the calf will quickly be able to sustain itself. With air in the lung the pulmonary vascular resistance will rapidly decrease as the vessels dilate in response to the increased oxygen and the decreased carbon dioxide tensions. The reduction in pulmonary vascular resistance and the concomitant increase in pulmonary blood flow are the second step of the cascade. Vasoactive kinins, which are released from the aerated lung, further cause the pulmonary vessels to dilate and also cause constriction of the ductus arteriosus and umbilical vessels.[3]

As the resistance to blood flow into the lungs decreases, right atrial pressure also decreases. Simultaneously, increased blood flow into the left atrium and increased systemic vascular resistance due to constriction in the umbilical arteries cause functional closure of the foramen ovale. At this point, the newborn calf has switched from the fetal circulatory pattern to the independent pulmonary and cardiovascular systems of the adult.

NEWBORN RESPIRATORY DISTRESS OF THE CALF

Full-term, normally developed calves may exhibit signs of respiratory distress immediately following birth. Some of the causes for this syndrome have been identified. As indicated previously, the respiratory center of the brain is stimulated by changes in the blood's oxygen and carbon dioxide levels. Dystocia can cause the calf to become severely hypoxic and acidotic. With severe hypoxia or acidosis the ability of the calf to respond and to initiate ventilation diminishes until the calf is unable to generate the large negative pressures needed to displace the lung fluid.[1] Weakened calves are often delivered following dystocias or when cesarean sections have been performed because of the large calf size.

Another cause of weak, ineffectively ventilating calves is the breech presentation. It is believed that placental blood flow becomes disrupted while the calf's head is still within the uterus or vagina. When delivery is prolonged, the blood gas changes become severe, resulting in the unresponsive weakened calf. Any factor that causes disruption of placental blood flow during the birth process will lead to fetal depression.

In humans, respiratory distress syndrome of the newborn is associated with immaturity of the lung. This is most frequently a problem with premature infants. The immature infant lacks sufficient amounts of surfactant in the lung. This deficiency causes the alveoli to be unstable. In order to sustain these infants, they are intubated and maintained on mechanical ventilators until the lungs produce enough surfactant to remain inflated. Some apparently full-term calves may be born lacking surfactant. The initial resuscitation procedures will be the same but continued mechanical ventilation will be required. This type of intensive neonatal support is beyond the scope of this article and of most veterinary hospitals. These calves not only fail to initiate adequate ventilation, but they also die if ventilation support is terminated.

RESUSCITATION PROCEDURES

As soon as the fetus has been delivered, a series of evaluations need to be performed. If the calf begins to fail in its conversion from a fetus to a neonate, resuscitation must be instituted immediately. After initially cleaning the face, nares and oral pharynx of mucous and fetal membranes, the heart rate, mucous membrane color and respiratory efforts should be evaluated.[2] The results of the initial evaluation will be quite variable, depending on the vitality of the calf, but it is important to establish the basis for future evaluations.

Calves with weak or slow heart beats and pale mucous membranes and lacking any ventilatory effort should be immediately resuscitated. If ventilation is shallow, erratic or labored, the calf should be closely monitored, and the veterinarian should be prepared to intubate the calf. Strong vigorous calves should be rechecked every 30 seconds and intubated if respiratory distress begins to occur. The success of the resuscitation is dependent upon early support before cardiovascular failure occurs.

The first step in ventilatory support is to place an endotracheal tube into the trachea.[1] Attempts to inflate the lungs by blowing through the calf's nose or by using a mask will result in air filling the stomach, since the resistance to stomach inflation is less than the resistance to displacement of the lung liquid.

In order to quickly and atraumatically intubate a calf it is important to understand the anatomy of the upper airway. The bovine larynx is dome shaped and easily moveable. The rounded edges of the arytenoid cartilages allow the endotracheal tube to slide into the esophagus. This is especially true if the alignment of the larynx and the endotracheal tube is not straight. The calf's head should be positioned so that the tip of the nose is in a straight line with the thoracic inlet. Extension of the head will straighten the airway. Care must also be taken to keep the head and chest in the same plane. Intubation around a bend is usually difficult to accomplish. Placement of the calf in sternal recumbency with the head pulled upward provides the best visualization for intubation. This position does require an assistant to hold the calf. Intubation of the trachea can be performed with the calf in lateral recumbency. The head and neck must still be extended to straighten the airway.

Blind intubation in the calf is more difficult than intubation done while visualizing the laryngeal opening. For this reason it is recommended that a simple laryngoscope be used to ensure rapid, atraumatic placement of the endotracheal tube. An equine sweat scraper can be used as the laryngoscope blade. The aluminum scraper should be straightened slightly and then covered with Elasticon tape to prevent the sharp edges from cutting the delicate tissues of the calf.

Several light sources are available to illuminate the larynx during intubation. A long-shaft pen light provides the best illumination without blocking the clinician's visualization of the larynx. Summitt Hill Labs (PO Box 1, Avalon, NJ 08202) and Concept Inc. (21707 US 19 South, Clearwater, FL 33516) each sell this type of light. The lighted tip of the laryngoscope blade should be placed on the base of the tongue. The epiglottis and larynx will be seen immediately in front of the light.

The endotracheal tube is passed through the mouth and placed on top of the epiglottis. Gentle but forceful advancement of the tube will place the endotracheal tube tip against the larynx. Often, the endotracheal tube will slide into the trachea without resistance, but occasionally gentle pressure and rotation are necessary for the tube to separate the vocal folds and to enter the trachea.

To facilitate manipulation of the tube, a rigid wire stylet inside of the endotracheal tube is necessary. Stylets can be made out of an aluminum splint rod or coat hanger wire. A rubber stopper should be used on the stylet to prevent the wire from extending beyond the cuffed end of the tube.

Most calves have tracheas large enough to accommodate a 7 mm ID (inside diameter) endotracheal tube. However, very small calves may require a 5.5 mm ID tube. Both size tubes are inexpensive and available from many sources.

Following intubation, the calf should be ventilated.[1] Inflation of the fetal lungs will be difficult until the lung liquid is absorbed through the alveoli. Several commercial ventilators are available and are described in this book in the section on resuscitation of foals. However, it is possible to inflate the lungs of the neonate by blowing through the endotracheal tube. This is often the only readily available source for positive pressure ventilation.

Most full-term calves will readily convert to the neonatal circulatory pattern following several deep breaths. A few calves will require sustained ventilatory support for the lungs to remain filled with air. Once the calf begins to breathe on its own and is able to move a sizable forceful volume of air through the endotracheal tube, ventilatory support can be stopped. The endotracheal tube should remain in place until the calf strongly objects to the presence of the tube. Swallowing, coughing and the ability to hold its head up are signs that the endotracheal tube is no longer needed.

Once intubation and lung inflation have been accomplished, additional methods of postpartum care can be utilized. Since heat loss can rapidly occur in newborns because of evaporation and convection, care should be taken to keep the calf warm and dry. Hypothermic infants are unable to respond to normal amounts of stimulation and frequently will not suckle or breathe adequately.

Dextrose-containing fluids can be given intravenously to the calf to provide a readily available energy source. Forced feeding of calves that lack strong reflex responses may result in pulmonary aspiration of the colostrum. Furthermore, if the calf is hypothermic, its ability to digest and to absorb milk-based nutrients will be markedly slowed.

In summary, weak calves should be intubated and ventilated to facilitate the conversion from the fetal to the neonatal circulatory pattern. Newborns must be kept at their normal body temperature and may require intravenous dextrose fluids for energy support.

References

1. Brunson DB: Ventilatory support of the newborn calf. Com Cont Ed 3:S47, 1981.
2. Drost M: Perinatal care of the calf. In Current Therapy in Theriogenology. Philadelphia, WB Saunders Co, 1980, pp 274–276.
3. Murray JF: The Normal Lung. Philadelphia, WB Saunders Co, 1976, chap 1, pp 1–14.
4. Oxender WD, Newman LE, Morrow DA: Factors influencing dairy calf mortality in Michigan. JAVMA 162:458, 1973.

Passive Transfer of Immunity in Calves

Michelle M. LeBlanc
University of Florida,
Gainesville, Florida

IMPORTANCE OF COLOSTRAL IMMUNOGLOBULIN TRANSFER

The importance of passive immunity through colostral absorption from the mother to the newborn calf during the first hours of life cannot be overemphasized. It is so critical that it is likely to determine how well or how poorly the individual will perform during its life. Calves are born essentially agammaglobulinemic, since transplacental transfer of immunity from the dam does not occur. Immunologic competence is present at birth, but endogenous antibody production does not reach protective levels in the calf until 1 month of age, with maximum levels at 2 to 3 months. Initial protection against disease is provided by passive transfer of immunoglobulins from the dam via colostrum.

Colostrum consists of the accumulated secretions of the mammary gland over the last few weeks of pregnancy together with proteins transferred from the maternal blood stream under the influence of estrogens and progesterone. Concentration of immunoglobulins in the mammary gland begins 5 weeks prior to parturition, reaching maximum levels approximately 3 weeks later. Colostrum contains the immunoglobulins IgG_1, IgM and IgA. IgG_1 accounts for 75 to 85 per cent of the total, and most of it is transferred from the serum of the dam. Sixty per cent of IgA is locally synthesized, while IgM comes from both serum and the mammary gland.

Circulating immunoglobulins are necessary for protection against septicemia. They do not prevent diarrhea, since they presumably do not reach the lumen of the intestine in protective amounts. However, high serum levels of IgG and IgA reduce the severity of diarrhea by preventing massive outpouring of fluids and electrolytes into the intestinal lumen.[1] Conversely, high amounts of intestinal immunoglobulins protect the calf against diarrhea but not against septicemia. Neutrophil phagocytosis is much more active in colostrum-fed calves, and these calves have higher total leukocyte counts than those deprived of colostrum. Finally, colostrum is high in vitamins A, D and E, which are present in very low levels in the newborn calf.

ABSORPTION OF IMMUNOGLOBULINS

Immunoglobulins are absorbed intact through the wall of the small intestine of the neonatal calf. Absorption is most efficient in the jejunum and ileum and occurs by pinocytosis on the gut side of the epithelial cells and by exocytosis on the lamina propria side.[4] The ability of the calf's intestine to absorb immunoglobulins is time dependent, decreasing from 100 per cent open at birth to closure, approximately 24 hours later. Gut closure time is different for each class of immunoglobulins. Although immunoglobulin can be absorbed for varying amounts of time, this absorption occurs at a decreasing rate. IgG can be absorbed for 27 hours, IgA for 22 hours and IgM for only 16 hours. A calf that nurses for the first time at 10 to 12 hours of age could acquire high levels of IgG and IgA but little IgM.[2] Since serum IgM is required for protection against septicemia due to *Escherichia coli,* those calves with low IgM levels are very susceptible to septicemia. Pinocytosis is not specific for immunoglobulins, hence a variety of macromolecules can be absorbed. In studies in which enterotoxigenic *E. coli* bacteria were fed prior to colostrum feeding, immunoglobulin absorption was inhibited. This suggests that ingestion of macromolecules, including immunoglobulins, may activate the closure process.[6] Almost all colostrum-deprived calves that die do so because of *E. coli* septicemia.[9] The same is true of calves that have received colostrum but fail to absorb immunoglobulins.

Studies have shown that 2 liters may be the amount of colostrum needed to activate closure of all absorption sites. The calf should receive the colostrum as soon as possible after parturition, with a second feeding within 12 hours of birth. It appears that a second feeding displaces colostrum from the higher parts of the gastrointestinal tract into the jejunum and ileum, where maximum absorption takes place.

Factors That Influence Absorption

The ultimate level of serum immunoglobulins obtained will depend on the total mass of immunoglobulins absorbed. This mass is a function of concentration of immunoglobulins in colostrum and the total amount ingested during the maximum period of absorption. Concentration is affected by leakage of colostrum prior to parturition, parity, length of dry period and poor husbandry. Higher levels of immunoglobulins have been measured in colostrum from pluriparous dams versus first-calf heifers. A marked depressant effect on colostrum yield due to poor husbandry has been reported in beef cows.[1, 3] Several factors affect ingestion of colostrum. Calves, weak and traumatized at birth as a result of dystocia, will be unable to suck. Abnormal teat conformation, a pendulous udder or poor mothering ability will cause the calf to spend more time teat-seeking before suckling, thereby receiving colostrum at a much later hour. Increased efficiency of immunoglobulin absorption has been reported when the calf is allowed to remain with its dam for the first 24 hours.[11] Ingestion of adequate quantities of colostrum within a few hours of birth is necessary owing to progressive gut closure.

DETERMINATION OF IMMUNOGLOBULIN LEVELS

Several procedures are available for evaluation of serum immunoglobulin levels in the neonatal calf. The most accurate measurements are obtained by direct measurement of immunoglobulins using single radial immunodiffusion or paper electrophoresis. Indirect assessment of serum immunoglobulins by means of the refractometer, zinc sulfate turbidity test, sodium sulfite precipitation test or glutaraldehyde coagulation test provides accurate results in the field. These procedures are most valuable if used before calves become ill. They are excellent tools in epidemiologic investigations to determine if newborn calves are receiving sufficient good quality colostrum early enough.

Reliable immunoglobulin estimations may be obtained in the field with use of the refractometer. A direct linear correlation exists between the refractive index of serum and immunoglobulin concentration.[1] Hemoconcentration will give artificially high readings. Total protein concentration over 6.0 gm/dl is considered adequate immunoglobulin absorption in the absence of dehydration. Calves with a protein concentration of less than 5.0 gm/dl have minimum absorption, while levels between 5 and 6 gm/dl are marginal.[4]

The zinc sulfate turbidity test estimates immunoglobulin levels by means of their precipitation. Interpretation is made in units (0 to greater than

20) by visually evaluating the degree of turbidity, which is proportional to immunoglobulin concentration. Hemolyzed blood samples, hemoconcentration and use of plasma will give artificially high readings. The sodium sulfite precipitation test is similar to the zinc sulfate turbidity test, but its results are not significantly altered when hemolyzed serum is used. Reagents can be obtained as a commercial kit from Veterinary Medical Research and Development, Pullman, WA 99163.[5]

The 10 per cent glutaraldehyde coagulation test has been proposed for use as a field screening test to diagnose colostrum-deprived calves. Ten per cent gluteraldehyde fails to coagulate serum immunoglobulins in concentrations of less than 400 mg/dl, gives equivocal results between 400 and 600 mg/dl and coagulates sera with concentrations greater than 600 mg/dl. Experimental test-negative calves (no coagulation) had significantly higher mortality rates than test-positive calves.[11]

MANAGEMENT OF COLOSTRUM FEEDING

Immunoglobulins are most important in *preventing* bacterial septicemia and diarrhea and have little effect after infection is established. Normal passive transfer of immunoglobulin is best accomplished by feeding 2 liters of colostrum to calves within 6 hours of birth, with continuation of colostrum feedings for the first 3 days. Although absorption of globulin is greatly reduced after 24 hours, its local protective action in the intestine against diarrhea justifies its maximal utilization. Warmed colostrum (39°C) may be fed from a nipple bottle that has an orifice small enough to require effort by the calf when sucking. Force feeding should be implemented only when necessary, by means of an esophageal probe or stomach tube. At 5 days of age, calves should be fed from an individual open-faced pail to discourage their nursing one another. Due to the excellent nutritive value of nonmastitic fresh milk (milk taken during the second through sixth milking postpartum), it should be fed to the calf for at least the first week following colostrum consumption. Colostrum and fresh milk must be measured prior to feeding to avoid diarrhea due to overconsumption. Calves need to be fed 2 liters daily. Colostrum may be fed soured, which seems to reduce the incidence and severity of this diarrhea. Offensive odors, putrefaction and calf refusal are problems encountered with feeding of fermented colostrum.

Although colostrum is slowly produced over a 5-week dry cow period, at calving the immunoglobulin supply is rapidly diluted. As early as 6 hours after the first milking, 33 per cent of the immunoglobulin is lost and after 24 hours up to 66 per cent.[7] Only colostrum taken from the first milking can be considered immunoglobulin rich. Management systems, tailored to fit the individual needs of farms, should be improvised to collect and to store this colostrum. Low bacterial count, nonmastitic, high quality colostrum pooled from several pluriparous cows may be frozen and stored in labeled and dated half-gallon or gallon containers. Immunoglobulin content of colostrum may be quantitated with a colostrometer, a hydrometer that measures the specific gravity of colostrum. Specific gravity greater than 1.046 indicates adequate globulin content.[10]

References

1. Blood DC, Henderson JA, Radostits OM: Veterinary Medicine. 5th ed. Philadelphia, Lea & Febiger, 1979, pp 66–74.
2. Drost M: Perinatal care of the calf. *In* Morrow DA (ed): Current Therapy in Theriogenology. Philadelphia, WB Saunders Co, 1980.
3. Logan EF: The influence of husbandry on colostrum yield and immunoglobulin concentration in beef cattle. Br Vet J 133:120, 1977.
4. McGuire TC, Adams DS: Failure of colostral immunoglobulin transfer to calves: Prevalence and diagnosis. Comp Cont Ed 4:35, 1982.
5. Pfeiffer NE, McGuire TC, et al.: Quantitation of bovine immunoglobulins: Comparison of single radial immunodiffusion, zinc sulfate turbidity, serum electrophoresis and refractometer methods. Am J Vet Res 38:693, 1977.
6. Proceedings, Seminars on Recent Advances in Neonatal Diarrhea in Farm Animals. Presented Oct. 27, 1980, University of Florida, Gainesville, Florida. Bristol, Beecham Laboratories, 1980.
7. Roy JH: Symposium: Disease prevention in calves. J Dairy Sci 63:650, 1980.
8. Selman IE: The absorption of colostral globulins by newborn calves. Ann Rec Vet 4:213, 1973.
9. Selman IE, McEwan AD, et al.: Serum immune globulin concentration of calves left with their dams for the first two days of life. J Comp Pathol 80:419, 1970.
10. Stott GH: New device measures disease protection in colostrum. Hoards Dairyman 126:149, 1981.
11. Tennant B, Baldwin BH, et al.: Use of the glutaraldehyde coagulation test for detection of hypogammaglobulinemia in neonatal calves. JAVMA 174:848, 1979.

The Metritis-Pyometra Complex

Jerry D. Olson, D.V.M., M.S.
Katherine N. Bretzlaff, D.V.M., M.S.
University of Illinois,
Urbana, Illinois

Robert G. Mortimer, D.V.M., M.S.
Leslie Ball, D.V.M., M.S.
Colorado State University,
Fort Collins, Colorado

Uterine infections are a major cause of economic loss to the cattle industry, with both short- and long-term losses occurring. Short-term losses are associated with systemic disease of the cow and occur mostly in cows during the first few weeks postpartum. In most herds only a small percentage of cows acquire a life-threatening toxic or septic metritis. However, 50 to 75 per cent may develop pyrexia and anorexia, resulting in weight loss and decreased milk production. A 20 to 30 per cent reduction of intake in dry matter and a 15 to 20 per cent decrease in milk production are typical.

Long-term losses are associated with decreased reproductive efficiency, which includes more days open, more services per conception and increased culling for poor reproductive performance. These factors increase losses from reduced milk production, higher insemination costs, increased replacement costs and reduced genetic progress within herds because of forced culling of superior dams and loss of voluntary culling.

The incidence of uterine infection is influenced by calving management, general sanitation, pathogenic organisms, endocrine factors, lactation, nutrition and other environmental stress factors. The incidence of severe endometritis has ranged from 6 to 26 per cent in California dairy herds. In selected dairy herds in Colorado the incidence of pyometra has varied from 2 to 13 per cent.

DEFINITION AND CLASSIFICATION OF THE POSTPARTUM PERIOD

In this article the postpartum period is defined as the period from parturition to complete uterine involution. Most classification schemes for uterine infections have considered only the character of the uterine discharge. Palpation findings, interval from parturition to examination, endocrine status and character of discharges are also important because they influence prognosis and therapeutics. Consequently, the following intervals of the postpartum period are used for definition and discussion of uterine infections.

The puerperal period begins at the time of calving and continues until the pituitary gland becomes responsive to GnRH at 7 to 14 days postpartum. The diseases commonly seen during this period include retained fetal membranes (RFM) and puerperal metritis. Puerperal metritis varies from a mild to severe, life-threatening disease. Severe forms are described as septic, toxic or even gangrenous, and most delay involution of the uterus. This period is critical because diseases incurred during this time may result in chronic disease and infertility later in the postpartum period.

The intermediate period begins with increased pituitary sensitivity to GnRH and continues until the first postpartum ovulation. Its length is variable, depending on many factors that influence time of ovulation, such as age, nutrition, puerperal infections, uterine bacterial ecology and endocrine status. During this time, infections with pathogenic bacteria are reduced or eliminated in normal cows. Uterine infections that persist are often referred to as metritis or endometritis and are usually signaled by a purulent vulvar discharge and an enlarged uterus, which may contain palpable fluid.

The postovulatory period begins at the time of the first ovulation and lasts until involution is complete, at about 45 days postpartum in normal cows. Diseases of the postovulatory period include chronic metritis, endometritis and pyometra.

FACTORS IN UTERINE DISEASE

Bacteriology. The uterus of the cow has been cultured extensively. Uterine cultures have been taken from cows with abnormal vulvar discharges and from both gravid and nongravid uteri following slaughter. These approaches to bacteriology have varied but until recently have used only aerobic culture techniques. Recent evidence shows that the uterus is an anaerobic environment. Consequently, pathogenic anaerobic bacteria were overlooked in earlier studies. We have studied 20 cows with RFM and 20 normal postpartum dairy cows. The results are presented in Figures 1 to 5 and in Table 1. Bacteria were grouped for discussion according to their cultural characteristics (Table 1).

The number and type of bacteria recovered by culture varied with interval from calving. Coliforms and incidental bacteria were frequently isolated in the early postpartum period but decreased over time (Figs. 1 and 2). Isolations of *Corynebacterium pyogenes* (now *Actinomyces pyogenes*) first increased then decreased over time except in cows that developed pyometra (Fig. 3). In these animals

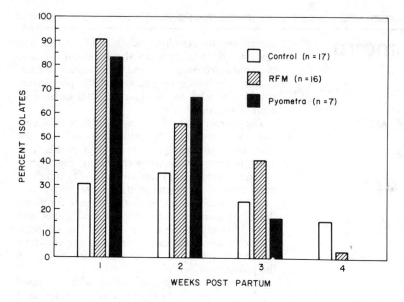

Figure 1. Incidence of coliforms.

Figure 2. Incidence of incidental bacteria.

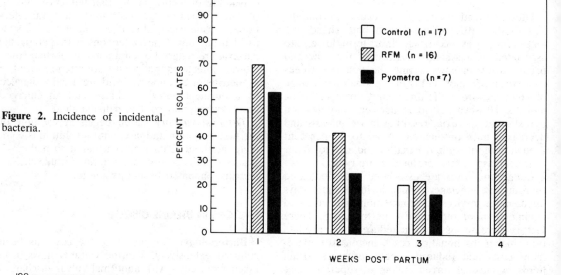

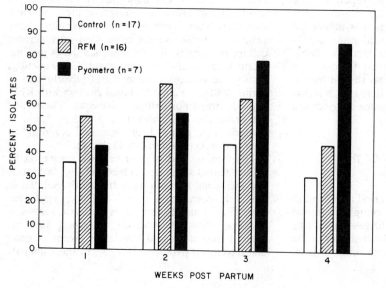

Figure 3. Incidence of *C. pyogenes*.

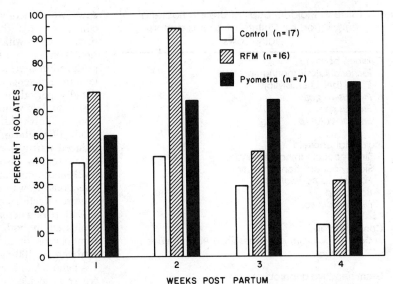

Figure 4. Incidence of gram-negative anaerobes.

isolations increased first then reached a high-level plateau, where they remained.

The frequency of isolation of gram-negative and gram-positive anaerobic bacteria is presented in Figures 4 and 5. Gram-positive anaerobic bacteria were isolated significantly more often in cows that later developed pyometra than in controls or in cows with RFM that did not develop pyometra.

Isolation of gram-negative anaerobic bacteria followed the same pattern as isolation of *C. pyogenes* (Figs. 3 and 4). This parallel relationship is evidence that these organisms work together in causing severe disease of the uterus. In addition, pyometra is more consistently produced in experimental cows when combinations of these bacteria are infused together into the uterus.

Thus, the flora of the postpartum uterus form an ecological system. Within this system, *C. pyogenes*, *Fusobacterium* and *Bacteroides* sp. act synergisti-

cally to enhance disease. Histopathology and aerobic bacteriology have demonstrated that *C. pyogenes* is the most significant pathogen of the intermediate and postovulatory periods. The bacterial ecology of extrauterine anaerobic disease in cattle and other species may be similar to that of the uterus of the cow; consequently, insight might be gained by studying anaerobic models of pathogenic bacteria that flourish in anaerobic environments outside the uterus. Such comparisons and experimental animal models have demonstrated a synergism between *C. pyogenes*, *Fusobacterium*, and *Bacteroides* sp. Many other bacteria intermittently inhabit the uterus in the postpartum period, but most have little effect on fertility. However, they can influence responses of pathogenic bacteria to therapeutic agents, since some elaborate substances such as penicillinase protect other sensitive organisms.

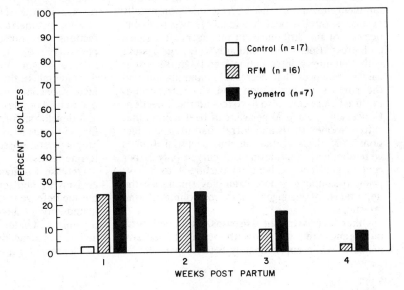

Figure 5. Incidence of clostridia.

Table 1. Major Groups of Uterine Bacteria Recovered by Culture of 40 Postpartum Dairy Cows

Coliform bacteria
 Escherichia coli (nonhemolytic)
 E. coli (beta-hemolytic)
 Proteus vulgaris
 Proteus sp.
 Enterobacter sp.

Incidental bacteria
 Streptococci (alpha hemolytic)
 Staphylococci (nonhemolytic)
 Pasteurella haemolytica
 Bacillus sp.
 Diphtheroid sp.

Corynebacteria
 Corynebacterium pyogenes (now *Actinomyces pyogenes*)

Gram-negative anaerobic bacteria
 Bacteroides sp. *(fragilis)*
 Bacteroides sp. *(nonfragilis)*
 B. melaninogenicus
 B. oralis
 Fusobacterium sp.
 Veillonella sp.

Gram-positive anaerobic bacteria
 Clostridium perfringens
 C. sporogenes
 Clostridium sp.

Unsanitary Calving Conditions. If the calving environment is dusty or wet or is often used without sanitation, pathogenic bacteria increase in numbers. Damp, cold calving quarters also stress the cow and lower her resistance to disease. Under such conditions, the likelihood of invasion of the uterus and multiplication of large numbers of pathogenic bacteria is increased. Specific bacteria such as *Clostridium* sp., *C. pyogenes* and gram-negative anaerobic bacteria may become seeded in an area, making it difficult to intervene in a dystocia without introducing them into the uterus. Uterine infection usually occurs less often in beef than in dairy cows, probably because of the differences in management systems and stress. Beef cows frequently calve on pasture with minimal intervention and nurse their calves—practices that decrease contamination and the stresses of parturition and the puerperium. Pastured dairy cows also have less uterine infection. Conversely, nearly 50 per cent of beef heifers that calved in open sheds and corrals had uterine infections at 25 days postpartum, but bacterial isolates were obtained from uterine contents of only 29 per cent of beef cows calving on pasture 1 to 8 days prior to sampling. These examples emphasize the importance of management in controlling uterine infections.

Other Periparturient Diseases. Retained fetal membranes are associated with increased puerperal metritis. While approximately 5 to 15 per cent of cows with uncomplicated deliveries may acquire clinical metritis, disease rates of 50 to 90 per cent occur in cows with RFM. Consequently, periparturient conditions that increase RFM also increase postpartum uterine disease, e.g., vitamin A or selenium deficiencies, excessive weight gain during the dry period, multiple births, heat stress, short gestation, late winter and early spring calving, abortions, stillbirths, dystocia, increasing age, high milk production, uterine atony, milk fever, hydrops and induced parturition. These cause uterine subinvolution that is associated with increased infection levels and hinderance of uterine ability to eliminate infections. Cows with RFM are also more likely to acquire infections because RFM have a wick effect.

Endocrine Factors. Endocrine patterns have been evaluated in both pre- and postpartum cows. A combination of low progesterone (<3 ng/ml) and estrogen (< 100 pg/ml) or of high progesterone (> 7.9 ng/ml) alone are associated with a tenfold increase in incidence of RFM. Lower levels of prostaglandin $F_2\alpha$ ($PGF_2\alpha$) also occurred in the cotyledons of cows with RFM. Thus, endocrine chemistry plays an important role in release of the placenta and the associated risk of more metritis and pyometra. Once parturition occurs, reproductive hormones are decreased until the pituitary gland becomes sensitive to the gonadotropin-releasing factors, which may occur as early as 7 or as late as 14 days after calving.

Suckled beef cows have a different postpartum physiology than dairy cows. Recovery of pituitary responsiveness to GnRH is delayed until about 14 days postpartum in suckled beef cows. Yet plasma levels of luteinizing hormone (LH) do not rise and fluctuate in beef cows until 2 to 3 weeks before the first postpartum estrus, which ranges between 30 to 100 days after parturition. Suckling probably suppresses the release of pituitary LH needed to stimulate the first postpartum ovulation. This would explain the prolonged interval between calving and first ovulation in beef cows. Because they cycle late, beef cows might be expected to be less able to rid themselves of postpartum uterine infections. The reverse is true. Dairy cows that have RFM and develop pyometra ovulate early, before uterine infections are controlled and uterine fluids are expelled (Fig. 6). In cows with an aberrant puerperium, a longer preovulatory period may not be detrimental. In the postovulatory period, endocrine factors become important again in the metritis-pyometra complex. Then some cows ovulate early and develop a corpus luteum (CL), and the uterus fills with purulent exudate. This creates a pseudopregnant state associated with high blood progesterone levels.

Defense Mechanisms. Phagocytosis of microorganisms by neutrophils is important in the bovine uterine defense system. This defense system is stimulated about 2 days postpartum by invading microorganisms. Under pathologic conditions, such as delivery of dead or weak calves, phagocytosis can be depressed for several days to several weeks.

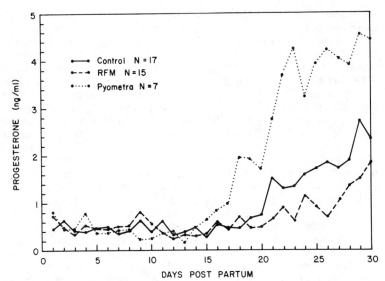

Figure 6. Serum progesterone in postpartum cows, including normal, pyometritic and RFM cows.

Trauma to the genital tract by removal of RFM and by obstetric procedures also depresses phagocytosis. Possibly a number of antibiotics commonly placed in the uterus might also depress phagocytosis because of irritation. In vitro the tetracyclines and chloramphenicol both depress phagocytic activity of neutrophils isolated from milk.

Leukocytosis is stimulated by estrogen and inhibited by progesterone, contributing to the ability of the uterus in the follicular phase to resist infection. This is the basis of recommendations of some workers to treat the cow with exogenous estrogens during the puerperium, a practice now proven unproductive.

Poorly Selected Uterine Treatments. Many of the antimicrobials and disinfectants infused into the bovine uterus lower the uterine defense mechanisms and irritate and denude the endometrium. Irritation of an inflamed postpartum uterus is of questionable value. It is difficult to document exact effects of infusing various substances into the postpartum uterus because their effects are confounded by other processes that occur in the uterus during the puerperium. However, exacerbation of localized metritis into perimetritis with adhesions sometimes occurs following intrauterine infusion. Irritating substances in the oviducts may also result in tubal inflammation and perimetritis. Severe straining occurs if compounds containing irritating substances such as iodine either are placed in or reflux into the vagina. Although this effect is usually transient, the added stress and local irritation may prolong genital disease.

Physical Manipulation. Excessive manipulation of the postpartum genital tract, either per rectum or per vagina should be avoided, especially in cows with systemic signs of illness. The inflamed uteri of these cows are more friable and subject to transudation and adhesions. Local examination of the reproductive tract is risky in cows or heifers with severe vaginal swelling or lacerations. If local examination is necessary, strict hygiene should be used and repeated manual entries should be avoided. Movement of the hand inside the uterus may abrade the epithelium and reduce its ability to wall off infection; generous lubrication helps reduce damage, discomfort and stress to the cow.

Nutritional Aspects. Metritis and RFM are more prevalent in overfed cows that become excessively fat before calving. Improper ratios of calcium to phosphorus fed prior to calving and deficiencies of vitamins A and E and selenium increase the incidence of RFM and metritis. The effects of underconditioning are less well defined unless they are extreme, but debilitated cows are probably less resistant to puerperal infections.

UTERINE INVOLUTION

Because veterinarians are often asked to examine cows in early stages of involution, they must be able to appreciate and to evaluate the rapid changes that take place in uterine and cervical size and in character of discharges and judge whether or not involution is progressing normally. Otherwise, normal cows are often treated needlessly.

Physical Involution. The entire uterus is impossible to palpate per rectum at the beginning of the postpartum period, but if involution is normal, the uterine wall is thick and longitudinal rugae can be palpated on its surface. The diseased uterus is more likely to be smooth, flaccid and thin walled. By 10 to 15 days the entire uterus can usually be palpated. At first the uterus is larger than the cervix, but by about 15 days both uterus and cervix are about 70 mm in diameter. The uterus continues to involute more rapidly than the cervix. The horns usually vary between 20 and 30 mm by days 30 to 40 postpartum. Grossly, the cervix is the last structure to involute completely. In primigravid cows, it is usually between 25 and 30 mm and in older cows, 30 to 45 mm in diameter by 40 to 50 days postpartum. Epithelization of caruncular sites is usually complete between 40 and 50 days postpartum.

Uterine Fluids. Uterine fluids are expelled quite rapidly during the first 15 days after parturition. Normally, all palpable fluids are expelled by 18 days postpartum; however, some cows may continue to expel abnormal fluids 20 to 30 days postpartum.

The character of the uterine fluids also gives insight into the normality of involution. For a day or two after calving, the expelled fluids are serosanguineous, but when caruncular dissolution begins, their character changes. As caruncular sites degenerate, variable amounts of blood are expelled into the uterine lumen, and discharges become thicker. If fluid expulsion is delayed, the color of the blood may change from red to dark brown and be interlaced with white material from dissolution of caruncles. This white material may be confused with purulent discharges. Discharges expelled early may be fairly red and may contain small amounts of exudate as well, since most cows have some bacterial infection. As long as the discharge does not become foul smelling or fetid from putrefaction, involution usually proceeds without complication.

Too often an enlarged uterus and cervix palpated early in the postpartum period and lochial discharges containing some white material are interpreted to be abnormal when involution is normal. If fluids are gone by 18 days postpartum, it is unlikely that intrauterine treatment will be necessary but reexamination may be indicated in slow-involuting cows to make certain pyometra does not develop.

PATHOPHYSIOLOGY OF METRITIS AND PYOMETRA

The Puerperal Period. During the puerperal period, mixed populations of bacteria are present in the uterus (Figs. 1 to 5). Their numbers increase for several days then decrease as involution progresses. If conditions are favorable, *C. pyogenes, Fusobacterium necrophorum* and *Bacteroides* sp. become established (Figs. 3 and 5). Coliform and incidental bacteria are decreased in number or eliminated from the uterus during the puerperal period, especially in cows that develop more persistent infections with *C. pyogenes* and gram-negative anaerobes (Figs. 1 and 2).

Life-threatening infections occur almost exclusively during the puerperal period when cows become affected by septic, toxic or gangrenous metritis. Toxic and gangrenous metritis are often associated with clostridial infections. Eventually, infections with *C. pyogenes* and gram-negative anaerobic bacteria can become localized and cause a more chronic type of metritis. The coliform and incidental bacteria apparently play no significant role in causing chronic infertility, although in the early stages they may be associated with septic or toxic metritis.

The Intermediate Period. In the intermediate period bacterial populations are reduced in the uterus of normal cows, but in abnormal cows fluids and pathogenic bacteria remain until the first ovulation takes place. If large numbers of bacteria persist during the intermediate period and fluids are not expelled, subinvolution results. Existing metritis becomes chronic in the intermediate period.

The Postovulatory Period. In the postovulatory period chronic metritis may persist long after the causative bacteria are eliminated from the uterus. The bacteria that seem to be associated with more severe infertility are *C. pyogenes, Fusobacterium necrophorum* and *Bacteroides* sp. These bacteria stimulate exudation of large numbers of leukocytes, resulting in purulent exudate. If ovulation occurs before the uterus has expelled all of the exudate and debris that is present in cases of subinvolution, the corpus luteum that develops may be retained, the purulent exudate may be increased in volume, the estrous cycle may be interrupted and pyometra may be perpetuated.

DISEASES OF OTHER REPRODUCTIVE ORGANS

Oviducts. Primary lesions of the oviducts are uncommon, but up to 70 per cent of cows with purulent endometritis and pyometra have histologic evidence of involvement of the oviducts. These lesions are consequences of infection ascending from the uterus.

Ovaries and Bursa. Ovaritis and ovarian bursitis are also sequelae to uterine infection. The combined prevalence of involvement of these extrauterine structures usually ranges from 10 to 15 per cent. This is greater by more than half than the percentage that can be detected by per rectum palpation.

Course of Extrauterine Infection. Inflammation of the oviducts, ovaries and ovarian bursa may be resolved, and fertility may be restored in many cows. However, permanent functional impairment of oviductal epithelium may prevent successful fertilization and ova transport in other cows. Intratubal or bursal adhesions or inspissated pus may provide physical barriers to fertilization.

Occasionally, extragenital adhesions occur following septic metritis, generalized peritonitis or rough manipulations of the tract. Adhesions incorporating ovaries, oviducts and surrounding structures may also impose physical restrictions on the genital tract and cause sterility.

PHARMACOLOGICAL CONSIDERATIONS

Penicillin. Penicillin acts by interfering with bacterial cell wall synthesis. The primary mechanism of resistance to penicillin is production of penicillinase, an inducible enzyme that is released into the environment. This has therapeutic implications. In the mixed bacterial environment of the early post-partum bovine uterus, penicillin-resistant organisms can provide protection for penicillin-sensitive pathogens. Therefore, intra-uterine administration of penicillin in the early and intermediate postpartum period is not likely to be effective, since populations with penicillin-resistant bacteria often exist.

However, by 25 to 30 days postpartum, only *C. pyogenes* and gram-negative anaerobes remain in the uterus of most cows with metritis (Figs. 3 and 4). These bacteria are usually sensitive to intrauterine infusion of penicillin. One million units of intrauterine penicillin G procaine provides therapeutic levels for 30 hours in both the uterine lumen and the endometrium. Dosages of 10,000 to 20,000 IU/lb (dosage recommendations are based upon bacterial susceptibility testing and exceed FDA approved dosages) given systemically provide serum levels higher than 1 μg/ml for 6 to 12 hours in the wall of the uterus. The average minimum inhibitory concentration (MIC) for *C. pyogenes* isolated from the bovine uterus is 1 μg/ml. Clinical observation indicates that once-daily dosage with penicillin is usually effective in treatment of septic puerperal metritis even though serum levels may drop lower than 1 μg/ml for 6 to 12 of the 24 hours. Its effectiveness under these conditions may be the result of a pulse-dose effect.

Oxytetracycline. Oxytetracycline is the tetracycline most commonly used in food animal practice. Its mechanism of action is inhibition of protein synthesis at the level of the ribosome. Resistant bacteria decrease oxytetracycline uptake, an individual cell phenomenon, so one resistant bacterium does not affect adjacent bacteria. Consequently, tetracyclines are likely to be effective in treatment of most of the mixed bacteria that exist in the early postpartum uterus.

Practical considerations in the use of tetracyclines include pharmacokinetics, route of administration and their MIC for various pathogenic bacteria. The average MIC for uterine isolates of *C. pyogenes* was 20.4 μg/ml in one study. Pharmacokinetic studies demonstrate that intravenous dosages of 5 mg/lb administered b.i.d. are necessary to maintain a serum concentration of 5 μg/ml in cattle. Since plasma to uterine tissue concentrations are only slightly higher than 1:1, the pharmacologically desirable concentration of 5 μg/ml is well below the average MIC for uterine isolates of *C. pyogenes,* so systemic therapy would likely be ineffective. In contrast, effective levels of tetracyclines can be easily achieved within the uterine lumen by local therapy. However, the actions of locally administered tetracyclines are limited primarily to the uterine lumen and the endometrium. Therefore, local therapy with tetracyclines alone is of questionable value in the treatment of uterine infections associated with systemic involvement. A second consideration is the vehicle in which the tetracycline is dissolved. Propylene glycol vehicles are less desirable for local treatment because of endometrial irritation than are povidone or polyvinyl pyrrolidine

vehicles. Finally, tetracyclines are active under anaerobic conditions and are not inhibited by pus and blood; both conditions are common to the early postpartum uterus.

Aminoglycosides. Gentamycin, kanamycin, streptomycin and neomycin are examples of aminoglycosides that have been used in treatment of uterine infections. The mechanism of action for aminoglycosides is inhibition of protein synthesis at the level of the ribosome. However, the mechanisms of resistance to aminoglycosides are varied and include not binding the antibiotic to the ribosome, inhibition of antibiotic uptake into the bacterial cell and production of enzymes of degradation. However, the most important consideration in the use of aminoglycosides is that they enter the cell across a proton gradient generated by oxidative phosphorylation, so they work well only under aerobic conditions. In general anaerobic bacteria are resistant to aminoglycosides because the drugs do not enter cells without the required redox-established charge differential across the cell membranes. The important bacteria of puerperal metritis are anaerobic or facultative anaerobes. Comparative field studies of postpartum uterine treatments using neomycin boluses have demonstrated a reduction of fertility in treated animals. Basic pharmacology and results of field trials with aminoglycosides both suggest that these drugs are also poorly suited for intrauterine treatment of anaerobic infections.

Nitrofurazone. Nitrofurazone has, at various times, been available for use in treatment of intrauterine infections as a solution, in suppositories with estradiol and in boluses with urea. One of the primary bovine uterine pathogens, *C. pyogenes,* is very resistant to nitrofurazone; average MIC exceed 590 μg/ml. Commercially available nitrofurazone solutions contain 0.2 per cent of nitrofurazone, which is equivalent to 2000 μg/ml. Thus, the average MIC for *C. pyogenes* is near the concentration of commercial nitrofurazone with no dilution! Furthermore, nitrofurazone is markedly inhibited by blood, pus and bacteria, all factors common to the postpartum uterus. In addition, nitrofurazone is irritating to the endometrium and causes shortened estrous cycles when infused into the uterus of cows in diestrus. In a field trial evaluating treatment of pyometritic cows, nitrofurazone infusion had a significant adverse effect on fertility. Consequently, nitrofurazone is contraindicated in the treatment of uterine infections.

Sulfonamides. Sulfonamides in combination with urea were among the earliest anti-bacterial preparations marketed specifically for intrauterine therapy. The mechanism of action for sulfonamides is competition with para-aminobenzoic acid in the formation of folic acid. Bacterial resistance to sulfonamides is either from increased production of essential metabolites or from development of alternate metabolic pathways for synthesis of essential metabolites. Para-aminobenzoic acid combines with pteryolglutamic acid to form folic acid, which is a coenzyme in several major metabolic pathways.

However, in the postpartum uterus with necrotic tissue debris and dead leukocytes, most of the metabolites derived through para-aminobenzoic acid pathways are readily available in the environment. Consequently, sulfonamides are ineffective therapeutic agents in the postpartum uterus because their effectiveness is negated by available metabolites.

TREATMENT AND CONTROL OF UTERINE INFECTIONS

General Discussion. It is difficult to devise routine treatments for the postpartum cow because of variation in severity of disease and the ability of different cows to resist infection. Economics may dictate routine treatment of cows with metritis, but individual attention would result in optimum response. The majority of cows with mild puerperal metritis do not need treatment. However, in some dairies, individual attention is not practical, so all cows are treated to cover those that would be significantly affected. These treatments are not always best for individual cows.

Several factors are involved when evaluating a cow for treatment. A history of calving date and difficulties, appetite and periparturient disease is essential. A general physical examination is required to determine the severity of the condition. Determination of uterine size and volume of contents, uterine consistency and character of uterine discharges and presence or absence of RFM all aid in choice of proper treatment.

It is a common practice to treat cows on the basis of empirical evidence or simply because treatment in a particular way or with a particular drug is possible. Examples include infusions or placement of boluses containing certain sulfa drugs, neomycin, dilute iodine or nitrofurazone (Furacin) into the uterus. These are detrimental, but each has been widely used in its time as a uterine medication. When a new or untested treatment of the uterus is contemplated, one should at least doubt its efficacy until its effect on fertility is tested in a well-controlled study. Probably many of the concoctions placed in the uterus actually decrease fertility without sterilizing cows. Consequently, many eventually become pregnant, encouraging a continuation of detrimental treatment.

Many factors determine the outcome of antimicrobial therapy in the treatment of uterine disease. An ill-defined factor is the immune response of the host. Another is the ability to attain therapeutic concentrations of the antimicrobial agent in the blood, the uterine wall and the uterine lumen. This is affected by route of administration, form of the agent and pharmacokinetics. Generally, compounds placed in the uterus result in higher concentrations in its lumen and endometrium over longer periods of time than if they are administered parenterally. However, concentrations in the remainder of the uterine wall are lower than those obtained with parenteral administration. To maintain adequate drug concentrations in all tissues, including the oviducts and ovaries, both local and parenteral administration are often needed.

The desired quantity of drug infused is debatable. Small quantities of concentrated solutions infused into the puerperal uterus may not be evenly distributed, especially in cows with RFM. Large quantities may stimulate straining and reflux of some infusate back through the cervix. Therefore, the size of the uterus should be determined before infusion of quantities greater than approximately 120 ml.

Many different formulations of drugs are used for intrauterine infusions. Aqueous solutions are more rapidly and completely absorbed than long-acting preparations, making one-time treatments with aqueous compounds of questionable value. Both Lugol's iodine and oxytetracycline in some vehicles are irritating to the endometrium, while others, such as penicillin, are not. Generally, treatment with excessively irritating substances should be avoided. Some boluses fail to dissolve and act as foreign bodies, retarding involution. Frequently, gelatin capsules filled with antimicrobial powders are inserted into the uterus, but little is known about how well these are dissolved and distributed. A common practice is to use tetracycline powder, directly applied or in gelatin capsules. Yet oxytetracycline, when dissolved in water in a concentrated solution, has an acidic pH and may cause necrosis of the epithelium of the uterus. In spite of this, fertility in most studies has improved following use of tetracyclines in the uterus of postpartum cows with RFM.

Another consideration is the character of uterine contents. There are large volumes of fluid and necrotic tissue in the infected postpartum uterus. This proteinaceous fluid can buffer some compounds such as oxytetracycline, which otherwise might be irritating. This, coupled with the higher pH of metritic exudates and the massive population of microorganisms, can cause antimicrobial dilution, ionization, binding and metabolic inactivation. Consequently, the reduced dosages of antimicrobials frequently used for local treatment of the uterus may be inadequate in puerperal cows.

The Puerperal Period. Retained fetal membranes are a common problem of the early postpartum period and increase the risk of uterine infections. The question of whether to remove RFM manually is not resolved. Some practitioners think it desirable to remove RFM because they act as foreign bodies and can hinder drainage of uterine contents. However, excessive manipulations are stressful to the cow and may traumatize the endometrium, caruncles, and subendometrial tissues and delay involution more than that would occur by leaving them unmolested. Several studies have shown decreased fertility in cows in which RFM were removed, and other studies have shown little benefit. It is generally accepted that removal is contraindicated if RFM are complicated by septic or toxic metritis because in these cows the uterus is friable and more subject to damage. However, a hygienic vaginal examination is appropriate to determine whether or not

RFM are loose in the uterine cavity. If so, gentle removal is probably beneficial.

There is probably no best way to treat all cows with RFM because of variation in their amount and character, the ease of removal, the amount of preexisting trauma and the occurrence of concurrent metabolic or infectious diseases. Individual attention is ideal, with the final decision on handling based on the practitioner's evaluation of the situation. However, in large herds, routine treatments must be devised that can be worked into daily routines. Clearly, the trend in recent years is to make no attempt at removal. However, the goals of suppressing bacterial growth and establishment of uterine drainage must be met by judicious use of antimicrobial agents and gentle traction when indicated.

Whether or not RFM are removed, cows should be treated with 2 to 6 gm of the tetracyclines, the antibiotics of choice for intrauterine therapy in the puerperal period. The vulvar area and the operator's arm should be cleaned and disinfected before powders or boluses are administered. If solutions or suspensions are administered by infusion, care should be taken to prevent traumatization of the uterine wall by the tip of the pipette. Otherwise, abscessation of the body of the uterus can occur.

Treatment should begin immediately on cows with membranes retained more than 12 hours postpartum and should be continued daily until the membranes are expelled. Attempts to remove the membranes should be limited to gentle traction; any greater force is detrimental to fertility. The fact that some dairies are successful with treatment administered every second or third day suggests that some dairies have minimal uterine contamination because of the hygienity of the maternity area.

Cows with puerperal metritis can be divided into two categories: those with and those without systemic involvement. If a cow is anorectic, depressed and febrile, she should be treated systemically as well as locally. Most organisms that cause septic puerperal metritis are susceptible to penicillin, so it is the antibiotic of choice for systemic treatment of affected cows. Clinically, dosages of 10,000 IU or more per pound of body weight have given good results. However, this dose exceeds recommendations on the label of the drug. The uterus of cows with puerperal metritis should also be treated locally with tetracyclines as discussed under RFM. In cows with puerperal metritis without systemic involvement, local therapy with tetracyclines alone is usually adequate. Administration and dosage regimens are the same as those for RFM.

The Intermediate Period. In the intermediate postpartum period uterine infections are primarily localized. The predominant discharge, if observed, is purulent. A common problem of this period is identification of the cow with the uterine infection. Deposits of purulent discharge are often left on the ground when a diseased cow lies down; otherwise, she may have few external signs to identify her. Intrauterine infusion of 1 gm of tetracycline in 20 to 40 ml of sterile water or physiological saline

solution (PSS) is indicated because the uterus of many cows still contains mixed populations of bacteria that may produce penicillinase. Therapy should be continued for a minimum of 3 days.

The Postovulatory Period. The primary diseases of the postovulatory period are either pyometra or metritis caused most often by a mixed infection of *C. pyogenes* and gram-negative anaerobes. The first objective of therapy for pyometra is to cause regression of the corpus luteum and to stimulate uterine evacuation. Estrogens have been used in the past, with estradiol 17β-cypionate (ECP) having a single treatment success rate of 50 to 60 per cent. More recently, treatments with luteolytic prostaglandins have had success rates varying from 80 to 90 per cent. Fertility of cows following evacuation appears to be related to the postpartum interval to treatment. Cows treated at the time of a postpartum examination 21 to 35 days after calving have better overall fertility than contemporaries treated 2 weeks later. Cows that conceive usually do so only after a 60-day lapse following treatment because of the protracted uterine healing time.

The role of local therapy in the treatment of pyometra has not been well defined. However, infusion of nitrofurazone into the uterus following evacuation of pyometritic fluid reduced subsequent fertility. No comparative studies have evaluated the effectiveness of local therapy with penicillin, but penicillin should be the antibiotic of choice if any is used.

Metritis is the other common disease of the postovulatory period. Since most metritis of the late postpartum period is the result of penicillin-sensitive *C. pyogenes* and gram-negative anaerobes, and most other bacteria have been eliminated, penicillin is the antibiotic of choice for treatment. Intrauterine infusion of 1 to 1 1/2 million IU of penicillin provides therapeutic levels in the lumen and the entire wall of the uterus for a minimum of 24 hours. Since normal healing of the endometrium following elimination of *C. pyogenes* requires about a month, early post-treatment inseminations are often unproductive. In bull-bred herds conception is delayed about 20 days compared with herdmates even though treatment is initiated fairly early in the postpartum period.

Prophylactic Treatment. Cows with complicated deliveries and RFM have increased risk for metritis-pyometra. Therefore, numerous prophylactic treatments of these high risk cows have been applied, with inconsistent results. Some studies indicate that routine antimicrobial administration can be detrimental to fertility, others demonstrate no improvement and still others show that fertility of treated cows approaches that of normally calving herdmates. Unfortunately, these studies frequently lack untreated controls. Certainly, any treatment should have a logical pharmacologic and therapeutic basis.

The benefit derived from prophylactic administration of antibiotics may vary from herd to herd. Consequently, selection of treatment should be made after careful evaluation of each situation. Prophylactic antibiotics are more beneficial when genital infection rates are initially high. However, antibiotics should not be used in lieu of good management.

Single intrauterine applications of antimicrobials early in the puerperium seldom give an optimal response, especially in cows with RFM. Consequently, multiple treatments with antibiotics of the tetracycline family should be administered at least every other day until the membranes are expelled.

The economics of prophylactic antimicrobials should be considered before subscribing to this method of treatment. Ideally, milk production and reproductive performance of treated and untreated abnormal cows and healthy contemporaries should be compared. Any apparent benefit of treatment should be evaluated relative to the cost of the drug, cow mortality from lack of treatment, loss of salable milk, costs of repeated handling of cows and effect upon subsequent fertility.

Hormone Therapy. Hormone therapy has been used with variable success both alone and with other agents to treat cows with RFM, metritis and pyometra. Estrogens used in treatment of RFM are ineffective and may be detrimental in some cows. Gonadotropin-releasing hormone (GnRH) administered in the intermediate period has improved the fertility of cows with uterine subinvolution but has not enhanced fertility of normal cows. However, it must be given between 12 and 18 days postpartum to shorten the calving interval. Earlier or later administration is ineffective. In addition, if cows are not to be bred back before 60 days after calving, potential benefits for shortening the calving interval are lost.

Luteolytic prostaglandins and estrogens both stimulate evacuation of pus in cows with pyometra, but luteolytic prostaglandins perform best. In addition, luteolytic prostaglandins and estrogens have been evaluated for therapeutic efficacy in treatment of chronic metritis of the post-ovulatory period. In one study, estrogens increased and luteolytic prostaglandins decreased days open in treated cows compared with controls. However, blanket treatment of all postpartum cows with luteolytic prostaglandins does not improve overall reproductive performance; it is apparently only effective in cows with metritis and pyometra. Luteolytic prostaglandin therapy for metritis has the advantage of not requiring milk withdrawal, whereas antibiotic therapy does.

Adverse Effects of Faulty Treatment. Faulty treatment of metritis-pyometra may have adverse consequences. Vigorous manipulations of the genital tract are at times associated with perimetritis and uterine adhesions to surrounding structures. Obstetric operations and manual removal of RFM are often implicated. Excessive irrigation can rupture the uterus with similar sequelae. Intrauterine application of irritating substances, especially into a traumatized or lacerated uterus, often causes local tissue reaction and subsequent infertility.

Traumatic removal of RFM may allow pyogenic organisms to localize in the uterine wall and cause abscesses. Abscesses and perimetrial adhesions may also form following manipulation of the uterus and following trauma induced by infusion pipettes. Fluids from uterine irrigation, especially early in the puerperal period, may ascend the oviducts and cause salpingitis and ovarian bursitis. Rarely, treatment of pyometra with estrogens initiates pyosalpinx and peritonitis and their excessive use may also delay postpartum ovulation.

Because routine use of antimicrobials can lead to development of resistant strains of microorganisms, efficacy of treatment may require periodic reevaluation. Resistance to economical antimicrobials may require use of expensive ones that render prophylactic treatment economically impractical.

Etiology and Pathogenesis of Retained Bovine Placenta

Eberhard Grunert, M.D., Ph.D.
Clinic of Obstetrics and Gynecology of Cattle, Hanover, Germany

DEFINITION

In cattle the fetal membranes are physiologically expelled within 12 hours after delivery of the fetus. Retention of the entire afterbirth or of parts of the fetal membranes for longer periods must be considered a pathologic condition. Partial retention is observed particularly on the placentomes in the ovarian end (apical section) of the pregnant horn. It is, however, not always possible to establish a sharp time limit between the end of the physiological and the beginning of the pathologic state in every case of retained bovine afterbirth. In most cases placental retention should be considered as a clinical symptom of a more generalized disease, e.g., infections, metabolic diseases, nutritional deficiencies, allergies or other disorders, and seldom as a primary disease.

OCCURRENCE AND INCIDENCE

Retention of the fetal membranes is observed more frequently in cattle than in other species, with dairy cattle affected more commonly than beef cattle. In brucellosis-free areas the frequency of retained placenta after apparently normal parturition is reported to be between 3 and 12 per cent, with an average of 7 per cent. The incidence of retained afterbirth in cattle following abnormal deliveries (e.g., twin parturition, cesarean section, fetotomy, forced extraction of the fetus, abortion and premature calving) and in herds infected with brucellosis is high, ranging between 20 and 50 per cent or even more. The same is true for other infections that may cause abortion or premature parturition, e.g., infectious bovine rhinotracheitis (IBR) virus, epizootic bovine abortion and *Salmonella*.

An enzootic outbreak of retained placenta in herds that are free of the common enzootic infections causing abortion is observed when calf diarrhea or acute mastitis or both are common and when management problems or nutritional deficiencies or both can be found. Cows that have had a previous retained afterbirth have an increased chance of the placenta being retained after subsequent calvings.

ETIOLOGY

The retention of the afterbirth is positively correlated with the duration of pregnancy (Figs. 1 and 2), which influences subsequent prophylactic and therapeutic measures. Therefore, animals with retention of the fetal membranes can be divided into those that deliver within the expected physiological range of time and those that deliver outside the normal range of time. However, additional factors that cause retention of the afterbirth must be considered under physiological as well as under pathologic conditions of the gestation period.

Causes of retained placenta that can lead to changes in the placentomes (see Pathogenesis) are summarized in Table 1.

PATHOGENESIS

In the majority of cases placental retention in cattle is caused by a disturbance of the loosening mechanism in the placentomes. Some of the processes that lead to retained placenta should have taken place in the placentomes days or weeks or even months before parturition or premature delivery, e.g., in instances of metabolic and deficiency diseases (Fig. 3).

The Loosening Process in Placentomes

An undisturbed loosening mechanism (Fig. 3) is essential for timely, spontaneous expulsion of the afterbirth. This mechanism is already apparent during the last months of pregnancy when preparatory changes take place in the placental epithelium and connective tissues. The maternal and fetal connective tissues in the placentomes become progressively collagenized up to the time of parturition. The maternal epithelial lining of the crypts nearest the caruncular stalk becomes flattened. In addition, many binuclear giant cells appear, whose resorptive and phagocytic activities are manifested by the development of polynuclear giant cells shortly before the detachment process. With the onset of parturition and following hormonally induced imbibition, the tissues of the placentomes become loose—a process that appears to be essential for the undisturbed expulsion of the fetal membranes.

During the steps of dilation and particularly during the contractions of the uterus, there is a constantly changing uterine pressure that leads to al-

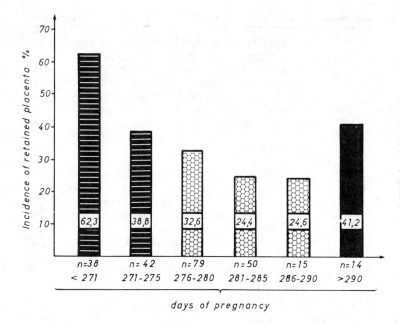

Figure 1. Relationship between length of gestation and incidence of retained placenta in German black pied cattle. (The high incidence of retained placenta even in cows with a normal gestation period is due to the high percentage of dystocia in the control animals.)

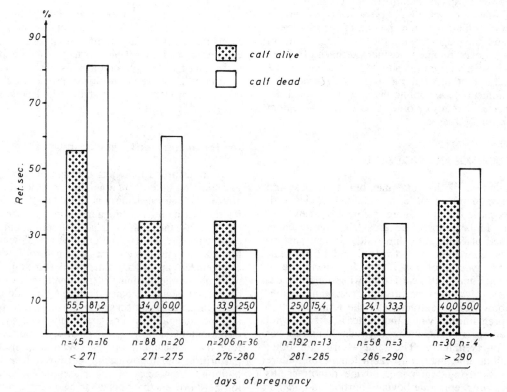

Figure 2. Relationship between length of gestation and incidence of retained placenta in German black pied cattle after parturition of a live or a dead calf. (The high incidence of retained placenta even in cows at normal term is associated with dystocia.)

Table 1. Causes of Retained Placenta in Cattle

Retained Placenta in Cattle after Physiological Duration of Gestation
  Factors causing primary or secondary uterine inertia during the different stages of labor (nutritional, circulatory, hormonal, hereditary)
    Metabolic diseases (e.g., parturient hypocalcemia, ketosis)
    Chronic diseases
    Infectious diseases (e.g., mastitis caused by *C. pyogenes)*
    Dystocia (uterine torsion; fetal oversize due to delivery by forced extraction, cesarean operation, fetotomy; incomplete dilatation of cervix; stillbirth; trauma of the uterus with secondary infection during dystocia)
    Age of the dam (particularly in older cows)
    Insufficient exercise
  Miscellaneous causes
    Breed differences
    Different years
    Seasonal influences
    Rate of daylight change
    Too rapid closure of the umbilical blood vessels

Retained Placenta in Cattle After Shortened or Prolonged Gestation Period
  Shortened gestation period
    Stress or allergy from vaccination or other manipulation (panic)
    Hormonal induction of abortion or premature birth
    Infections that may cause abortion or premature parturition (particularly brucellosis)
    Toxic causes (some chemicals and drugs, e.g., heavy metals, chlorinated naphthalenes)
    Allergies and anaphylactic reactions (warble fly allergy, brucella antigens)
    Urticaria from different sources (e.g., green or rotten potatoes)
    Trauma of the uterus
    Excessive distention of the uterus (multiple birth, hydrallantois and hydramnios, fetal giants and fetal double monsters)
  Prolonged gestation period
    Aplasia or severe hypoplasia of the adrenal gland or of the pituitary gland of the fetus
    Hereditary factors

Retained Placenta in Cattle After Shortened, Prolonged or Physiological Gestation Period
  Intensive stress (especially in older animals usually associated with a shortened gestation period)
    Management problems (e.g., short dry period less than 4 to 5 weeks in dairy cattle, handling or transport stress, heat stress, calving in a herd with a large number of other cows, change of locality in advanced pregnancy)
    High milk production
  Nutritional factors
    Metabolic disorders induced by imbalanced feeding
    Underfeeding (low levels of TDN)
    Overfeeding (high levels of energy and/or protein of dairy cows in the dry period)
    Fat cow syndrome (hepatic lipidosis, increased serum glutamic-oxaloacetic transaminase (SGOT), increased serum bilirubin, decreased blood glucose leading to ketosis, which in turn leads to uterine inertia)
    Vitamin deficiencies (e.g., carotene, vitamins A and E)
    Mineral deficiencies (e.g., imbalances in calcium and phosphorus (Ca:P ratio $< 1.4{:}1$)
    Calcium and phosphorus deficiency
    Trace element deficiencies in certain areas (e.g., selenium, iodine)
    Increased use of by-products (e.g., citrus pulp, whey, cottonseed)
    Toxins in feedstuffs (e.g., nitrate)
  Hormonal disturbances (asynchrony of hormonal mechanisms that normally synchronize birth and release of fetal membranes)
    Subnormal concentrations of plasma or serum 17β-estradiol and estrone at least until 4 days prior to parturition alone or in combination with either abnormally high or abnormally low progesterone. (Physiologically, estrogens rise sharply, late in the third trimester of the gestation period, reaching peak levels at term)
    Decreased plasma concentrations of 17β-estradiol and increased concentrations of 17α-estradiol from days 6 to 1 before calving
    Increased estrogen levels from day 1 prepartum to day 1 postpartum together with reduced fall in the progesterone levels
    Chronically low progesterone levels (days or weeks prior to calving)
    Increased plasma levels of progesterone on the day of parturition
    High androgen plasma levels on the day of parturition
    Decreased prolactin in plasma during the periparturient period (?)
  Hereditary factors (higher incidence of retained placenta in daughters of dams that have shown retained placenta)

Pathogenesis of retained bovine placenta

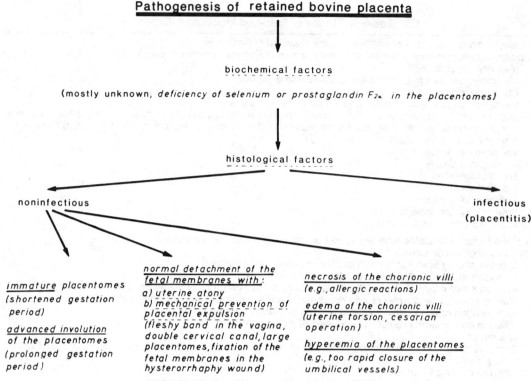

Figure 3. Pathogenesis of retained bovine placenta.

ternating ischemic and hyperemic conditions and temporary changes in the surface area of the fetal chorionic villi. As a result, the attachment of the chorionic epithelium in the maternal crypts becomes impaired. During the expulsion period, the first signs of the mechanical processes of detachment become evident in the vicinity of the caruncular stalk. These processes are probably facilitated by the fact that the caruncles are pressed against the fetus following uterine contractions.

A placentome that is not pathologically altered will therefore expand peripherally as a result of this flattening. This change in shape is apparently possible only if the hormonally induced relaxation of the maternal connective tissue allows the sideward expansion of the caruncular stalk, which was more compact before parturition. An essential factor after expulsion of the fetus and rupture of the umbilical cord is the ischemia of the fetal villi, which results from lack of blood circulation into the fetal capillaries. By shrinking of the blood vessels, the surface area of the chorionic epithelium also becomes greatly reduced. The postpartum uterine contractions complete the process of detachment of the membranes. The reduction in size of the uterus leads to a decrease in size of the caruncular stalk. These purely mechanical processes of detachment of the fetal membranes should not be underestimated.

Disturbance of the Loosening Process in Placentomes

A disturbance of the detachment mechanism in the placentome can be infectious or noninfectious. Among the causes of retained placenta are the following:

Immature Placentomes. This important cause of retention of fetal membranes occurs mostly in noninfectious abortions or premature parturition, i.e., in instances of a shortened gestation period. The average duration of pregnancy could depend on the breed and might be influenced by specific bulls. The frequency of placental retention is dependent upon the duration of pregnancy up to the time of expulsion of the fetus (Fig. 1). The incidence has been found to be nearly 15 per cent in cows that abort between days 121 and 150 of pregnancy, whereas it rises to 50 per cent or higher in those animals that expel the fetus between days 240 and 265 of pregnancy. The afterbirth is expelled normally as long as abortion occurs before day 120 of gestation.

Changes that are normally induced by estrogens, such as the imbibition of the maternal connective tissue and the swelling of the connective tissue fibers as well as the absorption of water by the cells, are found to be absent in immature placentomes removed immediately after parturition and examined histologically. The histologic study reveals deficient

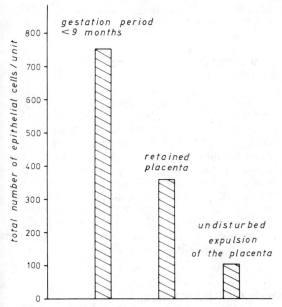

Figure 4. Number of epithelial cells (mean value) per unit of the maternal crypt epithelial layer in the vicinity of the caruncular stalk.

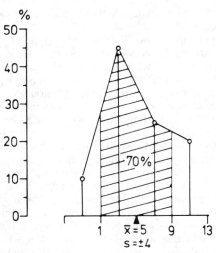

Figure 5. Number of epithelial cells (mean value and standard deviation) per crypt (longitudinal section) in cows with normal expulsion of the placenta. (Ziegler U: Hannovoer, Tierarztl. Hochschule, Diss, 1978.)

hormonal preparation of the maternal placental connective tissue. The collagen fibers of the caruncles are wavy and clearly contoured, particularly in the caruncular stalk. They become swollen, acquire indistinct contours and become nearly linear after hormonal sensitization. These caruncles, which are not prepared for detachment, do not seem to permit mechanical loosening in the area of the stalk during the expulsion period. Maturity occurs approximately 2 to 5 days before the end of breed-dependent average gestation length. Therefore, the earlier premature parturition occurs, the higher the percentage of retained placenta. The transformation of placental connective tissue is thought to be an important prerequisite for uncomplicated delivery of fetal membranes. In addition, the advanced disappearance of the maternal crypt epithelium is decisive for the correct timing of the expulsion of the placenta (Figs. 4, 5, 6). The number of epithelial cells in cases of retained placenta after premature parturition corresponds approximately to the number of epithelial cells during the eighth month of gestation.

Edema of the Chorionic Villi. Often one finds severe, noninflammatory edema of the fetal cotyledons. This can be seen in placentomes recovered shortly after calving, especially in cows following cesarean section or in animals that have had a long-standing uterine torsion. In these cases the edema extends to the ends of the chorionic villi, and the fetal membranes therefore remain firmly attached to the surface of these placentomes.

Necrotic Areas Between the Chorionic Villi and the Cryptal Walls. The presence of small areas of necrotic epithelium between the chorionic villi and

the cryptal walls is observed in animals with retained placenta. These alterations presumably occur antepartum and are often the main symptom of a more generalized disease. The observation of blood extravasations preceding the necrosis in a firmly attached placenta indicates the presence of a weak hemorrhagic diathesis. Thus, necrosis might be an effect of an allergic reaction.

Advanced Involution of the Placentomes. An additional cause of retained fetal membranes is an already advanced involution of the placentomes. In these cases placentomes recovered shortly after delivery show proliferative processes in the maternal connective tissue when examined histologically. Because the maternal septal tissue becomes thicker,

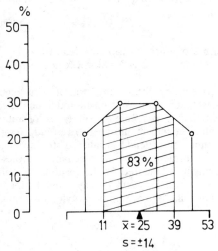

Figure 6. Number of epithelial cells (mean value and standard deviation) per crypt (longitudinal section) in cows with retained placenta. (Ziegler U: Hannovoer, Tierarztl. Hochschule, Diss, 1978.)

fetal villi can be trapped within it, thus complicating the process of detachment.

Hyperemia of the Placentomes. Hyperemia of the placentomes is seldom considered to be the cause of placental retention. This could occur before parturition or perhaps could even be caused by the too rapid closure of the umbilical blood vessels. The surface area of the fetal capillaries increases as a result of their congestion with blood. The villi may therefore remain incarcerated in the crypts.

Placentitis and Cotyledonitis. In placentitis and cotyledonitis the degree of the inflammatory reaction may vary from slight alterations to severe necrosis. The lesions may be localized in the cervical or apical part of the pregnant horn or may be diffuse. The nongravid horn is not always involved, and the degree of placentitis in this horn is usually not as severe as in the gravid horn. Affected cotyledons or portions of them are necrotic and of a yellow-gray color. In mold infections the placentomes are greatly enlarged and necrotic, have swollen margins and are firmly incarcerated. The inflammation may involve only the villi, small localized portions of the cotyledon or all of the placentome. The edematous placental stroma contains increased numbers of leukocytes.

Infectious agents are transmitted to the placenta during gestation from primary foci that may be localized in various parts of the body of an infected animal. For example, pyogenic bacteria such as *Corynebacterium pyogenes,* coliform bacteria, cocci and other organisms come from diseased udders or infected claws or from wounds or peritonitis. Infections of the placenta may also originate from disorders of the gastrointestinal tract, such as diarrhea caused by bacteria, molds and other organisms, particularly when spoiled feed is fed or the diet has been changed suddenly. If the placentitis develops before parturition, the fetal membranes are edematous, necrotic or leathery and sometimes hemorrhagic.

Uterine Atony Associated with Normal Detachment of the Fetal Membranes

Uterine atony without any form of disturbance of the detachment process is considered to be the cause of less than 1 per cent of all cases of retained placenta. The fetal membranes are already detached and cannot be expelled because of the absence of uterine contractions, or the mechanical process of detachment is hindered by the insufficiency of the uterine contractions and muscle tone. In this case it is possible to remove the cotyledons from the caruncles without causing any harm by pulling slightly on the fetal membranes.

Mechanical Prevention of Placental Expulsion

This occurs in isolated instances, in less than 0.5 per cent of all cases of placental retention. The fully or nearly detached cotyledon becomes trapped in a rapidly closing portion of the nonpregnant or invaginated uterine horn, in a double cervical canal or behind a fleshy band in the vagina. Such complications are usually caused by very large cotyledons. Occasionally, the retention occurs because membranous parts of the placenta wrap around the caruncles. Very seldom retention may also occur after cesarean section when parts of the membranes become sutured within the uterine incision.

Selected Readings

1. Arthur GH: Retention of the afterbirth in cattle: A review and commentary. Vet Ann 19:26, 1979.
2. Bostedt H, Schramel P: Vergleichende untersuchungen über die selenkonzentrationen im blutserum, in der plazenta, im myometrium und in der milch von kühen mit oder ohne retentio secundinarum. Zbl Vet Med A 28:259, 1981.
3. Chew BP, Keller HF, Erb RE, Malven PV: Periparturient concentrations of prolactin, progesterone and the estrogens in blood plasma of cows retaining and not retaining fetal membranes. J Anim Sci 44:1055, 1977.
4. Chew BP, Erb RE, Randel RD, Rouquette FM Jr: Effect of corticoid induced parturition on lactation and on prepartum profiles of serum progesterone and the estrogens among cows retaining and not retaining fetal membranes. Theriogenology 10:13, 1978.
5. Du Bois PR, Williams DJ: Increased incidence of retained placenta associated with heat stress in dairy cows. Theriogenology 13:115, 1980.
6. Grunert E, Schulz LCl, Ahlers D: Retained placenta problems with induced labor in cattle. Ann Rech Veter 7:135, 1976.
7. Grunert E, Zaremba W: Untersuchungen über negative einflüsse von endogenen und exogenen faktoren auf das frühpuerperium des rindes. Dtsch Tierärztl Wschr 86:461, 1979.
8. Leidl W, Hegner D, Rockel P: Investigations on the PGF$_{2\alpha}$ concentration in maternal and fetal cotyledons of cows with and without retained fetal membranes. Zbl Vet Med A 27:691, 1980.
9. Schulz LCl, Merkt H: Morphologische befunde an exstirpierten plazentomen, zugleich ein beitrag zur ätiologie der retentio secundinarum beim rind. Mh Vet Med 11:712, 1956.
10. Schulz LCl, Grunert E: Physiologie und pathologie der puerperalen involution des rinderuterus. Dtsch Tierärztl Wschr 66:29, 1959.
11. Schulz J, Wilhelm G, Richter A: Der nachgeburtsabgang und seine beziehungen zum verlauf von geburt and puerperium beim rind. Mh Vet Med 34:931, 1979.
12. Ziegler U: Zytologische untersuchungen an plazentomen im hinblick auf nachgeburtsverhaltungen beim rind. Hannover, Tierärztl. Hochschule, Diss., 1978.

Cystic Follicular Degeneration in the Cow

R. S. Youngquist, D.V.M.
University of Missouri—Columbia
Columbia, Missouri

Cystic follicular degeneration is a cause of abnormal estrous behavior and infertility in cows. The various synonyms for the disease include cystic ovarian disease, cystic ovarian degeneration, cystic graafian follicles, ovarian cysts, luteal ovarian cysts and "cystic cows."

DEFINITION OF THE CONDITION

Ovarian cysts are defined as folliclelike ovarian structures that are 2.5 cm in diameter or larger and persist for 10 days or more in the absence of a corpus luteum. Pathologic ovarian cysts are further divided into two types: (1) follicular cysts and (2) luteal cysts.[1]

Follicular cysts are thin-walled structures that may occur as single or multiple structures on one or both ovaries. Luteal cysts tend to be single structures occurring on one ovary and have a thicker wall than do follicular cysts. Both types of cysts arise following ovulatory failure.

Cystic corpora lutea are nonpathologic ovarian cysts. They arise following ovulation and are defined as corpora lutea that contain a fluid-filled central cavity of variable size. Cystic corpora lutea have a palpable ovulatory papilla, are capable of normal progesterone synthesis and do not alter the length of the estrous cycle.

INCIDENCE

The incidence of ovarian cysts in dairy cows is variously reported as ranging from 10 to 20 per cent, with some authors estimating that since not all ovarian cysts are detected, the incidence may approach 30 per cent. While the incidence of ovarian cysts in beef cattle is low, the condition is occasionally diagnosed and may be more common in the dual-purpose breeds.

Various factors are reported to influence the incidence of ovarian cysts; however, not all reports are in agreement. Factors that have been suggested include season, age, level of milk production, nutrition, heredity, length of the postpartum interval, exogenous estrogens (ingested and parenteral), frequency of examination of the reproductive tract and stress around the time of parturition, such as trauma, retained placenta and hypocalcemia. Ovarian cysts are a significant cause of reproductive failure because of prolongation of the interval from parturition to the first estrus and because of postservice anestrus, if the cyst develops following mating.

ETIOLOGY

While most authors agree that ovarian cysts are caused by an endocrine imbalance and/or ovarian dysfunction, the mechanism by which ovarian cysts develop is not well-defined. The development of ovarian cysts prior to the first postpartum ovulation may be explained by the hypothesis that the hypothalamic-pituitary axis may not be responsive to estradiol from follicles that may begin to develop as early as 1 week postpartum in the dairy cow. The lack of an ovulation-inducing luteinizing hormone (LH) surge in response to estradiol would then result in ovulatory failure. This hypothesis does not, however, explain the development of an ovarian cyst in a cow that had previously experienced normal ovarian cycles.[2] Thus, it is apparent that there is probably no single cause of all ovarian cysts; abnormal functions of the hypothalamus, pituitary ovary and/or adrenal glands may all contribute to the development of ovarian cysts.

CLINICAL SIGNS

The behavior of cows with ovarian cysts includes anestrus (lack of detectable estrus behavior) or nymphomania (intense and/or frequent sexual desire). While early descriptions of the condition indicate that the primary behavorial change associated with ovarian cysts is nymphomania, more recent reports indicate that approximately 80 per cent of cows with ovarian cysts are anestrous, with the remaining 20 per cent displaying nymphomaniac behavior.

The apparent difference in clinical signs reported over time is probably not due to a change in the disease process but to the widespread practice of examining the ovaries of cows during the early postpartum period, allowing the detection of cases that might have otherwise gone unnoticed. In cows that are not routinely examined, the clinical signs of nymphomania are more apparent to the herdsman and these cows are more likely than anestrous cows to be brought to the attention of a theriogenologist.

The physical appearance of cows with ovarian cysts depends upon the length of time the condition has existed. In acute cases there are no observable changes, whereas in cows in which the condition has become chronic relaxation of the pelvic ligaments resulting in the appearance of a prominent tail head, along with the development of masculine characteristics such as a crested neck and changes in voice, often occur.

DIAGNOSIS

The diagnosis of ovarian cysts is usually based on a history from accurate reproductive records and on a clinical examination. A history of nymphomania, short or irregular estrous cycles or anestrus is consistent with a diagnosis of ovarian cysts.

On per rectum palpation ovarian cysts are found to be fluid-filled, smooth, rounded structures, raised above the surface of the ovary. They are larger than a preovulatory follicle, with a diameter greater than 2.5 cm. Cysts up to 5 cm in diameter or larger are not uncommon. The thickness of the wall of the cyst is variable, ranging from an easily ruptured thin-walled follicular cyst to a thick-walled luteal cyst. Cysts may occur as single or multiple structures on one or both ovaries. It may not be possible for the examiner to differentiate between a single large cyst or several smaller cysts occurring on the same ovary. While it may be possible to differentiate between follicular and luteal cysts on the basis of the palpable characteristics of the cyst wall, in most cases no effort is made to determine the type of cyst, since both respond similarly to treatment with human chorionic gonadotropin (hCG) or gonadotropin-releasing hormone (GnRH).

Ovarian cysts appear to be dynamic structures. Those that occur early in the postpartum period may regress without treatment, and the cow may develop a normal estrous cycle or the cysts may be replaced by another cystic structure (see the following section on spontaneous recovery).

Endocrine Profile. Plasma progesterone concentrations are low in cows with follicular cysts and are higher in cows with luteal cysts. Cysts may undergo various degrees of luteinization, and progesterone concentrations may increase over time but remain lower than those in cows with normal corpora lutea. Estrogen concentrations in plasma of cows with ovarian cysts are variable and have been reported to be similar to and higher than those of normal cows. Testosterone concentrations in the plasma of cows with follicular and luteal cysts are similar to those during the normal estrous cycle. Concentrations of LH in cows with ovarian cysts are generally reported to be higher than those of normal cows and are inversely correlated to concentrations of plasma progesterone.

Differential Diagnosis. Several normal ovarian structures may complicate the diagnosis of ovarian cysts by palpation of the ovaries per rectum. A normal preovulatory follicle may approach 2.5 cm in diameter. Its palpable characteristics of being a thin-walled, fluid-filled, smooth structure raised above the surface of the ovary may be confused with those of a small cyst.

The palpable uterine changes associated with estrus may aid in differentiating between the two structures. The uterus of a cow in estrus is characterized by increased tone and responsiveness to palpation, while the uterine tone of a cow with an ovarian cyst varies from that similar to a cow in diestrus to flaccid. Mucometra may develop in chronic cases of ovarian cysts accompanied by varying degrees of uterine enlargement, which must be differentiated from pregnancy.

Corpora lutea in various stages of development and regression may be confused with ovarian cysts. During the first 5 to 7 days of the estrous cycle, the developing corpus hemorrhagicum may be smooth and soft. As the corpus luteum continues in development, it becomes more liverlike in consistency and may be more easily differentiated from an ovarian cyst. Sequential examinations 7 to 10 days apart may be useful in differentiating between an ovarian cyst and a corpus luteum. Both normal and cystic corpora lutea are characterized by an ovulation papilla, which is frequently palpable.

Other causes of ovarian enlargement that must be considered in the differential diagnosis of ovarian cysts include adhesions between the ovary and surrounding structures, salpingitis, hydrosalpinx, oophoritis, ovarian abscesses, neoplasia (primarily granulosa cell tumors) and cysts of the fimbria.

TREATMENT

Various approaches to the treatment of ovarian cysts have been used since the disease was first described in 1831. Most approaches are directed toward luteinization of the cyst, which is followed by reestablishment of a normal estrous cycle. Drugs used in treatment regimens are listed in Table 1.

Spontaneous Recovery. The number of cases in which spontaneous recovery occurs varies with the time postpartum at which the condition is diag-

Table 1. Drugs Used to Treat Cystic Follicular Degeneration in Cattle

Name of Drug	Dose
Follutein (hCG)	5000 to 10,000 IU
PLH	25 mg
Cystorelin (GnRH)	100 μg
Lutalyse (PGF$_{2\alpha}$)	25 mg
Estrumate (Cloprostenol)	500 μg
Repogest (Repository Progesterone)	750 to 1000 mg

nosed. As many as 60 per cent of cows in which ovarian cysts develop prior to the first postpartum ovulation are reported to develop normal estrous cycles spontaneously. In contrast, spontaneous recovery may be expected to occur in only about 20 per cent of cows that develop ovarian cysts after the first postpartum ovulation. The phenomenon of spontaneous recovery may confound the evaluation of therapeutic agents.

Manual Rupture. One of the earliest procedures described for the treatment of ovarian cysts is manual rupture of the cystic structure by palpation per rectum. In the case of thin-walled follicular cysts, this procedure may be relatively easy and require little pressure. Unintentional rupture of the cyst may, in fact, occur during examination of the ovary.

Various rates of recovery are reported following manual rupture of ovarian cysts. Most rates are in the range of those reported for spontaneous recovery, and it is difficult to attribute any beneficial effect to intentional rupture of ovarian cysts. Ovarian hemorrhage and adhesions may follow manual rupture, which could further contribute to infertility. More effective pharmacologic forms of treatment are available, and it is the opinion of the author and others that manual rupture of ovarian cysts is an archiac form of treatment and should be discouraged.

Exogenous Luteinizing Hormone. Biologic preparations high in LH-like activity have been widely and effectively used for the treatment of ovarian cysts. Human chorionic gonadotropin (hCG) and pituitary extracts (PLH) from sheep and swine are common sources of exogenous LH. Successfully used doses of hCG range from 5000 IU given either intravenously (IV) or intramuscularly (IM) to 10,000 IU given IM. PLH doses of 25 mg IM are recommended.

In cows that respond positively to exogenous LH, luteal tissue develops by either luteinization of the cysts or by luteinization of other follicles with or without ovulation. Development of luteal tissue and secretion of progesterone in response to LH treatment may be monitored by measurement of progesterone concentrations in milk or plasma.

Recovery rates of 65 to 80 per cent following a single dose of LH are reported. Cows that respond to LH usually develop a normal estrous cycle within 20 to 30 days after treatment. A second or third treatment may be required in a few cases. Cases of ovarian cysts are not usually retreated until at least 3 to 4 weeks have elapsed unless signs of nymphomania persist. Cows that exhibit a normal estrus following treatment should be inseminated at the first opportunity. Those cows that do not conceive or those from which service is withheld may develop subsequent ovarian cysts.

Since LH is a protein hormone, the possibility of anaphylaxis following administration to sensitized animals exists. No accurate information on the incidence of acute untoward reactions is available but they appear to be uncommon. Another unde-

sirable response to the administration of protein hormones is the development of antibodies that may diminish the effectiveness of subsequent treatments. Again, accurate information on the magnitude of this phenomenon in cows is lacking, but several authors suggest that consideration be given to the utilization of different products in subsequent treatments.

Gonadotropin-Releasing Hormone. The most recently introduced product for treatment of ovarian cysts is synthetic gonadotropin-releasing hormone (GnRH). Exogenous GnRH acts on the pituitary gland to cause the release of endogenous LH. Response of cows with ovarian cysts appears to vary with the dose administered. The standard dose of GnRH in the United States is 100 µg/cow. Following treatment with this dose, concentrations of plasma progesterone increase in cows with ovarian cysts that respond to treatment. In most cases response to 100 µg GnRH is characterized by luteinization of the cysts. When GnRH is used at doses of 0.5 to 1.5 mg, some cows respond with luteinization of the cyst, while others respond with ovulation and luteinization of graafian follicles present at the time of treatment. Most cows that respond to GnRH enter estrus 18 to 23 days after treatment.

When GnRH is compared with hCG on the basis of the proportion of cows that respond to treatment and the interval from treatment to the first estrus and fertility following treatment, the results are similar.

GnRH is a small molecule and thus may have an advantage over hCG in the treatment of ovarian cysts, since it is unlikely to stimulate an immune response that might reduce the effectiveness of subsequent treatments. Anaphylaxis following GnRH treatment has not been reported.

The practicing theriogenologist must determine the optimum time for treating ovarian cysts based on the expected frequency of spontaneous recovery, the time postpartum at which the condition is diagnosed and the interval between scheduled examinations. If ovarian cysts are diagnosed in the early postpartum period (< 30 days), spontaneous recovery may be expected in up to 60 per cent of the cases. Affected cows in herds in which examinations are scheduled for every 2 weeks may be conveniently examined at that time and treated if the ovarian cysts persists. If examinations are conducted at less frequent intervals or if ovarian cysts are diagnosed later in the postpartum period, immediate treatment should be instituted.

White and Erb[4] reported on the application of a decision analysis to determine at what time postpartum it becomes less expensive to treat ovarian cysts with GnRH than to wait for spontaneous recovery. Under the conditions of their model, they determined that it is more expensive to depend on spontaneous recovery and recommended that an ovarian cyst be treated whenever it is diagnosed.

Sequential GnRH and PGF$_{2\alpha}$. Ovarian cysts that luteinize in response to GnRH administration appear to undergo regression at a time similar to that of normal corpora lutea. The luteolytic activity of prostaglandin $F_{2\alpha}$ ($PGF_{2\alpha}$) or its synthetic analogs may be used to advantage in reducing the interval from treatment with GnRH to the first estrus from 18 to 23 days to an average of 12 days by administering a luteolytic dose of $PGF_{2\alpha}$ on day 9 after GnRH treatment. Fertility in cows given $PGF_{2\alpha}$ 9 days after GnRH is similar to that of cows given only GnRH.

Progesterone. The administration of exogenous progesterone has been shown to be useful in reestablishing estrous cycles in cows with ovarian cysts. The daily administration of 50 to 100 mg progesterone in oil for 14 days or a single dose of 750 to 1000 mg repository progesterone is reported to result in the development of estrous cycles in 60 to 70 per cent of cows with ovarian cysts. Conception rates in cows that respond to progesterone treatment are approximately 50 per cent, which are lower than those reported following treatment with hCG and GnRH. The mechanism by which progesterone causes regression of the ovarian cyst is not well established.

PROPHYLAXIS

Selective Breeding. The heritability of ovarian cysts is low; however, the incidence of ovarian cysts could be reduced by breeding only to bulls whose daughters have been shown to have a low incidence of ovarian cysts. This information is, unfortunately, not easily available. If replacement animals are available, consideration should be given to the removal of cows that develop ovarian cysts and their daughters from the herd.

Pharmacologic Control. Several studies have been reported that show the incidence of ovarian cysts in dairy cows may be reduced and fertility improved by the administration of GnRH during the early postpartum period. In one trial cows that ovulated in response to GnRH administration at 12 to 14 days postpartum did not develop ovarian cysts, and fewer GnRH-treated cows were culled owing to infertility than control cows. When cows were given GnRH 8 to 23 days after parturition, the incidence of ovarian cysts was reduced, and fertility was increased.

The mechanism by which GnRH treatment during the early postpartum period reduces the incidence of ovarian cysts is thought to depend on the stimulation of ovulation by a GnRH-induced LH release. Kesler and colleagues[3] have demonstrated that while the administration of GnRH will induce the release of LH during the very early postpartum period, ovulation is not induced with GnRH until days 12 to 13 postpartum. Thus, it is recommended that GnRH treatment for the prevention of ovarian cysts be given on days 12 to 14 postpartum.

SUMMARY

Ovarian cysts develop as a result of ovulation failure in dairy cows and are a significant cause of pre- and postservice anestrus. Economic loss due to ovarian cysts can be minimized by early diagnosis during routine reproductive and herd health examinations and by early treatment with an effective drug such as GnRH. The incidence of ovarian cysts may be reduced by the administration of GnRH on days 12 to 14 postpartum, selective breeding and culling of affected cows and their daughters.

References

1. Bierschwal CJ, Garverick HA, Martin CE, et al.: Clinical response of dairy cows with ovarian cysts to GnRH. J Anim Sci 41:1660, 1975.
2. Kesler DJ, Garverick HA: Ovarian cysts in dairy cattle: A Review. J Anim Sci 55:1147, 1982.
3. Kesler DJ, Garverick HA, Youngquist RS, et al.: Ovarian and endocrine responses and reproductive performance following GnRH administration in early postpartum dairy cows. Theriogenology 9:363, 1978.
4. White ME, Erb H: Treatment of ovarian cysts in dairy cattle, a decision analysis. Cornell Vet 70:247, 1980.
5. Zaied AA, Garverick HA, Bierschwal CJ, et al.: Effect of ovarian activity and endogenous reproductive hormones on GnRH-induced ovarian cycles in postpartum dairy cows. J Anim Sci 50:508, 1980.

Bovine Anestrus

Steven M. Hopkins, D.V.M.
Iowa State University,
Ames, Iowa

Anestrus is a broad term that indicates the lack of estrous expression at an *expected* time. Estrus detection failures that appear to be cases of anestrus are extensively covered in other articles in this section. The exact meaning of anestrus as it relates to an individual animal or to a group of animals depends on age, weight, breed and history. A prepubertal heifer that has sufficient body size at the appropriate age but fails to cycle is different from a mature cow that is anestrous following parturition. For convenience and accuracy, the discussion of anestrus will be covered under the separate headings of prepubertal, postpartum and postservice anestrus.

PREPUBERTAL ANESTRUS

Pubertal estrus represents the initiation of the reproductive cycle, and this first estrus generally occurs by a certain age relative to the animal's weight. Heifers must attain approximately two thirds of their adult size before they will reach puberty. With good nutritional management, most *Bos taurus* heifers attain their pubertal weight between 8 and 13 months of age. Failure of estrous expression past this time is prepubertal anestrus.

To begin the investigation of an anestrous problem, the history of the individual or of the group of heifers often provides the key to the etiology. Clinically, heifers generally fall into one of two categories: The acyclic heifer of the same age as the rest of a cycling group or several acyclic heifers in a group of the same age or a group of mixed ages.

The etiology of anestrus in a heifer in the first category frequently is related to an abnormal reproductive tract. Cyclicity of herdmates indicates that the problem does not affect the entire group. Cases of freemartins, hermaphrodites and aplasia are readily diagnosed by palpation. Three cases of X-trisomy have been reported in cattle[1]—one animal was fertile and two animals had protracted periods of anestrus. Since diagnosis of trisomy requires chromosome analysis, the condition has been infrequently reported but may be considered. Finally, any debilitating disease such as chronic pneumonia can delay puberty by decreasing rate of gain, and this appears to be a functional dietary problem.

Management practices play a major role in the second category, which comprises acyclic heifers of similar or diverse ages. Since the onset of puberty is influenced by the level of available nutrition, heifers of similar ages that are fed a suboptimal energy diet will show a prolonged prepubertal anestrous period. Likewise, groups of heifers of diverse ages that are housed together and given a balanced ration may contain several acyclic animals. Larger or more aggressive herdmates consume a greater portion of the available nutrition and tend to cycle first. Puberty, however, is not postponed indefinitely, and eventually the entire population cycles. There is an inherent danger in breeding these late heifers before they have developed adequate body size. They tend to have more dystocia problems and are prone to very long postpartum anestrous periods.

Certain infectious diseases can also produce anestrus in heifers. Blue tongue and bovine diarrhea virus are capable of causing an acute ovaritis, which leads to varying degrees of ovarian atrophy.[4, 5] Animals with complete atrophy are anestrous unless stimulated with exogenous hormones. They promptly return to the anestrous state when hormone therapy is withdrawn.

Growth-stimulating implants must be used with caution in prepubertal heifers that will be used as breeding animals. Synovex-H and zeranol (Ralgro) can delay pubertal estrus and may affect future fertility.

POSTPARTUM ANESTRUS

A period of anestrus following parturition is a normal physiological event, and ovarian cyclicity resumes as the uterus involutes. The anestrous period becomes abnormal when its duration extends past the accepted average. The duration of the average anestrous interval is influenced by age, breed, environmental factors and genetic background.

It is necessary to understand the mechanism of the hypothalamo-pituitary-gonadal axis to appreciate the causes of anestrus and to be able to initiate therapy to promote estrus. For the sake of simplicity, systems that promote postpartum follicular development and then luteinization will be considered as two interrelated mechanisms. The normal postpartum cow undergoes surges of follicle-stimulating hormone (FSH), which promotes follicular growth that may be detected as early as 9 to 15 days postpartum in the dairy cow. Plasma estradiol levels are variable but are closely timed with the FSH surges and follicular growth. The estradiol surges interact with the neuroendocrine centers, which results in increased sensitivity to gonadotropin-releasing hormone (GnRH). Concurrently, the plasma luteinizing hormone (LH) levels rise, and the number and magnitude of episodic LH peaks tend to increase during the first 2 weeks postpartum. This correlates with the fact that the quantity of LH at the pituitary level increases after parturition and that GnRH sensitivity returns at about 8 to 10 days postpartum. At approximately 2 to 3 weeks postpartum the LH levels are able to induce ovulation of one of the ovarian follicles. The corpus luteum of this first ovulation has a lower progesterone content and may not be as responsive to LH, which results in a shorter lifespan. Also, due to the absence of progesterone prior to this ovulation the estrus is generally silent. Normal behavioral estrus generally develops at successive heats.

Factors that modify this course of events can be divided into three categories: lactational effects, nutritional effects and organic disease. Anestrus may be due to a combination of the above factors, which makes therapy relatively more difficult. First-calf beef or dairy heifers generally have a protracted postpartum anestrous period because of the demands of continued growth plus lactation. This was illustrated in a study in which 85 per cent of the 2-year-old dairy heifers were anestrous at 60 days postpartum as compared with only 47 per cent of the mature cows for the same time period. A clinical examination of a true anestrous animal typically reveals ovaries that range from small and firm with no palpable structures to those that have multiple medium size follicles (5 to 10 mm). Although most cases of anestrus will eventually resolve themselves, this leads to a prolonged calving interval, which is economically unsound.

Lactation has been shown to cause an extension of the anestrous period. In a controlled experiment 3-year-old Angus cows were fed a balanced diet to limit any nutritional effects and were divided into three groups: mastectomized, intact nonsuckled and intact suckled.[3] It was shown that suckling decreased the average plasma LH concentrations and lengthened the interval to the development of episodic LH secretion. This prevented the first postpartum ovulation and blocked the return to cyclicity. Comparison of milked and suckled cows incriminated circulating cortisol levels as a possible component to the block of LH secretion. Corticoids were shown to depress episodic elevations of LH and decrease the sensitivity of the pituitary gland to GnRH. Plasma cortisol levels were highest in suckled cows and lowest in cows machine milked twice per day. Furthermore, cortisol levels were higher in high producers as compared with low producers, which were machine milked. Both clinically and experimentally, high producers tend to have a longer anestrous period.

Specific nutritional problems that influence the reproductive cycle and fertility are well documented and are presented in this section under the articles Effects of Nutrition on Reproduction in Beef (and Dairy) Cattle. There is, however, a general relationship between a balanced nutritional intake and anestrus. Energy balance, which is the difference between net energy requirements and net energy consumed, appears to be an accurate indicator of the length of the anestrous period. Energy balance is closely related to milk production, which is the greatest single drain on the postpartum cow. An individual cow has a finite capacity for feed intake, so additional energy requirements are met by the catabolism of body stores. Since the capacity and endogenous metabolism varies between animals, daily feed intake alone or body weight changes do not accurately predict the duration of the anestrous period. Ovulation has been associated with the return of the individual from the maximum negative energy balance. The cows were, however, still in a negative energy state when the first ovulation occurred. This model then suggests that within a group of cows on the same diet, the lower producers will tend to cycle first when compared with the high producers. While the exact mechanism of the effect of energy balance remains obscure, LH secretion is suppressed. Extension of the normal anestrous period can be caused by a deficient diet, particularly one low in energy. The low producers would still cycle first; however, the length of anestrus would become protracted. Clinically, this herd of cows would appear as a heterogeneous group, depending on production and days postpartum. Examination of individual estrus records would indicate that the first ovulation for the cycling cows has been delayed.

Organic dysfunctions in the postpartum cow that cause anestrus may be related to a primary uterine disease or a secondary systemic problem. A cow that undergoes delayed uterine involution because of placental retention, metritis, twinning, hydrops or uterine disease has a longer anestrous period. Recent evidence indicates that prostaglandins of uterine origin are markedly elevated during postpartum involution, suggestive of a role for prostaglandins in the decrease of uterine size.[2] In an abnormal cow undergoing delayed uterine involution, prostaglandin levels are elevated for a prolonged period of time. Concurrent with the increased prostaglandin release, plasma progesterone levels remained low, indicating the lack of functional luteal tissue.

Chronic debilitating diseases, such as leg injuries, displaced abomasum or hardware disease, are associated with the anestrous state. The etiologic agent may be chronic stress, or it may be related to the reduction in nutrient intake due to a decrease in the animal's desire and ability to eat properly. This is further supported by a concurrent decrease in milk production, indicating the inability to support lactation.

A retained corpus luteum without the presence of uterine pathology does not occur in cattle. Careful palpation over two estrous periods reveals the regression of the previous corpus luteum and the formation of new luteal tissue.

POSTSERVICE ANESTRUS

Postservice anestrus is a normal event following insemination if the animal has conceived. Approximately 5 per cent of the pregnant cows or heifers may exhibit behavioral signs of estrus early in the gestation period. Following breeding, the animals are closely observed for estrous activity, which should occur 18 to 23 days after breeding if they failed to conceive or to maintain the embryo past day 12 after ovulation. If the animal remains anestrous, she is presented for a pregnancy exam at 35 to 40 days after breeding. If the cow or heifer is nongravid at this time, the next estrus is expected in a few days, and reinsemination is advised. Cases of anestrus other than pregnancy most frequently are due to estrus detection failure, cystic follicular degeneration, pyometra, early embryonic death and uterus unicornis, rarely granulosa cell tumors or leiomyomas. True cases of postservice anestrus, in which the ovaries are nonfunctional or only have multiple small follicles, are uncommon and reflect a severe nutritional deficiency and/or systemic disease. These animals tend to remain in the anestrous state until the underlying illness is resolved.

THERAPY

Therapy for the induction of cyclicity in the anestrous animal has been attempted with a variety of exogenous hormones and management practices. For economic considerations it is important to have heifers calve at 2 years of age and cows calve every 12 months. Many hormone treatments have been utilized to hasten the onset of puberty or to decrease the interval from calving to conception. Unfortunately, due to the number of variables, including age, weight, diet and management, hormones do not always give consistent results. The overriding considerations for correcting an anestrous problem are that the animal be healthy, have palpable follicular development and have access to good feed.

Induction of a pubertal estrus in heifers depends largely on the weight of the animal after she reaches 13 months of age. Optimum results will be obtained if the heifer is near the average weight at puberty for her breed. When a heifer is over 13 months of age but has insufficient body weight she can be induced into estrus; however, the pregnancy rate is unacceptably low. If a heifer is very light she may not continue to cycle after an attempt at puberty induction. The treatment with Syncro-Mate B, which combines a 6 mg Norgestomet ear implant with an injection of 3 mg Norgestomet plus 5 mg estradiol valerate, has given the best results. The implant is removed 9 days later, and estrus ensues in 50 to 94 per cent of the animals within 120 hours. Pregnancy rates following insemination during this induced estrus have been reported to be as high as 50 per cent. The mechanism behind this therapy attempts to mimic the short luteal phase associated with the "silent" pubertal estrus. The estradiol valerate causes luteal regression if a functional corpus luteum (CL) is present but not detectable by palpation. The injectable Norgestomet prevents luteinization of additional follicles by the progesterone negative feedback mechanism. The 9-day period of implantation is important in promoting estrous expression by causing progestogen priming

necessary for a psychic estrus. Also, the implant helps decrease the incidence of induced corpora lutea having a reduced lifespan by promoting a normal LH release pattern following implant removal. Finally, using a progestogen for only 9 days does not appear to depress post-treatment fertility as would longer courses of progestogen.

The use of hormonal therapy in the anestrous suckling beef or lactating dairy cow has been researched extensively. Beef cows are usually treated 45 to 90 days postpartum, and as with heifers, success depends on their nutritional status and body condition. Hormone therapy is the same as that described for acyclic heifers; however, best results are obtained by removing the nursing calves for 48 hours at the time of implant removal (Shang treatment). Estrus occurs 24 to 48 hours later, and first service conception rates have been reported to range from 40 to 70 per cent under ideal conditions. As with heifers, the progestogen implants decrease the incidence of short luteal lifespans following the induced estrus, although the implants do not completely eliminate this phenomenon.

Weaning without prior hormone therapy results in a higher expression of estrus when compared with nonweaned cows; however, the incidence of short cycles has been reported to be as high as 84 per cent.

GnRH has been used extensively in beef cows. When there were palpable follicles at 4 weeks postpartum, 250 mcg GnRH IM resulted in a 50 per cent ovulation rate. Additionally, calf removal for 48 hours tended to improve the ovulatory response but many of the cows exhibited a shortened estrous cycle.

GnRH is used in lactating dairy cows to shorten the anestrous interval and increase the number of estrous cycles prior to breeding. By increasing the number of estrous periods before breeding there is a decrease in the number of services per conception. Dose levels have been 100 mcg or 250 mcg of GnRH at 2 weeks postpartum. A favorable response occurred when there was a follicle of $\leq$ 15 mm when compared with cows that had follicles of $\leq$ 10 mm. Generally, there is a decrease in the interval from calving to conception in abnormal cows and in those with a slower involution rate and an extended anestrous period. Normal cows showed no significant decrease in the open period.

Cows and heifers with completely smooth, nonfunctional ovaries respond very poorly when hormones are used to shorten the anestrous interval. Therapy for these cows must be approached first by correcting the underlying nutritional deficiency or systemic disease.

Estrogens and follicle-stimulating hormone have been used extensively for the treatment of anestrous animals, even though there is a lack of scientific evidence to support this practice. It is well known that estrogens promote a behavioral estrus in an anestrous animal, but this is rarely accompanied by ovulation. The addition of FSH and/or estrogens at the time of an induced estrus does not improve fertility.

CONCLUSION

The application of hormonal therapy for the treatment of an anestrous problem should be approached with caution. In too many instances hormones are used in an attempt to correct management errors. The results are unsatisfactory and economically unsound. Hormone therapy for the treatment of an anestrous problem can, however, be a useful tool in selected herds when used in healthy, well-nourished animals.

References

1. Buoen LC, Seguin BE, Weber AF, Shoffner RN: X-Trisomy karyotype and associated infertility in a Holstein heifer. JAVMA 179:808, 1981.
2. Lindell JO, Kindahl H, Jansson L, Edquist LE: Postpartum release of prostaglandin $F_{2\alpha}$ and uterine involution in the cow. Theriogenology 17:237, 1982.
3. Short RE, Bellows RA, Moody EL, Howland BE: Effects of suckling and mastectomy on bovine postpartum reproduction. J Anim Sci 34:70, 1972.
4. Ssentongo YK, Johnson RH, Smith JR: Association of bovine viral diarrhoea-mucosal disease virus with ovaritis in cattle. Aust Vet J 56:272, 1980.
5. Williams DJ: Blue tongue in cattle. Proc Soc Theriogenology Sept. 1979.

Effects of Infectious Bovine Rhinotracheitis on Reproduction

Robert F. Kahrs, D.V.M., Ph.D.
University of Missouri, Columbia, Missouri

Infectious bovine rhinotracheitis (IBR), a herpesvirus infection with widespread geographic distribution, produces a diversity of clinical manifestations. These can have profound effects on reproduction in both male and female cattle.

ETIOLOGY

IBR virus, sometimes called the IBR-IPV virus, has physical, biochemical, epidemiologic and immunologic properties of the herpesvirus group. The virus grows readily in a variety of cell cultures, producing distinctive cytopathologic changes useful for virus isolation, virus titration and neutralization tests for presence of antibody in serums. This ease of laboratory manipulation has expedited studies on pathogenicity, epidemiology, diagnosis and vaccine technology and helps to make IBR one of the best described of cattle diseases.

EPIDEMIOLOGY

The infection is easily transmitted by virus exteriorized in respiratory, ocular and reproductive secretions of infected cattle. The virus is perpetuated in individuals and populations by latent infections, sometimes localized in trigeminal ganglia. These are occasionally reactivated, causing shedding of virus.

Cattle are probably the principal reservoir, although most ruminants can be infected. The virus is widely distributed among cattle populations, and unless they are extremely isolated, cattle have a high probability of eventual exposure.

PATHOGENICITY AND PATHOLOGY

Initial exposure and primary infection can cause clinical signs and lesions or a mild inapparent or unobserved infection. The characteristic lesions are adherent, whitish, necrotic material raised above mucosal surfaces. These lesions, frequently referred to as plaques, result from coalescence of discrete pustules. They consist of leukocytes, fibrin and necrotic epithelial cells. Intranuclear inclusion bodies are a histologic feature. The lesions may appear at the site of inoculation or at other target organs after systemic distribution by macrophages. When lesions are present in the respiratory tract, they cause upper respiratory disease. When they involve reproductive mucosa, they cause infectious balanoposthitis in the male and infectious pustular vulvovaginitis (IPV) in the female. Focal necrosis is the classic lesion found in the parenchyma of body organs. Fetuses and newborn calves are more likely to suffer serious systemic effects than are mature animals. Following primary infection, latent infections may develop.

Abortion can occur following or concurrently with inapparent infection, respiratory disease, conjunctival infection or IPV. The principal clinical signs and diagnosis of each form will be discussed briefly.

FORMS OF IBR

IBR as a Respiratory Disease. The respiratory form of IBR is manifested by elevated temperature, reduced appetite, rapid respiration and upper respiratory dyspnea. Occasionally, blockage of the upper airways causes open mouth breathing.

Affected cattle may have profuse nasal discharge that is clear in the early stages and later becomes mucopurulent. There is hyperemia of the nasal turbinates and sometimes the muzzle. This explains the former nickname "red nose."

The visible portions of the nasal mucosa frequently have adherent, white, necrotic debris that results from the coalescence of pustules. These lesions, although not pathognomonic, are very highly suggestive of IBR.

Some cattle with respiratory IBR have conjunctivitis and excess ocular secretions that change from clear to mucopurulent as the disease progresses. Usually, auscultation with a stethoscope reveals no abnormal lung sounds other than an increased vesicular murmur (the reasonant sound of normal breathing) or referred sound due to occlusion of the upper air passages. If rales or other lung sounds are heard, the clinician should suspect another respiratory disease (particularly pulmonic pasteurellosis) or other complications.

The death rate in respiratory IBR is low unless secondary bacterial infections, superimposed viral infections or other complications occur. Occasionally, a severely infected animal will suffocate from mucopurulent material in the trachea, and pulmonic pasteurellosis may be a sequela.

When respiratory IBR is present in a herd containing pregnant cattle, abortions may begin while clinical signs are present in the herd and may continue for 90 to 100 days. Most fetuses are aborted during the last 4 months of gestation, and the belief exists that fetuses are more susceptible to abortion during late gestation. This may be true. However, the difficulty of finding small aborted fetuses and the variable exposure-abortion interval raise the question of whether this is true age susceptibility or an artifact of observation.

IBR Conjunctivitis. Inflammation of the conjunctiva accompanies the respiratory form of IBR. Occasionally, in outbreaks in which respiratory signs are not evident, conjunctivitis is the principal manifestation of IBR infection. Such outbreaks may be misdiagnosed as pinkeye. The diagnosis of IBR conjunctivitis should be considered when corneal opacities originate at the corneoscleral junction (limbus). In contrast, classic pinkeye, caused by the bacterium *Hemophilus bovis,* produces a corneal opacity that originates in the center of the cornea and spreads centrifugally.

Abortion rates may be high or low in outbreaks manifested primarily as conjunctivitis. Sometimes a cluster of aborted fetuses occurs, and it is learned that the herd experienced an outbreak of "a peculiar form of pinkeye" a month or two earlier. When the abortions are subsequently identified as IBR by virus isolation, histopathologic examination, or fluorescent antibody assay, the diagnosis of IBR conjunctivitis is arrived at retrospectively.

The diagnosis of IBR conjunctivitis is strengthened by finding pustules or plaques of white, necrotic debris on the conjunctiva. Such conjunctivae are frequently edematous and painful, and affected cattle object to the careful conjunctival examination needed to see the lesions. The diagnostic significance of isolating IBR virus from the conjunctivae of cattle with ocular disease must be carefully evaluated, since IBR virus can exist as a latent infection with reactivation by stressors such as those that might be associated with outbreaks of other eye conditions.

Infectious Pustular Vulvovaginitis (IPV). The disease known as IPV is caused by the IBR virus. The viruses isolated from the reproductive and respiratory tracts are immunologically similar but may be distinguished by DNA fingerprinting technology. There may be subtle differences between strains, with a predilection for reproductive mucosa and biotypes with an affinity for the respiratory tract. Although IPV is usually not observed during respiratory outbreaks (and vice versa), occasionally both respiratory IBR and IPV occur simultaneously when nose-to-vulva contact is common. This observation fosters the belief that the etiologies of these two "diseases" are similar and that the location of the lesions is determined primarily by the route of inoculation.

Usually, IPV is first noticed because of the unusual tail position. The owner observes that the cow's tail fails to return to the normal relaxed position after defecation or urination because of pain in the perineal area. Frequently, IPV is accompanied by edema and mucopurulent discharge from the vulva. Internal examination reveals pustules or plaques of white, necrotic material on the wall of both the vulva and vagina and pools of mucopurulent, usually odorless material on the vaginal floor.

Infectious pustular vulvovaginitis can be transmitted by natural breeding and probably by the sniffing habits of cattle. In one outbreak a dog with a habit of licking the vulva of cattle as they lay in stanchions was implicated epidemiologically as the mode of transmission.

In diagnosing IPV it should be remembered that not all pustular or necrotic lesions on vulva or vaginal mucosa are caused by this virus. Necrotic vaginitis (secondary to parturition injuries), sadism and application of caustic materials must also be considered. In addition, every clinician should be familiar with the disease known as granular vaginitis, which produces elevated granular lesions on the vulvar mucosa. These lesions sometimes have a brownish or off-orange color and can be found in many normal cattle. They are probably a hypoplasia of lymphoid follicles in the mucosa. The individual lesions are smaller than those produced by IPV and do not increase in size on subsequent days. Furthermore, they are usually not associated with mucopurulent discharge or discomfort.

Mycoplasmal infections and infections associated with the disease known as catarrhal vaginitis of cattle have similar lesions. Examination of the vulvar mucosa is often neglected as a diagnostic aid in respiratory IBR because vulvar lesions are frequently not severe enough to produce discomfort or otherwise attract attention. When these lesions are found, they add to the evidence of IBR.

Bulls bred to cows with IPV can acquire the infection, develop a severe balanoposthitis with lesions similar to those seen in IPV and transmit the disease during breeding. The shedding of virus from these lesions into semen can occur, and if the semen is frozen, viral infectivity can be preserved. The artificial insemination industry is also concerned about contamination of semen with IBR from bulls with latent infections.

IBR Abortion. In order for abortion to result from IBR, the female must be both pregnant and susceptible at the time of primary infection. Under field conditions, with cattle of various stages of gestation, susceptibilities and variations in the severity of exposure, about 25 per cent of pregnant cattle may abort following an outbreak. In experimental situations with known seronegative animals inoculated with large doses of virus, higher percentages of abortions have been reported. Most fetuses aborted as a result of IBR are in the last third of gestation when expelled, but fetuses exposed to IBR at any time during gestation can be aborted. Although the interval between exposure and abortion is sometimes prolonged, abortion can follow infection by a few days. That is, fetuses may be expelled while clinical IBR is present in the herd or shortly thereafter, or abortion may be delayed for as long as 100 days after infection of the pregnant cow.

Occasionally, fetuses exposed in late gestation are carried to term. These may be dead at birth or may succumb within a few days with lesions of fatal systemic IBR.

Fetuses aborted because of IBR are usually dead in utero for several days before expulsion. This explains the presence of autolysis, the brownish-stained, friable tissues and the fluid in both body cavities as well as the lack of obvious gross lesions. Such fetuses are frequently reported as being too decomposed for an adequate diagnostic work-up. While gross lesions are difficult to find under these conditions, astute pathologists can find focal necrosis and intranuclear inclusions in the autolyzed fetal liver and adrenal gland.

Diagnosis of IBR Abortion. Fetuses aborted as a result of IBR usually have no characteristic gross lesions other than indistinct petechiation throughout and marked autolysis manifested as brownish-stained tissue discolorations and serosanguineous fluids in both body cavities. Some diagnosticians suggest that finding fetuses in this autolyzed condition is highly suggestive of IBR. However, this condition can result from retention of a fetus in utero following death from a number of reasons, and, therefore, further evidence for a diagnosis of IBR must be found.

To diagnose abortion, the entire placenta and fetus should be submitted refrigerated to the laboratory, enabling the diagnostician to do a complete work-up for a variety of abortifacient agents. The virus of IBR can sometimes be isolated from the fetal liver, adrenal, kidney, placenta and other tissues. Likewise, virus can be demonstrated in these areas by fluorescent antibody assay.

The focal necrosis and inclusions in the fetal adrenal and liver can be found after careful histopathologic search. Serologic examination of fetal cardiac blood or of fluids found in body cavities has not been a productive method for the diagnosis of IBR. It is speculated that the fetal disease is so acute that the fetus dies before it can respond immunologically with antibody.

Some clinicians attempt to base a diagnosis of IBR abortion on paired serologic tests on the dam. This approach is productive only if the fetus is aborted in the early stages of the disease. Usually, by the time the fetus is aborted, the dam's antibody titer is elevated enough that a further rise is not demonstrable when a second (convalescent) sample is collected.

Effects of IBR on Fertility. Reports, which have not been substantiated by controlled studies, suggest that a period of temporary infertility follows intramuscular vaccination or natural infection of IBR. The credibility of such speculation is enhanced by the finding that large doses of IBR virus inoculated into the uterus cause a mild endometritis and temporary failure of conception. For this reason, the prohibition concerning intramuscular vaccination of pregnant cattle should be extended to cover the period 1 month prior to breeding.

Fatal Systemic IBR in Neonates. The birth of a healthy calf capable of surviving to maturity is the culmination of the reproductive process. Thus, the fatal systemic form of IBR in neonatal calves is included in theriogenology. Fetuses that acquire primary IBR infection in late gestation or calves that acquire the infection shortly after birth sometimes experience an acute febrile form of IBR that usually terminates fatally. Such fetuses or calves have respiratory distress and may have necrotic lesions on the mucosa of the mouth, tongue and esophagus and on all four stomach compartments. In addition, a diffuse peritonitis may be present. Such calves may have diarrhea and may be misdiagnosed as having colibacillosis, but the lesions are so characteristic that they indicate IBR to the experienced pathologist.

IBR Associated with Metritis. Belgian workers have isolated a virus resembling IBR from the uterine exudate of postparturient cows delivered by cesarean section. These cows had fever, metritis and mucopurulent uterine discharge, and a crepitant feel to the uterus on palpation per rectum was also present. The source of infection was not determined.

TREATMENT OF IBR

Like most viruses, IBR is unaffected by the available antimicrobial agents, thus treatment is directed toward controlling complications. Therefore, the welfare of affected cattle is maintained by good nursing care, supportive therapy and antibiotics when clinical judgment indicates bacterial complications are significant. Antibiotic therapy must be evaluated with respect to its value to the patient as weighed against withdrawal times and residue potential.

Infectious pustular vulvovaginitis can be treated locally with soothing antiseptic or antibiotic ointments. By and large, IPV is self-limiting and without complications. In bulls, severe cases of balanoposthitis may produce preputial adhesions. Treatment with antibiotic or antiseptic ointments may be necessary to reduce the likelihood of this sequela.

PREVENTION OF IBR

The prevention and control of IBR is difficult. Preventing exposure by rearing animals in isolation is impractical because of the ubiquity of the virus and the ever-present hazard of virus exteriorization from reactivated latent infections in clinically normal cattle.

Vaccination is currently the most logical means of control. IBR vaccines are obtainable from many manufacturers, come in many combinations and are available for intramuscular or intranasal inoculation. Inactivated vaccines are intermittently available, and they lack the hazards of live vaccines.

In using any IBR vaccine it is important to study the label and the package insert for contraindications against vaccinating pregnant cattle and for precautions about vaccinating cattle that are in contact with pregnant cattle. In general the vaccine should be used on healthy, well-nourished cattle that have not recently been moved or exposed to disease.

To prevent the effects of IBR from affecting reproductive efficiency, it is recommended that cattle be vaccinated well before their first breeding. Since maternal antibody may persist for 4 to 6 months, it is best to vaccinate cattle after 6 months of age and prior to breeding. If carried out in the area where calves are raised, such a program will result in repopulation of herds with partially resistant cattle. The protection induced by vaccines has variable effectiveness and duration. Although some animals may lose their vaccine-induced humoral antibody, it will persist in others. In some cases restimulation may occur by natural exposure or by reactivation of vaccine virus infection. An additional percentage of vaccinated cattle can probably develop an anamnestic response in sufficient time to resist systemic distribution of virus to the fetus following exposure. The duration of immunity is controversial, and many veterinarians and vaccine producers recommend annual revaccination.

The intramuscular live vaccines may be less attenuated than vaccines prepared for intranasal use. Most can cause abortion and are contraindicated for use in pregnant animals and in cattle or calves that may come in contact with pregnant animals within 30 days following vaccination. Generally, it is accepted that most calves 4 months or older will have lost enough maternal antibody to respond satisfactorily to these vaccines. Calves can also be vaccinated at an earlier age. However, the conservative clinician who vaccinates before 4 months of age anticipates interference from maternal antibody in some vaccinated calves and therefore repeats the vaccination at a later date prior to breeding.

The intranasal vaccines appear to be more attenuated than those used intramuscularly, and most are approved for use in pregnant animals. Careful scrutiny of all labels and package inserts of each product is necessary because it cannot automatically be assumed that all intranasal vaccines are tested and approved for use in pregnant cattle. The proposed advantages of intranasal vaccines include the induction of local or secretory antibody and the prompt appearance of interferon in nasal secretions. It is suggested that interferon provides early protection and may be of some value in controlling early infection. In addition to eliciting a local immune response, the intranasal vaccines cause a humoral antibody response comparable to that of the intramuscular vaccines. There are suggestions that intranasal vaccines can override low levels of maternal antibody and thus be effective for very young calves. However, those attempting to prevent adverse effects on reproduction will be thinking of long-term immunity or anamnesis and will not rely on inducing active immunity in calves under 4 to 6 months of age. When management situations dictate early vaccination, a second vaccination should be administered before breeding.

Intranasal administration is difficult in mature animals unless restraint is excellent. However, vaccination of younger animals is less difficult. Precautions must be taken to see that restraint is excellent and that both nostrils are inoculated with viable vaccine. In addition care must be taken to see that the cattle do not blow out the vaccine following its administration.

Because of uncertainty about the duration of immunity and a desire to be on the safe side, most manufacturers usually recommend annual revaccination. Annual revaccination is indicated for the bovine parainfluenza-3 vaccine, which is usually combined with intranasal IBR vaccines. Also, annual revaccination affords the opportunity to immunize cattle that failed to respond to earlier inoculations. In addition, such vaccination could conceivably "boost" waning vaccine-induced titers, assuring greater protection and higher colostral antibody titers for passage to nursing calves.

The clinician must decide if the advantages of annual revaccination outweigh the expense of vaccination and the problems of restraint. One properly administered vaccination in the lifetime of each animal should be adequate to provide herds with enough herd immunity so catastrophic episodes of IBR abortion can be avoided.

The question of whether to vaccinate purebred bulls for IBR is difficult to answer because of its many ramifications. When all things are considered, the safest course is to avoid vaccination of breeding bulls and purebred bulls. Importers of bulls and semen discriminate against seropositive individuals because of their potential for exteriorizing virus from reactivated latent infections. Thus, vaccination may limit the opportunity for sale of a purebred bull for export or to an artificial insemination unit. In a total herd health program involving IBR vaccination, the impact of leaving a few bulls unvaccinated would probably be minimal when regarded on a population basis.

In the management of bull studs a decision on the use of IBR vaccine must be based on the serologic status of the population, the requirements of foreign importers of semen and the disease control philosophies of the management. These considerations must be tempered by the arguments that the virus is virtually ubiquitous and may eventually gain entrance to the stud. The exclusion of bulls because of IBR serotiters constitutes a serious loss of genetic material that may not be justified by the minimal hazard associated with transmission of virus by semen.

Effects of Bovine Viral Diarrhea on Reproduction

Robert F. Kahrs, D.V.M., Ph.D.
University of Missouri, Columbia, Missouri

Bovine viral diarrhea (BVD) is widely known as a systemic disease that produces lesions in the gastrointestinal mucosa. However, in animals kept for breeding purposes its most serious economic impact can result from damage to the developing fetus. These reproductive manifestations usually follow inapparent or undiagnosed BVD. Thus, its significance as a reproductive disorder is unappreciated.

Clinical manifestations occur most commonly in young cattle and can be acute or chronic. The disease appears sporadically and is characterized by fever, diarrhea and erosions or necrosis of the mucous membranes of the gastrointestinal tract. The erosions may be almost imperceptible or quite severe (resembling rinderpest). Unless oral erosions are observed, the disease usually goes undiagnosed. In herd outbreaks with minimal diarrhea or mucosal involvement, BVD is frequently diagnosed as "undifferentiated respiratory disease" because fever, nasal discharge and rapid breathing are prominent signs.

ETIOLOGY

The BVD virus is classified with the pestiviruses of the family Togaviridae as are the viruses of hog cholera and equine viral arteritis, with which it shares many characteristics. It grows readily in a variety of cell cultures, and many strains produce distinctive cytopathogenic changes. Other strains of the virus are not readily cytopathogenic and require other techniques for identification. Cytopathogenic strains are utilized in neutralization tests for detection of serum antibody.

EPIDEMIOLOGY

Epidemiologically, BVD is characterized by widespread distribution, easy transmission, high antibody prevalence, frequent inapparent or undiagnosed infection and a very variable incubation period. Although sheep and swine can be infected, the epidemiologic significance of these infections is not known, and cattle are usually considered the principal reservoir. Chronic persistent infections in some cattle help the virus survive in populations. When susceptible cattle or sheep are infected during pregnancy, a variety of fetal abnormalities can occur. These are usually not evident until months after infection.

The pathogenesis of postnatal BVD is usually explained by the virus' predisposition to replicate in lymphoid tissues, with resulting lymphoid depletion, leukopenia and profound immunosuppression at the cellular level, which is manifested by degeneration, necrosis and ulceration of mucosa. In the fetus, hypoplasia or degeneration of ocular and brain tissue occurs.

The virus of BVD is virtually ubiquitous in cattle populations. Even cattle raised under relatively isolated conditions seem to become infected ultimately. The consequences of these infections vary from a mild inapparent or undiagnosed infection to an acute or chronic fatal illness. Fatal cases succumb before effects on the developing fetus are evident, and those with chronic infections are usually culled. Therefore, the inapparent infections probably have the greatest impact on reproduction. This makes the economic loss insidious. Before discussing the effects of BVD on reproduction, the clinical forms of the infection will be reviewed.

FORMS OF BVD

Acute Systemic BVD. In early reports attack rates were high, all ages were affected and most sick cattle survived. Today (at least in the eastern United States) the disease occurs sporadically and is frequently fatal. Most cattle are between 6 and 24 months of age. Herdmates usually appear normal, but careful examination of the oral mucosa may reveal mildly affected penmates or herdmates with sparse mucosal erosions or blunted, reddened buccal papillae.

The typical case is characterized by an elevated temperature, salivation, gingivitis and erosion of the lips, gums and palate. Although not always present, diarrhea is a common finding and is frequently intractable, leading to severe dehydration that signals death. Rapid respiration occurs, and the animal is leukopenic. In some cases acute laminitis may be present and corneal opacities occasionally develop.

Chronic BVD. The chronic form of BVD is sometimes called classic mucosal disease. It may appear in cattle recovering from recognized acute disease or in cattle in which no prior evidence of infection was observed. The chronically infected animal is unthrifty and there is loss of weight and failure to grow or gain weight at the same rate as penmates of the same age. Such cattle are frequently culled as "poor doers" without a diagnosis of the etiologic agent being made. Chronic BVD is frequently manifested by an intermittent diarrhea followed by periods of recovery and relapse. Chronically infected cattle may have any of the lesions seen in the acute form. Erosions heal rapidly, and new erosions may appear throughout the course of the disease, which may be several months. Cattle with chronic BVD may have dry, scruffy skin, lameness, cracking or skin necrosis in the interdigital spaces and erosions or necrosis around the coronary band. Protracted cases may show overgrowth and malformation of hooves, prompting a diagnosis of chronic laminitis.

Cattle with chronic BVD usually have a persistent infection, and virus may be isolated from blood or from ocular and nasal secretions for prolonged periods. They frequently fail to develop detectable circulating antibody. Such animals may be inept at handling the BVD virus and incapable of immunologic response of a magnitude sufficient to tip the host-parasite relationship in favor of the animal. With the virus prevailing, the animal's physical state declines, and it eventually dies or is culled.

Mild Clinical BVD. Because the severely ill animals (both acute and chronic cases) are usually removed from herds, it is mild, undiagnosed and inapparent infections that account for most reproductive losses. Some inapparent and mild cases appear in herds when severe acute or chronic cases are present. In other herd infections, there is only mild diarrhea or "undifferentiated respiratory disease," and the association with BVD is not suspected unless careful examination of the oral mucosa is performed or thorough necropsy or laboratory studies are conducted.

Mild clinical BVD is characterized by fever and leukopenia. These may go undetected. Affected animals frequently have an increased respiratory rate and a few scattered erosions of the oral mucosa or blunted, reddened buccal papillae, but these lesions are hard to find unless the mouth is examined carefully. Such cases are usually not fatal unless mild fever, metritis, acute mastitis, peritonitis or another infectious disease occurs concurrently. Because of the mild symptomatology and the similarity to other diseases, these mild cases frequently are not diagnosed. Thus, the vast majority of reproductive damage from BVD is undiagnosed or unreported.

Inapparent BVD Infection. Most commonly, BVD infections are unobserved. Such infections cause leukopenia, transient biphasic temperature elevation and occasional oral erosions or blunted buccal papillae. They occur in susceptible cattle and sometimes in animals with low levels of colostrally derived humoral antibodies. Immunologically, normal cattle with low levels of actively induced antibody can be expected to elicit an anamnestic immune response adequate enough to prevent serious clinical disease and dissemination of virus to the fetus.

Postvaccination BVD. All the forms of BVD infection just discussed can occasionally occur following vaccination with modified live virus (MLV) vaccines attenuated by serial passage in cell cultures. The probability of postvaccination reactions other than mild inapparent infection is relatively low, unless the vaccine contains contaminating field strains of virus or the cattle are incubating the infection when vaccinated.

When pregnant susceptible cattle are vaccinated with MLV vaccines, abortion can result, and such vaccination of pregnant cattle is clearly contraindicated. These are several possible explanations for BVD-like disease within a "reasonable incubation period" after vaccination; the diagnosis may be inaccurate, the BVD infection may have been acquired before vaccination or the animal may be unable to tolerate the vaccine virus. This inability to respond immunologically to the virus explains why some calves succumb to the natural infection, while herdmates have a subclinical infection. Some explanations for postvaccination BVD are innate immunologic deficiencies, vaccination of "stressed" animals, vaccination of corticosteroid-treated animals, vaccination of animals under other immunosuppressive influences, the immunosuppressive effect of the vaccine virus, "immune tolerance" due to in utero infection and immune paralysis from an antigen excess.

When investigating postvaccination BVD, the first question to be asked should be "why were these cattle vaccinated?" Frequently, the answer is "because BVD was present in the herd." Use of inactivated vaccines eliminates this concern.

DIAGNOSIS OF BVD

Clinical diagnosis is based on clinical signs and lesions. Virus isolation, fluorescent antibody assay for virus and serologic examination are additional diagnostic aids.

At necropsy, the typical BVD-infected carcass is

thin, dehydrated and soiled with feces. The nasal orifices are usually encrusted. Erosions or ulcerations may be present in the oral mucosa, esophagus, rumen, abomasum and rarely on vulvar mucosa. A characteristic finding is lymphoid depletion, hemorrhage or necrosis of Peyer's patches. An occasional fatal case has necrotic areas around the skin of the lower limbs, particularly the coronary band.

The diagnosis can be confirmed by isolation of the virus from the spleen, lymph nodes or bone marrow. These must be harvested aseptically because bacterial contaminants readily overgrow cell culture systems. In the live animal, virus can be isolated from blood and nasal or ocular discharges. Some laboratories rely heavily on fluorescent antibody (FA) assay to identify BVD virus in tissues taken at necropsy.

Serologic diagnosis is usually based on a neutralization test performed in cell cultures. In most bovine populations there is a high antibody prevalence from previous infection or vaccination. Thus, a single serum specimen is inadequate for diagnosing the disease in an individual animal. Paired serum specimens are useful if the first specimen (taken during the acute stages of the disease) is negative and the second specimen (taken from the same animal 3 to 4 weeks later) is positive, indicating seroconversion around the time of clinical disease. Many acutely infected cattle die before the second specimen is collected, and many chronic cases fail to have demonstrable humoral antibody. Therefore, serologic diagnosis is severely limited.

Early leukopenia is an additional diagnostic aid.

ABORTIONS AND CONGENITAL ANOMALIES FROM BVD

For BVD infection of the developing fetus to occur, the cow or heifer must be both pregnant and susceptible at the time of infection. Fetal BVD frequently occurs in herds in which BVD was never diagnosed, and the etiologic agent remains unknown because of the obscure nature of the maternal infection. Because of the variable amount of time between maternal infection and abortion or birth of anomalous calves, a variety of abnormal pregnancy terminations can occur over many months without arousing suspicion of a common etiologic origin.

Abortion is more likely to occur if the dam is infected in the early months of gestation, but it can occur following infection at other stages of gestation. Expulsion of the infected fetus can occur close to the time of maternal infection or many months afterward.

The most clearly delineated syndrome resulting from fetal BVD infection is cerebellar degeneration with ocular defects. These do not always occur in the same calf, but their concurrent appearance is suggestive of congenital BVD. Affected fetuses may be aborted, but many are carried to term. Individual cases are frequently regarded as curiosities or genetic defects. However, birth of these calves tends to cluster in time, becoming evident with calving of cows that were in the middle trimester of pregnancy at the time the infection was active in the herd.

Calves with congenital ataxia from cerebellar deficiency produced by in utero BVD infection are usually normal except for ocular and visual deficiencies and motor incoordination. Severely affected calves are unable to rise after birth and eventually die. The mildly affected calf will have difficulty in rising and walking after birth. All reflexes are usually normal, and if the calves are hand-fed, they can survive. They may have a head tilt and a stilted basewide gait and may stumble easily, but by the time they are several weeks of age, mildly affected calves can appear normal.

In addition to damage to the developing cerebellum, such calves frequently have congenital cataracts, microphthalmia or other ocular anomalies. The diagnosis of congenital BVD is confirmed by finding an ataxic, partially blind calf with cataracts and BVD humoral antibody demonstrable in serum collected before nursing and cerebellar degeneration present at necropsy.

Aside from abortion and the cerebro-ocular syndrome, brachygnathia and other musculoskeletal defects and alopecia are occasional sequelae to fetal infection with BVD.

Fetal mummification can also occur after infection of the pregnant cow with BVD. Mummified fetuses can develop following fetal death from many causes. Therefore, the presence of a mummified bovine fetus is no assurance that BVD was the cause.

When BVD infection is introduced into a totally susceptible herd, about 25 per cent of the pregnancies may be expected to terminate abnormally.

In pregnant sheep experimental infection with BVD is inapparent but can be followed by low fertility, fetal death with abortion or mummification, cerebellar hypoplasia, hydrocephalus and congenital malformation of the limbs. Like BVD in cattle, the actual economic impact in sheep remains to be elaborated.

Diagnosis of BVD Abortions and Congenital Anomalies

Serologic specimens collected from the dam at the time of abortion or at the birth of anomalous calves are usually worthless as tools for confirming BVD except that absence of BVD antibodies tends to eliminate BVD from consideration.

On the other hand, antibody in presuckle serum collected from anomalous or stillborn calves or aborted fetuses provides convincing evidence that the fetus was infected in utero and supports the hypothesis of BVD as the etiologic agent. If the calf is ambulatory, the diagnostician must have assurance that it did not nurse and acquire colostral antibody. Serum antibody in a calf that has nursed indicates only that the dam had been vaccinated or exposed to BVD at some time in her life, and like a specimen of the dam's serum, this fact adds very little to the diagnostic picture. Assurance that the calf had not nursed can be obtained if the calf was dead at birth, if the clinician was present at birth or if the calf was unable to stand up and therefore could not have suckled. In cases in which diagnostic tests are anticipated on presuckle serums, the cow's udder should be examined for evidence of suckling. Sometimes owners report the calf has not nursed, but the cow's teats are clean, wet and covered with foamy milk and saliva, and presence of slack quarters suggest the calf did suckle. Also, the stomach must be free of milk at necropsy. Serums from anomalous calves and aborted fetuses should be sterile to avoid bacterial overgrowth of the cell cultures in which the serologic tests are performed.

Attempts to isolate virus from aborted fetuses and anomalous calves are usually unsuccessful. Some develop antibody, which neutralizes the virus, and some are heavily contaminated. In addition, some BVD virus strains are noncytopathogenic.

Fluorescent antibody assay on aborted fetuses can be a useful diagnostic tool. This procedure should be performed by well-trained, experienced, skillful and patient technicians using high quality reagents.

Other Effects of BVD on Reproduction

Early embryonic death may occur in cattle experiencing systemic infection immediately after breeding, but this is not a widely observed or a well-documented phenomenon. There are indications that BVD infections have immunosuppressive activity and suggestions that this contributes to susceptibility to postparturient metritis and placental retention.

TREATMENT OF BVD

Specific therapeutic measures are not available for treating BVD. It is usually treated empirically with supportive therapy. Although fluid therapy, antibiotics and antidiarrheals are used, most veterinarians agree that the outcome of the acute systemic disease is not greatly influenced by therapeutic regimens and supportive measures. The infections resulting in congenital anomalies are usually unrecognized and thus untreated. By the time abortion occurs or an anomalous calf is recognized, the damage is done.

PREVENTION OF BVD

Rearing cattle in isolation has proved inadequate for preventing infection with BVD virus. Thus, preventive methods are limited to the use of vaccines. In 1982 inactivated vaccines appeared for the first time. They avoid the safety problems associated with MLV vaccines, but they must be repeated frequently. The MLV vaccine is widely used alone or in combination with infectious bovine rhinotracheitis (IBR) and/or parainfluenza-3 vaccines.

Successful immunization with MLV products requires that the vaccinated animal be infected with the vaccine virus and subsequently respond immunologically. Most findings suggest that previously infected animals usually have enough resistance to ward off fetal BVD infection. Thus, the approach to the control of BVD-induced reproductive disease is vaccination prior to breeding, reduction of the herd's susceptibility and avoidance of catastrophic reproductive losses. It is unrealistic to expect any procedure to eliminate all abortions and other reproductive disorders.

The maternal antibody acquired from colostrum may persist from 6 to 8 months of age and sometimes longer and may interfere with successful vaccination. Therefore, vaccination of heifers should be carried out some time after 6 to 8 months of age and before breeding.

Calfhood vaccination programs for BVD can be maintained on an ongoing basis. One successful vaccination prior to the first breeding probably will markedly reduce the probability of BVD interfering with reproductive efficiency, but some experts recommend annual revaccination.

In addition to being abortifacient, the MLV BVD vaccines have a reputation for inducing postvaccination mucosal disease in a small percentage of vaccinated cattle. Therefore, only healthy, well-nourished, unstressed and socially adjusted heifer calves should be vaccinated. The use of MLV BVD vaccine on lactating animals is not recommended. Inactivated products overcome these concerns.

Because the major benefit derived from BVD vaccine is prevention of fetal damage, there appears to be no advantage to vaccinating bulls.

Each veterinarian should evaluate the management scheme on each farm or ranch and make a decision regarding a BVD vaccination program.

Effects of Blue Tongue Virus on the Reproductive Performance of Cattle

Thomas H. Howard, D.V.M., Ph.D.
American Breeders Service,
DeForest, Wisconsin

Blue tongue virus (BTV) is the prototype of the genus *Orbivirus*. At least 21 serotypes of this virus and two of the related orbivirus of epizootic hemorrhagic disease (EHD) have been identified. These viruses are distributed worldwide in equatorial and warm temperate regions. They are transmitted by a biologic vector, biting midges of the genus *Culicoides*. At least five blue tongue and two EHD virus serotypes are present in the United States.

EPIDEMIOLOGY

Prevailing winds and movement of major weather systems may be important to the movement of virus-laden midges from enzootic regions in the tropics and warm temperate regions. Such movement can produce blue tongue epizootics in ruminants within adjacent areas. Likewise, introduction of viremic animals into regions containing a competent vector population may result in outbreaks of blue tongue virus.

These viruses infect many wild and domestic ruminant species. Infection by BTV produces clinical disease only in sheep, antelope and deer. In North America, cattle and possibly elk are the important reservoir species from which the midges disseminate virus. Cattle experience a 30- to 90-day viremia without concurrent clinical signs of disease.

Blue tongue virus infection of pregnant females may result in fetal disease, a phenomenon that could be an overwintering adaptation of BTV outside the tropics. Overwintering of the virus in areas where continuous vector activity is not possible is not completely understood. There are seasonal peaks of infection in late summer and autumn in both the blue tongue–enzootic and –epizootic zones of the United States.

In North America serologic evidence indicates infection by blue tongue virus is prevalent in the western states, lower Great Plains, and Southeast. The upper Great Lakes and northeastern states are free of the virus. Limited studies of *Culicoides* native to the northeastern United States indicate those midges are not highly competent blue tongue vectors. Canada is presently free of blue tongue, although the virus has appeared in British Columbia at least once. Within blue tongue–enzootic, –epizootic, or –free zones there may be specific local ecosystems that differ so substantially from the surrounding areas that they present completely different obstacles or opportunities to the vector and virus. The epidemiology of epizootic hemorrhagic disease is more poorly understood than that of blue tongue virus, but EHD does appear to have a more northerly distribution, including several of the BTV-free states and Canada. The virus of EHD is pathogenic only in whitetail deer and exhibits low infectivity for sheep, while cattle are readily infectable.

PATHOGENESIS

In cattle, blue tongue virus infects hematopoietic and reticuloendothelial cells. However, clinical blue tongue disease in cattle is very rare and has not been experimentally reproduced. It appears that the absence of a significant cell-mediated immune response to BTV by the bovine species may be the reason clinical blue tongue disease of cattle is so rare.

While BTV does not cross the bovine placenta with consistency, it can produce arteritis in the caruncle. If the fetus becomes infected during the first trimester of gestation, infection of the developing brain and/or fetal death may result. The fetal immune response system is not fully developed at this stage of development, so a prolonged fetal viremia may ensue. Blue tongue virus serotypes 10, 13 and 17 are neuropathogenic for early fetal calves, producing porencephalia and hydranencephaly, which result in the birth of "dummy calves" having little or no functional cerebral cortex. Serotype 11 of BTV, as well as EHDV, produced fetal death when inoculated into first trimester bovine fetuses.

EFFECTS ON BOVINE REPRODUCTION

In vitro blue tongue viruses have a demonstrated capability to produce cytocidal infection of preimplantation bovine embryos. The virus cannot penetrate the zona pellucida. Presumably, embryos within viremic females could be destroyed by the virus once hatched from the zona on day 9 of development. Such a circumstance would be most likely when the breeding season of a herd of non-immune cows coincided with the seasonal peak of BTV infections, that is, in the months of August, September and October.

Seminal contamination is a sporadic consequence of BTV viremia in the bull. Seminal virus titers may be very high in some bulls, but more often such contamination is characterized by the sporadic presence of low titers of virus in the semen. Seminal contamination is possible only during the period of viremia. Limited histopathologic and immunofluorescence studies indicated that BTV contamination of semen is a consequence of BTV permissive lymphocytes and macrophages infiltrating the epididymal epithelium. Seminal contamination seems unlikely to result in significant amplification of vector-borne BTV outbreaks in herds using natural service. However, both the potential for BTV infection via the uterus and the survival of BTV through seminal processing, freezing and thawing have been verified; hence, the possibility of BTV transmission through artificial insemination does exist. Bulls used in artificial insemination programs should be proved to be nonviremic prior to collection of their semen. Nonimmune bulls should be housed in a vector-free environment. Immune (seropositive) bulls may be safely used as semen donors if proved to be no longer viremic. Isolation of blue tongue virus from blood is not only technically easier than isolation from semen but is a more sensitive indicator of the possibility of the presence of BTV in semen. The potential for seminal contamination by EHDV is presently unknown.

CONTROL OF BLUE TONGUE VIRUS

No blue tongue vaccines are available for cattle. Since blue tongue immunity is largely serotype specific, an effective vaccine should include antigens of all blue tongue serotypes to which an animal might be exposed. The possible use of a modified live virus vaccine in cattle is confounded by the dangers of fetal infection, vector transmission of vaccine virus during the long viremia, and the possibility of reassortment among vaccine serotypes in animals vaccinated with polyvalent vaccines, producing new BTV viruses with greater virulence and different serologic determinants. Inactivated or subunit blue tongue vaccines would appear to be better candidates for use in cattle.

Studies of vector-control procedures are under way, but widespread control of *Culicoides* seems unlikely. The midge breeds along shallow streams and irrigation ditches contaminated by fecal matter or in manure moistened by water trough overflow or feedlot runoff.

Cattle raisers should refrain from moving very valuable pregnant females into blue tongue endemic areas during the first half of gestation. Native cattle in endemic areas usually acquire immunity to at least one BTV serotype before reaching breeding age. Young stock destined for export or artificial insemination markets requiring negative BTV serologic response should be moved from endemic areas before passive immunity is lost, which is usually at about 6 months of age.

SEROLOGIC TESTS FOR BLUE TONGUE VIRUS

The official test in current use is the agar gel immunodiffusion (AGID) test. This test detects antibodies to all BTV serotypes and in some instances antibodies to epizootic hemorrhagic disease virus. Seroconversion of cattle tested with AGID follows infection by 14 to 35 days. The test is interpreted as either "positive" or "negative." The AGID responses of some animals are inconsistent between different serum samples and/or laboratories. More sensitive serologic tests can be used to resolve inconsistent AGID responses. These tests include serum neutralization, which is serotype specific; hemolysis-in-gel; and enzyme-linked immunosorbent assay (ELISA). However, none of these tests are presently accorded official regulatory recognition in the United States. Standardization of blue tongue serologic tests and their performance, as well as the interpretation of the significance of serologic responses to BTV, should be an urgent priority of international veterinary regulators, as the monetary losses to cattle breeders associated with the performance and interpretation of the present tests probably exceed that resulting from the infection itself.

Epizootic Bovine Abortion

Paul B. Kimsey, Ph.D.
*Massachusetts Institute of Technology,
Cambridge, Massachusetts*

DEFINITION

Epizootic bovine abortion (EBA), or foothill abortion, is an arthropod-borne, last trimester abortion disease of unknown etiology. The only known vector is the argasid tick *Ornithodoros coriaceus* Koch (*O. coriaceus*) (Figs. 1 and 2). The disease is geographically limited to the oak woodland or chaparral life zones that rim the Central and San Joaquin Valleys of California.

HISTORY

In 1956 field and laboratory studies of an abortion disease designated as EBA were described. The disease was characterized as having a sudden onset, high fetal mortality and annual occurrence, once it was established in a herd. Abortions were confined to first-calf heifers, except during the first year of its introduction into a herd, when cows of all ages were affected. An etiologic agent was not determined.[2]

In 1959 organisms of the genus *Chlamydia* were isolated from two cases of EBA in California, and a syndrome similar to EBA was later reproduced experimentally by inoculation of the chlamydial agent into pregnant cattle.[13]

The strict geographic limitations of the disease suggested that the disease was transmitted by a vector with a similar geographic distribution.[2] This presumed vector was not identified until 1976 when the argasid tick *Ornithodoros coriaceus* Koch was shown to inhabit ranges that were geographically coincidental with areas in which EBA was enzootic. Also, feeding of *O. coriaceus* to pregnant susceptible cattle resulted in abortion of fetuses that had lesions characteristic of EBA.[12]

Because of the following information, EBA and bovine chlamydial abortion (BCA) at this time are felt to be two separate abortion syndromes.

1. *Chlamydia* has been implicated as a cause of bovine abortions (BCA) in North America, Europe, South Africa and Asia.[14] The only known vector of EBA is the Argasid tick *O. coriaceus* Koch, which in the United States is essentially limited to California (see distribution under vector) and then only in areas of specific life zones.[7]

2. Several experimental chlamydial vaccines have failed to protect susceptible cows from subsequent EBA abortion when challenged by natural field exposure.[9, 10] Heifers experimentally immunized with an intradermal vaccine were protected against homologous parenteral challenge with a bovine chlamydial abortifacient.[11] Thus, the causative agent of EBA would appear to be other than *chlamydial*.

3. The initial experimentally induced chlamydial

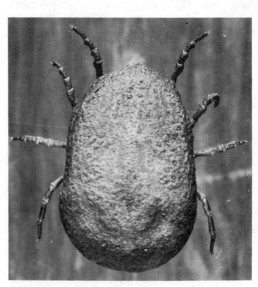

Figure 1. Adult female, unfed (top view).　　　　**Figure 2.** Adult female, blood fed (top view).

abortions were believed to reproduce the pathologic lesions of EBA.[4, 13] More recent in-depth pathologic examinations have shown differences between BCA and EBA.[5, 6]

4. Maternal and fetal serologic assays do not support the role of *Chlamydia* in EBA. Cows experimentally inoculated with chlamydial organisms show an increase in group-specific antibodies using the complement-fixation (CF) test as do the experimentally infected fetuses. These results are in contrast with the pathogenesis of EBA in the field. Cows exposed to ticks that transmitted EBA failed to show an increase in chlamydial antibody titer, and the diseased fetuses show no CF antibody to *Chlamydia*.[6, 15]

5. A commercially available monoclonal antibody to a genus-specific antigen was used in an indirect fluorescent antibody test. *Chlamydia* were not detected in tissues from EBA fetuses diagnosed to be in the early, middle or late stages of the disease.

VECTOR

The *O. coriaceus* Koch tick has been found in 52 of 58 counties in California and in western Nevada and southern Oregon. The tick lives in the coarse soils and sands mixed with tree litter from nearby chapparal species that serve as cover for deer and range cattle. These habitats are common in coastal and foothill areas at elevations of 0 to 3000 feet. Above these elevations to about 8000 feet the tick is commonly found under juniper, yellow and pinion pine and bitterbrush.[8]

The tick's life cycle involves four stages: egg, larva, nymph and adult. Eggs hatch in 10 to 20 days. Larvae may live for 5 months without a blood meal. Once attached to a host, larval feeding time is usually 7 to 10 days. Nymphs pass through three to seven molts (instars), each requiring a blood meal that takes 8 to 100 minutes. Adults feed in 5 to 50 minutes. The average life cycle from egg to adult is 1 year. Females lay 150 to 300 eggs at a time and produce about four batches per year during a 5-year lifespan. The short-term feeding habits of this tick explain why few are ever seen attached to cattle, and since the tick does not defecate during feeding or produce coxial fluid until after detachment, the transmission of an abortifacient agent apparently occurs during the feeding process.[8] Techniques and devices for CO_2 entrapment, laboratory maintenance and feeding of ticks on experimental animals and media are available.[3, 4]

MICROBIOLOGY

Since the initial isolations of *Chlamydia* in the late 1950s, very few subsequent documented chlamydial isolations have been made from EBA enzootic areas. Numerous attempts have been made to duplicate the isolation of *Chlamydia* from these fetuses, including use of recently developed techniques that have proved helpful in isolating the organism from other known chlamydial diseases. All attempts have been negative.[6]

The etiology of EBA is unknown. The significance of nine recent isolations of a virus and eight isolations of a nonchlamydial agent that kills eggs intermittently from EBA fetuses is as yet uncertain. Work is continuing on these agents to determine their relationship to each other and to EBA.[6]

CLINICAL SIGNS

The dam infected with EBA shows no clinical signs of disease or of impending abortion, and the abortion occurs most commonly during the last trimester. Susceptible cows exposed before the sixth month of gestation are at risk. Susceptibility is based solely on lack of prior exposure to the tick. There is no information on the incidence of the agent in the tick, so consequently, little is known about the minimum number of ticks necessary for EBA transmission. Experimentally, the disease has been transmitted with as few as 36 ticks.[6]

PATHOGENESIS

With the identification of *O. coriaceus* as a vector of EBA, it became possible to study the disease in a prospective experimental manner. Studies on the pathogenesis have shown lesions characteristic of EBA in fetuses recovered 100 days or more after maternal tick exposure. Fetuses surgically collected between 50 and 100 days showed mild to moderate lymphoid and mononuclear cell hyperplasia. This fact reveals one of the unique aspects of EBA, namely the chronic progressive nature of the disease in the fetus. The early stages of EBA infection are characterized by lymphocytic transformation and proliferation. At the same time, cells of the mononuclear macrophage system become activated and undergo a parallel proliferation. These proliferative responses are associated with plasma cell formation and result in elevated immunoglobulin levels. The frequency with which necrosis and vasculitis are seen in fetuses that are aborted in both field and experimental cases suggests that it may be the conversion of the disease from a chronic, largely proliferative one to an acute necrotizing phase that triggers the premature parturition. The mechanisms involved in this shift are not known, but the pattern and timing of the acute necrotizing lesions suggest that they may be immune mediated. Unlike the changes in the lymph node, spleen and liver, which are progressive throughout the course of the disease, the thymic lesion develops later in the disease.[5, 6]

PATHOLOGY

Gross. Although EBA fetuses often appear quite fresh, having died just prior to, during or shortly after delivery, autolysis, though usually not severe, may also be present. The placenta can be edematous, but this is not diagnostic except for the lack of a fibrinopurulent placentitis associated with bovine chlamydial abortion.

Hemorrhages, ranging from petechiae seen on the skin and the conjunctival and oral mucous membranes to ecchymoses seen on the entire ventral surface of the tongue, are quite prominent. Petechiae are also regularly seen in the thymus, salivary glands, lymph nodes and pericardium. Linear hemorrhages are seen in skeletal muscle and are associated with a yellow gelatinous infiltrate that separates muscle bundles. Straw-colored peritoneal and pleural effusions are common; in some cases the ascites is sufficient to cause distension of the abdomen. The subcutaneous tissues are quite often edematous, particularly the head and neck regions.

The most prominent lesions are the swollen, coarsely nodular liver, enlarged spleen and edematous, enlarged lymph nodes. Some supracervical (prescapular) lymph nodes weigh as much as 14 to 16 gm in EBA fetuses (normal = 4 to 6 gm). In many instances the fetus has breathed prior to death, and in these the partially aerated lung is outlined by the thickened edematous septa.[4]

In cases in which an EBA fetus survives parturition, the weak calf may exhibit lymphadenopathy, especially of the supracervical lymph node and oral/conjunctival petechial hemorrhages.

Histology. The histologic lesions seen in EBA abortions include the following:

Liver. Large numbers of mononuclear cells are found around the majority of portal vessels, with foci in other locations. Granulomatous foci are often more than 100 μm in diameter.

Spleen. Widespread infiltration of macrophages is found, forming sheets and granulomas, some with necrotic centers.

Lymph Node. Widespread severe macrophage infiltration is found throughout the lymph nodes. Sinuses are congested with macrophages, which form sheets in medullary regions. Focal areas of necrosis, occasionally in centers of granulomatous reaction, are also found. An inflammatory reaction often extends outside the node.

Brain. Widespread inflammatory foci, some of which are granulomatous, and granulomatous meningitis are present.

Heart, Kidney and Skin. Numerous foci of inflammation, some more than 150 μm in diameter and granulomatous in appearance, are present.

Lung. Alveolar septa are markedly increased in thickness. Granulomatous inflammation is present in interlobular septa or lung parenchyma.

Thymus. Cortical thymocytes are reduced to 20 per cent or less of the lobule. Widespread macrophage infiltration is present in both the medulla and septa. Occasionally, edema and hemorrhage occur.[4, 5]

DIAGNOSIS

Based on geographic location in California, the established presence of the vector or its habitat, the herd history and the evaluation of the gross fetal pathology, the presumptive diagnosis of EBA can often be made. A histopathologic evaluation along with the above information is preferred for a definitive diagnosis.

The herd histories that would support an EBA diagnosis would include the following:

1. Moving newly purchased replacement cows of any age from the valley (a nontick exposure area) to the foothills or mountains (a known tick exposure area).

2. Changing calving seasons, e.g., putting the bulls in earlier or later or changing from fall calving to spring calving, thereby exposing pregnant susceptible cows to the most active tick season—the cow would be in a susceptible part of her gestation at a time when the tick is active.

3. Movement of pregnant susceptible animals on the same ranch, e.g., moving susceptible cows from an irrigated pasture (nontick exposure area) to a nonirrigated pasture (tick exposure area).

4. Having a 30 to 80 per cent abortion rate in first-calf heifers each year.

5. Changing the heifer calving program, e.g., breeding yearlings instead of 2-year-olds.[1]

EBA needs to be differentiated from other late-term abortions caused by *Brucella abortus*, *Leptospira pomona* and *Chlamydia psittaci*.

PREVENTION

Preventing or reducing the impact of the disease can be achieved by various management procedures. Avoiding areas where the tick is established is the most obvious, but not always the most practical strategy.

Based on field observations, exposing open yearlings or 2-year-old heifers to summertime brush areas containing ticks seems to confer immunity. These animals are then bred during the fall and are therefore immune at the first calving season as 2- or 3-year olds.

Changing spring calving to fall calving on some ranches in northern California tends to expose pregnant cattle to the tick after they are 6 months pregnant. Since the disease has a long incubation period, the disease process does not have time to proceed to abortion.

On ranches in the warmer areas of central and southern California where tick exposure begins earlier (May to June), backing the calving season up by 2 months in susceptible cattle will also produce maximum tick exposure after the susceptible gestation period and thereby reduce abortion. This means a September calving rather than a November calving for most of the herd.[1] It should be remembered that fetuses exposed late in gestation can still be affected congenitally (i.e., weak, poor doer calves) even though abortion is avoided.

References

1. Bushnell RR: Foothill abortion update. Nev Calif Beef Conf Proc February 1977.
2. Howarth JA, Moulton JE, Frazier LM: Epizootic bovine abortion characterized by fetal hepatopathy. J Am Vet Med Assoc 128:441, 1956.
3. Howarth JA, Hokama Y: Studies with *Ornithodoros coriaceus* Koch (Acarina:Argasidae), the suspected vector of epizootic bovine abortion. In Wilde JKH (ed): Proc Conf Tick-borne Dis Their Vectors. Edinburgh, Edinburgh University Press, 1976, pp 168–176.
4. Kennedy PC, Olander HF, Howarth JA: Pathology of epizootic bovine abortion. Cornell Vet 50:417, 1960.
5. Kennedy PC, Casaro AP, Kimsey PB, et al.: Epizootic bovine abortion: Histogenesis of fetal lesions. Am J Vet Res 44:1040, 1983.
6. Kimsey PB, Kennedy PC, Bushnell RB, et al.: Studies on the pathogenesis of epizootic bovine abortion. Am J Vet Res 44:1266, 1983.
7. Loomis EC, Schmitmann ET, Oliver MN: A summary review on the distribution of *Ornithodoros coriaceus* Koch in California. Calif Vect Views 21:57, 1974.
8. Loomis EC, Furman DP: The pajaroello tick. Div Agri Sci Univ Calif Vet Med Extension Leaflet No. 2503, Univ Calif Davis, May 1977.
9. McKercher DG, Wada EM, Howarth JA: Epizootiologic and immunologic studies of epizootic bovine abortion. Cornell Vet 56:433, 1966.
10. McKercher DG, Robinson EA, Wada EM: Vaccination of cattle against epizootic bovine abortion. Cornell Vet 59:211, 1969.
11. McKercher DG, Crenshaw GL, Theis JH: Experimentally induced immunity to chlamydial abortion of cattle. J Infect Dis 128:231, 1973.
12. Schmitmann ET, Bushnell RB, Loomis EC, et al.: Experimental and epizootiologic evidence associating *Ornithodoros coriaceus* Koch (Acari:Argasidae) with exposure of cattle to epizootic bovine abortion in California. J Med Entomol 13:292, 1976.
13. Storz J, McKercher DG, Howarth JA, Straub OC: The isolation of a viral agent from epizootic bovine abortion. J Am Vet Med Assoc 137:509, 1960.
14. Stortz J, Whiteman CE: Bovine chlamydial abortions. Bov Prac 16:71, 1981.
15. Wada EM, McKercher DG, Castucci G, Theis JH: Preliminary characterization and pathogenicity studies of a virus isolated from ticks (*Ornithodoros coriaceus*) and from tick-exposed cattle. Am J Vet Res 37:1201, 1976.

Bovine Genital Campylobacteriosis

Paul J. Dekeyser, D.V.M.
National Institute of Veterinary Research,
Brussels, Belgium

Campylobacteriosis is an infectious venereal disease of cattle mainly caused by the bacterium *Campylobacter fetus* subspecies *venerealis*. The infection is introduced at the time of coitus or artificial insemination with infected semen and results in a uterine infection that prevents conception or causes an early termination of pregnancy. In a relatively small number of animals abortion will occur.

In 1973 the results of a taxonomic study of the genus *Campylobacter* were published by Veron and colleagues. They proposed that *Vibrio fetus intestinalis* should be renamed *Campylobacter fetus* ss. *fetus* and that *Vibrio fetus venerealis* should be renamed *Campylobacter fetus* ss. *venerealis*.[7]

PATHOGENESIS AND CLINICAL SIGNS

Enzootic Infertility: Venereal Bovine Campylobacteriosis

Bulls most commonly become infected by serving infected female animals, but contact with infected bedding can also lead to infection. This contact infection is the basic reason why more than 50 per cent of the bulls in an artificial insemination center may be affected. Bulls 4 years old or older are more susceptible than younger ones. A possible explanation for this is that the crypts in the epithelium of the penis become deeper and more numerous with age and thus provide a more favorable milieu for *Campylobacter*. Infection of the prepuce always remains strictly localized and produces no local or general symptoms. Spontaneous recovery from a natural infection occurs very rarely. This could be due to the very slight antigenic variation undergone by the organisms so that, because only a local and minimal immunologic response occurs, infected bulls may become lifelong asymptomatic carriers.

Campylobacter multiplies rapidly in the vagina of a susceptible female animal served by an infected bull. In a week the organisms traverse the cervix into the uterus and there continue to spread over a period of 6 to 8 weeks. In 25 per cent of naturally infected heifers the organisms reach the oviducts. They can survive in the cervix and even more easily in the vagina for months and sometimes for the duration of the pregnancy, during which time it is very difficult for the animal to get rid of the infection.

Histologic examination shows a progressive endometritis with inflammatory damage that reaches a peak about the eighth to thirteenth week after infection. It can be described as a subacute diffuse mucopurulent endometritis, characterized by the accumulation of exudate in the lumen of the uterine glands and by periglandular infiltration by lymphocytes.

Because of this inflammatory reaction the embryo finds itself in a very hostile environment, and the oxygen supply to the embryo may become so restricted that it dies, resulting in a prolonged cycle of 24 to 40 days or more in a large percentage of the animals. The symptoms are most pronounced in heifers, more than 75 per cent of whom return to heat, usually after a prolonged cycle. Sometimes a 2- to 3-month old fetus is expelled with its membranes intact, or abortions may occur at a still later stage, usually around the fourth to sixth month. The entire process of recovery requires 4 to 5 months. Thereafter, the animals are relatively immune. Nevertheless, fertility never returns to its normal level, and in individual animals bilateral salpingitis leads to permanent sterility. On rare occasions a female animal remains a permanent vaginal carrier of *Campylobacter fetus* ss. *venerealis*.

Sporadic Abortion Due to *C. fetus* ss. *fetus*

This form of genital infection is much less spectacular because it arises from an accidental dissemination of *Campylobacter* that is present in the gut or gallbladder. When such an occasional bacteremia occurs, the already well-formed placenta of the pregnant uterus is a selective target for any organisms such as *Mycobacterium pyogenes, Salmonella,* and *Listeria* as well as *Campylobacter fetus* ss. *fetus* that may be circulating in the blood. The placentitis caused by these organisms leads to the death of the fetus through anoxia, and this is inevitably followed by a late abortion. This is the only symptom of the infection, of which the female genital system rapidly rids itself. In contrast to its pathogenic role in the sheep, *Campylobacter jejuni* does not interfere in any way with reproduction in cattle.

CAUSAL AGENTS

The cause of enzootic infertility is *Campylobacter fetus* ss. *venerealis* in more than 95 per cent of cases. The biochemical variants that produce hydrogen sulfide in cysteine-enriched media are also included. In addition, some of these variants are relatively tolerant of glycine, but none of them reduce selenite. Antigenically, they all belong to serotype A. *Campylobacter fetus* ss. *fetus* is responsible for less than 5 per cent of cases. They all belong to serotype B.

During extensive investigations carried out on farms with normal fertility, the only vibrios that could be frequently isolated either from bulls or from heifers were catalase negative. This is in direct contrast to the pathogenic vibrios, which are all catalase positive. These saprophytic vibrios were originally called *Vibrio bubulus* but are now named *Campylobacter sputorum* ss. *bubulus*.

Morphology and Colonial Characteristics

Campylobacter fetus ss. *venerealis* and *C. fetus* ss. *fetus* cannot be differentiated with certainty by microscopic examination. They are gram-negative, slender, short, comma- or S-shaped rods that may form a helix. They do not form spores. The proportion of short and S-shaped forms to the longer spirals is very much influenced by the composition of the medium on which they are grown. These microorganisms are best examined under phase-contrast illumination, which shows not only their shape particularly well but also the rapid to and fro movement characteristic of the shorter forms.

Colonies of *C. fetus* ss. *fetus* are already well developed by 48 hours, but *C. fetus* ss. *venerealis* needs at least 72 hours. They have a diameter of 1 to 2 mm, and they are grayish white to light brown in color and are nonhemolytic.

Culture

Campylobacter fetus is a microaerophilic organism that will grow only on solid media in an atmosphere with reduced oxygen and increased carbon dioxide; this is particularly important for primary isolation. The best results are obtained when two thirds of the normal air is replaced by a mixture of 95 per cent nitrogen and 5 per cent carbon dioxide. When these organisms are grown in a rich broth the resulting turbidity is only moderate and cannot be seen except in good lighting. They are often grown in semi-solid media where a ring of growth appears just below the surface.

The optimum temperature for development is about 37°C. Growth always takes place also at 25°C, but at 42°C the growth of most strains is completely inhibited.

Antigenic Studies

Using "whole cells antigen," *C. fetus* strains can be divided into five serologic groups. However, based on heat-stable somatic antigens, they can be divided into only two groups.

All the strains that belong to serotype A can be venereally transmitted and cause enzootic infertility with the exception of those strains that reduce 0.1 per cent sodium selenite and are tolerant of 1.3 per cent glycine.

All the strains of serotype B can be found as commensals in the gastrointestinal tract and belong to *C. fetus* ss. *fetus*. They can cause sporadic abortion and in occasional rare cases of enzootic infertility are encountered either in the prepuce of the bull or in the vaginal mucus of the animal served by the infected bull. An experimental vaginal infection with serotype B can also be set up but usually disappears within a few weeks. The fact that there is little sharing of antigens between serotype A and serotype B means that immunization with a vaccine prepared from a strain of serotype A can usually neither prevent nor cure an infection in the bull due to a strain of serotype B.

Sensitivity of Antibiotics

In the diffusion test C. fetus ss. venerealis is sensitive to gentamicin, neomycin, chloromycetin, kanamycin, erythromycin, tetracycline, penicillin and streptomycin. Streptomycin-resistant strains were isolated from preputial washings in rare cases. C. fetus ss. venerealis is resistant to bacitracin and novobiocin, and most strains are also resistant to polymyxin B. The minimal inhibitory concentrations (MIC) of bacitracin, novobiocin and polymyxin B were also greater than 50 μg/ml. These three antibiotics are used in selective media designed for the isolation of C. fetus ss. venerealis from heavily contaminated material. C. fetus ss. fetus shows the same pattern of antibiotic sensitivities except that it is not sensitive to penicillin.

TRANSMISSION AND DISSEMINATION

From the many publications on enzootic infertility, whether dealing with field cases or experimental infections, it is clear that transmission of the infection occurs principally by the venereal route. For female animals it is the only way in which they become infected. However, bulls may be indirectly infected by contact with infected material or by equipment used in the artificial insemination (AI) centers for the collection of semen as well as by contact with infected bedding. Schutte reported that three of the six bulls placed on bedding that had been used previously by infected bulls became positive for C. fetus ss. venerealis in 39, 42 and 55 days respectively.[6]

This observation provided a logical explanation for the fact that in many AI centers a number of bulls have been found to be infected before they had ever served a single cow or heifer. The infection can be very easily spread if artificial insemination is carried out with infected semen. The addition of penicillin and streptomycin to semen, whether used fresh or stored deep frozen, proved to be very effective in preventing spread of the disease by artificial insemination.

In the sporadic cases of abortion due to C. fetus ss. fetus, dissemination of the organisms at the time of the abortion itself and for a week afterward is extensive, but only rarely do other cattle in the herd abort as a result.

DIAGNOSIS

Careful investigation of a farm affected by enzootic infertility often leads to a clinical diagnosis, but it must be confirmed by laboratory examination of preputial smegma, vaginal mucus and fetal and placental tissues.

Approximately 40 ml of phosphate-buffered saline (PBS, pH 7.1), a sterile rubber tube (1.2 m long and 1 cm in diameter) attached to a sterile plastic funnel, and disposable gloves are needed for the collection of smegma. The tube is introduced 10 cm into the sheath and the PBS allowed to flow into the preputial cavity. With one hand the preputial opening is tightly closed while with the other hand the liquid is thoroughly massaged for at least 1 minute. The material is then drained back into the funnel and dispensed into two sterile test tubes: one sample is to be used for immediate bacteriologic examinations, the other for the fluorescent antibody test.

Preputial samples can also be obtained by the swab procedure or by aspirating smegma into an AI pipette using a syringe. In both cases the sample is to be mixed with a few milliliters of PBS.

When the preputial washing cannot be processed immediately, PBS must be replaced by a selective transport and enrichment medium such as thioglycollate broth USP-alternative (Oxoid CM 391) containing 40 mg of vancomycin, 5000 IU of polymyxin B sulfate, 10 mg of trimethoprim, 100 mg of cycloheximide (Actidione) and 100 mg of 5-fluorouracil per liter.

The viability of C. fetus ss. venerealis is maintained for at least 1 week in this medium when held at 22°C. Lower temperatures must be avoided because they increase the absorption of oxygen from the atmosphere.

Direct Culture

Campylobacter, whether in the prepuce or the vagina, is in an environment containing large numbers of other organisms. The growth of a wide variety of these possible contaminants is inhibited or suppressed on the following medium, which is routinely used for the isolation of Campylobacter fetus: brain-heart infusion agar or fluid thioglycollate agar medium containing 10 per cent ox or sheep blood; to this is added, per milliliter, 25 IU bacitracin (Nutritional Biochemicals Corp., Cleveland, Ohio), 0.005 mg novobiocin (Merck, Sharpe and Dohme), 1 I.U. polymyxin-B sulfate (Pfizer) and 0.05 mg Actidione (Upjohn).

Preputial washings must first be centrifuged at 1500 × g for 5 minutes. Four milliliters of the surface liquid is then aspirated into a syringe for subsequent filtration through a 0.65-Millipore filter. The first 3 ml are discarded; 0.3 ml of the remaining liquid is filtered directly into each of two Petri dishes, one containing the above-described medium and the other containing the same medium without polymyxin, the latter permitting the growth of saprophytic C. sputorum ss. bubulus. Vaginal mucus samples and fetal abomasal contents can be plated directly.

Immunofluorescence

Immunofluorescence is a convenient, quick and accurate method for detecting carrier bulls. A combination of culture and isolation procedures and a fluorescent antibody (FA) test will detect 98 per cent of infected bulls. The test will of course give a false-negative result if a serum against only serotype A is used and the infection is due to *C. fetus* ss. *fetus* serotype B. Similarly, it will give a false-positive result if the bull's prepuce has been colonized by *C. fetus* ss. *fetus* serotype A.

Vaginal Mucus Agglutination Test

Following a natural infection, female animals produce local antibodies, which may be detected in cervical mucus from 6 weeks to 7 months afterward. These antibodies will agglutinate a suitable antigen in a tube test. This technique also allows an anti-bovine globulin test to be carried out, whereby the possible presence of "incomplete" antibodies may be demonstrated and the sensitivity of the test increased.

In the individual animal a negative result does not exclude infection. Furthermore, the sample of mucus must be free of blood and transudate because the commonly used antigens usually give a fairly high titer if the test is carried out on serum instead of vaginal mucus. Nevertheless, when the mucus agglutination test, together with the antibovine globulin test, is carried out on a large number of samples from all the animals in a herd in which there has been a serious and recent infertility problem, a decisive answer as to the presence or absence of enzootic infertility will be obtained.

Vaginal infection has no influence on serum antibody titers. It does give rise, however, to the formation of local antibodies belonging to immunoglobulin classes A, G and M.

TREATMENT AND PREVENTION

When a diagnosis of enzootic infertility has been made, there is no point in trying to treat infected female animals unless they were served less than 3 weeks earlier. In curative treatment of bulls with antibiotics the best results are obtained by applying an ointment containing 10 gm neomycin and 4 gm erythromycin in 200 gm carbowax to the surface of the exteriorized penis and to the prepuce after both have been thoroughly washed with 8 liters of warm water containing 1 per cent hydrogen peroxide. Bulls that were known to have been treated unsuccessfully earlier with streptomycin or tetracycline were cured after this combined therapy. The presence of multiresistant *Escherichia coli* in the prepuce was considered to be responsible for the production of enzymes that inactivated the streptomycin and tetracycline, as has been demonstrated in vitro.

The great problem with bulls serving cattle naturally is reinfection. In countries where extensive pasture breeding is practiced, preventive and curative vaccination has been given since 1961 to female animals but not to bulls. Clark and associates, however, successfully treated four infected bulls

with two injections of their vaccine.[3] Bouters and associates were able to cure infected bulls with an experimental vaccine, 30 animals after one dose and 11 animals after two doses 6 weeks apart.[2] These bulls continued to serve regularly in an infected area and remained free of infection for more than a year. In the same infected area, 288 bulls negative for *C. fetus* were given one dose and similarly remained free of infection for more than a year. After vaccination, the preputial secretion contains antibodies of classes IgG, IgM and IgA. The objection to vaccinating bulls was that they continue to be able to transmit the infection from the vagina of an infected cow to that of an uninfected one during coitus. This objection was removed by the work of Clark and his colleagues.[4] Frank and associates confirmed that vaccination of heifers produced a significant improvement of their breeding efficiency, although protection against infection was not obtained.[5]

Vaccinated heifers that have been served by a naturally infected bull have an almost normal fertility in spite of the fact that 90 per cent may acquire a vaginal infection. That they do in fact become pregnant can be explained only by the uterus being absolutely resistant, mainly due to the more ample supply of antibodies from the blood.

Inoculated pregnant animals also can apparently rid themselves of a vaginal infection only with great difficulty. Berg and associates[1] recommend the vaccination of all bulls and cows in breeding herds. The first time an animal is vaccinated protective immunity can be obtained only after two doses of the vaccine injected about 6 weeks apart, the second dose being given a few weeks prior to the start of breeding time. For previously vaccinated bulls and cows Berg and associates[1] recommend giving an annual booster vaccination approximately 10 days before breeding begins. This will maintain a high degree of protection in the herd.

References

1. Berg RL, Firehammer BD: Effect of interval between booster vaccination and time of breeding on protection against campylobacteriosis (vibriosis) in cattle. J Am Vet Med Assoc 173:467, 1978.
2. Bouters R, Dekeyser J, Vandeplassche M, et al.: *Vibrio fetus* infection in bulls: Curative and preventive vaccination. Br Vet J 129:52, 1973.
3. Clark BL, Dufty JH, Monsbourgh MJ: Vaccination of bulls against bovine vibriosis. Aust Vet J 44:530, 1968.
4. Clark BL, Dufty JH, Monsbourgh MJ, Parsonson IM: Studies on venereal transmission of *Campylobacter fetus* by immunized bulls. Aust Vet J 51:531, 1975.
5. Frank AH, Bryner JH, O'Berry PA: The effect of *Vibrio fetus* vaccination on the breeding efficiency of cows bred to *Vibrio fetus* infected bulls. Am J Vet Res 28:1237, 1967.
6. Schutte AP: Some aspects of *Vibrio fetus* infection in bulls. Meded Veeartsenijschool Rijksuniversiteit Gent 13, 1969, 88 p.
7. Veron M, Chatelain R: Taxonomic study of the genus *Campylobacter* Sebald and Veron and designation of the neotype strain for the type species, *Campylobacter fetus* (Smith and Taylor) Sebald and Veron. Int J Syst Bact, 23:122, 1973.

Effects of Leptospirosis on Bovine Reproduction

W. A. Ellis, Ph.D., B.V.M.S., F.R.C.V.S.
Veterinary Research Laboratory,
Belfast, Northern Ireland

Leptospirosis is a common zoonotic disease, occurring in most mammals throughout the world. It causes economic losses to the cattle industry primarily by its effect on reproductive performance and secondarily by decreased milk production and occasionally death. However, many aspects of bovine leptospirosis are still inadequately defined owing to limitations inherent in the clinical, epidemiologic and microbiologic techniques that have been used in the study of both naturally occurring and experimental infections.

The disease can be caused by any of the parasitic spirochetes classified within the genus *Leptospira*. For taxonomic purposes and as an aid to epidemiologic studies the parasitic leptospires are subdivided into serogroups on the basis of antigenic relationships as determined by cross-agglutination reactions and further subdivided into serovars by agglutinin-absorption patterns.[9] The last official list[48] recognized 16 serogroups, and more than 150 serovars have now been identified.

EPIDEMIOLOGY

Distribution. While a large number of serovars have been identified throughout the world, only a small proportion of these will be endemic in any particular region or country. Furthermore, leptospirosis is a disease that shows a natural nidality, and each serovar tends to be maintained in specific maintenance hosts.[4] Therefore, in any region cattle are infected by the following:

1. Serovar *hardjo*, which is the cattle-maintained serovar. It has a worldwide distribution, and high serologic[1] and/or microbiologic[16, 32, 47] prevalences have been identified in many countries.

2. Strains maintained by other domestic and free-living animals. What these incidental infections are is determined by what other animal species are present in the area and by what serovars they maintain. The relative importance of these incidental infections to cattle is determined by the opportunity and by the prevailing management and environmental factors that allow for contact and transmission of leptospires between incidental hosts and cattle.

Serovar *pomona*, which is maintained by pigs and a variety of free-living animals, is the most important incidental infection of cattle in North America, Australia and New Zealand. In parts of Africa, U.S.S.R. and Israel, infection by *grippotyphosa* constitutes the most important incidental leptospiral infection of cattle. In parts of the Caribbean this role is filled by *autumnalis*.

Transmission. Direct transmission among cattle can occur via infected urine, post-abortion uterine discharge, infected placenta, sexual contact, or *in utero* infection. It is probably of greatest importance with serovar *hardjo* where infection appears to be largely independent of rainfall and cattle management systems, transmission having been reported in both housed[28] and pastured animals.[34]

Indirect transmission plays a much greater role in the transmission of incidental infections. It occurs through exposure to an environment contaminated with infective material from cattle or incidental hosts. This is favored by an environment that permits the maximum survival of leptospires outside the host and a management system that facilitates close contact between carrier and susceptible animals. Survival of leptospires outside the host is favored by warm moist conditions and a pH close to neutral. Areas such as waterholes where cattle and other animals congregate are frequently incriminated in outbreaks of bovine leptospirosis.

PATHOGENESIS

Infection of susceptible cattle occurs through mucous membranes and abraded or water-softened skin and is followed after a 4- to 10-day incubation period by a bacteremic phase that may last from a few hours to 7 days. This phase is characterized by pyrexia, excretion of leptospires in milk, and, with some serovars, by functional damage to the internal organs, especially in younger animals. Acute clinical infection occurs at this stage.

With the appearance of circulating antibody, bacteremia ceases but leptospires localize and persist in a number of organs, especially the proximal renal tubules and the genital tract of sexually mature females.[13, 40, 45] Relapses of pyrexia may occur.[13] Whether these are associated with persistent foci of infection giving rise to recurring bacteremia or possibly toxemia is unknown.

Leptospires are excreted in urine for a variable period depending on the infecting serovar and the age of the animal. In incidental infections urinary excretion usually lasts only for several weeks, but excretion of *pomona* has been observed for up to 102 days following experimental infection.[24] Prolonged urinary excretion is a feature of serovar *hardjo* infections; mean shedding times of 215 ± 26 days have been reported,[33] while in individual animals shedding times of up to 542 days have been observed.[45] It is probable that some animals continue to shed *hardjo* throughout their lives. Higher renal carrier rates have been observed in younger cattle than in old cows.[16]

Localization of leptospires in the pregnant and nonpregnant uterus has been shown to persist for up to 142 days and 97 days post-infection respectively.[45] Localization in the pregnant uterus may in turn be followed by fetal infection with subsequent chronic reproductive wastage and excretion of the leptospires in the post-calving uterine discharge for up to 8 days, with persistence in the oviducts for up to 22 days after calving.[12] Infection persists in both the oviduct and the body of the uterus of pregnant and nonpregnant cows.[12]

Whether localization of leptospires occurs in the male genital tract has not been definitely established; however, leptospires of the *pomona* serovar[42] and *hebdomadis*[36] serogroups have been demonstrated in bull semen. These isolations indicate either urinary contamination of semen or infection of the genital tract. Leptospiral antibodies (mostly *hebdomadis* serogroup) have been detected in the semen of bulls,[46] suggesting possible local antibody production in the genital tract.

A recent report[45] has indicated that strains belonging to the *hebdomadis* serogroup may also localize and persist in the mammary gland; serovar *hardjo* was recovered from the milk of an experimentally infected cow on days 30 and 91 postinfection.

CLINICAL SIGNS

Clinical bovine leptospirosis can be divided into two distinct phases: first, an acute phase whose onset coincides with the bacteremic phase of infection, and second, a chronic phase that occurs much later and whose effects are most noticeable on the reproductive tract.

Acute Infection. The clinical signs exhibited in the acute phase can vary markedly in severity. The most severe form is usually observed in young calves,[22] although outbreaks may occasionally occur in adult cattle. The clinical signs are those of severe septicemia with pyrexia, anorexia, an acute hemolytic anemia, hemoglobinuria and jaundice. The mortality can be high, and if recovery does occur there is a prolonged convalescent period. In lactating cows milk production almost stops, and the small amount of milk present is pink or red in color and contains blood clots. Occasional cases may be characterized by signs of meningitis.[22] A necrotic dermatitis may occur in some animals infected with *grippotyphosa* serovar.[5] Such acute outbreaks are associated with incidental infection of cattle by hemolysin-producing serovars of *pomona, grippotyphosa, icterohemorrhagiae* and *autumnalis.*

There is a gradation of clinical signs from those observed in very acute cases to the mildest form of acute infection, which is that most commonly seen in dairy cattle. This is characterized by pyrexia, which is frequently undetected, and by a marked drop in milk flow. This mild clinical syndrome is commonly associated with serovar *hardjo,* although it can be caused by serovar *pomona.* All four quarters of the udder are affected, and the udder feels soft and flabby and not hard as it does in most mastitis cases.[21, 34] Milk from affected cows appears thick, yellow and colostrum-like. It contains clots and has a high white cell count. Agalactia lasts for 2 to 10 days, after which production usually returns to almost normal; although if infection occurred late in lactation, milk production may not return.

The number of animals affected on a farm will vary from more than 50 per cent of cows over a 2-month period of an epizootic in a susceptible herd to sporadic cases in animals in their first or second lactation in enzootically infected herds.[31]

While agalactia is not readily recognized in beef cattle, it may become apparent by the presence of weak calves that do not receive proper nutrition.[26]

Subclinical Infection. In many animals, especially nonpregnant, nonlactating cattle, infection is subclinical; however, in lactating cattle some reports suggest that subclinical infection may be more apparent than real. During epidemics, drops in milk production have been observed[35] that cannot be explained by the number of clinically affected cows. A comparison of computer milk production predictions with actual production figures in infected herds[34] and a comparison of pre- and post-vaccination milk production figures[6] suggest that there may be considerable losses in milk production associated with such apparently subclinical infections.

Chronic Infection. The most important chronic sequelae to leptospirosis are seen in the pregnant cow, in which consequent fetal infection with resultant abortion, stillbirth or premature live birth of weak calves may occur. While such reproductive wastage can occur in cattle infected by many parasitic leptospires, it is particularly a feature of *pomona* and *hardjo* infections. Abortion and the other effects usually occur 1 to 6 weeks (*pomona* infection) and 4 to 12 weeks (*hardjo* infection) after the acute phase of infection; however, such animals have frequently shown no clinical evidence of acute infection.

With *pomona* infections these events usually occur in the last 3 months of gestation. Abortion has been observed in the second trimester in cases of *autumnalis* infection.[7] With *hardjo* infection, abortion has been diagnosed at all stages from the fourth month through to term, and circumstantial evidence indicates that it may also cause early embryonic death.[11]

It has been very difficult to define the importance of leptospirosis relative to other factors in the etiology of bovine abortion, stillbirth and premature live birth because of difficulties in diagnosis. Recent studies suggest that this role may be considerable. Leptospiral infection (almost entirely serovar *hardjo*) was demonstrated in 49.7 per cent of 348 aborted fetuses examined in Northern Ireland.[17] In that study 9.8 per cent of the aborted fetuses examined had leptospiral antibodies. Studies in the United States[39] and in the U.S.S.R.[2] have reported finding leptospiral antibodies in the sera of aborted fetuses.

The incidence of abortion on individual farms can be very high following an epizootic of *pomona* infection; incidences of up to 50 per cent have been reported.[37] With *hardjo* infection abortion rates tend to be much lower (3 to 10 per cent), but occasionally rates of more than 30 per cent can occur.[11] However, *hardjo* is the most important leptospiral infection because it is associated with long-term herd infections on farms with new infections occurring year after year.[25]

This recurring loss is most noticeable where management practices regularly ensure the introduction of susceptible animals into an infected herd.[14] In one study,[31] out of a group of 13 second-calf heifers, 3 aborted (*hardjo* was isolated from the two fetuses examined) and another delivered a premature live calf. This episode occurred approximately 14 months after an outbreak of acute *hardjo* agalactia in the herd.

An association between *pomona* infection and infertility has not been shown.[38] However, infertility has been a common field observation in *hardjo* infected herds[27] in the United States, and improvements in breeding efficiency have been noted in herds following *hardjo* vaccination.[29] The infertility noted in *hardjo* infected herds may possibly be associated with the ability of *hardjo* to colonize the oviducts.[12, 15] Colonization of the oviduct has not been reported in *pomona* infection.

FETAL AND UTERINE PATHOLOGY

Most findings at necropsy of aborted fetuses are nonspecific and result either from autolysis or cannot be differentiated satisfactorily from autolytic changes. Autolysis is a particular feature of fetuses aborted before 6 months. Occasionally, jaundice may be observed in the subcutaneous tissues of infected fetuses aborted in the last stages of gestation whereas stillborn fetuses frequently exhibit lesions similar to those produced by anoxia, i.e., petechial hemorrhages on the surface of the thymus, thyroid, lungs and heart and in the parietal pleura and mesentery.

The only consistent histologic changes observed in experimental leptospiral abortion have been in the fetal kidney.[13, 23, 40] These have consisted of foci of tubular necrosis with interstitial and perivascular infiltration of lymphocytes along with a few plasma cells and polymorphonuclear leukocytes.

Severe vascular lesions were a feature of the histopathologic findings in two reports of *hardjo* and *icterohemorrhagiae* infection in aborted fetuses.[19, 20] These lesions were particularly severe in the liver and to a lesser extent in the thymus, cerebral meninges, and the interlobular septa of the lungs. The vessels were often congested and exhibited mural edema and necrosis. Perivascular hemorrhage was noted.

Polyarthritis has been reported in a live calf born to a cow experimentally infected with *hardjo*.[45]

In cases of *pomona* abortion the cotyledons appear light tan to yellow in color and avascular and are affected uniformly.[8] However, a controlled serial kill experiment[40] failed to demonstrate any histologic changes in the pregnant uterus or fetal membranes of infected heifers that were not present in control heifers and that have not been reported in so-called normal placentae.[3]

DIAGNOSIS

Diagnostic methods for leptospiral abortion, stillbirth, and other sequelae of infection are somewhat unsatisfactory, particularly for serovar *hardjo*. Diagnosis should be based on a combination of the clinical history and laboratory results. Unfortunately, leptospiral abortions frequently occur without any previous clinical evidence of leptospirosis having been observed in a herd, and the veterinarian then has to rely on laboratory diagnosis alone.

Microbiologic Investigation. Ideally, laboratory diagnosis should be based on the isolation of the organism from fetal tissues or by demonstrating its presence by immunofluorescence;[17] however, these techniques are not generally available in diagnostic laboratories. Other methods such as silver impregnation staining techniques and dark field microscopy have been used to demonstrate leptospires in tissues, but these are of only limited value.

Isolation of leptospires from the urine of recently aborted cows has been widely used as a diagnostic method in the past. This technique has limited value since it may identify renal carriers, and many cattle may be carriers.[16, 32, 47]

Serologic Investigation. Serologic testing using the microscopic agglutination test (MAT) is the most frequently used laboratory procedure in the diagnosis of leptospiral abortion. It is best used as a herd test rather than as a test for an individual animal, although it still has a limited role when only individual animal samples are available.

Because of individual variations in antibody responses, serum from at least 10 per cent of a herd should be tested. This sample should include sera from different age groups, management groups and clinical groups within the herd. This herd approach is particularly useful in the investigation of *pomona* and other incidental leptospiral infections. Most recently infected cases will have MAT titers of 1:100 or greater.

The herd sample test approach is not very useful for the diagnosis of *hardjo*-associated abortion in endemically infected herds because of the insidious and chronic nature of herd infections and the very low levels of antibody (especially as determined by the plate test) that may be found in post-abortion cow sera.[18] The limited reliable information available suggests that if a high MAT titer (1:1000 or greater) is found in a serum sample taken from a cow shortly after abortion then there is a very good probability (approximately 80 per cent) that the fetus will be infected.[18] Unfortunately, the converse is not true; approximately one third of aborting cows with low levels of antibody (less than 1:100) have been shown in one study[18] to have had leptospiral infected fetuses.

There is no value in examining post-abortion paired serum samples from individual cows because titers are either static or falling.[18]

Examination of fetal sera by the MAT should always be carried out when possible. As many as one in six of infected fetuses[17] may have developed MAT titers. These will range from 1:10 upward. The plate test is not sufficiently sensitive for examining fetal sera.

TREATMENT AND CONTROL

Control measures must be directed toward the following:

1. Minimizing the risk of incidental infection of cattle by leptospires maintained by other hosts. To prevent this, there should be strict separation of cattle from pigs and fencing off of cattle pastures from streams, ponds and marshes to reduce contact with potentially contaminated water. However, the wide host reservoir range of some serovars that involve many species of wildlife makes it virtually impossible to avoid some exposure to leptospires in surface waters.[26] Strict rodent control should be carried out around farm buildings.

2. Minimizing the risk of infection from other cattle and the clinical effect of exposure to infection by vaccination or combined vaccination and dihydrostreptomycin therapy.

Within the herd, control can most economically be achieved by vaccinating all members of the herd. In closed herds vaccination should take place annually, while in open herds vaccination should be repeated every 6 months. New additions to the herd should be given a single dose of dihydrostreptomycin (25 mg/kg) and vaccinated immediately on arrival on the farm.

During an outbreak of leptospiral abortion, vaccines containing the appropriate serovar can be administered simultaneously with dihydrostreptomycin (25 mg/kg), whereas in outbreaks of agalactia vaccination alone is more cost-effective.

Infertility problems related to enzootic hardjo herd infections usually decrease following vaccination with a specific bacterin. This improvement may be due to transduction of serum IgG into the uterus, resulting in elimination of uterine infection.[26]

Vaccination of cattle has also been reported to be a significant factor in reducing the risk of associated human infection.[41]

There are dangers inherent in faulty vaccination programs, particularly with serovar hardjo. The highly efficient parasitic adaption of hardjo to cattle and the relatively low immunogenicity of leptospiral vaccine means that hardjo vaccination programs, once initiated, must be continuous.[30] By disrupting the enzootic cycle, natural immunization is prevented. The reintroduction of hardjo into a herd where vaccination has been discontinued or poorly applied might result in particularly severe outbreaks of clinical disease.

RISK TO MAN AND OTHER ANIMALS

All serovars of Leptospira pathogenic to cattle can also cause disease in man and other domestic animals. Transmission to man is most likely to occur from urine splashing in milking parlors, removal of retained infected placentae, handling aborted fetuses or contact with urine-contaminated ponds or streams. Although relatively small numbers of cases have been reported in the United States and Britain, much higher prevalences have been recorded in New Zealand,[41] and consequently, infections may be more common in the former countries than currently diagnosed.

The cattle-adapted serovar hardjo can cause clinical disease in other farm species, and hardjo has now been recovered from aborted horse, sheep, pig and dog fetuses[12]; in all instances cattle appeared to be the source of infection.

Cattle owners should be informed of the risk of infection to farm personnel and other livestock that may come into close contact with infected cattle.

References

1. Amatredjo A, Campbell RSF: Bovine leptospirosis. Vet Bull 43:875, 1975.
2. Belousov VI: Diagnostic significance of antibodies to Leptospira in the serum of cows that have aborted. Sborn Nauch Trud Mosk Vet Akad, 108:105, 1979.
3. Bjorkman N, Sollen P: Morphology of the bovine placenta at normal delivery. Acta Vet Scand 1:347, 1960.
4. Blackmore DK, Schollum LM: Leptospirosis: A neglected health hazard in the meat industry? In Proceedings of the 26th European Meeting of Meat Research Workers, Colorado Springs, 31 August–5 September 1980. 2:313, 1980.
5. Burdin ML, Froyd G, Ashford WA: Leptospirosis in Kenya due to Leptospira grippotyphosa. Vet Rec 70:830, 1958.
6. Carroll RE: Leptospirosis in California dairy cattle: A seven year study. In Proceedings 69th Annual Meeting U.S. Livestock Sanitation Association, 1965. 1966, pp. 153–154.
7. Damude DF, Jones CJ, Myers DM: A study of leptospirosis among animals in Barbados. Trans R Soc Trop Med Hyg 73:161, 1979.
8. Dennis SM: Diagnosis of infectious abortion in cattle. Vet Med Sm Anim Clin 64:423, 1969.
9. Dikken H, Kemety E: Serological typing methods of leptospires. In Bergan T, Norris JR (eds): Methods in Microbiology, vol. 2. London, Academic Press, 1978, pp. 259–306.
10. Elder JK, Zard WH: The prevalence and distribution of leptospiral titres in cattle and pigs in Queensland. Aust Vet J 54:297, 1978.
11. Ellis WA: Recent developments in bovine leptospirosis. In Grunsell CSG, Hill FWG (eds): The Veterinary Annual, 23rd issue. Bristol, Scientechnica, 1983, pp. 91–95.
12. Ellis WA: Unpublished data.
13. Ellis WA, Michna SW: Bovine leptospirosis: Experimental infection of pregnant heifers with a strain belonging to the Hebdomadis serogroup. Res Vet Sci 22:229, 1977.
14. Ellis WA, Michna SW: Bovine leptospirosis: Infection by the Hebdomadis serogroup and abortion—a herd study. Vet Rec 99:409, 1976.
15. Ellis WA, Neill SD, O'Brien JJ, et al.: Bovine leptospirosis:

Microbiological and serological findings in normal fetuses removed from the uteri after slaughter. Vet Rec 110:192, 1982.

16. Ellis WA, O'Brien JJ, Cassells J: Role of cattle in the maintenance of *Leptospira interrogans* serotype *hardjo* infection in Northern Ireland. Vet Res 108:555, 1981.

17. Ellis WA, O'Brien JJ, Neill SD, et al.: Bovine leptospirosis: Microbiological and serological findings in aborted fetuses. Vet Rec 110:147, 1982.

18. Ellis WA, O'Brien JJ, Neill SD, Hanna J: Bovine leptospirosis: Serological findings in aborting cows. Vet Rec 110:178, 1982.

19. Ellis WA, O'Brien JJ, Neill S, et al.: The isolation of a leptospire from an aborted bovine fetus. Vet Rec 99:458, 1976.

20. Ellis WA, O'Brien JJ, Neill S, et al.: The isolation of a strain of *Leptospira* serogroup Icterohaemorrhagiae from an aborted bovine fetus. Br Vet J 133:108, 1977.

21. Ellis WA, O'Brien JJ, Pearson JKL, Collins DO: Bovine leptospirosis: Infection by the Hebdomadis serogroup and mastitis. Vet Rec 99:368, 1976.

22. English AW: Sudden death. In Proceedings of the 42nd Refresher Course for Veterinarians: The J.D. Stewart Memorial Course in Cattle Diseases. Sydney, Australia 3:26, 1979.

23. Fennestad KL, Borg-Peterson C: Foetal leptospirosis and abortion in cattle. J Inf Dis 102:227, 1958.

24. Ferguson LC, Ramge JC, Sanger VL: Experimental bovine leptospirosis. Am J Vet Res 18:43, 1957.

25. Hanson LE: Control of bovine leptospirosis. Bovine Pract, 7:17, 1972.

26. Hanson LE: Effects of leptospirosis on bovine reproduction. In Morrow DA (ed): Current Therapy in Theriogenology. Philadelphia, W.B. Saunders, 1980, pp. 488–492.

27. Hanson LE, Brodie BO: *Leptospira hardjo* infections in cattle. Proceedings 71st Annual Meeting U.S. Livestock Sanitation Association, 1967. 71:210, 1968.

28. Hanson LE, Mansfield ME, Andrews RD: Epizootiology of enzootic leptospirosis in a cattle herd. In Proceeding 68th Annual Meeting U.S. Livestock Sanitation Association, 1964. 68:136, 1965.

29. Hanson LE, Tripathy DN, Killinger AH: Current status of leptospirosis immunization in swine and cattle. J Am Vet Med Ass 161:1235, 1972.

30. Hathaway SC: Leptospirosis in New Zealand: An ecological view. NZ Vet J 29:109, 1981.

31. Hathaway SC, Little TWA: Epidemiological study of *Leptospira hardjo* infection in second calf dairy cows. Vet Rec 112:215, 1983.

32. Hellstrom JE: Studies on some aspects of the epidemiology of bovine leptospirosis. Ph.D. Thesis, Massey University, Palmerston North, New Zealand, 1978.

33. Hellstrom JS, Blackmore DK: A cohort analysis study of bovine leptospirosis within a dairy herd. In Proceedings 2nd Internat. Symposium Vet. Epidem. Econ. May 7–11, 1979, Canberra, Australia. 1980, pp. 214–219.

34. Higgins RJ, Harbourne JF, Little TWA, Stevens AE: Mastitis and abortion in dairy cattle associated with leptospira of the serotype *hardjo*. Vet Rec 107:307, 1980.

35. Hoare RJ, Claxton PD: Observation on *Leptospira hardjo* infection in New South Wales. Aust Vet J 48:228, 1972.

36. Kiktenko VS, Balashov NG, Rodina VN: Leptospirosis infection through insemination of animals. J Hyg Epidem Microbial Hyg, 20:207, 1976.

37. Knott SG, Dadswell LP: An outbreak of bovine abortions associated with leptospirosis. Aust Vet J 46:385, 1970.

38. Lingard ER, Hanson LE: Effect of *Leptospira pomona* on the reproductive efficiency of cattle. J Am Vet Med Assoc 139:449, 1961.

39. Moojen V, Roberts AW, Carter GR: Microbial causes of bovine abortion in Michigan. Vet Med Sm Anim Clin 78:102, 1983.

40. Murphy JC, Jensen R: Experimental pathogenesis of leptospiral abortion in cattle. Am J Vet Res 30:703, 1969.

41. Ryan TJ, Hellstrom JS, Penniket JH: Leptospirosis in dairy farmers: Prevention by vaccination of cattle. N Z Vet J, 30:107, 1982.

42. Sleight SD, Atlallah OA, Steinbauer DJ: Experimental *Leptospira pomona* infection in bulls. Am J Vet Res 25:1163, 1964.

43. Stoenner HG: Application of serologic findings to the diagnosis of leptospirosis. In Proceeding 67th Annual Meeting U.S. Animal Health Association 1972, pp. 622–624.

44. Stoenner HG: Bovine leptospiral abortion. In Faulkner LC (ed): Abortion Diseases of Livestock. Springfield, Ill., Charles C Thomas, 1968, pp. 35–50.

45. Thiermann AB: Experimental leptospiral infections in pregnant cattle with organisms of the Hebdomadis serogroup. Am J Vet Res 43:780, 1982.

46. Vaz AK, Oliveira SJ de: Leptospira agglutinating titres of bulls used in artificial insemination in Rio Grande do Sul, Brazil. Bol Inst Pe Squish Vet Desiderio Finamere 5:23, 1978.

47. White FH, Sulzer KR, Engel RW: Isolation of *Leptospira interrogans* serovar *hardjo, balcanica* and *pomona* from cattle at slaughter. Am J Vet Res 43:1172, 1982.

48. World Health Organization: Technical Report Series 380, 1967, p. 7.

Effects of Brucellosis on Bovine Reproductive Efficiency

Paul Nicoletti, D.V.M., M.S.
University of Florida, Gainesville, Florida

Brucellosis is a zoonosis that causes heavy economic losses in most countries of the world. The prevalence varies widely between herds, areas and countries. In most areas of the United States, brucellosis is not a factor in bovine reproductive performance. This is due to a test and slaughter program that includes the widespread use of vaccine. In some regions the incidence has changed little. The percentage of reactors among cattle tested has been reduced from 1.06 per cent in 1962 to 0.91 per cent in 1982. The USDA estimates that the disease costs the cattle industry between 35 and 50 million dollars annually.

Nearly all cattle infections are caused by one of the eight biotypes of *Brucella abortus*. Three biotypes (1, 2 and 4) are known to exist in the United States. There are no apparent differences in antigenicity or pathogenicity, and biotypes are important only in epidemiologic studies. In countries where *B. melitensis* exists, cows sometimes become infected with this species, and there may be spread to other cows and to humans.

PATHOGENESIS

Brucellosis is characterized by abortion after the fifth month of pregnancy with the sequelae of retained placenta and acute or chronic metritis. Only a small percentage of infected cows abort more than once, and many do not abort. The percentage of abortions within herds varies widely and depends on many factors.

The infection begins by ingestion, and, if the cow is not pregnant, it is localized, and serologic tests may be negative. If the cow is pregnant, the production of the carbohydrate erythritol by the fetoplacental unit results in rapid multiplication of the bacteria. Large numbers of the organisms (10^{12} per ml or more) are expelled with the fetus and its associated membranes and fluids, contaminating the environment and allowing transmission to other susceptible cattle. Excretion ceases as fluids disappear, usually by 2 to 3 weeks. In subsequent pregnancies the uterus may again be infected but with reduced severity. Calves born from contaminated uteri usually do not retain infection, but a small number (approximately 5 per cent) may retain the infection for life and be seronegative until the first calving (latency).

The incubation period is highly variable and is inversely related to the stage of pregnancy at the time of infection.[1] Transmission of brucellosis from infected bulls to susceptible cows by natural service has not been demonstrated in controlled experiments. Intrauterine insemination with semen containing virulent organisms may result in infection.

Course of Infection in the Cow

The initial infection occurs in the lymph nodes nearest the point of invasion. The organisms have a predilection for the udder and supramammary lymph nodes, which are usually permanently infected. Shedding from the udder occurs in a high percentage of cows, but the degree varies considerably.

Infection of the uterus occurs during the second trimester of pregnancy. The earliest lesion is inflammation of the connective tissue between the uterine glands, which leads to ulcerative endometritis. The cotyledons become involved by spread of exudate along the allantochorion. Large numbers of organisms appear in the endothelial cells lining the fetal blood vessels of the chorionic villi. There is tissue destruction, and eventually entire villi are destroyed. The cause of fetal death and abortion is interruption of fetal function of the placenta and the effects of endotoxin. The fetus usually remains in utero for 24 to 72 hours after its death, and autolysis of tissues is common. There are no pathognomonic lesions of the fetus, but bronchopneumonia is commonly present. The placenta is characteristically edematous with lesions of inflammation and necrosis.

Course of Infection in the Bull

Bulls are apparently more resistant to brucellosis than cows but may be infected at younger ages. They also become infected by ingestion of *B. abortus*. Plant and associates[7] have reviewed published literature on brucellosis in bulls and suggested two clinical syndromes. One involves the testes and epididymides and is characterized by orchitis. The other involves the seminal vesicular glands and ampullae.

There may be focal areas of adhesions between the tunica vaginalis and the testicle. Sperm granulomas may be formed with chronic fibrosis of interstitial tissue and accumulations of phagocytes (mostly macrophages) and lymphocytes. In the ampulla of the ductus deferens, connective tissue may be found with necrosis of tubular epithelium. Infection is often unilateral. The presence of *B. abortus* in genital organs seems to have a variable effect on libido and semen quality, and organisms may or may not be shed in the semen.

A diagnosis is based on blood serum and semen plasma tests, clinical examinations, cultures of the semen and herd history. The presence of agglutinins in seminal plasma is of diagnostic value and indicates that brucella organisms are located in one or more parts of the genital system. Some authors suggest that all bulls from infected herds should be considered infected regardless of serologic and clinical examinations. In another study,[4] several bulls that reacted to serologic tests were culture negative, and the author concluded that they may have recovered. It appears that either many bulls recover from mild infections or the infections become localized so that semen quality and libido are unaffected and serologic tests become negative.

Effects of Fertility

There have been few controlled studies on the effects of brucellosis on individual cattle and herds. The need to include large numbers and to exclude other factors are important reasons.

Ogden and associates[6] studied 3005 cows in 123 herds and concluded that vaccination reduced brucellosis in herds to the point that the disease was not a major factor in fertility. There was a poorer reproductive performance among 56 ring test and vaginal mucus test–positive cows when compared with 2390 negatives with a 7.6 per cent difference in failure to conceive following insemination. (Similar findings have been observed by others.[2]) Hignett and associates[3] compared infected and noninfected cows and concluded that there was no significant difference in the number of services per conception but there was a difference in percentage of abortions. In another study,[2] 74 per cent of naturally infected cows had dead or weak calves, and milk production was significantly reduced.

In an extensive review of the effects of brucellosis on reproduction, Plommet[8] cited several studies. In one there was a difference of 5.4 per cent between infected and noninfected cows in conception at first insemination and a 3.1 per cent difference in sterility. In another, there was a 2.8 per cent difference between rates of abortion and a 13-day average

Table 1. Effects of Brucellosis on Reproduction

	Noninfected Herds	Infected Herds
Per cent of nonrepeat breeders at 120–150 days	61.6 (2388)	57.7 (1710)
Number inseminations per conception	1.65 (2394)	1.88 (1711)
Number inseminations per live births	2.02 (1153)	2.24 (1414)
Number inseminations per viable calves	2.11 (1104)	2.34 (1346)

(   ) = number of cows
(From Plommet M: Brucellose bovine et reproduction. Bull Techn d'Info 257:121, 1971.)

difference in calving interval between infected (n = 825) and noninfected (n = 584) cows. Other criteria are compared in Table 1.

The author concluded that there is a difference of about 4 per cent between conception rates of infected and noninfected cows. He further stated that the study of the effects of brucellosis on fertility is difficult. There are degrees of infection that vary from recovery, chronic infection without effects on reproduction, and mild to severe infection of the reproductive organs with clinical symptoms such as abortion, retained placenta and sometimes metritis. These infections are affected by the degree of exposure to and virulence of the organisms and the physiological status, age, sex, and natural or vaccine-induced resistance of the animal. The stage of gestation and the dose of inoculum are the most important factors.

DIAGNOSIS

The diagnostic methods for brucellosis can be divided into those used for a herd and those used for an individual. The latter may be serologic or bacteriologic.

In the United States, dairy herds are surveyed by the ring test, which is conducted at least three to four times per year. Beef herds are monitored through a marketed cattle system at markets and slaughterhouses. Both surveillance methods may be slow to detect infections. Brucellosis should be considered when abortions occur during the latter part of gestation. (A list of diseases and diagnostic methods has been published elsewhere.[1])

Many diagnostic tests are available for individual cattle. Serologic tests have varying degrees of sensitivity, specificity, and limitations.[5] None is absolutely accurate. The standard plate and tube agglutination tests are quantitative measurements of antibodies and are affected by many factors. Many studies have shown that qualitative tests are superior to quantitative tests. The card or rose bengal test is an effective screening procedure and should be followed by less sensitive methods, especially in vaccinated cattle.

Antibodies in blood serum, milk, whey, vaginal mucus or seminal plasma are presumptive evidence of brucellosis. Blood serum tests may be negative before and a few days following an abortion or full-term infected calving.[5] If possible, antibody tests should be supported by cultures. *Brucella abortus* may be isolated from uterine fluids, milk, colostrum or nonlactating udder secretions, placental tissues, and stomach contents or lungs of the fetus.

In summary, a diagnosis of brucellosis begins at the herd level. Many methods are available for individual animals. The results may be affected by type of test, stage of infection, vaccinal history, age, and heterospecific antigens. When proper methods are used and the results evaluated using pertinent data, the limitations of the tests can be minimized.

TREATMENT

Brucellae are intracellular parasites and therefore are protected from host defenses and activity of most antibiotics. At the present time, brucellosis in cattle is considered an incurable disease, although approximately 15 per cent of cattle recover from naturally acquired infections.

An effective therapy has been the goal of many studies. Some workers have been quite successful in reducing the severity or preventing infections in experimentally exposed cattle through the use of antibiotics. Many other workers have tried nonantibiotic therapy. Controlled experiments have largely failed to confirm the early claims of success.

With the development and widespread use of artificial insemination and embryo transfer, individual cattle have become increasingly valuable. Therefore, development of an effective and practical treatment would be very useful. In addition to salvage of these cattle, many countries cannot afford to sell infected animals for immediate slaughter.

Studies are underway to re-evaluate treatment as an alternative to slaughter of diseased cattle. Novel drug delivery mechanisms as well as prolonged antibiotic therapy are being investigated.

CONTROL

Brucellosis is a regulatory disease in many countries, and prerogatives for its control are limited. Several countries have eradicated brucellosis, and others have made considerable progress toward that goal. In the United States, a program of control began in the 1930's and was accelerated in the 1950's. Approximately 150 million dollars of federal and state funds are spent annually in this effort.

Progress in reducing the incidence of brucellosis in some areas of the world has been somewhat offset by increased incidence in others. The demands for animal protein, especially dairy products, have led to development of large units of highly susceptible cattle. Economic circumstances prevent immediate sale of seropositive cattle. Vaccination of all cows is the logical control measure under these circumstances.

The best control of brucellosis combines flexible herd plans that include vaccination, slaughter of diseased cattle and hygienic measures. In acute phases of the disease in unvaccinated populations, the immediate slaughter of seropositive cattle may be economically devastating as well as unsuccessful. It is frequently impossible to follow recommendations for isolation and replacement of parturient cattle. Infected cattle may abort without early detection.

Until recently, strain 19 was limited to usage in sexually immature cattle in the United States. This was due to the limitations of diagnostic tests in differentiating titers caused by vaccination and natural infection. Much recent research has confirmed earlier limited studies that a reduced dosage (at least 5×10^8 organisms) provides protection equal to that of a standard dose with fewer persistent titers. The use of a reduced dose combined with cultures and supplemental serologic tests permits high accuracy in identification of infected cattle. The length of protection from the reduced dose is largely unknown, and revaccination of some herds is necessary.

The benefits of vaccination are cumulative. It practically eliminates clinical disease and thus reduces the numbers of organisms excreted from infected cows. While the protection resulting from vaccination is not absolute, a much higher exposure is necessary to infect vaccinates. A small percentage of cows in advanced pregnancy may abort following vaccination. Strain 19 can sometimes be isolated from the fetus and placenta, but the virulence is unchanged and there is no further spread. There is no deleterious effect on subsequent conception rates.[1]

Since strain 19 may produce permanent infections in bulls with lesions similar to those of natural disease, vaccination of bulls is not recommended and may be prohibited.

Many decisions about brucellosis control depend on the types of herd management, prevalence in the area, the purpose of cattle, and government regulations.

EPIZOOTIOLOGY

In a previous review,[5] I have listed intrinsic and extrinsic factors that complicate the control of bru-

cellosis. The variable incubation period and the difficulties that arise from it are most important in epizootiology. A single negative test is unreliable for a diagnosis, and herd (population) status is paramount. This is difficult to establish under many management conditions.

The trends toward larger herds and increased livestock movement have contributed to an increase in brucellosis within herds as well as geographic spread. The larger herds usually have a greater density, which increases exposure potential. The degree of shedding is the most critical factor within herds. It was found that the greatest effect on persistence and prevalence of brucellosis in large dairy herds was the vaccinal status of reactors.[9] The presence of one or more reactor cows increases the percentage of reactors in the herd by eightfold.

The epizootiology of brucellosis is complicated by many aspects of a host-parasite relationship. The principles of management should try to balance the measures that are applicable to control of infection within populations with the least possible interference with cattle management and commerce.

References

1. Blood DC, Henderson JA, Radostits DM: Veterinary Medicine, 5th ed. Philadelphia, Lea & Febiger, 1979, pp. 500–509.
2. Crawford RP, Williams JD, Childers AB, et al.: The effects of *Brucella abortus* on serology, bacteriology, and production in three Texas cattle herds. Proc 82nd Anim Health Assoc 89:89, 1978.
3. Hignett PG, Nagy LK, Ironside CJT: Bovine brucellosis: A study of an adult-vaccinated *Brucella*-infected herd. I. The effect of *Brucella abortus* infection on infertility. Vet Rec 79:886, 1966.
4. Hill BD: The cultural and pathological examination of bulls serologically positive for brucellosis. Aust Vet J 60:7, 1983.
5. Nicoletti P: The epidemiology of bovine brucellosis. Adv Vet Sci Comp Med 24:69, 1980.
6. Ogden AL, Sellers KC, Crabb WE: The incidence of brucellosis in a random sample of dairy herds in East Anglia and its effects on fertility. Res Vet Sci 5:385, 1964.
7. Plant JW, Claxton PD, Jakovljevic D, deSaram W: *Brucella abortus* infection in the bull. Aust Vet J 52:17, 1976.
8. Plommet M: Brucellose bovine et reproduction. Bull Techn d'Info 257:121, 1971.
9. Vanderwagen LC, Sharp J, Meyer M: A retrospective study on the relationships of vaccination status of reactor animals, management practices at calving and herd size to eradicating brucellosis in 79 dairy herds. Proc 81st Anim Health Assoc 83:83, 1977.

Bovine Trichomoniasis

Paul B. Kimsey, Ph.D.

Massachusetts Institute of Technology,
Cambridge, Massachusetts

DEFINITION

Bovine trichomoniasis is a contagious venereal disease of worldwide distribution characterized by infertility, abortion and pyometra. The causative agent, *Tritrichomonas fetus (T. fetus),* is a piriform protozoan of the family Trichomonidae (Fig. 1).

PATHOGENESIS

Trichomoniasis is a true venereal disease. Infection is confined to the genital tract, and, with one exception, transmission occurs through sexual contact. Spread of the disease in artificial insemination (AI) bull studs is presumed to have occurred through contact of the penis with the rump or escutcheon of the teaser animal that had been contaminated through similar contact by an infected animal. With this exception, control measures may be based on the assumption that transmission is by coitus. Although there are documented cases in the literature of the transmission of *T. fetus* through AI, present-day regulations and standards maintained at AI bull stud centers minimize the chance of transmission by this procedure.[4]

In bulls *T. fetus* is found only on the penis and the preputial membranes, localizing in the secretions (smegma) of the epithelial lining of the penis, prepuce and the distal portion of the urethra.[20] It causes no lesions of diagnostic significance, affects neither semen quality nor sexual behavior, and is asymptomatic. Thus the infected bull serves only as a carrier of this agent. Older bulls tend to become permanent carriers. This is felt to be a result of the increased number of crypts in the epithelial lining of older bulls, providing a site for localization of the protozoan.[5, 14] With the possible exception of Brangus, Texas Longhorn and Santa Gertrudis breeds, young bulls (less than 4 years) are thought either to recover spontaneously or to be refractory to infection.

In cows the organism colonizes the vagina, uterus and oviduct but does not prevent conception.[21] The protozoan can be found in the secretions from these organs and in the mild mucopurulent discharges associated with vaginitis and endometritis. *T. fetus* does not affect ciliary activity of cells from the oviduct in vitro.[24] The inflammatory response of the uterus, approximately 1.5 to 2 months post-infection by the bull, may be responsible for embryonic wastage and death.[21]

CLINICAL SIGNS

Pyometra and abortion are often the first signs of trichomoniasis that are noticed in a herd, but they occur in relatively few animals, perhaps 5 per cent or less. Infertility is the most prevalent and economically damaging symptom and occurs in a high percentage of cows in a recently infected group. As a result, an abnormally long interservice interval (2 to 5 months) is frequently seen in cows with trichomoniasis.

The infertility associated with *T. fetus* infection may be the result of early embryonic death followed by a period of failure of conception or nidation due to an inflamed uterus (see earlier section, Pathogenesis). After a variable period of infertility following the initial exposure, cows may regain their fertility, even though they are bred by infected bulls. On subsequent exposures cows appear not to be as susceptible. These animals will conceive and carry the fetus to term, although calving intervals may be prolonged.[2]

The cow can maintain an infection through a

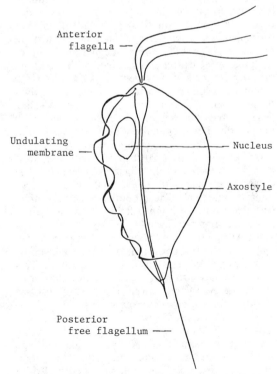

Figure 1. *Tritrichomonas fetus:* approximate size is 10 to 25 mcg in length by 5 to 10 mcg in width.

normal gestation period.[18, 19] This is an unusual occurrence, and the incidence of this postpartum infection decreases during the succeeding estrous periods. But such cows do represent a potential female carrier state. Abortions due to *T. fetus* occur in the first half of gestation, although a very few abortions have been reported in the seventh month of gestation. The fetal membranes may be expelled with the fetus or retained. In the latter case a chronic catarrhal or purulent endometritis usually results. The affected cow may become sterile owing to the resultant destruction of the uterine mucosa.[12]

DIAGNOSIS

In extensively managed beef herds the possibility of trichomoniasis is often not suspected until the herd is examined for pregnancy, at which time a lower than expected pregnancy rate is encountered with gestational ages widely spread among those who are pregnant. In intensively managed herds, delayed returns to estrus are suggestive of venereal disease. Isolation and identification of the protozoan establishes the definitive diagnosis. The organism can be observed microscopically or cultivated from fluids associated with pyometra and abortion. Since pyometra and abortion are not frequently observed, the collection of preputial smegma has become the most common means of isolating *T. fetus*.

Samples of smegma can be collected by the following two methods: (1) *Pipette:* A "dry" AI pipette with a 10- to 15-ml syringe attached is introduced into the fornix of the bull's prepuce. Negative pressure is applied with the syringe while the pipette is simultaneously scraped and slid back and forth in the sheath. The milky white smegma at the tip of the pipette (at least 1 ml) is mixed with 3 to 5 ml of transport medium (see below). A "wet" pipette technique is similar to the dry technique but involves the infusion of 5 to 10 ml of physiological saline (PSS) or transport medium into the prepuce with the pipette. The preputial orifice is then held so as to allow no fluid to escape. The sheath is then massaged vigorously (100 strokes), and the fluid is then drawn back into the pipette. (2) *Douche:* The sheath is infused with 100 to 200 ml of PSS or transport medium. The preputial opening is then occluded while the trapped fluid is vigorously massaged and then recollected.[9]

An AI pipette can be used to collect cervicovaginal mucus from a cow bred to an infected bull or from a pyometra. This mucus can be cultured. This procedure may also prove useful as an indicator of impending embryonic loss. A recent study using a small number of cows has shown that 50 per cent of pregnant exposed cows with positive cultures subsequently aborted.[1]

Collection of materials for isolation should be done as cleanly as possible with minimal aeration and exposure to sunlight. Samples should also be protected from extreme changes in temperature. Ideally, samples should be put onto culture medium as soon as possible. Once samples are on culture medium the layers should not be mixed (see below).

Various fluids and culture preparations can be centrifuged (2000 rpm for 10 minutes) and the sediment examined microscopically or cultured. This concentration procedure has proved useful in conjunction with the douche and pipette techniques.

Transport media have been used to carry the sample to the laboratory, where under more controlled conditions the sample can be processed. Lactated Ringer's (LR) solution has proved to be the most useful transport medium due to its availability and its superiority to PSS. Buffered physiological saline (PBS) with 5 per cent fetal calf serum and LR are effective as transport media for up to 48 hours if refrigerated. Transport times of up to 84 hours have been achieved with Kupferberg medium.[13]

Diamond's medium (Table 1) is a very effective culture medium.[7] The medium is inoculated by layering 1 ml of preputial smegma in transport medium on the surface of the culture medium. This is done with a Pasteur pipette, and care should be taken to prevent mixing. The anaerobic, motile

Table 1. Preparation of Diamond's Medium (100 ml)

Ingredient	Gm
Trypticase peptone	2.0
Yeast extract	1.0
Maltose	0.5
L-cystine hydrochloride	0.1
L-ascorbic acid	0.02
Distilled water to make 90 ml	
K_2HPO_4*	0.08
KH_2PO_4*	0.08

1. Mix all ingredients and check to see if pH is 7.2 to 7.4. If not, adjust pH with NaOH or HCl.
2. Add 0.05 gm of agar and autoclave to 10 minutes at 121°C.
3. Cool to 49°C and aseptically add 10 ml of inactivated (56°C for 30 minutes) bovine serum,* 100,000 units of penicillin G (1 ml of a stock solution prepared by adding 10 ml of sterile H_2O to 10^6 units of penicillin G) and 0.1 gm of streptomycin in sulfate (0.5 ml of stock solution prepared by adding 5 ml of sterile H_2O to 1 gm of streptomycin sulfate).
4. Aseptically dispense 10 ml per sterile 16 × 125 mm screw cap vial. Check for sterility by incubating 24 hours at 37°C.

*Original media, as reported by L. S. Diamond, did not contain K_2HPO_4 or KH_2PO_4, were adjusted to a pH of 6.8 to 7.0 and contained 10 ml per 100 ml of inactivated sheep serum. All asterisks refer to slight modifications in media. The modifications are a result of experience in field and laboratory use of the media in conjunction with the diagnosis of *Trichomoniasis* by Dr. C. P. Hibler of the Pathology Department, College of Veterinary Medicine and Biomedical Sciences, Colorado State University, Fort Collins, Colorado, 80523.

trichomonads swim to the bottom of the tube and multiply, leaving the bacteria and fungi to multiply in the upper layers. The medium is incubated at 37°C and evaluated at 1, 2, 4, 6, and 10 days post-inoculation. If contaminating growth (descending cloudiness in the tube) threatens to reach the bottom of the tube, the clear layer at the bottom of the tube should be transferred and layered onto fresh medium.

To determine if a culture is positive a Pasteur pipette is inserted to the bottom of the tube, and a small aliquot is placed on a microscope slide with a coverslip and viewed under a microscope. Phase or dark-field illumination makes identification easier.

T. fetus must be distinguished morphologically from contaminating protozoans that may be encountered. Suspected positive preparations should be examined at 1000 X magnification for morphologic criteria, including an undulating membrane, three anterior flagella, and a posterior flagellum. Subsequent identifications can be made at 400 × magnification on the basis of the organism's irregular, jerky movement and its continuous rolling.[19]

A quick screening method involves viewing the bottom of the culture medium tube through an inverted microscope. This method requires a larger population of organisms for a positive diagnosis.

Several laboratories have noticed a certain variability between batches of media and its ability to grow *T. fetus*. It has been our experience that the quality of water is extremely important for consistency in media. The use of glass-distilled water has alleviated a number of these problems. We also recommend that each batch of media be checked for its ability to grow *T. fetus* from positive control cultures.

Schneider's medium has proved useful for long-term cultures of *T. fetus* in the laboratory.[23] Freezing of the organism has also been reported.[11] This provides the opportunity for the practitioner to purchase the media, receive a frozen culture, grow the organism and do his or her own diagnostic work with a known positive control culture.

The dry pipette method used in conjunction with LR as a transport medium and Diamond's culture medium has been shown to be 90 to 100 per cent accurate in diagnosing an infected bull.[6,13] If a sensitivity of 90 or 99 per cent is assumed, then with three tests run on a bull (which has been sexually rested for at least 2 weeks) at weekly intervals, the chances of misdiagnosing an infected animal are 1 in 1000 and 1 in 1,000,000 respectively.

CONTROL

Depending on the management procedures that can be applied to a beef herd, the prognosis for reducing the impact of the disease is fair. With a general knowledge of the epizootiology of the disease, the practitioner can adopt a control program for each particular herd situation. These control measures usually involve some combination of the following areas.

Identification

Identifying infected or exposed animals and culling them from the herd is an obvious solution but is not always economically feasible. All bulls should be sexually rested for at least 2 weeks (preferably longer) and then cultured at weekly intervals for a minimum of 3 weeks. Valuable cows can also be cultured, but negative cultures are difficult to interpret. Bulls and cows with positive cultures can be treated (see later section on Treatment) or culled. Cows exposed to infected bulls should be palpated, and cows with abnormal reproductive tracts should be culled. Those with involuted uteri and those who have been pregnant more than 5 months may be retained in the herd. A more severe program involves retaining only pregnant cows.

Quarantine

A quarantine system can also be implemented in which females are divided into exposed and unexposed herds. "Clean" replacement cows can be added to the unexposed group, whereas the exposed group is eliminated over a period of time due to natural attrition, or cows can be added back to the unexposed group after sexual rest and isolation (see below). The drawbacks to this program are generally that record-keeping is not sufficient to identify two such groups of animals or the facilities are not conducive to a quarantine system.

Sexual Rest and Isolation

A method of sexual rest and isolation has been reported to be effective for controlling trichomoniasis.[3] Cows suspected of being bred to infected bulls can be removed and sexually rested for a minimum of three normal estrous periods before being bred to uninfected bulls. Pregnant cows can be rebred 90 days after calving. Such a practice gives the cow the opportunity to clear the organism. This decreases the risk from the chronically infected cows mentioned earlier. A program of physical examination of the genitalia in conjunction with culturing may be beneficial prior to resumption of breeding.

Artificial Insemination

AI is a proven method of avoiding infected bulls and is often used on a certain percentage of affected cows. The practicality of changing from natural service to AI has proved difficult for many management systems. Synchronization of the cows' estrous cycles may make AI more feasible. If AI is used as an emergency measure, care should be taken to identify carrier cows, and some surveillance system should be initiated when the herd returns to natural service.

Young Bulls

The use of younger bulls to lower the prevalence of trichomoniasis in large intensive operations is documented.[6] A surveillance program is initiated, and infected bulls are culled. Only bulls younger than 4 years of age are used as replacements. Cows that have not calved or conceived before the next breeding season are culled. The success of this and any combination of the control programs listed above depends on a continued surveillance program. Such a program includes culturing the bulls before the breeding season, allowing enough time for treatment, and/or finding replacement animals.

Control measures involving natural service require the removal of infertile cows due to the possibility that they may serve as a reservoir for reinfection of the herd. Bulls should be pastured separately from cows after the breeding season. Once infected bulls are identified, they should be isolated prior to treatment or culling because of the possible spread of the organism by homosexual behavior.

The more extensive beef operations present the greatest challenge for the practitioner. Common ranges, year-round breeding and the large numbers of animals involved are representative problems. The introduction of minimal control measures will have to depend on the economic benefits that the rancher can expect to receive.

TREATMENT

In treating an individual bull, the prognosis for a cure is good (a cure being defined as three negative weekly cultures after a post-treatment period of 45 days). Treatment for bulls can be either local or systemic. Cows can be treated systemically.

Local Treatment

Local treatment in the bull consists of applying trichomonadicidal compounds directly or via douche onto the penis, prepuce or distal portion of the urethra. These compounds include (1) acriflavine[8, 25] (a mixture of 2,8-diamino-10-methyl-acridinium chloride and 2,8-diaminoacridine), (2) a proprietary compound, Bovoflavin Salve, containing trypaflavine,[3, 25] (3) the compound diminazene aceturate (p,p'-diguanyldiazoaminobenzene diaceturate,[8] and (4) metronidazole [1-(β-hydroxyethyl)-2-methyl-5-nitroimidazole].[9] These treatments are cumbersome, difficult to apply and have given inconsistent and conflicting results. They are mentioned here because of the possible development of resistant strains of trichomonads to the currently used systemic imidazole drugs. The spontaneous recovery and the lack of a reliable diagnostic method in the cow have hindered the development of local treatment for the female.

Systemic Treatment

Dimetridazole (1,2-dimethyl-5-nitroimidazole) is effective orally at 50 mg/kg of body weight daily for 5 days.[15] The compound can be given as an oral drench, via boluses or mixed into feed rations. Bulls often go "off feed" for several days following initial intake of the drug. Dimetridazole in subtherapeutic amounts can lead to resistant populations of trichomonads.[16] This is a drawback in combining the drug in the feed. Rumen stasis is frequently observed during or following treatment. Animals with existing rumen disorders should be observed closely for adverse side effects.

Intravenous administration of dimetridazole is also effective, but due to the vehicle needed to dissolve the drug (10 to 70 per cent sulfuric acid), severe side effects have been noted. The dissolved drug is administered in dosages ranging from 10 mg/kg of body weight daily for 5 days to 50 to 100 mg/kg of body weight in a single intravenous injection.[17] Side effects have included respiratory difficulty, ataxia, recumbency for up to 15 minutes, and weakness for periods up to 2 days. One author recommends the oral treatment via boluses or drench to ensure adequate dosages.

Ipronidazole, 30 gm soluble powder dissolved in 40 ml water given as a single dose intramuscularly, has been shown to be 80 per cent effective in treating bulls. A broad-spectrum antibiotic administered parenterally for a few days before treatment begins apparently lowers the commensal population of bacteria in the sheath, preventing the breakdown of the imidazole drug. This pretreatment step is felt to make treatment with ipronidazole more efficacious. Treatment regimes of 10 to 30 gm of ipronidazole injection for 2 to 3 days in combination with long-acting antibiotics are being evaluated. A systemic treatment for cows of 15 gm of ipronidazole dissolved in water given intramuscularly has been shown to be effective.[22]

Metronidazole is effective when given intravenously at dosages ranging from 75 mg/kg of body weight for three successive injections at 12-hour intervals to 10 mg/kg of body weight given once daily for 2 days.[10]

The above compounds, dimetridazole, ipronidazole and metronidazole are imidazole derivatives and are not approved for use in the bovine species in the United States. Trichomonads resistant to one of the compounds will be resistant to the other related drugs.[16] This brings up the necessity of instituting adequate treatment regimes to ensure their effectiveness in the future. As of this writing ipronidazole is less expensive than dimetridazole, which is less expensive than metronidazole.

PREVENTION

With proper screening and culturing of new arrivals in a herd, trichomoniasis can be prevented.

Replacement cows should be limited to virgins or animals from herds known to be free of the disease. Culturing of cows may be useful but can be expensive and time-consuming given the uncertainty of culture results in the female. Ideally, all cows should be put through a 90-day postpartum isolation period before breeding and should be culture negative for *T. fetus*. Open cows should go through three normal estrous cycles before being cultured. Sexually rested bulls should be cultured for 3 weeks at weekly intervals before being added to a beef herd. Older bulls should be replaced with young animals (3 years old or younger).

References

1. Abbitt B, Ball L: Diagnosis of trichomoniasis in pregnant cows by culture of cervical-vaginal mucus. Theriogenology 9:3, 1978.
2. Bartlett DE: *Trichomonas foetus* infection and bovine reproduction. Am J Vet Res 8:343, 1947.
3. Bartlett DE: Further observations on experimental treatments of *Trichomonas foetus* infection in bulls. Am J Vet Res 9:351, 1948.
4. Certified Semen Services. CSS minimum requirements for health of bulls producing semen for A.I. Columbia, MO, Certified Semen Services, 1980.
5. Clark BL, Parsonson IM, White MB, et al. Control of trichomoniasis in a large herd of beef cattle. Aust Vet J 50:424, 1974.
6. Clark BL, White MB, Banfield, JC: Diagnosis of *Trichomonas foetus* infection in bulls. Aust Vet J 47:181, 1971.
7. Diamond LS: The establishment of various trichomonads of animals and man in axenic cultures. J Parasitol 43:488, 1957.
8. Fitzgerald PR, Johnson AE, Hammond DM: Treatment of genital trichomoniasis in bulls. JAVMA 143:259, 1963.
9. Fitzgerald PR, Hammond DM, Miner NL, Binns W: Relative efficacy of various methods of obtaining preputial samples for diagnosis of trichomoniasis in the bulls. Am J Vet Res 49:452, 1952.
10. Gasparini G, Vaughi M, Tardani A: Treatment of bovine trichomoniasis with metronidazole (8823 R.P.). Vet Rec 75:940, 1963.
11. Jeffries L, Harris M: Observations of *Trichomonas vaginalis* and *Trichomonas foetus*; the effects of cortisone and agar on enhancement of severity of subcutaneous lesions in mice. Parasitology 57:321, 1967.
12. Kendrick JW: An outbreak of bovine trichomoniasis in a group of bulls used for artificial insemination. Cornell Vet 43:231, 1953.
13. Kimsey PB, Darien BJ, Kendrick JW, Franti CE: Bovine trichomoniasis: Diagnosis and treatment. J Am Vet Med Assoc 177:616, 1980.
14. Ladds PW, Dennet DP, Glazebrook JS: A survey of the genitalia of bulls in Northern Australia. Aust Vet J 49:335, 1973.
15. McLoughlin DK: Dimetridazole, a systemic treatment for bovine venereal trichomoniasis. I. Oral administration. J Parasitol 51:835, 1965.
16. McLoughlin DK: Dimetridazole, a systemic treatment for bovine venereal trichomoniasis. II. Intravenous administration. J Parasitol 54:1038, 1968.
17. McLoughlin DK: Drug tolerance by *Trichomonas fetus*. J Parasitol 53:646, 1967.
18. Morgan BB: Studies on the trichomonad carrier-cow problem. J Anim Sci 3:437, 1944.
19. Morgan BB: Bovine Trichomoniasis. Minneapolis, Burgess Publishing Co., 1964, pp. 1–150.
20. Parsonson IM, Clark BL, Dufty JH: Early pathogenesis of *Tritrichomonas foetus* infection in the bull. Aust Vet J 50:421, 1974.
21. Parsonson IM, Clark BL, Dufty JH: Early pathogenesis and pathology of *Tritrichomonas fetus* infection in virgin heifers. J Comp Pathol, 86:59, 1976.
22. Retief GP: Trichomoniasis treatment in cattle. Vet Clinician June/July 1978.
23. Schneider MD: A new thermostabile medium for the prolonged bacteria-free cultivation of *Trichomonas foetus*. J Parasitol 28:428, 1942.
24. Stalheim OHV, Gallagher JE: Effects of *Mycoplasma* spp., *Trichomonas fetus*, and *Campylobacter fetus* on ciliary activity of bovine uterine tube cultures. Am J Vet Res 36:1077, 1975.
25. Thorne JL, Shupe JL, Miner ML: The diagnosis and treatment of trichomoniasis in bulls. Proceedings of the 92nd Annual Meeting of the American Veterinary Medicine Association, 1955, pp. 374–377.

Chlamydial Infection of the Bovine Reproductive System

Patricia E. Shewen, B.Sc., D.V.M., M.Sc., Ph.D.

Ontario Veterinary College
Guelph, Ontario

Chlamydiae are obligate intracellular parasites belonging to a single order, Chlamydiales, and genus, *Chlamydia,* in which two species are recognized: *C. trachomatis,* a human pathogen, and *C. psittaci,* the cause of a number of diseases in both man and animals. *C. psittaci* isolated from cattle are of two antigenic types: type 1, associated with epizootic bovine abortion (EBA), seminal vesiculitis syndrome (SVS), pneumonia, and enteritis, and type 2, the agent of sporadic bovine encephalomyelitis (SBE), polyarthritis, or conjunctivitis. Bovine isolates are antigenically indistinguishable from ovine chlamydiae recovered from similar syndromes. The intestinal tract is apparently the natural habitat for both chlamydial types, and although persistent intestinal infections are common in some herds, overt enteritis is rare. Up to 60 per cent of animals in individual herds may shed organisms for several years, in levels that vary from minimally detectable to 10^4 to 10^6 infectious units per gram of feces. Thus fecal excretion provides a potential source of massive environmental contamination that may be important in the transmission of infection.

The actual mode of transmission in infection of the reproductive tract is unknown. Disease in heifers and bulls has been reproduced experimentally by parenteral inoculation of organisms, with genital infection occurring after a phase of chlamydemia.

Ticks have been proposed as possible vectors. Chlamydia-infected ticks *(Ornithodoros coriaceus)* were recovered from enzootic areas in California, and experimentally infected ticks were shown to be capable of inducing abortion in pregnant heifers. Venereal transmission is also a possibility, since chlamydiae have been demonstrated in the semen of bulls.

INFECTION OF THE FEMALE REPRODUCTIVE SYSTEM

Chlamydiae were first suspected as the cause of abortions in cattle in Germany in 1956. Since then they have been implicated by isolation from fetuses or placentae, as well as by serologic evidence, as the cause of reproductive failure in cattle in North America, most countries of western and eastern Europe, South Africa and many parts of Asia.

Epizootic bovine abortion (EBA), as it is frequently termed in North America, occurs most commonly in the intermountain regions of California and Colorado. The onset of abortion in a herd is sudden, and almost all primiparous heifers and previously unexposed cows introduced into enzootic areas abort. The rate of abortion depends on the number of first-calf heifers in the herd. There is no clinical evidence of systemic disease in cows that subsequently abort, usually in the seventh to ninth month of gestation. Occasionally, infection results in the delivery of dead calves at term or the birth of weak calves that die later. The placenta is commonly retained, and milk production drops in dairy cows, but overall there is little adverse effect on the dam. There is no apparent breed predisposition. The seasonal incidence observed in California beef cattle most likely reflects breeding practices designed to ensure calving in the late summer and early fall, although seasonal variation in arthropod vectors may be a factor.

The initial infection with chlamydiae is virtually undetectable clinically. Experimentally infected animals develop fever and leukopenia for 3 to 5 days following inoculation, but understandably, these signs have not been observed in naturally occurring infections. Infection results in chronic disease, abortion in experimental trials occurring 40 to 126 days after exposure. An episode of chlamydemia is necessary for infection of the placenta and fetus. After experimental inoculation this occurs during a secondary blood-infectious phase following replication of chlamydiae in somatic organs. The uterine infection progresses independently, and organisms appear to be eliminated from other organs soon after multiplication. The fetus becomes infected hematogenously, although uterine fluids may contain organisms.

Chlamydiae produce placentitis and generalized infection of the fetus. Placental lesions, described in most detail after experimental infection, are patchy in distribution and characterized by edema, necrosis, hyperemia and hemorrhage. The intercotyledonary tissue may have a leathery, tough consistency and a reddish-white opaque color on the uterine surface. The margins of the cotyledons in affected areas have small, round focal areas of necrosis. Chlamydiae have a predilection for the hilar region of the ovine placentome but affect the interplacentome regions of the bovine placenta. The corresponding areas of the fetal placenta are edematous. A superficial resemblance to *Brucella abortus* placentitis has been noted.

The most striking change in aborted fetuses is hepatopathy, perhaps reflecting hematogenous spread. The liver is enlarged and has a coarsely nodular surface and a firm consistency. It is red-yellow and may appear mottled. In some epizootics this lesion is seen in approximately 50 per cent of fetuses. Ascites, extensive enough to cause distention of the abdomen and pleural effusion, have also been observed. Petechial hemorrhages are found on the mucous membranes of the oral cavity, the tongue and eyes. The subcutis may reveal petechiae after skinning, and petechiae can also be found in the thymus, salivary glands and lymph nodes. Small gray foci (5 to 10 mm in diameter), found irregularly distributed in all tissues, can best be seen in kidney cortices and ventricular myocardium. Histologically, these reflect reticuloendothelial cell hyperplasia characteristic of a granulomatus response.

Chlamydial elementary bodies (infective particles) or intracytoplasmic inclusions may be demonstrated in smears of infected placenta or fetal organs. Fetal brain, lungs, liver, spleen, kidney, stomach and lymph nodes as well as pleural and peritoneal fluid should be used in attempts at isolation. Chlamydemia usually follows abortion, and a diagnostic rise in complement fixation titer can be demonstrated in dams in paired serum samples taken at the time of abortion and 2 or 3 weeks later.

INFECTION OF THE MALE REPRODUCTIVE SYSTEM

Chlamydia psittaci has been isolated from semen and epididymal tissues of bulls with unsatisfactory semen quality in the United States, Poland, Czechoslovakia, Turkey and South Africa. Organisms of the type isolated from aborted fetuses have also been implicated in the seminal vesiculitis syndrome (SVS), which may affect up to 10 per cent of bulls in herds where EBA is enzootic. SVS is characterized by chronic inflammation of the seminal vesicles, accessory sex glands, epididymides and testes and results in inferior semen quality and, in some cases, in testicular atrophy. Semen from affected bulls has a large number of leukocytes and a low concentration of sperm with poor motility and a high percentage of primary and secondary sperm cell abnormalities. Chlamydiae have been isolated from the semen of affected bulls and also from "carrier" bulls in the same herd. These bulls were clinically normal and had satisfactory semen quality.

An SVS-like disease has been reproduced in bulls by parenteral or intratesticular inoculation of EBA *Chlamydia* isolates. Experimental inoculation results in an early febrile phase, corresponding to primary chlamydemia, followed in 2 to 4 days by a second chlamydemia. During this second phase, organisms localized in genital tissues and may be isolated from semen intermittently for the next 3 weeks. In one study control bulls housed with infected animals also excreted chlamydiae in semen 14 days after infection, but no signs of SVS developed in the following year nor was semen quality affected.

The natural route of infection for SVS is unknown, and the role of contaminated semen in transmission of SVS and EBA has not been determined. Evidence from experimental trials suggests two possible mechanisms for reproductive failure associated with *Chlamydia*-infected semen: first, fertilization failure due to poor quality semen, as seen in clinical SVS, and second, early embryonic death resulting after fertilization with contaminated normal semen. This latter situation might occur with chronically infected carrier bulls and is believed to result from infection of the endometrium rather than of the embryo per se.

Chlamydial elementary bodies or inclusions may be seen in impression smears of genital tissues obtained from affected bulls at postmortem examination. Organisms may be isolated from semen samples and occasionally from urine specimens, but failure of isolation does not rule out infection since shedding occurs intermittently. The complement fixing (CF) titer in serum rises after experimental infection, but the level of antibody bears no relationship to the presence of organisms in semen. The use of the CF test to screen for potentially infected bulls has not been examined.

DIAGNOSIS

Definitive diagnosis of chlamydial infection depends on isolation and identification of the organisms from discharges, placenta, fetal fluids, the aborted fetus, semen, or postmortem tissues. Isolation is carried out in embryonated hens' eggs or more recently, in cell cultures. Criteria used for identification include demonstration of elementary bodies and group antigen in the indicator system. Because chlamydiae are fastidious intracellular organisms, they may be inactivated during the chronic course of intrauterine events that lead to expulsion of the fetus or rapidly lost from fetal and placental tissues following abortion. Consequently, *Chlamydia* as a cause of abortion may be underdiagnosed.

A presumptive diagnosis may be made on the basis of clinical signs and recognition of elementary bodies or inclusions in Giemsa-stained impression smears or exudates. However, this technique is a relatively insensitive method for the detection of infection.

Other causes of abortion, particularly brucellosis, listeriosis, and *Campylobacter* and *Mycoplasma* infections should be ruled out.

All *Chlamydia psittaci* organisms possess a common group-specific lipopolysaccharide antigen that is detected in the complement fixation test. Although the CF test has been used to screen herds for chlamydial infection, its usefulness as a diagnostic tool is limited. Possibly as a result of inapparent intestinal infection, as many as 20 per cent of adult cattle have complement-fixing antibody, although it is found only rarely in animals under 2 years of age. The CF test is relatively insensitive in detection of antibody due to localized infections such as those of the genital tract, in which positive results occur in only 50 per cent of proven cases. It may be used in cases of abortion to establish a diagnosis of current infection when a rising titer can be demonstrated in paired serum samples. The microimmunofluorescence test appears to be more sensitive than the CF test in diagnosing genital infection in humans, but its usefulness in cattle is as yet unexplored.

CONTROL AND PREVENTION

To control chlamydial abortion, all pregnant animals should be segregated during calving. Infected fetuses and placentae should be carefully disposed of and pens disinfected. Tetracycline (2.5 to 5 gm orally or 350 mg intravenously daily) is effective in preventing abortion only if given prior to secondary chlamydemia. Since this cannot be predicted unless the onset of infection is known, its clinical usefulness is doubtful.

Tetracycline treatment could be potentially useful in clearing chlamydiae from infected bulls, but this method has not been evaluated. If such therapy is attempted, treatment should be continued for at least 2 weeks after the disappearance of clinical signs to minimize the induction of a latent carrier state. In any case it would be prudent to exercise caution in proclaiming a cure on the basis of semen culture, particularly in normal carrier bulls, since natural shedding occurs only intermittently.

Under field conditions immunity to abortion develops as a result of natural infection and is thought to be due to a cell-mediated immune response. Immunization trials have produced variable results dependent on the route of artificial challenge used. Commercial vaccines available in Europe but not in North America are apparently effective in preventing abortion if given to nonpregnant animals or early in gestation. No information is available regarding prevention of SVS by vaccination.

References

1. Bowen RA, Spears P, Storz J, Seidel GE: Mechanisms of infertility in genital tract infections due to *Chlamydia psittaci* transmitted through contaminated semen. J Infect Dis 138:95, 1978.

2. Shewen PE: Chlamydial Infection in animals: A review. Can Vet J 21:2, 1980.
3. Storz J: Chlamydia and Chlamydia-Induced Diseases. Springfield, Ill.: Charles C Thomas, Publisher, 1971.

4. Storz J, Whiteman CE: Chlamydia-induced bovine abortions: Cause, pathogenesis, and detection. Reports and summaries. XIth International Congress on Diseases of Cattle, Tel-Aviv, 1980, pp. 560–565.

Effects of Ureaplasma Infection on Bovine Reproduction

Paul A. Doig, D.V.M. M.Sc.,
Syntex Agribusiness, Mississauga, Ontario

H. Louise Ruhnke, B.S.A. M.Sc.,
Ontario Ministry of Agriculture and Food,
Guelph, Ontario

Ureaplasmas (formerly called T-strain mycoplasma) were first isolated from the bovine reproductive tract in 1967.[21] A number of subsequent studies demonstrated that the organisms could be recovered from the lower genital tract of bulls and cows that showed no indication of associated genital disease. For this reason, ureaplasmas were considered for a number of years to be part of the nonpathogenic microflora of the lower reproductive tract. More recent studies have demonstrated an association between ureaplasma and disease, and it is now apparent that ureaplasmas may play a more important role in bovine reproductive failure than had previously been recognized. The organisms have been isolated from field cases of bovine granular vulvitis, endometritis, salpingitis, abortion and seminal vesiculitis. In each instance, the disease has been reproduced following experimental inoculation.

ETIOLOGY

Ureaplasmas are part of the group of microorganisms designated the Mycoplasmatales, more often simply referred to as the mycoplasmas. The Mycoplasmatales group contains three families, Mycoplasmataceae, Acholeplasmataceae and Spiroplasmataceae.

The Mycoplasmataceae family, which requires sterol for growth and is the most important family with respect to animal disease, is further divided into two genera. The first of these is the so-called large-colony *Mycoplasma* genus; these organisms have been recognized for many years as disease-causing agents. Mycoplasmas produce the well-known fried-egg colony growth on agar and have been divided into over 80 species according to various biochemical and serologic criteria.

The second genus in the family Mycoplasmataceae is *Ureaplasma*, so-named because of its ability to hydrolyze urea. Thus far, 11 bovine *Ureaplasma* serotypes have been serologically identified and appear to be distinct from the eight serotypes of *Ureaplasma urealyticum* isolated from humans. For this reason, a new name, *Ureaplasma diversum*, has been proposed for the bovine isolates.[10]

Ureaplasmas share many of the characteristics of other mycoplasmas, which are the smallest free-living organisms. They are characterized by the absence of a rigid cell wall and are therefore resistant to many antibiotics, most notably penicillin. Like other bacteria, they can live and reproduce on synthetic media, although their growth requirements are very specific.

Both virulent and avirulent strains have been demonstrated by intramammary inoculation,[9] but a reliable method of identifying pathogenic serotypes by serologic or other means has not yet been developed.

OCCURRENCE AND INCIDENCE

Following the first reported isolation of *Ureaplasma* from the bovine urogenital tract in England in 1967, a number of subsequent studies confirmed that the organisms could be isolated from the lower reproductive tract of apparently healthy animals. Recovery rates of 11 to 14 per cent were reported from the cervicovaginal mucus of fertile cows and heifers,[13, 18, 21] with a slightly higher (27 per cent) but not significantly different isolation rate being reported for repeat breeders.[18] The failure to recover the organism from the uterus of infertile animals and the fact that apparently fertile bulls in artificial insemination (AI) units carried ureaplasma in the prepuce (29 to 100 per cent) and raw semen (23 to 84 per cent) led to the conclusion that ureaplasmas were merely commensals and were not involved in bovine reproductive disease.[17, 22]

Due to the recently recognized chronic, persistent nature of the disease and its often devastating effect on herd fertility, *Ureaplasma* should be viewed as one of the potentially most important infectious causes of infertility in dairy cattle. Fewer studies have been carried out on beef cattle to determine the possible role of *Ureaplasma* as a cause of infertility under these management conditions, but evidence would indicate similar pathogenic potential.

PATHOGENESIS

Cow

In the cow, ureaplasmas appear to colonize principally the vulva and vagina and are only rarely found in the upper reproductive tract of normal animals. This appears to be true for both pathogenic and nonpathogenic strains.[2, 8] A granular vulvitis isolate,[19] used to reproduce the disease by vulvar inoculation, did not appear to colonize the uterus or oviducts actively.[6] However, when experimentally introduced into the uterus of virgin heifers, the organisms were found to persist for up to 7 days and produced a mild endometritis and salpingitis. After day 7, the organisms were cleared from the uterus but were still present in large numbers in vulvar swabs. One experimentally inoculated heifer was found to carry ureaplasmas in the vulva for up to 7 months.[7]

Uterine lesions have also been produced in one of five heifers receiving uterine inoculation with a *Ureaplasma* strain previously isolated from the bladder and urethra. The organism was recovered from the uterus, in the absence of bacteria or viruses, at necropsy 3 weeks after inoculation.[3]

The localized vulvar infection is believed to be a possible source of recontamination of the uterus at each breeding through mechanical transmission on the insemination pipette. If the organisms are mechanically introduced or repeatedly reintroduced into the uterus at breeding, the persistence for up to 7 days may be sufficient time to create an abnormal uterine environment for the fertilized egg. A number of field observations support this concept. Ureaplasmas are rarely found in uterine swabs taken 21 days postbreeding at the time of return to estrus. The organisms have been recovered in pure culture from embryo transfer flushings containing fertilized but degenerate ova. Guarding the insemination pipette as it passes through the vulva and/or infusing the uterus postbreeding with an appropriate antibiotic have been associated with significant improvement in herd fertility rates.

Although the organisms appear to be cleared from the uterus of virgin heifers approximately 7 days following uterine inoculation, it is apparent from field studies that on occasion ureaplasmas may overwhelm the uterine defenses and colonize the uterus. The ability to colonize the uterus for a prolonged period of time and produce disease may be related to the degree of uterine resistance, the number of previous exposures to the organism, or the strain of *Ureaplasma*.[8] The latter may be particularly important because all nine field cases of abortion and prematurely delivered calves evaluated thus far have been associated with *Ureaplasma* serotype known as D48.[20]

Once uterine exposure has occurred, one of three clinical syndromes can result: (1) loss of the fertilized egg prior to day 14 and a return to estrus at the normally expected time, (2) early embryonic death occurring between 40 and 90 days postbreeding, and (3) abortion at any stage of pregnancy or the delivery of weak infected calves.

Abortion appears to result from a placentitis and fetal pneumonitis.[16, 20] It is not known at this time whether the abortions result exclusively from direct uterine exposure at breeding or whether the hematogenous route may be involved subsequent to aerosol exposure.

Bull

Ureaplasmas have been found to be common contaminants of the preputial cavity. Recovery rates of 29 to 100 per cent have been reported from preputial swabs taken from bulls at AI centers. Raw semen samples from carrier bulls were also commonly contaminated (23 to 84 per cent), and the organism was found to survive routine processing and freezing, being present in at least 14 per cent of samples.[17] *Ureaplasma* contamination of semen appears to result mainly from the penile and preputial mucous membranes. However, in one study 6 of 10 bulls examined were found to have urethral colonization, and at least half of them were carrying the organism in the urinary bladder.[25]

Although venereal transmission no doubt can occur, it is also apparent that even virgin bulls can be *Ureaplasma* carriers. In most cases, preputial and semen contamination has no significant detrimental effect on fertility, suggesting that the organisms are nonpathogenic commensals. However, in clinically normal carrier bulls it has been demonstrated that there is a significant and unpredictable variation in the number of organisms present in the semen collected at different times from the same bull.[25] Additional variation can occur due to dilution, processing and freezing of semen resulting in only a small percentage of processed straws from a given collection containing the organisms. Not only may a limited number of straws from any one ejaculate be positive, but the sample should be quantitated because positive samples may contain only a few organisms or more than 1000 colony-forming units. With this appreciation of the shedding characteristics, it is also apparent that even if a bull were shedding a potential pathogen, the number of infective straws may be sufficiently low that the 60-day nonreturn rate of the bull may appear normal.

In most cases *Ureaplasma* does not appear to cause clinical disease in carrier bulls. Although seminal vesiculitis has been produced experimentally following direct inoculation, it is unknown whether or under what conditions ureaplasmas may spread from the preputial cavity to the upper reproductive tract to cause infection and disease.[25]

CLINICAL FORMS

Granular Vulvitis (Infertility) Syndrome

Bovine granular vulvitis is a relatively old clinical syndrome, first described in the veterinary literature in 1887. The disease is characterized by the formation of discrete, raised, red to brownish-colored granules in the vulvar mucosa.

Over the years, there has been controversy about the role of disease in infertility. Part of the apparent disagreement may be due to a failure to correlate the severity of the lesion with the effect on fertility. The mild form characterized by only a few granules may have little or no effect on fertility, whereas the acute form with associated hyperemia and a purulent discharge can have a severe effect.

The granular vulvitis syndrome associated with *Ureaplasma* infection differs somewhat from the previous descriptions in the literature, namely, in the amount of purulent material produced and the formation of epithelial inclusion cysts.[5] When the disease first appears in a herd, the predominant clinical feature is a profuse, sticky, mucopurulent vulvar discharge.[1, 5] In the most acute form, the discharge may pool in the vagina and empty behind the recumbent cow in 60- to 100-ml amounts. In many cases rectal palpation may precipitate an emptying of the purulent material in the absence of palpable abnormalities. Less severe discharges may be noted on the tail or vulvar hair or occasionally may appear only as purulent flecks in otherwise clear estrual mucus.

The vulvar epithelium during the acute purulent stage is inflamed, sensitive and hyperemic. Small 1- to 2-mm raised granules are evident, usually most prominent around the clitoris. Purulent material may often be observed in the ventral commissure. In severe cases the granularity may extend dorsally along the lateral walls of the vulva and occasionally may involve the dorsal commissure. Coalescence of the granules produces raised ridges, resulting in a corrugated and pebbled vulvar mucosa. The granularity does not appear to extend cranially to involve the vaginal epithelium.

The vulvar discharge persists for 3 to 10 days before the disease progresses to a chronic form. In many cases the acute form will reappear at subsequent heats.

The chronic form is characterized by an absence of purulent discharge and a gradual decline in the severity of both the hyperemia and granularity. Occasionally, there may be an excessive discharge of clear mucus, which makes heat detection difficult for many owners. The granularity gradually disappears over the next few weeks, and the vulvar epithelium returns to normal within 6 weeks to 3 months. Reinfection, however, is common. The disease may become enzootic within many herds, and numerous infections can be observed over a prolonged period. The clinical signs are generally less severe during reinfection, with the acute stage being short or apparently absent.

A characteristic finding observed in approximately 10 per cent of affected animals is the presence of discrete, raised, white epithelial inclusion cysts, 2 to 5 mm in diameter and usually arranged in rows or clustered on the dorsolateral wall of the vulva or in the dorsal commissure. The cysts do not appear to form around the clitoris but have been observed on occasion in small numbers on the lateral vaginal wall and outer cervical ring. A creamy white exudate can be expressed from the nodules during the acute stage. The contents tend to become inspissated later in the chronic form.

The effect on fertility appears to be directly proportional to the severity of the disease. When the acute purulent stage of the disease predominates in a herd, there can be a severe effect on fertility. First service conception rates often drop to below 20 per cent and may remain low for a 4- to 6-month period. When the disease progresses to the chronic form, herd conception rates usually increase gradually but may remain 10 to 15 per cent lower than normal for the herd.

The incidence of the disease in affected herds is generally between 40 and 75 per cent. A slightly higher number of cows are affected during winter months with close confinement.

Early Embryonic Death and Abortion

The initial studies carried out on herds affected with granular vulvitis gave no indication of an increase in pregnancy loss even in cows conceiving during the acute stage of the disease. More recently, however, there have been indications that in some herds, the infection may be associated with a high incidence of early embryonic death.[7]

In herds in which the syndrome was observed, cows confirmed to be pregnant by palpation per rectum at 40 to 45 days returned to estrus between 60 and 80 days, usually with evidence of a purulent vulvar discharge. Uterine cultures taken from cows returning to estrus have been positive for *Ureaplasma*, in some cases in pure culture. Endometrial biopsies taken from affected cows have also demonstrated an inflammatory response in the endometrium.

Abortions determined to be due to *Ureaplasma* infection have occurred sporadically in affected herds. The abortions appear to occur primarily in the third trimester of pregnancy and are associated both clinically and experimentally with a chronic placentitis and fetal pneumonitis. The latter finding, although not specific, is sufficiently characteristic of *Ureaplasma* infection to alert the pathologist to culture for the organism. The lung, stomach contents, cotyledons and maternal caruncles appear to be the culture sites of choice.[14, 16, 20]

The clinical and experimental observations that calves infected in utero can be carried to term and appear weak after delivery suggest that further studies are needed on the role of the infection in neonatal calf disease.

Infection in the Bull

Although a correlation has been made between impaired spermatozoan motility and the presence of mycoplasmas (primarily *M. bovigenitalium*) and ureaplasmas in the semen,[11] specific clinical signs attributable to *Ureaplasma* infection have not been observed in bulls. Experimentally, both acute and chronic inflammatory lesions have been observed at necropsy in the distal and proximal urethra of carrier bulls in association with positive *Ureaplasma* culture. Clinical signs, however, were not apparent.[25]

Clinical signs suggestive of urethritis have been observed in bulls being used for "clean-up" breeding in *Ureaplasma*-infected herds with the onset being associated with a decrease in both libido and fertility.

Experimentally, *Ureaplasma* has been found to be pathogenic for the seminal vesicle following direct inoculation, and positive cultures have also been made from field cases of seminal vesiculitis.[4, 25] These findings suggest that *Ureaplasma* may play a role in the seminal vesiculitis syndrome, but field studies to confirm this have not been done. The experimental finding that *Ureaplasma* persists in an inflamed gland for only 4 weeks suggests that cultures must be done early in the course of the disease if the organism is to be recovered. For this reason, establishing a cause-and-effect relationship between *Ureaplasma* infection and field cases of chronic seminal vesiculitis may be difficult.

DIAGNOSIS

Difficulties should not be encountered in differentiating granular vulvitis from the other common cause of vulvitis—namely, infectious pustular vulvovaginitis (IPV) (due to infectious bovine rhinotracheitis virus infection). The only similarity is that both diseases may be associated with a profuse purulent vulvar discharge. IPV is an acute erosive disease characterized by pustules or white necrotic plaques on the walls of both the vulva and vagina. A purulent discharge is usually seen only for 5 to 7 days and is associated with pain and discomfort. The disease is explosive, of short duration and not usually associated with herd infertility.

Granular vulvitis, on the other hand, is a raised productive lesion limited to the vulva and associated with infertility and recurrent episodes of a purulent vulvar discharge. The vulva, although slightly edematous and tender, is not as painful. It should be noted that granular vulvitis associated with *Ureaplasma* infection has been observed to follow outbreaks of IPV and may therefore appear to be part of the same syndrome.

Specimen collection and submission must be carried out properly to confirm a diagnosis. In cases of infertility or early embryonic death associated with granular vulvitis, samples should be taken from the vulva. Additional samples should be taken from the cervicovaginal mucus or, more preferably, the uterus. Care should be exercised in interpreting negative uterine samples because the organism can be rapidly cleared from this location and may no longer be present at the time of the sampling.

Conversely, positive vulvar samples in the absence of granular vulvitis or a purulent discharge should be viewed with caution because of the 10 to 15 per cent carrier rate in apparently normal fertile animals. In abortion cases, however, signs of granular vulvitis may not be present at the time abortion occurs. It is also notable that the D48 abortion isolate may not cause the degree of granular vulvitis observed with other strains. The development of techniques that can serotype pathogenic strains accurately will greatly facilitate interpretation of positive cultures.

Cultures should always be submitted to the laboratory in a commercial transport medium. If placed on ice, the samples should reach the laboratory in 24 hours. Samples that are not chilled must be submitted within 6 hours.

In cases of abortion the fetus and placenta should be submitted as soon as possible. If samples are submitted, the minimum submission should include the placentome, lung and stomach contents on ice (or in transport media) for culture as well as lung and placentome fixed for histopathologic examination.

Samples from bulls should be submitted in a similar manner in transport media or, in the case of semen samples, in liquid nitrogen. In the absence of serotyping to identify pathogenic strains, preputial samples are almost impossible to interpret due to the high carrier rate of apparently fertile bulls. Positive necropsy samples from cases of seminal vesiculitis can be viewed with more significance because the organisms are rarely found in this location in normal animals.

Interpretation of positive semen samples also presents difficulties due to the current inability to identify pathogenic strains. Quantitative assessment of positive semen samples should be carried out because levels may vary from only a few organisms to more than 1000 colony-forming (CFU) units.[8, 12]

Until laboratory methods of determining pathogenic strains are developed, a "safe level" of ureaplasmas in semen cannot be determined. However, due to the demonstrated pathogenic potential of bovine ureaplasmas, all processed semen isolates should be viewed as potentially significant, especially those from bulls with a suspicious history or if present in levels of at least 100 CFU. Due to the variability that can occur between straws, a number of samples of processed semen should be evaluated to determine the bull's shedding characteristics.

TREATMENT AND CONTROL

Cows

Because *Ureaplasma* infection appears to be primarily localized in the vulva, treatment and control procedures should be directed at minimizing the potential for mechanical transmission to the uterus at the time of breeding. Eliminating the infection

Table 1. Drugs

Name of Drug	Company Name and Address	Species	Dose (mg or IU/kg)
1. Spectinomycin	Diamond Laboratories Inc. Des Moines, Iowa 50304	Bovine	1–2 gm intrauterine
	Syntex Agribusiness Mississauga, Ontario L4V 1R5		
	Ceva/Abbott Laboratories Inc. Overland Park, Kansas 66212		
2. Rolitetracycline (Reverin suspension)	Hoechst Pharmaceuticals Montreal 383, Quebec	Bovine	1 gm intrauterine
3. Lincospectin	UpJohn Kalamazoo, Michigan	Bovine	300 μg of lincomycin plus 600 μg of spectinomycin per ml of semen extender
	TUCO, Division of Upjohn Orangeville, Ontario		
4. Minocycline hydrochloride (Minocin)	Cyanamid Canada Ltd. Montreal, Quebec	Bovine	500 μg per ml of semen extender

from a herd is extremely difficult due to the recurrent nature of the disease.

Minimizing uterine transmission can be attempted in a number of ways:

1. In all animals in which the disease is diagnosed, all insemination or treatment pipettes should be protected as they pass through the vulva through a "double-rod" technique. This technique using plastic drinking straws or a commercial double pipette system is usually effective in increasing the herd fertility rate.

2. Antibiotic therapy directed locally at the vulva or in the form of uterine infusions has also been used with apparent success. Based on field experience, the antibiotics of choice for the treatment of *Ureaplasma* infection appear to be nonirritating tetracycline formulations such as rolitetracycline or spectinomycin (Table 1). Both can be used locally in the vulva and the vagina or as uterine infusions. The usual uterine infusion dosage used is 1 to 2 gm. Practitioners should be aware that in many areas products containing these antibiotics may not be cleared for uterine use, and withdrawal periods appropriate for the specific antibiotic group should be followed.

Local treatment of the vulva in late diestrus using douches or creams is designed to control the infection and minimize the number of organisms present at the time of breeding. Uterine infusions are designed to treat an existing endometritis or, when used 24 hours postbreeding, to minimize potential uterine transmission that may have occurred. Rigorous antibiotic therapy in the form of postbreeding infusions is usually needed only during acute infections when herd fertility rates are extremely poor. During chronic infections, the double-rod technique coupled with treatment of repeat breeders will usu-

ally achieve fertility rates close to the previous farm average. Unfortunately, in many instances appropriate therapy is not instituted until the disease has been present in the herd for some time. In such cases a number of cows may not respond owing to the presence of chronic and occasionally irreversible lesions in the endometrium or oviducts. Sham embryo transfer flushings with warm saline have been found to be of value in some individual animals in which chronic productive endometritis is present.

Nutritional deficiencies, although not incriminated as a predisposing factor in any of the Ontario studies, should be considered and corrected if present. New York researchers found a correlation between selenium and vitamin E deficiency and the incidence of the disease. An improvement in fertility with fewer clinical signs appeared to follow supplementation of herds with these deficiencies.[15]

Bulls

To date an effective treatment for eliminating the carrier state in bulls has not been developed. On-farm bulls have been treated with sexual rest and preputial flushes in an attempt to reduce transmission of the disease and improve fertility. As yet there are insufficient response data to allow specific recommendations.

In AI centers in Ontario the approach has been to control any *Ureaplasma* contamination that might occur in processed semen through the addition of antibiotics. Initially, the antibiotics lincospectin and spectinomycin were added to extenders to control mycoplasmas. More recently, the further addition of minocycline hydrochloride appeared to control both mycoplasmas and ureaplasmas effectively without being detrimental to sperm quality. Unfortunately, at the present time this antibiotic appears to be compatible only with milk extenders.[23, 24] Additional studies are under way to develop methods of controlling the organism in other extenders, and it is hoped that in the near future it will be possible to control *Ureaplasma* in all processed semen marketed in North America.

References

1. Anderson NG: Mycoplasma genital tract infections in cattle. Can Vet J 15:95, 1974.
2. Ball HJ, McCaughey WJ: Distribution of mycoplasmas within the urogenital tract of the cow. Vet Rec 104:482, 1979.
3. Ball HJ, McCaughey WJ, Mackie DP, Pearson GR: Experimental genital infection of heifers with ureaplasmas. Res Vet Sci 30:312, 1981.
4. Blom E: Studies on seminal vesiculitis in the bull. I. Semen examination methods and postmortem findings. Nord Vet Med 31:193, 1979.
5. Doig PA, Ruhnke HL, MacKay AL, Palmer NC: Bovine granular vulvitis associated with ureaplasma infection. Can Vet J 20:89, 1979.
6. Doig PA, Ruhnke HL, Palmer NC: Experimental bovine genital ureaplasmosis. I. Granular vulvitis following vulvar inoculation. Can J Comp Med 44:252, 1980.
7. Doig PA, Ruhnke HL, Palmer NC: Experimental bovine genital ureaplasmosis. II. Granular vulvitis, endometritis and salpingitis following uterine inoculation. Can J Comp Med 44:259, 1980.
8. Doig PA, Ruhnke HL, Waelchi-Suter RO, et al.: The role of *Ureaplasma* infection in bovine reproductive disease. Compend Continuing Education 3:S324, 1981.
9. Howard CJ, Gourlay RN, Brownlie J: The virulence of T-mycoplasmas, isolated from various animal species, assayed by intramammary inoculation in cattle. J Hyg Camb 71:163, 1973.
10. Howard CJ, Gourlay RN: Proposal for a second species within the genus *Ureaplasma, Ureaplasma diversum* sp. nov. Int J Syst Bact 32:446, 1982.
11. Jurmanova K, Sterbova, J: Correlation between impaired spermatozoan motility and mycoplasma findings in bull semen. Vet Rec 100:157, 1977.
12. Jurmanova K, Mazurova J: Quantitative findings of mycoplasmas and ureaplasmas in bovine semen doses. Proc Int Org Mycoplasmology (IOM), Freiburg 1:260, 1978.
13. Langford EV: Mycoplasma species recovered from the reproductive tracts of western Canadian cows. Can J Comp Med 39:133, 1975.
14. Langford EV: Mycoplasma recovered from bovine male and female genitalia and aborted feti. Proceedings of Meeting American Association Veterinary Laboratory Diagnosis 18:221, 1975.
15. Lein DH: Bovine reproductive disorders associated with *Ureaplasma, Mycoplasma, Hemophilus somnus* and *Chlamydia.* Proceedings Annual Meeting of the Society for Theriogenology 1982, pp 118.
16. Miller RB, Ruhnke HL, Doig PA, et al.: The effect of *Ureaplasma diversum* inoculated into the amniotic cavity of cows. Theriogenology.
17. Onoviran O, Truscott RB, Fish NA, et al. The recovery of mycoplasmas from the genital tracts of bulls in artificial breeding units in Ontario. Can J Comp Med 39:474, 1975.
18. Panangala VS, Fish NA, Barnum DA: Microflora of the cervico-vaginal mucus of repeat breeder cows. Can Vet J 19:83, 1978.
19. Ruhnke HL, Doig PA, MacKay AL, et al.: Isolation of ureaplasma from bovine granular vulvitis. Can J Comp Med 42:151, 1978.
20. Ruhnke HL, Palmer NC, Doig PA, Miller RB: Bovine abortion and neonatal death associated with *Ureaplasma diversum.* Theriogenology 20:367, 1983.
21. Taylor-Robinson D, Haig DA, Williams MH: Bovine T-strain mycoplasma. Ann NY Acad Sci 143:517, 1967.
22. Taylor-Robinson D, Thomas M, Dawson PL: The isolation of T-mycoplasmas from the urogenital tract of bulls. J Med Microbiol 2:527, 1969.
23. Truscott RB, Abreo C: Antibiotics for elimination of mycoplasmas and ureaplasma from bovine semen. J Dairy Sci 21:295, 1984.
24. Truscott RB: A comparison of the in vitro activity of two antibiotics against bovine ureaplasmas. Can J Comp Med 45:113, 1981.
25. Waelchi-Suter RO, Doig PA, Ruhnke HL, et al.: Experimental genital ureaplasmosis in the bull. Schweiz Arch Tierheilk 124:273, 1982.

Effects of Mycoplasma and Acholeplasma Infection on Bovine Reproduction

Paul A. Doig, D.V.M. M.Sc.,
Syntex Agribusiness,
Mississauga, Ontario

H. Louise Ruhnke, B.S.A. M.Sc.,
Ontario Ministry of Agriculture and Food,
Guelph, Ontario

Organisms belonging to the mycoplasma group were first isolated from the bovine genital tract in 1947.[5] The initial isolates were placed in two serologic groups, the P or pathogenic group, believed to be associated with disease, and the S or saprophytic group, which appeared to be nonpathogenic contaminants. The P strain was later identified as *Mycoplasma bovigenitalium* and the S group as *Acholeplasma laidlawii*.

Subsequent studies throughout the world have resulted in the recovery of a number of other *Mycoplasma* species from the genital tracts of both cows and bulls. Many of the reported recoveries were made from apparently healthy animals and, in the absence of experimental transmission studies, the true role of many of the isolates in reproductive disease has remained in doubt. It is clear, however, from experimental and field studies that a number of *Mycoplasma* species have pathogenic potential and should be considered in any reproductive evaluation involving infertility or abortion.

GENERAL CHARACTERISTICS OF MYCOPLASMAS

The mycoplasmas are the smallest free-living organisms, being smaller than some of the large viruses. Like bacteria, but unlike viruses and chlamydiae, they can live and reproduce on synthetic media.

An important characteristic of the organisms is that they do not have a rigid cell wall and are therefore resistant to penicillin. Both pathogenic and nonpathogenic strains have been identified, and with few exceptions, infections tend to be specific for a particular animal species.

The organisms generally cause chronic rather than acute disease. Infections most often involve the lung, joints, urogenital tract, mammary gland and eyes.

ROLE IN BOVINE INFERTILITY

Although up to 19 species of *Mycoplasma* have been identified in cattle, only a few have been experimentally evaluated to assess their potential reproductive pathogenicity.

Mycoplasma bovigenitalium

Following the first isolation in 1947, *M. bovigenitalium* has been the subject of numerous experimental evaluations. The organism has been recovered from field cases of granular vulvitis, endometritis, infertility, abortion and the seminal vesiculitis syndrome.[1, 2, 3, 7, 15, 16, 24]

Although a number of experimental studies have failed to demonstrate pathogenicity,[4, 6] it is apparent from other studies that some isolates are pathogenic and may be involved in specific cases of reproductive failure.

In bulls *M. bovigenitalium* is a common preputial inhabitant, and although it is also present in semen, there has not, in general, been an apparent detrimental effect on fertility.[4, 18] In specific instances, however, definite pathogenicity has been established. Seminal vesiculitis has been reproduced in a number of studies, usually by direct inoculation of the gland but also by urethral inoculation.[4, 7, 21]

Decreased sperm motility has been observed in European studies in semen samples contaminated with *M. bovigenitalium* and/or ureaplasmas under natural conditions.[13] Cornell researchers reported reduced post-thaw motility of sperm from young 1- to 2-year old bulls positive on culture for *M. bovigenitalium*. Clinical signs of disease were not evident, but the organism could be isolated regularly from vesicular gland secretions derived by a technique that excluded contamination by the preputial flora. High concentrations of specific antibodies were also detected in the secretions of affected bulls but not from normal bulls. At necropsy, most affected bulls had histologic lesions in the vesicular glands consistent with mild mycoplasmal disease.[9]

Further studies on the effect of adding washed suspension of *M. bovigenitalium* to bovine semen showed a reduction in motility after 48 to 72 hours that was dose dependent. Immunofluorescent staining revealed that the organisms were associated with the head of the spermatozoa, particularly the acrosome.[20]

On the basis of these findings, some strains of *M. bovigenitalium* appear to be capable of suppressing sperm motility with or without associated clinical evidence of disease. For this reason, the organisms should be viewed as significant if isolated from abnormal semen or diseased portions of the upper reproductive tract. Preputial isolates may be less significant because they appear to be common in bulls with apparently normal fertility.

In the cow M. bovigenitalium has been recovered from up to 11 per cent of cervicovaginal mucus samples taken from healthy animals.[4, 14] Slightly higher isolation rates have been reported from infertile cows and those with granular vulvitis, but a consistent cause-effect relationship with disease had not been made.[1, 19, 24]

Although there has been evidence serologically of a correlation with M. bovigenitalium infection and infertility,[24] culture studies on samples taken from infertile cows have been inconclusive. In one study only 3 of 80 uterine samples from infertile cows were found to be positive. The organism could be isolated from 1 of 65 samples taken from cotyledons and fetal kidney tissue of pregnant cows.[14, 15]

Experimentally, M. bovigenitalium isolated from a low percentage of field cases was found to reproduce granular vulvitis but only if the vulvar epithelium was scraped prior to the inoculation.[1] Other investigators were unable to demonstrate pathogenicity following uterine inoculation.[6]

Venereal transmission of M. bovigenitalium has been reported in cows bred naturally to a carrier bull. A purulent vulvar discharge and granular vulvitis were observed, and conception rates were poor. When the bull was test bred to three first-calf heifers, a purulent discharge was observed within 4 days, and all heifers developed a necrotizing endometritis of sufficient severity to cause an early return to estrus within 11 to 12 days. When rebred with semen from AI bulls following sexual rest for one cycle and intrauterine infusions, apparently normal fertility rates were obtained.[16] The possible involvement of Ureaplasma in the syndrome was not determined because the study was carried out prior to their recovery from the bovine reproductive tract.

The role of M. bovigenitalium as a cause of infertility in the cow appears, therefore, to need further clarification. The development of criteria to identify pathogenic and nonpathogenic strains may be required before the true role of the organism in infertility can be determined.

Mycoplasma bovis

Although M. bovis is a well-known bovine pathogen producing mastitis, polyarthritis and pneumonia,[8] it has not been shown to be a significant cause of bovine reproductive failure. However, definite pathogenic potential has been demonstrated in experimental inoculation studies.

In the bull, M. bovis has been isolated from one natural case of seminal vesiculitis and epididymitis. Seminal vesiculitis has been reproduced experimentally following direct inoculation.[16] In the cow definite pathogenicity has also been established under experimental conditions.

Varying degrees of endometritis, salpingitis and salpingoperitonitis were produced in seven of eight mature virgin heifers following uterine inoculation.[10]

Subsequent studies showed that M. bovis remained viable in frozen bull semen for as long as 18 months when added prior to extension and freezing in liquid nitrogen.[11a] Ten of 12 heifers inseminated with contaminated frozen semen became repeat breeders, and at necropsy four of eight had varying degrees of chronic suppurative salpinigitis, chronic endometritis and ovarian adhesions.[11a]

Others have experimentally induced abortion with M. bovis following direct inoculation into the amniotic fluid.[23]

Although serologic evidence of a correlation between M. bovis infection and infertility has been made,[24] there is little evidence at present from culture studies that the organism plays an important role in bovine reproductive disease. Isolations from aborted fetuses have been made only infrequently, and the organism has rarely been recovered from the uterus or cervicovaginal mucus of infertile cows or semen of bulls.[4]

Acholeplasma laidlawii

Acholeplasma laidlawii has been isolated on a number of occasions from the lower genital tracts of both cows and bulls as well as aborted fetuses. Although generally regarded as a nonpathogenic saprophyte, there have been reports implicating the organism in disease conditions. Possible pathogenicity was suggested following isolations from the oviducts of infertile cows. Positive isolations were made from 71 per cent of 73 repeat breeder cows and only 24 per cent of 179 cows slaughtered for other reasons. A high incidence of salpingitis and bursal adhesions was found in culture-positive animals.[12]

Other studies, however, have demonstrated that Acholeplasma laidlawii may be a common contaminant on the serosal surface of oviducts following removal of the tracts at slaughter.[4] Care is therefore needed during sampling to ensure that oviduct flushings have not been inadvertently contaminated.

Although studies have associated Acholeplasma laidlawii with infertility, and production of disease following uterine inoculation has also been reported, other investigators have been unable to demonstrate pathogenicity. This failure, plus the infrequent recovery of Acholeplasma laidlawii from infertile cows in field studies, suggests that the organisms do not play an important role in bovine infertility at this time. However, there have been a sufficient number of recoveries from aborted fetuses to justify additional investigation into the possible role of the organism in bovine abortion.[4]

Other Mycoplasmas

A number of other Mycoplasma species have been isolated from the bovine urogenital tract or aborted fetus, but experimental studies have not been carried out to establish their role in reproductive disease. These include M. bovirhinis, M. can-

adense, M. sp. Group 7, *M. alkalescens, M. alvi, M. arginini* and *M. verecundum.*[4, 8]

ROLE IN ABORTION

A number of studies have incriminated mycoplasmas, including ureaplasmas, as possible causes of abortion. In only two instances, however, have experimental inoculation studies been conducted to determine pathogenicity. *Mycoplasma bovis,* when inoculated directly into the amniotic fluids of two heifers, resulted in abortion by 11 and 18 days, respectively. The placentae were retained, and both fetuses (approximately 100 and 150 days of age) were decomposed. The same organism was given by intraperitoneal injection to two other pregnant cows (130 and 180 days, respectively). At necropsy of the latter 36 days later, placentitis was severe. *M. bovis* was recovered from the placentae of both cows, and from the fetus of one cow. One of the heifers inoculated intraperitoneally developed arthritis, which led to speculation that hematogenous dissemination might be a prerequisite for colonization of the placenta.[17]

Direct inoculation of the amniotic fluid with *Ureaplasma* was also found to produce abortion. As with *M. bovis,* the abortions were associated with placentitis and retained fetal membranes. However, the interval between inoculation and abortion was considerably longer (up to 117 days), and fetal pneumonitis was a consistent finding.[17]

Studies comparing isolation rates from aborted and nonaborted fetuses have provided evidence that mycoplasmas may play a role in field cases of abortion. Extremely low isolation rates have been reported in each of three studies from fetal tissues and placentae from apparently healthy animals.[3, 14, 15] In one Canadian study no isolations were made from 33 normal fetuses and 74 normal placentae. A second study recovered mycoplasmas in only 1 of 65 normal fetuses. A third study in Ireland also found a low incidence in samples taken from normal pregnancies—1.3 per cent of fetal samples, 1.3 per cent of amniotic fluid samples and 0 per cent of placental samples.

Considerably higher isolation rates were made in cases of abortion. In the Canadian study, seven species of "mycoplasmas" were recovered—namely, *Ureaplasma, M. bovigenitalium, A. laidlawii, M. bovirhinis, M. bovis, M.* sp. Group 7 and *M. arginini.* The highest recovery rates were from the fetal membranes (37.5 per cent) followed by the lung, liver and stomach contents. *M. bovigenitalium* and *M. bovis* were recovered from both the placenta and the fetal tissues, suggesting that these organisms were causes of the abortions. Similarly, dams in cases in which *Mycoplasma* sp. Group 7 was isolated were also serologically positive.[15]

In the Irish study, three species of Mycoplasma, *A. laidlawii, M. bovigenitalium* and *Ureaplasma,* were isolated from aborted fetuses, placental tissues or vaginal mucus of the dam. Positive recoveries were made from 23.7 per cent of aborted placental material, 10.2 per cent of vaginal mucus samples and 4.4 per cent of the fetuses. *Acholeplasma laidlawii* was the predominant placental isolate, whereas *Ureaplasma* was the most common in vaginal fluid.[3]

More recent Canadian studies have reported positive *Ureaplasma* recoveries from the lungs of aborted fetuses. A fetal pneumonitis similar to that seen following experimental inoculation was also observed. The *Ureaplasma* isolate in all cases appeared to belong to serogroup D48.[22]

On the basis of these findings and in view of the relatively low diagnostic rate currently being achieved in cases of bovine abortion, consideration should be given to including *Mycoplasma* culture as part of the routine diagnostic procedure.

References

1. Afshar A, Stuart P, Huck RA: Granular vulvovaginitis of cattle associated with *Mycoplasma bovigenitalium.* Vet Rec 78:512, 1966.
2. Al-Aubaidi JM, McEntee K, Lein DH, Roberts SJ: Bovine seminal vesiculitis and epididymitis caused by *Mycoplasma bovigenitalium.* Cornell vet 62:581, 1972.
3. Ball HJ, Neill SD, Ellis WA, et al.: The isolation of mycoplasmas from bovine fetuses and their dams. Br Vet J 134:584, 1978.
4. Doig PA: Bovine genital mycoplasmosis. Can Vet J 22:339, 1981.
5. Edward DG, Hancock JL, Hignett SL: Isolation of pleuropneumoniae-like organisms from the bovine genital tract. Vet Rec 59:329, 1947.
6. Erno H, Philipsen H: Mycoplasmosis: Cervical and uterine inoculation of heifers with a Danish strain of *Mycoplasma bovigenitalium.* Acta Vet Scand 10:108, 1969.
7. Erno H, Blom E: Mycoplasmosis: Experimental and spontaneous infections of the genital tracts of bulls. Acta Vet Scand 13:161, 1972.
8. Gourlay RN, Howard CJ: Bovine mycoplasmas. In Tully JG, Whitcomb RF (eds): The Mycoplasmas. II. Human and Animal Mycoplasmas. New York, Academic Press, 1979, pp. 49.
9. Hall CE, McEntee K: Reduced post-thawing survival of sperm in bulls with mycoplasmal vesiculitis. Cornell Vet 71:111, 1981.
10. Hartmann HA, Tourtellotte ME, Neilson SW, Plastridge WN: Experimental bovine uterine mycoplasmosis. Res Vet Sci 5:303, 1964.
11. Hirth RS, Neilsen SW, Plastridge WN: Bovine salpingo-oophoritis produced with semen containing a mycoplasma. Path Vet 3:616, 1966.
11a. Hirth RS, Plastridge WN, Tourtellotte ME: Survival of mycoplasma in frozen bovine semen. Am J Vet Res, 28:97, 1967.
12. Hoare M: A survey of the incidence of mycoplasma infection in the oviducts of dairy cows. Vet Rec 85:351, 1969.
13. Jurmanova K, Sterbova J: Correlation between impaired spermatozoan motility and mycoplasma findings in bull semen. Vet Rec 100:157, 1977.
14. Langford EV: Mycoplasma species recovered from the reproductive tracts of western Canadian cows. Can J Comp Med 39:133, 1975.
15. Langford EV: Mycoplasma recovered from bovine male and female genitalia and aborted feti. Proceedings Annual Meeting American Association Veterinary Laboratory Diagnosis 18:221, 1975.
16. Lein DH: Bovine reproductive disorders associated with *Ureaplasma, Mycoplasma, Hemophilus somnus* and *Chlamydia.* Proceedings Annual Meeting of the Society for Theriogenology 1982, pp. 118.
17. Miller RB, Ruhnke HL, Doig PA, et al.: The effect of *Ureaplasma diversum* inoculated into the amniotic cavity of cows. Theriogenology 20:367, 1983.

18. Onoviran O, Truscott RB, Fish NA, et al.: The recovery of mycoplasmas from the genital tracts of bulls in artificial breeding units in Ontario. Can J Comp Med 39:474, 1975.

19. Panangala VS, Fish NA, Barnum DA: Micoflora of the cervico-vaginal mucus of repeat breeder cows. Can Vet J 19:83, 1978.

20. Panangala VS, Winter AJ, Wijesinha A, Foote RH: Decreased motility of bull spermatozoa caused by *Mycoplasma bovigenitalium*. Am J Vet Res 42:2090, 1981.

21. Parsonson IM, Al-Aubaidi JM, McEntee K: *Mycoplasma bovigenitalium:* Experimental induction of genital disease in bulls. Cornell Vet 64:240, 1974.

22. Ruhnke, HL, Palmer NC, Doig PA, Miller RB: Bovine abortion and neonatal death associated with *Ureaplasma diversum*. Theriogenology 21:295, 1984.

23. Stalheim OH, Proctor SJ: Experimentally induced bovine abortion with *Mycoplasma agalactiae subsp. bovis*. Am J Vet Res 37:879, 1976.

24. Tourtellotte ME, Lein DH: Infertility of cattle caused by mycoplasmas. Hlth Lab Sci 13:152, 1976.

Bovine Abortion

R. B. Miller, D.V.M.

Ontario Veterinary College, Guelph, Ontario

The terminology used in this discussion will coincide with that recommended by the Committee on Bovine Nomenclature.[20] Early embryonic death refers to deaths occurring from the day of conception until about 42 days of gestation, which coincides with the end of the stage of differentiation. Embryos lost during this period may be either absorbed or aborted. Fetuses discharged from day 42 until approximately 260 days are generally called abortions, and from day 260 until term, premature deliveries.

MAGNITUDE OF REPRODUCTIVE LOSS

The magnitude of reproductive loss has been found by David and associates to be approximately 37 per cent of all first breedings in which healthy cows and fertile bulls are used.[7] The majority of these losses occur in the first 45 days. Fourteen to 20 per cent of the ova are not fertilized, and up to 20 per cent of embryos die by 45 days.[37] Approximately 3 to 4 per cent of cows identified as pregnant between 30 and 50 days after breeding will abort or deliver a dead calf prematurely. Four to six per cent of pregnancies are presented as stillbirths, and of these 7 to 28 per cent have congenital abnormalities (that is, 0.5 to 1 per cent of all calves), 84 per cent die because of neonatal asphyxia, and 9.1 per cent have evidence of infection.[24]

PATHOGENESIS OF ABORTION

Genetic Factors

Abortions associated with genetic factors are beyond "routine diagnostic capability" except for those that occur near term and have some recognized phenotypic abnormality—for example, "congenital osteopetrosis," which is inherited as a simple autosomal recessive trait in Angus calves.[25] Losses due to genetic factors are most completely recorded in human pregnancies. Of 100 human pregnancies 17 spontaneous abortions were observed, and 7 of these 17 had an abnormal chromosomal constitution. Approximately 0.4 per cent of humans are born with a chromosomal abnormality.[4] The portion of abortions caused by genetic factors is not known in animals.

Environmental Factors

Environmental factors is a general term that includes the effects of nutrition, season, exogenous hormones and toxic compounds.

Nutrition

Mineral or vitamin deficiencies may be an important factor. Iodine deficiency may result in the birth of weak or dead, hairless and goitrous calves.[15] A correlation between vitamin E and selenium deficiency and abortion in cattle has not been documented experimentally; however, lesions typical of vitamin E and selenium deficiency are not uncommon in aborted bovine fetuses.[15, 28] Vitamin E and selenium deficiency is associated with the birth of weak and dead lambs.[14] Vitamin A deficiency is associated with defective bone growth, birth of weak calves and/or abortion.[32, 42] Dietary protein may be of some importance. One group of workers found that when feeding two levels of protein to pregnant beef cows there was an increased calf mortality in the low-protein group. This was associated with either dystocia or prematurity. They concluded that protein malnutrition in late pregnancy may be a factor contributing to neonatal mortality in beef calves.[43]

Temperature

There is some evidence to suggest that pregnant cows exposed to sudden rises in environmental temperature may abort; however, this manifestation is probably rare. Experimentally, extreme maternal hyperthermia causes profound fetal hypotension, hypoxia and acidosis. The fetal temperature is higher than the maternal.[30] High fetal temperatures may be more important as a cause of abortion when cows develop fever as a result of infection rather than from high environmental temperatures.

Toxins

Certain plants and toxic chemicals are capable of causing abortion. Abortion associated with eating the needles of *Pinus ponderosa* occurs in cattle during the last trimester and is characterized by desultory labor, excessive uterine hemorrhage, incomplete dilatation of the cervix and usually retained placenta and metritis. Cows may become very sick and die.[40] Until the factor resulting in abortion has been clearly identified, diagnosis in cattle will be presumptive and associated with animals consuming pine needles. Nitrate or nitrites are commonly incriminated as a cause of abortion, but experimental results have been equivocal.[8] Ingestion of warfarin will produce abortion in cattle and is thought by some to be teratogenic for human infants. In cattle it is uncommonly seen as an abortifacient, occurring only following ingestion of food contaminated by rat bait. The pathogenesis of the abortion and the usual trimester in which abortions occur have not been investigated. A related compound, coumarin, occurring naturally on some moldy sweet clover, has been associated with neonatal death.[13]

Locoism is a disease produced by toxic varieties of plants in the genera *Oxytropis* and *Astragalis*. Poisoning by locoweeds occurs particularly in the western United States and Canada and is most prevalent when pastures are poor, as in winter feeding. The toxic principal, an indolizidine alkaloid, can cause abortion or fetal abnormalities. Many tissues are affected including the corpus luteum, chorioallantois and neurons, resulting in lesions resembling mannosidosis, a hereditary storage disease occurring in Angus calves.[22] In the hereditary disease lysosomal alpha-mannosidase is absent because of a genetic deficiency. In locoweed poisoning indolizidine alkaloids inhibit the enzyme.

The use of intravenous sodium iodide in pregnant cattle is customarily avoided because of the threat of abortion. In a recent trial to test this premise, ten clinically normal pregnant cows were given a single intravenous dose of 50 gm of sodium iodide, and no adverse effects on pregnancy were noted.[27]

Infectious Causes of Abortion

The last category of abortions are those associated with infectious causes. The proportion of abortions attributable to infectious agents is not known; however, of those abortions in which the cause is determined, approximately 90 per cent are due to infection.[21]

Infections in the cow commonly travel to the placenta and/or the fetus and may result in abortion.

Several factors in infections not strictly associated with the reproductive tract may result in abortion in cattle. Any cause of high fever, such as mastitis or pneumonia, may result in abortion. Maternal hypoxia may result in fetal hypoxia and subsequent abortion. This may occur with severe chronic pneumonia or may be associated with circulatory failure as in traumatic pericarditis. Hemoconcentration and concurrent acidosis such as that occurring in grain overload may contribute to fetal hypoxia and acidosis with subsequent abortion. Endotoxemia may result from any maternal gram-negative bacterial infection in the feet, udder, pharynx, lung or intestine. Endotoxemia may produce abortion directly by evoking a generalized synthesis of F-prostaglandins[39] or indirectly through substances such as serotonin that may be released by endotoxin.[16, 35] Endotoxin also induces intravascular coagulation, which results in fetal hypoxia by interfering with placental circulation.[31] Maternal endotoxemia has also been shown to produce central nervous system (CNS) anomalies in the fetus. Fetal CNS anomalies associated with maternal endotoxemia have been produced experimentally in rats and occur naturally in women early in pregnancy associated with coliform infections of the kidney.[33, 34]

DIAGNOSIS OF THE CAUSES OF BOVINE ABORTION

Using conventional methods, the diagnostic rate in bovine abortion is usually between 25 and 40 per cent.[21] The causes for this low diagnostic rate are many. Three compartments are involved: maternal, placental and fetal, and disease in each, individually or together, may result in abortion. In order to increase the percentage of abortions diagnosed, each compartment must be thoroughly examined. The owner must have complete records of the breeding history, exposure to diseases, travel and other stresses to which the dam has been subjected. Records of feedstuff content, treatments and the general health of the animal are desirable. The clinician must examine the animal carefully at the time of abortion and take adequate samples to discover other reasons besides those related to the fetoplacental unit that may have been associated with abortion. On examination of the fetus and placenta at necropsy the pathologist must take complete samples because the system involved cannot be identified by the clinician. This is necessary so that later, if the disease is not the one originally suspected, another approach may be utilized and the diagnosis reached. The pathologist's knowledge of the specificity of lesions related to the causes of abortion is incomplete. In a survey conducted by Miller and Quinn, as many tissues with lesions were examined in which the cause of the abortion was not diagnosed as those in which it was. This places a heavy weight on the clinician and microbiologist, and if samples and history are inadequate, a diagnosis will not be reached.

MANAGEMENT OF ABORTION

The management of a single abortion or an outbreak may be conducted in the following manner. First, the laboratory preference has to be considered. Some laboratories, especially in the early spring, may be so inundated with fetuses that they do not wish to conduct investigations in which only a single abortion has occurred but prefer to have specimens only from cases of second and third abortions submitted. When submitting specimens, a complete history is important. A suggested individual and herd history is outlined in Table 1. Systems to be examined in the cow that aborted and possibly in other cows in the herd are tabulated in Table 2. The longer after abortion that samples for bacteriology are taken from the cervicovaginal mucus, the greater the variety of contaminating bacteria.[18] Samples that may be collected from the cow are listed in Table 3 and those from the herd are listed in Table 4.

With regard to a retained placenta, a caruncle with retained cotyledon should be removed intact. Submit one third of this, frozen, one third chilled, and one third fixed, preferably in Bouin's fixative. If the placenta is not available, then perhaps even preferably, a large caruncle from the pregnant horn should be removed and proportioned similarly. A cotyledon and/or caruncle obtained from deep within the uterus is generally cleaner and more representative of the disease than the portion of placenta hanging at the vulva. The importance of the placenta (cotyledon and caruncle) cannot be overemphasized, and a clear relationship between placental submission and an increased proportion of abortions diagnosed has been shown.

Examination of the fetal membranes should include a description of their condition, degree of autolysis, weight and whether or not they were retained. Normal weight may range from 9 to 18 pounds in the cow.[36] Increased weight of the placenta may be caused by edematous fluid as well as by inflammatory exudates. The cause of edema usually goes unrecognized and may be observed with a viable as well as a nonviable birth, whereas exudates are usually related to infection. An excessively light placenta may reflect placental insufficiency. The number of cotyledons may be important and normally ranges from 75 to 120.[36] The presence of adventitial placentation probably indicates a need for more placental area. This may be associated with placental insufficiency, as evidenced by decreased numbers of cotyledons, hypoxia in the uterine circulation, uterine fibrosis, or twin births. Cows with excessive adventitial placentation should be considered carefully before rebreeding because this may reflect inadequate caruncular reserve. Sometimes the size of individual cotyledons may be

Table 1. History

Individual History	
General	**Prophylaxis**
Age	Previous exposure
Breed	Vaccination
Lactation status	**Nutritional**
Illness during pregnancy	Water
Previous illness	Vitamin
Types	Mineral
Dates	Protein
Health during and after abortion	Carbohydrate
Purchased: Yes _____No _____	Fat
Before breeding	Other substances
After Breeding	
Transport	
Date	
Distance	
Condition	**Herd History**
Reproductive	**Number of breeding females**
Age	*Category of herd*
Breeding: Artificial _____Natural _____	Beef
Embryo transfer _____	Dairy
Dates _____	*Calving interval*
Parturitions	*Signs of disease in herd*
Number _____	During abortions
Date of last _____	Prior to abortions
Abortion	*Other abortions*
Infertility	This season
Retained placenta	Last season
Dystocia	*Additions*
Biopsy	During gestation
Other	Previous to breeding
Treatments	*Other animals on premises in association with cows*
Previous to abortion	Other age groups
After abortion	Other species

Table 2. Examination

Examination of Cow
  Temperature, pulse, respiration
  General body condition
  Respiratory system
  Ocular signs
  Digestive system
  Genitourinary system
    Urine
    Mammary
    Vulva
      Inflammation
      Discharge
    Vaginal
      Scope
        Inflammation in vagina or cervix
        Condition of vagina and cervix
          Tears
          Prolapse of cervical rings
          Retention of fetal membranes
  Examination per rectum
    Cervix
    Uterus
    Ovaries

Examination of Herd
  General body condition
  Ocular
  Mammary
  Lactation
  Vulvar discharges
  Examinations per rectum
    Pregnancy
    Mummified fetus
    Pyometra

Table 4. Samples to Be Collected from the Herd

Blood
Vaginal swabs
Urine
Milk

---

increased excessively. This may reflect too few caruncles or placental disease. Roberts states that placentome diameters exceeding 15 cm are abnormal. Retention of the placenta may result from inadequate preparation for parturition, or it may be due to inflammation in the maternal septa. The placenta should also be examined for uniformity of cotyledonary size. The largest cotyledons are usually just inside the pregnant horn and correspond to the site of umbilical vessel attachment. Uniformity in size and state of the cotyledons may be a clue to whether or not they are diseased. Fresh and rela-

Table 3. Samples to Be Collected from the Cow

Clotted blood	Another sample should be obtained in 2 to 3 weeks
Urine	Culture
	Cytology (need fresh sample for dark-field examination)
Vagina	Cervical or uterine swab (the longer after abortion the greater the increase in contaminants)
Placenta and/or caruncle	Even if retained remove a portion for culture (freeze one third for virology, chill one third for bacteriology, and fix one third for histologic examination)

tively healthy cotyledons and caruncles are dark red or hemorrhagic immediately following separation. Diseased cotyledons may retain portions of caruncular material, as is commonly observed in mycotic abortions, and may also be tan in color, indicating necrosis. A V-shaped area of infarction, either red or tan, may be seen on a cut surface of the caruncles. So-called cupping is frequently observed in the cotyledon and is caused by infiltration of inflammatory cells or exudates into the interstitium, causing the cotyledon to retain the same conformation as when it is attached to the caruncle. It is important to examine the clarity and texture of the intercotyledonary placenta as well. Lesions present in the immediate pericotyledonary region may be observed as slight thickenings, changes in color, or unevenness.

Autolytic changes in the placenta may be confusing. Following a moderate degree of autolysis, the cotyledons become a dull uniform red to tan, and the intercotyledonary zone loses its normal translucency, becoming opaque and a uniform dark red or gray. This is associated with the breakdown of red blood cells and imbibition of pigments by tissues adjacent to vessels. So-called amniotic plaques are present on the inner surface of the amnion and are most conspicuous in the region of the umbilicus. They are white to yellow, multifocal to coalescent, raised, firm regions that on microscopic examination consist of heaped-up mounds of epithelial cells that are frequently keratinized. They are normal structures that are usually most conspicuous at 3 to 7 months of gestation. The extremities of the chorioallantoic placenta in the tips of each of the uterine horns in cattle have a region of necrosis; this is normal and is due to failure of vascularization. Mineralization of the placenta may occur normally in the first few months of gestation and should not be considered pathologic during that period. Toward the end of gestation, however, mineralization may reflect previous placental injury associated with bacterial, mycotic or viral infection.

Samples, ideal and essential, to be obtained from the fetus are shown in Table 5. Examination of the fetus should include measurements of the crown-rump length, hair pattern and color, all of which may be used to estimate the age of the fetus. The condition of the fetus, whether fresh, decomposed or mummified, should be recorded. Examination of the teeth may reveal pitting as a result of in utero viral infection such as with bovine viral diarrhea virus. Edema around the jaw and face, conjunctival hemorrhage and swelling of the tongue occur commonly with dystocia. One of the causes of dystocia, of course, may be illness in the calf.

Table 5. Samples to Be Collected From the Fetus and Placenta

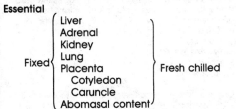

Ideal
  Entire placenta (caruncle collected from cow)
  Amniotic fluid
  Entire fetus

Essential
  Fixed { Liver / Adrenal / Kidney / Lung / Placenta / Cotyledon / Caruncle / Abomasal content } Fresh chilled

Careful examination of the newly haired regions over the eyelid, ears, withers or tail head may reveal slightly raised white crusts typical of mycotic dermatitis. White puttylike precipitates are frequently observed on the hair of aborted fetuses and newborn calves. These are of unknown significance and have not been associated with any specific disease.

The container in which an animal is submitted to the laboratory may be very important. Fertilizer bags containing small amounts of fertilizer produce gross lesions on the skin of fetuses and may be confusing to the pathologist. Mineralization occasionally occurs in the epidermis and may be associated with a chronic infectious process or other unrecognized cause of dermatitis.

The skin should always be examined for the presence of meconium staining as evidence of in utero fetal distress. Fetuses aborted as a result of a slowly developing placentitis or circulatory problem may be meconium stained and frequently are fresh because the slowly developing lesion results in fetal hypoxia, which stimulates premature delivery. An estimate of the chronicity of fetal distress may be made based on the intensity and degree of penetration of meconium into the fetal hair. This should not be mistaken for the normal progression of staining that occurs in the fetal eponychium of the developing fetal hoof. At 3 months' gestation the eponychium is becoming yellow; this color increases in intensity until 5 months, when it becomes a brilliant gold. By 7 months the color decreases, and by term only a faint yellow remains. This correlates with the color of the amniotic fluid and the stomach contents; however, these clear more rapidly than the eponychium. Failure to lose this staining indicates in utero distress. The eponychium is shed immediately as the calf starts to walk and may be eaten by birds in stillborn calves. The color of the conjunctiva should be observed; if white, it may reflect excessive bleeding. This may be caused by prolonged disruption of umbilical vessels; in pigs it has been associated with ascorbic acid deficiency.[38] This condition has not been described in cattle, but neither was it expected in pigs because primates

and guinea pigs are the only mammalian species known to require exogenous ascorbic acid.[5] Other causes such as a decrease in vitamin K–dependent coagulation factors should be considered in calves. This has been observed in aassociation with moldy sweet clover poisoning.[13]

Internal findings of subcutaneous thoracic and abdominal serosanguineous fluid are consistent with autolysis; this fluid is usually due to prolonged retention in utero following death of the fetus.[9] It is not a lesion associated with any specific disease. Fetal kidney is one of the first organs to show marked autolysis and may be surrounded by blood-stained fluid. Hemorrhage around the umbilical vessels indicates that the animal was alive shortly before or during parturition.[26] Inflation of the lungs generally indicates that the animal has breathed; however, vigorous resuscitation such as mouth-to-nose breathing has been shown to partially inflate the lungs in an already dead fetus. Stomach contents should always be examined. If the stomach contains meconium swallowed when the fetus was alive, in utero fetal distress is indicated; if it contains white material, the animal may have been given colostrum. Mucus present in the abomasum may be difficult to distinguish grossly from milk in some instances. Trauma in utero with severe injury to the fetus, such as broken ribs, can occur but is a rare event. Healed rib fractures have been observed in aborted fetuses, verifying severe trauma in utero. Whether this was the cause of the abortion occurring some weeks later, however, was not determined. Hemorrhage around the liver may occur as the fetus is being discharged, especially in a fetus less than 5 months old, and would not be related to the cause of abortion. A ruptured liver in a newborn calf that has breathed is frequently observed and is associated with trauma during or following birth.

Criteria used for the diagnosis of fetal abortion include the history, isolated agents, lesions and the development of fetal antibody.

The fetus is immunologically competent at a relatively early age, and chronic in utero infections result in antibody production. Many researchers have demonstrated that fetuses have substantial quantities of immunoglobulins in the fetal fluids. It was thought that these immunoglobulins would be useful as specific indicators of in utero infection and presumptive evidence of the cause of abortion. There is increasing evidence, however, that antibodies to many agents are present in these fluids. The passage of immunoglobulins from the cow to the fetus following placental injury has been suggested by different authors.[1, 10, 29] Experiments to determine whether or not this occurs are being conducted, and until this problem is clarified, antibodies in fetal fluids, unless titers are very high, will be of doubtful use in the diagnosis of the cause of abortion.

The commonly recognized causes of abortion and some of the associated findings are listed in Table 6. Details of the most commonly recognized conditions are discussed elsewhere in this book.

Table 6. Common Causes of Abortion

Agent and Common Names	Prevalence	Source of Agent	Incubation to Abortion	Probable Pathogenesis	Usual History	Abortion Rate
BACTERIAL *Brucella abortus* Brucellosis Bang's disease	All countries in which cattle are raised	Aborted fetus, uterine discharge, placenta, infected premises, milk	2 weeks to 5 months or longer	Organism enters through mucous membranes (e.g., alimentary tract), go to lymph nodes, udder and uterus; grows well in placenta, causing placentitis	Abortion, birth of weak or dead calves, retained placenta, infertility	80 per cent of unvaccinated cows infected in first or second trimester will abort
Campylobacter fetus ss. *venerealis*, Vibriosis Bovine genital vibriosis	Throughout the world	Infected crypts of the penis and fornix of the prepuce. Infected bulls to heifers approximately 100 per cent; infected cows to susceptible bulls considerably lower; bull to bull unlikely but can occur in groups of bulls; cow to cow highly unlikely	3 to 8 months	Organism produces endometritis in progestational phase following breeding	Infertility and failure of conception	Usually less than 10 per cent
Campylobacter fetus ss. *fetus*	Widely distributed	Possibly intestine	Not established	Ingested; may cause a bacteremia from intestine to liver with subsequent infection of uterus and placentome	Rarely infertility, sporadic abortion	Sporadic
Mycobacterium (*Corynebacterium pyogenes*)	Worldwide	Common on many of the mucous membranes and in the tonsils of normal cattle	—	Probably hematogenous to caruncle, adjacent endometrium and placenta	Usually no signs before or after infection, occasionally preceded by systemic illness, mastitis, and/or followed by endometritis	Sporadic or multiple up to 64 per cent
Leptospira pomona, hardjo, canicola, icterohemorrhagiae, grippotyphosa, Leptospirosis	Most areas of the world, related to geographic areas	Infected cows, wildlife, swine, etc. contamination of water or feed by urine	2 to 5 weeks after initial infection, maybe 3 months	Penetration of abraded skin and mucous membranes; localizes in renal tubules and placenta	Usually no observed premonitary signs; may be mastitis, icterus or anemia; fever may accompany or precede the abortion	5 to 40 per cent may be sporadic or epidemic
Salmonella spp. *dublin, typhimurium, muenster, newport, anatum,* many others	Throughout the world; *Salmonella dublin* abortion not yet reported in Canada or U.S.A. but organism reported in U.S.A.	Excreted in feces, urine and milk by sick or carrier cows; unsterilized bone meal; birds may carry it and contaminate feed	—	In intestine of cow, hematogenous to placenta	May be febrile; enteric disease or no clinical signs in cows; human disease may be present	Usually sporadic but may be herd outbreak
Listeria monocytogenes Listeriosis	Widespread throughout the world	Wide host range of carrier animals; birds and fish that excrete the organism in	May be very long because it appears to be stress-related	Penetrates intact mucous membranes of respiratory or alimentary tract; latent	Pyrexia, depression and retained placenta may occur in the dam	Sporadic or multiple up to 50 per cent

Table 6 Common Causes of Abortion *Continued*

Stage of Gestation in Which Abortion Occurs	Diagnostic Method Preferred: Microbiology (1) Serology (2) Lesions (3)	Duration of Carrier State	Recurrence of Abortion	Prevention and Control	Samples to be Submitted
6 to 9 months	(1) Isolation of organism from uterine fluids, milk, placenta, fetal lung, fetal stomach contents (2) Tube agglutination titer of 1:100 or greater is evidence of infection and presumptive evidence of abortion	Spread by milk for prolonged periods, possibly for life	High rate of infertility; majority abort only once	Vaccination of females at 3 to 10 months with Strain 19; remove infected animals; depopulate	Fetus and placenta paired serum samples
6 to 8 months	(1) Culture from fetus, placenta or abomasal contents; darkfield examination of abomasal contents (2) Obtain vaginal mucus antibodies on a herd basis or for culture	May survive on cervix for a full gestation; bulls may carry for 18 months	Uncommon; convalescent cows resistant to reinfection	Vaccination at 4½ months prior to breeding followed by a booster 10 days before breeding; revaccinate yearly (both bulls and cows); artificial insemination with antibiotic treated-semen	Placenta and fetus for culture; vaginal mucus on herd basis; use transport media
4 to 9 months	(1) Culture from placenta, abomasal contents	Survives in intestine for an extended period	Not established	Sporadic, usually not necessary	Placenta and fetus for culture
Usually in the last trimester	(1) Culture from placenta or lung; organism may not be present in fetal tissues	Unknown	May be sterile with endometritis or salpingitis; recurrence unknown	No vaccines used	Placenta and fetus
Usually in last trimester	(1) Cultures and fluorescent antibody tests can be conducted successfully on aborted fetuses and, when done properly, more accurately detect infection than serologic tests; culture urine from cow commonly up to 10 days, may be 3 months—also milk (2) Microscopic agglutination test on serum in herd	Shed in urine for 2 to 3 months; also in milk	Immune to serotype causing the abortion but susceptible to the other types; infertility common after abortion	Isolate affected animals; bacterins available	Placenta and fetus, fresh urine or milk, paired serum samples
Any time, 6 to 9 months	(1) Isolation from placenta or fetus	Prolonged latent, passive or active carriers	Unknown	Autogenous killed bacterins may be beneficial; isolate carriers	Placenta and fetus
Most in latter portions of last trimester	(1) Isolation from fetus or placenta	May be in feces and milk; healthy carrier may be important reservoir	May recur in same animal and on same farm from year to year	No commercial bacterin; isolate known infected animals	Placenta and fetus for culture and histologic studies

Table 6. Common Causes of Abortion *Continued*

Agent and Common Names	Prevalence	Source of Agent	Incubation to Abortion	Probable Pathogenesis	Usual History	Abortion Rate
Listeria monocytogenes Listeriosis *Continued*		feces; survives in dried feces for 2 years; organism resistant to adverse environmental conditions; propagates in high pH silage		infection established, and stress results in placentitis and fetal septicemia		
Ureaplasma diversum, T-strain mycoplasma	Probably widespread but not recognized	Semen, vulvar discharges, possibly respiratory	Probably several months	Unknown, may be introduced with semen or contamination from vulva; lives in uterus and infects fetus; also possibly respiratory and hematogenous to fetus	Abortion may be preceded by suppurative vulvitis; fetal membranes frequently retained	Sporadic; may be more important cause of infertility
FUNGAL *Aspergillus* sp. 60 to 80 per cent Mucorales 10 to 15 per cent	Worldwide	Ubiquitous in nature, wet hay or straw	28 days after intravenous inoculation of spores; probably weeks or months after natural infection	Molds are taken into lungs or mouth and then invade through lesions, travelling to the placenta hematogenously	Tends to be seasonal in northern hemisphere; peak incidence in January, February or March where cattle are confined: usually no prodromal signs	Sporadic to 5 to 10 per cent of herd
PROTOZOAN *Trichomonas fetus* Trichomoniasis *Trichomonas fetus*	Worldwide	Infected bulls at breeding only; artificial insemination transmission from infected bulls is 1 per cent	From breeding, any time up to 7 months	Inflammation of vagina, cervix and endometrium produces a hostile intrauterine environment	Natural breeding and infertility most common with pyometra and abortion, abortions may be most common in older cows with partial immunity	Very low
VIRAL Blue tongue virus	Widespread but not worldwide	*Culicoides* spp. from infected sheep or cattle; also by infected semen	Variable, may be very long; at least 16 autogenic strains that vary widely in their virulence for cattle	Viremia and infection of fetus	Signs in cow mild or absent	Probably low, not established
Bovine viral diarrhea BVD–MD virus BVD	Widespread throughout the world	Infected cattle housed or pastured together	4 days to 3 months after an outbreak	Viremia crossing the placenta as early as 58th day and up to day 120	Febrile disease in herd prior to abortion and calves born with brain damage	Usually very low but in utero infection may cause severe intrauterine growth retardation in surviving fetus
Infectious bovine rhinotracheitis Red nose IBR, IBR–IPV	Widespread throughout the world	Infected cows; any animal with a positive titer may be carrying the virus	2 weeks to 4 months	Virus carried in blood leukocytes is localized in placental vessels; on entering fetus, kills fetus within 24 hours	Commonly follows respiratory, conjunctival form of the disease; may be no signs in the cow; introduction of infected animals	5 to 60 per cent
UNKNOWN Epizootic bovine abortion EBA	Probably localized to one area in California	Unknown	Not established	Not established	Occurs in cows pastured on native vegetation in foothills and mountains of California	Up to 75 per cent

Table 6. Common Causes of Abortion *Continued*

Stage of Gestation in Which Abortion Occurs	Diagnostic Method Preferred: Microbiology (1) Serology (2) Lesions (3)	Duration of Carrier State	Recurrence of Abortion	Prevention and Control	Samples to be Submitted
Anytime but usually last trimester	(1) Isolation and (3) histologic demonstration of alveolitis and chronic nonsuppurative placentitis	May be 2 months	Unknown	Use clean or treated semen; double-rod artificial insemination	Placenta and fetus
May be from 4 months gestation to term	(3) Mycotic elements in typical placental, skin or lung lesions (1) yeast and molds may be present in abomasal contents and not be the cause of abortion—care must be taken in interpretation	Probably not a factor	Recovery in severe cases may be slow and prolonged; permanent sterility may follow	Keep off moldy feed at least while pregnant	Placenta and fetus for culture and histologic studies; caruncle or placentome invaluable
Usually in first half of gestation but may be up to 7 months	(1) Must find the organism in pyometra discharge, placental fluids or stomach contents	Males remain carriers for a long period; cows may retain the organism for 150 days	As animals lose immunity, they may become reinfected	Artificial insemination from noninfected bulls; use only bulls 1 to 3 years old in infected herd	Uterine sample; placenta and fetus for culture; transport sample in lactated Ringer's and refrigerate—will keep up to 48 hours
Variable may be born at term with congenital deformity including hydranencephaly	(1) Virus isolation from fetus or from blood of dam (2) Antibody in fetal serum	Calves infected in utero may be permanently infected	Unlikely	None	Blood samples from dam for culture, paired serum samples, fetus for culture and serum for antibody
Usually early but may be up to 4 months	(2) Febrile, enteric disease in cows with a two- to fourfold titer rise (3) serum-neutralizing antibody in calves with brain and eye abnormalities (1) culture virus from uterine biopsy	May remain up to 56 days in respiratory tract or in urine for 2 days; could be transmitted in semen	Unlikely because animals are immune	Vaccination, after 8 months of age; don't vaccinate pregnant cows; may be unfavorable reactions with some vaccines	Placenta and entire fetus; acute and convalescent sera from cow; sera from colostral-free calves with congenital abnormalities
4 months to term	(1) Fluorescent antibody test on fetal kidney; (3) lesions in the fetal liver and adrenal gland may be diagnostic; (2) fourfold rise in titer from abortion to 2 weeks	Probably for life of animal	Unlikely	Vaccinate heifers at 6 to 8 months of age	Placenta and fetus; paired sera from cow
Last trimester	(3) Lesions consistent with the condition in a localized area (2) elevated fetal immunoglobulin G	Not established	Seldom abort more than once	No vaccination	Complete history; placenta and fetus

References

1. Brown TT, Schultz RD, Duncan JR, Distner SI: Serological response of the bovine fetus to bovine viral diarrhea virus. Infect Immun 25:93, 1979.
2. Bruner DW, Gillespie, JH: Hagan's Infectious Diseases of Domestic Animals, 6th ed. Ithaca NY, Cornell University Press, 1973.
3. Bulgin MS: *Salmonella dublin:* What veterinarians should know. J Am Vet Med Assoc 182:116, 1983.
4. Carr DH: Chromosomal anomalies as a cause of spontaneous abortion. Am J Obstet Gynecol 97:283, 1967.
5. Chatterjee IB, Kar NC, Ghash NC, Guha BC: Aspects of ascorbic acid biosynthesis in animals. Annal NY Acad Sci 92:36, 1961.
6. Clark BL, Parsonson IM, White MB, et al.: Control of trichomoniasis in a large herd of beef cattle. Aust Vet J 50:424, 1974.
7. David JSE, Bishop MWH, Cembrowicz HJ: Reproductive expectancy and infertility in cattle. Vet Rec 89:181, 1971.
8. Davison KL, Hansel W, Krook et al.: Nitrate toxicity in dairy heifers. I. Effects on reproduction, growth, lactation, and vitamin A nutrition. J Dairy Sci 47:1065, 1964.
9. Dillman RC, Dennis SM: Sequential sterile autolysis in the ovine fetus: Macroscopic changes. Am J Vet Res 37:403, 1976.
10. Dunne HW, Ajinkyas SM, Bubash GR, Griel LC Jr: Parainfluenza-3 and bovine enteroviruses as possible important causative factors in bovine abortion. Am J Vet Res 34:1121, 1973.
11. Ellis WA, O'Brien JJ, Neill SD, et al.: Bovine leptospirosis: Microbiological and serological findings in aborted fetuses. Vet Rec 110:147, 1982.
12. Ellis WA, O'Brien JJ, Neill SD, Hanna J: Bovine leptospirosis: Serological findings in aborting cows. Vet Rec 110:178, 1982.
13. Fraser CM, Nelson J: Sweet clover poisoning in newborn calves. J Am Vet Med Assoc 135:283, 1959.
14. Hartley J, Dodd DC: Muscular dystrophy in New Zealand livestock. NZ Vet J 5:61, 1956.
15. Hidiraglou M: Trace elements in the fetal and neonate ruminant: A review. Can Vet J 21:328, 1980.
16. Hinshaw LB: The release of vasoactive agents by endotoxin. In Bacterial Endotoxins. Rutgers, The State University, 1964, pp. 118–125.
17. Hinton M: Salmonella abortion in cattle. Vet Bull 41:973, 1971.
18. Hinton M: Bovine abortion associated with *Corynebacterium pyogenes.* Vet Bull 42:753, 1972.
19. Hoffer MA: Bovine campylobacteriosis: A review. Can Vet J 22:327, 1981.
20. Hubbert WT: Recommendations for standardizing bovine reproductive terms. Cornell Vet 62:216, 1971.
21. Hubbert WT, Booth GD, Bolton WD, et al.: Bovine abortions in five northeastern states 1960–1970. Evaluation of diagnostic laboratory data. Cornell Vet 63:291, 1973.
22. Jolly RD, Hartley WJ: Storage diseases of domestic animals. Aust Vet J 53:1, 1977.
23. Kimsey PB, Darien BJ, Kendrick JW, Franti CE: Bovine trichomoniasis: Diagnosis and treatment. J Am Vet Med Assoc 177:616, 1980.
24. Leipold HW: Genetics and disease in cattle. Proceedings 11th Annual Convention American Association Bovine Practitioners, Baltimore, Maryland, December 11–14:1978, pp. 18–31.
25. Leipold HW, Doige LE, Kay MM, Cribb PH: Hereditary osteopetrosis in Aberdeen Angus calves. I. Pathological changes. Annals Genet Sel Anim 3:245, 1971.
26. McFarlane D: Perinatal lamb losses. I. An autopsy method for the investigation of perinatal losses. NZ Vet J 13:116, 1965.
27. Miller V, Drost M: Failure to cause abortion in cows with intravenous sodium iodide treatment. J Am Vet Med Assoc 172:466, 1978.
28. Miller RB, Quinn PJ: Observations on abortions in cattle: A comparison of pathological, microbiological and immunological findings in aborted foetuses and foetuses collected at abattoirs. Can J Comp Med 39:270, 1975.
29. Miller RB, Wilkie BN: The indirect fluorescent antibody technique as a method for determining antibodies in aborted fetuses. Can J Comp Med 43:255, 1979.
30. Morishima HO, Glaser B, Niemann WH, James LS: Increased uterine activity and fetal deterioration during maternal hyperthermia. Am J Obstet Gynecol 121:531, 1975.
31. Morrison DC, Ulevitch R: The effects of bacterial endotoxins on host mediation systems. A review. Am J Pathol 93:527, 1978.
32. Moustgaard J: Nutritive influences upon reproduction. In Cole HH, Cupps PT (eds): Reproduction in Domestic Animals, 2nd ed. New York, Academic Press, 1969, pp. 489–516.
33. Niswander KR, Gordon M: The Women and Their Pregnancies. Philadelphia, W.B. Saunders, 1972, pp. 252–256.
34. Ornay A, Altshuler G: Maternal endotoxemia, fetal anomalies and central nervous system damage. A rat model of a human problem. Am J Obstet Gynecol 124:196, 1976.
35. Parant M, Chedid L: Protective effect of chlorpromazine against endotoxin-induced abortion. Proc Soc Exp Biol Med 116:906, 1964.
36. Roberts SJ: Gestation period—embryology, fetal membranes, and placenta-teratology. In Veterinary Obstetrics and Genital Diseases (Theriogenology), 2nd ed. Ithaca, SJ Roberts, 1971, pp. 45–47. Distributed by Edwards Bros, Inc, Ann Arbor, MI.
37. Roche JF, Boland MP, McGeady TA, Ireland JJ: Reproductive wastage following artificial insemination of heifers. Vet Rec 109:401, 1981.
38. Sandholm M, HonKanen-Buzalski T, Rasi V: Prevention of navel bleeding in piglets by preparturient administration of ascorbic acid. Vet Rec 104:337, 1979.
39. Skarnes RC, Harper MJK: Relationship between endotoxin-induced abortion and the synthesis of prostaglandin F. Prostaglandins 1:191, 1972.
40. Stevenson AH, James LF, Call JW: Pine-needle *(Pinus ponderosa)* induced abortion in range cattle. Cornell Vet 62:519, 1972.
41. Thiermann AB: Experimental leptospiral infections in pregnant cattle with organisms of the *hebdomadis* serogroup. Am J Vet Res 43:780, 1982.
42. Thomas DD: Nutritional aspects of calf losses. National Academy of Science Publication 1685. Washington, D.C., National Academy of Sciences, 1968, pp. 45–76.
43. Waldhalm DG, Hall RF, DeLong WJ, et al.: Restricted dietary protein in pregnant beef cows: I. The effect on length of gestation and calfhood mortality. Theriogenology 12:61, 1979.

Effects of Climate on Bovine Reproduction

William W. Thatcher
and Robert J. Collier*
University of Florida
Gainesville, Florida

ENVIRONMENTAL EFFECTS ON REPRODUCTIVE PERFORMANCE

Seasonal climatic effects on reproductive performance influence herd management efficiency and management programs and are becoming more important as tropical, subtropical and arid areas of the world take on an even greater role in supplying man's food. The veterinarian's understanding of thermal stress effects on reproductive physiology, endocrinology and overall animal performance is essential for providing proper recommendations for treatment and management of cattle during periods of thermal stress. Suppression of conception rates during certain months of the year has been well documented and is illustrated clearly in Figure 1. Results represent analysis of 6555 inseminations during a 3-year period (1975–1977) with three breeds (Jersey, Brown Swiss and Holstein) within a commercial dairy herd in Florida (subtropical environment).

Several points are clear from Figure 1: Heifers had a higher conception rate than lactating cows (47 per cent compared with 32 per cent); conception rates of cows decreased much more in the summer months of June through August; conception rates did not recover until November, suggesting a carry-over effect during the months of September and October. Of practical significance is the question of whether specific climatic measurements could be related quantitatively to fertility on an insemination-to-insemination basis. Maximum environmental temperature on the day after insemination was associated negatively with conception rates, and the relationship is shown in Figure 2. A clear difference in conception rates was detected between lactating dairy cows and heifers as maximum environmental temperature increased the day after insemination. Conception rates decreased in cows, and the decrease was accelerated when the maximum environ-

mental temperature exceeded 30°C. In contrast, conception rates increased for heifers. Decrease in conception rates of lactating cows is probably due to an inability to maintain a normal body temperature under heat stress conditions because of a high rate of internal heat production associated with production of milk. In contrast, nonlactating heifers are more likely to have a higher critical environmental temperature beyond which body temperature is elevated, but not to the point where fertility is diminished. This does not imply that heifers are not sensitive to thermal stress. In fact, in a study performed with an environmental chamber, none of 23 heifers conceived when exposed to a constant 32.2°C environmental temperature for 72 hours following breeding, whereas 12 of 25 heifers conceived when maintained at a 21.1°C environment.[3] Heifers in the 32.2°C group had elevated rectal temperatures of 40°C. Relationships of maximum temperature on the day following insemination with conception rates do not represent exposure of animals to a constant environmental temperature, but instead reflect maximum temperatures achieved under natural conditions of constantly changing circadian temperature fluctuations. Under these conditions, the fertility of lactating cows is affected more adversely than that of heifers (Fig. 2). Furthermore, the differences in conception rates noted among breeds (Jersey versus Holstein and Brown Swiss: 45 per cent versus 39 and 41 per cent, respectively) probably also reflected differences associated with milk production and thermoregulatory responses during summer thermal stress periods. In relating various climatologic measurements (e.g., maximum, minimum and average daily temperatures; average daily rainfall; average wind movement; average daily solar radiation; average maximum and minimum daily atmospheric pressure) with fertility, the maximum environmental temperature on the day after insemination was the most potent environmental measurement associated with fertility in the subtropical environment of Florida.[6] Obviously, many of the environmental measurements are correlated, and the most potent environmental measurement may vary depending on geographic location. For example, in northern Israel during summer, minimum ambient temperature was associated negatively with conception rates.[4] Likewise, in Israel conception rates for heifers were unchanged during the summer months, whereas fertility was suppressed for cows.

Changes in climatic measurements represent alterations in the animal's microenvironment that are related to conception rates. A logical question is whether similar associations can be detected within the potential embryo's microenvironment, i.e., the uterus. Uterine temperatures recorded the day of insemination (UT_0) and the day after insemination (UT_1) were related negatively to conception rates.[5] An increase of 0.5°C above the mean UT_0 (38.6°C) and UT_1 (38.3°C) decreased conception rates 12.8 and 6.9 per cent, respectively.

*The authors acknowledge the close cooperation of Mr. Lokenga Badinga, Dr. H. H. Head and Dr. C. J. Wilcox, whose research efforts partially contributed to this manuscript.

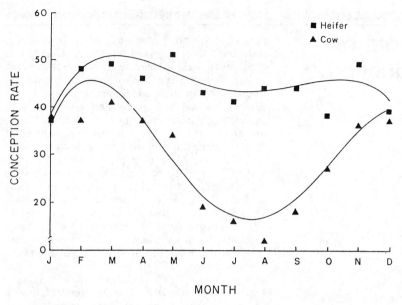

Figure 1. Least squares means for monthly conception rates (%) in heifers and cows, unadjusted for environmental effects.

Evidence is abundant that thermal stress can influence reproductive performance in female dairy cattle. An offspring at term represents successful function of a series of sequential physiological events. Thermal stress could act by influencing sexual behavior, the quality of the ova ovulated and the ova after fertilization and could elicit specific responses by the dam that may subsequently affect the embryo's environment, rate of fetal growth, postnatal development and performance responses of the dam (e.g., reproductive and lactational) after birth of the calf.

EFFECT OF THERMAL STRESS ON REPRODUCTIVE PROCESSES OF THE FEMALE

Early Pregnancy

Herd reproductive inefficiency results from two main problems: (1) an absence of expressed estrus or inefficient detection of estrus, and (2) infertile services, of which embryonic mortality in dairy cattle is estimated to be approximately 15 per cent.[8] The magnitude of these problems is amplified during hot seasonal periods. One of the most consistent gross observations during thermal stress exposure is a reduction in the duration of estrus to approximately 10 hours and a lower intensity of estrous behavior. This reduced sexual activity lowers metabolic heat production and reduces the heat load that must be dissipated by the cow. If estrous activity occurs during the night, it may be easily missed by persons responsible for estrous detection. If estrus occurs during the hot periods of the day, cattle are reluctant to become active because they need to leave the shade. Thus, estrus may easily remain undetected. Such behavioral alterations contribute to a reduction in success of heat detection

for artificial insemination programs. This is documented in Table 1 for a large commercial dairy herd of Jersey cows. Approximately 66 per cent of potential heats were not detected for the calendar year of 1982. The striking observation is that the hypothetical percentage of potential heats not detected increased to a plateau of approximately 80 per cent during the hot summer months of June through September. This, coupled with the lower conception rates to detected heats (Fig. 1), accounts for a tremendous amount of herd infertility during the summer period of June to October.

It seems reasonable that heat stress would alter the hormonal balance of the animal, which may interfere with reproductive processes that culminate in a successful pregnancy. We followed daily changes in plasma hormonal concentrations (estradiol, LH, progesterone and corticoids) throughout the estrous cycle of five cows maintained in a shade management system versus four cows managed under a stressful no-shade management system.[14] The transitory hormonal concentrations between the two groups indicated that thermal stress, of the magnitude observed in this experiment, did not inhibit recurrence of estrous cycles (Fig. 3). In both groups, a fall in progesterone concentrations associated with corpus luteum regression and a proestrous rise in estradiol were sufficient to induce a preovulatory surge of LH and heat followed by ovulation. However, in cows managed with no-shade, slight elevations were detected in progesterone and corticoids during the luteal phase, whereas the proestrous rise in estradiol concentrations was slightly lower. A smaller proestrous rise of estradiol in heat-stressed heifers (32°C versus 21°C) was detected also when samples were collected at 6-hour intervals in an environmental chamber.[7] The biologic importance of these subtle but statistically significant differences in both luteal progesterone concentrations and

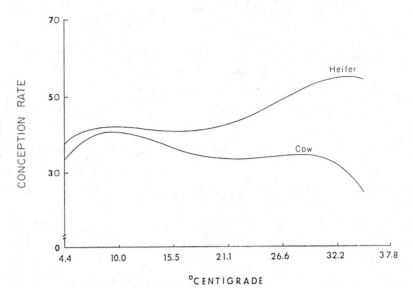

Figure 2. Least squares regression curves for conception rates (%) and maximum environmental temperatures on the day after insemination for heifers and cows.

proestrous estradiol/progesterone ratios (Fig. 3) may be related to the quality of the developing preovulatory follicle, the intensity of estrous behavior, and the subsequent microenvironment of the uterus and oviduct that controls such processes as capacitation, sperm and ova transport and fertilization.

There is a paucity of data defining the period of thermal sensitivity during early pregnancy in cattle. Various in vivo and in vitro experiments in other domestic farm animals (e.g., sheep) indicate that exposure of the newly fertilized ovum and/or zygote during early cleavage divisions markedly increased subsequent rates of embryonic death.[14] Because rectal and uterine temperatures near the time of insemination are related to conception rates, and elevated environmental temperatures (32.2°C) for 72 hours after breeding completely blocked concep-

tion, then a similar period of thermal sensitivity probably exists in cattle. In fact, recent research with dairy cattle by Arizona investigators indicates that fertilization occurs normally in summer heat-stressed cows (Monty DE, Jr., personal communication). Flushing the oviducts 3 to 5 days after insemination revealed a high incidence of cleaving embryos (80 per cent). Thus exposure of cow and zygote (early cleavage divisions) to thermal stress induces embryonic death after the embryo arrives in the uterus but before pregnancy is recognized ($\cong$ day 16). Extensive studies are needed to document the duration of the thermal sensitive period and when embryos perish in their later development. Death probably occurs early since in both nonparous and parous beef cattle, a large proportion of reproductive failure normally occurs by day 8 of gestation and has no noticeable effect on the length

Table 1. Monthly Per Cent of Possible Breedings That Were Inseminated After 60 Days Postpartum in a Commercial Florida Dairy Herd of Jersey Cows

Year, 1982 Month	Number of Cows	Per Cent of Possible* Breedings Inseminated	Estimate for Per Cent† Nondetected Heats
January	191	36	64
February	167	36	64
March	145	35	65
April	126	35	65
May	106	34	66
June	132	24	76
July	160	18	82
August	191	19	81
September	218	21	79
October	254	38	62
November	258	54	46
December	228	56	44
Mean	181	33.8	66.1

*Per cent of possible breedings that were inseminated. See Dairyman's DHI Manual 1981, Dairy Records Processing Center at Raleigh, NC, North Carolina State University.
†Estimate of per cent nondetected heats (100 − per cent of possible breedings inseminated).

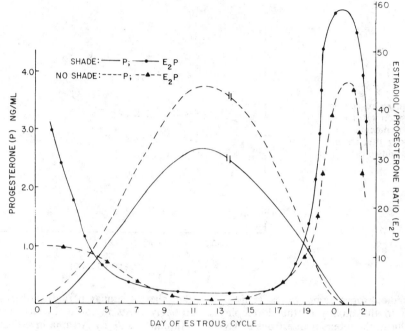

Figure 3. Least squares regressions of plasma progesterone and ratios of estradiol/progesterone concentrations during the estrous cycle in shade and unshaded cattle during summer.

of the estrous cycle.[11] The situation may be somewhat different in normal dairy cows,[8] in which embryonic deaths apparently occur after day 16, whereas in repeat breeder dairy cows[1] it occurs by day 8.

Because elevated environmental and uterine temperatures near the time of fertilization are related to conception rates, factors controlling uterine temperature are important. The greatest rate of uterine blood flow during the estrous cycle occurs during the periestrous period in association with high ratios of estradiol/progesterone concentrations. In cows exposed to the sun with no shade during the summer, an increase in uterine blood flow induced by estradiol (200 μg) was less than that in the same cows treated with estradiol (200 μg) but exposed to an effective shade structure.[13] Thus during the animal's thermoregulatory response to thermal stress, there is a decreased rate of blood perfusion to the uterus after injection of estradiol. Such a thermal stress–induced reduction in uterine blood flow would preferentially elevate uterine temperature and would probably affect the availability of water, electrolytes, nutrients and hormones to the uterus. This may be critical during the periods of elevated uterine blood flow that normally occur during the periestrous period or early pregnancy at 14 to 16 days (the localized conceptus–induced increase in uterine blood flow occurs at this time). As a consequence of thermal stress such induced inhibitory responses would have a high probability of increasing rates of embryo death during early pregnancy.

Collectively, these results indicate that the "infertility heat stress syndrome" is due to a potential combination of factors that compromise the well-being of the embryo in its uterine microenvironment. Direct elevation in temperature of the reproductive tract, slight but possibly important physiological changes in hormonal balance, and reduction in blood flow to the reproductive tract may alter the delicate synchrony required between embryo and mother. The importance of this synchrony is documented by embryo transfer experiments showing that if the donor is more than one day earlier or later in gestation than the recipient, the probability of maintaining a pregnancy is markedly reduced.

Periparturient Period

Several reports indicate that thermal stress during late pregnancy in sheep causes a reduction in uterine blood flow, decreased placental weight, and a retardation of fetal growth.[16] Approximately 60 per cent of bovine fetal growth occurs during the last 90 days of pregnancy, and coupled with fetal growth is simultaneous development of the mother's mammary gland. Conceptus growth and development therefore clearly are controlling maternal function to some degree. This is further substantiated by two additional lines of evidence. Part of the variation in postpartum milk production is influenced by the sire of the fetus, which is exerting some intrauterine environmental influences via the conceptus (fetus, placental membranes and fetal fluids) on the maternal unit, which ultimately influences subsequent milk production. Second, the birth weight of the

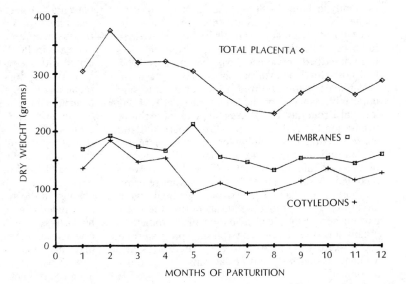

Figure 4. Least squares means for dry weight of total placenta, membranes, and cotyledons in cattle undergoing parturition in different months (1 = January, 12 = December).

calf is positively associated with the subsequent milk yield of the mother.[16] Analysis of a large herd data set for a 23-year period indicated that the birth weight of Holstein calves was lower during hot summer months than cool winter months (range, 6 kg) in the subtropical environment of Florida. These observations led to further studies to characterize the placenta (n = 187), collected within 24 hours of parturition, from Holstein and Jersey cows during a 1.5-year period. As expected, the total placental dry weight from Holstein cows was greater than that from Jersey cows (332.2 versus 212.6 gm), and placentae associated with male calves tended to have a greater total placental dry weight than those with female calves (292.9 versus 272.8 gm). Clear month effects were detected on total placental dry weight and on the dry weight of cotyledonary tissues (Fig. 4). Cows undergoing parturition in July and August had reduced weights of total placental dry

tissue, whereas cotyledonary dry weights appeared to be lower during the months of May to September.

Collectively, these results indicate that the late pregnant cow and conceptus are sensitive to seasonal changes in environment. The ultimate size of the placenta and calf are influenced by seasonal periods of heat stress, and these reductions may partially contribute to the seasonal depression in milk production. Cows undergoing parturition during the winter months produce more milk in a 305-day lactation than those undergoing parturition in the hot summer months.

We designed an experiment to test whether a stressful thermal environment would alter conceptus (placental function and calf birth weight) and maternal (postpartum milk production and restoration of reproductive function) functions during the periparturient period (also endocrine responses).[2] Twenty-one cows and 10 heifers were assigned

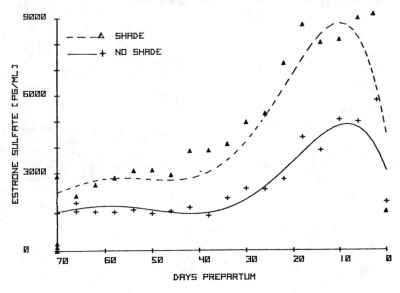

Figure 5. Least squares regressions and day means of plasma estrone sulfate concentrations prepartum in shade- and no-shade-treated cows.

randomly in June, 1978, to shade (S; n = 16) or no shade (NS; n = 15) treatments during the last trimester of pregnancy. Animals in S were provided full access to a shade management system that has been described previously,[12] whereas animals in NS had no natural or artificial shade. At parturition, all animals were removed from treatments and uniformly managed in the milking herd. At 4-day intervals from day 199 of pregnancy to parturition, respiration rate, rectal temperature, heart rate and environmental black globe temperature were recorded and blood samples collected. Birth weight of the calf and subsequent milk yield also were recorded. A subsample of 20 animals were selected for hormonal analyses prepartum. Animals were monitored for reproductive status during the postpartum period by rectal palpation of reproductive organs and blood sampling (plasma progesterone and 15-keto-13, 14-dihydro-$PGF_{2\alpha}$ [PGFM]) each Monday, Wednesday and Friday until day 50 postpartum.[9]

As expected, black globe environmental temperature, rectal temperature and respiration rates were higher in NS cows prior to parturition. Thus animals in the NS area were exposed to a higher effective heat load. Calf birth weights were depressed in the NS group (36.6 versus 39.7 kg), and the decrease was associated with lower concentrations of E_1SO_4 in maternal plasma (NS = 2505 pg/ml versus S = 4433 pg/ml) during the entire prepartum sampling period (Fig. 5). Since E_1SO_4 is produced by the cotyledon (fetal placenta) and was lower, it is an indication of reduced conceptus function during thermal stress and is consistent with a lower calf birth weight in the NS group.

No difference in gestation length was detected between the two groups ($\bar{X}$ = 281.3 days). Postpartum concentrations of PGFM were monitored in the maternal peripheral circulation (thrice weekly), and concentrations in the NS group were appreciably higher than those in the S group (472 versus 197 pg/ml; Fig. 6). This response in PGFM (NS > S) may reflect a functional difference in the maternal placenta (caruncle) between treatment groups that was established prepartum and expressed postpartum as a difference in PGFM profiles (Fig. 6). A decrease in PGFM postpartum appears to be associated with the process of uterine involution (reduction in size, loss of tissue and repair), of which tissue loss may be related to the dynamics of PGFM concentrations in maternal plasma.

The difference postpartum in PGFM between groups (NS > S) may represent an associated compensatory vascular adjustment within the placentome that occurred during late gestation. Total uterine blood flow is reduced in response to thermal stress in late gestation of sheep and probably contributes to the syndrome of "fetal stunting." There may indeed be a conceptus-induced adaptation to heat stress. This may result in a greater degree of arteriole branching and capillary density within the maternal septa that are adjacent to the fetal villi and its vascular network within the placentome. Such an arrangement, in NS animals, would increase vascular exchange and extraction between conceptus and maternal units under conditions in which total uterine blood flow is reduced during heat stress. This would permit continued growth of the fetus and completion of a successful pregnancy. Of course, such a compensatory process would not be totally efficient because the final birth weight of calves born to NS cows was reduced by approximately 7.8 per cent. Following parturition, the more richly vascularized caruncle of NS animals would contribute to a greater production of $PGF_{2\alpha}$. Although cotyledonary weight is reduced in the summer months (Fig. 4), the vascular composition (arteriole mass, arteriole branching and capillary density) of the cotyledon and caruncle is not known. Another possible explanation for increased concentrations of PGFM postpartum is that no shade-treated cows have metabolic alterations that result in increased concentrations of nonesterified fatty acids pre- and postpartum. Such an altered metabolic state may alter or enhance prostaglandin synthesis by the postpartum uterus.

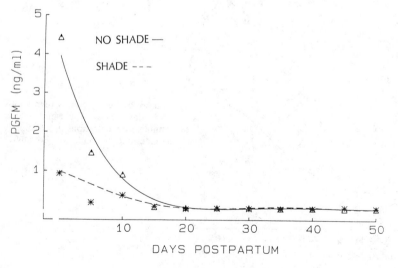

Figure 6. Least squares regressions and day means for postpartum concentrations of 15-keto-13, 14-dihydro-$PGF_{2\alpha}$ (PGFM) in shade- and no-shade-treated cows.

Part of the process of uterine involution is movement of the uterus to its normal nonpregnant position within the pelvic canal. Animals in the NS group had a greater percentage of their uteri within the pelvic canal earlier in the postpartum period. The constrictor action of $PGF_{2\alpha}$ on smooth muscles of blood vessels and myometrium may have induced the earlier rate of uterine involution in NS cows that also had higher concentrations of PGFM (Fig. 6). Swedish workers found that the rate of uterine involution in cows with no clinical signs of genital tract disturbances was increased in cows with higher concentrations of PGFM.[10]

At each palpation per rectum, the following observations were recorded: cervical diameter, diameter of each uterine horn at external bifurcation, location of uterus, uterine tone, size of ovary (length, width and thickness), size of follicle on each ovary and the size and location of the corpus luteum. In the S animals, luteal activity was greater on the ovary adjacent to the previous nonpregnant horn. This agrees with previous research in which 92 per cent of first ovulations in postpartum dairy cows occurred from the ovary adjacent to the previous nonpregnant horn. These findings suggest that the previous pregnant uterine horn exerts a local inhibitory effect on the ovary that influences ovarian responsiveness. However, this local control appeared to be reduced in animals of the NS group. Both ovaries (adjacent and opposite to the previous pregnant horn) were equally responsive in the early postpartum period during evaluation of either the diameter of the largest follicle or the occurrence of CL.

Perhaps differences in postpartum uterine function (PGFM of NS greater than S) or chronic prepartum endocrine status (E_1SO_4 of NS less than S) influenced subsequent postpartum ovarian function relative to local control of ovarian responsiveness. Such factors as utero-ovarian blood flow, intraovarian receptors for gonadotropins and other factors regulating follicle recruitment and growth warrant additional investigation. Although the mechanisms are not known currently, it is clear that environmental modification altered the conceptus and placental function prepartum, which subsequently influenced uterine and ovarian function postpartum. Although these specific biologic responses were detected, various management measures of postpartum reproductive efficiency were not altered between groups (S versus NS): days to first progesterone concentrations of more than 1 ng/ml (13 versus 12 days), days to first estrus (28 versus 36 days), days open (114 versus 92 days) and services per conception (2.6 versus 2.4). However, these latter responses do not reflect local control of ovaries adjacent to the previous pregnant or nonpregnant uterine horns.

Alteration in E_1SO_4 concentrations (NS less than S) was associated with reduced calf birth weight (NS less than S), and calf birth weight was associated with postpartum milk yield ($Y = 221.54 + 70.76$ X; X = calf birth weight in kilograms and

Y = the actual 100-day milk yield in kilograms, r = 0.54; P < 0.05). Thus a reduction in birth weight induced by a thermal stress may indirectly influence postpartum milk yield, presumably by altering the degree of mammary development or the process of lactogenesis.

Results of this study indicate that environmental heat stress prepartum has pronounced effects on the conceptus and mother that influence the well-being and subsequent performance of each unit. The pregnant cow during the dry period should not be ignored because her physical environment and nutritional management program to some degree affect her postpartum performance.

MANAGEMENT STRATEGIES AND PERSPECTIVES THAT IMPROVE REPRODUCTIVE EFFICIENCY DURING HEAT STRESS

Lactating dairy cattle are extremely sensitive to periods of thermal stress. The basic problem is that the environmental temperature is too high for maintaining the normal internal heat production that results from body metabolism. Therefore, adjustments in rate of metabolism are made by reducing feed intake, milk production, estrous behavior and, inadvertently, fertility. Such responses indicate that environmental modification should be a means of increasing animal performance. However, consideration of environmental modification should be complemented with better feeding and management systems. Such alterations with cattle of good genetic potential will allow considerable future increases in both production and efficiency of production in arid, subtropical and tropical areas of the world. This conclusion is supported by the high levels of milk production obtained by certain dairy herds and systems in Arizona, California, Israel and Florida.

Various practical and economical systems that modify the microclimate of the cow are needed to improve fertility. Arizona workers have been very successful in reducing air temperature 10 to 12°C with the use of evaporative cooling under practical farm conditions in large herds.[15] Both milk production and fertility are improved in cows exposed to cooled shades.

Environmental conditions in tropical and subtropical areas are not ideally suited for evaporative cooling systems due to the high relative humidity. Evaporative cooling requires the addition of moisture to the air, and its effectiveness is limited by the ability of air to absorb additional water. Consequently, evaporative cooling systems cool more effectively in dry arid climates than in areas with higher relative humidities. Several alternative systems combined with proper management are useful in these environments. In a Florida project, daily total air conditioning or partial air conditioning during different portions of the day allowed for gradient increases up to 9.4 per cent in production of 4 per cent fat-corrected milk.[17] Cows cooled either during daylight hours or throughout a 24-hour period produced more milk and had a higher level of fertility. However, the producer felt that the benefits of increased milk production and fertility were indeed not sufficient to pay for the expense of operating the unit.

Perhaps the simplest environmental modification is the use of shade structures. The principal function of shade is to reduce the heat load of animals by reducing the incident solar radiation. If this reduction is sufficient to maintain a near normal body temperature, then increases in production should be detected. However, the type of shade and the associated management of animals will be critical in obtaining a production benefit. Exposure of cows managed as a group to an insulated shade structure in which they also had access to feed, water and an adjacent sod area for loafing resulted in a distinct alteration of the animal's microenvironment, lowered respiration rate and rectal temperature, and improved milk yield and reproductive performance. Cows exposed to the shade management system produced 10.7 per cent more milk and their percentage of conception was 44.4 per cent versus 25.3 per cent for controls without shade.[12]

Environmental modifications such as air conditioning, evaporative cooling, zone cooling and various shade structures have been used with different degrees of success to reduce the detrimental effects of heat stress. However, use of various systems to alter the environment should be coupled with management that provides an adequate feed supply (quantity and quality) and readily available drinking water. Use of a particular system to alter the environment depends on the severity of that environment, the characteristics of the climate and economic considerations.

Recently, workers in Arizona and Israel have upgraded systems of environmental control by utilizing intermittent upper body sprinkling (overhead sprinklers) with large fans that run continuously to keep air moving in order to evaporate the water from the body surface. Fan spray nozzles must dispense the water with sufficient pressure to beat the water into the hair. Thus the water is retained for evaporation and is not shed from the hair surface. These systems can be utilized in holding lots or in holding pens prior to milking. Such a system reduces surface temperatures and aids in removing excess heat from the body.

Additional physiological strategies should be combined with environmental modification. In dairy systems, utilization of frozen semen from proven bulls is essential for improving genetic merit. Furthermore, heat stress effects on the bull are avoided completely through the use of artificial insemination in which semen can be collected and frozen during cooler times of the year. Sperm exposed to high temperatures (e.g., 36°C vs 40°C) will fertilize ova but will produce abnormal embryos that subsequently die. Therefore, if sperm are harvested under ideal conditions, summer periods of infertility are attributable largely to the female through the environment she provides. Prostaglandin $F_{2\alpha}$ works effectively in heat-stressed cattle,[7] and effective synchronization systems should be implemented with environmental management systems. Parts of the herd could be synchronized and bred to avoid the heat stress season. Alternatively, groups of cows could be synchronized during hot weather to intensify the accuracy of heat detection, and these synchronized groups could be managed under shade management systems for a limited time (e.g., 20 to 40 days) to maximize conception rates. Although the early period around ovulation is sensitive to heat stress ($\cong$ 3-day period from estrus), the duration of this sensitivity is not known. Embryo preservation and subsequent embryo transfer may be a means of bypassing the early postovulation period of thermal sensitivity. However, advances in this area will come when the time period of thermal sensitivity for the conceptus-maternal unit is accurately identified; the biochemical and physiological processes associated with pregnancy recognition are elucidated; the physiological, hormonal, biochemical and molecular processes associated with development of the early blastocyst are understood and the factor or factors that ensure its in utero survival when exposed to heat stress are known. At present, management systems have not been developed that integrate reproductive management programs with environmental management systems.

SUMMARY

Conception rates are suppressed during hot seasonal periods of the year, and lactating cows are more adversely affected than heifers. Certain climatic measurements, such as maximum environmental temperature on the day after insemination, are related to conception rates. Likewise, variations in uterine temperatures are also associated with conception rates. Seasonal increases in frequency of nondetected heats during heat stress months also contribute to the decrease in herd reproductive efficiency. Hormonal measurements indicate that lactating dairy cows exposed to practical field conditions of heat stress in a subtropical environment have recurring estrous cycles. Slight alterations in hormonal concentrations and the animals' normal thermoregulatory response to heat stress may reduce blood flow to the reproductive tract. Such reductions in blood flow would contribute to a more hostile in utero environment and increase the probability of subsequent embryo death. Seasonal periods of heat stress reduce the birth weight of calves and placental weights. Heat stress prepartum has pronounced effects on the conceptus-maternal unit and must be considered when evaluating various conceptus (calf birth weight, prepartum maternal E_1SO_4 concentrations) and maternal (postpartum PGFM concentrations, uterine involution, ovarian activity and milk yield) responses. Several systems of environmental modification and management are described that improve reproductive performance of lactating dairy cows during periods of heat stress.

SPECIFIC RECOMMENDATIONS

The following recommendations are intended to maximize reproduction and production efficiencies during periods of thermal stress:

1. Provide access for lactating cattle to a system of environmental modification (type depends on location) that reduces exposure to environmental climatic factors known to reduce fertility.

2. Provide ready access to water and feed within the modified environment.

3. Allow cattle free access to loafing areas away from the environmental structure so they can more effectively radiate their heat loads during the evening and night hours.

4. Make intensive management efforts to obtain greater frequency and accuracy of heat detection and proper timing of insemination, because intensity of estrous behavior is thereby reduced.

5. Incorporate a system of pregnancy diagnosis per rectum in order to maintain intensive management awareness to maximize reproductive efficiency.

6. Dry cows also should be protected from periods of thermal stress because chronic exposure to conditions that cause hyperthermia reduces calf birth weight and subsequent milk yield of the mother during the ensuing lactation.

7. Because prepartum thermal stress causes postpartum carry-over effects on restoration of postpartum reproductive function, cows should be examined postpartum in a routine "reproductive veterinary herd health program."

8. These recommendations will improve both herd reproductive efficiency and milk production.

References

1. Ayalon N: A review of embryonic mortality in cattle. J Reprod Fertil 54:483, 1978.
2. Collier RJ, Doelger SG, Head HH, et al.: Effects of heat stress during pregnancy on maternal hormone concentrations, calf birth weight and postpartum milk yield of Holstein cows. J Anim Sci 54:309, 1982.
3. Dunlap SE, Vincent CK: Influence of postbreeding thermal stress on conception rate in beef cattle. J Anim Sci 32:1216, 1971.
4. Francos G, Mayer E: Observations on some environmental factors connected with fertility in heat stressed cows. Theriogenology 19:625, 1983.
5. Gwazdauskas FC, Thatcher WW, Wilcox CJ: Physiological, environmental, and hormonal factors at insemination which may affect conception. J Dairy Sci 56:873, 1973.
6. Gwazdauskas FC, Wilcox CJ, Thatcher WW: Environmental and managemental factors affecting conception rate in a subtropical climate. J Dairy Sci 58:88, 1975.
7. Gwazdauskas FC, Thatcher WW, Kiddy CA, et al.: Hormonal patterns during heat stress following $PGF_{2\alpha}$—tham salt induced luteal regression in heifers. Theriogenology 16:221, 1981.
8. Hawk HW: Infertility in dairy cattle. In Hawk HW (ed): Beltsville Symposia in Agricultural Research. vol 3. Animal Reproduction. Montclair, Allanheld, Osmum and Co., 1979, pp. 19–29.
9. Lewis GS, Thatcher WW, Bliss EL, et al.: Effects of heat stress during pregnancy on postpartum reproductive changes in Holstein cows. J Anim Sci 58:174, 1984.
10. Lindell JO, Kindahl H, Jansson L, Edqvist LE: Postpartum release of prostaglandin $F_{2\alpha}$ and uterine involution in the cow. Theriogenology 17:237, 1982.
11. Maurer RP, Chenault JR: Fertilization failure and embryonic mortality in parous and nonparous beef cattle. J Anim Sci 56:1186, 1983.
12. Roman-Ponce H, Thatcher WW, Buffington DE, et al.: Physiological and production responses of dairy cattle to a shade structure in a subtropical environment. J Dairy Sci 60:424, 1977.
13. Roman-Ponce H, Thatcher WW, Caton D, et al.: Thermal stress effects on uterine blood flow in dairy cows. J Anim Sci 46:175, 1978.
14. Roman-Ponce H, Thatcher WW, Wilcox CJ: Hormonal interrelationships and physiological responses of lactating dairy cows to a shade management system in a subtropical environment. Theriogenology 16:139, 1981.
15. Stott GH, Wiersma F: Response of dairy cattle to an evaporative cooled environment. Proc Int Livestock Environment Symp ASAE SP09174. St. Joseph, American Society of Agricultural Engineers, 1974, pp. 88–95.
16. Thatcher WW, Collier RJ: Effect of heat on animal productivity. In Recheigl M (ed): CRC Handbook of Agricultural Productivity, vol 2. Boca Raton, CRC Press, 1982, pp. 77–105.
17. Thatcher WW, Gwazdauskas FC, Wilcox CJ, et al.: Milking performance and reproductive efficiency of dairy cows in an environmentally controlled structure. J Dairy Sci 57:304, 1974.

Effect of Nutrition on Reproduction in Dairy Cattle

Brian J. Gerloff, D.V.M., Ph.D.
David A. Morrow, D.V.M., Ph.D.
Michigan State University
East Lansing, Michigan

Many practicing veterinarians are convinced that there are profound interrelationships between the nutritional status of dairy cattle and their reproductive performance. Very few, though, by virtue of their knowledge and training are able to determine what the nutritional cause of reduced fertility might be. In many cases regular reproductive examinations alone are not adequate to ensure good herd reproductive health. If there is an underlying nutritional problem, herd reproductive health and profitability may also suffer. This review is a brief discussion of some specific areas where nutrition has been documented to have an effect on reproduction in cattle as an aid to the practicing veterinarian.

Different physiological processes have different priorities in receiving nutrients. Depending on the age and physiological status of the animal, nutrients may be preferentially partitioned for lactation, growth or fattening. Reproductive functions, especially in conditions of scarcity, have a relatively low priority for nutrient partitioning; thus in some instances, subclinical deficiencies may manifest themselves as impaired reproduction. Requirements for normal reproductive function in the male are considerably less than in the female. In addition, the added demands of lactation are not present, so borderline nutritional deficiencies are less likely to contribute to decreased male fertility.

There are several time periods in which nutritional deficiencies are more likely to affect reproduction. They correspond to times when metabolic demands or other physiological processes are greatest, yet reproductive function is also at a critical time period. These include the period of rapid growth during puberty, parturition, and peak lactation, the last of which corresponds to the time to rebreed following calving. Peak lactation, especially, is the time when it is very difficult to meet the nutrient requirements of the dairy cow and to impose on her the necessity of having a fertile estrus and conceiving. First calf heifers that are still growing have an additional demand.

Nutritional deficiencies may impair reproduction by producing their primary effect on a variety of tissues. Theoretically, a nutrient deficiency or toxicity may affect a variety of organs and still result in nonspecific decreased reproductive performance. Deficiencies or toxicities may primarily affect the anterior pituitary or hypothalamus, thus interfering with normal luteinizing hormone (LH) or follicle-stimulating hormone (FSH) production. Alternatively, other endocrine glands could be affected as well, as is the case with iodine and the thyroid gland. Some other deficiencies and toxicities may have a direct effect on the gonads. Inadequate intake and utilization of some nutrients may result in decreased formation of luteal tissue and thus decreased progesterone, which would have a detrimental effect on fertility. Nutrient imbalances may also produce a direct effect on the genitalia. This could result in altered sperm development and survival in the male or decreased ovum or embryo survival in the female. The net result of any of these deficiencies is suboptimum fertility or repeat breeders. Clinically, it may be extremely difficult to distinguish between these different effects.

In reviewing the experimental data, it is often difficult to determine the different effects on reproduction that may be due to nutrition. Frequently the nutritional treatments result in differences in milk production, which may interact with direct nutritional effects on fertility. It is also difficult to design rations in which only one nutrient is varied. Often there are multiple nutrient imbalances. Clinically, more than one nutrient is also frequently deficient. In clinical situations, it is difficult to separate nutritional reasons for infertility from other management effects such as poor heat detection. Because of these reasons, well-controlled studies demonstrating a clear effect of nutrition on reproduction are scarce.

It is also important to remember that nutritional causes are only one possible reason for breeding troubles; infectious and management factors should also be evaluated when dealing with a herd reproduction problem.

PUBERTY

Normal diary heifers should come into their first estrus and begin cycling at 10 to 11 months of age, be large enough to breed at 14 to 15 months, and subsequently, calve at 24 months. The onset of puberty is closely related to energy intake in both males and females. Large breed dairy heifers (Holstein and Brown Swiss) will usually weigh 550 to 600 pounds at the beginning of puberty, with smaller breeds weighing less. In a Cornell University study, 102 Holstein heifers were fed at the rate of 62, 100 or 146 per cent of required digestible nutrients. Onset of puberty occurred at 20, 11 and 9 months of age, respectively; however, all three groups weighed approximately 600 pounds when cyclic activity began, suggesting that weight was the most important factor.

Housing and management of breeding age heifers are frequently less than optimum, and this may be the first or only group of animals showing signs of energy deficiency. Clinical signs related to an energy deficit include thin animals with very small, inactive ovaries and a delay in puberty. Such a deficit may be seen when heifers are maintained on poorer quality pasture or roughages, or in late winter or early spring when good quality feed is in short supply. To reach puberty before 12 months of age, breeding weight of 750 pounds by 14 to 15 months, and to calve at 24 months weighing 1200 pounds, heifers need to be fed a diet sufficient to allow for 1.5 pounds of body weight gain per day. To achieve these gains, it may be necessary to supplement the roughage with 5 pounds of grain daily. Once cyclic activity begins, feeding level does not appear to affect estrous activity unless severe restrictions occur. National Research Council (NRC) energy requirements should not be exceeded on prepubertal heifers, however. Animals that are fed excessively before and around the time of puberty appear to have inadequate mammary secretory tissue development and lower subsequent milk production. Normally, this is the period of very rapid or allometric mammary growth, but heifers fed a high plane of nutrition at this time have increased mammary fat deposition and decreased secretory tissue.

Males also are affected by dietary energy levels. In an early Pennsylvania study, dairy bulls were reared at 70, 100, 115 and 130 per cent of NRC total digestible nutrient (TDN) requirements. Those animals receiving 70 per cent of their energy requirements did not begin semen production until 61 weeks of age, while the other groups averaged 43 weeks. The low-energy group also had only 50 per cent of the motile sperm output per ejaculate of the high-energy group. By 112 weeks of age, however, there was no difference in motile sperm output per ejaculate due to level of energy intake. Between 3 and 4 years of age, though, the bulls on a high-energy intake became more sluggish in sexual response. These same bulls also showed increased feet and leg weaknesses. These and similar findings suggest that liberal or high-energy feeding early in life hastens the onset of sperm production, but moderate dietary restriction after 2 years of age is desirable. More recent evidence from Alberta, Canada, suggests that high-energy diets until 2 years of age are undesirable. Hereford bulls on a high plane of nutrition after weaning (0.9 kg weight gain/day) initially displayed a more rapid increase and larger scrotal circumference than bulls on a lower plane of nutrition (0.6 kg weight gain/day). However, with a moderate reduction in energy intake beginning at 21 months of age, the high-energy group showed a decrease in scrotal circumference and 59 per cent lower epididymal sperm reserves than bulls on the low-energy rations, suggesting that high-energy diets should not be continued past 1 year of age.

Recent research may indicate a relationship between onset of puberty and other nutritional factors. Monensin, an ionophore commonly used as a feed additive in beef cattle rations to improve average daily gain (ADG) and feed efficiency, has been reported by researchers in Wyoming and Montana to decrease the age of onset of puberty in beef heifers. One hundred and forty cross-bred heifers were categorized as heavy or light based on weaning weight. Within each weight class three diets were fed: (1) restricted diet, (2) restricted diet plus 200 mg/head/day monensin, and (3) ad lib diet plus monensin. In the heavy group, age at puberty was decreased by monensin supplementation independent of weight and ADG. In one Pennsylvania trial with diary heifers, monensin supplementation at 200 or 600 mg/head/day did not increase blood LH concentrations but did improve conception rates in pubertal heifers. Monensin supplementation increases the GnRH and estrogen-induced LH response in prepubertal heifers, which may be related to its effects on puberty. These effects have been hypothesized to be related to the decreased ruminal acetate:propionate ratio present when monensin is fed; however, the reason for the specific effects of monensin has yet to be determined.

NUTRITION, FERTILITY AND LACTATION

Energy

Dairy cows in early lactation draw upon their body energy reserves to produce large volumes of milk. Because maximum feed intake lags behind peak milk yield by several weeks, in early lactation it is nearly impossible to achieve adequate energy intake to sustain production. Production is maintained by using body reserves, primarily fat. Thus there is considerable weight loss during early lactation. This period of weight loss precedes and sometimes overlaps the time during which the cow must be bred successfully to achieve a calving interval approaching 12 months. Energy status has frequently been thought to be related to postpartum fertility.

In one Louisiana study, 1145 pregnancies from 1912 inseminations were analyzed. Animals were divided into two groups—those gaining weight and those losing weight. For those animals gaining weight at the time of breeding, 1368 services resulted in 911 pregnancies, for a conception rate of 67 per cent and 1.5 services per conception. For those animals losing weight, 544 services resulted in 234 pregnancies, for a conception rate of 44 per cent with 2.32 services per conception. These results suggest that dairy cows gaining weight are more likely to conceive.

Fertility appears to be related to progesterone concentrations in the cycle preceding the insemination, greater fertility being associated with higher blood progesterone concentrations. There is some evidence that progesterone concentrations may be related to energy balance. In an Israeli study, 14 dairy cows were placed on high and standard planes of nutrition. Those cows on a high plane of nutrition required fewer inseminations and conceived 19 days earlier than cows on a standard level of nutrition. Cows on a high intake also had a postpartum blood progesterone peak 23 days earlier than those animals on a standard intake, suggesting an earlier return to cyclic ovarian activity. There was a tendency for animals gaining weight to have higher progesterone concentrations preceding the first insemination as well as higher conception rates. These results are similar to those in a North Carolina study in which 212 Jersey and Holstein cows were monitored from calving to conception or culling. Conception rate at first service was primarily related to blood progesterone concentration preceding insemination. In this study Jerseys gaining weight had higher progesterone concentrations than those losing weight. In Holsteins, however, progesterone concentrations appeared to be unaffected by weight changes.

The mechanism of reduced progesterone concentrations in animals with declining weight has not been well determined. In one Cornell study, Holstein heifers were fed at 65 or 100 per cent of maintenance TDN allowances. Heifers on the lower energy diet had lower serum and corpus luteum progesterone concentrations and elevated serum LH concentrations, suggesting that LH release was not impaired and that there may be a decreased ovarian response to LH with restricted dietary intake. In contrast, results of another Cornell study with the same dietary treatments showed that animals on the restricted energy diet had significantly lower serum LH concentrations with only a slight decrease in progesterone. In vitro, however, the ovaries from the restricted energy heifers were less responsive to LH stimulation as measured by progesterone production.

A common negative association between high production and fertility is frequently made by veterinarians and owners. In one New York study of 9750 cows, those producing 907 or more kg of milk above herdmates had a first service conception rate 20.5 per cent lower than those animals producing 907 kg below herdmates. This relationship may not be due to high production per se, though; instead, it may be present because higher producers are probably more likely to be suffering from an energy deficit, or there may be other management differences between high and low producers. Indeed, in a recent Cornell study with 13 cows, there was a strong negative correlation between average energy balance and days to first ovulation. Many other studies have shown no direct relationship between high production and reduced fertility. These and other results suggest that it is important to maximize dry matter intake of high-energy feed early in lactation, both for maximum milk production and for best reproductive performance. Maximal energy intake should not extend beyond peak lactation, because this may lead to overconditioning of the cow with severe consequences to health and fertility.

Excess grain consumption has been reported to have adverse effects on fertility in several studies. In the New York study in which heifers were fed low, medium and high planes of nutrition, these treatments were maintained over a 3-year period. Those cows on a high plane of nutrition had more breeding problems with a greater number culled for infertility. In another Cornell study, 50 cows were studied for three lactation periods. They were assigned to one of four groups: (1) controls fed a maximum of 20 pounds of grain and forage ad lib, (2) larger amounts of grain plus forage ad lib, (3) liberal amounts of grain with restricted forage and (4) liberal amounts of grain with corn silage as the only forage offered ad lib. The interval from parturition to first estrus and ovulation was unaffected by liberal concentrate feeding, but those animals receiving liberal concentrate had significantly longer calving intervals and required more services per conception than the controls. Other studies have shown no effect of high-energy diets on reproduction. In a 4-year Michigan study, 170 cows were fed concentrates varying from 464 kg to 4790 kg per lactation. There was no effect of level of concentrate feeding on conception rate or occurrence of other diseases.

One possible explanation for these contradictory results may be that in some cases the high concentrate feeding resulted in overconditioning while in others it did not. The Cornell cows mentioned above, for example, were overconditioned. Overconditioned cows are predisposed to develop the "fat cow syndrome" and a variety of periparturient diseases that have an adverse effect on fertility. These overconditioned cows also have a tendency to mobilize large amounts of body fat and develop excessive amounts of fat deposition in the liver. This fatty infiltrated liver may be associated with reduced fertility. Clinical reports suggest that overconditioned cows have slower uterine involution and a longer postpartum interval than cows with normal condition. British workers, among others, have begun a number of studies on bovine fatty liver syndrome. In one report, 100 dairy cows from three herds had liver biopsies taken 1 week after calving. Those with excessive hepatic fat infiltration had a 33-day longer calving interval than those cows that did not develop fatty liver. These and other data, though, show only an association, not a causative role for fatty liver in infertility.

To maximize reproductive performance, then, one should strive for high-energy intakes in the postpartum period to avoid excessive weight loss. In practice, one must increase the energy density and amount of the diet gradually to avoid causing the cows to go off feed. Energy intake should increase until the cow's production peaks and then decline with the normal decline in production. Energy intakes in late lactation and the dry period should not be excessive, because this will result in fat, overconditioned cows.

High-quality forage availability is essential to maximize dry matter and energy intake, so forage production and harvest should be of top priority for the dairyman. There is a wide natural variation in forage quality, and it is important to have the forages tested. Some average nutrient values and ranges for forages are shown in Table 1. Good dry cow rations can be achieved using most forages, but if corn silage or very high quality hay is used, intake must be limited to avoid overconditioning. Frequently, medium quality hay can be fed with 2 to 5 pounds of grain as a supplement to balance mineral requirements. Table 2 shows nutrient requirements of dry Holstein cows and several diets that can achieve them. Table 3 shows recommended nutrient concentrations and toxic amounts in dry matter of dairy cattle diets.

Protein

Protein deficiency can result in a delay in onset of puberty, increased days open and decreased dry matter intakes. The decreased intakes are due to poor digestibility of the ration, and thus, some of the signs of a severe protein deficiency could be related to an energy deficit. Adequate protein intake is also necessary for normal fetal growth and development.

When determining the protein requirement in ruminants, it is important to remember that two protein requirements must be fulfilled: readily available protein that can furnish ammonia for the growth and multiplication of the rumen microbes, and protein required by the whole animal that is digested in the small intestine. This protein digested in the small intestine is furnished by a combination of microbial protein synthesized in the rumen and protein that is not readily available to ruminal degradation. Different protein sources vary in the amounts that are soluble and available for use by the rumen microbes and the portions that will bypass microbial action. Soybean meal is a readily soluble protein source, while brewer's grains and corn gluten meal are relatively insoluble. The amount and composition of the protein reaching the small intestine determines the productive capacity of the cow in terms of protein supplementation. Urea and other nonprotein nitrogen (NPN) sources furnish ammonia that the rumen organisms can synthesize into protein provided adequate energy, vitamins and minerals are present.

Eleven to 12 per cent of crude protein is required to sustain adequate rumen ammonia levels for normal rumen fermentation, digestion and dry matter intakes. These levels are adequate for normal reproductive function in bulls, heifers and dry cows. Higher protein levels should be fed for growth and lactation.

Optimum protein concentrations and amounts for peak lactation have not been precisely determined. There is evidence that protein concentrations at the upper end of current recommendations may have a negative effect on fertility. In one Oregon study reported in 1979, 45 dairy cows were divided into three groups and fed isocaloric rations of, respectively, 12.7, 16.3 and 19.3 per cent crude protein beginning 4 days postpartum. Days open were 69, 96 and 106 days for cows on the three dietary protein concentrations, respectively. Services per conception were 1.47, 1.87 and 2.47, increasing with increasing protein concentration. Some authors have suggested that elevated rumen ammonia concentrations with high-protein feeding may have a toxic effect on the embryo and/or other direct negative effects on fertility. However, in this study, intakes were not reported, nor were weight loss and milk production, although the authors suggested that lower protein did not diminish milk production.

An Israeli study compared feeding crude protein levels of 16 or 20 per cent to cows with very high milk production (greater than 40 kg/day). Cows fed the ration containing 20 per cent crude protein had higher rumen ammonia and blood urea concentrations, greater days open and services per conception, and a lower conception rate than cows receiving a 16 per cent crude protein. There is substantial evidence that in early lactation there will be an increased production response when 17 or 18 per cent crude protein is fed. However, results of these two studies suggested that higher protein levels were undesirable for reproductive efficiency. Recent Michigan State research demonstrated the opposite effect. Eighty-four cows were fed diets containing 11.5, 14.5 or 17.5 per cent crude protein. At the higher protein levels, different ingredients were used to vary the amounts of readily soluble protein and rumen bypass protein. In this study, days open and services per conception decreased as the protein concentration increased. Huber has recently summarized 11 different trials, involving 1109 cows in which protein levels were varied and fertility information recorded. Protein concentration ranged from 9 to 20 per cent, with most comparisons between 12 and 18 per cent. Five of the 11 studied showed decreasing fertility with increasing protein, while 5 of 11 demonstrated improved fertility with increasing protein. In this survey, there was a slight trend for cows receiving 16 to 18 per cent crude protein to have decreased services per conception compared with cows receiving 11 to 13 per cent crude protein. There was an apparent increase in days open and services per conception above 19 per cent crude protein. Taken as a group, the information indicates that 16 to 18 per cent crude protein for early lactation cows is acceptable for optimum reproductive performance, particularly if some bypass protein is fed so that rumen ammonia does not become excessive.

Urea is a highly soluble source of ammonia and has frequently been used as a protein source in ruminants. Research from Purdue associated high-levels (290 gm daily) with increased abortion rates, increased incidence of retained placentae and increased calving intervals. Cows fed 145 gm daily showed no difference from controls. Data from 85,281 calving intervals in 3157 herd-year observations in Michigan DHI herds showed that urea

Table 1. Mean (and Range) of Nutrient Values for Common Michigan and New York Feedstuffs, 1977–1979

Feed	Dry Matter (per cent)	Crude Protein (per cent)	Net Energy Lact. (Mcal/kg)	ADF (per cent)	Calcium (per cent)	Phosphorus (per cent)	Potassium (per cent)	Magnesium (per cent)
Legume hay	87 (73–99)	17.0 (9.9–37.9)	1.0 (0.6–1.4)	36.1 (22.6–43.7)	1.34 (0.36–2.18)	0.28 (0.12–0.52)	2.12 (0.53–3.94)	0.28 (0.03–0.50)
Legume grass hay	89 (75–94)	14.5 (7.9–23.3)	0.9 (0.7–1.2)	42.1 (40.6–43.6)	1.17 (0.30–2.85)	0.27 (0.13–0.48)	1.90 (0.92–3.75)	0.27 (0.09–0.56)
Grass hay	88 (81–94)	10.2 (4.3–18.5)	0.8 (0.6–1.1)	36.1 (19.6–46.3)	0.65 (0.29–1.88)	0.25 (0.12–0.43)	1.72 (1.07–2.99)	0.19 (0.06–0.42)
Legume silage	51 (22–74)	17.8 (6.3–26.4)	1.1 (0.6–2.0)	37.4 (18.2–51.1)	1.45 (0.60–2.59)	0.30 (0.12–0.54)	2.31 (0.72–4.26)	0.29 (0.13–0.56)
Ear corn	77 (70–92)	9.1 (8.0–10.1)	1.8 (1.7–1.8)	5.3	0.14 (0.10–0.18)	0.22 (0.10–0.38)	0.67 (0.39–2.73)	0.13 (0.06–0.21)
Untreated corn silage	38 (28–48)	8.2 (7.2–9.1)	1.5 (1.5–1.6)	25.5 (20.9–30.0)	0.22 (0.11–0.32)	0.20 (0.16–0.23)	0.85 (0.60–1.09)	0.13 (0.08–0.17)
NPN-treated corn silage	40 (32–48)	11.7 (9.2–14.1)	1.5 (1.4–1.7)	23.3 (19.5–27.0)	0.37 (0.17–0.57)	0.26 (0.19–0.32)	0.79 (0.57–1.00)	0.14 (0.08–0.19)

Table 2. Sample Diets and Requirements for 600 kg Dry Cow

	Dry Matter (kg)	Crude Protein (kg)	NE₁ (Mcal)	Crude Fiber (kg)	Calcium (gm)	Phosphorus (gm)	Vitamin A (IU)	Vitamin D (IU)
Diet 1								
11.4 kg corn silage	4.3	0.35	6.65	1.00	9.5	8.6		
8.4 kg medium quality mixed hay (free choice)	7.4	1.1	6.85	2.24	87.2	20		
70 gm monosodium phosphate	0.07	—	—	—	—	18.2		
30 gm TMS with selenium	0.03	—	—	—	—	—		
Vitamin A and D supplement	—	—	—	—	—	—	46,000	23,000
	11.8	1.45	13.50	3.24	96.7	46.8	46,000	23,000
Diet 2								
10 kg grass hay (free choice)	8.8	0.9	6.6	2.65	57.2	21.8		
29.5 kg ground ear corn	2.5	0.23	4.6	0.17	3.6	5.4		
0.60 kg soybean meal	0.6	0.30	1.1	0.02	2.3	4.5		
30 gm TMS with selenium	0.03	—	—	—	—	—		
Vitamin A and D supplement	—	—	—	—	—	—	46,000	23,000
	11.93	1.43	12.3	2.84	63.1	31.7	46,000	23,000
Requirements	12	1.32	12.6	2.40	45–100	30–50	46,000	10,000

TMS = trace mineral salt

intake averaged 81 gm in 1709 herd-year observations. There were no differences in calving intervals or number of cows sold for sterility in the urea- or nonurea-fed herds. At very high levels, rumen ammonia concentrations may interfere with normal fertility as well as being stressful to the animal. Limiting urea feeding to NRC recommendations of 1 per cent of dry matter intake, however, appears to have no effect on fertility. When urea is introduced to a ration it should be done gradually over a 2- to 3-week period to allow for rumen adaptation.

In conclusion, a severe protein deficiency can interfere with normal reproductive processes. An 11 to 12 per cent protein diet is necessary for normal rumen microbial growth and digestion, and this should be considered a minimum. Higher protein levels can be fed to high producers as well as soluble NPN sources such as urea and ammonia. When feeding higher levels of protein or NPN, it is best to provide some bypass protein so that rumen ammonia levels do not become excessive.

Vitamins

Ruminants depend on several sources for their vitamin needs: (1) dietary intake of preformed vitamins; (2) tissue synthesis of a variety of vitamins and (3) rumen microbial synthesis of several major vitamins. Most commercial feeds also contain sup-

plemental vitamins, so the chances of cattle developing infertility due to a vitamin deficiency are not great.

Vitamin deficiencies are most likely to occur in one of two basic situations: (1) Vitamins may be depleted in feeds stored for long periods of time, or (2) tissue synthesis may be reduced where housing prevents exposure to sunlight or where cattle are placed in a very stressful situation.

Vitamin A. Vitamin A is necessary for normal epithelial development in all species. Failure of epithelial development with vitamin A deficiency is responsible for signs of infertility. Clinical signs of infertility related to vitamin A deficiency include (1) delayed onset of puberty in the male and female, (2) abortion or birth of weak, blind or incoordinated calves, (3) increased incidence of retained placenta with keratinization and degeneration of the placenta and metritis, and (4) suppressed libido in the male. In the male a deficiency provokes testicular atrophy and loss of germinal cells in the seminiferous tubules, but this is not expressed until an advanced stage. In adult cows one of the first signs of a vitamin A deficiency may be shortened gestation with increased incidence of retained placentae. Deficient cows have normal estrous cycles and conceive with normal early fetal development. Vitamin A deficiency is most likely to develop in colostrum-deprived calves or older cattle fed forages damaged by weather or storage or stored for long periods of

Table 3. Recommended Nutrient Concentrations in Dry Matter of Dairy Cattle Diets and Toxic Amounts

Nutrient	Units	Milking Cow	Dry Cow	Toxic or Maximum	Amount per Cow per Day*
Protein	%	13–17	11	22	2.7–3.2 kg
Energy NE₁	Mcal/kg	1.4–1.8	1.2	—	30–35 Mcal
ME	Mcal/kg	2.3–2.9	2.2	—	—
TDN	%	63–75	60	—	13–15.5 kg
Crude fiber	%	15–17	>20	—	3.2 kg
Acid detergent fiber	%	18–22	23–40	—	4.1 kg
Crude fat	%	2	2	—	0.45 kg
Minerals					
Ca	%	0.65–0.84	0.4	2.0	145 gm
P	%	0.35–0.40	0.25	0.7	72 gm
Mg	%	0.22	0.16	2	40 gm
K	%	0.8	0.8	5	163 gm
NaCl	%	0.46	0.25	5–9	95 gm
S	%	0.2	0.17	0.35	40 gm
Fe	ppm	100	100	1000	2 gm
Co	ppm	0.1	0.1	10	2 mg
Cu	ppm	10	10	80	200 mg
Mn	ppm	40	40	1000	800 mg
Zn	ppm	40	40	500	800 mg
I	ppm	0.5	0.25	50	4 mg
Mo	ppm	?	?	6	—
Se	ppm	0.2	0.1	3–5	4 mg
F	ppm	?	?	30	—
Vitamin A	IU/day	50,000	50,000	+ +	—
Vitamin D	IU/day	10,000	7,500	+ +	—
Vitamin E	IU/day	(± 300)	(± 100)	?	—

*Assuming a DM intake of 20 kg and producing about 27 kg milk.
Table prepared by J. W. Thomas, Michigan State University, as adapted from National Research Council-National Academy of Sciences: Nutrient Requirements of Dairy Cattle. Washington, D.C., National Academy of Sciences, 1978.
DM = dry matter
ME = metabolized energy
TDN = total digestable nutrients

time. Animals on an all corn silage forage program may also develop a vitamin A deficiency.

No positive effects on production or fertility were observed in a recent Cornell study in which injectable vitamins A, D and E were administered to alternate cows in nine herds at drying off and parturition. Each injection contained 2,500,000 USP units of vitamin A, 500,000 USP units of vitamin D, and 250 IU of vitamin E. The vitamin status of the rations was not reported, but these results suggest that under normal field conditions where no deficiency is present, vitamin A injections provide no added benefit.

Vitamin A can be supplied in the diet as preformed vitamin A or as carotene. Carotene is con-

verted by the intestinal epithelial cells to vitamin A. One mg of carotene provides 400 IU of vitamin A in dairy cattle rations. Most nutritionists recommend supplementing all diets with the vitamin A requirement as inexpensive insurance against a deficiency. Current NRC requirements are 1900 IU per 100 pounds body weight for growth and 3500 IU per 100 pounds body weight for pregnancy and lactation. This is equivalent to 1500 IU of vitamin A activity per pound of ration dry matter or 30,000 to 50,000 IU per cow per day. Excessive supplementation should be avoided because it may impair normal metabolism of carotene.

β-**Carotene.** Recent reports have suggested that there is a vitamin A–independent role for β-carotene in bovine reproduction. Carotene accumulates in the corpus luteum of cattle, and several reports have suggested that a carotene deficiency may result in decreased progesterone output, delayed ovulation, lower estrous intensity and an increased incidence of cystic ovaries, early embryonic deaths and abortions. These effects occurred even with adequate dietary vitamin A.

In one German study, 17 cows were fed a carotene-deficient diet and 15 were fed the same diet supplemented with 400 to 600 mg per cow of β-carotene, depending on milk production. Preformed vitamin A was supplied to the cows in both groups. The carotene-supplemented group received enough preformed vitamin A to furnish their requirement. The carotene-deprived group received this plus the vitamin A equivalent of the carotene supplied to the supplemented group. The authors reported that the carotene-deficient cows had (1) delayed involution of the uterus; (2) delayed ovarian activity; (3) delayed ovulation after onset of estrus and LH peak; and (4) a 43.8 per cent incidence of early embryonic deaths and abortion compared with 0 per cent in the supplemented cows.

An Israeli study, however, failed to demonstrate any benefit for supplemental β-carotene. Seven heifers were fed a carotene-restricted diet and 11 heifers were supplemented with β-carotene beginning at 7 months of age. The basal diet contained 0.1 mg carotene per kg dry matter. The β-carotene supplemented heifers received this plus 30 mg carotene per 100 kg body weight daily. Both groups received adequate levels of preformed vitamin A. In this study there were no differences in age of first ovulation, sexual behavior, LH peaks, plasma progesterone or conception rate between the groups, despite very low serum carotene concentrations in the unsupplemented groups.

Other, more recent Canadian and United States trials have presented conflicting results with some showing a positive effect of carotene supplementation while most have shown no beneficial effect. Many of these trials have been field studies and have failed to report the basal carotene content of the diet or serum carotene concentrations in depleted versus supplemented animals. One recent Nebraska study did report lower serum carotene levels in the control cattle with no apparent effect of β-carotene supplementation on reproductive performance.

It is possible that some of the conflicting results may be due to breed differences in carotene and vitamin A metabolism. At this point all that can be said is that there may be a unique requirement of carotene for reproduction, independent of its role as a vitamin A precursor. Under some circumstances, when large amounts of stored and ensiled feed with little green forage are fed, carotene supplementation may aid fertility. Under most circumstances, however, when legumes and grasses are a significant part of the forage, B-carotene supplementation is probably not necessary.

Vitamin D. Vitamin D is essential for normal calcium and phosphorus metabolism including their absorption from the intestine and bone, normal bone growth, and prevention of rickets. It is normally formed from cholesterol in the skin upon exposure to sunlight and is present in large quantities in sun-cured forages. Vitamin D deficiency may result in delayed onset of estrus and ovarian inactivity, although under normal circumstances it is unlikely to develop.

In one Kansas State University study 37 cows were used to compare the effect of weekly supplementation of vitamin D on reproduction with and without added calcium. The experiment extended over 3 years, and half of the observation cows received 300,000 IU of vitamin D_3 weekly. Both groups were further divided so that half had calcium intakes of 100 gm per day and half had 200 gm. Phosphorus intakes were constant, 80 to 100 gm per day. In the vitamin D–supplemented cows, first postpartum estrus occurred 16 days earlier and conception 37 days earlier than in the unsupplemented group. With high calcium intake, uterine involution was more rapid with vitamin D supplementation; however, with moderate calcium intakes (100 gm), vitamin D appeared to delay uterine involution.

Adequate vitamin D is necessary in the dry period to ensure that calcium mobilization ability is adequate to help prevent milk fever. The vitamin D requirement for growth is 300 IU per 100 pounds of body weight, and for lactating cattle it is 150 IU per pound of ration dry matter, or 6000 to 12,000 IU per cow. Excessive supplementation should be avoided. Two to four times NRC requirements appear to be safe, but amounts as little as 100,000 IU per head per day have been reported to produce signs of toxicity.

Vitamin E. Vitamin E, along with selenium, functions as an antioxidant and is important in the prevention of white muscle disease in calves. There is no documented evidence that vitamin E is essential for reproduction in cattle.

Minerals

Mineral imbalances frequently are thought to be associated with infertility in cattle. It is often difficult under clinical conditions to determine if a specific mineral is responsible for a given infertility problem. There are many interrelationships between the absorption and utilization of many of the essential minerals, and it is frequently difficult to assess whether an excess or deficiency of a specific mineral is responsible for a given problem. In clinical situations it is also unlikely to see a deficiency of a specific mineral; more frequently, several nutrients would be likely to be deficient at the same time.

Calcium. Calcium is the mineral needed in the greatest amount for both growth of the skeletal system and lactation. Its effect on reproduction appears to be primarily an indirect one because it affects the incidence of parturient paresis. Common sequelae to parturient paresis include dystocia, prolapsed uterus and retained placentae, which tend to have negative effects on fertility. To prevent milk fever, it is important to restrict calcium intake during the dry period, particularly the last 3 weeks. Current recommendations generally suggest that calcium intake should be less than 100 gm per head per day for Holstein dry cows or less than 0.5 percent of dry matter intake. The calcium-phosphorus ratio is not generally believed to be as important as the absolute levels of calcium.

There is some evidence that calcium intake affects uterine involution, although it is not clearly established. In the Kansas State University study previously cited, milking cows receiving 200 gm of calcium and vitamin D supplementation involuted to normal 8 days earlier than cows receiving 100 gm of calcium and vitamin D. Cows on the high-calcium diet also ovulated 6 days earlier. A recent case report suggests that too narrow a calcium-phosphorus ratio may increase incidence of postpartum metritis and fertility. Controlled studies have, however, failed to show any effect of calcium-phosphorus ratio on fertility. Absolute amounts of calcium, phosphorus and vitamin D in the diet are more important than the ratio.

Calcium content of forages varies greatly, and in order to formulate a balanced ration it is important to have a feed analysis done that gives this information. Because the calcium availability in some forages may be limited, some nutritionists recommend a greater level of supplementation in the lactating cow's diet than the 0.6 per cent recommended by the NRC. The calcium-phosphorus ratio should be between 1.5:1 and 2.5:1.

Phosphorus. Phosphorus is the mineral most frequently associated with reproductive abnormalities in cattle. It is necessary for normal energy and phospholipid metabolism as well as normal skeletal development and milk production. Serum phosphorus values generally reflect intake, although they can be modified by vitamin D and calcium status. Clinical signs of a deficiency may include a delayed onset of puberty and postpartum estrus. Milder deficiencies have been reported to be associated with repeat breeding. Some clinicians have suggested that an increased incidence of cystic follicles may also be associated with a phosphorus deficiency, although documented reports are not available.

In a study with 27 dairy heifers on a phosphorus-deficient diet, services per conception were 2.8. With phosphorus supplementation in 26 heifers, services per conception declined to 1.3.

An Oklahoma study of 48 dairy cows suggested that an increased incidence of cystic follicles and more services per conception resulted after feeding cows a diet of 0.4 per cent phosphorus over 2 years compared with 0.6 per cent phosphorus. Most other studies have found 0.4 per cent to be adequate for normal reproduction, including a recent Michigan study in which 48 2-year-old heifers fed either 98 per cent of the NRC phosphorus requirement or 138 per cent of the NRC requirement did not differ in reproductive performance.

Phosphorus is present in fairly high quantities in the seed fraction of plants, with lower amounts in the rest of the plant. A deficiency is most likely to be present when cattle are on all-forage diets, particularly hay, haylage or pasture. This situation is most apt to apply to dry cows or heifers, so these groups are usually the most susceptible to a phosphorus deficiency.

Current NRC recommendations suggest that phosphorus content should be 0.4 per cent of the ration on a dry matter basis for the high producing cow. Amounts greatly exceeding this may have a depressing effect on milk production and may interfere with calcium and other nutrient availability. Phosphorus content of the dry cow diet should be 0.26 per cent of dry matter intake.

Selenium. Selenium is a component of the glutathione peroxidase system and interacts with vitamin E to prevent tissue damage due to peroxide production. Deficiency signs include a muscular dystrophy known as white muscle disease, decreased fertility and an apparent increase in the incidence of retained placenta.

Several studies have shown a positive effect of selenium and vitamin E injections 20 to 30 days prepartum as an aid in the prevention of retained placenta. In one British trial, 49 cows on a selenium-deficient diet received one of three treatments: (1) no injection, (2) injection of 15 mg of selenium and 680 IU of vitamin E, and (3) injection of 15 mg of selenium 1 month prepartum. Incidence of retained placenta was 26.5, 0, and 7 per cent, respectively. In several Ohio trials injection of 50 mg of selenium and 680 IU of vitamin E 3 weeks prepartum or consumption of 0.1 ppm of selenium daily during the dry period were both effective in preventing retained placentae. A recent Ohio study suggested that selenium and vitamin E injections resulted in faster uterine involution as well.

Other studies have found that selenium injections or supplementation are ineffective in reducing the incidence of retained placenta. It is certainly only one of many possible causes. In selenium-deficient areas (see Fig. 1), additional supplementation with or without selenium injections is recommended. Current NRC recommendations suggest that selenium content of the ration should be a minimum of 0.1 ppm. Many nutritionists feel that even greater concentrations, up to 0.3 ppm, may be necessary to achieve desired serum levels of 0.07 mg/ml. Minimum toxic levels are 3 to 5 ppm.

Iodine. Iodine is required for synthesis of the thyroid hormones. Its effects on fertility are related to the effects on the thyroid gland and hormone synthesis. Signs of an iodine deficiency related to reproduction include delayed puberty, cessation of estrus activity and anovulatory estrus periods. When an iodine-deficient diet is fed during pregnancy, cows may deliver weak or dead, hairless calves. Cows may also abort and have an increased inci-

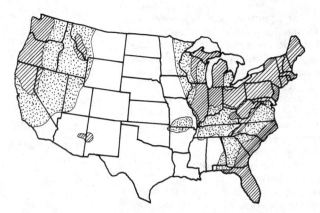

Figure 1. Selenium content of grains and forages in the United States. (With permission of Dairy Cattle: Principles, Practices, Problems, Profits. Lea & Febiger, 1972.)

▨ MOST GRAINS AND FORAGES LOW OR VERY LOW IN SELENIUM

▦ VARIABLE LEVELS OF SELENIUM-LOW AND ADEQUATE

☐ MOST GRAINS AND FORAGES ADEQUATE TO HIGH IN SELENIUM

dence of retained placenta, and calves may be born with goiter.

While iodine supplementation is necessary in many areas of the country, excessive feeding of organic iodine for therapeutic uses may result in toxicity. Excessive iodine intakes have been reported to result in abortion, especially in the first trimester, as well as a generalized decrease in resistance.

The dietary requirement for lactating cows is 0.5 ppm. This can be achieved by feeding trace mineralized salt, which contains 0.005 to 0.01 per cent iodine. When goitrogenic feeds such as kale are utilized, higher levels of iodine will be necessary. Excessive supplementation (greater than 50 mg per head per day) should be avoided.

Copper. Copper is necessary for normal connective tissue maturation and normal hemoglobin and red blood cell development. The mechanism of impaired fertility due to copper deficiency is unknown but may be related to anemia and unthriftiness.

Signs of copper deficiency related to reproduction in cattle are a general decline in fertility. An increased incidence of inactive ovaries and a greater incidence of retained placentae have been reported in animals receiving inadequate copper. There are numerous reports of copper supplementation improving fertility; however, fertility has been reported to be related to serum copper levels in some studies and unrelated in others. Copper is stored in the liver, and serum levels may not always accurately reflect copper nutrition.

The requirement for dairy cattle is 10 ppm. Copper availability is also strongly affected by other minerals, and in areas where sulfur or molybdenum is high, copper supplementation should be increased.

Cobalt. Cobalt is required for the microbial synthesis of vitamin B_{12}. Many areas of the world are endemically deficient. Signs of cobalt deficiency include a general unthriftiness and anemia as well as delayed uterine involution, irregular estrus cycles and decreased conception rate. Dietary cobalt requirement for lactating cows is 0.1 ppm of the ration dry matter intake.

Manganese. Manganese is required for activation of many enzyme systems and may be specifically involved in luteal tissue metabolism. A deficiency has been reported to result in anestrus or delayed return to estrus postpartum as well as decreased conception and delayed ovulation. Increased abortions and small birth weights are also reported to result from inadequate manganese intake. Neonatal deformities may also result from insufficient manganese, including twisted legs and enlarged joints as well as general weakness.

The dietary requirement for manganese is not well defined, but 40 ppm of the ration dry matter has been suggested. Corn silage is relatively low in manganese.

Zinc. Signs of zinc deficiency include delayed testicular development in the young bull and testicular atrophy in the adult. There is atrophy of the seminiferous tubules and cessation of spermatogenesis. Lower conception rates have also been reported in zinc-deficient cows. These symptoms may be present before there are other signs such as impaired growth or parakeratosis.

The dietary requirement for zinc in lactating dairy cattle is 40 ppm of ration dry matter. This is also adequate for normal testicular function. Feeding trace mineral salt should provide adequate amounts of copper, cobalt, manganese and zinc for normal reproduction.

CONCLUSIONS

Nutritional deficiencies or imbalances are only one possible source or cause of a herd reproductive problem. In dealing with a problem, other areas such as infectious agents, a vaccination program, hygiene and overall management should not be neglected. If nutrition is responsible, it is frequently difficult to pinpoint a specific cause; usually more than one nutrient deficiency or excess will be responsible.

The best approach is to evaluate the ration and feed in relation to the animal's requirements for maintenance, growth, lactation and gestation. In most cases these requirements should be adequate to ensure normal reproductive function. Several time periods are especially critical: (1) the time around puberty and breeding, (2) the dry period or just before calving, and (3) the immediate postpartum period when lactation peaks and the cow is being rebred. Challenge feeding in early lactation should be beneficial for this latter group.

The ration should be balanced for energy, protein, vitamins and minerals based on laboratory analysis of feedstuff content. An analysis of the forages is especially critical because they vary so much.

First and second lactation animals should be provided additional feed for growth as well as lactation and maintenance. Twenty and 10 per cent above maintenance is usually recommended for first and second lactation, respectively.

To identify or prevent nutritional problems, it is important that an effective working relationship exists between the dairyman, his veterinarian, nutritionist and feed salesman. Effective communication of knowledge should serve to minimize problems and maximize fertility and production.

Selected Readings

1. Hidiroglou M: Trace element deficiencies and fertility in ruminants: A review. J Dairy Sci 62:1195, 1979.
2. Huber JT: Influence of ration protein percent and feeding of nonprotein nitrogen during early lactation on reproductive efficiency of cows. Animal Science Newsletter, Cooperative Extension Service, Michigan State University, February 1982, pp. 11–13.
3. Moseley WM, Dunn TG, Kaltenbach CC, et al.: Relationship of growth and puberty in beef heifers fed monensin. J Anim Sci 55:357, 1982.
4. Moutgaard J: Nutritive influences upon reproduction. In Cole HH, Cupps PT (eds.): Reproduction in Domestic Animals. New York, Academic Press, 1969, pp. 489–516.
5. National Research Council-National Academy of Sciences: Nutrient Requirements of Dairy Cattle. Washington, D.C., National Academy of Sciences, 1978, pp. 1–76.
6. Otterby DE, Linn JG: Effects of nutrition on reproduction in dairy cattle. Comp Cont Educ Pract Veterinarians 5:S85, 1983.

Influences of Nutrition on Reproduction in Beef Cattle

John C. Spitzer, B.S., M.S., Ph.D.
Clemson University, Clemson, South Carolina

Beef herds in the United States are managed under conditions varying from confinement cow-calf production units to the more common grazing systems. Furthermore, conditions in the southwest, where it may take 30 or more acres to support a cow-calf unit, are vastly different from situations in the east and southeast, where one or two intensively managed acres will support a cow-calf unit. However, all areas have certain production criteria in common. This chapter will expand on these common factors, especially as they relate to nutrition. Obviously, it will be a condensed discussion and the reader is directed to reference textbooks and articles where appropriate. One essential reference is Nutrient Requirements of Beef Cattle from the National Research Council (NRC).[6]

Significance of Reproductive Performance in Beef Cattle

A simplified formula of beef-herd economics is Income = *(number of calves weaned × weaning weight × price per pound) − (annual costs)*. Price per pound of calf sold is something over which individual producers have little control, so we will limit our discussion to the other variables. Annual costs are obviously of paramount importance, and producers should constantly search for ways to reduce costs. However, many producers reduce costs so much that the number of calves weaned and weaning weight suffer as a result—certainly not a profitable situation. In many cases costs can be judiciously increased, and the increases in number of calves weaned and weaning weight will justify the added expense.

The greatest factor influencing the number of calves weaned is cows failing to become pregnant in a 12-month production year (12 to 22 per cent) followed by neonatal and postnatal deaths (8 to 11 per cent) and abortion losses (3 to 4 per cent).[9] Weaning weight depends on three factors: Weaning weight = *(birth weight) + (average daily gain × age at weaning)*. Increasing birth weight has severe limitations associated with dystocia and concomitant postpartum infertility. Average daily gain can be increased through selection or crossbreeding of cows, both of which will increase milk production, or by creep feeding. However, these are long-range changes; therefore, altering the average age of calves weaned offers the most potential for increasing weaning weight.

A study in which 8742 calves were divided into three groups based on weaning weight is summarized in Table 1. Calves in the top third weighed 52 kg more than calves in the bottom third and 26 kg more than calves in the middle group. Notice that 70 per cent of the heavier calves were born in *the first 20 days* of calving and were therefore older at weaning time. The average age of calves at weaning can be increased only by having calves born early in the calving season, which is a direct reflection of the reproductive performance of the cow herd.

If we go back to our original equation, the two variables, number of calves weaned and weaning weight, are both controlled by reproductive performance. While many factors besides nutrition can lower reproductive performance, inadequate nutrition is the most frequent cause.

Nutritional Philosophy

The beef cow is a ruminant, and generally the majority of the diet is obtained from forages—the beef cow is a "harvesting machine" for a grass farmer. However, there are circumstances that make nonforage feeds more economical than conventional grass systems, especially when considering supplemental feeding. Cow-calf producers should constantly be searching for nonconventional, cheap feeds regardless of whether these are components of traditional diets for beef herds. In other words, meet the nutritional needs of the cow, but do it as cheaply as possible without preconceived constraints of what should and should not be fed to the beef cow. What cows eat is far less important than the *quality* and *quantity* of the nutrients furnished in diets available to them.

GENERAL NUTRITION

Nutrient Categories

Any brief scheme of nutrient description will be oversimplified, but we can divide nutrients into five general though not completely discrete categories. The reader is referred to the textbook of Jurgens[4] for a more complete discussion.

Water. Water is generally the cheapest and most abundantly supplied nutrient but is critical since it comprises 45 to 60 per cent of the body weight of the animal. Water is distributed intracellularly, extracellularly and as fill in the urinary and digestive tracts. Functions include transport of nutrients and excretory products, solvent properties involved in chemical reactions and maintenance of cell size and shape. Additionally, water and water movement play a critical role in regulating body temperature as well as providing lubrication for joints and cushioning the joints and organs of the body.

Deficiency symptoms include reduced feed intake, weight loss (both as a result of reduced feed intake and dehydration) and increased nitrogen and electrolyte losses. Always ensure an adequate, clean water supply. A mature nonstressed animal will consume 35 to 55 liters per day—more under heat stress.

Vitamins. Vitamins are organic entities distinct from water, protein, carbohydrates and fats. They are essential for normal cellular and tissue function and regulate many metabolic pathways. However, vitamins do not enter into structural components of the body. Vitamins can be subdivided into water-soluble vitamins (B-complex and C) and fat-soluble vitamins (A, D, E and K). All of the water-soluble vitamins and vitamin K can be synthesized by microorganisms in a healthy rumen environment, leaving only vitamins A, D and E for supplementary considerations in adult cattle.

Vitamin A requirements of beef cattle are generally adequately provided by the carotene content of actively growing or well-cured forages. If the forages consumed have any green color, vitamin A requirements will be supplied. The amount of vitamin A or its precursor beta-carotene present in a roughage is generally proportional to the amount of green color in the forage. Excess vitamin A is stored in the liver and will supply the need of the animal for 3 to 6 months of decreased vitamin A intake. Even during winter, most diets provide some vitamin A, which, along with dietary-acquired liver stores, prevents vitamin A deficiency. However, some rations are devoid of vitamin A. In this case a 3- to 6-month hepatic supply is enough to maintain the cow to the last trimester of gestation before it is depleted. Problematic is that vitamin A requirements during late gestation are increased, not only for bodily function but also to enrich colostrum for the neonate.

Vitamin A is necessary for maintaining the mem-

Table 1. Relationship Between Actual Weaning Weight of Calves and Their Time of Birth During a 60-Day Period

Weaning Weight Rank	Number of Calves	Average Weaning Weight (kg)	Average Weaning Age (days)	Calves Born During		
				First 20 days	Second 20 days	Third 20 days
Top third	2910	189	207	70%	24%	6%
Middle third	2916	163	195	42%	39%	19%
Bottom third	2916	137	181	19%	33%	48%

branes lining the respiratory, intestinal and reproductive tracts. Deficiency symptoms in cattle include night blindness, locomotor problems, excessive lacrimation, nutritional problems, and reproductive problems in males and females. Pregnant cows may abort (retained placenta and uterine infection are common sequelae) or give birth to weak, dead, or blind calves. Bulls produce abnormal and fewer spermatozoa due to degeneration of seminiferous epithelium. In practice, vitamin A deficiency should be considered during drought years or after prolonged feeding of bleached grasses and hay or silage feeding. Vitamin A in feedstuffs (natural or exogenous) decreases with storage, and losses are accelerated with processed feeds or upon mixing with oxidizing materials such as minerals and organic acids. The most practical supplementation of vitamin A appears to be through injection of emulsified vitamin A at the rate of 2 to 4 million IU, which will maintain hepatic stores for 3 to 6 months.

Even though cows may have ample vitamin A, the newborn calf is deficient in vitamin A. Vitamin A deficiency of the neonate is corrected only if colostrum contains adequate vitamin A and if sufficient quantities of colostrum are ingested. If the cow has sufficient vitamin A reserves, the colostrum will contain ten times more vitamin A than milk.

Vitamin D is synthesized in vivo from direct exposure to sunlight or supplied by ingestion of sun-cured forages. It is difficult to envision deficiencies occurring in most beef herds. Additionally, deficiency symptoms develop very slowly in adult animals, and even intermittent exposure to sunlight will supply adequate vitamin D. However, vitamin D deficiency has been observed in confinement housing where diets contain little forage. Deficiency symptoms include digestive disturbances, stiff gait, labored breathing, weakness, locomotor problems and possibly tetany and convulsions. Severe deficiencies in pregnant animals may result in weak, dead or deformed calves.

Vitamin E requirements for mature cattle are minute, and commonly ingested feedstuffs contain adequate supplies for normal reproduction. There is no evidence to show that vitamin E supplementation is of value in increasing reproductive performance. White muscle disease occurs in calves in some areas of the United States and may be due to deficiency of selenium, vitamin E or both. Supplemental vitamin E may be added to the diet or injected intramuscularly in calves. Deficiency is not of general concern in mature cattle, since deficiencies have not been known to occur in the adult population.

Recommendations. Except for unusual situations, there is no need to be concerned with vitamin D or E deficiencies in adult animals. Because most vitamin A deficiencies in mature cows will occur during late gestation or the subsequent breeding season, the following procedures are recommended: (1) Evaluate dietary intake of the cow at weaning time. If cows (or bulls) have grazed forages that appear to be lacking in vitamin A and will not receive feeds

adequate in vitamin A through calving, inject 2 to 4 million IU of vitamin A. (2) Routinely administer 2 to 4 million IU of vitamin A to all cows, yearling heifers and bulls in conjunction with the prebreeding vaccination schedule for the cow herd. Cost is minimal for this insurance program against possible vitamin A deficiency and its related reproductive problems. If vitamin A is incorporated into a ration, provide the cow with 20,000 IU per day. This may be supplied by feeding a mineral mix or other supplement containing vitamin A.

Injecting 200,000 to 300,000 IU of vitamin A into calves at birth may again be inexpensive insurance even though most calves ordinarily receive sufficient vitamin A through the colostrum. Replacement heifers and bulls should receive 1 to 2 million IU of vitamin A at weaning, which will provide hepatic stores to carry them through until they are covered under the routine recommendations for the cow herd.

Minerals. Minerals are inorganic, solid, crystalline chemical elements important in many body structures and functions. Minerals are rather loosely divided into major (macro) elements (present or needed in larger amounts in the body) and minor (micro) elements (present or needed in smaller amounts in the body). Generally considered major elements are calcium, phosphorus, sodium and chloride. In some geographical areas magnesium should be considered in this group. Minor (trace) elements are potassium, sulfur, cobalt, copper, fluorine, iodine, iron, manganese, molybdenum, selenium and zinc. Functions include skeletal structure (calcium, phosphorus, magnesium, copper, manganese); protein synthesis (phosphorus, sulfur, zinc); oxygen transport (iron, copper); and acid/base and fluid balance (sodium, choride, potassium, calcium). Additionally, many minerals are activators and/or components of enzyme systems, and there are mineral-vitamin interrelationships (vitamin E and selenium are but one example).

In general, most forages contain adequate calcium but are deficient in phosphorus, sodium chloride and possibly magnesium while most grains are good sources of phosphorus but are deficient in calcium, sodium and chloride. Except for regionalized deficiencies, beef herds do not generally receive feedstuffs deficient in minor elements (for example, iodine deficiency in the northwest and Great Lakes area; copper deficiency in Florida and areas of the southeastern coastal plains; cobalt in Florida, the Great Lakes area and New England). Selenium is unique because it can be present in toxic amounts in forages in the Rocky Mountains–Great Plains area and deficient in some southeastern coastal areas. Other mineral deficiencies or toxic concentrations may also appear in other regions or under unusual circumstances and are of local concern.

Phosphorus deficiency symptoms in calves are reduced feed intake and a concomitant reduction in growth rate. In the brood cow, weight loss, decreased milk production and delayed conception are generally inconspicuous deficiency symptoms. Severe phosphorus deficiency causes abnormal habits such as chewing on wood and metal, eating dirt and hair of herd mates and abnormal gait. However, by the time these symptoms are exhibited, reproductive performance has already been compromised.

Grass tetany is due to a hypomagnesemia. Grass tetany occurs most commonly in older, heavily lactating cows during cool damp weather in the spring when they are consuming either actively growing pastures or winter wheat pastures. However, it can occur in any cattle at any time, particularly around parturition. Affected animals have a decreased appetite, are dull and lethargic and may isolate themselves from the herd. They progressively develop a staggering gait, become highly excitable, nervous and often belligerent and have muscular tremors that progress to collapse and tetany. Death may occur within several hours from onset of symptoms.

Recommendations. For breeding herds, allow ad libitum consumption of a loose mineral supplement containing 10 to 12 per cent phosphorus with a 1:1 calcium-phosphorus ratio. A 1:1 ratio *in the mineral supplement* is desired because with forage diets it is possible to have calcium-phosphorus ratios of 6:1 or 8:1. A calcium-phosphorus ratio of greater than 4:1 is detrimental, since excess calcium appears to prevent absorption of phosphorus from the intestine, thereby creating a phosphorus deficiency in spite of adequate dietary phosphorus. The 12 per cent phosphorus, 1:1 calcium-phosphorus ratio supplement fed free choice will help balance the total dietary intake. Although some studies refute the need for phosphorus intakes of this magnitude, many others have confirmed it as necessary. It is a fairly cheap insurance program to protect against phosphorus deficiency. Calcium is not necessary in the mineral supplement with forage diets, but it increases palatability, prevents caking and reduces cost of the supplement. In a few areas of the United States, it may be advantageous to further reduce calcium so that there is a 0.5:1 calcium-phosphorus ratio. If diets are fed that contain high levels of concentrates (such as bull gain test or replacement heifer rations), the calcium-phosphorus ratios can be relaxed to 2:1 and the phosphorus level lowered to 4 to 6 per cent. The mineral supplement should be in a loose form because consumption may not be sufficient if the supplement is fed in block form. In addition to the phosphorus-mineral supplement, provide salt blocks free choice to correct the sodium and chloride deficiencies of most diets. Blocks are advisable in this situation, because many cows overconsume salt.

In areas where grass tetany due to magnesium deficiency is apparent the aforementioned loose minerals and salt blocks should be replaced with a single mineral supplement containing 14 per cent magnesium in addition to the requirements of 10 to 12 per cent phosphorus and a 1:1 calcium-phosphorus ratio previously specified. Withhold salt blocks and begin feeding this mineral several months in advance of when the problem will be manifest and

through the problem months. If an emergency arises, a mixture composed of equal proportions of salt, magnesium oxide, dicalcium phosphate and soybean or cottonseed meal fed free choice will generally give positive results.

There has been a great deal of discussion concerning "home mixed" versus commercially prepared mineral formulations. In general, it is just as economical and certainly more convenient to feed a premixed mineral. For large operators, buying in several ton lots may result in a better price on a commercially available mineral, or a mineral can be mixed to his specifications. An additional benefit is that these mineral formulations will also contain the minor (trace) elements that give added insurance against deficiencies. Given that a cow will consume only 18 to 23 kg of a good mineral mix in a year's time, buying commercially prepared minerals is not a large portion of the annual cost. However, cheap minerals with high calcium-phosphorus ratios are generally not a good buy at any price.

Protein. Proteins are made up of carbon, hydrogen, oxygen and nitrogen with small amounts of sulfur and phosphorus. Proteins are the principal constituent of the organs and tissues of the body and are themselves made up of units of 22 amino acids linked through peptide bonds. Proteins function as structural units—collagen, elastin, contractile proteins, keratin proteins, and blood proteins—and in metabolism, enzymes, hormones and immune antibodies, and they can serve as a source of energy after deamination. However, deamination is a very wasteful process from an energy standpoint. Proteins are digested to amino acids and peptides for absorption from the digestive system except during early neonatal life, i.e., under 24 hours of life, when whole proteins are absorbed across the intestinal epithelium.

Protein deficiency symptoms include decreased growth and feed efficiency, anorexia, fatty liver, infertility, reduced fetal weight and reduced milk production. Part of the reason for these effects is that protein deficiency results in reduced total feed intake and therefore depresses intake of all nutrients.

Crude protein (CP) is a term quantifying total protein and is a calculated value (CP = 6.25 × %N) based on the estimate that proteins contain approximately 16 per cent nitrogen. This nitrogen is total nitrogen, and no differentiation is made as to source. In the case of young, actively growing plants, considerable nitrogen can be present in the form of amides, nitrates and amino acids. Although the value of 16 per cent is not totally accurate, it is a sound estimate of nitrogen content of proteins in most feeds. Digestible protein (DP) is a measure of the protein absorbed by the animal (DP = CP of feed − CP of feces).

We will assume that there are no essential amino acids for ruminants because essentially all protein ingested is catabolized and resynthesized into microbial protein, which goes to the lower digestive tract and is absorbed to meet the protein needs of the animal. In light of more current research, this may not be absolutely correct, but it is workable for beef cows.

True proteins are composed only of amino acids, whereas nonprotein nitrogen (NPN) compounds are not proteins but contain nitrogen that can be converted to protein by bacterial action in the rumen. The most common source of NPN is urea, which may be used in certain diets to replace a portion of the crude protein. Urea is converted to ammonia in the rumen and is then utilized by rumen microorganisms for synthesis of microbial protein, which is utilized by the ruminant animal. However, this microbial protein synthesis from NPN necessitates a readily available source of energy. NPN compounds work well when used in high concentrate feedlot diets but have worked poorly in diets for range cattle. There is just not enough available energy in a primarily forage ration for good utilization of NPN. Feeding molasses or a few pounds of grain is of little benefit in enabling the animal to utilize the NPN as a protein source. A maximum of 2 to 3 per cent urea or 5 to 8 per cent crude protein equivalents from an NPN source is not harmful, but for cattle on forages it is of little benefit. Therefore when supplementing range cattle, the protein provided by NPN should be subtracted from the total protein of the supplement to obtain the true protein content of the feed.

Numerous studies have demonstrated that poor results will be obtained when a urea-molasses supplement is fed to cattle that consume primarily roughages if the urea it contains is the sole source of protein. Because of this fact, some manufacturers make a big advertising point that their supplements do not contain urea. However, close inspection of ingredients will reveal that the supplement contains some other source of NPN—i.e., ammonia, biuret, IBDU (isobutyl diurea), nucleic acids, and so on. In spite of claims to the contrary, numerous studies have failed to show any better utilization of these sources of NPN than of urea.

Two problems arise with protein supplementation on dry winter forages. First, as forage quality decreases, cows consume less rather than more pounds of forage. As winter progresses, cows actually consume less total feed. Second, although addition of protein does stimulate forage intake, often this does not compensate for total dietary shortages; in this case, other feeds beside protein supplement should be provided. Recommendations for protein supplementation will be discussed further in the section on nutrient requirements.

Energy. Defining energy as a nutrient is a misnomer, but for practical purposes carbohydrates and fats are used as energy and will be discussed as such. Carbohydrates and fats are composed of carbon, hydrogen and oxygen. Carbohydrates, which include simple sugars, starches, cellulose and gums, mono-, di-, and polysaccharides and mixed polysaccharides, are formed by photosynthesis in plants. In ruminants complex carbohydrates are broken down to monosaccharides by enzymes from micro-

flora in the rumen. Rumen microbes also synthesize volatile fatty acids (VFAs) by anaerobic fermentation. These VFAs (mainly acetic, propionic and butyric acids) provide a large portion of the total energy requirement of the ruminant. There is little free carbohydrate in the animal body, and there is rapid conversion to fats for energy storage, although carbohydrates and fats are constantly being interconverted.

Fats are composed of (1) simple lipids—triglycerides (esters of fatty acids with glycerol) and waxes (esters of fatty acids with alcohols other than glycerol); (2) compound lipids—phospholipids, glycolipids and lipoproteins; and (3) derived lipids—fatty acids and sterols. Carbohydrates and fats function as sources of energy for bodily functions, heat, and (carbohydrates) as building blocks for other nutrients. Fats further provide insulation and protection (cushioning) to the body. Upon oxidation, fats provide 2.5 times more energy than carbohydrates.

A discussion of commonly used terms in energy nutrition is required before continuing our discussion of nutrition. Gross energy (GE) is the heat of combustion of a feedstuff and is expressed as kilocalories per gram (Kcal/gm) or megacalories per kilogram (Mcal/kg). Digestible energy (DE) is a measure of the energy absorbed by an animal (DE = GE of feed − GE of feces). Metabolizable energy (ME) is an even more specific measure because it accounts for energy lost not only in feces but also in urine and combustible gases.

Net energy (NE) may be the most precise method of measuring the energy content of feedstuffs (NE = ME − heat increment or specific dynamic effect*). NE is actually the energy available to the animal for useful purposes such as maintenance, growth, fattening, reproduction or milk production (see Fig. 1).

While the net energy system is quite precise and very useful in calculating well-balanced diets for many classes of animals, it has severe limitations for beef herds. One major shortcoming is that each feedstuff has a specific NE value for a specific function. For example, alfalfa hay at mid-bloom has 1.99 Mcal ME per kilogram. When used for maintenance, its NE value is 1.17 Mcal/kg, whereas its NE value for milk production is 1.21 Mcal/kg, for weight gain it is 0.48 Mcal/kg, and for fetal growth it is 0.28 Mcal/kg. Second, the NE value of all feedstuffs has not been determined for all functions involved in beef production since this involves costly

---

*Heat increment or specific dynamic effect represents the difference between absorbed energy and energy that is actually captured by the metabolic processes of the animal. For example, if glucose is oxidized to generate adenosine triphosphate (ATP), 44 per cent of the gross energy of a molecule of glucose is converted to high-energy phosphate compounds, and the remainder (56 per cent) is lost as heat. Other processes contributing to specific dynamic effect include mastication, the work of moving food through the gastrointestinal tract and the heat of fermentation in the rumen.

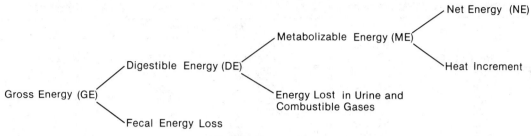

Figure 1. Energy terms.

digestion trials. Most of the NE values have been estimated from other measures. Finally, and most limiting, is the fact that sufficient information is not available for using NE formulations for grazing, reproducing or lactating beef cows, and net energy requirements for reproduction have not been determined.

For practical purposes, the total digestible nutrients (TDN) system used for estimating energy content of feeds is the system of choice for reproducing grazing cattle. The percentage of TDN in a feedstuff equals the percentage of digestible crude protein plus the percentage of digestible crude fiber plus the percentage of digestible nitrogen-free extract (lipids) × 2.25. The TDN system obviously is not as precise, but it is simpler and is certainly accurate enough when we consider our usually crude estimations of intake of grazing beef cattle or even their consumption of bulk-fed supplements. TDN and DE can be roughly interconverted (1 kg TDN = 4.4 Mcal DE).

Nutrient Requirements Generalized

Nutrient requirements for the various classes of animals represented in most beef herds have been adapted from NRC recommendations[6] and will be individually discussed. While these values are good estimates of minimum nutrient levels, they do not consider all environmental variables encountered and may need to be adjusted.

Table 2 is adapted from NRC recommendations for growing steer calves and yearlings. Weight ranges from 200 to 500 kg are presented along with average daily gain (ADG) of 0.7 to 1.3 kg/day. Requirements for animals of intermediate weights and/or intermediate ADG can be interpolated (see example 2 in the section on ration formulation). In most progressive beef herds, bulls will be placed on some type of a gain test following weaning and will be performance tested through roughly yearling age. The range in weights and ADG presented in Table 2 seems practical since bulls weighing less than 200

Table 2. Nutrient Requirements for Growing Bull Calves and Yearlings*

| Weight (kg) | Desired ADG (kg) | Minimum Consumption | | |
		Dry Matter (kg)	CP (kg)	TDN (kg)
200	0.7	5.7	0.61	3.6
	0.9	4.9	0.61	3.7
	1.1	4.6	0.63	3.9
250	0.9	6.2	0.69	4.5
	1.1	6.0	0.73	4.7
	1.3	6.0	0.76	5.2
300	0.9	8.1	0.81	5.4
	1.1	7.6	0.82	5.6
	1.3	7.1	0.83	6.0
350	0.9	8.0	0.80	5.8
	1.1	8.0	0.83	6.2
	1.3	8.0	0.87	6.8
400	1.0	9.4	0.87	6.8
	1.2	8.5	0.87	7.0
	1.3	8.6	0.90	7.3
450	1.0	10.3	0.96	7.4
	1.2	10.2	0.97	7.9
	1.3	9.3	0.97	8.0
500	0.9	10.5	0.95	7.5
	1.1	10.4	0.96	8.1
	1.2	9.6	0.96	8.2

*Adapted from National Research Council: Nutrient Requirements of Domestic Animals, No. 4. Nutrient requirements of beef cattle. Washington, D.C., National Academy of Sciences, National Research Council, 1976.

Table 3. Nutrient Requirements for Bulls for Growth and Maintenance—Moderate Activity*

| Weight (kg) | Desired ADG (kg) | Minimum Consumption | | |
		Dry Matter (kg)	CP (kg)	TDN (kg)
500	0.7	12.2	1.07	7.5
600	0.5	12.0	1.02	7.3
700	0.3	12.9	1.08	7.7
800	Maintenance	10.5	0.89	5.8
900	Maintenance	11.4	0.99	6.3
1000	Maintenance	12.4	1.05	6.9

*Adapted from National Research Council: Nutrient Requirements of Domestic Animals, No. 4. Nutrient requirements of beef cattle. Washington, D.C., National Academy of Sciences, National Research Council, 1976.

kg at weaning should be steers. An ADG from weaning to yearling age of 0.7 to 1.3 kg/day is certainly adequate to evaluate ability to gain and does not result in overly fat yearling bulls. Recommendations for yearling and mature bulls appear in Table 3.

Nutrient requirements for growing heifer calves and yearlings are presented in Table 4. Again, a range in weights and ADG practical for most beef herds is depicted. Few heifers weighing less than 150 kg will grow fast enough to reach puberty as yearlings, and weights of much over 350 kg are not generally necessary in yearling heifers.

Table 5 depicts nutrient requirements for pregnant yearling heifers during the last trimester of gestation. This 3-month period is critical because the fetus is making large absolute weight gains. The recommendations for 0.4 kg/day ADG do not allow for any growth of the heifer, only the conceptus. If heifers have not been well developed before this time, a higher ADG would be more appropriate.

Strict attention must be given to the body fat reserves of the pregnant heifer so she will calve in good body condition.

Nutrient requirements for brood cows are presented in Table 6. Note that requirements are listed for a dry cow in the last trimester of gestation. The same comments as discussed for the heifer during this last trimester are also appropriate here. Keep in mind that an ADG of 0.4 kg/day includes only the growth of the conceptus and does not allow for weight gain in the cow.

Dramatic changes occur in nutrient requirements once a cow has calved and initiated lactation (Table 6). The current edition of the NRC publication[6] contains two sets of requirements for cows nursing calves for the first 3 to 4 months of lactation. The first set, labeled *cows of average milking ability, should be totally ignored* because the levels of nutrients listed, especially TDN values, are inadequate to support lactation and satisfactory reproduction in most cows. Recommendations listed in

Table 4. Nutrient Requirements for Growing Heifer Calves and Yearlings*

| Weight (kg) | Desired ADG (kg) | Minimum Consumption | | |
		Dry Matter (kg)	CP (kg)	TDN (kg)
150	0.7	4.0	0.50	2.8
	0.9	4.0	0.54	3.1
	1.1	4.0	0.60	3.4
200	0.5	6.0	0.58	3.5
	0.7	6.0	0.61	3.8
	0.9	5.3	0.62	4.0
	1.1	5.0	0.64	4.3
250	0.3	6.4	0.57	3.5
	0.5	6.5	0.62	3.9
	0.7	5.8	0.62	4.1
	0.9	5.9	0.65	4.6
	1.1	6.5	0.74	5.2
300	0.3	7.4	0.63	4.0
	0.5	7.4	0.67	4.5
	0.7	6.6	0.67	4.7
	0.9	6.8	0.70	5.2
350	0.3	8.2	0.69	4.6
	0.5	8.3	0.73	5.1
	0.9	7.9	0.73	5.4
	0.9	8.1	0.77	6.0

*Adapted from National Research Council: Nutrient Requirements of Domestic Animals, No. 4. Nutrient requirements of beef cattle. Washington, D.C., National Academy of Sciences, National Research Council, 1976.

Table 5. Nutrient Requirements for Pregnant Yearling Heifers—Last Trimester*

| | | Minimum Consumption | | |
Weight (kg)	Desired ADG (kg)	Dry Matter (kg)	CP (kg)	TDN (kg)
325	0.4†	6.6	0.58	3.5
	0.6	8.5	0.75	4.5
350	0.4†	6.9	0.61	3.7
	0.6	8.9	0.78	4.7
375	0.4†	7.2	0.63	3.8
	0.6	9.3	0.81	4.9
400	0.4†	7.5	0.65	3.9
	0.6	9.7	0.84	5.1
425	0.4†	7.8	0.69	4.1
	0.6	10.1	0.88	5.3

*Adapted from National Research Council: Nutrient Requirements of Domestic Animals, No. 4. Nutrient requirements of beef cattle. Washington, D.C., National Academy of Sciences, National Research Council, 1976.
†Approximately 0.4 kg of weight gain is accounted for by growth of conceptus during last trimester of gestation. These requirements are estimates for quantities necessary for this conceptus development.

Table 6 are appropriate for cows of average milking ability and are actually the NRC set of values for *cows of superior milking ability* with CP levels calculated as 10 per cent of dry matter intake.

Recommendations in Table 6 are *not* adequate for cows of superior milking ability or for first-calf cows. Actual requirements for these two classes of animals are not accurately known, but a good estimate would be to increase DM and TDN levels by 15 to 25 per cent and increase CP to 12 per cent of the dry matter intake.

Note that several simplifications have been made that facilitate ration calculations. First, protein requirements are listed as crude protein because this value is generally more available for forage diets,

and for beef herds it provides enough accuracy in meeting nutrient needs. Second, no vitamin or mineral requirements are listed, and example rations in the following section do not include balancing for calcium, phosphorus or vitamin A. If the recommendations given in the previous sections on vitamins and minerals are followed, these requirements will be met with insurance, leaving only CP and TDN as considerations.

Ration Formulation

Rations for two classes of beef animals will be formulated as examples. The procedures for ration

Table 6. Nutrient Requirements for Brood Cows*

| | | Minimum Consumption | | |
Weight (kg)	Desired ADG (kg)	Dry Matter (kg)	CP (kg)	TDN (kg)
400 Dry†	0.4	7.5	0.44	4.0
Wet‡		10.8	1.08	6.1
450 Dry†	0.4	8.1	0.48	4.2
Wet‡		11.3	1.13	6.4
500 Dry†	0.4	8.6	0.51	4.5
Wet‡		11.8	1.18	6.7
550 Dry†	0.4	9.1	0.54	4.8
Wet‡		12.4	1.24	7.0
600 Dry†	0.4	9.7	0.57	5.1
Wet‡		12.9	1.29	7.3
650 Dry†	0.4	10.2	0.60	5.4
Wet‡		13.4	1.34	7.6

*Adapted from National Research Council: Nutrient Requirements of Domestic Animals, No. 4. Nutrient requirements of beef cattle. Washington, D.C., National Academy of Sciences, National Research Council, 1976.
†Requirements for last trimester of gestation. Approximately 0.4 kg of weight gain is accounted for by growth of conceptus during last trimester. These requirements are estimates of quantities necessary for this conceptus development.
‡Requirements for cows nursing calves in the first 3 to 4 months postpartum. These are estimates for cows of average milking ability. Protein requirements were estimated at 10 per cent of dry matter. *Note:* See discussion in text.

formulations for other classes are identical. By using Tables 2 through 6 and these examples, appropriate rations can be formulated for individuals in the beef herd. Several rules of thumb should be used in formulating rations. First, balance the ration for TDN, since this is the major portion of the total diet. Next, evaluate your available feedstuffs as to cost per pound of nutrient and use your cheapest source of TDN as the major portion of the diet. Forages will generally, but not always, be your cheapest source of TDN, and they usually offer the advantage of being "home grown." The *Composition of Feeds* tables in the NRC publication[6] can be used to evaluate the cost per unit of nutrient, which is considerably different from the cost per unit of feed. However, while these values are good average estimates of nutrient composition, there are tremendous variations in feed quality. Furthermore, all feedstuffs are not included in these tables. For these and other reasons it is imperative that samples of your feedstuffs be submitted to a laboratory for analysis. Most states have such services available through the County Extension offices, and the use of these services is encouraged.

Example 1. Assume you have weaned a group of bull calves with an average weight of 240 kg and a range of 225 to 250 kg. These bulls are on a performance-testing program, and you would like this group of bulls to average close to 450 kg as yearlings. Since the bulls average 240 kg, an ADG of 1.3 kg for 160 days (20-day warmup period plus 140-day performance testing period) will have the average bull weighing almost 450 kg. Obviously, the initial ration will not be adequate as the bulls grow. Therefore, we will make the following assumptions. The first assumption is that we will change the ration twice, or at day 50 and day 100 of the program. In this case we will calculate our initial ration for the heaviest bull in the group (250 kg) and feed that ration to all bulls. The requirements listed in Table 2 for a 250-kg bull to gain 1.3 kg/day are 6.0 kg of DM, 0.76 kg of CP and 5.2 kg of TDN.

For this problem, we will assume that corn silage and corn are the cheapest and most plentiful feed resources available. The nutrient composition of corn silage and corn was obtained from NRC[6] and appears in Table 7. The amount of corn and corn silage needed to meet the requirement for our ration can be calculated. There are two methods that can be utilized to solve this problem—simultaneous equations or the Pearson Square method. Simultaneous equations will be used for this example.

To set up these equations, X equals the amount of DM from corn silage and Y equals the amount

of DM from corn. The sum of these two feedstuffs equals the minimum DM requirement (6.0 kg). In the second equation, the percentage of TDN in corn silage and the percentage of TDN in corn equal the TDN requirement (5.2 kg).

Solution

Set up:

$$X + Y = 6.0$$
$$0.70X + 0.91Y = 5.2$$

Solve the first equation for X:

$$X = 6.0 - Y$$

Substitute this volume for X in the second equation and determine value for Y:

$$0.70(6.0 - Y) + 0.91Y = 5.2$$
$$Y = 4.76$$

Substitute this volume for Y in the first equation and determine the value for X:

$$X + 4.76 = 6.0$$
$$X = 1.24$$

The solution to this pair of simultaneous equations shows that 4.76 kg of DM from corn and 1.24 kg of DM from corn silage will meet the TDN requirement. To convert the DM values to as-fed values, divide each by the DM per cent in the ingredient:

4.76/0.89 = 5.35 kg of corn on an as-fed basis
1.24/0.279 = 4.44 kg of corn silage on an as-fed basis

The next step is to determine if the amounts of corn and corn silage that meet the TDN requirement will also meet the requirements for CP. In our example, the CP requirement was 0.76 kg and our ration of 5.35 kg of corn and 4.44 kg of corn silage will provide only 0.58 kg of CP; we are deficient 0.18 kg of CP. Assume that the cheapest protein supplement available is soybean meal (SBM). Again, we look to NRC for the nutrient composition of soybean meal (Table 7). We will need to add 0.35 kg of DM from SBM to meet our deficiency for CP. The total ration is shown in Table 8. This assumes that phosphorus and calcium requirements as well as vitamin A requirements will be met with supplementation as discussed elsewhere in this chapter. Also it assumes that the animal can consume the additional DM provided by the soybean meal. As a general rule, animals on moderate to high-energy

Table 7. Composition of Feeds Used in Example Rations

Ingredient	DM (per cent)	CP (per cent)	TDN (per cent)
Corn silage	27.9	8.4	70
Corn	89.0	10.0	91
Soybean meal (solv. extd.)	89.0	51.5	81
Coastal Bermuda grass hay	91.5	9.5	49

Table 8. Example Ration for 250-kg Bull Calves to Gain 1.3 kg/day (to Be Fed First 50 Days of 160-Day Period)

Item	DM (kg)	CP (kg)	TDN (kg)
Requirements	6.0	0.76	5.2
Ration (as fed)			
5.35 kg corn	4.76	0.48	4.33
4.44 kg corn silage	1.24	0.10	0.87
0.39 kg SBM	0.35	0.18	0.28
Totals	6.35	0.76	5.48

diets will consume 2.75 to 3.0 per cent of their body weight. The 250-kg bull could consume up to 6.9 to 7.5 kg of feed dry matter. Of course, as with all the high-concentrate diets, an adjustment period will be necessary before providing this level of corn.

Example 2. Assume you have a weaned heifer calf weighing 220 kg and you would like her to gain 0.5 kg/day. Again, you would need to change rations as the heifer grows, and I would recommend recalculating a ration at no more than 50-kg weight increments. There are no values listed in Table 4 for a 220-kg heifer, so we will need to calculate these requirements.

The values for the requirements are calculated by interpolation of values in Table 4:

$$\frac{220 - 200}{250 - 220} \times \begin{array}{l}\text{Difference in values} \\ \text{between 200-kg and} \\ \text{250-kg heifer}\end{array} + \begin{array}{l}\text{Values for a} \\ \text{200-kg} \\ \text{heifer}\end{array}$$

For dry matter (DM):

$$0.67 \times (6.5 - 6.0) + 6.0 = 6.3 \text{ kg}$$

Similar calculations give the requirements for a 220-kg heifer to gain 0.5 kg/day of 6.3 kg of DM, 0.60 kg of CP and 3.8 kg of TDN.

For this problem, assume that you will feed corn and coastal Bermuda grass hay. The nutrient composition is again obtained from NRC (Table 7). In this example, we will use the Pearson Square method of determining the amounts of corn and hay needed to meet our TDN requirement (3.8 kg).

First, we must determine what percentage of the total requirements are TDN:

$$\frac{3.8 \text{ kg TDN}}{6.3 \text{ kg DM}} = 60\% \text{ TDN in ration}$$

Then set up a Pearson Square with per cent TDN from corn and hay on the left, top to bottom, and the required per cent TDN in the middle. Subtract (absolutely) across the diagonals, giving proportions for each ingredient that can be converted to per cent DM and kg DM from each ingredient:

TDN from		*Portion of ration from*
corn 91		11 parts corn
	60	
hay 49		31 parts hay

Ration requires

$$\frac{11}{11 + 31} = 26\% \text{ of ration DM from corn}$$

or 26% of 6.3 = 1.64 kg of DM from corn

$$\frac{31}{11 + 31} = 74\% \text{ of ration DM from hay}$$

or 74% of 6.3 = 4.66 kg of DM from hay.

The solution to this Pearson Square shows that 1.64 kg of DM from corn and 4.66 kg of DM from hay will meet the TDN requirement. To convert the DM values to as-fed values, divide each by the DM per cent in the ingredient:

1.64/0.89 = 1.84 kg of corn on as-fed basis
4.66/0.915 = 5.09 kg of hay on as-fed basis

Again, determine if our amounts of hay and corn that meet the TDN requirement will also meet the requirement for CP. In this example, the CP requirement is met and the complete ration is given in Table 9 with the same assumptions for calcium, phosphorus and vitamin A as in example 1.

NUTRITION OF THE BEEF COW

Any producer not weaning a 90 per cent plus calf crop is not really in the cattle business. A definition of a 90 per cent calf crop is that for every 100 cows exposed at breeding, there are 90 calves to sell at weaning 15 to 17 months later. To achieve a 90 per cent calf crop, the nutritional needs of the cow must be met every day and under changing circumstances. If a cow is not adequately fed during the last trimester of gestation, she will use her body reserves to nourish the fetus. Consequently, she will calve thin and will fail to rebreed. After calving, the priorities for nutrients are maintenance of life, milk production and lastly, reproduction. If a cow is not a good milk producer, she should have been culled. If she is a good milk producer, she must have nutrients to meet her genetic capabilities for milk production plus the nutrients to reproduce. Reproduction will be the first function to suffer with poor nutrition.

Table 9. Example Ration for 220-kg Heifer Calf to Gain 0.5 kg/day

Item	DM (kg)	CP (kg)	TDN (kg)
Requirements	6.3	0.60	3.8
Ration (as fed)			
5.09 kg coastal bermudagrass hay	4.66	0.44	2.28
1.84 kg corn	1.64	0.16	1.49
Totals	6.3	0.60	3.77

General

Calving Season. A finite calving season is a pre-requisite to any nutritional consideration in a cow herd. With prolonged or even year-round calving seasons, gestating cows are overfed and lactating cows are underfed. The nutrient needs of a cow vary dramatically over a production year (Table 6), and cows should be grouped so requirements for all stages of production are met. Otherwise, a sensible nutritional program is impossible. Unfortunately, available data and experiences indicate that many producers have no finite calving season, or have one of too long a duration. In one study of 166 herds in western Canada, only 7 per cent of the herds had calving seasons of 65 days or less, only 44 per cent had calving seasons of 105 days or less, and 41 per cent had calving seasons of more than 125 days—over 4 months long!

Many producers feel that they need to have a long breeding season to get all cows pregnant. However, a logical argument can be constructed that a short calving season (60 days) would increase the pregnancy rate over time. With a 4-month calving season, a cow could have an average interval between calves of 405 days and stay in the herd for six calf crops. If her daughters were selected as herd replacements, they potentially would also have long calving intervals. Even if heritabilities for reproductive traits are low, which recent data dispute, continual selection for a long calving interval can certainly reduce overall herd pregnancy rate.

Environment. A short calving season also has advantages when fitting a calving season to the local environment. Figures 2 and 3 illustrate the effects of environment on weaning weight and average calving interval (Boleman LL, Unpublished data, Texas A&M University) from data collected in south central Texas. The difference between the highest birth-month weaning weight and the lowest birth-month weaning weight was 42 kg (Fig. 2). The heaviest weaning weights occurred with the birth-months of December through April, and the average weaning weight of calves born during these five birth-months was 216 kg, while the average weaning weight of calves from the remaining seven birth-months was 193 kg—a 23-kg difference due to the season in which calves were born.

Cows calving in November and December maintained an average calving interval of approximately 365 days, while cows calving in August had an average calving interval of 514 days (Fig. 3). Cows

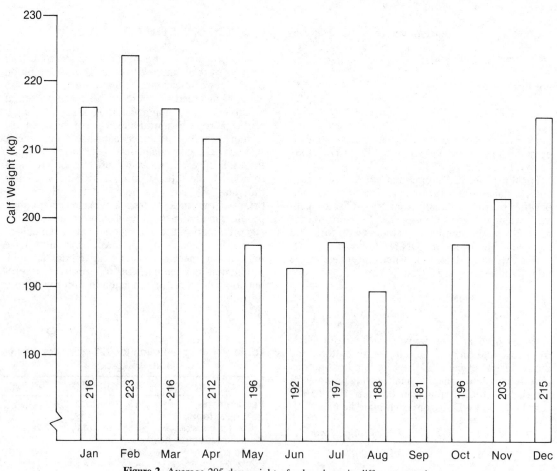

Figure 2. Average 205-day weight of calves born in different months.

calving in the months from November through April had an average calving interval of 376 days, and cows calving in the months of May through October had an average calving interval of 431 days. Note the close agreements between the calving season months that resulted in the heaviest weaning weights (December to April) and the months that resulted in the shortest calving interval (November to April). In these studies, herds received very limited supplemental feeding, and the majority of differences observed were nutritionally related.

All areas of the country obviously will not fit these data exactly, but other studies also indicate that there are months of calving that favor increased weaning weights and decreased calving intervals. Figures similar to those in Figures 2 and 3 could be created for all geographic regions of the United States—the months will shift, but the principles remain the same.

Couple these data with those previously discussed on nutritional management and the effect of calf age on weaning weight, and the argument for a short calving season—60 and certainly no more than 90 days—becomes overwhelming. Generally, this

calving season will best fit into the late winter and early spring months so that the calving season will be about 2 months ahead of grass in your area. Other options require more management and certainly more supplemental feed.

Supplemental Feeding. All nutritional considerations for the beef herd should fit around forage production in a particular area. Advice should be sought from competent forage and range management specialists in the locality. As a general rule, forages harvested by the cow are the most economical feed, but a knowledge of forage characteristics for a local area is essential for planning a feeding program for a beef herd. Again, if a calving season is planned to fit around the forage system so that high-quality "cow-harvested" forages are available when the cow has her greatest nutritional needs, supplemental feeding can be kept to a minimum and costs kept in line.

When considering supplemental feeds, do not get trapped into a "forage only" or even traditional nonforage supplements. For example, consider a situation in which cows must be supplemented (for whatever reason) with 0.45 kg of CP/day. Either 3

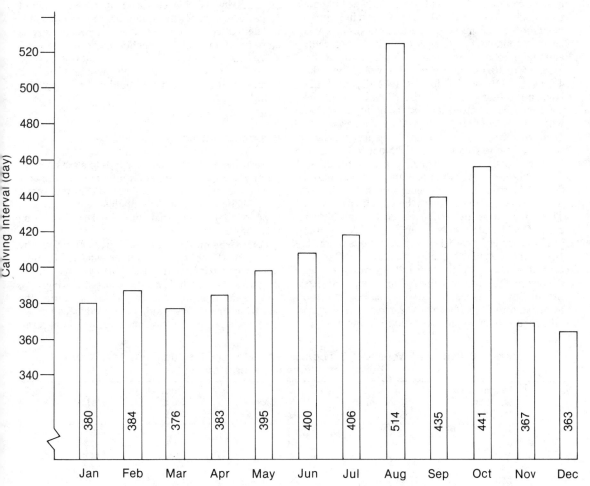

Figure 3. Average calving interval of cows calving in different months. (From Boleman LL, Texas A&M University, College Station, Texas, unpublished material.)

kg of mid-bloom alfalfa hay or 2 kg of whole cottonseed will meet this level of supplement. If alfalfa hay costs 13.2¢/kg and whole cottonseed costs 11¢/kg, it would cost 40¢/cow/day to supplement with alfalfa and 22¢/cow/day to supplement with whole cottonseed.

Consider another example in which cows must be fed 4.5 kg of TDN/day. Either 10.1 kg of coastal bermudagrass hay or 5.6 kg of corn will meet this TDN requirement. If coastal Bermuda grass hay costs 8.8¢/kg and corn costs 13.2¢/kg, it would cost 89¢/cow/day to supplement with hay and 74¢/cow/day to supplement with corn. Cows cannot function on concentrates alone, so some roughage must be fed, and grains will not always be cheap. However, the point of these two examples is that *forages are not always cheap supplements.* Individual costs should be appropriately figured for all supplemental programs. Even more exotic ingredients can sometimes be economical cattle supplements— cookie and bread crumbs, canary wastes and poultry litter are just a few examples.

One other point needs to be emphasized about supplemental feeding. Many producers attempt to winter dry pregnant cows on cured native range or in some cases cured bermudagrass. They will initiate this feeding program with proper protein supplementation, since many of these cured forages will have reasonable TDN levels (usually 40 per cent) and marginal levels in CP (4 to 6 per cent). In this case, 9.5 to 10.5 kg of cured forage would meet the 4.2 kg of TDN needed for a 450-kg dry cow. But later in the year problems arise. First, some of the cows may have calved and be lactating, and now, with a TDN requirement of 6.4 kg, the cow would need to consume 14 to 16 kg of this forage. Since cows are able to eat only 2.0 to 2.5 per cent of their body weight in DM with this type of feed, about 9.5 to 11 kg of DM is the maximum consumption. Second, protein and TDN values of these types of forages continue to decline as the season progresses. They may get as low as 2 per cent CP and 30 per cent TDN. In late winter, even our dry cow would have to consume over 13 kg of this low-quality feed. Now, with the lower quality feed, 1.5 to 2.0 per cent of her body weight or 7 to 9 kg would be her maximum DM consumption. Third, not only has the quality of these forages decreased, but the available forage also becomes scarce in late winter. Although protein supplementation will increase digestibility of low-quality forages, there is a limit, and in the situations described, protein supplementation will not alleviate the nutritional deficiencies.

Cow Size. It is important to recognize that when we use weight to designate cow size, we are talking about a cow in moderate body condition, neither thin nor fat. A starved-down cow who weighs 450 kg is not a 450-kg cow but is still the size of cow her frame size dictates. When making nutritional recommendations, consideration must be given to the size of cows in the herd and possibly even sorting cows if there are drastic differences in size. The DM, CP and TDN requirements generally used for rule-of-thumb guidelines are for a 450-kg cow. From Table 6, the requirements of such a cow during the last third of gestation are 8.1 kg of DM, 0.48 kg of CP and 4.2 kg of TDN. If cow size is changed to a 550-kg cow, DM requirements increase 15 per cent, CP requirements increase 12 per cent and TDN requirements increase 13 per cent.

Milk Production. Milk production is seldom taken into serious consideration by producers when evaluating nutrient requirements. However, more attention should be given to level of milk production than to cow size. If cow size is increased from 450 kg to 550 kg, TDN level must be increased by about 13 per cent to meet the additional requirements for the 550-kg cow. However, if the same cow size is considered and milk production increases from 4.5 kg/day to 9.0 kg/day, TDN levels need to be raised 20 to 25 per cent to meet the increased nutrient requirement to support the additional milk production.

Prepartum Nutrition

Ensuring next year's calf depends to a great extent on meeting the nutritional requirements of the cow during the last trimester of gestation for this year's calf. Viability and vitality of this year's calf also depend on the maternal nutritional status during this period.

Fetal Growth. As can be seen from Table 10, the conceptus (fetus, fetal membranes and fetal fluids) weighs approximately 14 kg at 180 days of gestation. By parturition (280 days) the conceptus weighs 58 kg—a gain of approximately 0.45 kg/day during the last trimester of gestation. Fetal weight comprises the largest portion of this conceptus weight at term.

Table 10. Predicted Weights of Conceptus, Fetal Membranes and Fluids, and Fetus During Last Trimester of Gestation

Length of Gestation (days)	Conceptus (kg)	Fetus Membranes (kg)	Fetal Fluids (kg)	Fetus (kg)
180	13.9	1.1	6.8	5.9
200	18.9	1.4	7.8	9.7
220	25.5	1.8	8.9	14.8
240	33.9	2.2	10.2	21.6
260	44.6	2.6	12.4	29.6
280	57.9	3.0	16.4	38.4

An approximation of conceptus weight can be made by multiplying the weight of the calf at birth by 150 per cent.

Once pregnancy is initiated, it will be maintained even under severe nutritional deprivation of the dam. The conceptus has a high priority for nutrients, and the maternal system will sacrifice body reserves to meet this demand. Weight of the conceptus at term will be reduced somewhat under severe nutrient restriction, but the major portion of this weight gain will be maintained at all costs to the maternal system. The underfed cow will, in essence, lose weight proportional to the weight gain of the conceptus.

Calf Mortality and Morbidity. Cows underfed during the prepartum period produce less colostrum of lower quality (Table 11) and less milk, which can have a dramatic effect on mortality, morbidity and subsequent growth rate of the calf.[1] The single most important factor in preventing neonatal disease is to ensure that the calf receives adequate quantities of good quality colostrum immediately after birth. When calves receive less than 90 gm of total colostral immunoglobulins and are exposed to a pathogenic agent, they will develop an acute, severe diarrhea and, regardless of treatment, will generally die. Thus, inadequate nutrition during the prepartum period dramatically increases the incidence and severity of disease in calves exposed to pathogenic organisms.

In a study where cows received a diet meeting only 70 per cent of their energy needs during the last 100 days prepartum, 52 per cent of the calves required treatment for scours, whereas only 33 per cent of calves from cows fed adequately prepartum required treatment.[1] All cows and calves comingled and received the same feeding regime after parturition. Nineteen per cent of calves from nutritionally deprived dams died prior to weaning, whereas there was no calf loss in the group fed adequately during the prepartum period. Additionally, milk production was decreased by 1.4 kg/day and weaning weights reduced by 11.8 kg when the cows were restricted in energy intake.

Body Condition and Nutrition. Determination of adequate levels of prepartum nutrition is difficult, since cows differ in their response to a given level of nutrition due to differences in age, size, milking

Table 12. Effect of Body Condition at Calving on Rebreeding

Condition at Calving	Pregnant After Breeding (per cent)	
	20 days	80 days
Thin	25	72
Moderate	35	89
Good	39	92

ability, stage of pregnancy, environment, body condition and probably other factors we fail to recognize. The nutrient requirements in Tables 5 and 6 are only good approximations. Reproductive rate in beef herds might be increased by evaluating body condition as a criterion for determining nutritional status. This is in no way contradictory to previous discussions of prepartum nutrition since *body condition score (BCS) at calving is a direct measure of prepartum nutritional status.*

A significant relationship has been shown between BCS at calving and subsequent pregnancy rate. Only 72 per cent of cows that were thin at calving were pregnant after an 80-day breeding season that started 82 days after the first cow calved. This compares to 89 and 92 per cent, respectively, of cows in moderate and good condition at calving being pregnant after 80 days of breeding. Note also the decrease in cows pregnant early in the breeding season when they were thin at calving (Table 12).

The main reason for the lowered pregnancy rate in thin cows in this study was a decreased incidence of return to estrus after calving. If a cow herd is to average a 12-month calving interval, very few cows can fail to return to estrus by 80 days postpartum. In fact, in most herds maintaining a 12-month calving interval, there will be very few individual cows with calving intervals outside of the range of 345 to 385 days. Most of the cows in moderate and good condition at calving returned to estrus by 80 days after calving, whereas only 62 per cent of cows that were thin at calving had shown estrus by this time (Table 13). There must be adequate condition on the cow at parturition if we expect her to be in estrus within 80 days after calving.

These data certainly are well supported if we

Table 11. Effect of Malnutrition on Colostrum and Immunoglobulin Production Postpartum

		Adequately Fed Cows	Inadequately Fed Cows
Body weight at calving	(kg)	473	345
Condition at calving		good	thin
Colostral immunoglobulin concentration	IgG	57	56
immediately after	IgM	5.2	6.4
calving (mg/ml)	IgA	5.4	7.0
Total colostrum			
produced in first 6 hours after	mean	2500	1200
calving (ml)	range	1700–4900	150–1900
Total immunoglobulins secreted in the			
first 6 hours after calving	(gm)	144	76

Table 13. Cows Showing Estrus as Related to Body Condition at Calving

Condition at Calving	In Estrus Postpartum (cumulative per cent)					
	40 days	*50 days*	*60 days*	*70 days*	*80 days*	*90 days*
Thin	19	34	46	55	62	66
Moderate	21	45	61	79	88	92
Good	31	42	91	96	98	100

recognize that weight gain or loss during the last trimester of gestation and BCS are directly related. Large net weight losses during the last trimester of gestation cause cows to calve in low BCS, which results in a decreased percentage of cows in estrus early in the subsequent breeding season.[2, 10] In fact, cows with extreme weight losses prepartum often fail to show estrus at any time during the breeding season. The converse also appears to be true. Preliminary data (Spitzer JC, Unpublished data, Clemson University) from an on-going project involving 130 cows over 2 years are depicted in Table 14. *All* of these cows received a high level of nutrition during the last trimester of gestation and calved with moderate to good BCS. A high proportion showed estrus early in the breeding season regardless of how they were fed postpartum.

The key to early return to estrus in beef cows is adequate prepartum levels of nutrition, which result in cows calving in moderate to good BCS. As previously discussed, this is also the key to a healthy calf and a milk supply capable of supporting heavy weaning weights.

By recognizing differences in body condition we can plan a supplemental feeding program more intelligently so that cows are maintained in satisfac-

Table 14. Effect of Postpartum Nutrition on Occurrence of Estrus When Cows Calved with Moderate to Good BCS*

Group†	In Estrus Postpartum (cumulative per cent)		
	20 Days	*40 Days*	*60 Days*
High	82	96	100
Moderate	90	97	100
Low	81	91	100
Low-flush	86	96	100

*From Spitzer JC: Unpublished data, Clemson University, 1984.
†High: Fed to gain 0.45 to 0.68 kg per day from calving through the breeding season. Moderate: Fed to maintain body weight from calving through the breeding season. Low: Fed to lose 0.45 to 0.68 kg per day from calving through the breeding season. Low-flush: Fed to lose 0.45 to 0.68 kg per day until 14 days prior to the start of the breeding season and then fed a flushing ration calculated to ensure rapid weight gains for a 28-day period.

tory condition at calving. Table 15 depicts the 1 through 9 scoring system utilized in evaluating cow condition. These scores describe the body condition of fatness of a cow and have no implication as to quality or merit. Any cow could vary in condition over the 9-point system depending on lactational status and feed supply. Additional research has demonstrated that a 450-kg cow can gain or lose 25 to 35 per cent of her body weight. This would allow a range in weight of 290 to 610 kg, and with our 9-point system allows approximately 35 kg between body condition scores. On-going studies suggest that 35 kg is indeed needed to change condition by 1 point in a 450-kg cow.

Satisfactory or acceptable condition cannot be precisely defined at this time, because it will vary with the environment and type of cattle. Additional research is needed, but the practical implications of the effect of body condition at calving on return to estrus after calving make it imperative that we develop and utilize some system in managing beef herds.

Probably the most efficient way to utilize these data would be to sort cows by condition 90 to 100 days prior to calving. It is then possible to feed each group in an attempt to control body condition to have all cows with condition scores of 5, 6, and 7 at calving (Table 16). These appear to be the most logical scores to maximize reproductive performance while minimizing supplemental feeding.

Postpartum Nutrition

As previously discussed in the section on nutrient requirements, parturition signals dramatic changes in the nutritional needs of the cow. The reproductive tract of the cow is undergoing involution, and she must re-establish endocrine function, cyclicity and lactation. There are also many interacting and additional facets affecting postpartum reproductive performance.

Suckling. While the nutrient requirements to maintain lactation are large, there appears to be a compounding of this effect because the suckling stimulus depresses the return to postpartum estrus even when these nutritional needs for milk production are satisfied. This neuroendocrine depression of reproductive performance is independent of lactation. If the suckling stimulus is eliminated or altered, the interval to first postpartum estrus is shortened. Complete removal of lactational stress results in a marked increase in rebreeding efficiency. The effects of early weaning of calves on the reproductive performance of their dams and subsequent calf performance to weaning are shown in Table 17. Even removing only a portion of the suckling stress by creep feeding calves enhanced the pregnancy rate. However, early weaning may cause more problems than it cures, such as the problem of management and rearing of early weaned calves. The cost of feeding the early weaned calf from 60 days to 7 months of age is often too high to be

Table 15. System of Body Condition Scoring (BCS) for Beef Cattle

Group	BCS	Definition
Thin condition	1	EMACIATED. Cow is extremely emaciated with no detectable fat over spinous processes, transverse processes, hip bones or ribs. Tail-head and ribs project quite prominently.
	2	POOR. Cow still appears somewhat emaciated but tail-head and ribs are less prominent. Individual spinous processes are still rather sharp to the touch, but some tissue cover exists along spine.
	3	THIN. Ribs are still individually identifiable but not quite as sharp to the touch. There is obvious palpable fat along spine and over tail-head with some tissue cover over dorsal portion of ribs.
Borderline condition	4	BORDERLINE. Individual ribs are no longer visually obvious. The spinous processes can be identifed individually on palpation but feel rounded rather than sharp. Some fat cover over ribs, transverse processes and hip bones.
Optimum moderate condition	5	MODERATE. Cow has generally good overall appearance. Upon palpation, fat cover over ribs feels spongy, and areas on either side of tail-head now have palpable fat cover.
	6	HIGH MODERATE. Firm pressure now needs to be applied to feel spinous processes. A high degree of fat cover is palpable over ribs and around tail-head.
	7	GOOD. Cow appears fleshy and obviously carries considerable fat. Very spongy fat cover over ribs and over and around tail-head. In fact "rounds" or "pones" beginning to be obvious. Some fat around vulva and in crotch.
Fat condition	8	FAT. Cow very fleshy and overconditioned. Spinous processes almost impossible to palpate. Cow has large fat deposits over ribs, around tail-head and below vulva. "Rounds" or "pones" are obvious.
	9	EXTREMELY FAT. Cow obviously extremely wasty and patchy and looks blocky. Tail-head and hips buried in fatty tissue and "rounds" or "pones" of fat are protruding. Bone structure no longer visible and barely palpable. Animal's mobility may even be impaired by large fatty deposits.

Table 16. Recommendations for Feeding Cows in Varying Condition 90 to 100 Days Prior to Calving to Have Good Postpartum Reproductive Performance*†

Condition 90 to 100 Days Prior to Calving		Desired Condition at Calving	Recommendations
Too Thin	1	5	Needs to gain in excess of 160 kg. Economics questionable
	2	5	Needs to gain 135 to 160 kg. Economics questionable.
	3	5	Needs to gain 90 to 135 kg.
Borderline	4	5	Needs to gain 70 to 90 kg.
Optimum	5	5–7	Needs to gain weight of fetus—45 kg.
	6	5–7	Needs to gain weight of fetus—45 kg.
	7	5–7	No weight gain needed
Too Fat	8	5–7	Can probably lose 20 to 70 kg.
	9	5–7	Can probably lose 45 to 90 kg.

*Assumes a cow weighing 450 kg with a body condition score of 5.
†An allowance of 45 kg has been made for growth of the conceptus during the last trimester. This occurs regardless of body condition, and this weight gain needs to be satisfied.

Table 17. Effect of Early Weaning or Creep Feeding Starting 60 Days After Calving on Pregnancy Rates in a 90-day Breeding Season

	Control	Calves Creep-Fed	Calves Weaned
Pregnant	29%	57%	100%
Calf weight @ 60 days	52 kg	45 kg	61 kg
Calf weight @ 205 days	160 kg	171 kg	171 kg

economical except under severe drought or other extreme conditions.

Since the effect of suckling is more dependent on udder stimulation than on absolute milk production, a study investigating once-daily suckling as a management alternative has been recently reported. Once-daily suckling was initiated at 30 days postpartum and continued until first estrus in first-calf cows. Once-daily suckling decreased the postpartum interval to estrus by 99 days, and 74 per cent of the once-daily suckled cows had returned to estrus prior to 90 days postpartum, while only 6 per cent of the normally suckled cows had returned to estrus by 90 days postpartum. Milk production of the cow and total calf gain from birth to weaning were not altered by once-daily suckling, and no difference was noted in health problems.

Interaction of Postpartum Nutrition with BCS and Return to Estrus. As previously discussed, cows that are thin at calving are more likely to have an extended postpartum interval to estrus, whereas cows that are in moderate to good condition will have a shorter postpartum interval to estrus. Cows calving in moderate to good body condition returned to estrus at a satisfactory rate regardless of postpartum nutrition. However, if the weight loss after calving is severe, even cows calving in good body condition may not cycle or may initiate cyclicity and then become anestrous. These effects are compounded if cows receive low levels of nutrition both before and after calving (Table 18).

Pregnancy Rate. Note also from Table 18 that first service pregnancy rates are dramatically reduced when cows are receiving low levels of nutrition after calving. Based only on cows showing estrus, the first service pregnancy rate was halved by low levels of feed after calving. In general, evidence points to maximum pregnancy rates when cows are gaining weight during the breeding season. However, all of this is dependent on adequate BCS at parturition.

First-Calf Heifers

Heifers calving for the first time tend to have lower pregnancy rates and breed back later in the breeding season following their first calf. Many first-calf heifers take longer to return to estrus following calving than do mature cows and fail to rebreed or breed late during their second breeding season. It has been clearly shown that heifers that calve early with their first calf have higher lifetime production than do heifers that calve late with their first calf.[7] Table 19 shows the delay in return to estrus after calving in first-calf heifers.[11] This delay is caused by the greater stress that calving places on the first-calf heifer. In addition to performing all of the body functions of mature cows—body maintenance, calving, lactation and rebreeding—heifers must continue to grow and develop. The heifer has a limited capacity for feed intake because of her smaller size and because her incisor teeth are being shed at this time. Consequently, the ability of the heifer to consume feed, particularly low-quality roughages, is limited. Thus, some body functions are sacrificed, and reproductive capability suffers first. Additional stress is added if dystocia occurs.

Three management practices have evolved to overcome problems in rebreeding first-calf heifers successfully. One management practice is to breed virgin heifers 20 days earlier than the rest of the cow herd to ensure early calves. If it is recognized that first-calf heifers take longer to return to estrus and that many will not be able to maintain a 12-month calving interval, these facts need planning. Calving early gives heifers extra time to return to estrus during the second breeding season, which corresponds to that of the regular cow herd. In one study this practice increased the weight of the calf weaned by 15 kg per cow and increased the number of cows in estrus and pregnant during the first 25 days of breeding by 17 and 14 per cent, respectively.[7] A second management practice is to separate

Table 18. Reproductive Performance of Mature Cows on Low Levels of Energy Both Before and After Calving*

Energy		Cows Pregnant		Cows Showing Estrus (per cent)			Pregnant First Service (per cent)
Before	After	20 days	80 days	50 days	70 days	90 days	
High	High	60	95	65	90	95	67
Low	Low	15	20	22	22	22	33

*From Wiltbank JN, Rowden WW, Inglis JE, et al.: Effect of energy level on reproductive phenomena of mature Hereford cows. J Anim Sci 21:219, 1962.

Table 19. Per Cent of Cows Showing Estrus at Various Times After Calving*

| Group | In Estrus Postpartum (Cumulative per cent) | | | | | |
	40 days	50 days	60 days	70 days	80 days	90 days
Mature cows	30	53	72	82	89	94
First-calf heifers	15	24	47	62	68	79

*From Wiltbank JN: Research needs in beef cattle reproduction. J Anim Sci 31:755, 1970.

heifers from mature cows and provide higher quality feeds during the last 2 to 3 months of pregnancy and through the breeding season. Sorting cows may be one of the best (but most infrequently used) management tools to increase the reproductive rate in first-calf heifers. If wintered with the older cow herd during late gestation, heifers will be underfed because they are too small and not aggressive enough to compete for their portion of the feed. The result is that the animals having the greatest need for supplemental feed (first-calf heifers) receive less than needed and animals with a lesser need (mature cows) receive more than their share.

A third management practice, used less often but gaining in popularity, is to alter the suckling status as described in the section on suckling. If faced with a group of thin or late calving first-calf heifers, early weaning or once-a-day suckling may be the only salvation for reproductive performance.

PUBERTY IN THE BEEF FEMALE

Heifers should be bred 20 days ahead of the regular cow herd. However, heifers cannot be bred early unless they reach puberty prior to, or early in, their first breeding season. One alternative is to calve heifers as 3-year-olds. However, in our present economic climate, it is only in extreme circumstances that calving heifers as 3-year-olds would be economical. Heifers bred to calve at 2 years produce more calves in a lifetime, with higher average weaning weights, than those bred to calve first at 3 years. In addition, high monthly maintenance costs make

it necessary to get heifers into production as early as possible.

Age and Breed Effect. To calve at about 2 years of age, a heifer must reach puberty by 13 to 16 months of age. There is much variation in age at puberty among heifers, and breed, environment, nutrition and other factors must be considered. Genetic selection definitely plays a role in determining the age and weight at puberty among and within breeds of cattle. Most heifers show estrus between 13 and 16 months of age if they are of sufficient size and weight. Exceptions to this include Brahman heifers, Brahman crossbred heifers and heifers from some breeds derived from crosses with Brahman. Approximately 90 per cent of Brahman crossbred heifers show estrus, provided sufficient weight is attained, at 15 to 17 months, while purebred Brahman heifers may be close to 20 months of age before 90 per cent reach puberty. Heritability estimates for age and weight at puberty are moderate to high. This means that selection for heifers reaching puberty between 13 and 16 months of age would eventually reduce the average age at puberty within a herd or breed.

Nutrition Effect. In practical breeding situations, the nutrition of the heifer, or weight achieved, is the greatest factor in determining onset of puberty. A summary of data available on weight necessary for 50, 70 or 90 per cent of heifers reaching puberty appears in Table 20. For example, 50 per cent of Angus × Hereford heifers 13 to 16 months of age could be expected to have reached puberty at 260 kg body weight. This is the average weight at puberty. To expect 90 per cent of these Angus ×

Table 20. Estimates for Heifers Reaching Puberty at Various Weights

| | Heifers Reaching Puberty | | |
	50 per cent in Estrus	70 per cent in Estrus	90 per cent in Estrus
Angus	250	272	295
Brahman	306	329	340
Brangus	272	295	318
Charolais	318	340	352
Hereford	272	295	318
Santa Gerturdis	306	329	340
Shorthorn	226	249	272
Brahman × British	306	329	340
British × British	261	283	306
Charolais × British	306	329	352
Jersey × British	226	249	272
Limousin × British	295	318	352
Simmental × British	283	306	340
S Devon × British	272	295	329

Hereford heifers to be in estrus, each would need to weigh 306 kg. These weights should be considered as target weights to be achieved prior to the start of the breeding season. Information is presented for other breeds for which there are sufficient data to make recommendations. If a particular breed or crossbreed is not represented on this chart, a rule-of-thumb is that each heifer should achieve a minimum of 65 per cent of her mature weight before the first breeding season.

Management and Feeding Groups. Consider, for example, a producer who has 100 Angus × Hereford heifers with an average weaning weight of 214 kg on September 1. These heifers will be on winter pasture until April 1, the start of the breeding season, and past performance on this ranch indicates that the heifers will gain 0.45 kg per day. These heifers would then weigh 310 kg on April 1, an adequate weight to expect 90 per cent or more to come into estrus during the breeding season. But 214 kg was the average weight at weaning. The lightest heifer weighed 160 kg and the heaviest heifer weighed 250 kg at weaning. If all heifers gained 0.45 kg per day for 211 days, the lightest heifer would weigh 255 kg and the heaviest heifer 346 kg. Some of the heifers would be too light and other much heavier than necessary to achieve puberty. Averages will not get the job done. For 90 per cent of these Angus × Hereford heifers to be in estrus during the breeding season, each individual should weigh the target weight of 306 kg.

Ideally, selecting only replacement heifers with heavy actual weaning weights would be the most efficient way to achieve economical beef production. Heavy heifers would need to gain less weight from weaning to the start of breeding to reach target weights discussed above. Additionally, heavy actual weaning weights reflect a dam with good milk production who calved early in the calving season, both highly desirable traits that will be passed on to the heifer.

The ideal, however, is seldom realized because many variables influence heifer selection programs. Long, extended calving seasons, the need for a large number of replacement heifers and value as a registered animal are a few considerations that may cause retention of lightweight heifers. But these heifers still must reach target weights to have satisfactory reproductive performance.

Recent work has shown an increase in reproductive performance when heifers were sorted into light and heavy groups and fed to reach target weights. Heifers fed separately were more similar in weight at the start of the breeding season than were heifers fed together. Sorting heifers into feed groups resulted in a 19 per cent increase for light heifers cycling at the start of the breeding season and an increase of 15 per cent in total heifers pregnant after 45 days of breeding.

A projection for the previous 100 Angus × Hereford heifers when fed together or sorted is summarized in Table 21. If fed together, the projection is that 57 per cent of the heifers would be pregnant after 20 days and 81 per cent would be pregnant after 40 days of the breeding season. This assumes a 70 per cent conception rate to a single breeding.

Sorting the heifers into three groups based on weight gain needed to reach a target weight would increase the proportion of heifers pregnant to 63 per cent in 20 days and 90 per cent in 40 days of breeding. More heifers would be pregnant and more would be pregnant early in the breeding season if the heifers were sorted. The diets necessary for these weight gains could be calculated by using the data listed in Table 4 and the examples in the section on ration formulation.

Feed costs would be similar—the average daily gain is 0.45 kg per day for both groups. However, when heifers are sorted, feed dollars have been more judiciously allocated. Reproductive performance in the heifers fed as a group would probably be less than indicated in this example. The light heifers would not gain as much as the heavy heifers because of competition for available feed.

Feeding virgin heifers to appropriate weights prior to first breeding also influences rebreeding after the first calf. There are two problems with heifers being too light at first breeding. Not many get pregnant as virgin heifers, and they have a

Table 21. Projections for Reproductive Performance When Heifers are Sorted or Fed as a Group

Feeding Group	Number of Heifers	Weaning Weight (kg)	Daily Gain to Breeding (kg)	Projected Wt. at Breeding (kg)	Expected in Estrus (per cent)		Expected Pregnant (per cent)	
					20 days	40 days	20 days	40 days
Fed together								
Heavy	50	228	0.45	323	100	100	70	92
Moderate	30	210	0.45	305	70	90	49	77
Light	20	186	0.45	282	50	70	35	60
Average		214	0.45	310	81	91	57	81
Fed separately								
Heavy	50	228	0.39	309	90	100	63	90
Moderate	30	210	0.50	315	90	100	63	90
Light	20	186	0.59	311	90	100	63	90
Average		214	0.45	312	90	100	63	90

greatly reduced chance of getting pregnant while nursing their first calf. In a study involving Hereford heifers, 90 per cent of the heifers weighing more than 272 kg at the start of breeding were pregnant, while 56 percent of the heifers weighing less than 249 kg were pregnant. In the subsequent breeding season, only 18 per cent of those calving from the lightweight group were pregnant. Only 8 per cent of the lightweight heifers exposed the first year did not skip a calf. A few heifers get pregnant at very light weights, but calving problems will be increased and their chances of being rebred while nursing their first calves are practically nonexistent.

NUTRITION OF THE BEEF BULL

Most producers at least recognize a relationship between nutrition and reproduction in the cow herd. Unfortunately, most fail to recognize the importance of nutrition to the bull, even though many can relate cases in which reductions in overall herd fertility seemed caused by nutritionally related bull failures. Lack of data compounds the problems in making specific recommendations on the effects of nutrition on reproduction in bulls. Additionally, what reports are available generally have confounding influences and/or are not applicable to modern beef production practices. However, the available data will be discussed here and conclusions reached where appropriate.

General

There are few data indicating relationships between specific nutrients and reproduction in *mature* bulls. Spermatozoa production and semen quality or quantity in mature bulls are not affected by diets varying widely in carbohydrate or protein content.[3] However, there does appear to be some reduction in spermatozoa production if TDN levels are below 60 to 70 per cent of NRC requirements (refer to Table 3). Severe protein deficiency can reduce spermatozoa production and ejaculate volume, although some motile sperm cells are ejaculated even up to death of the bull from protein deprivation.[3] A reduction in libido and increases in abnormal mating behavior have been reported in severely undernourished bulls and in obese bulls. It appears to be prudent management practice to maintain breeding bulls in moderate to good body condition analogous to the 5 to 7 BCS for cows.

Although high levels of supplemental vitamins and minerals have been advocated, data are scarce to support these recommendations. Providing levels of vitamin A and E supplementation above those already recommended for the entire cow herd (see earlier section on vitamins) does not seem efficacious in enhancing male reproductive capabilities. Although vitamin A has been shown to be essential for maintaining the integrity of seminiferous tubule epithelium, other deficiency symptoms are manifest prior to the appearance of abnormal sperm cells in the ejaculate. Therefore, warning signals are broadcast long before reproduction is impaired.

Again, data are lacking on the specific effects of mineral deficiencies on bull reproduction. Again, the recommendations made for the entire cow herd in the earlier section on minerals also seem to be adequate for the bull.

Calving Seasons. When producers have a finite breeding season, bulls are commonly allowed to fend for themselves between breeding seasons. If a finite breeding schedule is not practiced, it is assumed that bulls will "get along" on the same diet as that of the cow herd they accompany. In all probability, neither of these practices will meet the nutritional needs of the bull on a year-round basis and may affect fertility. Due to the spermatogenic cycle, if a bull is severely undernourished and spermatozoa production is affected, viable spermatozoa will not appear in the ejaculate until approximately 60 days following reinitiation of sperm production. It certainly appears to be more feasible to maintain bulls in good condition year-round to ensure that the bull will go into service immediately upon being turned with cows.

Bulls will lose weight during the breeding season. It is not uncommon for a bull to lose over 1.4 kg/day during a finite breeding season. This weight loss would probably occur even if he were provided a diet meeting all NRC requirements, since his interest is usually diverted to topics other than nutrition. Generally, bulls with the highest level of libido lose the most weight. Again, if BCS of 5 to 7 are maintained prior to breeding, bulls can lose weight during the breeding season without becoming excessively thin and without showing an effect on reproductive capabilities. Of course, the benefits of a short breeding season are apparent here; bulls are removed before becoming too thin. Conversely, while overfat *mature* bulls do not appear to have reductions in seminal quantity or quality, obese bulls will have decreased libido and a propensity to increased feet and leg problems.

Environment. Changes in environment, at least when bulls are initially purchased, can have a drastic effect on the ability of a bull to get cows pregnant. Bulls coming from a Central Performance Test Station or even from an on-farm test situation or from the show string will not be accustomed to forages or foraging. Generally, it will take 4 to 6 weeks to condition these bulls. Radical changes in diet should be avoided, and these bulls should be supplemented on pasture, with the supplement gradually reduced during the 4 to 6 weeks so that the bull becomes accustomed to a forage diet.

In yearling bulls it may be necessary to continue supplemental feeding since only very lush pasture will meet nutritional needs and allow for continued growth. An alternative is to rotate bulls so that they can be fed away from the cows. The best way is to have a short breeding season so young bulls can lose weight and then be "rescued" with a better diet between breeding seasons.

Puberty in Beef Bulls

It is now generally accepted by the industry that all bull calves intended for breeding be performance tested to evaluate comparative rate of gain from weaning to approximately a year of age. There is a widely held belief that level of feed on test affects reproduction and that overfeeding during this period causes infertility. However, the few experimental reports available give no support to this theory. There are some data indicating decreases in libido, but generally seminal production parameters are in fact enhanced by high levels of feed during the time of normal attainment of puberty.[3] Underfeeding may also influence capacity for semen production later in life, reducing testicular size, ejaculate volume and seminal concentration. In one study, undernourished bull calves were less efficient in replenishing spermatozoal reserves in depletion tests conducted periodically between puberty and 4 years of age.[8]

Defining puberty in bulls is more difficult than in heifers, since the latter is an all-or-none response while onset of puberty in bulls is a graduated response. Puberty has been defined as appearance of the first sperm or the first motile sperm in the ejaculate. However, the most common definition from a research standpoint and for practical measures of fertility is an ejaculate containing 50×10^6 spermatozoa with at least 10 per cent motility.

As in heifers, puberty in bulls is dependent on both age and weight. Bulls generally reach puberty (as defined) about 2 months earlier than their heifer counterparts. Therefore, as in heifers, from a practical beef production standpoint weight becomes the critical factor in attainment of puberty. Weight at puberty in bulls has not been as well defined for various breeds as weight at puberty in heifers. An estimate is that bulls need to be about 10 per cent heavier than the maximum weights presented in Table 20 for heifers. This weight appears to be adequate to enable bulls 12 to 15 months of age to reach puberty. It is then obvious that if a sound performance testing program is followed, few bulls gaining 0.9 to 1.4 kg/day will not attain the age and weight necessary for onset of puberty prior to the time they are used as yearlings. Data have been presented that show that scrotal circumference (SC) at puberty is surprisingly similar across various breed types differing in age and weight at puberty (SC at puberty = 27.9 ± 2 cm). Obviously a complete breeding soundness evaluation (BSE) will evaluate pubertal problems in a bull or population of bulls.

Growth and Development

Prior to the era of performance testing, most bulls were simply grown out and not put into service until they were 2 years of age or older. Now with the higher level of feeding, bulls can be and should be successfully used as yearlings. While it is essential to provide a level of nutrition that will allow for weight gains required for puberty, the young growing bull cannot be neglected. These bulls still have high nutritional requirements for additional growth and development (Table 3) but, like the yearling heifer and first-calf heifers, have limited size and capacity for feed intake. Additionally, changes in dentition during this time further impair consumption of an adequate diet. Either inadequate energy or inadequate protein during this time will retard growth and development of the reproductive tract, especially testicular size. Since spermatozoa output is directly related to SC in young bulls, anything that retards or decreases SC is undesirable.

SUMMARY

It is important that producers recognize the nutrient requirements of the various classes of cattle and with the brood cow recognize that her requirements change during the reproductive cycle. Emphasis should be on matching inexpensive feed resources (usually forages) with these requirements to optimize productivity at costs that will maximize profits.

Several things are prerequisite to planning a nutritional program for a beef herd: (1) a calving season of 60 days ideally, but certainly no longer than 90 days; (2) feeding of heifers so that they will reach puberty to be bred approximately 20 days ahead of the regular cow herd; (3) separation of various classes of cattle according to their requirements (i.e., virgin heifers, first-calf heifers, dry cows, lactating cows).

When these management practices have been met, recognize that the last trimester of gestation and the breeding season are the critical times of the reproductive cycle. Provide supplements of vitamin A and minerals as insurance and be concerned with balancing rations for energy and protein. Brood cows should calve with a BCS of 5 to 7 and gain weight during the breeding season.

Nutritional needs of the bull must be met for proper development of the reproductive tract. Underfeeding a young, growing bull will delay puberty and may affect capacity for spermatozoa production later in life. A high-quality diet is essential, but do not allow mature bulls to become obese. Bulls (especially young bulls) lose weight during the breeding season, so anticipate this weight loss by getting bulls in a BCS of 5 to 7 prior to the breeding season.

References

1. Corah LR, Dunn TG, Kaltenbach CC: Influence of prepartum nutrition on the reproductive performance of beef females and the performance of their progeny. J Anim Sci 41:819, 1975.
2. Dunn TG, Ingalls JE, Zimmerman DR, Wiltbank JN: Reproductive performance of 2-year-old Hereford and Angus heifers as influenced by pre- and post-calving energy intake. J Anim Sci 29:719, 1969.

3. Hentges RJ Jr.: Level of feeding and bull performance. *In* Cunha TJ, Warnick AC, Kroger M (eds): Factors Affecting Calf Crops. Gainesville, University of Florida Press, 1967.
4. Jurgens MH (ed): Animal Feeding and Nutrition, 5th ed. Dubuque, Iowa, Kendall/Hunt Publishing Company, 1982.
5. Maynard AB, Loosli JK, Hintz HF, Warner RG (eds): Animal Nutrition, 7th ed. New York, McGraw-Hill Book Company, 1979, p. 193.
6. National Research Council (NRC): Nutrient Requirements of Domestic Animals, No. 4. Nutrient requirements of beef cattle. Washington, D.C., National Academy of Sciences, National Research Council, 1976.
7. Spitzer, JC, Lefever DG, Wiltbank JN: Increase beef cow productivity by increasing reproductive performance. Colorado State University Experiment Station Bulletin, Gen. Series 949, 1975.
8. VanDemark NL, Fritz GR, Mauger RW: Effect of energy intake on reproductive performance of dairy bulls. II. Semen production and replenishment. J Dairy Sci 47:898, 1964.
9. Wiltbank JN, Warwick EJ, Vernon EH, Priode BM: Factors affecting net calf crop in beef cattle. J Anim Sci 20:409, 1961.
10. Wiltbank JN, Rowden WW, Ingalls JE, et al.: Effect of energy level on reproductive phenomena of mature Hereford cows. J Anim Sci 21:219, 1962.
11. Wiltbank JN: Research needs in beef cattle reproduction. J Anim Sci 31:755, 1970.

Genital Surgery of the Cow

Robert S. Hudson, D.V.M., M.S.
Auburn University, Auburn, Alabama

The knowledgeable veterinarian approaches surgical intervention involving the reproductive system of the cow with caution, always considering whether the condition at hand materially detracts from the potential performance of the patient, whether the condition merits a reasonably good prognosis and whether the anticipated expense is justified. Keeping these factors in mind and considering the actual and potential values of the animal, the operator decides whether to recommend temporary or minimal repair to facilitate salvage or permanent and perhaps extensive repair to restore useful reproductive function. Although it is folly to instigate a complicated, and therefore expensive, procedure for an animal of marginal worth, the valuable animal and its owner deserve the benefit of the best the profession can offer.

Many of the indications for elective surgery arise from injuries sustained during assisted parturition. Far fewer injuries occur when birth is unassisted, indicating the need for prudence and patience in all obstetrical manipulations.

Injuries associated with dystocia frequently are multiple, and thorough examination is required to avoid overlooking one or more serious conditions while concentrating on a more obvious defect. Heroic restoration is a failure if the animal ceases to perform economically. The purpose of this portion of the text is to present some of the currently useful techniques for protection from injury and for restoration to reproductive health and function.

EPISIOTOMY

Surgical incision of the vulva is indicated during an obstetrical procedure when the vulva interferes appreciably with mutation or delivery of the fetus. Specific indications include marginal fetal oversize or insufficient dilation of the vulva due to hypoplasia or juvenility.[3, 5] Induration of the vulva or vestibule caused by previous trauma may also preclude sufficient dilation. The premise is that surgical incision is preferable to bursting or laceration. Considering the advantages of avoiding serious and costly injury to the perineum of the parturient heifer or cow, episiotomy, when indicated, is a simple and rewarding procedure.

An episiotomy may be elected when the fetal head or, rarely, the gluteal prominence is presented at the vulva and it appears likely that further traction will result in tearing of the vulva. It is usually difficult to assess the need for episiotomy prior to actual presentation of the fetal part. In the presence of a decomposing fetus, partial fetotomy is preferable to episiotomy because of the difficulty in securing first intention healing in the presence of gross contamination.

Surgical Technique. Choice of the mode of anesthesia presents a unique situation. Epidural anesthesia may be sluggish in onset, particularly if the patient is recumbent. Additionally, the effect of epidural anesthesia may adversely inhibit the desired abdominal pressing of the animal once delivery is resumed. Provided the limiting fetal part, for example, the head, is stretching the vulva, local infiltration of an anesthetic agent is probably ineffective and superfluous. Careful observation has revealed no evidence of reaction to pain from incision of the grossly stretched tissues. The stretching may provide insensitivity to pain. Following delivery, anesthesia may be required in order to suture the incision.

Since the objective of episiotomy is to avoid vulvar tearing, which tends to begin at the dorsal commissure and to extend dorsally into the anus and rectum, the incision is begun at a point along the free edge of the stretched vulva 3 to 5 cm from the dorsal commissure, using a scalpel or a sharp, straight scissors. Incising entirely through the vulvar lip, the incision is continued in a dorsolateral direction, the length of the incision depending on the need for enlargement of the orifice. A 7-cm incision is usually sufficient to allow delivery of the fetus without tearing of the vulva.

Following delivery, the incision is cleansed of foreign material such as fetal fluid and is sutured with a modified vertical mattress suture pattern, the deep thrusts of the pattern passing through skin, fibrous tissue and vestibular submucosa and the superficial thrusts passing through skin alone. If the patient is to receive little or no postoperative attention, absorbable suture material such as No. 1 chromic gut is used. Otherwise, nonabsorbable suture is preferred. Careful cosmetic closure is indicated to reduce the probability of excessive fibrosis and disruption of the symmetry of the vulvar cleft, which could predispose to pneumovagina. Aftercare includes the initial application of a topical antibiotic powder and examination of the patient by the veterinarian prior to the next breeding season.

PERINEAL LACERATIONS

Lacerations of the perineum have been classified according to location and degree of tissue disruption.[8] First-degree lacerations are superficial wounds of the mucosa of the vagina or vestibule. Second-degree lacerations involve the entire wall of the vagina or vulva, or both. Third-degree defects result from laceration of the vagina and rectum as well as the anus, perineal body and vulva.

Torn or lacerated mucosa without further complications seldom requires specific treatment, and rapid healing is expected. Disruption of mucosa alone is unlikely to result in stenosis. If, however, the laceration is complicated by deep bruising of perivaginal or perivulvar tissues, severe necrosis often follows, with ascending infections of the genital or urinary tract and sometimes stenosis of the vagina. These sequelae can be avoided at times by vigorous attention to hygiene and by administration of systemic and topical antibacterial therapy.

Second-degree lacerations involving the entire vaginal wall frequently accompany forced delivery in undersized or overfat beef heifers but also may result from any obstetrical delivery when impatience or excitement guides the operator. Often the immediate effect is protrusion of perivaginal fat through the laceration. This protruding fat should be removed. Failure to do so may allow a pedunculated mass of fat to persist as the laceration heals, causing tenesmus and perhaps being mistaken for a neoplasm. The laceration, however recent, should not be sutured. Occasionally, severely bruised perivaginal fat becomes necrotic and fibrotic, causing persistent vaginal irritation, which in turn encourages tenesmus and vaginal prolapse. When irregular fibrotic masses are palpated in the perivaginal area, suggesting the condition just described, surgical

removal is indicated. Under epidural anesthesia the vagina is manually prolapsed, the vaginal wall is incised, and the mass is removed by blunt dissection. The incision is sutured with No. 1 absorbable suture material, using a vertical interrupted mattress pattern.

Occluding Adhesions of the Vagina

Severe trauma deep in the vaginal vault sometimes includes circumferential tearing of the vaginal wall. Unattended healing may lead to extensive adhesion formation, which occludes a portion of the lumen.

Diagnosis. If the adhesions form following calving injury, fluid accumulates proximal to the occlusion, eventually causing a feeling of fullness for the cow. This may result in tenesmus, which is often the first sign of the problem. Upon manual examination of the vagina, the occlusion is readily evident. In most instances the adhered tissues are relatively weak and can be separated with moderate manual force, thus releasing the trapped fluid. The ease of separation and the ragged adhesions, together with a history of calving, should help differentiate the condition from congenital segmental aplasia.

Rarely, the laceration is located in the fornix of the vagina. The occlusion then forms just caudal to the external os of the cervix, effectively sealing the cervix. The anterior end of the vagina appears as a smooth blind pouch.

Prognosis. If the occlusion has caused excessive fluid accumulation in the uterus with accompanying endometrial atrophy or obstructive bilateral salpingitis, the prognosis is poor. Adhesions in the midportion of the vagina without serious lesions anterior to that point are amenable to correction. The primary problem is preventing recurrence of the adhesions. The following technique for maintaining re-established patency has proved to be of value in some cases.

Surgical Technique. After epidural anesthesia and preparation of the perineum and accessible portion of the vagina, it is well initially to attempt manual separation of the adhered surfaces, especially if the injury is recent and the adhesions are still formative. It may be necessary to force closed forceps centrally through the area of adhesion, opening the forceps to tear open the occlusion. Any irregular pockets that have formed are flattened by incision of the mucosa. It is better to avoid excision of large areas of mucosa. Suturing is quite difficult and is not necessary.

Various pessaries have been designed for maintaining patency and preventing reformation of the adhesions. None of these has worked as well for the author as an inflatable rubber beach ball, 25 cm long when deflated, that has a grommet on the end opposite the inflation tube. Following medication of the vagina with a lanolin-based antibiotic ointment, the grommet of the beach ball is drawn snugly against the cervix by a suture through the edge of the external cervical os, using No. 3 polyamide nonabsorbable suture (Supramid). Once in place, the beach ball is inflated minimally, just enough to smooth the surface of the ball but not enough to cause severe pressure on the dilated vagina or to stimulate tenesmus when anesthesia wears off or to interfere with urination. Retention of the ball is ensured by closing the vulva with interrupted vertical mattress tape sutures at the perineal hairline. The inflation tube should be easily accessible for the convalescent period.

Aftercare consists of daily cleansing of the perineum, deflation of the beach ball, infusion of the vagina with a lanolin-based antibiotic ointment and reinflation of the ball. The vulvar sutures and the ball can be removed in 7 to 10 days. The daily topical medication should be continued until healing is near completion.

Incompetence of the Constrictor Vestibuli Muscle

A properly functioning constrictor vestibuli muscle is a primary barrier to ascending contamination of the vagina.[4] Located at the junction of the vestibule and vagina, the muscle, if undamaged, forms a constriction that is evident by its resistance when a cylindrical speculum is passed into the vagina.

Extensive lacerations in the area of this muscle or severe repeated stretching of the muscle at parturition may disrupt its function, predisposing to pneumovagina, chronic vaginitis and infertility. The condition often becomes apparent when there is additional dysfunction, such as malocclusion of the vulvar cleft caused by vulvar laceration, excessive episiotomy scars or innate conformational defects.[6]

The veterinarian who is concerned with the effects of pneumovagina must decide whether to disregard the incompetent constrictor vestibuli muscle and depend on episioplasty alone. This is the preferred approach when pneumovagina is not severe enough to cause persistent ballooning and dilation of the vaginal vault and when there is no concomitant surgical problem of the anterior vagina or cervix. Conversely, when pneumovagina is severe in spite of a properly aligned vulvar cleft, a rapidly performed alleviating technique involves placement of a deep circumferential suture (Buhner suture) to create the competence originally provided by the constrictor vestibuli muscle. Episioplasty consists of some form of the classic Caslick's operation. Both procedures are described later in the section on retention of vaginal prolapse.

Formerly, it was thought that partial closure of the vulvar cleft would necessitate artificial insemination. However, experience has demonstrated that natural service is quite possible.

Third-Degree Perineal Lacerations

Rectovaginal or rectovulvar lacerations usually occur when traction is applied to a fetus by an overzealous, excited or impatient operator. Most often the operator fails to allow sufficient time for dilation of the soft tissues of the birth canal once delivery is begun. Predisposition to injury may include a hypoplastic or stenotic vulva or an oversized fetus. It is extremely rare for a cow to sustain third-degree lacerations when calving is unassisted.

Most lacerations commence as the head of the fetus in the anterior longitudinal presentation approaches the vulvar cleft. The incidence of third-degree laceration with posterior presentation is low. The tearing begins at the dorsal commissure of the vulva and extends dorsally and cranially for a variable distance, dividing the anus, anal sphincter and rectum as well as the perineal body, vestibule and vagina. The divided tissues are severely bruised and devitalized. The immediate result will be a variable amount of tissue loss.

Management of Third-Degree Lacerations. When the operator, whether layman or veterinarian, discovers the extent of injury, there is an inclination to make immediate repair. However, the devitalized tissues do not allow for optimum healing. In fact, immediate repair, which is often unsuccessful, may cause added loss of tissue, making subsequent repair more difficult. It is better to postpone surgical correction for 4 to 6 weeks, allowing for resolution of tissue damage.

Rectovaginal defects in cattle are not always a cause of infertility. In fact, it sometimes is difficult to render an accurate prognosis. It is likely that the affected commercial cow in a herd with a limited breeding season will fail to conceive on schedule, with or without surgical repair. When breeding schedules are nonexistent, a cow of marginal value may be kept in the herd for a time without repair in hopes that she will eventually conceive against the odds. Valuable purebred animals should be restored surgically.

Once satisfactory resolution of inflammation is obtained, the cow is ready for surgery. There is little need for extensive preoperative preparation. Fasting to reduce fecal volume is contraindicated. Feces that is neither firm nor diarrheic is desirable to obviate immediate postoperative irritation. One last thorough examination of the entire reproductive tract is in order.

The patient is confined in a chute or stanchion in the standing position. If there is a calf at the side, it should be in full view of the dam. Epidural anesthetic (2 per cent procaine) in volume just sufficient to produce anesthesia of the perineum is administered, being careful to avoid anesthesia of the pelvic limbs. The tail is tied to one side by a neckrope. The perineal region and vaginal vault are cleansed by repeated flushing with a mild povidone iodine surgical detergent (Betadine Scrub). Care must be taken to avoid excessive infusion of the detergent or rinse water into the rectum because this may reflux during the procedure.

There is no need for the special longhandled instruments employed in similar procedures in the mare. The usual assortment of instruments used in routine general surgery is sufficient.

At the operator's option a tampon of 5-cm stock-inette stuffed loosely with cotton and tied with a 25-cm length of umbilical tape may be placed in the rectum cranial to the rectovaginal defect. The loose end of the tape is secured to one side of the perineal region outside the operative area, to be used after surgery for removing the tampon.

The operative area is exposed by placing tension sutures in the perineal skin near the mucocutaneous margin on each side of the disrupted dorsal commissure of the vulva and at the lacerated edges of the anus. These four sutures are anchored laterally near the tubera ischii to hold open the common cavity of the defect The cranial limit of the defect is thus revealed as a "shelf" separating the rectal and vaginal lumina, caudal to which is the common cavity created by the laceration.[6] The healed junctions of bright red rectal mucosa and pale vaginal and vestibular mucosa form a seam on each side of the common cavity extending to the perineal skin (Fig. 1). The free edge of the shelf is incised to a depth of 3 cm and extended laterally and caudally on each side, following the lines of junction of the rectal and vaginal (or vestibular) mucosae (Fig. 2). The horizontal dissection is intended to provide flaps of tissue sufficient to allow reconstruction of the rectal floor and vaginal roof. Occasionally, especially following previously unsuccessful attempts at repair, excessive fibrous scar tissue may lie along the lines of dissection. The fibrous tissue is carefully removed with minimal excision of normal tissue in order to preserve as much tissue as possible to bridge the defect.

Synthetic nonabsorbable No. 3 polyamide (Supramid) and a No. 2 or No. 3 half-circle cutting edge needle (fistula needle) are used in the modified vertical mattress suture pattern after the method of Goetze as described by Rosenberger (Fig. 3). A surgeon's knot is tied snugly by hand. Following each tie the defect is inspected carefully for proper

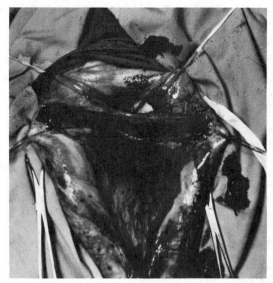

Figure 2. Dissection along margins of rectum and vagina forming flaps for reconstruction of rectal floor and vaginal roof. (From Hudson, R. S.: The Bovine Practitioner, 7:34, 1972.)

alignment and apposition because there is no opportunity for placement of sutures as an afterthought once the suture line is completed. The two tag ends of each suture are left long (8 cm) and are tied together at their ends to aid in identification of each surgical knot during removal. Both natural and synthetic absorbable suture materials have proved to be inferior to nonabsorbable sutures for this procedure, and the added effort of nonabsorbable suture removal is considered worthwhile.

It is important that the suture pattern effects abutment closure of the edges of the rectal mucosa. The suture must not penetrate the rectal mucosa. While the edges of vestibular mucosa are everted, excessive flap formation is of no value and tends to exert undue tension on the suture line.

The first one or two sutures are placed in the shelf cranial to its free edge in order to establish the pattern of tissue relationship prior to suturing the actual defect. The cranial limit of the defect is most vulnerable to dehiscence. Sutures are placed at 1-cm intervals until the rectum and vestibule are reconstructed, with the perineal body in between, to within 1 cm of the perineal skin. Vertical dissection is then made, beginning at the anus and extending ventrally to the point of the original dorsal commissure of the vulva, or, if there is an indication of malocclusion of the vulvar lips, the dissection is extended farther, along the edges of the labia. The closure of the horizontal dissection is completed, after which the vertical perineal incision is closed with interrupted vertical mattress sutures of 0.4-mm nonabsorbable material (Fig. 4).

Aftercare consists of the initial application of an antibacterial powder, furazolidone (Topazone), to the perineal suture line and administration of systemic antibiotics for 5 days. Little advantage is

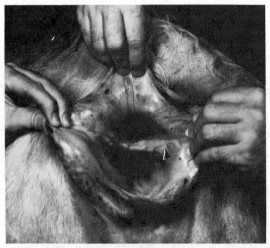

Figure 1. Third degree perineal laceration in a cow. Note common opening of rectum and vagina. Arrow marks healed junction of rectal and vaginal mucosae.

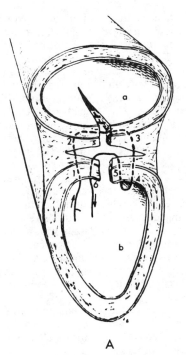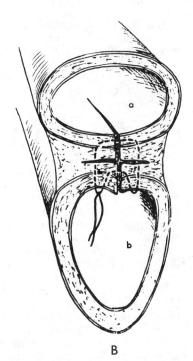

A   B

Figure 3. *A,* Pattern for closure of perineal laceration. (1) Deep thrust through left vaginal flap, (2) thrust through left perirectal tissue and rectal submucosa, (3) thrust through right rectal submucosa and perirectal tissue, (4) deep thrust through right vaginal flap into vaginal lumen, (5) superficial thrust through right vaginal flap and (6) superficial thrust from deep side of left vaginal flap to vaginal lumen. *B,* Closure of perineal laceration. Suture must not penetrate rectal mucosa. (From Hudson, R.S.: The Bovine Practitioner, 7:34, 1972.)

gained by curious exploration of the horizontal closure during healing. Sutures are removed with long scissors in 10 to 14 days, following digital palpation of the individual knots in the vestibular

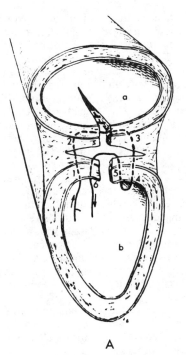

Figure 4. Closed perineal skin; vertical mattress sutures. Temporary guy sutures are holding anus open for visualization.

mucosa. The cow may be serviced naturally at any time after the thirtieth postoperative day. Manual rectal examination of the internal genitalia or artificial insemination should be postponed until the fortieth day. There is no evidence of an increased incidence of dystocia after or related to the restoration.

Rectovaginal fistulae in the cow apparently are rare. The mode of perineal laceration in the cow, i.e., from the vulva cranially, does not provide for fistula formation. The fistulae in cows that have been encountered by the author have resulted from partial failure of repair of complete perineal disruption. The method of repair of fistulae has been surgical conversion to a complete disruption and repair as just described.

UROVAGINA

General Considerations. Pooling of urine in the anterior portion of the vagina is a rare but extremely serious cause of infertility. The condition is instigated by either congenital or acquired cranioventral tipping of the pelvis, so that the external urinary meatus is higher than the anterior pelvic floor, thus directing the urine flow inward. The collection of increasing volume of urine in the anterior part of the vaginal vault induces sacculation and eventual drooping of the dilated vaginal vault into the abdominal cavity. Hence, a vicious circle is formed, which is aggravated by pneumovagina. The external cervical os is bathed in urine that may permeate the cervical canal and fill the uterus. As much as 3.5 liters of urine has been formed in the vaginal pool in some patients.

In order to avoid procreation of heritable conformational defects, the veterinarian should try to determine whether the abnormal pelvic structure is due to heritable influence or trauma. In many instances there will be a history of trauma, such as sacroiliac luxation acquired during extreme traction in delivering a fetus, and occasionally after violent struggling by an animal that has been cast. The condition will be evident by noticeable protrusion of the tubera sacrale above the spinal column. The tipped pelvis gives the appearance of a "weak loin."

Correction of urovagina is quite successful. However, if the condition has persisted for a prolonged period, the prognosis for restoration of fertility is guarded. Fortunately, the surgical procedure is relatively simple and inexpensive, justifying an attempt at complete restoration.

Surgical Technique. A transverse dam composed of a fold of vaginal mucosa is established cranial to the external urinary meatus in order to prevent cranial flow of urine (Fig. 5). Surgery is done under low epidural anesthesia with the cow in the standing position. Urine and debris are scooped from the vagina by hand. The perineal region and vaginal vault are thoroughly and repeatedly flushed with a povidone iodine surgical detergent. In order to deflate the greatly enlarged vagina, the cranial limit of the vagina is depressed, grasped with one hand and retracted, thus forcing out the air. Deflation is transitory, but it is helpful in elevating a transverse fold of mucosa on the vaginal floor. The fold should include the ventral 120° of the circumference of the vagina and is fixed in position by using a 12-cm half-curved, cutting-edge needle and No. 2 nonabsorbable suture material (Supramid) in a continuous horizontal mattress pattern through the base of the fold. Approximately 8 cm of vaginal floor should be elevated to form the fold. The suturing is laborious, and, provided the vagina is large enough, the use of both hands is helpful. Alternatively, vulsellum forceps may be helpful in maintaining the fold during establishment of the suture pattern. As the pattern is carried across the midline, the urethra must be avoided. The continuous suture is drawn taut, thus forming a semilunar dam about 5 cm high. The intent is to cause adhesion of the base of the fold for permanent structural change. Fortunately, the free edge of the dam tends to lean cranially, a safety factor for both cow and bull during coitus, should natural services be used. The suture is removed in 30 days. The vagina is infused daily with a bland, oil-based antibiotic ointment.

If concomitant perineal injury causes pneumovagina, repair is required using the applicable techniques previously described. In the absence of primary pneumovagina, when only the dam is employed, the pooling of urine should cease immediately. This may be checked by manual rectal examination. The vagina, relieved of the continuing insult, should return to normal condition and tone.

PROLAPSE OF THE VAGINA

General Considerations. Protrusion of all or part of the everted vagina through the vulva is a common condition in certain pluriparous cows, especially those of the Hereford, Santa Gertrudis and Holstein breeds. Predisposing factors include vaginal injury at previous parturition; obesity, with a heavy dep-

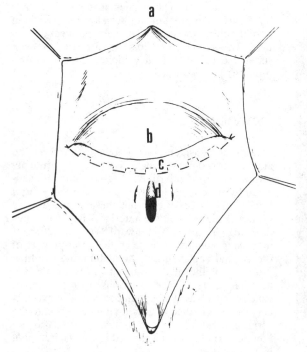

Figure 5. Surgical management of urine pooling in anterior vagina. Posterior view of open vulva showing technique of construction of transverse fold of vaginal floor: (a) dorsal commissure, (b) vaginal lumen, (c) transverse fold of vagina constructed by placement of continuous mattress sutures through base of fold and (d) suburethral diverticulum. (From Hudson, R. S.: The Bovine Practitioner, 7:34, 1972.)

osition of perivaginal fat; extended intake of large volumes of low quality roughage; severe cold weather and poor conformation, including an excessively large and flaccid vulva. Studies have confirmed the influence of heredity on vaginal prolapse in some instances, particularly in certain bloodlines of Hereford cattle. Although this is cause for concern, it would be injudicious to diagnose every case of vaginal prolapse as being hereditary.

It is interesting to note that the common denominator in virtually every instance of vaginal prolapse is incompetence of the constrictor vestibuli and constrictor vulvae muscles.

Typically, vaginal prolapse is a condition of advanced gestation, occurring a few days to 2 to 3 months prior to parturition. This period coincides with increasing intra-abdominal volume and pressure and with gradual slackening of the pelvic ligaments. An excessive amount of estrogenic substances in the diet may stimulate vaginal prolapse.

Walker[13] has classified vaginal prolapse based on progression, severity and prognosis.

First-Degree Prolapse. The floor of the vagina protrudes intermittently through the gaping vulvar cleft, usually only when the cow is lying down. This stage may go unnoticed. The vagina becomes irritated by exposure to sun, wind, dust, cold temperature and fecal contamination. If parturition is not imminent, the continued vaginal irritation may produce tenesmus, which leads to the next stage.

Second-Degree Prolapse. The floor of the vagina is in continuous prolapse. If neglected, the bladder may be reverted into the prolapsus, kinking the urethra and interfering with urination. Exposure to external irritants is protracted. The problem is obvious even to the casual observer.

Third-Degree Prolapse. The cervix and almost the entire vagina are prolapsed. This may happen without progression through the first and second stages and is dependent on flaccidity of the vagina and lack of support of the perivaginal tissue. Third-degree prolapse is common in Santa Gertrudis cows with chronic cervical enlargement. If the cervical seal is materially disturbed, there is danger of imminent septic abortion. Regardless of the method of repair, the cow should be kept under close observation. Repeated attempts to detect viability of the fetus may aggravate the irritated vagina but may be worthwhile. Signs of toxemia indicate fetal death.

Fourth-Degree Prolapse. The prolapse is of prolonged duration. Deep necrosis has ensued, and there are adhesions between perivaginal tissue and adjacent organs, especially the bladder. Peritonitis is present or imminent. The prognosis for the dam is poor.

Frequently, unattended prolapse is complicated by prolapse of the rectum. Some authors favor amputation of the prolapsed rectum in these cases. This author chooses to dispense with amputation if at all possible, depending instead on replacement and purse-string suture.

Replacement of Vaginal Prolapse. Using epidural anesthesia, the cleansed vagina is firmly but gently returned to its natural position with the hands. The fingers are kept together, or the fists are used in order to prevent bruising with the fingertips. The use of probangs is discouraged. Prolapse of long duration with severe edema may require patient and extended effort. Repeated covering of the exposed mucosa with a hygroscopic material such as sulfa urea powder is helpful.

Selection of Method of Retention. There are virtually dozens of ways of retaining the replaced vaginal prolapse. These depend on (1) the ingenuity of practitioners in a vexing situation and (2) the continued pursuit of the comprehensive "perfect" method. Vaginal prolapse characteristically appears during late gestation but sometimes occurs or recurs in the nongravid cow. Selection of a method of retention is somewhat dependent on the nearness to parturition and the frequency of observation that the convalescent patient will receive.

Lacing of the Vulva. This technique is preferred by some operators when parturition or abortion is expected in a few days. Paired loops of doubled wide umbilical tape are placed in the thick skin at the hairline on each side of the vulva, and the loops are laced with 1-inch gauze. The advantages are simplicity and the intentional breaking of the lacing if the animal calves unattended. The disadvantages are that retention is temporary and may have to be replaced, the lacing tends to collect feces and the irritation may induce resumption of tenesmus and prolapse.

Halsted Pattern. A series of umbilical tape sutures using the Halsted pattern is placed just dorsal to the dorsal commissure and along the vulvar cleft (Fig. 6). The sutures enter and exit through the thick skin at the hairline lateral to each vulvar lip. The area remains relatively free of gross fecal

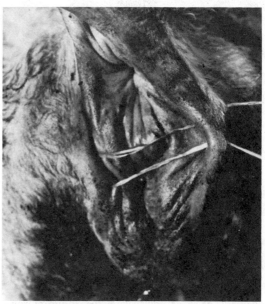

Figure 6. Halsted pattern for closure of vulva. Note sutures placed laterally at hairline.

contamination. Sutures can be expected to last 3 weeks.

Modified Quill Technique. Widely placed mattress sutures encircle vertically placed "quills" of rubber tubing or rope (Fig. 7). This is one of the most secure external fixation patterns.

Buhner Method. The objective is to insert a loop of tape that in effect simulates the action of the constrictor vestibuli muscle. Thus it can be used for correction of mild pneumovagina as well as retention of the replaced vagina.[1, 2, 11] The technique is not to be confused with superficial purse-string sutures. The special equipment needed includes a Buhner needle with the eye in the point and Buhner suture tape (tubular woven, flattened, nonabsorbable synthetic material).

After onset of epidural anesthesia, the perineal region is scrubbed and disinfected. A horizontal skin incision approximately 1 cm long is made midway between the anus and the dorsal commissure of the vulva. Another horizontal incision approximately 1.5 cm long is made at the same level as the ventral commissure of the vulva (cranial to the normally projecting ventral commissure).

The Buhner needle is introduced through the lower incision with the curvature directed in a lateral-medial direction (Fig. 8). With one hand in the vagina for guidance, the needle is forced as far cranially as possible and then dorsally through the dorsal incision until the needle eye is well exposed.

An antibiotic-soaked Buhner suture tape approximately 40 cm long is threaded through the needle (Fig. 9). While one end of the tape is held, the needle is withdrawn ventrally and the tape is removed from the eye of the needle. The needle

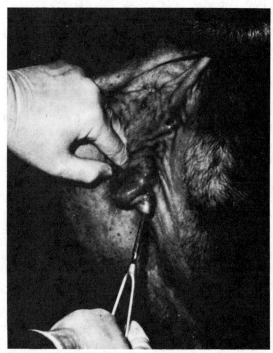

Figure 8. Buhner suture technique. Needle is directed through incision at ventral commissure of vulva and is forced as deeply cranially as possible before exiting through incision dorsal to dorsal commissure.

without tape is introduced into the ventral incision and is forced dorsally on the opposite side, again emerging from the dorsal incision. The tape is again threaded into the eye of the needle, and the needle is withdrawn ventrally through the ventral incision (Fig. 10).

Tension is applied to each end of the tape, thus forcing the dorsal loop beneath the skin of the upper incision. The suture is tightened to permit entry of two or three fingers into the vulva, and a square knot or bow knot is used to maintain closure (Fig. 11). The constriction thus formed is circular (Fig. 12). When the square knot is used, it will actually be under the skin. The incisions may or may not be closed with simple interrupted sutures, depending on the individual surgeon's preference.

If the cow is close to calving (within 30 days), the bow knot is preferred. Prior to calving this technique has disadvantages because extremely close observation of the patient and removal of the tape are necessary just prior to or at the time of parturition. The knot can be untied and gentle digital dilatation of the vulva will reduce tension.

For postpartum prolapse the square knot is used and is embedded under the skin. If the cow is left in the breeding herd, normal copulation may occur and no hindrance to artificial insemination has been noticed. Often after the tape has been retained for 2 months or more, a moderate deposit of connective tissue is stimulated by the buried tape. The connective tissue band that is formed may be strong enough

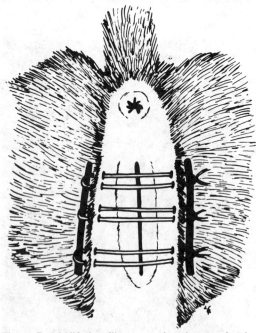

Figure 7. Modified quill pattern for closure of vulva. Rubber tubing is incorporated in suture line.

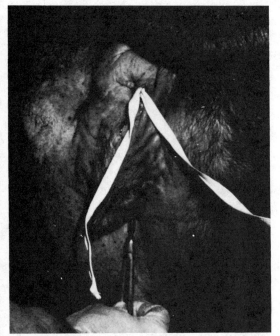

Figure 9. Buhner suture technique. Buhner suture material is threaded through exposed eye of needle. Note depth of tissue traversed.

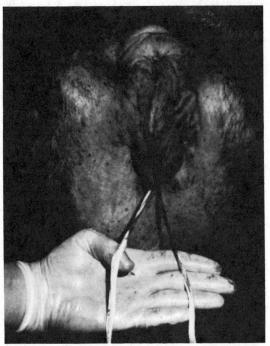

Figure 11. Buhner technique. The suture is pulled taut and tied at the ventral incision.

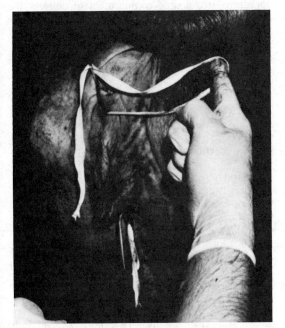

Figure 10. Buhner suture technique. Second limb of suture is carried around left side of vulva.

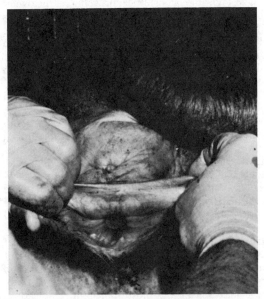

Figure 12. Completed effect of Buhner suture. Constriction resembles that of constrictor vestibuli muscle.

to prevent future prolapse, even after removal of the suture tape, and infrequently the stenosis may cause dystocia. In such cases, episiotomy may be required.

Cervicopexy. Winkler[14] has described a technique in which the external os of the cervix is sutured to the prepubic tendon with a large U-shaped needle and nonabsorbable suture. This technique has not received the popularity that it deserves primarily because of initial discouragement of some of those who are trying it for the first time. One of the primary advantages is that postanesthesia tenesmus is minimal.

EPISIOPLASTY

Closure of the vulvar lips (Caslick's operation) alleviates pneumovagina and continued irritation. A 1.8-cm band of mucosa is removed from the mucocutaneous junction of the dorsal commissure and each vulvar lip to about 4 cm above the ventral commissure. The opposing denuded surfaces are closed with vertical mattress sutures of nonabsorbable material. Unfortunately, the closure may not hold against severe tenesmus and should be reinforced with the Halsted or quill patterns described above.[7]

CESAREAN SECTION

Cesarean section, when truly indicated, generally meets acceptance by cattlemen as well as veterinarians. Since the operation frequently commands the highest fee among obstetrical procedures, the owner of a patient appreciates consideration of alternatives and even initial attempts at conventional delivery. However, the confident obstetrician wastes little time in deciding when cesarean section is indicated, thus avoiding further deterioration of the condition of dam and fetus.

Indications. Ideally, cesarean section is indicated when a live fetus cannot be delivered otherwise, when the dam presents a good surgical risk and when environmental factors are favorable for a major surgical procedure.[12] Realistically, many cases in which the operation is indicated are less than ideal and require complexities of judgment.[9, 10] Cesarean delivery of a dead calf unduly upsets the cost-benefit ratio when a less costly alternative procedure (e.g., fetotomy at the hands of a skilled operator) would serve as well. This is particularly true with large dairy cows, less so with small beef heifers. Commonly in bovine practice, the patient is a poor surgical risk because of general debilitation or prolonged neglected dystocia, but cesarean section may still be the most appropriate indication. Perhaps the most important disadvantage is that the novice owner may unfairly condemn the procedure if an unfavorable termination ensues. Surgical invasion of the abdomen at low ambient temperature

or when a brisk wind is stirring heavily contaminated air compounds the surgical risk.

Fetal oversize is one of the most common indications for cesarean section. Among the causes are relative immaturity of the dam, genetic mismatching and prolonged gestation. The novice may presume that a fetus is too large for conventional delivery when the overall physical size or pelvic diameters of the dam are categorically small. This may not be the case; many very young heifers produce extremely small calves. In order to determine accurately whether a calf can be delivered by traction, the operator may attempt to draw the appropriate fetal parts, usually the head and extended forelimbs, into the pelvic canal. That is, the critical measurement of fetus versus maternal pelvis can be made by trying to deliver the calf. Good judgment dictates that this effort be done as quickly and gently as possible to avoid undue trauma to dam or fetus should the final indication be cesarean section.

If the fetal head and extended forelimbs can be brought into the pelvic canal, delivery by traction is probable. One notable exception to this test is fetal muscular hypertrophy, "double muscling," in which the fetal hips and buttocks have the greatest transverse diameters of all fetal parts. This partial oversize allows the anterior parts of the fetus to be delivered with impunity, but then the extremely large hindquarters become impacted in the birth canal. Continued traction usually results in permanent unilateral femoral paralysis of the calf and may induce calving paralysis in the dam. Unfortunately, the condition is difficult to anticipate prior to the operator's irreversible commitment to delivery by traction. When the condition is perceived as a herd problem, the veterinarian and owner or herdsman may instigate elective cesarean sections, or perhaps pelvic symphysiotomy.

A grossly putrescent and emphysematous fetus may be an indication for cesarean section, particularly if the uterine and cervical musculature are contracted, so that mutation is not accomplished safely. Again, this is a matter of good judgment. If the fetus can be removed readily by other than cesarean section, one avoids the high risk of peritonitis.

Cesarean section is clearly indicated when the uterus is ruptured in order to avoid further trauma to the uterus, major uterine vessels and small intestines. Prolonged instances of torsion of the uterus, seen particularly in beef herds under careless surveillance, present a probable indication for cesarean section. While detorsion may be quite possible, the accompanying edema of the torsion area renders the tissue very friable and subject to rupture on delivery by traction.

Advanced hydrallantois suggests immediate cesarean section in the author's experience. While a more conservative means of inducing labor, such as use of estrogens and oxytocin, is a subjective alternative, the patient is usually physically weakened owing to the reduced feed intake into the crowded rumen and the heavy weight of excessive intrauterine fluid. Every effort should be made to relieve the cow of the burden before involuntary recumbency, an extremely poor prognostic sign, develops.

The experienced obstetrician will encounter numerous other valid indications for cesarean section.

Choice of Surgical Approach. Certainly experience and personal preference influence each operator's selection of surgical approach. Key considerations include availability of restraint devices, operator control of the actions of the patient and accessibility to the gravid uterus. Some operators feel that the alert, even frenzied, beef heifer is an ideal candidate for the standing position, left flank approach in a squeeze chute, whereas a phlegmatic or exhausted cow might elect to lie down. The large, mature beef or dairy cow may also be amenable to a standing position.

The flank approach may be used for animals in lateral recumbency. A distinct advantage of the left flank approach is that the rumen helps to hold the small intestine in place. In addition, should the animal develop rumen tympany during the operation, the opened left flank reduces respiratory embarrassment, and the rumen is readily accessible for deflation.

Ventral approaches include longitudinal midline and paramedian incisions, the latter being located either medial or lateral to the course of the left or right subcutaneous abdominal vein. The midline site is less vascular and probably can be incised and sutured more rapidly than paramedian locations. Unless there is a specific contraindication, left paramedian incisions are preferable to those on the right, in that during preparation and in the final stages of the operation the animal can rest in right lateral recumbency. The flank and ventral midline approaches will be described in detail.

Preoperative Considerations. Once a decision is made to perform cesarean section, the physical condition of the patient should be assessed. Although the procedure may be an emergency, haste should not preclude supplying any necessary antishock therapy, which can be continued during and after the surgery as needed.

Anesthesia. Usually epidural anesthesia and regional or local anesthesia are sufficient for most patients. General anesthesia and deep sedation are to be avoided when the fetus is alive. Xylazine is used extensively by some veterinarians but has the reported disadvantage of adversely increasing myometrial tone.

A muscle relaxant drug, isoxsuprine 230 mg IM, is used in Australia to simplify manipulation of the uterus at the laparotomy incision. Oxytocin is used after surgery to neutralize the action of the relaxant.[10] Isoxsuprine is expensive in the injectable form and is unapproved for this use in the United States.

Flank Operation—Standing Animal. The patient should be of a temperament and physical condition that indicate that the animal will remain standing during the procedure. Fractious animals should be confined in a clean chute with only a moderate amount of "squeeze," thus discouraging the animal's resting on the sides of the chute. Excessive restraint encourages the animal to lie down. All personnel should be warned to stay away from the patient's head to avoid causing the animal to charge and perhaps fall.

Epidural injection of 5 to 10 ml of 2 per cent procaine hydrochloride will reduce abdominal straining, defecation and tail movement and preserve the standing position. Next, left paralumbar fossa and adjacent areas are clipped and scrubbed. Linear infiltration of the dorsal and cranial boundaries of the operative field with 2 per cent procaine hydrochloride provides satisfactory anesthesia. Paravertebral thoracolumbar block is an alternative.

If the animal is unruly, only the side bar of the chute should be draped. With tractable patients the operative field is covered with a waterproof absorbent shroud with a 30- to 40-cm incision opening.

Beginning at a point approximately 10 cm ventral to the lumbar transverse processes, all layers of the abdominal wall are incised along a 25- to 40-cm vertical line. Small heifers may require an oblique incision along the direction of the fibers of the external oblique muscle to gain adequate length of incision above the chute side.

Usually the pelvic limbs of the fetus are in the cranial portion of the gravid uterine horn, i.e., anterior fetal presentation. Grasping one or both pelvic extremities through the uterine wall, the appropriate portion of the uterus is rotated up and out through the incision. Avoiding placentomes and selecting the least vascular area of the exposed portion of the uterus, a longitudinal incision is made over the line from fetal foot to hock. A fetus with large buttocks may require a somewhat longer incision. Certainly the incision should be of sufficient length to prevent tearing of the uterus as the fetus is removed. The fetal membranes are incised or torn and the fetus is withdrawn, preferably by an assistant, so that the operator can control the uterus and avoid intraperitoneal or intraincisional spillage of fetal fluid. As the fetus is removed, the umbilical cord is stretched and allowed to break 10 cm or so from the umbilicus, holding the cord at its abdominal end. The operator ensures that a living calf receives adequate neonatal care.

If the fetus is alive, the placenta should be left undisturbed except for trimming frayed edges that could interfere with suturing the uterine incision. The serosal surface of the uterus is cleansed of blood clots and fibrin accumulation by rinsing with physiological saline. The operator may elect to place a broad-spectrum antibiotic in the uterus, particularly if the uterus is obviously septic.

A variety of inverting suture patterns are suitable for closing the uterine incision. Continuous patterns are preferable to interrupted sutures in their speed of application and exactness of closure. Patterns that completely bury the suture material including knots are preferred to reduce adhesions.[11] De Bois described a recurrent suture pattern that is successful. Oxytocin (40 IU) may be given after suturing to hasten uterine contraction.

The abdominal incision is closed by simple continuous suture of the peritoneum and transverse abdominal muscle combined using No. 1 chromic gut or polyglycolic acid suture, by simple continuous or interrupted sutures of No. 2 or 3 chromic gut or polypropylene in the internal oblique muscle and the external oblique muscle and fascia, and by a continuous interlocking pattern in the skin, using nonabsorbable suture material. The procedure as described is suitable for the recumbent flank approach as well.

The weakened animal with advanced hydrallantois but with ability to stand should be operated on with all haste in the standing position. Once an animal in this state becomes recumbent, the prognosis is poor. One may consider the right flank approach if the uterus distends the upper portion of that side. The unusually voluminous uterus may resist exteriorization. However, the fetus is usually small in such cases and can be removed intraabdominally through a small uterine incision. As much fetal fluid as possible is left in the uterus, which is carefully sutured. One should anticipate spontaneous dilation of the cervix with gradual escape of the fluid within 24 hours. The patient should be observed and treated with intravenous fluids as needed.

Ventral Midline Approach. The young beef heifer is particularly suited to the ventral midline approach. This site is also useful when the operator encounters a large, greatly distended, septic uterus.

Low epidural anesthesia aids in preventing abdominal straining during the procedure. The patient is cast and restrained at an angle between right lateral and dorsal recumbency by tying the head and forelimbs anteriorly and the left hindlimb posteriorly. The right hindlimb is secured dorsally.

The ventral surface of the abdomen is clipped or shaved and scrubbed from the udder to a transverse line 12 cm anterior to the umbilicus. The midline is infiltrated with 2 per cent procaine hydrochloride from a point 7 cm anterior to the umbilicus to the base of the udder. A waterproof, absorbent shroud of sufficient size to cover the abdomen, udder and hindlimbs is put in place.

The skin incision is begun 5 to 7 cm anterior to the umbilicus and is carried posteriorly as needed. Following incision of the subcutaneous fascia, the abdominal tunic and peritoneum are incised longitudinally.

Upon opening the abdominal cavity, the free edge of the greater omentum is identified internal and posterior to the posterior commissure of the abdominal incision. This free edge is drawn anteriorly, thus exposing the uterus. The gravid horn is exteriorized by grasping a fetal part, usually one or both pelvic limbs.

Incision of the uterus, removal of the fetus and suturing of the uterine incision are performed much the same as in the flank approach. Following return of the uterus to the abdominal cavity, the greater omentum is drawn posteriorly over the exposed viscera.

The peritoneum and abdominal tunic together are closed, using a continuous overlapping mattress pattern with No. 3 or larger nonabsorbable synthetic suture. Care should be taken not to damage the suture material, which reduces its tensile strength. The closure is completed by applying a simple continuous pattern of the same suture material to the free overlapping edge and the underlying tunic. The skin and fascia are sutured with a continuous interlocking pattern, again using nonabsorbable synthetic suture.

Aftercare. The dam is encouraged to rise as soon as possible. If the fetus is alive, it is often wise to milk some colostrum from the dam and give it to the calf via stomach tube with the idea that the intervention of the obstetrical procedure may delay natural acceptance of the calf by the dam.

Uncomplicated cases indicate a good prognosis. If the uterus is particularly debilitated and septic, one should anticipate possible severe septicemia for up to 1 week postdelivery.

References

1. Bierschwal CJ, DeBois CHW: The Buhner method for control of chronic vaginal prolapse in the cow. Vet Med/Sm Anim Clin 66:230, 1971.
2. Buhner E: Simple surgical treatment of uterine and vaginal prolapse. Tieraerztl Umsch 13:183, 1958 (in German).
3. Friermuth GJ: Episiotomy in veterinary obstetrics. J Am Vet Med Assoc 113:23, 1948.
4. Habel RE: Topographic anatomy of the muscles, nerves and arteries of the bovine female perineum. Am J Anat 19:79, 1966.
5. Horney FD: In Jennings PB Jr. (ed): The Practice of Large Animal Surgery, Vol 2. Philadelphia, WB Saunders Co, 1984, pp. 1109-1118.
6. Hudson RS: Repair of perineal lacerations in the cow. Bovine Pract 7:34, 1972.
7. Roberts SJ: Veterinary obstetrics and genital diseases. In Theriogenology, 2nd ed. Ann Arbor, SJ Roberts, 1971.
8. Rosenberger G: Krankheiten Des Rindes. Berlin, Paul Purey, 1970 (in German).
9. Sloss V, Dufty JH: Elective cesarean operation in Hereford cattle. Austral Vet J 53:420, 1977.
10. Sloss V, Dufty JH: Handbook of Bovine Obstetrics, Baltimore, Williams & Wilkins Co, 1980, p. 160.
11. Turner AS, McIlwraith CW: Techniques in Large Animal Surgery. Philadelphia, Lea & Febiger, 1982, pp. 227-283.
12. Vandeplassche M: Embryotomy and cesarotomy. In Oehme FW, Prier JE (eds): Textbook of Large Animal Surgery. Baltimore, Williams & Wilkins Co, 1974.
13. Walker DF: In Walker DF, Vaughan JT. Bovine and Equine Urogenital Surgery. Philadelphia, Lea & Febiger, 1980, pp. 73-76.
14. Winkler JK: Repair of bovine vaginal prolapse by cervical fixation. J Am Vet Med Assoc 149:768, 1966.

Surgical Procedures of the Reproductive System of the Bull

Dwight F. Wolfe, D.V.M., M.S.
Auburn University, Auburn, Alabama

PENILE PAPILLOMATOSIS

Etiology

Fibropapilloma of the penis, caused by the bovine papilloma virus, is a common clinical entity in young bulls. The virus, a host-specific papovavirus, gains entrance into the skin through wounds and causes neoplastic growth of fibroblasts. The lesions do not metastasize and are not locally invasive.

Papillomas are most frequently seen in bulls between 1 and 3 years of age, and bulls presented with penile papillomas often do not have papillomas on other parts of the body. The habit of young bulls mounting penmates can lead to penile abrasions and provide an avenue for virus infection of penile skin. This behavior may lead to an epizootic of penile fibropapillomatosis in a group of young bulls maintained in the same pen. The papillomas may occur singly or as multiple growths on the penis. The pedunculated or sessile growths are usually located on the glans and free portion of the penis and rarely occur on the prepuce.

Diagnosis

Scant hemorrhage from the preputial cavity following copulation is frequently the earliest sign of penile fibropapillomatosis. The bull may display reluctance or refusal to breed. At times the lesion is first noted when the young bull is presented for breeding soundness evaluation. Continued growth of the papilloma mass with the penis retracted within the preputial cavity may preclude penile protrusion, resulting in phimosis. Large masses of fibropapillomas may interfere with complete retraction of the penis, resulting in paraphimosis. Other neoplastic growths of the penis are extremely rare. Diagnosis is confirmed by visual examination of the characteristic warty growth on the free portion of the penis (Fig. 1*A*). Histopathologic examination of the excised tissue mass may be utilized if the owner or practitioner desires laboratory confirmation.

Surgical Procedure

Surgical excision of bovine penile fibropapilloma is readily accomplished with the bull restrained in a squeeze chute with a drop side. (A general list of equipment needed for surgery is included in Table 1.) Table restraint, if available, makes the procedure more convenient for the surgeon. The penis is manually extended, secured by placing a towel forcep beneath the apical ligament on the dorsum of the penis (Fig. 1*B*), and thoroughly scrubbed in preparation for surgery. Small growths (less than 5 mm) may simply be excised with surgical scissors or a scalpel blade and topical antibacterial medication applied. For larger lesions local anesthesia and suture closure are preferred.

Anesthesia is attained by a ring block proximal to the lesion or by local infiltration around the

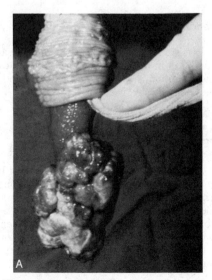
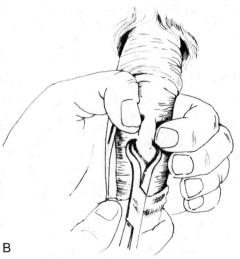

Figure 1. Penile papilloma. *A*, Penile papilloma. *B*, Towel forceps placed beneath apical ligament.

Table 1. Equipment Needed for Reproductive Surgery of the Bull

Name	Company
1. Extension set, 51 cm (cat. no. 2c0065)	Travenol Laboratories, Inc. Deerfield, Ill.
2. Betadine Solution	Purdue Fredrick Co. Norwalk, Conn.
3. Betadine Surgical Scrub	Purdue Fredrick Co. Norwalk, Conn.
4. Vetafil	S. Jackson, Inc. Washington, D.C.
5. Heimlich chest drain valve	Wyatt Oxygen Supply Birmingham, Ala.
6. Newberry castrating knife	Jorgenson Laboratories Loveland, Colo.
7. Latex tubing 1/4-inch ID × 3/32-inch	American Hospital Supply McGraw Park, Ill.
8. Elasticon	Johnson & Johnson New Brunswick, N.J.
9. Foley catheter	American Hospital Supply McGraw Park, Ill.
10. Technovit Hoof Acrylic	Jorgenson Laboratories Long Island City, N.Y.
11. Conray 60	Mallinckrodt, Inc. St. Louis, Mo.

dorsal nerves of the penis with 5 to 10 ml of 2 per cent lidocaine hydrochloride injected subcutaneously and on the tunica albuginea across the dorsum of the penis near the preputial orifice while the penis is held in extension. The penis is again scrubbed and a gauze tourniquet applied proximal to the surgical field. Frequently papillomas are encountered adjacent to or overlying the urethra. Urethral catheterization with a sterile male dog catheter is helpful for clearly defining the limits of the urethra. The urethra should be carefully avoided because incision into this structure may lead to urethral fistula formation.

The papillomas are excised by dissecting through the moist skin at the base of the growth with surgical scissors or a scalpel and bleeders are ligated. The skin is sutured with No. 0 chromic gut.

Postoperative Care and Prophylaxis

A topical antibacterial agent should be applied to the incision and the penis should be allowed to return to the preputial cavity. Wart vaccine should be administered at the time of surgery to help reduce recurrence of the growth. Recurrence of the growth is common because the bull may be in an active state of the disease at the time surgery is performed. The bull should be re-examined for new growths in 3 weeks. If no new growths occur the bull should be ready for service at that time.

Commercial and autogenous wart vaccines appear to be more beneficial prophylactically than thera-peutically. Vaccination is recommended at least 3 weeks before young bulls are grouped together.

PERSISTENT FRENULUM

Etiology and Diagnosis

The moist skin of the penis and prepuce of bulls are fused at birth. Under the influence of male hormones the penis and prepuce begin to separate at about 4 months of age, and the separation should be completed by 8 to 11 months of age. The frenulum is a fine band of connective tissue that extends from the prepuce to near the tip of the glans on the ventral aspect of the penis. The frenulum normally ruptures during separation of the penis and prepuce. Failure of complete separation of the connective tissue band produces a persistent frenulum that causes a marked ventral bending of the free portion of the penis when erection is attained. The ventral bending may not occur in bulls with excessive preputial length. The condition is usually noticed when the young bull begins to masturbate or attempt breeding. Occasionally the frenulum is first noticed when the young bull is presented for semen evaluation.

Surgical Procedure

Correction of persistent frenulum is easily accomplished with the bull restrained in a squeeze chute. The penis is manually extended and an assistant grasps the penis with a gauze sponge. The penile and preputial attachments of the frenulum are infiltrated with 2 ml of 2 per cent lidocaine hydrochloride. The frenulum, which usually contains a large vein, is ligated at each end and excised. A topical antibacterial agent is applied, and the bull should be ready for breeding service in 2 weeks.

Recommendations

Persistent frenulum is suspected to be a heritable condition in bulls. Breeders should be advised that the condition is easily surgically corrected but these bulls should be used in herds where their male offspring will be castrated.

PENILE HAIR RINGS

A problem occasionally seen in young bulls is an encircling hair ring just proximal to the glans penis. The formation of a penile hair ring is a sequela of the previously described homosexual activity of young bulls. Body hair from the bull being ridden accumulates on the penis of the aggressor bull and forms a firm band when the penis is retracted into the preputial cavity (Fig. 2). The hair ring may

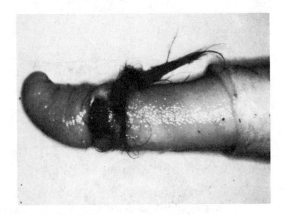

Figure 2. Penile hair ring.

cause pressure necrosis of the urethra, leading to urethral fistula formation. Avascular necrosis and sloughing of the glans penis may occur if the condition goes unnoticed. Treatment consists of removal of the hair ring and the application of a topical antibacterial agent unless extensive damage has occurred.

URETHRAL FISTULAE

Etiology and Significance

Fistulae into the urethra occasionally occur from injuries to the free portion of the penis. The urethra is located on the ventral aspect of the penis and is surrounded by the corpus spongiosum penis. From the junction of the penis and prepuce the urethra becomes more superficial as the size of the corpus spongiosum penis diminishes and terminates near the glans penis.

The fistulae may occur following any trauma that causes a laceration into the urethra. Penile hair rings may cause pressure necrosis of the urethra leading to fistula formation. Infertility is due to inadequate semen deposition near the cervix due to leakage through the fistula. The degree of infertility is determined by the location and size of the fistula. Large lesions or lesions located proximal to the glans penis are more deleterious than small lesions or lesions near the tip of the penis. Additionally, blood from freshly formed fistulae may become admixed with semen, causing seriously reduced fertility. The fistulae are of little consequence in bulls used for artificial insemination, but surgery is often necessary to restore fertility in bulls used in natural service.

Surgical Procedure

Urethral fistulae are difficult to repair successfully due to the forceful urination of the bull. The forceful urination produced by contraction of the bulbospongiosus muscle encourages leakage of urine through the suture line, and dehiscence is common. Best results are obtained by performing an ischial urethrostomy and inserting a catheter into the bladder before attempting fistula repair. This procedure diverts urine flow so that the fistula may heal without urine pressure on the suture line.

For closure of the fistula, table restraint of the bull is desirable. Extend the penis and apply towel forceps under the apical ligament to prevent penile retraction. Prepare the penis for aseptic surgery and administer a local block of the dorsal nerves as previously described (see earlier section, Penile Papillomatosis). Carefully debride the urethral mucosa at the edge of the fistula and dissect it free from the skin of the penis. Insert a 10 or 12 French catheter up the urethra to a point 5 cm above the fistula to serve as a stent during the surgical procedure. The urethral edges are approximated with simple interrupted 3–0 chromic gut sutures spaced 2 mm apart. The skin edges are apposed with closely spaced nonabsorbable suture, the catheter is removed and a topical antibacterial agent is applied.

If excessive tension is required to appose the urethral edges, a 2-mm gap may be left and the urethral catheter sutured to the tip of the penis and left for 7 days. This procedure is useful to reduce urethral stricture when a wide urethral defect exists and can only be achieved when an ischial urethrostomy has been performed.

Postoperative Care

Management of the patient postoperatively is dictated by the method of repair. If an ischial urethrostomy has been performed systemic antibiotics should be administered for 10 days. The author prefers procaine penicillin G at 10,000 IU per pound. The urethrostomy site should be gently cleaned daily. The Foley catheter may be removed

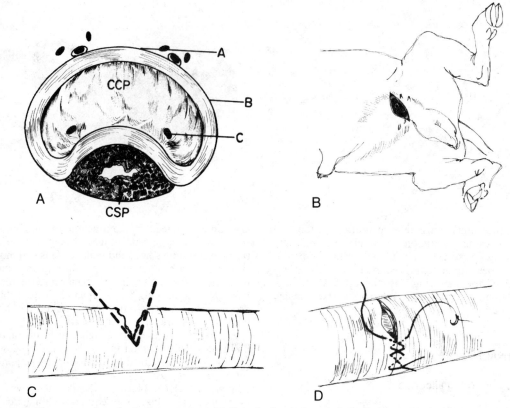

Figure 3. Hematoma of penis. *A*, Cross section of bull penis. Surgical procedure: *B*, 20 cm skin incision over hematoma swelling and anterior to teats. *C*, Excision of thin wedge of tunica albuginea at rupture site. *D*, Suture of tunica albuginea with bootlace pattern.

2 weeks following surgery and the wound allowed to heal by granulation.

The penis should not be disturbed for 10 days following surgery. Skin sutures are removed 10 days postoperatively and the bull should have 30 days sexual rest.

HEMATOMA OF THE PENIS

Etiology

Hematoma of the penis occurs commonly in bulls used in natural service. The condition is also referred to as broken penis, ruptured penis and fractured penis. The hematoma occurs during coitus when the cow slips or goes down under the weight of the bull or when the penis is thrust against the escutcheon of the cow. By definition, any injury that results in a blood clot surrounding the penis is classified as hematoma of the penis. However, a more specific meaning applies to hematoma of the penis in bulls. Penile hematoma in the bull results from a tear of the tunica albuginea into the corpus cavernosum penis and subsequent peripenile clot formation.

The bovine penis is composed of fibrocartilage, and the corpus cavernosum penis consists of cavernous spaces within the fibrocartilage framework. The tunica albuginea, the thick fibrous outer layer of the penis, surrounds the corpus cavernosum penis (Fig. 3A). During the erection process momentary peak blood pressure within the corpus cavernosum penis may exceed 14,000 mm Hg. The corpus cavernosum penis is a closed system at that time, and sudden angulation of the erect penis increases the high intracorporeal blood pressure to produce the tear in the tunica albuginea and the resultant clot formation. The mean rupture pressure of 25 penile specimens obtained from a slaughterhouse was found to exceed 76,000 mm Hg. The tear usually occurs on the dorsum of the penis at the distal curvature of the sigmoid flexure opposite the initial attachment of the retractor penis muscles. The tear is usually transverse to the long axis of the penis and is 2 to 7 cm in length.

The swelling of the hematoma is due to blood from the corpus cavernosum penis being forced into the peripenile tissue. Although the penis contains only about 250 ml of blood during erection, blood clots of several liters may accumulate around the penis. The size of the hematoma is determined by the number of breeding attempts the bull makes following the injury and is not related to the size of the tear in the tunica albuginea.

Diagnosis

Diagnosis of penile hematoma is not difficult and is based on physical examination. Frequently the owner first notices that the bull has a prolapsed prepuce. Swelling and blood accumulation in the peripenile elastic tissue often cause a preputial prolapse, the surface of which appears edematous and dark red from congestion. A large, cool symmetrical swelling occurs immediately anterior to the scrotum of affected bulls. The swelling may surround the penis or lie primarily on the dorsum of the penis. The swelling is fluctuant until the clot begins to organize by 10 days postinjury, when the swelling becomes quite firm. Fibrous tissue begins to replace the blood clot at this time and the rent in the tunica albuginea begins to heal by granulation. Due to the explosive force of blood escaping the corpus cavernosum penis at the time of tunica albuginea rupture, skin discoloration over the hematoma may be vivid the first few days following the injury (Fig. 3B).

Conditions that must be differentiated from penile hematoma include retropreputial abscess, preputial laceration with or without abscess, or posthitis. Generally, a retropreputial abscess feels warm to the touch and may not be symmetrical around the penis. The swelling should not be aspirated by needle puncture through the sheath to confirm the diagnosis. This procedure may create a tract of infection from the skin to the peripenile elastic tissue that could create adhesions between the sheath and elastic tissue that would prevent penile extension.

Conservative Therapy

Spontaneous recovery occurs in more than 50 per cent of the bulls that are given 90 days sexual rest. Parenteral antibiotics should be administered for 10 days to prevent possible abscessation. Sexual rest should be enforced for a minimum of 60 days postinjury.

Surgical Procedure

Many authors believe that surgical repair of a penile hematoma reduces the incidence of complications resulting from the injury. Surgery should be performed as quickly after the injury as possible. Surgery is not recommended after day 10 because the extent of fibrous tissue surrounding the hematoma makes exteriorization of the penis difficult. After a 48-hour fast the bull is tabled in right lateral recumbency and general anesthesia attained. The left rear leg is secured in flexed abduction to allow greater surgical exposure and a 40 by 40 cm site over the hematoma swelling is prepared for aseptic surgery.

Make a 20-cm skin incision over the swelling anterior and parallel to the rudimentary teats (Fig. 3C). Deepen the incision through the subcutaneous tissue and into the elastic layers until the hematoma is visible. The hematoma is organized as black clotted blood within the elastic layers. Ligate all bleeders and pay strict attention to hemostasis. Incise the connective tissue over the hematoma and manually remove the clotted blood. Only the large, easily removed clot fragments are extracted. Rinse the hematoma cavity with warm 3 per cent povidone iodine in normal saline solution to remove small detached clot fragments.

Exteriorize the penis with its surrounding elastic tissue through the skin incision. Note the attachment of the retractor penis muscles on the ventral aspect of the distal curvature of the sigmoid flexure. Palpate the urethral groove to identify the ventral aspect of the penis and, using this as a landmark, make a left lateral longitudinal incision through the elastic layers to expose the tunica albuginea of the penis. Carefully reflect the elastic layers dorsally by blunt dissection to expose the rent in the tunica albuginea. This approach to the dorsum of the penis is made to avoid surgical trauma to the dorsal vessels and nerves of the penis.

Excise a thin wedge of tunica albuginea on either side of the tear to establish healthy wound edges (Fig. 3D). Overzealous excision of the wound edge may lead to incomplete straightening of the distal sigmoid flexure and resultant restriction of penile extension. Carefully appose the edges of the rent in the tunica albuginea with No. 1 polyglycolic acid sutures in a bootlace pattern (Fig. 3E). Appose the elastic tissues over the penis and close the longitudinal incision by placing closely spaced simple continuous 3–0 chromic gut sutures in the superficial elastic layers. Return the penis to its normal position and flush the cavity with warm 3 per cent povidone iodine solution. Swab the cavity with sterile surgical sponges to remove small fragments of clotted blood that may have been loosened by the surgical procedure. Suture the subcutaneous tissue with No. 0 chromic gut in a simple continuous pattern and close the skin with 0.6-mm synthetic nonabsorbable suture.

Postoperative Care

Administer prophylactic intramuscular antibiotics for 5 days postoperatively. A seroma normally occurs in the hematoma cavity and should begin to subside about 10 days after the surgery. Remove the skin sutures on the tenth postoperative day and enforce sexual rest for at least 60 days.

Complications

Several severe complications may develop as sequelae to hematoma of the penis. Penile hematomas commonly recur in a subsequent breeding season but surgical repair reduces this risk. The hematoma and traumatized tissues are quite susceptible to abscessation. Bacterial contamination of the traumatized tissue may occur by surgical sepsis or hematogenous spread. If the penis and elastic tissue become involved, adhesions frequently develop. Adhesions of the elastic layers to the tunica albuginea or the skin may prevent complete penile extension.

Analgesia of the penis may occur due to damage to the dorsal penile nerves. The analgesia may occur immediately at the time of the tunica albuginea rupture if the dorsal nerves are damaged by the explosive release of blood from the corpus cavernosum penis. In other cases, bulls recovering from penile hematoma may breed successfully and then develop analgesia of the penis. Fibrous tissue formation may impinge on the dorsal nerves, and when the bull returns to breeding, stretching or tearing of the scar tissue may disrupt the nerves, thus resulting in delayed loss of sensation to the glans penis.

Erection failure occasionally occurs subsequent to penile hematoma. Bacterial infections of the cavernous tissue deep to the rent in the tunica albuginea may occur, producing a septic cavernositis that may interrupt blood flow to the distal corpus cavernosum with resultant inability to attain erection. More commonly, erection failure following hematoma is due to the development of vascular shunts between the corpus cavernosum penis and the peripenile vessels. In the healing process following penile hematoma neovascularization occurs and occasionally anastomotic vessels form that allow blood flowing into the corpus cavernosum penis to exit through the tunica albuginea and into the peripenile vasculature. This vascular shunt prevents the formation of a closed system within the corpus cavernosum penis and consequently sufficient erection pressure cannot be achieved. Surgical repair of post-hematoma vascular shunts consists of careful wedge excision of the involved portion of the tunica albuginea and suture closure as described for penile hematoma repair.

ERECTION FAILURE

Mechanism of Erection

The process of erection in the bull depends on the corpus cavernosum penis being a closed system. Blood is supplied to the corpus cavernosum penis by two large vessels from the distal end of the crura. These two vessels converge into a single dorsal canal that extends distally to the sigmoid flexure. Two ventral canals extend distally from the sigmoid flexure to the distal portion of the corpus cavernosum penis. The dorsal and ventral canals communicate with the cavernous spaces of the corpus cavernosum penis throughout the entire length of the penis. Normally there are no vascular communications from the cavernous spaces through the tunica albuginea to peripheral vessels during the erection process.

On sexual stimulation active rhythmic contractions of the ischiocavernosus muscles force blood from the crura into the dorsal canal and subsequently into the cavernous spaces of the corpus cavernosum penis. The ischiocavernosus muscle contractions also cause occlusion of the small, thin-walled crural veins that drain blood from the corpus cavernosum penis. Thus, intracorporeal blood pressure rapidly increases and full erection is attained. Vascular communications from the corpus cavernosum penis would therefore prevent the establishment of sufficient intracorporeal blood pressure to produce and maintain erection.

Etiology

The most common cause of erection failure in the bull is defects in the tunica albuginea that prevent the function of a closed system within the corpus cavernosum penis. In the presence of these defects blood escapes the corpus cavernosum penis, and high intracorporeal blood pressure cannot be attained.

Defects in the tunica albuginea are most often associated with hematoma of the penis. The tear in the tunica albuginea predictably occurs on the dorsum of the penis at the distal curvature of the sigmoid flexure. Vascular anastomoses may develop as the tunica albuginea heals following the injury so that blood from the corpus cavernosum penis escapes to peripenile vessels. The author has also seen one case of vascular anastomosis from the corpus cavernosum penis to the corpus spongiosum.

A less frequent cause of erection failure is multiple defects in the tunica albuginea in the free portion of the penis. With this condition blood escapes from the corpus cavernosum penis through numerous sites near the distal end of the penis. This condition has been described as a congenital weakness of the tunica albuginea. The bull may have a history of one or more successful breeding seasons before the shunts develop.

Diagnosis

Diagnosis of erection failure should begin with a thorough history and physical examination followed by a closely observed test mating. If necessary, the veterinarian should attempt to palpate the penis during the test mating to determine whether engorgement occurs. In the presence of multiple shunts in the free portion of the penis, a distinct "blush" may be noted in the distal end of the penis due to ecchymotic hemorrhages from ruptured vessels as the bull attempts intromission.

Contrast radiography is useful to confirm and locate the presence of vascular shunts through the tunica albuginea. The bull should be tabled in right lateral recumbency, the penis manually extended, towel forceps placed under the apical ligament near the distal end of the penis, and a surgical scrub applied. Palpate the junction of the retractor penis muscles at the ventral aspect of the distal sigmoid flexure, and with a large cutting needle pass a double strand of 0.6-mm suture through the skin of the sheath, between the retractor penis muscles and the penis, then out through the opposite side of the sheath. This suture will serve as a retractor to pull the penis away from the abdominal wall when radiographs are taken.

With the penis extended, insert a 16-gauge needle into the corpus cavernosum penis about 5 cm from the tip and inject sterile physiological saline solution to ascertain a patent flow. A 51-cm extension set is utilized to connect the needle to a 30-ml syringe filled with Conray 60. Position the penis over the cassette with the aid of the towel forceps and the previously placed suture. Serial radiographs should be taken 5 seconds apart. Inject 15 ml of the contrast media and take the first exposure. The subsequent exposures should each be taken after additional 15-ml injections.

Because the corpus cavernosum penis is a closed system, in a normal penis the contrast medium stays entirely within the tunica albuginea. The single dorsal and double ventral canals observed on the contrast radiograph lie within the corpus cavernosum penis. If a shunt exists, the contrast material will be seen in the tortuous nutritional vessels of the penis and prepuce outside the tunica albuginea. If a shunt exists in the corpus spongiosum penis, it will become filled with contrast media.

Surgical Procedure

Surgical repair of the corpus cavernosal shunts is recommended only when the shunt develops following hematoma of the penis. Shunts that develop into the corpus spongiosum penis are inaccessible surgically without creating excessive trauma. Multiple distal shunt repair has been uniformly unsuccessful. Therefore, the following surgical procedure describes repair of post-hematoma shunts that develop between the tunica albuginea and peripenile vessels following hematoma of the penis.

The bull should be tabled in right lateral recumbency and general anesthesia attained. The left rear leg is fixed in flexed abduction and a 40- by 40-cm site anterior to the rudimentary teats is prepared for aseptic surgery.

Make a 20-cm skin incision anterior and parallel to the rudimentary teats and deepen the incision through the subcutaneous tissue until the elastic layers are visible. Meticulous hemostasis should be attained throughout the procedure. Exteriorize the penis with its surrounding elastic tissue through the skin incision. Note the attachment of the retractor penis muscles on the ventral aspect of the distal sigmoid flexure. Palpate the urethral groove, and using this as a landmark to identify the ventral aspect of the penis, make a left lateral longitudinal incision through the elastic layers to expose the tunica albuginea of the penis. Carefully reflect the elastic layers dorsally by blunt dissection to expose the shunt on the dorsum of the penis. This approach is used to avoid surgical trauma to the dorsal nerves and vessels of the penis.

The shunt is repaired by careful wedge excision of the affected area of tunica albuginea. The surgeon should excise only sufficient tissue to remove the defect because excessive excision may prevent complete straightening of the sigmoid flexure postoperatively. The edges of the tunica albuginea are carefully apposed and sutured with No. 1 polyglycolic acid sutures in a bootlace pattern. The excised portion of tunica albuginea is ligated and removed from the peripenile vessels. Appose the elastic tissues over the penis and close the surgical site as previously described for hematoma of the penis.

Postoperative Care

Administer prophylactic intramuscular antibiotics for 5 days postoperatively. Remove skin sutures on the tenth postoperative day and enforce sexual rest for at least 60 days.

DEVIATIONS OF THE PENIS

Etiology

Penile deviation is a common cause of copulation failure in bulls. Deviations occur in three forms: spiral, ventral and the S-shaped curvature. The spiral deviation occurs most commonly and is usually seen in bulls between 2.5 and 5 years of age; the bulls usually have a history of successful breeding prior to the occurrence of the deviation.

Penile deviations may occur following traumatic injuries with resultant scar tissue formation that prevents normal penile extension. Deviations of this nature must be diagnosed by test breeding and careful physical examination. Correction usually depends on revision of scar tissue or adhesions. Surgical technique depends on the specific etiology of the particular case.

The more typical penile deviation develops insidiously and no previous trauma has been noted. The fibrous architecture of the tunica albuginea of the penis causes the normal penis to deviate 30° right laterally during erection. The apical ligament of the penis counteracts the deviation tendency of the erect penis and holds the normal penis in a straight position. The apical ligament consists of a thick band of collagen fibers arising from the outer longitudinal layer of the tunica albuginea. The ligament originates on the dorsal midline of the tunica albuginea about 2.5 cm proximal to the distal end of the prepuce, and the fibers fan out at its insertion into the tunica albuginea near the distal end of the corpus cavernosum penis (Fig. 4A).

Diagnosis

Diagnosis of penile deviation due to inadequate apical ligament function should begin with a thor-

ough physical examination of the bull. The penis and prepuce should be carefully inspected for evidence of trauma and scar tissue that might cause the deviation. Specific methods of diagnosis for the three forms of penile deviation caused by inadequate apical ligament function follow. Heritability of apical ligament inadequacy is unknown.

Spiral deviation occurs at the peak of erection in the bull, and with the aid of a transparent artificial vagina up to 50 per cent of normal bulls have been shown to develop spiral deviation during copulation.

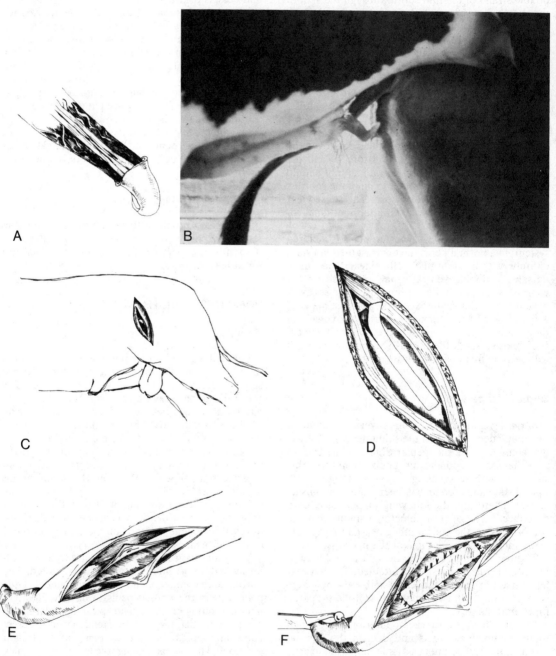

Figure 4. Penile deviations. *A*, Apical ligament of the penis. *B*, Spiral deviation of the penis. Surgical procedure: *C*, Incision through skin and superficial fascia lata. *D*, Excision of long rectangular strip of deep fascia lata. *E*, Incised apical ligament reflected laterally to expose tunica albuginea. *F*, Interrupted sutures placed along margins of fascia lata implant.

The deviation is also frequently seen during electroejaculation and masturbation in apparently normal bulls. Therefore, spiral deviation should be considered pathologic only when it prevents intromission. Spiral deviation occurs when the apical ligament slips to the left side of the penis at peak erection and the penis usually spirals to the left (Fig. 4B).

Spiral deviation should be diagnosed only by observing the bull during test breeding. The condition is insidious in nature and several matings may be necessary because the condition does not consistently occur, especially during the early stages of the disease.

Occasionally spiral deviation may be difficult to diagnose in bulls with Bos indicus breeding such as Beefmaster, Santa Gertrudis and Brangus. If spiral deviation develops in these bulls the pendulous sheath and excessively long prepuce may serve as a shroud and preclude penile extension leading to an erroneous diagnosis of erection failure. Careful observation of the test breeding possibly including palpation or manual retraction of the sheath during the breeding act may be necessary to determine if spiral deviation is present.

Ventral penile deviation is less common than spiral deviation and it is likely that the normal suspensory structures fail to compensate for the normal ventral curvature of the erect penis. Stretching or deterioration of the apical ligament fibers allow the ventral deviation to develop.

With ventral deviation a long gradual curvature of the penis develops and becomes more evident as the extent of erection increases. Ventral deviation can satisfactorily be diagnosed with the aid of an electroejaculator but test breeding is recommended to ascertain that the bull has acceptable libido and is free from musculoskeletal deficits that might prevent successful breeding.

The S-shaped curvature of the penis is the least common of the deviations caused by inadequate apical ligament function. This condition usually occurs in older bulls and is thought to be due to inadequate apical ligament length or excessive penile length with a normal apical ligament. This condition may develop following trauma to the apical ligament with subsequent cicatricial shortening of the ligament. No therapy is recommended for this condition but the bull could be utilized by artificial insemination if the deviation prevents intromission.

Surgical Procedure

The fascia lata implant technique is currently used for repair of both spiral and ventral penile deviations. This procedure has proved to provide more effective and longer lasting results than alternative methods. A strip of fascia lata is harvested from the thigh and sutured between the tunica albuginea of the penis and the apical ligament in this procedure. The graft becomes homogeneous with the adjacent structures and serves to strengthen and stabilize the ligament on the dorsum of the penis. The reorganization process is not complete for 90 days but sufficient healing occurs by 60 days after surgery to permit breeding. Autogenous grafts are usually utilized but homologous fascia lata preserved in 70 per cent ethyl alcohol is satisfactory.

Following a 48-hour fast the bull is restrained in right lateral recumbency and general anesthesia is attained. A surgical site 20 cm wide and 40 cm long is clipped and prepared dorsal to the left patella and extending toward the tuber coxae. The preputial hairs are clipped, the penis manually extended and the towel forceps is applied under the distal end of the apical ligament to aid in holding the penis in extension. The penis and prepuce are scrubbed and prepared for aseptic surgery and then returned to the retracted position with towel forceps in place while the fascia lata implant is harvested.

The fascia lata implant is harvested first and placed in warm normal saline while the graft bed is prepared. Beginning 10 cm proximal to the anterior lateral margin of the patella, the incision is extended 20 cm toward the tuber coxae. The incision is deepened through the superficial fascia until the thicker deep layer of fascia is exposed (Fig. 4C). Excise a rectangular strip of fascia lata 3 cm wide and at least 12 cm long and place it in warm saline while the incision is closed (Fig. 4D). The deep and superficial fascial layers are each closed with No. 1 polyglycolic acid suture in a bootlace pattern. The skin is closed with a continuous interlocking pattern of 0.6-mm synthetic suture. This incision should be meticulously closed to prevent muscle herniation that might make the bull quite lame following surgery. Loose connective tissue and fat are removed from both surfaces of the fascia lata strip and it is returned to the normal saline.

The penis is again extended and held in extension by an assistant for the rest of the surgical procedure. Beginning just caudal to the glans penis extend a 20-cm skin incision on the dorsum of the penis. Deepen the incision through the loose fascial layers in the area of the free portion of the penis and the thin elastic layers in the preputial portion to expose the apical ligament.

Incise the apical ligament in its thickest portion throughout its length along the dorsum of the penis. Reflect the margins of the ligament laterally in either direction to expose the tunica albuginea and create a bed for the fascia lata implant (Fig. 4E). Two large veins draining the corpus spongiosum penis lie deep to the apical ligament on the right ventral aspect of the penis and should be avoided.

Place the fascia lata implant between the apical ligament and tunica albuginea beginning as far proximally as possible. Place four simple interrupted No. 0 polyglycolic acid sutures through the fascia lata and into the tunica albuginea on the proximal border of the implant. Avoid penetrating the tunica albuginea because corpus cavernosal vascular shunt development could occur, producing erection failure. Place interrupted sutures along the lateral margins of the implant at 2-cm intervals, stretching the fascia lata in both directions (Fig. 4F). Trim the implant to fit at the distal end of the incision and suture it under mild tension with three interrupted sutures. Pull the apical ligament over the implant and suture the incised edges with No. 1 polyglycolic acid suture using a simple interrupted pattern. These sutures should also engage the fascia lata strip.

Suture the elastic layers of the preputial portion of the incision with No. 3–0 chromic gut using closely spaced sutures in a simple continuous pattern. Close the skin with closely spaced simple interrupted sutures of No. 0 chromic gut. Apply liquid nitrofurazone to the incision and remove the towel forceps, allowing the penis to retract into the preputial cavity.

Postoperative Care

Prophylactic procaine penicillin G is administered 5 days postoperatively and the penile skin sutures are removed on the tenth postoperative day. Thigh skin sutures are not removed until 3 weeks following surgery to reduce the risk of painful muscle herniation. The bull should be withheld from breeding for 60 days.

PREPUTIAL PROBLEMS

Preputial problems are among the most common causes of impotence in bulls. A variety of clinical conditions occur due to the varying etiology and pathogenesis of preputial maladies. A thorough physical examination, including age, breed and history, is important in determining the diagnosis and prognosis of clinical cases. Trauma is the most common etiologic agent in the development of preputial pathology.

Anatomy of the Prepuce

Familiarity with the anatomy of the prepuce is necessary to understand the pathogenesis of preputial injury and the physiological goals of medical or surgical therapy. The sheath is the hair-covered skin appendage that supports and protects the penis on the ventral abdomen. The sheath extends from just caudal to the scrotum and terminates anteriorly as the preputial orifice, the preputial attachment to the sheath. The prepuce is the hairless moist skin joining the sheath to the penis. The preputial attachment to the penis, caudal to the glans and free portion of the penis, is the preputial ring. The prepuce is firmly attached only at the preputial ring and the preputial orifice. When the penis is retracted, the preputial cavity is formed, and the only visible portion of the prepuce is the orifice.

As the penis extends, the prepuce everts onto the penis. Beneath the moist preputial skin a complex series of elastic tissue layers is continuous with the elastic layers surrounding the penis. Stretching and gliding of the elastic layers is essential to normal penile and preputial extension. The elastic layers extend from the preputial ring to caudal to the scrotum. The extent and nature of elastic tissue damage usually determines the prognosis and mode of therapy for preputial trauma.

The protractor prepuce muscles, the paired cranial muscles of the prepuce, raise and constrict the preputial orifice. The retractor prepuce muscles, the caudal muscles of the prepuce, arise from the abdominal tunic and insert into the insertion of the protractors. These muscles are frequently absent or vestigial in polled bulls and their absence may be associated with the development of habitual preputial prolapse. When the retractor prepuce muscles are absent, preputial retraction is a passive act and occurs secondarily to penile retraction by the retractor penis muscles. Because of this, polled bulls commonly prolapse the prepuce during relaxation.

Bulls of the *Bos indicus* breeds have a more pendulous sheath and prepuce that averages 5.5 cm longer than that in *Bos taurus* breeds. Occasionally *Bos indicus* bulls will be impotent due to inability to elevate an extremely pendulous sheath so that the penis cannot be raised to the level of the vulva of the cow. The size of the preputial orifice and the effectiveness of the protractor prepuce muscles vary between breeds and individuals within a breed. It has been suggested that culling bulls with preputial prolapse could reduce the incidence of the condition.

PREPUTIAL LACERATIONS

Etiology

Preputial lacerations frequently occur during coitus and usually occur in a longitudinal manner on the ventral aspect of the prepuce. The injuries occur as a longitudinal bursting of the ventral prepuce as the bull makes the ejaculatory lunge and the prepuce is forced against the bony pelvis of the female. These injuries are seldom noticed in the fresh state, and swelling of the sheath or preputial prolapse is usually the first indication that injury has occurred. Occasionally blood will be noticed at the preputial orifice or on the hindquarters of the female immediately following the injury. The severity of preputial laceration varies according to the extent of elastic layer damage that occurs. Lacerations that deeply invade elastic tissue are more serious than superficial lacerations.

Nonsurgical Therapy

Lacerations that involve the preputial epithelium with minimal elastic tissue damage frequently heal spontaneously with at least 30 days sexual rest. If little or no prolapse of preputial tissue occurs, daily irrigation of the preputial cavity with 3 per cent povidone iodine solution is recommended to aid in the control of superficial infections and reduce the risk of abscessation. No attempt should be made to extend the penis manually during the early treatment period. Premature penis extension may disrupt granulation tissue formation and prolong the convalescent period. The bull should not be returned to breeding services until the preputial laceration has healed and all swelling has subsided so that the penis can be easily extended completely.

PREPUTIAL LACERATIONS WITH PROLAPSE

Pathogenesis

More extensive lacerations that deeply involve the elastic layers often lead to preputial prolapse. This situation is most prevalent among bulls of *Bos indicus* breeding. Under these conditions the longitudinal laceration assumes a transverse orientation as the penis is retracted (Fig. 5*A*, *B*, *C*). Injuries of this nature require more intensive therapy if breeding soundness is to be restored.

Nonsurgical Therapy

Bulls that present with preputial laceration with prolapse often display extensive preputial edema and gross contamination of the laceration (Fig. 5*D*). The prolapse should be thoroughly but gently washed with antiseptic surgical soap being careful not to create additional elastic tissue damage at the laceration site. The preputial cavity should then be liberally irrigated with 3 per cent povidone iodine solution. An oily antibacterial ointment should be applied to reduce bacterial contamination and maintain pliability of the moist preputial skin. An ointment consisting of 60 ml scarlet oil and 2 gm tetracycline powder in 500 gm of anhydrous lanolin has proved effective.

Treatment of preputial edema with prolapse requires the application of a pressure bandage. Insert a firm latex tube, 6.3 mm ID × 2.4 mm wall into the preputial cavity before applying the bandage so that urine flow will remain patent. The prolapsed prepuce should be coated with the antibacterial ointment and a protective stockinette applied. A snug elastic tape wrap is applied over the stockinette and the latex tube secured to the elastic bandage with 2.5 cm adhesive tape. The bandage should be changed every 2 to 3 days until edema subsides and the prolapse can be reduced. If healing occurs with the prepuce prolapsed, the prepuce will be shortened due to the transverse orientation of the laceration. A pendulous portion of tissue will be formed on the dorsum of the prepuce due to the ventral shortening. Surgery may be necessary to reconstruct the prepuce to allow normal copulation.

Following reduction of the prepuce into the preputial cavity an alternate bandaging technique may be needed to prevent the prolapse from recurring. After cleansing and ointment application, the latex tubing should again be inserted into the preputial cavity. Elastic tape is applied directly on the sheath beginning at the preputial orifice and wrapping toward the abdominal wall. This bandage should be changed every 2 to 3 days until the preputial prolapse no longer recurs.

CHRONIC PREPUTIAL PROLAPSE

Habitual prolapse of the prepuce is a common clinical entity. The predisposition to preputial prolapse involves the interplay of four anatomic factors: size of the preputial orifice, pendulousness of the sheath, length of the prepuce and the presence of retractor prepuce muscles. *Bos indicus* bulls have a higher incidence of habitual preputial prolapse than other breeds, although the condition also occurs in Angus and polled Hereford bulls.

Preputial prolapse does not interefere with copulation unless the prolapsed portion becomes traumatized. Small abrasions occur on the prolapsed prepuce that quickly lead to edema formation, which in turn produces further prolapse. The edematous prolapsed prepuce frequently sustains more extensive trauma and infection with possibly abscessation and ultimately fibrosis or hypertrophy of the preputial tissue.

The same clinical condition also occurs in young bulls owing to two different causes. Young bulls occasionally are infected with bovine herpesvirus and develop the clinical syndrome of infectious pustular balanoposthitis. This disease first becomes manifest as vesicles on the penis and prepuce that rupture and are replaced by pustules. Additionally, young bulls may repeatedly mate estrual females until the penis and prepuce become erythematous and excoriated, creating a traumatic balanoposthitis. Following either of these conditions the irritated prepuce prolapses and gravitational edema develops, leading to chronic preputial prolapse.

Nonsurgical Therapy

Treatment of chronic preputial prolapse is the same as previously discussed for preputial laceration with prolapse.

Surgical Therapy of Preputial Prolapse

Restorative preputial surgery is frequently necessary to return bulls to breeding soundness following preputial prolapse. Surgery is indicated if fibrous tissue development prevents normal excursion of the prepuce. Presurgical conditioning of the prepuce is very important when surgery is contemplated. Edema should be reduced, infections eliminated and lacerations allowed to establish healthy granulation tissue before surgery is attempted. Failure to attain these objectives jeopardizes surgical success, and delayed healing, dehiscence and sepsis occur frequently. The presurgical conditioning is achieved

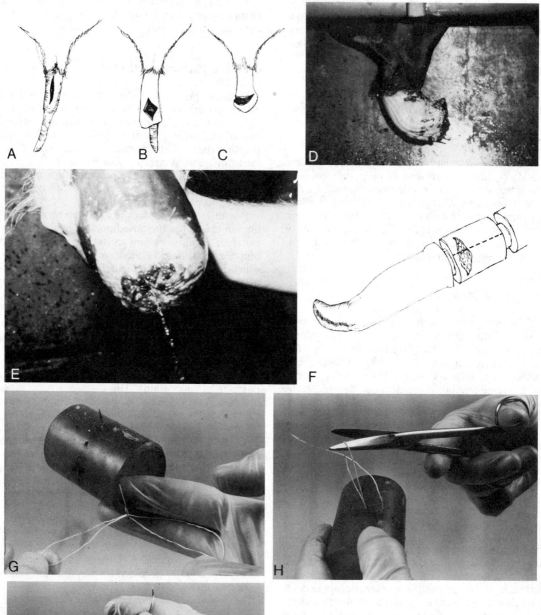

Figure 5. Preputial laceration. *A*, Longitudinal preputial laceration. *B*, Longitudinal preputial laceration beginning to assume transverse orientation. *C*, Transverse orientation of preputial laceration. *D*, Edematous preputial prolapse with contaminated laceration. *E*, Preputial stenosis. Surgical procedure: *F*, Circumferential preputial incision. Ring technique for circumcision. *G*, Loop of suture threaded on needle and placed through ring and prepuce. *H*, Suture cut and tied. *I*, Second suture placed through ring and prepuce.

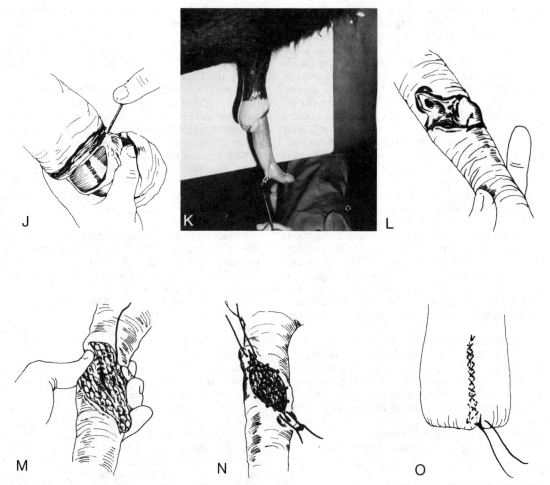

Figure 5. *Continued. J,* Amputation of prepuce distal to ligating sutures. Preputial scar tissue revision. *K,* Healed preputial laceration with excessive scar tissue. Surgical procedure: *L,* Excision of fibrous tissue of preputial skin. *M,* Longitudinal closure of elastic layers. *N,* Loosely placed bootlace suture pattern. *O,* Tightened bootlace suture pattern with prepuce retracted.

by judicious cleansing of the prepuce and firm bandaging as described under Nonsurgical Management of Preputial Laceration with Prolapse.

Circumcision is the surgical procedure most frequently employed for repair of damaged preputial tissues following preputial prolapse. The chief indications for circumcision are chronic prolapse with fibrosis or irreversible stenosis of the lumen of the preputial cavity (Fig. 5E). The surgical technique of choice is resection and anastomosis whereby damaged tissue is excised and healthy preputial skin is apposed.

With the bull restrained in right lateral recumbency general anesthesia is induced and the preputial bandage is removed. The sheath is clipped and prepared for aseptic surgery. Manually extend the penis and place a towel forceps under the apical ligament to aid in holding the penis in extension. A final surgical scrub is applied and sterile drapes are placed around the surgical field. A sterile 2.5-cm latex drain tube is used as a tourniquet placed

around the prepuce at the preputial orifice. A circumferential incision is made through the moist skin of the prepuce proximal to any lesion (Fig. 5F). A second circumferential incision is made distal to any lesions, and these two incisions are joined by a longitudinal incision. Care must be taken to ensure that the length of prepuce remaining after the surgery is at least twice the length of the free portion of the penis. If the prepuce is excessively shortened complete penile extension will not be possible. *Bos indicus* bulls frequently experience recurrence of the injury if insufficient prepuce is removed. On the other hand, when operating on a *Bos taurus* bull, the surgeon may be unable to excise all affected preputial tissue owing to the inherent shortness of the prepuce.

The preputial skin is bluntly excised, removing elastic tissue only as deeply as necessary to remove pathologic lesions. All visible vessels are ligated, the tourniquet is removed and all other bleeders are ligated. Thorough hemostasis is essential for satisfactory postoperative healing. Following completion of ligation the surgical field is liberally irrigated with warm 3 per cent povidone iodine solution.

Close the incision in two layers utilizing No. 0 chromic gut. Four simple interrupted sutures are placed in the elastic layers at 90° intervals around the incision. Simple continuous sutures are placed between the interrupted sutures to complete elastic layer closure. The preputial skin is closed with interrupted cruciate mattress sutures. A 2.5-cm Penrose drain is placed over the glans penis and sutured to the skin of the free portion of the penis with four to six simple interrupted No. 0 chromic gut sutures. The urethra and corpus spongiosum penis must be avoided when placing these sutures. The purpose of the Penrose tubing is to ensure that urine bypasses the incision during the convalescent period. A 16-cm length of sterile 3-cm semiflexible polyethylene tubing is placed over the Penrose tubing and into the preputial cavity as the penis is allowed to retract. A snug elastic tape bandage is applied to hold the large tube in place and to keep pressure on the incision site, thereby reducing seroma formation.

Intramuscular antibiotics are administered once daily for 5 days. The elastic bandage is removed 5 days postoperatively and the large tubing withdrawn from the preputial cavity, leaving the Penrose tubing attached to the penis. Ten days after surgery the penis is extended, the Penrose tubing removed and the sutures removed. Avoid excessive traction while extending the penis. Sixty days sexual rest is advised before returning the bull to breeding service.

Preputial Amputation by the Ring Technique

A polyvinylchloride ring 7 cm long and 5 cm in diameter is prepared before performing surgery. A series of 2-mm diameter holes are drilled 8 mm apart, circumscribing the midpoint of the tubing. Smooth the edges of the ring and place it in a cold sterilization solution.

The procedure can be performed with the bull restrained in a squeeze chute with a drop side but is more easily accomplished with the bull tabled in right lateral recumbency. After applying a surgical scrub to the prolapsed prepuce, the ring is place in the preputial cavity so that the line of suture holes is located at the intended level of amputation. The ring is secured to the prepuce with 0.6-mm Vetafil so that absolute ligation of the prepuce is achieved by adjacent simple interrupted sutures according to the following technique. Thread a 10-cm half-curved cutting needle onto the free end of the suture and introduce it into the lumen of the ring through one of the holes in the ring and through the prepuce (Fig. 5G). Remove the needle from the suture and form a loop of suture between the prepuce and the suture container and thread this loop through the needle eye (Fig. 5H). Introduce this double strand

of suture through the adjacent hole in the ring and through the prepuce (Fig. 5J). Remove the needle and identify the side of the loop that is continuous with the free end of the suture. Tie very tightly, making sure to crush the preputial tissue and cut above the knot.

Repeat the suture process until the circumference of the prolapse has been ligated, including overlapping one hole in the ring. Amputate the prepuce by cutting through the prepuce against the plastic ring 1 cm distal to the suture line (Fig. 5K). Apply a 2.5-cm Penrose drain over the glans penis and suture it to the skin of the free portion of the penis to prevent urine contamination of the surgical site. Return the penis and prepuce to the retracted position, apply a topical antibacterial liquid and bandage the prepuce.

Remove the bandage and ring 10 days postoperatively. A ring of necrotic tissue will be attached to the ring at this time. The Penrose drain is left attached to the penis for several more days and a topical antibacterial is applied daily until the preputial epithelium is healed. The bull should have enforced sexual abstinence for a minimum of 30 days. The penis should be extended and the prepuce examined for healing and stenosis before returning the bull to service.

This procedure is less tedious and less time-consuming than the resection and anastomosis technique of circumcision, but it is also less successful. The ring technique provides eversion of the skin edges that heal by granulation and fibrosis compared with the first-intention healing achieved by the abutment closure of the resection and anastomosis technique. The resultant granulation and fibrous tissue are less pliable and more prone to tearing as the bull attempts to extend the penis. This tearing promotes additional scar tissue formation so that an unacceptably high incidence of preputial stenosis follows the procedure. The technique is a viable alternative as a salvage procedure for a bull of low economic worth but is not recommended for valuable bulls.

Reconstructive Preputial Surgery

Reconstructive surgery of the prepuce is utilized to remove fibrous tissue from the elastic layers following preputial lacerations. This procedure is employed when excessive scar tissue formation prevents normal penile extension and the prepuce length is inadequate to allow circumcision. Usually this situation occurs when a longitudinal laceration has healed in a transverse manner with subsequent shortening of the prepuce.

The bull is tabled in right lateral recumbency, inhalation anesthesia is attained and the prepuce is prepared for aseptic surgery. The penis is manually extended and a towel forceps is placed beneath the apical ligament. A sterile 2.5-cm Penrose drain tube is utilized as a tourniquet placed at the proximal end of the prepuce. The scar on the ventrum of the prepuce is generally cross-shaped and the deformity produces a dorsal bulging of the prepuce (Fig. 5L). Excise the fibrous tissue of the preputial skin in both a longitudinal and transverse manner (Fig. 5M). Remove scar tissue from the elastic layers of the prepuce and ligate visible vessels. Remove the tourniquet and ligate all bleeders to achieve complete hemostasis.

Completely extend the penis, allowing the prepuce to resume its normal length. The elastic layers are closed in a longitudinal manner using No. 0 chromic gut in a simple interrupted pattern (Fig. 5N). Suture a 2.5-cm Penrose drain over the free portion of the penis before attempting to close the preputial skin. With the penis fully extended, place No. 0 chromic gut in a bootlace pattern on the longitudinal axis of the skin incision. The suture should be loosely placed with the free ends toward the preputial orifice (Fig. 5N). With the penis extended the moist skin will not stretch sufficiently to achieve apposition when sutured on the longitudinal axis due to the prolonged contraction. This contracted tissue will relax several weeks following surgery because no loss of skin has occurred. Remove the towel forceps and allow the penis and prepuce to retract into the preputial cavity. Tightening the bootlace suture with the penis retracted will allow apposition of the edges of the preputial incision (Fig. 5O). Tie the free ends of the suture.

This procedure creates a planned temporary stenosis of the prepuce. Two weeks postoperatively begin to attempt manual extension of the penis. Repeat the penile extension every 2 or 3 days until the penis can extend normally. The bull should be ready for breeding 60 days following surgery.

AVULSION OF THE PREPUCE

Etiology

Avulsion of the prepuce from its attachment to the free portion of the penis is a condition most frequently sustained when bulls have semen collected by artificial vagina. The injury occurs when the artificial vagina contacts the preputial attachment to the free portion of the penis when the ejaculatory thrust is made, consequently interfering with penile extension. Alternatively, an ill-fitting artificial vagina might be snug enough to squeeze the prepuce and not provide sufficient pressure on the free portion so that overextension occurs at the time of ejaculation. The injury occasionally occurs in bulls used in natural service.

Diagnosis

When bulls sustain the injury on an artificial vagina the operator should immediately notice hemorrhage on the penis and perhaps the artificial vagina when the bull dismounts. Blood may contaminate the semen sample just collected. Hemorrhage from the prepuce or blood on the preputial hairs may be the first indication of injury in bulls in natural service. Definitive diagnosis is made by physical examination of the penis with the bull restrained in a squeeze chute. The avulsion typically appears as a transverse separation of the prepuce from the dorsum of the penis.

Surgical Procedure

Preputial avulsion should be surgically repaired immediately after the injury occurs. Surgical closure is indicated to prevent the formation of a dorsal transverse bulge of scar tissue at the preputial ring. This scar tissue would increase the risk of further avulsion when the bull returns to service or semen collection. Repeated injury to this area could lead to anesthesia of the penis due to disruption of the dorsal penile nerves overlying the tunica albuginea immediately beneath the elastic layers of the prepuce. If the injury occurs in natural service, hours or days may elapse before the condition is noticed. If such is the case a different therapeutic approach is dictated. These wounds are contaminated and possibly infected when presented to the veterinarian and must be conditioned before surgical closure is attempted. Presurgical conditioning of contaminated wounds consists of daily gentle extension of the penis, gentle application of surgical scrub and a nonirritating topical antibacterial ointment. Care should be exercised not to further disrupt exposed preputial elastic tissue and create a more extensive area of infection. The therapy is continued daily until the wound is covered with healthy granulation tissue and there is no threat of abscessation. The bull is now ready for surgical closure of the defect.

The surgery may be performed with the bull restrained in a squeeze chute but table restraint makes the procedure more convenient for the surgeon. Either general anesthesia or a ring block of the prepuce and dorsal nerves proximal to the injury will suffice. Extend the penis manually and affix towel forceps under the apical ligament to aid in holding the extended penis. The penis and prepuce are surgically scrubbed and prepared for aseptic surgery.

Carefully debride the wound edges, removing only friable or devitalized tissue in preparation for surgical closure. If the wound has been allowed to granulate before surgery, excise the granulation tissue carefully to prepare the surgical field. Close the defect carefully by using closely spaced simple continuous sutures of 3–0 chromic gut to appose the elastic layers of the prepuce and penis. Appose the skin of the prepuce and penis with No. 0 chromic gut sutures in a closely spaced simple interrupted or horizontal mattress pattern. Apply a topical antibacterial ointment to the suture line and return the penis to the retracted position.

Postoperative Care

Administer prophylactic intramuscular antibiotics once daily for 5 days following surgery. No other therapy is indicated until the sutures are removed in 10 days. The bull should have a minimum of 30 days sexual rest.

URETHRAL CALCULI

Etiology

Urethral calculi are caused by the interaction of several factors. The accumulation of an organic matrix consisting of mucoprotein, peptides, and epithelial debris serves as the nidus for calculi formation. Nephritis, cystitis, or administration of diethylstilbestrol all result in excessive epithelial debris in the urine. Highly concentrated diets result in increased mucoprotein and peptides in the urine. Mineral salts bind with the organic matrix to form calculi.

The composition of the calculi varies with the diet. Grain concentrates are high in phosphorus content, and smooth-surfaced phosphate calculi are most common in feedlot or show cattle. Grazing cattle more commonly develop oxalate or silicate calculi. Oxalate calculi occur in cattle grazing pasture plants containing high oxalate content, and silicate calculi develop in cattle grazing pastures with acid, sandy soils that favor plant uptake of silicone. Silicate calculi are usually rough-surfaced.

Additional management factors are involved in the development of obstructive urethral calculi. Steers castrated at an early age have a small urethral size compared to bulls. The use of diethylstilbestrol also causes small urethral size in steers and lambs. Inadequate water intake produces urine concentration and resultant increased calculi formation. This problem is most notable in winter months.

The calculi form in the bladder and are excreted with urine into the urethra. The urethra becomes progressively smaller from the ischial arch toward the tip of the penis. The distal sigmoid flexure creates an additional constriction of the urethra and is the most common location where calculi become lodged.

Diagnosis

When calculi lodge in the urethra bladder distention develops and mild signs of abdominal pain may be noted. The bull or steer may stretch or occasionally kick at the abdomen, but the most characteristic sign is frequent unsuccessful attempts to urinate. The tail will pump up and down and contractions of the bulbospongiosus muscle can be seen or palpated over the ischial arch. Rectal examination reveals bladder distention and the preputial hair may be covered with crystals.

If the blockage is unrelieved the bladder or urethra will rupture, and signs of abdominal pain will subside and attempts at urination cease. The patient may remain nearly asymptomatic for several days and in the event of bladder rupture the owner may notice abdominal enlargement due to urine accumulation within the abdominal cavity. The animal will become dehydrated and abdominal paracentesis will reveal copious quantities of clear fluid that may be difficult to identify as urine without laboratory analysis. Upon rectal palpation the veterinarian usually finds a thickened, partially filled bladder.

Urethral rupture is more common in steers than in bulls and produces more obvious clinical lesions. Urine permeates the peripenile tissue and edematous swellings develop that may encompass a large portion of the ventral abdominal wall. Urea and ammonia in the urine initiate necrosis in the involved tissues and large areas may slough. A urine or ammonia odor may be noted and the steer is usually anorectic and quite depressed.

Ischial Urethrotomy

Indications. This surgical procedure is used primarily for introducing a catheter into the bladder. It may be the procedure of choice when dealing with urolithiasis in feedlot steers until they are in acceptable slaughter condition. This procedure is also utilized to divert urine flow when attempting surgical repair of urethral fistulae in bulls or in the management of bladder rupture in bulls.

A ruptured bladder in the bovine will heal spontaneously if subsequent bladder distention is prevented. Peritonitis following bladder rupture is not a severe problem and can be managed by antibiotic therapy. With the animal restrained in a chute, drain the urine from the abdominal cavity by inserting a trocar and cannula just medial to the subcutaneous abdominal vein; then remove the trocar and insert a 20-cm section of sterile gum rubber tubing into the cannula. Remove the cannula and fix the drain tube in place with a simple suture to the abdominal skin. The ischial urethrotomy should now be performed with the animal in the standing position.

Surgical Procedure. Administer epidural anesthesia, tie the tail away from the surgical field and prepare a 25-cm by 25-cm area over the ischial arch for aseptic surgery. Beginning 5 cm below the anus, make a 10-cm incision through the skin on the midline. A dense fascial plane will be encountered beneath the subcutaneous tissue; this is incised to expose the retractor penis muscles (Fig. 6A). Dissect between the muscles until the bulbospongiosus muscle is encountered. Palpate the urethral groove immediately below the muscle and incise through the corpus spongiosum and into the urethra (Fig. 6B). Hemorrhage from the corpus spongiosum may be reduced by digital pressure applied dorsal to the incision. Inserting forceps easily in both directions

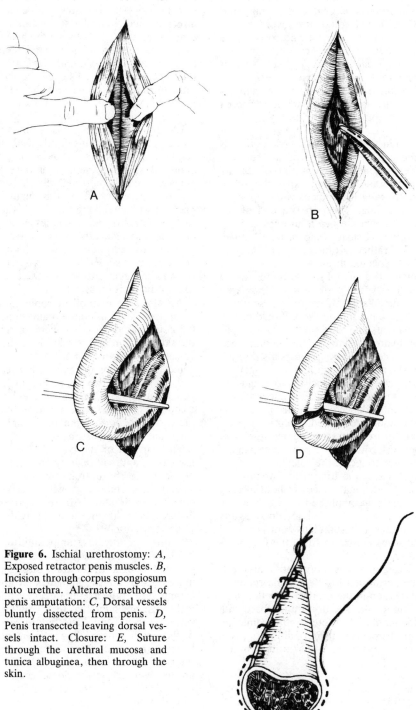

Figure 6. Ischial urethrostomy: *A*, Exposed retractor penis muscles. *B*, Incision through corpus spongiosum into urethra. Alternate method of penis amputation: *C*, Dorsal vessels bluntly dissected from penis. *D*, Penis transected leaving dorsal vessels intact. Closure: *E*, Suture through the urethral mucosa and tunica albuginea, then through the skin.

from the incision will verify location of the urethra and a urinary catheter may now be inserted.

A Foley catheter is inserted into the bladder and the cuff is inflated. Grasp the tip of the catheter with curved hemostats to aid catheter passage into the urethra. Care should be taken to avoid overinflation of the cuff so that pressure necrosis of the neck of the bladder does not occur. A one-way valve should be attached to the catheter so that aspiration of air into the bladder is prevented. If the animal is destined for slaughter the catheter is left in place until the urine contamination is cleared and the steer is acceptable for slaughter.

In bulls that may be restored to breeding soundness a sterile 3-mm × 200-cm polyethylene tube is utilized for the catheter. Passage of the catheter into the bladder is achieved by grasping the tubing with curved forceps and directing it over the ischial arch, then withdrawing the forceps while applying pressure on the tubing. The opposite end of the tubing is directed down the penile urethra and out the preputial orifice. Calculi removal may be necessary before this catheter is inserted. This may be accomplished by repeated flushing.

Stone Removal. The animal should be restrained in dorsal recumbency and a surgical site prepared on the midline immediately anterior to the scrotum. General anesthetics and tranquilizers should not be used in these patients and local infiltration of 2 per cent procaine hydrochloride on the midline will suffice for the procedure. Grasp the penis through the skin and make a 10-cm longitudinal skin incision over the penis. Deepen the incision through the subcutaneous tissue until the penis is encountered. The penis is bluntly dissected free from the surrounding tissue and exteriorized. Identify the attachment of the paired retractor penis muscles at the distal sigmoid flexure of the penis and palpate the urethral groove to locate the calculi.

The preferred technique for calculus removal is to crack the stone into small pieces without incising the urethra. This is accomplished by crushing the stone between the tips of towel forceps. Lightly massaging the penis will stimulate contraction of the bulbospongiosus muscle to force the fragments from the urethra.

If the calculi cannot be easily crushed, a urethrotomy should be performed to effect stone removal. Make a small incision in the urethra over the stone and tease the stone out. The urethra is closed with closely spaced, simple interrupted 3-0 chromic gut sutures. Return the penis to its normal location and close the subcutaneous tissue and skin in a routine manner.

Penile Amputation

Indications. Amputation of the penis is indicated following urethral rupture in steers and bulls. The animals generally require several weeks healing time to become acceptable for slaughter.

Surgical Procedure. With the animal restrained in a squeeze chute attain epidural anesthesia and prepare an area from the perineum to the scrotum for aseptic surgery. The desired location for the skin incision should allow the penile stump to be directed caudoventrally so that urine flow will be directed at an angle between the hocks and the tail. Make a 12-cm skin incision on the midline beginning at the point where the anterioventral curvature of the perineum begins. Deepen the incision through the subcutaneous tissue and the dense connective tissue between the semimembranosus muscles to expose the penis.

Bluntly dissect the penis from the surrounding tissue, grasp the penis firmly and apply traction caudally and dorsally. If necrosis has begun the penis will separate from the prepuce and the entire penis can be pulled through the incision. If the penis cannot be separated in this manner, incise the prepuce while applying traction to the penis. Transect the retractor penis muscles as far proximally as possible and ligate the dorsal vessels of the penis proximal to the point of amputation. Transect the penis 5 cm distal to the dorsal apex of the skin incision and generously open the urethra with scissors to the incision apex.

An alternate method of penile amputation may be utilized when minimum damage has occurred to the peripenile tissues. The penis is grasped through the skin incision and traction is applied. The dorsal vessels are bluntly dissected from the penis and hemostatic forceps are placed between the vessels and the body of the penis (Fig. 6C). Transect the penis leaving the vessels intact (Fig. 6D). This technique preserves the nutrient blood supply to the distal portion of the penis and may be used when minimal necrosis exists.

The cut end of the corpus cavernosum penis is not closed and will heal by granulation. There will be no hemorrhage from this cavernous tissue in steers, but hemorrhage will occur in bulls when erection is stimulated. In order to minimize hemorrhage in bulls the stump may be closed after wedge resection.

Suture the penile stump and form a urethral fistula using nonabsorbable monofilament suture material. Begin the suture through the urethral mucosa and tunica albuginea at the left dorsal commissure of the urethral opening and then extend it through the skin (Fig. 6E). Continue the pattern ventrally to a point 1 cm before reaching the end of the penile stump. At this point pass the suture beneath the penile stump and through the skin on the right side of the incision. Continue the pattern up the right side to the dorsal commissure and tie. Close the skin incision below the stump with interrupted sutures.

Hemorrhage from the corpus spongiosum penis will occur during urination. To control hemorrhage in bulls and large steers insert a 15-cm length of 1-cm diameter tubing into the urethra and fix it in place with a single suture through the tubing and penile stump. This tubing will compress the corpus spongiosum penis and reduce hemorrhage. The tubing should be removed in 5 days.

Postoperative Care. Administer antibiotics for 5 days postoperatively and give supportive care as indicated. Adequate water intake should be ensured. The sutures may be removed in 10 days. The animal should be observed for urethral stenosis, but this should not occur if the fistula was made sufficiently large.

INGUINAL HERNIA

Etiology

Hernias may be congenital or acquired, but in the bovine a congenital inguinal hernia is uncommon. Congenital hernias are evident early in calfhood and are occasionally encountered as intestinal evisceration following castration.

Acquired inguinal hernias may be of traumatic origin or may result from management practices in the development of young bulls. Traumatic inguinal hernias have occurred in bulls that have become entangled when attempting to jump fences. Perhaps in these cases increased intra-abdominal pressure allows the intestines to perforate the peritoneum near the vaginal ring and descend through the inguinal canal alongside the spermatic cord. The intestines frequently become strangulated.

The most common inguinal hernia is acquired and nontraumatic in origin. This management-induced hernia occurs primarily in beef bulls over 3 years of age and is the result of feeding practices in young bulls. As bulls are fattened for show or sale extraperitoneal fat deposits develop in the inguinal region. Large pendulous deposits may extend into the inguinal canal, stretching the internal abdominal oblique muscle anteriorly, thus dilating the inguinal ring. As the bull ages and loses excess fat the extraperitoneal fat deposit atrophies, allowing a loop of intestine to dilate the vaginal ring and descend into the tunica vaginalis. Most of these hernias develop on the left side, probably due to the habit of bulls of lying on the right side with the left rear leg extended, thereby allowing the left inguinal ring to dilate. This type of hernia is decreasing in frequency as producers become more performance conscious and bulls are not as heavily fattened.

Diagnosis

Congenital inguinal hernias are diagnosed by palpation of the scrotum and inguinal region for swelling. The hernial contents will be fluctuant and not painful to the calf. By careful digital palpation the external inguinal ring will be found to be dilated and the hernial mass may be reducible through the ring.

Acquired inguinal hernias are diagnosed by history and physical examination. The hernial contents, usually the small intestine, do not descend into the area of the testicle but remain proximal to it, producing an hourglass appearance of the scrotum (Fig. 7A). Palpation of the scrotum reveals a fluctuant mass within the neck of the scrotum that is not hot or painful to the bull. The hernial mass may consist of the previously described extraperitoneal fat mass and is difficult to differentiate from intestinal mass. If the hernia is of traumatic origin and the intestines are strangulated, considerable inflammation and pain may be evident.

On rectal palpation the internal inguinal ring is found to be dilated and filled with abdominal contents. Traction on the mass produces visible movement of the hernia within the neck of the scrotum with little or no movement of the testicle.

Surgical Procedure

Congenital Inguinal Hernia

The congenital inguinal hernia is considered to be heritable and therefore the calf should be castrated at the time of hernia repair. Repair of a congenital hernia is accomplished with the calf restrained in dorsal recumbency. Sedation with thiamylal sodium or xylazine facilitates the procedure. After surgically preparing the area over the inguinal ring, a skin incision is made over the hernial mass. The tunica vaginalis is isolated and by firm traction the testicle and hernial mass are exteriorized. The tunica vaginalis is twisted from the testicular end, forcing the intestines back into the abdominal cavity. The tunica vaginalis is ligated with No. 1 chromic gut near the inguinal ring and excised distal to the ligature, thus removing the testicle and a portion of the cremaster muscle and spermatic cord. The stump of the tunica vaginalis is forced into the abdominal cavity and the same suture material is used to close the inguinal ring. The margins of the aponeurosis of the external abdominal oblique are apposed with simple interrupted sutures to achieve closure of the ring. The skin is closed with 0.4-mm Vetafil in a simple continuous pattern.

Acquired Inguinal Hernia

The presence of an inguinal hernia interferes with the thermoregulation of the testicle and testicular degeneration ensues. This testicular degeneration is reversible unless fibrosis develops within the testicle. Surgical correction of the hernia is designed to preserve the fertility of the bull. Unilateral castration is indicated if orchitis of periorchitis accompanies the hernia. Following unilateral castration in these cases the inguinal ring is closed as described for congenital inguinal hernias.

The bull is fasted for 48 hours prior to surgery to reduce the risk of bloat and regurgitation during anesthesia. Table the bull in lateral recumbency

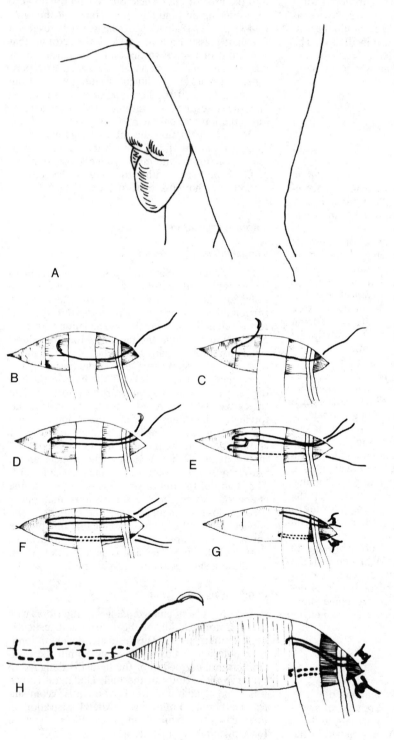

Figure 7. Inguinal hernia: *A*, Hour-glass appearance of scrotum in bull affected with inguinal hernia. Inguinal ring closure: *B*, Beginning suture closure of inguinal ring. *C*, Suture bite through internal abdominal oblique muscle. *D*, Completion of first suture closing inguinal ring. *E*, Placement of second suture closing inguinal ring. *F*, Completion of second suture closing inguinal ring. *G*, Reduction of lumen of inguinal ring. *H*, Second layer of closure of inguinal ring.

with the affected side up and achieve inhalation anesthesia. The upper rear leg is secured in flexed abduction to expose the inguinal area and the surgical site is clipped and prepared for aseptic surgery. Sterile drapes are applied to expose the neck of the scrotum and inguinal area.

Beginning 6 cm dorsal to the inguinal ring, incise the skin over the distended cord distally to the top of the scrotum. Deepen the incision through the subcutaneous tissue and tunica dartos until the tunica vaginalis is exposed. Ligate all bleeders encountered to this point.

Bluntly dissect the tunica vaginalis containing the hernial mass until it is free from the proximal pole of the testicle to the internal inguinal ring. If the large mass of adipose tissue is present along the anterior margin of the inguinal ring it should be bluntly dissected from the ring and tunica vaginalis. This mass may be excised by placing a transfixed ligature around its base as far proximal as possible and amputating below the ligature. The stump is then allowed to retract, thereby exposing the entire inguinal ring.

The inguinal rings are slitlike openings in the posterior abdominal wall. The inguinal canal is merely a potential space between the muscles and fascia of the internal and external inguinal rings. The external ring is a slit in the aponeurosis of the external abdominal oblique muscle. The internal inguinal ring is the abdominal opening of the canal and is bounded cranially by the internal abdominal oblique muscle, caudally by the inguinal ligament, which consists of iliac fascia reinforcing a portion of the aponeurosis of the external abdominal oblique muscle, medially by the lateral border of the prepubic tendon and laterally by the attachment of the internal abdominal oblique muscle to the inguinal ligament. Transverse fibers of the internal abdominal oblique muscle lie deep to the external ring and anterior to the tunica vaginalis and form the anterior border of the inguinal canal. This layer has been forced forward due to the hernial mass and will be pulled posteriorly during repair of the dilated ring. The caudolateral wall of the inguinal canal is formed by the inguinal ligament. Identify the external pudic vessels at the posterior margin of the ring.

Incise the tunica vaginalis to expose the hernial contents and examine for adhesions between the tunic and intestines. If adhesions are encountered they must be separated. Collateral circulation develops between the tunica vaginalis and intestine at sites of adhesions and all vessels must be completely ligated to control all hemorrhage and subsequent fibrin formation in the vaginal cavity. After all adhesions are separated and absolute hemostasis is obtained, the intestines are returned to the abdominal cavity. If a strangulated loop of intestine is found intestinal resection and anastamosis may be necessary. The reader should consult an appropriate text for this procedure.

Closure of the inguinal ring will be made utilizing 0.6-mm nonabsorbable suture. Insert an atraumatic needle from the outside through the medial edge of the external ring beginning 2 cm from the posterior apex of the ring (Fig. 7B). Carry the suture forward deep to the tunica vaginalis and pass the needle through the edge of the internal oblique muscle from the inside out (Fig. 7C). Now pass the suture posteriorly deep to the tunica vaginalis and again through the edge of the inguinal ring from inside out 1 cm anterior to the first suture (Fig. 7D). Both suture ends are grasped with a forceps for identification and will be tied later. A second suture is similarly placed in the lateral margin of the ring. Beginning 2 cm from the posterior apex of the ring insert the suture from the outside through the edge of the ring and carry it forward over the tunica vaginalis and through the edge of the internal oblique from the inside out (Fig. 7E). Return the suture again passing over the tunica vaginalis and pass it from the inside out through the lateral margin of the ring 1 cm anterior to the first bite (Fig. 7F). The two sutures through the internal oblique muscle should be at least 3 cm apart and should straddle the cord. Be sure that the hernia is reduced and draw the internal oblique muscle posteriorly by tightening the preplaced sutures. When these sutures are tied the lumen of the inguinal ring is reduced so that the hernia cannot recur (Fig. 7G).

Close the incision in the tunica vaginalis with No. 0 chromic gut in a simple continuous pattern. To strengthen the inguinal ring closure an overlapping mattress suture is placed in the anterior portion of the external ring utilizing 0.6-mm nonabsorbable suture. Begin the pattern by securing the suture 2.5 cm medial and anterior to the cranial apex of the ring. Introduce the suture from the inside outward through the anterior lateral lip of the inguinal ring, exiting 1 cm from the edge. Pass 2 cm posteriorly and parallel to the edge of the ring and introduce the suture inward through the lateral lip of the ring. Insert the suture from the outside inward 2 cm from the medial edge of ring and exit 2 cm posterior to the entry point. Carry the suture outward through the lateral lip of the ring and repeat the process until the external ring is sufficiently closed to permit the easy insertion of three fingers (Fig. 7H).

Antibiotics should be administered for 5 days postoperatively. Postoperative edema is expected in the area and may persist for 10 days. Semen quality should be examined 60 days following surgery; if found to be acceptable the bull is ready for breeding service.

SURGERY OF THE SCROTUM

Castration

Calf castration is the most common bovine surgical procedure. Various techniques are described in many surgery texts and will not be discussed here.

Unilateral Scrotal Disease

Etiology. Orchitis, inflammation of the testicle, occurs in a small percentage of bulls and is usually a unilateral condition. Systemic infections, the most common cause of orchitis, reach the testicle by hematogenous spread, but extension of infection from the urogenital tract may occur. Epididymitis, inflammation of the epididymis, occurs more frequently than orchitis and more frequently in the bull than in other domestic animals. Numerous bacteria, viruses, and fungi may cause orchitis ·or epididymitis but *Corynebacterium pyogenes*, *Chlamydia* sp. and *Brucella abortus* are the most frequent causative agents. Noninfectious causes of pathologic changes in scrotal contents are less common in the bull and usually include trauma or neoplasia. Trauma may produce hematocele or hydrocele, consisting of accumulation of hemorrhage or fluid in the vaginal cavity. Primary tumors of the scrotum are rare but metastatic lesions occasionally occur.

In the bull inflammation of the peritesticular tissues, periorchitis, frequently accompanies epididymitis or orchitis. This condition is more common than orchitis.

Diagnosis. Diagnosis of scrotal disease is based on physical examination. The scrotum usually is greatly distended and one side of the scrotum may be many times its normal size. Palpation of the affected scrotal half will reveal edema in the skin and, in the case of periorchitis, hematocele or hydrocele, considerable fluid accumulation between the testicle and the scrotal wall. In the case of orchitis the testicle will be enlarged and firm. All bulls considered for surgical or medical therapy for scrotal disease should be proved negative for brucellosis before treatment is initiated. Testicular biopsy is strongly discouraged because disruption of the tubular integrity of the testicle or epididymis will allow extravasation of sperm and a resulting autoimmune reaction that will cause the formation of sperm granulomas.

The veterinarian should realize that unilateral scrotal disease usually results in degenerative changes in the contralateral testicle. This testicular degeneration is due to disruption of the thermoregulatory mechanism of the testicle by the inflammatory response. The degeneration is usually temporary and normal testicular function can be expected to return approximately 8 weeks following resolution of the insult.

Surgical Procedure. The bull is restrained in right lateral recumbency and general anesthesia is achieved. The left rear leg is secured in flexed abduction and the scrotum is clipped and disinfected with povidone iodine.

A vertical skin incision is made on the lateral surface of the scrotum beginning near the base and extending 15 cm toward the apex. The incision is deepened through the skin, tunica dartos and scrotal fascia, leaving the tunica vaginalis parietalis intact. Bluntly dissect the testicle in the parietal tunic from the scrotal fascia and make a 12-cm incision through the parietal tunic beginning proximally and ending at the cranial pole of the testis. Exteriorize the testicle through this incision and expose the spermatic cord (Fig. 8A).

Bluntly divide the spermatic artery, vein and ductus deferens 8 cm proximal to the pampiniform plexus and individually double ligate them with No. 0 chromic gut. Transect these structures between the ligatures. Ligate the external cremaster muscle and transect the muscle and tunica vaginalis parietalis just distal to the spermatic cord. Close the tunic with a Connell pattern using No. 0 chromic gut (Fig. 8B).

Close the tunica dartos with No. 0 chromic gut in a simple continuous pattern. Skin closure is made with 0.4-mm Vetafil using a continuous interlocking pattern. The incision is coated with a topical antimicrobial spray.

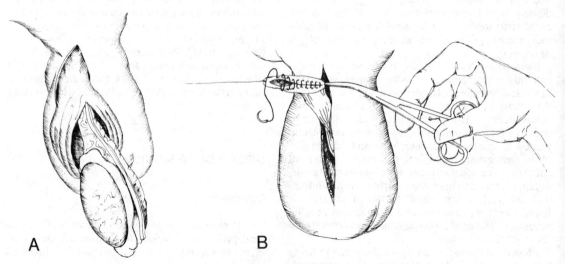

Figure 8. Unilateral castration. *A*, Testicle and spermatic cord exteriorized. *B*, Closure of parietal tunic.

Postoperative Care. Intramuscular systemic antibiotics should be administered for at least 5 days after surgery. Sutures may be removed in 2 weeks and the bull will be ready for breeding when semen quality returns to normal in the remaining testicle. Volume of sperm production following unilateral castration can be expected to approach 75 per cent of that from bulls with both testicles.

SURGICAL PREPARATION OF ESTRUS-DETECTOR BULLS

Philosophy and Liabilities

Many veterinarians feel that the best method of estrus detection is frequent observation of the cow herd by experienced personnel. Others feel that bulls are superior to man in heat detection and that estrus-detector bulls reduce the time expended by farm personnel in detecting estrous females.

Various techniques have been used in preparing bulls for estrus-detection but regardless of the technique utilized two objectives should be satisfied. The first objective is to render the bull incapable of intromission. This should be performed in a manner that does not make copulation attempts uncomfortable for the bull. This criterion is necessary so that the spread of venereal and nonspecific disease is prevented and so that the bull will maintain his libido.

The second objective is to render the bull incapable of impregnation. This precautionary step is necessary in the event that the bull learns to achieve intromission or if the surgery to prevent intromission fails. The veterinarian should be cognizant that there is a legal obligation to render the bull sterile and incapable of coitus.

Bulls chosen for estrus detection should be healthy, show obvious male characteristics and have a vigorous nature with a high level of libido. Size of the bull is important, and well-grown yearlings are usually used so that they will be growing and represent a financial return when they have completed their usefulness. Very large bulls should be avoided with yearling heifers.

Nonsurgical Methods for Preparing Estrus-Detector Animals

Cull cows, heifers or steers may be utilized as estrus detector animals without surgical alteration. Testosterone-treated females or steers may be as efficient as surgically altered bulls and may be more desirable for some producers. Advantages of using testosterone-treated animals for heat detection include their ready availability within the herd, avoiding the need to raise or purchase a bull for surgical alteration. Additionally, treated cows or steers are less expensive to prepare than teaser bulls and may be safer to handle. Disadvantages of testosterone-treated teaser animals include failure of some animals to show male behavior following treatment, the tendency for some treated animals to lose weight due to excessive sexual activity in the herd, and the possibility that some treated animals may mount nonestrual females.

Various treatment regimes are utilized to produce estrus-detector animals. One popular program utilizes testosterone propionate, 0.2 gm intramuscularly, on the initial treatment day. This same dosage is administered on treatment day 4 through 9 and on day 10 when 1 gm of testosterone propionate is administered, a chinball marker is attached and the teaser is put with the breeding herd. Every 10 to 14 days a 1-gm booster injection is administered to maintain the teaser. Recent reports indicate that testosterone enanthate given as a single 2-gm treatment is as effective, requires less labor and prepares the teaser more quickly than the more common testosterone propionate program. The treatment schedule is as follows: 0.5 gm testosterone enanthate intramuscularly and 1.5 gm subcutaneously divided in two locations. After 4 days a chinball marker is attached and the teaser is put with the breeding herd. Testosterone enanthate should be given at the rate of 0.5 to 0.75 gm subcutaneously every 10 to 14 days to maintain the libido of the teaser animal.

Surgical Procedures

Preputial Pouch Technique. The preputial pouch technique consists of closing the preputial orifice after creating a small ventral midline fistula 5 cm posterior to the orifice for urine drainage. This procedure produces a teaser bull that is quickly ready for service and that maintains libido for a long period of time. The size of the fistula is critical. If the opening is too large, paraphimosis may result, if too small, excessive urine collection in the preputial cavity may develop. One objection to the technique is that calculi tend to form in the preputial pouch, leading to inflammation and infection if not washed out periodically.

The bull is restrained in right lateral recumbency and tranquilized or sedated if the surgeon desires. The preputial orifice and sheath are clipped and prepared for aseptic surgery for a distance of 30 cm posteriorly. A local anesthetic agent should be infiltrated around the preputial orifice and at the site of the fistula.

Manually extend the penis and suture a 2.5-cm Penrose drain over the free portion of the penis using three or four simple interrupted No. 0 chromic gut sutures and being careful to avoid the urethra. This tube is placed to provide for drainage of urine out of the blind preputial pouch during the healing period.

Introduce the left index finger into the preputial cavity to the depth of the previously prepared site and make an elliptical skin incision on the ventral midline (Fig. 9A). This opening should not be large enough to allow the penis to extend through it postoperatively because paraphimosis may result.

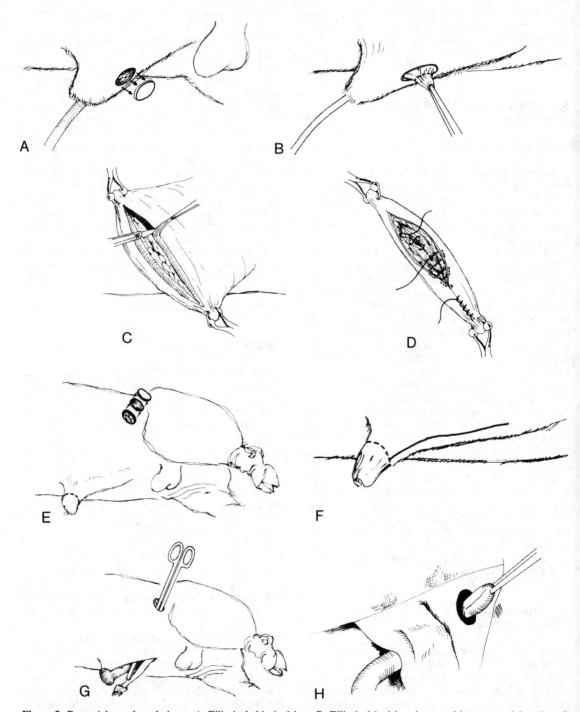

Figure 9. Preputial pouch technique: *A*, Elliptical skin incision. *B*, Elliptical incision deepened into preputial cavity. *C*, Excision of 5-mm ring of tissue from preputial orifice. *D*, Closure of preputial orifice. Preputial translocation: *E*, Excision of 7-cm circle of skin and cutaneous trunci muscle. *F*, 20-cm longitudinal skin incision on ventral midline. *G*, Dissection tunnel deep to the cutaneous trunci muscle. *H*, Preputial orifice pulled through the flank incision.

Deepen the incision through the elastic tissue and into the preputial cavity, avoiding large vessels (Fig. 9B). Suture the moist skin of the prepuce to the skin of the sheath utilizing interrupted nonabsorbable suture to create the fistula. Pull the free end of the previously placed Penrose tubing through the fistula.

Excise a 5-mm wide ring of tissue from the preputial orifice at the junction of sheath skin and preputial skin. This step is facilitated by using towel forceps to stretch the orifice (Fig. 9C). Close the preputial skin with No. 0 chromic gut with closely spaced sutures in a Cushing pattern to effect a watertight seal. This step is important to prevent urine seepage into the incision with subsequent dehiscence. Another row of sutures is similarly placed in the connective tissue and the skin is closed with monofilament nonabsorbable suture in a continuous interlocking pattern (Fig. 9D). A caudal epididymectomy should be performed to ensure sterility.

Prophylactic antibiotics may be given for 5 days postoperatively. Ten days after the surgery the skin sutures should be removed from the preputial orifice and fistula. Remove the Penrose tubing by applying firm gentle traction to the tubing and removing the sutures in the free portion of the penis. The bull should be ready for service 4 week postoperatively, and the owner should be admonished to flush the preputial cavity every 3 to 4 weeks to avoid the accumulation of calculi.

Preputial Translocation. The preputial translocation technique consists of relocating the preputial orifice just above the left flank fold. This procedure requires general anesthesia and entails more surgical trauma than some other methods of teaser preparation. The relocation site is critical. If the opening is placed too high on the flank urine pooling in the preputial cavity occurs and urine scald will occur ventral to the opening. If the opening is placed too low on the flank the action of the cutaneous trunci muscle will not function to help evacuate urine from the preputial cavity.

The bull is restrained in right dorsal recumbency and general anesthesia or heavy sedation is attained. Clip and surgically prepare the lower left flank and the abdominal floor including the preputial orifice. Excise a 7-cm circle of skin above the left flank fold so that the lower edge of the resulting hole is 3 cm above the flank fold. Remove a corresponding circle of the underlying cutaneous trunci muscle to expose the abdominal wall (Fig. 9E). Ligate all bleeders and cover the opening with a sterile surgical sponge while the next phase of the procedure is performed.

Make a skin incision 3 cm caudal to the preputial orifice that circumscribes the sheath. Beginning 40 cm caudal to the preputial orifice make a longitudinal skin incision on the ventral midline of the sheath that intersects the circumscribing incision (Fig. 9F). Deepen the incision through the subcutaneous tissue to expose the elastic layers of the prepuce and bluntly dissect the penis, prepuce and elastic tissue free from the abdominal wall. Avoid traumatizing the large vessels in the elastic tissue. Continue the dissection anteriorly to the circumscribing incision around the preputial orifice. Ligate all bleeders encountered. Place a single simple interrupted skin suture in the dorsal aspect of the preputial orifice to serve as a reference point when suturing the orifice into the new opening. When the penis, prepuce, and preputial orifice are completely free, exteriorize the entire mass through the ventral midline incision.

Introduce a long blunt forceps such as a Knowles' forceps into the circular skin incision above the flank. Begin deep to the cutaneous trunci muscle and bluntly dissect a tunnel to the ventral midline incision (Fig. 9G). The fascial tissue will have to be incised in the area of the penis to expose the end of the forceps. This tunnel should be sufficiently large to allow redirection of the penis and prepuce without restriction. Grasp the preputial orifice with the forceps and pull the prepuce through the circular opening, carefully avoiding torsion of the tissue (Fig. 9H).

Align the dorsum of the preputial orifice with the dorsal aspect of the circular opening using the previously placed reference suture. Place a simple interrupted suture of No. 0 chromic gut at each quadrant of the opening to appose the subcutaneous tissue and muscle of the preputial orifice and the cutaneous trunci muscle. Additional interrupted sutures are now placed around the periphery of the incision to complete the deep layer closure. The skin is closed in a similar manner using 0.6-mm nonabsorbable suture. Remove the reference suture from the preputial orifice.

Close the ventral sheath incision with 0.6-mm nonabsorbable suture using a continuous interlocking pattern, occasionally catching the abdominal fascia to reduce tissue sagging and seroma formation. Leave the circular incision at the end of the sheath open to allow serum drainage. A caudal epididymectomy should also be performed. Prophylactic antibiotics may be administered for 5 days postoperatively. The surgeon should be aware that the translocated preputial orifice may undergo severe skin discoloration until revascularization occurs. Skin sutures are removed in 14 days and the bull should be ready for service in 4 weeks.

Corpus Cavernosal Block. This technique consists of injecting soft hoof acrylic in a liquid form into the corpus cavernosum penis to create a thrombus, thereby preventing erection. Failures with this technique have resulted when inadequate thrombus formation was achieved due to small-volume acrylic injection or perhaps injecting the acrylic too slowly. The surgeon should be aware that hoof acrylic has not been approved for injection in cattle in the United States. Advantages of this technique are that the surgical procedure is performed with the bull standing in a chute, obviating the need for general anesthesia.

Restrain the bull in a squeeze chute, administer epidural anesthesia and prepare a surgery site 15 × 25 cm on the midline caudal to the scrotum. Make

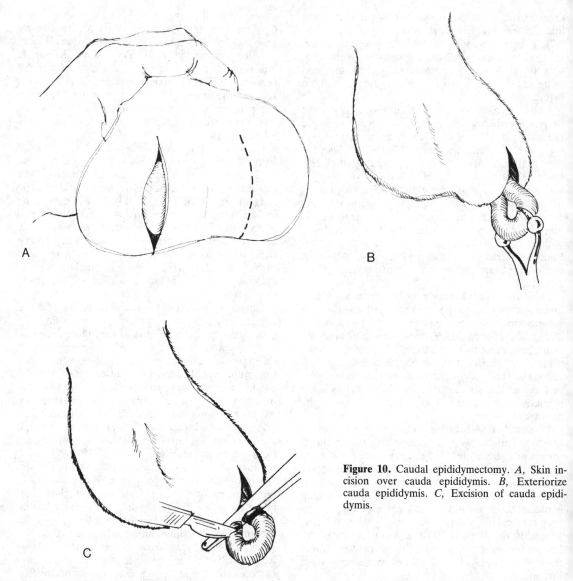

Figure 10. Caudal epididymectomy. *A,* Skin incision over cauda epididymis. *B,* Exteriorize cauda epididymis. *C,* Excision of cauda epididymis.

a 15-cm midline skin incision ending posterior to the scrotum and deepen the incision by blunt dissection until the distal sigmoid flexure of the penis is exposed. Exteriorize the retractor penis muscles and palpate the ventral urethral groove. Utilizing the urethral groove as a landmark, insert a 14-gauge needle into the corpus cavernosum penis from the lateral aspect of the penis proximal to the attachment of the retractor penis muscles. The surgeon should avoid inserting the needle into the corpus spongiosum penis surrounding the urethra. Inject sterile saline through the needle to verify placement and patency of the needle. The saline will flow freely when the needle is placed in the corpus cavernosum penis. Remove the syringe and leave the needle in place. An assistant should fill a 10-ml syringe with freshly prepared hoof acrylic and inject 6 ml of the mixture through the 14-gauge needle into the corpus cavernosum penis. The surgeon

should feel the enlargement of the penis as the injection is made. The acrylic hardens almost immediately.

Place a retaining suture in the penis to hold the penis in the retracted position while healing occurs. Beginning near the ventral commissure of the skin incision pass a single suture of 0.6-mm nonabsorbable suture through the skin 1 cm lateral to the incision. Take a bite into the tunica albuginea on the lateral aspect of the penis just proximal to the point where the retractor penis muscle attaches to the penis, exit the skin 1 cm above the original suture bite and tie. A caudal epididymectomy should be performed next.

The bull should be allowed sexual rest until healing is complete. Prophylactic antibiotics may be administered at the surgeon's discretion but are generally not necessary. The sutures are removed after 2 weeks and the bull is ready for service.

EPIDIDYMECTOMY

Bilateral caudal epididymectomy is recommended to sterilize the bull when any method of surgical teaser bull preparation is performed. This procedure is easier to accomplish than vasectomy in the bull. Surgically prepare the distal third of the scrotum and infiltrate the ventral scrotal skin with local anesthetic. Force the testicle to the bottom of the scrotum and make a 2.5-cm skin incision directly over the tail of the epididymis (Fig. 10A). Deepen the incision through the scrotal fascia and vaginal tunic until the epididymis protrudes through the incision. Grasp the epididymis with towel forceps and apply traction to exteriorize the entire epididymal tail (Fig. 10B). Apply hemostatic forceps across the tail of the epididymis and excise the tissue with a scalpel (Fig. 10C). The surgeon should avoid traumatizing the tunica albuginea of the testis because excessive hemorrhage will result. Remove the hemostatic forceps and repeat the procedure on the other side. Ligatures or skin sutures are not necessary and the wound is allowed to heal by second intention.

Selected Readings

1. Ashdown RR, Pearson H: The functional significance of the dorsal apical ligament of the bovine penis. Res Vet Sci 12:183, 1971.
2. Beckett SD, Walker DF, Hudson RS, et al.: Corpus cavernosum penis pressure and penile muscle activity in the bull during coitus. Am J Vet Res, 35(6):761, 1974.
3. Hudson RS: The effect of the penile injuries on breeding ability of bulls. Annual Meeting Society for Theriogenology, 1978, pp. 83-86.
4. Humphrey JD, Ladd PW: Pathology of the bovine testis and epididymis. Vet Bull 45:787, 1975.
5. Young SL, Hudson RS, Walker DF: Impotence in bulls due to vascular shunts from the corpus cavernosum penis. J Am Vet Med Assoc 171(7):643, 1977.

Induction of Lactation in Cattle

R. J. Collier, Ph.D.
University of Florida
Gainesville, Florida

S. R. Davis, Ph.D.
Ruakura Animal Research Station
Hamilton, New Zealand

Estrogen and estrogen-progesterone in combination have been used for many years to induce lactation in cattle. Prior to 1973, induction attempts were characterized by long injection regimens (60 to 180 days) that produced variable success rates and relatively low milk yields. Smith and Schanbacher in 1973 greatly improved procedures to induce lactation by shortening the injection period to 7 days and changing the dose of estradiol and progesterone to mimic concentrations found just prior to parturition in cattle.

METHOD OF SMITH AND SCHANBACHER

Smith and Schanbacher used a daily dose of 0.1 mg per kg body weight estradiol and 0.25 mg per kg body weight progesterone dissolved in absolute alcohol and administered in split daily injections at 12-hour intervals for 7 days. Injections were given subcutaneously at sites on the dorsal aspect of the rib cage behind the scapula. Approximately 70 per cent of animals given this treatment achieve a peak milk production of 9 kg per day or greater (Table 1). However, this technique shared with previous methods the disadvantage of variability of response to treatment. Peak milk production ranged from 1 kg per day to 32 kg per day. Approximately 70 per cent of animals given this treatment produced greater than 9 kg per day (Table 1).

Reproductive performance following treatment varied as well. Ovaries of all animals given the injections became inactive, and animals displayed intense estrous behavior for 2 to 3 weeks. Occasionally, pelvic injuries occurred in some animals due to estrous behavior. First estrus following treatment was observed an average of 43 days following the last injection. Cystic ovaries developed in approximately 30 per cent of animals given this treatment. The treatment of cystic animals with 10,000 units human chorionic gonadotropin (hCG) resulted in resumption of normal estrous cycles. Conception rate to first service in noncystic animals was 56 per cent in one study.[1]

MODIFICATIONS OF SMITH AND SCHANBACHER TECHNIQUE

Following initial reports of this method, studies were conducted to modify the induction scheme to improve milk yields and reduce variability. Inclusion of dexamethasone (Azium, Shering, Kenilworth, NJ, 20 mg/day) on days 17, 18 and 19 in the treatment scheme, as suggested by Chakriyaret and

Table 1. History and Lactation Performance of Cows and Heifers Hormonally Induced into Lactation*

| | | | Induced Lactation | | |
| | | | | 305 Day† | |
Animal	Breed	Previous Lactations (Number)	Peak Milk Yield (kg/day)	Milk Yield (kg)	Time to Peak Milk Yield (wk)
1	Holstein	2	32	5765	6
2	Holstein	1	31	5615	9
3	Holstein	0	18	5070	8
4	Holstein	0	17	4060	8
5	Holstein	0	16	3485	12
6	Holstein	0	14	3065	12
7	Holstein	0	13	2610	6
8	Holstein	4	10	2600	12
9	Brown Swiss	2	10	2220	10
10	Holstein	0	13	2190	8
11	Brown Swiss	6	9	1510	6
12	Jersey	1	4	830	
13	Holstein	4	4	610	
14	Holstein	3	2	380	
15	Holstein	4	1	—	
16	Holstein	3	1	—	

*305-day production for unsuccessful animals (Cows 12, 13 and 14) were predicted from partial records.
†From Collier RJ et al.: J Dairy Sci 58:1525, 1975.

Table 2. Comparison of Induced Lactation Treatments on Mature Equivalent Basis

| | Previous Lactation 305-Day (kg) | Treatments | | | | Induced Lactation (Per Cent of Previous) | |
Number		E_2	P_4	Dex	Reserpine Days	Peak Yield	100 Day
14	6580 ± 370	+	+	+	—	37.1 ± 9.0	36.4 ± 7.9
9	6490 ± 370	+	+	+	—	37.0 ± 8.3	30.7 ± 7.1
5	6320 ± 750	+	+	+	13, 14, 15, 16	54.7 ± 2.6	49.2 ± 3.1
5	6540 ± 690	+	+	+	8, 10, 12, 14	62.7 ± 2.8	55.4 ± 8.6
3	8600 ± 200	+	+	+	8, 10, 12, 14	57.1 ± 6.4	50.7 ± 8.6
4	7970 ± 850	+	+	+	8, 10, 12, 14	63.9 ± 12.5	55.1 ± 12.1
4	7730 ± 1000	+	+	+	2, 5, 9, 11, 14	79.6 ± 2.9	74.1 ± 2.8

All milk yields expressed as mature equivalent basis and represent mean ± SE.
E_2 = estrogen; P_4 = progesterone; Dex = dexamethasone.

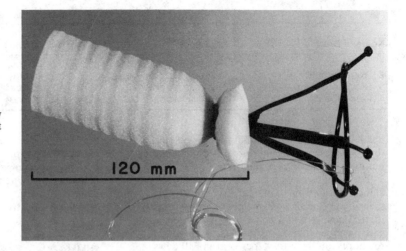

Figure 1. Intravaginal sponge ready for insertion. (From David SR et al.: J Dairy Sci: 66:451, 1983.)

associates,[1] improved yields only slightly (Table 2). Collier and his colleagues[3] hypothesized that prolactin might be the limiting component in the induction scheme. Inclusion of reserpine (Sandril) at a dose of 5 mg per day to cause prolactin release in addition to the administered dexamethasone markedly improved milk yields and reduced variability of response (Table 2).

Subsequently, Kensinger and associates[5] demonstrated that the time of year when the animals were given the treatment dramatically influenced prolactin release in response to reserpine and the subsequent milk yield of animals (Table 3). Prolactin release in response to reserpine was highest in spring, and milk yield following treatment was twice as high as in animals injected during the winter. Thus, prolactin concentrations during induced lactation markedly affect subsequent milk yield.

The Use of Intravaginal Drug Delivery for the Induction of Lactation

The steroid injection regime developed by Smith and Schanbacher and improved by others has dis-

advantages, some of which diminish its potential for practical application.

1. Reduced production (60 to 70 per cent) relative to that found following normal calving.
2. Nymphomaniac behavior with associated management problems (mainly lameness) due to high estrogen dosage.
3. Repeated veterinary visits required to inject drugs twice daily for 7 days.
4. Opposition of regulatory authorities to the use of estrogen depot injections.

The delivery of estrogen and progesterone from intravaginal devices has been achieved successfully in studies conducted in New Zealand. Of a number of devices examined, a steroid-impregnated sponge (Fig. 1) has been most thoroughly evaluated. Another device is composed of Silastic coils, which suffer from low efficiency of drug release.

With an intravaginal device the need for steroid injections is obviated, with the added advantage that the steroid source is removed following treat-

Table 3. Mean Temperature, Serum Prolactin and Milk Yields of Cows Induced Into Lactation During Two Seasons*

	Season	
	Winter	Spring
Mean daily temperature‡	-6.5	11.9
Basal prolactin prior to reserpine (ng/ml)†	10	43.6
Reserpine-stimulated prolactin three postinjection (ng/ml)†	203	482.3
Peak daily yield (kg)‡	13.2	24.5
100-day yield (kg)‡	863	1985.3

*From Kensinger RS et al.: J Dairy Sci 62:1884, 1979.
†Data represent means of three treatment groups for each season.
‡Treatment means are expressed on a mature equivalent basis.

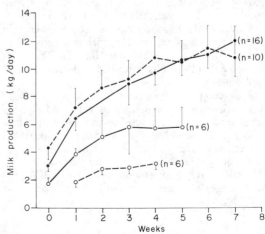

Figure 2. Milk production following induction of lactation by intravaginal sponge in spring (●) and autumn (○) of 1979 (—) and 1980 (---). (From David SR et al.: J Dairy Sci: 66:454, 1983.)

Table 4. Drugs

Name of Drug	Company Name and Address	Species	Dose (mg or IU/kg)
1. 17β Estradiol	Sigma, St. Louis, Missouri	bovine	0.1 mg/kg body wt.
2. Progesterone	Sigma, St. Louis, Missouri	bovine	0.25 mg/kg body wt.
3. Dexamethasone (Azium)	Schering, Kenilworth, N.J.	bovine	20 mg/day
4. Reserpine (Sandril)	Eli Lilly, Indianapolis, Indiana	bovine	not to exceed 2.5 mg/day

ment, minimizing contamination by residues. Further, any residues would remain a part of the body not used for human consumption.

Studies of cows with steroid-impregnated sponges alone indicated unsatisfactory retention rates; less than 50 per cent of treated cows retaining the sponge for 10 days. A nylon collar attached to the sponge with a rubber ring overcomes this problem, and the retention rate rose to 95 per cent in 310 cows.

The sponge was loaded with 500 mg estradiol-17β and 100 mg progesterone by injection of a solution of these in acetone/ethanol (in a ratio of 30:70 v/v). The sponge was inserted via a speculum (sponge first), and the presence of the sponge in the vagina was indicated by an exposed loop of nylon line. Six days after sponge insertion an intramuscular injection (20 mg) of mixed dexamethasone esters (Opticortenol, Ciba-Geigy, N.Z.) was given, or intramuscular injections of reserpine (2.5 mg) were made on days 6, 8 and 10. Sponges were removed on day 10.

Response rates (cows in milk) to treatment with the sponge alone, the sponge plus dexamethasone injection and the sponge plus reserpine injections were 25, 89 and 96 per cent, respectively, the responses to dexamethasone and reserpine not differing statistically, but both being significantly better treatments than the sponge alone. Treatment with both dexamethasone and reserpine was not tested on this study.

Cows induced to lactate did so within 2 days of sponge removal, and milk production increased slowly from this time to peak production 6 to 8 weeks later. However, there was a marked seasonal variation in response to treatment, cows induced in the spring being considerably more productive than those induced in the autumn (Fig. 2). This is in agreement with results published by Kensinger and colleagues.[5]

Milk composition of cows induced to lactate by this technique was essentially normal and showed an absence of estrogen residues in milk even at first milking. Further advantages were that the incidence of lameness arising from steroid treatment was less with sponge treatment than with injected steroids. More recently, a lower dose of estradiol-17β (250 mg/sponge) has been found to be as efficacious as the 500-mg dose, and although this has not been vigorously tested, increasing the ratio of progesterone to estrogen in the sponge should reduce the incidence of riding activity and its associated animal health problems. Following sponge removal the frequency of estrus activity rapidly diminishes.

SUMMARY

Highest success rates of treatments to induce lactation were found when dexamethasone and reserpine were included in a steroid treatment regimen. Estradiol and progesterone may be administered by subcutaneous injection or intravaginal sponge. Dramatic seasonal effects were also detected in two studies indicating that the highest success was achieved during spring and early summer. Doses of reserpine exceeding 2.5 mg per day result in extreme drowsiness and loss of appetite in some animals. However, adverse reactions have not been detected in doses of 2.5 mg per day or less (R. J. Collier, unpublished observations).

It should also be noted that these treatments are not presently cleared for use in farm animals by the U.S. Food and Drug Administration except on a research basis. Drug dosages are summarized in Table 4.

References

1. Chakriyaret S, Head HH, Thatcher WW et al.: Induction of lactation: lactational, physiological and hormonal responses in the bovine. J Dairy Sci 61:1715, 1978.
2. Collier RJ, Bauman DE, Hays RL: Milk production and reproduction performance of cows hormonally induced into lactation. J Dairy Sci 58:1524, 1975.
3. Collier RJ, Bauman DE, Hays RL: Effect of reserpine on milk production and serum prolactin of cows hormonally induced into lactation. J Dairy Sci 60:89, 1977.
4. Davis SR, Welch RAS, Pierce MG, Peterson AJ: Induction of lactation in nonpregnant cows by estradiol:17β and progesterone from an intravaginal sponge. J Dairy Sci 66:450, 1983.
5. Kensinger RS, Bauman DE, Collier RJ: Season and treatment effects on serum prolactin and milk yield during induced lactation. J Dairy Sci 62:1881, 1979.
6. Smith KL, Schanbacher FL: Hormone induced lactation in the bovine. I. Lactational performance following injections of 17β-estradiol and progesterone. J Dairy Sci 56:738, 1973.

Reproductive Management Programs for Large Dairies

Leon D. Weaver, V.M.D.
University of California
Tulare, California

OBJECTIVES

Dairying has become big business in many parts of the world. Dairy operations often exceed 500 to 1000 cows, employ 10 to 20 people, and have capital investments and annual revenues exceeding 2 million dollars. The owner of a large dairy must manage people and finances effectively if he wishes to be successful in the management of cows.

The basis for all dairy health programs must be their economic return to ownership. The pursuit of optimal animal health and productivity cannot be justified except by increased profit. This goal requires the consultant and herd owner to continually seek new, more efficient production methods. All proposed diagnostic, therapeutic and management procedures must be scrutinized for economic viability.

The economic success of the dairyman is the most important objective of a program, but it is seldom the only one. The owner's degree of personal involvement, pride in ownership, innovative nature, financial portfolio and tax structure all markedly affect program development and implementation. Large dairies frequently involve several family members as partners, management apprentices and employees. Not infrequently, choices are made to sacrifice short-term productivity to nurture an individual within the organization. Reproductive and herd health programs are likely to fail if they do not recognize the unique character of each dairy operation.

Finally, reproductive management programs must be economically rewarding to the consultant. Successful programs include both professional health care services and management consultation. Ideally, ranch workers, AI and animal health technicians, herdsmen, and veterinary professionals will all be able to contribute as much as they can. If properly trained ranch personnel and technicians are not used for routine reproductive and health delivery procedures, costs for technical services will increase, and the veterinarian will have less time for consultation. The veterinarian's role should be one of program designer, team leader, instructor and performance evaluator. The veterinarian is often an important communicator between owners and the people who do the work. If the veterinarian is not compensated for management services, he is unlikely to provide them effectively.

Dairy profitability is directly related to the level of milk production. With few exceptions, higher production levels yield higher returns for labor and management. Due to the effect of scale, large dairies are profoundly affected by the quality of management. Projected gross revenues from the sale of milk on a 500 milking cow dairy can vary as much as $40,000 per month or $500,000 per year (Table 1.) The herd health consultant can affect profitability by designing, implementing and supervising programs that achieve maximum daily production levels while minimizing expenditures.

Reproductive management and health care can increase productivity and profits by providing for optimum calving intervals, reduced culling for reproductive failure, and efficient utilization of labor. Optimal calving intervals produce the maximum daily milk production over the lifetime of the cow. Disease prevention, early diagnosis and timely treatment are justifiable if they optimize calving intervals. If culling for reproductive failure is reduced, genetically superior animals can be kept and inferior ones culled. Expenditures for labor can be minimized by grouping cows and defining specialized job assignments.

FACILITY DESIGN AND UTILIZATION

Large dairies typically have from 4 to 20 corrals or pens where the herd is housed and fed. Each pen must be designed to allow for efficient, accurate feeding, effortless cow handling, and protection from environment, injuries, and pathogens. Geographic conditions and individual cow groupings dictate pen specifications. Some pens (e.g., maternity and breeding pens) require more facilities, protection and space than others.

Implementation of a reproductive program will require an inspection of all facilities available. It is helpful in planning a reproductive program to diagram the entire dairy facility, indicating the location and capacity of each pen, presence or absence and type of locking stanchions, and any other limitations such as milking order required for orderly cow

Table 1. Production Level Effect on Gross Income (500 milking cows)

Production Level	No. Cows	Price/cwt		Annual Milk Income
65/lb/day	500	$14.00 × 365 days	=	$1,660,750
45/lb/day	500	$14.00 × 365 days	=	$1,149,750
		Annual difference	=	$ 511,000
		Monthly difference	=	$ 42,583

movement. Cows may already be grouped for production feeding, mastitis control, or other purposes. Existing grouping objectives may conflict with ideal groupings for reproductive management. In such cases, relative cost-benefit comparisons and compromises must be considered.

Facilities with fewer corrals have fewer options than those with many corrals. It is essential that an adequate number of corrals with sufficient capacity and facilities (e.g., locking stanchions) be available from the outset. Ideally, every animal of weaning age and older should have a lock-up stanchion. Individual animal restraint and access is vital to management procedures for all age and lactation groups. Inadequate facilities should be changed. Failures in reproductive programs commonly result from overcrowding, disrepair or lack of stanchions, or labor inefficiencies due to poorly conceived cow groupings. Smaller dairies seldom find it feasible to provide pens for all desired cow groups. These dairies may be able to substitute more individual animal care to compensate for fewer cow groups. Very large herds (over 1000 cows) are often best managed as multiples of smaller ones. For the purposes of this discussion, a maximum number of pens available will be assumed.

Dry cows should be divided into four groups. A small pen near the milking barn is desirable to house cows for approximately 2 weeks immediately following drying. When the mammary gland is fully involuted, these cows can be moved into one of two dry cow pens. Cows that are at or above ideal body weight and cows that are expected to have a dry period of more than 60 days can be placed in one corral while thin cows can be placed in a second corral. These two corrals should be located at the most distant area from the milking facility since these dry cows require less intensive observation than other cow groups. In hot climates, provision of shade for dry cows will improve calf birth weights and milk production in the subsequent lactation. A fourth pen receives cows from the two dry pens approximately 2 to 3 weeks prior to the expected date of parturition. This close-up corral should be located adjacent to the calving area to allow intensive observation and should have mangers suitable for concentrate feeding.

Parturient cows must have access to a sanitary, uncrowded, well-attended, and lighted area. A clean pasture, a deeply bedded, covered group maternity pen, or an individual box stall will each serve adequately. The calving area should have restraint facilities with lights, water, electricity, and adequate drainage for obstetric manipulations and surgical procedures. A cabinet containing all obstetric equipment, lubricant and disinfectant should be located adjacent to the restraint facility.

Postparturient cows are grouped together for colostrum collection, feeding, mastitis detection, and intensive daily observations for health problems. This corral should have lock-up stanchions and easy access to a catch chute since many cows will be reluctant to come to the manger in the first days postpartum.

The fresh cow corral should have a capacity equal to the number of cows that will normally calve in a 4- to 6-week period. A corral of this capacity will allow a weekly or biweekly postpartum examination schedule and provide for the retention of cows in the fresh cow string until they are determined to be normal and "OK to breed."

A suitable number of pens to house the balance of the milking herd must be available to accept cows discharged from the fresh string. Depending on the number of corrals available, groupings for production feeding, mastitis segregation and parity may be desirable. Production feeding schemes tend to group cows by stage of lactation. Such groupings are equally desirable for breeding management since they allow for concentration of heat detection and AI breeding, achieve labor efficiency, and minimize the daily standing time for cows restrained in locking stanchions for AI service. Confirmed pregnant cows can be moved into pregnant cow or natural service strings later in lactation. Natural service strings can be used for problem breeders beyond a certain stage of lactation or below a set production level. Pens for AI breeding of milking cows and replacement heifers should have locking stanchions, preferably of the self-locking type. Geographic orientation should ideally have the sun away from the herdsman's line of sight during heat detection and breeding times. Adequate manger space and stanchions must be available to allow each animal to be locked in daily. It is often desirable in the interests of labor efficiency to designate one milking corral a to-cull/to-dry corral. Cows can be moved to this string to await the optimum drying or culling date. Additionally, cows judged unsuitable to rebreed as a result of conformation or disease processes can be retained in this corral until culling is warranted.

A most important part of the dairy is the hospital area. This pen must be close to a milking and treatment facility. It can be near the maternity, postpartum and fresh cow pens but should be distinctly separate from them. The hospital corral should have a capacity equal to 2 to 5 per cent of the milking herd. The hospital area provides a place to retain animals that are clinically ill from any cause for diagnosis, treatment, disease containment, and residue avoidance procedures.

An examination of the cow identification and record systems must precede the implementation of a herd reproductive program. During the past two decades the dairy industry has rapidly progressed from a state of few or no individual cow records to a confusing duplication of record systems. It is not uncommon for a modern dairy to have as many as four or five record systems! Typically, some information (such as fresh dates and breeding dates) is written directly on the cow with livestock crayon. This information is written simultaneously in one or more herdsman's diaries and is subsequently transferred into the working herd files. Data are transferred monthly from the herd files onto the DHIA barnsheet for EDP (electronic data processing). DHIA-EDP records are returned and filed in notebooks with a page registering all known information for each cow in the herd. Microcomputers with software for herd health records are now beginning to appear in large commercial dairies, potentially adding still another layer to the herd record system. Before implementing herd reproductive management schemes, it is essential that data collection deficiencies and duplication be minimized. Duplicate or overlapping record systems greatly increase the probability that no one system will be complete and reliable. Additionally, each transfer of information represents an opportunity for errors. On-farm microcomputer systems or a mainframe-modem connection through a DHIA center are the only systems that can provide current daily information, list and report generating capability, and replace separate working herd files. Such a system should be seriously considered for any dairy of more than 500 cows.

Accuracy of records must be verified. Commonly, the person recording the data is the same person that is evaluated by the analysis of those data. Breeding data omissions or modifications can be a serious problem in herds in which ownership and veterinary control are distant. Employee job security may take precedence over integrity when data are recorded or analyzed. This problem can be addressed by appointing a specific individual to enter data, by implementing routine data verification procedures, or by instituting internal controls matching semen usage, cow inventories and conception rates. Program evaluations and modifications based on inaccurate or omitted data are doomed to failure.

REPRODUCTIVE HEALTH PROGRAMS FOR COW GROUPS

Dry Cows. Optimal reproductive efficiency begins with proper dry period management. Ideally, cows with known serious health problems, locomotor weakness, and pendulous or injured udders are culled before entering the dry period. There is some evidence that cows with chronic mastitis may have decreased conception rates, although it has not been proved. Retention of an excessive number of cows with chronic mastitis may adversely affect breeding efficiency. Dry periods of 45 to 60 days minimize economic loss while providing dry cows their necessary rest phase. Dry periods of less than 40 or more than 70 days are detrimental to the next lactation.

Cows should be dried off at least every other week. Prior to drying off, each cow should have been reconfirmed for pregnancy by rectal palpation or external abdominal ballottement. Most herdsmen are competent to "bump" cows at 200+ days gestation, and many can be taught pregnancy diagnosis by rectal palpation at advanced stages of gestation. Animals not reconfirmed by lay personnel must be submitted for veterinary palpation prior to drying. Management supervision at this time of drying off ensures accurate cow identification, provides an·

opportunity to observe the animal, and encourages adherence to proper dry treatment procedures. Dry cow vaccination programs for the control of neonatal calf diarrhea and other diseases can be instituted at this time when indicated by local conditions. In deficient areas, injections of selenium and vitamin E preparations at drying off may be indicated for the control of retained placenta and postpartum metabolic disease.

Grouping cows immediately following drying facilitates observation for mastitis and dietary disorders that might occur following the abrupt cessation of grain feeding and daily milking. Cows in the recently dried corral should be looked at daily for proper involution of the udder during the first week. Enlarged quarters should be palpated and undergo strip plate examination to appraise the need for culture and further treatment. Dry period infections should be rare. If not, a review of the mastitis control program, culling practices, and dry treatment procedures is indicated.

Proper nutrition during the dry period is extremely important. Fat cows have more reproductive problems than properly conditioned cows. When cows are dried, concentrate intake should be abruptly curtailed. Intake of energy and calcium must be limited to prevent metabolic diseases and milk fever in the subsequent lactation. Ideally, cows should enter the dry period in good body condition. Cows that are thin at drying off may require energy supplementation (e.g., corn silage or grain plus hay), while cows that are overconditioned may be allowed to lose some body condition during the dry period. In the close-up corral, 3 to 8 pounds of milk cow concentrate ration should be introduced to prepare the rumen microflora for the onset of lactation and heavy concentrate feeding. Professional management of the dry cow nutrition program to achieve NRC requirements for energy, protein, calcium, phosphorus and vitamin A is essential.

Parturient Cows. Close-up dry cows should be observed daily for signs of impending or actual labor. If calving pastures or maternity pens are utilized, animals should be taken from the close-up dry corral to the maternity area within a day or two of calving. When utilizing a larger group maternity pen it may be helpful to have two adjoining pens—one holding cows due to calve and the other for cows actually in labor. This arrangement allows for very low cow densities at the time of calving. More than two or three cows in a large maternity pen sets the stage for deficiencies in sanitation and observation. Maternity box stalls and group maternity pens must be covered, well-bedded and zealously cleaned to optimize their benefits. Unless sufficient manpower is assigned to the maternity area, a breakdown in sanitation and observation will occur. The more individualized the maternity facilities are designed, the more labor-intensive they become, increasing the potential for mismanagement. Properly managed, individual calving pens are the most desirable maternity facility.

Individual cow records should be checked prior

to calving for conditions from previous lactations that may affect the animal at parturition. Milk fever in a prior lactation, reconstructive vulvar or vaginal surgery or sutures, and birth canal abnormalities should be noted. Cows should be free of manure and filth on their flanks, udder and underside upon entering the calving area. Individuals should be assigned primary responsibility for the maternity area on each shift, providing 24-hour supervision. Since attention and sanitation in the periparturient period and colostrum management affect calf mortality, it is often practical to assign primary responsibility of the maternity area to an individual associated with calf rearing. Salary incentives based on percentage of live births, colostral absorption scores and calf mortality can markedly affect performance in the calving area. Calving dates and complications or conditions of significance at calving should be recorded on the health record and the cow herself. Suggested codes to be written on the dam's hips are OB (dystocia), RP (retained placenta), MF (milk fever), TW (twins) and ABO (abortion). These cows will receive special attention in the postpartum period.

Within 12 to 24 hours postpartum, the newborn calf should be removed to the calf facility and the fresh cow placed in a pen for postparturient cows. Grouping of cows immediately postpartum allows for the accurate collection and separation of first milking colostrum and other fresh cow milk for the calf program. Cows immediately postpartum should be housed in pens containing approximately 10 to 20 per cent excess square footage and manger space. Low population density is important for sanitation, and adequate manger space is crucial for getting cows "on-feed" after calving. Moderate amounts of concentrate can be fed in this postpartum pen until the animals are fully adapted. Each postpartum cow should be locked in a stanchion and examined daily for signs of fever, depression, mastitis and abnormal uterine discharges. Cows with known complications at calving can be medicated on a daily basis if necessary. Before the cow leaves the postpartum pen (usually in 4 to 7 days) she should be on-feed and found free of clinical illness including mastitis and metritis.

Cows leaving the postpartum pen can be congregated in a large fresh cow string awaiting postpartum examination, treatments and vaccinations. Schedules for postpartum examinations will vary. Cows with known complications at calving should be examined early in the postpartum period (10 to 21 days). Cows without complications may be examined later, perhaps 3 to 4 weeks postpartum. Procedures for diagnosis and therapy of reproductive disease are outlined in detail elsewhere in this text. Emphasis should be placed on early diagnosis and prompt attention to the small percentage of cows with known problems. Lay personnel should be provided instructions for treatment of cows with dystocia, retained placenta, and so on. Indiscriminate intrauterine medication is potentially detrimental, labor intensive and unnecessary for efficient

reproduction. Reproductive herd problems are rarely if ever associated with epizootic, nonvenereal uterine infections. More commonly, uterine infections seriously impair fertility in a small group of cows. Emphasis should be placed on identification and treatment of this small group.

Animals in the fresh cow string should be kept under close observation for acetonemia, displaced abomasum and other clinical disease. These cows are most susceptible to disease and can be monitored closely by being grouped together. Sick animals should be removed from the fresh string and placed in the hospital string for treatment and recovery evaluation. The hospital, postpartum and fresh cow strings should be kept separate. Cows with mastitis and other clinical disease will not compete successfully in the large fresh cow pen. Additionally, if sick cows are not segregated from fresh cows, disease detection, treatment and recovery will be delayed and disease transmission opportunities enhanced.

Heat detection should be performed in the fresh cow pen, even though these cows are not ready to be bred. Records of early heats or the lack thereof provide important data for diagnosing reproductive dysfunction and making decisions to begin breeding. When cows have been declared fully involuted and OK to breed, they can be moved into the breeding corrals.

Breeding Cows. Successful AI breeding in large herds is dependent on the ability to restrain large numbers of cattle with minimal effort. Lockable stanchions are useful in accomplishing this task under a variety of housing conditions ranging from drylots to freestalls. Breeding-age heifers and cows are locked once or twice daily for application and observation of heat detection aids, genital examinations, and AI breeding. Heat detection aids should include crayon markings on the tail-head as well as the date of the last observed estrus written on the animal's hip. Proper stanchion facilities and feeding practices should ensure that 98 to 100 per cent of the animals are locked in daily for reproductive management. Heat detection accuracy and high conception rates are positively correlated with the percentage of animals that are locked up daily. A breeding cart containing breeding records, equipment and a semen tank encourages proper breeding decisions, improved labor efficiency, and decreases daily standing time for cows.

Herdsmen and AI technicians must be provided instructions concerning postpartum waiting periods, timing-of-service, and actions to be taken when abnormal heats or uterine discharges are observed. Waiting periods in commercial herds should be no less than 40 nor greater than 60 days. Breeding of nonestrous cows is a more common cause of decreased conception rates than improper timing during estrus. A once-daily schedule of breeding all animals with heats observed during the past 24 hours achieves results comparable to twice-daily breeding because accurate determination of estrus onset is difficult. Recommendations for postbreeding uterine infusion and use of LH-releasing hormones should weigh the potential benefits of prompt treatment of clinical disease against data supporting these practices and frequency of veterinary examinations. Obvious nymphomania (three heats within 14 days) should be treated immediately by dairy personnel. Likewise, endometritis manifested by purulent discharge at AI service can be treated 12 to 36 hours postservice with infusion of a nonirritating, broad-spectrum antibiotic such as procaine penicillin. Cows in heat that have passed the desired postpartum waiting period should always be inseminated unless grossly abnormal heat intervals or discharges are observed. When veterinary visits are weekly, follow-up on these animals is enhanced. Firm, written guidelines and constraints for lay procedures and treatments will promote rational actions, encourage cooperation, control drug costs, and improve reproductive efficiency.

Labor should concentrate maximum heat detection and AI breeding effort on cows in the first 150 days in lactation. Placing confirmed pregnant and chronically infertile cows in pens separate from the breeding corrals may facilitate this concentration of effort. Cows with delayed conception may be grouped and placed in a bull string. Natural service "clean-up" breeding is economically justifiable if it intensifies and improves the AI breeding effort, reduces labor requirements, and yields pregnancies that result in decreased culling for reproductive failure. Young, owner-raised, semen-tested, *Vibrio*-vaccinated bulls are ideal sires for natural service. *Vibrio* immunization of cows prior to natural service is indicated when infection is present.

REPRODUCTION/ HERD HEALTH INTEGRATION

Reproductive tract palpation schedules are ideally integrated into scheduled weekly herd visits encompassing a full spectrum of dairy health and management services. The need to perform palpation on many animals in large herds provides an opportunity to visit the dairy at frequent intervals. Visits of longer duration at extended intervals are less conducive to early diagnosis and limit follow-up evaluations. Implementation and supervision of programs for sick cow care, calf management, mastitis control, and nutrition are greatly facilitated by a relatively continuous professional presence in the dairy. Diagnoses and treatments of cows retained in the hospital string can be reviewed on each herd visit. Similarly, frequent visits facilitate milk sample procurement (from bulk tank milk and clinical mastitis) as well as surveillance of milking practices and equipment function. Postmortem examinations, personnel training, and collection of disease prevalence data are also conveniently incorporated into regularly scheduled visits.

Animals selected for reproductive examinations should include all animals overdue to calve, those who have aborted and those marked with complications at parturition (RP, MF, OB, etc). Additionally, all fresh cows should be examined for normal uterine involution and ovarian structures not later than 30 days postpartum. Cows with delayed involution, metritis, or other pathology may be marked to be rechecked at a subsequent visit. If no estrus is observed within 23 days following palpation, the cow should be re-examined. All cows more than 23 days past the AI service waiting period or diagnosed nonpregnant on a previous visit should be palpated for ovarian structures and estrus prediction or synchronization unless an AI service has been recorded. Nonpregnant animals with irregular heats, pregnant animals with observed heats, and repeat breeders should be examined. All cows inseminated 30 or more days previously should be diagnosed for pregnancy. Distinctively marking the tailheads of confirmed pregnant cows with green livestock crayon (contrasting with orange color on nonpregnant animals) provides a convenient visible record of

Table 2. Conception Rates—Bulls and Technicians on Model Dairy Farms

			Technicians			
			Joe		Bob	
Bull No.	No. Services	Per Cent Conception	No.	Per Cent	No.	Per Cent
443	76	39.4	40	50.0	36	38.8
6563	64	40.6	40	45.0	24	33.3
205	36	66.7	14	71.4	22	63.6
801	34	23.5	18	33.3	16	12.5
4139	34	41.1	26	46.1	8	25.0
452	32	50.0	14	57.1	18	44.4
800	22	18.1	14	28.5	8	0.0
4100	22	0.0	16	0.0	6	0.0
635	20	50.0	10	60.0	10	40.0
Total	340	38.8	192	43.8	148	32.4

Time period: Beginning date: 2/1/84
           End date: 4/15/84
Service number: Combined first, second, third columns

pregnancy status. Reconfirmation of pregnancy status at 90 to 120 days in gestation and prior to drying is indicated. Desirable intervals for reproductive examinations are weekly for postpartum examinations, every other week for AI breeding strings, and every 30 to 60 days for natural service pens. Comprehensive veterinary programs for herds larger than 600 to 800 cows usually require weekly herd visits. Smaller herds and herds that are geographically remote may be scheduled less frequently. In such cases, genital tract examination schedules must be adjusted accordingly.

Routine examination and treatment of cows that have had complications at birth or postpartum metritis and pregnancy diagnosis may be within the capabilities of properly trained herdsmen. Programs using dairy personnel for palpation and treatment must be monitored closely to ensure timely and accurate execution. Integration of competent dairy personnel into the reproductive program may decrease the professional requirement for routine examinations and permit more intensive veterinary involvement with problem animals and program evaluation.

The development of an accurate list of cows to be examined, complete with reproductive histories, is essential to the efficient reproductive management program. Ideally, records are segregated into groups corresponding to cow groups or pens. Such segregation of records provides quality control on cow movement and allows for selected strings to be examined on specific dates. Computerizing herd records allows daily updating and access and rapid and precise preparation of these lists.

CONTROL

Reproductive efficiency is ultimately determined by three factors: election of postpartum waiting period, heat detection efficiency, and conception rate. Poor heat detection renders the elected waiting

Table 3. Reproductive Summary Model Dairy Farm

Criteria	No. Cows	Actual	Goal
Calving interval	179	12.3	12.2
HRS index (100 days)	161/931	80	80
Average days open	278	108.7	95
Average days in milk	760	155.2	155
Per cent open > 150 days	16/429	3.7	< 5.0
Heifers			
Average age at calving	98	25.2	24.0
Average wt at calving	25	1300#	1250#
Conception rates			
Per cent first service	103/279	36.9	45.0
Per cent second service	60/169	35.5	50.0
Per cent third service	40/99	40.4	50.0
Per cent projected—total first three		76.7	88.0
Services/conception (all)	672/251	2.7	2.0
Services/conception (preg)	363/161	2.3	1.9
Natural service			
Average days exposure/conception	0	0	0
Per cent cows in heat by 60 days	230/315	73.0	90.0
Per cent cows bred by 90 days	239/296	80.7	95.0
Per cent cows pregnant at pregnancy exam	331/351	93.5	95.0
24-day heat trial percentage (1/24/84)	139/183	75.9	90.0
Heat intervals:			
<18 days	65	11.8	<10.0
19–24 days	284	51.4	65.0
25–37 days	105	19.0	<10.0
38–46 days	51	9.2	<10.0
>46 days	47	8.5	< 5.0
Per cent abortion rate—annualized	21/490	4.3	< 8.0
Per cent this period	7/490	1.4	
Culls			
Per cent infertile vs herd	40/798	5.0	< 5.0
Per cent infertile vs all culls	40/186	21.5	<25.0
Per cent all culls vs herd	186/798	23.3	<30.0

Comments: Low conception rates and heat detection scores are probably interrelated. Suggest heat detection review and milk progesterone surprise test.

Time Period: 10/1/83—12/31/83   Group: all cows
Strings used: Entire herd

period meaningless and often results in reduced conception rates due to services of cows not in heat. Since poor heat detection equals reproductive inefficiency, it is important to calculate the percentage of cows in heat by 60 days, percentage bred by 90 days, average interestrous interval, percentage presented for pregnancy diagnosis and found open, and percentage of 24-day heat trial.

Conception rate statistics should be calculated for each technician, service number and service sire (Table 2). Low conception rates can be a result of poor semen quality, low fertility sires, semen handling errors, and poor estrus detection, as well as pathological conditions of the cow. Good technicians often experience less reduction in conception rates with poor fertility sires than do technicians with marginal abilities. Technicians with decreasing or low conception rates require immediate retraining, and if they fail to improve, reassignment to more appropriate responsibilities. Conception rate data must be interpreted in conjunction with heat detection data and with measurements of sire and technician performance. Without these data the female reproductive tract may be falsely incriminated, leading to excessive treatments and continued reproductive failure. Detailed statistics such as incidence of dystocia and complications at calving, evaluation of postpartum treatments, and age-specific abortion rates can help reveal the causes of reproductive failure. Comprehensive herd reproductive indices include calving interval, Herd Reproductive Status (HRS), average days open, percentage infertile at 150 days in milk, and reproductive culling percentage.

Proper training, periodic review, and performance recognition are key elements in maintaining herdsman and inseminator efficiency. Principles of examination, sanitation, and intervention with cases of dystocia, retained placenta, and metritis are best taught by combining didactic "herdsman schools" with individualized "wet-lab" instruction. Training in insemination techniques should be supplemented by annual semen handling and placement evaluation including a dye test in cows to be slaughtered or in extirpated tracts. Right-left pregnancy ratios can be calculated to further evaluate placement technique. Milk progesterone testing of cows presented for AI service can provide data that can be used to assess heat detection accuracy.

Graphics of monthly herd and technician performance indices such as average days open, HRS, conception rates, and heat detection efficiency can promote awareness of individual and program deficiencies. Economic incentives linked to performance indices should be limited to a few parameters that are directly influenced by the individual's performance (e.g., heat detection efficiency and first service conception rates). Public recognition of outstanding performance can be beneficial and complement financial incentives. Scheduled monthly meetings bringing together owners, herdsmen, and technicians from many herds can be an effective vehicle for dissemination of information, procedural reviews, and the establishment of the health management program as a team effort with the veterinarian firmly in control.

Herd reproductive records have little value unless they are summarized, evaluated and used for planning management changes. Review of performance indices should occur monthly. Computer-assisted and graphic displays are invaluable for the presentation of data from a large herd (Table 3). Commonly, owners of large herds have little contact with their employees and cows compared with dairymen who own smaller herds. Monthly reports provide reference material for meetings with dairy owners. Concise summaries of reproduction program status, employee performance, and recommendations can be incorporated into a full herd management report. These summaries become the foundation for future planning and continuing veterinarian-client communications. A poorly informed owner represents the most serious threat to sound health management; formal communication and documentation are the strongest allies.

SUMMARY

The achievement of excellent reproductive efficiency in large dairy herds must focus first on the organization and training of labor; second, on the grouping of cows for intense reproductive management; and finally, on procedures for collecting and analyzing data pertinent to the breeding program. Reproductive failure is more often a result of human error than of reproductive dysfunction of the cow. Recognition of the interdependence of human programs and healthy cows is essential for effective reproductive management.

Reference

1. Wilcox CJ, Van Horn HH (eds): Large Dairy Herd Management. Gainesville, University Press of Florida, 1978.

Reproductive Management of Small Dairy Farms

Chester L. Rawson, D.V.M.
Hazel Green, Wisconsin

The objective of an organized approach to reproductive management initiated and directed by the veterinarian is to maximize client profit. This goal will be realized if the results of the program increase the number of quality herd replacements, decrease the number of reproductive failures and increase the percentage of the herd in peak production at any given time. In order to justify the effort and expense involved in an ongoing reproductive program, measurements of herd performance must be generated and evaluated and the economic impact of these values determined on a routine basis. Losses of up to 5 dollars per head per day are incurred by cows that do no calve yearly. Losses of up to 6 dollars per head per day are incurred by heifers that do not calve by 24 months of age.[1]

The steps essential for producing and maintaining an economic response include:

1. Client education
2. Routine examination of all eligible animals
3. Collection and processing of data
4. Assessment of reproductive performance
5. Establishment of herd reproductive goals
6. Implementation of management changes to obtain goals
7. Monitoring herd response.

CLIENT EDUCATION

The client must be made aware that all increases in reproductive efficiency, hence profit, depend largely on improving his management skills. Areas of special emphasis include estrous detection, breeding practices, vaccination programs, herd nutrition, calving practices and heifer management.

ROUTINE EXAMINATIONS

On a monthly basis the following animals should be examined per rectum, appropriate individual treatments administered and all results recorded:

1. All cows fresh 14 days or more
2. Cows with abnormal discharges
3. Cows with abnormal estrous cycles

4. Any cows fresh 60 days and not observed in estrus
5. Any cow bred three or more times
6. All cows bred 32 days or more ago that did not return to estrus.

In addition, at least twice a year, evaluations should be made of heifer growth rates. Age, height, and weight values need to be recorded and compared to breed standards

COLLECTION AND PROCESSING DATA

A simple and accurate method of collecting and processing herd reproductive information must be established. Items of interest include calving interval, days open, services per conception, first service conception rate, days in milk to first service, percentage of cattle observed and recorded in estrus by 60 days fresh and average age of heifers at freshening.

ASSESSMENT OF REPRODUCTIVE PERFORMANCE

Evaluation of the herd reproductive data enables one to establish a herd baseline. The terminal indicator of herd reproduction is the calving interval. All other indices represent areas that support or deny an acceptable calving interval.

Breeding management decisions often are made that create an acceptable calving interval but reduce overall reproductive efficiency and herd profitability. Figure 1 represents a 100-cow herd with a conception rate of 40 per cent whose owner chose to start breeding at 42 days to obtain a 12-month calving interval. His calving interval is 11.9 months.

Figure 2 represents a 100-cow herd with a 50 per cent conception rate whose owner made the same choice as that in herd 1 with even better results—a calving interval of 11.5 months. Figure 3 represents a dairyman with a 60 per cent conception rate who elected to start breeding at 63 days postpartum. His calving interval is 12 months.

Production records show that cows will maximize lifetime milk yields with lactation periods that are 305 to 365 days in length when allowed a dry period of 42 to 60 days.

Table 1 shows the comparison between herds 1, 2, and 3.

REPRODUCTIVE GOALS

Achievable reproductive goals are:
1. A 12-month calving interval
2. 85 days open
3. 1.6 services per conception
4. 60 per cent first service conception rate
5. 85 per cent of cows observed in estrus and recorded by 60 days fresh

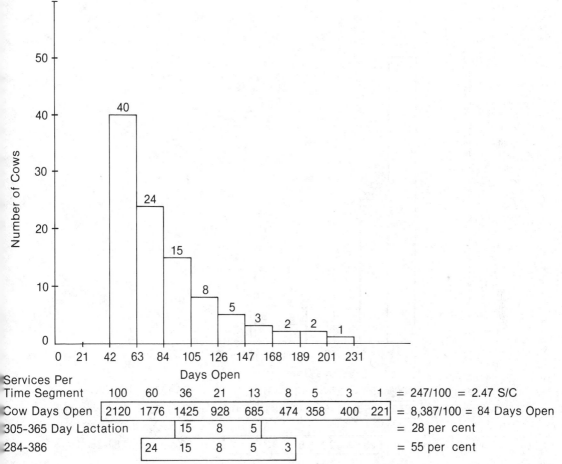

Services Per									
Time Segment	100	60	36	21	13	8	5	3	1	= 247/100 = 2.47 S/C
Cow Days Open	2120	1776	1425	928	685	474	358	400	221	= 8,387/100 = 84 Days Open
305–365 Day Lactation			15	8	5					= 28 per cent
284–386		24	15	8	5	3				= 55 per cent

Figure 1. Cows conceiving during different time segments. It is assumed that breeding starts at 42 days postpartum and that the conception rate is 40 per cent in a l00-cow herd.

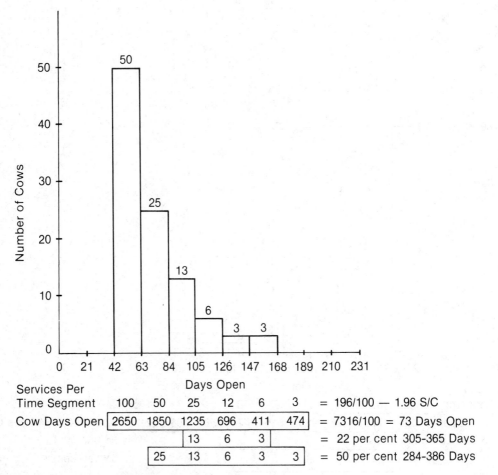

Figure 2. Cows conceiving during different time segments. It is assumed that breeding starts at 42 days and that the conception rate is 50 per cent in a 100-cow herd.

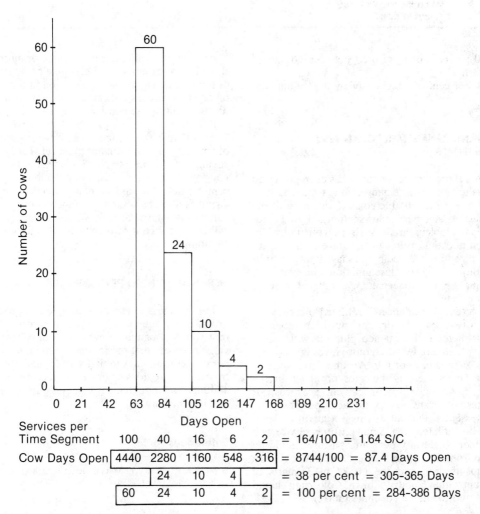

Figure 3. Cows conceiving during different time segments. It is assumed that breeding starts at 63 days and that the conception rate is 60 per cent in a 100-cow herd.

Table 1. Comparison of Reproductive Efficiency

	Herd 1	Herd 2	Herd 3
Calving interval (months)	11.9	11.5	12.0
Services per conception	2.47	1.96	1.64
Semen cost per pregnancy at $20 per insemination	$49.40	$38.00	$32.00
Conception rate (per cent)	40	50	60
Per cent cows 305–365 days in milk	28	22	38
Per cent cows 284–386 days in milk	55	50	100

6. 90 per cent of cows bred between 60 and 84 days fresh

7. 90 per cent of heifers calving at 24 months of age.

IMPLEMENT MANAGEMENT CHANGES TO OBTAIN GOALS

After a reproductive summary has been produced and evaluated, management changes may be necessary to reach acceptable goals. Evaluation of the reproductive summary allows attention to be focused on problem areas such as cow nutrition, lactation nutrition, calving environment, periparturient procedures, breeding management, estrous detection, timing of insemination, insemination techniques, bull management, venereal disease or heifer management.

An increased incidence of retained placenta demands a review of the dry cow nutrition program, whereas increases in retained placenta with weak, dead or premature fetuses require investigation into possible causes of abortion. An unacceptable level of postpartum metritis indicates problems in the calving environment, poor calving practices, or problems with transition to the lactation ration.

It is essential that all calvings occur in a clean, dry, well-ventilated area. Small pastures service well in summer. Maternity pens and pasture should be isolated from the rest of the herd. Neonates require navel disinfection and the intake of 3 quarts of colostrum within 6 hours of birth. Colostrum should be hand fed to ensure adequate intake.

All cows returning to service three or more times should be re-examined to determine possible causes of infertility. An abnormal elevation in the number of repeat breeders indicates problems with timing of insemination, semen handling, semen quality or bull fertility.

Age at first freshening is the final measurement of young stock management practices. Factors influencing age at first freshening include sanitation, housing, ventilation, disease prevention, parasite control, nutrition and breeding practices. Because age at first estrus is largely a function of size, dairy heifers must grow at a rate that ensures that they will be 65 per cent of their mature body weight by 14 months of age.

MONITORING HERD PERFORMANCE

The key to success in a complete reproductive program is frequent continuous monitoring of current values. Regular re-evaluation of calving interval, days open, first service conception rate, services per conception, days to first service, and age at first freshening provides a basis for recommendations and management changes made in pursuit of maximal productivity.

References

1. MacKay RD: The economics of herd health program. Vet Clin North Am 3 (2):347, 1981.

Reproductive Management Programs for Dairy Bulls

William D. Hueston, D.V.M., M.S., Ph.D.
The Ohio State University, Columbus, Ohio

The role of the dairy bull in American agriculture has changed dramatically in the past 50 years. The once ubiquitous individual dairy herd bull has been gradually replaced, first by bull pools, then by regional artificial insemination (AI) centers. These regional bull studs began merging after the transition from fresh to frozen semen in the 1950's, so that now the major AI organizations maintain hundreds of bulls. Today the dairy herd bull is increasingly uncommon, with approximately 65 per cent of dairy cattle being bred by AI. In 1982, American AI organizations sold 12.8 million breeding units of frozen semen for domestic use.

Herd health management is a dynamic process. The development of a realistic reproductive management program for dairy bulls requires careful evaluation of each of the following: the objectives of the dairy bull enterprise, the number of bulls involved, the value of the individual animals, the available resources, the geographic location, and specific medical considerations. An appropriate program for a dairyman with an individual bull differs greatly from that of a large AI station. Similarly, the collection of semen for AI entails regulatory and management constraints not found for bulls used only in natural service. Finally, continuous herd health surveillance is required when semen is to be exported. Tables 1 and 2 list equipment and drugs, with dosages, helpful in devising a reproductive management program.

HANDLING THE INDIVIDUAL BULL

Physical restraint begins with control of the head and neck, the bull's most powerful and coordinated muscle mass. The best control is provided by a nose ring, whereas little control is gained by a halter or

Table 1. Equipment

Name	Company Name and Address
1. Ritchey Eartagger	Available through Nasco, Inc., Fort Atkinson, Wisconsin

neck chain, especially for the bull that is seldom handled. Brass or steel rings are available in various sizes. Most bull rings do not meet the marketing claim of being "self piercing." Proper placement of the ring can be facilitated by first piercing the noncartilaginous rostral portion of the nasal septum with a rumen trocar. The trocar is then withdrawn, leaving the cannula in place. The sharp end of the opened bull ring can be guided through the nasal septum by placing it in the cannula as the cannula is withdrawn. Similarly, a Ritchey eartag trocar can be used to guide the ring through the nasal septum.

The muzzle cannot withstand excessive strain without tearing. If torn, the nasal septum will rarely reunite sufficiently to allow replacement of the ring as before. In this case, a vertical ring of a smaller diameter can be placed, but it will withstand less abuse than a properly placed horizontal ring.[5] The bull should be led with both a halter and a lead rope attached to the nose ring. The ring is used to control, whereas only the halter should be used to pull or tie the bull. Alternatively, the halter lead, a horn rope or a neck chain can be passed through the nose ring to the handler. Capture of a bull loose in a box stall is facilitated by attaching four to six links of plastic boat chain to the ring. A capture hook can be easily made from a 2-meter piece of 3/8-inch (9.5-mm) aluminum rod. Metal chain should not be attached to the nose ring because it creates a very dangerous weapon.

The sheer size and strength of bulls demand larger and heavier handling facilities than those used for cows. In designing bull handling facilities, the head squeeze is less important because the bull often cannot be caught by the head alone due to the large neck mass. A bar run behind the bull is a better way to confine a bull in a chute. Head restraint is more effectively accomplished with a halter or neck collar and nose ring than with a head squeeze. If individual collars are used, the bull can be restrained in the chute by attaching a chain to a heavy ring on the collar and anchoring the chain in front of the chute.

HOUSING

Bulls less than 3 years old can generally be housed in cow facilities, including tie stalls, box stalls or loose housing. Group housing is widely used for young bulls; however, disease transmission and injury due to trauma are more frequent in this type of housing. The increased animal-to-animal contact in group housing can lead to rapid transmission of conditions such as venereal diseases, leukosis, warts, and ringworm.

Individual housing for the mature dairy bull requires more space than for a cow. Tie stalls should be at least 1.5 meters wide and 2.5 meters long for large breed dairy bulls (Holstein, Brown Swiss and Guernsey). The minimum size for box stalls is 3.7

Table 2. Drugs

Name of Drug	Company and Address	Species	Dose (mg or IU/kg)
1. Nasalgen	Wellcome, Kansas City, Missouri	Bovine	2 ml intranasally (1 ml in each nostril)
2. Vibrin	Norden, Lincoln, Nebraska	Bovine	Bulls: 5 ml SQ (Note: Approved for use in cows and heifers only at 2 ml SQ)
3. Dursban 44	Dow Chemical, Midland Michigan	Bovine	Not approved for dairy bulls
4. Phenylbutazone 1 gm tablets	The Butler Company, Columbus, Ohio	—	Bulls: 2–6 gm PO daily (Note: Not approved for food animal use)
5. Dihydrostrepto-mycin 50% solution	The Butler Company, Columbus, Ohio	Bovine	Bulls: 22 mg/kg SQ q.i.d. for three treatments (Note: Approved for use at 11 mg/kg b.i.d. for 3–5 days)
6. Wart vaccine	Norden, Lincoln, Nebraska	Bovine	Calves: 10–15 ml SQ Mature cattle: 20–25 ml SQ

meters by 3.7 meters for mature Jersey bulls and 3.7 meters by 4.3 meters for mature large breed dairy bulls. Designs for bull pens are available from the Cooperative Extension Service.[4] Whichever housing design is used, special provision should be made for the safe catching and handling of the bull.

The individual farm bull running loose with the cow herd poses a potential threat to the safety of farm workers. Individual housing and the use of a breeding chute or corral reduces this risk. Selective breeding in this way also facilitates the blending of an AI program with a "clean-up" bull.

NUTRITION

Nutritional guidelines for growing and mature dairy bulls are available from the National Research Council (NRC).[6] The requirements of growing dairy bulls are similar to those of growing dairy heifers, although bull calves grow faster. Large breed dairy bull calves gain approximately 0.9 kg a day. Low-energy rations during the first year of life delay the onset of semen production and result in a smaller sized bull at puberty. Sperm cell production is also lower in underfed bulls up to 2 years of age. It appears that protein levels have little or no effect on the onset of semen production.[2]

After the rapid growth phase of the bull's life (i.e., the first 3 years), continued high-energy diets result in a decrease in sexual activity.[2] Overweight bulls may accumulate adipose tissue at the base of

the scrotum that can adversely affect its thermo-regulatory function. Furthermore, excessive weight places an additional strain on the bull's feet and legs, which can contribute to reduced sexual activity. The NRC guidelines for mature bull diets most closely approximate dry cow rations, with a calcium level of 0.24 per cent and a phosphorus level of 0.18 per cent. The role of calcium-phosphorus levels in the pathogenesis of ankylosing spondylosis in dairy bulls is still debated. Providing at least 15 per cent crude fiber is important in decreasing the frequency of abomasal displacements, rumen acidosis and episodes of simple indigestion.

FEET AND LEGS

Regular examination of feet and legs is essential to maintaining soundness. Without sound feet and legs, a bull cannot serve a cow or an artificial vagina. Furthermore, overgrown hooves can accentuate conformational weaknesses and existing disease conditions such as tarsitis or neurologic problems. Annual hoof trimming of the entire herd can help prevent lameness.

There are several neurologic conditions of older bulls that can affect soundness. The rear limb spasms and "stretches" seen with spastic syndrome can reduce mounting ability. These spasms are often responsive to oral phenylbutazone therapy at doses of 3 to 6 gm per day. Progressive spinal paralysis is the gradual loss of conscious proprioception in the hind legs, increasing weakness and eventual collapse. While there are no specific treatments available, reduction of the bull's activity level may slow the deterioration. Spastic syndrome or progressive spinal paralysis may prevent natural service and require electroejaculation or ampullar massage for collection of semen.

PARASITES

Internal parasite control is important for young bulls and bulls maintained on pasture. For control of external parasites, caution is needed in the use of insecticides. Dose levels are not routinely extrapolated for the 1000- to 1300-kg animal. Furthermore, testosterone has been suggested to increase the sensitivity of bulls to certain insecticides. A notable case involved chlorpyrifos (Dursban), which, when used at the extrapolated dose, proved fatal to some of the treated bulls.[3] This resulted in the withdrawal of the label indication for dairy bulls. Therefore, dose relationships are not always linear (e.g., the dose for 1300 kg does not necessarily equal twice the dose for 650 kg). In practice, it is often both effective and safe to treat mature bulls with the recommended dose for a 650- to 800-kg cow. The manufacturer's advice should be sought before exceeding label dosage.

INFECTIOUS DISEASES

Most of these diseases are discussed more extensively in other chapters. Only those specifically important for dairy bulls will be mentioned here.

Blue Tongue. Active infection or past exposure to blue tongue virus or other antigenically related viruses can cause long-term seropositive reactions to blue tongue virus. It appears that blue tongue virus shedding in the semen occurs only during the period of viremia; thus virus isolation testing of blood can be as diagnostic as semen virus isolation. Blue tongue virus infected semen can infect susceptible females through natural service or AI. Serial culturing of blood and semen suggests that most blue tongue virus seropositive bulls are not viremic or shedding blue tongue virus in semen. Semen from seropositive bulls is ineligible for export to many foreign countries.

Brucellosis. Infection of the male genitalia with brucellosis may result in the shedding of *Brucella* organisms in semen. Natural service with *Brucella*-infected semen is not considered a major factor in the transmission of brucellosis due to the protective barrier offered by the cervix. However, the technique of artificial insemination greatly enhances the potential for brucellosis transmission because the insemination catheter or syringe is passed through the cervix.

The vaccination of bulls with Strain 19–modified live *Brucella* organisms at any dosage is contraindicated because (1) there is a small risk of persistent strain 19 infection that might result in seminal shedding; (2) the increased *Brucella* titers resulting from vaccination may negatively affect the disposition of the bull; and (3) for semen export, some countries require that there be no bulls vaccinated with a modified live *Brucella* vaccine in the AI station herd.

There are documented cases of bulls with genital brucellosis infections but no detectable serologic response. Consequently, seminal plasma *Brucella* agglutination tests are required for all bulls used in AI.

Campylobacteriosis (Vibriosis). As an inhabitant of the prepuce and therefore a potential semen contaminant, *Campylobacter fetus* ss. *venerealis* was widely disseminated in the early days of fresh semen AI. Reliable diagnostic tests and treatments are presently available for campylobacteriosis. The recommended diagnostic test is repeated cultures of preputial smegma. Dihydrostreptomycin administered subcutaneously at 22 mg/kg body weight and/or 5 gm infused in the sheath with vigorous massage has been shown to be effective treatment for campylobacteriosis.[9] Research suggests that vaccination with Vibrin at a 5-ml dose may be a successful treatment as well as preventive for the bull.[11] However, a vaccinated bull mating infected and susceptible cows can still serve as a mechanical vector of campylobacteriosis, even though the bull may not become infected. Today many AI studs maintain *Campylobacter*-free herds. In addition, most frozen semen is specifically treated for *Campylobacter* by the addition of antibiotics, primarily dihydrostreptomycin and polymixin B sulfate.

Enzootic Bovine Leukosis. Leukosis virus is associated with circulating lymphocytes; therefore, lymphocyte contamination of semen represents a theoretical route for transmission of this disease. Multiple studies, however, have been unable to demonstrate actual AI transmission. A seronegative leukosis status is important for some semen export markets. Control of leukosis within a herd rests chiefly on limiting contact between infected and noninfected bulls. Iatrogenic transmission via any equipment contaminated by infected lymphocytes may also play a role.

Infectious Bovine Rhinotracheitis (IBR)/Infectious Pustular Vulvovaginitis (IPV)/Infectious Balanoposthitis (IBP). This herpes virus can be shed sporadically in the semen of infected bulls. Shedding increases in the presence of clinical IBP. No treatment is available for IBR virus either in the bull or in semen. However, vaccination of unexposed bulls with modified live intranasal vaccine (Nasalgen) has been shown to prevent preputial shedding of the virulent virus subsequent to exposure.[8] Intranasal vaccination of exposed bulls or any intramuscular vaccination of bulls fails to prevent shedding, especially during times of stress. Specific foreign countries require that semen-producing bulls be seronegative to IBR virus, and therefore a vaccination program may be contraindicated in those bull studs with export markets.

Leptospirosis. As common and often latent pathogens of the urinary tract, leptospires may be transmitted by natural service or by fresh semen AI. Serologic surveillance for leptospirosis may not identify all infected bulls. Multivalent vaccines, which are useful in reducing the clinical signs and effects of leptospirosis, have been shown to reduce urine shedding by as much as 50 per cent. The treatment of bulls with dihydrostreptomycin at 22 mg/kg subcutaneous (SQ) every other day for three treatments also aids in reducing the renal carrier state. Addition of dihydrostreptomycin to semen has been shown to be effective in controlling *Leptospira pomona.* Certain foreign countries require that individual bulls and/or the entire herd be seronegative to leptospirosis, a requirement that may preclude vaccination within a bull stud.

Paratuberculosis (Johne's Disease). Genital paratuberculosis infections in bulls can result in the shedding of *Mycobacterium paratuberculosis* organisms in the semen; however, research suggests that cows inseminated with paratuberculosis-contaminated semen do not become infected. Negative paratuberculosis tests of semen donor bulls are required by many foreign countries as well as some states. Additionally, clinical paratuberculosis usually affects bulls at 4 to 6 years of age, when initial progeny test data are first available.

Fibropapillomatosis. Fibropapillomas (warts) are common in young bulls and are most frequently observed in bulls in group housing. Warts can affect breeding soundness if located on the penis. Commercially available killed wart vaccines and autogenous killed wart vaccines have been shown to be efficacious in reducing the incidence of penile warts in young group-housed bulls.[7]

Trichomoniasis. Bovine venereal trichomoniasis still represents a major venereal and semen-borne disease problem. Unlike *Campylobacter,* there are no semen additives available for the control of trichomoniasis. Therefore, control rests on the testing and treatment of infected animals. Culture of preputial smegma is currently the most sensitive test, although direct examination of preputial flushings is still widely practiced despite the tedious nature of the test.

Tuberculosis. Despite the present low incidence of this disease in the United States, surveillance in the bull is essential due to the documented potential for semen transmission of tuberculosis. The bull must be included in testing for accreditation of the herd.

THE INDIVIDUAL HERD BULL

The individual herd bull is as important to a successful reproductive herd health program as all the cows. Additionally, in terms of disease transmission, the bull occupies a unique position more important than that of any individual cow. Through the act of natural breeding, the bull is exposed to every communicable disease within the herd. This exposure may result in infection of the bull and/or the spread of disease to cows subsequently served. Therefore, maintenance of a high level of disease resistance in the individual herd bull is a key to disease control within the entire herd. Optimally, vaccinations should include semiannual boosters for IBR (intranasal), leptospirosis (5 serotypes) and campylobacteriosis (vibriosis).

Regular reproductive examinations of postpartum, pregnant and repeat breeder cows, combined with adequate record keeping, can be more important in the bull-bred herd than in the AI-bred herd owing to the role of the bull in disease transmission through direct sexual contact. To reduce herd reproductive failures, regular physical and breeding soundness examinations of the bull are as necessary as disease surveillance. Observation of breeding behavior and semen evaluation are essential components of a thorough breeding soundness examination. Examination of the bull should occur several weeks prior to the breeding season in order to allow for a replacement if the bull is unsatisfactory. The experience of AI industry veterinarians indicates that one out of every ten bulls is potentially not a satisfactory breeder.

Careful selection of a new herd sire should minimize the introduction of new diseases to the cow herd. This involves a complete breeding soundness examination and health testing prior to purchase, strict isolation for 30 to 60 days and retesting before the bull is allowed to enter the herd. Before breeding cows, the bull should be tested for brucellosis and tuberculosis, and vaccinated for IBR (intranasal), leptospirosis (5 serotypes) and campylobacteriosis. Prophylactic treatment with dihydrostreptomycin at a dose of 22 mg/kg body weight subcutaneously every other day for three treatments will further reduce the risk of introducing campylobacteriosis or leptospirosis into the herd.

THE BULL STUD

The goal of a bull stud is maximum production of high-quality semen that is free of specific pathogens. Optimal production requires a healthy animal that is trained for semen collection procedures. Precollection stimulation through "warm-up stalls" (where a bull can observe other bulls being collected) and false mounts (mounting without allowing ejaculation) will increase semen volume and total sperm production. Collection technique and equipment must be tailored to the individual bull.

Semen of high quality requires constant monitoring of collection, processing, handling, sperm abnormalities, semen contaminants and post-freeze motility to ensure adequate spermatozoa per insemination dose for optimal fertility. The testicles and secondary sex organs of the bull have no normal flora, but the contamination of the prepuce and distal urethra make routine aseptic collection of semen impossible. The level of semen contamination may be decreased by strict adherence to guidelines for sanitary collection and processing. The addition of antibiotics in semen processing minimizes the effects of bacterial contamination and protects against certain semen-transmissible diseases. Screening of semen for cells other than sperm is also a good monitor for abnormality of the reproductive tract such as seminal vesiculitis.

The production of specific pathogen-free semen depends on individual bull and herd health surveillance, prophylaxis and possibly vaccination. Surveillance begins on the farm of origin of each herd addition. Examination of the bull should identify potential heritable defects, acute or chronic disease, or any other limitations on breeding soundness. Pre-entry disease testing provides an initial screening for bulls whose serologic tests indicate health risks or regulatory constraints for the bull stud.

The disease-free status of the herd is far more important than that of any individual animal. The disease-free herd requires maintenance of healthy individuals and strict control over herd additions. This includes strict isolation upon arrival of all acquisitions, including teaser animals. Ideally, isolation means physical separation from the resident herd, separate equipment and waste disposal, and strict adherence to sanitation and disinfection of personnel and machinery between different facilities. All of the pre-entry examinations and testing must be repeated during the isolation period to ensure their reliability. Completion of the isolation program requires 45 to 60 days in order to identify any disease possibly acquired since the pre-entry testing.

Intense disease surveillance replaces vaccination as the key to disease control in the bull stud. While detectable titers may be protective for the individual herd bull, they may limit semen marketability. A comprehensive review of disease diagnostics and control in the AI setting has been written by Bartlett.[1]

REGULATORY CONSIDERATIONS FOR SEMEN COLLECTED FOR ARTIFICIAL INSEMINATION

Unlike many countries, notably Canada, the United States has no federal regulation of semen collection for domestic AI use. Furthermore, there is no federal regulation of interstate movement or export of semen. Despite the absence of federal regulations, five states (Mississippi, Montana, Virginia, Washington, and Wisconsin) have established regulations governing intrastate use and interstate movement of semen for AI. Copies of the appropriate regulations are available from each state's Department of Agriculture. In these states, bovine semen must be accompanied by an interstate health certificate or a "Uniform Certificate for Interstate or Intrastate Shipment of Bovine Semen for Artificial Insemination" as adopted by the subcommittee on AI, Committee of Infectious Diseases of Cattle, United States Animal Health Association in 1962.[10] Alternatively, copies of the uniform certificate may

be filed with the appropriate state veterinarian as each bull enters service. These uniform certificates must be updated yearly.

The AI industry, through its trade organization, the National Association of Animal Breeders (NAAB), has long recognized the need for health guidelines for the bulls and semen used in artificial insemination. In 1954 NAAB adopted a set of recommendations, drafted by the American Veterinary Medical Association, which addressed general sanitary practices for semen collection and handling as well as disease testing or treatment for brucellosis, tuberculosis, trichomoniasis and campylobacteriosis. In 1976 NAAB established a subsidiary organization, Certified Semen Services (CSS),* whose explicit purpose was AI industry self-regulation. Among the stated goals of CSS are to create confidence in the use of frozen semen and to prevent the need for governmental regulation in the AI industry. In 1979, CSS implemented a program of Recommended Minimum Standards for the Health of Bulls Producing Semen for Artificial Insemination, which covers six diseases: brucellosis, campylobacteriosis, leptospirosis, paratuberculosis, trichomoniasis and tuberculosis.

To facilitate semen exportation, good communication and cooperation among the bull owner, veterinarian, USDA District Veterinarian, diagnostic laboratory and exporter are required. All export certification is handled through the local federal veterinarian-in-charge. At the national level, veterinarians in the export division of the Animal and Plant Health Inspection Service (APHIS) have knowledge of semen export requirements. However, on a day-to-day basis, most updated requirements for a particular receiving country are relayed by that country to the exporter when the export permit is obtained. Export requirements can serve multiple purposes, not all of them with veterinary justification. Health requirements may provide very effective trade barriers. All export health testing must be done at federally approved laboratories.

In caring for the purebred bull calf that is destined for sale, export or semen collection, both the farmer and the veterinarian must be very careful not to administer any vaccine or treatment that might jeopardize the suitability of the calf. If the bull has been contracted by a specific AI organization, that organization should be contacted about pertinent health care. As a general rule, the unvaccinated and seronegative bull is the most marketable, whatever the disease(s) involved.

References

1. Bartlett DE: Health management of bulls used in AI. In Morrow DA (ed): Current Therapy in Theriogenology. Philadelphia, WB Saunders Co, 1980, pp. 405–410.
2. Flipse RJ, Almquist JO: Effect of total digestible nutrient intake from birth to four years of age on growth and repro-

*Certified Semen Services, P.O. Box 1033, Columbia, Missouri 65201

ductive development and performance of dairy bulls. J Dairy Sci 44:905, 1961.

3. Haas PJ, et al.: Effect of chlorpyrifos on Holstein steers and testosterone-treated Holstein bulls. Am J Vet Res 44:879, 1983.
4. Midwest Plan Service: Dairy Housing and Equipment. Iowa State University, Ames, Iowa 1976.
5. Monke DR: Local nasal anesthesia in the bull. Vet Med/Sm Anim Clin 76:389, 1981.
6. National Research Council: Nutrient Requirements of Domestic Animals. Number 3, Nutrient Requirements of Dairy Cattle. 5th ed. Washington DC, National Academy of Sciences, 1978.
7. Olson C, Robl MG, Larson LL: Cutaneous and penile fibro-

papillomatosis and its control. J Am Vet Med Assoc 153:1189, 1968.
8. Schultz RD, Sheffy BE: Current status of viral infections of the bovine genital tract. In Morrow DA (ed): Current Therapy in Theriogenology. Philadelphia, WB Saunders Co, 1980, pp. 503–509.
9. Seger Cl, Lank RB, Levy HE: Dihydrostreptomycin for treatment of genital vibriosis in the bull. J Am Vet Med Assoc 149:1634, 1966
10. U.S. Animal Health Association: Proceedings of the Annual Meeting, Richmond, 1962, pp. 170.
11. Vasquez LA, et al.: Bovine genital campylobacteriosis (vibriosis): Vaccination of experimentally infected bulls. Am J Vet Res 44:1553, 1983.

Reproductive Health Management in Beef Cows

Lawrence E. Rice, D.V.M., M.S.
Oklahoma State University
Stillwater, Oklahoma

REPRODUCTIVE EFFICIENCY

Criteria such as interval to first estrus, interval to first breeding, days open, first service conception rate, services per conception, calving interval and others are often used as measures of reproductive efficiency by dairymen and veterinarians involved in dairy herd health programs. Such measures are important for economic control of the reproductive cycle and milk production of dairy cattle.

Beef cattle are not as intensively managed, and there are neither the economic importance nor the management opportunities required to maintain the necessary records. Many beef operations with low input–low output management use only the number of calves weaned or sold as their measure of reproduction and production.

The objectives of this chapter are to discuss a philosophy that reproduction is production and to present a plan whereby production is increased by improved reproductive efficiency. Items discussed include production and reproduction goals, production losses and a total reproductive program.

Reproduction Goals

High reproduction goals must be set to achieve production goals. Every phase of breeding, calving and nursing must be managed at maximum efficiency to avoid loss of beef production. Increased

reproductive efficiency by use of more intensive management is necessary to increase weight of the calves weaned.

The following criteria and their respective goals are suggested as measures of reproduction and production for intensive beef reproductive management.

Adult Cow Breeding Efficiency

1. Per cent cows cycling during first 21 days breeding =

$$\frac{\text{Number cows in estrus first 21 days}}{\text{Total cows}} \times 100$$

(Goal = 90%)

This criterion is important and easy to measure in beef artificial insemination (AI) herds. It is of equal economic importance in herds using natural service, but observations of estrus are less accurate and therefore unreliable in measuring estrus activity.

2. First service conception rate =

$$\frac{\text{Number cows pregnant first service}}{\text{Number bred first service}} \times 100$$

(Goal = 70%)

This criterion is especially important for all beef herds. The combination of high conception rates and high cycling rates ensures a high percentage of calves born early in the calving season (90 per cent cycling first 21 days × 70 per cent conception = 63 per cent pregnant first 21 days).

3. Per cent cows pregnant =

$$\frac{\text{Number cows pregnant}}{\text{Total cows}} \times 100$$

(Goal = 95%)

This value is the one most commonly used to measure reproductive performance in beef cows. The goal of 95 per cent has greater significance when the breeding season is short. The goal should be a breeding season of 63 days (three cycles) to ensure ideal weaning weights. Each rancher must set his own goals, but his veterinarian can provide much help in shortening the breeding season to 63 days.

Replacement Heifer Breeding Efficiency

Heifers that calve late the first year always tend to calve late in subsequent years or have a greater tendency not to get pregnant. Replacement heifers must cycle early and be bred during a 42-day breeding season to prevent late calving the first and subsequent years. High reproductive performance must be demanded from replacement heifers:

1. Per cent cycling first 21 days (Goal = 85%)
2. Per cent pregnant after 42 days (Goal = 85%)

Calf Survival

The best measure of calf survival at birth is expressed as the percentage of palpated pregnant cows that have live calves 24 hours after birth. This percentage reflects losses due to abortions and perinatal calf mortality.

1. Calf survival at birth =

$$\frac{\text{Live calves at 24 hours}}{\text{Number pregnant cows retained}} \times 100$$

(Goal = 95%)

The percentage of calves weaned from the total cows exposed to breeding during the previous breeding season measures: (1) breeding efficiency, (2) calf survival at birth and (3) nursing survival. This figure can be no greater than the lowest of the three exponents involved. Therefore, nursing survival must have a high goal:

2. Nursing survival =

$$\frac{\text{Calves weaned}}{\text{Calves alive at 24 hours}} \times 100$$

(Goal = 95%)

3. Per cent calf crop weaned =

$$\frac{\text{Calves weaned}}{\begin{array}{c}\text{Total cows exposed to breeding}\\ \text{previous season}\end{array}} \times 100$$

(Goal = 85%)
(95% breeding efficiency × 95% survival at birth × 95% nursing survival = 86% calf crop)

Achieving each of these reproductive efficiency goals is difficult; however, herd records prove it is possible. High goals must be set as the first step toward making progress.

LOSS OF PRODUCTION

Genetic Management

Loss of production can be due to poor genetic management. Careless selection of both cows and bulls will result in low weaning and yearling weights, especially if replacements are selected for factors other than production. Cattlemen have too often selected bulls that have "eye appeal," popular blood lines, and impressive pedigrees. Physical soundness should always guide bull selection, but visual appraisal has little objective value beyond soundness and size for age comparison.

An evaluation including three criteria—pedigree, performance test and progeny test—would meet the ultimate goal in sire selection. A pedigree will tell how a bull is expected to perform on the basis of the performance of his ancestors. A performance test will tell how the bull actually did perform. A progeny test will tell how a bull's offspring perform and is therefore the most important of the three factors. Unfortunately, very few bulls are selected on the basis of all three values. Some bulls in AI studs have accurate progeny information, but bulls in natural service are primarily selected by visual appraisal with perhaps either pedigree or performance test evaluation.

Cattlemen participating in production testing programs are those making the most genetic progress in producing replacements with better growth rates. Production records are useful in (1) identifying the top producing individuals and blood lines within a herd, (2) helping the producer evaluate the genetic progress of his herd and (3) identifying cattlemen who are producing superior quality cattle. Veterinarians should encourage their clients to (1) select bulls on the basis of performance, production records, and breeding soundness examination; (2) incorporate reproductive performance in the selection of replacements; (3) record reproductive performance of cows and bulls and include this data into their herd records. This information may then be used in culling and selection.

Artificial insemination has long been recognized as being responsible for increased milk production in dairy cattle. Beef cattle breeders who utilize AI have also demonstrated genetic progress. While less than 10 per cent of all beef cows are bred by AI, purebred breeders now rely heavily on AI for genetic progress. Breeders who have herds with good reproductive performance find AI to be a useful management tool and many incorporate embryo transfer to utilize superior females.

The significant point is that progressive producers have recognized the importance of good reproductive performance. Veterinarians should now provide the leadership by promoting and evaluating beef cattle reproductive and genetic performance for their clients.

REPRODUCTIVE MANAGEMENT

Causes of decreased weight of calf weaned per animal unit can be classified into three categories: (1) increased calf mortality, (2) reduced weaning weights and (3) reduced pregnancy rates.

Increased Calf Mortality

High calf mortality means that there have been excessive deaths at or near birth or from birth to weaning, or both. Although control of losses from birth to weaning is crucial in a herd health program, this topic will not be discussed as part of reproductive health management.

Perinatal calf deaths from dystocia have been reported to range from 4 to 16 per cent. Reports indicate that cows experiencing dystocia have subsequent conception rates reduced by 15 per cent. Calf losses and breeding problems following dystocia are most commonly seen in replacement heifers.

Studies have been conducted to attribute various maternal and fetal traits as causes of dystocia. In all studies, calf birth weight was determined to be the single most important trait related to dystocia. Data from the United States Meat Animal Research Center show that as birth weight increases, the dystocia rate and the perinatal calf mortality rate also increase. Dystocia and calf mortality increase markedly in the common English beef heifers when birth weights exceed 32 kilograms. Large European breeds have considerably heavier birth weights and higher dystocia rates than do the English breeds.

Breed association and artificial insemination organization progeny test records have demonstrated large differences in birth weights and dystocia rates among different sire progeny groups. These records indicate that bulls can be selected to sire calves that cause relatively fewer dystocias.

Dam size has been shown to affect birth weights and dystocia. Restricted prepartum nutrition will reduce calf birth weights but will not reduce the dystocia rate in heifers. This is because maternal growth is stopped early in poorly grown heifers, which will be weak and have small pelvic areas at calving. Conversely, excessively fat heifers will have increased dystocia rates due to pelvic fat, but calf birth weights will be no greater than those from properly grown heifers.

Properly grown replacement heifers with roomy pelves will have lower dystocia rates, and losses will be minimized when these heifers are bred to bulls known to be "easy calvers." Replacements produced under very intensive management may be selected even more critically by performing pelvic area measurements at breeding time or during pregnancy testing. The very best replacements will be selected when 20 to 30 per cent of heifers with the smallest pelvic measurements are culled.

Reduced Weaning Weights and Pregnancy Rates

Low weaning weights and reduced pregnancy rates can be directly attributed to poor reproductive efficiency. Too few cows in estrus during the first 21 days of the breeding season and low first service conception rates directly affect weaning weights and pregnancy rates. Assuming that a calf will gain from 0.7 to 0.9 kilograms per day from birth to weaning, one can calculate that a weaned calf will weigh from 14 to 18 kilograms less for every 21-day cycle delay in getting pregnant. Table 1 shows the effects of

Table 1. Kilograms of Calf Weaned Per Cow Bred

Age of Calf (days)	Calf Crop (kilograms)			
	90%	80%	70%	60%
220	206	184	160	138
200	190	169	148	125
180	174	155	135	116
160	157	140	123	105
140	141	125	110	94

percentage of calf crop and age of the calf on kilograms of calf weaned per cow bred.

Note that a 20-day reduction in age at weaning is nearly as devastating to weaning weight as a 10 per cent reduction in calf crop. These weights were calculated on the assumption that growth rate throughout the suckling period was similar for all calves; however, this is not true because calves born late in the calving season may not have as high an average daily gain as calves born early in the calving season. Consequently, late calves will always be lighter at weaning regardless of when they are weaned. This phenomenon is not fully understood or completely accepted, but one explanation is that most ranchers tend to select the calving season that results in the best weaning weights for their particular area. Therefore, late calves will be out of phase with maximum growth for the environment and will have lower weaning weights regardless of age at weaning. This reduction in average daily gain for calves in the bottom third of weaning weights could be due to (1) late calving cows not milking as well when they are out of phase with the most productive forage and (2) calves not being old enough to get maximum utilization of the most productive forage. In South Dakota the best grass season is in May, June and July, and the early calves can receive the benefit of that forage.

A cow must have a calf every 12 months to be an efficient production unit. The very nature of a beef cow's reproductive physiology is a major obstacle to that 12-month goal. The gestation period averages 283 days, so a cow must become pregnant by 80 days after calving to produce a calf every 12 months. Cows most likely to cycle and become pregnant early are those in good condition at calving, regardless of nutrition level. Many cows in thin body condition do not become pregnant. In one study the percentage open varied from 77 in very thin cows to 5 in cows in good body condition.

The main reason why thin cows calve late or are open is that the interval from calving to first estrus is greatly delayed. This was shown in a Nebraska study in which only 46 per cent of thin cows were in heat by 60 days compared to 91 per cent of cows in good condition (Table 2). By 100 days after calving only 70 per cent of the cows in thin body condition had shown heat. The final result is fewer pregnancies among thin cows. Cows in moderate or good condition at calving had acceptable pregnancy

Table 2. Body Condition at Calving and Per Cent Cycling in the Postpartum Period

Body-Condition at Calving	No. Cows	Per Cent Cycling 50 to 100 Days after Calving					
		50 Days	60 Days	70 Days	80 Days	90 Days	100 Days
Thin	272	44	46	55	62	66	70
Moderate	364	45	61	79	88	92	100
Good	50	42	91	96	98	100	100

rates, but only 72 per cent of thin cows were pregnant after 80 days of breeding.

Details on the effect of body condition on beef reproduction are discussed in the article Influences of Nutrition on Reproduction in Beef Cattle, and the reader should refer to that article for details on body condition scores. However, the subject is so important that a brief review of body condition at calving is necessary.

1. Body condition scores (BCS) of 1 to 3 apply to emaciated and thin cows. Tailheads, ribs and spinous processes are visible and obviously palpable. These cows will not return to estrus.

2. Body condition score 4 is borderline. Ribs are palpable but not obviously visible unless hair is short. Special care such as early weaning, flushing and short-term (48-hour) calf removal may improve cycling and pregnancy rates.

3. Body condition scores of 5 to 7 indicate moderate to good body conditions and are probably the most cost-effective. These cows have acceptable reproductive rates after 60 days postpartum rest.

4. Cows with body condition scores of 8 and 9 are fat. Reproductive performance is usually good, but feed has been wasted to maintain such conditions if the cows are calving every year. Often many cows with these scores calve only every other year.

A comment must be made that fat rarely causes poor reproductive performance, but poor reproductive performance will result in fat cows.

Wiltbank has suggested two approaches to keeping cows in moderate body condition. First, cows should be carefully observed 1 or 2 months before calves are scheduled to be weaned. If cows are thin, calves should be weaned early. This will give cows a few months of good feed before the quality of the forage declines, or, if supplementation is required, feed costs can be minimized. Calves are probably growing at a slow rate because of the low quality of feed available, and a weaning ration will improve their growth.

The second approach that could be used is to sort cows by body condition at weaning time. Cows should be scored for body condition from 1 (thin) to 9 (fat). The type of ration necessary to meet the required average daily gain can then be fed (Table 3). Note that all cows must gain 45 kilograms to offset fetal and uterine weights, and body condition improvement must be in addition to fetal growth. Also, thin cows must be fed high-energy rations, whereas fat cows can be maintained on low energy forages.

Table 4 illustrates the importance of energy levels after calving. Cows fed a high level of energy after calving achieved a higher first service conception rate and overall pregnancy rate. This emphasizes that *postcalving* energy level will be a major determinant of conception rates.

Feeding thin cows (BCS of three or less) for short periods of time after calving to initiate estrus or improve conception rates is not practical. A minimum of 0.91 kg a day must be gained by the cow with a body condition score of 3 at calving if we want her to have enough body condition to show heat early in the breeding season. If in addition to scoring 3 she has only 60 days from calving to breeding, she must gain 1.2 kg per day. As soon as her feed level is increased, she will increase her milk production; therefore, only a small amount of the nutrients fed go to weight gain. It is difficult if not impossible for her to gain 0.91 kg a day while nursing a calf. This means that we need to put the condition on the cow before calving.

The onset of estrus following calving is delayed in beef cows that are suckling calves. The interval from calving to first estrus has been reported to be from 35 to 54 days longer in cows suckling calves than in dry or milked cows.

Table 3. Weight Needed to Increase Body Condition Score (BCS)

BCS at Weaning	BCS at Calving	Weight Gain Needed (kg)			Days Weaning to Calving	ADG	TDN Value of Rations
		Fetal Fluids	Fat or Muscle*	Total			
5	5	45	0	45	130	0.35	50
3	5	45	73	118	130	0.90	70
3	5	45	73	118	200	0.95	60
3	5	45	73	118	100	1.18	70
2	5	45	109	154	130	1.18	70
7	5	45	−73	−27	130	−0.21	45

*Difference between body condition scores = 37 kg.

Table 4. Effect of Energy on Post-Calving Pregnancy Rate

| Calving Time to Breeding | Pregnant | | | Cows Not Showing Heat (%) |
	From First Service (%)	20 Days After Breeding (%)	90 Days After Breeding (%)	
Losing weight (3.6 kg TDN)	43	29	72	14
Gaining weight (7.3 kg TDN)	60	57	82	0
Difference	17	28	10	14

Other methods that might be used to decrease the interval from calving to first heat are to wean the calves early or decrease the frequency of suckling. A study at Oklahoma State University showed that weaning calves at 6 to 8 weeks of age markedly improved reproductive performance of beef cows. The calves were weaned on a high-energy calf starter. The roughage content was increased as the calves consumed more dry matter. There were no problems encountered with the early weaning but feed costs were greatly increased. However, cost-effectiveness analysis of the data indicated that early weaning of calves could salvage a reproductive program facing an environmental crisis such as drought or severe shortages of natural forage. The increased pregnancy rate and weaning weight of subsequent calf crops following early weaning returned more income per cow than did supplementing lactating cows that faced severe feed shortages.

Cows that score a 4 or greater at calving will respond to a flushing ration fed for 3 weeks prior to breeding *if* the calves are removed for 48 hours at the beginning of the breeding season. A study conducted in South Texas with first-calf heifers that were in borderline condition at calving time demonstrates this principle (Table 5). Pregnancy rate was increased only in the group in which flushing and calf removal were both used.

Suckling inhibits the release of gonadotropins, and this effect is greatest in (1) cows shortly postpartum, (2) thin to marginal body condition cows, and (3) cows frequently nursed. The removal of this inhibitory effect for 48 hours permits the buildup and release of gonadotropins from the pituitary if

Table 5. Pregnancy Rates Following Calf Removal and Flushing

	Control	FI*	CR†	FI + CR
No. cows	18	21	21	21
Pregnant (per cent)				
21 days	28	14	38	57
24 days	56	52	62	72
63 days	72	76	62	86

*Flushed with 10 lb corn for 2 weeks before breeding and first 3 weeks of breeding.
†Calf removal for 48 hours at start of breeding.

the cows have a body condition score of at least 4 and are 50 days or more postpartum.

Sickness or undue stress has not been encountered in the calves. Tight fences, fresh water, and a high-energy calf starter are all that are necessary for the calves. Neither udder problems nor mothering up problems have occurred when the calves are returned to the cows.

The important point is that we expect cows to become pregnant by 90 days or less after calving, but 60 to 80 days of postpartum rest is necessary for 80 per cent of beef cows to start cycling. Cows that calve late have two distinct disadvantages. First, they have fewer chances to cycle and therefore make up the greater number of open cows. Second, even when cows show estrus at less than 50 days postpartum, conception rates are below 50 per cent. Remember, cows must be in moderate or better condition at calving and have adequate postpartum rest to have high reproductive rates.

After 80 or 90 days of breeding, the total conception rate exceeds 90 per cent, but cows that calve in the third and fourth 21-day period of the calving season are the poorest producers. Eighty per cent of the cows that calve in the first 21-day period are pregnant at the end of 42 days breeding, whereas only 20 per cent of those calving in the fourth 21-day period are pregnant at the same time. Many of the late calving cows will be open or will continue to calve late and wean lighter calves in successive years.

Variation in bull fertility has a marked effect on the reproductive efficiency of the cow herd. Studies involving 3700 cows and 150 bulls in multiple sire pastures at the King Ranch in Texas showed that bulls with greater than 32 cm scrotal circumference and more than 70 per cent normal sperm cells increased herd pregnancy rates by 6 per cent. Do not compromise on questionable bulls. Reevaluate them but *do not* put them with the cows until they are satisfactory.

The following conclusions are valid: (1) cows tend to calve at the same time every year if conditions are favorable, (2) unfavorable conditions tend to extend calving intervals or cause pregnancy failures and (3) the probability of early calving increases when replacement heifers calve early and when the calving season is short. A short calving season can be attained during a 4- or 5-year period if all replacements calve early in the first two calving seasons.

Three-Year Heifer Control Program

The first-calf heifer has more difficulties cycling and conceiving than all other cows. At calving she still has high growth requirements and is then suddenly subjected to two new stresses, calving and nursing. These three stresses require the first-calf heifer to have 20 more days of postpartum rest than older cows to start cycling. Therefore, the breeding of the replacement heifer must be controlled throughout the first 3 years of her life. Control thereafter is much easier since the calving pattern of adult cows is established in the first two reproductive years and rarely changes unless adverse conditions cause her to calve later.

What is the controlled 3-year heifer program? The goals are:

1. To breed 13- to 15-month old virgin heifers for 42 days, starting 21 days before the regular breeding season. Eighty-five per cent of the heifers should be cycling and bred during the first 21 days and 95 per cent by the end of 42 days. Eighty-five per cent of the heifers bred should become pregnant.

2. To enable 2-year-old heifers nursing their first calves to be cycling at a rate of 85 to 95 per cent during the first 42 days of the regular breeding season, and 85 per cent or more should be pregnant at the end of 63 days breeding.

To accomplish these breeding goals, three growth requirements should be met at specific times:

1. First year (from birth to breeding). Heifers should reach 65 per cent of their mature weight at 13 to 15 months of ages.

2. Second year (from first breeding to first calving). Heifers should reach 85 per cent of their mature weight at 2 years of age.

3. Third year (from second breeding to second calving). Heifers should reach 95 per cent of their mature weight at 3 years of age.

The 65 per cent of mature weight for puberty at 14 to 15 months of age is only an approximation. Table 6 shows more specific weights for various breeds.

How to Establish a Heifer Program

The following steps are required to establish a 3-year controlled heifer program:

1. Select approximately 1.5 times as many heifers as will actually be needed for replacements. These heifers should be selected so that they will be between 13 and 15 months of age at the beginning of the heifer breeding season. Younger heifers will not be old enough or have sufficient weight by the start of breeding. Less than 30 per cent of properly

fed heifers will be cycling at 12 months of age, whereas 85 to 90 per cent of the same heifers will be cycling at 15 months of age. Zebu breeds will require 3 to 6 months longer to reach puberty. However, there are records of these cattle reaching puberty as early as English cattle through selection for early puberty.

2. Weigh all heifers as a group and determine average weights. If there are wide ranges between the smaller and the larger heifers, they should be divided into two feeding groups in order to reach their desired weight by breeding time. Achieving this goal is very important. Less than 50 per cent of heifers that reach 50 per cent of their mature weight at 15 months of age will be cycling.

3. Calculate the days between initial weighing and beginning of the breeding season. Determine the average daily gain necessary to reach the desired breeding weight, and feed to attain that average daily gain.

4. Weigh a random sample of the heifers every 30 days to check growth rates. If growth rates aren't being attained, the ration must be adjusted.

5. At 1 year of age, it may be necessary to remove approximately 10 per cent of heifers as undesirable for replacement breeding. These heifers should be fattened for slaughter or sold to reduce carrying costs.

6. Breed for 42 days, starting 21 days before breeding the cows. Well-grown replacement heifers are ideal candidates for estrus synchronization, which facilitates a short breeding season. Preferably, all breeding should be by artificial insemination, using semen from a progeny-tested bull proved to be an "easy calving" bull. Such a bull should also have the genetic ability to transmit above average growth rates to his offspring.

7. The heifers may be pregnancy tested any time after 35 days following the end of the 42-day breeding season. The sooner the heifers are pregnancy tested, the sooner it will be possible to sell all open heifers. Pelvic measurements may be taken at this time, and the bottom 20 to 30 per cent of heifers may be removed from the replacement group to decrease calving problems. Pelvic measurements, however, are of no value unless the heifers are properly grown by breeding and calving time. Culling the bottom 20 to 30 per cent from a group of small heifers will not significantly reduce calving difficulties. Second, selecting replacement heifers with large pelvic areas is not helpful if they are bred to bulls with unknown dystocia rates. The use of the pelvimeter is recommended only in herds that are under intensive management and in instances when it will provide the additional selection pressure necessary to select the very best replacement heifers.

8. Once the pregnant replacement heifers have been selected, maintain their growth rate to reach 85 per cent of mature cow size at calving. This will help ensure proper cycling rates for the second breeding and will decrease the incidence of calving problems.

Table 6. Estimates for Heifers Reaching Puberty at Various Weights

| | Heifers Reaching Puberty | | |
Breed	50% in Estrus	70% in Estrus	90% in Estrus
Angus	250	273	295
Brahman	307	330	341
Brangus	273	295	318
Charolais	318	341	352
Hereford	273	295	318
Santa Gertrudis	307	330	341
Jersey × British	227	250	273
Limousin	295	318	341
Simmental	284	307	341

Table 7. Calving Pattern*

Calving Group	1	2	3	4	5	6	No. Calves	No. Open
Days of Calving Season	21	42	63	84	105	126		
First-calf heifers	3	4	1	1			9	1
Adult cows	14	27	27	13	4	2	87	3
Total	17	31	28	14	4	2	96	4

*Number of pregnant adult cows, 90.
Number of pregnant heifers, 10.

9. Maintain growth through 3 years of age (95 per cent of mature body weight).

The culling rate in an intensive management program may seem severe, but cull heifers will become cull cows if not eliminated. Intensive culling at early stages permits sales at peak value, not at 3 to 4 years of age when the inferior cows will be sold for lower prices. The practice of early severe culling will produce maximum performance in the herd and avoid carrying costs for poor producing females.

Maintaining control of replacement heifers through the first 3 years of life results in a herd of early calving, high-producing mother cows. After having been on a controlled heifer replacement program for approximately 5 years, calves from first-calf heifers could have weaning weights equal to the herd average. This is possible because the heifers' calves will be weaned at an average age of approximately 20 days older than the rest of the calves. Also, if artificial insemination has been used, the genetic merit of replacement heifers will exceed the average genetic merit of the cow herd.

TOTAL REPRODUCTIVE MANAGEMENT PLAN

An overall reproductive management plan should be decided upon by a producer and his consulting veterinarian. The plan should have enough flexibility to allow for year-to-year economic variations and differences in management abilities of producers. For example, some ranchers may not find feeding of replacement heifers to calve at 2 years of age to be cost-effective. It may be necessary for replacements to calve first at 3 years of age, but all replacements should be bred to calve in a short time interval early in the calving season.

A 5-year projection of reproduction should be

calculated initially and then updated each year. The projection will not always be accurate each year but will be helpful in establishing and evaluating both short- and long-range goals. Goals may change with economic changes in the beef cattle business and, in turn, alter projections.

A 5-year reproductive projection simply involves determining the number of cows eligible to breed during any 21-day segment of the breeding season. This is done by analyzing the postpartum interval and the levels of prepartum and postpartum nutrition, and by evaluating body condition to estimate cycling rates.

The following data are required:

1. Calving dates. When calving dates are not recorded, the veterinarian and the rancher can estimate the number of calves born during each 20 or 30 days of the calving season. This is often necessary for the first year in the initial 5-year projection, but calving dates should be available after that for yearly updates.

2. Nutritional levels before and after calving. These are often estimates during the first year, but subsequent years' records should be readily available to determine feed consumed.

3. Estimate of body condition before and after calving. Currently, this is the best estimation of the cows' well being and is the best measure of nutritional status. Cows may be fed according to the best recommendations of nutrition guidelines but still may not be in the desirable body condition for suitable reproductive performance.

In the following herd example, the calving pattern has been similar for many years. The cows have been on low nutrition levels before calving and in relatively poor condition at calving (body condition scores 3 to 5). Nutrition has improved to moderate levels following calving, especially as summer pas-

Table 8. Five-Year Reproduction Plan

First-calf Heifers		21-Day Calving Groups						Total Calves	Total Open
		1	2	3	4	5	6		
		21 Days	42 Days	63 Days	84 Days	105 Days	126 Days		
This year	0	17	31	28	14	4	2	96	4
Next year	10	32	26	22	5			95	5
2	10	39	27	16	8			95	5
3	10	44	27	14				95	5
4	10	46	27	12				95	5
5	10	46	28	11				95	5

ture improved. Ten per cent replacements have been added annually and have been bred at the same time as the cows. Note that 70 per cent of the replacement heifers calved in the first 42 days of the calving season, but only 47 per cent of the adult cows calved at that time. Control of the replacements was lost at the first calving (Table 7).

Projections for the 5-year reproductive plan should include the following changes:

1. Plan 15 per cent replacements each year.

2. Maintain the same number of animal units in the herd but reduce the number of late calving cows to permit adding more early calving replacements each year.

3. Feed and manage replacement heifers to start breeding 21 days before older cows. Select herd replacements from those becoming pregnant in a 42-day breeding season. This applies to heifers that calve first at 3 years of age as well as to those that calve first at 2 years of age.

4. Maintain first-calf heifers separately from older cows and on a higher level of nutrition through their second breeding season while nursing their first calves.

5. During the last trimester, feed cows to be in body condition score 5 or 6 at calving. This condition should be maintained during the postpartum period. Remember, cows should be at condition score 5 and gaining slightly at the beginning of the breeding season for the best conception rates.

6. Be prepared to flush cows starting 3 weeks before breeding and remove calves for 48 hours at the beginning of breeding. This can increase the cycling rate in body condition score 4 cows or in better condition cows with short postpartum intervals. Good condition cows with more than 50 days postpartum rest will not need this extra care.

7. Evaluate bulls for breeding soundness during the 30-day period before breeding and observe bulls for mating ability during the breeding season. Any bull that does not breed or becomes injured should be replaced. Bulls should have minimum scrotal circumference of 32 cm and 70 per cent or more normal sperm cells.

Three-year control of replacement heifers is the key to maintaining the program. Twenty-two heifers will be exposed to breeding to acquire 15 pregnant

replacements. Ten heifers would be expected to become pregnant 21 days before the cows. Approximately seven more heifers should become pregnant in the second 21 days of heifer breeding. Five of these would be selected to complete the 15 replacements. The combination of controlled replacement breeding and improved nutrition for the adult cows should increase the number of calves born in the first 21 days from the current 17 to a projected 42 calves next year.

The projection calls for shortening the cow breeding season to 63 days during the third breeding season. However, this cannot be accomplished unless at least 50 per cent of the calves are born within the first 21 days of calving. Little change will occur in the calving season once it has been reduced to 63 days (Table 8). Management failures will lengthen the breeding and calving season and will cause a return to previous unsatisfactory patterns of performance.

Wiltbank initiated this system including flushing and 48-hour calf removal at the O'Connor Ranch in Texas. Pregnancy rates after 21, 42, 63, and 84 days were 80, 87, 87, and 93 per cent, respectively. He subsequently used the O'Connor system in a controlled study in Utah. Cows selected for the O'Connor system were all early calvers while the control cows represented a 150-day calving pattern that had existed on the ranch for years. Cows in both groups had body condition scores ranging from 4 to 7 at calving. Calving started the last of January, and breeding began April 22. First-year results are shown in Table 9.

The question that every consulting veterinarian must answer is "Will it pay?" More management and feed costs must be accrued by the O'Connor system. All costs were known and weaning weights were estimated for both groups. Additional cost for the O'Connor system was $1095. The estimated increase in weaning weights for the O'Connor system was 2329 kilograms of calf or 26 kilograms of calf per cow bred. If calves sold for $1.32 per kilogram ($0.60 per pound) the additional income would be $3,070.00, a 181 per cent return of the investment of $1095.

Controlled reproduction can result in excellent production when a plan is made and adhered to.

Table 9. Reproductive Performance at Elberta, Utah, Using O'Connor System

	Cows Managed Under		
	O'Connor System	Control System	Difference
No. cows	89	86	
Showing heat after breeding (%)			
25 days	95	59	36
46 days	98	72	26
Pregnant after one breeding	80	50	30
Calved (%)			
After 20 days	80	28	52
After 40 days	91	52	39
After 60 days	99	72	
After 120 days	99	93	8

Cows that are well managed will calve every 12 months in a short season. Late calving cows will not move up to an earlier calving date easily, but the 3-year heifer control program and the O'Connor system will maintain reproductive efficiency and increase profitability.

References

1. Lusby KS, Pama AA: Effect of early weaning on calf performance and reproduction in mature cows. Oklahoma State University Anim Sci Res Report M-P 108, 1981, p. 64.
2. Rice LE: Coping with calving difficulties. Proceedings 2nd Annual OK Cattle Conference, Oklahoma State University, 1976, pp. 11–12.
3. Whitman RW, Remmega EE, Wiltbank JN: Weight change, condition and beef cow production. J Anim Sci 41:387, 1975 (Abstr).
4. Wiltbank JN, Faulkner LC: The management of beef breeding programs. Proceedings of Conference on Reproductive Problems in Animals. ASSBS and University of Georgia Center for Continuing Education, 1969, pp. 1–15.
5. Wiltbank JN: Personal communication, 1983.
6. Wiltbank JN: Evaluation of bulls for potential fertility. Proceedings, Society for Theriogenology, 1982, p. 141.

Vaccination to Maximize Bovine Fertility

Steven M. Hopkins, D.V.M.
Iowa State University, Ames, Iowa

A planned vaccination regime is a vital component of a herd health program even though vaccination cannot prevent or control all potential reproductive diseases. There are pathogens (e.g., *Ureaplasma*) for which no vaccines are available, and some vaccines are not marketed in the United States.

The ability of a vaccination program to prevent the clinical appearance of a specific disease depends heavily on management practices. Consideration must be given to the current health, reproductive status and age of the animal as well as to population density and handling facilities.

To maximize the benefits of vaccination the veterinarian must understand the differences between types of vaccines, expected biologic responses, duration of immunity, storage requirements and potential hazards from vaccination.

A vaccination program cannot remain static if it is to provide maximum protection. Population changes, introduction of new pathogens and development of new vaccines require careful monitoring and adjustment of the program (Table 1).

VACCINE TYPES AND STORAGE

Vaccines may be classified into three general types: modified live (MLV), killed and subunit. The antigenicity of each type is different, and therefore the duration of the immune period depends on the vaccine and the number of injections.

Modified live vaccines, like the *Brucella* Strain-19 and infectious bovine rhinotracheitis (IBR) types are attenuated or modified to minimize pathogenicity yet are live agents that promote a long-lasting immune response. MLV vaccines generally require fewer inoculating doses to obtain an adequate immune response since they stimulate the host's immune system like field strains. Live antigenic material does not require the use of adjuvants to enhance immune stimulation, resulting in fewer hypersensitivity reactions.

Killed products are safer than MLV vaccines because the disease agent itself cannot infect another susceptible host. Because these bacterins are less stimulatory to the host's immune system, however, higher antigenic concentrations, multiple injections and adjuvants are required with the use of killed products. The duration of immunity also tends to be shorter than that with MLV products. The necessity for multiple injections may increase the potential for type 1 (inflammation) and type 3 (immune complex) hypersensitivity reactions.

Subunit vaccines are composed of protein particles that produce an immune response that is protective against the intact organism. The humoral antibody response is different from that which occurs under natural infective conditions, allowing for the differentiation between vaccination and natural titers. Subunit vaccines are administered at higher antigenic doses because they are not as efficacious as MLV vaccines.

As biologic agents, all vaccines require temperature controlled storage and handling. Only dry, sterile needles and syringes should be used for vaccination. Manufacturers are required by the United States Department of Agriculture (USDA) to demonstrate that the vaccine is sufficiently antigenic to protect against clinical manifestation of a disease when administered under optimal conditions. Protection from clinical manifestations, except for brucellosis, does not imply that vaccination titers will provide maximum protection for reproductive functions. This concept is applicable to both vibriosis and bovine viral diarrhea (BVD). The immunoglobulin G response from a vibriosis bacterin declines rapidly and may not be completely protective months later.[1] Similarly, vaccination ti-

Table 1. Immunizations

Disease (Agent)	Vaccine (Type Route)	Initial Vaccination/Booster Ages
Brucellosis (Brucella abortus)	Strain-19: MLV* subcutaneous	Dairy: 2 to 6 months. Beef: 2 to 10 months. 65 to 75 per cent protected. Do not vaccinate bulls.
Leptospirosis (Leptospira pomona) L. grippotyphosa (L. hardjo) (L. icterohaemorrhagiae) (L. canicola)	Bacterin: killed† intramuscular	Dairy or beef: 30 to 60 days prebreeding. Revaccinate annually in a closed herd. Revaccinate every 6 months in a high risk herd. Vaccinate bulls at the same rate.
Vibriosis (Campylobacter fetus ss. fetus)	Bacterin: killed intramuscular	Dairy or beef heifers or unvaccinated adults: two injections 3 to 4 weeks apart, second injection 10 to 14 days before breeding in enzootic areas. A single injection in low-risk areas 10 to 14 days prebreeding. Annual booster 10 to 14 days before breeding. Bulls: Vaccinate twice initially at 6-week intervals, annual revaccination thereafter.
Infectious bovine rhinotracheitis (herpes 1)	MLV Intramuscular	Calves: If vaccinated before 6 months, then revaccinate at 6 months of age. Nongravid cows and heifers: 30 to 45 days prebreeding (do not co-mingle with susceptible pregnant cows for 30 days). Annual revaccination.
	MLV intranasal	Calves: At birth. Revaccinate at 6 months of age, annually thereafter. Cows: Safe for pregnant animals. Vaccinate cows 30 days prebreeding. Annual revaccination. Bulls: Vaccinate bulls every 4 to 6 months.
	Killed intramuscular	Calves: If vaccinated before 6 months, then revaccinate at 6 months of age. Cows, heifers: Initial injection 30 to 60 days prebreeding followed by booster 14 to 28 days later. Revaccinate annually. Safe for pregnant females.
	Subunit experimental	Potentially applicable to young calves and gravid females. Probable annual revaccination
Bovine viral diarrhea (Toga virus)	MLV intramuscular	Calves: (nonstressed) 4 to 6 months of age. Bulls, cows: 30 days prebreeding. Annual revaccination. 2 to 5 per cent remain seronegative.
	Killed intramuscular	Calves: If vaccinated before 6 months revaccinate at 6 months of age. Cows, heifers, bulls: Two injections 14 to 28 days apart. Annual revaccination. Safe in pregnant females.

*45 states participate in a reduced dosage program at this time.
†Available in three (L. pomona, L. grippotyphosa, L. hardjo) and five (L. grippotyphosa, L. hardjo, L. pomona, L. icterohaemorrhagiae, L. canicola) serovar combinations.

ters of 1:32 will protect a pregnant dam against abortion from BVD, but a titer of 1:128 is necessary for maximum fertility in an open animal. The shelf-life of the product must be validated, and these tests are conducted under the same conditions that the manufacturer recommends for storage and usage of the product. Deviation from the recommendations may render the vaccine less protective or ineffective as the antigenic material is destroyed or altered. Antigenicity may also change with improper use of multiple dose vials. The chemicals or antibiotics employed to control bacterial contamination may be overwhelmed by unsanitary techniques that lead to gross contamination. Similarly, MLV vac-

cines may be rendered inactive if they contact disinfectants that are commonly used to sterilize reuseable syringes.

POTENTIAL VACCINATION HAZARDS

There are vaccination risks that must be considered before the initiation of a vaccination program.

Brucellosis. The vaccination of males for breeding purposes is contraindicated because the Strain-19 bacteria can localize in the testes and epididymides. This produces a localized infection that results in the shedding of the vaccine bacteria in the ejaculate.

Another hazard with Strain-19 is accidental human inoculation, which can result in the development of undulant fever.

Leptospirosis. Vaccination with one serovar does not produce immunity to another serovar, so protective immunity is conferred only for the type of leptospira in the vaccine.

Vibriosis. The vaccination of bulls against vibriosis is still controversial. Studies have indicated that infected bulls will eliminate an active infection following an initial multiple dose vaccination with an annual booster. They can, however, still become passive carriers and act as vectors for susceptible females.

Infectious Bovine Rhinotracheitis. The major problem with IBR vaccination is the ability of the host to become infected with the virulent virus and serve as a latent carrier. Stress, prolonged corticosteroid therapy or parturition may lead to the shedding of the virulent virus with subsequent exposure of susceptible females to IBR. Bulls vaccinated intranasally appear to resist viral recrudescence for up to 6 months following vaccination. Vaccination of purebred bulls for export may be contraindicated because seropositive bulls may fail the export requirements. Vaccination titers could prevent the identification of an IBR infected bull, which could potentially be a latent carrier.

Bovine Viral Diarrhea. MLV BVD vaccines have been incriminated as an agent causing the appearance of mucosal disease and abortions in the field. Because the MLV BVD vaccine virus can cause abortions in controlled experiments, prebreeding inoculation is indicated. It is difficult, however, to ascertain whether vaccination problems were produced by the vaccine, by failure of seroconversion or by the concurrent incubation of the disease at the time of vaccination. Killed BVD vaccine is safe in pregnant animals.

All vaccinations have the potential to produce anaphylactic reactions, although reported cases are rare. The manufacturers recommend the use of epinephrine as the treatment for anaphylaxis.

INCOMPATIBILITIES

Vaccinations, to be effective, must be able to stimulate the host's immune system effectively. Stress, nutritional mismanagement and antibiotics can be incompatible with the development of adequate protection. Vaccination of stressed cattle has the potential to block the development of protective antibody titers.[3] Likewise, low-energy diets prevent the host from producing antibody levels comparable to those in an animal on a balanced diet.[2] The use of antibiotics has the potential to mask the expression of diseases. Animals receiving antibiotics may be actively infected, and apparent vaccination failure ensues when the drugs are withdrawn.

References

1. Berg RL, Firehammer BD: Effect of interval between booster vaccination and time of breeding on protection against *Campylobacter* (vibriosis) in cattle. J Am Vet Med Assoc 173:467, 1978.
2. Spire MF: Bovine immunizations. Bov Pract 16:101, 1981.
3. Weiser RS, Myrvik QN, Pearsall NN: Fundamentals of Immunology. Lea and Febiger, Philadelphia, 1970.

The Economics of Reproductive Herd Health Programs for Dairy Herds

Norman Bruce Williamson, M.V.S.C.
University of Minnesota
St. Paul, Minnesota

Herd reproductive health programs are now an accepted and established part of veterinary practice. Programs operate in large dairies of several thousand head in the western United States, in small midwestern herds of 40 cows where cows calve year round and in the typically 100-cow herds that calve seasonally in Australia, New Zealand and England.

The assumption is that reproductive health programs are profitable. Studies of various types and at various times have indicated that they may be very profitable. However, reproductive health programs vary greatly. Planned pregnancy diagnosis visits every few months represent a reproductive health program to some. Others consider goal setting, client education, record maintenance, record monitoring, nutritional advice and vaccination programs to be essential components of reproductive health programs in addition to the regular genital examination and treatment of cows.

With such a wide variation in the location and style of programs, no generally applicable specific conclusions can be made about their value. Any attempt to calculate a dollar value for the application of reproductive health programs in general would be futile owing to differences in enterprise size, environment levels of performance, program style and costs, milk prices and so forth.

Reproductive health programs are an important aspect of a total herd health approach and are widespread and growing. Producers participate in reproductive health programs primarily to increase their net farm income. Clients who consider participation in programs understandably seek estimates of the economic impact of the programs before they finally decide to participate. Estimates of the economic impact of reproductive health programs have come from three types of study: (1) partial farm budgets of the effect of altered reproductive performance on income, (2) computer models of changes in reproductive performance and (3) controlled studies on farms where programs were applied and their impact evaluated. This paper will demonstrate the budgeting approach to the evaluation of reproductive health programs.

DETERMINATION OF REPRODUCTIVE HEALTH PROGRAM PROFITABILITY BY BUDGETING

A common assumption is that participation in a reproductive herd health program will improve the reproductive performance of a herd. A budgeted assessment of the costs of suboptimal reproductive performance or of the benefits from improved reproductive performance is the most popular way to determine the benefits from improved reproductive performance. To develop budgets, information is needed on the cost of services, the effect of lactation length on yield, the influence of calving interval on calf numbers, the influence of yield, concentrate use and calf output on profitability, changes in heifer selection and replacement intake, and the cost of veterinary services.[2]

The production levels of cows that have various calving intervals have been determined from official herd production recording information. Olds and associates[7] estimate milk losses at 9.04 pounds for heifers and 18.96 pounds for cows for each day conception is delayed between 40 and 140 days after previous calving.

Another benefit of reducing calving intervals is the increased rate at which calves are born. Fortunately, this can readily be estimated. The number of calves born per year is

$$\frac{365}{G + C} \times H$$

where G days is the gestation length, C days is the interval from calving to conception and H cows is the nominal herd size. Changes in calf production for given changes in calving interval can be readily estimated using this formula. The value of calves produced can then be determined on the basis of expected sex ratios, estimates of calf survival and sale prices for male and female calves. The fate of additional calves cannot be predicted because it will vary between enterprises. If herds raise their own replacements, it is appropriate to consider the impact of additional calves born by calculating the costs and returns until they reach the milking herd. A greater selection differential would also occur in herds with a higher rate of calf births, but this is difficult to value. For herds in which calves are not raised it would be more appropriate to value calves at sale when approximately 1 week old.

An effective means of reducing calving intervals is by breeding cows earlier.[6, 8] Each 1-day reduction in the interval from calving to breeding results in about 0.8 to 0.9 days decrease in calving interval. The impact of a health program on the number of services required per conception may vary. Early breeding may cause conception rates to fall and semen costs to rise, or the converse may occur when improved heat detection, insemination technique, herd nutrition or disease control may result in improved conception efficiency and lower semen costs.

The changes in calving interval that influence production and calf numbers also influence feed usage, since increased production and calves both require additional feed. Thus improved reproductive efficiency will cause changes in feed consumption and costs. However, the efficiency of feed conversion into saleable product is likely to increase with improved reproductive efficiency.

Culling patterns can be changed markedly by improvements in reproductive performance achieved by health programs through introduced management techniques.

If changes in reproductive performance are achieved as a consequence of participation in a herd health program, the cost of conducting the program and implementing the changes necessary to make it work must be considered when evaluating the worth of the program.

EVALUATION OF HERD HEALTH PROGRAM PROFITABILITY USING PARTIAL BUDGETING

To illustrate the use of partial budgeting to evaluate the potential impact of a reproductive health program on herd profitability, consider a hypothetical Minnesota herd. Participation in a health program could and should change the herd's performance, as shown in the following Table 1.

A decrease in the culling rate will change the average lactation age of the herd, which would increase from an estimated 2.2 to 3.5 lactations.[4] Lactation production will increase from 92.8 to 97.8

Table 1. Herd Profitability with a Reproductive Herd Health Program

Characteristic	Before Program	After Program
Herd size	50 cows	50 cows
Open interval	115 days	90 days
Cull cows	16	10
Calf losses		
Males before sale	3	2
Females	3	2
Services per conception	2.2	2.0
Veterinary costs ($)	1250	1800
Average age at first calving	28 months	25 months

per cent of peak mature levels if herd age is increased from 44 to 60 months, the expected ages at 2.2 and 3.5 lactations.[5] The 25 days earlier conception of the herd after program implementation would result in (25 × 18.96 × 40) pounds of extra milk from the cows and (25 × 9.04 × 10) pounds of extra milk from the heifers, totalling 21,220 pounds of additional milk from decreasing the calving-to-conception interval if the production effects observed by Olds *et al.* are achieved.

Decreasing the culling rate also affects the number of replacements required for the herd. We can budget the impact of the program on livestock numbers as shown in the following Table 2.

Calf losses of 13 per cent are typical of Midwestern dairy herds. A reduction to 8 per cent after program introduction would be modest and likely to result from counselling regarding the use of bulls with a suitable calving ease index on heifers, improved assistance for dystocia and better vaccination and calf raising procedures. An assessment of the economic impact of improving reproductive performance needs to consider conception, pregnancy, parturition and also the growth of a newborn calf to breeding age. In this example it is assumed that the dairyman retains all females and grows them until they are bred and ready to enter the milking herd. Heifer raising costs were estimated by Fuller and colleagues[3] to be $756 for 24 months or $1.05 per day. Heifers take 28 months until first calving occurs before the program and 25 months after the program. Excess heifers are then sold for $1100 as replacements. Cull cows average 1200 pounds and are sold for $500, and bull calves sell for $50.00.

Feed costs for milk production are generally estimated at around 40 per cent of the value of milk produced. However, the increased production achieved as a result of health program participation results from increased feed conversion efficiency due to milking older, more efficient cows and milking cows proportionately more in early than in late lactation, which doubles the conversion efficiency

of concentrate to milk.[1] This analysis will assume that the extra feed cost for the extra production due to increasing the age of cows is 30 per cent of the value of the increased production obtained; the extra feed cost for increased production due to a shorter calving interval is 20 per cent of the value of the increased production that results.

A farmer must invest something to achieve the production changes that have been outlined. Veterinary fees for an average 50-cow herd would be approximately $1400, but costs would rise when a program was introduced. A 50 per cent increase in veterinary costs due to participation in a reproductive health program would not be excessive. Thus, veterinary fees would be $2100 per year. It is estimated that extra record keeping and heat detection required after program implementation takes 1 hour per day extra labor at $6.00 per hour.

The herd, before participation in the program, is taken as an average Minnesota herd that participates in DHIA. Thus production is at 14,900 pounds of milk per cow per year (the 1982 average). Milk price received is set at $12.50 per 100 pounds.

A partial farm budget can be used to estimate the expected net return if the above outcomes are achieved (Table 3). In the partial budget approach we look at the difference in the economic situation of the farm before and after participation in the program, according to the formula: (additional returns + costs no longer incurred) − (additional costs + returns no longer obtained). For simplicity, this analysis will ignore the effects of the time between investing in the program and the time when results are achieved. In conducting the partial farm budget, only the differences in costs and returns between the groups need to be considered.

This budget presents the net return that may be achieved by improving herd reproductive performance through participation in a dairy reproductive health program. Studies have emphasized the influence of calving interval on herd productivity. Although this significantly influences herd profitability,

Table 2. Livestock Numbers with a Reproductive Herd Health Program

	Before Program	After Program
No. calves born/year	$\frac{365}{115 + 282} \times 50 = 46$	$\frac{365}{90 + 282} \times 50 = 49$
No. males born/year	$\frac{46}{2} = 23$	$\frac{49}{2} = 24.5$
No. males died	3	2
No. males sold	20	22.6
No. females born/year	23	24.5
No. females died	3	2
No. females raised	20	22.5
No. replacements available per year	$\frac{24}{28} \times 20 = 17.1$	$\frac{24}{25} \times 22.5 = 21.6$
Heifers required as replacements	16	10
Heifers sold	1.1	11.6

Table 3. Partial Farm Budget

I. Additional Returns

1. Increased milk production
   a. Increased production due to calving interval difference — $ 2652.50
   b. Increased production due to increased average herd age from 43.6 months to 55.4 months — $ 4643.75

   Total from increased milk production — $ 7296.25

2. Replacements for sale
   An additional (11.6 − 1.1 = 10.5) heifers at $1100.00 each — $11,550.00

3. Bull calves for sale, 2.5 at $50.00 each — $ 125.00

   Total additional returns — $18,971.25

II. Costs No Longer Incurred

1. Semen costs
   2 doses × 50 cows at $10.00 per dose — $ 100.00

2. Raising costs for 20 heifers from 25 to 28 months
   (20 heifers × 90 days at $1.05 per day) — $ 1890.00

   Total costs no longer incurred — $ 1990.00

III. Additional Costs

1. Increased veterinary costs — $ 550.00

2. Increased labor
   (1 hour per day at $6.00 per hour) — 2190.00

3. Increased feed for increased production
   $(2652.5 \times 0.2) + (4643.75 \times 0.3)$ — 1923.62

   [20% of the value of extra production due to decreased calving interval + 50% of the value of extra production due to increased herd age]

4. Cost of raising an additional 2.2 heifers to 25 months (2.2 heifers × 760 days at $1.05 per day) — $ 1755.60

   Total additional costs — $ 6419.22

IV. Returns No Longer Obtained
   6 cull cows at $500 each — $ 3000.00

NET RETURN
   (I + II) − (III + IV) — $11,542.03

it can be seen that changes in culling and replacement patterns in herds that improve reproductive performance also have major impacts and should be considered in any evaluation of the profitability of reproductive herd health programs.

CONCLUSION

This section has examined the profitability of herd reproductive health programs using the technique of partial farm budgeting. This study indicates that effective reproductive herd health programs can lead to more efficient production of milk and livestock and to improved herd profitability. Improved estrus detection or control is the major means of achieving improved reproductive performance, followed by factors influencing conception efficiency. Increases in herd productivity that result from participation in herd reproductive health programs can result in financial returns of 500 per cent to even greater than 1000 per cent over invested funds. Thus there is a great incentive for farmers to participate in this type of program to improve the productivity and profitability of their herds.

References

1. Broster WH, Broster VJ, Smith T: Experiments on the nutrition of the dairy heifer. VII. Effect on milk production of level of feeding at two stages of the lactation. J Agric Sci 72:229, 1969.
2. Esslemont RJ: Economic and husbandry aspects of the manifestation and detection of oestrus in cows. Part 1. Economic aspects. ADAS Q Rev 12:174, 1974.
3. Fuller EI, Thomas KH, Freeman ML, Appleman RD: Dairy herd planning guide. Farm management series FM-520. University of Minnesota, Agricultural Extension Service, 1982.
4. Morris RS: The economics of bovine mastitis control systems. Master of Veterinary Science thesis. University of Melbourne, Australia, 1974.
5. Norman HD, Miller PD, McDaniel BT, et al.: USDA-DHIA factors for standardizing 305-day lactation records for age and month of calving. ARS-NE-40. Washington DC, Agricultural Research Service. U.S. Department of Agriculture, 1974.
6. Olds D: An objective consideration of herd fertility. J Am Vet Med Assoc 154:253, 1969.
7. Olds D, Cooper T, Thrift FA: Effect of days open on economic aspects of current lactation. J Dairy Sci 62:1167, 1979.
8. Williamson NB, Quinton FW, Anderson GA: The effect of variations in the interval between calving and first service on the reproductive performance of normal dairy cows. Aust Vet J 56:447, 1980.

Analysis of Reproductive Records Using DHIA Summaries and Other Monitors in Large Dairy Herds

R. Kenneth Braun
University of Florida, Gainesville, Florida

Zemjanis recognized some 20 years ago that apparent anestrus was the major factor limiting optimal reproductive performance.[4] He also found that only 10 per cent of this problem was organic and the remainder was due to inadequate management. In spite of these findings, little progress has been made in improving reproductive efficiency on many dairy farms in terms of increasing conception rate, improving estrus detection rates and decreasing days open.

Veterinarians have achieved considerable technical expertise in palpating skills and are adept in identifying ovarian structures, fetal membranes and amniotic vesicles at 30 to 35 days postconception. Veterinarians can evaluate the uterus and synchronize the reproductive cycle with hormones. Considerable progress has also been made in embryo transfer, freezing and splitting embryos, genetics, nutrition, milk quality control and metabolic diseases.

Reproductive performance is determined by the interplay of management and environmental and biologic factors. Other aspects of dairy production such as nutrition, replacement rearing, udder health and milk quality control are likewise heavily dependent upon management for success. If veterinarians want to meet the challenge as consultants for herd health and production control of today's large-scale, highly mechanized dairy enterprises, they must broaden their interest and knowledge to include healthy animals and train themselves to include an agricultural management and economic thought mode.[1] Veterinarians who want to maintain and strengthen their role as herd health–related consultants in reproduction must be competent in analyzing and evaluating herd performance records so that deficiencies can be recognized and appropriate changes recommended for implementation by management.[3] Only by performing much of the physical work (physical examinations, treatment, necropsy) of gathering information on which they base their advice can they advise clients to make appropriate adjustments when goals are not being attained. Accurate and complete record keeping is a prerequisite to the optimal function of a reproductive program. The Dairy Herd Improvement Association (DHIA) has been in the dairy records business for over 50 years. The state or regional[1] and national DHIA organization provides up-to-date records to dairymen on individual cows and bulls as well as a herd summary.[2] Presently, DHIA record systems are the most widely used and nationally popular record systems among dairymen. Stand-alone farm computers have been gaining in popularity, but availability of software programs remains a major drawback when compared to DHIA programs.

Dairymen, with assistance from veterinarians and other agricultural consultants, have to maintain an accurate up-to-date record system on individual cows as well as the herd. These data must be handled and processed to make the information relevant. Dairymen, as well as their consultants, must be able and willing to monitor herd performance in relation to attainable goals.

Personally, I like to set individual performance goals for each of my dairy farms. These goals must meet three criteria: First, they must be economically justified and provide comfort for cattle; second, they must be attainable; and third, they must be measurable. Veterinarians and dairymen should realize that production goals will vary with regions of the country, herd size, and the level of management intensity that the owner wishes to or can attain.

The object of this section is to identify parameters that are of assistance to the management team in increasing reproductive efficiency and to provide information on how to analyze data in relation to realistic goals attainable by dairymen.

Average Days Open. This is the average number of days that cows have been open from their most recent calving date to the reported breeding date, or to date of test for cows that are open 60 days or more without breeding date, or to date of test for cows not bred that are open 60 days or more. Cows with no breeding date, in milk less than 60 days, are not included.

> Goal: Temperate regions of U.S. = 100 days
> Southeastern U.S. = 115 days

Projected Minimum Calving Interval. This is the average minimum calving interval for cows with breeding dates and cows open 60 days or more without breeding dates. The interval for each cow is determined using the last calving date and projected due date for all cows with breeding dates. Cows without breeding dates and open 60 days or more on test day are assumed bred and pregnant on test day, and the earliest due date is projected as 280 days. Actual calving date may be a month or more later.

> Goal: Temperate regions of U.S. = 12.4 months
> Southeastern U.S. = 13.0 months

Per Cent of Possible Breedings that Were Serviced. This is an indication of the success of heat detection in the herd. This percentage is calculated as follows:

1. The average days open is calculated for all cows in the breeding herd that are in milk longer than the dairyman's goal for first breeding plus 10 days.
2. Dairyman's goal to first breeding (usually between 45 and 60 days) plus 10 days (to account for half of the next heat period) is subtracted from average days open.
3. Divide this value by the number of days between normal heats (21 days).
4. This results in the number of possible heats.
5. Possible heats divided into the number of breedings × 100 = per cent of possible breedings that were serviced.

Goal: Temperate regions of U.S. = > 85%
       Southeastern U.S. = > 70%

Preservice Estrus Detection Trial. Estrus detection rate can also be evaluated by the 24-day trial. This trial consists of a list of cows meeting the following criteria when breeding begins at 45 days postpartum.

1. Cows examined okay-to-breed by 45 days postpartum.
2. 45 days plus 24 days = 69 days.
3. Count the number of cows with a breeding date during the first 24 days (45 to 69) and divide by the total number of cows eligible to be bred during this period.
4. Number of cows bred between 45 and 69 days = per cent detected of total number of cows eligible.

Goal	Cows	Virgin Heifers
Temperate regions of U.S. =	> 85%	> 95%
Southeastern U.S. =	> 70%	> 90%

Preservice Detection of Estrus. Interestrous intervals on herds that record all preservice estruses can be used as a measure of estrus detection efficiency. The normal interval between estruses is 18 to 24 days. The expected level of achievement is:

30 to 52 days postpartum
Goal: Temperate regions of U.S. = > 75%
       Southeastern U.S. = > 60%

53 to 75 days postpartum
Goal: Temperate regions of U.S. = > 85%
       Southeastern U.S. = > 70%

Postservice Detection of Estrus (distribution of cycle length).
1. Another measure of efficiency of heat detection is to examine the breeding records. When *repeat breedings* are performed, the percentage bred between 18- to 24-day cycles should be:

Goal: Temperate regions of U.S. = > 75%
       Southeastern U.S. = > 60%

2. Repeat breedings performed between 18 and 24 days plus multiples of these days—i.e., 36 and 48 days:

Goal: Temperate regions of U.S. = > 90%
       Southeastern U.S. = > 75%

3. Number of cows rebred within 3 days of previous insemination:

Goal: Temperate regions of U.S. = < 5%
       Southeastern U.S. = < 10%

4. Number of cows rebred following estrus intervals of 3 to 17 days and/or 25 to 35 days:

Goal: Temperate regions of U.S. = < 10%
       Southeastern U.S. = < 15%

5. The ratio of estruses detected at normal intervals and at multiples of these intervals can be compared and used as a gauge for measuring estrous detection efficiency:
Ratio of repeat breeding performed between
$$\frac{18 \text{ and } 24 \text{ days}}{36 \text{ and } 48 \text{ days}}$$

Goal: Temperate regions of U.S. = 6:1
       Southeastern U.S. = 4:1

Cows Conceiving with Three or Fewer Services. The number of cows conceiving with three or fewer services is dependent on the interval between calving and first breeding date, condition of the reproductive tract, accuracy of estrus detection, semen quality, handling of semen, expertise of inseminator and nutritional status of herd. When breeding begins at 45 days postpartum, the number of cows conceiving with three or fewer services is:

Goal: Temperate regions of U.S. = > 90%
       Southeastern U.S. = > 80%

Proportion of Cows Confirmed Pregnant by Rectal Palpation. This proportion confirmed pregnant between 35 and 60 days postbreeding is another monitor for estrus detection. If cows are examined and found not pregnant, their return to estrus was not observed. For herds in which pregnancy status is monitored between 35 and 60 days postbreeding by rectal palpation, the number of cows found to be open is:

Goal: Temperate regions of U.S. = < 10%
       Southeastern U.S. = < 20%

Pregnant Cows Presented for Insemination. Another consequence of poor heat detection is presenting pregnant cows for insemination. Rebreeding cows may cause them to abort. Under optimum conditions the number of pregnant cows presented for insemination is:

Goal: Temperate regions of U.S. = < 5%
       Southeastern U.S. = < 5%

Average Days to First Breeding. This is calculated from the average days open for all first services of cows in the current breeding herd. Days open are summed and averaged for these cows.

1. When breeding begins at 45 days and heat detection rate is 70 per cent for southeastern U.S. and 85 per cent for more temperate regions of U.S.:

   Goal: Temperate regions of U.S. = < 59 days
   Southeastern U.S. = < 65 days

2. When breeding begins at 60 days:

   Goal: Temperate regions of U.S. = < 74 days
   Southeastern U.S. = < 80 days

3. When breeding begins at 45 days postcalving and average length of estrous cycle is 21 days, then, if 100 per cent of cows are detected in heat, the average days to first breeding would be 45 + ½ × 21 = 55.5 days. If estrus detection rate is 70 per cent, then the following equation is used:

$$100 \text{ cows} \times 70\% = 70 \text{ cows} \times (45 \text{ days} + 10.5 \text{ days}) = 3885.0 \text{ cow days}$$
$$30 \text{ cows} \times 70\% = 21 \text{ cows} \times (66 \text{ days} + 10.5 \text{ days}) = 1606.5 \text{ cow days}$$
$$9 \text{ cows} \times 70\% = 6 \text{ cows} \times (87 \text{ days} + 10.5 \text{ days}) = 585.0 \text{ cow days}$$
$$3 \text{ cows} \times 70\% = 2 \text{ cows} \times (108 \text{ days} + 10.5 \text{ days}) = 237.0 \text{ cow days}$$
$$1 \text{ cow} \times 70\% = 1 \text{ cow} \times (129 \text{ days} + 10.5 \text{ days}) = \underline{139.5 \text{ cow days}}$$
$$Total = 6453.0 \text{ cow days}$$

$$\frac{6453.0}{100} = 64.5 \text{ days to first service when heat detection rate is 70 per cent.}$$

Percentage Problem Cows. This percentage is identified by dividing the number of cows in the current breeding herd open over 100 days by the total cows in the herd on test day, times 100. (Example: cows with no breeding dates—(1) 101–140 days, (2) > 140 days, plus days open at last breeding for cows not yet checked pregnant, (3) 101–140 days, (4) > 140 days; 1 + 2 + 3 + 4 divided by total number of cows in herd (open + pregnant) × 100 = per cent problem cows.

   Goal: Temperate regions of U.S. = < 15%
   Southeastern U.S. = < 20%

Cows Bred Four or More Times as of Last Breeding. These cows are an indication of problem breeders in the current breeding herd. If the number and percentage of these cows become excessive, it may be a reflection of the insemination technique of the person doing the artificial insemination, the fertility of bulls used, the fertility of cows, or a reproductive disease/infection in the herd.

   Goal: Temperate regions of U.S. = < 12%
   Southeastern U.S. = < 20%

Breeding for Past 12 Months. This is a summary of (1) the number of breedings, (2) the percentage successful, (3) the number of breedings per conception, and (4) the first breeding conception rate included in all test intervals used in computing rolling year herd averages. This information is very valuable in evaluating the reproductive efficiency of the herd breeding program. An excessive number of breedings, or a low successful percentage indicates poor fertility of cows or sires used, early embryonic death (due to heat stress), poor artificial insemination technique, or a reproductive herd health problem. Bulls are rated by the breeding organizations on first service conception rate, and the average for the herd can be compared with these ratings for sires used.

1. Per cent successful is calculated by dividing the number of pregnancies during the past 12 months by the number of breedings:

   Goal: Temperate regions of U.S. = 50%
   Southeastern U.S. = 40%

2. Number of breedings per conception:

   Goal: Temperate regions of U.S. = < 2.5
   Southeastern U.S. = < 3.5

3. First breeding conception rate (when breeding begins at 45 days postpartum)

   Goal: Temperate regions of U.S. = > 55%
   Southeastern U.S. = > 45%

4. Average number of breedings for pregnant cows:

   Goal: Temperate regions of U.S. = < 1.5
   Southeastern U.S. = < 2.5

Breedings for the Test Interval. This is a summary of the services and percentage that was successfully compiled for the test interval each test day. Extreme variation in the per cent successful from month to month should be analyzed as to possible cause(s). Conception rate of sires used, semen quality, technique in breeding, fertility of cows and bulls as well as general herd health should all be examined. Extremes in temperature as well as inadequate or unbalanced nutrition programs also affect breeding efficiency and conception.

   Goal: Temperate regions of U.S. (Summer)
   = > 40% success
   Southeastern U.S. (Summer)
   = > 20% success

Summary of Service Sires with PD$. The average predicted difference in dollars (PD$) of sires of cows is a genetic measurement value. Evidence of genetic progress is an increase in this value from older cows to younger cows and to service sires used in the current breeding program. The sires of calves and heifers to be used as future herd replacements have a major influence on genetic improvement.

1. Service sires used in current breeding programs (1983)

   Goal = PD$ > $100.00

2. Percentage of herd with sire identification

   Goal = > 85%

Sire Selection Plus Culling Plus Nutrition of First Lactation Heifers Compared to Second and Later Lactations. Raising replacement heifers should be based on improving herd production level with yearly increases of > 100 pounds of milk (projected mature equivalent 305 days) for first lactation heifers during the past 12 months compared with the previous 12 months.

ME of second and later lactations compared with first lactations, when genetic value is equal, usually favors the former by approximately 500 pounds. If a yearly genetic improvement of 100 pounds of milk is to be realized we should expect:

Goal: First lactation heifers ME not less than 400 pounds compared to ME for second and later lactations.

Culling for Reproductive Reasons

Goal: Temperate regions of U.S. = < 8%
      Southeastern U.S. = < 12%

Abortion. Losses from 45 to 270 days gestation:

Goal: Temperate regions of U.S. = < 8%
      Southeastern U.S. = < 12%

Goal after 120 days gestation:
    Temperate regions of U.S. = < 2%
    Southeastern U.S. = < 2%

Retention of Fetal Membranes. Cows retaining their fetal membranes for greater than 12 hours are considered abnormal.

Goal: Temperate regions of U.S. = < 8%
      Southeastern U.S. = < 15%

Dry Cow Profile. This includes average days dry for all cows that have a complete dry period. The length of dry period has a significant effect on the production level of subsequent lactation. The dry cow period is not the end of previous lactation but rather the beginning of subsequent lactation.

Goal:
Dry < 40 days	< 1%
Dry more than 70 days	< 5%
Average days dry (herd)	50–55 days

Condition Scoring. Condition scoring will indicate the average body condition of cows in a herd and in addition will provide an index for evaluating whether cattle are gaining or losing weight. Optimum body condition scores have been established for the breeding period, at drying off, and at calving. Using a scoring system of 1 (thin) to 5 (fat), the recommended body condition scores are:

Goal:
Dry cows	3.5–4.0
At calving	3.5–4.0
At breeding	2.5–3.0
Heifers	
At calving	3.0–3.5
At breeding	2.5–3.0

Calf Mortality. Calves born dead and those that have died by 24 hours after birth give a good indication of calving area management. Factors contributing to calf mortality are: (1) condition score of heifers and cows, (2) sire selection and ease of calving, (3) observation of cows in early stages of parturition, (4) cleanliness of calving area, hands, and equipment if calving difficulties arise, (5) ability and training of individuals working in calving area, and (6) colostral management.

Number of calves born dead and those that have died within 24 hours of birth:

Goal:
Cows	< 6%
Heifers	< 8%

Percentage of Calves with Enlarged Umbilical Stumps that survive the first 24 hours following birth. Environmental factors (sanitation) can be monitored by assessing the percentage of calves having abnormally enlarged (> 10 mm) umbilical stumps.

Goal: Temperate regions of U.S. = < 10%
      Southeastern U.S. = < 10%

Reproductive Efficiency Summary of Virgin Heifers

Number of heifers in breeding herd bred	Average age at first breeding	Number of heifers over 18 months and not bred

Number of pregnant heifers	Number of breedings	Number of breedings per conception	Summary of service sires with PD$
			Number | Average

Replacement Heifers (Holstein-Friesian). These heifers should be inseminated at first heat beginning at 14 months of age at a body weight of 340 kg (750 pounds) and pelvic height of 128 cm (51 inches).

Replacement Heifers (Holstein-Friesian). These should calve at 25 months of age, weight 525 kg (1150 pounds) after calving with a pelvic height of 143 cm (56 inches).

Conclusion

The implementation of a reproductive program must be adjusted to specific farm conditions and management goals. Accurate and complete record keeping is a prerequisite to the optimal function of a reproductive program. Within this framework, data collected by the dairyman, veterinarian and other agricultural consultants must be handled and processed to provide relevant information. This information will show a momentary profile of the herd reproductive status and assist in making farm management more transparent. It will allow advice given on farm management practices regarding reproductive performance, treatment and prevention of reproductive disorders to be justified. This information must be transferred to the dairyman with a minimum loss of time in order to be functional for daily decision making.

Without the assistance of computers, this information will be retrospective in nature. Computerization of data handling and analysis is an important management tool. Through its use, unwanted situations regarding reproductive control can be prevented or identified early so that optimum farm income can be realized.

References

1. Braun RK, Noordhuizen JP, Donovan GA, Brand A: A goal oriented approach to herd health and production control. Proceedings 15th Annual Convention AABP, December 1–4, 1982.
2. Dairyman's DHI Manual. Dairy Records Processing Center (DRPC) Raleigh, North Carolina, 1981.
3. Williamson NB: The use of records in reproductive health and management programs for dairy herds. Vet Clin North Am, November 1981.
4. Zemjanis R, Fahning ML, Schultz RH: Anestrus—The practitioners dilemma. Vet Scope 14:14, 1969.

Programmable Calculator Uses in Herd Reproductive Health Programs for Dairy Cattle

John H. Kirk, D.V.M.
Michigan State University, East Lansing, Michigan

PROGRAMMABLE CALCULATORS

The programmable calculator can perform all the functions of most advanced calculators and can be programmed to do the computations in a precise order. In addition, the program order can be stored for future use on magnetic cards. The low cost and portability of programmable calculators make them very useful for on-farm estimations of reproductive parameters. Programmable calculators reduce the time necessary to make these calculations and therefore increase the likelihood that they will be done. The records available on the farm for management decision making are enhanced, and the producer's ability to use and interpret their records is improved.

The dairyman should record calving, heat, breeding and pregnancy dates for his herd: however, the amount and types of records kept by dairymen vary from farm to farm. At present, a minority of dairymen convert these records into meaningful indicators of reproductive performance by such systems as the Dairy Herd Improvement Association (DHIA) record keeping system. Many of these indicators of reproductive efficiency can be calculated on a programmable calculator if the proper records are kept on the farm. (See the article Analysis of Reproductive Records using DHIA Summaries and other Monitors in Large Dairy Herds.)

CALVING INTERVAL

Calving dates can be converted to calving intervals, which give an indication of the reproductive performance of the herd over a given period of time. An illustration of a program using only calving dates is shown in Tables 1 and 2. Using this program, the veterinarian can quickly calculate the calving interval for each cow that has calved at least twice and compute the average calving interval for the herd. Grouping of cows by calving interval is also displayed by the program. It should be pointed out that a method of monitoring overall reproductive performance that is more responsive to current changes in herd performance is a calculation of days open. An accurate diagnosis of pregnancy must be available to calculate days open. This program can be used to make this computation by substituting the breeding date when pregnancy occurs for the second calving date and changing the interval headings in the output section of the program.

Table 1. Example of Calving Interval Program Input Dates

| | Dates | |
Cow	Previous Calving	Recent Calving
1	602.1982	629.1983
2	529.1982	601.1983
3	401.1982	623.1983
4	324.1982	227.1983
5	415.1982	429.1983

The inputs are the cow numbers and the respective calving dates in the numerical form acceptable to the calculator. For example, the initial calving date for Cow 1 is June 2, 1982.

Table 2. Example of Outputs for Calving Interval Program

	316.1984	—Today's date, March 16, 1984
Calving Intervals		
	392	—Calving interval for first cow
	368	—Calving interval for second cow
	448	
	340	
	379	
1	− 350	—1 cow with fewer than 350 days calving interval
0	− 364	—0 cows with calving interval between 351 and 364 days
2	− 389	
1	− 420	
1	420 +	
	385.4	—Average calving interval for herd

The first date shown in the output section is the date the program was executed. Under the heading "Calving Intervals" are the calving intervals in days for each cow printed in the order in which they were entered into the program. The next series of numbers is the number of cows grouped according to calving interval. The interval − 350 is a period ranging from 0 to 350 days; the interval − 364 ranges from 351 to 364 days, and so on. The final number of 385.4 is the average calving interval in days for all the cows entered in the program.

SERVICE INTERVALS AND HEAT DETECTION ACCURACY

When dairymen record breeding dates as well as calving dates, the interval from calving to first service and the intervals between services can be calculated. These computations can be used to determine heat detection accuracy from several standpoints. The printout for a program to make these calculations is shown in Table 3.

Table 3. Heat Detection Accuracy for Individual Cows

Cow 103		—Cow number 103
84	DT1S	—84 days to first service
22	D12S	—22 days first to second service
24	D23S	—24 days second to third service
Cow 121		—Cow number 121
88	DT1S	—88 days to first service
0	D12S	—no second service
0	D23S	—no third service

The breeding intervals for each cow are given in days followed by an abbreviated interval heading. DT1S stands for the days to first service, whereas D12S represents the days from first to second service. Individual cow performance can be compared with projected days to first service to identify problem breeders, while interservice intervals may help to explain reasons for poor reproductive performance due to infectious disease.

Table 4. Herd Heat Detection Accuracy— Service Interval Section

Herd Stats		
69.9	AD1S	—Average 69.9 days to first service
45.2	AD12	—Average 45.2 days first to second service
22.5	AD23	—Average 22.5 days second to third service
37.6	ADAS	—Average 37.6 days all services
Vol Wait		
55		—Waiting 55 days before breeding
Proj Ave DT1S		
69		—Projected days to first service to give a yearly calving interval
Act DT1S		
69.9		—Actual days to first service of 69.9

Under Herd Stats, AD12 is the average number of days for the herd from first to second breeding. The last figure under this heading is the average number of days between all services.

To use this program, the veterinarian enters the calving date and breeding dates for each cow. The length of the voluntary waiting period from calving to first service is also entered. From these dates, the calculator computes the intervals to first service and between services for each cow. Once all the cow information has been entered, the average days to first service and between services are calculated for the herd (Table 4). Based on the stated volun-

Table 5. Heat Detection Accuracy— Accuracy Section

Heat Detection		
46.4	%1–2	—46% heat detection first to second service
93.3	%2–3	—93% heat detection second to third service
55.7	%ALL	—55% heat detection all services
Breeding Interval		
1	47 −	—1 service interval over 47 days
2	− 46	—2 service intervals between 46 and 39 days
0	− 38	—service intervals between 38 and 25 days
3	− 24	—3 service intervals between 24 and 18 days
0	0–17	—0 service intervals less than 17 days
% 18–24 TOTAL		
60		—60% of interval between 18 to 24 and 39 to 46 days in the 18 to 24 day interval

In the Breeding Interval section, the intervals are grouped by the days, and the number of cows in each interval is shown. The final estimate of heat detection accuracy is the % 18–24 TOTAL, which is the comparison of the number of cows with breeding intervals of 18 to 24 days and 39 to 45 days. The last figure is the percentage of cows with intervals falling in the 18 to 24 day interval of the total in both intervals.

tary waiting period, the projected days to first service are estimated. To reach this projected goal, 85 to 90 per cent accuracy of heat detection is necessary.[1] Another estimate of heat detection accuracy is made by analyzing the length of the intervals between breedings. The percent of detections based on normal intervals of 21 days is shown in the program output.[2] Groupings of cows by intervals are also shown. A final analysis of heat detection accuracy is calculated by comparing the number of breeding intervals 18 to 24 days long with the number between 39 and 45 days[2] (Table 5).

For most dairy herds, production is optimized when the calving interval for the herd is less than 12.5 months. To achieve this, an organized heat detection system must be used. The measure of such a program is the accuracy of detection. This calculator program measures heat detection accuracy by analyzing the days to first service and the days between services. The projected days to first service can be compared to the actual days to first service for the herd. To meet the projected goal, heat detection must be greater than 85 per cent. If the goal is not met, the heat detection system should be evaluated to increase efficiency of heat detection. Likewise, if the days between breedings indicate less than optimal detection rates, changes should be suggested. Optimal detection requires two to three observation periods at least 20 minutes each per day with one of the periods at dusk and another at dawn. One person should be specifically in charge of the system, and records must be kept. The best

Table 6. Example of Individual Cow Statistics

428.84		—Today's date, April 28, 1984
235.00	COW	—Cow number 235 (open/not pg chekd)
5.00	LC	—Milking in fifth lactation
110.00	MLK	—110 pounds of milk
205.83		—Fresh date, Feb. 5, 1984
82.00	DIM	—82 days in milk today
315.83		—Date of first service
38.00	DYS	—Days in milk on above date
2.00		—Number of services and last entry for this cow
789.00	COW	—Cow number 789 (pregnant)
1.00	LC	—Heifer in first lactation
89.00	MLK	—Milk weight (optional)
105.83		—Fresh date
113.00	DIM	—Days in milk today
215.83		—Date of first service
41.00	DYS	—Days in milk at first service
321.83		—Date of service for pregnancy
75.00	DO	—Days open on above service date
294.00		—Projected lactation (60 days dry)
11.64	CI	—Projected calving interval (months)
38.00	DPG	—Days pregnant today
3.00		—Number of services (must be an integer 0, 1, 2, etc.)

Table 7. Example for Herd Statistics

		Herd Statistics
41.00	TOT	—Total number entered
193.07	DIM	—Average days in milk for herd
2.93	LAC	—Average lactation number
86.00	SVS	—Total number of services entered
29.00	PRG	—Total number pregnant in herd
Cows OPN		**Open Cow Statistics**
8.00		—Number of cows in the category
95.37	DIM	—Average days in milk (DIM)
34.87		—Standard deviation of DIM
1.00		—No. cows with no services
30.00	DIM	—Average DIM for above cows
2.00		—No. cows with one service
75.50	DIM	—Average DIM for above cows
2.00		—No. cows with two services
110.00	DIM	—Average DIM for above cows
3.00		—No. cows with three or more services
120.33	DIM	—Average DIM for above cows
Cows PG		**Pregnant Cows Statistics**
9.00		—Number of cows in this category
105.14	DO	—Average days open (DO) for this group
29.30		—Standard deviation of DO
0.00		—No. cows pregnant with one service
1.00	? DO	—Average days open for above cows
4.00	?	—No. cows pregnant with two services
90.00	? DO	—Average days open for above cows
3.00	?	—No. cows pregnant with three or more services
125.33	? DO	—Average days open for above cows
196.25	DPG	—Average days pregnant for above cows
55.33		—Standard deviation for DPG
12.82	ACI	—Average calving interval for above cows
1.27		—Standard deviation for calving interval
2.71	S/C	—Services per conception (approximate)
0.00	FS%	—First service conception rate
65.25	DYS	—Average DIM first service, open and pregnant cows
21.90		—Standard deviation of DYS
Hfrs OPN		**Open Heifer Statistics**
4.00		
61.50	DIM	(above format repeats for heifers)
1.00		
10.00	DIM	

true indicator of heat is one animal standing to be mounted by another.

DHIA-TYPE STATISTICS FOR DAIRY HERDS

Although the usefulness of the DHIA record keeping system is well documented, many dairymen do not presently use this sytem. Most dairymen could benefit from evaluation of their herd's reproductive efficiency. It will show them the strengths and weakness of their heat detection and artificial insemination programs as well as the progress being made by their routine herd health program with their veterinarian.

As with the DHIA records, this program requires that good records be kept on all animals, including the cow number, lactation number, first service date, pregnancy date and the number of services. Once the program is loaded into the computer, the information on each cow is entered individually (Table 6). After all the data on cows have been entered, the program computes and categorizes the herd statistics and characterizes the open and pregnant heifer and cow groups. The output is shown in Table 7.

This program has been used under field conditions by its originator, Dr. John Gay, Box 506, Gooding, Idaho, as a part of his herd health programs for dairymen. For complete details on the program and magnetic cards contact Dr. Gay.

HERD FERTILITY INDEX

Once the DHIA-type statistics have been computed, a herd fertility index can be calculated using an equation developed by Esslemont and Eddy.[3] The equation is shown below:

$$\text{Fertility Index} = \frac{\text{First service conception rate}}{\text{Average services/conception}}$$
$$- [(\text{days open}) - 125] - [(\% \text{ cull rate}) - 25]$$

Herds with efficient reproductive programs will score greater than 70 on the index. Herds with an index of greater than 86 have excellent programs with usually fewer than 90 days open, first service conception rates of 60 per cent or better and overall cull rates of around 20 per cent. This index includes the cull rate that allows for a measurement of the cows culled for reproductive reasons. This is important because many of the reproductive culls are not pregnant and do not calve and for that reason do not enter into the days open or calving interval. The program also estimates the dollars lost due to less than optimal reproductive efficiency. A loss of $3.00 is currently used for each day open over 85. Example calculations are shown (Tables 8 and 9).

CALF MORTALITY AND HEIFER REPLACEMENTS

The availability of heifer replacements for a dairy herd markedly affects the ability of the dairyman to

Table 8. Example of Herd Fertility Index

Fertility Index	
87.5	—Index for the herd
Est Dol Loss	
30.00	—Estimated dollars loss/cow

This calculation is for a herd with a 60 per cent first service conception rate, a 1.6 total services per conception rate, an average of 70 days open and an overall cull rate for the herd of 25 per cent. Due to fewer than 85 days open, the dollar loss estimate is a negative number that indicates a savings over what would be expected for a herd with a yearly calving interval.

Table 9. Example of Herd Fertility Index

Fertility Index	
40.04	—Index of the herd
Est Dol Loss	
−57	—Estimated dollars loss/cow

This herd had a 40 per cent first service conception rate with a total services per conception of 2.1. The days open averaged 104 for all the cows in the herd, and the overall cull rate was 25 per cent. This herd is losing $57 dollars for each cow compared to a herd with a 12-month calving interval.

increase production by allowing him to practice elective culling of low-producing cows. When calf mortality is excessively high, culling for production may be impossible if cow numbers are to remain constant. This program calculates the effect of preweaning calf mortality on the number of available replacements. The computations allow dairymen to become increasingly aware of the devastating effect of calf mortality. They can also see the benefits of reducing the preweaning mortality loss to a level of 5 per cent, which should be attainable in all dairy herds under veterinary supervision. This goal is used as a conservative estimate because it is well known that many herds have losses under 1 or 2 per cent.

The program calculation assumes that all cows are pregnant and that live-born calves will be equally divided as to sex. The number of calves available is reduced to reflect the calving interval, abortions, death in dystocia (5 per cent) and losses between weaning and first calving (5 per cent). Due to early sale on most farms, preweaning bull calf loss is figured at half the declared preweaning loss.

Table 10. Example Calf Mortality and Heifer Replacements Program

Heifer Replacements	
31.1	—Number of replacements available
Sale (−Buy)	
1.1	—1.1 Heifers available for sale; a negative number indicates a need to buy heifers to keep cow numbers constant
Bull Dollar Lost	
1091.34	—Loss due to dying bull calves
Heifers 5%	
8.2	—Number of heifers gained by reducing mortality to 5 per cent
Dollar Save Heifers	
8294.23	—Dollars saved by reducing mortality
Dollar Save Bull	
873.07	—Dollars saved by reducing mortality
Total Savings	
9167.30	

Table 11. Equipment List

Product	Supplier
TI/59 Programmable calculator	Texas Instruments Inc, Dallas, Texas 75221
Print/Security cradle, PC-100C	Texas Instruments Inc, Dallas, Texas 75221
TI/59 Magnetic Cards	Texas Instruments Inc, Dallas Texas 75221
TI/59 Programs (calving interval, service interval and heat detection, herd fertility index, calf mortality and heifer replacements)	IMC Marketing Service, Michigan State University, E Lansing, MI 48824
TI/59 Program (DHIA-type statistics)	Dr. John Gay, Box 506, Gooding, Idaho 83330

When the program is executed, estimated values for the replacement heifer and a 3-day old bull calf are entered into the calculation. The overall cull rate must also be entered. By comparing the present situation to the loss at a goal of 5 per cent preweaning mortality, the dairyman can fully appreciate his economic loss above that of an acceptable level. An example of the program is shown (Table 10). Through the calculations, the program points out the three major factors that influence the number of heifers available for replacements. These are preweaning calf mortality, calving interval and overall cull rate for the herd. Controlling these factors will result in availablity of a maximum number of heifers.

The sources for program codes and detailed instructions for use of these programs and other programs concerning food animal medicine are listed in Table 11. Other TI/59 programs can be found in the Updated Inventory of Agricultural Computer Programs, Circular 531, Food and Resource Economics Department, Cooperative Extension Service, Institute of Food and Agricultural Science, University of Florida, Gainesville, Florida 32611.

References

1. Smalley SA.: Management problems of large dairies. Vet Clin North Am 3(2):289, 1981.
2. Williams NB: Monitoring reproductive health records. Vet Clin North Am 3(2):279, 1981.
3. Esslemont RJ, Eddy RG: The control of cattle fertility; the use of computerized records. Br Vet J 133:346, 1977.

Uterine Cultures and Their Interpretation

C. H. W. de Bois
State University at Utrecht, Utrecht, The Netherlands

Uterine secretions and, to a lesser extent, endometrial biopsy specimens are used for the microbiologic examination of the uterus. Concurrent sensitivity tests can be of importance for a possible treatment. Collection and processing of the material to be examined must be done extremely carefully and with the use of the appropriate instruments; only then can reliable results be expected. Unfortunately, the techniques described in the literature are often inadequate and frequently give rise to false positive results.

COLLECTION OF UTERINE SECRETIONS

Over the years several types of instruments have been developed for the collection of uterine secretions. Most of the instruments are based on the principle described by Folmer Nielson, who developed an instrument consisting of two concentric tubes. The proximal portion of the inner tube contains a space for the collection of uterine secretions, and the distal portion is equipped with a handle. The author recommends the use of a slightly modified model contained in a single cylindrical speculum. The proximal portion of the speculum is covered with freezer paper, and the entire instrument is wrapped and autoclaved. Just before the apparatus is introduced, the freezer paper is moistened with 5 per cent iodine. The vulva and surrounding area are carefully cleansed, the tail wrapped with sterile gauze, the lips of the vulva parted and the mucosa sprayed with an iodine solution. The instrument is guided per rectum as far as possible through the cervix. Next, the iodine-treated paper is perforated with slight pressure, and the instrument is guided into one of the horns of the uterus by withdrawing the external portion. The space in the inner tube is exposed, permitting collection of uterine secretions by rotating the inner portion of the instrument. This method of exposure of the collection space, instead of advancing the inner portion of the instrument, practically eliminates the danger of perforation. The method of introduction, which has been tested experimentally, prevents the introduction of microorganisms, which are nearly always present in the vagina and caudal portion of the cervix.

Minocha and associates (1964) pointed out the

risk of contamination and used a set of four tele-scoping metal tubes. The outer one serves as a vaginal speculum, the second tube is inserted well into the cervix, and the two inner units constitute the sampler (cotton swab). The tips of the tubes are capped with sterile gelatin capsules to protect the inner tubes from contamination during placement. Many instruments and procedures described in the literature do not eliminate the possibility of contam-ination of the uterine lumen.

EXAMINATION OF THE UTERINE SECRETIONS

Uterine secretions should be inoculated on a suitable medium or in a transport medium imme-diately after collection. It is well to remember that certain microorganisms, such as the group of *Bac-terioides,* die quickly when the uterine secretions are exposed to the air. The choice of the culture media is strongly dependent on the organisms that are anticipated (e.g., for the culture of specific infectious agents such as *Campylobacter fetus*) spe-cial nutrient media and culture techniques are re-quired. In cattle that are free from *Trichomonas foetus* and *Campylobacter fetus* infection and such conditions as tuberculosis and brucellosis, the oc-currence of everyday infectious organisms such as streptococci, staphylocci, *Escherichia coli* and *C. pyogenes* should be considered. However, the type and degree of these infections can vary consider-ably.[3] The greatest quantity and variety of micro-organisms may be expected during the first 14 days postpartum, particularly in animals in which the fetal membranes were retained and/or parturition was abnormal. Reliable follow-up of the culture results requires experience and is not usually the forte of the average practitioner. After 2 to 3 weeks postpartum, almost completely pure cultures are frequently recovered from cows that have not re-covered spontaneously from parturition. The ma-jority of these consist of *C. pyogenes.* Such micro-organisms can be cultured relatively simply, generally under aerobic conditions. In cases of chronic purulent metritis we can expect difficult-to-culture microorganisms such as *Hemophilus somnus*[2] or a combination of *Hemophilus* with *Fu-sobacterium necrophorum*[7] in addition to *C. py-ogenes.* From these facts it follows that expertise in processing the material is required to obtain reliable information. In addition to the culture, a direct smear should be made and stained with methylene blue and Gram stain. Hematoxylin-eosin staining may also be used for cytologic examination. Ac-cording to some investigators endometritis may be diagnosed this way.[4] Such staining procedures are of course well suited to practice conditions.

SIGNIFICANCE OF THE MICROORGANISMS

In the presence of *C. pyogenes,* with or without strict anaerobes, and of *Hemophilus somnus* there nearly always is moderate to severe inflammation of the endometrium. Significant signs of inflamma-tion may also be expected when *Streptococcus uberis* and *Streptococcus dysgalactiae* are encountered. In a number of cases nonpathogenic microorganisms may be encountered in the uterine secretions with-out significant signs of inflammation in the endo-metrium. It is not always possible to demonstrate microorganisms in the uterine secretions in the presence of significant inflammatory signs of the endometrium, or, when microorganisms are present under these circumstances, they cannot always be considered pathogenic. During the healing process of an endometritis the microorganisms disappear first and later the inflammatory signs.

SIGNIFICANCE OF THE MICROBIOLOGIC EXAMINATION OF UTERINE SECRETIONS IN EVERYDAY PRACTICE

If one is a proponent of timely treatment of postpartum endometritis with antibiotics, it is nec-essary to perform regular bacteriologic examina-tions of uterine secretions and to test the sensitivity of the microorganisms that occur on the farm in question (because of the danger of the development of antibiotic resistance). Furthermore, microbio-logic examination of uterine secretions may be useful in cases of outbreaks such as a sudden increase in incidence of repeat breeding. As a rule, examination of uterine secretions from individual cows that fail to conceive for unknown reasons and that are on farms where the average fertility is acceptable is not productive.

SIGNIFICANCE OF THE BACTERIOLOGIC EXAMINATIONS OF UTERINE SECRETIONS FOR RESEARCH

Like endometrial biopsy, bacteriologic examina-tion of uterine secretions provides important infor-mation for (1) the incidence of microorganisms during the postpartum period and their influence on the course of uterine involution and on fertility, (2) the occurrence of microorganisms in normal fertile animals, repeat breeders and cows with en-dometritis, and (3) the course of certain specific infections such as *Campylobacter fetus* infection.

References

1. Bois CHW de: Endometritis en vruchtbaarheid bij het rund. Thesis, University of Utrecht, 1961.
2. Corboz L, Nicolet J: Infektionen mit sogenannten *Haemophilus somnus* beim Rind: Isolierung und Charakterisierung von Stam-men aus Respirations—und Geschlechtsorganen. Arch Tier-heilk 117:493, 1975.
3. Luginbühl A, Kupfer U: Unspezifische bakteriologische Be-funde und Endometritis beim Rind. (Eine Literaturübersicht). Schweiz Arch Tierheilk 122:151, 1980.

4. Manser H, Berchtold M: Untersuchungen über die Eignung von Schleimhautabstrichen zur Diagnose der chronischen Endometritis des Rindes. Berl Munchen Tierarztl Wochenschr 88:41, 1975.
5. Minocha HC, Marion GB, Gier HT, McMahon KJ: An instrument for obtaining aseptic bacteriologic and histologic samples from the bovine genital tract. Am J Vet Res 25:1051, 1964.
6. Nielsen F: Cited by Rasbeck NO: Den normale involutio uteri hos koen. Nord Vet Med 2:655, 1950.
7. Ruder CA, Sasser RG, Williams RJ, et al.: Uterine infections in the post-partum cow. II. Possible synergistic effect of *Fusobacterium necrophorum* and *Corynebacterium pyogenes*. Theriogenology 15:573, 1981.

Endometrial Biopsy of the Bovine

C. H. W. de Bois
State University at Utrecht, Utrecht, The Netherlands

Joe E. Manspeaker, V.M.D.
University of Maryland, College Park, Maryland

Endometrial biopsy, first reported in the cow by Zurgilgen (1948),[10] is a relatively easy procedure for the practicing veterinarian to perform. Its use in conjunction with a detailed history, rectal and vaginal examinations and microbial cultures can lead to a more accurate prognosis of difficult breeders and greater therapeutic efficiency by the clinician.

TECHNICAL ASPECTS

Endometrial biopsy sampling is a safe procedure. Repeated biopsies have been shown to cause no adverse effects on a cow's reproductive capacity. The lesions resulting from the biopsy heal rapidly. Hemorrhages, which invariably occur, are of little or no clinical significance and are quickly resorbed. The biopsy specimen should be of sufficient size (4 × 6 mm).

Specimens should be taken from the left and right horns and the body of the uterus due to the variability of pathology in each section.

The instrument's cutting edge should be sharp so that the endometrial tissue is cut and not unduly compressed. Artifacts are easily produced when using dull instruments. These artifacts are difficult to evaluate microscopically. The biopsy instrument should be so designed that it can easily pass through the cervix with little risk of perforation.

The biopsy instrument used by the first author is in essence the one designed by Miller (1951).[6] It consists of two concentric tubes. The outer tube is made of stainless steel, whereas only the proximal portion of the inner tube is made of stainless steel. This proximal exchangeable piece is equipped with a sharp cutting edge for cutting the endometrium. The outer tube has a small window near its tip that can be opened by withdrawing the inner tube. This allows one to press a portion of the endometrium into the opening so it can be cut off. The instrument is placed in a cylindrical speculum that is covered at one end by freezer paper to prevent infection. The entire assembly is sterilized with dry heat in a manner described in the section on uterine cultures and their interpretation.

Other biopsy instruments, including the alligator type forceps with a basket approximately 4 × 8 mm in size or a biopsy punch, are available for use in the cow.

Proper care, disinfection and sterilization of the biopsy instrument are necessary to prevent microbial contamination of the uterus. The instrument is introduced into the vagina in the same manner as that described for the culture instrument in Chapter 53.

FIXATION AND PROCESSING

Care is of utmost importance in removing the delicate tissue from the biopsy instrument because artifacts that may be produced will hinder true evaluation of any histopathologic changes present. The tissue specimen should be removed with fine forceps or a hypodermic needle and immediately immersed in a fixing solution to prevent drying out. A 10 per cent buffered formalin or Bouin's solution may be used for fixation. When using Bouin's solution, the tissue sample should be removed from the solution after 12 to 24 hours and placed in 70 per cent alcohol or the tissue will become too hard for easy sectioning. The amount of fixing solution used should be at least 10 times the volume of the sample.

The biopsy specimens are cut in their entirety with a microtome at approximately 6 microns in thickness. Every twenty-fifth section is caught and stained with hematoxylin and eosin. Other stains can be used for specific purposes, such as the demonstration of connective tissue or certain enzyme activities.

HISTOPATHOLOGIC EVALUATION

The bovine endometrium can be evaluated histologically for periglandular fibrosis, cystic glandular changes, and cellular infiltration of the endometrial stroma.

Periglandular fibrosis (scarring or encapsulation), cystic glands and lymphoid nodules are considered pathologic lesions of the uterus. Periglandular fibrosis is the most frequent abnormality found in the bovine.[7] Cellular infiltration is the most striking feature of acute endometritis.

A grading system has been established in the bovine as in the mare categorizing the degree and extent of periglandular fibrosis. The degree of fibrosis varies from mild to moderate to severe with some sections showing ranges in between. This system is based on the visibility and clarity of the fibroblasts surrounding the endometrial glands in the connective tissue stroma. The connective tissue is hypertrophied and distinctly modified. The fibroblasts become spindle-sharp and are closely packed parallel to each other and slender nuclei. As the fibroblasts and their nuclei become more spindle-shaped and more closely packed together, the classification changes.

Varying degrees of fibrosis between each horn and body of the uterus may exist simultaneously. Also, fibrosis may exist independent of the more recent pregnant horn or of the more recent pregnant horn with placental retention. As the number of normal sections in a cow's uterus decreases and the degree of fibrosis increases, there is a trend toward poorer conception.

Cystic glands occur much less frequently than periglandular fibrosis with wide branched lumina and low cuboidal or flattened epithelium. Usually with cystic glands, the periglandular connective tissue is not altered. In a study of first-calf heifers, in which cystic glands were present, varying degrees of fibrosis or scarring occurred during subsequent pregnancies. The occurrence of cystic glands showed no significant relationships to breeding performance.

In studying the sections, special attention should be paid to the occurrence of the various types of free cells present. The total number of cells observed, the interrelationship of the different types, the manner of distribution (diffuse or focal) and their locations (periglandular or perivascular) in the endometrium are meaningful. Functional cellular cyclic variations are most marked in the surface epithelium and the adjacent layer, the stratum compactum, and are less marked in the stratum spongiosum. These free cells include neutrophils, lymphocytes, eosinophils, plasma cells, mast cells and pigment-bearing macrophages, and are present only in small numbers (cyclic variation occurs) in "normal" cows.

Lymphoid nodules are masses of small round cells (lymphocytes) with dense nuclei that often have a fibrous connective tissue capsule around them and are actually focal infiltrations of mononuclear cells. They are distributed at random throughout the entire uterus within otherwise normal endometrial stroma. They do not appear to interfere with normal pregnancy, although in one study these lesions appeared to be more prevalent in poor breeders than in normal breeders. There is a possibility that the nodular (focal) formation of these lymphocytes is a sequel to puerperal infections.

Continual degenerative or regenerative changes are noted in the surface epithelium, the stroma, the lumina of the glands, the capillaries and the blood vessels. These changes are considered normal.

Mild endometritis may be readily missed due to the few inflammatory cells usually occurring in the more dense epithelial and stratum compactum areas. Moderate and severe cases of endometritis are much easier to diagnose on the basis of the increased number of inflammatory cells spread throughout the stratum compactum and spongiosum layers compared with the few cells seen in mild endometritis.

The significance of inflammatory cells in the endometrium must be considered in relation to the estrous cycle at the time of biopsy. The first author prefers to take the biopsy specimen during estrus when chances for the development of endometritis due to contamination are minimal. The second author recommends that endometrial biopsies be taken approximately 5 days postestrus in the bovine for the best histologic detail. Neutrophils may be present in high numbers during normal estrus, erroneously suggesting an acute endometritis. Neutrophils present during the luteal phase are definitely indicative of an acute endometritis.

Mild chronic endometritis (lymphocytes) has long been regarded as one of the most common causes of repeat breeders. The great majority of cows with clinical deviations of the reproductive tract show endometritis in varying degrees. In some instances, cows with mild endometritis, and a few with moderate disease are able to conceive and maintain a pregnancy.

Additionally, it should be pointed out that in the initial phases of endometritis, the diffuse and possibly the periglandular and perivascular cellular infiltrations are dominated by neutrophils and lymphocytes. Accumulations of cellular infiltrates develop gradually. The severity of the inflammatory signs depends on the nature of the infection. As soon as the microorganisms are eliminated, the neutrophils disappear fairly rapidly and diffuse infiltration of other inflammatory cells (lymphocytes) disappears more gradually. The disappearance of the focal cellular infiltrates takes several months. This implies that in the endometrium of cows less than 92 to 100 days postpartum, focal cellular infiltrates may be found that are the remnants of an endometritis that developed during or shortly after parturition.

REPRESENTATIVENESS

Various investigators have studied the question of representativeness of the endometritis biopsy specimen. Assuming that the biopsy specimen is quantitatively and qualitatively correct and that more than one section is examined, then the biopsy specimen is highly representative of the uterine horn from which it is taken. However, considerable differences can occur between the histopathology of the endometrium of the two uterine horns and that of body. It is advisable to take tissue samples from both uterine horns and the body to evaluate more effectively the complete histopathologic condition of the entire uterus.

SIGNIFICANCE OF THE ENDOMETRIAL BIOPSY IN EVERYDAY PRACTICE

Endometrial biopsy is not warranted in bovine practice on a routine basis, but it can be extremely useful with the repeat breeder. The endometrial biopsy is valuable for the practicing veterinarian who is interested in a complete evaluation of the reproductive tract of high-priced cattle. This includes cows that do not conceive and those that do conceive but do not maintain a full-term pregnancy. To completely analyze a reproductive problem in a herd, specific infections such as leptospirosis, brucellosis and trichomoniasis should be under control.

When clinical deviations of the reproductive tract are obvious on vaginal and rectal examination, a biopsy specimen may not be necessary. In clinically "normal" cows that are repeat breeders, the use of the endometritis biopsy is imperative for a complete diagnosis and a more valid prognostic evaluation of individual animals.

The correlation between clinical and histopathologic findings is greater than that obtained between clinical and bacteriologic findings, or between histopathologic and bacteriologic findings. Mild inflammatory changes in the endometrium, such as focal areas of cellular infiltration, have little effect on fertility. Diffuse cellular infiltration does diminish the chances of conception. Chronic signs of inflammation such as dilation of endometrial glands and periglandular fibrosis can lead to an increase in the number of services per conception.

SIGNIFICANCE OF THE ENDOMETRIAL BIOPSY IN RESEARCH

In the last 10 to 20 years the endometritis biopsy has been a useful tool in various research projects including the study of (1) cyclic micromorphologic and cytochemical changes of the endometrium, (2) the prevention and resolution of endometritis, (3) the presence of specific infections due to *Campylobacter*, viruses, mycoplasmas, and so on, (4) tissue levels of various antibiotics, (5) the significance of endometritis and the incidence and degree of periglandular fibrosis on fertility, and (6) immunologic aspects of the endometrium.

References

1. Aria G: Technique and indications for biopsy and endoscopic examinations of the uterus of cows. At tidella Societa Italiana di Buiatria 8:216, 1976.
2. Bois CHW de: Endometritis en vruchtbaarheid bij het rund. Thesis, University of Utrecht, The Netherlands, 1961.
3. Brus DGJ: Biopsia uteri of cows. Report to the Second International Congress on the Physiology of Animal Reproduction 2:175, 1952. Thesis, University of Utrecht, The Netherlands, 1954.
4. Manspeaker JE, Haaland, MA: Implementation of uterine biopsy in bovine reproduction: A practitioner's diagnostic tool. Vet Med Small Anim Clin 5:760, 1983.
5. Manspeaker JE, Haaland, MA, Davidson JP: Incidence and degree of endometritis periglandular fibrosis in parity I dairy cows. Vet Med Small Anim Clin 6:943, 1983.
6. Miller JG: A technique of endometrial biopsy in the bovine animal. J Am Vet Med Assoc 119:368, 1951.
7. Moss S, Sykes JF, Wrenn TR: Some abnormalities of the bovine endometrium. J Anim Sci 15:631, 1956.
8. Sagartz JW, Hardenbrook HJ: A clinical bacteriologic and histologic survey of infertile cows. J Am Vet Med Assoc 158(5):619, 1971.
9. Schmidt-Adamopoulou B: Diagnosis of endometritis in cows. A comparison of clinical features and histopathologic findings in uterine biopsy specimens. Dtsche Tieraerztl Wochenschr 85(12):476, 1978.
10. Zurgilgen H: Die brunstauslosende Wirkung des oestradiolpropionates (Ovocyclin) und dessen Einfluss auf die Uterusschleimhaut beim Rinde. Inaugural. Dissertation, Zurich, 1948.

Blood Types of Cattle and Their Application

Jerry Caldwell, Ph.D.

Imm Genn Inc., College Station, Texas

The almost endless array of differences among plants and animals is most essential in our lives. Responsible for this astounding degree of variation are both environmental and genetic forces that interact to form highly complex and intricate organisms. It is primarily genetic variation that yields a constantly changing spectrum of animals from which man can select and propagate for his own purposes.

Many facets of genetics have been studied ranging from multivariate genetic control of quantitative traits such as body size to single gene control of qualitative conditions such as polledness or hornedness. This paper will discuss the highly variable genetic base that determines blood types of cattle. Although blood types are classified as qualitative owing to the nature of their detection, the complete blood type of an animal is multigenically controlled. It is hoped that this discussion will help in understanding this complex system and the uses to which it may be applied.

BLOOD TYPE–ANTIGEN AND ANTIBODY

The blood type of an animal denotes a combination of factors known as antigens on the surface of red blood cells (erythrocytes) that are detected by tests with a complementary reagent (antibody). In cattle, blood types are divided into ten systems. Each blood group system comprises a series of antigens controlled by alleles at a particular chromosomal locus. The ten systems used in blood typing by this laboratory are designated as A, B, C, F, J, L, M, S, Z and R', which represent ten different pairs of chromosomes.

Whereas a blood group system denotes a particular pair of chromosomes involved, the term blood group or phenogroup implies one or more antigens coded for by genes linked on the same chromosome.

In some systems, such as the B system, from 1 to 14 antigens constitute a single blood group. Thus, blood types are controlled by a cluster of loci rather than by a single locus. The complete blood type of an animal is noted by the combination of antigens controlled by genes on each pair of chromosomes.[18]

Erythrocyte antigens are designated by letters with superscripts and subscripts such as A, H, Z', B, G_1, G_2, G_3, E'_1, E'_2, Z, and so on. The symbolic identification of antigens began by applying the letters A through Z. However, after antigen Z was identified other antigens discovered were assigned the prime superscript such as A', B', and C', to distinguish A from A', B from B', and so on. In these cases the two antigens may not be related either serologically or genetically. However, the subscript series (I_1, I_2 and E'_1, E'_2, E'_3, etc.) denotes a serologic relationship such that I_1-positive cells will be hemolyzed by both I_1 and I_2 antibody but are not affected by I' antibody. Even though the subtype series are serologically related they represent different genetic products and are inherited independently.

The substances used to detect specific antigens are protein molecules of the gammaglobulin class commonly called antibodies. These protein molecules are produced by cattle (recipient) that have been injected with blood from another animal (donor) possessing erythrocyte antigens foreign to the recipient. The immunologic mechanism of animals responds to unlike objects (in this case blood antigens) by producing antibodies that neutralize, destroy or otherwise render the foreign antigen harmless to the recipient. By utilizing this phenomenon one can force cattle to produce a large array of different antibodies that could be used to detect specific antigens.

It was exactly this principle that allowed scientists to develop a bank of reagents to perform cattle blood typing. During the late 1930's and early 1940's a group of workers at the University of Wisconsin noted that after blood transfusions, the serum from recipient cows lysed red cells of the donor and other cows, but not all, cattle tested. Those early immunizations were blind whereby neither the antigen nor the corresponding antibody had as yet been identified. However, with a battery of typing reagents it is now somewhat easier to plan immunizations to produce specific reagents. An example of antibody production is shown in Table 1.

Note that antigens A', O' and P' of donor cow 371 do not exist in the recipient 285. Thus, after immunizing cow 285 for several weeks with blood from 371 one would expect to observe antibodies

Table 1. Antibody Production

	Blood Type									
Donor 371	AH/	A'O'P'/I_2E'$_1$	C$_1$/E	F/F	J/	L/	M$_1$/	SH'/	Z/	S'/S'
Recipient 285	AH/	I_2E'$_1$/Q'	C$_1$EW/	F/F	J/	L/	M$_1$/	SH'/	Z/	S'/S'

against each of these antigens. Should more than one antibody type be produced, then all but one must be removed via absorptions in order to make a typing reagent. Needless to say, a number of steps are necessary in reagent preparation; however, once made, these typing sera become quite useful in genetic studies.

INHERITANCE OF BLOOD TYPES

Cattle blood types are the most complex of any species known. Given the number of chromosomes involved and the number of alleles observed, it is not unreasonable to postulate that close to two trillion blood types are possible. Thus, blood types tend to yield a unique identification for cattle. The knowledge of blood types increases constantly as new antigens and phenogroups are discovered. However, the individual's blood type is fixed and unchanging.[19]

Table 2 lists the antigens currently being identified in this laboratory. Note that they are grouped by system—A system, B system, etc., which indicates that antigens A, H and Z' are controlled by genes on one pair of chromosomes while antigens B, G_1, G_2, G_3, I_1, I_2, K, etc. are coded for by genes on a separate pair. The system designated as ? (bison) is known to control erythrocyte antigens in the American buffalo. However, bison possess certain antigens that are also common to cattle such as A, E'_3, Q', C_2, W, and so on.

Each antigen may be inherited as a single unit or in combination with other antigens of the same genetic system such as A/, AH/ or AZ'/. These

Table 3. Number of Known Phenogroups by System in Several Breeds

System	Number of Allelic Determinants (Phenogroups)
A	6
B	614
C	83
F	2
J	2
L	2
M	3
S	20
Z	2
R'	2

combinations are referred to as phenogroups and show that rather than a single locus we are detecting a set of linked loci on a given chromosome. This genetic structure increases the number of phenogroups that can exist in the cattle population.

Given the B system (Table 2) with 32 unique antigens and the possibility of various phenogroups, it becomes obvious that a tremendous array of genetic variation can exist in cattle with respect to the B system alone. Indeed, we have already identified 614 phenogroups in this system (Table 3), and additional groups are being added to the list as new segments of the population are tested. Also note in Table 3 that a large number of phenogroups are also known for the C and S systems.

Examples of the 614 B-system phenogroups are shown in Table 4, and some of the 83 C-system phenogroups are listed in Table 5. Note that while an antigen may be inherited by itself it may

Table 2. Blood Type Factors by Genetic System

A System	B System (cont.)	J System
A	F'	J
H	G'	
Z'	I'	L System
	J'	L
B System	K'	
B	O'	M System
G_1	P'	M_1
G_2	Q'	M'
G_3	Y'	
I_1	A''	S System
I_2	B''	S_1
K	G''	S_2
O_1		U
O_3	**C System**	H'
P	C_1	U'
Q	C_2	S''
T	E	U''
Y_1	R	
Y_2	W	Z System
A'	X_1	Z
B'	X_2	
D'	L'	R' System
E'_1		R'
E'_2	**F System**	S'
E'_3	F	? System
	V	(Bison)
		156–1

Table 4. Examples of Phenogroups in the B System of Cattle Blood Types

Code No.*	Phenogroup	Code No.	Phenogroup
1	B	72	QE'_1I'
2	BI_1	74	$G_3TE'_3F'$
3	BO_1	76	$Y_1A'Y''$
4	$BI'Q'$	78	$I_2Y_2E'_1Y'$
5	BO_1B'	79	$Y_1E'_3G'Y'G''$
7	$BPY_2G'Y'$	81	$Y_1D'I'$
12	$BG_2KE'_2F'O'A''$	84	$D'E'_3F'G'O'$
16	BO_1Y_2D'	85	E'_1
18	$BI_2A'D'G'Q'$	93	$A'O'P'$
25	$BG_2KA'E'_3O'A''G''$	96	O'
28	$BG_2KO_3Y_1A'B'$	98	$BTE'_1O'P'$
	$E'_3G'O'Y'A''G''$	101	Y_2A'
30	G_1I_1A''	103	$BG_2KA'A''$
31	G_1O_1A''	111	$G_3TY_1A'E'_3G'G''$
38	$G_2Y_1D'A''$	173	BI_1Q'
39	$G_2Y_2E'_1Q'$	174	$BG_2KY_2A'E'_3I'O'A''G''$
43	$I_1E'_1G''$	202	$III2$
44	$I_1QE'_1$	232	E'_3G''
45	O_1Q'	283	$BQG'P'B''$
46	O_1A'	296	$Q_4E'_1P'$
54	$G_3O_1TE'_3F'K'$	340	$BI_1O_1QD'I'$
61	O_3K'	449	$PY_1A'Y'$
62	$O_3J'K'O'$	506	$BG_2KA'O'A''B''$
70	$QI'Q'$	513	$G_3TE'_3F'Q'$

*The numbers 1, 2, 3, etc. are numerical codes assigned to each phenogroup to facilitate ease of handling in the data bank.

Table 5. Examples of Phenogroups in the C System of Cattle Blood Types

Code No.	Phenogroup
1	C_1
2	C_1E
3	C_1EW
4	C_1EWX_2
5	C_1ER
6	C_1RW
9	C_1EL'
16	C_2EW
18	C_2ERX_1
21	C_2W
23	EW
24	EWL'
26	RWX_2
31	X_1
32	X_2
33	X_2L'
39	C_2EWX_2
49	C_1ERW
63	C_1EWX_2L'
67	$ERWX_1L'$
79	C_1EX_1L'
83	C_2ERWX_1L'

also be inherited in combination with other antigens such as in phenogroups B, BI_1, BO_1, $BG_2KA'E'_1O'A''G''$, and so on. This indicates that different clusters of genes are responsible for these groups, and each group would be inherited as a single unit (except in cases of crossover). For example, an individual with a B system type of $BO_1Y_2D'/O_3J'K'O'$ would transmit to each of its progeny either the group $BO_1Y_2D'/$ or $O_3J'K'O'/$ at the expected 1:1 ratio. Similarly, the same animal that is C_1E/X_2L' in the C system would transmit either $C_1E/$ or $X_2L'/$; however, the segregation of these phenogroups in the C system is completely independent of the B system. The inheritance of blood types was well established by Stormont.[19]

DISTRIBUTION OF BLOOD TYPES IN CATTLE

Although each antigen of a given system could occur in different breeds of cattle, the units in which they are inherited may differ considerably between breeds. For example, the antigens O_1, Y_1, D', E'_1, I' and P' exist in alternative phenogroups such that $Y_1D'I'/$ occurs in Herefords but not in Angus while $O_1E'_1P'$ occurs in Angus but not in Herefords. In both cases these groups may occur in breeds developed from crossing with the parent breed.

After blood typing significant numbers of cattle per breed, it is possible to estimate the frequency and distribution of phenogroups in the population. By using this type of information population studies have been conducted using blood type data to determine breed origins and relationship between breeds and herds that have been isolated for long periods of time.[8, 10, 13, 19] Table 6 includes data on 18 of the 614 B system groups as observed for some breeds.

Some phenogroups appear to be common to several breeds (note those coded as 12, 22, 39 and 307), while others seem to have a more limited distribution. For example, group 33 occurs in Holstein, Jersey and Brown Swiss at 0.0001, 0.1292 and 0.0002 frequency, respectively. The 340 group $(BI_1O_1QD'I')$ exists in Brahman and breeds derived from crosses with Zebu cattle but does not appear to occur in other breeds. There are numerous examples of blood types with limited breed distribution or those even unique to a given breed. However, one must be careful not to totally exclude a particular phenogroup as a component of any breed because of the possibility that it exists in very low frequency and simply has not been observed to date. On the other hand, when large numbers of each breed are tested, the argument for uniqueness becomes more convincing.

Differentiation of cattle breeds has occurred over long time spans, within varied geographic locations

Table 6. Estimated Frequency of a Few B System Phenogroups in Some Breeds

Code	Phenogroup	Holstein	Jersey	Guernsey	Brown Swiss	Hereford	Angus	Brahman	Brangus	Charolais	Texas Longhorn
5	BO_1B'	.0359	.0001	.0005							
7	$BPY_2G;'Y'$				.0516					.0001	
12	$BG_2KE'_2F'O'A''$	.0097	.0004	.1415	.0173		.0000		.0031	.0059	.0484
16	BO_1Y_2D'	.0202				.0008	.1594		.0156	.0868	
22	$BO_3Y_1E'_3G'P'Q'G''$	.0135		.0017	.0017		.0245	.0142	.0179	.1137	.0224
28	$BG_2KO_3Y_1A'B\ 'E'_3$ $K'O'Y'A''G$		.2134	.0367							
33	$G_2D'A''$	.0001	.1292		.0002						
38	$G_2Y_1D'A''$	.0152	.0012								
39	$G_2Y_2E'_1Q'$	.2600	.0004	.0010	.0010	.0029	.1977		.0281	.0002	
46	O_4A'	.0312					.0005		.0031		
74	$G_3TE'_3F'$		.1364	.0002	.0010						
81	$Y_1D'I'$					.3700				.0085	
283	BQG'P'B''										.0288
296	$O_1E'_1P'$						.0079		.0218		
307	Q'	.0650	.0065	.0090	.0340	.0211	.0011		.0101	.0042	
340	$BI_1O_1QD'I'$							.1302	.0218		
346	$G_3QTB'P'$									.0167	
506	$BG_2KA'O'A''B''$										.0825

Table 7. Parentage Analysis—No Exclusion

				System							
	A	**B**	**C**	**F**	**J**	**L**	**M**	**S**	**Z**	**R'**	
Sire:	A/−	$O_3J'K'O'/G_2Y_2E'_1Q'$	C_1E/WX_2	F/F	−/−	L/	M'/−	H'/U'	Z/	S'/S'	
Dam:	H/−	$BO_1Y_2D'/I_2Y_2E'_1Y'$	RWX_2/X_2L'	F/V	J/	L/	−/−	SH'S''/	−/−	S'/S'	
Calf:	A/H	$BO_1Y_2D'/O_3J'K'O'$	C_1E/X_2L'	F/V	J/−	L/	M'/−	SH'S''/U'	Z/−	S'/S'	

and under selection pressure by man. Thus it is likely that certain genetic markers remained with some breeds yet were lost from others. An example of this point concerns the $Y_1D'I'$ phenogroup (Table 6), which has a 0.3700 frequency in Herefords. Thus far this combination has been observed only in that breed or in breeds derived by upgrading with Herefords. Note the frequency of 0.0085 for $Y_1D'I'$ in domestic Charolais in the United States; however the same group has not been observed in Full French Charolais.

These data yield significant information relative to breed differentiation and can be used to reveal inconsistency in pedigree records. Although the determination of purity or impurity on the basis of blood types must be made with some caution, this information has been used for both breeding stock and show steers. However, should questions arise concerning ancestry (either because of purity or just uncertainty about the sire, for example) it is advisable to perform a parentage verification check.

PARENTAGE ANALYSIS

Given the various phenogroups that exist in different breeds it becomes possible to determine whether the reported sire and dam qualify as the parents of a calf or whether there is an exclusion. Consider in Table 7 the blood type of a calf and its sire and dam as listed on the pedigree.

In this case it is obvious that A/, $O_3J'K'O'/$, $C_1E/$, F/, −/, L/, M'/, U'/, Z/ and S'/ could have been inherited from the reported sire while H/, $BO_1Y_2D'/$, $X_2L'/$, V/, J/, L/, −/, SH'S/, −/ and S'/ groups could have been transmitted by the listed dam. Thus, the conclusion to be drawn is that according to blood types the reported sire and dam would qualify as the parents.

Given another case, in which the blood types of the reported family are in Table 8, it is obvious that the listed parentage of this calf is not correct. Upon close examination the dam would qualify as a par-

ent; however, the listed sire is excluded since neither B nor C system group of the bull occurs in the calf.

Quite often multiple sire problems are encountered, either because of artificial insemination or natural service to more than one bull. An example of problem solving in these type situations is given in Table 9.

An examination of this problem shows that bulls 1 and 3 must be excluded since neither of their B system groups occur in the calf. Although not proof of parentage, bull 2 and the listed cow would qualify as parents.

MOSAICISM AND FREEMARTIN DETERMINATION

Approximately 95 per cent of all male-female cattle twins result in a sterile female. During early embryonic development the placental membranes fuse, allowing tissue and hormones to be transported from twin to twin. This allows the male hormones to affect the female's reproductive development adversely. Concurrent with the hormonal exchange, primordial erythrocytes can transfuse from twin to twin and become fixed in the bone marrow (the site of red blood cell production) of the co-twin. After this transplantation, a twin may exhibit its own genetic blood type as well as that of its twin. This condition is generally noted by weak and partial reactions, and in some cases the animals appear to possess three or four phenogroups per system rather than the normal two expected of diploid organisms.

Tables 10 and 11 show examples of blood typing twins.

In the first example there is no evidence of admixture; however, the second example clearly shows admixture between the twins, and thus the female would be classified as a freemartin. This information may be available for a female as young as 3 months old and could be beneficial to the owner who otherwise may keep her at some expense for

Table 8. Parentage Analysis—Exclusion

				System							
	A	**B**	**C**	**F**	**J**	**L**	**M**	**S**	**Z**	**R'**	
Sire:	−/−	G_1I_1A''/Y_2A'	E/WX_2	F/F	−/−	L/	−/−	H'/	Z/	S'/S'	
Dam:	H/	$BO_1B'/G_2Y_1D'A''$	C_1E/X_2	F/V	J/	−/−	−/−	SH'/−	−/−	S'/S'	
Calf:	H/	$G_2Y_1D'A''/I_2$	C_1E/X_2L'	F/V	J/	−/−	−/−	U'/−	−/−	S'/S'	

Table 9. Parentage Analysis—Multiple Sires

				System						
	A	*B*	*C*	*F*	*J*	*L*	*M*	*S*	*Z*	*R′*
Bull 1	AH/	I_2/Q'	C_1E/W	F/F	J/	–/–	–/–	H′/	Z/	S′/S′
Bull 2	H/	$BG_2KE'_2F'O'A''/I_2$	C_1E/X_2L'	F/F	J/	L/	–/–	U′/	Z/	S′/S′
Bull 3	A/	$G_2Y_2E'_1Q'/O_3J'K'O'$	$WX_2/$	F/V	–/–	L/	M′/	SH′S″/	–/–	S′/S′
Cow	A/	$O_1A'/D'E'F'G'O'$	E/X_2	F/F	–/–	–/–	–/–	SH′/	Z/	S′/S′
Calf	A/H	$BG_2KE'_2F'O'A''/O_1A'$	E/X_2L'	F/F	J/–	L/–	–/–	SH′/U′	Z/	S′/S′

two or more years only to learn by her failure to conceive that she is sterile.

BLOOD GROUPS, DISEASES AND PRODUCTION TRAITS

Many attempts have been made to discover associations between genetic markers and production traits or disease resistance. Different workers have studied tissue proteins such as transferrins and cellular blood groups both on white and red blood cells.

Since white blood cells are directly involved in the immune response mechanism and are charged with maintaining a relatively healthy state in animals, they have become prime targets for investigation. The initial work in this area, however, is related to identification of lymphocyte antigens to determine their specificity and inheritance.[1, 3, 5, 6, 17] Although the thrust of research will probably be directed toward studying the effect of lymphocyte type and function on disease resistance, data on this question are limited to the report by Caldwell and Cumberland.[4] However, the future in this field appears quite promising in attempts to identify genetic markers that are associated with disease resistance.

Whereas few data are presently available on the association between white blood cells and different traits, numerous studies have been reported on the association between red blood cell phenogroups and production traits (particularly in dairy cattle). One of the earlier studies by Mitscherlick and colleagues[11] indicated a strong depression of milk yield in cattle with the M blood gene. Heifers with the M allele produced 332 kg less milk than did their M-negative paternal half sibs. Niemann-Sorensen and Robertson[12] found no significant effects of blood group alleles on birth weight, age at first calving, service period or milking time. However, significant differences were found between blood types in milk yield and fat percentage. Rendel[14] also observed a relationship between blood types of the B system and fat percentage. He further observed that, whereas the J allele had an increasing effect on fat percentage, the L allele was negatively associated. Other workers[2, 7] indicated significant associations with the F system blood groups and transferrin types for fat yield.

Little research has been reported on beef production and blood groups or transferrin types. However, a study by Makarechian and Howell[9] with feedlot steers showed no significant differences among transferrin types with respect to either gain or carcass characteristics. On the other hand, possible relationships between blood groups and live weights of cattle at birth, 6, 12, 18 and 24 months of age was studied by Salerno.[15] Phenogroups of the F, L, M and S systems appeared to be associated with weights at different ages.

Sanders[16] studied an Angus herd over a 10-year period, obtaining data on blood types, weaning and postweaning weights and gains and body measurements. During this period the herd became infected with brucellosis, and data on reactors vs nonreactors to the brucellosis test were included in the study. The results of that study indicated reasonably strong evidence for some association of reactors with blood type. With respect to production traits, there appears to be some relationship between blood types of the S system and average daily gain and postweaning weights, between the Z system and weaning weights, and between blood types of the F, J and S systems and various body measurements.

These studies on the relationship of red cell blood types and production traits appear promising from the standpoint of being able to select for greater production based on qualitative genetic markers. However, one should not be overly optimistic about this prospect. First, the observed associations may be transient in that linkages to other genes affecting

Table 10. Blood Typing Twins—Example 1

			System						
A	*B*	*C*	*F*	*J*	*L*	*M*	*S*	*Z*	*R′*
Twin 1									
AH/	BO_1/I_2	$C_1E/$	F/F	–/–	L/	–/–	SH′/	Z/	S′/S′
Twin 2									
–/–	$G_2Y_2E'_1Q'/O_3K'$	–/–	F/V	J/	–/–	M′/	–/–	–/–	S′/S′

Table 11. Blood Typing Twins—Example 2

A	B	C	System F	J	L	M	S	Z	R'
Male Twin									
AH/	B̈O'/Ï₂G̈₂E'₄/O̊₃	C₁E/	F/F	−/−	L/	−/−	SH'S"/	Z/	S'/'
Female Twin									
A/	G̈₂Y₂E'/Q'/B/O₃K'	−/−	F/	J/	L/	M'/	H'/	−/−	S'/S'

these traits may have been responsible for the associations. Second, it is unlikely that single genes have very large effects on quantitative traits that are multigenically controlled. However, studies considering several genetic systems simultaneously with production traits may be useful in determining whether genetic markers would be useful as selective tools.

The area that does seem promising is the study of the immune response system involving the white blood cells and disease resistance/susceptibility. Studies in humans, mice, chickens and cattle indicate that future cattlemen may be able to select animals with a higher level of resistance when sufficient knowledge of the white blood cell system becomes available.

SUMMARY

Studies on qualitative genetics of cattle have resulted in identification of a wide array of genes. A broad genetic base is exemplified by results obtained on blood typing, from which it is estimated that approximately two trillion blood types exist in the bovine population. This information is used to do the following:

1. Produce a permanent record of identification for each animal.

2. Aid breed registry associations in maintaining accurate pedigree records through parentage analysis.

3. Determine the bull that qualifies in multiple sire problems that arise in artificial or natural service situations.

4. Indicate those females born twin to males that are nonfertile because of blood admixture.

5. Indicate cases of crossbreeding in both breeding stock and show steers.

6. Derive the blood type of dead bulls whose semen is to be used.

7. Assist in special investigations ranging from gross errors in records of a given herd to theft or other fraudulent practices.

Research on associations of blood types with production traits has indicated a possible relationship with fat percentage, milk yield and growth traits; however, the data also suggest that red blood cell types may not be very useful as selection criteria. On the other hand, the research on white blood cells appears promising in identifying genetic markers associated with disease resistance.

References

1. Amorena B, Stone WH: Serologically defined (SD) locus in cattle. Science 201:159, 1978.
2. Brum EW, Rausch WH, Hines HC, Ludwick TM: Association between milk and blood polymorphism types and lactation traits of Holstein cattle. J Dairy Sci 51:1031, 1968.
3. Caldwell J, Bryan CF, Cumberland PA, Weseli DF: Serologically detected lymphocyte antigens of Holstein cattle. Anim Blood Grps Biochem Genet 8:197, 1977.
4. Caldwell J, Cumberland PA: Cattle lymphocyte antigens. Transplant Proc 10:889, 1978.
5. Caldwell J: Polymorphism of the BoLA System. Tissue Antigens 13:319, 1979.
6. Caldwell J, Cumberland PA, Weseli DF, Williams JD: Breed differences in frequency of BoLA specificities. Anim Blood Grps Biochem Genet 10:93, 1979.
7. Kiddy CA, Miller RH, Stormont C, Dickinson FN: Transferrin type and transmitting ability for production in dairy bulls. J Dairy Sci 58:152, 1975.
8. Larsen B, Gruchy CL, Moustgaard J: Studies on blood groups and polymorphic protein systems in Jersey cattle on the Isle of Jersey. Acta Agric Scand 24:99, 1974.
9. Makarechian M, Howell WE: Relationship between transferrin type and productive traits in beef steers. J Anim Sci 26:27, 1967.
10. Miller WJ: Blood groups in Longhorn cattle. Genetics 54:391, 1966.
11. Mitscherlich E, Tolle A, Walter, E.: Untersuchungen über das Bestehen von Beziehungen zwischen Blutgruppenfaktoren und der Milcheistung des Rindes. Zeitschr Tierzucht Zuchtbiol 72:289, 1959.
12. Neimann-Sorensen A, Robertson A: The association between blood groups and several production characteristics in three Danish cattle breeds. Acta Agric Scand 11:2, 1966.
13. Rausch WH, Hines HC, Brum EW: A blood type comparison in three beef breeds in America. Immunogenetics Lett 2:43, 1967.
14. Rendel J: Relationships between blood groups and the fat percentage of the milk in cattle. Nature 189:408, 1961.
15. Salerno A: Relationships between blood groups and beef production in Chiana breed cattle. Ninth European Annual Blood Group Conference, 1964, p. 463.
16. Sanders NE: A study of blood type frequencies and association of blood types with other traits in an Angus herd. M.S. Thesis. University of Tennessee, 1981.
17. Spooner RL, Leveziel H, Grosclaude F, et al.: Evidence for a possible major histocompatibility complex (BLA) in cattle. J Immunogenet 5:335, 1978.
18. Stormont CR, Owen D, Irwin MR: The B and C systems of bovine blood groups. Genetics 36:134, 1951.
19. Stormont C: Contribution of blood typing to dairy science progress. J. Dairy Sci 50:253, 1967.

Bovine Hybrids

Parvathi K. Basrur
Ontario Veterinary College,
Guelph, Ontario

Ever since the early days of domestication, livestock breeders have attempted to breed males of one species with females of another species in the hope of combining the desirable traits of both species in the offspring (hybrids). Hybridization occurs occasionally in the wild and frequently under conditions of semi-isolation where males and females of closely related species live in proximity to each other. Successful matings have occurred from time to time between members of various species of the major family Bovidae. Among these are cattle, yak and bison, all of which are different species of the genus *Bos*.

The most successful interspecific hybridization is that which occurs between the two subspecies of domestic cattle, i.e., the Asiatic domestic cattle, Zebu *(Bos indicus)* and the European domestic cattle *(Bos taurus)*. However, both types of domestic cattle could also be crossed with yak *(Bos grunniens),* or bison *(Bos bison),* and yak could be crossed with bison. These interspecific matings produce viable offspring, although they also lead to varying degrees of reproductive problems.

YAK

Yak, which occupies an intermediary position between cattle and bison in evolution, is one of the heaviest of the subfamily. It is the most valuable beast of burden and draft in the mountainous terrain of central Asia including the Himalayas, central China and Mongolia. It also serves as a source of milk, meat, manure, hide and hair in these areas of the world, where other animals do poorly.

Yak is a nocturnal breeder. The male yak reaches sexual maturity at about 6 years of age and shows a decline in vigor and reproductive efficiency after 5 to 6 years of service. The female yak (cow) reaches sexual maturity at 2 years of age, has a gestation period of 250 to 270 days and a calving interval of 330 days. The yak cow has a lactation period of 200 days. Her milk yield is poor, but her fat content is the highest (12 per cent) of all mammalian milk.[7]

Yak cows are sensitive to temperature and altitude changes and often lose fecundity at altitudes lower than their preserves in the upper reaches of mountains 4000 to 6000 meters above sea level. They have a life span of 15 to 20 years.

BISON

The North American bison, which includes the wood bison and the plains bison, is often referred to as buffalo. Both types are believed to have originated in central Asia, from which region they arrived in North America through the Bering Strait.[3] They ranged in areas extending from south of Lake Ontario to eastern Florida and up to New Mexico, and along the Rocky Mountains as far as the Northwest Territories. The bison is hardy and thrifty. It is considerably larger than domestic cattle, has a massive and low-slung head and relatively small hindquarters. Bison meat is dark and coarse in grain, and the large hump, which houses the elongated spinous process of the vertebrae (from the lumbar to the cervical vertebrae) is a source of good quality meat. The thick coat, made up of fine, abundant hair, renders bison capable of facing the severe cold and blizzards prevailing in some parts of North America. They are also resistant to blackflies and other ectoparasites, which often take a toll from domestic cattle through arthropod-borne diseases.

The bull calves follow their mothers for 2 years even though they are fully weaned by 7 months. They reach sexual maturity between 2½ and 3 years of age. The rutting season is July to late September. The female is sexually mature at 2 years. She is a seasonal breeder with a tendency to stay in peak breeding state for 3 to 4 days. The gestation period is 285 days, and calving is generally uneventful and quick, lasting 20 minutes from the time the cow lies down.[3] Twinning is not uncommon in bison. In one survey, approximately 6 per cent of bison breeders reported twinning in their herds, and in another case a rate of 0.35 per cent of twinning was recorded for a herd of 1700 bison.[3] Bison calves may be raised on domestic milk cows, since the bison cow often tends to accept only one of the calves. The bison has a long life span (over 40 years) and a relatively long reproductive span. The bison cow, which generally delivers a calf every other year, is capable of reproduction till she is 28 to 30 years of age.

CATTLE-BISON HYBRIDS

The potential of creating a new line of beef cattle that combines the size, hardiness, and strength of the bison with the growth rate, carcass quality and reproductive efficiency of the beef cattle has long been recognized by cattle breeders in North America. Hybrids of European cattle and American bison existed since 1750 in various parts of North America including California and Virginia. However, it is only since the latter part of the last century that serious attempts were made to cross domestic cattle with bison. The centers that were actively involved in cattle-bison hybridization were Texas[5] and Ontario[2] and later the prairie provinces of Canada.[4]

Domestic cows of different breeds, including Shorthorn, Angus, Hereford, Holstein and Charolais, have been crossed with bison bulls to produce hybrids. A striking feature of this hybridization is that because the male hybrids are sterile, combinations of bison and domestic cattle can be made only through back crossing the female hybrid. The female hybrid is generally fertile and may be mated to domestic bull or to bison bull to decrease or increase the bison percentage in the progeny.

The results of the first cross (50 per cent bison, 50 per cent domestic cattle) are called hybrids regardless of the sire species. The backcross progeny of the hybrids that are greater than 50 per cent bison (or greater than 50 per cent cattle) are called cattaloes. Other names suggested for these animals include catalo if they are 50 per cent bison, or catfalo if the bison percentage is greater than 50 per cent[2, 4] However, the name cattalo is traditionally used for a bison-cattle cross that is less than 50 per cent of one parent species with a corresponding increase in the other.[2] More recently, the name beefalo has been used for part bison-part cattle cross to imply the beef characteristic of these crossbred animals.

General Features

The hybrid (50 per cent bison) at birth is of yellowish brown coat and black nose, resembling a bison calf more closely than a domestic bull calf. The color changes to dark brown by autumn and exhibits fluctuations in coat color intensity before and after shedding. The animals exhibit remarkable vigor, size, stamina and longevity, the latter traits being similar to those of the bison parent. The hybrids show greater feed lot gains than bison but lower than those of beef cattle.[4, 9]

Conception rates among cattalo cows are similar to those of beef (Hereford) cattle, and the length of gestation is somewhat similar to that in cattle, the mean being 264 days. Cattalo cows give more (and richer) milk and wean heavier calves than beef cattle, indicating the better maternal ability of the former. The udder is larger than that of bison and domestic cattle; however, the total milk yield of cattaloes (within the range of 10 to 25 per cent bison parentage) decreases significantly as the bison percentage of the dam increases.[8] The resemblance to cattle increases as the percentage of domestic cattle is increased through back crossing. Unlike the bison cow and like the beef cow, cattalo cows breed as yearlings. Hybrid males, which are generally steerlike in appearance, are smaller and of poorer conformation than hybrid females.

Reproductive Problems

In spite of some of the superior traits of cattaloes, the hybridization venture is not practical. The setbacks are mating indifference, pregnancy wastage through abortion, stillbirths and neonatal mortality, and sterility of the male hybrid and cattalo bulls.

Mating Indifference. Mating indifference is a common problem in attempts to cross bison bulls to domestic cows because the latter refuse the approaches of bison bulls. One method used to reduce mating indifference is to raise bison bull calves on domestic cows before they are used for hybridization. Behavioral repulsion is more pronounced in the reverse cross because the domestic bull is more averse to mating with a bison cow. This tendency is more striking in older than in younger domestic bulls. Even in this case, separation of the bull calf from domestic cows reduces the mating indifference.

Hybrid females, which are generally fertile, are occasionally indifferent to bison bulls and domestic bulls. In many instances, domestic bulls also have been known to refuse to serve the hybrid cows in season. Hybrid males, on the other hand, show no indifference to bison cows or domestic cows.

Pregnancy Wastage. Although conception rates in cattalo cows are similar to those in beef cattle,[8] the number of calves weaned is lower than that in the latter mainly because of abortion, stillbirths, and perinatal mortality of the male cattaloes. Abortion takes place between 175 and 180 days of gestation. Stillbirths are related to the size of the calves. The calves of bison cows and cattaloes are relatively small at birth. However, hybrid calves sired by bison tend to be larger than domestic calves, and the male hybrid calves offer calving difficulties. As a rule, if the sire is a bison and the bull calf is larger than a domestic calf, stillbirth occurs probably because of cephalopelvic or respiratory distress to the fetus and the inability of the mother to expel the fetus in time.

Hydramnios is the most common cause of cow and calf mortality in cattalo pregnancies. The hybrids and cattalo cows are often unable to stand on their feet because of the weight of the amniotic fluid. A common sequel is rupture of the amniotic membranes and fetal death, which may or may not be followed by the expulsion of the fetus. This condition is generally more frequent in pregnancies sired by the bison than in the reverse cross. The sex of the calf has no influence on the incidence of hydramnios.

The reason for the difference in the incidence of hydramnios between the two types of cross is not known. It may be related to the tendency of bison cows to resorb fetuses rather than abort them because remnants of fetal bones indicative of resorption attempts have been detected in the uteri of some slaughtered bison cows. Thus, it is possible that the incidence of fetal death is similar in both types of crosses but occurs earlier in bison cow–domestic bull matings than in the reverse cross. In the former, the loss of a conceptus may not be detected because the dead hybrid fetus is often resorbed early.

The birth weight of the hybrid calf is greater than that of beef cattle. However, in back cross progeny,

Table 1. Pregnancy Wastage in Domestic Cows and Cattalo Cows Mated to Bison
or Domestic Bulls

Experiments	No. Impregnations	Abortions	Stillbirths	Cow Mortality	Live Births	
					Male	Female
Boyd; Ontario 1884–1915	102	63	4*	11	2	33
Agr. Canada† 1916–1935	62	12	14	20	19	17

*Stillborn were all bull calves.
†Agriculture Canada, Research Station, Alberta.

the birth weight of the calf drops and the incidence of neonatal mortality increases as the percentage of bison in cattalo cows is increased.[8] The incidence of neonatal mortality and stillbirth is greater if the hybrid fetus is a male (Table 1). The mortality of the male hybrid was once thought to be due to the hump, which the hybrid is expected to inherit from the bison parent. However, this assumption is erroneous because the hump does not develop until several months after birth.

The sex ratio (percentage of males born) of hybrids when the sire is a domestic bull is normal. However, in the reverse cross, it is very low, varying from 0 to 15 per cent in trials using cows of different breeds of domestic cattle as the dam.

In one report[3] on 29 pregnancies in cattaloes and hybrids mated to domestic bulls, pregnancy wastage from abortion and stillbirth and cow mortality at calving amounted to 10 per cent. However, of 53 pregnancies in the reverse cross (cattaloes and hybrids mated to bison bulls), the incidence of abortion and stillbirth rose to 45 per cent and cow mortality was 36 per cent. In general, a 50 per cent to 70 per cent pregnancy wastage and 10 to 32 per cent cow mortality are common in cattle-bison hybrid experiments. It is noticed that the loss is greater in bison bull–domestic cow crosses. However, early fetal mortality is generally high in bison cows, and pregnancy wastage through fetal resorption may be more frequent than noticed in the domestic bull–bison cow crosses. Mortality of the dam also is considerably higher in bison bull–domestic cow matings than in the reverse cross. The cow loss could be minimized by the use of big, mature cows instead of smaller cows or heifers.

Male Sterility. In crosses of domestic cows with bison bulls, bull calves born alive are fewer than heifer calves and hybrid bulls from both types of crosses are sterile. Newborn hybrid bull calves show a few germ cells in the seminiferous tubules, and a few primary spermatocytes are encountered in yearlings. However, in adults, a majority of the tubules lined by Sertoli cells are devoid of germ cells.

In back crosses with less than 50 per cent bison, spermatogenic activity varies according to the bison percentage. For example, in cattalo bulls of 31 per cent bison, the seminiferous tubules resemble those of 50 per cent hybrids, whereas bulls of 25 per cent bison exhibit spermatogenic activity and some fully differentiated spermatozoa in some tubules. The

number of tubules showing spermatogenic activity is generally low, and spermiophages are frequently encountered in the lumen. The epididymis is generally devoid of spermatozoa, indicating that a majority of the spermatozoa noted in the seminiferous tubules of cattalo bulls with 25 per cent bison do not reach the epididymis. In comparison, cattalo bulls with less than 25 per cent bison show nearly normal spermatogenesis and occasionally fertility, although spermatozoa with abnormal morphology are abundant even in cattalo bulls with 18 per cent and 22 per cent bison.[1]

The interstitium is generally expansive, and the Leydig cells appear to be active in cattalo bull testes. These bulls exhibit testosterone levels and male libido similar to those of normal beef bulls of corresponding age. However, some of these cattalo bulls are more aggressive than domestic beef cattle.

Semen samples of cattaloes vary in quality depending on their bison percentage. Cattalo bulls that are over 30 per cent bison consistently show no spermatozoa in the semen, whereas those between 20 and 30 per cent bison exhibit some motile spermatozoa, although a majority of these bulls are sterile. Cattalo bulls with less than 20 per cent bison generally show no overt difference from beef cattle in semen quality. The testicles of these cattalo bulls are pendulous with a well-defined neck, a short scrotal pouch, thick skin and a dense, short hair coat. The weight of the testicles ranges from 8 ounces in 50 per cent hybrids to 9 ounces in 25 per cent bison, whereas in 12.5 per cent bison, the average weight is 13 ounces compared to the 8 to 9 ounces in domestic bulls of corresponding age. The accessory sex glands of cattalo bulls weigh, on an average, 2 ounces in 50 per cent hybrids and 2 and 6 ounces respectively in 25 per cent and 12.5 per cent bison.

CATTLE-YAK HYBRIDS

Hybridization between yak and Asiatic Zebu generally occurs in settlements along the trade routes connecting India with Russia, China and Tibet. The hybrid cow, called churi, is fertile, yields larger quantities of milk than the Zebu cows and has a higher milk fat content than either the Zebu or the yak cow. Hybrid cows can withstand extremely cold

Table 2. Pregnancy Wastage and Sex Ratio in Cattle-Yak Matings

Matings					Live Births	
Sire	Dam	Abortions	Still-births	Mortality	Male	Female
Domestic	Yak	0	0	0	1	1
Domestic	½ yak, ½ domestic	2	1	0	10	3
Yak	Domestic	3	2	1	3	8
Yak	½ yak, ½ domestic*	0	0	1	11	0
	Total	5	3	2	25	12

*West Highland cow.

or warm climates, unlike the parental species, and can be maintained on low-value feed.[7]

The male hybrid, called churu, is smaller than the female hybrid. His physical appearance, the differentiation of the external genitalia and libido are male-like although he is sterile. The female hybrid can be used for back crossing with yak bull or domestic ox. After repeated back crossing with yak or with oxen for three generations or more, fertile male progeny may be obtained.

Crossing yak with European cattle gives results similar to those obtained with Asiatic cow. The hybrids are heavier and larger than beef cattle and cattaloes, but they do not exhibit the stamina and speed characteristic of cattle-bison hybrids. Abortions and stillbirths occur in such crosses (Table 2), although even in this type of cross, the reverse cross (domestic bull mated with yak cow) is more productive. The sex ratio is not reduced in yak-cattle crosses. Furthermore, there appears to be a preponderance of bull calves in domestic bull-yak cow crosses.

There is no overt mating indifference in yak bulls or yak-cattle hybrid bulls toward domestic cows. However, domestic bulls are generally unwilling to mate with yak cows. This reaction is progressively reduced as the domestic cattle percentage in the cows is increased through back crossing the female hybrid cow with domestic bulls.

YAK-BISON HYBRIDS

Hybridization of yak and bison yields much better results than mating bison with cattle or yak with European cattle. Yak-bison hybrids have more stamina and speed than all the hybrids described previously. However, even in this cross, the hybrid bulls (50 per cent bison, 50 per cent yak) are sterile, even though an alleged hybrid bull is reported to have produced a stillborn calf in one study.[4]

In addition to the hybrids already described, there are some less well known bovine hybrids. The Zebu and the Southeast Asian Banteng have hybridized and produced Madura cattle, which are more resistant to extremely hot weather, prolonged dry spells and tickborne diseases than cattle. These hybrids are also reputed to be the fastest of all

bovines and the most intelligent. Other Asiatic species of Bovidae including the Mithan, Gaur and Kouprey are also known to hybridize with domestic cattle. Incorporation of their genes into domestic cattle may be beneficial. However, this may be achieved only through the use of female hybrids for back crossing with domestic cattle, since the F_1 male hybrid in all these crosses is likely to be sterile.

PARTIAL STERILITY OF HYBRIDS

A common feature of all interspecific bovine hybrids described above is partial sterility characterized by the normal fertility of the female hybrid and total sterility of the male hybrid. This phenomenon, which is widespread in mammalian hybrids,[6] is recognized as one of the isolating mechanisms that preserves the integrity of different species. Reproductive isolation between species is achieved by the preservation of the various gene mutations and chromosomal rearrangements that have proved advantageous to each species during its evolution. Although cattle, yak and bison have evolved in different regions as genetically distinct species, all of them originated in central Asia. They carry 60 chromosomes and show no overt morphologic differences in autosomes and X chromosomes. The difference between cattle and bison resides in the morphology of the Y chromosome, which is a small submetacentric entity in European cattle and a small acrocentric entity in bison.[1] This difference has been considered the probable cause of sterility in hybrid bulls, since the hybrid females, which are karyotypically indistinguishable from bison cow or domestic cow, are fertile. However, this theory does not explain the partial sterility of the yak-Zebu hybrids (or bison-Zebu hybrids), since the Y chromosome in these species are morphologically identical. In fact, the male hybrids are either inviable or sterile in interspecific crosses of all mammals, regardless of the morphologic features of the Y chromosome.[6] Among the other explanations offered for male sterility are differences between species in testicular position and seasonality of spermatogenic activity. However, since the phenomenon of male sterility is present in hybrids of species that do not differ much in seasonal response, the explanation for partial sterility of the hybrid progeny of closely related species has to be sought elsewhere.

The source of male sterility in hybrids may be the divergent gene loci in the parental chromosomes. These divergent loci may reduce the synaptic affinity between the "homologous" chromosomes of the parental species during spermatogenesis or interfere with the function of other gene loci coding for proteins essential for spermiogenesis. These divergent loci are not harmful in somatic tissue cells where the co-adapted genes of different species could work in relative harmony, whereas they could interrupt the specific processes of the germ line. The effect of these loci is more severe in males because of the intricate process of spermiogenesis that takes place while the male nucleus is in the haploid state. The haploid state is practically nonexistent in females in which second meiosis is completed after the entry of sperm in most mammals.

References

1. Basrur PK: Hybrid sterility. In Benirschke K (ed.): Comparative Mammalian Cytogenetics. New York, Springer-Verlag, 1968, p. 107.
2. Boyd, MM: Crossing bison and cattle. J Hered 5:189, 1914.
3. Dary DA: Cattalo. In The Buffalo Book. Chicago, Swallow Press, 1974, p. 271.
4. Deakin A, Muir GW, Smith AG: Hybridization of domestic cattle, bison and yak. Publication 479: Technical Bulletin 2,5, Canada Dept of Agriculture, 1935.
5. Goodnight C: My experience with bison hybrids. J Hered 5:194, 1914.
6. Haldane JBS: Sex ratio and unisexual sterility in hybrid animals. J Genet 12:101, 1922.
7. Kalia HR: Appraisal of cow *(Bos indicus)* × yak *(Bos grunniens)* cross breeding work in cold and elevated regions of Himachal Pradesh (India). International Symposium on Genetics Applied to Livestock Production. 1974, p. 723.
8. Keller DG, Lawson JE: Influence of bison percentage on pre- and post-weaning traits of cattalo calves. Can J Anim Sci 58:537, 1978.
9. Lawson JE, Peters HF: Growth and carcass traits of cattalo, Hereford and 1/4-Brahman bull calves. Can J Anim Sci 56:193, 1976.

Reproduction in Zebu Cattle

V. R. Vale-Filho

Federal University of Minas Gerais,
Belo Horizonite, Brazil

L. E. L. Pinheiro

Faculty of Veterinary Medicine,
UNESP, Jaboticabal, Brazil

P. K. Basrur

University of Guelph,
Guelph, Ontario

The Asiatic Zebu cattle *(Bos indicus)* and the European taurine cattle *(Bos taurus)* exhibit divergence in various morphologic and physiologic traits, even though both of them originated from the same ancestral stock. The Zebu, adapted to the tropical areas of the world, has emerged with a larger skin area with folds on the neck and brisket, a larger prepuce, and larger and more numerous sweat glands to facilitate heat loss. Also, the Zebu cattle are hardier and more resistant to ectoparasites common to tropical areas, and they are good grazers even in rough land by virtue of their long legs and hard hoofs. On the other hand, they are slow to grow, their food conversion rate is lower than that of taurine cattle and they attain sexual maturity 12 to 18 months later than taurine cattle. However, the Zebu has a longer life span, and bulls over 10 years old produce good quality semen and cows of that age routinely produce normal calves.

CLINICAL EXAMINATION OF THE FEMALE

The vulvar lip of the external genitalia of the Zebu cow is bigger and more protuberant than that of the taurine cow. Similarly, the cervix of the Zebu cow appears two to three times bigger than that of the taurine cow on rectal palpation. This difference is more pronounced after the first parturition, when prolapse of the first ring generally occurs. In Zebu heifers, the cervix is smaller than in cows, and it is easily localized on the pelvic floor. In cows, the cervix can be localized on the pubic symphysis or slightly projected into the abdominal cavity. Ovaries of Zebu cows are smaller than those of taurine cows, and the proper assessment of corpus luteum by rectal palpation is often difficult because it is embedded deep within the ovary. The pelvic cavity of Zebu is smaller than that of taurine cows. However, rectal palpation of the uterine horns for pregnancy diagnosis or for the detection of mucometra or pyometra does not pose any difficulty.

For pregnancy diagnosis at 45 to 90 days, slipping of the chorioallantoic membranes is relatively easy for trained individuals. At 90 to 100 days of gestation, placentomes of 2 cm in diameter are palpable. The descent of the uterus into the abdominal cavity begins at 50 to 60 days' gestation in cows and at 80 to 90 days in heifers. By the fourth month of gestation, the fetus and uterine horns have moved far forward into the abdominal cavity.

ESTRUS AND ESTRUS DETECTION

The clinical and physiological aspects of estrus manifestation in Zebu heifers and cows are similar to those of taurine cows. The age of onset of puberty varies greatly between different breeds of Zebu cattle raised in different parts of the world. In the dairy breeds of Zebu raised in Brazil, the mean age at puberty is 32.5 to 32.7 months,[13] and in another breed (Nelore) it is generally 2 months earlier.[13] In India and Pakistan the age at which the first heat is detected is 36 months or more, and some of the heifers may be bred at the first heat.[6] However, the results of a 10-year study show that less than 50 per cent of the heifers (41 per cent) settle at the first estrus, and the others take an average of 55.5 ± 46 days from the onset of pubertal heat before they become pregnant.[9, 11]

The length of the estrous cycle varies from breed to breed and from animal to animal within a breed. In a study of 38 heifers belonging to five different breeds of Zebu maintained under the same environment, a total of 574 observations over a 12-month period showed that the mean length of estrous cycle was 21.16 ± 2.26 days.[5]

The duration of estrus and estrous cycle length is shorter in heifers than in cows. Estrus occurs at any time during the day. In heifers, 43 per cent of estrus occurs during the morning, 21 per cent during the afternoon and 36 per cent during the night. However, in cows a majority of estrus (61 per cent) occurs after sunset and before sunrise.[5, 6] The intensity and the secondary signs of estrus vary greatly, although hyperactivity, bellowing, nervous symptoms and copious flow of cervicovaginal secretions characteristic of pronounced estrus are relatively rare in many breeds of Zebu cattle. Normally intense estrus with detectable excitement and weak intensity with no overt secondary signs of estrus are more common. In cows, 50 per cent of the animals show normal estrus intensity, 16 per cent show weak intensity and 34 per cent show pronounced estrus intensity. In contrast, more than 54 per cent of heifers show weak estrus intensity and 43 per cent show normal estrus intensity, whereas pronounced estrus is detected only in 3 per cent of heifers. The first and second estrus manifestations are generally weak in that only 33 to 37 per cent of the first and second estrus are of normal intensity. Pronounced estral symptoms are generally not evinced by Zebu heifers at the first or second estrus. Also, only 26 per cent of the first and second estrus is ovular, whereas the rest (76 per cent) is anovular. Approximately 11 per cent of heifers exhibit gestational estrus between 69 and 180 days of pregnancy, and in some cases it recurs a second time approximately 23 days after the first gestational estrus.[5, 6, 9]

Ovulation occurs in both ovaries. However, the right ovary appears to be more active than the left since implantation takes place more frequently from ova shed from the right ovary. In a survey of 916 pregnant Zebu cows, 568 had a fetus on the right horn, 346 had a fetus on the left horn, and two had a fetus on both horns. In this study the corpus luteum of gestation was noted in the left ovary in two cows in which implantation was noted in the right horn, suggesting that intercornual migration of the blastocyst occurs in Zebu as it does in taurine cows.[12]

The size and weight of corpora lutea in some breeds of Zebu cattle, including Brahman, are lower than those of taurine cows, although the luteal concentration or total content of progesterone is not significantly different[10] in the breeds compared (Brahman vs Hereford). The preovulatory surge of luteinizing hormone (LH) and the pituitary response to exogenous gonadotropin-releasing factor (GnRH) are also lower in this breed of Zebu compared to those in taurine cattle.[15] It is not known whether the smaller size of the corpus luteum is due to the low ovulatory LH surge or to a lower ovarian response to gonadotropin. The low preovulatory LH surge may be responsible for the poor estrous symptoms generally evinced by some Zebu cattle.[16]

BREEDING

In a majority of countries where Zebu cattle are found in abundance, natural mating is the method practiced. However, artificial insemination is being carried out increasingly in countries that now have facilities for this service. The relatively short estrus period (15 to 18 hours' duration) and the poor manifestations of secondary signs pose some problems for the practice of artificial insemination for Zebu. If the cow shows estrus before 7 o'clock in the morning, insemination should be done on the same day after 5 in the afternoon, and if estrus is detected in the afternoon, insemination must be carried out by 7 the next morning. Two types of teasers may be used to detect heat. One of them is left with the females in pasture to detect the onset of heat, while the other is kept in the pen with the cows already separated after detecting estrus. When a female in the pen starts to reject the second teaser, indicating the end of estrus, she is ready to be separated from the teaser for insemination.

In the tropical areas of the western hemisphere more than 60 per cent of conceptions take place during June to August when the pastures are generally in top condition. When nutrition and management are good, a rate of more than 80 per cent conception to first insemination is relatively common in some breeds of Zebu cattle. The use of SHANG treatment for interrupted suckling and effective selection for reproductive efficiency contribute to the success rate. When the calf is kept with the cow suckling all day, the first postpartum estrus is delayed, occurring sometimes 4 to 6 months after calving. First estrus is further delayed if the cows are on poor pasture, deficient in phosphorus and other essential minerals. In some cases, the ovary is extremely small, and no tertiary follicle or corpus luteum can be detected by palpation until 4 to 6 months after calving.[8]

ESTRUS CONTROL

Estrus response of Zebu and taurine cows maintained under similar environmental conditions to prostaglandin ($PGF_{2\alpha}$) treatment has been compared by workers in various countries. The regimen of $PGF_{2\alpha}$ treatment, the time of insemination and the specific breeds examined vary between these studies. A study comparing the White Fulani breed of Zebu with German Brown and Holstein breeds of taurine cattle[1] showed that 50 per cent of the cycling Zebu heifers and 38 per cent of the taurine heifers were in estrus after one intramuscular injection of 25 mg of prostaglandin ($PGF_{2\alpha}$) and 100 per cent were in estrus after a second injection 12 days later. The duration of estrus in this study was similar in Zebu and taurine heifers, both showing 17.5 hours estrus duration in synchronized heifers compared to 14.6 hours in nonsynchronized heifers. Conception in estrus-synchronized heifers, as confirmed by rectal palpation at 90 days postinsemination, was 66.6 per cent in Zebu heifers and 58.3 per cent in taurine heifers, suggesting that the estrus response to $PGF_{2\alpha}$ and the conception rate are comparable in cycling taurine and Zebu heifers. In contrast, the first-calf Fulani heifers, with a long postpartum anestrus of 3.5 to 5.4 months, did not respond to prostaglandin treatment.[1] Similar studies carried out in Brazil indicate that estrous synchronization efficacy of prostaglandin $F_{2\alpha}$ in Zebu breeds is comparable to that in taurines and ranges between 70 and 95 per cent in cycling cows.[3, 17] This treatment is effective only in less than 25 per cent of the cases if cows at 50 to 90 days postpartum are included in

the experiment (Table 1). Pregnancy outcome in these estrus-synchronized cows is generally low. The results can be improved considerably if the cows selected are all in good health and nutritional plane and have functional ovaries. Conception rate is far better if synchronization is attempted sooner than 50 to 90 days after parturition (Table 1). Superovulation response of Zebu cows to gonadotropin (FSH) is generally inconsistent. However, in some experiments with proper selection of the donor cows, five to nine embryos have been recovered with FSH administration prior to nonsurgical embryo collection. Successful pregnancies with these embryos in synchronized recipients to date has been low.[20]

CALVING AND CALVING INTERVAL

The mean gestational length is 295 days for single births and 7 to 10 days shorter for twins.[11] The age at first calving varies greatly between breeds and within a breed maintained in different countries. Thus, the mean age at first calving in Red Sindhi in Brazil is 46.7 ± 1 month,[13] but for the same breed maintained in India, it is 47.0 ± 4 months.[11] In the latter group only 10 per cent of the heifers calve when they are below 40 months of age. The age at first calving has a heritability estimate of 0.39. Because of this relatively high genetic component, it is easy to lower the age at first calving by selective breeding.

There is a slight seasonal trend in calving, 65 per cent of the calvings occurring between December and June in Asiatic countries. Since both cows and bulls exhibit marked reduction in activity during the rainy season (November to February), the conception is low at this time. Furthermore, cows conceiving during the 3 months following the cessation of

Table 1. Estrus Synchronization with Prostaglandin F_2 (500 μg/animal)* and Conception Rate in Zebu (Nelore) Cows, in Brazil

| | | | Estrus Manifestation | | | | | |
| | | | 2 to 7 Days after Treatment | | Random Within 24 Days | | Conception | |
Experiment†	Groups	No. Cows	Number	Percentage	Number	Percentage	Number	Percentage
Experiment 1	Control	50	—	—	44	88.0	32	72.7
Nanuque-MG[17]	T 1	50	40	80.0	—	—	16	40.0
	T 2	50	35	70.0	—	—	10	28.6
Experiment 2	Control	44	—	—	43	97.7	16	37.2
Marilandia-PR[2]	T 1	44	42	95.4	—	—	15	35.7
Experiment 3	Control	38	—	—	9	23.6	5	55.5
Brotas-SP‡	T 1	40	7	17.5	—	—	6	85.7
	T 2	40	10	25.0	—	—	10	100.0

*Cloprostenol (ICI-80.996) twice at 11 days apart.
†In experiments 1 and 2, the interval between calving and treatment was over 6 months and in experiment 3 it was closer to calving (50 to 90 days). Cows of test group 2 (T 2) in experiments 2 and 3 were inseminated twice at 72 and 96 hours after the second prostaglandin treatment and in T 1, once at estrus.
‡Vale-Filho, V.R., unpublished data.

monsoon exhibit the longest calving intervals in the herd.

Calving interval is 14.7 to 15 months in Red Sindhi and 17.2 months in Hariana breeds. Among the Brazilian breeds it is 16.4 months in Gir and 15.3 months in Nelore.[9, 13] The heritability estimate of the calving interval, like age at first calving, is also above 0.30.[9]

The birth weight of calves varies greatly between breeds, As a rule, the bull calves weigh more than heifer calves. In Red Sindhi breeds, the mean weight of bull calves is 39.0 ± 5 pounds and that of the heifer is 34.0 ± 0.6 pounds.[11]

DISEASES OF THE FEMALE REPRODUCTIVE SYSTEM

The pathologic conditions observed in taurine cows and heifers are also observed in Zebu. However, the frequencies of these conditions vary between different breeds of Zebu and within the breeds selected for different geographic and climatic conditions. For example, the most common conditions detected in the Zebu cattle of the Sindhi breed in Pakistan are prolapse of the cervix and kinked and pyosalpinx,[19] whereas these conditions are seen only occasionally in the Zebu breeds in Brazil. Common types of anomalies noted in Brazilian breeds of Zebu are unilateral or bilateral ovarian hypoplasia, segmental aplasia of the mullerian ducts[7] and cystic ovaries. Tumors of the ovary and uterus are relatively rare in Zebu cows. Among those present, granulosa cell tumors and teratomas are the most common. Among the reproductive tract malfunctions, imperforate hymen and hymenal obstructions are the most common (Table 3).

The third category of problems (cystic ovary) is generally seen in inbred lines of Zebu. In one study of a highly inbred dairy type of Zebu cattle exhibiting subfertility, cystic ovaries with nymphomania were detected in 90 out of 150 cows over 3 years of age. Fifty-four of these were nulliparous, while the other 36 (pluriparous) cows exhibited prolonged calving intervals up to 31 months. Out of these two lots, 34 animals exhibiting irregular estrus and nymphomania were slaughtered at random to study the lesions. Clinical symptoms included enlargement and induration of the vulva and cervix, congestion of the vagina with mucus, enlargement of the uterus with a thin and flaccid wall, and mucometra. Microscopic examination showed follicular cysts in all 34 cases. In one case a tumor was detected in both ovaries, the right and left ovaries weighing 172 and 167.5 grams respectively. Hyperplasia of the adrenal cortex, which approached approximately four times the size of normal, was also detected in some of the cows exhibiting nymphomania.[4]

The incidence of vaginal prolapse or postpartum endometritis is low in Zebu cattle. This may be related to the ease with which the Zebu expels the calf and placenta. In some cases of severe uterine infections, periovarian adhesions or oviductal obstructions may be observed. In a survey of histo-pathologic lesions in 478 nonpregnant cows, 40 (8.3 per cent) showed various lesions of the uterus. Endometritis was noted in 16 (3.3 per cent) of these cows.[14]

Abortions occur as a result of brucellosis, leptospirosis, toxoplasmosis, listeriosis and trichomoniasis. In addition, leukosis and pustular vulvovaginitis have also been observed in Zebu cattle.

MALFORMATIONS OF THE CALF

Anomalies of the newborn are prevalent in some inbred lines. The most frequently detected malformations in some dual-purpose lines of Gir breed include cleft palate, umbilical hernia and hypospadias. Congenital anomalies including hydrocephaly, excessively straight limbs with short extensor tendons, and muscular incoordination also occur relatively frequently in some lines of Nelore breed. In addition, abnormal pigmentation of the face and around the eyes and nose is recognized in some inbred calves in association with other multiple congenital anomalies.

CLINICAL EXAMINATION OF THE MALE

There is no difference between the genital tract of the Zebu and taurine bulls except in the size of some of the organs. The testes in adult Zebu bulls are slightly smaller than those of taurine bulls, the mean length being approximately a centimeter shorter. The mean scrotal circumference is 38.9 cm for Zebu and 39.9 cm for taurine bulls. Between Zebu breeds, however, there is a great variation in testicular size, with the milk breed having the smallest testicle. The size and type of the prepuce also vary greatly between Zebu breeds. In some breeds the prepuce is short while in others it is large and pendulous and has a generally ventral projection of the orifice. This trait often leads to trauma, which may result in fibrosis, stenosis or paraphimosis. Since the large size and the more pendulous nature of the prepuce in Zebu bulls are highly heritable, these preputial diseases should be avoided by selective breeding. The prognosis of corrective surgery for bulls with stenosis of the prepuce depends on the extent of the lesion. Sometimes surgery may lead to shortening of the preputial lining, thereby causing difficulty in extension of the penis.

The glands and the sigmoid flexure of the penis are similar in size, and the accessory glands of the genital tract are similar in consistency and size in Zebu and taurine bulls.

LIBIDO AND SEMEN COLLECTION

Zebu bulls show libido and mating ability later in life than taurine bulls. At sexual maturity, the reaction of the Zebu bull to the cow is similar to that of the taurine bull, although the former has often been reported to show little "libido." Assess-

Table 2. Comparative Frequencies of Functional Disturbances Detected in the Genital Organs of 218 Zebu Bulls and 175 Taurine Bulls Raised in Similar Environment*

Description	Bos indicus†		Bos taurus‡	
	No. of Cases	Per cent	No. of Cases	Per cent
Testicular degeneration	46	21.1	102	58.2
Retarded sexual maturity	82	37.5	26	14.9
Orchitis	6	2.8	4	2.3
Testicular fibrosis	2	0.9	9	5.1
Testicular hypoplasia	25	11.5	12	6.9
Cryptorchidism	1	0.5	1	0.6
Abnormal spermatogenesis	11	5.1	3	1.7
Epididymal dysfunction	17	7.8	4	2.3
Sperm decapitation (consistent)	4	1.8	1	0.6
Sperm granuloma	—	—	1	0.6
Seminal vesiculitis	13	6.0	4	2.3
Posthitis	7	3.2	2	1.1
Penis defects (deviation, torsion)	4	1.8	6	3.4

*Pasture-bred in Brazil (at 14° to 24° latitudes, 40° to 60° longitudes) of standard pedigree
†Total examined 538
‡Total examined 278

ment of the bulls used in AI centers for libido and mating ability indicates that the mating behavior of the Zebu bull is subject to misinterpretation. As the first sign of interest in the cow in estrus, the Zebu bull touches her (or even another male) from behind and emits intermittent grunting noises, followed by the Flehmen response. After that, he suddenly mounts the cow or the teaser mount with the penis completely extended and ready to ejaculate. Sometimes an abbreviated pre-ejaculation behavior may be confused with mating indifference.

The interval between the libido manifestation and completion of ejaculation in bulls used in AI centers is longer in Zebu compared with that in taurine bulls, the former taking 10 to 20 minutes while the latter take 5 to 10 minutes after the signs of preliminary excitement are detected. Artificial insemination centers with 100 to 200 Zebu bulls regularly collect semen twice a week using an artificial vagina with two ejaculations each time.

SEMEN QUALITY

It is possible to divide Zebu bulls that produce usable semen for AI into three categories. The first category consists of bulls that show 80 to 90 per cent motile spermatozoa, with high vigor and con-

Table 3. Comparative Frequencies of Functional Disturbances Detected in the Genital Organs of 213 Zebu Bulls and 155 Taurine Bulls Belonging to Highly Selected and Well Managed Herds from Similar Environment*

Description	Bos indicus†		Bos taurus‡	
	No. of Cases	Per cent	No. of Cases	Per cent
Testicular degeneration	64	30.0	78	50.3
Retarded sexual maturity	22	10.3	8	5.2
Orchitis	1	0.5	1	0.6
Testicular fibrosis	8	3.9	2	1.3
Testicular hypoplasia	31	14.5	22	14.2
Abnormal spermiogenesis (knobbed; diadem)	13	6.0	16	10.4
Epididymal dysfunction (mid piece and tail defects)	36	16.9	5	3.2
Sperm decapitation (consistent)	5	2.3	2	1.3
Abnormal sperm maturation (proximal cytoplasmic droplets)	9	4.3	8	5.2
Sperm granuloma	1	0.5	1	0.6
Low sperm motility (with normal morphology)	19	8.9	8	5.2
Seminal vesiculitis	1	0.5	1	0.6
Posthitis	3	1.4	—	—
Penis defects (deviation, torsion)	—	—	3	1.9

*Examined for selection at Artificial Insemination Center in Sertaozinho, Brazil (14° to 24° latitudes, 40° to 60° longitudes)
†Total examined 511
‡Total examined 320

centration of 1.0 to 1.2 million sperm cells per ml and a 5- to 10-ml ejaculate. This category exhibits good sperm morphology with less than 5 per cent of head anomalies and no more than 10 per cent total spermatozoal abnormalities. This type of semen freezes well and is produced by 25 per cent of the bulls. The second category presents an intermediate pattern of semen quality, with 60 to 80 per cent of semen usable after freezing, and comprises 50 per cent of Zebu bulls. In the third group of Zebu bulls, only 40 to 60 per cent of the semen is usable after freezing, although the spermatozoa may be physiologically and morphologically normal.

PATHOLOGY OF THE MALE REPRODUCTIVE TRACT

Pathologic conditions seen in taurine bulls have generally been diagnosed in Zebu bulls as well. Reproductive pathology in Zebu and taurine bulls raised under similar environmental conditions in central Brazil was compared to study the impact of nutrition and management on the type and incidence of lesions detected in these two species. The most frequent problems detected in Zebu bulls were delayed sexual maturation, degeneration and hypoplasia of the testes and spermatozoal abnormalities remniscent of epididymal dysfunction.[18] In the taurine bulls of this study, testicular degeneration was the most common lesion observed (Table 2), while other types of lesions were relatively rare. A similar comparison of highly selected bulls of Zebu and taurine species showed (Table 3) that testicular hypoplasia and testicular degeneration increased in frequency in the Zebu bulls with inbreeding while the incidence of problems related to nutrition and management were relatively low. The incidence of testicular hypoplasia is increased in bulls of both species despite good nutrition and management when intense genetic selection is used.

References

1. Adeyemo O, Akpokodje UU, Odili PI: Control of estrus in *Bos indicus* and *Bos taurus* heifers with prostaglandin $F_{2\alpha}$. Theriogenology 12(5):255, 1979.

2. Basile JR: Genital anomalies of development in Zebu cows, in Minas Gerais State. MS Thesis, Veterinary College, UFMG, Belo Horizonte-MG, Brazil, 1971.

3. Basile JR, Benedito VA: Estrus cycle synchronization in Nelore cows with prostaglandin F_2 analogue (ICI-80.996-Cloprostenol) by intramuscular route. Rev Bras Reprod Anim 3(4):7, 1979.

4. Bezerra CA: Clinical, histopathologic and genetic aspects of the follicular cysts, in a Gir herd. MS Thesis, Veterinary College, UFMG, Belo Horizonte-MG, Brazil, 1981.

5. Bhattacharya S, Chowdhury TM: Observations on oestrus cycle in five breeds of Indian dairy heifers. Indian Vet J 42:503, 1965.

6. Chowdhury G, Luktuke SN, Sharma UD: Studies on the pattern of oestrous cycle in Hariana heifers. Indian Vet J 42:581, 1965.

7. Costa AC, Megale F: Occurrence of ovarian pathological changes in the genital tracts of slaughtered Zebu cows of Goias and Minas Gerais States. Arq Esc Vet-UFMG, Brazil 30(3):376, 1978.

8. Fonseca VO, Norte AL, Chow LA, Lima OP: Effects of suckling intensity on postpartum reproductive efficiency of Zebu cows. Arq Esc Vet-UFMG, Brazil, 33(1):165, 1981.

9. Gurnani M, Bhatmagar DS, Nair PG: Performance of crossbreds as compared to their Zebu dams at the National Dairy Research Institute, Karnal. Indian Vet 48:1131, 1971.

10. Irvin, HJ, Randel RD, Haensly WE, Sorensen AM Jr: Reproductive studies of Brahman cattle. III. Comparison of weight, progesterone content, histological characteristics, and 3β-hydroxy-steroid dehydrogenase activity in corpora lutea of Brahman, Hereford and Brahman × Hereford heifers. Theriogenology 10(6):417, 1978.

11. Kumar SSR: A report on some important economic traits on Red Sindhi and Jersey Grades. Indian Vet J 46:965, 1969.

12. Megale F, Conto GS: Anatomical aspects of the genital tract of slaughtered Zebu cows. Arq Esc Vet UFMG, Brazil 12:529, 1959.

13. Pereira JCC: Genetic improvement applied to domestic animals. Ed Esc Vet UFMG, Brazil 1983.

14. Pires MFA: Alterations in the body and horns of uterus of slaughtered Zebu cows, in Minas Gerais. MS Thesis, Veterinary College UFMG, Belo Horizonte MG, Brazil, 1981.

15. Randel RD: LH and ovulation in Brahman, Brahman × Hereford and Hereford heifers. J Anim Sci 43:300, 1976.

16. Randel RD, Mosely WM: Serum luteinizing hormone surge and progesterone near estrus in Brahman compared to Brahman × Hereford and Hereford heifers. Proc Soc Anim Sci 199, 1977.

17. Simplicio AA, Chow LA, Santiago ED, Resende HS: Control of the estrus cycle in the bovine. II. Treatment with "Estrumate" by intramuscular route. Rev Bras Reprod Anim 2(3):37, 1978.

18. Vale-Filho VR, Pinto PA;, Megale F, et al.: Fertility of the bull in Brazil. Proceedings of the Ninth International Congress Animal Reproduction and AI, Madrid 2:273; 4:545, 1980.

19. Vighio GH: Gross pathological studies on the female genitalia of cattle and buffalo. MS Thesis, Sind Agriculture University Tandojam, Pakistan, 1980.

20. Warmling I: Annual Report of Agricultural Ministry of Brazil, DFIMA (Brasilia-DF), 1982.

Reproduction in the Water Buffalo

M. R. Jainudeen, B.V.Sc., M.S., Ph.D.
University Pertanian Malaysia,
Serdang, Selangor, Malaysia

The water buffalo *(Bubalus bubalis),* the African wild buffalo *(Syncerus caffer)* and the North American "buffalo" *(Bison bison)* are in the same family Bovidae but belong to different genera, have different chromosome numbers, and interbreeding between them appears not to be possible.

As a source of draft power, milk and meat, water buffaloes are among the most important domestic ruminants in more than 40 countries. The world buffalo population is approximately 150 million or one-eighth the population of cattle. The water buffalo has a predilection for water and is classified as swamp or river buffalo according to its wallowing habits. The swamp buffalo, with a diploid chromosome number of 48, serves as a draft animal in the eastern half of Asia, whereas the river buffalo, with a diploid chromosome number of 50, is primarily a dairy animal in the western half of Asia.

EXAMINATION OF THE REPRODUCTIVE SYSTEM

Female

Rectal Palpation. The female internal reproductive organs of water buffalo are similar to those of cattle in structure and location, but the cervix is less conspicuous, the uterine horns are more coiled, and the ovaries are firmly attached.

Physiological changes in the ovaries and the uterus may be detected by rectal examination. The cyclic corpus luteum of the buffalo is smaller and more difficult to palpate than in cattle. Follicles can be palpated, but some protrude above the surface of the ovary and may be mistaken for a corpus luteum. Rectal diagnosis of ovarian contents in the buffalo is 60 to 80 per cent accurate. The uterine horns are turgid and coiled and have marked tone during estrus but are flaccid and lack tone during diestrus. Rectal examination is the preferred method for the diagnosis of pregnancy and involution of the postpartum uterus.

Among the pathologic conditions that can be diagnosed per rectum are inactive smooth ovaries, follicular or luteal cysts, adhesions and inflammation of the ovarian adnexa, pyometra, metritis and cervicitis.

Laparoscopy. A more detailed examination of the ovaries, ovarian bursa and oviduct can be made by laparoscopy through the right paralumbar fossa with the cow in the standing position using a zero degree vision laparoscope (10 mm diameter and 600 mm long).

Male

The clinical examination of the male buffalo consists of inspection and palpation of the penis, prepuce and scrotum and its contents (testes and epididymis) followed by rectal palpation of the prostate gland, seminal vesicles and ampulla. Most males can be examined with minimal restraint. In the normal buffalo male, the location and clinical findings of the various reproductive organs are similar to those in the bull, but the testes and scrotum are smaller in size.

Semen Evaluation

Semen for evaluation is obtained with a bovine artificial vagina or by electroejaculation. For collection with the artificial vagina, the teaser may be either a female or a castrated buffalo male. At collection, the water jacket temperature of the artificial vagina should be 40 to 42°C, and the pressure within the artificial vagina is adjusted by blowing air. Allowing the animal two to three false mounts before the actual collection increases sperm concentration. Erection, extension and mounting occur in quick succession, followed by intromission and ejaculation lasting 20 to 30 seconds.

Although difficult, semen samples may be obtained by electroejaculation with a tubular rectal probe that has three electrodes on the ventral surface (Lane, Pulsator IIB). With experience, semen samples can be collected that are similar both in quality and quantity to those obtained with an artificial vagina. Electroejaculation is useful for collection from buffalo males under range conditions. Recently, rectal massage of the ampullae has yielded semen samples from buffaloes. This collection technique should be further investigated.

Much more information pertaining to semen characteristics is available for the river than the swamp buffalo (Table 1). The normal ejaculate collected with an artificial vagina is grayish to milky white in color, rarely exceeds 5 ml and has a concentration of 500 to 1500 million spermatozoa per milliliter. Sperm motility is lower in buffalo semen than in cattle semen.

Normal ejaculates frequently contain 5 to 20 per cent abnormal spermatozoa. In the past, breeding soundness examinations were based on semen char-

Table 1. Semen Characteristics of Water Buffalo

Characteristic	River Buffalo	Swamp Buffalo
Age at first collection (months)	24–72	24–72
Volume of ejaculate (ml)	3–5	2–4
General motility (%)	70–90	60–80
Progressive motility (%)	65–85	60–70
Live spermatozoa (%)	70–85	60–70
Normal acrosome (%)	80–95	80–90
Sperm concentration ($\times 10^9$/ml)	0.6–1.5	0.3–1.5
Sperm abnormalities (%)	2–14	6–15

acteristics, but a breeding soundness examination system is needed that includes scrotal circumference as an indicator of potential sperm production, the percentage of abnormal spermatozoa and sperm motility.

PUBERTY

The buffalo reaches puberty at a later age than cattle. Female puberty or age at first estrus and ovulation is difficult to establish due to problems of estrus detection. Most estimates have been extrapolated from age at first calving. First estrus occurs at 15 to 18 months in the river buffalo and 21 to 24 months in the swamp buffalo, but conception does not occur until an average body weight of 250 to 275 kg is attained at about 24 to 36 months for river and swamp buffaloes respectively (Table 2). In the male, spermatogenesis commences at 12 to 15 months in both buffalo types, but the appearance of viable spermatozoa in the ejaculate is delayed until males are around 24 months of age. Because of the faster growth rates, F_1 river × swamp crossbreeds attain puberty at an earlier age than the slower growing swamp buffalo.

ESTROUS CYCLE

The buffalo female is polyestrous, with the estrous cycle lasting 21 days and estrus lasting approximately 19 to 21 hours (Table 3). Overt signs of estrus are less obvious than in cattle. Estrus is detected either by visual observation for mounting behavior or by a vasectomized buffalo fitted with a chinball marking device. Other than the acceptance of the male, signs such as swollen vulva, mucous discharge, increased frequency of urination and homosexual behavior are not reliable indicators of estrus. Estrus commences toward late evening with peak sexual activity between 6 P.M. and 6 A.M. Matings continue until late morning in the river buffalo but usually cease during daylight hours in the swamp buffalo.

It is commonly believed that "silent estrus"—ovulation not preceded by estrus—is a major problem in buffalo breeding. Those who believe in silent estrus often fail to recognize the efficiency of estrus detection in the affected herds. To state that a buffalo experienced silent estrus is incorrect unless the animal was observed carefully and frequently by competent observers in the days preceding ovulation. Since the incidence of silent estrus appears to be higher in herds using artificial insemination than in those using natural breeding, most cases may be related to management problems of estrus detection.

BREEDING

The breeding season in the buffalo is complex and confusing. The buffalo breeds throughout the year, but seasonal calving patterns do occur. Among the factors identified are rainfall, feed supply and high ambient temperatures. Both natural mating and artificial insemination (AI) are employed, but AI has not been widely practiced owing to difficulties in estrus detection and lowered fertility.

Table 2. Diagnosis of Cyclic Changes in the Ovaries of Water Buffalo

Day of Cycle	Ovarian Structure*	Rectal Diagnosis	Plasma Progesterone (ng/ml)
0 (Estrus)	Graafian follicle thin walled, translucent bulge on surface	Soft fluctuation	<0.02
1–2	Ovulation point raised, light red spot	Depression	0–0.6
2–4	Corpus luteum I (early) red elevation	Not palpable	0.5–0.7
4–8	Corpus luteum II (developing) dark red protrusion	Soft protrusion	0.8–2.4
8–16	Corpus luteum III (mature) a sharply demarcated red to orange protrusion	Firm, well-defined protrusion	1.2–2.3
16 ff.	Corpus luteum IV (regressing) shrunken yellow to white protrusion	Hard nodular protrusion	<0.02

*Description based on laparoscopy.

Table 3. Reproductive Parameters of the Female Water Buffalo

Parameter	River Buffalo		Swamp Buffalo	
	Mean	Range	Mean	Range
Age at puberty (months)	24	15–18	36	21–24
Estrus duration (hours)	21	11–30	19	12–24
Estrous cycle length (days)	21	18–24	21	17–24
Ovulation from beginning of estrus (hours)	30	18–45	35	27–44
Twin ovulations (%)	<1	—	1	—
Gestation length (days)	315	305–320	330	320–340
Age at first parturition (months)	40	30–48	47	39–56
Calving interval (days)	504	340–675	532	373–700
Postpartum interval to:				
Uterine involution (days)	45	15–60	28	16–39
First estrus (days)	75	35–185	90	40–275
First ovulation (days)	59	35–87	96	52–140
Conception (days)	125	85–150	180	40–400

Male sexual behavior is similar to that of domestic bulls but is less intense. Libido is suppressed during the hotter part of the day, particularly in the swamp buffalo. Sniffing of the vulva or urine and the "Flehmen" reaction precede mounting of the receptive female. Mating is brief and lasts less than 20 to 30 seconds. The ejaculatory thrust is less marked than in the bull. After ejaculation, the male dismounts slowly, and the penis is retracted gradually into the sheath. Breeding males run with the female herd either continuously throughout the year or for two restricted mating periods of 3 to 4 months. One male should be assigned to not more than 20 breeding females.

Artificial Insemination

AI is one method by which extensive breeding of buffaloes with a few proven males is possible. The availability of frozen semen with good fertility and a technique for induction of estrus has led to an international trade in semen from superior males for the improvement of indigenous populations and for crossbreeding of the swamp and river buffaloes.

Frozen Semen. Most semen for freezing is normally collected with an artificial vagina, extended in a Tris buffer containing 7 per cent glycerol and 20 per cent egg yolk, packed in 0.25 or 0.5 ml French straws, frozen over nitrogen vapor at $-120°$ to $-140°$ C for 7 minutes and stored in liquid nitrogen. The post-thaw progressive motility varies from 35 to 60 per cent. The principles and precautions for handling frozen buffalo semen and bovine semen are similar. Frozen semen is best thawed at $37°$ to $40°$ C and should be used within 5 to 10 minutes.

Insemination. Semen is deposited in the uterine body with a French inseminating gun by the rectovaginal technique. Insemination time in relation to ovulation is not well defined, but animals are usually inseminated 12 to 24 hours after the onset of estrus.

Induction of Estrus

The difficulty of detecting estrus, a major limitation to the widespread use of AI, could be overcome by two methods of estrus induction: (1) premature regression of the corpus luteum by injection of prostaglandin $F_{2\alpha}$ ($PGF_{2\alpha}$) or its synthetic analogs, or (2) prolongation of the life-span of the corpus luteum by a progesterone-releasing intravaginal device (PRID). Buffaloes are usually inseminated at a fixed time following estrus induction. However, the conception rates are low (20 and 40 per cent) and need improvement if fixed-time insemination is to replace insemination at detected estrus. These techniques depend on the presence of a corpus luteum and are of limited value in lactating or suckled buffaloes due to the high incidence of nonfunctioning ovaries (true anestrus).

Conception Rates

Most previous estimates of conception rate in the water buffalo were based on the nonreturn rate, which is unreliable due to the inherent difficulty of estrus detection. Accurate figures on conception rate based on pregnancy diagnosis are presently available for both natural service and AI. The conception rate for swamp buffaloes in a 3- to 4-month breeding season may range from 20 to 75 per cent depending on the nutritional and lactational status of the females at joining. The first service conception rate for natural service in the river buffalo has varied from 50 to 75 per cent. In AI programs conception rate is higher with chilled than with frozen semen. The conception rate for first insemination is 50 to 60 per cent with chilled semen and 25 to 45 per cent with frozen semen. Also, conception rate is lower with fixed-time inseminations than at detected estrus.

Crossbreeding

In several southeast Asian countries, attempts are being made to improve the milk yield, size and draught ability of the swamp buffalo by inseminating with chilled or frozen semen from river-type buffaloes. Cytogenetic studies have cast doubt on the fertility of the F_1 river × swamp cross because of its diploid chromosome complement of 49, which is intermediate to that of its parents—the swamp buffalo (2n = 48) and the river buffalo (2n = 50). The female F_1 hybrid is fertile and readily conceives and produces viable offspring. The male F_1 is also fertile, has normal testes, produces semen with normal quality and sire-viable calves. Present evidence favors the view that fertility is not adversely affected by crossbreeding of the two types of water buffaloes.

GESTATION

Pregnancy Maintenance

The corpus luteum of pregnancy is maintained throughout gestation, but its role in the maintenance of pregnancy is not known. Plasma progesterone levels remain elevated during pregnancy but decline to basal levels on the day of parturition. Estrus is generally suspended with the onset of pregnancy, but a small percentage of cows may exhibit one or more periods of anovulatory estrus.

Placenta

The epitheliochorial placenta is of the cotyledonary type. The convex maternal caruncles fuse with fetal cotyledons to form 60 to 90 placentomes, which are distributed in both gravid and nongravid uterine horns. As gestation advances, placentomes change from flat, plaquelike bodies to rounded, pedunculated, mushroomlike structures 5 to 7 cm in diameter.

Pregnancy Diagnosis

Rectal examination is widely used for pregnancy diagnosis. It is accurate and can be performed after 6 weeks of gestation, and the result is known immediately. The rectal findings, like those in cattle, are based on the detection of uterine enlargement, fetus or fetal membranes and fremitus in the uterine arteries. As a nonpregnancy test, the assay of progesterone levels in milk or plasma 22 to 24 days after service is expensive and has limited application under field conditions.

Length of Gestation

Compared with cattle, water buffaloes have longer gestational periods ranging from 305 to 320 days for the river buffalo and 320 to 340 for the swamp buffalo (Table 3). A swamp female carrying a fetus sired by a river type has an intermediate gestational length—315 to 325 days. Extremely short or long gestational lengths are questionable and are indicative of abortions or early embryonic mortality followed by a conception.

PARTURITION

Prepartum Changes

Among the external signs of approaching parturition are mammary enlargement and activity, hypertrophy and edema of the vulval lips, relaxation of the pelvic ligaments resulting in an elevation of the tailhead, and a string of clear mucus hanging from the vulva. The endocrine mechanism initiating parturition in the buffalo is not known, but about 15 days prior to parturition, plasma levels of both estrone and $PGF_{2\alpha}$ metabolite increase and reach peak values at 3 to 5 days prepartum. Whereas plasma progesterone levels that remained elevated through gestation decline abruptly on the day of parturition, both estrone and $PGF_{2\alpha}$ metabolite levels decline more gradualy, reaching baseline values 7 to 14 days after parturition.

Stages of Labor

The act of parturition in water buffalo resembles that in cattle. The first stage of labor—onset of uterine contractions and dilation of the cervix—lasts 1 to 2 hours and is longer in primiparous than in pluriparous buffaloes. During the second stage of labor, lasting 30 to 60 minutes, strong abdominal contractions cause the rupture of the amnion and delivery of the fetus. The fetus is delivered in anterior presentation and dorsal position with extended limbs. With the onset of the third stage of labor, abdominal straining ceases, and fetal membranes are expelled within 4 to 5 hours after delivery of the fetus.

Complications

Dystocia. Dystocia is not a serious problem in the water buffalo. The incidence of dystocia is higher in the river than in the swamp buffalo and also in primipara than in pluripara. Most cases of dystocia are due to postural abnormalities arising from flexion of the distal joints of the front limbs or deviations of the head and neck of the fetus. Fetopelvic disproportion is uncommon, but primiparous swamp buffaloes carrying river × swamp fetuses may require assistance at parturition. Torsion of the uterus may occur in river buffaloes kept in close confinement due to slipping, falling or rolling during late gestation.

Retention of Fetal Membranes. Failure of fetal membranes to be expelled within 12 to 24 hours after parturition is associated with abortions, dystocia or uterine inertia. The incidence varies from 5 to 10 per cent of calvings. A higher incidence in the river than the swamp type suggests that differences in management may be implicated. The incidence is also higher in Brucella-positive herds. The control measures for retained fetal membranes are the same as for cattle.

Uterine Prolapse. Excessive straining immediately following delivery can lead to a complete prolapse of the uterus. The condition in the swamp buffalo is very rare, but in the river buffalo the incidence in certain herds may be as high as 5 per cent. Treatment involves epidural anesthesia and replacement of the uterus to its normal position.

POSTPARTUM PERIOD

The postpartum period extends from parturition until the female returns to her normal nonpregnant state and experiences a fertile estrus. The most important physiological events are uterine involution and resumption of estrous cycles.

Uterine Involution

Immediately after delivery, lochia or uterine discharge contains mucus, blood, shreds of fetal membranes and caruncular tissue. Approximately 500 ml of lochia are discharged on the first day. It gradually decreases in volume, changes to a white mucoid discharge and ceases by day 14 to 18 postpartum. Involution of the uterus is completed by 28 to 45 days (Table 3). The rate of uterine involution is more rapid in the suckled swamp buffalo than in the milked river buffalo and is delayed in abnormal parturition.

Ovarian Activity

The corpus luteum of pregnancy regresses very rapidly and is palpable as a small hard protuberance by day 14 postpartum, secreting no progesterone. An increase in follicular activity occurs during the second month postpartum, but only a small percentage of animals ovulate. Plasma progesterone levels remain at basal levels for a variable time until the resumption of ovarian cyclicity (Fig. 1). The interval from parturition to first ovulation is approximately 35 to 87 days for milked river buffaloes and 52 to 140 days for suckled swamp buffaloes (Table 3). Once ovarian cyclicity resumes, plasma progesterone levels exhibit a cyclic pattern. The first postpartum ovulation may or may not be associated with overt signs of estrus.

REPRODUCTIVE EFFICIENCY

Over 95 per cent of buffaloes belong to small-holder farmers who do not consider it an economic

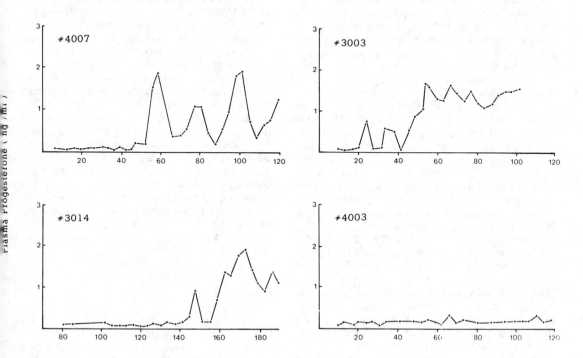

Figure 1. Plasma progesterone profiles of suckled swamp buffaloes illustrating postpartum anestrus (Buffalo no. 4003) and resumption of estrous cycle and luteal activity at day 40 (Buffalo no. 3003), day 45 (Buffalo no. 4007) and day 155 (Buffalo no. 3014) postpartum. Note that buffalo no. 3003 conceived at day 40 postpartum.

necessity to maintain breeding records. Many farmers use only the number of calves born, weaned or sold as their measures of reproductive efficiency. Lack of proper identification makes the adoption of even the simplest of recording systems difficult. In recent years, many buffalo research stations have used beef cattle fertility criteria such as conception, pregnancy or calving rates, calving intervals or calving-to-conception intervals (Table 3).

The interval between the birth of two offspring, commonly called the calving interval, is the most widely quoted fertility criterion for buffalo (Table 3). It is stated that a buffalo produces, on the average, two calves every 3 years. Conception rates are used for measurement of reproductive efficiency in AI programs (see earlier section on Artificial Insemination).

REPRODUCTIVE FAILURE

Reproductive rates in buffaloes are generally lower than those in cattle. Both infectious and noninfectious factors contribute to the long calving interval through repeat breeding, abortion, anestrus, poor semen quality and reduced male libido.

Repeat Breeding and Abortion

Of the diseases causing reproductive failure in cattle, brucellosis, leptospirosis, vibriosis, trichomoniasis and infectious bovine rhinotracheitis (IBR) are prevalent in the buffalo. Brucellosis caused by *Brucella abortus* is characterized by abortions during the latter half of gestation. Buffaloes are as susceptible to the disease as cattle. Brucellosis in buffaloes is prevalent worldwide and is an important zoonotic disease in India and Italy.

Campylobacter fetus and *Trichomonas fetus* occur in the reproductive tract of the buffalo. Also, several serologic surveys have confirmed the existence of leptospirosis *(L. pomona, L. hardjo)*. Of the viral infections, the IBR virus was isolated from buffaloes in Australia and Malaysia. These infections are recognized in cattle as causes of repeat breeding/early embryonic death, pyometra and abortion, but their role in reproductive failure in the buffalo has not been clearly defined.

Abattoir studies of river buffaloes discarded for infertility indicate a high incidence of endometritis (20 to 30 per cent) and pathologic conditions of the ovarian bursa and oviducts (5 to 20 per cent). Whether these conditions are due to nonspecific infections or to the infections mentioned earlier needs to be ascertained. The practice of inserting the hand or implements to stimulate milk letdown in some countries or the unhygienic conditions under which animals are allowed to calve could account for a considerable proportion of reproductive infections.

Postpartum Anestrus

Postpartum anestrus, or a state of ovarian acyclicity, occurs during lactation in many mammalian species. It also affects 30 to 40 per cent of lactating buffaloes and persists until calves are weaned naturally or are separated from their dams. Anestrus has been erroneously attributed to the maintenance of the corpus luteum of the previous pregnancy or the "persistence" of the corpus luteum of the first postpartum estrous cycle.

Recent studies have provided convincing evidence that the anestrus seen during suckling in the swamp buffalo is due to a failure in resumption of ovarian cyclicity (true anestrus), not to a failure of estrus detection (apparent anestrus). Plasma progesterone remains at basal levels throughout this period, and luteal levels of plasma progesterone occur after the first postpartum ovulation, which may or may not be preceded by estrus.

Postpartum anestrus has long been recognized as a serious cause of infertility in the swamp buffalo. Among the physiological factors, body condition, lactation, suckling, and age, either alone or in combination, adversely affect ovarian function. Buffaloes in poor body condition and young females in their first lactation have inactive ovaries. Anestrus is more common is suckled (swamp) than milked (river) buffaloes. The endocrine mechanism mediating this effect is unknown, but recent evidence suggests that the block to ovulation resides at the ovarian level rather than at the pituitary level.

Various hormonal preparations have been used in the treatment of postpartum anestrus—pregnant mare serum gonadotropin, human chorionic gonadotropic hormone, GnRH and progesterone—but results have been disappointing due to failure to initiate a fertile ovulation.

Management strategies are more likely to succeed in reducing the incidence of postpartum anestrus than use of hormonal therapy. Early weaning reduces the incidence of postpartum anestrus, but it may not be applicable under existing systems in which calves are used to stimulate milk let-down (river buffalo) or left unweaned (swamp buffalo). Temporary calf removal (72 hours) in the suckled buffalo, as in cattle, induces an anovulatory estrus that could be overcome by pretreatment with PRID for a 10- to 12-day period. Improvements in plane of nutrition or body condition are necessary if any method is to be effective in reducing the postpartum interval in the buffalo.

Male Infertility

Less attention has been directed toward male infertility in the swamp buffalo. Except for limited studies on semen quality of males maintained for semen collection, information is scanty on pathologic conditions of the male reproductive system. Perhaps opportunities of studying male reproduction are limited because most males are castrated at an early age for tractability, particularly the swamp buffalo. Several sperm defects have been noted, but their significance has not been established. Apparently, no significant monthly variations occur in semen characteristics of buffaloes maintained in pens provided with water sprinklers for cooling.

REPRODUCTIVE MANAGEMENT PROGRAMS

Reproductive management programs used for dairy and beef cattle could be applied with some modifications to the river (dairy) and swamp (beef) buffaloes. Such programs have been successfully adopted in well-managed, large buffalo herds in several countries.

In a reproductive management program designed for milking buffaloes (river type), animals are grouped according to lactation and pregnancy status. The lactating group includes postpartum, recently bred and pregnant animals, whereas the nonlactating group contains pregnant and problem cows. In such herds, twice-daily observations for estrus, artificial insemination and pregnancy diagnosis at 60 to 90 days after insemination can be practiced.

Buffaloes used for meat production can be subjected to breeding practices similar to those used for beef cattle. Two 3-month mating seasons can be designed to coincide with the times of the year when there is an abundance of feed combined with pregnancy diagnosis 2 months after the end of the mating season to separate pregnant from nonpregnant animals. Males should be regularly tested for breeding soundness and assigned to not more than 20 breeding females.

Developing a reproductive management program for small herds (5 to 10 animals), which account for more than 95 per cent of the buffaloes in the world, is beset with problems ranging from poor animal identification and record keeping to a lack of farmer interest. Herein lies the challenge for increasing reproductive efficiency so that the water buffalo can fulfill its potential as a source of draft, beef and milk.

References

1. Bhattacharya P: Reproduction. In Cockrill WS (ed.): The Husbandry and Health of the Domestic Buffalo. Rome, Food and Agriculture Organization of the United Nations, 1974.
2. Jainudeen MR, Bongso TA, Bashir Ahmad F, Sharifuddin W: A laparoscopic technique for *in vivo* observation of ovaries in the water buffalo *(Bubalus bubalis)*. Vet Rec 111:32, 1982.
3. Jainudeen MR, Bongso TA, Tan HS: Postpartum ovarian activity and uterine involution in the suckled swamp buffalo *(Bubalus bubalis)*. Anim Reprod Sci 5:181, 1983.
4. Singh M, Matharoo JS, Chauhan FS: Preliminary results with frozen buffalo semen using Tris extender. Theriogenology 13:191, 1980.

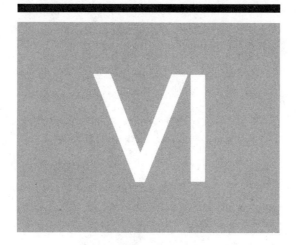

SECTION

VI

CANINE

**Shirley D. Johnston, D.V.M., Ph.D.,
Patricia N. Olson, D.V.M., Ph.D.**

Consulting Editors

Reproductive Endocrinology and Physiology of the Bitch

Patricia N. Olson, D.V.M., Ph.D.
Terry M. Nett, Ph.D.
Colorado State University, Fort Collins, Colorado

Much has been learned about the reproductive endocrinology and physiology of dogs since Heape[10] first described the "sexual season" of the bitch over 80 years ago. The reproductive cycle of the bitch, classified as monestrus, is unique in several aspects. The follicular phase, period of sexual receptivity and luteal phase are longer than those found in most other domestic animals. After a lengthy luteal stage (diestrus), the bitch enters a stage of sexual quiescence (anestrus). Although some other domesticated species have an anestrous stage in their reproductive cycles, the dog is unique in that anestrus in the bitch occurs independent of season[24-26] except for the basenji,[15] which cycles annually in the fall.

DEFINITIONS

The classical stages of the canine estrous cycle introduced by Heape in 1900 were proestrus (the beginning of the sexual season), estrus (the period of sexual receptivity), metestrus (the period of subsiding activity) and anestrus (the period of reproductive quiescence). In recent years the term metestrus has been largely replaced by the term diestrus. Diestrus is the period following estrus, when the uterus is under the primary influence of progesterone. Therefore, the term diestrus more appropriately describes the luteal phase of the canine reproductive cycle, since metestrus denotes either the time when concentrations of progesterone in the serum are increasing at the greatest rate (which occurs during estrus in the bitch) or the time when leukocytes rapidly invade the vaginal wall (which occurs only for a few days in early diestrus for most dogs). Conversely, Heape described diestrus as that period of the reproductive cycle immediately followed by another follicular phase (e.g., proestrus), which does not occur in the bitch. Although it may be scientifically more correct to refer to the follicular, luteal and quiescent stages of the canine estrous cycle, identifying proestrus, estrus and diestrus is clinically important in determining stages relating to sexual receptivity and breeding management. For the purpose of this article, *behavorial diestrus* will be used to describe the stage of the canine estrous cycle that begins the first day after a period of receptivity (estrus) when a bitch refuses a male. *Cytologic diestrus* will be used to describe the stage that begins the first day when a significant change occurs in vaginal smears from smears obtained during estrus (see the article Vaginal Cytology in the Bitch).

The duration of diestrus, based on luteal function, is similar for nonpregnant and pregnant bitches. Therefore, all nonpregnant bitches (whether mated or not) are considered to be pseudopregnant. Breast development may be noted, since progesterone is elevated in both the nonpregnant and pregnant dog and enhances alveolar development of mammary tissue in both groups of animals. Other than enlarging mammae (which can vary considerably among bitches), the owner may be unaware of the false pregnancy.

Once serum progesterone concentrations fall to less than 1 or 2 ng/ml, diestrus and pseudopregnancy cease. It is at the termination of pseudopregnancy that overt signs of motherhood may begin. As progesterone falls, concentrations of prolactin dramatically increase in pregnant dogs[6] and are also elevated in some pseudopregnant dogs (unpublished observation). Prolactin aids in initiating lactation and is probably responsible for a bitch mothering toys or other small objects. Since signs of motherhood begin at the *termination* of pseudopregnancy, such overt signs should probably be referred to as pseudoparturition rather than pseudopregnancy. It is still unclear why some nonpregnant bitches manifest few or no signs of motherhood at the termination of pseudopregnancy, whereas others intensely lactate and nest.

PUBERTY

The bitch enters puberty between 6 and 24 months of age; however, most animals do not reach their maximal reproductive potential until the third or fourth estrus. Individuals of small breeds enter puberty earlier than larger breeds, with the onset of a season correlating with the time an animal reaches a growth plateau.[26]

The estrous cycle in puberal bitches may differ from that of mature dogs. "Split heats" are occasionally observed in puberal bitches and rarely in adults. Bitches manifesting split heats exhibit vulvar swelling and a serosanguineous discharge passing from the vagina, and they may or may not become receptive to mating. This is followed by regression of vulvar size and cessation of the vaginal discharge for a few weeks until the bitch enters her "true" season and ovulates. Conception frequently follows a mating during the second (ovulatory) but not the first (anovulatory) part of a split heat.

Lack of sexual receptivity and reduced or inconsistent patterns of circulating concentrations of 17-β estradiol, luteinizing hormone (LH) or progesterone also reportedly occur in some puberal cycles.[29] The ability of puberal bitches to display normal cycles appears to be related to age, since animals that exhibit normal sexual behavior and endocrine profiles tend to be older than females with aberrant patterns. Although puberal bitches may refuse to be mated, ovulation frequently occurs.[29] It is probably wise to advise owners to delay breeding a bitch until at least her second estrus. This assures that a physically mature bitch will be mated during a normal estrous cycle.

THE CANINE ESTROUS CYCLE

Proestrus

In dogs proestrus has been defined as that stage of the reproductive cycle prior to estrus when a bitch attracts males, but is not receptive to mating. Frequently, a serosanguineous discharge passes from a swollen, turgid vulva. The average duration of proestrus is 9 days but can range from 0 to 17 days. Concentrations of 17-β estradiol rise in the serum of proestrous bitches and usually peak before late proestrus. Most investigators agree that peak concentrations of 17-β estradiol occur 1 to 2 days before the end of proestrus and are declining when acceptance is first observed[4,8,12,17,18,28] (Fig. 1). Serum concentrations of progesterone remain low prior to and during the first few days of proestrus. During the 2 to 3 days prior to acceptance there is a slight increase in concentrations of progesterone[2,4,9,13,18,21,28] (Fig. 2). This increase appears to be related to the preovulatory luteinization of ovarian follicles.[5,21] Concentrations of testosterone also increase in the

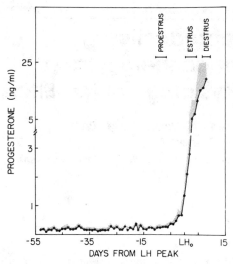

Figure 2. Concentrations of progesterone in canine serum throughout late anestrus, proestrus, estrus and early diestrus. Stippled area is SEM. (⊢—⊣ = range of proestrus, estrus and diestrus). (Reprinted with permission, Olson PN, et al.: Biol Repro 27:1196, 1982.)

serum of bitches during late proestrus and estrus, and may approach concentrations found in stud dogs[19] (Fig. 3). Whether such an increase merely reflects increased steroidogenesis or is important for normal physiological events (e.g., behavioral estrus, target tissue proliferation) is still unclear. Serum concentrations of LH remain near baseline during most of proestrus although increased concentrations of LH above basal levels have been reported to occur during late anestrus[18] or early proestrus[27] in some bitches (Fig. 4). Serum concentrations of follicle-stimulating hormone (FSH) appear to be at their lowest during late proestrus[18] and again follow-

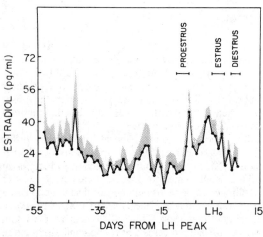

Figure 1. Concentrations of estradiol in canine serum throughout late anestrus, proestrus, estrus and early diestrus. Stippled area is SEM. (⊢—⊣ = range of onset of proestrus, estrus and diestrus). (Reprinted with permission, Olson PN, et al.: Biol Repro 27:1196, 1982.)

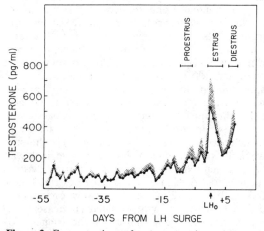

Figure 3. Concentrations of testosterone in canine serum throughout late anestrus, proestrus, estrus and early diestrus. Stippled area is SEM. (⊢—⊣ = range of onset of proestrus, estrus and diestrus). (Reprinted with permission, AJVR. Accepted, 1983.)

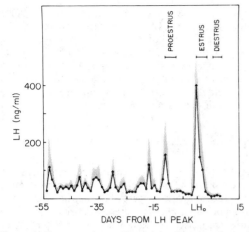

Figure 4. Concentrations of luteinizing hormone in canine serum throughout late anestrus, proestrus, estrus and early diestrus. Stippled area is SEM. (⊢—⊣ = range of proestrus, estrus and diestrus). (Reprinted with permission, Olson PN, et al.: Biol Repro 27:1196, 1982.)

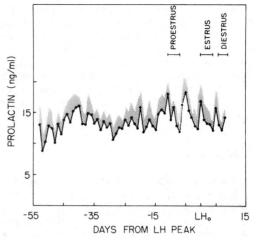

Figure 6. Concentrations of prolactin in canine serum throughout late anestrus, proestrus, estrus and early diestrus. Stippled area is SEM. (⊢—⊣ = range of proestrus, estrus and diestrus). (Reprinted with permission, Olson PN, et al.: Biol Repro 27:1196, 1982.)

ing the FSH surge (Fig. 5). Prolactin appears variable throughout proestrus,[18] although one report suggested that a prolactin surge might occur near the end of proestrus,[14] possibly increasing coincident with elevated concentrations of estradiol at this time (Fig. 6).

Estrus

Estrus is that period of the reproductive cycle characterized by the bitch's acceptance of the male. This period normally lasts for about 9 days but can range from 3 to 21 days. The bitch appears to become receptive to the male after serum concentrations of 17-β estradiol are beginning to fall and concentrations of progesterone are beginning to

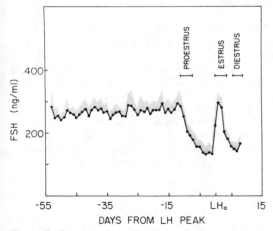

Figure 5. Concentrations of follicle stimulating hormone in canine serum throughout late anestrus, proestrus, estrus and early diestrus. Stippled area is SEM. (⊢—⊣ = range of proestrus, estrus, and diestrus). (Reprinted with permission, Olson PN, et al.: Biol Repro 27:1196, 1982.)

rise. This hypothesis is supported by data obtained after administration of 17-β estradiol alone or followed by progesterone to ovariectomized bitches.[3] Behavioral estrus was not displayed until after the administration of the 17-β estradiol was halted, and the onset of estrous behavior was more synchronous when progesterone was administered at the time of estrogen withdrawal. Similarly, the preovulatory surge of LH appears to be mediated by the decline in serum concentrations of 17-β estradiol with a concomitant rise in concentrations of progesterone.[7] Some investigators have reported that the preovulatory surge of LH occurs on the first day of estrus.[17,22] Others have found no correlation between the preovulatory surge of LH and the onset of estrus.[16,27] The duration of the preovulatory surge of LH in the bitch appears to vary, with periods ranging from 24 to 96 hours reported.[9,13,18,20,24,26] There is a surge in serum concentrations of FSH that occurs coincidentally with or 1 or 2 days after the preovulatory LH surge.[18,22]

Ovulation in the bitch can occur from 0 to 96 hours after the LH peak, although most ovulations occur between 24 and 72 hours after maximum serum concentrations of LH are noted. Whether ovulations occur only after the onset of estrus in mature bitches, or whether some can occur during late proestrus, has not been resolved. Although puberal bitches may refuse to be mated, ovulations reportedly can occur.[29]

As mentioned previously, serum concentrations of progesterone begin rising during late proestrus. This gradual rise continues until after the LH surge, when serum concentrations of progesterone undergo a more rapid increase for approximately 10 days.[5,17,18,22,23,27] The bitch appears unique in that behavioral estrus is exhibited in the face of high concentrations of progesterone. There is no corpus hemorrhagicum formed in the bitch at ovulation, possibly owing to the rather extensive luteinization prior to ovulation. Unlike most other species, the bitch ovulates a primary oocyte rather than a secondary oocyte. The first meiotic division begins about 1 day after ovulation, usually in the midportion of the oviduct. Oocyte maturation is complete within 3 days after ovulation. Once maturation is complete, the viable life span of the secondary oocyte is approximately 24 hours.

DIESTRUS

Behaviorally, the onset of diestrus is defined as the first day after a period of estrus that a bitch refuses a male. There is a sharp decline in superficial cells on vaginal smears obtained from bitches about 3 days prior to the end of estrus. It has been suggested that the onset of diestrus be defined by the decline in superficial cells rather than by behavior. There is merit to this suggestion, since the LH peak, ovulation, oocyte maturation and whelping can be timed more accurately using the disappearance of superficial cells from the vaginal epithelium as a marker rather than using breeding or the end of behavioral estrus.[11]

During early diestrus, serum concentrations of progesterone continue to increase until approximately day 15 of diestrus. After this time serum concentrations of progesterone begin a gradual decrease that continues for 5 to 6 weeks. The progesterone profile is very similar for pregnant, nonmated and hysterectomized bitches[20] (Fig. 7). Therefore, it is unlikely that the canine uterus plays a vital role in maintenance or regression of the corpora lutea. The exact mechanism(s) for luteal regression in the dog are unknown. Although luteal function ceases in hypophysectomized bitches, the regression that normally occurs at the end of the luteal phase does not occur as a result of LH withdrawal, since concentrations of LH appear to increase in the serum near the end of diestrus.[1,20] Similarly, uterine prostaglandins are unlikely mediators of luteal maintenance or regression, since hysterectomized dogs have a luteal phase similar to that seen in intact bitches. Clearly, this is one area of canine reproduction requiring more study.

ANESTRUS

Although for years anestrus has been referred to as the quiescent phase of the canine reproductive cycle, recent work suggests that neither the ovary nor the pituitary gland is quiescent during anestrus.[18] Concentrations of estradiol may decrease prior to the onset of proestrus from those earlier in anestrus (Fig. 1). The decrease in estradiol appears to occur at about the same time concentrations of LH increase (10 to 15 days before the preovulatory LH peak) (Fig. 4). Concentrations of FSH are high in the serum of anestrous bitches, comparable to those found during the FSH surge (Fig. 5). Concentrations of progesterone and testosterone are at baseline levels during late anestrus, and concentrations of prolactin are variable in the serum of bitches sampled throughout anestrus, proestrus and estrus (Figs. 2, 3 and 6). Although the mechanisms for terminating anestrus and initiating a new follicular phase are still not completely understood, concentrations of LH appear to increase prior to the onset of proestrus and may be important in inducing a new follicular phase. Clearly, concentrations of FSH are high during anestrus. Therefore, the dog appears to have sufficient FSH present during anestrus for follicular growth. This may explain the apparent lack of success in inducing a fertile estrus in the bitch with FSH.

SUMMARY

There are many aspects of canine reproductive physiology that are still incompletely understood. If the mechanism of luteal regression could be established, perhaps a safe and efficacious abortifacient could be developed for use in mismated bitches. If the exact mechanisms for terminating anestrus were known, a method for inducing a fertile estrus might be established. If canine pituitary cells producing gonadotropins could be manipulated, a better contraceptive might emerge. Clearly, more research is needed in the area of canine reproduction.

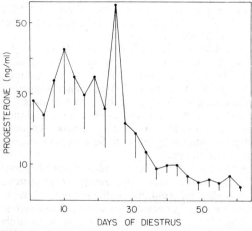

Figure 7. Concentrations of progesterone in the serum of six hysterectomized bitches during the luteal phase following surgery. (Standard deviation given at each point with vertical lines.) (Reprinted with permission from AJVR.)

References

1. Chakraborty PK, Panko WB, Seager SWJ: Hormone levels during the estrous cycle, pregnancy and pseudopregnancy in the Labrador bitch. Proc 70th Ann Am Soc Anim Sci Mtg (abstr). 337:349, 1978.
2. Chakraborty PK, Panko WB, Fletcher WS: Serum hormone concentrations and their relationships to sexual behavior at

the first and second estrous cycles of the Labrador bitch. Biol Reprod 22:227, 1980.

3. Concannon PW, Hansel W: Effects of estrogen and progesterone on plasma LH, sexual behavior, and pregnancy in Beagle bitches. Fed Proc 34:323, 1975.
4. Concannon PW, Hansel W, Visek WJ: The ovarian cycle of the bitch: Plasma estrogen, LH and progesterone. Biol Reprod 13:112, 1975.
5. Concannon PW, Hansel W, McEntee K: Changes in LH, progesterone and sexual behavior associated with preovulatory luteinization in the bitch. Biol Reprod 17:604, 1977.
6. Concannon PW, Butler WR, Hansel W, et al.: Parturition and lactation in the bitch: Serum progesterone, cortisol and prolactin. Biol Reprod 19:1113, 1978.
7. Concannon PW, Cowan R, Hansel W: LH release in ovariectomized dogs in response to estrogen withdrawal and its facilitation by progesterone. Biol Reprod 20:523, 1979.
8. Edqvist LE, Johansson EDB, Kasstrom H, et al.: Blood plasma levels of progesterone and oestradiol in the dog during the oestrous cycle and pregnancy. Acta Endocrinol 78:554, 1975.
9. Hadley JC: Total unconjugated oestrogen and progesterone concentrations in peripheral blood during the oestrus cycle of the dog. J Reprod Fertil 44:445, 1975.
10. Heape W: The sexual season of mammals and the relationship of "pro-estrus" to menstruation. Part I. Quart J Micro Sci 44:1, 1900.
11. Holst PA, Phemister RD: Onset of diestrus in the Beagle bitch. Definition and significance. Am J Vet Res 35:401, 1974.
12. Holst PA, Phemister RD: Temporal sequence of events in the estrous cycle of the bitch. Am J Vet Res 36:705, 1975.
13. Jones GE, Boyns AR, Cameron EHD, et al.: Plasma oestradiol, luteinizing hormone and progesterone during the oestrus cycle in the beagle bitch. J Endocrinol 5:331, 1973.
14. Jones GE, Brownstone AD, Boyns AR: Isolation of canine prolactin by polyacrylamide gel electrophoresis. Acta Endocrinol 82:691, 1976.
15. McDonald LE: Reproductive patterns in dogs. In McDonald LE (ed): Veterinary Endocrinology and Reproduction. Philadelphia, Lea & Febiger, 1969, pp 377–385.
16. Mellin TN, Orczyk GP, Hichens M, Behrman HR: Serum profiles of luteinizing hormone, progesterone and total estrogens during the canine estrous cycle. Theriogenology 5:175, 1976.
17. Nett TM, Akbar AM, Phemister RD, et al.: Levels of luteinizing hormone, estradiol and progesterone in serum during the estrous cycle and pregnancy in the Beagle bitch. Proc Soc Exp Biol Med 148:134, 1975.
18. Olson PN, Bowen RA, Behrendt MD, et al.: Concentrations of reproductive hormones in canine serum throughout late anestrus, proestrus and estrus. Biol Reprod 27:1196, 1982.
19. Olson PN, Bowen RA, Behrendt MD, et al.: Concentrations of testosterone in canine serum throughout late anestrus, proestrus, estrus and early diestrus. Am J Vet Res 45:149, 1984.
20. Olson PN, Bowen RA, Behrendt MD, et al.: Concentrations of progesterone and LH in the serum of diestrous bitches before and after hysterectomy. Am J Vet Res 45:149, 1984.
21. Phemister RD, Holst PA, Spano JS, Hopwood ML: Time of ovulation in the Beagle bitch. Biol Reprod 8:74, 1973.
22. Reimers TJ, Phemister RD, Niswender GD: Radioimmunological measurement of follicle stimulating hormone and prolactin in the dog. Biol Reprod 19:673, 1978.
23. Smith MS, McDonald LE: Serum levels of luteinizing hormone and progesterone during the estrous cycle, pseudopregnancy and pregnancy in the dog. Endocrinology 94:404, 1974.
24. Smith WC, Reese WC Jr: Characteristics of a Beagle colony. I. Estrous cycle. Lab Anim Care 18:602, 1968.
25. Sokolowski JH: Reproductive features and patterns in the bitch. JAAHA 9:71, 1973.
26. Sokolowski JH: Reproductive patterns in the bitch. Vet Clin North Am 7:653, 1977.
27. Wildt DE, Chakraborty PK, Danko WB, Seager SWJ: Relationship of reproductive behavior, serum luteinizing hormone and time of ovulation in the bitch. Biol Reprod 18:561, 1978.
28. Wildt DE, Panko WB, Chakraborty PK, Seager SW: Relationship of serum estrone, estradiol 17-β, and progesterone to LH, sexual behavior, and time of ovulation. Biol Reprod 20:648, 1979.
29. Wildt DE, Seager WJ, Chakraborty PK: Behavioral, ovarian and endocrine relationships in the pubertal bitch. J Anim Sci 53:182, 1981.

Vaginal Cytology in the Bitch

Phyllis A. Holst, M.S., D.V.M.

Longmont, Colorado

Vaginal exfoliative cytology is the most useful clinical laboratory tool we have to understand and to manage breeding in dogs. When we are misled by the bitch's behavior, are in doubt about the significance of her discharge or wonder whether she is really in estrus because of a marginal amount of vulvar swelling, cytology can always help to define her reproductive status.

The principle of vaginal cytology is simple. The vaginal epithelium is responsive to levels of estradiol, and it changes from a bistratified cuboidal epithelium to a stratified squamous epithelium of greater than 30 cell layers with every estrous cycle. Early in proestrus, undoubtedly before proestrus is detectable clinically, the number of cell layers increases, and a gradual transition to a mature stratified squamous epithelium occurs. During late proestrus and most of estrus the epithelium is maintained. Presumably, the function of the epithelium is similar to that of the skin or some other similar membranes—mechanical protection, in this case for coitus. Late in estrus, at a constant interval following ovulation,[6] and because of the loss of estradiol stimulation, the epithelium returns rather quickly to its interestrous condition. When we examine a vaginal smear we are seeing cells exfoliated from the surface of the epithelium at that particular time. The stage of the cycle, whether or not the cycle is normal, the presence of infection and the presence of spermatozoa (to confirm breeding or a misalliance) are easily determined by vaginal cytology.

PREPARATION OF VAGINAL SMEARS

Materials Needed

1. Glass microscope slides, frosted-end preferred
2. Blunt-ended glass pipette with rubber bulb (Pasteur pipette with tapered end cut off and fire-polished is ideal) or sterile cotton-tipped swabs
3. Isotonic saline solution
4. Stain, any suitable for blood smears
5. Microscope, 100 × magnification

Procedure

Labelling of Slide. Write on the frosted slide with a lead pencil. Include the full date, bitch's name and other helpful information, such as day of heat and bred that day.

Sample Collection

Pipette Method. A small column of saline (approximately 1 ml) is drawn up into the pipette. The pipette is slipped its full length into the caudal vagina, taking care not to squeeze the bulb (Fig. 1). Ideally, the bitch should be lying on her side to avoid the need to hold the pipette upside down. Squeeze the bulb quickly, gently and only partially several times, to make the fluid column wash rapidly back and forth and pick up cells. Withdraw the pipette, being careful not to put pressure on the bulb. Most of the fluid may have been lost, but

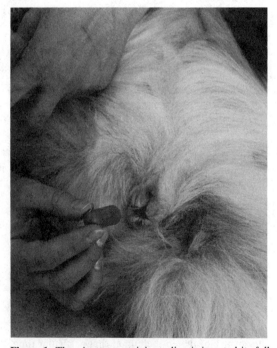

Figure 1. The pipette containing saline is inserted its full length into the caudal vagina, the bulb gently and partially squeezed several times to collect a sample of cells, and then withdrawn. The bitch is in dorsal or lateral recumbency.

even a single small drop is enough to make an excellent smear.

Place a small drop of fluid on the slide near the labelled end. Tip the slide vertically to allow the drop to run down the length of the slide. Blot the excess fluid from the end of the slide and stand it upright to air dry.

Swab Method. The cotton swab should be moistened with saline solution. A speculum should be used to prevent contact between the swab and the lips of the vulva and vestibule. Insert the swab into the caudal vagina and twist a full turn to pick up a sample of cells. Withdraw the swab. Place the swab on the slide and roll it across the surface. Air dry. This method is somewhat more uncomfortable for the bitch and may have the disadvantage of actually rubbing the vaginal epithelium and picking up deeper cells. This could confuse our interpretation, which is based on examining recently exfoliated cells. The cells collected in this manner often tend to be folded compared with those collected in a pipette (Figs. 2 and 3).

Staining of Slide. The smears can be held after air drying and without fixation for an indefinite time. Fix them for several seconds in methyl alcohol, then air dry before staining. Any blood or general cytology stain, such as Giemsa, Wright's, or new methylene blue can be used. Quick-staining kits such as Diff-Quik (Harleco Diff-Quik Stain Set, Gibbstown, NJ 08027) are ideal. Identification of intracellular structure is not particularly important in canine vaginal cytology. The epithelial cells must be stained adequately to identify them according to type and maturity. It is important to be able to identify red and white blood cells and to recognize bacteria.

INTERPRETATION OF THE SMEARS

Cells Seen in the Smear

Epithelial Cells. Parabasal cells are the least mature epithelial cells. They are small ovoid cells with a large nuclear-to-cytoplasmic ratio. Parabasal cells are seen when the epithelium is low: in anestrus, in early proestrus and again in diestrus. Their numbers are never high, and in many individuals true parabasal cells may never appear in the smear.

Intermediate cells include a wide range of sizes and types because they represent all stages of maturation between parabasal and fully mature superficial cells. The less mature intermediate cells are small and rounded, with a relatively large nucleus. They become more angular, enlarge and flatten as they mature. The relative size of the nucleus decreases as the cells enlarge. Some intermediate cells contain cytoplasmic granules, and they are often seen in clusters or sheets of several cells. Superficial intermediate[5] or large intermediate cells have a nonpyknotic nucleus and the mature superficial configuration of the cytoplasm.

Superficial or cornified cells are the fully mature

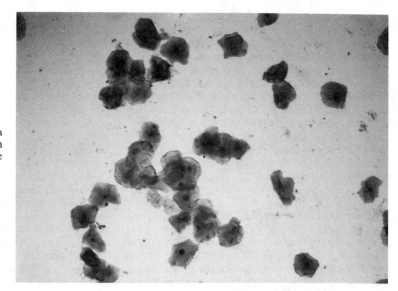

Figure 2. A smear made with a pipette and saline from a bitch in estrus. All of the epithelial cells lie flat on the slide.

squamous epithelial cells. These cells have keratin incorporated into the cytoplasm, which can be demonstrated with special stains, and are thus often called cornified cells. The nucleus may be pyknotic, barely visible as a shadow or absent. Superficial cells are dead cells, incapable of further change.

Leukocytes. During anestrus and early proestrus and again in diestrus, varying numbers of leukocytes, almost exclusively neutrophils, are seen in the smear. They appear to migrate from the subepithelial vasculature through the vaginal epithelium and are then released into the lumen. During late proestrus and estrus the many layers of the stratified squamous epithelium block the migration of the leukocytes, and they accumulate in the submucosa. With the breakdown or sloughing of the cornified epithelium, which occurs late in estrus, leukocytes again appear in the lumen. Thus, white blood cells

in variable numbers will be seen during anestrus and proestrus. They are absent during most of estrus and reappear at the end of estrus or early in diestrus. In some bitches in early diestrus the numbers are so great that the smear may resemble pus. When vaginitis is present, however, the neutrophils are degenerate in appearance, and toxic, with abundant ingested debris and/or bacteria. In normal diestral smears the neutrophils show none of the signs of reactivity or toxicity, in spite of their abundance.

Erythrocytes. Red blood cells are usually present during proestrus, estrus and early diestrus, having entered the uterus and vagina by diapedesis. They are seen microscopically in many cases before the clinical appearance of proestral bleeding. The number of erythrocytes varies proportionately with the depth of color of the sanguineous discharge.

Generally, it is best to ignore the erythrocytes in

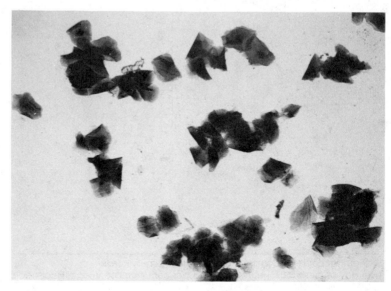

Figure 3. A smear from the same bitch illustrated in Figure 2, made with a cotton swab. Many of the epithelial cells are folded.

a smear except to note their presence. There are so many normal patterns, from virtually no red cells in the smear ("silent heat") to huge numbers throughout proestrus, estrus and early diestrus, that no reliable correlation can be made with the other more important patterns seen in the epithelial cells.

Bacteria. The vagina is not a sterile chamber, and it is normal to see various kinds of bacteria. The numbers vary but are usually fairly low when estradiol levels are high and the vaginal epithelium is cornified. Large numbers of bacteria along with many reactive or degenerating white blood cells may be evidence of vaginitis.

Patterns During the Estrous Cycle

The simplest way to understand the patterns of vaginal cytology during the stages of the estrous cycle is to do a differential count of parabasal, intermediate and superficial cells from smears collected daily, beginning as early as possible in proestrus. To simplify further, parabasal and intermediate cell numbers can be combined and compared with numbers of superficial (including superficial intermediate) cells. Table 1 gives a daily differential count for a typical bitch.

During proestrus the percentage of superficial cells increases until it is nearly 100 per cent. The percentage plateaus for a period of 10 to 14 days, during which time virtually no change is seen.

Examining a single random smear during this time period, one cannot know exactly at what point the bitch is in her cycle. Other signs, including behavior, vulvar swelling, turgidity and discharge must be taken into account. In breeding management it is important to examine enough smears to know when the period of maximum epithelial maturity (cornification) begins or ends or preferably both. After 10 to 14 days of the maximum percentage of superficial cells, the number of superficial cells drops dramatically in a single day and continues to drop to a low level within 48 hours. This simple pattern— a rise in superficial cells to nearly 100 per cent, a 10 to 14 day plateau, a sudden return to immature cells—is seen in bitches of all breeds, sizes and ages that are having a normal heat.

The technique used to prepare the smear may have some influence on the percentage of superficial cells counted at its peak. With the pipette and saline method it will approach 100 per cent and no small intermediate cells should be seen. Using a swab some intermediate cells may remain, presumably because the swab may abrade the epithelium during collection. With gentle handling this need not be the case. Thus, it is important to become familiar with the results of the technique being used.

The sudden decline in superficial cell numbers observed late in estrus correlates closely with the time of ovulation, the time of fertilization and subsequent embryo transport and development, all stages of prenatal development and whelping (Table

Table 1. Daily Differential Count of Vaginal Epithelial Cells in an 18-Month-Old Shetland Sheepdog

Day Relative to Onset of Proestrus	Cell Type (Per Cent Total)				
	Parabasal	Small Intermediate	Superficial Intermediate	Superficial	Leukocytes
3	0	69	16	15	+
4	0	13	14	73	few
5	0	15	21	64	few
6*	0	2	5	93	0
7	0	0	4	96	0
8	0	0	0	100	0
9	0	0	0	100	0
10	0	0	1	99	0
11	0	0	1	99	0
12	0	0	1	99	0
13	0	0	3	97	0
14	0	0	1	99	+
15	0	0	2	98	few
16	0	4	10	86	0
17	0	5	7	88	0
18	0	1	9	90	0
19	0	0	7	93	few
20†	2	14	1	83	+ + +
21	27	63	3	7	+
22	17	81	2	0	+ +

*First day smear is predominantly superficial epithelial cells.
†First day of diestrus (D1) signaled by 16 per cent increase in small intermediate and parabasal cells.

2).[3, 4] The reason for the close correlation is that the change is hormonally regulated and follows ovulation (and the accompanying decline in serum estradiol concentration) by a consistent interval of 6 days. The reason that the change in cell type occurs so suddenly has not been explained. One day prior to the change, in many bitches sheets and clusters of superficial cells are seen, and the bitch's discharge takes on a thick creamy consistency, indicating that the stratified squamous epithelium sloughs quite suddenly.

The first day of the reappearance of intermediate cells and the decline of superficial cells is by definition referred to as the onset of diestrus (D1).[3] The standards for defining the day D1 are (1) a drop in the percentage of superficial cells by 20 per cent or more and (2) a rise in small intermediate cell numbers from less than 5 to more than 10 per cent. In reality the changes are usually much greater than the minimums required by definition. Diestrus may also reasonably be defined as the bitch's first refusal of breeding. Behavior, however, does not correlate nearly as well as vaginal cytology with hormonal events and ovulation. First refusal may occur from 3 days before to 9 days after D1 but usually occurs from D1 to D4.[3, 4]

THE USE OF CYTOLOGY IN BREEDING MANAGEMENT

Successful breeding has been shown to occur in bitches bred from 4 days before until 3 days following ovulation. Since fertilization occurs 3 days after ovulation in the bitch, this means that maximum conception rates can be achieved by breeding any time during the 7 days prior to fertilization.[1, 3] Expressed another way, the bitch's fertile period extends from D-10 to D-3, 10 to 3 days before the onset of diestrus. The vaginal smear will be of the fully mature, cornified pattern during this entire fertile period in normal bitches.

An important principle of management, then, is that breeding must occur while the smear is fully cornified, regardless of other observations, including behavior.[5] One need not pinpoint ovulation, and in fact smears cannot be used to determine the time of ovulation except in retrospect, after D1 has been determined. In a bitch whose smear remains fully cornified for 10 days, the desired breeding time (equivalent to D-10 until D-3) will be the first to the eighth day of the cornified smear (Table 3). In the bitch with an 11-day cornified period the corresponding fertile period will be the second to ninth day of her cornified smear. A similar estimate can be made for bitches whose smears remain cornified for 12, 13 and 14 days. Any normal bitch, whether her period of cornification lasts 10, 11, 12, 13, or 14 days, can be bred between the fifth and eighth day of complete cornification with excellent prospects for conception. This information is useful in a prospective way and can be helpful in management when other signs during the estrous cycle are misleading or difficult to interpret. Each bitch tends to have a constant duration of cornification from one cycle to the next.

Misalliance

Examination of a smear following every suspected mismating should be considered mandatory. In many cases it will eliminate the need to give an abortifacient.

First, it is important to determine whether the bitch's smear was fully cornified at the time of the possible misalliance. If it was not, because she was in proestrus or diestrus, there is no need to worry

Table 2. Time Schedule of Events in the Estrous Cycle Related to D1*

Day	Event
D-17	Average first day of proestrus
D-12	Average first day smear is fully cornified (approaching 100 per cent superficial cells)
D-9	Peak level of estradiol
D-8	Surge of LH—average first day of estrus
D-6	Ovulation
D-3	Fertilization
D-2	Cleavage to two-cell embryo in oviducts
D-1	Four-cell stage
D1	Eight-cell stage
D2–4	Morula stage—first refusal usually occurs D1 to D4
D4	Morula enters uterus, becomes blastocyst
D12	Blastocyst begins attachment
D13–18	Early organogenesis—individual locules too small for abdominal palpation
D19	Locules marble-sized, may be palpable
D20–28	Locules palpable—completion of organogenesis
D28–55	Fetal stage—growth and maturation, pregnancy palpation difficult
D56–58	Whelping—85 per cent of bitches whelp during this time

*D1 is the first day of diestrus as defined by a sudden decline in superficial vaginal epithelial cells. D-1 is the day preceding D1.

(Reprinted with permission from Holst PA, Phemister RD: Onset of diestrus in the Beagle bitch: Definition and significance. Am J Vet Res 35:401, 1974.)

Table 3. The Use of Vaginal Cytology to Estimate Breeding Time in the Bitch

	Day of Cycle Related to D1*										
	D-10	D-9	D-8	D-7	D-6	D-5	D-4	D-3	D-2	D-1	D1
a			1	2	3	4	5	6	7	8	9	10
b				1	2	3	4	5	6	7	8	9	10	11
c			1	2	3	4	5	6	7	8	9	10	11	12
d		1	2	3	4	5	6	7	8	9	10	11	12	13
e	1	2	3	4	5	6	7	8	9	10	11	12	13	14

*Consecutive days on which the smear approaches 100 per cent superficial epithelial cells.

a = Bitch in which the period lasts 10 days.
b = Bitch in which the period lasts 11 days.
c = Bitch in which the period lasts 12 days.
d = Bitch in which the period lasts 13 days.
e = Bitch in which the period lasts 14 days.

The area outlined by a broken line (– – –) represents the breeding days on which optimum conception rate can be expected. Bitches in all categories can be bred between the fifth and eighth days of maximum vaginal epithelial maturity, represented by the portion of the chart outlined by a solid line (————).

about the occurrence of a fertile mating. The second reason is to check for the presence of spermatozoa. They can be seen on a fresh wet smear with reduced illumination, or on a stained smear for many hours after a mating. It is normal to see an occasional spermatozoon 24 to 48 hours after breeding. During proestrus and diestrus, even if the bitch allowed breeding, sperm survival in the vagina is poor.

Vaginitis

Vaginitis is diagnosed by a combination of clinical signs and cytology. The character of the discharge and its color and odor along with visible inflammation of the vaginal epithelium are important findings. The vaginal smear will support the diagnosis by the presence of degenerative epithelial cells and reactive or toxic neutrophils that have ingested bacteria or cellular debris. Large colonies of bacteria may also be present and in greater concentration than seen in the normal vaginal smear.

References

1. Doak RH, Hall E, Dale HE: Longevity of spermatozoa in the reproductive tract of the bitch. J Reprod Fertil 13:51, 1967.
2. Holst PA, Phemister RD: The prenatal development of the dog: Preimplantation events. Biol Reprod 5:194, 1971.
3. Holst PA, Phemister RD: Onset of diestrus in the Beagle bitch: Definition and significance. Am J Vet Res 35:401, 1974.
4. Holst PA, Phemister RD: Temporal sequence of events in the estrous cycle of the bitch. Am J Vet Res 36:705, 1975.
5. Olson PN, Husted PW, Nett TM: The Management of a Successful Mating Between The Bitch and The Stud Dog. Kal Kan Forum, 1983, pp 15–21.
6. Phemister RD, Holst PA, Spano JS, Hopwood ML: Time of ovulation in the Beagle bitch. Biol Reprod 8:74, 1973.

Breeding Management for Optimal Reproductive Efficiency in the Bitch and Stud Dog

Patricia N. Olson, D.V.M., Ph.D.
Paul W. Husted, V.M.D., M.S.
Colorado State University, Fort Collins, Colorado

Several unique features of canine reproductive physiology ensure that conception occurs after a normal stud dog and bitch mate. The canine oocyte is viable for several days after ovulation, since the bitch ovulates a primary rather than a secondary oocyte like most other species.[6] The primary oocyte is viable throughout its maturation into a secondary oocyte (approximately 3 days), and the fertilizable life span of the secondary oocyte is similar to that in other species (approximately 24 hours). The life span of the primary oocytes, which lasts several days, probably aids in assuring that conception results following a mating, since capacitated canine spermatozoa can penetrate the zona pellucida, enter the vitellus and undergo nuclear decondensation in primary oocytes in vitro, with pronuclei forming after oocyte maturation has completed.[4] Although comparable in vivo studies have not been reported, it is likely that a canine spermatozoon can penetrate the zona pellucida of either a primary or secondary oocyte over a 4-day period, whereas this must occur during a 24-hour period in many other species. Since spermatozoa can survive in the bitch's reproductive tract for 4 to 11 days after a mating,[2] conception will follow a single mating in many instances. Because most bitches will allow a stud dog to mate multiple times over several days during estrus, conception is further ensured to occur.

The relationship among behavioral events, hormonal events and physiological changes of the reproductive tract has been established for "average" bitches (Fig. 1). While it is helpful to know when most bitches (i.e., "average" bitches) enter and leave estrus, many fertile bitches vary from this so-called average. If such animals are inappropriately managed and fail to conceive, they may be erroneously considered infertile. Therefore, a thorough, systematic approach must be utilized in managing a breeding between a bitch and a stud dog to ensure that inadequate breeding management is not the cause of reproductive failure.

THE ESTROUS CYCLE AND UTILIZATION OF VAGINAL CYTOLOGY FOR STAGING ESTRUS

The endocrinologic and physiological events of the canine estrous cycle have been described in detail in the article Reproductive Physiology and Endocrinology of the Bitch. The following discussion will serve to emphasize only those aspects that are crucial in managing a successful breeding between a bitch and a stud dog. Likewise, the use of vaginal cytology is discussed in detail in the article Vaginal Cytology in the Bitch and will be referred to in the following discussion as it relates to breeding management.

Proestrus. Proestrus is the stage of the canine estrous cycle characterized by a swollen and often turgid vulva. Uterine and vaginal serosanguineous discharges are frequently observed passing through the vulva. Although the bitch attracts males during proestrus, she is not receptive to mating. The average length of proestrus is approximately 9 days in mature bitches but can range from 0 to 17 days. Although one study[1] suggested that the average length of proestrus was shorter for puberal (x = 3.9 days) than for mature bitches, a subsequent investigation[7] failed to substantiate this finding. The concentration of estradiol increases in the blood during proestrus and results in hyperplasia of vaginal cells and diapedesis of red blood cells through uterine capillaries. This vaginal proliferation and movement of blood into the uterine lumen accounts for the type of vaginal cells and the red blood cells seen in vaginal smears taken during proestrus.

Estrus. Estrus is the stage of the reproductive cycle characterized by the bitch's acceptance of a male. The average length of estrus is approximately 9 days but can range from 3 to 21 days. Two studies have reported that the duration of estrus is shorter for puberal (4.2 to 5.6 days shorter) than multiparous bitches.[1,7] The serosanguineous discharge observed passing through the vagina during proestrus usually clears during estrus but can persist throughout estrus and on into diestrus in some individuals. The vulva remains swollen during estrus but may lose some of the turgidity that was present in proestrus. When a male attempts to mount, most estrous bitches will deviate the tail from the midline (flag), present the perineum and stand to be bred. Reportedly, some puberal bitches will not stand to be bred even though ovulation occurs normally.[7] Since increasing concentrations of progesterone along with declining concentrations of estradiol appear necessary for optimal behavioral receptivity, puberal or mature bitches that fail to allow a male to mate may have hormone profiles that deviate from "average." Other causes that result in estrous bitches being nonreceptive to a male include persistent hymen, vaginal hyperplasia, vaginal hypoplasia, vaginal tumors, vestibulovaginal strictures, vestibulovulvar strictures, clitoral enlargement and aberrant behavior (see Diseases of the Vagina and Vulva in the Bitch). Frequently, owners may present non-receptive bitches for artificial insemination that have not been correctly staged. Vaginal smears obtained from such animals confirm that the bitches are not in estrus. Similarly, a bitch with vaginitis may be presented for artificial insemination. Bitches with vaginitis or anal sac infections frequently attract male dogs. Owners may interpret this to mean that the bitch is in proestrus. When the bitch fails to enter a receptive period, owners may present the animal to be artificially inseminated. A vaginal smear obtained from such bitches verifies genital vaginitis inflammation.

Diestrus. Diestrus (occasionally referred to as metestrus) may be behaviorally defined as that stage of the reproductive cycle that begins the first day after a period of estrus when a bitch refuses to allow a male to mate. During diestrus the reproductive tracts of the nonmated and pregnant bitch alike are under the influence of progesterone. The duration of diestrus, based on concentrations of progesterone being elevated in the blood, is approximately 2 months.

Anestrus. Anestrus is the period extending from the end of diestrus to the next proestrus. This stage ranges from 2 to 10 months among various breeds.

VAGINAL CYTOLOGY

Vaginal cytology is an extremely valuable tool in correctly managing a breeding between a bitch and a stud dog. The method of obtaining and staining vaginal smears is described in the article Vaginal Cytology in the Bitch.

The cell types found in vaginal smears during the estrous cycle have been referred to as "cornified" and "noncornified" in the past. These terms are not adequate in differentiating all the epithelial cell types found on a vaginal smear. Naming them beginning with the cells of the deepest vaginal layer observed in vaginal smears and progressing to the layer nearest the lumen of the vagina seems more appropriate: parabasal, intermediate, superficial intermediate and superficial cells (nucleated and anucleated).

The following are epithelial cells observed in vaginal smears:

1. Parabasal cells. Parabasal cells are the smallest epithelial cells observed on vaginal smears. They are round and have the largest nuclear/cytoplasmic ratio of the vaginal cells.

2. Intermediate cells. Intermediate cells vary in size but are generally about twice the size of parabasal cells. These cells still have a circular shape and a nucleus similar to that of parabasal cells.

3. Superficial intermediate cells. Superficial intermediate cells have nuclei similar to those of parabasal and intermediate cells. These cells differ in that the cell borders are angulated and/or folded. These cells are nearly as large as superficial cells.

4. Superficial cells. Superficial cells are the largest epithelial cells in the vaginal smear. The nuclei are either pyknotic, faded or absent. These cells line the luminal surface of the estrogen-stimulated vagina and have angulated and/or folded cytoplasmic borders.

Vaginal Cell Types During a Normal Estrous Cycle

In early proestrus neutrophils, erythrocytes, parabasal, intermediate, superficial intermediate and superficial epithelial cells may be seen on vaginal smears. By midproestrus the neutrophils decrease in number and are usually absent in smears taken during late proestrus. Erythrocytes usually decrease in number by late proestrus but may occasionally persist throughout estrus and early diestrus. By late proestrus the predominant epithelial cells on a vaginal smear are the superficial intermediate and superficial cells. Bacteria are often abundant in smears obtained during proestrus or estrus.

Vaginal smears taken from normal estrous bitches contain no neutrophils. Conversely, large numbers of bacteria are often observed in estrous smears from normal bitches and *do not* indicate genitourinary tract infection unless accompanied by neutrophils. The predominant epithelial cell type during estrus is the superficial cell. Frequently, greater than 90 per cent of the vaginal cells observed in estrous smears are superficial cells. Superficial cells can be present in clumps or in sheets on vaginal smears taken near the end of estrus.

An abrupt change in relative numbers of epithelial cell types has been reported to signal the onset of diestrus in the beagle bitch. The number of parabasal, intermediate and superficial intermediate cells that were previously absent or made up less than 5 per cent of the total number of cells increases to more than 10 per cent and is often greater than 50 per cent on the first day of diestrus when defined cytologically.[3] The abrupt change in epithelial cell types usually occurs about 3 days before the end of behavioral estrus. Neutrophils reappear in variable numbers; the time of appearance may coincide with the increased numbers of parabasal and intermediate cells but occasionally precedes or lags behind these changes.

It has been suggested that the onset of diestrus be defined by the cytologic change on vaginal smears rather than by behavior. There is some merit to this suggestion, since the LH peak, ovulation, oocyte maturation and whelping can be timed more accurately using the decline of superficial cells in vaginal smears as a marker rather than by using breeding dates or the first refusal of a male.[3] Identifying the onset of diestrus is also important, since conception rates dramatically decline if bitches are bred only after diestrous smears are obtained.

Parabasal and intermediate cells are the predominant cell types present in vaginal smears during anestrus. Neutrophils may be present or absent but are generally fewer in number than during early diestrus.

MANAGING A BREEDING

Bitches failing to conceive because of inappropriate breeding management may be presented for infertility. If a bitch fails to conceive after a breeding has been managed properly, both the stud dog and the bitch should be evaluated for infertility. The best way of finding evidence of fertility in the male dog is to establish that normal litters were sired with other bitches near the time that a pregnancy failure occurred with the bitch under evaluation for infertility (see Infertility in the Male Dog).

Many fertile bitches are presented for reproductive failure because of estrous cycles that vary from "average." Such animals should be examined the first day or so that the owner recognizes the onset of proestrus. A blood sample should be obtained, with the serum harvested and frozen for later hormone analysis if the estrous cycle fails to progress normally or if the bitch again fails to conceive. Similar blood samples should be obtained on a weekly basis for 5 weeks. By the end of the 5-week period, or shortly thereafter, the veterinarian should be able to determine if the bitch is pregnant. If the bitch has again failed to conceive, selected serum samples can be assayed for sex hormones to determine whether the cycle is endocrinologically normal. For example, if a bitch fails to ovulate or fails to maintain luteal tissue after ovulation, concentrations of progesterone in the serum may not increase or may decrease prematurely during estrus or diestrus. Persistent elevations of estradiol for several weeks may suggest cystic ovaries. This would generally be accompanied by vulvar swelling, persistent estrous or estrous-appearing vaginal smears and estrous or proestrous behavior. Slight but persistent elevations of progesterone and testosterone may also be present in some bitches with cystic ovaries. Any animal with abnormally prolonged elevations of sex hormones should also be evaluated for hepatic disease, since many hormones are conjugated in the liver and persistent elevations of estradiol and testosterone have been observed in few animals with portal-caval shunts.

When a bitch is presented in early proestrus, the veterinarian should demonstrate the method of obtaining vaginal smears from the bitch for the owner. Most owners can perform this task with relative ease. The owner should be instructed to obtain daily smears until the bitch enters a cytologic diestrus or for at least 28 days in those cases in which a veterinarian is unavailable to determine the onset of diestrus. The owner should be given a package of sterile cotton-tipped applicator sticks, a box of microscope slides with a frosted edge for dating each smear and a small jar of methanol. The owner should be instructed to dip each slide once in the methanol after the slides have air-dried. This will fix the cells and prevent cellular distortion prior to evaluation. This is especially important when there will be a several-day delay prior to the evaluation. If the bitch is to be bred locally, the owner may have a veterinarian evaluate the slides on a daily basis or at frequent intervals (slides obtained over a 2- to 3-day period) to determine the optimal time of breeding. The bitch should be bred as soon as she will allow a male to mate or as soon as 90 per cent or more of the vaginal epithelial cells are of a superficial type. Since high fertility can be attained from a single breeding that occurs any time during the interval from 4 days before to 3 days after ovulation,[3] breeding a bitch every 7 days may be sufficient. Reportedly, motile canine spermatozoa are present in undiminished concentrations in the uterine lumen for 4 to 6 days after a breeding.[2] Therefore, breeding a bitch every fourth day beginning at the onset of receptivity (or when 90 per cent or more of the vaginal epithelial cells are of the superficial type) might be a better approach. Some breeders may want to breed their bitch every 48 hours. While this appears to offer no advantage over breeding every fourth day, it is an acceptable plan as long as the bitch is bred *until* she enters diestrus. Daily breeding may result in decreased numbers of spermatozoa in the ejaculate[5] and should probably not be considered with males having low sperm numbers.

Some bitches have a very short discernible proestrus and will allow a male to mate soon after the owners observe a swollen vulva or a bloody discharge passing from the vagina. Vaginal smears obtained from these bitches reveal greater than 90 per cent of the vaginal epithelial cells to be of the superficial type. Concentrations of progesterone in the serum of such bitches are already elevated, also suggesting that these animals enter estrus sooner than most females (Fig. 1). If the owner is unaware of this possibility, the bitch may not be presented to a stud dog for several days or until she is in diestrus and unreceptive to mating. The owner may then request a veterinarian to artificially inseminate the nonreceptive bitch. Inseminating such diestrous bitches will generally not result in pregnancy, as the ova are no longer capable of being fertilized.

Conversely, some normal bitches may have extremely long periods of proestrus and estrus. Although motile spermatozoa can be present in the uterus in undiminished concentrations for 4 to 6 days after a single mating, numbers progressively decline after that time (especially when the bitch enters diestrus) although some may be observed as late as 11 days following copulation.[2] If a normal bitch has a 21-day estrus, several breedings at the beginning of estrus may not be sufficient for conception if ovulation occurs late in estrus. Although most bitches ovulate within the first several days of estrus, the exact time of ovulation in bitches with prolonged periods of receptivity is unknown. Likewise, the longevity of spermatozoa in the reproductive tract of such bitches is unknown. Therefore, these bitches should be mated every fourth day during estrus until a diestrous smear is obtained.

Occasionally, a bitch enters proestrus but fails to progress into a normal estrus. Although many *superficial intermediate epithelial cells* may be present in vaginal smears obtained from these animals,

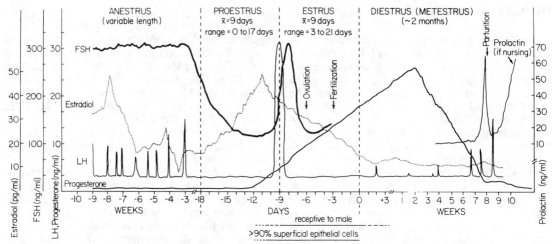

Figure 1. Behavioral, physiological and endocrinologic events of the canine estrous cycle.

superficial cells rarely approach 90 per cent of the total, suggesting an abnormal cycle. Although such animals attract males, they may never become receptive to mating. In a study evaluating various methods of inducing estrus in the bitch, we found that such abnormal seasons were frequently observed. Superficial epithelial cells did not always approach 90 per cent of the total, induced bitches frequently refused to be mated, bitches often failed to ovulate, although several developed luteinized follicles, and premature luteal regression occurred in animals that did ovulate. Unfortunately, the exact endocrinologic profiles of spontaneously occurring cycles that fail to progress normally is unknown. Until such cycles are characterized, it will be impossible to select a treatment that is efficacious in treating such aberrant cycles.

In cases in which reproductive failure has occurred as a result of atypical estrous cycles, it should be apparent that the owner and veterinarian need to work together in managing a breeding between a bitch and a stud dog. Although many typical bitches conceive if mated on the ninth, eleventh and thirteenth days after entering proestrus, other animals may be in proestrus or diestrus at these times.

References

1. Chakraborty PK, Panko WB, Fletcher WS: Serum hormone concentrations and their relationships to sexual behavior at the first and second estrous cycles of the Labrador bitch. Biol Repro 22:227, 1980.
2. Doak RL, Hall A, Dale HE: Longevity of spermatozoa in the reproductive tract of the bitch. J Reprod Fertil 13:51, 1967.
3. Holst PA, Phemister RD: Onset of diestrus in the beagle bitch: Definition and significance. Am J Vet Res 35:401, 1974.
4. Mahi CA, Yanagimachi R: Maturation and sperm penetration of canine ovarian oocytes in vitro. J Exp Zool 196:189, 1976.
5. Olar TT, Amann RP, Pickett BW: Relationships among testicular size, daily production or output of spermatozoa, and epididymal spermatozoal reserves of the dog. Biol Reprod 29:1114, 1983.
6. Phemister RD, Holst PA, Spano JS, Hopwood ML: Time of ovulation in the beagle bitch. Biol Reprod 8:74, 1973.
7. Wildt DE, Seager SWJ, Chakraborty PK: Behavioral, ovarian and endocrine relationships in the pubertal bitch. J Anim Sci 53:182, 1981.

Infertility in the Bitch

Cheri A. Johnson, D.V.M., M.S.
Michigan State University, East Lansing, Michigan

Successful management of the infertile bitch is dependent upon a thorough understanding of normal reproductive physiology and endocrinology.

The initial diagnostic and therapeutic approach is determined primarily by whether or not the bitch has normal estrous cycles. The history should establish the interestrous interval, the length of proestrus, the length of estrus (first day of acceptance to first refusal) and previous breeding dates. Previous pregnancies, abortions or whelpings should be noted, as should overall health and results of *Brucella canis* testing.

Breeding management must also be investigated. Were breeding dates based on vaginal cytology, behavioral changes in the bitch or stud or merely the number of days in-season? Was breeding accomplished by artificial insemination or natural service, with or without "tie"? Has the stud sired any litters and what was his status in regard to testing for *Brucella canis*? If breeding management is questionable, the owner should be instructed on proper canine breeding techniques and the evaluation of infertility postponed until the bitch has been properly bred.

A complete physical examination should be done. Systemic illness or nongonadal endocrine disorders may have infertility as a sign. The vulva is inspected for structural abnormalities and the presence or absence of a discharge. Abnormal placement of the vulva or an enlarged clitoris may be present in intersex conditions. Karyotyping may be indicated in these patients. The uterus is palpated per abdomen. Rectal examination will help evaluate the bony pelvis and may be useful in delineation of vaginal lesions. If indicated, vaginal culture should be obtained before the vestibule and posterior vagina are examined. The majority of the length of the vagina is inaccessible to digital examination but can easily be visualized using a human anoscope or proctoscope (adult or pediatric), depending upon the size of the bitch. The character of the vaginal mucosa and source of any discharge should be noted. Samples for vaginal cytology may be obtained at this time.

A complete blood count, urinalysis and serum biochemical profile are helpful in detecting extra-reproductive disease, which might affect fertility. Testing for *Brucella canis* should be routinely included in the examination of an infertile bitch. Evaluation for hypothyroidism or hyperadrenocorticism may be indicated in some infertile bitches.

NORMAL ESTROUS CYCLE

The normal estrous cycle is dependent upon interactions among the hypothalamus, pituitary, ovaries and other endocrine organs. The presence of normal cycles implies that these organs are functioning in a normal manner. Poor breeding management is the most common cause of infertility in normally cycling bitches. If breeding techniques have been appropriate, the stud dog should be investigated as the potential cause of infertility. Proven ability to sire litters is the best evidence of fertility in the male. However, semen evaluation is recommended for studs that have not recently sired litters and for unproven studs.

Examination of the bitch that has been properly bred to a fertile stud should proceed with evaluation for the presence of infection or obstruction in the reproductive tract. The canine cervix is very difficult to catheterize; thus, samples are rarely obtained directly from the uterus. Therefore, cultures for evaluation of uterine flora are usually obtained during times when the anterior vagina should contain material originating from the uterus, such as during proestrus. Ascending infection is thought to be the most common source of uterine infection. Interpretation of culture results is difficult because

the vagina has a normal resident population of bacteria. If bacterial infection is thought to play a role in the patient's infertility, culture and sensitivity testing should be done, and appropriate antibiotic therapy should be administered for 3 to 4 weeks.

Brucella canis can cause apparent conception failure as well as the more characteristic abortion at 45 to 55 days of gestation. The organism has fastidious growth requirements and is usually *not* recovered from vaginal cultures in the absence of vaginal discharge. Serologic testing using a rapid slide agglutination test (Pitman Moore's plate test for *Brucella canis*) is recommended. The test is very sensitive, so false-negative reactions are rare; however, false-positive reactions are possible. Positive results must be confirmed by additional tests such as the tube agglutination test and blood culture. Recovery of the organism is the only definitive diagnostic test. Recent antibiotic therapy can interfere with serologic and culture results, making them both negative. At present, there is no effective treatment for *Brucella canis* and no vaccine. Infected animals should be eliminated from the kennel.

Herpesvirus infection has been associated with infertility in several species, including dogs. Parvoviruses adversely affect fertility in some species. Canine parvovirus has been incriminated by dog breeders as the cause of reproductive problems in their kennels. However, Meunier and colleagues[2] found no change in conception rate, incidence of stillbirth, average litter size or average number of pups weaned per litter for 1 year after introduction of canine parvovirus into a kennel containing approximately 2000 brood bitches.

Obstruction of the tubular organs (oviduct, uterus, vagina) can be caused by congenital, inflammatory or neoplastic lesions. The vagina is easily evaluated for such lesions by digital examination and vaginoscopy.

Survey radiography is likely to demonstrate only gross enlargements of the reproductive tract or surrounding tissue. Contrast radiography (hysterosalpingography) can be done in the bitch but is limited by the difficulty of cervical catheterization and poor visualization of the oviducts. Most procedures are simplified by injecting contrast material directly into the vagina.

If noninvasive diagnostic methods have been exhausted, exploratory laparotomy or laparoscopy can be considered. These procedures will allow direct visualization of the reproductive tract. If excessive periovarian fat is present, the oviduct may not be visible, but it may still be palpable. The surface of the ovary will not be visible because of the surrounding bursa and fat. Uterine biopsy (to include the endometrium) and uterine culture should be obtained during laparotomy. Oviductal patency has been difficult to demonstrate in the bitch because the ovarian bursa obstructs cannulization of the oviduct in situ. Retrograde flushing (via the uterus) using sterile saline, dye or radiographic contrast media has been suggested but is not always possible if the tubouterine junction is tightly closed and resists retrograde flow.

Hyperplastic, inflammatory or infiltrative lesions within the uterine wall may adversely affect fertility. Histopathologic examination of biopsy specimens should establish such diagnoses. Antibodies to sperm have been found in the serum and vagina of some infertile women; it is unlikely that this will have clinical significance in dogs because repeated exposure is necessary to maintain titers, and the length of canine anestrus provides long periods of "abstinence." Also, changing male mates is easily done in cases of canine infertility in contrast to human infertilities.

Immune responses directed against the placenta and fetus, resulting in fetal death, have also been identified in women. These and other placental or implantation disorders have yet to be described and evaluated in the bitch.

ABNORMAL ESTROUS CYCLE

The onset of the puberal estrus is quite variable and may not occur until 18 months of age. Therefore, evaluation for infertility is usually postponed until the bitch is 2 years old. If complete anestrus is present, the following should be considered in the differential diagnosis: previous ovariohysterectomy, previous progestin or androgen therapy, gonadal hypoplasia, pituitary abnormality, intersex, hypothyroidism and hyperadrenocorticism. Exogenous glucocorticoid administration, such as in cancer chemotherapy or for chronic dermatopathy, can also suppress estrus. Several other endocrinopathies such as hyperprolactinemia have been described in amenorrheic women but have not been adequately studied in the bitch.

Some bitches appear to have normal estrous cycles but refuse to accept the male for breeding. These bitches should be examined for structural abnormalities such as vestibulovaginal stricture, which may make breeding painful or impossible. If no abnormalities are found, breeding time should be determined by vaginal cytology. These bitches may then be muzzled or physically restrained for natural service or artificially inseminated. Some bitches will refuse one stud but accept another. Progesterone (as well as estrogen) is necessary for normal behavioral estrus in the bitch, and measuring serum progesterone concentrations may identify some bitches with abnormal luteal phases.

Beagle bitches that continue to accept mating for longer than 10 days have decreased fertility compared with those that stand for 10 days or less. If prolonged acceptance is documented on more than one cycle, ovulation induction early in estrus may be considered. The following drugs have been suggested: human chorionic gonadotropin (hCG), 1000 units intramuscularly for a 40 lb bitch, and gonadotropin-releasing hormone (GnRH), 50 µg intramuscularly for an approximately 60 lb bitch. Breeding should be initiated 24 hours later.

Some bitches exhibit "split heats" that begin with what appears to be normal proestrus, which does not progress into estrus. Four to six weeks later, a normal, fertile cycle occurs. This usually happens only once, generally during the puberal cycle, but is occasionally seen in an older bitch. There is no adverse effect on fertility if the bitch is bred during the normal, second part of the "split heat."

Complete endometrial repair from the preceding, nonpregnant cycle requires about 120 days (150 days postpartum). Bitches with interestrous intervals of less than 4 months are often infertile, perhaps because the uterus has not completely recovered from the previous cycle. Some authors have suggested treatment of short interestrous intervals with a synthetic androgen (mibolerone, Cheque Drops, Upjohn) to postpone the next cycle for 6 months.

Interestrual intervals longer than 8 months are usually considered abnormal. Hypothyroidism is a common cause. Hypothyroidism has familial tendencies, and affected animals may not be the most desirable brood stock. This should be discussed with the owner. If any endocrinopathy is identified, it should be appropriately treated and the bitch's fertility reevaluated during the next cycle. Breeding during a natural estrus is much preferred to breeding during an induced estrus.

Estrus induction should be reserved for those bitches that have undergone a thorough evaluation (especially of the endocrine system) and have been found to be otherwise normal. Although many therapeutic regimens have been reported, none are consistently effective for inducing fertile estrous cycles in the bitch. Until a safe and reliable method is found, estrus induction should be considered only as a last resort.[1] Some normal bitches will begin cycling if they are housed with other cycling bitches (dormitory effect).

Once the cause of infertility has been found and corrected, the bitch should be bred to a proven fertile stud using optimal breeding management. Pregnancy examination should be performed at 25 to 30 days. If the bitch is not pregnant at that time, serum progesterone concentrations can be measured to determine adequacy of luteal function.

References

1. Johnston SD, Larsen RE, Olson PS: Canine theriogenology. J Soc Theriogenology 11:1, 1982.
2. Meunier PC, Glickman LT, Appel MJG: Canine parvovirus in a commercial kennel: Epidemiologic and pathologic findings. Cornell Vet 71:96, 1981.
3. Pollock RVH: Canine brucellosis: Current status. Comp Cont Ed 1:255, 1979.

The Use and Misuse of Vaginal Cultures in Diagnosing Reproductive Diseases in the Bitch

Patricia N. Olson, D.V.M., Ph.D.
Colorado State University, Fort Collins, Colorado

R. L. Jones, D.V.M., Ph.D.
Edward C. Mather, D.V.M., Ph.D.
Michigan State University, East Lansing, Michigan

Whenever inflammatory disease of the reproductive tract of the bitch is diagnosed, the veterinarian must attempt to identify the causative agent before appropriate therapy can be instituted. Frequently, vaginal cultures are obtained in an attempt to correlate various reproductive diseases (e.g., inflammation of the clitoral fossa, vestibule, vagina, cervix or uterus; infertility; abortion; neonatal deaths) with specific infectious agents. Since a variety of microorganisms are present in the vaginas of bitches with and without reproductive diseases, it is often difficult to associate disease with a specific microbial isolate. Approximately 60 per cent of normal bitches harbor aerobic bacteria in the cranial vagina and approximately 90 per cent of normal bitches harbor similar organisms in the caudal vagina.[16] Therefore, merely isolating bacteria from the vagina does not constitute a basis for diagnosis of reproductive disease. Conversely, organisms known to cause infertility, abortion, stillbirths or neonatal deaths (e.g., herpesvirus, *Brucella canis*) are often difficult to isolate. Hence, a negative vaginal culture does not ensure that a bitch is free of infectious disease involving the reproductive system.

Although the owners of stud dogs may require a "negative" vaginal culture before accepting a bitch for a mating, most male dogs also harbor microorganisms in the prepuce and penile urethra that are similar to those present in the vagina of healthy females.[12] Therefore, it is unreasonable to refuse to breed a bitch to a stud dog merely because aerobic bacteria have been isolated from the vagina.

Vaginal cultures are useful in diagnosing and treating certain diseases of the reproductive tract as long as they are carefully interpreted and they correlate with other clinical findings. Although isolating bacteria from the vagina of a healthy bitch does not constitute a diagnosis of reproductive disease, "normal" bacteria may become pathogenic if uterine or vaginal defense mechanisms are altered. For example, diestrous uteri appear more susceptible to bacterial infection, since *Escherichia coli* can be isolated from nearly 65 per cent of the uteri removed from bitches with pyometra.[8] It has been postulated that *E. coli* may adhere via the K-antigen to the progesterone-stimulated endometrium and myometrium.[19] Similarly, bacteria are frequently associated with postwhelping metritis. Bacterial overgrowth in the uterus can follow a prolonged labor, retained puppies or retained membranes, which predisposes the uterus to developing metritis.

Anomalies of the reproductive tract can also predispose the bitch to infection and inflammation when urine or vaginal secretions pool in aberrant locations. Likewise, mechanical irritation or ulceration from clitoral hypertrophy or foreign bodies may render the vagina more susceptible to secondary bacterial infections. Therefore, utilizing vaginal cultures as an aid for diagnosing and treating reproductive diseases can be very useful as long as the veterinarian is aware of the limitation of the test.

VAGINAL MICROFLORA

Aerobic Bacteria. In a study of 81 postpuberal healthy bitches, aerobic bacteria were isolated from 51 (63 per cent) of the cranial vaginas and from 74 (91 per cent) of the caudal vaginas.[16] Therefore, most normal bitches have an established bacterial flora that can be isolated from vaginal swabs. The types of organisms isolated may vary with the age of the bitch. A higher percentage of prepuberal bitches have coagulase-positive staphylococci present in the vagina than postpuberal animals (Tables 1 to 3). The types of bacteria do not appear to vary with different stages of the estrous cycle (Tables 4 to 6),[15] but an increased number of organisms appear to be present during proestrus and estrus.[1,3]

Frequently, many bacteria can be observed on vaginal smears obtained from estrous bitches. This is not an abnormal finding unless the bitch has overt signs of vaginitis (inflamed vaginal mucosa, purulent-appearing or foul-smelling vaginal discharge, pollakuria, licking of the vulva), and the vaginal smear contains many toxic-appearing neutrophils. Although many bacteria are frequently present in vaginal smears obtained from normal estrous bitches, neutrophils should be absent or few in number until the bitch enters diestrus.

Anaerobic Bacteria. Vaginal microflora from healthy and infertile bitches were cultured by Osbaldiston and colleagues.[18] The aerobic bacteria isolated were similar to those reported later by other investigators.[1,3,11,12,16,20] Anaerobic organisms isolated included *Bacteroides melaninogenicus*, *Corynebacterium* spp., *Haemophilus aphrophilus*, *Bacteroides* spp., anaerobic enterococci, *Peptostrepto-*

Table 1. Classification of Vaginal Isolates from 20 Pups, 1 to 11 Weeks Old

Type of Isolate	No. of Isolates	Per Cent of Total Isolates	Pups with Isolate (%)
Escherichia coli	9	18.0	45.0
Coagulase + staphylococci	13	26.0	65.0
Coagulase − staphylococci	6	12.0	30.0
Alpha-hemolytic streptococci	3	6.0	15.0
Beta-hemolytic streptococci	6	12.0	30.0
Nonhemolytic streptococci	4	8.0	20.0
Proteus	3	6.0	15.0
Bacillus	3	6.0	15.0
Corynebacterium	2	4.0	10.0
Pseudomonas	1	2.0	5.0
Total	50 (2.5 isolates/pup)		

(From JAVMA 172:708, 1978.)

coccus spp. (hemolytic and nonhemolytic). No correlation could be made by the authors between bacterial flora and infertility. This suggests that canine infertility is not necessarily associated with bacterial infection of the vagina.

Mycoplasma and Ureaplasma. Doig and colleagues[5] attempted the isolation of genital mycoplasmas and ureaplasmas from 136 dogs with varied reproductive histories. Mycoplasma spp. were recovered from 88 per cent of vulvovaginal swabs, 85 per cent of preputial swabs and 72 per cent of semen samples. There was no significant difference in isolation rates among infertile dogs, dogs with evidence of genital disease and fertile animals.

Ureaplasmas were recovered from half of the bitches sampled. Higher, but not statistically significant, isolation rates (75 per cent) were obtained from infertile females with purulent vulvar discharge than for those that were clinically normal and fertile (40 per cent).

In the male dog a significantly higher number of ureaplasmal isolates were obtained from swabs of the prepuce of infertile animals (69 per cent) than fertile dogs (0 per cent), but isolations from semen samples were similar for the two groups. The role of Ureaplasma in infertility in the bitch and stud dog needs further evaluation.

BRUCELLA CANIS

Brucella canis can infect bitches and cause infertility, fetal or neonatal deaths and persistent uterine or vaginal discharges. Since the infection can also exist without overt manifestations, inapparently infected animals are an important source of transmission. The isolation of Brucella canis from blood, vaginal discharges, lymph nodes, placental or fetal tissues is the definitive method of diagnosis. Although bacteremia can persist for long periods of time, nonbacteremic intervals of variable lengths can follow bacteremic phases. Therefore, a negative blood culture cannot rule out a diagnosis of canine brucellosis.[7] Similarly, a negative vaginal culture does not eliminate the possibility of canine brucel-

Table 2. Classification of Vaginal Isolates from 21 Pups, 12 Weeks to 6 Months Old

Type of Isolate	No. of Isolates	Per Cent of Total Isolates	Pups with Isolate (%)
E. coli	8	17.0	38.1
Coagulase + staphylococci	14	29.8	66.7
Coagulase − staphylococci	5	10.6	23.8
Alpha-hemolytic streptococci	4	8.5	19.0
Beta-hemolytic streptococci	3	6.4	14.3
Nonhemolytic streptococci	2	4.3	9.5
Proteus	1	2.1	4.8
Bacillus	3	6.4	14.3
Corynebacterium	2	4.3	9.5
Micrococcus	3	6.4	14.3
Neisseria	1	2.1	4.8
Klebsiella	1	2.1	4.8
Total	47 (2.2 isolates/pup)		

(From JAVMA 172:708, 1978.)

Table 3. Classification of Vaginal Isolates from 81 Postpuberal Bitches

Type of Isolate	Cranial Vaginal Swabbings			Caudal Vaginal Swabbings		
	Number of Isolates	Per Cent of Total Isolates	Bitches with Isolate (%)	Number of Isolates	Per Cent of Total Isolates	Bitches with Isolate (%)
E. coli	15	19.0	18.5	25	13.2	30.9
Coagulase + staphylococci	5	6.3	6.2	15	7.9	18.5
Coagulase − staphylococci	5	6.3	6.2	16	8.4	19.8
Alpha-hemolytic streptococci	8	10.1	9.9	18	9.5	22.2
Beta-hemolytic streptococci	12	15.2	14.8	15	7.9	18.5
Nonhemolytic streptococci	3	3.8	3.7	10	5.3	12.3
Pasteurella	8	10.1	9.9	26	13.7	32.1
Proteus	4	5.1	4.9	5	2.6	6.2
Bacillus	3	3.8	3.7	13	6.8	16.0
Haemophilus	1	1.3	1.2	0	0	0
Corynebacterium	2	2.5	2.5	12	6.3	14.3
Pseudomonas	0	0	0	2	1.1	2.5
Moraxella	1	1.3	1.2	7	3.7	8.6
Acinetobacter	0	0	0	3	1.6	3.7
Flavobacterium	1	1.3	1.2	4	2.1	4.9
Lactobacillus	0	0	0	1	0.5	1.2
Micrococcus	1	1.3	1.2	3	1.6	3.7
Neisseria	2	2.5	2.5	7	3.7	8.6
Enterobacter	1	1.3	1.2	1	0.5	1.2
Klebsiella	0	0	0	0	0	0
Nonclassified spp.	7	8.9	8.6	7	3.7	8.6
Total	79 (0.975 isolate/bitch)			190 (2.35 isolates/bitch)		
No growth	30 (37% of total dogs)			7 (9% of total dogs)		

(From JAVMA 172:708, 1978.)

Table 4. Classification of Vaginal Isolates from 34 Anestrous Bitches

Type of Isolate	Cranial Vaginal Cultures			Caudal Vaginal Cultures		
	Number of Isolates	Per Cent of Total Isolates	Dogs with Isolate (%)	Number of Isolates	Per Cent of Total Isolates	Dogs with Isolate (%)
E. coli	6	26.1	17.6	8	10.5	23.5
Coagulase + staphylococci	2	8.7	5.9	8	10.5	23.5
Coagulase − staphylococci	1	4.3	2.9	9	11.8	26.5
Alpha-hemolytic streptococci	3	13.0	8.8	8	10.5	23.5
Beta-hemolytic streptococci	5	21.7	14.7	9	11.8	26.5
Nonhemolytic streptococci	0	0	0	3	3.9	8.8
Pasteurella	1	4.3	2.9	8	10.5	23.5
Proteus	1	4.3	2.9	1	1.3	2.9
Bacillus	1	4.3	2.9	6	7.9	17.6
Haemophilus	1	4.3	2.9	0	0	0
Corynebacterium	1	4.3	2.9	6	7.9	17.6
Pseudomonas	0	0	0	1	1.3	2.9
Moraxella	0	0	0	4	5.3	11.8
Acinetobacter	0	0	0	1	1.3	2.9
Flavobacterium	0	0	0	1	1.3	2.9
Lactobacillus	0	0	0	1	1.3	2.9
Nonclassified spp.	1	4.3	2.9	2	2.6	5.9
Total	23 (0.7 isolate/dog)			76 (2.2 isolates/dog)		
No growth	18 (52.9% of total dogs)			3 (8.8% of total dogs)		

(From Olson PNS: M.S. Thesis, University of Minnesota; 1976.)

Table 5. Classification of Vaginal Isolates From 25 Proestrous-Estrous Bitches

Type of Isolate	Cranial Vaginal Cultures*			Caudal Vaginal Cultures		
	Number of Isolates	Per Cent of Total Isolates	Dogs with Isolate (%)	Number of Isolates	Per Cent of Total Isolates	Dogs with Isolate (%)
E. coli	4	18.2	18.2	10	17.2	40.0
Coagulase + staphylococci	1	4.5	4.5	6	10.3	24.0
Coagulase − staphylococci	1	4.5	4.5	3	5.2	12.0
Alpha-hemolytic streptococci	3	13.6	13.6	6	10.3	24.0
Beta-hemolytic streptococci	2	9.1	9.1	3	5.2	12.0
Nonhemolytic streptococci	0	0	0	3	5.2	12.0
Pasteurella	4	18.2	18.2	7	12.1	28.0
Bacillus	0	0	0	4	6.9	16.0
Corynebacterium	0	0	0	2	3.4	8.0
Moraxella	0	0	0	1	1.7	4.0
Acinetobacter	0	0	0	1	1.7	4.0
Flavobacterium	1	4.5	4.5	3	5.2	12.0
Micrococcus	0	0	0	2	3.4	8.0
Neisseria	2	9.1	9.1	4	6.9	16.0
Enterobacter	1	4.5	4.5	1	1.7	4.0
Nonclassified spp.	3	13.6	13.6	2	3.4	8.0
Total	22 (1.0 isolate/dog)			58 (2.3 isolates/dog)		
No growth	6 (27.3% of total dogs)			1 (4.0% of total dogs)		

*Cranial vaginal cultures were obtained on 22 of 25 dogs in this group.
(From Olson PNS: M.S. Thesis. University of Minnesota, 1976.)

Table 6. Classification of Vaginal Isolates From 19 Diestrous or Pregnant Bitches

Type of Isolate	Cranial Vaginal Cultures			Caudal Vaginal Cultures		
	Number of Isolates	Per Cent of Total Isolates	Dogs with Isolate (%)	Number of Isolates	Per Cent of Total Isolates	Dogs with Isolate (%)
E. coli	3	13.6	15.8	4	8.7	21.1
Coagulase + staphylococci	2	9.1	10.5	2	4.3	10.5
Coagulase − staphylococci	3	13.6	15.8	4	8.7	21.1
Alpha-hemolytic streptococci	1	4.5	5.3	3	6.5	15.8
Beta-hemolytic streptococci	2	9.1	10.5	2	4.3	10.5
Nonhemolytic streptococci	2	9.1	10.5	3	6.5	15.8
Pasteurella	2	9.1	10.5	7	15.2	36.8
Proteus	2	9.1	10.5	2	4.3	10.5
Bacillus	1	4.5	5.3	4	8.7	21.1
Corynebacterium	1	4.5	5.3	4	8.7	21.1
Pseudomonas	0	0	0	1	2.2	5.3
Moraxella	1	4.5	5.3	2	4.4	10.5
Acinetobacter	0	0	0	1	2.2	5.3
Micrococcus	0	0	0	1	2.2	5.3
Neisseria	0	0	0	3	6.5	15.8
Nonclassified spp.	2	9.1	10.5	3	6.5	15.8
Total	22 (1.2 isolates/dog)			46 (2.4 isolates/dog)		
No growth	6 (31.6% of total dogs)			5 (26.3% of total dogs)		

(From Olson PNS: M.S. Thesis. University of Minnesota, 1976.)

losis, since the organism localizes in deeper tissues and is not consistently shed.

HERPESVIRUS

Canine herpesvirus (CHV) is a fatal infection of neonatal pups characterized by hemorrhage and necrosis in various tissues. Earlier investigations suggested that puppies are infected with the virus during passage through the birth canal,[4] while later studies suggested that transplacental infection can also occur.[9,10] CHV has been cultured from the vaginas of experimental bitches for as long as 2 weeks after oral-nasal inoculation.[2] In one naturally occurring case CHV was cultured from the cranial vagina of a bitch 18 days postwhelping.[13] Information is not available that indicates the maximum time at which CHV can be isolated from the vagina after naturally occurring infections; clearly, a positive CHV culture from the vagina is abnormal, whereas a negative culture may be harder to interpret. Viral isolation requires fastidious sampling and culturing techniques; therefore, a negative culture for CHV might be due to inadequate methodology.

MICROORGANISMS FOUND IN THE HUMAN VAGINA BUT NOT REPORTED TO OCCUR IN THE CANINE VAGINA

Frequently, owners bring bitches to veterinarians for treatment of vaginitis and ask whether agents that cause vaginal inflammation in humans can also result in canine vaginitis. The veterinarians should be aware of normal and pathogenic microorganisms found in the human vagina, so that such questions may be answered.

Lactobacillus acidophilus (Döderlein's bacillus) is a frequent vaginal isolate from healthy women[14] but has not been identified in the majority of healthy bitches.[1,3,12,16,18] Döderlein's bacilli are speculated to play an important role in suppressing the growth of pathogenic microorganisms in the human vagina.

A frequent cause of vaginal discharge and odor in women is *Gardnerella vaginalis (Haemophilus vaginalis)* infection. Cervicitis may also be caused by *G. vaginalis.*[6] Although *Haemophilus* has been isolated and associated with one case of canine vaginitis,[17] it is rarely isolated from either healthy bitches or from bitches with genital diseases.[11,12,16,18]

Other pathogens which cause genital diseases in women but not yet reported to cause similar disorders in dogs include *Neisseria gonorrhoeae, Chlamydia trachomatis, Trichomonas vaginalis, Candida* (yeast) and *Treponema pallidum* (syphilis).

INTERPRETATION OF VAGINAL CULTURES

Vaginal cultures can be a valuable examination procedure for infectious diseases of the reproductive system as long as the veterinarian is aware of their limitations. A positive culture for an obligate pathogen such as *B. canis* is a definitive diagnosis.

However, the successful isolation of opportunistically pathogenic aerobic bacteria, anaerobic bacteria or mycoplasmas from the vagina is not primafacie evidence of infection. These organisms can frequently be isolated from normal animals. If the organism is a significant pathogen, it will be recovered in very large numbers and in nearly pure culture because it will have gained some competitive advantage as a pathogen and have overgrown the normal flora. Normal flora will usually be recovered in mixed cultures of light to moderate growth.

Clinical microbiology is the most subjective of the laboratory sciences. Absolute rules for positive and negative cultures are unacceptable when culturing sites that are not normally sterile. Therefore, each specimen must be individually evaluated, including a direct examination of stained smears, semiquantitative cultures and other clinical signs compatible with infectious disease in order to make the best judgmental decisions.

References

1. Allen WE, Dagnall GJR: Some observations on the aerobic bacterial flora of the genital tract of the dog and bitch. J Small Anim Pract 23:325, 1982.
2. Apple MJG, Menagus M, Parsonson IM, Carmichael LE: Pathogenesis of canine herpesvirus in specific-pathogen-free dogs: 5 to 12 week old pups. Am J Vet Res 30:2067, 1969.
3. Baba E, Hata H, Fukata T, Arakawa A: Vaginal and uterine microflora of adult dogs. Am J Vet Res 44:606, 1983.
4. Carmichael LE: Canine herpesvirus: a recent discovered cause of death of young pups. Proc 15th Gaines Veterinary Sym (Missouri), 1965, p 24.
5. Doig PA, Ruhnke HL, Bosu WTK: The genital mycoplasma and ureaplasma flora of healthy and diseased dogs. Can J Comp Med 45:233, 1981.
6. Fleury FJ: Adult vaginitis. Clin Obstet Gynecol 24:407, 1981.
7. Flores-Castro R, Carmichael LE: Canine brucellosis: Current status of methods for diagnosing and treatment. Proc 27th Gaines Veterinary Sym (Texas), 1977, p 17.
8. Hardy RM, Osborne CA: Canine pyometra: Pathophysiology, diagnosis, and treatment of uterine and extra-uterine lesions. JAAHA 10:245, 1974.
9. Hashimoto A, Hirai K: Studies on canine herpesvirus infection III. Transplacental transmission by intravaginal inoculation of pregnant dogs. Fac of Agri, Gifu Univ, Japan, Res Bull 34:157, 1982.
10. Hashimoto A, Hirai K, Yamaguchi T, Fujimoto Y: Experimental transplacental infection of pregnant dogs with canine herpesvirus. Am J Vet Res 43:844, 1982.
11. Hirsh DC, Wiger N: The bacterial flora of the normal canine vagina compared with that of vaginal exudates. J Small Anim Pract 18:25, 1977.
12. Ling GV, Ruby AL: Aerobic bacterial flora of the prepuce, urethra, and vagina of normal adult dogs. Am J Vet Res 39:695, 1978.
13. Love DN, Huxtable CRR: Naturally occurring neonatal canine herpesvirus infection. Vet Rec 99:501, 1976.
14. Mikat DM, Mikat KW: A Clinician's Dictionary Guide to Bacteria. Indianapolis, Eli Lilly and Co., 1974.
15. Olson PNS: Canine vaginal flora. M.S. Thesis, University of Minnesota, 1976.
16. Olson PNS, Mather EC: Canine vaginal and uterine bacterial flora. JAVMA 172:708, 1978.
17. Osbaldiston GW: Vaginitis in the bitch associated with *Haemophilus* sp. Am J Vet Res 32:2067, 1971.
18. Osbaldiston GW, Nüru S, Mosier JE: Vaginal cytology and microflora of infertile bitches. JAAHA 8:93, 1972.
19. Sandholm M, Vasenuis H, Kivisto AK: Pathogenesis of canine pyometra. JAVMA 167:1006, 1975.
20. Stockner PK, Brudvik AM, Baker D: Canine vaginal flora: A technique for sampling and clinical observation. Canine Pract 6:18, 1979.

Diseases of the Vagina and Vulva in the Bitch

Peggy M. Wykes, D.V.M., M.S.
Colorado State University, Fort Collins, Colorado

The vagina is a long tubular and very expansile structure that extends from the uterus to the vulva, with measurements of 10.5 to 23.5 cm for bitches weighing 6.5 to 27 kg.[2] This length usually prevents complete visualization of the canine vagina with otoscopic specula or standard vaginal specula. The use of endoscopic equipment will allow a more thorough examination and can also be used to obtain cytologic samples for staging the estrous cycle.[9]

The vaginal lining is composed of a series of prominent mucosal folds. The dorsal median postcervical fold can be observed to originate from the vaginal aspect of the cervix and gradually blend with smaller longitudinal folds caudally. This structure can occlude the cervical os during vaginoscopy. The function of the postcervical fold is not known.[12]

The external genitalia, or vulva, includes the vestibule, clitoris and labia.[11] The vestibule connects the vagina with the vulvar labia. On the floor of the vestibule, just caudal to the vestibulovaginal junction, the urethral tubercle is found. The vestibulovaginal margin is easily identified by the change in mucosal conformation from a smooth surface (vestibule) to one containing many longitudinal folds (vagina). The labia, or lips of the vulva, originate from the embryonic genital swellings. These structures are homologous to the male scrotum, and in the female they function to form the external boundary of the vulva (vulvar cleft). The clitoris, the homolog of the penis in the male, arises from the floor of the vestibule and extends into the clitoral fossa. The clitoris and clitoral fossa are readily visualized when the lips of the vulva are separated. The clitoris is normally a few millimeters in diameter and does not contain any structure comparable to the os penis unless the bitch is exposed to anabolic steroids (e.g., drug therapy, intersex states, Cushing's disease).

To appreciate some of the diseases of the vagina and vulva, an understanding of the embryologic development of these organs is necessary. The canine vagina and vulva are primarily derived from the paired müllerian ducts and the urogenital sinus, respectively. The cranial portion of the müllerian ducts forms the uterine horns, while the caudal portion fuses longitudinally to form the uterine body, cervix and vagina. The cranial region of the vestibule originates from the urogenital sinus and ultimately unites with the vagina to form the vestibulovaginal junction. A membranous partition, the hymen, identifies this junction in the fetus, but normally disappears by the time of birth of the animal.

During fetal life the external genitalia arise from an undifferentiated phallic tubercle. The central portion of the phallus contains a ventral groove that later forms the caudal vestibule. The clitoris also arises from the phallus, and the genital tubercles become the labia of the vulva.[5]

DISEASES OF THE VAGINA

Congenital Abnormalities

Congenital abnormalities of the vagina probably develop often in the bitch, but only occasionally are they associated with clinical disease. Abnormal development of the müllerian ducts and/or urogenital sinus account for most of the anomalies recognized. There exists either a developmental inhibition of a portion of the müllerian ducts or an aberration in the pattern of their fusion to each other or to the urogenital sinus (vestibule).

Segmental Vaginal Aplasia, Hypoplasia. Segmental aplasia of the müllerian duct system is seen most commonly in women and cattle (called "white heifer disease" in cattle). It has also been reported in dogs.[6,16] The occlusion created may be partial (hypoplasia) or complete (aplasia) and can occur anywhere along the vaginal wall. Hypoplastic conditions may only become apparent in bitches during natural breeding or parturition. Complete partitioning of the vagina (aplasia) causes retention of uterine or vaginal fluids during the estrous cycle and may easily be confused both clinically and radiographically with a closed-cervix pyometra. The etiology of segmental aplasia of the müllerian duct system in cattle is considered a sex-linked trait, but a genetic correlation has not been established in the dog.[6]

In breeding animals caudal and midvaginal strictures have been successfully resected, with the vaginal segments anastomosed.[6] No treatment is required for a nonbreeding, asymptomatic female with partial obstruction. Nonbreeding symptomatic animals are treated by ovariohysterectomy and/or vaginectomy.

Persistent Hymen. A hymen may persist because of incomplete fusion of the caudal müllerian ducts or a failure of the müllerian ducts to cannulate completely with the urogenital sinus. An incomplete perforation of the hymen, taking the form of a vertical septum (band) (Fig. 1A) or annular fibrous stricture (Fig. 1B), results in stenosis at the vestibulovaginal junction. Annular hymens may be confused with hypoplasia of the genital canal at the vaginal entrance (Fig. 1C). Both conditions demonstrate a narrowing of the tubular lumen—the

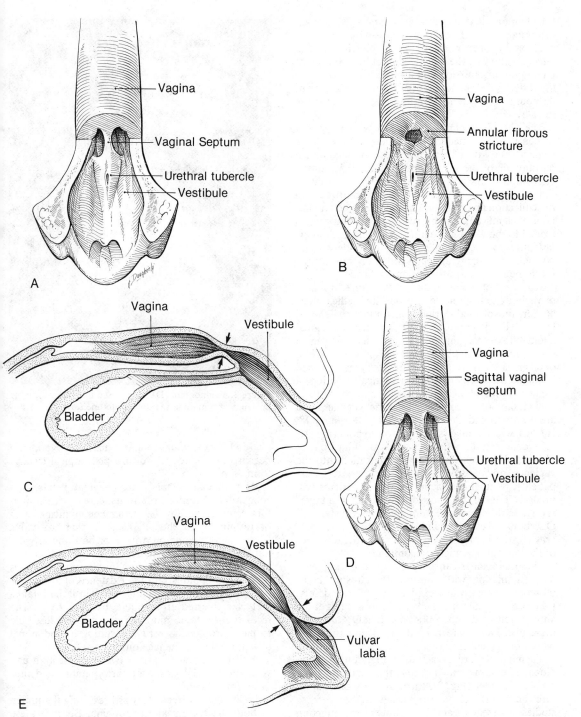

Figure 1. *A,* Vertical septum (band); a form of persistent hymen. *B,* Annular fibrous structure, a form of imperforate hymen. *C,* Hypoplasia of the vestibulovaginal junction. *D,* Retention of a sagittal vaginal membrane due to incomplete fusion of the caudal müllerian ducts. *E,* Congenital stenosis at the vestibulolabial junction.

hypoplastic state resulting in a reduction of total wall circumference, whereas the annular hymens have a circular, often fibrous, membrane that extends from the vaginal wall and results in a reduced stomal size at the vaginal entrance.[18]

Incomplete fusion of the caudal müllerian ducts can lead to retention of a midline sagittal membrane

(Fig. 1*D*). If this partition completely compartmentalizes the vagina (i.e., extends from vaginal opening to cervix) a double vagina or bifid vagina is formed.[4]

Those bitches that develop clinical problems associated with various forms of persistent hymen usually present to the veterinarian for difficulty in breeding or whelping, chronic vaginitis or "urinary incontinence." Affected females usually cycle normally and express normal mating behavior by flagging and allowing the male to mount but experience pain upon intromission and are unable to complete the "tie." The male may also experience pain, dismount or refuse further attempts to mount the female.

The chronic vaginitis associated with persistent hymen is due to inadequate drainage of uterine or vaginal fluids or of urine because of incomplete partitioning of the vagina and vestibule. Abnormal angulation of the vagina in a cranial ventral direction ("up and over" vagina) may also contribute to the collection and retention of fluids.[8] Some animals pool a significant volume of urine in the vagina cranial to the vestibulovaginal stenosis, which intermittently overflows when the dog changes body positions. This may appear similar to true urinary incontinence due to urologic anomalies.[7]

A history of breeding difficulty, failure of a case of vaginitis to respond to appropriate medical therapy or unexplained "urinary incontinence" should lead the clinician to suspect the presence of a vaginal anomaly. A simple digital examination of the vagina is the most informative and least expensive method of diagnosis. When a small vestibulovaginal foramen is palpated on either side of a vertical partition, a vaginal band, elongated vaginal septa or double vagina should be considered. Some vaginal septa are "rubberband-like" and can be "strummed." Bitches with annular strictures or hypoplastic defects demonstrate a single vaginal opening, but of reduced size, such that digital penetration into the vagina is prevented (depending on the size of the patient). Normal contraction of the constrictor vestibularis muscle (at the vestibulovaginal margin) should be differentiated from an abnormal stenosis. Questionable cases require examination under general anesthesia or during estrous when the diameter of the vaginal opening is maximum.

These anomalies can be overlooked during vaginal examination with routine vaginal specula or otoscopic cones, which tend to bypass the defect. Likewise, vaginal septa and strictures are not easily appreciated with fiberoptic equipment, although these instruments are helpful for examination and biopsy of vaginal mucosa.

Vaginograms are obtained by injection of a radiopaque contrast material into the vagina through a Foley catheter (Fig. 2). Intravaginal septae, strictures and mural lesions can be detected with these studies, but stenoses at the vestibulovaginal junction are difficult to define.[18]

Surgical removal of annular strictures and thick hymen bands is necessary in many cases to eliminate the clinical signs. Some smaller bands may be resected per vaginum with the assistance of a vaginal speculum; however, most vaginal anomalies cannot be adequately visualized without an episiotomy.

Enlarging the vaginal opening in cases of hypoplasia requires vaginal reconstruction through the use of a vaginoplasty procedure. Prognosis is more

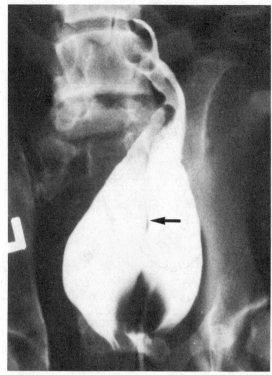

Figure 2. Vaginogram (DV view) used to demonstrate the presence of a midline sagittal membrane (*arrow*).

guarded for cases of annular hymens or hypoplasia because of a tendency toward postsurgical cicatrix formation.

Rectovaginal Fistula. Rectovaginal fistula is a congenital condition, often associated with imperforate anus, whereby the rectum communicates with or terminates in the vagina such that the vulva functions as a common orifice for both the urogenital and gastrointestinal tracts. Barium sulfate can be administered via the vagina (if atresia ani is present) to demonstrate the existence of a fistula.

The condition may go unnoticed until the infant's diet is converted from liquid to solid food. The feces then become more formed and are less able to pass through the fistula, resulting in abdominal distention due to megacolon.

A fistula can also exist between the rectum and vestibule (caudal to the urethral papilla) and produce similar signs.

Treatment is directed toward restoring the lumen of both the rectum and the vagina. Because these infants frequently lack an anal sphincter, fecal incontinence tends to persist even after surgical closure of the fistula and reconstruction of the anal opening.[13]

Acquired Abnormalities

Vaginal Hyperplasia. The vaginal and vulvar mucosae normally become very edematous during the follicular phase of the estrous cycle. An exaggeration of this estrogenic response can result in excessive mucosal folding of the vaginal floor just cranial to the urethral papilla such that redundant mucosa begins to protrude through the vulvar labia (Fig. 3). The exposed tissue rapidly becomes edematous and inflamed and is easily traumatized. The urethra does not become exteriorized and can still be catheterized. Vaginal hyperplasia is most frequently seen during the first estrous period and usually spontaneously regresses during the luteal phase. Recurrence is common during succeeding estrous periods. Affected bitches usually require artificial insemination, since the hyperplastic tissue tends to interfere with natural breeding. The hyperplastic state may also occur at parturition and interfere with normal whelping.

Saint Bernards, English bulldogs, boxers and other brachycephalic breeds are most commonly afflicted, and breeders should be aware that the etiology of this condition may have a hereditary component.[2]

Treatment. In bitches known to have a history of vaginal hyperplasia, megestrol acetate (1.0 mg/lb per os daily for 7 days) can be administered in early proestrus in an attempt to prevent vaginal hyperplasia from developing. Megestrol acetate is a synthetic progestogen that may be antagonistic to estrogens at the target tissue level and will prevent ovulation during the current cycle.[19]

Gonadotropin-releasing hormone (GnRH) has also been used to treat vaginal hyperplasia in the bitch (50 mcg GnRH IM once per 40 lb).[20] Administration of GnRH should result in release of luteinizing hormone (LH) and cause a subsequent rise in the serum concentration of progesterone. Since progesterone is antagonistic to the effects of estradiol, treatments that increase serum concentrations of progesterone might be beneficial in treating cases of estrogen-dependent vaginal hyperplasia. However, frequently by the time vaginal hyperplasia is diagnosed, concentrations of progesterone are already elevated as progesterone increases in canine serum during late proestrus. Administration of GnRH in early proestrus, during a period when ovarian follicles are still immature, could result in preovulatory luteinization of follicles or ovarian cysts.

Since the exposed hyperplastic tissue is aesthetically displeasing to many owners, in addition to interfering with coitus, surgical resection is the treatment of choice in breeding animals. Recurrence can occasionally appear during the following heat cycle, even after previous surgical resection. Permanent relief is achieved with ovariohysterectomy.

Vaginal Prolapse. Vaginal prolapse is not as commonly seen as vaginal hyperplasia in the dog. In contrast to vaginal hyperplasia, the entire circumference of the vaginal wall (including urethral papilla) protrudes through the vulvar labia, giving the exposed tissue a "donut-shaped" appearance (Fig. 4). The cervix is exteriorized in cases of complete vaginal prolapse but not with partial prolapses. The everted tissue often becomes discolored and edematous and is easily traumatized. Displacement of abdominal or pelvic organs into the prolapse is rare, although vaginal prolapse may act as a prelude to prolapse of the uterus.[15]

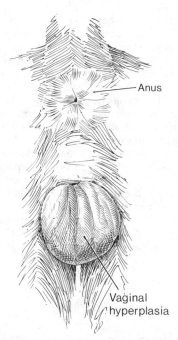

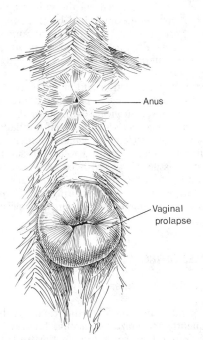

Figure 3. Vaginal hyperplasia. Redundant vaginal mucosa, arising from the vaginal floor, protrudes through the vulvar labia.

Figure 4. Vaginal prolapse: 360° eversion of the vaginal mucosa giving a "donut-shaped" appearance to the exteriorized tissue.

Brachycephalic breeds (boxers, Boston terriers) appear predisposed to vaginal prolapse and may possess a hereditary weakness of the perivulvar tissue.[15] Constipation, forced separation during coitus and size discrepancy between breeding animals may contribute to the development of this disease.[1] This condition occurs rarely during pregnancy in the bitch and occasionally may be secondary to dystocia.[15]

Both vaginal prolapse and vaginal hyperplastic states must be differentiated from polyps and neoplasias that arise from the vagina and vulva. Suspicious masses protruding from the labia, especially in the geriatric patient, should be biopsied.

Treatment. Mild prolapse cases often require no treatment, since spontaneous regression occurs during diestrus. More severe prolapses require protection of exposed tissues until estrus is completed. Attempts to reposition the vaginal mucosa usually require general anesthesia or an epidural block. The everted tissue is cleansed prior to reduction. If severe tissue edema prevents manual reduction, application of hypertonic solutions (50 per cent dextrose) in addition to manual compression of the tissue may help diminish tissue swelling. A lubricated plastic syringe case can assist in replacing the inverted tissue. An episiotomy will provide additional exposure for easier reduction. Once the vaginal tissue is replaced, a urinary catheter is inserted and the vulvar labia are temporarily sutured until the swelling resolves. Placement of a urinary catheter prevents refluxing of urine into the vagina while vaginal mucosal edema exists. Iatrogenic urinary tract infections can be minimized if a closed collection system is utilized. If repositioning of the vaginal tissue cannot be restored via the vulvar approach, reduction can be accomplished by traction on the uterus through a ventral midline abdominal approach. Recurrent prolapses can be minimized by suturing the uterine body or broad ligaments to the abdominal wall.

Hemorrhage, infection and/or necrosis of tissue may exist in severe acute or long-standing cases of vaginal prolapse. Surgical resection of the devitalized tissue is necessary to avoid self-mutilation and sepsis and to restore the vaginal lumen. Future breeding is seldom impaired following surgical resection of tissue. However, because the etiology of this condition is felt to have a hereditary component, future breeding is discouraged.[15] Ovariohysterectomy is recommended and provides permanent relief.

DISEASES OF THE VULVA

Congenital Anomalies

Congenital anomalies of the canine vulva are infrequently recognized clinically; however, when present, they may contribute to the formation of vaginitis, cystitis and difficulty in breeding. Some of the vulvar diseases include vestibulovulvar stenosis,

anovulvar cleft, vulvar atresia and clitoral hypertrophy. Very rare conditions include total vulvar agenesis and double vulvar development.

Vulvar Stenosis. Vulvar stenosis is usually detected at the junction between the vestibule and the vulvar labia and is thought to be the result of an imperfect fusion of the genital folds or genital swellings (Fig. 1E).[7] The author has identified this condition in several collie dogs. These animals were presented because they experienced pain when they attempted coitus.[18]

An episiotomy can be performed to enlarge the strictured region permanently in order to prevent dyspareunia (difficult mating) and potential dystocia.[10] Without surgical correction affected bitches require artificial insemination.

Anovulvar Cleft (Vulvar Vaginal Cleft). Anovulvar cleft is recognized in bitches as an incomplete fusion of the skin from the anus to the dorsal vulvar commissure. Failure of the urogenital folds to fuse dorsally allows direct visualization of the vestibular floor and clitoris. Inflammation of the vestibular mucosa and clitoris occur secondary to environmental exposure and fecal contamination. Surgical closure offers a good prognosis.[3,17]

This anomaly has been recognized both in sexually normal females as well as in association with intersex states. The rarity of this defect would imply that it is not hereditary.[3]

Atretic Vulva. With either vulvar hypoplasia or atrophy, the vulva appears small or infantile and is frequently retracted into the perineal skin folds.[14] The condition is usually recognized in spayed females, who clinically present with a moist, perivulvar dermatitis caused by the retention of urine within the skin folds.

Estrogen therapy has been effectively used to maintain normal vulvar size. However, continual estrogen administration is required for its effectiveness, which may result in fatal bone marrow suppression. Exteriorization of the vulva using an episoplasty procedure is the treatment of choice.

Clitoral Hypertrophy. Clitoral hypertrophy can be recognized in sexually normal females but is usually seen in conjunction with hermaphroditic or pseudohermaphroditic states secondary to anabolic steroid administration or in bitches with hyperadrenocorticoidism. Protrusion of the hypertrophied clitoris through the vulvar labia may result in clitoritis. Similarly, the mechanical irritation of an enlarged clitoris can cause vaginitis. If an os (baculum) is present, clitoral enlargement may persist even after removal of the source of anabolic steroids. Therefore clitoral resection must accompany neutering.[19]

Acquired Vulvar Abnormalities

Vulvar Hypertrophy. The canine vulva normally becomes swollen and edematous in response to estrogen stimulation during the follicular stage of the estrous cycle. The vulvar enlargement may become excessive and persist beyond the normal estrous period in animals possessing cystic ovaries or granulosa cell tumors. The labia become thickened, pigmented and hairless in chronically untreated cases. Permanent relief can be achieved with ovariohysterectomy.[14]

References

1. Alexander JE, Lennok WJ: Vaginal prolapse in the bitch. Can Vet J 2:428, 1961.
2. Burke TJ, Reynold HA: The female genital system. In Bojrab MJ (ed): Pathophysiology in Small Animal Surgery. Philadelphia, Lea & Febiger, 1981, p 425.
3. Burke TJ, Smith CW: Vulvovaginal cleft in a dog. Am Anim Hosp Assoc 11:774, 1975.
4. Capel-Edwards K: Double vagina with perineal agenesis in a bitch. Vet Rec 101:57, 1977.
5. Evans HE, Christensen GL: Miller's Anatomy of the Dog. 2nd ed. Philadelphia, WB Saunders Co, 1979, p 31.
6. Gee BR, Pharr JW, Furneaux RW: Segmental aplasia of the müllerian duct system in a dog. Can Vet J 18:281, 1977.
7. Holt PE, Sayle B: Congenital vestibulovaginal stenosis in the bitch. J Small Anim Pract 22:67, 1981.
8. Jones DE, Joshua JO: Reproductive Clinical Problems in the Dog. Boston, PSG Wright, 1982.
9. Lindsay FEF: The normal endoscopic appearance of the caudal reproductive tract of the cyclic and noncyclic bitch: Postuterine endoscopy. J Small Anim Pract 24:1, 1983.
10. McConnell DA: Correction of vaginovestibular strictures in the bitch. JAAHA 13:92, 1977.
11. Miller ME, Christensen GC, Evans HE: Anatomy of the Dog. 2nd ed. Philadelphia, WB Saunders Co, 1964, p 790.
12. Pineda MH, Kainer RA, Faulkner LC: Dorsal medial postcervical fold in the canine vagina. Am J Vet Res 34:1487, 1973.
13. Rawlings CA, Capps WF: Rectovaginal fistula and imperforate anus in a dog. J Am Vet Med Assoc 159:320, 1971.
14. Smith KW: Female Genital System. In Archibald J (ed): Canine Surgery. Santa Barbara, American Veterinary Publications Inc, 1974, p 751.
15. Troger CP: Vaginal prolapse in the bitch. Mod Vet Pract 53:73, 1972.
16. Wadsworth PF, Hall JC, Prentice DE: Segmental aplasia of the vagina in a beagle bitch. Lab Anim 12:65, 1978.
17. Wilson CF, Clifford DH: Perineoplasty for anovaginal cleft in the dog. J Am Vet Med Assoc 159:871, 1971.
18. Wykes PM, Soderberg SF: Congenital abnormalities of the canine vagina and vulva. Am Anim Hosp Assoc 19:995, 1983.
19. Wykes PM, Olson PN: Diseases of the vagina. In Slatter D (ed): Textbook of Small Animal Surgery. Philadelphia, WB Saunders Co, 1985.
20. Johnston SD: Personal communication. University of Minnesota, St. Paul, January 1984.

Prostaglandins in Small Animal Reproduction

Donald H. Lein, D.V.M., Ph.D.
Cornell University, Ithaca, New York

Prostaglandins of the F series ($PGF_{2\alpha}$) are used in the bitch and queen for the luteolytic and smooth muscle effect that results in cervical dilatation and uterine contraction. This effect is used to cause luteolysis and abortion in midpregnancy, which is approximately from 30 days and 40 days to parturition in the bitch and queen, respectively. The current popular clinical use is to treat pyometra-endometritis in the bitch and queen. Studies have also shown prostaglandin analogs to cause luteolysis and abortion in the bitch. The right analog could become a very important drug for small animal use because analogs are usually much more potent and long acting, with lower dosage and less side effects.

TOXICITY AND SIDE EFFECTS

The median subcutaneous lethal dose for $PGF_{2\alpha}$ in the bitch has been reported to be 5.13 mg/kg.[11]

Clinical signs of side effects and toxicosis include excessive salivation, vomiting, diarrhea, hyperpnea, ataxia, urination, anxiety and pupillary dilatation followed by constriction. Severity of side effects is dose dependent. At low dosages defecation is more frequent, while at intermediate dosages, hyperpnea, anxiety, hypersalivation, vomiting as well as defecation have been observed. Higher doses have caused ataxia and slight depression.[8] The dose range used has been from 0.02 to 1.0 mg/kg (20 μg to 1000 μg/kg) in the bitch[1,2,4-8,10] and 0.220 to 1.0 mg/kg (220 to 1000 μg/kg) in the queen[6,9] when $PGF_{2\alpha}$ is administered intramuscularly or subcutaneously.

Side effects are seen 20 to 120 minutes after injection. Death in animals given lethal doses occurs from 2 to 12 hours after injection.[11] Bitches seem to adapt to $PGF_{2\alpha}$ with side effects diminishing by the fourth or fifth treatment. Prostaglandin $F_{2\alpha}$ or analogs should not be used in dogs or cats with asthma or liver, kidney or cardiac problems. Prostaglandins have not been approved for use in small animal medicine and should be considered experimental by clinicians, and owners of pets should be warned that these are not approved drugs.

LUTEOLYSIS AND ABORTION

Early researchers thought that $PGF_{2\alpha}$ was not luteolytic in the dog. Concannon and Hansel were the first to show that 20 μg/kg every 8 hours or 30 μg/kg every 12 hours for 3 days caused abortion in

4 of 7 bitches started on treatment on days 33 to 53 of gestation, with abortion occurring 56 to 80 hours after the initial treatment.[2] Progesterone plasma levels were 0.6 to 1.4 ng/ml when abortion occurred. The three bitches that did not abort had a mean low value of 2.1 ng/ml of plasma progesterone during $PGF_{2\alpha}$ treatment beginning on days 31 to 40 of gestation. Their plasma progesterone concentrations then increased to 5 to 10 ng/ml and were maintained until normal antepartal decline. In this study eight nonpregnant bitches in the mid-to-late luteal phase were also treated, and all eight had complete luteolysis with low anestrous baseline plasma progesterone levels afterwards. Two nonpregnant bitches in the early luteal phase (days 5 and 20) were also treated, and plasma progesterone levels were not drastically altered.

Concannon and Hansel also reported that a transient fall in rectal temperature occurred within 15 minutes; maximal temperature drop occurred at 45 to 60 minutes after inoculation and averaged 1.39°C. No change in temperature was seen in ovariectomized bitches treated with $PGF_{2\alpha}$. It was concluded that hypothermia was caused by the 20 to 45 per cent fall in plasma progesterone levels within the 15 minutes after inoculation of $PGF_{2\alpha}$.

Paradis and colleagues reported on 10 mated bitches that were given 250 µg/kg of $PGF_{2\alpha}$ bid; five were given $PGF_{2\alpha}$ between 1 and 5 days of metestrus and five were given it between 31 and 35 days of metestrus.[8] Dogs in early metestrus were not affected and appeared the same as the five nontreated controls, whereas all five in midgestation had complete luteolysis, hypothermia following the initial injection of $PGF_{2\alpha}$ and abortion following the fourth to eighth injection.

Prostaglandin analogs fluprostenol (Equimate) and cloprostenol (Estrumate) were administered to 42 beagle bitches at gestational periods of 4 to 35 days at doses of 10 to 40 µg/kg.[3] A slow-releasing formula of both analogs (48 to 72 hours) and a 24-hour-release intravaginal device of both analogs showed minimal acceptable side effects compared with the aqueous marketed form of cloprostenol. Sustained depression of plasma levels and pregnancy termination were seen in 6 of 22 bitches (27 per cent) treated before day 25 of gestation and 16 of 20 bitches (80 per cent) treated on or after day 25. An interesting effect was that two bitches whose pregnancies and/or corpora lutea were terminated at 14 days by the 40 µg/kg cloprostenol showed clinical estrus 10 to 14 days after treatment, with normal mature ovarian follicles at necropsy. This suggests that a bitch could possibly be remated in a few weeks after correction of a misalliance in the first 2 weeks instead of having to wait until the next cycle at 4 to 12 months.

Eleven pregnant bitches were treated with a single subcutaneous injection of 20 µg/kg of synthetic prostaglandin analog (TPT) in an aqueous buffer.[12] Five bitches treated between days 30 to 43 of pregnancy aborted 5.4 ± 1.4 days following treatment. Two of four bitches treated on days 20 to 22 of gestation continued to normal term, while the other two appeared to resorb their fetuses following diagnosis by palpation on day 28. Two others treated on day 9 had successful pregnancies.

In further work by this group, bitches were given TPT subcutaneously in different treatments on days 20 to 22 of pregnancy: minipump at a rate of 10 µg per hour for either 24 or 48 hours, single injection of 200 µg in either aqueous or polyethylene glycol 400 and the methyl ester of TPT in polyethylene glycol 400.[13] All treatments caused abortion or resorption, with the best treatments being those that had the longest administration of analog. After 48 hours with the minipump, five sixths aborted; with the methyl esther of TPT, three fourths aborted.

This research indicates that the early corpora lutea (to days 25 to 30) are quite resistant to exogenous prostaglandins. The author has treated six mismated bitches with $PGF_{2\alpha}$ to attempt to induce abortion; they were of the following breeds: Labrador retriever, Chesapeake Bay retriever, Siberian husky, vizsla, cocker spaniel and coonhound. Their ages ranged from 8 months to 5 years, and gestations ranged from 31 to 60 days, with a range of 2 to 8.5 days of $PGF_{2\alpha}$ treatments used to attempt to cause abortion.

Treatment consisted of 25 to 50 µg/kg of $PGF_{2\alpha}$ (Lutalyse) intramuscularly, given twice a day. All bitches were hospitalized, secluded in a quiet area and observed for signs of abortion. The lower dose was given the first day or two to allow for observation of the severity of side effects and to relax the cervix. These bitches showed nesting signs 24 to 48 hours prior to abortion. Vaginoscopic examination of three of six revealed daily changes in the anterior vagina, with increasing edema of the vaginal and cervical folds, fluid and dilatation of the cervix 24 to 48 hours prior to abortion. The two late gestation bitches, 57 and 60 days of gestation, aborted at 2 and 4.5 days of treatment, respectively, and both had live pups. The bitch at 31 days of gestation aborted three pups 6 days after the initial treatment and appeared to have completed abortion. She was given 10 IU of oxytocin intramuscularly the following day to enhance uterine involution. Two weeks later, two retained viable fetuses were noted on palpation and on radiographs. The bitch whelped two normal live pups and has since had three normal litters. All bitches returned to estrus at normal intervals. One bitch had prolonged postpartum hemorrhage for 6 weeks that was diagnosed as subinvolution of placental sites. All bitches showed varying individual slight side effects for the first 15 to 60 minutes after injection, including increased salivation, diarrhea, emesis and panting.

This research shows that $PGF_{2\alpha}$ can be used to induce abortion in healthy bitches from midgestation to term, and a dosage range of 25 to 250 µg/kg given intramuscularly, bid to effect can be used. Hospitalization and close observation are necessary and the later the stage of gestation, the quicker the effect. More research is needed on the analogs different routes of administration such as the intravaginal route, possible early-gestation luteolysis and early return to estrus.

Luteal function in the pseudopregnant and pregnant queen can also be altered by $PGF_{2\alpha}$. Pregnancy was terminated in 13 queens after day 40 of gestation, with one or two injections of either 0.50 or 1.00 mg/kg of $PGF_{2\alpha}$.[6] Two injections of 0.25 mg/kg aborted three of six queens. Parturition or abortion occurred within 8 to 24 hours in nine cats and within 8 to 24 hours after the second injection in four queens. Queens with gestation times prior to 40 days were not affected. Minimal side effects were seen in these queens. Longer dose schedules need to be studied in queens in the earlier gestation period.

A luteolytic effect was seen in pseudopregnant queens administered either 220 or 440 µg/kg every 12 hours on days 21 to 25, but minimal depression of plasma progesterone levels occurred in queens treated on days 11 to 15. A significantly higher concentration of plasma progesterone levels was found in the refractory early-treated queens when compared with controls on days 33 and 36 after coitus.[9]

PYOMETRA-ENDOMETRITIS

Several investigators have reported on the clinical treatment of bitches with pyometra or endometritis.[1,4,5,7,10] Prostaglandin $F_{2\alpha}$ is very effective in causing luteolysis, cervical dilatation and myometrial contraction in late-metestrus bitches when closed-cervix pyometra is diagnosed. It is also effective in uterine evacuation in open pyometra or endometritis showing varying degrees of vaginal discharge. Usually within 48 to 96 hours of treatment, marked reduction in size of the uterus, increased myometrial tone and increased vaginal discharge occur.

Bitches are usually treated for 3 to 5 days or to effect with $PGF_{2\alpha}$ until vaginal discharge is scant or absent and the uterus is reduced to a very firm small size. Parenteral antibiotic therapy should always be given during treatment and carried out for at least 10 to 30 days, depending on the severity of the condition. Deep vaginal or cervical swabs for bacterial, mycoplasmal and ureaplasmal culture and sensitivity should be taken for the most beneficial antibiotic therapy. Before results are known, parenteral chloramphenicol or ampicillin is given. Chloramphenicol is the author's drug of choice, if the bitch can tolerate it, because it is a broad-spectrum antibiotic and is usually highly effective against *Escherichia coli*, *Mycoplasma* and *Ureaplasma* infections. Daily deep vaginal douches with 200 to 500 ml warm 1 per cent tamed iodine solutions (Betadine) are beneficial during the $PGF_{2\alpha}$ treatment.

Various subcutaneous and intramuscular dosages of $PGF_{2\alpha}$, 25 to 1000 µg/kg, and schemes of treatment have been reported. Success has been seen with single doses at 250 to 1000 µg/kg as well as with a scheme of multiple injections every 12 hours

at 25 to 50 µg/kg. Most of these schemes were given to effect (usually 3 to 5 days). The lower the dosage, the more minimal the side effects. Burke[1] recommends that 3 to 5 days after the last dose of $PGF_{2\alpha}$ a final dose be given to ensure that the uterus is not refilling with exudate. The author uses multiple dosages of 25 to 250 µg/kg every 12 hours to effect. Dosage depends on the clinical condition and side effects exhibited by the individual dog. The lower dosage is used first.

Bitches that develop pyometra as a sequela to cystic endometrial hyperplasia–endometritis should be bred the next estrus after treatment, since pyometra following nonpregnant cycles may recur. If further litters are not desired, an ovariohysterectomy should be performed.

Prior to the next estrus the bitch should have a deep vaginal culture and cytology while in late anestrus or early proestrus and should be treated with appropriate antibiotics parenterally prior to breeding. Bitches highly susceptible to postcoital infections should also be considered for artificial insemination with antibiotic-treated extenders to reduce the number of potential infectious organisms. In these bitches cultures should also be done after breeding and treatment given as indicated. donebe treated accordingly.

Prognosis depends on the age of the bitch, the severity of degenerative lesions in the uterus and the quality of aftercare prior to breeding. Old bitches with severe uterine degenerative conditions or renal, pulmonary or cardiac disorders are poor risks. Pyometritis in some cases of cystic hyperplasia can be a positive factor, since the suppuration and necrosis of the uterine lining acts as a curettage and results in regrowth of a new endometrium after treatment. Several of these bitches will conceive if bred the next estrus following treatment. Bitches with minimal degenerative endometrial conditions, such as the young bitch with a pyometra following a mismating injection of estradiol, are highly successful breeders following treatment with $PGF_{2\alpha}$.

Queens with pyometritis can be treated similarly to bitches, following the same dosages of $PGF_{2\alpha}$ and use of antibiotic therapy. The prognosis for queens undergoing these treatments is similar to that for the bitch.

Besides the use of prostaglandins for the treatment of pyometra-endometritis and abortion in small animal reproduction, future studies and research may lead to their successful use as mismating injections early in metestrus and as controls in the length of luteal function throughout the estrous cycle of the bitch and queen.

References

1. Burke TJ: Prostaglandin $F_{2\alpha}$ in the treatment of pyometra-metritis. Symposium Hormone and Corticosteroid Therapy. Vet Clin North Am: Small Anim Pract 12:107, 1982.
2. Concannon PW, Hansel W: Prostaglandin $F_{2\alpha}$ induced luteolysis, hypothermia, and abortions in Beagle bitches. Prostaglandins 13:533, 1977.
3. Jackson PS, Furr BJA, Hutchinson FG: A preliminary study of pregnancy termination in the bitch with slow-release for-

mulation of prostaglandin analogues. J Small Anim Pract 23:287, 1982.
4. Johnson SD: Use of prostaglandins in reproduction. DVM 10:18, 1979.
5. Lein DH: Pyometritis in the bitch and queen. In Kirk RW (ed): Current Veterinary Therapy VIII, Small Animal Practice. Philadelphia, WB Saunders Co., 1983, pp 942–944.
6. Nachreiner RF, Marple DN: Termination of pregnancy in cats with Prostaglandin $F_{2\alpha}$. Prostaglandins 7:303, 1974.
7. Nelson RW, Feldman EC, Stabenfeldt GH: Treatment of canine pyometra and endometritis with prostaglandin F. J Am Vet Med Assoc 181:899, 1982.
8. Paradis M, Post K, Mapletoft RJ: Effects of Prostaglandin $F_{2\alpha}$ on corpora lutea formation and function in mated bitches. Can Vet J 24:239, 1983.
9. Shille VM, Stabenfeldt GH: Luteal function in the domestic cat during pseudopregnancy and after treatment with Prostaglandin $F_{2\alpha}$. Biol Reprod 21:1217, 1979.
10. Sokolowski JH: Prostaglandin F_2 alpha-THAM for medical treatment of endometritis, metritis and pyometritis in the bitch. JAAHA 16:119, 1980.
11. Sokolowski JH, Geng S: Effect of Prostaglandin $F_{2\alpha}$-THAM in the bitch. J Am Vet Med Ass 170:536, 1977.
12. Vickery BH, McRae GI: Effect of synthetic prostaglandin analogue on pregnancy in Beagle bitches. Biol Reprod 22:438, 1980.
13. Vickery BH, McRae GI, Kent JS, Tomlinson RV: Manipulation of duration of action of a synthetic prostaglandin analogue (TPT) assessed in the pregnant Beagle bitch. Prostaglandins Med 5:93, 1980.

Pyometra in the Bitch

R. W. Nelson, D.V.M.
Purdue University, West Lafayette, Indiana

E. C. Feldman, D.V.M.
University of California, Davis, California

PATHOPHYSIOLOGY

Pyometra in the bitch is a hormonally mediated diestrual disorder. The disease results from bacterial interaction with an endometrium that has undergone pathologic changes from prolonged or repeated progesterone stimulation.[3] The plasma progesterone concentration in the anestrous bitch is less than 0.5 ng/ml.[4] For approximately 2 months following ovulation the plasma progesterone concentration is increased, often exceeding 40 ng/ml. During this period progesterone promotes endometrial growth and glandular secretion while suppressing myometrial activity, thus allowing accumulation of uterine glandular secretions. These secretions provide an excellent environment for bacterial growth. Bacterial growth is further enhanced by inhibition of the leukocyte response to infection in the progesterone-primed uterus.

Progesterone-induced endometrial hyperplasia usually precedes the development of pyometra.[2] Endometrial thickening is caused by an increase in the size and number of endometrial glands, which may show secretory activity. The mucosal epithelial cells are typically tortuous with hypertrophic, clear cytoplasm. The stroma becomes edematous, and an inflammatory cell infiltration is present. Occasion-ally, endometrial gland secretion results in an accumulation of thin or viscid fluid within the lumen of the uterus. This fluid-filled uterus is referred to as hydrometra or mucometra, with the degree of hydration of the mucin determining its description. These conditions are typically sterile.

Bacterial infection is a secondary problem. Bacteria from the vagina is the most likely source for a uterine infection. These bacteria ascend through the cervix into the uterus during estrus. A predominance of *Escherichia coli* in uterine infections may be secondary to the ability of this organism to adhere via specific antigenic sites to receptors in the progesterone-stimulated endometrium and myometrium.[5]

Estrogen, by itself, is not usually associated with the development of cystic endometrial hyperplasia or pyometra. However, estrogens enhance the stimulatory effects of progesterone on the uterus. Pharmacologic concentrations of estrogen (e.g., mismate shots) during the diestrual phase of the estrous cycle may increase the risk of developing pyometra.

SIGNALMENT AND HISTORY

Historically, pyometra is a disorder of middle-aged bitches (8 to 10 years old), developing after years of repetitive progesterone stimulation of the uterus. However, with use of estrogens for mismating in young bitches, we have seen open-cervix and closed-cervix pyometras developing at an increasingly younger age. A mean age of 3 years was reported by the authors for 17 bitches with pyometra recently treated with protaglandin $F_{2\alpha}$ ($PGF_{2\alpha}$) (Lutalyse).[4] Several of these dogs were less than 1 year of age. Pyometra should be considered in any bitch with consistent clinical signs appearing during or shortly after diestrus, regardless of her age.

Signs reported by the owner depend on the patency of the cervix. A bitch with open-cervix pyometra has a sanguineous to mucopurulent discharge from the vulva. The discharge is usually first noticed 4 to 8 weeks after standing heat but can be observed as early as the end of standing heat or as late as 12 to 14 weeks after the end of standing heat. Other signs include lethargy, depression, inappetence, polyuria, polydipsia and vomiting. It is also common for bitches with open-cervix pyometra to be relatively healthy except for the presence of an abnormal vaginal discharge.

Signs in bitches with closed-cervix pyometra include depression, lethargy, weakness, inappetence, polyuria, polydipsia and vomiting. Occasionally, an owner will have noticed a discharge from the vulva prior to the onset of the other signs, which lasts only a few days. Vomiting and anorexia, in conjunction with polyuria, will cause progressively worsening dehydration, shock, coma and eventually death. The severity of illness at the time of presentation is dependent on the ability of the owner to recognize the problem. Signs of illness usually begin 4 to 10 weeks following standing heat.

PHYSICAL EXAMINATION

Abnormalities found on physical examination include depression, dehydration, uterine enlargement and a sanguineous to mucopurulent discharge from the vulva if the cervix is patent ("open"). Fever is a variable sign and, when present, is associated with uterine inflammation and secondary bacterial infection as well as septicemia or bacteremia. With septicemia or bacteremia, shock may ensue.

Uterine enlargement may be difficult to detect by palpation, especially if the uterus is draining much of its contents or if the uterus is enlarged but flaccid. Abdominal radiography can be used to confirm uterine enlargement. Overzealous palpation should be avoided to prevent rupture of the uterine wall. Occasionally, open-cervix pyometra will drain enough uterine contents to prevent marked uterine enlargement; however, the organ may still be inflamed and infected.

CLINICAL PATHOLOGY

The total white blood cell count is usually increased in the bitch with closed-cervix pyometra, often exceeding 30,000 cells per mm^3. An absolute neutrophilia with variable degrees of cellular immaturity may progress, with subsequent infection and septicemia, to a degenerative left shift with toxic neutrophils. Similar total white blood cell counts may be found in the bitch with open-cervix pyometra; however, normal white blood cell counts may be encountered. Six of eleven bitches with open-cervix pyometra treated with PGF$_{2\alpha}$ by the authors had total white blood cell counts within the normal range.[4]

A mild normocytic, normochromic, nonregenerative anemia (packed cell volume 28–35 ml/dl) is often associated with pyometra. The anemia should resolve once the pyometra is corrected. Concomitant hyperproteinemia (total protein of 7.5 to 10.0 gm/dl) and hyperglobulinemia result from dehydration and chronic antigenic stimulation of the dog's immune system.

Results of a serum biochemical panel are usually unremarkable except for hyperproteinemia. Serum urea nitrogen concentration may be increased if dehydration is present. Occasionally, alanine aminotransferase and alkaline phosphatase concentrations are mild to moderately increased from hepatocellular damage caused by septicemia and/or diminished hepatic circulation and cellular hypoxia in the dehydrated bitch.

Urine specific gravity is variable. Early in the disease process, the urine specific gravity may be greater than 1.030. With secondary bacterial infection, especially with *E. coli*, toxemia develops that may interfere with the resorption of sodium and chloride in the loop of Henle.[1,3] This reduces renal medullary hypertonicity, impairing the collecting tubules' ability to resorb free water. Polyuria and compensatory polydipsia result. Others claim that a specific cause for the loss of concentrating ability has not been established but propose a renal tubular insensitivity to the action of antidiuretic hormone (ADH) as a sequel to tubular damage caused by *E. coli* endotoxins.[3] Tubular immune complex injury may also have a role. Prolonged polyuria and polydipsia cause renal medullary solute washout, further impairing the kidney's ability to conserve water. As a result, urine becomes progressively more dilute. Hyposthenuria (urine specific gravity < 1.006) is not uncommon in a bitch with pyometra. Prerenal azotemia may also be present if water consumption inadequately compensates for the polyuria.

Urinary tract infections may be suspected if pyuria, hematuria and proteinuria are found in the urinalysis. However, urine obtained by a midstream collection may be dramatically altered if a vaginal discharge is present. We do not recommend cystocentesis on dogs with suspected or known pyometra. There is a risk of puncturing the infected uterus, with subsequent leakage of uterine contents into the abdomen, causing peritonitis. We do not routinely culture the urine unless quantitative evaluation of the bacterial growth from a midstream collection is performed, and then, only if there is no vaginal discharge.

Proteinuria without pyuria or hematuria may also be found with pyometra. Immune complex deposition in the glomeruli causes a mixed membranoproliferative glomerulonephropathy and leakage of plasma proteins into the glomerular filtrate. The proteinuria gradually resolves with correction of the pyometra.

RADIOGRAPHY

The uterus can be visualized radiographically beginning with the fourth week of gestation, continuing through pregnancy and for 2 to 4 weeks after whelping. Radiographic visualization of the uterus at other times is abnormal. Abdominal radiographs should be assessed in a bitch with suspected pyometra to confirm the diagnosis. With pyometra, a fluid-dense tubular structure should be seen in the ventral and caudal abdomen, displacing loops of intestine dorsally and cranially. In addition to confirming the diagnosis of pyometra, radiographs may provide important information regarding the medical status of a bitch. Two major concerns in a dog with pyometra are the presence or absence of peritonitis from a uterine rupture and retained fetal tissue from a previous pregnancy. Abdominal compression may be of value using a belly band or wooden spoon to displace the intestines away from the uterus. This procedure may enhance radiographic contrast and often allows improved visualization of the uterus. Inability to radiographically visualize the uterus does not rule out pyometra associated with an open cervix and significant drainage of uterine contents through the vagina.

ULTRASONOGRAPHY

Ultrasonography has greatly enhanced the clinician's ability to document pyometra, especially when abdominal radiographs are inconclusive. Ultrasound allows determination of uterine size, the thickness of the uterine wall and the presence of fluid accumulation within the uterus. In some cases the character of the fluid within the uterus (serous versus viscid) can be determined.

DIAGNOSIS

The diagnosis of pyometra is confirmed when the appropriate clinical signs reported by the owner are present in conjunction with abnormalities on physical examination, laboratory studies and radiographic evaluation. A definitive diagnosis becomes a challenge when the history is vague, especially in regard to estrous activity and breeding, when a vulvar discharge is present yet the uterus feels normal, when no vaginal discharge is observed or when the dog has been previously "spayed" yet clinical signs and pathology suggest pyometra. Pyometra should be considered in any older, intact bitch presenting with vague signs of illness, polyuria/polydipsia or a neutrophilic leukocytosis present on a hemogram. Evaluation of a hemogram, serum biochemical panel, urinalysis and abdominal radiographs may be necessary in differentiating the various causes of polyuria and polydipsia.

It may be difficult to differentiate renal failure from pyometra with prerenal azotemia. If urine specific gravity is less than 1.006 or greater than 1.030, prerenal azotemia and not primary renal failure should be considered. If isosthenuria is present, the clinician must rely on the history and presence or absence of other biochemical abnormalities (e.g., serum calcium, phosphorus concentration), abdominal radiographs (evaluating uterus and kidneys), response to fluid therapy and perhaps renal function tests to make an accurate diagnosis. Occasionally, pyometra and concomitant primary renal failure will occur.

Vaginal cytology and bacterial cultures are not definitive in diagnosing pyometra. Neutrophils in a vaginal smear may be associated with vaginitis or uterine inflammation, especially if the cervix is patent. Vaginal bacteria can be caused by normal flora (Table 1), vaginitis or drainage from open-cervix pyometra. Vaginal bacterial growth does not imply similar organisms are present in the uterus unless the cervix is patent and the culture is taken from within the cervix with a guarded culture swab. Anterior vaginal cultures are useful when treating a bitch with open-cervix pyometra medically with $PGF_{2\alpha}$. Results of antibiotic sensitivity can be used to make a rational choice of antibiotics. We do not routinely culture the anterior vagina of a bitch suspected of having closed-cervix pyometra.

A healthy bitch may present with a copious vaginal discharge without uterine enlargement. A carefully obtained history and results of a hemogram, vaginal examination and, if possible, an ultrasound examination of the uterus should be used to differentiate open-cervix pyometra from a vaginal problem. Systemic signs of illness such as lethargy, inappetance and depression may be subtle with open-cervix pyometra and may suggest uterine rather than vaginal disease. Mild fever, neutrophilic leukocytosis and hyperproteinemia are also supportive of a uterine problem. Vaginoscopy allows visualization of the vaginal mucosa for inflammation, masses, foreign bodies, congenital abnormalities and determination of the origin of the vulvar discharge. If the discharge appears to be coming from the anterior vaginal/cervical area, a uterine problem should be suspected. If doubt still exists, the bitch is not severely ill or a valuable breeding animal and the owners will not consider surgery, the bitch may be treated for vaginitis and reevaluated. If the reproductive potential of the dog is to be saved, medical therapy with $PGF_{2\alpha}$ can be instituted. Pyometra will usually respond to $PGF_{2\alpha}$ therapy, while vaginitis will not respond.

Stump pyometra refers to inflammation and bacterial infection of a remnant of the uterine body. If ovarian tissue also remains following ovariohysterectomy, estrous cycles, progesterone secretion and

Table 1. Bacterial Isolates from Clinically Normal Canine Vagina

Escherichia coli
Sreptococcus sp.
Staphylococcus sp.
Pasteurella sp.
Corynebacterium sp.
Bacillus sp.

(From Olson P, Mather E: Canine vaginal and uterine bacterial flora. JAVMA 172:708, 1978.)

uterine stimulation and inflammation will occur. Owners may assume the estrous behavior is normal in a spayed dog and will not seek veterinary assistance until clinical signs consistent with pyometra develop. Clinical signs and laboratory abnormalities are the same as those previously discussed. Forming a diagnosis can be difficult if a discharge from the vulva is not present. Caudal abdominal radiographs with abdominal compression or an ultrasound examination may demonstrate the diseased uterine stump. Many bitches require surgical exploration for a definitive diagnosis. Stump pyometra may also occur without the presence of remnant ovarian tissue. A thorough exploration of the abdomen for ovarian tissue is recommended if a uterine stump is surgically removed.

SURGICAL TREATMENT

Ovariohysterectomy is the preferred treatment for pyometra unless the reproductive potential of the bitch must be saved. Severely ill bitches should be vigorously treated with intravenous fluids and should be closely monitored. Abnormalities in serum electrolytes, acid-base status, cardiac rhythm and fluid status, in addition to septicemia, bacteremia and azotemia, are common. One cannot always wait for stabilization of the animal before surgery is performed. In some dogs surgery may not be postponed more than a few hours. Septicemia originating from the diseased uterus is often responsible for the severe illness, and only surgical removal of the uterus will resolve the septic state of the bitch.

Injectable broad-spectrum antibiotics and intravenous polyionic fluids with appropriate electrolyte supplementation should be given immediately. Initiating these procedures will improve the chances of survival. Supportive therapy should be continued during and after surgery. Oral antibiotics should be continued for 7 to 10 days after the removal of the infected uterus.

MEDICAL TREATMENT

Medical therapy utilizing estrogens, androgens, ergot alkaloids, quinine and oxytocin is inconsistent and often unsuccessful. In addition, systemic antibiotics are generally ineffective as the sole therapy for canine pyometra. However, results using prostaglandin $F_{2\alpha}$ ($PGF_{2\alpha}$) have been encouraging and offer a medical alternative for therapy.

Prostaglandin $F_{2\alpha}$ has several physiological effects on the female reproductive system, including contraction of the myometrium. This effect results in expulsion of the exudate accumulated in the uterus. Synthesis and secretion of progesterone are the primary functions of the corpora lutea. Lysis of the corpora lutea or transitory inhibition of ovarian steroidogenesis result from administration of $PGF_{2\alpha}$. These actions are partially dependent on the dosage,

route and frequency of administration and the timing within the bitch's luteal cycle. The resultant decreased plasma progesterone concentration reduces the stimulus for endometrial growth and glandular secretion (Fig. 1).

When deciding whether to use $PGF_{2\alpha}$, the clinician should consider the age of the bitch, the owner's desire to save this animal's reproductive potential, the severity of the illness at the time of presentation, the presence or absence of other concurrent disease and the patency of the cervix. Medical therapy utilizing prostaglandins should be discouraged in older bitches (> 8 years) or in bitches whose owners are unsure about or not interested in maintaining the reproductive capabilities of their dog.

Clinical response may not be observed for 48 hours after beginning prostaglandin therapy. Therefore, this drug is not ideal for use in severely ill animals that are poor anesthetic risks, unless the owner refuses to allow surgery. Concurrent illness or disease (e.g., uncontrolled congestive heart failure) may increase the surgical risk to an unacceptable level. The use of $PGF_{2\alpha}$ may be necessary in these cases.

Prostaglandin $F_{2\alpha}$ should be used with caution in bitches with closed-cervix pyometra because of the potential for uterine exudate being expelled into the peritoneal cavity, causing peritonitis. Although estrogens may relax the cervix, their use prior to $PGF_{2\alpha}$ therapy is not recommended because of estrogen enhancement of the progesterone effects on the uterus.

Prostaglandin $F_{2\alpha}$ is not approved for use in the bitch, but it is available for use in the cow and the mare. Owners should be informed that the use of $PGF_{2\alpha}$ for treating canine pyometra is experimental.

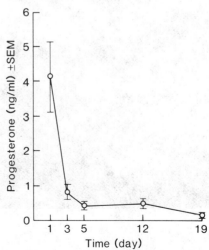

Figure 1. Plasma progesterone concentrations in nine bitches with pyometra and open cervix before (day 1), during (days 2–5) and after (days 12–19) treatment with $PGF_{2\alpha}$. The bars represent SEM. (Reprinted with permission from Nelson RW, Feldman EC, Stabenfeldt GH: JAVMA 181:899, 1982.)

The bitch should not be pregnant because the depressive effects of $PGF_{2\alpha}$ on progesterone synthesis/secretion may induce abortion. We have seen two bitches referred for $PGF_{2\alpha}$ therapy because of a copious mucopurulent discharge from the vulva; both were pregnant and both had severe vaginitis that responded to appropriate therapy. Both bitches whelped healthy litters. Because of the drug's myotonic effects, its use is contraindicated in bitches with mummified fetuses because of the potential for tearing a uterine wall, resulting in peritonitis.

Only naturally occurring prostaglandin $F_{2\alpha}$ (Lutalyse, Prostin) should be used at the following recommended dosage. Synthetic prostaglandin $F_{2\alpha}$ analogs (cloprostenol, fluprostenol, prostalene) are much more powerful than the natural prostaglandin $F_{2\alpha}$. Use of these synthetic products at our recommended dosage will result in shock and possibly death. The LD_{50} for $PGF_{2\alpha}$ in the bitch is 5.13 mg/kg.[6]

We recommend the following protocol for $PGF_{2\alpha}$ therapy: 0.25 mg/kg $PGF_{2\alpha}$ SQ daily for 5 days. In addition, concomitant, broad-spectrum antibiotics effective against *E. coli* should be administered for 7 days. This will help prevent bacteremia following contraction of the uterus around potentially infected uterine luminal contents. When treating a bitch with closed-cervix pyometra, a discharge from the vulva should be seen by the third $PGF_{2\alpha}$ injection. If such a discharge is not seen, a thorough physical examination and abdominal radiographs should be performed to ensure peritonitis is not developing.

The bitch should be reevaluated 2 weeks later. If sanguineous or mucopurulent vulvar discharge, uterine enlargement or clinical signs are still present, treatment with $PGF_{2\alpha}$ and antibiotics should be reinstituted for an additional 5 days. If there is no discharge and the uterus is not enlarged, or if the discharge appears clear and serous, further treatment is not required. We have only had one bitch out of forty treated with $PGF_{2\alpha}$ that required a third series of injections. The bitch had closed-cervix pyometra, did not respond to $PGF_{2\alpha}$ therapy and eventually required ovariohysterectomy.

Several reactions will be observed after the subcutaneous injection of $PGF_{2\alpha}$. Initially, the bitch may be restless and may begin pacing. Hypersalivation and occasional panting then occurs, followed by vomiting and defecation. These reactions diminish within 20 to 60 minutes of the injection. Observance of uterine evacuation after an injection is variable.

Indications of a successful response to $PGF_{2\alpha}$ therapy include a decrease in clinical signs, a development of a serous vulvar discharge, which then stops completely, a decrease in the palpable uterine diameter (Figs. 2 and 3) and a return to a normal leukogram. After a pyometric uterus is surgically removed, the peripheral white blood cell count often increases dramatically. This is believed to be caused by the loss of the "sink" into which white blood cells flood. With medical management of pyometra, the sink remains but the infection clears. Thus, with this form of treatment the white blood

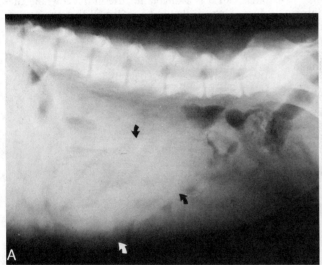
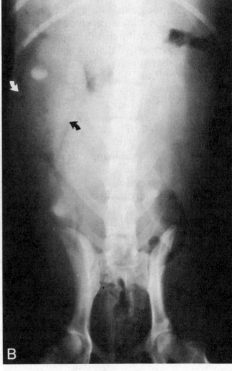

Figure 2. Lateral *(A)* and ventrodorsal *(B)* abdominal radiographs of a bitch with pyometra and open cervix, illustrating an increased diameter of the uterus (arrows).

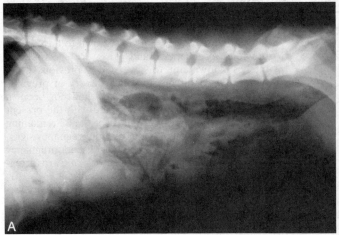

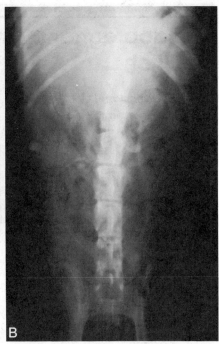

Figure 3. Lateral *(A)* and ventrodorsal *(B)* abdominal radiographs of the bitch in Figure 2 two weeks after completing 5 days of $PGF_{2\alpha}$ therapy. The previously enlarged uterus is no longer visible radiographically.

cell count quickly diminishes (Fig. 4). Of 19 bitches with open-cervix pyometra treated by the authors, all responded favorably. Fourteen of these bitches (74 per cent) have since whelped healthy litters.

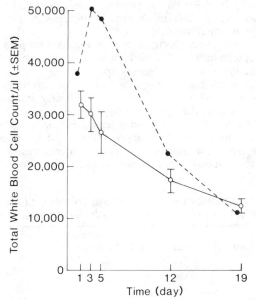

Figure 4. Total white blood cell counts in 11 bitches with pyometra before (day 1), during (days 2–5) and after (days 12–19) treatment with $PGF_{2\alpha}$ (solid line), and in four bitches with pyometra following surgical removal of the uterus on day 1 (dotted line). The bars represent SEM.

One bitch has had three litters. Owners have not reported any behavioral changes in their bitches.

Results in treating bitches with closed-cervix pyometra have not been as successful. Only three bitches of the first seven treated responded favorably and whelped healthy litters. Because of the potential complications during $PGF_{2\alpha}$ therapy and the poor response, a guarded prognosis should be provided for a bitch with closed-cervix pyometra when medical therapy is being considered.

Pyometra has recurred in subsequent heat cycles in a few of the treated bitches. Because it is impossible to predict if or when pyometra may recur, owners of treated bitches should breed their bitches during the estrus immediately following treatment. The reproductive potential of a treated bitch may be limited and mating on the following estrus increases the opportunity of obtaining a litter.

References

1. Asheim A: Pathogenesis of renal damage and polydipsia in dogs with pyometra. JAVMA 147:736, 1965.
2. Dow C: The cystic hyperplasia-pyometra complex in the bitch. Vet Res 69:1409, 1957.
3. Hardy RM, Osborne CA: Canine pyometra: Pathophysiology, diagnosis and treatment of uterine and extra-uterine lesions. JAAHA 10:245, 1974.
4. Nelson RW, Feldman EC, Stabenfeldt GH: Treatment of canine pyometra and endometritis with prostaglandin $F_{2\alpha}$. JAVMA 181:899, 1982.
5. Sandholm M, Vesenius H, Kivisto AK: Pathogenesis of canine pyometra. JAVMA 167:1006, 1975.
6. Sokolowski JH, Geng S: Effect of prostaglandin $F_{2\alpha}$-THAM in the bitch. JAVMA 170:536, 1977.

Pseudopregnancy in the Bitch

Shirley D. Johnston, D.V.M., Ph.D.
University of Minnesota, St. Paul, Minnesota

Pseudopregnancy (pseudocyesis, false pregnancy) in the bitch is a syndrome of clinical signs that occur in the nonpregnant bitch following cessation of progestational stimulation.

Pseudopregnancy is a normal phenomenon in the intact nonpregnant bitch, which undergoes a luteal phase of approximately 60 days after every season. Signs of pseudopregnancy mimic signs of parturition and lactation in the pregnant bitch; they include mammary gland development and secretion of serous, sanguineous or milky fluid, nesting behavior, personality change, depression and anorexia. Mammary gland secretion is the most frequent sign (Table 1). One or more clinical signs may occur concurrently.

Onset of signs of pseudopregnancy occurs after decline in concentrations of serum progesterone approximately 2 months following onset of estrus in all intact bitches. Signs may also occur 3 to 4 days following diestrual ovariohysterectomy (OHE) when surgical removal of ovaries and functional corpora lutea causes a decline in progesterone or following cessation of exogenous progestogen therapy.

In a survey of 59 cases of canine false pregnancy diagnosed at the University of Minnesota Veterinary Teaching Hospital, dogs ranged from 7 months to 10 years of age and represented 28 different breeds. One bitch had been treated with medroxyprogesterone acetate in the preceding month, and 2 bitches had undergone diestrual OHE in the 7 days preceding presentation; the others had been in estrus within 3½ months preceding onset of signs.

Fifteen presented within 3½ months after onset of their first estrus. Eleven were known to have had a previous pregnancy, and 11 were postpuberal bitches known not to have had a previous pregnancy. Of 37 bitches in which history of previous pseudopregnancy was known, 15 had not been in heat prior to the estrus associated with the present admission (puberal bitches); 21 of the 22 remaining animals had shown previous pseudopregnancy signs, suggesting a high recurrence rate. Pseudopregnancy is not associated with increased risk of estrus irregularity, pyometra or mammary neoplasia.[1, 3]

The most common clinical sign in our survey was presence of mammary gland development and fluid secretion (Table 1). The characteristics of the secretion varied from serous to sanguineous to milky, and both sanguineous and milky secretions could sometimes be expressed from a single gland. One bitch had concurrent mastitis, and another had concurrent staphylococcal dermatitis over several mammary glands secondary to self-nursing. Other signs included nesting behavior and personality change, which included mothering of toys or other animals, depression and irritability. Several bitches demonstrated destructive nesting behavior, such as chewing holes in upholstered furniture. Five bitches were anorexic. One bitch showed panting and contraction of uterine and voluntary abdominal musculature as well as lactation.

Diagnosis is based on clinical signs and history of estrus within the preceding 3 to 4 months, OHE during diestrus or progestogen therapy. The major differential diagnosis is pregnancy, which can generally be ruled out by abdominal palpation and/or radiography late in diestrus when signs of false pregnancy commence.

No treatment is currently recommended for pseudopregnancy in the bitch because it is a normal phenomenon that resolves spontaneously. Severe mammary gland engorgement can be treated with a 3- to 4-day decrease in food and water intake. Androgenic therapy (1 mg/kg reposital testosterone IM once; or 40 µg/kg mibolerone PO daily for 5 days) may be used to suppress signs in bitches with destructive nesting behaviors or concurrent mastitis. Progestational steroids will suppress signs during

Table 1. History and Signs in 59 Bitches with Pseudopregnancy Diagnosed at the University of Minnesota Veterinary Teaching Hospital (Ages 7 Months to 10 Years, with 28 Breeds Represented)

History/Sign	Present	Absent	Not Reported/ Unknown
Previous pregnancy	11	26*	22
Previous pseudopregnancy	21	16*	22
Bred at previous estrus	8	51	—
Lactation/mammary gland development	54	5	—
Nesting behavior	5	—	54
Personality change/depression	12	—	47
Anorexia	5	22	32
Concurrent mastitis	1	—	58

*Fifteen were seen within 3½ months after the onset of their first estrus.

treatment, but relapse following cessation of therapy is common. OHE is the only permanent preventative measure. Prognosis for recovery is excellent in all animals in the absence of mammary gland disease.

References

1. Brodey RS, Fidler IJ, Howson AE: The relationship of estrous irregularity, pseudopregnancy, and pregnancy to the development of canine mammary neoplasms. JAVMA 149:1047, 1966.
2. Concannon PW, Hansel W, Visek WJ: The ovarian cycle of the bitch: plasma estrogen LH and progesterone. Biol Reprod 13:112, 1975.
3. Fidler IJ, Brodey RS, Howson AE, Cohen D: Relationship of estrous irregularity, pseudopregnancy, and pregnancy to canine pyometra. JAVMA 14:1043, 1966.
4. Hadley JC: Unconjugated estrogen and progesterone concentrations in the blood of bitches with false pregnancy and pyometra. Vet Rec 96:545, 1975.
5. Whitney JC: The pathology of the canine genital tract in false pregnancy. J Small Anim Pract 8:247, 1967.

Physiology and Endocrinology of Canine Pregnancy

Patrick W. Concannon, M.S., Ph.D.
Cornell University, Ithaca, New York

LENGTH OF GESTATION

The interval from a fertile mating to parturition can range from 57 to 68 days, with an average of 64 days. In some instances parturition may not occur until 71 or 72 days after the first of a series of matings. The variation is not a reflection of any inconsistency in the timing of the physiological events of pregnancy but rather reflects the large variation that can occur among pregnancies in the intervals from mating to ovulation, to oocyte maturation and to passage of blastocysts through the tubouterine junction. Canine sperm can retain the ability to fertilize for 6 to 7 days after mating.[12] Because of variability in the onset of behavioral estrus and/or in husbandry practices, fertile matings may occur as late as 5 days after ovulation or as early as 5 days before ovulation. Ova are ovulated as primary oocytes about 2 days after the preovulatory surge release of luteinizing hormone (LH) and do not undergo oocyte maturation until 2 or 3 days later. A limited period follows, starting 4 to 5 days after the LH peak and ending with degeneration of oocytes in the oviduct 2 to 3 days later, in which canine oocytes can be fertilized by either previously deposited or freshly deposited sperm. This limited period for fertilization, along with an apparently consistent time for the opening of the tubouterine junction late in estrus, contributes to the low variability in the timing of events of canine

gestation when related to the time of ovulation or of the preovulatory LH surge. For nearly all normal pregnancies parturition occurs 64, 65 or 66 days after the LH peak.[12]

EVENTS OF PREGNANCY

With a relatively consistent gestation length of 65 ± 1 days when measured relative to the LH peak, it is reasonably possible to time some of the individual events of pregnancy accurately relative to one another. However, many aspects of pregnancy in the dog have only been studied in relation to the time of mating or onset of estrus, including implantation, and the development of the fetus, placenta and fetal membranes. For these events, estimates must be made based on the fact that the average breeding date is about 1 day after the LH peak and 1 day before ovulation. Canine embryology and fetal development have been well summarized,[13, 24] and will not be reviewed here. The timing of many of the clinically relevant events of pregnancy in the dog are indicated in Table 1 and discussed in more detail in sections below.

ENDOCRINOLOGY OF PREGNANCY

Except for the dramatic changes in hormone levels associated with parturition, the patterns of peripheral levels of hormones during pregnancy are very similar to those observed during nonpregnant cycles and their associated prolonged phases of luteal progesterone secretion. Serum or plasma levels of estradiol and progesterone have been reasonably well characterized during canine pregnancy; those of the pituitary hormones LH, follicle-stimulating hormone (FSH), prolactin and growth hormone have been less so. Hormone profiles during canine pregnancy are summarized schematically in Figure 1.

Estrogen. In late proestrus estradiol reaches peak levels of 50 to 100 pg/ml about 1 to 2 days before the preovulatory LH surge. Estradiol levels decline during and following the LH surge and throughout

Table 1. Estimated Times of Various Events of Canine Pregnancy in Relation to the Preovulatory LH Peak and Potential Times of Fertile Matings

Event of Pregnancy	Days after LH Peak	Days after Fertile Mating
Proestrus onset	−25 to +3	
Estrus onset	−4 to +5	
Preovulatory LH peak	0	−7 to +3
First of multiple matings	−5 to +7	−12 to 0
Fertile mating	−3 to +7	0
Ovulation of primary oocytes	2	−5 to +5
Oocyte maturation	4	−3 to +7
Fertilization	4 to 7	0 to 7
Vaginal cornification reduced	7 to 9	0 to 12
Morulae in distal oviducts	8 to 10	2 to 13
Blastocysts enter uterus	9 to 11	2 to 14
Zonae pellucidae shed	15 to 17	8 to 20
Attachment sites established	16 to 18	9 to 21
Swelling of implantation sites	18 to 20	11 to 23
Palpable 1 cm swellings	22 to 24	15 to 27
Pregnancy anemia onset	27 to 29	20 to 31
Uterine swellings detectable on x-ray	30 to 32	23 to 35
Reduced palpability of 3 cm swellings	32 to 34	25 to 37
Hematocrit below 40 per cent PCV	38 to 40	31 to 43
Fetal skull and spine radiopaque	44 to 46	37 to 49
Earliest x-ray pregnancy diagnosis	45 to 47	39 to 50
Hematocrit below 35 per cent PCV	48 to 50	41 to 53
Fetal pelvis radiopaque	53 to 57	46 to 60
Fetal teeth radiopaque	58 to 63	51 to 66
Prepartum luteolysis and hypothermia	63 to 65	56 to 68
Parturition	64 to 66	57 to 69

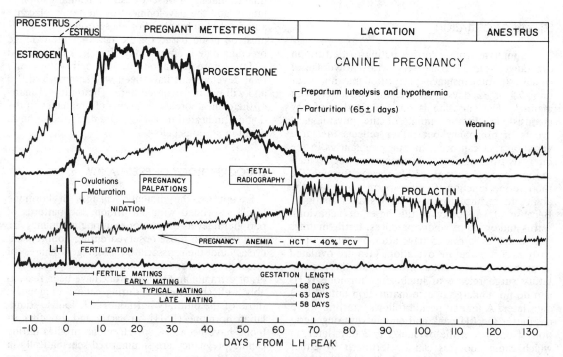

Figure 1. A schematic representation of typical endocrine changes reported to occur in association with ovulation, pregnancy, parturition and lactation in the bitch, shown in relation to the day of the preovulatory peak in luteinizing hormone and various events of gestation. (From Concannon PW: In Kirk R (ed): Current Veterinary Therapy, Small Animal Practice. Philadelphia, WB Saunders Co, 1983, pp 886–901.)

most of estrus and then rather undramatically increase during pregnancy to reach elevations (20 to 30 pg/ml) prior to parturition that are considerably below those seen in late proestrus.[10] The changes in estrogen secretion and/or metabolism responsible for the late pregnancy rise are probably of greater magnitude than those reflected in peripheral levels, since the latter are "dampened" by an increase in volume of distribution associated with increased body weight and decreased red blood cells (RBC) packed cell volume.[11] Estradiol falls abruptly to basal levels (5 to 10 pg/ml) following parturition; levels throughout lactation and postlactation anestrus have not been determined, but considerable elevations in estradiol levels have been reported during anestrus following nonpregnant cycles.[25] Changes in estrone levels reported tend to parallel those of estradiol. Circulating levels of estrogen metabolites, such as estrone sulfate, have not been rigorously studied during canine pregnancy.

Progesterone. During proestrus and before the preovulatory surge in LH, progesterone levels remain low and sporadically fluctuate between 0.5 and 1.0 ng/ml, probably as a result of the effects of sporadic pulses of LH acting on follicles as they mature and undergo variable degrees of minor but detectable proestrual luteinization.[9] Progesterone levels rapidly increase over 1 ng/ml during the onset of the preovulatory LH surge and continue to increase throughout estrus to reach initial peak levels of 15 to 85 ng/ml by 15 to 30 days after the LH peak. However, throughout the period of elevated progesterone levels, considerable fluctuations can be encountered from day to day, and even within days. Following implantation and placental development, when progesterone levels are either near their initial apex or declining, there is a second increase in progesterone levels that either rises to a second peak[32] or produces a broadening of the ongoing decline during the fourth and fifth weeks of gestation.[10, 11] During the last third of pregnancy progesterone levels slowly decline to a plateau of 4 to 16 ng/ml, which is maintained for 1 to 2 weeks until the abrupt decline to 1 to 2 ng/ml, which occurs 1 to 2 days before parturition.

While progesterone levels are on average higher during the second half of pregnancy than during the comparable period in nonpregnant bitches, serum progesterone levels cannot be used to diagnose pregnancy, since the range in absolute progesterone levels in both pregnant and nonpregnant bitches is quite large. Whatever the extent of pregnancy-specific changes in progesterone secretion or metabolism during the second half of gestation, like those of estrogen they are apparently only poorly reflected in peripheral levels owing to the increased volume of distribution associated with the progressive, post-implantation anemia characteristic of canine pregnancy.

Pituitary Hormones. During proestrus, FSH levels decrease,[25] and pulses of LH drive follicles to full maturation and maximal estrogen secretion. In late-proestrus/early-estrus levels of both gonadotropins surge simultaneously as the ratio of estrogen to progesterone rapidly declines. The LH surge lasts 1 to 3 days and causes luteinization and ovulation of the follicles, with ovulation occurring 2 days after the peak in LH.[9] FSH levels decline less rapidly than those of LH owing to the longer half-life of FSH in the circulation. LH levels continue to fluctuate near basal levels throughout pregnancy, and no dramatic changes in either LH or FSH have been reported. However, following implantation, FSH levels are somewhat higher than those in nonpregnant cycles and apparently remain so throughout gestation. This increase in FSH has been suggested as a basis for the elevated estrogen levels reported in late pregnancy.[27]

Prolactin levels appear to fluctuate undramatically during proestrus and estrus and prior to implantation, although a transient surge in prolactin levels during a concomitant decline in progesterone levels has been observed in a few bitches shortly prior to implantation.[17] As in nonpregnant cycles, prolactin levels increase during the protracted period of declining progesterone levels after days 35 to 40 of pregnancy. The broad rise in prolactin levels during the second half of pregnancy appears to be greater than that in nonpregnant cycles,[27] and terminates with a transient, large surge during the rapid decline in progesterone 12 to 36 hours prior to parturition.[8] While prolactin levels are usually reduced for 1 to 2 days postpartum, they are then elevated and fluctuate during lactation in response to suckling. Prolactin levels decline slowly during the second half of lactation and fall abruptly following weaning.[8]

PREIMPLANTATION EVENTS

The timing of pre- and postimplantation events appears to be relatively consistent among bitches when viewed relative to the preovulatory LH peak and ovulation, which are considered herein as day 0 and day 2, respectively, of the "pregnant cycle." Under clinical conditions the expected times of various events of gestation can be reasonably estimated for bitches in which the late-estrus decrease in vaginal cornification is monitored by means of daily vaginal cytology[18] and/or daily vaginal endoscopy.[20] The initial, discrete reappearance of non-cornified cells in the vaginal smear and the late-estrus regression of the vaginal mucosa, recognized grossly in terms of patchy areas of visible underlying vasculature, both occur 7 to 8 days after the LH peak in the majority of bitches.[6, 19]

Fertilization is probably limited to a 3-day period, from days 4 to 7, i.e., 2 to 5 days after ovulation, based on the assumptions that oocyte maturation occurs 2 days after ovulation (day 4) and that unfertilized oocytes degenerate by day 8. These estimates are prompted by reports that canine oocytes require 48 hours to undergo spontaneous maturation in vitro[21] and that fertilization by extremely short-lived, previously frozen sperm is limited to the 3-day period prior to the late-estrus decrease in the number of cornified cells in vaginal smears,[33] i.e., day 7 or 8 of the cycle. Embryos accumulate as morulae in the distal segments of the oviducts and develop into 32 to 64 cell blastocysts. Their passage into the uterine horns is permitted by the opening of the tubouterine junctions around day 10. This is followed by 3 days in which 1 mm blastocysts are free floating in their ipsilateral uterine horns and another 3 days in which 2 mm blastocysts freely migrate from one horn to another. The zonae pellucidae are shed, and rather equally spaced attachment sites are established around day 16. Distinct swellings of implantation sites become evident by day 18 during formation of the embryonic primitive streak and initial development of the placenta.

POSTIMPLANTATION EVENTS

Uterine swellings at implantation sites are about 1 cm in diameter by day 20 and represent localized uterine edema, expansion of the embryonic membranes and early placental development. The canine placenta is endotheliochorial in composition and zonary and circumferential in morphology. The girdle of fetal trophoblast tissue develops marginal hematomas, while the chorioallantoic poles remain thin and transparent. The marginal hematomas contain large pools of stagnant maternal blood from which the extraembryonic circulation absorbs various metabolites, particularly iron. In the dog there is also the somewhat unique persistence of an elongated yolk sac often attached to both ends of the paraplacental zones and not attached to the zonary placenta.

The maternal hematocrit slowly declines following implantation and is usually below 40 per cent packed cell volume (PCV) by day 35 and below 35 per cent at term. It has been suggested that as in humans much of the anemia of canine pregnancy represents the hemodilution effects of increased plasma volume.[11] If so, the potential increase in blood volume of distribution must be considered when measuring peripheral levels of hormones or metabolites during late pregnancy. Total body weight of a bitch may increase 20 to 55 per cent over the course of gestation; the average increase is about 36 per cent.[11] During the second half of pregnancy there is also a decrease in hemoglobin levels and an increase in sedimentation rate. The potential for the development of a moderate immunosuppression during pregnancy, as reflected in serum IgG levels below 500 mg/dl, has been described.[14] Plasma levels of fibrinogen and other proteins involved in coagulation increase following implantation. Fibrinogen levels increase rapidly and become maximal at day 30, decline towards term and increase again at parturition.[15] Pregnancy has also been reported to increase systemic and pulmonary vascular resistance in the dog.[23] Interestingly, the pregnant canine uterus produces large amounts of prostacyclin, which may act as a circulating vasodepressor substance.[16]

The extent to which pregnancy alters general metabolism or the efficiency of metabolic hormones in the bitch has not been extensively studied. The effects may be considerable, since as early as mid-pregnancy (days 30 to 35) at least minor alterations in metabolic hormone responses have been demonstrated relative to anestrus and/or to the comparable period in the luteal phase of nonpregnant bitches.[26] In addition, pregnancy may aggravate a pre-existing subclinical diabetic state, as in humans. It has been recently demonstrated that sensitivity to insulin, but not glucagon, is reduced as early as day 35 of pregnancy in comparison to that in nonpregnant metestrous bitches or in bitches in any other reproductive state.[22] Pregnancy in the bitch increases the insulin requirements for the ongoing management of diabetes to a greater extent than does the luteal phase of nonpregnant cycles.[31] Pregnancy also increases the requirement for available carbohydrate in the diet. Bitches maintained on a carbohydrate-deficient diet during pregnancy became hypoglycemic during the last 2 weeks of gestation, had a 7-fold increase in dead pups in litters and had an abnormally high incidence of postnatal mortality among their pups during the first 3 days postpartum.[30]

PREGNANCY DIAGNOSIS AND RADIOGRAPHY

Palpation. By days 20 to 25 uterine swellings at placental sites are detectable by deep abdominal palpation as 1 to 2 cm enlargements along the uterine horns in all but the most obese bitches if the abdomen is relaxed and a careful examination of the entire length of the reproductive tract is performed. However, the swellings remain readily palpable for only 7 to 10 days. After day 30, the horns drop to a more ventral position and the anterior ends are pushed forward under the caudal ribs. By day 35 the fetal swellings are over 3 cm in diameter, elongated, nearly confluent and pliable rather than firm and in all but the leanest of bitches become difficult to palpate as distinct entities diagnostic of pregnancy. At about the same time mammary gland development starts to become prominent but no more so than in many nonpregnant cycles. When pregnancy diagnosis is a matter of concern, palpations at weekly intervals or more frequently should be initiated by day 20 after breeding with an appreciation of the potential range in the time of implantation in relation to the time of mating (Table 1). The application of two ultrasonographic techniques in the detection of pregnancy has been reported in detail.[1]

Radiography. Conventional radiography can be used for diagnosis of pregnancy (versus pseudocyesis or uterine disease) or for evaluation of fetal development—but only during the last 3 weeks of gestation. The fetal skeletons do not become radiopaque until after day 44 (at 21 days antepartum) and become distinct only after day 46 (at 18 days prepartum). Due to the variation in timing of gestational events in relation to the time of mating, radiography of fetal skeletal elements in some bitches may not be possible until 50 days postcoitus, whereas in others it may be possible by 39 days.[7] The stage of fetal development in the last 2 weeks of gestation can be estimated reasonably well radiographically, based on the sequence and timing of the appearance of distinct calvaria, proximal and then distal limb bones, pelvis, caudal ribs and, finally, teeth (Table 1).

A radiographic analysis of changes in uterine morphology during canine gestation has been recently reported[29] and provides useful information. However, it is important to note that fetal skeletal elements after day 45 are required for an unequivocal radiographic diagnosis of pregnancy, and earlier changes in uterine morphology as detected radiographically can have counterparts in various uterine diseases. Enlargements of implantation sites viewed by conventional radiography progress from small and ovoid at day 30, to larger and spherical at day 35 and then to large and ovoid at day 40. The spherical shapes seen around day 35 are usually, but not necessarily, distinct from enlargements associated with mucometra, pyometra or other uterine disease states. The methodology and details for radiography of the pregnant uterus and of the dead fetuses in the bitch have also been reviewed.[28] In late pregnancy fetal death can be diagnosed radiographically based on deformed calvaria, intra- or perifetal gas spaces or abnormal fetal postures, including excessive flexion of the body or extension of the hind limbs.

Pregnancy Tests. There are no validated assay procedures for the diagnosis of pregnancy in bitches either before or after implantation. The existence or presence of any placental gonadotrophin or fetoplacental-specific protein on which such a test might be based have not been demonstrated in dogs. The extent of the anemia seen late in canine pregnancy might be useful for the differential diagnosis of pregnancy from overt pseudopregnancy, but this has yet to be demonstrated by evaluation of hematocrits during pseudocyesis. A concomitant decrease in serum creatinine and a decrease in serum gammaglobulin (IgG) levels at 21 days after breeding compared with prebreeding levels have been reported as characteristic of pregnancy in the bitch and are useful in the determination of pregnancy.[14]

PREGNANCY MAINTENANCE AND LUTEAL FUNCTION

Elevated peripheral levels of progesterone are required for the maintenance of pregnancy throughout gestation, although the levels normally present are probably well in excess of the minimum required. The major if not only source of progesterone is the corpus luteum; ovariectomy at any time during pregnancy results in either resorption or abortion.[34]

Progesterone appears to be the only sex steroid required for pregnancy maintenance in the bitch, since the synthetic progestin medroxyprogesterone acetate (MPA) can maintain pregnancy in the ovariectomized bitch.[11] However, MPA has a greater affinity for uterine progesterone receptors than does progesterone itself, and under physiological conditions the presence of estrogen during pregnancy may contribute to the synthesis or availability of intracellular progesterone receptors. The fact that estrogen levels do not increase to any great extent during pregnancy in the bitch is probably critical. Abnormally high levels of estrogen are not only antinidatory but can also terminate a fully established, postimplantation pregnancy.[11] The requirement for progesterone during pregnancy is probably multiple, with progesterone supporting endometrial development, promoting placental integrity and reducing myometrial activity and sensitivity to oxytocin.

Luteal secretion of progesterone and thus the maintenance of pregnancy are dependent on pituitary secretion of luteotrophic hormones, and pregnancy at any stage is terminated by hypophysectomy.[2] Both LH and prolactin appear to be required luteotrophic hormones in the pregnant as well as nonpregnant bitch. Administration of anti-LH serum dramatically reduces progesterone levels; administration of bromergocryptine, a dopamine agonist that reduces prolactin secretion, can produce complete luteolysis and cause abortion in the bitch.[3] The possibility that elevated prolactin levels serve to promote synthesis or secretion of progesterone during the second half of pregnancy in the bitch has not been investigated.

The corpora lutea of pregnancy, like those of nonpregnant cycles, are sensitive to the luteolytic effects of prostaglandin $F_{2\alpha}$ ($PGF_{2\alpha}$), although not as sensitive as in most other species of domestic animals studied. Repeated administrations of $PGF_{2\alpha}$ are required to induce complete luteolysis and abortion, even after day 30 when the corpora lutea are more sensitive than during early pregnancy.[5] Administration of 30 to 50 μg/kg body weight two or three times daily or of 100 μg/kg daily for 3 to 6 days IM causes luteolysis, with resorption or abortion occurring after suppression of progesterone levels to basal levels for 3 or more days. A single administration of a long-acting $PGF_{2\alpha}$ analog has been reported to terminate pregnancy at any stage of gestation.[36] Pregnancy can also be terminated by administration of a steroidal competitive inhibitor of the enzyme that converts pregnenolone to progesterone, d5,3β hydroxysteroid dehydrogenase. Such a compound might find application as an abortifacient in the bitch. The fact that $PGF_{2\alpha}$ is luteolytic in the bitch is important in considering the finding that uterine release of $PGF_{2\alpha}$ during late pregnancy is negligible, while that of other products of arachidonic acid, PGE_2 and PGI_2 (prostacyclin), is considerable.[16] The high PGE_2-to-$PGF_{2\alpha}$ ratio may represent a protective mechanism for the maintenance of luteal function a well as provide for the maintenance of myometrial and uterine vascular tone during gestation.

PARTURITION

The normal delivery of an average or large litter can be rapid and completed within 4 hours or may take up to 18 hours for completion. The delivery of the first pup in nearly all normal pregnancies occurs 64 to 66 days after the preovulatory LH peak; it can range from 57 to 72 days after the first of multiple matings and 57 to 68 days after a single fertile mating. Gestation is reportedly longer in bitches bearing small litters, but supporting data are lacking. There is, however, ample, albeit, incidental evidence that bitches can actively postpone the delivery of pups for up to 1 day if stressed and/or moved to a strange environment.

The trigger for parturition and the mechanisms involved have not been clearly delineated in the dog, but the endocrine information available suggests they are not unlike those proposed for several other species. The major endocrine event involved is a rapid and dramatic increase in the peripheral and/or local (uterine) estrogen-to-progesterone ratio. In the bitch this is accomplished by a rapid decline in progesterone levels 24 to 36 hours before parturition, while moderately elevated levels of estrogen remain unchanged and then decline after parturition. The decline in progesterone reflects an abrupt functional lysis of the corpora lutea, although alterations in progesterone metabolism could also be involved. Since exogenous $PGF_{2\alpha}$ is luteolytic in the bitch, it has been suggested that the fetoplacental unit initiates a prepartum release of luteolytic amounts of uterine and/or placental $PGF_{2\alpha}$, as has been suggested for several other species.[11] Direct evidence is lacking, and prepartum changes in $PGF_{2\alpha}$ levels or secretion rates have not been determined for the bitch.

Maternal cortisol levels are variable but within the normal range during the last week of gestation (23 ± 1 ng/ml) and, in most bitches, are clearly elevated (63 ± 7 ng/ml) on the day prior to parturition and then reduced (20 ± 4 ng/ml) at the time of parturition.[11] The observations are consistent with the hypothesis developed for other species that the trigger for the timing of parturition involves the maturation of the fetal pituitary-adrenal axis at the completion of fetal development, with the increase in maternal cortisol levels reflecting a far greater increase in fetal cortisol secretion, which acts locally at the level of the uterus to promote the release of luteolytic amounts of $PGF_{2\alpha}$.

Prolactin levels increase to peak levels shortly prior to parturition, and it has been suggested that the rise in prolactin occurs in response to the simultaneous decline in progesterone; $PGF_{2\alpha}$ could also be involved, since $PGF_{2\alpha}$ can cause prolactin release in other species. The extent to which the rise in prolactin is incidental to the events of par-turition or plays a role in accelerating the mechanism of parturition has not been evaluated, although the potential for prolactin to stimulate fetal corticoid secretion has been noted.

The prepartum decline in progesterone levels is required for normal parturition to occur, and its prevention by administration of exogenous progesterone blocks parturition and results in death of the pups in utero.[11] Progesterone withdrawal and the resulting increase in the estrogen-to-progesterone ratio is probably the major cause of placental dislocation, dilation of the cervix and increased uterine contractility, but other factors probably are involved. As myometrial sensitivity to oxytocin is increased during progesterone withdrawal, basal oxytocin levels would be expected to play an increasingly important role in uterine contractions, as would any increases in oxytocin released reflexively in response to fetal pressure on the cervix or vagina. However, measurements of oxytocin or relaxin levels around the time of parturition have not been reported for the bitch. Increases in relaxin levels and the contribution of relaxin to cervical dilation and relaxation of the pelvis have been documented for several species.

The occurrence of prepartum luteolysis can be monitored by observing the prepartum decline in rectal temperature that parallels the decline in progesterone with a delay of about 12 hours. Rectal temperature falls about 1°C between 12 and 36 hours prior to the onset of parturition.[8] The hypothermia is transient; temperatures rise during or immediately after parturition and remain slightly above normal for several days. Based on the known hyperthermic effects of exogenous progesterone and the transient hypothermia observed during $PGF_{2\alpha}$-induced luteolysis, it has been suggested that the prepartum hypothermia represents a transient failure to compensate for a rapid withdrawal of the hyperthermic effects of progesterone.[5]

For 2 to 3 days prior to parturition bitches usually become restless, seek seclusion and reduce food intake, possibly in response to elevated prolactin levels. During the 12 to 24 hours prior to parturition when prolactin levels are highest, there are usually observed increased restlessness, panting, scratching, chewing and nesting behavior. This is the period of stage I labor, during which uterine contractions increase but are not accompanied by voluntary abdominal contractions. During stage II labor the fetuses are delivered through the cervix and vagina. Individual pups may present with or without complete rupture of the membranes. In pregnancies that are not equilateral, delivery is usually initiated from the horn containing most pups. The incidence of alternation between uterine horns in the delivery sequence has been studied in detail for the bitch and is relatively high.[35] While the delivery of a litter is usually completed within 6 hours it may extend to 24 hours without complications. The intervals between delivery of individual pups may be 2 to 3 hours, particularly between the first and second pups, but subsequent intervals are usually shorter.

Normal maternal behavior includes breaking of intact fetal membranes, intensive licking of the pups and obsessive chewing of the umbilicus (at times to the point of perforating the abdomen) and eating of the placentae. Placentae are delivered attached to the umbilical cords or, when detached, within 5 to 10 minutes after the delivery of individual pups. Endocrine factors regulating peripartum and post-partum maternal behavior in the bitch have not been determined but probably involve elevations in prolactin and oxytocin.

References

1. Allen WE, Meredith MJ: Detection of pregnancy in the bitch: A study of abdominal palpation, A-mode ultrasound and Doppler ultrasound techniques. J Small Anim Pract 22:609, 1981.
2. Concannon PW: Effects of hypophysectomy and of LH administration on luteal phase plasma progesterone levels in the beagle bitch. J Reprod Fert 48:407, 1980.
3. Concannon PW: Discussion. In Rothchild I (au): The regulation of the mammalian corpus luteum. Rec Prog Horm Res 37:287, 1981.
4. Concannon PW: Reproductive physiology and endocrine patterns of the bitch. In Kirk R (ed): Current Veterinary Therapy, Small Animal Practice. Philadelphia, WB Saunders Co, 1983, pp 886–901.
5. Concannon PW, Hansel W: Prostaglandin $F_{2\alpha}$ induced luteolysis, hypothermia and abortions in Beagle bitches. Prostaglandins 13:533, 1977.
6. Concannon PW, Lindsay FEF: Unpublished data.
7. Concannon PW, Rendano V: Radiographic analysis of canine pregnancy: Onset of fetal skeletal radiopacity in relation to times of breeding, preovulatory luteinizing hormone release, and parturition. Am J Vet Res 44:1506, 1983.
8. Concannon PW, Butler WR, Hansel W, et al: Parturition and lactation in the bitch: Serum progesterone cortisol and prolactin. Biol Reprod 19:1113, 1978.
9. Concannon PW, Hansel W, McEntee K: Changes in LH, progesterone and sexual behavior associated with preovulatory luteinization in the bitch. Biol Reprod 17:604, 1977.
10. Concannon PW, Hansel W, Visek WJ: The ovarian cycle of the bitch: Plasma estrogen, LH, and progesterone. Biol Reprod 13:112, 1975.
11. Concannon PW, Powers ME, Holder W, Hansel W: Pregnancy and parturition in the bitch. Biol Reprod 16:317, 1977.
12. Concannon PW, Whaley S, Lein D, Wissler R: Canine gestation length: Variation related to time of mating and fertile life of sperm. Am J Vet Res 44:1, 1983.
13. Evans HE: Reproduction and prenatal development. In Evans HE, Christensen GC (eds): Miller's Anatomy of the Dog. Philadelphia WB Saunders Co. 1979, pp 13–77.
14. Fisher T, Fisher D: Serum assay for canine pregnancy testing. Mod Vet Pract 62:466, 1981.
15. Gentry PA, Liptrap RM: Influence of progesterone and pregnancy on canine fibrinogen values. J Small Anim Pract 22:185, 1981.
16. Gerber JG, Hubbard WC, Nies AS: Uterine vein prostaglandin levels in the late pregnant dogs. Prostaglandins 17:623, 1979.
17. Graf KJ: Serum oestrogen, progesterone and prolactin concentrations in cyclic, pregnant and lactating beagle dogs. J Reprod Fert 52:9, 1978.
18. Holst PA, Phemister RD: Onset of diestrus in the Beagle bitch: Definition and significance. Am J Vet Res 35:401, 1974.
19. Holst PA, Phemister RD: Temporal sequence of events in the estrous cycle of the bitch. Am J Vet Res 36:705, 1975.
20. Lindsay FEF: The normal endoscopic appearance of the caudal reproductive tract of the cyclic and non-cyclic bitch: Post-uterine endoscopy. J Small Anim Pract 24:1, 1983.
21. Mahi CA, Yanagimachi R: Maturation and sperm penetration of canine ovarian oocytes in vitro. J Exper Zool 196:189, 1976.
22. McCann JP, Concannon PW: Effects of sex, ovarian cycles, pregnancy and lactation on insulin and glucose response to exogenous glucose and glucagon in dogs. Biol Reprod 28:41, 1983.
23. Moore LG, Reeves JT: Pregnancy blunts pulmonary vascular reactivity in dogs. Am J Physiol 239:H297, 1980.
24. Noden D, Delahunta AI: The Embryology of Domestic Animals. Philadelphia, Williams & Wilkins Co, 1984.
25. Olson P, Bowen R, Behrendt M, et al.: Concentrations of reproductive hormones in canine serum throughout late anestrus, proestrus and estrus. Biol Reprod 27:1196, 1982.
26. Reimers RJ, Mummery LK, Cowan RG: Effects of reproductive status on adrenal function in dogs. Biol Reprod 28:41, 1983.
27. Reimers T, Phemister R, Niswender G: Radioimmunological measurement of follicle stimulating hormone and prolactin in the dog. Biol Reprod 19:673, 1978.
28. Rendano V: Radiographic evaluation of fetal development in the bitch and fetal death in the bitch and queen. In Kirk R (ed): Current Veterinary Therapy, Small Animal Practice. Philadelphia, WB Saunders Co, 1983, pp 947–952.
29. Rendano V, Lein D, Concannon PW: Radiographic evaluation of prenatal development in the beagle: Correlation with times of breeding, LH release and parturition. Vet Radiol 25:132, 1984.
30. Romos D, Palmer H, Muirvri K, Bennink M: Influence of a low carbohydrate diet on performance of pregnant and lactating dogs. J Nutrit 111:678, 1981.
31. Siegel ET: Endocrine Diseases of the Dog. Philadelphia, Lea & Febiger, 1977.
32. Smith MS, McDonald LE: Serum levels of luteinizing hormone and progesterone during the estrous cycle, pseudopregnancy and pregnancy in the dog. Endocrinology 94:404, 1974.
33. Smith and Johnson, U. of MN, personal communication, 1984.
34. Sokolowski JH: The effects of ovariectomy on pregnancy maintenance in the bitch. Lab Anim Sci 21:696, 1971.
35. van der Weyden G, Taverne M, Okkens A, Fontijne P: The intrauterine position of canine fetuses and their sequence of expulsion at birth. J Small Anim Pract 22:503, 1981.
36. Vickery B, McRae G: Effect of synthetic PG analogue on pregnancy in beagle bitches. Biol Reprod 22:438, 1980.

Management of the Pregnant Bitch

Frances O. Smith, D.V.M., Ph.D.
University of Minnesota, St. Paul, Minnesota

THE PREBREEDING EXAMINATION

The bitch should be examined during proestrus in anticipation of breeding during that season. A thorough physical examination including a fecal examination should be conducted. The bitch's vaccinations should be brought up to date prior to breeding. Serum should be drawn for serologic testing for *Brucella canis* antibodies. If the slide agglutination test (Pitman Moore Rapid Slide Agglutination Test, Washington Crossing, New Jersey) is positive, the tube agglutination test should be performed, as it is more specific than the slide test. A vaginal smear should be collected and stained with an appropriate cytology stain such as new methylene blue or Diff-Quik to assess the type of epithelial cells present. A rectal examination should be done to estimate the size of the bony pelvis. A digital vaginal examination should be performed to check for vaginal strictures or other anomalies or vaginal hyperplasia that may interfere with natural mating. Vaginal culture for aerobic bacteria should be obtained before collection of the vaginal cytology specimen and before the digital vaginal examination in bitches with historical infertility, pyometra or abnormal vaginal discharge. Total plasma protein may be measured prospectively, as a bitch with a total protein of less than 5.0 gm/dl is unlikely to whelp a litter of vigorous puppies.[7]

DIET AND NUTRITION

Proper diet for the pregnant bitch begins before pregnancy. The bitch should be maintained in proper body condition with good muscle tone. Overweight bitches have lower conception rates and may have more difficulty in whelping. Prior to breeding, the bitch may be fed any commercial dog food meeting National Research Council (NRC) standards as a complete food.

Supplementation with vitamins and/or minerals is unnecessary when complete food is provided. Following breeding, little change is necessary in feeding during the first 4 to 6 weeks of a bitch's pregnancy. A protein level of 25 per cent or more is necessary for optimal reproductive performance.[9] Liver (raw or cooked) is an excellent addition to the diet. One half to 1 oz per 30 lb body weight two to three times weekly starting in the second half of gestation may result in improved neonatal vitality and increased milk production during lactation.[7]

During pregnancy the quantity of food should be gradually increased. Major caloric increases are necessary after the first six weeks of gestation, which result in improved neonatal vitality and increased milk production during lactation.[7]

The average weight gain for a well-nourished bitch carrying a normal-size litter for her breed is 36 per cent over the gestation period. The bitch should be 5 per cent over her ideal nonpregnant weight immediately following whelping to allow for peak lactation. It is nearly impossible to overfeed the lactating bitch. Food intake may be from two and one half to three times greater than maintenance intake during lactation. A bitch that is losing body condition in response to heavy lactation demands may have 10 per cent meat added to the dry diet to increase palatability and food intake. Water consumption is likewise increased during lactation. Fresh water should be available at all times.

PREGNANCY DIAGNOSIS

The bitch should be palpated for pregnancy by abdominal palpation of the uterus approximately 28 days after the first breeding. In lean relaxed bitches, it may be possible to detect discrete swellings in the uterus of a pregnant bitch as early as 21 days after breeding. After day 35, uterine swellings have enlarged, resulting in a confluent and more pliable uterus, making pregnancy diagnosis by palpation difficult.

Real time ultrasonography (linear array or sector scan) can be of value both in early pregnancy diagnosis and in diagnosis of fetal distress at term. Fetal heart beats have been detected as early as 24 days after breeding.[2]

Fetal distress at term may be detected by a decrease in fetal heart rate to less than 100 beats/minute. Fetal ultrasound can be used to differentiate uterine enlargement as a result of pyometra from uterine enlargement due to pregnancy prior to fetal calcification.[6]

Radiography of the abdomen may be used to differentiate pregnancy from other causes of abdominal enlargement, such as pyometra or hydrometra. The difficulty in the use of radiology is the apparent variability in gestation length, which is due to variation in the time of mating in relation to the time of ovulation. Fetal skeletons are first radiographically apparent 20 to 21 days before parturition (42 to 52 days after mating).[1] For definitive pregnancy diagnosis, the bitch must be radiographed for fetuses 17 to 20 days before parturition (43 to 54 days after mating).

TERATOGENS

A teratogen is an agent that can induce congenital defects when administered to a pregnant animal. There are three critical periods of development between conception and whelping: pregastrulation, the embryonic stage and the fetal stage. During pregastrulation, the conceptus is relatively resistant to teratogens. The embryonic stage is the most vulnerable to teratogens (days 13 to 30 in the dog). During the fetal stage resistance to teratogens and embryotoxic agents increases. As the embryo matures into a fetus, gross structural defects seldom occur except in structures undergoing rapid growth and maturation, such as the palate, the cerebellum and parts of the cardiovascular and urogenital systems.

Agents used in veterinary medicine that are known teratogens include carbaryl (may cause brachygnathia, taillessness, extra digits, failure of skeletal formation and dystocia in bitches due to uterine atony), diazinon and dichlorvos. Fungicides such as methyl mercury chloride and griseofulvin may cause cleft palate and other abnormalities. Hormones such as progesterone and androgens may cause masculinization of fetuses. Corticosteroids may cause cleft palates or late-term abortions. Phenobarbital and primidone are suspected human teratogens, as are trimethadione and paramethadione (anticonvulsants). In general all drugs should be avoided in pregnant bitches, including modified live virus vaccines unless they are necessary for maintenance of the bitch's well being and unless the drug is documented as safe to administer during pregnancy.

PREPARATION FOR WHELPING

Approximately 1 week prior to whelping, the bitch should be moved to the quarters in which whelping is desired. Preparation of a whelping box includes cleaning, disinfecting and thorough rinsing. Wooden whelping boxes should be painted with lead-free paint. Disposable whelping boxes minimize litter-to-litter parasite or disease transmission. A molded child's wading pool makes an ideal whelping box, as it is easy to clean, malleable (to reduce crushing of puppies by awkward bitches) and inexpensive.

The owner should have a scale to weigh puppies daily. A supplementary heat source is a necessity for most litters. Heat lamps suspended above the whelping box are preferable to heating pads, so that the puppies and the bitch may seek comfortable heat levels. Scissors, suture material or dental floss for tying umbilical cords, iodine and clean terry cloth towels are useful.

The bitch should be bathed and have excess hair trimmed away from the mammae and vulva. In long-haired breeds the coat may be braided to protect it and to prevent strangulation of the puppies.

THE HIGH-RISK PREGNANCY: DIAGNOSIS AND PROPHYLACTIC THERAPY

Certain bitches may show increased frequency/incidence of high-risk pregnancy. These are brachycephalic breeds, which may have cephalopelvic disproportion of fetal head and maternal pelvis, slack abdominal musculature and "walrus" or "water" puppies (fetal anasarca); toy breeds with small litter size; the bitch with a single-puppy litter and the primiparous bitch over age 6. Bitches with a history of previous spontaneous abortion, pyometra or dystocia may be included in the high-risk group.

A high index of suspicion can be formed by a thorough history and physical examination. Bitches in the risk group should be examined at approximately 28 days for pregnancy diagnosis by abdominal palpation and at approximately 55 days for radiographic evidence of number of fetuses and fetal viability. Any vaginal discharge during pregnancy warrants examination of the bitch. Anorexia, depression, weakness, trembling, polydipsia and polyuria are signs warranting examination. Hypocalcemia may occur in the prepartum bitch and cause signs of elevated body temperature, trembling and weakness. Partial abortion of a litter due to trauma has been known to occur. Uterine torsion, while rare, may present as acute abdomen, sudden collapse and shock.

Prevention of dystocia is designed to maintain overall body condition of the bitch and proper breeding management. The bitch should be bred early in standing heat and every other day throughout standing heat to maximize litter size. Maximum litter size occurs with breedings on days 4 to 5 prior to cytologic onset of diestrus.[3] Daily walks and exercise improve muscle tone and aid in easier delivery. The bitch should be well fed during pregnancy but not allowed to become obese. Careful monitoring of body temperature during the last week of gestation will aid in the diagnosis of impending parturition and possible primary uterine inertia if overt labor does not follow the temperature drop within 24 hours. If body temperature drops to 99°F or below without signs of stage I labor within 24 hours, the bitch should be examined. Following temperature drop, the temperature returns to normal prior to onset of delivery. When the fetus or fetuses are known to be nonviable through radiography (gas in the uterus, collapse of the calvarium or axial skeleton) or through ultrasonography (lack of fetal motion or heart beat), monitoring of the bitch's temperature is important. If the temperature drops and labor does not begin within 24 hours, a cesarean section should be performed.

References

1. Concannon P, Rendano V: Radiographic diagnosis of canine pregnancy: Onset of fetal skeletal radiopacity in relation to times of breeding, preovulatory luteinizing hormone release, and parturition. Am J Vet Res 44:1506, 1983.

2. Feeney DA: Personal communication, 1983.
3. Holst PS, Phemister RD: Onset of diestrus in the beagle bitch. Definition and significance. Am J Vet Res 35:401, 1974.
4. Johnston SD: Diagnostic and therapeutic approach to infertility in the bitch. JAVMA 176:1335, 1980.
5. Johnston SD, Larsen RE, Olson PS: Canine Theriogenology, Vol. XI. Soc. Theriogenol, 1982.
6. Johnston SD, Smith FO, Bailie NC, et al.: Prenatal indicators of puppy viability at term. Comp Cont Ed 5:1013, 1983.
7. Mosier JE: Nutritional recommendation for gestation and lactation. Vet Clin North Am 7:683, 1977.
8. Mohrman RK: Gestation and lactation of dogs. In Nutrition and Management of Dogs and Cats. St. Louis, Ralston Purina, 1979.
9. Sheffy BE: Nutrition and nutritional disorders. Vet Clin North Am 8:7, 1978.
10. Schneider NR: Development and genetic toxicology. In Kirk RW (ed): Current Veterinary Therapy, Small Animal Practice. Philadelphia, WB Saunders Co, 1983, pp 128–139.
11. Sokolowski JH: Normal events of gestation of the bitch and methods of pregnancy diagnosis. In Morrow DA (ed): Current Therapy in Theriogenology. 1st ed. Philadelphia, WB Saunders Co, 1980, pp 590–592.

Parturition and Dystocia in the Bitch

Shirley D. Johnston, D.V.M., Ph.D.
University of Minnesota, St. Paul, Minnesota

NORMAL PARTURITION

Onset of normal parturition in the bitch occurs approximately 63 days after ovulation or approximately 57 days after the change in the vaginal cytology smear from predominantly cornified to predominantly noncornified cells (the first day of diestrus).[10, 11] Normal parturition may occur from 58 to 71 days after a single breeding because of the long period of receptivity (estrus) in the bitch, the great variation between onset of estrus and ovulation in individual bitches (from 11 days before to 3 days after ovulation) and long survival of sperm in the uterus of the estrous bitch.[5–7, 10–12, 14, 15] The bitch that conceives after being bred a single time 8 days before ovulation will have an apparent gestation length (breeding to whelping) of 71 days; the bitch that conceives after being bred a single time 5 days after ovulation will have an apparent gestation length of 58 days. In both cases, however, time from ovulation to whelping is approximately 63 days.

If rectal temperature is monitored twice daily, an abrupt prepartum temperature drop can be detected in most pregnant bitches; onset of normal parturition occurs within the 24 hours following the abrupt drop. In 40 canine pregnancies mean rectal temperature drop was $0.8 \pm 0.1°C$ $(1.4 \pm 0.2°F)$ and mean low prepartum rectal temperature was $37.1 \pm 0.06°C$ $(98.9 \pm 0.11°F)$.[4] The temperature drop has been demonstrated to occur 10 to 14 hours following decline in plasma progesterone to less than 2 ng/ml.[3, 4]

The prepartum temperature drop in the bitch is transient; temperature returns to the normal range before onset of parturition.[4]

Stages of parturition in the bitch include stage 1, which starts at the onset of regular uterine contractions and ends with complete cervical dilation; stage 2, which starts with movement of the first puppy through the cervix and ends with complete delivery of the last puppy of the litter; and stage 3, which is the time of placental delivery.

Stage 1, which may last from 6 to 12 hours in the bitch, is associated with clinical signs of restlessness, panting and nesting behavior. As these signs may occur intermittently during the last week of pregnancy, onset and duration of stage 1 labor in the dog may be difficult for the owner to detect.

At the onset of stage 2 labor, fetal stretching of the maternal cervix causes a neuroendocrine reflex leading to increased maternal oxytocin secretion; uterine contractions are strengthened, and the bitch may strain and push, contracting her voluntary abdominal musculature. Abdominal contractions, straining and/or presence of fetal membranes or the fetus itself at the vulva are signs of the onset of stage 2 labor. Duration of stage 2 labor varies with breed and litter size. At normal whelping a first puppy should be delivered within 4 hours of onset of stage 2 labor, and subsequent puppies are generally delivered at intervals of less than 2 hours each. Many bitches will deliver 2 puppies within minutes of each other and then rest. Some bitches deliver their entire litter in 2 to 4 hours; others take 6 to 12 hours.

Stage 3 labor, or delivery of placentae, usually occurs following delivery of every 1 or 2 puppies.

DYSTOCIA

There are many causes of dystocia in the dog.[1] These can be categorized into three general groups of causes: inadequate size of the maternal birth canal (bony callus impingement from a healed pelvic fracture, vaginal stricture, prolapse or neoplasia), absolute fetal oversize (fetal monster, anasarcous fetuses, one-pup litters) and inadequate uterine contractions (primary or secondary uterine inertia).

In most cases of canine dystocia the diagnosis is made by observing failure of the bitch to start labor at the appropriate time (primary uterine inertia) or by her failing to progress appropriately through the three stages of labor.

Primary Uterine Inertia. The diagnosis of primary uterine inertia is based on the knowledge of the expected date of parturition and by the bitch's failure to start labor appropriately. Because normal gestations may range from 58 to 71 days in length from a single breeding, gestation length calculated from breeding date is a very inexact indicator of parturition date. Better indicators are gestation length timed from the first day of diestrus (Dl, 57 to 59 days) or parturition date timed from the prepartum rectal temperature drop, which should occur less than 24 hours before labor onset.

On physical examination the bitch with primary uterine inertia is generally bright and alert; cervical dilation may be detected vaginoscopically in small- to medium-sized bitches. A green-tinged vaginal discharge may be present. These patients are generally normocalcemic and show no response (uterine contractions, pushing behavior) to administration of oxytocin or calcium. Treatment is cesarean section, and prognosis for puppy survival is good if treatment is instituted on the date of expected parturition. Primary uterine inertia may, but does not always, recur at subsequent pregnancies.

Failure to Progress. Bitches that begin labor normally but fail to deliver their first or subsequent puppies in a timely manner constitute the second group of bitches with dystocia seen in veterinary practice. These may have obstructive dystocias (absolute or relative fetal oversize) or inadequate uterine contractions to expel the fetuses completely (asynchronous or ineffective contractions, uterine fatigue). Some of these animals may be identified prior to the onset of parturition by digital examination of the vagina and by radiographic examination of the maternal abdomen to examine fetal size and pelvic conformation. Ultrasound is also useful in monitoring fetal viability prior to or at parturition.[2, 9] Failure to progress is generally defined temporally as occurring when the bitch has been in second stage labor for more than 4 hours prior to birth of her first pup or for more than 2 hours between pups. While occasional bitches exceed these time constraints during normal delivery, most do not.

Clinical examination should include careful abdominal palpation to confirm that fetuses are present in the uterus, digital examination of the vagina and abdominal radiographs to assess fetal number, size and conformation of the maternal pelvis. Radiography may also help diagnose fetal death if signs of intrafetal or intrauterine gas, skeletal collapse or overlap of cranial bones are present.[8]

Plasma glucose and serum calcium concentrations should be measured, and a complete blood count and chemistry profile are useful preoperative tests if cesarean section becomes necessary.

Treatment of bitches with failure to progress is determined by results of physical examination and diagnostic tests. Relative or absolute fetal oversize is treated by cesarean section. Ineffective uterine contractions may be treated with oxytocin (3 to 20 units IM) and/or with 10 per cent calcium gluconate (3 to 5 ml, IV, given slowly) in the presence of low total or ionized serum calcium concentrations. Oxytocin administration may be repeated at 30-minute intervals; if there is no progress after three treatments, cesarean section is recommended. Possible adverse effects of oxytocin therapy over time (such as placental separation and fetal compromise) have not been well quantified in the dog but may occur. Most domestic female mammals become refractory to oxytocin after repeated injection, and cesarean section may be necessary to deliver some pups in a litter that was partially delivered vaginally. Prognosis for puppy survival depends on elapsed time of the dystocia.

References

1. Bennett D: Canine dystocia—a review of the literature. J Small Anim Pract 15:101, 1974.
2. Bondestam S, Alitalo I, Karkkainen M: Real-time ultrasound pregnancy diagnosis in the bitch. J Small Anim Pract 24:145, 1983.
3. Concannon PW, Hansel W: Prostaglandin F$_2$ alpha induced luteolysis, hypothermia and abortions in beagle bitches. Prostaglandins 13:533, 1977.
4. Concannon PW, Powers ME, Holder W, Hansel W: Pregnancy and parturition in the bitch. Biol Reprod 16:517, 1977.
5. Concannon P, Rendano V: Radiographic diagnosis of canine pregnancy: Onset of fetal skeletal radiopacity in relation to times of breeding, preovulatory luteinizing hormone release, and parturition. Am J Vet Res 44:1506, 1983.
6. Doak RL, Hall A, Dale HE: Longevity of spermatozoa in the reproductive tract of the bitch. J Reprod Fertil 13:51, 1967.
7. Evans HE: Prenatal development in the dog. 24th Gaines Vet. Symp, Ithaca, 1974.
8. Farrow CS, Morgan JP, Story EC: Late-term fetal death in the dog: Early radiographic diagnosis. J Am Vet Radiol Soc 17:11, 1976.
9. Feeney DA: University of Minnesota, personal communication, 1983.
10. Holst PA, Phemister RD: Onset of diestrus in the beagle bitch: Definition and significance. Am J Vet Res 35:401, 1974.
11. Holst PA, Phemister RD: Temporal sequence of events in the estrous cycle of the bitch. Am J Vet Res 36:705, 1975.
12. Johnston SD: Personal observation, 1983.
13. Phemister RD, Holst PA, Spano JS, Hopwood ML: Time of ovulation in the beagle bitch. Biol Reprod 8:74, 1973.
14. Rendano VT: Radiographic evaluation of fetal development in the bitch and fetal death in the bitch and queen. In Kirk RW (ed): Current Veterinary Therapy, Small Animal Practice. Philadelphia, WB Saunders Co, 1983, pp 947–952.
15. Wildt DE, Chakraborty PK, Panko WB, Seager SWJ: Relationship of reproductive behavior, serum luteinizing hormone and time of ovulation in the bitch. Biol Reprod 18:561, 1978.

Anesthesia for the Pregnant Bitch

Mollie Wright, D.V.M., M.S.
River Valley Veterinary Clinic, Plain, Wisconsin

The bitch presents special problems when anesthetized at any time during pregnancy. Early in pregnancy the primary concerns are abortion and/or the teratogenic effects of the anesthetic agent. Later in pregnancy physiological changes occur in the bitch that must be considered for safe induction, maintenance and recovery from anesthesia. This article will deal primarily with anesthesia of the bitch as necessary for a cesarean section at or near term. It will include physiological characteristics that influence anesthesia safety in the pregnant bitch and fetus/neonate. The effects of anesthesia and specific anesthetic agents will also be discussed. Although anesthesia of any kind has increased risk during pregnancy and should be avoided unless absolutely necessary, the final section of this article will present several anesthetic regimens judged to be safe.

PHYSIOLOGICAL CHANGES DURING PREGNANCY

Cardiovascular System. As gestation progresses, maternal blood volume increases by 20 to 40 per cent and plasma volume by 40 to 50 per cent with a resulting decrease in erythrocyte count and hematocrit. Cardiac output increases by 30 to 50 per cent owing to increased blood volume and to decreased vascular resistance from hormonal influences. These effects result in a continuously increased workload on the heart and a decreased cardiac reserve to protect and to compensate for changes caused by anesthesia and surgery.

Respiratory System. During pregnancy the increased volume of the uterus causes anterior displacement of the diaphragm. At the same time hormones cause an increase in the diameter of the thoracic cage and a relaxation of bronchiolar smooth muscle. This results in decreased functional residual capacity (FRC) and expiratory reserve volume, with concomitant increase in inspiratory capacity and inspiratory reserve volume. There is also an increase in respiratory rate, tidal volume and minute volume, with alveolar ventilation increased by about 70 per cent in the pregnant animal. This increase is important because increased alveolar ventilation may has-

ten the rapidity of induction with gas anesthesia. Since FRC serves to allow gas exchange during the period between breaths, when anesthesia greatly reduces rate and volume of breaths, decreased FRC causes a decreased margin of safety from hypoxia.

PHYSIOLOGICAL DIFFERENCES IN THE NEONATE

The renal and hepatic systems of the newborn are much less efficient at detoxification and elimination than those of the normal adult, and it is important to minimize administration of agents to the bitch that will cross the placenta.

The ability of the blood in the neonate to carry oxygen is different from that of the adult's in several ways. Levels of hemoglobin are high and characterized by a greater affinity for oxygen—a "left shift" in the oxyhemoglobin dissociation curve. At the same time plasma is more acidic, causing a "right shift" and increased release of oxygen from hemoglobin at the tissues. If this balance is upset by drug effects or alkalosis (hyperventilation), oxygenation of the newborn can be impaired.

An additional physiological problem in the neonate is its inability to regulate body temperature. Danger of hypothermia is increased when drugs causing peripheral vasodilation (e.g., halothane, acetylpromazine) were administered to the mother and crossed the placenta prior to delivery.

MATERNAL HAZARDS DURING ANESTHESIA

Anesthetic Depth. As noted previously, circulatory and respiratory systems in the pregnant bitch do not have the same margin of safety that is present in the normal animal to protect the animal from the excessive depth of anesthesia. Maintaining the plane of anesthesia as light as possible is extremely important. Slight movements of the bitch should be tolerated if such movements appear random and not in response to surgical pain.

Respiratory Depression. Ventilation must be monitored carefully as anesthetic depth increases. With decreased FRC, administration of 100 per cent oxygen via face mask prior to induction will increase the margin of safety, should breathing diminish or cease during induction. After induction, the bitch should be intubated with a cuffed endotracheal tube, and controlled ventilation should be supplied as necessary. Placement of the patient in a head-down position will greatly compromise ventilation and should be avoided.

Hypotension. Chances for this anesthetic complication are increased in the pregnant patient because of the combination of several potential causes: the anesthetic agent, decreased venous return due to pressure of the uterus on the posterior vena cava and sympathetic blockade if epidural anesthesia is used. In addition, depletion of extracellular fluid volume and endotoxic shock can develop rapidly during dystocia or when dead fetuses are present.

To detect hypotension, pulse pressure and arterial pressure are important to monitor by taking lingual and/or femoral pulses frequently. Special attention should be paid during induction, positioning of the bitch on the table, and exteriorization of the uterus. After closure of the uterus, bleeding may occur but be hidden, so blood pressure is important to monitor at that time as well.

Prevention of hypotension is important for pups as well as the bitch, since decreased uterine perfusion can result in hypoxia to the fetus. Steps in its prevention and treatment include the following: (1) avoiding dorsal recumbency, tilting the patient slightly to one side if dorsal recumbency is necessary for surgery; (2) giving fluids prior to and during anesthesia (20 ml/kg/hour); (3) keeping anesthetic depth at the lightest possible plane; and (4) giving ephedrine as necessary for short-term vasopressor effects without reducing uterine blood flow.

Aspiration. Since time of parturition is unpredictable, the bitch may have been fed just prior to labor. In addition, in later pregnancy gastric emptying time has slowed. When these circumstances combine with the increased abdominal pressure during labor, hormonally caused relaxation of sphincters and internal surgical manipulation, emesis is very likely. Aspiration can be prevented or minimized if the trachea has been intubated with a cuffed tube to prevent leakage of fluids. Glycopyrrolate can be administered as a preanesthetic medication to reduce the chance of emesis and decrease the acidity of gastric contents. Other treatments, if emesis and aspiration occur, are suction and lavage of mouth, pharynx and trachea and, as necessary, controlled ventilation, drug treatment (steroids, antibiotics and bronchodilators) and general supportive therapy.

Convulsions. Hypocalcemia and drug toxicity may cause convulsions as another complication of anesthesia in the later stages of pregnancy. Calcium levels in the blood of less than 7 mg/dl may result in eclampsia and should be treated with administration of calcium. Toxicity from inadvertently high systemic doses of local anesthetics may cause convulsions, which must be treated symptomatically with barbiturates or diazepam. Harm to the fetus is a possible side effect of the treatment.

FETAL HAZARDS FROM ANESTHESIA

Hypoxia is the primary hazard to the fetus. It may begin before birth, as a result of maternal hypotension and decreased uterine perfusion. Increased and prolonged myometrial pressure, as may occur when oxytocin is administered, will also contribute to hypoxia.

After birth, the neonate can experience respiratory depression from anesthetic agents that have crossed the placenta and remain in the blood. This is a particular hazard when barbiturates, narcotics or high levels of inhalant anesthetics are given to the bitch prior to delivery. Prolonged passage through the birth canal and fetal aspiration of amniotic fluids may also result in hypoxia. In general, tracheal suction, intubation, administration of oxygen and controlled ventilation will help to reverse hypoxia and aid recovery of the pups. When narcotics are administered to the bitch, naloxone (1 drop sublingually) should be given to each pup. A respiratory stimulant (doxapram, 1 to 2 drops, sublingually) may also be administered.

PLACENTAL TRANSFER OF ANESTHETIC AGENTS

Transfer of agents from bitch to pups occurs through simple diffusion, with the rate limited primarily by concentration gradients. A concentration gradient is influenced by rate of uptake (how rapidly it is administered), distribution and excretion of the drug by the bitch and the amount of the drug that is protein bound or inactive. Molecular size, lipid solubility and ionization of the molecules also determine the amount that can cross the placenta, with small, highly lipid-soluble, nonionized molecules crossing most readily.

Barbiturates. Barbiturates have high lipid solubility and cross the placenta rapidly. Pentobarbital contributes to extreme depression and high mortality of pups, thus should be avoided for obstetric anesthesia. Thiobarbiturates (thiopental, thiamylal) have even higher lipid solubility and appear to achieve equilibrium across the placenta within 3 to 4 minutes. When small doses (less than 8 mg/kg) are given for induction only, the anesthetic is redistributed, and depression is minimal in pups delivered more than 10 minutes after induction. Administration should not be repeated, however.

Inhalants. Gas anesthetics (methoxyflurane, halothane and nitrous oxide) have small molecular size and high lipid solubility and are primarily nonionized in the maternal blood, so they readily achieve equilibrium across the placenta. Depression of the pups is proportional to depth of anesthesia in the bitch. For this reason inhalant anesthesia must be maintained at the lightest possible plane prior to delivery of the pups. Methoxyflurane has an advantage over other inhalants in that it provides some degree of analgesia at light planes, so it may allow maintenance at levels that cause little depression of pups. If depression does occur, however, methoxyflurane requires a longer time for recovery than other inhalants, so minimal use is very important. Halothane may cause some uterine relaxtion and increased bleeding though this has not been shown in dogs. Nitrous oxide will aid in producing analgesia at light planes and can safely be used at 50 per cent concentrations, although it does decrease the oxygen concentration given and may be hazardous in some dogs in which hypoxia is feared.

Narcotics. Narcotic analgesics such as morphine, oxymorphone and meperidine cross the placenta and cause varying degrees of respiratory depression in both bitch and pups. This is less important than with other agents, since that depression is reversible with narcotic antagonists.

Locals. Local anesthetics such as lidocaine, mepivacaine and bupivacaine have been shown to be present in the neonate when used for local or regional anesthesia in the mother. Lidocaine and mepivacaine cause some depression in the human neonate when used for epidural blocks; bupivacaine is the agent of choice.

Tranquilizers. Phenothiazine (acetylpromazine) and butyrophenone (droperidol, component of Innovar-Vet) tranquilizers cross the placenta easily and cause some general depression in the pups after delivery. With prolonged action (6 to 8 hours in adults, longer in neonates), hypotensive effects and a tendency to cause hypothermia in both bitch and pups, these agents are contraindicated for use as anesthetics in cesarean section. Other tranquilizers such as diazepam and xylazine also cross the placenta and appear clinically to cause depression in the neonate, although probably for a shorter period of time.

Ketamine. This dissociative agent that is used most frequently in cats can also be administered intravenously to dogs for a quick induction and good analgesia for a relatively short period of time (10 to 20 minutes in the healthy dog). It crosses the placenta rapidly but appears clinically to cause little depression in the neonate when used alone.

Muscle Relaxants. With the exception of gallamine, these agents are large molecules, highly ionized with low lipid solubilities, and do not cross the placenta to any significant degree. For this reason, they have no effect on the fetus or neonate and can be highly useful as an adjunct, quieting the bitch and allowing analgesic, but not anesthetic, dosages of other, more depressant agents. Examples of useful relaxants are succinylcholine and pancuronium. Disadvantages of muscle relaxants in obstetric anesthesia, as in other situations, include the requirement for controlled ventilation, since total paralysis, including respiratory, is induced. This may prohibit their use in many common emergency clinical situations.

Anticholinergics. Atropine is used routinely as a preanesthetic medication to control salivary secretions and to provide vagal blockade to prevent bradycardia. Its use is often unnecessary and, since it crosses the placenta, will cause increased fetal heart rate and perhaps other effects in the central nervous system. Glycopyrrolate is another anticholinergic that guards against bradycardia but does not cross the placenta. It has the additional advantage of increasing gastric pH (greater safety from damage should aspiration occur) and is the anticholinergic of choice for obstetric anesthesia.

SUGGESTED ANESTHETIC REGIMENS

With all anesthetic techniques, the safest may well be that with which the practitioner is most familiar. It is unwise to try a new technique in an already hazardous case. Recommended regimens are offered with the assumption they can be used in ordinary situations to gain familiarity prior to use in a high-risk animal.

Regional Anesthesia. Epidural anesthesia in the bitch is one of the safest regimens. Bupivacaine (1 ml/3.5 kg) can be injected slowly into the L_7–S_1 intervertebral space with a spinal needle. Total relaxation and analgesia to the level of midabdomen should be apparent within 10 minutes after administration. Duration of effects will vary, ranging from 3 to 5 hours. Dose should not exceed the recommended amount. Higher doses may cause respiratory depression or paralysis and should be avoided. Hypotension may result from sympathetic blockade and vasodilation in the hind legs, so fluids (20 ml/kg as a loading dose, then 20 ml/kg/hour) must be administered prior to and at the time of performing the epidural. This is particularly important when the bitch is already potentially capable of entering a state of shock.

If tranquilization is necessary for the patient to lie quietly, oxymorphone (0.1 mg/kg, IV) is recommended and may be reversed in the bitch and pups after surgery is complete. Small amounts of gas anesthesia may be administered by mask as well.

A line block is a simpler method for using local anesthetics and this, with light gas anesthesia or narcotics used for tranquilization, can be very successful in a quiet or very sick patient.

Inhalant Anesthesia. Sedation can be initiated with a narcotic (oxymorphone, 0.1 mg/kg, IV) and the bitch can be gently intubated. If she resists, a small dose of ultra-short-acting barbiturate (thiopental, 4 to 8 mg/kg, IV) may be added. Depth is then maintained at a very light plane until pups are delivered and can be deepened if necessary at that time without danger. Methoxyflurane (1 per cent early, decreasing as possible to less than 0.3 per cent) and N_2O (50 per cent) are agents of choice, but halothane may also be effective if used in light levels (1 per cent or less) with N_2O.

References

1. Datta S, Alper MH: Anesthesia for cesarean section. Anesthesiology 53:142, 1980.
2. Hartsfield SM: Obstetrical anesthesia in small animals. Calif Vet 79:18, 1979.

Acute Metritis in the Bitch

M. L. Magne, D.V.M.
Colorado State University, Fort Collins, Colorado

Acute metritis in the bitch is an infectious disorder of the early postpartum period, usually occurring within the first week after whelping. Predisposing factors include dystocia, obstetric manipulations and retained placentae or fetuses. Metritis may also occur following apparently normal parturitions, or more rarely, after natural or artificial insemination or abortions. The postpartum uterus is enlarged and flaccid and has a patent cervix. These factors allow an environment to exist that is conducive to bacterial invasion and growth. Gram-negative organisms such as *Escherichia coli* and *Proteus* are commonly isolated, although infections with *Staphylococcus* or *Streptococcus* are also seen. These organisms gain access to the uterus via the patent cervix, or less commonly, from hematogenous spread.

Clinically, an abnormal vaginal discharge is characteristic. This discharge may be foul smelling and thick and range from purulent to sanguinopurulent. A dark green discharge is reportedly seen in bitches with retained placentae. Systemic signs including depression, anorexia, pyrexia, dehydration and tachycardia are common. Hypothermia may occur in later stages as the patient becomes debilitated or septicemic. An enlarged, "doughy" uterus may be detectable through abdominal palpation. The dam loses maternal instincts, milk production is usually decreased and puppies become restless, cry frequently and fail to grow. Metritis is an acute, rapidly progressive condition necessitating immediate therapeutic intervention.

A leukocytosis characterized by a neutrophilia with a left shift is common, although occasionally leukopenia may be seen. The hematocrit and total proteins are elevated because of dehydration; prerenal azotemia characterized by an elevated blood urea nitrogen (BUN) and creatinine with a high urine specific gravity may also be seen. Urine specific gravity may be low in animals suffering endotoxemia, since endotoxins may interfere with the action of antidiuretic hormone. Elevated liver enzymes reflect toxemia with secondary hepatic involvement. Radiographically, uterine enlargement or retained fetuses may be detectable. Cytology of the vaginal discharge reveals degenerate neutrophils, intracellular and extracellular bacteria, amorphous cellular debris and mucus. Endometrial cells may also occasionally be seen. Rarely, muscle fibers from decomposing fetuses may be observed.

Since acute metritis is a bacterial disorder and lacks the underlying hormonal etiology seen in the pyometra complex, conservative medical management is a viable treatment option in some cases. Broad-spectrum, systemic antibiotics (chloramphenicol, cephalosporins, trimethoprim-sulfa, ampicillin) should be instituted immediately on presentation. Antibiotic therapy can be altered, if necessary, according to results of culture and sensitivity studies of material from the cranial vaginal (cervical) area. Antibiotics should be continued for a minimum of 2 weeks.

In cases with a patent cervix and good uterine drainage, uterine infusions may be used in conjunction with systemic antibiotic therapy, although cannulation of the canine cervix is very difficult, even after whelping. If cannulation of the cervix is possible, solutions such as sterile saline or 2 per cent Betadine can be instilled into the uterus via a catheter. The cervix occasionally can be visualized with a long speculum or vaginoscope. Ventral traction of the uterus by abdominal palpation may aid in identifying the cervix and placement of the pipette or catheter. Care must be taken when catheterizing the diseased uterus, and use of a soft rubber catheter is recommended to avoid possible uterine rupture. Although infusion with antibiotic solutions has been advocated in the past, dosages and efficacy are questionable, and their use remains controversial. Infusions of nitrofurazone solutions have been shown to reduce subsequent fertility in cattle.

Uterine ecbolic agents are utilized to promote uterine involution and evacuation. Oxytocin is most commonly used, at a dosage of 0.5 to 1.0 U/kg IM. This can be repeated in 1 to 2 hours. Oxytocin may be ineffective in stimulating uterine contractions if several days have passed since whelping because of inappropriate sensitivity of the myometrium to oxytocin at this time. Ergonovine stimulates a more intense myometrial contraction than oxytocin and may be used if repeated administration of oxytocin fails to stimulate uterine emptying. Ergonovine is given intramuscularly at a dosage of 0.2 mg/15 kg, and some authors advocate using this dose three times daily for 2 to 3 days. Since ergonovine stimulates a more intense response and has a longer half-life than oxytocin, the danger of uterine rupture must be considered. Although the use of estrogens has been widely recommended in the past, their potential side effects (bone marrow suppression, uterine disease, behavioral estrus, reduced lactation) preclude routine use in the treatment of acute metritis.

Prostaglandin $F_{2\alpha}$ ($PGF_{2\alpha}$) might aid in the treatment of metritis through acting to maintain cervical patency and stimulating uterine contractions, thus promoting uterine emptying. The recommended dosage of $PGF_{2\alpha}$ is 25 to 100 µg/kg once or twice daily, for 3 to 5 days. Side effects of $PGF_{2\alpha}$ may occur and include vomiting, defecation, hypersalivation, restlessness or pacing. These occur within 20 minutes after injection and are usually transient. Uterine rupture might also follow $PGF_{2\alpha}$ administration if a diseased, friable uterus is forced to contract. Prostaglandins are not approved for use in the bitch.

Intravenous fluid therapy may be an important adjunct to therapy for the dehydrated, severely ill patient. A balanced electrolyte solution (lactated Ringer's) is recommended. Dextrose should be part of the electrolyte solution if endotoxemia is suspected.

In certain cases ovariohysterectomy remains the treatment of choice. Retained fetuses or placentae, severe infection, uterine erosion or rupture and lack of breeding potential are definite indications for surgical removal. A large incision is recommended, allowing easy visualization and exteriorization of the large, friable uterus. The incision site should be thoroughly packed off to prevent contamination in case of uterine rupture. Uterine massage and lavage has been described for more chronic cases that are refractory to routine medical management. A hysterotomy may be utilized to allow manual removal of uterine debris. An incision is made at the uterine bifurcation, the uterus is thoroughly lavaged, antibiotic solutions are instilled and the incision is closed. The uterus should always be examined carefully before manipulation or lavage. Retained placentae may be associated with uterine wall necrosis. These can be recognized as dark, swollen, discolored areas, palpable craters or swellings in the uterine wall, and their presence indicates the need for surgical removal of the uterus.

Differential diagnoses for acute metritis include eclampsia (puerperal tetany, postparturient hypocalcemia), subinvolution of placental sites and mastitis. These conditions are easily distinguished based on clinical presentation, examination of vaginal discharges, milk evaluation (grossly and cytologically), blood cell counts and serum chemistries.

References

1. Burke TJ: Postparturient problems in the dog. Vet Clin North Am 7:693, 1977.
2. Fazeli M, Ball L, Olson JD: Comparison of treatment of pyometra with estradiol cypionate or cloprosterol followed by infusion or noninfusion with nitrofurazone. Theriogenology 14:339, 1980.
3. Larsen RE, Wilson JW: Acute metritis. In Kirk RW (ed): Current Veterinary Therapy, Small Animal Practice. Philadelphia, WB Saunders Co, 1977, pp 1227–1229.
4. Mosier JE: Disorders in the postparturient bitch. In Morrow DA (ed): Current Therapy in Theriogenology. 1st ed. Philadelphia, WB Saunders Co, 1980, pp 608–614.

Disorders of the Canine Mammary Gland

Jerry D. Olson, D.V.M., M.S.
Patricia N. Olson, D.V.M., M.S., Ph.D.
Colorado State University, Fort Collins, Colorado

Bitches with varying disorders of the mammary gland are frequently brought to veterinarians for examination. The diagnosis and treatment of these disorders can be a challenging problem. Recognition of the various disturbances is extremely important, since some "disorders" occur as a result of normal physiological events. For example, inappropriate lactation is a normal physiological consequence of pseudopregnancy and usually resolves without treatment. In contrast, septic mastitis or acute inflammatory adenocarcinomas are life-threatening conditions requiring immediate therapy if the bitch's life is to be saved. This article will describe various diagnostic and therapeutic approaches for common disorders of the canine mammary gland.

MASTITIS

Mastitis is primarily a disease of the lactating bitch involving one or more mammary glands. In severe cases, the glands may be hot and painful, with the bitch displaying signs of systemic illness (e.g., depression, anorexia, fever and failure to care for the puppies). Bacteria commonly isolated from the milk of bitches with septic mastitis include

Escherichia coli, staphylococci, and beta-hemolytic streptococci.[1-4] A leukogram usually reveals leukocytosis, although leukopenia may be seen with endotoxemia. In milder cases the bitch may be systemically asymptomatic but is brought to the veterinarian because her puppies are failing to thrive.[5,6] The clinician should always evaluate the bitch for abnormal milk and/or hypolactia and agalactia when presented with poorly developing neonates. Abnormal or toxic milk from asymptomatic bitches has frequently been cited as a cause of neonatal morbidity and mortality. However, no critical studies have been conducted that correlate milk composition to neonatal morbidity or mortality.

Cytologic examination of secretions from inflamed glands of bitches with septic mastitis frequently reveals bacteria and numerous degenerative neutrophils. Quantitative bacteriology of the secretion from mastitic glands often shows dense bacterial growth. In contrast cytologic smears from normal-appearing mammary glands usually have fewer total cells (Table 1).

Ideally, antimicrobial therapy for bitches with septic mastitis should be selected on the basis of bacteriologic culture and antimicrobial sensitivity testing. In addition, certain pharmacologic principles should be considered in the selection of antimicrobial therapy. Antimicrobials that are weak acids are distributed in body compartments on the basis of pH partitioning, with weak acids concentrating in body compartments that are more alkaline than serum. Conversely, antibiotics that are weak bases will tend to concentrate in a more acidic environment.[7] This is important in that normal milk is slightly more acidic than serum. Therefore, under normal circumstances weak bases will concentrate more in milk than in serum. As mastitis develops,

the secretion becomes more alkaline, and in a severely inflamed gland it will approach that of serum. Thus, in a severely inflamed gland pH partitioning may not be a serious consideration in initial antimicrobial selection. However, as inflammation subsides, the secretion will again become more acidic than serum and the role of pH partitioning becomes more important. Another principle to consider is lipid solubility. Antimicrobials that are poorly lipid soluble will fail to achieve projected concentration advantages because of an inability to cross cell membranes. The aminoglycosides are examples of basic antibiotics that fail to concentrate in the acidic compartment because of low lipid solubility.[8] Careful consideration should be given to the selection of the tetracyclines for treatment of mastitis or any disease in nursing bitches, as concentrations of tetracycline in the milk may be high enough to result in staining of the puppies' teeth. However, once mastitis is diagnosed, the current recommendations are to hand rear the puppies. Chloramphenicol, which is a dihydro-alcohol, is nonionized, and thus its concentration in milk is not affected by pH partitioning. Therefore, chloramphenicol is a good initial choice for antimicrobial therapy because it has a broad spectrum and its concentration in the mammary secretion is not affected by pH. Chemical classification of the antimicrobials and lipid solubilities are given in Table 2.

Local antibiotic therapy can be used in addition to systemic therapy. The teats of the bitch are short and thick, with the teat end displaying a sievelike complex of 8 to 20 papillary duct orifices. Individual duct orifices can be identified in most bitches by gently expressing the gland and watching drops of milk form at the duct orifices. The part of the gland producing an abnormal secretion can be identified

Table 1. Cell Numbers and Types in Canine Milk

	Total Cells	Macrophages	Polymorpho-nuclear Cells	Unidentified Mononuclear* Cells
Normal bitches with nursing pups (n = 13)	33 to 14,548†	0 to 14,088	0 to 1418	0 to 1942
Normal bitches postweaning (n = 3)	13,750 to 67,654	8054 to 8869	5303 to 54,402	1577 to 4875
Pseudopregnant bitches (n = 3)	7302 to 38,233	5448 to 27,211	844 to 8808	0 to 910
Abnormal bitches‡ (n = 6)	4302 to 363,000	157 to 76,230	2352 to 283,400	751 to 24,861

*Unidentified mononuclear cells probably are degenerative nuclei of fat cells.
†Range of means; cells/μl milk.
‡Abnormal bitches include those with mastitis, mammary duct ectasia and galactostasis and those having septicemic puppies.
(The authors thank AL Olson for technical assistance in collecting data for this table.)

Table 2. Properties of Antibacterial Drugs

Drug	Chemical Nature	Degree of Lipid Solubility	Able to Exceed Serum Concentration in Normal Milk
Sulfas	Acid	Moderate	No
Penicillin	Acid	Moderate	No
Cloxacillin	Acid	High	No
Ampicillin	Acid	High	No
Amoxicillin	Acid	High	No
Cephapirin	Acid	Moderate	No
Aminoglycosides Neomycin Kanamycin Gentamicin Amikacin	Base	Low	No
Polymyxin B, colistin	Base	Very low	No
Erythromycin	Base	High	Yes
Tylosin	Base	High	Yes
Lincomycin	Base	High	Yes
Clindamycin	Base	High	Yes
Chloramphenicol	Alcohol	High	Equal
Tetracycline	Amphoteric	Moderate	Equal

and treated locally by lavaging with sterile saline and/or infusing antimicrobials (e.g., 0.2 per cent nitrofurazone) directly into the duct orifice with a lacrimal duct cannula. Fluid therapy is indicated in cases of septic mastitis with dehydration or shock. Glucose may need to be given if hypoglycemia develops secondary to endotoxemia. Acute septic mastitis may progress to abscess formation; in such cases surgical drainage is indicated, followed by dilute (1 per cent) Betadine flushes.

In bitches with septic mastitis, the question arises as to whether the puppies should be removed or left with the bitch. Puppies are generally hand reared after mastitis has been diagnosed. Although the owner must expend great amounts of time bottle or tube feeding the puppies, hand rearing usually assures that the nutritional requirements of the puppies are met. Bitches with inflamed glands may not be able to provide adequate caloric need for growing puppies. Additionally, if pups are hand reared, the veterinarian can select the antibiotics deemed more appropriate for treating the mastitis without being concerned about the effect these drugs may have on the nursing neonates. Puppies allowed to continue nursing from dams with septic mastitis should be monitored for daily weight gains. Although human infants are generally allowed to nurse from mastitic glands, no critical study has been performed to evaluate this practice in canine pediatrics.

Little work has been done in the bitch to correlate milk cytology with stage of lactation, bacteriology and composition of milk. We have recently evaluated cell numbers and types from the milk of normal bitches with nursing puppies, normal postpartum bitches, normal pseudopregnant bitches, and bitches with mammary gland diseases or "fading" puppies. Inflammatory cells are frequently observed on smears containing milk from "normal" or healthy bitches. Increased numbers of total and inflammatory cells do not always correlate with neonatal morbidity or mortality. In fact, some of the highest cell counts were observed in the milk of pseudopregnant and postweaning bitches (Table 1).

GALACTOSTASIS

Galactostasis is an abnormal collection of milk in the mammary glands. It can be seen as part of the clinical signs associated with septic mastitis. However, in this section galactostasis will be discussed as a primary condition of the mammary gland not associated with septic mastitis.

Although bitches with primary galactostasis are not systemically ill, they may be uncomfortable because of engorged glands that are hot and painful. Galactostasis is usually observed after weaning or following a pseudopregnancy when the body is attempting to resorb secretion that is not being removed from the gland through the teat. Entrapped milk within the ducts results in inflammation of the glands. Cytologic evaluation of the milk usually reveals cell counts of greater than 3000 cells per microliter, with macrophages and neutrophils as the predominant cell types. However, counts can be extremely variable (0 to 136,000/μl). The macrophages frequently have engulfed milk fat within the cytoplasm. Neutrophil numbers vary with severity of the inflammation.

Treatment is directed at decreasing the formation of secretion and reducing inflammation. Cool towels or compresses may be applied to the glands to decrease the inflammation. Systemic administration of glucocorticoids, diuretics and analgesics may be beneficial. Reducing food intake of the bitch combined with gradual weaning of the puppies may reduce the severity of the condition. Owners should be instructed not to milk the gland nor to stimulate the gland further, as this will only serve to further increase the release of prolactin and oxytocin, which contribute to milk production and let down.

AGALACTIA

Primary agalactia is rare in bitches. Although inadequate nutrition can result in decreased milk production, rarely is this the cause of clinically observed cases of agalactia. Occasionally, young, inexperienced bitches or nervous bitches with adequate milk are reluctant to nurse. Such apprehensive animals may be treated with low doses of tranquilizers, although reassurances from the owner will frequently calm the nervous or inexperienced bitch. Oxytocin as nasal sprays or injectables may be efficacious in enhancing milk let down but will not enhance milk production. Bitches with congenital abnormalities of the mammary glands or with inappropriate hormonal stimulation may have true agalactia. Because the underlying disorder in most cases of agalactia is unknown and treatment is ineffective, the puppies will have to be hand reared.

GALACTORRHEA (INAPPROPRIATE LACTATION)

Many bitches will lactate at the termination of diestrus. Decreasing concentrations of serum progesterone at the termination of the luteal phase will trigger a prolactin surge.[9] This results in lactation in many bitches, but it is usually so minimal that it goes unnoticed. However, some bitches lactate profusely, nest and mother small objects. The exact reason for the difference between overt and covert galactorrhea in the dog is unknown. The lactation generally resolves in a few weeks and does not require treatment. In severe cases the administration of diethylstilbestrol (1 mg/30 lb orally sid for 7 days), megestrol acetate (Ovaban) (0.25 mg/lb orally sid for 7 days) or mibolerone (Cheque Drops) (8 to 18 µg/kg orally sid for 5 days) may aid in decreasing prolactin release from the pituitary gland.[10] However, once these drugs are discontinued, prolactin may again surge, and inappropriate lactation may again occur. Occasionally, a bitch spayed during diestrus begins lactation several days after ovariohysterectomy. Owners should be told that this is a normal manifestation of acute progesterone withdrawal and the condition will resolve in a few weeks. Such lactation *does not* imply that the surgery was incorrectly performed.

INFLAMMATORY MAMMARY ADENOCARCINOMA

Inflammatory adenocarcinoma is a highly malignant neoplasm of the canine mammary gland that can mimic mastitis. Bitches presented with severely inflamed mammary glands are frequently thrombocytopenic due to disseminated intravascular coagulopathy (DIC). The prognosis in these cases is extremely poor. Bitches with inflammatory adenocarcinoma are usually older animals, and the onset occurs without regard to the stage of the estrous cycle or, in spayed bitches, in contrast to mastitis, which usually occurs after whelping. Inflammatory adenocarcinoma is discussed in more detail in the article Tumors of the Canine Female Reproductive Tract. It is mentioned here only to alert the veterinarian to a serious disorder that can mimic mastitis.

References

1. Johnston SD: Management of the postpartum bitch and queen. In Kirk RW (ed): Current Veterinary Therapy VIII, Small Animal Practice. Philadephia, WB Saunders Co, 1983, p 959.
2. Johnston SD, Hayden DW: Non-neoplastic disorders of the mammary glands. In Kirk RW (ed): Current Veterinary Therapy VI. Philadelphia, WB Saunders Co, 1980, p 1224.
3. Mosier JE: Disorders in the postparturient bitch. In Morrow DA (ed): Current Therapy in Theriogenology, Philadelphia, WB Saunders Co., 1980, p 608.
4. Lage AL: Non-neoplastic diseases of the mammary glands of dogs and cats. In Kirk RW (ed): Current Veterinary Therapy VI. Philadelphia, WB Saunders Co, 1977, p 1237.
5. Mosier JE: The puppy from birth to six weeks, toxic milk syndrome. Vet Clin North Am 8:90, 1978.
6. Small E: Pediatrics. In Kirk RW (ed): Current Veterinary Therapy VII. Philadelphia, WB Saunders Co, 1980, p 80.
7. Baggot JD: Principles of drug disposition in domestic animals: The basis of veterinary clinical pharmacology. In Kirk RW (ed): Current Veterinary Therapy. Philadelphia, WB Saunders Co, 1977.
8. Ziv G: Pharmacokinetic aspects of mastitis therapy. Bovine Mastitis Regional Seminar, Beecham Laboratories, University of Wisconsin Veterinary Extension, 1978.
9. Concannon PW, Butler WR, Hansel W, et al: Parturition and lactation in the bitch: Serum progesterone, cortisol and prolactin. Biol Reprod 19:1113, 1978.
10. Sokolowski JH: Mibolerone for treatment of canine pseudopregnancy and galactorrhea. Canine Pract 9:6, 1982.

Canine Uterine Prolapse

Donald S. Wood, D.V.M.
Hermosa Beach, California

Uterine prolapse, protrusion of the uterine body and/or one or both uterine horns through the cervix, is a rare condition in the bitch. During the period 1963 to 1979, 1,294,969 canine visits were reported to the American Veterinary Data Program (AVDP) of Cornell University, New York. Out of this number of visits, a diagnosis of uterine prolapse was made 28 times.

Review of the AVDP data and the sporadic case reports in the veterinary literature does not reveal a specific cause, predisposing factors or breed/conformation susceptibilities. Suggested causes include excessive traction on retained fetal membranes, forced fetal extraction and excessive straining due to metritis or a retained placenta. Suggested predisposing factors include failure of uterine involution and long mesometrial attachments. These have not been substantiated.

Uterine prolapse occurs during or after parturition or abortion, when the cervix is dilated. The prolapse may be complete or partial. In complete uterine prolapse one or both horns and the uterine body are everted through the vulva. In partial uterine prolapse one horn or the uterine body is everted into the vagina. An isolated case of prolapse of one horn while fetuses remain in the other has been reported. The pathologic sequelae of this condition include congestion and edema, which may lead to ischemia and necrosis. Potential complications include rupture of a uterine or ovarian artery and infection of and trauma to the exposed uterine tissues.

DIAGNOSIS

Diagnosis is made on the basis of history and physical examination. Signs noted by the owner may include vaginal discharge, abdominal pain, straining, restlessness, abnormal posture or a mass protruding from the vulva in the postpartum or postabortion period. The affected animal may be primiparous or multiparous. If the prolapse is complete, diagnosis is obvious. Vaginoscopic or digital examination of the vagina and abdominal palpation are required for diagnosis of partial prolapse. The exposed tissues should be examined closely for evidence of necrosis, self-mutilation, laceration or ruptured blood vessels. Differential diagnoses include vaginal hyperplasia, neoplasia (e.g., leiomyoma, transmissable venereal tumor), metritis and retained placenta. These can be ruled in or out on the basis of the stage of the estrous cycle and careful physical examination.

TREATMENT

The objectives of treatment are to return the uterus to its normal anatomic position and to prevent or to eliminate uterine infection. Whether or not these can be accomplished is dependent upon the condition of the animal and the prolapsed tissue. Complete physical examination may indicate that therapy for hypovolemic or septic shock is needed before treatment of the prolapse itself. Following stabilization the prolapse may be treated. Epidural or general anesthesia is required in most cases to relieve pain, to prevent straining and to facilitate palpation. The vulva and perivulvar area should be thoroughly cleansed with an antibiotic or antiseptic solution. In partial prolapse this is followed by elevation of the perineum and application of digital pressure to the prolapsed uterus. Simultaneous application of traction to the uterus through abdominal palpation may aid in reduction. If doubt exists about the completeness of reduction or tissue viability, techniques described for the reduction of complete prolapse are required. In complete prolapse the exposed tissue must also be cleansed. The exposed uterus can be thoroughly evaluated while this is accomplished.

Debridement and suturing of necrotic or lacerated areas may be indicated. If the damage is extensive, it may not be possible to salvage the uterus. If reduction will be attempted, application of a hypertonic dextrose or mannitol solution in conjunction with gentle massage will aid in reducing edema. A sterile water-soluble lubricant is then applied, the hind quarters are elevated and reduction is attempted. One horn should be grasped at the point most distal to the uterine body and gentle pressure applied in an attempt to reduce it. If this is successful, the opposite horn is reduced, followed by the body. Traction on the uterus via external abdominal palpation may aid reduction. Reduction may also be facilitated by insertion of a sterile test tube or syringe. Infusion of an aqueous antibiotic solution under slight pressure has also been suggested as a method of ensuring that the uterine horns are completely reduced. Reduction should be confirmed via digital vaginal examination and abdominal palpation. If external reduction is not successful, laparotomy may be performed, and reduction may be attempted via a combination of gentle traction on the suspensory ligaments of the ovaries and external manipulation by an assistant. Laparotomy is also indicated if reduction or tissue viability is questionable. Ovariohysterectomy may be necessary. If reduction cannot be performed, or if tissue damage is extensive, amputation of the prolapsed portion of the uterus at the vulva is indicated. The urethra should be catheterized prior to making an incision.

A short longitudinal incision is then made through the uterine wall distal to the vulva. The ovarian arteries should be identified at this point and ligated. The uterine tissue can then be excised via a transverse incision. The uterine stump may be sutured with a Cushing or Lembert pattern. The remaining portion of the uterus is then reduced. This procedure should be followed by laparotomy and completion of the ovariohysterectomy, since removal of both ovaries and the entire uterine body is not possible through a vaginal approach.

Systemic antibiotics should be given pre- and postoperatively to prevent or to treat metritis. Oxytocin, 5 to 10 units intramuscularly, should be given after reduction to stimulate uterine involution. Vulvar sutures or hysteropexy is not needed, as prolapse is not reported to recur. Lactation will not be affected by ovariectomy, as it normally occurs in the presence of decreased circulating concentrations of progesterone and estrogen.

Eclampsia in the Bitch

Johanna Kaufman, D.V.M.
Colorado State University, Fort Collins, Colorado

Eclampsia, or puerperal tetany, is a hypocalcemic tetanic condition that occurs in postparturient and occasionally in preparturient bitches. It has also been reported in cats, although it is rare in that species.

The disease occurs most frequently in small breeds of dogs, and primiparous bitches are more highly represented. This may be due to the fact that many owners do not wish to breed animals again once they have had the disease. A large litter size does not seem to play a role in predisposing animals to the disease. While the majority of cases are seen 1 to 3 weeks postpartum, they may occur earlier or later. Episodes occurring after 40 days postpartum are extremely rare.

The initial signs include restlessness, whining and apprehension. This progresses to a stiff gait, which may appear ataxic. The signs continue until the animal is recumbent with extreme extensor rigidity in the limbs. It is usually 8 to 12 hours after the initial onset of signs that tetany occurs. The animal may also have convulsions at this time.

Physical examination findings usually include hyperthermia, with temperatures occasionally exceeding 107°F. This is primarily caused by increased muscular activity. Many dogs will have an increased respiratory rate and will pant. The pupils will be dilated and sluggish in their response to light. However, the most striking finding is that of muscular tremors, extreme muscular rigidity or tetany. Convulsions are not uncommon. Other findings from the physical examination will be normal for a lactating bitch.

A blood calcium below 7 mg/100 ml will support the diagnosis, although most animals are treated on the basis of history and clinical signs before any clinical chemistries are completed by the laboratory. There are also some cases in which the blood calcium is measured in the normal range (10 per cent in one study). Blood glucose is normal in most individuals, but a moderate hypoglycemia may be present in some dogs. If so, it is probably the result of prolonged muscular activity. Phosphorus may be normal to low. Other clinical chemistries are within normal limits, including serum magnesium.

A differential diagnosis for seizures should include epilepsy, hypoglycemia, meningoencephalitis and toxicities such as strychnine, lead or metaldehyde. However, the sudden onset of the classic signs in a lactating bitch should point to the diagnosis of eclampsia unless there is a history of exposure to toxins, systemic illness or something that might suggest another disease process. Moreover, the signs of puerperal tetany persist in the postictal phase.

The pathophysiology of eclampsia in the dog is different than that of postparturient hypocalcemia in the cow. Bovine "milk fever" presents as a flaccid paralysis. The difference in clinical presentation is due to dissimilarities in the neuromuscular junction. In the cow transmission of acetylcholine is blocked by decreases in calcium. Therefore, nervous impulses do not get transmitted across the motor end plates. Transmission of acetylcholine is not blocked by hypocalcemia in the dog, but there is a loss of membrane-bound calcium. This in turn affects the muscular membrane so that it is more permeable to ions and thus requires less stimulus to depolarize. Consequently, the signs of spontaneous and repeated muscle cell depolarization are seen in the dog. Aberrations in magnesium to calcium ratios play a role in grass tetany in cattle. This does not appear to be important in the pathogenesis of the disease in dogs, and the levels of magnesium are within normal limits.

Although the measured calcium is the total serum calcium, only the ionized form is important for normal neuromuscular function. Maintenance of homeostasis is the result of a balance between the inflow and outflow of calcium. The amount of calcium from bone resorption is dependent on an actively secreting parathyroid gland. Differences between dogs and cattle are also notable in terms of predisposition to lactational hypocalcemia caused by the diet during gestation. In cattle, high levels of calcium in the preparturient ration create more of a reliance on intestinal absorption of calcium than on the secretory capabilities of the chief cells of the parathyroid gland. There is less active bone resorption to maintain blood calcium, and the requirements cannot be met when the calcium drain becomes extreme during peak lactation. The dog's parathyroid gland does not seem to be as sensitive to perturbations of the diet, so that intestinal absorption is more consistently the factor that may determine changes in inflow patterns. However, dogs receiving calcium supplementation during gestation have an increased incidence of the disease.

Metabolic or respiratory alkalosis results in a decrease of ionized calcium in the blood. Respiratory alkalosis may occur in the dog with eclampsia that is hyperpneic. Such alkalosis can create a vicious circle and drive the level of physiologically important form of calcium even lower.

Phytates are contained in many dog foods, especially those that have a high content of soybean meal. Phytate combines with ionic calcium and thus makes it physiologically unavailable. A diet high in phytates could conceivably play a role in the manifestation of hypocalcemia in an animal that was only marginally normocalcemic. This relationship has not been proved in any studies, but it is believed that it may play a role in an animal that is maintaining a tenuous balance.

Treatment consists of slow intravenous administration of calcium. The most common preparation is calcium gluconate. Five to 10 ml of a 10 per cent solution administered intravenously is usually adequate for a 5 to 10 kg bitch. Signs of muscular rigidity and tremors should dissipate within 15 minutes, although usually they subside sooner. Slow administration is essential, and many clinicians prefer to monitor the patient by electrocardiograph or auscultation in order to avoid arrhythmias or cardiac arrest. The amount given must be titrated to the animal's signs and must be moderated by any cardiac abnormalities. Cardiac signs can include bradycardias, tachycardias or premature ventricular contractions. EKG findings demonstrate a prolonged QT interval.

The pups should be removed from the bitch for a minimum of 24 hours to curtail the lactational drain. If possible, they should be weaned or nursed by hand.

Several authors in the past have recommended the use of corticosteroids in the treatment and prevention of relapse. This is without basis and may even be contraindicated inasmuch as glucocorticoids decrease intestinal absorption and enhance renal excretion of calcium. Oral administration of calcium or vitamin D supplements may be of benefit after the initial intravenous treatment.

Methods of prevention have not been documented in the dog. However, it is true that certain dogs have a predisposition to eclampsia and that recurrence of the disease in subsequent litters is common. While dogs are not as sensitive as cows in dietary manipulation of parathyroid function, it is still recommended that the diet during gestation contain a calcium-to-phosphorus ratio of 1:1 or less without an excessive amount of calcium. However, it is only conjecture that this may help. Owners may also wish to avoid feeding diets that contain high amounts of phytates during peak lactation. These include dry dog food diets with a high percentage of soybean meal or bran.

Suggested Readings

1. Austad R, Bjerkas E: Eclampsia in the bitch. J Small Anim Pract 17:793, 1976.
2. Bjerkas E: Eclampsia in the cat. J Small Anim Pract 15:411, 1974.
3. Capen CC, Martin SL: Calcium regulating hormones and diseases of the parathyroid glands. In Ettinger SJ (ed): Textbook of Veterinary Internal Medicine. Philadelphia, WB Saunders Co, 1983, pp 1584–1587.
4. Martin SL, Capen CC: Purperal tetany. In Kirk RW (ed): Current Veterinary Therapy VII, Small Animal Practice. Philadelphia, WB Saunders Co, 1980, pp 1025–1027.
5. Mosier JE: Disorders in the postparturient bitch. In Morrow DA (ed): Current Therapy in Theriogenology. Philadelphia, WB Saunders Co, 1980, pp 613–614.
6. Resnick S: Hypocalcemic tetany in the dog. JAVMA 144:1115, 1964.

Subinvolution of Placental Sites in the Bitch

Steven L. Wheeler, M.S., D.V.M.
Colorado State University, Fort Collins, Colorado

Following parturition, the uterus undergoes a process of involution that requires approximately 12 weeks to be fully completed.[2] Normally, the bitch may exhibit a dark vaginal discharge containing lochia in the immediate postpartum period. A mild serosanguineous discharge may also be present and last for approximately 4 to 6 weeks following parturition.[5] Subinvolution of placental sites (SIPS) is diagnosed when there is a failure or retardation of this involutionary process to occur. The most prominent clinical sign is that of a chronic hemorrhagic discharge passing from the vulva. The first case of SIPS was reported in 1950 and describes uterine perforation secondary to necrosis at multiple placental sites in a 2-year-old spaniel bitch, 1 day following an uneventful whelping.[10] In 1951 a second case report described the problem in a 10-month-old boxer bitch following a normal whelping.[8] In 1940 a case of uterine chorioepithelioma was described in a 7-year-old bitch, which, upon reexamination, closely resembles subinvolution of placental sites.[13] In this report a 7-year-old boxer terrier underwent an ovariohysterectomy 30 days after whelping three normal puppies because of a persistent vaginal discharge. A detailed histopathologic description was not included in the report, but a photograph of the uterus shows three eliptical enlargements that are similar to the gross lesions seen in SIPS. The first report describing subinvolution of placental sites as a clinical and pathologic entity was in 1966.[4] The condition is not commonly seen; however, in two surveys in which histopathologic examinations were performed on reproductive tracts from postpartum bitches, SIPS was confirmed in 32 of approximately 450[6] and in 20 of 95[1] cases. In both surveys the uteruses were submitted from bitches with and without a history of uterine disease. These reports suggest that the condition may occur more frequently than was previously thought but is clinically unrecognized.

CLINICAL FINDINGS

Affected bitches are most likely to be under 3 years of age,[1, 5, 13] although SIPS can be seen at any age. In one of the retrospective studies cited above, 23 of 32 cases were under 3 years of age.[6] SIPS was seen in many different breeds, and although the majority of the dogs in the above study were small breeds, no breed predilection was inferred. In addition, it was noted that in all of except two of the cases in this study in which an accurate history relative to the previous whelping was obtained, no known difficulty during parturition was seen, and normal puppies were whelped. In the two cases with complications, one bitch required a cesarean section to remove a dead fetus after whelping two live pups, while the other bitch experienced considerable difficulty during parturition and aborted one dead pup 4 days prior to whelping six pups, four of which were born alive.

The most consistent sign reported by owners of bitches presented with SIPS is that of a persistent postparturient serosanguineous discharge.[6, 13] Usually, owners will report that their dogs are healthy in other respects. Progressive weakness and collapse has been noted in cases in which perforation of the uterus occurred with a resulting peritonitis. Fortunately, this complication is rarely seen with SIPS.[6] Physical examination of these animals revealed a discharge passing from the vulva. The amount of the discharge may vary, with some dogs showing only a minimal discharge and others having a copious discharge. Also, the discharge can range from predominantly serous to predominantly bloody in nature. Small blood clots and grayish flecks of necrotic debris may be observed, especially in animals displaying a more copious discharge.[6] Abdominal palpation frequently reveals discrete oblong uterine enlargements corresponding to the regions where involution has failed to occur, although in a few cases, a generalized uterine enlargement may be palpated.[4] Abdominal palpation may reveal pain, and free peritoneal fluid may be ballotted in those rare cases in which uterine perforation with subsequent peritonitis has occurred. Slight pallor of the mucous membranes may be seen in bitches displaying a copious serosanguineous vaginal discharge.[4] Moderate to severe pallor may be seen if uterine perforation has occurred.

LABORATORY FINDINGS

In the majority of cases laboratory evaluation of the bitch reveals no abnormalities. The hemogram may reveal anemia if sufficient blood loss has occurred.[4] Blood chemistries are usually within normal limits, while a voided urinalysis will usually show varying degrees of hematuria. Hematuria is not seen with a cystocentesis urine sample. Vaginal cytology is consistent with the animal's postpartum stage, and a mixture of erythrocytes, neutrophils and parabasal cells is seen. Careful examination may reveal syncytial trophoblast-like cells, which is very helpful in establishing the diagnosis. The significance of this finding is discussed below.

PATHOPHYSIOLOGY

In order to fully understand the pathophysiological processes occurring in SIPS, the normal involution of the canine uterus following parturition must first be understood. The entire process of involution requires approximately 12 weeks to be completed.[2] The placental sites appear as 1.5 to 2 cm in diameter; they are rough, granular, and covered with mucus and a few blood clots during the first postpartum week. By the fourth week, the placental sites have decreased in size and appear as nodular grayish-tan areas with a clear mucous covering. At week 7 postpartum the placental sites appear about 0.8 to 1.5 cm in length and are light brown in color. By the ninth week, the placental sites appear as narrow light bands. Histologically, during the first week postpartum the placental sites are covered by eosinophilic necrotic collagenous masses. By the ninth week, these necrotic masses have sloughed completely, and by 12 weeks postpartum replacement of the uterine epithelium is complete.

In SIPS there is failure of the eosinophilic masses of collagen to slough, and the surface of these lobulated collagen masses becomes necrotic and hemorrhagic (Fig. 1).[1, 5] These masses extend down to involve the entire mucosa and may even invade the myometrium. Trophoblast-like cells are seen in abundant numbers at the base of these collagenous masses and may be seen to invade into the myometrium. Frequently, these cells are observed to surround blood vessels. Trophoblasts are fetal in origin and function to attach the developing ovum to the uterine wall and supply nutrition to the developing embryo. The same uterus may display normal involution at some placental sites, while at others it displays failure of this process to occur. The interplacental endometrium and ovaries in SIPS display no significant differences when compared with the normal postpartum organs.[1]

The exact etiology of SIPS is unknown. Initially, a hormonal etiology was proposed, with the influences of progesterone on the uterus being responsible.[9] Hemorrhage secondary to estrogen-induced capillary fragility has also been proposed as an important factor in the etiology of SIPS.[3] However, no hormonal assays were performed to prove this hypothesis. Additionally, estrogens are probably not elevated in the serum of postpartum bitches.[10] Differences in the degree of involution between placental sites in the same uterus indicate that hormonal influences are probably not a major factor in the pathogenesis of this disease. Also, no significant differences in the ovaries of normal and affected bitches have been seen. Furthermore, the concentration of progesterone in serum has been found to be the same in both normal animals and in those affected with SIPS, constituting further evidence against progesterone being involved in the pathogenesis of SIPS.[1] The absence of an inflammatory infiltrate in this disease makes bacterial

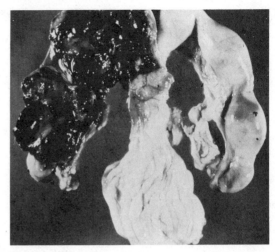

Figure 1. Uterus from a bitch affected with SIPS. Notice the elliptical enlargements in the left uterine horn and the lobated masses corresponding to the sites of subinvolution in the sectioned right horn.

infection an unlikely etiology.[1] Invasion of the endometrium and myometrium by trophoblast-like cells appears at present to be important in the pathogenesis of SIPS.[1] Invasion of the myometrium by fetal trophoblasts has also been shown to occur in pregnant women[7] and in the golden hamster.[12] Normally, these trophoblastic cells degenerate following abortion or parturition. In SIPS it appears as if these trophoblastic cells do not regress but continue to invade into the deeper aspects of the endometrium or even into the myometrium.[1] The reasons for the failure of these cells to regress and how their presence prevents the normal involution process from occurring remain unknown. Syncytial trophoblast-like cells may be observed on vaginal cytologic studies (Fig. 1).

DIAGNOSIS

Usually, this condition is diagnosed on the basis of a persistent postpartum vaginal serosanguineous discharge. The finding of syncytial trophoblast-like cells in the vaginal cytology helps to confirm the clinical diagnosis. Differential diagnoses for this condition include other conditions that may cause hemorrhage from the genitourinary tract such as metritis, vaginitis, endometrial hyperplasia, proestrus, trauma, bacterial cystitis, cystic calculi, coagulopathies and neoplasia of the genital or urinary tracts. However, these other conditions can usually be excluded with a history of recent whelping, a physical examination that reveals an otherwise healthy animal and a vaginal cytology showing trophoblast-like cells. In order to confirm the diagnosis it is necessary to perform a histopathologic study on an affected placental site.

TREATMENT

In the animal that is not desired for future breeding, ovariohysterectomy is the treatment of choice. Spontaneous recovery without medical or surgical therapy has been reported[14] and is the usual outcome. Others have recommended laparotomy and curettage of the placental sites as a treatment for bitches desired for future breeding; this has been successful in four cases as judged by later successful pregnancies,[6] although it must be remembered that spontaneous regression may have occurred without curettage. Posterior pituitary extracts, ergot derivatives and progesterone have been recommended but are usually not successful in treating SIPS.[3, 9]

Since spontaneous remission is likely, it is recommended that surgical or medical therapy be instituted only for those bitches showing signs of severe anemia, metritis or peritonitis. The owners should be instructed that because the cervix remains opened with SIPS, there is a small possibility for an ascending metritis to develop. Also, although very infrequent, the possibility that the uterine wall will perforate and a subsequent peritonitis will develop does exist. Animals showing any signs of systemic illness should be rechecked for complications.

PROGNOSIS

The prognosis for future reproductive success appears to be good if remission occurs. Affected bitches do not appear to be predisposed to developing SIPS in future pregnancies. In the case noted in which spontaneous remission occurred the bitch whelped a normal litter after being bred during the first estrus following the episode of SIPS.[14] There is evidence that reproductive success may also occur following laparotomy and curettage.

PROPHYLAXIS

Posterior pituitary extract administration after whelping has been recommended as beneficial in preventing this condition, but there are no studies to support this recommendation.

SUMMARY

Subinvolution of placental sites occurs when there is a failure or retardation of the normal involution process to occur. The most frequent clinical sign is that of a persistent bloody discharge from the vulva. A diagnosis can be confirmed on the basis of history, physical examination and vaginal cytology. If the animal is not desired for future breeding, ovariohysterectomy is the treatment of choice. If future breeding is desired, it is recommended that no surgical or medical therapy be instituted because spontaneous remission may occur. If surgery is performed, curettage of the affected placental sites may be attempted. Following spontaneous remission, the prognosis for future reproductive success is favorable.

References

1. Al-Bassam MA, Thompson RG, O'Donnell L: Involution abnormalities in the postpartum uterus of the bitch. Vet Pathol 18:208, 1982.
2. Al-Bassam MA, Thompson RG, O'Donnell L: Normal postpartum involution of the uterus in the dog. Can J Comp Med 45:217, 1981.
3. Arbeiter K: The use of progestins in the treatment of persistent uterine hemorrhage in the postpartum bitch and cow: A clinical report. Theriogenology 4:11, 1975.
4. Beck AM, McEntee K: Subinvolution of placental sites in a postpartum bitch: A case report. Cornell Vet 56:269, 1966.
5. Burke TJ: Postparturient problems in the bitch. Vet Clin North Am 7:695, 1977.
6. Glenn BL: Subinvolution of placental sites in the bitch. 18th Gaines Veterinary Symposium. White Plains, Gaines Dog Research Center, 1968, pp 7–10.
7. Hamilton JW, Boyd JD: Trophoblast in utero-placental arteries. Nature 212:906, 1966.
8. Jourdan RH, Hill HJ: A case of canine metorrhagia. JAVMA 118:377, 1951.
9. Kirk RW, McEntee K, Bentinck-Smith J: Diseases of the urogenital system. In Caticott EJ (ed): Canine Medicine. Wheaton, American Veterinary Publications, 1968, p 404.
10. Nett TM, Olson PN: Reproductive physiology of dogs and cats. In Ettinger SJ (ed): Textbook of Veterinary Internal Medicine, 2nd ed. vol 2. Philadelphia, WB Saunders Co, 1983, p 1698.
11. Nye SS: Even areas of uterine necrosis following parturition in the bitch. Vet Rec 62:118, 1950.
12. Orsinil NW: The trophoblastic giant cells and endovascular cells associated with pregnancy in the hamster, *Cricetus auratus*. Am J Anat 94:273, 1954.
13. Riger WH: Chorioepithelioma of the uterus of a dog. JAVMA 96:271, 1940.
14. Shall WD, Duncan JR, Finco OR, Knecht CD: Spontaneous recovery after subinvolution of placental sites in a bitch. JAVMA 159:1780, 1971.

Canine Herpesvirus Infection

Akira Hashimoto, D.V.M., Ph.D.
Katsuya Hirai, D.V.M., Ph.D.
Gifu University, Gifu, Japan

Canine herpesvirus (CHV) infection in neonatal pups is a fatal acute infectious disease characterized by generalized focal necrosis and hemorrhage. The disease is well known and has been recognized as one of the most important neonatal diseases encountered in the dog. The disease in adult dogs is usually mild or inapparent and generally restricted to the respiratory and genital tracts. However, CHV may cause genital lesions in the bitch that may be associated with infertility, abortion and stillbirths. Sexual transmission of CHV has also been suggested. Most recently, we have reported the effects of transplacental transmission of CHV on the fetus and newborn pups. The importance of this virus in canine theriogenology is now recognized, since various events caused by CHV infection of the dam have been investigated and clarified. Thus, it is reasonable to review briefly the available information associated with CHV infection of the bitch, especially during pregnancy.

EFFECTS OF CHV INFECTION DURING PREGNANCY

CHV has been isolated from the kidney of fetal and neonatal pups taken by cesarean section from apparently healthy pregnant dogs.[16] A spontaneous case of suspected intrauterine infection with CHV, indicated by the presence of placental lesions in the affected pups, has been reported.[6] This evidence suggests that transplacental transmission might serve as one of the routes of CHV infection in pregnant dogs. Recently, experimental transplacental transmission of CHV and its effects on the fetus and neonatal pups have been demonstrated.[8, 9] Results of one experiment suggested that transplacental transmission of CHV may occur in pregnant bitches during late gestation.[6] The pregnant bitches inoculated with CHV developed conjunctivitis, with serous or mucopurulent ocular discharge and serous nasal discharge between postinoculation days 2 and 5. Rectal temperature of the bitches generally remained normal before and after the inoculation. No abnormality was noticed in the bitches at or after parturition. Interestingly, immediately after publication of the first case of natural prenatal CHV infection, Dr. Carmichael at Cornell University observed a similar case (personal communication).

Results of a second experiment suggested that transplacental infection of fetal pups established by intravenous inoculation of pregnant bitches with CHV at 30 days gestation resulted in fetal death and subsequent mummification.[6] An interesting finding in this experiment was the occurrence of dead and mummified fetuses in the same litters as unaffected live pups (Fig. 1).

Abortion and premature birth may occur in pregnant bitches infected with CHV during the second trimester of gestation. Abortion occurred between the second and third weeks (44 to 51 days gestation) after CHV inoculation of the pregnant bitch on day 30.[6] These results suggest that abortion due to CHV infection may occur during a limited period of gestation, similar to that occurring with *Brucella canis* infection. Premature birth occurred at about 2 weeks after inoculation of the pregnant bitches at about day 40 of gestation. Delivery of the premature fetuses occurred approximately 5 to 7 days before the expected whelping date. These findings also indicate that effects of transplacental infection with CHV on the fetuses vary, depending on the stage of gestation at which infection occurs. Responses of the pregnant bitches after CHV inoculation were similar to those observed in the first experiment. Delay or lack of parturition may also be observed in pregnant bitches with CHV-induced mummified fetuses in the uterus. Therefore, fetal death, mummification, abortion, premature birth or abnormal parturition can be associated with prenatal CHV infection of bitches.[6]

PLACENTAL LESIONS CAUSED BY CHV IN THE PREGNANT BITCH

It is generally accepted that viral infection of the placenta is important principally because it may lead to infection of the fetus and that fetal damage may be more severe if placental lesions are also present. It is known that herpesvirus infections in cattle, swine and cats cause placental lesions. However, no information was available regarding placental lesions caused by CHV in the bitch until data on the placental pathology of natural and experimental CHV infection were published.[6, 8] The following description of placental lesions caused by CHV infection may be helpful in understanding the pathogenesis of transplacental transfer of CHV in pregnant bitches and in diagnosing the disease.

Placental Lesions with Spontaneous CHV Infection. Fetal placentae from a bitch with CHV infection are macroscopically underdeveloped and congested (Fig. 2). Several grayish-white foci ranging in size from miliary to rice grain can be observed in the placental labyrinth. Sometimes the lesions form zonal structures 2 to 3 mm wide. Histopathologically, the lesions are characterized by focal

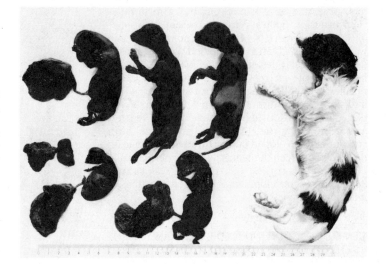

Figure 1. A litter of pups obtained by cesarean section from a bitch 31 days after maternal inoculation with CHV. Four mummified fetuses (with placentae), two partly mummified dead fetuses and one of three euthanized live-born pups (14 days old) are shown.

degeneration, necrosis and the presence of eosinophilic intranuclear inclusion bodies in the placental labyrinth. Generally, inflammatory cell reaction is slight or absent in these areas. Focal or segmental areas of fibrosis are scattered through the placental labyrinth.

Placental Lesions with Experimental CHV Infection. Placental lesions caused by experimental CHV infection are essentially the same as those of naturally occurring cases. Fetal placentae obtained from pregnant bitches inoculated with CHV during late gestation had gray-white foci on the cut surface of the placental labyrinth that were pinpoint to miliary in size. In addition to these lesions, pale gray-white foci formed zonal structures 2 to 3 mm in width that were located mainly near the marginal hematomas and on the cut surface of the placental labyrinth.

Microscopically, variable degrees of focal aseptic necrosis are observed in the placental labyrinth.

Walls of allantoic blood vessels have variable degrees of focal degeneration with or without mononuclear cell infiltration. Eosinophilic intranuclear inclusion bodies are detected in degenerating trophoblastic epithelial cells and in the cells of maternal and fetal blood vessels. Immunofluorescent studies reveal viral antigen in the trophoblastic epithelial cells of the placenta, with most being abundant in the junctional zone. Viral antigen is also found in the walls of maternal and fetal blood vessels, including allantoic blood vessels, and in epithelial cells of the chorioallantois covering the fetal margin of the placenta. Focal segmental areas of fibrosis in the placental labyrinth occurred when a pregnant bitch was inoculated intravaginally with CHV at midgestation. These areas were similar to those observed in placentae of spontaneous cases.

From results of both spontaneous and experimental cases of placental pathology associated with CHV infection, it has been determined that infected

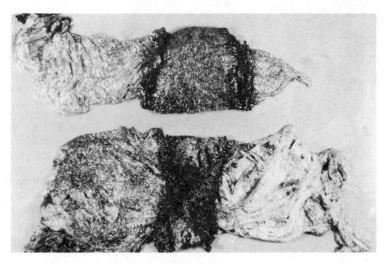

Figure 2. A placenta from a CHV-infected bitch (bottom) is poorly developed and decreased in width and has an irregular surface compared with a control placenta (top).

fetal placentae have necrotic lesions with intranuclear inclusion bodies. Virus is present in trophoblastic epithelial cells of the junctional zone and wall of maternal and fetal blood vessels; virus-induced vascular lesions of the placenta play an important role in transplacental transfer of CHV. Furthermore, placental lesions produced by CHV infection may disturb the normal function of the placenta and affect development of the fetuses, leading to stillbirths, abortion, premature birth and/or underdeveloped pups. Differences in placental lesions between the naturally and experimentally occurring cases suggest that placental lesions vary depending on developmental stages at the time of infection.

GENITAL INFECTION INDUCED BY CHV AND ITS EFFECTS ON THE FETUS AND NEONATE

Genital Lesions Caused by CHV. Poste and King reported the first isolation of CHV from genital lesions of female dogs in association with a clinical history of infertility, abortion and stillbirths.[15] Vaginal lesions were vesicular early in the course of the disease and later become circular and pocklike.[15] Lesions were found in the vestibule, commonly in the region of the urethral orifice, and on most surfaces of the vagina and mucocutaneous junctions. The lesions disappeared within 14 to 18 days and generally reappeared with the onset of proestrus. Vaginal lesions described by other authors are similar to those reported by Poste and King.[10] Several papulovesicular lesions, 2 to 3 mm in size, were observed on the mucosa of the vestibule and at the mucocutaneous junction of the vulva of a bitch with a history of CHV infection (Fig. 3). Several vesicles of variable size were observed immediately beneath

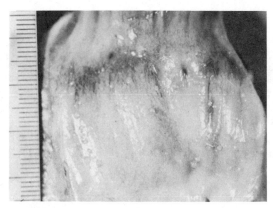

Figure 4. Multiple lymphoid nodules observed on the vestibular mucosa of a bitch inoculated intravenously with CHV.

the stratum corneum. A large number of neutrophils and a few mononuclear cells were present in and around these vesicles. Beneath the vesicular lesions, there was focal proliferation of epithelioid cells; marked ballooning degeneration was characteristic of some of the epithelioid cells. At the periphery of these degenerating cells, inflammation and hemorrhage were observed.

Severe vaginitis, characterized by petechial and submucosal hemorrhage, and multiple lymphoid nodules in the vagina of the bitches inoculated intravaginally with CHV have been described.[11] Multiple lymphoid nodules in the vaginal mucosa of the bitches inoculated intravenously with CHV may also occur (Fig. 4). Reasons for differences between lesions of naturally occurring and experimental cases are unknown. Different pathogenicities of genital and respiratory isolates for the genital tract of dogs may cause such variation in vaginal lesions.[11]

Effects of Maternal Genital Infection on the Fetus and Neonate. Decrease in number of pregnancies per mating (to 50 per cent of normal), decrease in number of pups per litter and abortion of near-term litters have been reported in spontaneous CHV infection of the pregnant bitch.[15] Stillbirths and underdeveloped pups have been reported after suspected intrauterine CHV infection in a bitch with vaginal lesions.[6] Intravaginal inoculation of pregnant bitches with CHV 1 to 2 weeks before whelping has been reported to produce vaginitis and death of all pups within 2 weeks of birth.[3] In our laboratory CHV infection was diagnosed in neonatal pups after natural whelping of bitches infected with CHV intravaginally 50 to 54 days after breeding. Although the exact route of infection of these pups is unknown, possible infection routes are as follow: (1) acquisition of infection during passage through the vaginal canal at birth, (2) neonatal infection from vaginal secretions by the dam after birth, and/or (3) fetal infection in utero via transplacental infection.

The first route was suggested when the virus was

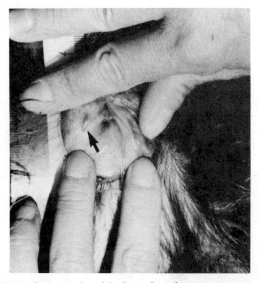

Figure 3. A papulovesicle (arrow) at the mucocutaneous junction of the vulva of a bitch with CHV infection.

isolated from vaginal swabs of infected bitches but not from uterine swabs or placental tissues.[3] Importance of the second route was suggested by isolation of CHV from the anterior vagina of a bitch at 18 days after whelping.[14] Bratberg reported a case of a bitch with signs of vaginitis during the last week of pregnancy and neonatal CHV infection later occurring in the pups.[2] CHV has been isolated from the vagina for periods as long as 2 weeks after oral-nasal inoculation.[1] Transplacental infection is supported by the evidence that such infection occurs in pregnant bitches after intravaginal CHV inoculation at mid-gestation.[7]

In summary, CHV genital infection in the pregnant bitch may play an important role in not only prenatal fetal infection but also in peri- and postnatal infection with this virus.

IMMUNOLOGIC AND PREVENTIVE ASPECTS

In breeding kennels CHV infection may result in sudden unexpected deaths of neonatal or infant pups. In addition CHV infection of the pregnant bitch at various stages of gestation may cause reproductive failure (fetal death, abortion, stillbirth, premature birth). Therefore, knowledge of virus source and mode of transmission (Fig. 5) from mother to infant is most important and may indicate useful preventive measures for CHV.

Maternal antibody apparently protects pups from fatal CHV infection, although it does not prevent inapparent infection and spread of virus.[12] Although protective levels of maternally transferred antibody are not known, the following prophylactic measures may be useful in order to provide the pups with maternal antibody in a kennel where CHV infection has been or may be a problem:[4]

1. Vaccination of bitches prior to breeding with 2 or 3 inoculations of an inactivated virus preparation in a suitable adjuvant.

2. Injection of serum from bitches that have lost litters previously as a result of CHV infection.

CHV is a poor antigen, and immune response to CHV has not been satisfactorily evaluated as yet. The antibody response in experimentally inoculated dogs is variable, ranging from an undetectable level to a marked increase in neutralizing antibodies to CHV. Nor is duration of immunity to CHV infection fully understood. Levels of neutralizing antibodies in dogs inoculated intranasally with CHV peaked at 1 month and persisted for at least 3 months.[13] Others have reported neutralizing antibodies persisting at low levels for at least 2 years.[5] In our work some bitches that were inoculated intravenously with CHV possessed a neutralizing antibody titer of 1:64 at 3 months after inoculation. Newborn pups that nurse bitches with a serum antibody titer of 1:4 or greater do not develop clinical signs of disease or die from experimental inoculation.[4] Thus, serial antibody titer determination in bitches may be use-

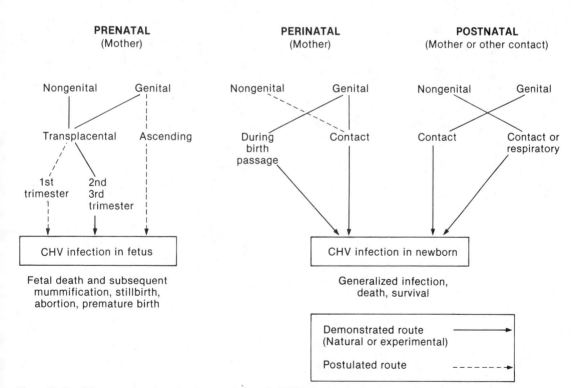

Figure 5. Possible sources and mode of transmission of CHV infection in the fetus and newborn pup demonstrated by natural and experimental cases.

ful in order to know whether that serum could be used effectively to prevent CHV infection of newborn pups.

Latent, persistent or recurrent infections are well-known features of herpesvirus infections in many species, including man. Available information suggests that this may also occur with CHV in the dog. If persistent CHV infection does occur, an infected bitch may pass virus to more than one of her litters. We have reported a case of a bitch losing a litter to CHV and subsequently whelping a second infected litter 7 months later.[6] This case suggests that continual transfer of infection from a bitch to successive litters may occur. Therefore, it is possible that this is a case of naturally occurring recurrent infection. The possibility of latent or persistent infection by intrauterine infection with CHV is also suggested by the presence of the virus in the neonatal pups. It has also been shown that CHV isolated from the genital tract of bitches may be able to produce latent and recurrent infection.[15] Thus, it seems reasonable to consider that latent, persistent and/or recurrent CHV infection of the bitch, especially the pregnant bitch, is possible, and separation of bitches with any infected litters from noninfected bitches is advisable.

Male dogs reared in a breeding kennel have been reported to develop preputial lesions after mating with a bitch known to have vaginal lesions caused by CHV.[15] This suggests that sexual transmission may occur and be important in the epizootiology of CHV infection. In breeding kennels in which CHV infection has occurred, examination of the genital organs of both male and female dogs is recommended to detect CHV-induced vesicular or lymphoid nodular lesions before mating. Bitches with such genital lesions should not be bred. It has also been demonstrated that bitches with genital CHV infection have a greater risk of fetal and neonatal viral infection, suggesting that when maternal genital CHV infection is detected, viral contamination of the fetus might be prevented by cesarean section.[7] Separation of neonatal pups from potential sources of infection, such as bitches with apparent herpetic vaginal lesions, should be considered.

References

1. Appel MJG, Menegus M, Parsonson IM, Carmichael LE: Pathogenesis of canine herpesvirus in specific pathogen free dogs: 5- to 12-week-old pups. Am J Vet Res 30:2067, 1969.
2. Bratberg B, Bjerkas I, Bjerkas E: Neonatal canine herpesvirus infection. Nord Vet Med 25:627, 1973.
3. Carmichael LE: Canine herpesvirus: A recently discovered cause of death of young pups. Proc 15th Gaines Vet Symp, Missouri, 1965, p 24.
4. Carmichael LE: Herpesvirus canis: Aspects of pathogenesis and immune response. J Am Vet Med Assoc 156:1714, 1970.
5. Carmichael LE: Canine herpesvirus infection. In Morrow DA (ed): Current Therapy in Theriogenology. 1st ed. Philadelphia, WB Saunders Co, 1980, p 632.
6. Hashimoto A, Hirai K, Okada K, Fujimoto Y: Pathology of the placenta and newborn pups with suspected intrauterine infection of canine herpesvirus. Am J Vet Res 40:1236, 1979.
7. Hashimoto A, Hirai K: Studies on canine herpesvirus infection. III. Transplacental transmission by intravaginal inoculation of pregnant dogs. Res Bull Fac Agric Gifu Univ 45:157, 1981.
8. Hashimoto A, Hirai K, Yamaguchi T, Fujimoto Y: Experimental transplacental infection of pregnant dogs with canine herpesvirus. Am J Vet Res 43:844, 1982.
9. Hashimoto A, Hirai K, Suzuki Y, Fujimoto Y: Experimental transplacental transmission of canine herpesvirus in pregnant bitches during the second trimester of gestation. Am J Vet Res 44:610, 1983.
10. Hashimoto A, Hirai K, Fukushi H, Fujimoto Y: The vaginal lesions of a bitch with a history of canine herpesvirus infection. Jpn J Vet Sci 45:123, 1983.
11. Hill H, Mare CJ: Genital disease in dogs caused by canine herpesvirus. Am J Vet Res 35:669, 1974.
12. Huxsoll DL, Hemelt IE: Clinical observation of canine herpesvirus. J Am Vet Med Assoc 156:1706, 1970.
13. Karpas A, Garcia FG, Calvo F, Cross RE: Experimental production of canine tracheobronchitis (kennel cough) with canine herpesvirus isolated from naturally infected dogs. Am J Vet Res 29:1251, 1968.
14. Love DN, Huxtable CRR: Naturally occurring neonatal canine herpes virus infection. Vet Rec 99:501, 1976.
15. Poste G, King N: Isolation of a herpesvirus from the canine genital tract: Association with infertility, abortion and stillbirths. Vet Rec 88:229, 1971.
16. Stewart SE, David-Ferreira J, Lovelace E, Landon J: Herpeslike virus isolated from neonatal and fetal dogs. Science 148:1341, 1965.

Tumors of the Canine Female Reproductive Tract

Stephen J. Withrow, D.V.M.
Steven J. Susaneck, D.V.M., M.S.
Colorado State University, Fort Collins, Colorado

Tumors of the female reproductive tract include tumors of mammary glands, ovaries, uterus, cervix, vagina and vulva. Mammary tumors represent the most common tumor type in the female and are frequently encountered by the veterinarian. Ovarian and uterine tumors are infrequently encountered by most veterinary practitioners compared with mammary gland tumors. The most common tumors of the vagina in the bitch are the transmissible venereal tumors and leiomyomas, depending on geographic locale.

CANINE MAMMARY TUMORS

Mammary cancer in the bitch has attracted much attention in the veterinary literature. In spite of voluminous writings, there is great controversy about the etiology, biology, pathology and treatment of this entity. Although the dog is generally a suitable model for the human disease, both over- and underextrapolation of human data have further confused the issues.

Incidence

Mammary cancer historically has been the most common cancer affecting the female dog. It is two to three times more prevalent than human breast cancer. However, this frequency will undoubtedly decline in coming years as a result of the common practice of early ovariohysterectomy.

The average age of affected dogs is 10 years.[9]

True breed incidence data are conflicting, but several authors believe that purebreds are at higher risk than mixed breeds. However, inbreeding of purebreds did not correlate with a higher cancer incidence in one study.[10]

Approximately two thirds of the tumors occur in glands 4 and 5, while one fourth to one-half of dogs have multiple gland involvement.

Supported in part by PHS grant no. l-PO1-CA-29582, awarded by the National Cancer Institute DHHS.

Etiology

Hormones play an important role in the initiation and/or promotion of mammary tumors. However, it is unclear which hormones, ratios of hormones and other exogenous (e.g., diet) or endogenous factors result in tumors.

Early ovariohysterectomy (before 2.5 years of age) will reduce the chances of mammary cancer developing to 12 per cent as compared with the number of tumors seen in the intact bitch.[27] Ovariohysterectomy at or before the first estrous cycle will reduce the risk to virtually zero. This implies that estrogen and/or progesterone may be involved in some latent initiation of the cancer, which is later promoted to clinically detectable cancer. There seems to be little preventative value in ovariohysterectomy after 2.5 years of age. Mammary cancer is seen four times more commonly in intact bitches than in those that have undergone ovariohysterectomy.[14]

Experimental and clinical studies have revealed several possible hormonal influences:

1. Sixty-six per cent of beagle dogs given oral contraceptives (progestin and mestranol) for 5 to 7 years developed mammary nodules (95 per cent benign).[16] Very few tumors developed in control dogs.

2. A pituitary-dependent increase in growth hormone and decrease in follicle-stimulating hormone (FSH), luteinizing hormone (LH) and thyroid-stimulating hormone (TSH) was seen in dogs with spontaneously developing mammary tumors.[12]

3. No statistical difference in prolactin levels was noted in tumor-bearing and nontumor-bearing bitches.[18]

4. Hypothyroidism has also been seen in bitches with mammary tumors and "may" be related to tumorigenesis.[13]

5. Medroxyprogesterone acetate was shown to increase the mammary cancer incidence when used clinically for estrus control.[31]

It seems clear that numerous hormones (in excessive or reduced amounts) may play a role in canine mammary tumorigenesis. A clearer understanding of the exact relationships involved will be difficult because of the long lag phase (5 to 10 years) between initiation of the tumor and actual clinical tumor formation. Hormone assays at the time the tumor is present may not indicate a cause and effect relationship. What can be said with certainty is that early ovariohysterectomy is preventative.

Further confusing the hormonal etiology is the fact that several hormonally regulated processes (irregular estrus, pseudocyesis, pregnancy, litter size and lactation) have not been correlated with a change in mammary cancer risk.[3] In addition, the influence of genetics, viruses and diet cannot be excluded as causative factors.

Pathology

No tumor type is fraught with more diversity of opinion regarding histopathologic classification than that of canine mammary cancer.[15, 19] Because of an almost complete lack of uniform reporting, comparison of treatment results is difficult.

Benign tumors are variously called benign mixed (fibroadenomas), simple adenomas, and benign mesenchymal tumors. Since little or no difference is seen in biologic behavior and since no conclusive data exist to show that these are premalignant, little help for the clinician evolves from further subclassification. Benign tumors comprise roughly 50 per cent of all mammary tumors. This figure is probably low because many studies are done at referral centers (small benign lesions not referred) and many small lumps are not surgically removed or subjected to biopsy in practice.

The malignant classifications include carcinoma (simple and complex), adenocarcinoma (tubular and papillary), anaplastic carcinoma, sarcomas and carcinosarcomas. Attempts to grade the various malignancies based on tubule formation, nuclear size, nuclear shape, nuclear staining, mitotic index and so on have been variously accepted as prognostic for in vivo behavior.[15] Because of the variable grading schemes published it is difficult to compare and contrast data from paper to paper. Histologic criteria of malignancy need to be correlated with clinical parameters to offer the most accurate prognosis.

Mammary cancer cells have been shown to contain estrogen (and progesterone) receptors. The presence of a significant level of estrogen receptors in human breast cancer implies the need for hormonal manipulation. This often involves antiestrogen drugs. The dog has been shown to be estrogen-receptor positive at roughly the same rate as women.[21] However, the test is not readily available, and the efficacy of antiestrogen drugs for therapy in the dog is largely untested.

Clinical Signs and Pretreatment Evaluation

The clinical signs of mammary tumors are generally obvious (single or multiple lumps in the breast). In some cases nonmammary tumors and inflammatory disease may mimic mammary neoplasia. On rare occasions animals will have signs relative to metastatic disease with an unnoticed primary in the breast. Paraneoplastic syndromes are rare, the most common being disseminated intravascular coagulation secondary to an anaplastic inflammatory carcinoma.

Important clinical criteria for primary tumors include size, ulceration, and fixation to skin or body wall. Regional lymph nodes can be aspirated when palpable and removed when positive. Although mammary cancer may metastasize anywhere, the lung is the predominant site of metastasis. For this reason, thoracic radiographs are advisable. Less than 10 per cent of all mammary tumors have a positive thoracic radiograph at presentation, however. Routine blood tests and urinalysis are also recommended as part of a comprehensive geriatric and anesthetic workup.

Owing to the mixed cell populations and necrosis present in many tumors, incisional biopsy and cytology may result in a significant number of false negative results. For this reason, it is advisable to remove all masses at surgery completely and confirm the histology postoperatively.

Treatment

Most mammary tumors should be removed surgically. The wait-and-see attitude may allow metastasis or inoperable growth to occur during the waiting time. Because "radical" mastectomy is only needed when multiple tumors need be removed, the surgery and anesthesia can often be done quickly, cheaply and safely.

The procedure of choice for a tumor-bearing dog has not been agreed upon. Much controversy exists, and no procedure has been objectively proved to be more beneficial than another. Procedures in common use are:

1. "Lumpectomy." This entails a small skin incision and removal of the mass for small (< 1 cm), firm, nonfixed nodules. This may be therapeutic if the tumor is benign, or it may be used as a biopsy technique.

2. Local mammectomy. This entails removal of the tumor and the affected gland. It is indicated for lesions confined to one gland with ill-defined margins and larger size, precluding lumpectomy.

3. Regional mastectomy. This surgery uses the proposed lymphatic draining route to predict which glands are at greatest risk for local spread. It generally means removal of the involved gland(s) and any gland that drains the tumor. This procedure may also be expanded to include the draining area and at least one gland on each side (i.e., a tumor of the fifth gland would require glands 4 and 5 to be removed). The underlying premise that in-transit tumor or spread from gland to gland occurs has not been proved, however.

4. Complete unilateral mastectomy. This procedure entails removal of glands 1 through 5 on one side regardless of where the tumor is located in the chain. Some surgeons routinely recommend removing the glands on the other side in 4 weeks.

5. Complete simultaneous bilateral mastectomy. This procedure entails removal of glands 1 through 5 bilaterally at one operation.[2]

Radical versus Local

The debate about which surgical procedure to perform will probably never be totally settled. The bottom line is to remove all tumor from the dog.

The "radical" procedures are advised for the

following reasons: (1) Nonpalpable multicentric primaries or metastasis within the chain are removed. (2) New primaries cannot occur because the site is gone. These concepts have not been proved in controlled clinical trials, however.

Why isn't radical surgery always curative or even indicated?

1. Bad tumors are bad before you can operate ("biological predeterminism"). This implies that the malignant tumor has regional skin involvement or distant metastasis at the time of surgery and that these problems lead to death at the same rate with lesser procedures. Radical surgery is not necessarily synonymous with curative surgery.

2. Long anesthesia and greater client cost are hard to justify when over half of the tumors are benign. A minor operation followed by a more "radical" procedure if the tumor is malignant might be a fair compromise.

3. Recent studies of various surgical procedures have shown no difference in survival in the dog.[20, 23]

Lymph Node Removal

The superficial inguinal lymph node is usually removed with wide skin margins along with gland 5 where it lies in close proximity. The axillary node is generally not removed because of the extensive anterior dissection necessary into the pectoral muscles and axillary region. The axillary node should be removed, however, if it is enlarged and is cytologically positive for tumor. Curative axillary dissection is rarely accomplished.

Adjuvant Treatments

Although largely untested in well-controlled clinical trials, chemotherapy, immunotherapy and irradiation have shown little reproducible benefit. More work on prognostic variables needs to be done to predict which animals are at high enough risk of recurrence or metastasis to warrant the expense and risk of adjuvant chemotherapy as is done in people.

Factors Affecting Prognosis

Survival. If the dog is going to die of metastatic or recurrent disease, death will probably occur within 2 years.

Histopathology. A histopathologic diagnosis is the most basic postoperative assessment that can be made. Sections should be requested of the tumor itself, including the skin margins as well as the lymph nodes. Additional information such as the presence of venous or lymphatic invasion may also be helpful in determining potential malignancy. The possibility of adding characteristics of nuclear morphology (grading) to the histologic evaluation is being investigated.[15]

Lymph Nodes. Evaluation of lymph node status

may not be as meaningful as was previously suspected. A recent report stated that dogs with histologically positive lymph nodes survived as well as dogs with negative lymph nodes.[23] This implies that mammary tumors in dogs metastasize by venous routes or that the regional node may be an effective local filtering system.

Size. Generally, malignant tumors are larger than benign tumors. The size of the tumor, however, should not deter or delay the surgeon from performing the mastectomy because the smaller tumors can be highly malignant.

Ulceration. The clinical sign of ulceration is generally thought to imply a worse prognosis. Some possible exceptions are the ulcerations resulting from trauma or pressure necrosis.

Ovariohysterectomy Status. The sparing effect of ovariohysterectomy on development of mammary tumors is well known. Once the tumor develops, however, there is no evidence that ovariohysterectomy will increase the length of survival.

The advent of hormone receptor assays (estrogen and progesterone receptors) on tumor tissue has been a breakthrough in individualized treatment of breast tumors in women. Patients in whom significant levels of estrogen and progesterone receptors are present benefit from antiestrogen therapy and/or estrogen ablation (oophorectomy, adrenalectomy and/or hypophysectomy). It has been established that some dog tumors (up to 40 per cent) do contain estrogen receptors. A prospective study is required to see whether reduction of estrogen levels after mastectomy will improve survival. Until the response of dogs to ovariohysterectomy is assessed objectively in relationship to receptors, the general statement that "ovariohysterectomy at mastectomy won't help survival" is true. Even with an ovariohysterectomy it should be remembered that an adrenal source of estrogen is possible. There are probably dogs that would respond favorably to ovariohysterectomy, but which ones is unknown at this time.

Rapid Growth. Tumors with a history of recent rapid growth carry a poor prognosis.

Mode of Growth. Tumors that are fixed to the body wall or skin carry a worse prognosis.

Factors Without Prognostic Significance. No significance has been shown for location of tumor, length of time the tumor has been present (as long as there is no recent rapid growth), type of surgery, multiple lesions, age of patient, or histologically positive lymph nodes.

OVARIAN TUMORS

Incidence

The incidence of ovarian tumors is low in the dog, accounting for 0.5 to 1.2 per cent of all neoplasms.[8, 20] In another study, Dow reported that ovarian tumors may constitute 6.25 per cent of canine tumors in the intact female population.[11] The mean age of occurrence is 8 years with a range of 1 to 17 years.

Pathology

Tumors of the ovaries may be of epithelial, germ cell, or sex-cord stromal origin. The epithelial tumors include papillary adenoma and adenocarcinoma, cystadenoma and cystadenocarcinoma, and undifferentiated carcinoma. Germ cell tumors include dysgerminoma and teratoma. The sex-cord stromal tumors include granulosa cell tumors, granulosa-theca cell tumors, thecoma and luteoma. The majority of ovarian tumors in the dog are epithelial or granulosa cell tumors, which occur with about equal frequency.[24]

Epithelial tumors are believed to originate from the ovarian surface "epithelium," which is really a coelomic mesothelium, and from epithelial cords in the underlying cortex.[24] Papillary adenomas frequently occur bilaterally and appear as cauliflower-like lesions on the ovarian surface. These tumors are benign and are confined to the ovarian stroma. The malignant counterpart of the papillary adenoma is the papillary adenocarcinoma. Papillary adenocarcinomas are common epithelial tumors that are often bilateral and have a histologic appearance that is similar to that of their benign counterpart. These tumors may be confined to the ovarian bursa early but often grow out of the bursa and exfoliate cells, resulting in transcoelomic metastasis. Malignant effusions resulting in ascites can be seen with carcinomas.

Cystadenomas are reported in one study to constitute 40 per cent of all ovarian tumors discovered at postmortem.[11] The tumors are made up of multiple thin-walled cysts containing fluid that varies from watery and clear to milky and viscid.

Undifferentiated carcinomas are a group of tumors made up of solid sheets of tumor cells separated by connective tissue. They are classified as undifferentiated because they lack morphology similar to that of the other epithelial tumors and do not produce hormones. Their exact site of origin is not known.

Germ Cell Tumors

With few exceptions, teratomas are benign, unilateral ovarian tumors. They may become very large in size, and mineralization is a prominent characteristic. They may contain teeth, hair, and/or skin. Occasional cases of metastasizing teratocarcinomas have been reported.[26]

Dysgerminomas are derived from undifferentiated germinal epithelium and account for about 10 per cent of canine ovarian tumors. All dysgerminomas are potentially malignant, but only about 10 to 20 per cent metastasize.[24] In the dog, dysgerminomas are usually soft masses 6 to 15 cm in diameter, round to ovoid in shape and well defined, with a smooth, lobulated external surface and a homogeneous grayish-white or brownish-yellow color. Dysgerminomas are similar to seminomas histologically but are rarely reported to produce hormones.

Sex-Cord Stromal Tumors

Sex-cord stromal tumors include granulosa cell tumors, luteomas, thecomas and combinations of these. In the bitch 10 to 25 per cent of sex-cord stromal tumors are malignant. These tumors may produce hormones, resulting in endocrine disturbances such as persistent or prolonged estrus, vaginal discharge, gynecomastia or cystic endometrial hyperplasia.

The most common ovarian tumor in the dog is the granulosa-theca cell tumor, accounting for 50 per cent of all ovarian tumors in the dog and the majority of sex-cord stromal tumors.[11] In the bitch the incidence of granulosa cell tumors increases with age, and only about 20 per cent will metastasize. Most of these tumors are unilateral and range in size from 4 to 16 cm in diameter. They can be smooth to coarsely nodular and are firm and grayish-white to yellow in color. The growth has solid or cystic areas and often hemorrhages. Granulosa cell tumors often grow large enough to cause abdominal distention or gastrointestinal upset.

Thecomas are usually unilateral and are often incidental findings at surgery or necropsy. The clinical behavior of thecomas is usually benign.

History and Clinical Signs

The history and clinical signs of ovarian tumors are variable depending on the type of tumor. Often the presenting sign is a large palpable mass in the abdomen or abdominal distention due to the tumor (cystadenoma, teratoma and granulosa cell tumors) or ascites (papillary adenocarcinoma, cystadenocarcinoma and granulosa cell tumor). The most common presenting sign of papillary adenocarcinomas is abdominal enlargement due to ascites. Some ovarian tumors cause signs of hormone imbalance on presentation (thecoma, granulosa cell tumor). Dogs with granulosa cell tumors are often presented with signs of abnormal hormone production. Signs of either excess progesterone production (cystic endometrial hyperplasia with a serosanguineous or mucopurulent discharge, or pyometra) or estrogen production (prolonged estrus, dermatologic changes, accessory sex organ changes or myelotoxicosis) may be seen. Another presenting sign of a large tumor may be gastrointestinal upset due to the tumor putting pressure on the bowel.

Diagnostic Techniques

The diagnosis of ovarian tumors is usually made through palpation of a large abdominal mass and radiographs of the abdomen. Exploratory laparotomy is often necessary to confirm a diagnosis of ovarian tumor. Histopathology is the only definitive way to determine the cell type in most cases. Thoracic radiographs should be taken to check for metastasis.

Suggested First Treatment

Surgery is always indicated if it is feasible. Oophorectomy should be performed with curative intent if spread has not taken place. All ovarian cancer and all omental spread should be removed if possible. Care should be taken not to rupture the tumor and to minimize transcoelomic spread.

Adjuvant Therapy

Little information is available on chemotherapy for metastatic ovarian tumors. Cyclophosphamide 50 mg/m^2 3 days per week has been recommended for advanced granulosa cell tumors and cystadenocarcinoma in dogs.[17] Drugs used for treatment of ovarian tumors in women that also may have clinical value in animals include vincristine and doxorubicin in addition to alkylating agents. The use of intra-abdominal triethylenethiophosphoramide (Thiotepa, Lederle Laboratories) for the control of intractable effusions has been recommended at a dose of 0.4 to 0.8 mg/kg body weight.

Radiation therapy may have some value in the treatment of residual disease following surgery. One report of successful immunotherapy using mixed bacterial vaccines to treat metastatic granulosa cell tumors has appeared in the literature.[20]

Prognosis

The prognosis for benign ovarian tumors is excellent. Prognosis for malignant tumors is good if complete oophorectomy can be performed and no evidence of metastatic disease exists but grave in all other cases. In the dog, most cases of malignant ovarian tumors are advanced at the time of diagnosis.

Unlike most metastatic tumors, metastatic ovarian tumors spread most often by transcoelomic implantation. For this reason, extreme care should be taken in palpation and during surgery of suspected ovarian tumors not to rupture the tumor.

NEOPLASIA OF THE UTERUS

Uterine tumors in the bitch are uncommon and account for 0.4 per cent of all canine tumors.[4] The most common uterine tumors are leiomyomas (fibroleiomyomas, 85 to 90 per cent) and leiomyosarcomas (10 per cent). Leiomyomas are benign firm, tan-colored nodular tumors of the myometrium. Leiomyosarcomas are the malignant counterpart of

the leiomyoma; they are rare in the uterus but are the most common malignant tumor in this organ. Leiomyosarcomas may be indistinguishable clinically from leiomyomas and may be multiple. Other rarely reported tumors include adenomas, adenocarcinomas and fibromas.

Most uterine tumors occur in older bitches and are rarely associated with clinical signs. Tumors of the uterus are often incidental findings at necropsy or surgery. In some cases the tumors are not diagnosed until signs relating to compression of the abdominal organs occur.

The treatment of choice for uterine tumors is ovariohysterectomy. Attempts should be made to remove all tumor and metastatic foci. The prognosis for leiomyomas is excellent, and the prognosis for leiomyosarcomas is good if metastasis has not occurred.

NEOPLASIA OF THE VAGINA AND VULVA

Neoplasias of the vagina and vulva represent about 2.5 to 3 per cent of all canine tumors.[4] Vaginal-vulvar tumors are most often benign (70 to 80 per cent) (fibroma, leiomyoma, polyp). At the Animal Medical Center (AMC) between 1978 and 1981, 99 tumors involving the vagina or vulva were seen. Of these, 72 were benign, 17 were malignant and 10 were transmissible venereal tumors.[28] The most common malignant vaginal tumor is the leiomyosarcoma.

The age incidence for leiomyoma is 5 to 16 years, with an average of 11 years. The breed most commonly affected is the boxer. In one study the boxer represented 16 per cent of the dogs with leiomyoma.[4]

Pathology

About 85 to 90 per cent of leiomyomas occur in the vagina and vulva. Leiomyomas originate from smooth muscle and may be intra- or extraluminal. Extraluminal leiomyomas produce a slow-growing perineal mass arising from the posterior smooth muscle wall of the vagina. About 70 per cent of leiomyomas of the vagina and vulva are extraluminal. Grossly, these tumors are grayish-white and firm to the touch. They are usually well encapsulated and poorly vascularized. Intraluminal leiomyomas usually arise from the vestibular wall and are attached by a thin pedicle that may protrude through the vulvar labia. They are firm to ovoid with intact mucosa, but they may ulcerate owing to exposure or irritation.

Leiomyosarcomas may be indistinguishable from leiomyomas in some cases. Some of these tumors are extensively necrotic, dark and cavitated, whereas others do not differ greatly from the uniform whitish-gray to pink color characteristic of leiomyoma.

Other tumors that have been reported to involve

the vagina and vulva are transmissible venereal tumors (which are covered in a separate section in this article), lipoma, mast cell tumor, epidermoid carcinoma, squamous cell carcinoma and fibromas. Pedunculated tumors arising from the vagina are sometimes referred to as polyps, but histologically they are usually leiomyomas or fibromas. Lipomas are sometimes seen arising from perivascular and perivaginal fat and may lie entirely in the pelvic canal.

History and Clinical Signs

Often the only clinical sign noticed is a mass protruding from the vulva. Bitches with extraluminal leiomyomas may be presented because of a slow-growing perineal mass. Tenesmus and dysuria frequently occur when extraluminal masses become very large.

In the study at the AMC it was found that pedunculated tumors were most often benign, whereas wide-based tumors were most often malignant.

Diagnostic Techniques, Workup and Treatment

Diagnosis of vaginal and vulvar tumors is often made by observing a mass protruding from the vulva. Abdominal radiographs and exploratory surgery may be needed to diagnose extraluminal vaginal tumors. Other signs may include dysuria or spotting blood, especially in dogs with transitional cell carcinomas from the bladder or urethra invading the vagina. The final diagnosis of cell type must be made by biopsy and histologic evaluation. Chest radiographs should be taken to rule out pulmonary metastasis.

Surgical excision of the tumor and all metastatic foci is the primary treatment. Intraluminal vaginal and vulvar tumors can often be surgically removed through the vulva; large tumors may necessitate an episiotomy. Radiation therapy may be used for inoperable tumors or metastatic foci.

The prognosis for benign tumors is good to excellent. The prognosis for leiomyosarcomas is good if metastasis has not occurred. The prognosis for adenocarcinomas and squamous cell carcinomas is poor because metastasis usually occurs before diagnosis of the primary tumor.

Leiomyomas are thought by some to be hormonally influenced. Ovarian cysts and estrogen-secreting tumors are often associated and endometrial hyperplasia usually coexists. About one-third of the patients with leiomyoma have mammary tumors as well. Nulliparous females may have a higher incidence. Because of the possible hormonal influence, ovariohysterectomy may be of value in preventing recurrence, but this is unproved.

In the study at the AMC, 91 per cent (69 of 76) of dogs with vaginal-vulvar tumors were intact, and all dogs with leiomyomas were intact. Thirteen of the dogs had concurrent mammary gland tumors, and 13 had had a recent estrus. Among the spayed dogs there appeared to be a higher incidence of malignant tumors.[28] Thirty-two of the dogs that had an ovariohysterectomy at the time of tumor surgery had no recurrence of the benign tumor, whereas 3 of 23 dogs that did not have ovariohysterectomy at the time of tumor removal did have a recurrence.[28] Although these figures indicate a possible hormonal component in vagina-vulvar tumors there is still no definitive proof of such a relationship. More work needs to be done to elucidate this question.

TRANSMISSIBLE VENEREAL TUMOR

Transmissible venereal tumor (TVT, "sticker" tumor, venereal granuloma, transmissible sarcoma, transmissible lymphosarcoma, contagious venereal tumor) is a naturally occurring, coitally transmitted neoplasm of the dog that usually affects the external genitalia of either sex. TVT has been reported in most parts of the world but appears to be more prevalent in large cities and temperate zones. The incidence of TVT varies within certain geographic regions, and the incidence within regions has changed over the years. TVT is enzootic in Puerto Rico and the Bahamas. TVT is seen most often in young, roaming, sexually active dogs. In a study of 71 dogs at the University of Georgia and the Animal Medical Center, the mean age was 4.2 years (2 to 10 years) with only 8 of 71 dogs older than 5 years of age.[7] Most affected dogs in that series weighed more than 20 kg, and the German shepherd dog accounted for 30 per cent of the cases.[7] There appears to be no sex predilection.

Pathology

The TVT is often cauliflower-like but may also be pedunculated, nodular, papillary and multilobulated. It ranges from a small nodule 5 mm in diameter to a large mass measuring more than 10 cm. The neoplasm is firm though friable and the superficial part is commonly ulcerated and inflamed. Some neoplasms are as large as 10 to 15 cm in diameter and, if located on the glans penis, may protrude from the preputial opening.

TVTs may be solitary or multiple and are usually located on the external genitalia. In the male dog the tumor is usually on the more caudal part of the penis from the crura to the bulbus glandis or the area of the glans penis, and is found occasionally on the prepuce. In the female dog the neoplasm is usually found in the posterior part of the vagina, often at the junction of the vestibule and the vagina. It sometimes surrounds the urethral orifice, and if it is just within the vagina it protrudes from the vulva.

Extragenital TVTs have been reported in the skin, face, scrotum and perineum, and in the buccal cavity, nasal cavity and brain. The metastatic rate is less than 5 per cent.

TVTs are round cell tumors of reticuloendothelial origin. The TVT is a unique tumor in that it usually has 59 chromosomes (57 to 64) compared with the normal canine complement of 78.

History and Clinical Signs

The presenting complaint is often a serosanguineous or hemorrhagic genital discharge. Licking of the external genitalia and/or protrusion of a mass are common complaints. A dog with a TVT of the nasal cavity may be presented for sneezing or epistaxis.

Diagnostic Techniques

Diagnosis is based on the history, location and typical appearance of the mass. Impression smears are often highly suggestive of TVT, but biopsy is needed for definitive diagnosis. Histologically and cytologically TVT cells appear histiocyte-like and are round to oval with large nuclei containing prominent nucleoli, and the cytoplasm often contains many vacuoles.

Suggested First Treatment

Once-weekly injections of vincristine at 0.025 mg/kg have been shown to give excellent results. Therapy should be continued until there is no visible evidence of disease. The course of therapy is usually 2 to 7 weeks (mean, 3.3 weeks).[6] Visible tumor regression is seen within 2 weeks.

Another method of therapy that has proved quite successful is a combination of vincristine (0.0125 mg/kg) weekly, methotrexate (0.3 to 0.5 mg/kg intravenously) weekly and cyclophosphamide (1 mg/kg orally) daily until no evidence of disease is present.[5] The same three drugs have also been used successfully by giving vincristine (0.025 mg/kg intravenously) weekly, cyclophosphamide (50 mg/m^2 orally) on days 2, 4 and 6 of each week and methotrexate (2.5 mg/m^2 orally) on days 3, 5, and 7 of each week.[29] Radiation is also very effective in the treatment of TVT. Thrall reported that 18 of 18 dogs treated with 10 to 30 Gray (Gy) were tumor-free at one year.[30] Seven of eight dogs were cured with 1 to 10 Gy treatment. Amber and Henderson reported that surgical excision of TVTs carried a 17.4 per cent recurrence rate at 6 months for dogs with only primary genital lesions. In contrast, the 6-month recurrence rate with combined primary and/or metastatic TVTs was 58.3 per cent.[1] Based on this information, surgical management of TVTs should be restricted to initial biopsy and the rare, small, solitary genital lesion.

The prognosis in most cases of TVT is good.

References

1. Amber EI, Henderson RA: Canine transmissible venereal tumor: Evaluation of surgical excision of primary and metastatic lesions in Zarla-Nigeria. J Am Anim Hosp Assoc 18:350, 1982.
2. Bartels KE, Ferguson HR, Gillette EL, Ferguson HL: Simultaneous bilateral mastectomy in the dog. Vet Surg 7(4):97, 1978.
3. Brodey RS, Fidler IJ, Howson AE: The relationship of estrous irregularity, pseudopregnancy, and pregnancy to the development of canine mammary neoplasms. J Am Vet Med Assoc 149(8):1047, 1966.
4. Brodey RS, Roszel JF: Neoplasms of the canine uterus, vagina and vulva: A clinicopathologic survey of 90 cases. J Am Vet Med Assoc 151:1294, 1967.
5. Brown NO, Calvert C, MacEwen G: Chemotherapeutic management of transmissible venereal tumors in 30 dogs. J Am Vet Med Assoc 176:983, 1980.
6. Calvert C, et al.: Vincristine for treatment of transmissible venereal tumor in the dog. J Am Vet Med Assoc 181(2):163, 1982.
7. Calvert CA: Transmissible venereal tumor in the dog. In Kirk RW (ed): Current Veterinary Therapy VIII, Small Animal Practice. Philadelphia, WB Saunders, 1983, pp. 413-415.
8. Cotchen E: Canine ovarian neoplasms. Res Vet Sci 2:133, 1961.
9. Dorn CR, Taylor DON, Frye FL, Hibbard HH: Survey of animal neoplasms in Alameda and Contra Costa Counties, California. I. Methodology and description of cases. J Natl Cancer Inst 40(2):295, 1968.
10. Dorn CR, Schneider R: Inbreeding and canine mammary cancer: A retrospective study. J Natl Cancer Inst 57(3):545, 1976.
11. Dow C: Ovarian abnormalities in the bitch. J Comp Pathol 70:59, 1960.
12. El Etreby MF, Muller-Peddinghaus R, Bhargava AS, et al.: The role of pituitary gland in spontaneous canine mammary tumorigenesis. Vet Pathol 17:2, 1980.
13. Fathy El Etreby M: Thyroid function in the dog and its possible relationship to mammary tumorigenesis. Pharmac Ther 5:403, 1979.
14. Fidler IJ, Abt DA, Brodey RS: The biological behavior of canine mammary neoplasms. J Am Vet Med Assoc 151(18):1311, 1967.
15. Gilbertson SR, Kurzman ID, Zachrau RE, et al.: Canine mammary epithelial neoplasms: Biologic implications of morphologic characteristics assessed in 232 dogs. Vet Pathol 20:127, 1983.
16. Giles AC, Kwapien RP, Geil RG, Casey HW: Mammary nodules in beagle dogs administered investigational oral contraceptive steroids. J Natl Cancer Inst 60(6):1351, 1978.
17. Greene JA, Richardson RC, Thornhill HA, Boon GD: Ovarian papillary cystadenocarcinoma: Case report and literature review. J Am Anim Hosp Assoc 16:352, 1979.
18. Hamilton JM, Knight PJ, Beevers J: Serum prolactin concentrations in canine mammary cancer. Vet Rec 102:127, 1978.
19. Hampe JF, Misdorp W: Tumours and dysplasias of the mammary gland. Bull WHO 50:111, 1974.
20. Hayes A, Harvey HJ: Treatment of metastatic granulosa cell tumor in a dog. J Am Vet Med Assoc 174:1304, 1979.
21. MacEwen EG, Patnaik AK, Harvey HJ, Panko WB: Estrogen receptors in canine mammary tumors. Cancer Res 42:2255, 1982.
22. MacEwen EG: Simple vs radical mastectomy for canine mammary tumors. Vet Cancer Newsletter, Summer, 1981, pp. 22.
23 Misdorp W, Hart AAM: Canine mammary cancer. I. Prognosis. J Sm Anim Pract 20:385, 1979.

24. Nielsen SW: Classification of tumors in dogs and cats. J Am Anim Hosp Assoc 19:13, 1983.
25. Owen LN: TMN classification of tumors in domestic animals. Geneva, World Health Organization, 1980.
26. Patnaik AK, Schaer M, Parks J, Liv SK: Metastasizing ovarian teratocarcinoma in dogs. J Sm Anim Pract 17:235, 1976.
27. Schneider R, Dorn CR, Taylor DON: Factors influencing canine mammary cancer development and postsurgical survival. J Natl Cancer Inst 43(6):1249, 1969.
28. Thatcher C: Vaginal and vulvar tumors. Proceedings American College of Veterinary Surgeons, 1983.
29. Theilen GH, Madewell RB: Tumors of the urogenital tract. In Veterinary Cancer Medicine. Philadelphia, Lea & Febiger, 1979.
30. Thrall DE: Orthovoltage radiotherapy of canine transmissible venereal tumors. Vet Radiol 23(5):217, 1982.
31. van Os JL, van Laar PH, Oldenkamp EP, Verschoor JSC: Oestrus control and the incidence of mammary nodules in bitches, a clinical study with two progestogens. Vet 3(1):46, 1981.

Population Control in the Bitch

Thomas J. Burke, M.S., D.V.M.
University of Illinois,
Urbana, Illinois

The 1960's saw an increasing public awareness of the dog overpopulation problem that has remained virtually unabated. It was realized that our companion animals, especially dogs, were creating serious problems to human health in both urban and rural areas. Also, they became a threat to wildlife and personal property. Dog bites remain a serious problem in urban areas with cost estimates for their treatment approximating $100 million per year. The majority of the overpopulation problem seems to stem from straying pets. Truly feral dogs are only able to maintain a stable population.[4]

The human health problem in the United States includes not only dog bites but also the spread of parasitic and bacterial diseases and the everpresent threat of rabies even though the latter is a rarity today. Also, there is a commensal relationship between straying dogs and rats because the foraging habits of dogs make food available to rats.[4] The esthetic insult to the environment has caused many municipalities to enact feces cleanup and leash laws. And we, as caring individuals, should be concerned that we must kill an ever-increasing number of animals who so freely give us their companionship and affection.

The reasons for the problem are complex but are related to the failure of the pet-owning public to become educated about their pets' reproductive biology and what can be done to prevent unwanted litters. There also exists a failure of pet owners to comply with existing laws and to avail themselves of current methods of population control. This latter problem may have a basis in owner bias—a reluctance to interfere with the pet's "sexual freedom" or its supposed "right" to roam. Human beings have become used to separating copulation from reproduction. Unfortunately, we have not made use of the same concept for our companion animals.

There are legitimate reasons for temporary birth control. The foremost is that the American Kennel Club forbids the surgical neutering of any animal entered in a competition sanctioned by that group. Also, sporting and working dogs are usually several years old before their value as breeding animals can be established. Estrus and breeding interfere with their training and performance. Many dog owners thus desire some means of eliminating estrus on a temporary basis.

The perfect contraceptive should have near 100 per cent efficacy with no risk to the patient. It should be acceptable and widely available at reasonable cost to the pet owner, preferably through currently established veterinary health care delivery systems. It has yet to be developed. The cheapest and most effective oral contraceptive is the word "no." For the pet owner this means confinement and/or physical control. This apparently is either unacceptable to or unattainable by a large segment of the pet-owning public.

SURGICAL METHODS OF BIRTH CONTROL

Ovariohysterectomy or spaying has been, and remains, the most widely practiced method of canine birth control. When performed correctly it eliminates estrus as well as the possibility of uterine disease. When performed early in life the risk of mammary neoplasia is reduced. Objections voiced by many owners include its cost, the risk of general anesthesia, and development of side effects such as obesity and urinary incontinence. The cost factor appears to be something that needs to be addressed by veterinarians in concert with governmental and private agencies while society decides whether pet ownership is a right or a privilege.

Oviductal ligation or resection can be performed with the use of operating laparoscopes in less time than traditional spaying. Like spaying, this method provides permanent contraception. Its disadvantages are the cost of instrumentation and acquisition of the skill necessary to become proficient in its use. It does not interrupt the normal estrous cycle, and the incidence of uterine disease and mammary neoplasia are unaffected.

IMMUNOLOGIC METHODS

Attempts have been made to induce antibodies to luteinizing hormone (LH) in dogs in order to prevent LH from reaching target organs (ovaries and testes).[10] This approach worked in dogs for varying periods of time with somewhat unpredictable success. Its efficacy was even lower in bitches. Similar attempts with gonadotropin-releasing hormone (LH-RH)[11] are more promising, but at present neither technique is close to being available to the practitioner.

Another technique being investigated is immunization with preparations of porcine zona pellucida, which either prevents sperm from binding to ova or masks sperm binding sites, thus preventing conception.[17]

Immunologic methods appear to be temporary,[10, 17] and a booster program will probably be required if these techniques become available for patient use. One must, however, consider the possibility that they may produce permanent infertility in some patients.

INDUCED ACYCLICITY

There is a point during fetal development (or the very early neonatal stage in some species) when the hypothalamus becomes either male (acyclic) or female (cyclic). Exposure of the animal to androgens during this critical phase creates an acyclic hypothalamus regardless of phenotypic sex.[3] In dogs this period apparently occurs in utero, and such treatment will produce anatomic abnormalities of the urogenital system. Also, in rodents, some of the treated females, although acyclic, stay in permanent behavioral estrus[3]—certainly an undesirable side effect.

INTRAVAGINAL AND INTRAUTERINE DEVICES

Because of its anatomic location, the cervix of the bitch is all but impossible to cannulate per vagina. Thus the placement of an IUD would require laparotomy, adding cost and the risks normally associated with major surgery and general anesthesia to the procedure. At this point in time IUDs are not feasible for the bitch.

An intravaginal device for the bitch was marketed at one time. Problems in properly fitting the device to the wide range of sizes of dogs, its cost, and the production of foreign body vaginitis, which many owners found objectionable, caused poor acceptance, and the device is no longer available.

The prospects for mechanical contraception meeting the criteria outlined in the introduction appear slim.

PHARMACEUTICAL AGENTS

Progestogens

The first hormone to be used to control estrus in animals was progesterone, and the first report of its use in the bitch appeared in 1952.[14] Since then a number of compounds possessing primarily progestational activity have been used for estrus inhibition in the dog and cat. The reader is referred to other reviews of the use of these compounds,[7, 9, 22] since several have not been widely used in the United States and only one, megestrol acetate (Ovaban), is currently approved for this use in this country. Compounds having the widest use, past or present, by American veterinarians are progesterone, hydroxyprogesterone acetate, medroxyprogesterone acetate and megestrol acetate.

The most severe side effect of chronic progestogen administration in dogs and cats is cystic endometrial hyperplasia, with or without subsequent infection. This is well recognized by most veterinarians[22] and need not be discussed further. Prolonged progestational therapy also has been correlated with the development of mammary neoplasia. Progestogens may also be diabetogenic. The injection of reposital forms of progestogens for suppression of estrus continues today, but the risk-benefit ratio dictates that this practice be discontinued.

Megestrol Acetate. Megestrol acetate is a potent, orally active progestogen with a relatively short half-life (8 days) in dogs.[6] It has been used by European veterinarians for prevention and postponement of estrus in the dog and cat since the mid-1960's and has been available to veterinarians in the United States since 1975.

There currently are two label indications for estrus control in the dog: stopping a cycle in proestrus (prevention of estrus) and postponement of an anticipated estrus prior to the onset of proestrus. Clinical trials have demonstrated 92 per cent and 97 per cent efficacy, respectively.[5] Treatment did not affect subsequent cyclicity and fertility.[5]

For prevention of estrus, megestrol is administered daily for 8 days at a dose of 2.2 mg/kg (1 mg/lb), beginning during the first 3 days after the onset of sanguineous discharge and vulvar swelling. Starting treatment too early results in an early post-treatment heat. A marked decrease in efficacy occurs if treatment is delayed beyond the third day of proestrus. Although timing of the first post-treatment heat cannot be accurately predicted, it will usually occur 4 to 6 weeks earlier than usual following administration of a correctly timed course of prevention therapy. British workers report that return to estrus can be delayed by administering megestrol at 2.2 mg/kg for 4 days beginning during the first 3 days of proestrus, followed by 0.55 mg/kg (0.25 mg/lb) for 16 days.[1]

If mating occurs during the first 3 days of treatment, megestrol therapy should be stopped and the bitch treated for mismating. If mating occurs after 3 days of treatment, therapy should be continued since the drug will prevent pregnancy in most cases.[1]

For postponement of an anticipated heat, megestrol is given at a dose of 0.55 mg/kg (0.25 mg/lb) daily for 32 days, beginning at least a week prior to the onset of proestrus based on the patient's history. British veterinarians have prescribed megestrol at a dose of 0.1 to 0.2 mg/kg twice weekly for up to 4 months following a postponement course of therapy for extended suppression.[1] Bitches so treated should be allowed to have a normal cycle before being retreated.

If postponement therapy is begun in late anestrus, the next heat should occur in 5 to 6 months. Treatment during early to midanestrus may have no effect on the occurrence of the next cycle.

Vaginal cytologic examination is often useful in timing megestrol therapy. If a sample, obtained atraumatically, shows erythrocytes, postponement therapy should not be given. Rather, that cycle should be treated with properly timed prevention therapy since proestrus is imminent.

Temporary minor side effects of increased appetite, decreased activity, weight gain and, rarely, lactation may occur during treatment. Changes in hair coat and olfaction have not been observed.

Bitches with grossly abnormal cycles are not candidates for megestrol therapy because correct timing cannot be ensured.

In summary, megestrol acetate appears to be a safe and efficacious drug for temporary estrus control in the bitch. Care must be exercised by the clinician to ensure proper timing and avoidance of gross overdosage.

Androgens

Testosterone. Testosterone propionate has been used to prevent estrus in working dogs, particularly racing greyhounds. Oral and parenteral routes have been used. Greyhound bitches given 25 mg of oral testosterone weekly have been kept out of estrus for as long as 5 years with apparent return to normal reproductive status.[15] Side effects of clitoral hypertrophy and vaginitis have been noted, the former being prominent enough in affected bitches to earn the term "tail-lighters." Silcone tube implants containing testosterone effectively prevented estrus in beagle bitches for as long as 840 days with return to normal cyclicity and fertility.[18] The effective dose released per day was calculated to be 168.6 µg/kg. Clitoral hypertrophy and vaginitis were observed in about 20 per cent of the treated bitches. Androstenedione at approximate doses of 200 to 450 µg/kg/day failed to inhibit estrus.[18]

Doses of testosterone sufficient to inhibit estrus may produce side effects that are undesirable to some owners. In addition, premature epiphyseal closure may occur if immature bitches are treated. Inadvertent treatment of pregnant bitches may cause severe urogenital anomalies in female puppies. Thus, testosterone cannot currently be recommended for estrus control.

Mibolerone. A synthetic 19-norsteroid compound, mibolerone, is approved for long-term estrus inhibition. Mibolerone is an androgenic, anabolic antigonadotropic steroid that does not possess progestational or estrogenic activity.[19] In purebred and mixed breed bitches treated for periods of up to 1300 days, estrus inhibition was more than 95 per cent successful.[19] Dosage ranged from 30 µg/day for dogs weighing 1 to 12 kg up to 180 µg/day for dogs more than 45 kg and for German shepherd dogs and German shepherd dog crossbreeds.[19] Observable side effects include clitoral hypertrophy and associated vaginitis that is more severe in prepuberal bitches, deepening of the voice in some patients, increased lacrimation, and seborrheic dermatitis in those patients predisposed to it. These disappear following cessation of therapy, with minor residual clitoral hypertrophy in some bitches. Mild to moderate increases in hepatic enzymes and decreased cholesterol are found in the serum during treatment.[13] Liver biopsies may show the presence of as yet unidentified crystalline structures in hepatocyte nuclei.[13] Overt hepatic dysfunction does not occur.[13] Conception rates are normal by the second posttreatment estrus. Administration of mibolerone to bitches in estrus did not interfere with conception or gestation.[21] However, female puppies were masculinized.[21]

Mibolerone will not arrest proestrus or estrus in the bitch, and therapy may need to be begun as early as 30 days prior to the onset of proestrus. Such therapy will effectively suppress estrus in dogs for long periods of time and may prove capable of being used for the lifetime of the animal.

MISMATING

Pregnancy can be avoided by treatment with estrogenic compounds administered within 3 to 5 days after coitus. Estrogens at low doses decrease oviductal transport time while higher doses prolong it.[16] They also alter the uterine biochemistry, especially carbonic anhydrase, in a manner unfavorable to fertilization and implantation.[12]

A careful history and physical examination are prerequisites to therapy. Many owners are ignorant about their pet's reproductive biology and may, for example, equate the presence of a male in the vicinity of the female with mating. It is important to obtain only the owner's observations. If necessary, vaginal cytology should be employed to determine if the dog is actually in estrus and the probability that mating has occurred. Because sperm rapidly disappear from the vagina, their absence is meaningless.

The owner should be apprised of the risk of using estrogens prior to commencing therapy. Estrogens have been shown to cause myelosuppression that may be fatal and to induce pyometritis.[16] The former appears to be dose-related in most cases with younger dogs being more resistant and more likely to recover. All estrogens, except for oral diethylstilbestrol (DES), should be given only once.[16]

DES, because of its nonsteroidal configuration, may be safer than the steroidal estrogens. Injectable DES is given once at a dose of 0.5 mg/kg (up to total dose of 25 mg) within 5 days of coitus.[16]

Estradiol-17-cyclopentyl propionate (ECP) is given as a single intramuscular injection within 72 hours of mating. The author's recommended dose is 0.02 mg/kg. Estradiol benzoate or valerate may be administered once at a dose of 0.1 mg/kg (not to exceed 3.0 mg total dose) up to 5 days following mismating.[16]

The owner should be informed about the signs of pyometritis. A reexamination is scheduled for 3½ weeks to palpate for pregnancy and to assess the general health status of the patient. A hemogram may be done at this time to look for evidence of myelosuppression or inflammatory uterine disease.

INDUCED ABORTION

Termination of an established pregnancy is difficult. Ovariectomy at any stage of gestation will result in abortion or resorption of the fetuses.[20]

Currently there are no drugs approved for therapeutic abortion in the bitch. Experimental work with prostaglandins and dexamethasone shows promise.

Two studies using dexamethasone have shown that it can cause either intrauterine death and resorption when given early in pregnancy or abortion when used during the last trimester. In both studies a 10-day treatment was used beginning on either day 30 or day 45 of pregnancy.[2,16] The drug was administered by intramuscular injection. In beagles the dose was approximately 0.5 mg/kg every 12 hours.[16] In Labrador retrievers the dose was about 0.15 mg/kg once daily.[2] The effect of this treatment on subsequent fertility has not been studied, but in the latter study one bitch that had been treated was rebred on her next estrus and conceived. She was retreated.

Prostaglandin $F_{2\alpha}$ given at 20 µg/kg three times a day for 2 days produced abortion in four of seven bitches that were at least 25 days pregnant.[8] Other prostaglandin analogs are being tested and appear promising.[23]

References

1. Anonymous: A Glaxo Guide to Ovarid. Greenford, England, Veterinary Division, Glaxo Laboratories Ltd, 1976.
2. Austad R, Lunde A, Sjaastad OV: Peripheral plasma levels of oestradiol-17β and progesterone in the bitch during the oestrous cycle, in normal pregnancy and after dexamethasone treatment. J Reprod Fert 46:129, 1976.
3. Barraclough CA: Alterations in reproductive function following prenatal and early postnatal exposure to hormones. In McLaren A (ed): Advances in Reproductive Physiology, Vol. 3. New York, Academic Press, 1968, pp 81-112.
4. Beck AM: The Ecology of Stray Dogs. A Study of Free-Ranging Urban Animals. Baltimore, York Press, 1973.
5. Burke TJ, Reynolds HA: Megestrol acetate for estrus postponement in the bitch. J Am Vet Med Assoc 167:285, 1975.
6. Chainey D, McCoubrey A, Evans JM: The excretion of megestrol acetate by beagle bitches. Vet Rec, 86:278, 1970.
7. Christie DW, Bell ET: The use of progestogens to control reproductive function in the bitch. Anim Breed Abstr 38:1, 1970.
8. Concannon PW, Hansel W: Prostaglandin $F_{2\alpha}$ induced luteolysis, hypothermia and abortions in beagle bitches. Prostaglandins 13:533, 1977.
9. Cox JE: Progestogens in bitches: A review. J Small Anim Pract 11:759, 1979.
10. Faulkner LC: Immunological control of fertility in dogs. In Morrow DA (ed): Current Therapy in Theriogenology. Philadelphia, WB Saunders Co, 1980, pp 677-678.
11. Fraser HM, Gunn A, Borthwick R, Fraser AF: Sterilising by immunisation. Vet Rec 96:323, 1975.
12. Friedley NJ, Rosen S: Carbonic anhydrase activity in the mammalian ovary, fallopian tube, and uterus: Histochemical and biochemical studies. Biol Reprod 12:293, 1975.
13. Johnston RL, Goyings LS: Effects of mibolerone on hepatic structure and function in the canine. In Lauderdale JW, Sokolowski JH (eds): Proceedings of the Symposium on Cheque for Canine Estrus Prevention. Kalamazoo, Mich, Upjohn Co, 1978, pp 54–60.
14. Murray GH, Eden EL: Progesterone to delay estrum in bitches. Vet Med 47:467, 1952.
15. Pegram L: Personal communication. St. Louis, Ralston Purina Co, 1976.
16. Shille VM: Mismating and termination of pregnancy. Vet Clin North Am 12:99, 1982.
17. Shivers CA, Sieg PM, Kitchen H: Pregnancy prevention in the dog: potential for an immunological approach. J Am Anim Hosp Assoc 17:823, 1981.
18. Simmons JG, Hamner CE: Inhibition of estrus in the dog with testosterone implants. Am J Vet Res 34:1409, 1973.
19. Sokolowski JH: The evaluation of efficacy of mibolerone for estrus prevention in the bitch. In Lauderdale JW, Sokolowski JH (eds): Proceedings of the Symposium on Cheque for Canine Estrus Prevention. Kalamazoo, Mich, Upjohn Co, 1978.
20. Sokolowski JH: The effects of ovariectomy on pregnancy maintenance in the bitch. Lab Anim Sci 21:696, 1971.
21. Sokolowski JH, Kasson CW: Effects of mibolerone on conception, pregnancy, parturition, and offspring in the beagle. Am J Vet Res 39:837, 1978.
22. Stabenfeldt GH: Physiologic, pathologic and therapeutic roles of progestins in domestic animals. J Am Vet Med Assoc 164:311, 1974.
23. Vickery B, McRae G: Effect of a synthetic prostaglandin analogue on pregnancy in beagle bitches. Biol Reprod 22:438, 1980.

Reproductive Physiology and Endocrinology of the Dog

Rupert P. Amann
Colorado State University,
Fort Collins, Colorado

An understanding of the reproductive capacity of the dog, familiarity with the normal range of concentrations for several hormones, and appreciation of how these characteristics can be influenced by the size of the dog, the environment, or medication are essential for an accurate andrologic evaluation. Despite decades of interest by clinicians in problems of dog reproduction and the utilization of countless dogs in research, until the past few years surprisingly little was known about the reproductive capacity of dogs.

Limitations of space preclude a consideration of the development of the male reproductive tract from the bipotential structures present in the young embryo, the role of testicular hormones and target tissue receptors in this development, or the process of testicular descent. Failure of these processes to occur normally, however, can affect the internal or external characteristics of the reproductive organs. Descriptions of the reproductive system in standard texts of anatomy and physiology provide insufficient detail on testicular function and reproductive capacity for a clinician interested in canine andrology. The goal of this chapter is to provide the necessary background using recent data for dogs, coupled with interpretations based on other species.[2, 3, 7, 16, 24] The discussion will be restricted to adult dogs, although changes occurring during puberty[26, 29] or in association with advanced age also are important to the clinician.

THE TESTES

Functional Compartmentalization. The two basic functions of the testes, production of spermatozoa and secretion of hormones, are intimately related even though they are spatially separated. The testis has three functional compartments.[3, 7, 16, 24] The interstitial tissue compartment includes the Leydig cells, which produce testosterone, estradiol and other hormones, intimately associated with blood vessels and lymphatic sinusoids or vessels (Fig. 1). Because of this arrangement, the seminiferous tubules are bathed with tissue fluid rich in testosterone.

The other two compartments are within the seminiferous tubules. The cytoplasmic processes of the Sertoli cells extend from the lamina propria of the seminiferous tubule around the developing germ cells and extend to the tubular lumen (Fig. 1). Junctional complexes between adjacent Sertoli cells serve as the major component of the blood-testis barrier that divides the seminiferous tubule into functionally separate basal and adluminal compartments.[7, 16] Spermatogonia divide by mitosis within the basal compartment. Meiosis of primary spermatocytes and secondary spermatocytes and development of spermatids occur in the unique isolated environment provided by the adluminal compartment. The blood-testis barrier excludes totally or partially from the adluminal compartment all macromolecules and many other compounds found in blood or interstitial fluid. Thus, proteins such as follicle-stimulating hormone (FSH) have access only to the basal portion of the Sertoli cells.

Leydig cells are the only cells in the testis specifically binding luteinizing hormone (LH),[3] and they respond to this stimulus by producing a number of steroids including testosterone. Leydig cells are active in early embryogenesis, regress during later fetal development and reactivate during the onset of puberty.[7] Leydig cells are the primary testicular source of progesterone, testosterone, other androgens, and probably estradiol. Steroid production by the testis is correlated with the total amount of smooth endoplasmic reticulum in the Leydig cells of a testis rather than with testicular size. The rate-limiting step in production of testosterone is the formation of pregnenolone from cholesterol.[7, 16] This step involves enzymatic cleavage of the side chain from cholesterol and occurs in the mitochondria. With stimulation by LH, formation of pregnenolone is increased, and this steroid is rapidly metabolized to testosterone in the smooth endoplasmic reticulum.

Sertoli cells have a pivotal role in the hormonal control of spermatogenesis and provide the microenvironment required for normal germ cell development.[24] Sertoli cells are the only testicular cells with specific binding sites for FSH,[3] and biochemical and morphologic changes in Sertoli cells are induced by FSH. FSH stimulates spermatogenesis indirectly by acting on Sertoli cells, rather than by a direct action on the germ cells. The normal function of Sertoli cells also is dependent on the availability of testosterone at a concentration far greater than that found in peripheral blood.[24] Sertoli cells secrete a number of specific products, which apparently are involved in coordination of spermatogenesis and normal development of spermatids.[7] These compounds have not been studied in dogs, but in other species the functions of Sertoli cells differ depending

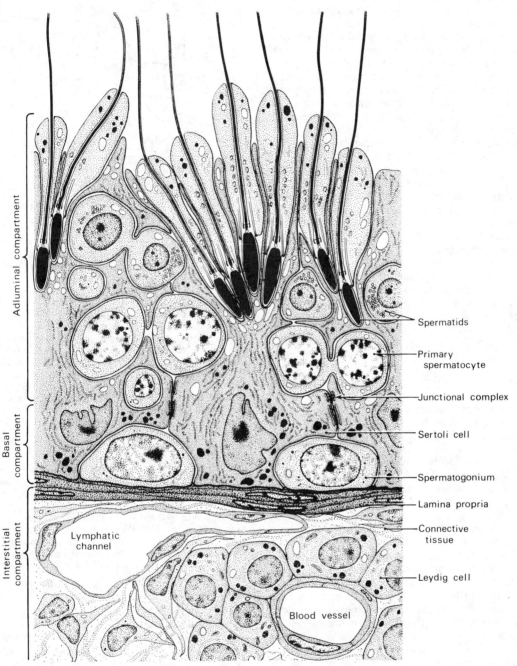

Spermatids

Primary spermatocyte

Junctional complex

Sertoli cell

Spermatogonium

Lamina propria

Connective tissue

Leydig cell

Lymphatic channel

Blood vessel

Adluminal compartment

Basal compartment

Interstitial compartment

Figure 1. The relationships among Leydig cells, the vascular system and a seminiferous tubule. Note the intercellular bridges between adjacent germ cells in the same cohort or generation and the relationship of the germ cells to the adjacent Sertoli cells. Formation of spermatozoa starts near the basement membrane when a spermatogonium divides to form other spermatogonia and ultimately primary spermatocytes. The primary spermatocytes are moved from the basal compartment, through the junctional complexes between adjacent Sertoli cells, into the adluminal compartment, where they eventually divide to form secondary spermatocytes (not shown) and spherical spermatids. The spermatogonia, primary spermatocytes, secondary spermatocytes and spherical spermatids all develop in the space between two or more Sertoli cells and are in contact with them. During elongation of the spermatid nucleus, the spermatids are repositioned by the Sertoli cells to become embedded within long pockets in the cytoplasm of an individual Sertoli cell. When released as a spermatozoon, a major portion of the cytoplasm of each spermatid remains as a residual body within a pocket of the Sertoli cell cytoplasm.

on the developmental stage of the germ cells with which they are associated. This observation means that germ cells also must have a role in modulating Sertoli cell function.

Especially during the prepubertal period, Sertoli cells in several species convert testosterone, produced by Leydig cells, to estradiol. In adults, however, most of the estrogens apparently are secreted by the Leydig cells. It remains to be established if the estradiol found in the testicular venous blood of the normal adult dog reflects production by the Leydig cells, the Sertoli cells, or both.

Sertoli cells secrete an androgen-binding protein (ABP) and a putative hormone called inhibin.[3, 7, 24] Androgen-binding protein is thought to attenuate changes in testosterone concentration within the seminiferous tubule or aid in the transport of testosterone to the epithelial cells lining the proximal epididymis. Inhibin is thought to act on the anterior pituitary gland to suppress FSH secretion.

Spermatogenesis. Spermatogenesis is the sum of the transformations that result in formation of spermatozoa from spermatogonia while maintaining spermatogonial numbers.[1, 2] In addition to the proliferating pool of spermatogonia, a seminiferous tubule contains a number of reserve or A_o-spermatogonia, which do not proliferate and are extremely resistant to radiation or toxic agents. Spermatogenesis may be suppressed by many known or unknown agents but usually will return to normal because of repopulation of the germinal epithelium by progeny of the A_o-spermatogonia. After transient exposure to an agent that alters function of the germinal epithelium and death of certain types of germ cells, several weeks may pass before a decrease in testicular size or an alteration of seminal characteristics is evident.[2, 17] More than 3 to 5 months may pass between termination of exposure to such an antispermatogenic agent and evidence in seminal characteristics of a marked improvement in spermatogenesis.

Cross sections through normal seminiferous tubules have different histologic appearances.[1, 9, 14, 15, 24] Eight or ten different "cellular associations" have been discerned for the dog.[9,14,15] Each cellular association contains four or five types of germ cells organized in a specific, layered arrangement (Fig. 2). Each layer represents one generation of germ cells with the most differentiated nearest the tubular lumen.[9, 14] The cells that should be present in a given cross section of a seminiferous tubule are listed in the eight columns shown in Figure 2. An alternative approach to defining cellular associations is based on the morphology of the acrosome in the developing spermatids; 10 cellular associations have been described for the dog.[15] The complete series of cellular associations is termed the cycle of the seminiferous epithelium.

Collectively, the germ cells at a given point within a seminiferous tubule sequentially acquire the appearance of each of the 8 or 10 cellular associations. The interval required for one complete series of cellular associations to appear at a point within a

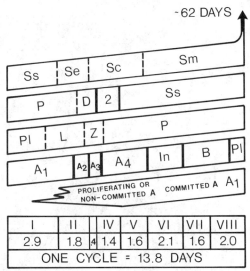

Figure 2. The cycle of the seminiferous epithelium in the dog. In this chart the basement membrane is at the bottom, and the lumen of the seminiferous tubule is at the top. Each of the five upper rows represents one generation of germ cells that are increasingly (from bottom to top) more mature. The columns represent the eight cellular associations that occupy all (or the major part) of a given cross section through a seminiferous tubule. The germ cells present in each cellular association (or tubule cross section) can be discerned by reading up each column. Germ cell types are A_1-, A_2-, A_3-, A_4-, In- and B-spermatogonia; preleptotene (P1), leptotene (L), zygotene (Z), pachytene (P), diplotene (D) and secondary (2) spermatocytes; and spermatids with a spherical (Ss), elongating (Se), condensing (Sc) or definitive (Sm) nuclear shape. The complete series of cellular association is termed the cycle of the seminiferous epithelium. In the dog the duration of one cycle of the seminiferous epithelium is 13.8 days. The duration of each cellular association is also shown. Since approximately 4.5 cycles of the seminiferous epithelium pass between commitment of an A-spermatogonium to differentiate and to produce more advanced types of spermatogonia and release of the resulting spermatozoa from the germinal epithelium, the duration of spermatogenesis is 62 days in the dog. (Based on published data of Davies PR: Ph.D. thesis, The University of Sydney, 1982; Foote RH, et al.: Anat Rec 173:341, 1972; Ibach B, et al.: Andrologia 8:297, 1976.)

tubule is termed the duration of the cycle of the seminiferous epithelium, which is 13.8 days for dogs.[9, 14] This duration is not influenced by hormonal changes and presumably is similar for all breeds of dogs. The duration of spermatogenesis is about 62 days in the dog.

For valid appraisal of testicular histology, fixation of small pieces (1 to 2 mm in the shortest dimension) of tissue in Bouin's or Zenker's fixative, or vascular perfusion, is essential. Use of buffered formaldehyde is unsatisfactory because vacuolization of the cytoplasm is induced by this fixative and preservation of nuclear detail is inadequate.[1, 2] A morphometric analysis[5] should be used to calculate the percentage of the testis occupied by seminiferous tubules, total tubular length, and the total numbers of primary spermatocytes of a specified developmental type and of spherical spermatids within the testis. Alternatively, appropriate cell types can be enumerated in a homogenate of fixed testicular tissue[19] obtained by biopsy[18] or at castration.

ENDOCRINE CONTROL OF TESTICULAR FUNCTION

The hypothalamic-pituitary-gonadal axis (Fig. 3) is a self-regulating system. Secretion of LH and FSH is controlled by a complex interaction of the sex steroids and gonadotropin-releasing hormone (GnRH).[3, 13, 20, 32, 33] GnRH is released from the hypothalamus[20] into the portal system in discrete pulses, and when GnRH reaches the cells in the anterior pituitary gland that produce LH and FSH (gonadotrophs), it causes secretion of gonadotropins. There are 5 to 20 randomly occurring discharges of LH per 24 hours.[10, 11] Whereas LH secretion is immediate and transitory after GnRH stimulation (10 to 40 minutes),[13, 23] the discharge of FSH is slow and gradual. FSH also is cleared more slowly from the blood than LH. Consequently, there is an attenuation of changes in blood concentration of FSH, whereas LH concentration increases rapidly from a baseline level and returns to baseline within 30 to 60 minutes after GnRH stimulation of the pituitary gland. In a mature male, the rise in the blood concentration of LH usually is followed within

60 minutes by a rise in serum testosterone.[10,11] It is likely that testosterone and estradiol act on the hypothalamus and possibly the anterior pituitary.[13, 20, 31, 32, 33] Estradiol, secreted by the testes or produced by local aromatization of testosterone, may alter hypothalamic function[33] and the response of the anterior pituitary to a given stimulus of GnRH.[13, 32] In studies with other species, it has been shown that Sertoli cells secrete the putative hormone inhibin, which is thought to suppress the discharge of FSH differentially by the anterior pituitary gland and regulate the ratio of LH to FSH secreted.[7, 16, 24] It also is possible, however, that the ratio of LH to FSH is dictated by the relative concentrations of testosterone and estradiol impinging upon the gonadotrophs.[32, 33]

Exogenous testosterone will suppress the discharge of LH by the anterior pituitary gland[28,31,32] and drastically reduce testosterone secretion by the Leydig cells. Reduced testosterone secretion is followed by a reduction in the concentration of testosterone around the seminiferous tubules, and this may be accompanied by a decline in spermatogenesis. Therefore, injections of testosterone or anabolic steroids are not recommended. In other species, testicular steroidogenesis may be abnormal for up to 10 days following injection of human chorionic gonadotropin (hCG). For this reason and because GnRH is not antigenic, injection of GnRH[13, 23] is preferable to injection of hCG[25] for testing the ability of the testes to secrete testosterone. If a

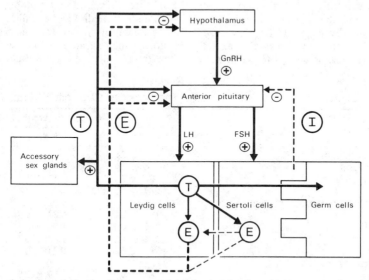

Figure 3. Diagram of the hypothalamic-pituitary-gonadal axis showing how hormones produced by Leydig cells are available to the germinal epithelium and feedback on the hypothalamus and anterior lobe of the pituitary gland. Stress can suppress discharge of luteinizing hormone (LH) and result in reduced secretion of testosterone. An increased concentration of testosterone in peripheral blood, either as a result of increased production by the testes or following injection of exogenous hormone, provides negative feedback on the hypothalamus to suppress pulsatile discharge of gonadotropin releasing hormone (GnRH) and, thus, to suppress discharge of LH from the anterior pituitary. Consequently, the Leydig cells receive less LH stimulation and produce less testosterone. Estrogens (E) are produced by the Leydig cells and to some extent by the Sertoli cells. The ratio of testosterone to estrogen reaching the anterior pituitary probably affects the relative amounts of LH and follicle-stimulating hormone (FSH) secreted by the gonadotrophs. Inhibin (I), a putative protein hormone secreted by Sertoli cells, may also suppress discharge of FSH from the anterior pituitary gland. The physiological role of prolactin in adult dogs remains conjectural.

Table 1. Frequency Distribution of LH and Testosterone Concentrations in Blood Serum from Adult Dogs*

LH		Testosterone	
ng/ml	Frequency (per cent)	ng/ml	Frequency (per cent)
0–<15	51	0–<1	21
15–<30	17	1–<2	17
30–<45	6	2–<3	18
45–<60	4	3–<4	16
60–<75	4	4–<5	10
75–<90	4	5–<6	7
≥90	13	≥6	11

*Data for 136 adult dogs ignoring the month when the blood sample was taken.

GnRH challenge is used to test pituitary sufficiency or testicular steroidogenesis, a dose of 125 to 250 ng/kg (55 to 115 ng/lb) should be adequate to bring about maximal discharge of LH.[13] Following such stimulation, it may require 24 to 48 hours for the gonadotrophs to resume normal function.

HORMONE CONCENTRATIONS IN PERIPHERAL BLOOD

Concentrations of LH and testosterone in blood are not stable because of episodic discharge of these hormones.[10, 11] Consequently, evaluation of a single sample will not provide accurate information on pituitary or testicular function. Although there apparently is no consistent diurnal rhythm for LH or testosterone secretion,[9] there is evidence for seasonal shifts.[12, 26] Basal levels of LH have been reported as less than 1.0 to 1.2 ng/ml, with maximal concentration during episodic secretion reaching 3.8 to more than 10 ng/ml.[11, 12, 17] During most of the year basal concentrations of testosterone are 0.5 to 1.5 ng/ml with peak concentrations of 3.5 to 6.0 ng/ml.[6, 10, 11, 12, 17, 26] In August and September, however, concentrations of testosterone are reported to be two to three times higher.[12, 26] Although most discharges of LH are followed by a discharge of testosterone, the seasonal variation in secretion of testosterone apparently is independent of the seasonal variation in secretion of LH.[12] The frequency distribution of values for testosterone concentration in dog blood follows a log curve rather than a normal distribution.[22] Data for LH and testosterone in blood serum for a group of 136 dogs are summarized in Table 1. Canine blood also contains FSH, prolactin, androstenedione, dihydrotestosterone, androstenediol and estradiol,[6, 8] but their physiological importance remains unknown.[32] It has been reported that estradiol is lower in young dogs with benign prostatic hyperplasia than in normal dogs.[8]

Table 2. Influence of Body Weight on the Reproductive Capacity of Adult Dogs*

Characteristic	Body Weight (lb)		
	10–34	35–39	60–84
Total scrotal testes width (mm)	36 ± 2§	50 ± 1¶	56 ± 1**
Paired testes weight (gm)	16 ± 1§	31 ± 1¶	44 ± 2**
DSP/gm parenchyma (10⁶)	20 ± 2	17 ± 1	20 ± 3
DSP/dog (10⁶)	287 ± 33	472 ± 32	750 ± 111
Extragonadal spermatozoal reserves (10⁹) at sexual rest			
Caput epididymidis	0.07 ± 0.01	0.23 ± 0.04	0.23 ± 0.05
Corpus epididymidis	1.10 ± 0.18	1.85 ± 0.16	2.27 ± 0.24
Cauda epididymidis	2.06 ± 0.31	3.30 ± 0.36	4.68 ± 0.39
Ductus deferens†	0.06 ± 0.02	0.21 ± 0.03	0.23 ± 0.04
Semen ejaculated after sexual rest			
Volume (ml)‡	2.4 ± 0.3	3.9 ± 0.5	5.4 ± 1.3
Concentration (10⁶/ml)‡	209 ± 42	359 ± 72	228 ± 58
Total sperm (10⁹)	0.4 ± 0.11	1.12 ± 0.13	1.43 ± 0.46

*Mean (± SEM) for 30, 53, and 32 dogs in the 10–34, 35–59 and 60–84 lb groups, but data on extragonadal spermatozoal reserves are for 17, 32 and 14 dogs and data for characteristics of a single ejaculate collected after ≥7 days of sexual rest are for 12, 14, and 11 dogs, respectively. DSP = daily spermatozoal production. For a characteristic, means without a superscript symbol (§, ¶, **) or with the same superscript symbol are not different (p>0.05).
†Not all of the ductus deferens was available for dogs castrated rather than euthanized.
‡The presperm and sperm-rich fractions were collected together, but ejaculation was terminated when ejaculation of the postsperm prostatic fluid started.

REPRODUCTIVE CAPACITY

Daily Spermatozoal Production. When evaluating spermatogenesis, the ultimate endpoint is the number of potentially fertile spermatozoa produced per day by the testes, and this value is highly correlated

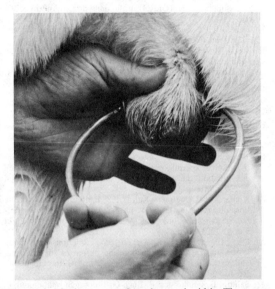

Figure 4. Measurement of total scrotal width. The testes are forced down into the scrotum and held parallel without distorting their breadth. This is best done by downward pressure of the thumb and forefinger directed on the dorsolateral aspect of the scrotum using a cranial approach. The calipers (hinge obscured by the technician's hand) are closed until snug against the scrotal skin at the widest point. Three to five measurements are made to the nearest millimeter and averaged; the scrotum is released and the testes are repositioned before each measurement. The 95 per cent confidence intervals for total scrotal width of dogs weighing 10 to 34, 35 to 59 and 60 to 85 pounds are 33 to 40, 49 to 52, and 54 to 58 mm, respectively.

with testicular weight ($r = 0.92$).[4, 9, 21] Thus, over 80 per cent of the variation in daily spermatozoal production is attributable to testicular weight or size. Because testicular size is influenced by body weight of a dog ($r = 0.75$),[4, 9] daily sperm production is much greater for large dogs than for small dogs (Table 2). However, age-associated changes in testicular size also affect daily sperm production. Beagle dogs are puberal by 6 months of age, but based on the total number of sperm in ejaculates collected weekly, they do not reach sexual maturity until at least 15 to 16 months.[30] The efficiency of spermatozoal production, the number of sperm produced per day per gram of testicular parenchyma (15 to 19×10^6),[4, 9] is independent of testicular weight, body weight or season. The efficiency of spermatozoal production is, however, lower in puberal dogs and may decline with advancing age. Administration of drugs also may influence the efficiency of spermatozoal production.

The efficiency of spermatozoal production is quite uniform in normal dogs, and testicular measurements are highly correlated with testicular weight. Thus, daily spermatozoal production can be estimated in a living animal by measuring total scrotal width (Fig. 4)[4, 21] or calculating testicular volume.[9] Such a measurement should be part of any andrologic examination. Correlations among total scrotal width, daily spermatozoal production and daily spermatozoal output of dogs are > 0.75.[9, 21]

Extragonadal Spermatozoal Reserves. The extragonadal spermatozoal reserves are the total number of sperm within the epididymis and ductus deferens.[1, 4] These numbers are influenced by size of dog (Table 2) and ejaculation frequency (Table 3). The number of sperm present in the caput and corpus epididymidis is not influenced greatly by ejaculation, but the number present within the cauda is considerably lower after a single ejaculation.[4, 9, 21] In dogs ejaculating once daily, the number of sperm in the cauda is stabilized at a level about 25 per cent below that in a sexually rested dog.[21]

Table 3. Influence of Ejaculation on Extragonadal Spermatozoal Reserves of Adult Dogs*

Characteristic	Sexual Rest (n = 63)	1 Ejaculate (n = 37)	1 Ejaculate/day (n = 15)
Testes	29.4 ± 1.5	30.6 ± 2.4	35.0 ± 2.7
Paired weight (gm)	490 ± 57	545 ± 66	435 ± 54
DSP/dog (10⁶)			
Extragonadal spermatozoal reserves (10⁹)			
Caput epididymidis	0.19 ± 0.02	0.19 ± 0.03	0.36 ± 0.11
Corpus epididymidis	0.87 ± 0.12	1.79 ± 0.21	1.95 ± 0.22
Cauda epididymidis	3.27 ± 0.24§	2.87 ± 0.39§	1.40 ± 0.18¶
Ductus deferens	0.18 ± 0.02	0.08 ± 0.02	0.05 ± 0.01
Ejaculated	0	1.02 ± 0.16§	0.24 ± 0.09¶
Total	5.38 ± 0.35	5.95 ± 0.68	4.90 ± 0.36

*Mean (± SEM) for dogs sexually rested for ≥7 days, sexually rested ≥7 days with one ejaculate collected 15 minutes before castration, or ejaculated daily for 10 or 20 days with the last ejaculation 15 minutes before castration or death. The data are confounded by body weight since the distributions of dogs weighing 10–34, 35–59 and 60–84 lbs were 17, 32 and 14 for the sexually rested group; 12, 24 and 11 for the one ejaculate group; and 1, 7 and 7 for the one ejaculate per day group. DSP = daily spermatozoal production. For a characteristic, means without a superscript symbol or with the same superscript symbol are not different (p<0.05).

Spermatozoal Output. The number of sperm in an ejaculate is influenced by many factors including age, testicular size, ejaculation frequency and interval since the preceding ejaculate, and possibly the degree of sexual arousal.[1, 4, 17, 21, 27, 29] Abstinence interval or ejaculation frequency profoundly influences the total number of spermatozoa per ejaculate.[1] If the interval between ejaculations is long, the excurrent ducts remain filled and the older spermatozoa are spontaneously discharged or voided in the urine as the new sperm are produced. If a series of ejaculates is collected over a period of time, daily spermatozoal production can be estimated accurately on the basis of daily spermatozoal output.[9, 21] However, the number of sperm in an isolated ejaculate, or even in several ejaculates collected at infrequent or irregular intervals, is not a satisfactory basis for calculating spermatozoal output or for evaluating testicular function.[1, 2]

In males ejaculating regularly, the number of sperm in the cauda epididymidis is reduced by 25 per cent relative to the number found in a male that has not ejaculated during the previous 7 days.[21] Consequently, fewer sperm are available for emission and fewer sperm are ejaculated. In most cases, a clinician will not have the opportunity to collect semen daily from a dog for 10 or 20 days. However, it would be desirable to ascertain the interval of abstinence prior to collection of an ejaculate. If this interval is $\geq$ 7 days, then the total number of sperm in a single ejaculate might be compared with values presented in Table 2. It is important to note that values for small dogs are less than those for large dogs (0.5 versus 1.4 × 10^9 sperm/ejaculate). If the interval of abstinence is less than 5 to 7 days, fewer sperm will be contained in a typical ejaculate than values given in Table 2.

References

1. Amann, RP: A critical review of methods for evaluation of spermatogenesis from seminal characteristics. J Androl 2:37, 1981.
2. Amann RP: Use of animal models for detecting specific alterations in reproduction. Fund Appl Toxicol 2:13, 1982.
3. Amann RP, Schanbacher BD: Physiology of male reproduction. J Anim Sci 57 (Suppl. 2):380, 1983.
4. Amann RP, Bowen RA, Behrendt M, Nett TM: Effects of body weight and season on reproductive capacity and hormone levels in dogs. Am J Vet Res (Submitted, 1985).
5. Bolender RP: Sterology and its uses in cell biology. Ann NY Acad Sci 383:1, 1982.
6. Boulanger P, Desaulniers M, Dupuy GM, et al.: Androgen levels in the liquid of the canine vas deferens and peripheral plasma. J Endocrinol 93:109, 1982.
7. Burger H, de Kretser D: The Testis. New York, Raven Press, 1981.
8. Cochran RC, Ewing LL, Niswender GD: Serum levels of follicle stimulating hormone, luteinizing hormone, prolactin, testosterone, 5α-dihydrotestosterone, 5α-androstane-3α,17β-diol, 5α-androstane-3β,17β-diol, and 17β-estradiol from male Beagles with spontaneous or induced benign prostatic hyperplasia. Invest Urol 19:142, 1981.
9. Davies PR: A study of spermatogenesis, rates of sperm production, and methods of preserving the semen of dogs. Ph.D. Thesis, University of Sydney, 272 pp, 1982.
10. de Coster R, Beckers JF, Wouters-Ballman P, Ectors F: Variations nycthémérales de la testostéronetet et de la lutropine plasmatiques chez le chien. Ann Med Vet 123:423, 1979.
11. DePalatis L, Moore J, Falvo RE: Plasma concentrations of testosterone and LH in the male dog. J Reprod Fertil 52:201, 1978.
12. Falvo RE, DePalatis LR, Moore J, et al.: Annual variations in plasma levels of testosterone and luteinizing hormone in the laboratory male mongrel dog. J Endocrinol 86:425, 1980.
13. Falvo RE, Gerrity M, Pirmann J, et al.: Testosterone pretreatment and the response of pituitary LH to gonadotropin-releasing hormone (GnRH) in the male dog. J Androl 3:193, 1982.
14. Foote RH, Swierstra EE, Hunt WL: Spermatogenesis in the dog. Anat Rec 173:341, 1972.
15. Ibach B, Weissbach L, Hilscher B: Stages of the cycle of the seminiferous epithelium in the dog. Andrologia 8:297, 1976.
16. Johnson AD, Gomes WR: The Testis, Vol.4. New York, Academic Press, 1977.
17. James RW, Crook D, Heywood R: Canine pituitary-testicular function in relation to toxicity testing. Toxicology 13:237, 1979.
18. James RW, Heywood R, Fowler DJ: Serial percutaneous testicular biopsy in the Beagle dog. J Small Anim Pract 20:219, 1979.
19. Johnson L, Petty CS, Neaves WB: A new approach to quantification of spermatogenesis and its application to germinal cell attrition during human spermatogenesis. Biol Reprod 25:217, 1981.
20. Kumar MSA, Chen CL, Kalra SP: Distribution of luteinizing hormone releasing hormone in the canine hypothalamus: Effect of castration and exogenous gonadal steroids. Am J Vet Res 41:1304, 1980.
21. Olar TT, Amann RP, Pickett BW: Relationships among testicular size, daily production and output of spermatozoa, and extragonadal spermatozoal reserves of the dog. Biol Reprod 29:1114, 1983.
22. Salutini E, Ghilarducci P, Biagi G: Il dosaggo radioimmunologico del testosterone plasmatico nel cane maschio in giovane eta. An Fac Med Vet Piza 30:245, 1977.
23. Schorner G, Choi HS, Bamberg E: Plasmatestosterongehalt beim Ruden nach Behandlung mit PMSG, HCG and LH-RH. Wien Tierarztl Mschr 64:153, 1977.
24. Setchell BP: The Mammalian Testis. Ithaca, Cornell University Press, 1978.
25. Sundby A, Ulstein T: Plasma concentrations of testosterone in the male dog and plasma testosterone profile following single intramuscular injection of HCG. Acta Vet Scand 22:409, 1981.
26. Taha MB, Noakes DE: The effect of age and season of the year on testicular function in the dog, as determined by histological examination of the seminiferous tubules and the estimation of peripheral plasma testosterone concentrations. J Small Anim Pract 23:351, 1982.
27. Taha MB, Noakes DE, Allen WE: The effect of season of the year on the characteristics and composition of dog semen. J Small Anim Pract 22:177, 1981.
28. Taha MB, Noakes DE, Allen WE: The effect of some exogenous hormones on seminal characteristics, libido and peripheral plasma testosterone concentrations in the male Beagle. J Small Anim Pract 22:587, 1981.
29. Taha MA, Noakes DE, Allen WE: Some aspects of reproductive function in the male Beagle at puberty. J Small Anim Pract 22:663, 1981.
30. Takeishi M, Tanaka N, Imazeki S, et al.: Studies on reproduction of the dog. XII. Changes in serum testosterone level and acid phosphatase activity in seminal plasma of sexually mature male Beagles (trans. title). Bull Coll Agri Vet Med Nilhon Univ (Jpn) 37:155, 1980.
31. Vincent DL, Kepic TA, Lathrop JC, Falvo RE: Testosterone regulation of luteinizing hormone secretion in the male dog. Int J Androl 2:241, 1979.
32. Winter M, Pirmann J, Falvo RE, et al.: Steroidal control of gonadotrophin secretion in the orchidectomized dog. J Reprod Fertil 64:449, 1981.
33. Worgul TJ, Santen RJ, Samojlik E, et al.: Evidence that brain aromatization regulates LH secretion in the male dog. Am J Physiol 241:E246, 1981.

Semen Collection and Evaluation in the Dog

S. W. J. Seager

Texas A&M University, College Station, Texas

Concurrent with the increase of purebred dog breeding and showing and the increased awareness and sophistication of dog breeders there has arisen over the past 5 years what seems to be an increase in reproductive failure in both the male and female dog. Veterinarians are routinely asked to perform fertility evaluations in the male dog for a variety of reasons. Among these reasons are AKC certification of the fertility of male dogs over 10 years of age, fertility evaluation prior to a stud dog's sale, and fertility evaluation for infertility. The last can be acutely important to the breeder who spends considerable time and financial resources in breeding a particular line of dog only to find that an important member of the male line is becoming or is infertile. This infertility or lack of breeding success may be a result of a variety of causes. Semen collection and evaluation play a vital part in overall diagnosis. This chapter deals with this technique in veterinary practice.

In our laboratory during the past 15 years, we have collected more than 11,000 ejaculates from more than 100 species of purebred dogs and many crossbred varieties. In all instances the semen was evaluated. In the majority of instances, the semen was either artificially inseminated directly or frozen and maintained in liquid nitrogen for subsequent insemination.

There are three requirements for a practicing veterinarian who performs fertility evaluation in the male.

1. Equipment needed to perform this function satisfactorily.
2. Experience and desire to learn collection techniques and subsequent evaluation.
3. Sufficient time for the procedure.

EQUIPMENT

1. Artificial vagina (AV) latex rubber cone.
2. Plastic graduated centrifuge tubes.
3. Small temperature-controlled incubator and/or slide warmer.
4. Disposable laboratory supplies (pipettes, microscope slides, cover slips, and examination gloves).

5. Binocular microscope with mechanical stage (preferably with phase contrast).
6. Low (4 to 10 ×), high (40 ×), and oil immersion eyepieces.
7. Sperm counting capability with a hemacytometer, spectrometer or cell counter.
8. Suitable stains and reagents to perform sperm morphology studies.

PROCEDURES

The dog should have a minimum of 4 days of sexual rest before semen evaluation. If the dog is not used regularly as a stud, three semen collections and examinations may be needed before a reliable evaluation can be made of the dog's ejaculate.

Veterinary hospitals or clinics are usually a strange environment to a male dog, and this may affect ejaculate quality. In a dog in which collection is particularly difficult, the veterinarian may decide to perform the collection and evaluation procedures at the dog breeder's home or kennel. In the majority of male dogs adequate collection can be done in a veterinary clinic. Time should be spent making the stud feel relaxed and establishing a rapport with him.

STUD'S REPRODUCTIVE HISTORY AND EVALUATION

Record the age, breed, number of times previously bred, conception rate, average litter size, the number of bitches that he failed to get pregnant and whether they were maiden bitches and became pregnant by other dogs subsequently. Also inquire about the reproduction history of the sire, dam and littermates.

Record the disease history, particularly any periods when the dog was off feed or showed a high temperature, orchitis or unusual licking of the prepuce and testicles, lameness in the hind legs, injuries or fight wounds, vaccination records and any previous tests for *Brucella canis* serology.

Record the length of his breeding "tie" and if this tie has decreased in length over the past year. Some stud dogs have a normal decrease in the length of tie during their reproductive life. As long as this decrease is not sudden, it should be considered normal.

Record the history of any previous semen examinations. If these have been done, the veterinarian may wish to call the client's former veterinarian.

EXAMINATION OF THE MALE DOG

When the male is presented for semen examination, before any attempt is made to collect the semen his exterior genitalia should be examined with care. A pair of examination gloves is put on, and the dog is approached and reassured by voice and gesture. He is restrained by a leash by the owner or veterinary assistant. The testicles are then examined for smoothness, adhesions, size, firmness and general "tone." At this time, ask the owner if there has been any noticeable decrease or thickening of the scrotal skin or any other change in the scrotal appearance, color or size. Once this initial examination has been made, the penis should be palpated in the preputial sheath and notation made of the amount of exudate at the preputial orifice. The dog's penis is then gently extruded from the sheath and examined to make sure that it is a bright pink, healthy color with no adhesions, injuries, scars, decolorization or spotting on the surface. Questions should be asked about the dog's micturition process and whether there has been any recent change. If the dog is not known to the practitioner, a minimum of a half an hour is required for the history taking, initial examination and getting to know the dog.

SEMEN COLLECTION

Prior to attempting semen collection, check to make sure that all collection utensils, pipettes, cover slips, and microscope slides are at body temperature. Ensure that the collection procedure will not be interrupted by telephone calls, people entering the examination room or conversation. In all instances, ask the owner to bring in an estrous teaser bitch to facilitate the semen collection. It is not necessary to have a bitch of the same breed, but it does help if they are the same general size. One may alternatively use Q-tip teasers, made by inserting a cotton tip applicator stick moistened in saline into the vagina of an estrous (*Brucella* negative) bitch. The Q-tip is then stored frozen in a sealed plastic container. It may be thawed 15 minutes prior to use and applied to the vulva of an anestrous bitch.

It is important for the dog to have secure footing in the examination room in order to obtain an optimum semen sample. Most males will not have adequate pelvic thrusts unless they have the reassurance of secure footing. Alternatively, one may use a rubber-backed mat for this particular purpose. It can also be used for breeding dogs naturally.

The mat is rolled out, and the bitch is led in and restrained by the handler. The handler should stand on the bitch's right side, and if there is any indication that she might snap or bite, she should be muzzled. The bitch handler restrains her head and then, kneeling, inserts his hand under her chest to maintain her in a standing position. He should not place his arm at right angles to the bitch, but at a more longitudinal angle in order to support her. Often, when the male dog is mounting, he may strike the arm of the bitch holder, and this will disturb him so that he may back off.

When everything is ready, the male dog is brought into the room on a short leash. Do not let him urinate and mark the area when he enters the room. This will usually result in urine in the ejaculate. If he does scent the area, allow the first couple of drops of the ejaculate to go on the ground. This will clear the urethra of urine residue. If the teaser bitch is not in standing estrus, a thawed Q-tip teaser is placed in front of his nose as he is led toward the bitch. If the bitch is suitably restrained, she may permit genital-nasal contact and even mounting; if not, the dog's semen can be collected approximately 1 foot from the bitch's rear end. The Q-tip can be dispensed with once the dog has obtained adequate erection and pelvic thrusts.

The artificial vagina is maintained in the pocket of the operator prior to use to keep it at approximate body temperature. The dog's penis is stimulated through the preputial sheath with digital manipulation and massage. When the penis has reached approximately 40 to 50 per cent of erection, the preputial sheath is slipped behind the bulbus glandis. If the dog's penis is allowed to expand more than this, there is difficulty in slipping the preputial sheath behind the glans. If this does happen, pull the dog away from the bitch and allow him to settle down for a couple of minutes. Allow him to approach the bitch again, and this time push the preputial sheath back over the glans before more than 50 per cent of erection has taken place. This is an important factor, particularly in a young dog that can get excited quickly and whose preputial sheath has not reached its maximum size.

Once the erect penis has been exteriorized, the artificial vagina is slipped on and up over the glans. A hand is placed between the dog's rear legs, and the glans (through the latex cone of the AV) is gripped between the thumb and forefinger in a circular fashion. Using a downward, holding pressure a tie is stimulated. The left hand holds the centrifuge tube. Observe the semen while it is being ejaculated. The first ejaculate fraction should be clear, 1 or 2 ml in a medium-size dog; the second sperm-rich fraction should then be seen entering the collection tube. This may amount to 1 to 3 ml. The third fraction will then follow and may be anywhere from 2 to 40 ml. Observe and record the dog's ejaculatory pattern. This pattern should remain stable; knowledge of how the dog ejaculates will assist in subsequent collections.

Once 1 to 2 ml of the third fraction has been collected, the artificial vagina is gently removed from the dog's penis. This gentle removal is necessary because at this time the dog's penis is engorged, and superficial vessels can be easily damaged. Such damage can cause pain, infection and subsequent lack of libido.

The male is kept in the room; if his engorged penis does not show signs of detumescence within 8 to 10 minutes, he should be walked until the penis withdraws back into the sheath. If this does not occur, gentle massage with cotton and tepid water can be done, or, the dog's penis can be immersed in a bowl of ice water. This is particularly important in dogs that seem to have a very large penis in relation to their size, such as bulldogs, basset hounds and other hounds. Do not put a stud dog with an engorged penis into a cage alone or into a run with other dogs. In long-haired breeds, ensure that no hairs come between the penis and artificial vagina.

SEMEN EVALUATION

Place the semen tube in a test-tube rack and cover the opening of the tube with parafilm. A warmed Pasteur pipette is removed from the incubator, and a representative drop of the semen is placed on a warmed microscope slide with a warmed cover slip. The semen is examined immediately for motility. The speed of progression is based on a scale of 0 to 5, 5 representing sperm moving rapidly across the microscope stage, and 0 representing motionless sperm. One expects to see 80 to 85 per cent of motile cells with a speed of progression of 5. This initial percentage of motility and motility status is recorded immediately after evaluation.

Next, observe and record the volume, pH and color. Semen of high quality should be milky white. A yellow color indicates urine in the ejaculate. A red or brown color can indicate either fresh or hemolyzed blood.

If the ejaculate is to be inseminated, it should be done so as soon as initial examination has taken place. *Never* inseminate a bitch without first examining the semen under the microscope.

SPERM COUNTING

With the parafilm over the tube, invert the sample gently three or four times. Fill a Unipette white blood cell dilutor pipette and dilute the pipette volume of semen in the reservoir provided in the kit. Write the dog's name, the owner's name and the date on the Unipette tube. Notation is made about the length of collection and libido. A further drop of semen is taken and put on a slide and prepared for staining. Sperm counting is normally done in a veterinary clinic with a hemacytometer. That is a routine procedure in most clinics and can be done proficiently. Sperm counts will range in the fertile dog from 200×10^6 to 1000×10^9. A medium-size dog with a sperm count below 200×10^6 has suspect fertility. If the dog has been sexually rested for more than 2 months, it may take as many as three semen collections and examinations over a period of 10 days to obtain reliable results.

Cryptorchidism in the Dog

Victor S. Cox, D.V.M., Ph.D.
University of Minnesota, St. Paul, Minnesota

DEFINITION

Cryptorchidism (cryptorchism) means cryptic or hidden testicles. When only one testicle can be palpated in the scrotum, the term monorchid is sometimes used, but this is incorrect because it implies the presence of a single testicle in the body, which, like anorchidism, is extremely rare. The correct term for the individual with a single descended testicle is unilateral cryptorchid or monocryptorchid. If neither testicle is in the scrotum, the dog is a bilateral cryptorchid. A less common term for the condition is ectopic testis.

PATHOGENESIS

In the fetus the developing testes lie immediately caudal to the kidneys. Testicular descent is brought about by contraction (shrinkage) of a gelatinous cord known as the gubernaculum testis, which extends from the caudal pole of the testis to the genital tubercle. The gubernaculum passes through the developing abdominal wall with the inguinal canal forming around it. The distal portion of the gubernaculum is the gubernacular bulb. Some authors believe that expansion of the gubernacular bulb outside the abdominal cavity may contribute to the traction that moves the testis caudally. Testicular descent is complete at birth in some domestic species, but not in the dog.[3]

There is disagreement in the literature concerning the time of testicular descent in the dog. Because of the small size of pups during the first few weeks of life, it is difficult to determine testicular position reliably by palpation. The small, soft, mobile immature testis is difficult to distinguish from adipose tissue, and the cremaster muscle may hold immature testicles in the inguinal region.[2] Recent dissection studies of beagle and mixed breed pups have revealed that at birth the canine testis is located midway between the kidney and the inguinal ring.[3] By the fifth day of postnatal life, the testis has passed through the canal. The gubernacular outgrowth continues until the fifth postnatal day and then begins to regress. Gubernacular growth is testis dependent.[4] The final scrotal position of the testis is reached by 7 weeks.[3] The testes cannot be palpated until 2 weeks of age, when they are midway between the inguinal ring and the scrotum. Until 3½ weeks of age the scrotum is filled with fat, which then regresses to allow space for the testicle. Most dissection studies on this subject used beagles or mixed breeds; other breeds may show testicular descent over a different time period. In particular, much slower descent has been observed in "normal" dogs from colonies with a high incidence of cryptorchidism.[5] At least three studies have indicated that descent may not be complete until 6 months of age.[5, 6, 12] In human studies many cryptorchid testicles descended from the superficial inguinal region at puberty, suggesting the influence of a hormonal factor; such a factor may be involved in late descent in response to gonadotropin treatment.

As the normal testis descends, the epididymis gathers around it, forming the close appositional relationship that is observed with the mature testicle. In a group of cryptorchid miniature schnauzers, bilaterally retained abdominal testicles were considerably more primitive in appearance than their unilateral counterparts, and only the heads of the epididymides were attached to the testes. In unilateral cases a more normal attachment between the testis and epididymis was observed.[5]

Cryptorchid testicles are always small and soft, especially when abdominal. Histologically, the seminiferous tubules are reduced to a single layer of spermatogonia, primary spermatocytes and Sertoli cells. The Sertoli cells are characterized by increased Golgi and smooth endoplasmic reticulum and a decrease in lysosomes.[7] The smooth endoplasmic reticulum is the site of steroidal synthesis. These observations are of interest because since cryptorchid testicles have an increased incidence of Sertoli cell tumors, which are associated with feminization.

Anatomic studies of perinatal pups have revealed defects of the gubernaculum as it passes through the abdominal wall. These defects may be the basis for some cases of cryptorchidism.

Canine cryptorchidism is generally considered to be a sex-limited inherited trait. The condition is often cited to be due to a single autosomal recessive gene. Mode of inheritance is difficult to establish. Parents of affected offspring are carriers, but it is difficult to determine whether a female carrier is homozygous or heterozygous for the trait. Noncarrier status is even more difficult to prove because the absence of affected offspring is meaningless unless a large number of offspring are available for analysis. This fact is illustrated in a study in which the ratio of cryptorchid to normal male offspring ranged from 1:1 to 1:20 among different carrier parents.[13] More than 40 pups (2 × 20) would have had to be produced from a dam and survive to 6 months to establish noncarrier status. This would require seven litters of six survivors each, and very

few canine genetic studies involve this amount of data.

Autosomal recessive genes have been postulated for the trait in boxers.[15] In a beagle colony an incidence of 22 per cent for carrier-to-carrier matings was close to the expected 25 per cent for a heterozygous recessive bred to the same (heterozygote recessive bred to another heterozygote).[13] Twenty-five per cent of the females from such a mating would be homozygous carriers and would constitute one-third of the carrier females mated in the next generation, resulting in an expected cryptorchid incidence of greater than 25 per cent. If, however, true noncarrier females are not recognized owing to insufficient progeny numbers, then the noncarrier and homozygous carrier effects would yield a balance closer to the previously mentioned 25 per cent.

Authors of the miniature schnauzer study reported that the high prevalence and the anatomic differences between bilateral and unilateral cryptorchids indicated a polygenetic trait.[5]

A third alternative was postulated based on data from the Veterinary Medical Data Program (VMDP).[11] These authors doubted the importance of a genetic etiology, owing to the large number of breeds affected and the heterogeneous breed makeup of the high-risk group. Predisposing factors such as the relative size of the testicle and the inguinal canal could explain the higher incidence in small breeds.[8, 11]

PREVALENCE

Cryptorchidism is a common developmental defect. Prevalence is higher in purebred dogs and varies widely from breed to breed; the true incidence is difficult to establish because local trends in breed distribution bias the incidence of cryptorchidism. The trait may be underreported by breeders or missed during incomplete physical examination. In a VMDP study the frequency of cryptorchid observation in male dogs was 0.8 per cent,[12] whereas in two smaller studies in which each dog was palpated, the frequency was 9.7 per cent for 108 male dogs and 10.9 per cent for 1494 male dogs.[6, 14] In experimental dog colonies even higher frequency figures have been noted. In a large beagle colony the frequency was > 15 per cent (556 male dogs), and 67 per cent of 12 male miniature schnauzers.[5] All of the above studies except the first were for dogs older than 6 months; a later VMDP report in 1975 dealt specifically with cryptorchidism, whereas the first covered all congenital defects.[11, 12] Although the defect was found in 68 breeds, only eight breeds were in a high-risk group with risk factors greater than one confidence interval from the norm of 1.0.

A recent study using a similar but larger data base found that among six breed groups the relative risk of cryptorchidism was always greater for the smaller close relative (e.g., toy poodle, 6.0; miniature poodle, 1.8; standard poodle, 1.1). A relative risk of 1.8 for boxers was the highest of all large breeds. Boxers are reported to have the highest frequency of cryptorchidism in Germany.[11,15] A frequency of 8.1 per cent for 1961–1965 was thought to be lower than actual because boxer breeders often culled cryptorchid pups.[15] Risk for beagles was 0.5 in one study,[11] placing them at low risk, while in a large colony mentioned earlier the frequency was greater than 15 per cent.[13]

Risk of cryptorchidism also has been correlated with other defects, especially patellar subluxation, hip dysplasia, penile/preputial defects, umbilical hernia and inguinal hernia.[11] Although both cryptorchidism and patellar subluxation are common in small breeds, the association was also strong in breeds not at high risk for the defect. The association with inguinal hernia could be the result of a gubernacular defect leading to formation of an oversized inguinal canal paired with lack of a spermatic cord to act as a "plug" in the canal.

Frequency of unilateral versus bilateral cryptorchidism has been reported in a few studies; generally, unilateral cryptorchidism is most common. If the condition is transmitted genetically, then the unilateral case would be expected to be more common, because bilateral cryptorchids are sterile. The right testicle is reported to be more commonly retained or smaller than the left in bilateral cases.[5] A right-left ratio of 27:14 has been reported for unilaterally retained testicles, and 41 of 55 cryptorchid dogs were unilateral.[14] In a highly inbred miniature schnauzer colony, four of eight dogs were bilateral cryptorchids, and in all four unilateral cases the testicle was retained on the right side.[5] The higher frequency of bilateral cryptorchidism (all abdominal) may have been due to the higher frequency of cryptorchidism in the colony as a whole. Figures on the relative occurrence of abdominal versus inguinal cryptorchidism have not been published. One author stated that the inguinal location was more common while another stated the reverse, but neither assertion was supported with data.[6,14]

In the scrotum of normal dogs the right testicle is usually more cranial than the left. Therefore, the right-sided predilection in cryptorchidism could be a reflection of a generally slower descent on the right side. The distance of descent may be greater because the right kidney is cranial to the left.

DIAGNOSIS

Cryptorchidism is diagnosed by palpation. If both testicles cannot be palpated in a young dog, he should be examined periodically until 6 months of age, when a definitive diagnosis can be made. Male dogs with feminization should be suspect for Sertoli cell tumor and hence for cryptorchidism as well. Torsion of the testes may be accompanied by abdominal pain and vomiting.

Major complications of cryptorchidism are neoplasia, feminization, blood dyscrasias and testicular torsion. Risk of testicular neoplasia has been determined to be 9.2 to 13.6 times greater in cryptorchid than in normal dogs.[8,11,14] Feminization and alopecia occur in 40 per cent of dogs with Sertoli cell tumors.[14] The greater mass of neoplastic testicles may predispose them to torsion. In a series of 13 torsions one affected testis was in the scrotum, one was inguinal, and the rest were abdominal; five of the affected testicles were neoplastic.[9]

TREATMENT AND RECOMMENDATIONS

Because of the risk of genetic transmission, neoplasia and testicular torsion, cryptorchid testicles should be surgically removed as should the remaining normal testicle in unilateral cases if the dog is a purebred and is likely to be bred. Because of the possibility of late descent, surgical treatment should not be undertaken in dogs less than 6 months of age. Descent has been reported to be aided by human chorionic gonadotropin treatment or gonadotropin-releasing hormone (GnRH) but without case reports or controlled studies.[1] The recommended dose of GnRH is 50 to 100 μg per pup given subcutaneously or intravenously.[1] If results are not observed after several days a second dose is recommended 4 to 6 days after the initial dose.[1] Since the inguinal canal is usually closed in abdominal cryptorchids, successful results with GnRH can only be expected for inguinal cryptorchids. When working with breeders an attempt should be made to correlate late descent with an increased incidence of cryptorchidism. Because of the strong evidence for inheritance of the trait, known carriers should not be used for breeding.

At the time of surgery, the scrotal testis should be pushed forward into its inguinal canal so that the side of the retained testicle can be determined. A ventral midline approach is usually used to remove abdominal testicles. A spay hook can be used to locate the ductus deferens, which is used to pull the retained testicle through the incision. If this is done, a small incision parallel to the prepuce may be sufficient to complete the procedure.[10]

References

1. Arbeiter K: Zum Maldescensus testis beim Hung. Tierarztl Prax 3:129, 1975.
2. Ashdown RR: The diagnosis of cryptochidism in young dogs: A review of the problem. J Small Anim Pract 4:216, 1963.
3. Baumans V, Dijkstra G, Wensing CJB: Testicular descent in the dog. Zbl Vet Med C Anat Histol Embryol 10:97, 1981.
4. Baumans V, Dijkstra G, Wensing CJB: The effect of orchidectomy on gubernacular outgrowth and regression in the dog. Int J Andrology 5:387, 1982.
5. Cox VS, Wallace LJ, Jessen CR: An anatomic and genetic study of canine cryptorchidism. Teratology 18:233, 1978.
6. Dunn ML, Foster WJ, Goddard KM: Cryptorchidism in dogs: A clinical survey. J Am Anim Hosp Assoc 4:180, 1968.
7. Goyla HO, Oliphant LW, Loewen RD: Fine structure of Sertoli cells in the normal and cryptorchid dog testes. Zbl Vet Med C Anat Histol Embryol 6:368, 1977.

8. Hayes HM, Wilson GP, Pendergrass TW, Cox VS: Canine cryptorchism and subsequent testicular neoplasia: Case-controlled study with epidemiologic update. Teratology 32:51, 1985.
9. Pearson H, Kelley DF: Testicular torsion in the dog: A review of 13 cases. Vet Rec 97:200, 1975.
10. Peddie JF: Removal of an intra-abdominal testis in the dog. Mod Vet Pract 62:231, 1981.
11. Pendergrass TW, Hayes HM: Cryptorchism and related defects in dogs: Epidemiologic comparisons with man. Teratology 12:51, 1975.
12. Priester WA, Glass AG, Waggoner NS: Congenital defects in domesticated animals: general considerations. Am J Vet Res 31:1871, 1970.
13. Rehfeld CE: Cryptorchidism in a large beagle colony. J Am Vet Med Assoc 158:1864, 1971.
14. Reif JS, Brodey RS: The relationship between cryptorchidism and canine testicular neoplasia. J Am Vet Med Assoc 155:2005, 1969.
15. Sittmann K: Cryptorchidism in dogs: Genetic assessment of published data. Ninth International Congress of Animal Reproduction and Artifical Insemination, Madrid, Spain 3:247, 1980.

Infertility in the Male Dog

Susan F. Soderberg, D.V.M.
Northeast Veterinary Hospital, Detroit, Michigan

The scientific literature provides little information on fertility of the male dog. Reports of semen evaluations from physically normal dogs are available in the literature, but breeding trials have not been performed to identify the significance of this information.

Infertile dogs may have never been fertile (primary infertility), may be infertile with a history of previous fertility (acquired infertility) or subfertile. A review of 200 dogs presented for reproductive evaluation found 158 with similar histories of reproductive failure and azoospermia beginning at 3½ years of age. The infertile males had three or four failures at stud and were not used for breeding until 2 or 3 years of age. During these 3 years, degenerative changes may have developed that were not recognized.

SUBFERTILITY

A subfertile stud dog is reported to have a poor conception rate owing to substandard spermatozoa in the ejaculate. Subfertile males are oligospermic or normospermic with poor motility or morphologic defects of spermatozoa in over 20 per cent of the sampled cells. Poor morphology, motility and concentration of sperm can result from an inguinal hernia with omentum or intestine in the scrotum, prostatic infection or retrograde ejaculation. Subfertility could reflect testicular damage progressing toward infertility, recovery of temporary infertility or partial, permanent testicular damage.

Decreased libido with low testosterone, hypothyroidism or psychological impotence may also account for some cases of subfertility.

PRIMARY INFERTILITY

Testicular hypoplasia is the result of poor gonadal development or maturation. Hypoplasia is generally suspected in young, postpuberal males with oligospermia or azoospermia. Different degrees of hypoplasia occur with a corresponding decrease in fertility. If a significant amount of tissue is hypoplastic, the testis size is also reduced. Libido is normal. Hypoplastic testes are reported to be more susceptible to degeneration in some domestic species.

Segmental aplasia of the epididymides may or may not be detected by careful palpation. This developmental defect will cause an azoospermia with normal ejaculatory reflexes. Agenesis of the testes and vas deferens has also been identified in dogs thought to be cryptorchid.

Prepuberal epididymo-orchitis can cause permanent damage to the epididymis or testicle. The inflammatory process generally is not detected by the owner but may be suspected in young dogs with testicular atrophy.

Defects in the hypothalamic-pituitary-gonadal axis must be suspected in animals with pituitary dwarfism or signs of other endocrine disease. Biochemical defects in androgen synthesis, eunuchoidism and hypogonadotropic hypogonadism are known to occur in man but have not been documented in dogs.

ACQUIRED INFERTILITY

Heat. Warming the testes to body temperature causes decreased sperm motility and eventual loss of sperm production. Increased testicular temperature may result from high fevers, scrotal dermatitis or inflammation of the testis and epididymis. Cryptorchid testes do not develop normally or rapidly lose their spermatogenic function, especially in the abdominal location. Scrotal testes warmed to body temperature for 10 days are not irreversibly damaged, however. Dogs appear to have the capacity to recover from degeneration caused by elevated scrotal temperatures to a greater extent than some other species.

Ischemia. Testicular ischemia has the potential to produce severe, permanent damage. Complete ischemia, as might be seen with testicular torsion, produces loss of spermatogenic capability within 1 to 2 hours. Some Leydig cells may remain after days of torsion if blood flow is not completely blocked.

Age. Senile atrophy of the testes may be found in dogs over 10 years of age. However, there is little evidence to suggest that age alone causes infertility. Debilitating systemic diseases and testicular neoplasia, more commonly found in older dogs, may contribute to the development of infertility observed in geriatric dogs.

Hyaline degeneration of testicular arteries and arterioles is identified in many old dogs with testicular degeneration. In advanced cases, the testes are small and soft. Testicular degeneration ranges in degree from a deficiency of germinal cells to complete disappearance of all epithelial elements, including Sertoli cells. Focal areas of infarction may occur as a result of severe vascular lesions.

Sexual Overuse. When dogs are ejaculated once or twice daily, the number of sperm per ejaculate declines rapidly during the first four collections. After the first four collections, the output per ejaculate remains fairly constant. Collection of semen every other day while maintaining sperm numbers is possible for indefinite periods in the normal dog. In some dogs semen quality deteriorates even with this management schedule, which then should be modified to allow efficient use of acceptable samples. Ejaculatory frequency does not influence daily sperm production; sperm are produced at a continuous rate, constantly pass into the epididymides, and are removed either by ejaculation or spontaneous discharge. Frequency of collection does not alter semen volume, sperm motility, morphology or libido.

Duct Occlusion and Epididymitis. Transport of sperm and seminal fluid into an ejaculate requires patency of efferent ducts, epididymal ducts, ductus deferentes, prostatic ducts and urethra. Occlusion within this duct network, with the exception of urethral obstruction, is rarely diagnosed. These lesions are commonly focal and would require contrast studies of the outflow tract for accurate antemortum diagnosis. Azoospermia or oligospermia result from an inability to transport sperm out of the testis into the ejaculate. Generally, testicular size and histology are normal.

Infectious agents causing epididymitis can originate in the vas deferens or seminiferous tubules, enter through the vaginal tunic from the peritoneal cavity, or be transported by hematogenous and lymphatic routes from infection sites elsewhere in the body. Prostatic disease may be a primary focus of infection or contribute to retrograde movement of infectious material from the urinary tract into the epididymis.

Chronic epididymitis can result in obstruction, distention of the ductules, fibrous scarring and obliteration or distortion of the duct lumen. Recurrent acute or sustained chronic infection may cause microabscesses, scrotal sinuses or sperm granulomas.

Orchitis. Acute orchitis may follow trauma, systemic infection, prostatitis and epididymitis. Routes of infection are the same as those causing epididymitis. Mild trauma results in decreased sperm output, which can be accompanied by poor motility. Common morphologic defects of spermatozoa observed following testicular trauma are bent tails, other tail defects and proximal cytoplasmic droplets. Minor traumatic injuries are usually followed by complete recovery. Traumatic episodes complicated by infection, hemorrhage or systemic exposure to sperm antigens may result in testicular atrophy or adhesions of the vaginal tunics.

Spermatozoa are antigenic to the male producing them as are certain other body tissues. Inflammatory responses initiated by trauma, infection or extreme temperatures can interrupt the integrity of the seminiferous tubule or epididymal duct wall and expose spermatozoal antigens to the body. The immune system will then form antibodies and sensitized lymphocytes against testicular tissue and spermatozoa. Spermatoceles and sperm granulomas develop from sperm stasis caused by congenital or acquired blockage of the ducts. Degeneration and rupture of these ducts commonly occurs, allowing further exposure of antigenic elements.

The Sertoli cells, acting as a sustentacular and transporting cell system between intertubular and interstitial circulations and the germinal cells, act to provide the blood-testis barrier. Rupture of the intercellular unions between Sertoli and germinal cells allows antibodies to reach antigens on the spermatogenic cells. Lymphocytic orchitis is characterized by lymphocytic infiltrations of the epididymis and testis. Focal degeneration, segmental atrophy and diffuse atrophy of the testis may be found with lymphocytic orchitis.

Brucellosis. *Brucella canis* will cause scrotal dermatitis, epididymitis or orchitis in 55 per cent of affected males. Abnormal sperm make up 30 to 80 per cent of the ejaculate within 2 to 5 weeks of acute infection. After the eighth week, large clumps of inflammatory cells, neutrophils and macrophages are commonly present with adherent and phagocytosed sperm. By week 15, bent tails, head-tail detachment and head-to-head agglutination predominate, resulting in infertility. A lymphocytic orchitis commonly develops with *Brucella canis* infection, leading to severe testicular damage.

Radiation. Exposure to radiation has been shown to adversely affect spermatogenesis in dogs. The spermatogonia are the most radiosensitive cells of the seminiferous epithelium. Older generations of germ cells continue to mature, disappearing in the order in which they were formed, until a point of maximum degeneration is reached. After a sublethal dose of whole body irradiation, males continue to void sperm derived from surviving spermatocytes and spermatids. Finally, after the epididymis has been emptied, maturation depletion results in temporary sterility. Multiple small doses of radiation damage the spermatogenic epithelium more efficiently and permanently than a single large dose of radiation.

Systemic Disease. Infectious diseases that induce prolonged fever cause temporary infertility of variable duration. During an active infection with distemper, dogs often lose the ability to produce seminal fluid, and serum testosterone drops to extremely low levels. Sperm production and testosterone secretion may return after recovery.

Systemic diseases such as renal failure, liver cirrhosis, diabetes mellitus or metastatic neoplasia alter hormone metabolism and have been shown to decrease fertility in man. These diseases are more commonly detected in elderly patients and may contribute to the development of senile testicular atrophy.

Up to 60 per cent of male dogs with hyperadrenocorticism have testicular atrophy. Healthy dogs caged in new surroundings may show a transitory drop in sperm count or complete azoospermia, possibly due to endogenous glucocorticoid elevation. These changes are reversible, returning to normal after 6 months in the new environment. Glucocorticoids have been shown to exert an antigonadotropic action on Leydig cell membranes and decrease levels of testosterone in humans. Marked tubular atrophy with moderate fibrosis may develop in humans with chronic hyperadrenocorticism.

Abnormal reproductive function has been identified in approximately 50 to 60 per cent of male hypothyroid dogs. Decreased fertility and libido is commonly encountered, while testicular atrophy and low sperm counts occur only in long-standing cases. Lymphocytic orchitis has been associated with lymphocytic thyroiditis in a beagle colony.

Hormonal Disturbances. Testicular degeneration and atrophy may occur because of tumors or abnormalities in the pituitary gland or hypothalamus that interfere with gonadotropin production and release. Androgen receptor deficiency may be responsible for as many as 40 per cent of the cases of human idiopathic infertility.

Tumors. The incidence of testicular tumors is higher in the dog than in any other species. Testicular tumors are found in dogs at an average age of 9.6 years. Sertoli cell tumors, seminomas and interstitial cell tumors reduce sperm cell production and fertility. Testicular degeneration is probably due to a combination of tumor compression of adjacent tissue and altered hormone production at both the pituitary and testicular levels.

Although normal seminiferous epithelium can be found in testicles containing a tumor, these individuals may have decreased numbers of spermatozoa in their ejaculate. The volume of functional tissue is diminished by the volume occupied by neoplastic tissue. If tumors expand within the central drainage area, flow of testicular fluid and spermatozoa through the ducts might become compromised. An outflow disturbance may be partial or complete. Often segmental tubular atrophy with pronounced dilatation is seen with tumors in or near the central drainage area of the testis.

The most frequent clinical sign associated with testicular neoplasia is prostatic disease, which may contribute to further inflammation and complications in the epididymis and testis. Prostatic enlargement and disease develops as a result of hormone production by the testicular tumor.

DIAGNOSIS

History and Physical Examination. The history is an extremely important part of the diagnosis and prognosis of infertility. The history should include all illnesses, injuries, treatments, management practices and owner observations related to development, behavior and mating experiences. Knowledge of previous reproductive examinations and number of nonconceptive breedings may indicate the duration of infertility.

A complete physical examination should always be performed to detect systemic disease or evidence of other organ malfunction. The reproductive examination should include evaluation of the prepuce, penis, scrotum, testicular size, shape and consistency, epididymides and prostate gland. Brucellosis tests and measurement of serum thyroid hormones may also be considered part of the routine physical examination of an infertile male.

Semen Evaluation. A semen sample should be collected from every male presented for a fertility evaluation, preferably in the presence of an estrous bitch. This will allow evaluation of the semen quality and the dog's sexual activity and libido. The first two fractions of the ejaculate, the presperm and sperm-rich fractions, appear milky in color and are collected in the same tube. The crystal-clear prostatic fraction follows and is collected separately. If blood appears in the ejaculate, it is of immediate importance to determine whether the hemorrhage is from the surface of the penis or from the urethra with the semen.

Owing to the large volume of prostatic fluid in the ejaculate, sperm cell concentration must be related to total numbers of spermatozoa. A minimum of 200 million spermatozoa has been suggested for fertility, but higher counts are expected. Most normal fertile dogs will have at least 80 per cent progressively motile cells. Abnormal movement often reflects a structural defect that can be found by morphologic examination of spermatozoa. Normal spermatozoa will maintain motility for several hours and are relatively resistant to cooling. Rapid loss of motility in collected semen may be an indicator of poor fertility.

Sperm morphology is easily visualized against the dark nigrosin background produced by an eosin-nigrosin stain. Oil immersion should be used to examine sperm morphology. An incidence of any morphologic abnormality of greater than 20 per cent can create subfertility. Because semen quality may improve with age, care should be taken in the evaluation of the young dog. A follow-up examination is frequently necessary to establish the diagnosis and prognosis of most reproductive tract disorders.

Semen that contains few sperm cells or has blood in the ejaculate should be examined for cellular content. The cells may be examined using a cytology stain. Neutrophils, macrophages and bacteria are found with infection in the reproductive tract. Unless infection is limited to the prostatic fluid, the location of infection generally is not identified. Degenerating spermatogenic cells are often found in azoospermic samples; they may be difficult to identify because of their pyknotic nuclei.

Retrograde ejaculation is diagnosed when semen is ejaculated into the urinary bladder instead of through the penile urethra. The concentration of spermatozoa in the urine is greater after than before ejaculation.

Cytology. Cellular components of the epididymis and testicle can be collected for examination by fine needle aspiration. An epididymal tap can be made into the tail of the epididymis using a 22- to 25-gauge needle and gentle suction by syringe. Generally less than 0.1 ml of material is obtained. Greater volumes of material may be obtained with epididymitis or conditions causing increased pressure and stasis. Azoospermic dogs with normal spermatozoa in the tail of the epididymis generally have a defect in spermatozoal transport in the reproductive tract. Epididymitis is detected with the presence of neutrophils, macrophages and bacteria.

The architecture of the seminiferous epithelium is disrupted when collecting cells by fine needle aspiration. Identification of specific cell types becomes very difficult. If mature spermatozoa or maturing spermatids cannot be identified, diagnosis should be made with a testicular biopsy.

Biopsy. Testicular biopsy provides a better analysis of spermatogenic function than semen evaluation or cytology. Complete azoospermia in the mature dog with no history of former sperm production carries a very negative prognosis, which in the absence of disturbances in other organ systems is unlikely to improve regardless of the biopsy findings. In dogs with acquired infertility, the biopsy may suggest both the etiology and the severity of the degeneration.

The testicular biopsy is obtained through a skin incision in the anesthetized dog. Surgical preparation is similar to that for castration. Several techniques for obtaining testicular tissue have been described. Fixation of the tissue should be in Bouin's fixative, glutaraldehyde or other solutions that have proved suitable for testicular tissue. Formalin should not be used since it distorts tubule walls.

Hormones. Testosterone, estradiol, luteinizing hormone (LH) and follicle-stimulating hormone (FSH) can be accurately measured by radioimmunoassay. Normal values have been established for each of these hormones by the various laboratories performing them.

Testosterone values ranging from 0.5 to 9.0 ng/ml have been observed in fertile dogs with normal semen. Infertile or azoospermic dogs often have testosterone concentrations within the normal range. Dogs with interstitial cell tumors may have testosterone concentrations above 5.0 ng/ml.

Estradiol values ranging from 1.1 to 8.8 pg/ml are found in dogs with normal semen. Only dogs with Sertoli cell tumors or seminomas located in an abdominal cryptorchid testis have estradiol levels above this range. These dogs show clinical signs of hyperestrogenism with feminization.

In one laboratory, LH values range from 0 to 174.7 ng/ml in dogs with normal semen. LH is secreted episodically, every 90 minutes, from the anterior pituitary gland; it is subsequently followed by testosterone secretion 50 minutes later. Consequently, dogs with LH levels of zero generally have normal levels of testosterone. LH levels are not related to testicular size or integrity of testicular cellular elements. When LH levels are above 150 ng/ml, testosterone levels are also increased. This may result from an androgen receptor deficiency in the pituitary gland or abnormal negative feedback.

FSH levels between 20 and 130 ng/ml are found in serum of normal dogs. FSH initiates spermatogenesis before puberty and after seminiferous epithelial damage. FSH levels above 250 ng/ml are found when the seminiferous epithelium is severely damaged and depleted. An active degenerative process in seminiferous tubules is generally present with FSH levels between 130 and 250 ng/ml. Azoospermia with FSH levels within the normal range suggests that an obstruction in the reproductive outflow tract is responsible for the infertility.

Behavior. Mating behavior and copulatory reflexes can be evaluated only by observation of the stud with an estrous bitch. Detailed descriptions of mating attempts can often be obtained from the owner and should include the dog's mounting attempts, receptiveness of the bitch, type of thrusting attempts and presence of an erection. When difficulty with intromission is noted, the genitalia of the bitch should also be examined for obstructions such as persistent hymen, vaginal hyperplasia or vaginal tumors. Males with adequate libido that are unable to mount or mate should be examined for physical defects causing pain or weakness.

TREATMENT

Treatment of Known Disease

Infection. Local infection of the testis and epididymis may be treated with appropriate antibiotic therapy. When only one testicle is seriously affected, unilateral orchidectomy is a valid approach. A male suffering from brucellosis should not be used at stud and should be neutered or destroyed. Other systemic diseases should be resolved and the dog allowed 10 to 12 weeks of sexual rest before a fertility evaluation is attempted.

Developmental Defects. Preputial stenosis, persistent ventral frenulum and inguinal hernias require surgical correction. The testis on the side of an inguinal hernia may swell for a week or more. Semen quality should return to normal 10 to 12 weeks after surgery.

Tumors. Neoplasia in scrotal testes is most often seen in older animals. Since semen quality will be affected by the presence of a tumor, fertility may be improved by the removal of the affected testis. If the dog is to remain at stud, unilateral orchidectomy with a 10- to 12-week rest period is the treatment of choice.

Systemic Disease. Renal failure, hepatic cirrhosis, metastatic neoplasia, diabetes mellitus, hyperadrenocorticism and cardiac disease should be managed with recommended treatment schedules. Because these diseases hold guarded prognoses, reproductive function should be of secondary concern. Fertility may return if the organ malfunction can be successfully controlled for 3 to 6 months.

Hypothyroidism may be corrected by providing thyroid supplementation. The seminiferous epithelium has a wide variation in functional ability prior to therapy, depending on the duration of hypothyroidism. Libido and semen quality may return to normal weeks to months after beginning thyroid supplements.

Treatment of Idiopathic Infertility

Historical Therapies. Many hormonal and nonhormonal preparations have been used to treat male sterility with variable results. Unfortunately, little documentation exists relating pretreatment fertility, semen quality and testicular structure to post-treatment values of the same parameters. Pregnant mare serum gonadotropin (PMSG) has been the most commonly advocated therapy for azoospermic and oligospermic dogs. It has been suggested that azoospermic dogs do not respond to PMSG but that males with oligospermia may benefit from 200 to 500 IU of PMSG intravenously at 3- to 6-day intervals. FSH has also been used at a dose of 25 mg subcutaneously once a week.

Untested Therapies. Because no hormonal treatment has received adequate study in canine infertility, any treatment is speculative. Treatment has to be considered absolutely empirical. Testosterone therapy does not cause a positive effect on and may be detrimental to spermatogenesis. Hormones with FSH and LH activity are often used but with questionable results. Prolonged stimulation is required for positive results, and antibody formation to these protein gonadotropins can be expected. Therapeutic agents stimulating spermatogenesis should be applied for at least 3 months before a significant improvement in sperm count can be expected. It must be remembered that virtually all azoospermic dogs remain azoospermic regardless of treatment, unless a specific cause can be identified and corrected.

Infertile men are generally subdivided into three groups by radioimmunologic methods:

1. Primary testicular failure with clearly elevated gonadotropin levels, particularly FSH. Pharmacologic treatment of these patients is unsuccessful.

2. Secondary testicular failure with decreased gonadotropin levels. In these men gonadotropin replacement therapy is successful.

3. Normogonadotropic men including those with andrologic disturbances, occlusion, retrograde ejaculation, acute and chronic male genital tract infections, other functional disorders of the male accessory sex glands and idiopathic forms of oligospermia. Treatment regimens that have proved effective for many of these men have used the kinin-releasing proteinase kallikrein or the antiestrogen tamoxifen.

If treatment of infertile stud dogs is to become more successful, radioimmunoassays and testicular biopsies must be used more efficiently to identify the etiology of infertility.

References

1. Boucher JH, Foote RH, Kirk RW: The evaluation of semen quality in the dog and the effects of frequency of ejaculation upon semen quality, libido and depletion of sperm reserves. Cornell Vet 48:67, 1958.
2. DePalatis L, Moore J, Falvo FE: Plasma concentrations of testosterone and LH in the male dog. J Reprod Fert 52:201, 1978.
3. Harrop AE: The infertile male dog. J Small Anim Pract 7:723, 1966.
4. Larsen RE: Infertility in the male dog. In Morrow DA (ed): Current Therapy in Theriogenology. Philadelphia, WB Saunders Co, 1980, pp 646–654.
5. Worgul TJ, Senten RJ, Samojlik E, et al.: Evidence that brain aromatization regulates LH secretion in the male dog. Am J Physiol 241:E246, 1981.

Disorders of the Canine Penis and Prepuce

Shirley D. Johnston, D.V.M., Ph.D.
University of Minnesota, St. Paul, Minnesota

Both congenital and acquired disorders of the penis and prepuce have been observed in the dog. With congenital abnormalities the disorder may be an incidental finding at physical examination, or it may be associated with signs referable to local urine scald or other genitourinary tract abnormality. Acquired penile-preputial disorders may also be asymptomatic or may be associated with signs of pain, local irritation, dysuria or reluctance to breed.

CONGENITAL DISORDERS

Congenital disorders of the penis and prepuce that have been observed in the dog include penile hypoplasia, incomplete ventral closure of the penile urethra or prepuce (hypospadias, preputial cleft), persistent penile frenulum, congenital stenosis or atresia of the preputial orifice with phimosis, and duplication of the penis and prepuce (diphallia).

Penile hypoplasia has been reported in the Great Dane, collie, Doberman pinscher, and cocker spaniel.[5, 20, 22] Patients were asymptomatic or showed dysuria, hematuria and dripping of urine secondary to urine pooling and infection inside the prepuce. Penile hypoplasia has been reported in female pseudohermaphrodites (78,XX individuals with ovaries and the presence of external genitalia that have been masculinized by prenatal androgen administration) and in a 78,XX cocker spaniel that produced HY antigen with bilaterally cryptorchid testes.[22] Initial diagnosis is by inspection; cytogenetic evaluation of the karyotype and histology of the gonad may be contributory in understanding the etiopathogenesis. Serum HY antigen assay is not generally available at present. Treatment is unnecessary in the absence of clinical signs; surgical enlargement of the preputial orifice by removal of a V-shaped wedge of tissue may prevent urine pooling and recurrent preputial infection in symptomatic dogs.[20]

Hypospadias and/or failure of preputial closure is diagnosed by inspection of the external genitalia and by catheterization of the urethra. The external urethral orifice opens on the ventral aspect of the penis (rather than at its tip) or in the perineum when hypospadias is present. Affected animals may be asymptomatic or may have urine scalding and infection of regional mucocutaneous surfaces. As with patients with penile hypoplasia, evaluation of the karyotype and gonadal histology may further characterize this disorder as an abnormality of sexual differentiation.[7, 9, 10, 16]

Persistent penile frenulum has been reported in several breeds.[2-5, 15, 21] In most cases a thin sheet of fibrous connective tissue attaches the ventral aspect of the glans penis to the prepuce, resulting in ventral or lateral deviation of the penile tip. Affected animals may be asymptomatic or may show discomfort during urination or at erection when attempting copulation. Dermatitis secondary to urination on the medial aspect of the hind legs has also been reported.[3] Diagnosis is by inspection. Treatment is surgical removal of the frenulum. Natural copulation by an affected dog has been reported after surgical correction.[21]

Congenital preputial stenosis with phimosis has been observed in the German shepherd dog and the golden retriever.[10, 13, 14] Severely affected puppies may develop balanoposthitis and septicemia and die within the first 10 days of life if not treated. When the preputial orifice is large enough to allow complete urination the puppies may be asymptomatic except for an inability to protrude the penis. Diagnosis is based on inspection, and treatment is surgical enlargement of the preputial orifice with topical and systemic antibacterial therapy if infection is present. This abnormality has been observed in at least four related golden retriever litters, suggesting a hereditary cause of the defect in this breed. One of the affected males, his mother, and his female sibling all had normal karyotypes.[14]

Duplication of the penis and prepuce has been observed in a 5-month-old pointer and a 6-month-old bilaterally cryptorchid cockapoo.[1, 19] The pointer was presented because the owner noticed two streams of urine at urination. The dog was later determined to have two patent urethras, a double bladder, and unilateral hydronephrosis.[19] The cockapoo was presented for urinating in the house; it was subsequently determined to be in renal failure with pyelonephritis of the left kidney and agenesis of the right kidney. At postmortem the descending colon was found to have bifurcated, the left branch continuing to the anus and the right branch connected with the cranial aspect of the right of two medially joined urinary bladders. The left penis contained a patent urethra draining the left urinary bladder; the right urethra extended from the tip of the right penis to a point approximately 3½ cm into the right penis. The dog had a 78,XY karyotype, and the cryptorchid testes were histologically normal.[1]

ACQUIRED DISORDERS

Acquired non-neoplastic disorders of the canine penis and prepuce include urethral prolapse, penile trauma (laceration, contusion), fracture of the os penis, balanoposthitis, paraphimosis and persistent erection.

Prolapse of the penile urethra is rare but has been described in the English bulldog and the Boston terrier.[4, 6] Affected individuals are usually less than 2 years of age and may be presented for hemorrhage from the everted urethral mucosa. One dog showed prolapse following manual stimulation of the penis for semen collection.[4] Although urethral prolapse in the male dog has been attributed to trauma, genitourinary tract infection and/or sexual excitement, there is no definitive evidence to support such etiology. Recommended treatment has generally been amputation of the everted tissue under general anesthesia. One affected male so treated was able to achieve natural erection and mating 8 months postoperatively without prolapse recurrence.[4]

Penile trauma due to accidents or fight wounds may result in contusion, laceration or puncture wounds. Clinical signs of trauma include hemorrhage, which may be profuse and recurrent, local pain or irritation. Treatment includes local pressure for hemorrhage, cleaning and debridement, and suturing as needed. The penis should thereafter be extruded at least twice daily for application of antibiotic ointment and to prevent formation of adhesions.

Fracture of the os penis may occur in any size or breed of dog and often follows penile trauma when the animal attempts to jump a barrier.[5, 11, 13, 23] Presenting signs include local pain, systemic depression, and variable signs referable to the urethra (dysuria, hematuria, oliguria/anuria, pollakiuria) depending on urethral involvement. Diagnosis is made by survey radiography; urethral involvement is characterized by passage of a urinary catheter and retrograde urethrography if necessary. If the urethra is intact and minimal bony displacement has occurred, surgical intervention may not be necessary. The fractured os penis with displacement may be stabilized with stainless steel surgical wires or by bone plating with soft tissue repair of the urethra and cavernous penile tissues as needed.[11, 23] Urethral stricture may occur following surgical correction.

Balanoposthitis, or inflammation of the penile-preputial mucosa, is generally caused by bacteria normally present in the preputial mucosa; infection may follow compromise of the dog's normal defense mechanisms. Inflammation of the penile-preputial mucosa has also been reported in association with herpesvirus or blastomycosis infection.[14, 18] Affected dogs may be asymptomatic or may show irritation and licking of the affected area. Diagnosis is based on gross appearance of the penis, exfoliative cytology and culture of the inflammatory lesions. Treatment is specific local and parenteral antimicrobial therapy (for bacterial infection) or systemic antifungal regimes (for blastomycosis).

Paraphimosis occurs when the extruded penis cannot be withdrawn back into the preputial cavity. It may occur following normal copulation or may be secondary to a constricting band of hair at the preputial opening. Treatment includes cleansing and lubrication of the penis and replacement inside the prepuce after lubrication or surgical enlargement of the preputial orifice.

Persistent erection has been observed in a dog with thromboembolism of the cavernous venous tissue at the base of the penis.[17] More frequently, this complaint refers to recurrent erection in excitable but otherwise normal dogs. Therapeutic amphetamine administration for narcolepsy may also result in persistent erection.

References

1. Bailie NC, Johnston SD, Hayden DW, et al.: Duplication of the penis, urethra, urinary bladder and descending colon in a dog with unilateral renal agenesis and bilateral cryptorchidism. (In preparation, 1985).
2. Balke J: Persistent penile frenulum in a Cocker Spaniel. Vet Med Sm Anim Clin 76:988, 1981.
3. Belkin PB: Persistence of penile frenulum in a dog. Mod Vet Pract 50:80, 1969.
4. Biondini J: Persistencia do "frenulum preputti" no cao. Arq da Esc Vet Univ Fed Minas Gerais 27, 1975.
5. Bloom F: Pathology of the Dog and Cat. Evanston, American Veterinary Publications, 1954.
6. Copland MD: Prolapse of the penile urethra in a dog. NZ Vet J 23:180, 1975.
7. Croshaw JE, Brodey RS: Failure of preputial closure in a dog. J Am Vet Med Assoc 136:450, 1960.
8. Hobson HP, Heller RA: Surgical correction of prolapse of the male urethra. Vet Med Sm Anim Clin 66:1177, 1971.
9. Fox MW: Brachyury and preputial cleft in the dog. Mod Vet Pract 44:68, 1963.
10. Jacobs D, Baughman GL: Preputial defect in a puppy. Mod Vet Pract 58:522, 1977.
11. Jeffery KL: Fracture of the os penis in a dog. J Am Anim Hosp Assoc 10:41, 1974.
12. Johnston DE: Repairing lesions of the canine penis and prepuce. Mod Vet Pract 46:39, 1965.
13. Johnston DE: Male genital system. In Canine Surgery, 1st Archibald ed. Wheaton, Ill., American Veterinary Publications, 1965, pp 611–640.
14. Johnston SD: Personal observation. St. Paul, University of Minnesota, 1983.
15. Joshua JO: Persistent frenulum. Vet Rec 74:1550, 1962.
16. Kipnis RM: Membranous penile urethra and preputial abnormality in a dog. Vet Med Sm Anim Clin 69:750, 1974.
17. Olson PNS: Personal communication. Fort Collins, Colorado, Colorado State University, 1982.
18. Poste G, King N: Isolation of a herpesvirus from the canine genital tract: association with infertility, abortion and stillbirths. Vet Rec 88:229, 1981.
19. Potena A, Greco G, Lorizio R: Su di una rarissima difallia in un cane. Acta Med Vet 20:125, 1974.
20. Proescholdt T, DeYoung D: Infantile penis in the canine. Iowa State Vet 2:59, 1977.
21. Ryer KA: Persistent penile frenulum. Vet Med Sm Anim Clin 74:688, 1979.
22. Seldon JR, Wachtel SS, Koo GC, et al.: Genetic basis of XX male syndrome and XX true hermaphroditism: Evidence in the dog. Science 201:644, 1978.
23. Stead AC: Fracture of the os penis in the dog—2 case reports. J Small Anim Pract 13:19, 1972.

Disorders of the Canine Testicles and Epididymides

Cheri A. Johnson, D.V.M., M.S.
College of Veterinary Medicine,
East Lansing, Michigan

Evaluation of the testicles and epididymides begins with a thorough history and physical examination. The history should include previous fertility, changes in testicular or scrotal size, shape and character, and previous illness and trauma. All past and current medications and *Brucella canis* test results should be recorded. The scrotum is examined for any lesions or evidence of trauma. The testicles and epididymides are carefully palpated for size, shape, symmetry and texture. The spermatic cord and pampiniform vessels are palpated to the inguinal ring. Examination of the prostate should be included because epididymotesticular disorders and prostatic disorders may occur concurrently. Reproductive physiology and endocrinology, and semen collection and evaluation are discussed in earlier articles.

Brucella canis testing, semen evaluation, semen culture, testicular aspirate, testicular biopsy, scrotal exploratory examination, hormonal evaluation and karyotyping may be indicated, depending on the individual case. Fine needle (25-gauge) testicular aspirate is easily obtained (see Infertility in the Male Dog). Material may be used for cytologic evaluation or culture. When azoospermia is present, testicular aspiration may be used to help differentiate lack of spermatogenesis from obstruction. Aspiration may also be helpful in evaluating discrete testicular masses for the presence of neoplastic or inflammatory changes. If spermatozoa are present in the ejaculate and/or if there are no discrete masses present, testicular aspiration is not likely to provide adequate information. Granuloma formation and hemorrhage are occasional complications associated with aspiration or biopsy. Techniques for testicular biopsy have been described.[3] Bouin's or Zenker's fixatives are recommended because formalin will distort testicular architecture. Hormonal evaluation is discussed in the article on male infertility.

Chromosomal abnormalities and disorders of sexual differentiation often result in abnormal testicles; these may or may not be descended into the scrotum and are usually smaller than normal. The histologic appearance will vary, depending on the underlying cause, such as ovotestes (true hermaphrodite) or sclerosis and Leydig cell hyperplasia (XXY karyotype). Spermatogenesis and steroid hormone production may be abnormal. Karyotyping may be diagnostic. There is no treatment (see Disorders of Sexual Development in the Dog).

Many factors can cause testicular atrophy or degeneration in the absence of inflammation. These include high temperatures, toxic chemicals and drugs, irradiation and hormonal imbalances. High environmental or endogenous temperatures have an adverse effect on spermatogenesis and sperm motility. The degree and reversibility of damage depend on both the degree and duration of hyperthermia. At temperatures of 38° to 40°C, as seen with cryptorchid testicles, testosterone production is maintained. Histologic changes consistent with heat damage in man are proportional hypoplasia of all germ cells (hypospermatogenesis) and maturation arrest.

Irradiation can cause permanent damage to the germ cells, but the Leydig cells are usually spared. Toxic chemicals such as lead, drugs such as amphotericin-B, and anticancer drugs such as cyclophosphamide can damage the testicle. Bunamidine hydrochloride (Scolaban) can cause reversible testicular lesions.[1] Hypospermatogenesis and maturation arrest can be seen with chemical as well as thermal injury.

Hypothyroidism, diabetes mellitus, glucocorticoid excess, estrogen, excess androgen and deficient gonadotropin can all cause decreased spermatogenesis and testicular atrophy. The mechanisms are variable and involve positive feedback inhibition of gonadotropin release (estrogen, glucocorticoids), inadequate gonadotropin production (hypogonadotropic hypogonadism) or possibly a direct effect on the testicle (glucocorticoids).

In most degenerative conditions of the testicle, the histologic appearance rarely indicates the underlying etiology. Hypospermatogenesis and maturation arrest are nonspecific changes. They are potentially reversible if the underlying cause can be identified and corrected. Occasionally, complete absence of germ cells is found, with only Sertoli cells remaining. This may occur in XXY males, in XX individuals producing HY antigen and in normal males after chemical or radiation insult. This testicular change is irreversible.

Orchitis/epididymitis may result from infection, immune-mediated disorders or trauma. Bacteria, fungi and viruses can infect these organs via hematogenous or ascending routes, or from penetrating scrotal wounds. Acute signs include swelling, warmth and pain. Fungal infections are unusual but can be seen with disseminated forms of the deep mycoses, such as blastomycosis. Viral orchitis has not been described in dogs, although dogs with distemper may have decreased spermatogenesis, decreased prostatic fluid and depressed testosterone production, which returns to normal after recovery from the acute illness. Canine parvovirus has not been associated with male infertility.[5]

Bacterial orchitis/epididymitis can occur with any generalized septicemia or as a sequel to prostatitis or scrotal wounds. *Brucella canis* should always be considered when orchitis is present. Epididymitis is the earliest and most pronounced pathologic change with *Brucella canis* infection. The histologic lesions include nonsuppurative inflammation with lymphocytes, plasma cells, macrophages and occasional giant cells. Multinucleated, sperm-containing cells are common. This inflammatory reaction diminishes with time. In the testicle, spermatogenesis is depressed early in the disease. Some dogs may regain fertility, but many develop testicular atrophy and sterility. Semen quality reflects epididymal dysfunction with immature sperm, bent tails, detached heads and inflammatory cells. High numbers of organisms are shed in the semen initially, but shedding decreases to nearly undetectable levels by 12 weeks after experimental infection.[2]

Serologic testing, using a rapid slide agglutination test, is recommended. The test is sensitive but lacks specificity, so false positive reactions are possible. False negative reactions are rare. Positive results must be confirmed by additional tests such as the tube agglutination test and blood cultures. Semen can also be cultured. The organism has fastidious growth requirements, so samples should be submitted to laboratories familiar with culturing *Brucella canis*. Recovery of the organism is the only definitive diagnostic test. Recent antibiotic therapy can affect the serologic and culture results, making them both negative. At present there is no effective treatment for *Brucella canis* and no vaccine. Infected animals should be eliminated from the kennel.[6]

Whatever infectious agent is involved, the initial prognosis for recovery of normal epididymal/testicular function should be guarded. In addition to the agent itself, heat and swelling associated with acute inflammation can cause damage. Therapy should be directed at all these aspects simultaneously.

Orchitis can occur in the absence of infection. Lymphocytic orchitis is an example. The pathogenesis is unknown, but in one beagle colony, lymphocytic orchitis and lymphocytic thyroiditis occurred simultaneously and were genetically related. An immune-mediated etiology has been implicated because it is known that the testicle and spermatozoa (like the thyroid) contain unique antigens that are normally protected from immune surveillance.

If sperm (or sperm antigens) are liberated into the epididymotesticular parenchyma, a granulomatous reaction can occur. Some disruption of tubular integrity is usually necessary to initiate the reaction. This could occur with any type of insult, but trauma is usually implicated. Granuloma formation is a risk associated with aspiration, biopsy or reconstructive surgery of the testicle or epididymis. Granulomatous reactions can also occur with some infectious agents, most notably *Brucella canis*, and the mycotic pathogens.

The testicles and epididymides may be trauma-tized. Usually there is concomitant trauma to the scrotum with scrotal lesions to alert the clinician. Besides direct epididymotesticular contusion, scrotal edema, hematoma formation and introduction of infection may complicate the situation. Therapy should attempt to relieve pressure, maintain normal scrotal temperature and prevent infection.

Torsion of a scrotal testicle is rare in dogs. Signs are acute pain and swelling. The spermatic cord and pampiniform vessels may be palpably abnormal, depending on the degree of torsion. Torsion of 360° for 24 hours will cause infarction. Ischemia for 1 to 2 hours will result in permanent damage with some recovery possible after 60 days. Treatment is hemicastration. For cosmetic purposes, the torsion could be surgically corrected. Even if this is done promptly, fibrosis usually occurs. Torsion of an abdominal testicle is much more common. Clinical signs are related to acute abdominal pain. Treatment is surgical removal of the testicle.

Spermatocele, varicocele (dilatation and thrombosis of the spermatic vein) and epididymal occlusion can cause oligospermia or azoospermia if bilateral. Scrotal exploration is usually necessary to identify these abnormalities. Congenital absence of the vas deferens and epididymis has been found in man. Epididymal occlusion may occur secondary to infection or iatrogenically during inguinal hernia repair. The closer the epididymal blockage to the testis, the more severe the damage. Therapy is surgical removal or bypass of the obstructive lesion. In man, success is dependent on location (the further from the testicle, the better the prognosis), size and duration of the lesion. Similar information is not available for dogs.

Functional abnormalities of the testicle have been identified in several species, including dogs under experimental conditions. Failure of the testicle to respond to gonadotropins can occur during periods of stress. This is reversible, provided other metabolic imbalances have not also occurred. There are many anecdotal clinical reports of apparent stress-related testicular failure in dogs that are heavily used for breeding or hunting or have recently changed environments. Recovery may occur after several months of rest. The testicular/epididymal disorders of cryptorchidism and neoplasia are discussed in separate articles in this section.

References

1. Burroughs-Wellcome Company: Report on Scolaban. Product insert. Kansas City, Burroughs-Wellcome Co.
2. George LW, Duncan JR, Carmichael LE: Semen evaluation in dogs with canine brucellosis. Am J Vet Res 40:1589, 1979.
3. Johnston SD, Larsen RE, Olson PS: Canine theriogenology. J Soc Therio 11 (part 2): 1982.
4. Larsen RE: Testicular biopsy in the dog. Vet Clin North Am 7:747, 1977.
5. Meunier PC, Glickman LT, Appel MJG: Canine parvovirus in a commercial kennel: Epidemiologic and pathologic findings. Cornell Vet 71:96–110, 1981.
6. Pollock RVH: Canine brucellosis: Current status. Comp Cont Ed 1:255, 1979.

Canine Prostatic Diseases

Jeanne A. Barsanti, D.V.M., M.S.
Delmar R. Finco, D.V.M., Ph.D.
University of Georgia, Athens, Georgia

The prostate gland is the major accessory sex gland in the male dog. It is located just caudal to the bladder in the area of the bladder neck and proximal urethra. Its purpose is to produce prostatic fluid as a transport and support media for sperm during ejaculation. Basal secretion of prostatic fluid is constantly entering the prostatic excretory ducts and prostatic urethra. When neither micturition nor ejaculation is occurring, urethral pressure moves this basally secreted fluid cranially into the bladder (prostatic fluid reflux).

Prostatic diseases are common in the older male dog. With aging, the prostate gradually enlarges owing to hyperplasia. Because of the prostate's glandular nature, prostatic fluid cysts may develop. The prostate is subject to infection from bacteria ascending the urethra. Hematogenous spread of bacteria and spread from the kidneys and bladder via urine or from the testicles and epididymis via semen are also possible. Bacterial prostatic infections can be acute and fulminant or chronic and insidious leading to abscessation. The aging prostate gland is also subject to neoplastic transformation, most commonly adenocarcinoma.

This chapter reviews canine prostatic diseases, describing the signs associated with prostatic diseases and the diseases that should be considered for each sign. Diagnostic techniques will be presented. Each disease will then be reviewed in regard to signs, diagnosis and treatment.

CLINICAL SIGNS OF PROSTATIC DISEASE

Clinical signs vary with the type and severity of prostatic disease (Table 1). Prostatic diseases can be present without causing any abnormal signs evident to the owner. These include prostatic hyperplasia, chronic bacterial prostatitis, early cyst and abscess formation and initial development of prostatic carcinoma. Probable avoidance of these problems is one reason for advocating neutering of young male dogs. Possible earlier detection of these diseases is one good reason for performing a yearly rectal examination on all mature male dogs.

Prostatic enlargement from any disease process can result in tenesmus by encroaching on the rectum in the pelvic canal. This is the only abnormal sign associated with uncomplicated prostatic hyperplasia. Prostatic enlargement also occurs with cyst and abscess formation and neoplasia. Detectable prostatic enlargement is uncommon with bacterial prostatitis alone.

If prostatic enlargement is marked, dysuria from urethral obstruction may result. This is an uncommon sign in dogs in contrast to man, since dogs have much less prostatic tissue lining the urethra. The dog's prostate tends to enlarge outward, away from the urethra. Partial urethral obstruction is usually noted only in dogs with abscesses, cysts or advanced neoplasia. If the partial obstruction continues, the bladder detrusor muscle and/or the external bladder sphincter may be damaged, resulting in urinary incontinence.

Blood or pus dripping from the urethral orifice is a classic sign of prostatic disease. This probably results from hemorrhage and/or exudation of pus from the prostatic acini through the prostatic ducts into the prostatic urethra in sufficient quantities not only to reflux into the bladder but also to drain out the urethral orifice. One must always rule out a preputial lesion as a cause of blood or pus from the prepuce. Urethritis is a potential cause of blood or pus dripping from the urethral orifice, but urethritis unassociated with primary inflammation of the bladder or prostate or urolithiasis is currently considered rare in the dog. Any disease that causes prostatic inflammation or hemorrhage can result in dripping of blood or pus. These diseases include bacterial prostatitis, prostatic cysts and abscesses, and prostatic neoplasia.

Systemic signs of prostatic disease include fever, depression, pain in the caudal abdomen, a stiff gait in the rear limbs, and leukocytosis. These signs are usually associated with acute bacterial prostatitis, prostatic abscessation (particularly if a localized or diffuse peritonitis has resulted) or prostatic adenocarcinoma. The systemic signs associated with neoplasia may be due to the necrosis and inflammation associated with tumor growth outstripping blood supply or with metastasis, particularly to vertebral bodies. Another systemic sign seen with suppurative prostatitis or prostatic abscessation is evidence of liver disease (icterus, elevated liver enzymes) and liver dysfunction (prolonged bromosulfophthalein (BSP) retention). This hepatopathy may be due to endotoxemia from prostatic infection.

Abdominal distention may be noted with very large prostatic cysts.

Recurrent lower urinary tract infection in male dogs is often due to chronic bacterial prostatitis. The major entities to rule out for recurrent cystitis in male dogs should be chronic bacterial prostatitis and chronic pyelonephritis. Recurrent urinary tract infection is often the only abnormal sign associated

Table 1. Clinical Signs Associated with Prostatic Diseases

	Tenesmus	Dysuria	Urethral Discharge	Systemic Signs*	Urinary Tract Infection
Prostatic Diseases that Can Cause the Abnormal Sign	Hyperplasia Cyst Abscess Neoplasia	Cyst Abscess Neoplasia	Cyst Bacterial prostatitis Abscess Neoplasia	Acute bacterial prostatitis Abscess Neoplasia	Bacterial prostatitis

*Signs including fever, depression, pain.

with chronic bacterial prostatitis. If the underlying cause of the cystitis is not suspected, routine antibiotic therapy will result in elimination of bacteria in bladder urine and resolution of the clinical signs. However, the prostatic infection will persist, reinfecting the bladder when antibiotics are stopped. Many dogs with prostatic adenocarcinoma also have bacterial prostatitis and abscessation.

DIAGNOSTIC TECHNIQUES FOR PROSTATIC DISEASE

The main diagnostic techniques for prostatic disease are history, prostatic palpation, cytologic examination of any urethral discharge, ejaculation, prostatic massage, prostatic aspiration, prostatic biopsy and radiography. Taking a complete history should be a standard veterinary practice and will not be reviewed here. During the physical examination, the rest of the urinary and reproductive tracts should also be carefully examined.

Prostatic Palpation. The prostate is best examined by concomitant rectal and abdominal palpation. The hand palpating the caudal abdomen can both evaluate the cranial aspects of the gland and push the prostate into or near the pelvic canal for better palpation per rectum. The dorsal median groove, the division between the two lobes, is palpable per rectum. The prostate should be evaluated for size, symmetry, surface contour, consistency, movability and pain. The normal prostate should be symmetrical, smooth, movable and nonpainful. The size in a 2- to 5-year-old, 25-pound dog was found to vary from ovoid, 1.7 cm in length by 2.6 cm tranverse by 0.8 cm dorsoventral, to spheroid, 2 cm in diameter in one study. However, because size varies with age, body size and breed, the judgment as to whether size is normal is subjective. If size is thought to be increased, approximate measurements should be recorded so that progression can be followed.

Urethral Discharge. If a urethral discharge is present, it should be examined cytologically. If sufficient urethral discharge is present or if the discharge increases with prostatic palpation, the discharge can be collected in a sterile container for culture after extending the penis and cleaning its surface. The culture should always be quantitative because of possible contamination from small numbers of the normal urethral flora.

Semen Evaluation. An ejaculate is valuable in assessing prostatic disease because prostatic fluid is the largest component of semen volume. The prostatic fluid is the last fraction of the ejaculate, following the sperm-rich fraction. To evaluate a dog for prostatic disease using an ejaculate, we first allow the dog to urinate to remove any urethral contents. Any preputial discharge is removed from the penis with gentle, minimal cleansing using sterile gauze sponges. The ejaculate is collected using a sterile funnel and test tube, a sterile large plastic syringe case or a sterile urine cup. If the ejaculate cannot be collected manually, a teaser bitch in estrus or an anestrous bitch with the dog phermone, methyl-p-hydroxybenzoate,* applied to the vulva is used. Part of the ejaculate is used for cytology and part for quantitative culture. Quantitative culture is essential because the distal urethra has a normal bacterial flora.

Both ejaculate cytology and culture must be assessed for accurate interpretation. Normal dogs have occasional white blood cells and positive bacterial cultures. Bacteria are present in amounts of less than 100,000/ml and are usually gram positive. High numbers (>100,000/ml) of gram-negative organisms with large numbers of white blood cells indicate infection. High numbers of gram-positive organisms with large numbers of white blood cells *probably* also indicate infection if preputial contamination did not occur. Lower numbers of gram-negative or gram-positive organisms must be correlated with clinical signs and ejaculate cytology to determine significance. Blood may be found in ejaculates in dogs with bacterial infection, prostatic cysts, prostatic neoplasia and possibly hyperplasia.

An abnormality in the ejaculate does not localize the problem to the prostate, since the testicles, epididymis, deferent ducts and urethra also contribute to or transport the ejaculate. Collecting and comparing the early fraction of the ejaculate, which is of testicular origin, with a late fraction of prostatic origin may help to localize an abnormal finding.

Prostatic Massage. Because of the dog's pain or temperament, it is not possible to collect semen in all cases of prostatic disease. An alternative to the collection of prostatic fluid is prostatic massage. The dog is allowed to urinate first to empty the bladder.

---

*Methyl-p-hydroxybenzoate, Eastman Kodak Co., Rochester, New York 14650.

A urinary catheter is then passed to the bladder using aseptic technique. The bladder is emptied and flushed several times with sterile saline to ensure that it is empty. The last flush of 5 to 10 ml is *saved* as the preprostatic massage sample. The catheter is then retracted distal to the prostate as determined by rectal palpation. The prostate is massaged rectally, per abdomen or both for 1 to 2 minutes. Sterile physiologic saline is injected slowly through the catheter with the urethral orifice occluded around the catheter to prevent reflux of the fluid out of the urethral orifice. The catheter is slowly advanced to the bladder with repeated aspiration, especially from the area of the prostate as determined by rectal palpation. Most of the fluid will be aspirated from the bladder. Both the pre- and post-massage samples are examined by cytology and quantitative culture. We consider it *very* important to compare the post-massage sample with the pre-massage sample to be sure that any abnormality is due to prostatic fluid and not to a pre-existing condition in the bladder or urethra. Prostatic massage in normal dogs produces only a few red blood cells and transitional epithelial cells.

Disadvantages of prostatic massage include the inability to know whether prostatic fluid has been obtained without comparing the sample to a pre-massage sample and the inability to detect abnormalities in prostatic fluid if the bladder or urine are abnormal. In these cases we administer antibiotics that enter the urine well but do not enter prostatic fluid (e.g., ampicillin) for a few days prior to massage. The samples obtained must be cultured immediately so that the antibiotic in the urine does not kill any bacteria in the prostatic fluid after collection.

Aspiration. Prostatic disease can also be evaluated by needle aspiration or biopsy. Needle aspiration is most easily done in the dog by the perirectal or transabdominal route, depending on the location of the prostate. The procedure is done aseptically using a long needle with a stylet such as a spinal needle. In the perirectal approach, the needle is guided by rectal palpation (Fig. 1). The procedure can be performed in most dogs with mild tranquilization. Needle aspiration is probably best avoided in dogs with abscessation since large numbers of bacteria may be seeded along the needle tract. We do not perform aspiration in dogs with fever or leukocytosis or before examining prostatic fluid obtained by ejaculation or massage. In spite of these precautions, we have inadvertently diagnosed abscessation in five dogs by aspiration. The absence of evidence of abscessation by the other diagnostic techniques in these cases suggests that the abscessed areas were not communicating with the urethra. No complications of aspiration occurred in three dogs; in two the aspirations were perirectal, and in one the aspiration was transabdominal. In two dogs evidence of a localized peritonitis developed after aspiration, requiring intravenous antibiotic and fluid therapy. Because of the possibility of an occult abscess, aspiration should always be performed prior to a closed biopsy. If an abscess is aspirated, intravenous antibiotics should be given and surgery performed as soon as possible.

Biopsy. Prostatic biopsy can be performed perirectally or transabdominally or can be done via a caudal abdominal surgical exposure. Closed biopsy can be performed with tranquilization and local anesthesia. We usually use a Tru-Cut needle.* If prostatic abscessation is being considered in the differential diagnosis, aspiration should always precede a blind biopsy technique. Large prostatic cysts and acute septic inflammation, as in acute bacterial prostatitis, are also contraindications to blind biopsy procedures. With these precautions, the only complication reported from blind biopsy is mild hematuria, although significant hemorrhage is possible as with any blind biopsy procedure. The dog should always be examined closely for several hours after biopsy. Biopsy samples can be cultured for bacteria as well as examined histologically.

---

*Travenol Laboratories, Deerfield, Illinois.

Figure 1. Perirectal aspiration of the prostate gland. (From Barsanti JA, Finco DR: Vet Clin North Am 9:686, 1979.)

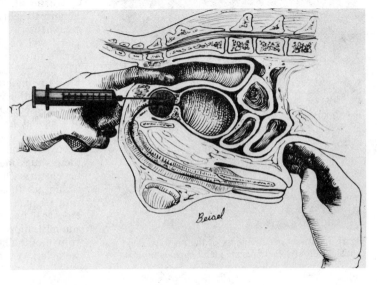

We often advise prostatic biopsy if castration is recommended as adjunctive therapy. A caudal abdominal incision with traction on the bladder will allow visualization of the prostate for biopsy (Fig. 2). An accurate diagnosis can be made and surgical therapy instituted if necessary.

Radiography. The size, location and contour of the prostate can be evaluated by caudal abdominal radiography. The prostate is often distinguishable on lateral and dorsoventral survey views. In some cases contrast cystography may be necessary to delineate the position of the bladder in order to locate the prostate. The normal gland is symmetrical with a smooth contour and is located near the cranial rim of the pelvic floor. As discussed, the size varies with age, body size and breed of dog. However, a normal-sized prostate does not displace the colon or the bladder from their normal positions.

Radiography is often of limited benefit in diagnosis of specific prostatic diseases. In many cases the prostate can be more accurately palpated on physical examination than visualized on survey radiographs. Changes in urethral size and the presence of reflux of contrast material into the prostate on retrograde urethrography were initially associated with specific disease processes. However, more recent surveys have found variable results with different diseases and in normal dogs.

The main benefits of radiography in prostatic disease are to define prostatic size and shape when the gland cannot be definitely palpated and to assess the effect of prostatic enlargement on the colon, bladder, urethra, ureters and kidneys. Excretory urography may be needed to evaluate the presence of ureteral obstruction by a markedly enlarged prostate. Radiographs are necessary to evaluate the thorax, vertebral bodies and sublumbar lymph nodes for the possibility of metastasis in cases of suspected prostatic neoplasia.

BENIGN PROSTATIC HYPERPLASIA

Benign prostatic hyperplasia is a change that occurs with aging of the male dog and is associated with an altered androgen-estrogen ratio. Because hyperplasia is an aging change, it occurs concomitantly with the other prostatic diseases to be discussed. This section will focus on uncomplicated benign hyperplasia.

Clinical Signs. Prostatic hyperplasia can be present without abnormal signs. In other dogs tenesmus may result from encroachment on the pelvic canal due to prostatic enlargement. We have noted an intermittent hemorrhagic urethral discharge in a few dogs in which hyperplasia was the only lesion on biopsy. Hyperplasia is not associated with any systemic signs of illness. The affected dog is alert, active and afebrile.

Diagnosis. On physical examination the prostate should be nonpainful and symmetrically enlarged with normal consistency. Hematology and urinalysis are normal. Abdominal radiographs confirm prostatic enlargement with dorsal displacement of the colon and cranial displacement of the bladder. If a urethral discharge is present, the discharge is hemorrhagic but not purulent. Semen and postprostatic massage samples may be normal or hemorrhagic. Definitive diagnosis is possible only by biopsy. A presumptive diagnosis can be made by the history and physical examination with support from hematology, urinalysis and prostatic fluid analysis, depending on the severity of the presenting complaint. We usually do not recommend biopsy for confirmation of the diagnosis unless the presenting complaint is a hemorrhagic urethral discharge; biopsy is then recommended in order to differentiate hyperplasia from more serious prostatic diseases that can also cause intermittent bleeding.

Treatment. Treatment is required only if related abnormal signs are present. The most effective treatment is castration. Involution of the prostate gland will begin within days, and a palpable decrease in prostatic size is expected within 1 week. The prostate gland will continue to decrease in size for 2 to 3 months after castration.

If castration is not feasible, low doses of estrogens can be used. Diethylstilbestrol administered orally at 1 mg/day for 5 days or estradiol cypionate at 0.1 mg/kg to a maximum total dosage of 2 mg have been recommended. The potential side effects of these drugs must be compared with their clinical benefit in each case before a decision is made to administer them. Severe bone marrow depression with resultant aplastic anemia is possible with overdosage or repeated administration. Repeated administration and overdosage can also cause growth of the fibromuscular stroma of the prostate, metaplasia of prostatic glandular epithelium and

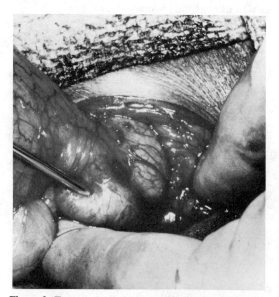

Figure 2. Tru-cut needle biopsy of the prostate gland via caudal celiotomy. The prostate gland appears normal.

secretory stasis. These changes can result in further prostatic enlargement and a predisposition to cyst formation, bacterial infection and abscessation.

An experimental drug that avoids the side effects of estrogens is the antiandrogen flutamide. When this drug was administered to research dogs at 5 mg/kg/day orally, prostatic size decreased with no change in libido or sperm production. Unfortunately, the drug is not currently available commercially.

PROSTATIC CYSTS

Prostatic cysts vary in size, number and location. Multiple, small cysts may be present in a hyperplastic gland, giving it a honeycomb appearance on a wedge biopsy. In other cases, a single cyst may become very large, approaching the size of a distended bladder.

Clinical Signs. With large cysts clinical signs such as dysuria and tenesmus may be related to increased prostatic size. If a single periprostatic cyst becomes very large, abdominal distention may be seen. With smaller intraprostatic cysts, there may be no abnormal signs or there may be a urethral discharge if the cysts communicate with the urethra. The discharge may be hemorrhagic, or it may be a clear light yellow fluid. Dogs with prostatic cysts have been misdiagnosed as having urinary incontinence because the cyst fluid appears similar to urine on gross inspection.

Diagnosis. Findings on rectal palpation will vary with cyst size. With a large cyst, a firm cystic structure associated with the prostate gland may be palpated in the caudal abdomen. With smaller intraprostatic cysts, the prostate gland may vary from mildly enlarged to markedly and asymmetrically enlarged. Fluctuant areas may or may not be palpable.

Hematology is normal. Urinalysis is usually normal. Mild hematuria may be present if hemorrhage occurs into the cyst and the cyst communicates with the urethra. If a urethral discharge is present, it should be examined cytologically to differentiate a urethral discharge from urine; a "urinalysis" can be performed on both and compared in regard to pH, specific gravity and dipstick analysis. Prostatic fluid collected by ejaculation or postprostatic massage should be examined. Prostatic cyst fluid is usually yellow to serosanguineous with only low numbers of white blood cells. Whether cyst fluid will be obtained by ejaculation or prostatic massage depends on whether the cyst communicates with the urethra.

With large periprostatic cysts, two "bladders" may be evident on survey radiography. A cystogram may be necessary to determine which structure is the bladder. With smaller cysts that communicate with the urethra, retrograde urethrography may indicate reflux of contrast agent into the prostate gland.

Treatment. The recommended therapy for prostatic cysts is drainage, surgical removal if possible, or marsupialization. Castration is recommended as adjunctive therapy. One potential complication of marsupialization is chronic infection.

ACUTE BACTERIAL PROSTATITIS

Acute bacterial prostatitis affects sexually mature male dogs. Infection usually results from ascent of bacteria up the urethra. *Escherichia coli* is the most frequent causative organism, but infection with other gram-negative and gram-positive organisms is also possible. Infection may also reach the prostate gland via blood, extension of infection from the bladder and urethra, and perhaps from the rest of the reproductive tract via semen.

Clinical Signs. Clinical signs include signs of systemic illness such as anorexia, depression and fever. Vomiting is possible due to an associated localized peritonitis. Caudal abdominal pain that can be localized to the prostate gland by palpation may be present. A low percentage of affected dogs will have a stiff, stilted gait. A constant or intermittent urethral discharge may be present.

Diagnosis. Prostatic palpation often elicits pain. The size, symmetry and contour of the prostate gland is often normal to mildly enlarged. The enlargement is often due to hyperplasia in the older dog rather than directly to the infection. Hematology often shows a neutrophilic leukocytosis with or without a shift to the left. Urinalysis usually shows blood, white blood cells and bacteria. If the urinalysis indicates a urinary tract infection, a quantitative urine culture and sensitivity testing should be performed on a sample collected by cystocentesis or catheterization. A presumptive diagnosis is based on the history, physical examination, hematology, urinalysis and urine culture.

Treatment. An antibiotic should be administered for 10 to 14 days. The choice of the antibiotic can be based on urine or prostatic fluid culture and antibiotic sensitivity testing. The blood-prostatic fluid barrier is usually broken in acute inflammation, allowing a wide antibiotic choice. If the presenting signs are severe, the antibiotic should initially be given intravenously along with parenteral fluid support. Oral antimicrobials can be used once the dog's condition stabilizes.

Since acute infections may become chronic, a recheck examination should be performed 3 to 4 days after antibiotic treatment is finished. This examination should include a physical examination, urinalysis and urine culture (if the urine was infected on initial presentation) and examination of prostatic fluid by cytology and culture.

CHRONIC BACTERIAL PROSTATITIS

Chronic prostatic infection may be a sequel to an acute infection or may develop insidiously without a prior bout of a clinically evident acute infection. It may be secondary to urinary tract infection or urolithiasis or due to changes in prostatic architecture that interfere with prostatic fluid secretion, such as cysts, neoplasia or squamous metaplasia from exogenous or endogenous (Sertoli cell tumor) estrogens.

Clinical Signs. Chronic bacterial prostatitis can be present without causing any signs referable to the prostate gland. Instead, the dog may have recurrent episodes of cystitis, or a urinary tract infection may be found on a routine urinalysis. Chronic bacterial prostatitis is the most common cause of recurrent urinary tract infection in men, and the same may be true in the dog. Other dogs may have a constant or intermittent urethral discharge.

Diagnosis. On palpation the prostate is not painful, and size is variable due to the degree of hyperplasia and of fibrosis. Chronic infection by itself causes no increase in prostatic size. The prostate gland may vary in symmetry and consistency owing to fibrous tissue deposition secondary to chronic inflammation. Areas of fibrous tissue will be firmer than areas of normal prostatic tissue. The areas of infection may be focal, multifocal or diffuse.

White blood cell count may be normal or increased. Urinalysis often shows evidence of infection with pyuria, hematuria and bacteriuria. Prostatic fluid collected by ejaculation or after prostatic massage is inflammatory, and quantitative bacterial cultures should be positive for significant numbers of one species of bacteria. As discussed earlier in the section on diagnostic techniques, results of prostatic massage are difficult to interpret in the presence of urinary tract infection. In order to utilize this technique, urinary tract infection must first be controlled.

A presumptive diagnosis is made by history, physical examination, hematology, urinalysis and prostatic fluid cytology and quantitative culture. In most cases if these techniques are carefully done and correctly assessed, a presumptive diagnosis is sufficient. Definitive diagnosis is accomplished by prostatic tissue culture and histopathology.

Treatment. Chronic bacterial prostatitis is very difficult to treat effectively because the blood-prostatic fluid barrier is intact. The blood-prostatic fluid barrier is based partly on the pH difference between the blood, prostatic interstitium and prostatic fluid, partly on the characteristics of the prostatic acinar epithelium and partly on the protein-binding characteristics of antibiotics.

The pH of blood and prostatic interstitium is 7.4. The pH of normal prostatic fluid is less than 7.4. The pH of prostatic fluid in dogs with prostatic infection is unknown. A few dogs with experimentally induced prostatitis had alkaline prostatic fluid, while others had acidic prostatic fluid. This unknown factor is very important. If infected prostatic fluid is acidic, basic antibiotics such as erythromycin, oleandromycin and trimethoprim will cross the barrier more effectively than other antibiotics. If infected prostatic fluid is alkaline, these drugs would be much less effective. Distribution of chloramphenicol is not affected by pH differences because it is nonionizable.

Lipid solubility is also an important factor in determining drug movement across prostatic epithelium. Drugs with low lipid solubility cannot cross into the prostatic acini. Many of these drugs are the acidic antibiotics such as penicillin, ampicillin and cephalosporins. Others include the aminoglycosides. Chloramphenicol, the macrolide antibiotics, trimethoprim and the sulfonamides are examples of lipid-soluble drugs that can potentially enter prostatic fluid.

Protein binding in plasma determines the amount of drug that enters prostatic fluid. The more protein bound the drug is, the less drug is available to cross the prostatic epithelium. This factor is probably less important than lipid solubility or pKa, since biologic systems rarely reach equilibrium. Examples of drugs with significant protein binding are clindamycin and chloramphenicol.

Current recommendations depend on whether a gram-positive or gram-negative organism is the infective agent. If the causative organism is gram positive, erythromycin, clindamycin, oleandromycin, chloramphenicol or trimethoprim/sulfonamide can be used based on sensitivity. If the causative organism is gram negative, chloramphenicol or trimethoprim/sulfonamide is best. Measurement of prostatic fluid pH is helpful in choosing a potentially effective drug.

Antibiotics should be continued for at least 4 to 6 weeks. Urine and prostatic fluid should both be recultured 3 to 4 days and 1 month after discontinuing antibiotics to be sure that the infection has been eliminated, not merely suppressed. The prognosis for cure, based on human medical experience, is only fair. The long-term cure rate in humans is only approximately 30 per cent. If the prostatic infection cannot be eliminated, antibiotics must be used continuously to prevent recurrent urinary tract infections. Trimethoprim/sulfonamide is most useful for this and can often be used effectively at 50 per cent of the usual daily dose every night. Supplementation with folic acid will help prevent folic acid deficiency with long-term use of trimethoprim/sulfonamide.

Castration has been recommended as adjunctive therapy to reduce the quantity of prostatic tissue. Used alone it will not eliminate infected prostatic tissue. It might be best to control the infection first, if possible, since prostatic blood flow (and thus antibiotic delivery) might decrease after castration.

Prostatectomy will eliminate infected prostatic tissue and can be used in cases that are refractory to antibiotic therapy. If castration is done a few weeks prior to prostatectomy, the reduction in prostatic size may make the surgery easier. However, this surgery is never easy. Severe hemorrhage is possible. The urethra must be meticulously sutured to prevent urine leakage. The presence of infection can lead to septic shock immediately postoperatively. Urinary incontinence is also a frequent sequel to prostatectomy.

PROSTATIC ABSCESSATION

Prostatic abscessation is a severe form of chronic bacterial prostatitis in which pockets of septic, purulent exudate develop within the parenchyma of the prostate gland.

Clinical Signs. The dog may have varying signs related to either prostatic enlargement or infection. Prostatic abscesses vary in size and number with each case. If the abscess or abscesses become very large, the dog may have tenesmus from incursion on the colon or rectum or dysuria from incursion on the urethra. Incursion on the urethra can lead to partial urethral obstruction causing a chronically distended bladder, eventual detrusor dysfunction and overflow urinary incontinence.

Clinical signs related to infection include a constant or intermittent urethral discharge that may be hemorrhagic or purulent. If the abscess ruptures on the outer surface of the prostate, a localized peritonitis results with fever, pain and possibly vomiting. Icterus due to an associated hepatopathy may also be present.

Diagnosis. On palpation the prostate gland may or may not be enlarged depending on the size and location of the abscess pockets. Occasionally a fluctuant area may be palpated. Inability to palpate such an area does not rule out abscessation because the abscess may be deeper within the gland or have a firm fibrous capsule. Pain on palpation is more often related to a localized peritonitis than to the abscess itself. Absence of pain does not rule out abscessation. The prostate gland is often asymmetrical and may vary in consistency (a cobblestone contour with firmer and softer areas).

White blood cell count may be normal, or a neutrophilic leukocytosis may be present. A neutrophilic leukocytosis is common with a localized peritonitis secondary to prostatic abscessation. A urinary tract infection is often present. Prostatic fluid collected by ejaculation or postprostatic massage is usually purulent and septic and may also be hemorrhagic. Refer to the section on diagnostic techniques for a discussion of the difficulty of accurately assessing the results of prostatic massage when urinary tract infection is present. Quantitative culture of urine and prostatic fluid should show significant numbers of the same organisms. Either aerobic or anaerobic bacteria may be involved in prostatic abscesses. Liver enzyme concentrations in serum may be elevated, and liver function such as BSP retention may be abnormal.

Prostatic enlargement, which may be asymmetrical, may be evident on survey radiographs. Reflux into the prostate gland may be noted on retrograde urethrography if the abscess communicates with the urethra.

The presumptive diagnosis is based on history, physical examination, hematology, urinalysis and prostatic fluid cytology and culture. The diagnosis should be confirmed by aspiration or exploratory celiotomy since the current treatment of choice is surgical. At surgery, the abscess contents should be collected for aerobic and anaerobic culture, and a tissue section should be obtained for histopathology.

Treatment. Surgical drainage is the current treatment of choice. There are many methods to accomplish this, including needle aspiration, use of tube or Penrose drains or marsupialization. Alternatively, the entire prostate may be removed. Complications are common with all methods. Drainage through the abdomen often results in oliguria and shock immediately after surgery, probably from the release of bacteria and their toxins. Intensive care is often required for several days after surgery. If drains are placed over the prostate, they may sever the urethra, leading to a urine fistula. Ascending infection with antibiotic-resistant bacteria is possible. Marsupialization leaves a chronic draining stoma in many dogs. If the stoma closes too early, the abscess may reform. Prostatectomy is difficult if the prostate is markedly enlarged and may result in urinary incontinence.

Polyuria and polydipsia, similar to that expected with nephrogenic diabetes insipidus, have been noted in a few dogs after surgical treatment for prostatic abscessation. Both polyuria and polydipsia and preoperative evidence of hepatic dysfunction resolved within 1 month of initiating treatment.

Castration is often recommended as adjunctive therapy to reduce the amount of prostatic tissue available for reabscessation. This is not necessary if prostatectomy is performed unless castration is done prior to prostatectomy in an effort to reduce prostatic size.

Regardless of which surgical therapy is elected, the dog must receive antibiotics. If the dog is systemically ill on presentation, intravenous antimicrobials should be used initially. Based on prostatic penetration, chloramphenicol or trimethroprim is the drug of choice. However, the choice should also be based on the causative organism, its antibiotic sensitivity and the degree of sepsis. After stabilization of clinical signs, the dog should be managed with antibiotics in the same way as a dog with chronic bacterial prostatitis.

If prostatic enlargement has resulted in partial urethral obstruction, bladder and urethral function should be carefully assessed. Prolonged bladder distention may have resulted in bladder atony so that the dog may have overflow incontinence. In such a case an indwelling urinary catheter is necessary to let the detrusor tight junctions reform. If the bladder wall has been chronically distended and infected, it may be irreversibly damaged.

Large prostatic abscesses are difficult and expensive to treat. The client should be made aware of these difficulties, so that a quick cure is not expected.

PROSTATIC NEOPLASIA

The most common prostatic neoplasm in the dog, as in man, is adenocarcinoma. Transitional cell carcinoma may also involve the prostate, but this section will focus on prostatic adenocarcinoma. This neoplasm is always malignant and tends to metastasize to sublumbar lymph nodes and the lumbar vertebral bodies as well as to the lungs.

Clinical Signs. Prostatic adenocarcinoma arises in old dogs. The presenting complaints by the owner are often related to increased prostatic size such as tenesmus and dysuria. Rear limb weakness or stiffness and pain in the hind quarters are common signs, present in 40 per cent of affected dogs in one survey. The pain may be related to necrosis and inflammation as the tumor outgrows its blood supply or to lumbar vertebral metastasis. Chronic weight loss may also be present. If the prostate gland is carefully palpated routinely in older male dogs, a firm neoplastic nodule may be felt prior to marked prostatic enlargement and prior to clinical signs.

Diagnosis. On prostatic palpation one or more firm nodules may be detected in early cases. In the majority of dogs presented with clinical signs, the prostate gland is markedly enlarged and asymmetrical with increased firmness. It may be painful on palpation and is often nonmovable. The sublumbar lymph nodes should be palpated rectally and may be enlarged.

A neutrophilic leukocytosis may be present depending on the degree of necrosis and inflammation associated with tumor growth. If the tumor has grown so that it obstructs both ureters, hydronephrosis and azotemia may result from such slowly developing obstruction. Urinalysis may show hematuria and pyuria due to prostatic necrosis and inflammation secondary to tumor growth. Infection may also be present. Prostatic fluid may vary from hemorrhagic to purulent, possibly with secondary infection. The prostatic fluid should also be examined for neoplastic cells, but falsely negative results are common.

Asymmetrical prostatic enlargement may be evident on survey abdominal radiographs. The lumbar vertebral bodies should always be carefully examined for areas of lysis suggestive of metastasis. The degree of enlargement of the sublumbar lymph nodes should also be determined. Thoracic radiographs are indicated to check for metastasis to the lungs.

A presumptive diagnosis is based on history, physical examination, hematology, urinalysis, cytology of prostatic fluid and radiography. Unless metastatic disease is evident radiographically, the diagnosis should always be confirmed by aspiration or biopsy because the prognosis is poor.

Treatment. Prostatectomy is the treatment of choice. The owner must be willing to accept the probable postsurgical development of urinary incontinence and the probability that metastasis has occurred even if it is not yet clinically or radiographically evident. In advanced cases with metastatic disease, euthanasia is often the most humane course because of lack of effective therapy. Palliative therapy includes castration, estrogen administration and various chemotherapy regimens designed for humans. Veterinary experience with these treatments is extremely limited. Castration in two dogs in our hospital did not halt or slow tumor growth.

References

1. Barsanti JA, Shotts EB, Prasse K, Crowell W: Evaluation of diagnostic techniques for canine prostatic diseases. J Am Vet Med Assoc 177:160, 1980.
2. Hardie EM, Barsanti JA, Rawlings CA: Complications of prostatic surgery. J Am Anim Hosp Assoc (In press, 1985).
3. Hornbuckle WE, MacCoy DM, Allan GS, et al.: Prostatic disease in the dog. Cornell Vet 68:284, 1978.
4. Ling GV, Ruby AC: Aerobic bacterial flora of the prepuce, urethra and vagina of normal adult dogs. Am J Vet Res 39:695, 1978.
5. Roberts SJ: Veterinary Obstetrics and Genital Diseases. Ithaca, New York, SJ Roberts, 1971, pp 607-613, 619-693.
6. Stone EA, Thrall OE, Barber DL: Radiographic interpretation of prostatic disease in the dog. J Am Anim Hosp Assoc 14:115, 1978.
7. Winningham DG, Nemoy NJ, Stamey TA: Diffusion of antibiotics from plasma into prostatic fluid. Nature 219:139, 1968.

Tumors of the Canine Male Reproductive Tract

Steven J. Susaneck, D.V.M., M.S.
Stephen J. Withrow, D.V.M.
Colorado State University, Fort Collins, Colorado

Tumors of the male reproductive tract include those of the testicle, penis, scrotum, prepuce and prostate. By far the most common of these are testicular tumors. Tumors of the penis, scrotum, prepuce and prostate are less common. Prostatic neoplasia is covered elsewhere (Canine Prostatic Diseases).

TESTICULAR TUMORS

The World Health Organization classifies testicular tumors into six categories: (1) germ cell tumors, which include seminomas, embryonal carcinomas and teratomas; (2) sex cord-stromal (gonadostromal) tumors, which include Sertoli (sustentacular) tumors, Leydig (interstitial cell) tumors, and tumors with intermediate Sertoli and Leydig cell differentiation; (3) multiple primary tumors (combinations of 1, 2 and 3 in the same testicle); (4) mesotheliomas; (5) stromal and vascular tumors; and (6) unclassified tumors.[9] Sertoli cell tumors, seminomas and interstitial cell tumors are the most common testicular tumors in the dog and are diagnosed with approximately equal frequency.[4] Other tumor types less frequently diagnosed are hemangioma, granulosa cell tumor, fibrosarcoma, carcinoma and neurofibrosarcoma.

Testicular tumors are the second most common tumor affecting the male dog, with a frequency second only to skin tumors. The incidence of canine testicular tumors is higher than in any other species including man. Determination of the true risk for canine testicular neoplasia is difficult because castration of young dogs is common. The mean ages of dogs with Sertoli cell tumors, seminomas and interstitial cell tumors are 9.7, 10.0 and 11.2 years, respectively.[9]

The location of the testes affects the cell type and clinical course of testicular tumors. Nearly 100 per cent of interstitial cell tumors and 75 per cent of seminomas are located in descended testicles, whereas only 40 per cent of Sertoli cell tumors occur in descended testicles. In cryptorchid testicles containing tumors, 60 per cent are likely to be Sertoli cell tumors and 40 per cent are likely to be seminomas. Ten per cent of cases of testicular tumors involve multiple tumors in one testis; usually an interstitial cell tumor occurs with a seminoma or a Sertoli cell tumor.

Interstitial Cell Tumors. Interstitial cell tumors are generally 1 to 2 cm in diameter and are usually surrounded by normal testicular tissue. On cut surface, the tumor is usually yellow to orange with a bulging dense fibrous capsule. On occasion interstitial cell tumors may be dark colored due to hemorrhage and necrosis and have only a thin capsule. Metastases of these tumors are rare.[4]

Sertoli Cell Tumors. Sertoli cell tumors are generally small tumors 1 mm to 5 cm in size and slow growing, but on occasion they may become much larger, especially when retained intra-abdominally. Grossly, these tumors are smooth and lobulated with a well-vascularized, intact tunica overlying them. On cut surface, they show a fine or coarse fibrous spongy network, which ranges from white to brown in color. These tumors are usually firm in consistency and may have cysts containing light brown fluid within them. In very large tumors, areas of hemorrhage and necrosis may be present. Between 10 and 20 per cent of these tumors metastasize to the lumbar or iliac nodes.[5]

Seminomas. In most cases seminomas are confined to the affected testes, although metastasis is reported in 6 to 11 per cent of seminomas.[8] Seminomas are usually homogeneous, white, gray or pinkish-gray and typically show no obvious coarse fibrous stroma. These tumors are generally not surrounded by an obvious capsule. Hemorrhage and necrosis may occur, resulting in a mottled appearance.

History and Clinical Signs. The history and clinical signs of testicular tumors vary depending on the location of the tumor and the cell type. The most common presenting signs are scrotal enlargement or inguinal masses. Dogs with intra-abdominal tumors may be presented for signs of abdominal enlargement or signs referable to abnormal hormone production or testicular torsion.

Interstitial cell tumors are usually found incidentally at elective castration or necropsy. These tumors rarely become large enough to cause clinical enlargement of the scrotum. Estrogen and testosterone levels may be elevated with interstitial cell tumors.[11] Associated clinical syndromes that "may" be related to testosterone production by interstitial cell tumors include perianal gland adenomas, perineal hernias and prostatic disease.[6] Although these associated clinical conditions have not been proved to be the result of hormone production by the tumor, their relationship to interstitial cell tumors cannot be overlooked. One case of pancytopenia, presumably from estrogen, was reported in a dog with an interstitial cell tumor, but the dog also had an adrenal adenocarcinoma and a bronchiolar carcinoma, so the pancytopenia cannot necessarily be attributed solely to the interstitial cell tumor.[7]

Patients with Sertoli cell tumors are most often presented for scrotal or inguinal enlargement. The morbidity of these tumors is more often related to estrogen production than to invasion or metastasis. Estrogen production is reported to be proportional to tumor size.[4] Approximately 25 to 50 per cent of dogs with Sertoli cell tumors are reported to show some type of pathology as a result of estrogen secretion.[7, 12] Clinical signs of hyperestrogenism include dermatologic changes (cutaneous and pilosebaceous atrophy, alopecia, increased cutaneous pigment, and sometimes pruritus), feminization (penile and contralateral testicular atrophy, decreased libido, attraction of males, gynecomastia and pendulous prepuce), prostatic enlargement (squamous metaplasia), and myelotoxicosis (anemia, thrombocytopenia, leukopenia). Signs of hyperestrogenism are much more common with large extrascrotal testicles than with intrascrotal tumors.

By far the most severe complication of hyperestrogenism is myelotoxicosis. Between 10 and 15 per cent of dogs with Sertoli cell tumors have signs of myelotoxicosis.[7, 10] Clinical signs are related to hemorrhagic diathesis caused by thrombocytopenia, severe anemia due to erythroid hypoplasia and infection due to granulocytic hypoplasia.

Patients with seminomas may present for scrotal or inguinal enlargement, although many seminomas may be found at elective castration in older dogs. Seminomas have been associated with estrogen/testosterone imbalance causing alopecia and myelotoxicosis, but this is rare.[1, 7] Perianal adenomas and perineal hernias have been reported in association with seminomas, but these associated conditions were not proved to result from hormone production by the tumor.

Diagnostic Techniques. Preoperative cytologic or histologic diagnosis of testicular tumors is generally not done because the treatment is usually castration. In the case of functional metastatic tumors, the tumor metastasis may still be functional after castration. Testicular tumors may be differentiated from orchitis by fine needle aspirate, cytology, needle biopsy and brucellosis titer. Incisional biopsies can also be used to differentiate tumor from infection. Because testicular tumors may be small, they may be missed on biopsy; therefore, a negative biopsy does not mean that the testicle is normal. Dogs with suspected testicular tumors should be carefully screened for thrombocytopenia, especially when an intra-abdominal or inguinal mass is present in a cryptorchid dog or when other signs of hyperestrogenism are present. Abdominal radiographs may be employed to check for sublumbar metastasis. Any intact male showing signs of bilateral alopecia or feminization should be evaluated for a testicular tumor.

Suggested First Treatment. Castration is the treatment of choice for testicular neoplasia. Dogs with myelotoxicosis as a result of hyperestrogenism should be treated with supportive care in addition to castration. Presurgical fresh whole blood or platelet-rich plasma transfusions should be given. In addition, prophylactic antibiotics should be given in animals with severe leukopenia. Hematinics and anabolic steroids may also be employed. In dogs that recover, recovery is often slow; improvement in hematologic values is first noticed 2 to 3 weeks postcastration, and complete recovery takes up to 5 months.

Adjuvant Secondary and Salvage Therapy. Surgical excision of solitary metastases, especially sublumbar lymph nodes, may be attempted. Chemotherapy using methotrexate, vinblastine, and cyclophosphamide has been reported.[12] In man cisplatinum is used to treat germ cell testicular tumors.

Prognosis. The prognosis for dogs with Sertoli cell tumors with myelotoxicosis is poor; two of seven (28 per cent) recovered in one study,[8] and two of six (33 per cent) recovered in another study.[7] The prognosis for most intrascrotal testicular tumors without metastasis is excellent. Larger tumors and abdominal tumors have the greatest tendency to metastasize, and the prognosis is fair. The prognosis for metastatic tumors should be guarded to poor.

PENILE TUMORS

Tumors of the penis are rare in the dog. The most common penile tumor is the transmissible venereal tumor. Squamous cell carcinomas are the second most common tumor. They are often ulcerated, and the dog may be presented for blood dripping from the penis. These tumors have a propensity for local invasion and extension to the prepuce as well as metastasis to superficial and deep inguinal lymph nodes and lungs. Other tumors that may be seen on the penis are squamous papillomas, fibromas, fibrosarcomas, hemangiomas, hemangiosarcomas, and histiocytic lymphosarcomas.

Diagnosis is based on a biopsy of the lesions. Nonhealing wounds and granulomas may mimic tumors on the penis. Small tumors may be treated with excisional surgery. In cases of more extensive lesions, penile and preputial amputation is indicated. A perineal urethrostomy should be performed prior to amputation. Radiation may also be used alone or in conjunction with surgery. Little information is available on the efficacy of radiation for tumors of the penis, but squamous cell tumors elsewhere in the body are often responsive to radiation therapy.

The most effective treatment of transmissible venereal tumors is once weekly injections of vincristine at 0.025 mg/kg. Therapy should be continued until there is no visible evidence of disease. The course of therapy is usually 2 to 7 weeks (3.3 week mean).[2] Visible tumor regression is seen within 2 weeks.

A thorough examination of the superficial and deep inguinal lymph nodes as well as a chest radiograph should be performed before therapy is instituted.

TUMORS OF THE PREPUCE AND SCROTUM

Any tumor arising from the skin or adnexa may involve the prepuce and scrotum. Mast cell tumors and melanomas are frequently seen on the scrotum. Mast cell tumors of the prepuce and scrotum tend to be malignant and highly aggressive in behavior. These tumors may present as a firm swelling or an ulcerated lesion in the inguinal area. Fine needle aspiration cytology is usually diagnostic for mast cell tumors. Careful examination and aspiration of inguinal and sublumbar lymph nodes are indicated prior to treatment. A bone marrow biopsy and buffy coat examination should be performed prior to surgery to detect systemic involvement. The scrotum and prepuce may be hot, swollen and bruised due to vasoactive amine release from the mast cells.

The treatment of choice for scrotal or preputial mast cell tumors is wide surgical excision. Surgery may include castration and scrotal ablation in addition to removal of the penis and preputial sheath. If surgery is incomplete, follow-up therapy using radiation or chemotherapy should be employed.[10] Recurrence is common following incomplete surgical removal.

Melanomas of the prepuce and scrotum are often benign. The treatment of choice is wide surgical excision. Squamous cell carcinomas involving the scrotum may arise from scrotal skin or from extension from the penis. The treatment of choice is wide surgical excision (see earlier section on penile tumors).

References

1. Barsanti JA, Duncan JR, Nachreiner RF: Alopecia associated with a seminoma. J Am Anim Hosp Assoc 15:33, 1979.
2. Calvert C, et al.: Vincristine for treatment of transmissible venereal tumor in the dog. J Am Vet Med Assoc 181(2):163, 1982.
3. Crow SE: Neoplasms of the reproductive organs and mammary glands of the dog. In Morrow DA (ed): Current Therapy in Theriogenology. Philadelphia, WB Saunders Co, 1980, p 64.
4. Hayes HM, Pendergrass TW: Canine testicular tumors: Epidemiologic features of 410 dogs. Int J Cancer 18:482, 1976.
5. Jubb KVF, Kennedy DC, McEntee K: The male genital system. In Jubb KVF, Kennedy DC (eds): Pathology of Domestic Animals, 2nd ed. New York, Academic Press, 1970.
6. Lipowitz AJ, et al.: Testicular neoplasms and concomitant clinical changes in the dog. J Am Vet Med Assoc 163(12):1365, 1983.
7. Morgan RV: Blood dyscrasias associated with testicular tumors in the dog. J Am Anim Hosp Assoc 18:970, 1982.
8. Moulton JE: Tumors of the genital system. In Moulton JE (ed): Tumors in Domestic Animals, 2nd ed. Berkeley, University of California Press, 1978, p 309.
9. Nielson SW, Lein DH: Tumors of the testis. WHO Bull 3168:71, 1974.
10. Sherding RG, Wilson GP III, Dociba GJ: Bone marrow hypoplasia in eight dogs with Sertoli cell tumor. J Am Vet Med Assoc 178:497, 1981.
11. Soderberg SS: Personal communication.
12. Theilen GH, Madewell BR: Tumors of the urogenital tract. In Veterinary Cancer Medicine. Philadelphia, Lee & Febiger, 1979.

Contraceptive Procedures for the Male Dog

Mauricio H. Pineda, D.V.M., Ph.D.
Iowa State University, Ames, Iowa

The canine population in the United States was estimated to be 41.3 million in 1975.[23] Survey data on the size and characteristics of the canine population are limited and restricted to certain geographic areas.[7, 11, 19, 20] Despite the limitations of this type of study, it is apparent that the canine population has not significantly decreased in size. At best, it has been projected to remain relatively stable in future years.[11]

Unwanted dogs and uncontrolled pets are primary sources of ecologic and social problems, including public exposure to zoonotic diseases, dog bites, pollution of parks and recreation areas and damage to livestock, wildlife, and public and private property. The increasing cost of capturing and disposing of free-roaming dogs and cats and unwanted pets obliges city and state governments and humane associations to divert funds from other important societal priorities to the handling and mass euthanasia of these animals.

The female dog and cat are still widely perceived as the primary targets for reproductive control on the premise that owners of fertile males are not likely to be concerned with pregnancies or the offspring of bitches and queens. As a consequence, the development of contraceptives for controlling the growth of the pet population has been primarily directed toward the female of the species. However, the participation of both sexes is an unavoidable requirement for pregnancy, and the contribution of the male to the overall growth of the pet population can no longer be ignored. Each intact male is reproductively active year round and therefore capable of siring a number of litters. The sterilization of a large number of males, particularly through the use of nonsurgical, inexpensive methods, would effectively contribute to curb the growth of the pet population.

Currently, the only proven means of contraception for the male dog are confinement and surgical sterilization. As effective as these two procedures are, neither has been widely embraced by the public, and the need for the development of suitable alternatives has been recognized by the veterinary profession and humane associations. Unfortunately, progress in the development of new contraceptive technology for the companion animal is hampered by the limited and inconsistent pattern of funding.

The involvement of the veterinary profession in all aspects of the population control of dogs and cats is a professional duty and a societal obligation. Veterinarians should not only be informed of the currently available and approved contraceptive procedures but also of those in different stages of development, offering potential for widespread application. This chapter is intended to provide information regarding contraceptive procedures applicable to the male dog.

SURGICAL STERILIZATION

Two surgical procedures are available to sterilize the male dog permanently: orchiectomy and vasectomy. Orchiectomy or neutering involves the surgical removal of the male gonads, and vasectomy is accomplished by sectioning vasa deferentia. Vasectomy is usually performed in the scrotal area, by removing a segment from each vas deferens and ligating the proximal and distal ends of the sectioned vas deferens. Both are safe and effective proven procedures to induce permanent sterilization in the male dog. However, they require anesthesia, surgical facilities and skilled veterinary surgeons. These requirements limit the applicability of these contraceptive procedures to extensive population control programs because of cost and diversion of veterinarians from other important professional activities.

Orchiectomy. Surgical castration is the most reliable method of contraception for the male dog because it eliminates both the source of spermatozoa and the testicular hormones that control the growth of androgen-dependent organs and influence sexual behavior. The behavioral changes induced by neutering are desirable from the point of view of contraception. Castrated dogs are less prone to fighting, territorial marking and roaming in pursuit of bitches in estrus. These behavioral changes caused by castration decrease or eliminate many of the hazards and nuisances to the public created by roaming dogs. Moreover, neutering has the added advantage of reducing or preventing diseases of the prostate gland that are common in the aged, intact male dog. Despite these advantages, neutering has not been widely embraced by the public as an acceptable contraceptive procedure. Survey studies indicate that the percentage of neutered dogs varies from 4.2 per cent[7] to 7.4 per cent[20] of the male dog population. Pet owners appear to be more willing to spay their bitches than to neuter their dogs. The percentage of spayed bitches varies from 31 per cent to 66 per cent of the bitch population, according to the study and the area surveyed.[7, 11, 19, 20] Cost of neutering, fear of surgery, anthropomorphic attachment to the pet, irreversibility of the procedure, the associated behavioral changes, and the fact that the bitch is the one that carries the pregnancy are all factors that contribute to make neutering a less acceptable procedure to pet owners than spaying.

Vasectomy. Compared to neutering, vasectomy is a relatively simpler surgical procedure but still requires anesthesia, surgical skills and facilities, and postoperative care. These requirements make vasectomy as costly as neutering without contributing any of its advantages, and surgical vasectomy is seldom used for contraceptive purposes in pets.

The ejaculates from a vasectomized dog may contain spermatozoa for as long as 21 days after vasectomy.[17] The viability and duration of the fertilizing capability of spermatozoa present in the postvasectomy ejaculates has not been critically evaluated for the dog. Therefore, it is advisable to recommend the confinement of vasectomized dogs for at least 4 weeks after vasectomy to prevent fertile matings. Ongoing studies from our laboratory indicate that flushing the vasa deferentia at the time of vasectomy resulted in azoospermic ejaculates 6 days after vasectomy in the dog.

Vasectomy by bilateral severance or occlusion by electrocoagulation of the abdominal vasa deferentia has been proposed as an alternative to the conventional procedure of scrotal vasectomy.[24] The proposed technique requires anesthesia, surgical preparation and procedure, postoperative care, and the investment and use of laparoscopic and electrocoagulation equipment by trained veterinarians. These requirements limit the application of this procedure. Abdominal vasectomy results in azoospermic ejaculates by 2 to 3 days after severance or occlusion of the vasa deferentia[24] as opposed to the 21 days required to clear the ejaculates of dogs vasectomized by conventional scrotal vasectomy.[17] The site of vasectomy must be taken into account by practitioners or researchers seeking early azoospermic ejaculates since the site of severance or occlusion of the vasa deferentia influences the length of time needed from vasectomy to azoospermic ejaculates.

CONTRACEPTIVES IN THE DEVELOPMENTAL STAGES

Public concern about the problems created by the growth of the pet population has stimulated research in the area of contraceptives for pets, and drug companies have begun to respond to the commercial potential of a growing market for an acceptable contraceptive for dogs and cats. Most of the developmental efforts have been addressed to the female of the species, and only isolated efforts have been made to develop contraceptives for the male.

Among these are the following approaches: (1) chemical vasectomy, (2) chemical orchiectomy, and (3) immunologic control of reproduction.

Chemical Vasectomy. The method of chemical vasectomy[13, 16, 18] was proposed as a nonsurgical alternative to neutering and vasectomy to overcome some of the major disadvantages of these surgical procedures: cost, postoperative care, low acceptability by pet owners, and unsuitability for large-scale sterilization programs. Chemical vasectomy involves bilateral injection of sclerosing agents into the cauda of the epididymides. The scarring reaction of the epididymal tubular and intertubular tissue at the site of injection blocks the passage of spermatozoa from the epididymides to the vasa deferentia, resulting in azoospermia.

The procedure for intraepididymal injection has been described.[13] Briefly, a sedative is given approximately 10 minutes prior to the intraepididymal injections. A disinfectant is applied to the scrotum, and the solution of the sclerosing agent is injected percutaneously through a 26-gauge, $\frac{3}{8}$- or $\frac{1}{2}$-inch long needle, depending on the size of the dog, into the cauda of each epididymis. The cauda of the epididymis is prominent and is easily located in both prepubertal and adult dogs. Paramedical personnel can be trained to administer the intraepididymal injections under veterinary supervision when large-scale male sterilization programs are contemplated.

The injection of 0.5 or 1.0 ml of an aqueous solution of 3.0 per cent chlorhexidine digluconate in 50 per cent dimethyl sulfoxide (DMSO) into each cauda of the epididymides of beagle dogs resulted in azoospermic ejaculates by 5 or 6 weeks after treatment, respectively.[16] These dogs were still azoospermic 952 days after treatment, when the seminal collections were discontinued.[16] Bilateral intraepididymal injection of 1.0 ml of an aqueous solution of 4.5 per cent chlorhexidine digluconate without DMSO was effective in inducing azoospermic ejaculates in mongrel dogs.[16]

Treatment of prepubertal and adult dogs with intraepididymal injections of solutions of chlorhexidine digluconate was not associated with undesirable clinical signs other than a transient swelling of the scrotum. Adhesions between the scrotum and the caudae of the epididymides develop when there is seepage of the chlorhexidine solution into the vaginal cavity of the scrotum, and some dogs may develop necrotic areas and ulcers in the scrotum. These lesions appear to be more frequent when the 4.5 per cent solution of chlorhexidine digluconate is used. Scrotal necrosis and localized ulcers do not interfere with ambulation and activity or with the general health of the dog; their occurrence can be prevented by careful intraepididymal injection. In my experience, topical treatment of the ulcers with antiseptics and protective ointments has been sufficient to produce a rapid and uncomplicated recovery.

The simplicity of the procedure makes the method of chemical vasectomy particularly well suited for large-scale sterilization programs. The method of chemical vasectomy is also suitable for the sterilization of males of other species.[12, 14]

Chemical Orchiectomy. Bilateral intratesticular injections of 1.0 ml of a 12 per cent solution of zinc tannate resulted in long-lasting sterilization of dogs by disrupting spermatogenesis and testicular steroidogenesis.[3] Blood testosterone levels after treatment were decreased to percentages varying from 27 per cent to 90 per cent of the pretreatment values. The published information[3] is preliminary, but if further testing proves the procedure to be effective and safe for the animal, it could have important applications in large-scale sterilization programs for dogs and other species.

Intratesticular injections of calcium chloride in concentrations ranging from 10 to 30 per cent in 90 per cent ethanol or in 70 per cent isopropyl alcohol have also been tested in dogs.[8] The pronounced tissue-irritating and necrotizing actions of calcium chloride and the potential for harmful post-treatment complications demand more studies before the suitability of the procedure can be assessed.

Immunologic Control of Reproduction. Immunization against gonadotropins, gonadotropin-releasing hormones, and gonadal steroids and the specific antibodies generated by the process of immunization have been and are used to elucidate mechanisms of hormonal action and can be applied to control reproductive processes in dogs and other species.

Active immunization of dogs against bovine luteinizing hormone (LH) and ovine pituitary gonadotropins resulted in atrophy of the testes and androgen-dependent organs[6, 9, 15] or delayed puberty in bitches.[6] The impairment of reproductive function was attributed to cross reaction between antibodies generated to the exogenous gonadotropins with the animal's own hormones. Active immunization against other hormonal factors such as gonadotropin-releasing hormone (GnRH), androgens or estrogens offers possibilities as potential contraceptive methods for pets.

The development of an acceptable contraceptive "vaccine" to selectively impair reproductive processes has long been sought by reproductive biologists in search of alternative methods to surgical contraception for humans and animals. Unfortunately, the procedure has several limitations, including variability in the qualitative and quantitative characteristics of the immune response between species and within individuals of the same species and the need for repeated immunizations. These limitations and the intense inflammatory reaction and abscessation at the site of injection of the immunogen and the adjuvant have precluded the application of this technique beyond the laboratory. The development of immune complex nephritis[22] in actively immunized animals further limits the applicability of this approach for large-scale sterilization programs.

Passive transfer of immunity, utilizing antibodies against gonadotropins, GnRH, or gonadal steroids for the short-term control of fertility has not been studied in the dog. This approach would allow the use of previously characterized and standarized antibodies and would have a greater potential for application in bitches to inhibit estrus and to block ovulation, to interfere with fertilization, and to prevent embryonic attachment and pregnancy. The production of monoclonal antibodies against hormones with enhanced specificity and affinity, compared with polyclonal antibodies,[5] may be the best source of specific antibodies for contraception.

OTHER POTENTIAL CONTRACEPTIVES

The use of ultrasound has been tested in dogs and cats for its contraceptive potential.[4] The procedure is said to induce temporary or long-lasting azoospermia, depending on dose and number of treatments, without apparent harmful effects to the animal.[4]

A series of compounds, such as tetramine, esters of methane sulfonic acid, dichloroacetylamines, and thio sugars (5-thio-D-glucose) have been tested in laboratory animals for potential contraceptives for the human male. Many of the compounds tested inhibited or disrupted spermatogenesis; however, they were also found to be either toxic or associated with undesirable side effects.

Gossypol, a polyphenolic yellow pigment extracted from cottonseed oil,[1] may have contraceptive potential for pets. In China, cottonseed oil has been used for centuries as an orally effective and reversible contraceptive for the human male. Recent evidence indicates that gossypol disrupts spermatogenesis and causes severe oligospermia or azoospermia by inhibiting the activity of lactate dehydrogenase X, an enzyme with a crucial role in the metabolism of spermatozoa.[10]

Prolonged feeding of cottonseed meal[21] or daily repeated high oral doses of gossypol[2] was associated with toxic reactions and death of dogs. However, the contraceptive potential of low doses of gossypol, administered for short periods, has not been determined for the dog.

Finally, psychological attitudes toward pets influence social attitudes toward pet control and methods to be used for controlling the population of pets. It is clear that surgical sterilization is not a popular solution to the overpopulation of pets, and it seems probable that no single method brought about by improved technology will be universally accepted as the solution. Therefore, several suitable alternatives should be made available to the public, coupled with a strong educational thrust to increase understanding and to encourage utilization of the available technology.

References

1. Abou-Donia MB: Physiological effects and metabolism of gossypol. Residue Rev 61:125, 1976.
2. Eagle E: Effect of repeated doses of gossypol on the dog. Arch Biochem Biophys 26:68, 1950.
3. Fahim MS, Fahim Z, Harman JM: Chemical sterilant for dogs. Arch Androl 9:13, 1982.
4. Fahim MS, Fahim Z, Harman J, et al.: Ultrasound as a new method of male contraception. Fertil Steril 28:823, 1977.
5. Fantl VE, Wang DY, Knyba RE: The production of high affinity monoclonal antibodies to progesterone. J Steroid Biochem 17:125, 1982.
6. Faulkner LC, Pineda MH, Reimers TJ: Immunization against gonadotropins in dogs. In Nieschlag E (ed): Immunization with Hormones in Reproduction Research. Amsterdam, North-Holland Publishing Co, 1975, pp 199-214.
7. Franti CE, Kraus JF: Aspects of pet ownership in Yolo County, California. J Am Vet Med Assoc 164:166, 1974.
8. Koger LM: Calcium chloride castration. Mod Vet Pract 59:119, 1978.
9. Lunnen JE, Faulkner LC, Hopwood ML, Pickett BW: Immunization of dogs with bovine luteinizing hormone. Biol Reprod 10:453, 1974.
10. Maugh TH: Male "Pill" blocks sperm enzyme. Science 212:314, 1981.
11. Nassar R, Mosier JE: Canine population dynamics: A study of the Manhattan, Kansas, canine population. Am J Vet Res 41:1798, 1980.
12. Pearson H, Arthur GH, Rosevink B, Kakati B: Ligation and sclerosis of the epididymis in the bull. Vet Rec 107:285, 1980.
13. Pineda MH: Chemical vasectomy in dogs. Canine Pract 5:34, 1978.
14. Pineda MH, Dooley MP: Surgical and chemical vasectomy in the cat. Am J Vet Res 45:291, 1984.
15. Pineda MH, Faulkner LC: Immunologic control of reproduction in dogs. Canine Pract 2:11, 1974.
16. Pineda MH, Hepler DI: Chemical vasectomy in dogs. Long-term study. Theriogenology 16:1, 1981.
17. Pineda MH, Reimers TJ, Faulkner LC: Disappearance of spermatozoa from the ejaculates of vasectomized dogs. J Am Vet Med Assoc 168:502, 1976.
18. Pineda MH, Reimers TJ, Faulkner LC, et al.: Azoospermia in dogs induced by injection of sclerosing agents into the caudae of the epididymides. Am J Vet Res 38:831, 1977.
19. Schneider R: Observations on overpopulation of dogs and cats. J Am Vet Med Assoc 167:281, 1975.
20. Schneider R, Vaida ML: Survey of canine and feline populations: Alameda and Contra Costa Counties, California, 1970. J Am Vet Med Assoc 166:481, 1975.
21. West JL: Lesions of gossypol poisoning in the dog. J Am Vet Med Assoc 96:74, 1940.
22. Wickings EJ, Nieschlag E: Inhibition of testicular steroids by antibodies—A feasible approach to male contraception. Int J Androl Suppl 2:384, 1978.
23. Wilbur RH: Pets, pet ownership and animal control: social and psychological attitudes, 1975. In Procedings National Conference on Dog and Cat Control. Denver, February 3-5, 1976, pp 21-34.
24. Wildt DE, Seager SWJ, Bridges CH: Sterilization of the male dog and cat by laparoscopic occlusion of the ductus deferens. Am J Vet Res 42:1888, 1981.

Disorders of Sexual Development in the Dog

Vicki N. Meyers-Wallen, V.M.D.
Donald F. Patterson, D.V.M., D.Sc.
University of Pennsylvania, Philadelphia, Pennsylvania

Normal development of the gonads, the internal duct systems and the external genitalia involves a complex series of steps that are under genetic and hormonal control. Abnormalities in the completion of these steps lead to a variety of congenital defects referred to collectively as disorders of sexual development. Our objective in this chapter is to provide a basic understanding of the processes of normal sexual development and to describe the pathogenesis, diagnostic features and management of the forms of abnormal sexual development known to occur in dogs.

NORMAL SEXUAL DEVELOPMENT

To understand disorders of sexual development, it is useful to view normal development in three major phases that occur in sequence, each dependent on successful completion of the previous step:

1. Establishment of *chromosomal sex*. Normally, an XX or XY sex chromosome constitution is established at fertilization and maintained by mitotic division in all cell types, including the primary germ cells.

2. Development of *gonadal sex*. In the early embryo, the gonad is undifferentiated. If the sex chromosome constitution is XX, an ovary will develop; if a Y chromosome is present, the indifferent gonad will develop as a testis. It is clear that testicular development is dependent on the presence of a Y chromosome, leading to the conclusion that the Y chromosome contains a gene or genes involved in initiation of testicular differentiation. According to a hypothesis advanced in 1975,[61] testicular induction depends on the presence of a phylogenetically conserved cell surface antigen (serologically detectable H-Y antigen) found in males but not in normal females. The way in which this antigen is controlled by genes on the Y chromosome and its exact role in sexual development are still a subject of controversy.[54] However, as will be discussed in the subsequent section on XX True Hermaphrodites and XX Males, serologically detectable H-Y antigen has provided special insight into the mechanisms involved in these defects.

3. Development of *phenotypic sex*. Once the gonad develops into a testicle or an ovary, differentiation of the internal and external genitalia follows (Fig. 1). The testis produces two factors, Müllerian inhibiting factor (MIF) and testosterone, which act to promote the formation of male structures. MIF, which is produced by Sertoli cells, acts locally to cause regression of the müllerian duct system. Testosterone, produced by the Leydig cells, stimulates the wolffian duct system, which becomes the epididymis and vas deferens. Testosterone is converted to dihydrotestosterone (DHT) by the enzyme 5-alpha-reductase in the tissues of the urogenital sinus and external genitalia. DHT induces the formation of the prostate and the closure of the urethral and labioscrotal folds, thus forming the penis, prepuce and scrotum. Descent of the testes into the scrotum completes the external genitalia. The controlling mechanism(s) for testicular descent are unclear at present.

In the absence of a testis and testis-dependent products (MIF, testosterone and dihydrotestosterone), the müllerian duct system persists, the wolffian duct system regresses, and the urogenital sinus and external genitalia retain their female characteristics. This results in a female genital tract (oviducts, uterus and cranial vagina) and external genitalia (vulva, caudal vagina and clitoris).

Intersexuality, that is, a condition in which the sex of the animal is ambiguous, can occur whenever any part of this complex sequence of events is disturbed. In evaluating disorders of sexual development, it is useful to think in terms of abnormalities of chromosomal sex (deviation from the normal XX or XY), gonadal sex (ovary or testis), or phenotypic sex (external and internal genitalia, exclusive of gonads). Our discussion of reported disorders of sexual development in the dog is arranged to follow this classification system:

I. Abnormalities of chromosomal sex
  A. XXY syndrome
  B. Triple-X syndrome
  C. Chimeras and mosaics
    1. True hermaphrodite chimeras
    2. XX/XY chimera with dysgenetic testes
II. Abnormalities of gonadal sex
  A. XX true hermaphroditism
  B. XX male syndrome
III. Abnormalities of phenotypic sex
  A. Female pseudohermaphroditism
  B. Male pseudohermaphroditism
    1. Hypospadias
    2. Persistent müllerian duct syndrome
    3. Other categories

Additional forms of abnormal sexual development are known to occur in man and other species but have not yet been reported in the dog.

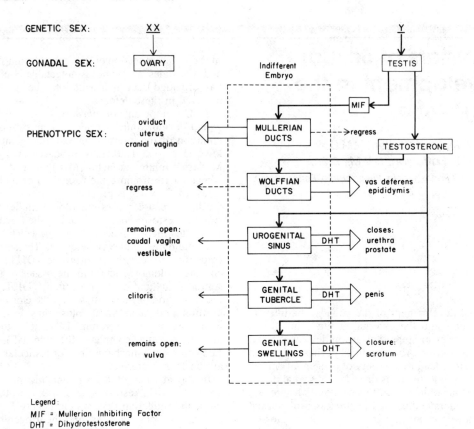

Figure 1. Differentiation of the internal and external genitalia after the gonad develops into a testicle or an ovary.

ABNORMALITIES OF CHROMOSOMAL SEX

With the exception of chimeras and mosaics, the abnormal sex chromosome constitutions reported in dogs give rise to males or females that have underdeveloped but not ambiguous genitalia. In chimeras and mosaics, the genitalia are often ambiguous.

The XXY Syndrome

The XXY syndrome, a condition analogous to human Klinefelter's syndrome, has been reported in the dog.[12] The dog was a phenotypic male, having a normal penis and prepuce and apparently normal male sexual behavior. Epididymides and small testes were present within the scrotum. Ejaculates contained no spermatozoa. Tubular dysgenesis of the testes with no evidence of spermatogenesis was present histologically. Cytogenetic studies revealed a 79,XXY chromosome constitution. An interventricular septal defect of the heart was also present in the affected dog, but this may have been unrelated to the XXY condition, since it has not been reported as a consistent component of the XXY syndrome in other species. The XXY syndrome should be suspected in any congenitally sterile male dog with small testes. Testicular histology and karyotype will confirm the diagnosis.

Human patients with multiple X chromosomes and a Y chromosome have a phenotype similar to individuals with Klinefelter's syndrome. The importance of the Y chromosome in directing male gonadal development is confirmed by these syndromes, since testicular differentiation occurs even in the presence of two or more X chromosomes. More than one X chromosome is apparently deleterious to normal spermatogenesis.

The XXY syndrome can arise by meiotic nondisjunction of the sex chromosomes during male or female gametogenesis or by mitotic nondisjunction in the early zygote. The incidence of Klinefelter's syndrome in human live-born infants is approximately 1 in 700 males.[60] Another common abnormality of chromosomal sex that can arise by nondisjunction, the XO syndrome, has not been reported in the dog but is known to occur in other domestic animals. The incidence of this syndrome (Turner's syndrome) in live-born human infants is 1 in 2500 females.[60] Affected individuals have a female phenotype but have dysgenetic ovaries and are usually examined for amenorrhea at the age of sexual maturity.

The Triple-X Syndrome

The triple-X syndrome has recently been observed in the dog,[28] and appears to be analogous to the triple-X syndrome in humans. The dog was a 4-year-old Airedale bitch presented with a history of failure to cycle. The external genitalia were those of a normal female except that the vagina was judged to be small by digital palpation. The internal genitalia consisted of small ovaries, oviducts and uterus. Histology of the ovaries showed no follicles, corpora lutea or primary oocytes. A 79,XXX chromosome constitution was found on chromosome analysis.

Though some human females with this condition are sterile, fertile triple-X females have been described.[15] The incidence of the triple-X syndrome in human live-born infants is 1 in 1000 females.[60] It is apparently rare in the general dog population, this being the only known case. Like the XXY and XO sex chromosome anomalies, the XXX condition is usually the result of an abnormality in chromosomal disjunction in meiosis.

Nondisjunctional events leading to abnormal sex chromosome constitutions generally are considered to occur randomly. There are thus no preventative measures and no effective therapy. Their chief importance in dogs is as a cause of sterility.

Chimeras and Mosaics

A chimera is an individual composed of two or more types of cells, each type arising from different sources and containing different chromosome constitutions. Fusion of two zygotes differing in sex chromosome constitution accounts for some XX/XY chimeras. A mosaic is an individual composed of two or more types of cells containing different chromosome constitutions, but the cells originate from the same source. A mosaic usually results from mitotic nondisjunction in a single zygote. This process could produce as many as three cell lines, but only two cell lines must survive in order to be defined as a mosaic. The sources of the cell lines in a chimera and a mosaic are different, but the end result is an animal composed of cells having different chromosome constitutions. Events producing these animals are random; familial aggregation is thus not expected.

The gonadal and phenotypic sex of chimeras and mosaics depends on the sex chromosome constitution of the separate cell lines and their distribution in the gonadal primordium. If one cell line contains a Y chromosome and the other does not, clearly demarcated ovarian and testicular tissue can develop in the same gonad, or the gonad can be dysgenetic, having a histologic architecture that has some features of both ovarian and testicular tissue but the typical appearance of neither.

True Hermaphrodite Chimeras. True hermaphrodites have both ovarian and testicular tissue. Ovotestes may represent one or both gonads, or one gonad may be an ovary and the other a testis, or there may be any combination of the above, such that ovarian and testicular tissue are both present. Several cases have been reported in the dog.[3, 21, 23, 29, 30, 32, 37, 40, 43, 44, 46, 52, 57, 58] In cases in which cytogenetic

studies were done, chimeras were rare.[3, 23] XX True hermaphrodites, which are more common, will be discussed with abnormalities of gonadal sex.

The three reported true hermaphrodite chimeras had either XX/XY or XX/XXY chromosome constitutions.[3, 23, 46] These dogs appeared externally to be females except that an enlarged clitoris was present in all, one dog having an os clitoris.[46] The dogs were presented with a history of failure to cycle or chronic vulvar irritation.

Internally, testicular and ovarian tissue and a uterus were present in all cases. The ovarian tissue contained follicles and in one case, graafian follicles were present.[46] Testicular tissue consisted of interstitial cells and seminiferous tubules with Sertoli cells. In only one case,[46] in which the ovotestis was in the inguinal canal, was there evidence of spermatogenesis.

XX/XY Chimera with Dysgenetic Testes. We have observed one XX/XY dog with dysgenetic testes and abnormal external genitalia. The animal was an Old English sheepdog with a history of failure to cycle by 2 years of age. The external genital opening was a cranially displaced vulvalike structure. A hypoplastic penis, classified as such because the urethral opening was at the cranial end, was contained within the vulvalike structure. No scrotum or testes was found on physical examination. At laparotomy, small gonads with the appearance of testes were located near the caudal pole of the kidneys. A small bicornuate uterus was present. Histopathology demonstrated dysgenetic testicular tissue lacking spermatogenesis. Chromosome analysis of blood lymphocytes showed approximately 1:1 XX/XY cells.

ABNORMALITIES OF GONADAL SEX

In this section, we will discuss primary abnormalities in gonadal sex determination. In affected individuals the chromosomal and gonadal sex do not agree. For this reason they are sometimes referred to as sex-reversed individuals.

XX True Hermaphroditism

In dogs, true hermaphrodites with an XX chromosome constitution have the external appearance of females but usually have an enlarged clitoris containing an os clitoris. The gonads are in an abdominal location and are usually ovotestes rather than separate ovary and testis. Some true hermaphrodites reproduce as females despite the presence of testicular tissue and clitoral enlargement.[52]

True hermaphroditism is apparently rare in the dog population. Thirteen isolated cases had been reported by 1976.[1, 23, 30, 32, 40, 43, 44, 57, 58, 62] Six cases were karyotyped,[1, 23, 57] and all were found to be 78,XX. Five of the 13 reported cases were cocker spaniels,[1, 30, 44, 52, 62] with a karyotype available in two cases.[1, 51] Recently a study of a large family of American cocker spaniels identified 9 XX true hermaphrodites and 2 XX males,[52, 52a] verifying that this is a genetically determined form of intersexuality.

The most common physical finding is an enlarged clitoris.[1, 30, 44, 57, 62] Attraction of male dogs was also reported in a few instances.[30, 44, 57] Diagnosis is obtained through (1) physical examination, which usually reveals an enlarged clitoris in an apparent female, (2) histologic examination of the gonads to confirm the presence of ovarian and testicular tissue, and (3) chromosome analysis, which will demonstrate a 78,XX chromosome constitution. In cocker spaniels and beagles XX true hermaphroditism occurs on a familial basis, and closely related dogs have the XX male syndrome. It is likely that the XX male syndrome and XX true hermaphroditism in these breeds are due to the same genetic defect, representing varying degrees of a common masculinizing event[52] (see following section).

The XX Male Syndrome

Individuals with this syndrome have a predominantly male phenotype, a 78,XX chromosome constitution, and are H-Y antigen positive.[52] The gonads are often cryptorchid testes and show no evidence of spermatogenesis. Seminiferous tubules with Sertoli cells are seen on histologic examination, but interstitial cells may[22] or may not[16] be evident. Although the penis is present, it is often malformed, sometimes being reported as a hypoplastic penis[16, 22, 56] with hypospadias.[52] In the cocker spaniel, affected dogs usually have persistent müllerian derivatives despite the presence of testicular tissue.[52a] Wolffian duct derivatives (vasa deferentia) may be found within the uterine myometrium.[22]

Diagnosis depends on the presence of bilateral hypoplastic, aspermatogenic testes in an animal with varying degrees of masculinization of the external genitalia and a 78,XX chromosome constitution. All of the XX male dogs we have seen had penile malformations, including hypoplasia and abnormal curvature.

This condition is apparently rare in the general dog population. However, nine of the eleven confirmed cases of XX male syndrome were cocker spaniels,[14, 16, 22, 52, 52a, 56, 66] and other intersex cocker spaniels have been described in which no cytogenetic studies were reported.[24, 43, 48] This, along with recent family studies,[52a] strongly supports an inherited etiology in cocker spaniels. It may be an inherited condition in the Chinese pug[56] and Kerry blue terrier,[66] because an XX male was one of three related intersex dogs described in each breed.

XX True hermaphroditism and the XX male syndrome may be partial and complete forms of sex reversal, the underlying defect being the same in both. XX True hermaphrodites and XX males have been shown to be H-Y antigen positive in both humans and dog.[52, 52a] This has led to the hypothesis that these conditions are due to the translocation of H-Y determining genes to the X chromosome or an autosome. Other explanations are also possible.

The mode of inheritance of XX true hermaphroditism and the XX male syndrome in cocker spaniels appears to be recessive, although it is not clear whether the gene is autosomal or X-linked recessive.[52a] At present, we do not recommend breeding affected dogs (fertile XX true hermaphrodites) or their parents. Although documentation of the familial nature of this condition and XX true hermaphroditism at present exists only for the cocker spaniel and beagle, the same or a similar defect probably occurs in other breeds.

ABNORMALITIES OF PHENOTYPIC SEX

In abnormalities of phenotypic sex, the chromosomal and gonadal sex agree, but there is some ambiguity in the genitalia. Affected animals are either female or male pseudohermaphrodites. A pseudohermaphrodite has the gonads of one sex with the internal or external genitalia of the opposite sex and is defined as male or female according to the gonadal sex. That is, a female pseudohermaphrodite has ovaries; a male pseudohermaphrodite has testes.

Female Pseudohermaphroditism

Naturally occurring female pseudohermaphroditism in the dog is rare.[23] In some cases the etiology is unknown,[1, 42, 49, 59] although the majority of reported cases are of iatrogenic etiology.[13, 23, 25, 38, 53, 65] With the exception of one possible chimera,[63] these dogs have an XX sex chromosome constitution and ovaries. They are masculinized females, the degree of masculinization ranging from mild clitoral enlargement (classified as such because the urethral meatus is not contained within the clitoris as it is in the penis) to nearly normal male external genitalia (penis and prepuce). Although a prostate may be present, there is a cranial vagina and uterus in all affected dogs.

Affected dogs have been presented as apparent males showing periodic signs of estrus, such as hematuria,[1, 36, 63] attractiveness to male dogs[1, 36, 63] or swelling of the vulvar/preputial tissues.[53] Cystic endometrial hyperplasia and pyometra may also be present.[53] Urethral abnormalities[5] and urinary incontinence, usually due to pooling of urine in the vagina or uterus,[18, 26, 27, 49, 59] have been associated with female pseudohermaphroditism.

A tentative diagnosis can be made from the gross appearance of a penis and prepuce externally, with uterus, vagina and ovaries internally. Confirmation of the classification of female pseudohermaphroditism requires cytogenetic studies showing a 78,XX chromosome constitution and histologic confirmation of bilateral ovaries. If signs of urinary tract disease are present, contrast studies should be done to establish the diagnosis and treatment of associated urinary tract complications.

The underlying cause of female pseudohermaphroditism may be difficult to determine. In humans, adrenogenital syndromes are a common cause of female pseudohermaphroditism. In general, these syndromes are due to metabolic errors that result in decreased cortisol production. Low cortisol levels allow an increase in ACTH production, which leads to an increase in cortisol precursors. Androgens are synthesized from the cortisol precursors because the metabolic error reduces the conversion to cortisol. The excess androgens masculinize the female genitalia. Adrenogenital syndromes have not been described as yet in the dog.

In some cases of canine female pseudohermaphroditism, the condition is known to be the result of androgen[38, 53] or progestagen[13] administration during gestation. If given during critical stages of development, female fetuses are virilized. In one study, female pseudohermaphrodites were produced when methyltestosterone was given throughout gestation.[53] In another report, mibolerone was given for the first 18 days of gestation.[38] In cases where progestagens were given, similar effects were produced when the hormones were given in the last trimester[13] or when given throughout gestation.[63] Few reports of this condition exist, and the prevalence in the general dog population is unknown. Prevention may be best achieved by avoidance of sex steroid administration during gestation.

Male Pseudohermaphroditism

Male pseudohermaphroditism was previously defined as a male individual with ambiguous genitalia and testes. With the advent of cytogenetics, we can now narrow the definition to individuals who also have an XY sex chromosome constitution. Many of the male pseudohermaphrodites previously reported were XX males.[23] In this discussion, we will limit the definition of male pseudohermaphrodites to dogs that have a Y chromosome, testes and internal or external genitalia with female characteristics. Excluding dogs that do not fit this description (e.g., XX males) leaves few cases of canine male pseudohermaphroditism. Included are individuals with unambiguous male external genitalia but female internal genitalia, and individuals with varying degrees of malformation of the penis, prepuce and scrotum. Male pseudohermaphroditism has been described in various breeds,[2, 4, 9, 10, 19, 33, 43] but chromosome analysis was not included in many of these reports. Two types of male pseudohermaphroditism that have been described in dogs are (1) various forms of hypospadias, and (2) the persistent müllerian duct syndrome.

Hypospadias. In uncomplicated cases of hypospadias, a normal male karyotype is expected and the external genitalia are abnormal but usually not ambiguous. The defect is an abnormality in the location of the urinary meatus, which is ventral and proximal to the normal site in the glans penis. Thus, the urinary orifice may be in the glans, the penile shaft, the penoscrotal junction or the perineum. The abnormality occurs as a result of incomplete closure of the urethral folds, which may be due to inadequate fetal testosterone or dihydrotestosterone production. A spectrum occurs from glanular hypospadias (mild) to perineal hypospadias (severe), which could be expected with variation in the severity of an androgen insufficiency.

Few reports of canine hypospadias are found in the literature, but this may not reflect the true prevalence in the dog population. As in man,[47] the condition may appear separately or in conjunction with other genital or somatic defects. Unilateral renal agenesis has been reported in association with one case of canine hypospadias.[35] Genital defects in association with hypospadias have included cryptorchidism, partial[35] or complete[9] absence of the scrotum, bifid scrotum[17] and persistent müllerian structures.[9]

In man, both familial and nonfamilial hypospadias occur. The probability of concurrent testicular abnormalities such as hypoplasia or cryptorchidism increases with the severity of the hypospadias. In the dog, familial hypospadias may be expected but has not been documented. Similarly, the probability of associated defects is unknown.

Male Pseudohermaphroditism—The Persistent Müllerian Duct Syndrome. The persistent müllerian duct syndrome in miniature schnauzers is a type of male pseudohermaphroditism in which müllerian derivatives persist in males having a Y chromosome. A number of cases have been reported in the veterinary literature.[8, 20, 31, 34, 50] Affected dogs are usually bilaterally or unilaterally cryptorchid but otherwise appear to be normal males externally. Internally, both testes are attached to the cranial ends of a bicornuate uterus. The testes may be in an ovarian position or within the inguinal ring or scrotum. If scrotal, the cranial uterine horn may be palpable. The cranial portion of the vagina[50] and a prostate[8, 50] are often present.

On histologic examination, the cryptorchid testes are hypoplastic without evidence of spermatogenesis. An epididymis is associated with each testis. Sertoli cell tumors in the cryptorchid testis are common.[8, 34] Squamous metaplasia of the prostate is also reported.[8] Common histologic uterine findings are cystic endometrial hyperplasia,[8, 34] pyometra[8, 20, 34, 50] and wolffian duct derivatives (vasa deferentia) within the myometrium.[34]

Most cases are presented for signs attributable to Sertoli cell tumor and/or pyometra. Bilaterally symmetrical alopecia, gynecomastia and abdominal discomfort were associated with Sertoli cell tumors in the cryptorchid testes.[8, 20, 31, 34] Acute onset of vomiting, polydipsia and abdominal enlargement due to pyometra were also common presenting signs.[8, 20, 34, 50] Diagnosis is confirmed by histologic examination of the testes, presence of müllerian structures and cytogenetic studies demonstrating a 78,XY karyotype, although one animal studied cytogenetically had a 79,XXY sex chromosome constitution.[34]

This syndrome appears to be the result of failure

of müllerian-inhibiting activity. The failure might occur by (1) an inability to synthesize müllerian inhibiting factor, (2) a defect in the timing of its secretion or transport, (3) synthesis of an inactive factor, or (4) nonresponsiveness of the ducts to the effects of the factor.[34] Synthesis of testosterone during development is presumably normal since Wolffian duct derivatives and the urogenital sinus develop normally.[34] An inherited etiology is likely because this disorder appears to occur predominantly in one breed, the miniature schnauzer.[8, 11, 20, 31, 34, 41, 50] There is evidence that the persistent müllerian duct syndrome in man is an inherited condition as well.[6, 55, 64] Prevention of this syndrome will rely on further studies to determine the mode of inheritance, which is presently unknown in the dog and man.[34]

Other Categories of Male Pseudohermaphroditism. At present it is unclear whether male pseudohermaphrodites in which a 78,XY chromosome constitution was reported in the beagle,[7] the German shepherd dog[11] and the Alsatian bull terrier[21] represent a condition(s) similar to the syndrome described in the miniature schnauzer. These other breeds had abdominal testes, uterus and vagina, but externally had an enlarged clitoris within a vulvalike structure. The external appearance of these dogs was that of masculinized females rather than normal males that were cryptorchid as seen in miniature schnauzers with persistent müllerian duct syndrome.

Two other forms of male pseudohermaphroditism in man that illustrate mechanisms of sexual development are the testicular feminization syndrome and 5-alpha-reductase deficiency.

The testicular feminization syndrome has been described in humans, mice and rats. The condition is inherited as an X-linked recessive trait. It is likely to occur in dogs as well but has not been documented. The syndrome is caused by a defect in the androgen cytosol receptor, resulting in an insensitivity to androgens. Thus, sexual differentiation that depends on testosterone or dihydrotestosterone does not occur. Müllerian regression occurs as expected, since müllerian-inhibiting factor is not affected. Humans with the testicular feminization syndrome have a normal male karyotype, bilateral (often cryptorchid) testes and female external genitalia. At puberty, these individuals become externally feminized as would be expected for normal females. They are usually presented for examination because they have an inguinal hernia or primary amenorrhea. This condition should be included in the differential diagnosis of apparent female dogs who fail to exhibit estrus.

Deficiency of 5-alpha-reductase, inherited as an autosomal recessive trait in humans, has not been described in dogs. This enzyme converts testosterone to dihydrotestosterone, the active cellular androgen. Tissues dependent on dihydrotestosterone for male sexual differentiation (Fig. 1) do not develop normally. The müllerian duct system regresses as expected. Affected individuals have a normal male karyotype, bilateral (often cryptorchid) testes

and ambiguous external genitalia. The term pseudovaginal perineoscrotal hypospadias has also been used to describe the syndrome of 5-alpha-reductase deficiency. The labioscrotal folds (genital swellings) do not fuse, and the urogenital sinus does not close in these individuals, resulting in perineoscrotal hypospadias and a blind pouch that resembles a vagina. The penis resembles a clitoris in size until puberty. Testosterone-dependent changes (e.g., phallic enlargement, increased facial hair, muscular hypertrophy and voice changes) do occur at puberty. There is no reason to doubt that this syndrome may occur in dogs, although it has yet to be described in this species.

DIAGNOSTIC AND THERAPEUTIC APPROACH TO CANINE INTERSEX CONDITIONS

In disorders of sexual development, definitive diagnosis rests upon the determination of phenotypic, gonadal and chromosomal sex. A thorough physical examination to establish phenotypic sex is the initial step in this investigation. The external genitalia should be described in detail. In particular, the site of the urethral meatus (at the tip of the penis or in the ventral vagina) should be noted so that the phallic structure can be properly termed a penis or a clitoris. The presence or absence of other structures, such as the scrotum, prostate, caudal vagina, vulva, prepuce and os clitoris should be noted. The position of the prepuce or vulva should also be described.

Laparotomy is often the next step taken in determining phenotypic sex. The presence or absence of urogenital sinus structures, such as the prostate and caudal vagina, should be noted. The gross appearance and location of the gonads should be described. Presence or absence of müllerian (oviduct, uterus, cranial vagina) and/or wolffian duct (epididymis, vas deferens) structures should be recorded. At this point, organs can be removed for diagnostic and therapeutic purposes.

With the exception of XX true hermaphrodites, most intersex dogs are sterile, and no therapy for infertility is indicated. Pyometra can occur in intersex animals having a uterus (see section on Persistent Müllerian Duct Syndrome), and for these, hysterectomy is recommended. Removal of the gonads is also indicated, since cryptorchid testicular tissue has an increased risk of Sertoli cell tumor development. Amputation of an enlarged clitoris is recommended in dogs in which the mucosal surfaces are exposed to drying or trauma. Plastic surgery of the prepuce and malformed penis may be required in dogs with the XX male syndrome or in dogs with hypospadias.

All excised tissues should be preserved for histologic examination. Histologic as well as gross examination of the gonads is essential for the diagnosis of gonadal sex. It may be necessary to section the gonad serially to identify an ovotestis.

In normal females, one of the two X chromosomes is inactivated in each cell and is seen as the sex chromatin body in interphase nuclei. The examination of buccal smears for sex chromatin bodies has been used as an adjunct to the diagnosis of chromosomal sex in humans and animals. The absence of sex chromatin bodies implies that less than two X chromosomes are present, while the occurrence of more than one sex chromatin body indicates the presence of more than two X chromosomes. Although this method does give preliminary information about the sex chromosome constitution, definitive diagnosis of the chromosomal status requires examination of the chromosomes directly. Chromosome preparations are usually derived from peripheral blood lymphocytes or fibroblasts that have been maintained in culture for a sufficient time to produce a large population of mitotic cells.[39, 45] A sufficient number of mitotic cells is examined to establish the presence or absence of more than one population of cells (chimerism or mosaicism), and a karyotype is constructed from at least one typical cell. Conventional methods of staining chromosomes usually are adequate for the identification of the X and Y chromosomes in the dog because they have unique morphologic characteristics, but the identification of minor structural defects requires the use of methods that have higher resolving power such as G-banding. This staining technique produces a pattern of banding along the chromosome arms that is characteristic of each chromosomal pair.[51]

A complete investigation of the dog with disorders of sexual development describing phenotypic, gonadal and chromosomal sex, as outlined above, is essential for a definitive diagnosis. A diagnosis is, in turn, essential if genetic counseling and preventive measures are to be undertaken. A complete family history should be taken in all cases. Pedigree analysis of the dog and related dogs is extremely helpful in establishing whether the condition is heritable. Genetic counseling and preventive measures for inherited disorders of sexual development depend on knowledge of the mode of inheritance. At present, knowledge of the mode of inheritance of most canine disorders of sexual development is incomplete. The description of accurately diagnosed cases with further pedigree analyses will lead to a better understanding of the inheritance of these conditions in dogs and other animals.

ACKNOWLEDGEMENT

Original observations described in this chapter were supported by the University of Pennsylvania Genetics Center Grant from the National Institutes of Health (GM 20138).

References

1. Allen WE, Daker MG, Hancock JL: Three intersexual dogs. Vet Rec 109:468, 1981.
2. Axelson RD: Pseudohermaphroditism in a dog. J Am Vet Med Assoc 172:584, 1978.
3. Bosu WTK, Chick BF, Basrur PK: Clinical, pathologic and cytogenetic observations on two intersex dogs. Cornell Vet 68:376, 1978.
4. Brodey RS, Martin JE, Lee DG: Male pseudohermaphroditism in a toy terrier. J Am Vet Med Assoc 125:368, 1954.
5. Brodey RS, McFarland LZ: Vulvar anomaly in a dog. J Am Vet Med Assoc 143:1326, 1963.
6. Brook CGD, Wagner H, Zachmann M, et al.: Familial occurrence of persistent Müllerian structures in otherwise normal males. Br Med J 1:771, 1973.
7. Brown RC, Swanton MC, Brinkhous KM: Canine hemophilia and male pseudohermaphroditism: Cytogenetic studies. Lab Invest 12:961, 1963.
8. Brown TT, Burek JD, McEntee K: Male pseudohermaphroditism, cryptorchism and Sertoli cell neoplasia in three Miniature Schnauzers. J Am Vet Med Assoc 169:821, 1976.
9. Browne TG: Hermaphroditism in a dog. Vet J Lond 81:144, 1925.
10. Carillo JM, Burk RL: Male pseudohermaphrodism associated with urinary incontinence in an Afghan. J Am Anim Hosp Assoc 13:80, 1977.
11. Chauffaux S, Mailhac JM, Cribiu EP, et al.: L'intersexualite chez le chien (*Canis familiaris*). A propos de quatre cas. Rec Med Vet 156:179, 1980.
12. Clough E, Pyle RL, Hare WCD, et al.: An XXY sex-chromosome constitution in a dog with testicular hypoplasia and congenital heart disease. Cytogenetics 9:71, 1970.
13. Curtis EM, Grant RP: Masculinization of female pups by progestogens. J Am Vet Med Assoc 144:395, 1964.
14. Dain AR: Intersexuality in a Cocker Spaniel dog. J Reprod Fertil 39:365, 1974.
15. Day RW, Larson W, Wright SW: Clinical and cytogenetic studies on a group of females with XXX sex chromosome complements. J Pediat 64:24, 1964.
16. Edols JH, Allan GS: A case of male pseudohermaphroditism in a Cocker Spaniel. Aust Vet J 44:287, 1968.
17. Finco DR, Thrall DE, Duncan JR: The urinary system. *In* Catcott EJ (ed): Canine Medicine. Santa Barbara, Am Vet Publ, 1979, pp 489.
18. Firth LK: What is your diagnosis? J Am Vet Med Assoc 166:93, 1975.
19. Fralick RL, Murray RC: Pseudohermaphroditism in an adult dog. Anat Rec 100:741, 1948.
20. Frey DC, Tyler DE, Ramsey FK: Pyometra associated with bilateral cryptorchism and Sertoli's cell tumor in a male pseudohermaphrodite dog. J Am Vet Med Assoc 146:723, 1965.
21. Gerneke WH, deBoom HPA, Heinichen IG: Two canine intersexes. J S Afr Vet Med Assoc 39:55, 1968.
22. Hare WCD, McFeely RA, Kelly DF: Familial 78XX male pseudohermaphroditism in three dogs. J Reprod Fertil 36:207, 1974.
23. Hare WCD: Intersexuality in the dog. Can Vet J 17:7, 1976.
24. Hernaman-Johnson K: Complex hermaphrodism in a Cocker. Vet Rec 15:1099, 1935.
25. Hinsch GW: Intersexes in the dog. Teratol 20:463, 1979.
26. Hoffman R: Pseudohermaphroditism (feminine) in a Shepherd dog. Dtsch Tieraerztl Wochenschr 79:393, 1972.
27. Jackson DA, Osborne CA, Brasmer TH, Jessen CR: Nonneurogenic urinary incontinence in a canine female pseudohermaphrodite. J Am Vet Med Assoc 172:926, 1978.
28. Johnston SD: Personal communication.
29. King NW, Garvin CH: Bilateral hermaphroditism in a dog. J Am Vet Med Assoc 145:997, 1964.
30. Lawrence J, Meisels R: A lateral canine hermaphrodite. J Am Vet Med Assoc 121:171, 1952.
31. Lederer HA: What is your diagnosis? J Am Vet Med Assoc 167:239, 1975.
32. Lee DG, Allam MW: True unilateral hermaphroditism in a dog. Vet Ext Q Univ Penn 128:142, 1952.
33. Leighton RL: Ablation of the penis and castration in a male pseudohermaphrodite dog. J Am Anim Hosp Assoc 12:664, 1976.
34. Marshall LS, Oehlert ML, Haskins ME, et al.: Persistent Müllerian duct syndrome in Miniature Schnauzers. J Am Vet Med Assoc 181:798, 1982.

35. McFarland LZ, Deniz E: Unilateral renal agenesis with ipsilateral cryptorchidism and perineal hypospadias in a dog. J Am Vet Med Assoc 139:1099, 1961.

36. McFeely RA, Biggers JD: A rare case of female pseudohermaphroditism in the dog. Vet Rec 77:696, 1965.

37. McFeely RA, Hare WCD, Biggers JD: Chromosome studies in 14 cases of intersex in domestic mammals. Cytogenetics 6:242, 1967.

38. Medleau L, Johnson CA, Perry RL, Dulisch ML: Female pseudohermaphroditism associated with mibolerone administration in a dog. J Am Anim Hosp Assoc 19:213, 1983.

39. Moorhead PS, Nowell PC: Chromosome cytology. *In* Eisen HN (ed): Methods in Medical Research. Chicago, Year Book Medical Publishers, 1964, pp 310.

40. Murti GS, Gilbert DL, Borgmann AR: Canine intersex states. J Am Vet Med Assoc 149:1183, 1966.

41. Norrdin RW, Baum AC: A male pseudohermaphrodite dog with a Sertoli's cell tumor, mucometra and vaginal glands. J Am Vet Med Assoc 156:204, 1970.

42. Perl S, Klopfer U, Nyska A, Bornstein S: A case of female pseudohermaphroditism in a dog. Refuah Veterinarith 36:143, 1979.

43. Phillips JM, Brief BJ, Sutton TS, Mills JW: Hermaphroditism. J Am Vet Med Assoc 95:663, 1939.

44. Potter WR, Riggott JM: A pseudohermaphrodite dog. Vet Rec 80:647, 1967.

45. Priest JH: Cytogenetics. Philadelphia, Lea & Febiger, 1969, p 192.

46. Pullen CM: True bilateral hermaphroditism in a Beagle: A case report. Am J Vet Res 31:1113, 1970.

47. Rimoin DL, Schimke RN: Genetic disorders of the endocrine glands. St. Louis, CV Mosby Co, 1971.

48. Robb JR: Pseudohermaphroditism in a Cocker Spaniel. North Am Vet 24:426, 1943.

49. Rothinzen J, Voorhout G, Okkens AC, Biewenga WJ: Urovagina associated with female pseudohermaphroditism in four bitches from one litter. Tijdschr Diergeneesk 103:1109, 1978.

50. Salkin MS: Pyometra in a male pseudohermaphrodite dog. J Am Vet Med Assoc 172:913, 1978.

51. Selden JR, Moorhead PS, Oehlert ML, Patterson DF: The giemsa banding pattern of the canine karyotype. Cytogenet Cell Genet 15:380, 1975.

52. Selden JR, Wachtel SS, Koo GC, et al.: Genetic basis of XX male syndrome and XX true hermaphroditism: Evidence in the dog. Science 201:644, 1978.

52a. Selden JR, Moorhead PS, Koo GC, Wachtel SS, Patterson DF: Inherited XX sex reversal in the cocker spaniel dog. Human Genetics 67:62, 1984.

53. Shane BS, Dunn HO, Kenney RM, et al.: Methyl testosterone-induced female pseudohermaphroditism in dogs. Biol Reprod 1:41, 1969.

54. Silvers WK, Gasser DL, Eicher EM: H-Y antigen, serologically detectable male antigen and sex determination. Cell 28:439, 1982.

55. Sloan WR, Walsh PC: Familial persistent Müllerian duct syndrome. J Urol 115:459, 1976.

56. Stewart RW, Menges RW, Selby LA, et al.: Canine intersexuality in a pug breeding kennel. Cornell Vet 62:464, 1972.

57. Tangner CH, Breider MA, Amoss MS: Lateral hermaphroditism in a dog. J Am Vet Med Assoc 181:70, 1982.

58. Vandevelde JE: True hermaphroditism in a dog. Can Vet J 6:241, 1965.

59. Van Schouwenburg SJEM, Louw GJ: A case of dysuria as a result of a communication between the urinary bladder and corpus uteri in a cairn terrier. J S Afr Vet Assoc 53:65, 1982.

60. Vogel F, Motulsky AG: Human Genetics: Problems and Approaches. Berlin, Springer-Verlag, 1979, p 67.

61. Wachtel SS, Ohno S, Koo GC, Boyse EA: Possible role for H-Y antigen in the primary determination of sex. Nature 257:23, 1975.

62. Walker RG: Hermaphroditism in a bitch. A case report. Vet Rec 73:670, 1961.

63. Weaver AS, Harvey MJ, Munro CD, et al.: Phenotypic intersex (female pseudohermaphroditism) in a dachshund dog. Vet Rec 105:230, 1979.

64. Weiss EB, Kiefer JH, Rowlatt UF, and Rosenthal IM: Persistent Müllerian duct syndrome in male identical twins. Pediatrics 61:797, 1978.

65. Wentink GH, Breeuwsma AJ, Goedegebuure SA, Teunissen GHB: Drie gevallen van hermaphroditismus bij de hond. Tijdschr Diergeneesk 98:437, 1973.

66. Williamson JH: Intersexuality in a family of Kerry Blue Terriers. J Hered 70:138, 1979.

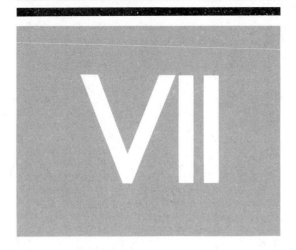

SECTION VII

CAPRINE

Mary C. Smith, D.V.M.

Consulting Editor

The Reproductive Anatomy and Physiology of the Female Goat

Mary C. Smith, D.V.M.
Cornell University, Ithaca, New York

ANATOMY

The ovaries of the goat may be round, oval, elongated or heart shaped. The longest dimension is approximately 2.2 cm in European goats[7] and the weight of each ovary varies from 1.8 to 3.5 gm, depending on the presence and number of corpora lutea. The ovaries are smooth and shiny. Large follicles near the surface (up to 1.2 cm diameter) often have a bluish tinge, while the corpus luteum gives the ovary a pink appearance. When several large follicles are present, the ovary may resemble a cluster of grapes. The right ovary is generally more active than the left.[8] Parovarian cysts in the bursa and mesosalpinx have been observed.

The uterine tubes (oviducts) are long and sinuous, and the uterine horns are also long and coiled. Approximately 115 to 120 caruncles with a concave surface, arranged in four rows in each horn, are very distinct, even in virgin does (Fig. 1). Older, parous animals commonly have melanin pigment in the caruncles and intercaruncular endometrium. The short body of the uterus joins with the firm and fibrous cervix. The cervix has a number of transverse folds or rings, often about five, and is commonly 5 to 6 cm long. Microscopic coiled glands within the cervix produce mucus.

The average length of the vagina is 7.3 cm, and the vestibule is an additional 3.6 cm long. A suburethral diverticulum is present on the floor of the vagina, and occasionally Gartner's ducts located ventrally on each side of the vagina are distended with thick, yellowish mucus. The vestibular glands have received little or no attention. Black pigmentation may be present in the vestibule. The clitoris normally should not be visible between the lips of the vulva. A large clitoris suggests that the doe is actually an intersex.

CLINICAL EXAMINATION

Clinical examination of the female goat's reproductive tract is limited by the impossibility of rectal examination in most animals. Laparoscopy has been used experimentally to allow observation of the ovaries and uterus in the living goat.[4] After tranquilization with 2.2 mg/kg of promazine hydrochloride, the animal is restrained on her back in a V trough. Under local anesthesia, a pediatric laparoscope is inserted through a trocar cannula. The abdomen is inflated with 5 per cent carbon dioxide in air or nitrogen, and a 5 mm tactile probe is used to manipulate the internal organs and expose them for observation. Examination with the animal in the standing position is usually unrewarding, especially without abdominal insufflation and without the use of a tactile probe.

For the average practitioner who would not have a laparoscope, an exploratory midline or flank laparotomy under halothane or ketamine plus xylazine anesthesia would be faster and easier. Visualization and palpation of the internal genitalia and acquisition of specimens from the uterus for biopsy and culture are readily accomplished. The intrapelvic position of the nongravid organs will hamper an ovariohysterectomy unless the incision is made as close as possible to the udder.

The vagina and cervical os can be examined either digitally or with a speculum, after careful cleaning of the vulva. See the article Semen Freezing and AI for details about the use of the speculum. If a short piece of rubber tubing is attached to a pipette, vaginal or cervical mucus can be aspirated for closer observation or culture.

Examination of the vulva is easy and should not be neglected. Neoplasms, ectopic mammary tissue, pox virus lesions or staphylococcal dermatitis may be evident. In addition, slight reddening and swelling of the vulva often accompany estrus.

PUBERTY

The well-fed female of one of the European breeds commonly reaches sexual maturity and begins to show signs of estrus at 6 to 8 months of age. In Pygmy goats this may occur as early as 3 months, and occasionally, even doelings of the larger breeds cycle this young. Generally, breeding should be delayed until the animal has attained 60 per cent or more of its adult weight. Angora goats should weigh a minimun of 27 kg; larger dairy goat breeds should weigh 32 to 41 kg before breeding. If these guidelines are followed, higher conception rates and safer parturitions will be achieved.

THE ESTROUS CYCLE

During the normal breeding season (August to March, and especially October to December in temperate latitudes), goats are polyestrous. Near the equator, they cycle year round. The normal

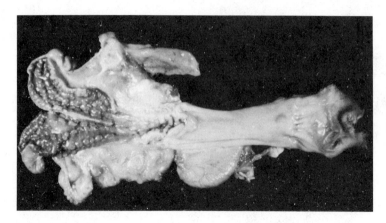

Figure 1. Normal female reproductive tract opened longitudinally to expose vagina, cervical rings and caruncles. (Courtesy of Dr. K. McEntee.)

estrous cycle of the dairy goat is approximately 20 to 21 days, while Pygmy goats are variously reported as having average cycles of 18- to 24-days. The estrous cycles are usually more erratic at the beginning and the end of the breeding season. Short cycles of less than 12 days, and often of only 5 to 7 days, are quite common, especially in young does. Estrus is occasionally observed during pregnancy.

Proestrus often lasts about 1 day. It is a period when the buck or teaser closely follows the doe, but she will not stand to be mounted. Estrus, or standing heat, lasts a variable time, often 12 to 24 hours. Metestrus is the time from refusal to mate until formation of one or more corpora lutea. Ovulation is variously reported to occur 12 to 36 hours after the onset of standing heat. Diestrus, the period of corpus luteum function, is the longest portion of the cycle.

Endocrinology. During estrus, as during seasonal anestrus, the plasma progesterone concentration is less than 1 ng/ml. Progesterone values reported during the luteal phase (typically 4 to 8 ng/ml) are variable and depend on the number of corpora lutea present and the assay procedure used.[6, 12] The progesterone concentration drops off precipitously 3 days before the next estrus. During the last 2 days of the cycle, 17-β estradiol rises from a baseline of about 8 to 10 pg/ml to a maximum of about 32 pg/ml at the beginning of standing estrus, only to fall to baseline again 12 hours later. Peak plasma levels of luteinizing hormone (LH), follicle-stimulating hormone (FSH) and prolactin are observed during estrus, within a few hours after the estradiol peak. A second FSH peak has been detected 48 hours after the first.[3] This sequence of hormonal events is quite similar to that reported for the ewe and the cow.

Estrus Detection. A teaser or breeding buck is best able to elicit and detect signs of estrus in the doe. If a buck is introduced into the herd at the beginning of the breeding season, the does will show heat in an average of 5 to 8 days. Standing and riding behavior among does is not as common as with cows. Many does will not cycle visibly unless a buck or another source of the buck odor, such as a burlap bag that has been rubbed all over the buck, is present in the environs. A common method of heat detection for small herds is to rub a rag on the rank buck's scent glands, caudomedial to his horns, and store this rag in a tightly covered container. The buck jar is opened and presented warm to the doe each day; when in estrus, she will be very interested in the jar. If the buck himself is present, the two animals will stay close together. If separated, they will restlessly search the perimeter of their enclosures for a means of escape.

The external genitalia may be more swollen, reddened and more moist during estrus, but these signs are not dependable with all does. Rapid side-to-side or up-and-down tail flagging is a good sign of heat that can often be detected in the absence of a buck. The behavior probably serves to spread odors from the doe's vulva to any nearby males. Restlessness and a tendency to be more vocal than usual are also commonly observed. Urination may increase in frequency. Milk production and appetite may decrease.

Vaginal smears have been used to identify the stage of the estrous cycle with only partial success.[5] The period of standing heat corresponds fairly well with the appearance of greater than 50 per cent desquamated, eosinophilic, polyhedral epithelial cells in the vaginal smear. These cells decline rapidly and are replaced by more basophilic and spherical epithelial cells, which continue to be present until just before the next estrous period. Metestrous leukocytes with compact nuclei appear in the smear at the time of ovulation.

A speculum examination of the cervix may be more helpful in detecting estrus. At the beginning of heat, the vaginal mucosa is reddened and moist, but little mucus is present. As heat progresses, a variable amount of transparent mucus is visible in the cervix and on the floor of the vagina. This mucus later turns cloudy and finally is cheesy white at the end of heat. Conception is best when the doe is bred at the stage at which her cervical mucus is cloudy and the cervical os is relaxed. Metestrous hemorrhage, as seen in the cow, is not reported to occur.

GESTATION

The percentage of multiple births seems to vary with the population under study. Twins or triplets are usually more common than single kids, except in primiparous animals. Quadruplets are not rare. In Angora goats, at least, the ovulation rate is 20 per cent higher on the second heat than on the first heat of the breeding season. Fertilized ova commonly migrate to the opposite horn in multiple births, allowing better spacing of conceptuses.

The plasma level of progesterone, which is produced almost entirely by the corpora lutea of the pregnant goat and not by the placenta, remains high until about 4 days before parturition. Estrone sulfate (from the fetus or placenta) begins to rise at 40 to 50 days of gestation, and can be used for pregnancy diagnosis after this time.[10] Peak estrogen levels are reached at parturition; a very low level is found 1 day after parturition.[2] Placental lactogen, which is also produced by the placenta and thus can be used for pregnancy diagnosis and prediction of litter size, follows a similar pattern. Placental lactogen is first detectable at about 60 days of gestation.[11] Prolactin levels are generally low during pregnancy but rise on the day of parturition. Oxytocin does not appear until the second stage of labor.

Although slight breed differences do exist, the average duration of gestation is generally reported as 5 months, or 150 days (varying from 147 to 155 days).[1] There is little effect of litter size on gestation length; quadruplets are born only 3 days earlier than single kids.[9]

References

1. Asdell SA: Variation in the duration of gestation in the goat. J Agric Sci 19:382, 1929.
2. Challis JRG, Linzell JL: The concentration of total unconjugated oestrogens in the plasma of pregnant goats. J Reprod Fert 26:401, 1971.
3. Chemineau P, Gauthier D, Poirier JC, et al.: Plasma levels of LH, FSH, prolactin, oestradiol-17 and progesterone during natural and induced oestrus in the dairy goat. Theriogenology 17:313, 1982.
4. Dukelow WR, Jarosz SJ, Jewett DA, Harrison RM: Laparoscopic examination of the ovaries in goats and primates. Lab Anim Sci 21:594, 1971.
5. Jarosz SJ, Deans RJ, Dukelow WR: The reproductive cycle of the African pygmy and Toggenburg goat. J Reprod Fert 24:119, 1971.
6. Jones DE, Knifton A: Progesterone concentration in the peripheral plasma of goats during the oestrus cycle. Res Vet Sci 13:193, 1972.
7. Lyngset O: Studies on reproduction in the goat. 1. The normal genital organs of the nonpregnant goat. Acta Vet Scand 9:208, 1968.
8. Lyngset O: Studies on reproduction in the goat. III. The functional activity of the ovaries of the goat. Acta Vet Scand 9:268, 1968.
9. Peaker M: Gestation period and litter size in the goat. Br Vet J 134:379, 1978.
10. Refsal KR, Marteniuk JV, Nachreiner RF, Williams CSF: Effects of gestation length and fetal number on serum estrone sulfate concentrations in pregnant goats. Proc. 10th Int Congr Anim Reprod AI. Illinois, June 10–14, V2:96, 1984.
11. Thomas CR, Forsyth IA, Hart IC: Goat placental lactogen: Levels through pregnancy and variation over 24 hour periods. J Endocrinol 75:51P, 1977.
12. Thorburn GD, Schneider W: The progesterone concentration in the plasma of the goat during the oestrus cycle and pregnancy. J Endocrinol 52:23, 1972.

Induction of Estrus in Does by Introduction of Buck or Photoperiod Manipulation

R.H. BonDurant, D.V.M.
University of California, Davis, California

Two nonhormonal methods for altering the breeding season of does include the sudden introduction of the buck and the use of an artificially altered photoperiod. In general the sudden introduction of a male to a group of mature females during the period of transition from anestrus to estrus can be expected to advance the breeding season by a matter of weeks, whereas the use of photoperiod alteration can allow for the breeding of does during the traditional "deep anestrous" time of year. It is also possible to combine the two techniques in order to achieve both "out of season" breeding and synchronization of estrus.

BUCK EFFECT

By analyzing kidding data from Angora does, Shelton[3] deduced that females apparently bred within 8 to 12 days of the introduction of a buck. Recently, prospective studies have shown clearly that the introduction of a normal or teaser male induces estrus and ovulation in mature transition-period does within 5 to 7 days. The induced estrus and ovulation are reasonably synchronized[2] (Fig. 1).

The precise mechanism for this induction is not completely understood, but seems to be mediated

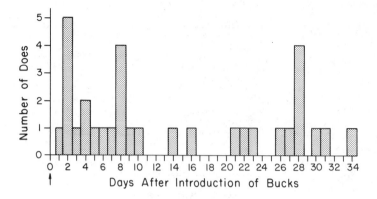

Figure 1. Number of does showing behavioral estrus after introduction of bucks on day 0. (↑ = bucks introduced.) Out of 17 does, 16 exhibited estrus within 21 days of exposure, with a mean of 5.5 days to first estrus. (From Ott RS, et al.: Theriogenology 13:187, 1980.)

Figure 2. Serum progesterone concentrations of four does experiencing short interestrus intervals after exposure to bucks. (Onset of estrus = ↓.) (From Ott RS, et al.: Theriogenology 13:189, 1980.)

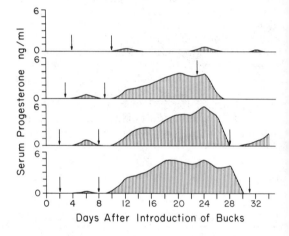

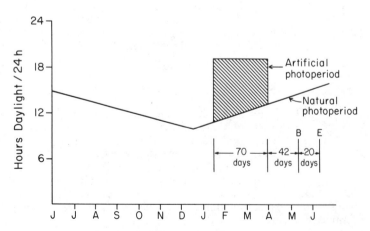

Figure 3. Lighting/management protocol for induction of estrus in yearling does (northern hemisphere). (B = buck introduced; E = first estrus.) (From Bon-Durant RH, et al.: J. Reprod. Fert. 63:2, 1981.)

through an induced surge of luteinizing hormone (LH). In any case, a group of does can be bred earlier (e.g., August in the northern temperate regions) if they are suddenly introduced to an *intact* male. If it is desirable to ascertain that the does are responding prior to breeding, as with an artificial insemination program, then the introduced male can be a surgically prepared teaser. The use of a marking harness, or simply painting the brisket of the teaser, should allow for the detection of responding does. Since the cycle induced by the buck is occasionally of abnormally short length and can be associated with insufficient luteal function (Fig. 2), this practice will preclude the possibility of breeding induced does at an infertile estrus. In cases studied to date an induced "short cycle" is usually followed by a cycle of normal length. Therefore, once it has been determined that the does are cycling in response to a male, the teaser can be removed and replaced by a breeding buck or by artificial insemination.

PHOTOPERIOD ALTERATION

Many studies have shown that the adult ewe is susceptible to induction of estrus by manipulation of length of daylight. Few controlled studies are available for mature goats, but it is known that yearling does can be induced into estrus at least 60 to 80 days early by providing feeding areas of a barn with 19 hours of artificial light per day, beginning in mid to late winter. An inexpensive timer is set to turn on the lights (a pair of 8-foot, 40-watt fluorescent tubes for each 36 to 40 square meters of pen space) at approximately 0500 and to turn them off 19 hours later. Animals should be fed in the evening, to encourage them to expose themselves to the augmented light. A protocol for lighting and animal management is shown in Figure 3. Note that "light tight" facilities are not necessary, since artificial light is merely added to the normal length of day. Apparently, the relative decrease in length of day when the artificial light is terminated, is the stimulus that induces hypothalamic events leading to estrus and fertile ovulation.

In the work so far reported the bucks have also been treated with supplemental light. It is not known if this measure is necessary, although seasonal changes in testicular function of sheep and goats are known to occur and may be reversed by photoperiod manipulation.

The physiological mechanisms that translate "decreased" length of daylight into estrus and ovulation are under study. When photoperiod-primed yearling does are suddenly exposed to bucks, there is a surge of LH within about 2 weeks. This first surge apparently does not induce ovulation, but may be responsible for the very slight rise in progesterone that follows and that precedes estrus by 2 to 4 days. This estrus may be tightly synchronized. It would appear, then, that the relative decrease in length of day may condition hypothalamic responses necessary to allow the "buck effect" in yearling does. The success of this method has not been examined in a controlled fashion for lactating does, but some producers have reported success rates similar to those achieved with yearlings.

References

1. BonDurant RH, Darien BJ, Munro CJ, et al.: Photoperiod induction of fertile oestrus and changes in LH and progesterone concentrations in yearling dairy goats (*Capra hircus*). J Reprod Fert 63:1, 1981.
2. Ott RS, Nelson DR, Hixon JE: Effect of presence of the male on initiation of estrous cycle activity of goats. Theriogenology 13:183, 1980.
3. Shelton M: The influence of presence of a male goat on the initiation of estrous cycling and ovulation of Angora does. J Anim Sci 19:368, 375, 1960.

Synchronization of Estrus and the Use of Implants and Vaginal Sponges

Mary C. Smith, D.V.M.
Cornell University, Ithaca, New York

There are several indications for manipulating the estrous cycle of the doe. Breeding outside the normal season may be desirable for animals that have failed to conceive or have aborted or for a percentage of a commercial herd when maintenance of a steady production level is necessary.[4] In season, some owners who are rarely home or who lack a buck have difficulty detecting natural estrus. At all times it would be convenient if estrus were to occur dependably when the buck could be available or when the doe could best be transported to it. Synchronization is also a helpful tool for embryo transfer.

SYNCHRONIZATION DURING THE BREEDING SEASON

During the breeding season synchronization may be achieved by inducing resorption of the corpus luteum and shortening of a cycle or by overriding the goat's system with exogenous progesterone to prolong a cycle. Prostaglandin would appear to be the drug of choice for shortening the cycle. Its use is described in a separate article.

Progesterone used to prolong the estrous cycle can be supplied in several forms. When fluoroge-stone acetate (FGA, 45 mg) impregnated vaginal pessaries are implanted for 16 to 21 days (preferably with administration of 400 to 500 IU of pregnant mare serum gonadotropin (PMSG) at the time of sponge removal, with or without administration of up to 500 IU of human chorionic gonadotropin (hCG) at the first sign of heat), ovulation has been successfully induced with 55 to 90 per cent fertility. Heat occurs 20 to 40 hours after sponge removal. The mucopurulent vaginal discharge that is evident when the sponge is pulled does not interfere with fertility but can be partially controlled by spraying the sponge with antibiotics at the time of insertion. Occasional adhesion of the pessary to the vagina in virgin does has been reported. On the other hand, sponges may be lost if the strings are not trimmed short to prevent extraction by other goats in the pen.

To avoid the difficulties sometimes associated with pessaries, removable subcutaneous implants of 375 mg progesterone or of 60 to 70 mg methylace-toxyprogesterone (MAP) in Silastic tubing have been used. A portion of a bovine norgestomet implant (3 mg/goat) is another alternative.[7]

Oral MAP at 50 mg/day for 16 days will bring does into heat on the third or fourth day after treatment ends, with acceptable fertility. (Pessaries impregnated with MAP have also been used.) Injectable progesterone, at 10 mg/day, or 20 mg every second day for 10 to 16 days, may be used if the labor involved is not prohibitive.

Although fertility may be decreased somewhat on the induced heat, it will usually return to normal on the subsequent cycle. It is also possible to administer prostaglandin during the luteal phase following the induced estrus, to synchronize a second estrus at a reduced interval.

SYNCHRONIZATION OUTSIDE THE BREEDING SEASON

Outside the normal breeding season, the average doe is not cycling, blood progesterone levels are very low (less than 1 ng/ml) and there is little ovarian activity. The use of artificial lighting to simulate decreasing day length and thereby initiate cycling is discussed in a separate article. The ability of a buck to trigger cycles during shallow anestrus should also be noted. Although these techniques do not actually synchronize estrous cycles, they permit out-of-season breeding and are readily available to all owners with no government restrictions.

Alternatively, hormones may be used in various dosages and combinations to induce follicle formation and ovulation. Progestogen vaginal pessaries have been used with variable results. Fluorogestone acetate (FGA) sponges implanted for 16 to 21 days can be used successfully outside the breeding season (40 per cent conception with artificial insemination) and administration of 400 to 600 IU of PMSG 48 hours before sponge removal improves fertility (65 per cent conception rate). Hormone dosage is an important consideration, as 45 mg FGA is superior to the 20-mg dose used in some studies. Increasing the number of live sperm per insemination also improves conception during the anestrous season, as will breeding twice 12 hours apart.[5] A newer technique involves the placement of a 45-mg FGA sponge for only 11 days, with administration of both PMSG (500 to 700 IU) and cloprostenol (200 µg) 48 hours before sponge removal. This permits a 65 per cent kidding rate after a single insemination.[6] Most published trials, except those from France, involve too few animals to permit statistical comparison of methods.

In several very small studies ovulation has been achieved outside the breeding season by daily injections of 100 μg of gonadotropin-releasing hormone (GnRH) for 4 or 5 days or by a single injection of 300 μg GnRH.[8] Heat began 2 days after the first treatment with the daily injections and was induced by estradiol injection in the other trial.

Unfortunately, almost all hormonal techniques proven to be effective outside the normal season require the use of PMSG. This product currently is not available commercially in the United States and its importation without special permit is illegal. The substitution of follicle-stimulating hormone (FSH, 2 mg repeated in 12 hours) is possible, but its comparative efficacy is unknown.

When hormones are administered for the purpose of ova transfer, higher doses of PMSG, FSH[3] or horse anterior pituitary extract (HAP)[9] will stimulate the production of more follicles. The fertilized ova are collected approximately 3 to 5 days after insemination by flushing the reproductive tract from the fimbriae to an incision in the uterine horn.[1] As handling the oviduct induces adhesions, other workers distend and drain each uterine horn via a cuffed catheter placed near the base of the horn. The ova are then surgically transferred to a synchronized recipient. Normally, fertilized eggs enter the uterus 4 days after mating. The early development of the caprine embryo has been described by Amoroso and colleagues.[2]

References

1. Agrawal KP, Mongha IV, Bhattacharyya NK: Collection and transfer of embryo in goats: Surgical method. Ind Vet J 59:298, 1982.
2. Amoroso EC, Griffiths WFB, Hamilton WJ: The early development of the goat (*Capra hircus*). J Anat Lond 76:377, 1942.
3. Armstrong DT, Evans G: Hormonal regulation of reproduction: Induction of ovulation in sheep and goats with FSH preparations. Proc 10th Int Congr Anim Reprod AI. Illinois, June 10–14, 1984, VII-8.
4. Barker CAV: Synchronization of estrus in dairy goats by progestin impregnated vaginal pessaries. Can Vet J 7:215, 1966.
5. Corteel JM: The use of progestagens to control the oestrus cycle of the dairy goat. Ann Biol Anim Bioch Biophys 15:353, 1975.
6. Corteel JM, Baril G, Leboeuf B, Boue P: A comparison of two hormonal treatments to provoke oestrus and ovulation in the anestrous dairy goat. Proc 10th Int Congr Anim Reprod AI. Illinois, June 10–14, 1984, p 313.
7. Corteel JM, Gonzalez C, Nunes JF: Research and development in the control of reproduction. Proc 3rd Int Conf Goat Prod Dis. Arizona, 1982, pp 584–601.
8. Mizinga KM, Verma OP: LHRH-induced ovulation and fertility of anestrous goats. Theriogenology 21:435, 1984.
9. Moore NW, Eppleston J: The use of embryo transfer in the Angora goat. Theriogenology, 6:638, 1976

Prostaglandins for Induction of Estrus, Estrus Synchronization, Abortion and Induction of Parturition

Randall S. Ott, D.V.M., M.S.
University of Illinois, Urbana, Illinois

Prostaglandin $F_{2\alpha}$ ($PGF_{2\alpha}$ or Lutalyse) manipulates reproductive events of goats very effectively. $PGF_{2\alpha}$ has been used successfully in dairy goats for the induction of estrus, synchronization of estrus, abortion and induction of parturition. Analogs of $PGF_{2\alpha}$ have also been demonstrated to induce estrus in the goat, but only limited data are available.

INDUCTION OF ESTRUS WITH $PGF_{2\alpha}$

$PGF_{2\alpha}$ has been shown to induce luteolysis effectively in the cycling doe during the breeding season. Endogenous $PGF_{2\alpha}$ is thought to be the naturally occurring compound that is released by the uterus to induce estrus in the doe. An injection of $PGF_{2\alpha}$ causes the corpus luteum of the cycling goat to regress and stop its production of progesterone. Does then come into estrus an average of 50 hours after the $PGF_{2\alpha}$ injection.

$PGF_{2\alpha}$ injection has been shown to be effective on any doe that is on days 4 to 17 of the estrus cycle. Does that are on day 18 or later will come into estrus soon anyway. $PGF_{2\alpha}$ will not cause does on days 1, 2 or 3 to come into estrus early. Successful induction of estrus with $PGF_{2\alpha}$ in goats treated as early as day 4 of the estrous cycle indicates that $PGF_{2\alpha}$ is luteolytic at an earlier stage of the cycle in goats than in sheep or cattle.

In early studies intramuscular administration of doses as large as 15 mg,[5] 8 mg[6] or 8 mg divided into two injections given 4 hours[7] apart were reported to be successful when given between days 4 and 16 of the estrous cycle. Clinical use of $PGF_{2\alpha}$ suggested that lower doses would be effective. In recent studies varying dosages of $PGF_{2\alpha}$ have been injected in cycling does during the luteal phase to determine the minimum dose effective for induction of estrus. As little as 1.25 mg $PGF_{2\alpha}$ was effective for the induction of estrus in the dairy goat.[4] Results of another study suggested that 0.0385 mg $PGF_{2\alpha}$/kg was effective for induction of estrus in the goat.[2] This is equivalent to 1.75 mg $PGF_{2\alpha}$/100 lb body weight. Based on this dosage, 2.5 mg $PGF_{2\alpha}$ (0.5 ml) would be effective in does weighing up to 65 kg (143 lb).

The onset of estrus in goats can be controlled with $PGF_{2\alpha}$ injections so that estrus will coincide with a time convenient to transport the doe to a distant site for artificial insemination or hand mating to a superior buck. Goat owners should be informed that some does may experience a short cycle, usually within 10 days after the induced estrus. Short cycling is a natural phenomenon in the goat, especially early or late in the breeding season. Multiple short cycles are more common following abortions induced during the breeding season.

SYNCHRONIZATION OF ESTRUS WITH $PGF_{2\alpha}$

Data pooled from two studies showed that when one injection of 8 mg $PGF_{2\alpha}$ was given to 37 cycling does, 78 per cent (29 of 37) were in estrus an average of 50 hours later.[6, 7] When a second injection was given 11 days after the first, 97 per cent (36 of 37) were in estrus 50 hours after the second series of injections. Control of the time of breeding allows for control of the time of kidding and milk production in does. Synchronization of estrus in cycling dairy goats during the breeding season can be used to facilitate the use of artificial insemination. Prostaglandins are not effective when administered to anestrous does during the nonbreeding season.

A most important aspect of estrus synchronization is the effect of the method on fertility at the synchronized estrus. Fertility of goats synchronized for estrus using two 8-mg injections 11 days apart and bred by natural service has been investigated.[6] The does were mated when they would first stand for the buck and every 12 hours until estrus subsided. The $PGF_{2\alpha}$-treated and control does were both mated an average of three times before going out of estrus. Thirteen of the 17 does in both groups did not return to estrus after the first breeding, giving a first-service conception rate of 76.5 per cent based on nonreturn to estrus. Radiography at midgestation revealed an overall pregnancy rate of 94 per cent for the treated does. Pregnancy rate in the control group was 82 per cent. It was concluded that estrus synchronization using $PGF_{2\alpha}$ treatments had no detrimental effects on pregnancy rate in goats.

INDUCTION OF ABORTION WITH $PGF_{2\alpha}$

A dosage of 20 mg $PGF_{2\alpha}$ has been shown to be effective in inducing abortion in goats bred at 30 and 65 days.[5] Abortion occurred within 42 to 76 hours after injection. Thus $PGF_{2\alpha}$ might be used therapeutically by practitioners to correct mismating.

However, in a recent study[3] most does induced to abort with 15 mg of $PGF_{2\alpha}$ during the breeding season experienced multiple consecutive interestrus intervals of 2 to 15 days. Progesterone concentrations associated with these short cycles suggested that ovulation did not occur. Therefore, does would not be expected to conceive if mated during an estrus period preceding a short cycle. Induction of abortion during the breeding season should be initiated with caution if immediate rebreeding of the doe is intended.

INDUCTION OF PARTURITION WITH $PGF_{2\alpha}$

$PGF_{2\alpha}$ is an excellent agent to induce parturition in goats as they rely on progesterone produced by the corpus luteum throughout gestation. In one study 15 mg $PGF_{2\alpha}$ was administered to pregnant does 140 or 142 days after breeding.[5] Parturition occurred 42 to 76 hours later. Live kids were delivered in all cases. It has been demonstrated that $PGF_{2\alpha}$ was more effective than dexamethasone for inducing parturition in goats.[8] Nine does were injected with 16 mg of dexamethasone and 9 does were injected with 20 mg of $PGF_{2\alpha}$ on day 144 in an attempt to induce parturition. A control group of eight does from the same management group was not injected and was allowed to kid naturally. The mean interval ($\pm$ SE) of the time from injection on day 144 to parturition was 196.5 $\pm$ 13.8 hours in the controls, 119.6 $\pm$ 29.8 hours in the dexamethasone-treated group and 31.5 $\pm$ 1.1 hours in the $PGF_{2\alpha}$-treated group. Retained fetal membranes, a problem associated with induction of parturition in the cow, were not present in the goats.

In a recent study[1] both 5.0 mg and 2.5 mg were effective in induction of parturition, but the interval from injection to parturition was not as predictable as that found in the earlier study, in which a 20 mg dose was given. Does receiving 5.0 mg $PGF_{2\alpha}$ and 2.5 mg $PGF_{2\alpha}$ kidded within a mean ($\pm$ SD) hours and range (hours) of 35 $\pm$ 9 and 28 to 48 and 43 $\pm$ 12 and 29 to 57, respectively. Results from control does receiving saline were 111 $\pm$ 79 and 41 to 200 hours.

Does should probably not be induced earlier than 144 days, as the kids from does with three or more fetuses might be too small for survival. Induction on days 145 to 149 should work satisfactorily.

References

1. Bretzlaff KN, Ott RS: Doses of prostaglandin $F_{2\alpha}$ effective for induction of parturition in goats. Theriogenology 19:849, 1983.
2. Bretzlaff KN, Hill A, Ott RS: Induction of estrus in goats with prostaglandin $F_{2\alpha}$. Am J Vet Res 44:1162, 1983.
3. Bretzlaff KN, McEntee K, Hixon JE, Ott RS: Short estrous cycles after $PGF_{2\alpha}$-induced abortions in goats. 3rd Int Con Goat Prod Dis. Tucson, 1982, p 498.

4. Bretzlaff KN, Ott RS, Weston PG, Hixon JE: Doses of prostaglandin F$_{2\alpha}$ effective for induction of estrus in goats. Theriogenology 16:587, 1980.
5. Bosu WTK, Serna-Garibay JA, Barker CAV: Peripheral plasma levels of progesterone in pregnant goats and pregnant goats treated with prostaglandin F$_{2\alpha}$. Theriogenology 11:131, 1978.
6. Ott RS, Nelson DR, Hixon JE: Fertility of goats following synchronization of estrus with prostaglandin F$_{2\alpha}$. Theriogenology 13:341, 1980.
7. Ott RS, Nelson DR, Hixon JE: Peripheral serum progesterone and luteinizing hormone concentrations of goats during synchronization of estrus and ovulation with prostaglandin F$_{2\alpha}$. Am J Vet Res 41:1432, 1980.
8. Ott RS, Nelson DR, Memon MA, et al.: Dexamethasone and prostaglandin F$_{2\alpha}$ for induction of parturition in goats. Proc 9th Int Congr Reprod AI. Madrid, 1980, vol IV, pp 659–662.

Anestrus, Pseudopregnancy and Cystic Follicles

Mary C. Smith, D.V.M.
Cornell University, Ithaca, New York

ANESTRUS IN GOATS

The sexually mature doe should show cyclic estrus during the normal breeding season. Failure to do so may be a sign of diverse problems. The intersex condition must be strongly considered if the nulliparous doe is naturally polled. The stimulatory effect of the buck odor for the doe has already been discussed. If the presence of a buck or a buck jar for 1 month in the fall does not result in observable estrus, then pregnancy, pseudopregnancy, nutritional deficiencies or other factors causing anestrus may be present.

Nutritional Influences. Starvation and parasitism usually appear together in goats and are important causes of reproductive failure, including anestrus. Good quality forage and adequate concentrates should be fed to the goat. Early cut grass hays should be accompanied by 16 to 18 per cent protein grain, while 12 to 14 per cent protein in the concentrate will be sufficient when legumes are fed. Approximately 1.4 kg of good hay is needed per day. A rough rule for determining grain feeding is 0.5 kg of grain per kg of milk production. More will be needed if the hay is poor. Many novice goat owners do not understand the progressive decrease in forage quality that occurs during maturation. September-cut weedy hay may not supply enough energy and protein for survival, let alone for reproduction. Those does that do cycle at the beginning of the winter will often abort if severe undernutrition continues.

Parasitism. Animals that are malnourished are usually also parasitized. The goat with many abomasal or intestinal strongyles or with liver flukes is often thin, pot bellied, anemic and diarrheic and has a rough hair coat that fails to shed in the spring.[1] Fecal examinations may confirm the diagnosis, but clinical signs may occur during the prepatent period. Thus, a diagnosis of parasitism cannot be eliminated on the basis of a single negative fecal examination. Every possible effort should be made to separate feed from feces. Hay and grain should be offered in feeders that cannot be contaminated by fecal pellets. Manure should be removed regularly. Barnyard drainage and pasture rotation are important. When many animals are present on a small, wet pasture, worming every 3 to 6 weeks may be necessary. Thiabendazole at a dose of 50 mg/kg is safe at any time. Fenbendazole, at 5 to 10 mg/kg, is also a safe wormer, although its use in goats is not approved in all countries. Paste is preferable to drenches when administered by unskilled owners who might otherwise induce inhalation pneumonia. Improper administration of boluses may cause injuries to the pharynx. The goat's milk is not suitable for human consumption for 4 days after administration of thiabendazole. Levamisole (Tramisol) at a dose of 8 mg/kg is commonly used to allow alternation of anthelmintics. This drug, however, is not approved for use with goats in the United States, and milk withdrawals have not been established. Tramisol has a reputation as being dangerous in late pregnancy, but researchers have been unable to induce abortions in goats being administered it.

Coccidiosis in goats is a serious problem under most management systems involving the intensive raising of kids. Diarrhea is typically prominent, but tenesmus and bloody feces are rarely observed. Treatment is with oral sulfonamides for 3 to 5 days at the recommended dosage level for sheep. Other coccidiostats, such as amprolium at 25 to 50 mg/kg, have also been used. Well-nourished adults rarely show clinical signs unless stressed or exposed to a species of *Eimeria* to which they are not yet immune. Coccidiosis should not be diagnosed in an adult in the absence of diarrhea, as heavy oocyst shedding occurs in many healthy goats.

When goats are housed in groups, the social dominance hierarchy will also affect estrus. Subordinate does eat less, lose weight, are more susceptible to parasites because they are forced to eat contaminated leftovers and show fewer heats. Separate housing and feeding are desirable any time an individual becomes unthrifty. Such an animal should also be closely examined for dental problems.

Mineral Deficiencies. Parasite-free goats with adequate dietary energy and protein may still fail to cycle if mineral deficiencies are present. Phosphorus deficiency may be associated with anestrus. Copper, iodine and manganese are among the trace minerals known to influence estrus. If the exact deficiency cannot be identified, a trace mineral salt should be supplied. Unfortunately, mineral requirements for goats are not yet established. Cattle salt is used by default. The common practice of offering goats both sodium chloride and trace mineral salt should be discouraged, as some animals may choose to consume only the plain salt. In localities in which selenium soil deficiencies are known to occur, injectable vitamin E-selenium preparations may improve reproductive efficiency. The mechanisms by which selenium affects caprine reproduction are not yet understood.

Infectious Diseases. Chronic debilitating infections such as paratuberculosis, internal abscesses and caprine arthritis-encephalitis may lead to anestrus in the goat.[4] While less common, neoplasia should also be considered.

PSEUDOPREGNANCY AND HYDROMETRA

Pseudopregnancy occurs rather frequently in the goat, whether or not exposure to a buck has occurred. The affected doe is anestrous, with elevated progesterone levels for a variable period of time, often approximating a normal 5-month gestation. Some does develop abdominal distention suggestive of pregnancy with multiple kids. The uterus is thin-walled and contains thin, clear to cloudy fluid (hydrometra). Several liters of liquid may be present. An enlarged uterus without fetal skeletons is evident radiographically, and amplitude-depth examination for pregnancy will be falsely positive. Hydrometra is confirmed by transabdominal aspiration of uterine fluids. Prostaglandin $F_{2\alpha}$ (2.5 mg, repeated if necessary) usually induces emptying of the uterus within 2 days. If a doe spontaneously voids the fluid, she is commonly said to have had a "cloud burst." The abdominal distention disappears, and lactation may begin, but the owner can find neither fetus nor placenta in the fluid-drenched pen. The doe may appear to search for the nonexistent kid.

Other does with pseudopregnancy do not develop noticeable hydrometra. Instead, at the end of a period of anestrus, a bloody vaginal discharge is observed. If the doe was bred 2 to 3 months earlier, the condition will be indistinguishable from early embryonic loss. In fact, one possible cause of a pseudopregnancy is prolongation of the progestational phase after death of the embryo. However, many affected animals have not been exposed to a buck prior to occurrence of the bloody discharge or cloud burst; therefore, other causes must exist.

The doe sometimes conceives during a heat that occurs a few days after the discharge is noted. She may carry a normal pregnancy to term even after a hydrometra, or she may have one or more subsequent false pregnancies. The unbred doe that does not return to heat after a first estrous cycle in the fall can be treated with prostaglandin for a possible false pregnancy. The sporadic nature of the condition makes scientific investigation difficult. Slaughterhouse studies have not shown any association with cystic follicles, fetal remnants or cervical obstruction. The prolonged elevation of progesterone levels has been documented in does that developed pseudopregnancy in the course of other endocrinologic studies.[2, 3]

CYSTIC FOLLICLES

A mature Graafian follicle in the goat averages 1.0 cm in diameter. "Follicles" larger that 1.2 cm in diameter, and ranging up to 3.7 cm in diameter, have been reported from slaughterhouse material and have been classified as cysts of the ovary. The size distinction between follicle and cyst is clearly arbitrary. The cysts are shiny and bluish if thin-walled or are milky white if thick-walled. Histologic examinations of these cysts have not been reported.

A clinical history of nymphomania may suggest the diagnosis of cystic follicular degeneration of the ovaries to the practitioner. Irregular estrous periods at the beginning or end of the normal breeding season may be assumed to be physiologically normal. When short cycles of 5 to 10 days are observed, determination of progesterone concentrations at estrus and in the middle of the interestrous period will often demonstrate development of functional, albeit short-lived luteal tissue. If persistent or irregular estrus is observed during the period from October to December, the clinician may attempt treatment with 250 to 1000 IU of human chorionic gonadotropin (hCG) given intravenously or intramuscularly. Progesterone therapy (10 mg/day for 18 days) or gonadotropin-releasing hormone (GnRH) might also be tried. The efficacy of these treatments in goats is unknown. Pen mating is recommended in preference to artificial insemination for does with irregularities of the estrous cycle.

Several etiologies for cystic follicles have been proposed, but experimental data are not available. Heredity and a relative phosphorus deficiency induced by high dietary calcium have both been implicated in herds with frequent infertility problems. Short cycles and temporary infertility have been reported to follow prostaglandin-induced abortion in goats.

References

1. Blackwell TE: Enteritis and diarrhea. Vet Clin North Am: Large Anim Pract 5:557, 1983.
2. Holdsworth RJ, Davies J: Measurement of progesterone in goat's milk: An early pregnancy test. Vet Rec 105:535, 1979.
3. Mizinga KM, Verma OP: LHRH-induced ovulation and fertility of anestrous goats. Theriogenology 21:435, 1984.
4. Sherman DM: Unexplained weight loss in sheep and goats. Vet Clin North Am: Large Anim Pract 5:571, 1983.

Pregnancy Diagnosis

Christine S. F. Williams, B.V.Sc., M.R.C.V.S.
Michigan State University, East Lansing, Michigan

Under extensive systems of management in which male and female goats are housed together during the breeding season, there is little reason to consider pregnancy diagnosis. As long as the males are healthy and fertile, most of the does will conceive. Those that do not may be culled when they do not kid. The cost of maintaining a few nonpregnant does is substantially less than the price of performing pregnancy tests for the whole herd.

Under more controlled conditions, such as commercial dairies or small hobby herds, there is justification for testing. The success of dairy operations depends on the ability to produce milk to meet market requirements. Unfortunately, the goat is a seasonal breeder and tends to produce milk on a supply curve that is the reverse of the fluid milk demand curve. Therefore, dairy herders attempt to even out the annual production by manipulating light cycles and by using hormonal treatments and delaying breeding until the end of the natural season so that does will deliver in the fall rather than in the spring. It is important for commercial dairy herders to know whether these maneuvers have been successful and whether they have enough pregnant goats to assure a winter milk supply.

The farmer with a hobby herd may also be interested in a year-round, constant milk supply but is more likely to be interested in showing goats. Milkers show best if they are at the peak of lactation, but this entails breeding them late in the season, leaving little time for corrective action if they do not conceive.

PHYSICAL METHODS OF PREGNANCY DIAGNOSIS

Traditional methods of pregnancy diagnosis used by hobbyists, such as a change in personality, drop in milk yield, tendency to fatten up and change in body outline, are not completely reliable, as they do not distinguish between true and false pregnancy.

Body outline change is more pronounced for primiparous animals, and by midgestation it is quite obvious. For adult goats it is not as reliable because many long, deep-bodied animals are quite capable of concealing a single fetus. Also obesity may be mistaken for pregnancy.

Drop in milk yield can only be used to detect pregnancy in individuals who are consistent, steady milkers. Does that normally show sharp drop-off lactation curves will decrease daily production regardless of their pregnancy status.

Udder development in doelings is not a good indicator of pregnancy, especially in doelings from heavy, persistent milking strains that have a tendency to develop precocious udders even before they are bred.

Absence of heat ought to be a useful indicator, but unfortunately many goats have a tendency to show some signs of heat during pregnancy. Considering that many owners do not keep a buck, it is difficult enough to catch the goat in heat without the added complication of the goat acting as if it were in heat while it is actually pregnant. Natural service of a pregnant goat should have no deleterious consequences, although artificial insemination might have negative effects. At the end of the breeding season absence of heat could be caused by pregnancy or anestrus.

Radiography is not practical for the on-farm diagnosis, but it is valuable for counting the fetuses in research projects. Fetuses can be seen as early as 75 days. However, it is not advisable to make a diagnosis of nonpregnancy until 90 days.

Abdominal palpation in late pregnancy is possible in slab-sided, thin, relaxed goats, but big-bodied, strong-willed goats will resist and tighten the abdominal muscles, making palpation very difficult. However, on the day of parturition, even these does can be palpated easily.

Owners are not particularly impressed with the balottement technique; nor do they look favorably on the rectal palpation rod technique used successfully by Hulet in sheep. Goats do not tip up as easily as sheep; nor do they relax when upside down. Furthermore, there is a definite possibility of injury to the goat or the handler during restraint. Sedation introduces the added complication of drug residues in the milk and the determination of a safe milk withdrawal time.

The Doppler ultrasound technique works well in the hands of skilled operators, but the cost of the machine and the length of time taken to become skilled may be a disadvantage. If very early diagnosis is required, the rectal probe should be used. With the doe positioned on a milking stand, the lubricated probe should be introduced into the rectum and positioned in the middle to detect the swooshing sound of blood flowing through the uterine vessels. A strong sound generally indicates pregnancy, a faint sound, nonpregnancy. No sound at all is often indicative of a false-negative pregnancy, and the probe should be moved to either side of the pelvis to detect the flow of blood in the pelvic vessels. If the sound is poor here, then transmission is not occurring properly, and most likely the probe is stuck in feces.

It is possible to test goats as early as 25 to 30 days with the Doppler ultrasound probe, but in the author's experience false-negatives are a problem. It is much more rewarding to perform the test at 35 to 40 days gestation. By this time it is very easy to detect the sound of the fetal blood flow, which is much faster than that of the dam. This confirms fetal viability and is a great source of satisfaction to the owner. Goats that become very nervous and shiver, or those that pant cannot be tested, as the constant movement produces too much background noise. Goats in their first pregnancy are easy to test to confirm fetal presence; old does with steep rumps are more difficult to test.

The external Doppler probe should be placed on a lubricated shaved area of the right flank, in front of the udder. The probe should be directed toward the last rib on the left side at an upward angle of 45°. The operator then listens for the characteristic swooshing sound of the uterine vessels and the faster fetal pulse. This technique works at 2 to 5 months gestation and is useful for confirming fetal viability prior to cesarean section. The ultrasonic external probe, which depends on the detection of fluid/solid interfaces, works well in midgestation but is less accurate in late gestation. It cannot differentiate between false pregnancy and true pregnancy and cannot indicate fetal viability.

Of all the mechanical methods listed, the rectal Doppler probe for detection of fetal sounds is the only one that does not give false-positives. Furthermore, it can be used in early gestation. The ultimate mechanical pregnancy test is real-time ultrasound with imaging, in which one can count the fetuses. However, these machines are expensive and therefore of limited availability.

CHEMICAL METHODS OF PREGNANCY DIAGNOSIS

The progesterone assay conducted 21 to 24 days after breeding has been used with both milk and serum samples. As a test for nonpregnancy it is very satisfactory.[2] However, high levels of serum or milk progesterone can indicate several different results other than pregnancy. The doe may have a shorter or longer cycle than 21 days and may have a diestrus corpus luteum. Hydrometra, pseudopregnancy or retained corpus luteum will give false-positives. The requirement for precise timing of the sample collection is an additional burden. Furthermore, the goat appears to metabolize progesterone to pregnanedione in the udder, therefore, the antiserum used for the goat milk test must cross react strongly with pregnanedione. This is not a requirement for the serum test.

Estrone sulfate radioimmunoassay* of the milk at 50 + days gestation overcomes the problems of the progesterone assay.[1] There is no precise date on which samples must be collected, and the test does not give false-positives with hydrometra or persistent corpus luteum.

A comparable estrone sulfate urine test* can be used for does that are dry or in their first pregnancy. The ultimate pregnancy test, which could be performed by the owner on any body fluid, does not yet exist.

---

*Probe-Tek, 3010 S. Washington, Lansing MI 48910.

References

1. Davies J, Chaplin VM: A caprine pregnancy test based upon measurement of oestrone sulphate in milk. 3rd Int Symp World Association of Veterinary Laboratory Diagnosticians. Ames, 1983, vol 1, pp 119–125.
2. Holdsworth RJ, Davies J: Measurement of progesterone in goats' milk: An early pregnancy test. Vet Rec 105:535, 1979.

Practical Management of Induced Parturition

Christine S. F. Williams, B.V.Sc, M.R.C.V.S.
Michigan State University, East Lansing, Michigan

There are a number of advantages to induced parturition: (1) improved kid survival, especially in severe weather, (2) reduced kid and doe mortality because of better observation by the owner and earlier intervention in cases of dystocia, (3) reduced stress on the owner because of the increased predictability of the time of parturition, and (4) increased ability to obtain kids free of colostrum and with minimal contact with the mother. This is important in disease control, e.g., caprine arthritis-encephalitis (CAE) and mycoplasma. There are also disadvantages. These include (1) owner reluctance to interfere with the natural process and (2) increased responsibility on the owner to maintain accurate breeding records and to *guarantee* no subsequent breedings, accidental or otherwise.

These advantages and disadvantages are magnified if induced parturition of synchronized does is undertaken. This, then, becomes a logistical exercise, which if it fails, will fail gloriously. Induction is not an easy way out for the disorganized. Preparations should begin 6 to 7 months prior to the induction date. Planned delivery should include a planned breeding date 145 days previously. Records should be kept of exact breedings, and bucks should not be allowed to run with does. Pregnancy confirmation is important. Any errors will soon be found when induced does abort 103- or 124-day fetuses instead of 145-day fetuses.

Many goats are not "bagged-up" at 144 days, and it requires confidence, based on accurate records, to inject these animals. However, the udder will rapidly develop in the 30 hours following the injection.

It is the author's practice to inject goats with prostaglandin (5 to 10 mg $PGF_{2\alpha}$ or 62.5 to 125 μg cloprostenol) at 144 days gestation at 7 to 8 AM and to expect the kids to be born during the afternoon on the succeeding day. Rarely does a goat deliver earlier than 27 hours following the injection, but the possibility of spontaneous delivery cannot be excluded. There is a peak of deliveries between 30 and 35 hours, and then the deliveries become sporadic. By 55 hours if an injected goat has not delivered, she will probably go to term and deliver spontaneously.

It is important when inducing parturition to maintain the goat in its usual surroundings, i.e., do not put it in a kidding pen, and to minimize all extraneous disturbances. Constant checking of the animal, especially by strangers, will inhibit parturition, and inviting all the local children to witness the birth practically guarantees failure. Synchronized induced goats should be penned individually after kidding; otherwise, they will steal kids from each other, and some kids will be disowned in the confusion. Kids to be hand-reared should be identified immediately after birth, either by tattooing or by temporarily placing wide rubber bands around the neck. A recording system should be used to ensure that every kid gets colostrum, either by nipple or stomach tube. Kids should be sorted by size and vigor into groups of three to four and kept in small pens or large cardboard appliance boxes for the first few days. In conclusion, prior preparation and attention to details are the keys to success in a synchronized induction program.

Periparturient Care of the Doe

Mary C. Smith, D.V.M.
Cornell University, Ithaca, New York

Goats, like cows, need a 6- to 8-week dry period for best milk production during the subsequent lactation. Does with a history of mastitis should be dry treated with one dry cow mastitis tube in each half of the udder. Culture and sensitivity testing will assist in the selection of appropriate antibiotics. Four weeks before the due date the doe should receive tetanus and enterotoxemia vaccinations to boost her own and her colostral immunity. This is also a suitable time for prophylactic vitamin E-selenium injections in localities in which white muscle disease occurs.

PREGNANCY TOXEMIA

The pregnant doe should not be allowed to become obese. However, high-quality forage and increasing concentrates must be supplied during the last month of gestation. Otherwise, pregnancy toxemia (ketosis) may occur in the doe carrying multiple kids; her energy demands are very high, and there is little room in the abdomen for feed. Early signs of pregnancy toxemia are twitching of the ears, muscular spasms and loss of appetite. Rapid respiration, ataxia, frequent urination, coma and death follow. Prevention requires feeding at least 0.25 kg of grain per day during the last month, and more, if the hay is of poor quality. Even obese does will need the grain. Any disease or condition that might cause the pregnant doe to go off feed should be treated promptly to avoid secondary ketosis.

Ketone bodies in the urine are diagnostic of pregnancy toxemia. Most does will urinate shortly after getting up or after being released by the examiner. Blood glucose levels can be high, normal or low. Treatment must be given early if the doe is to be saved. Mild cases may be controlled by hand feeding and oral dosing with 3 mg/kg of glycerol or 60 ml of propylene glycol twice a day. More severely affected animals are given 200 ml of 5 per cent dextrose intravenously. (Avoid 50 per cent dextrose in goats.) Recumbent animals should be treated with antibiotics and 20 mg of dexamethasone to combat endotoxic shock and to stimulate parturition. Three liters of fluid given intravenously, together with 150 mEq of bicarbonate, will help to correct the severe dehydration and acidosis that accompany advanced cases. A cesarean section is indicated if the doe does not respond promptly to medical treatment. Waiting for hormonally induced parturition to occur in the severely toxic doe is rarely prudent, as both the kids and the doe often die.

PARTURITION

As normal parturition approaches, the udder fills. It is occasionally necessary to milk out the doe to relieve pressure in the udder. The vulva also enlarges. This is most noticeable in does with ectopic mammary tissue in the lips of the vulva. When parturition is imminent, the doe should be placed in a clean, well-bedded and roomy box stall. The water pail is removed to prevent accidental drowning of the kids.

The expectant doe is restless and may hollow out a nest. After parturition, she licks the membranes off the kid and may eat part of the placenta. The kid is usually on its feet in 10 to 30 minutes. It is common to remove kids immediately at birth and raise them artificially to control diseases such as caprine arthritis-encephalitis, caseous lymphadenitis, paratuberculosis and coccidiosis. If the kid is left with its dam, it locates the udder after diffuse sucking activity. Once nursing begins, the kid wags its tail, and the doe sniffs underneath the tail. There is a critical period of about 2 hours after birth during which time the doe must be exposed to her kid if she is to accept it. Licking for 5 to 10 minutes is usually adequate for acceptance.

NORMAL INVOLUTION

Although the postpartum uterus never returns to its original pregestational size, involution is rapid. The placenta is normally passed within 1 to 2 hours after parturition. The caruncles degenerate during the first week and are re-epithelialized by 3 weeks. Lochia, normally red and odorless, persists for a maximum of 3 weeks. Uterine involution is complete by 6 weeks postpartum.

Dystocia and Obstetrics in Goats

Jessica S. Franklin, D.V.M.
Dundee Veterinary Clinic, Dundee, Michigan

The kidding process is considered dystocic when the doe has more than 1 hour of active abdominal contractions without producing a kid.[1] Normal parturition usually commences with a restless period of uterine contractions of 1 to 10 hours. This is followed by rupture of the placental membranes and presentation of a fetus. Normally, the fetus is positioned dorsosacrally with limbs extended; initial presentation of head and forelimbs is more common than posterior presentation. Usually, all kids are born within 3 hours, and the placenta is passed within 2 hours of the last kid.

There are many causes of dystocia. The most common and easily corrected dystocia results from two or more kids in the birth canal simultaneously. Frequently, a fetus is malpositioned with head or limbs retained. Hypocalcemia in the doe may cause nonproductive uterine contractions and failure of the cervix to dilate. Although less important than in cattle, a correctly positioned fetus may be too large in relation to the maternal pelvis and vulva. More unusual causes of dystocia include uterine torsion and tail ankylosis blocking the birth canal.

DIAGNOSIS

It is very important to recognize and correct dystocias early because the cervix will begin to close after 2 or 3 hours of nonproductive labor. Usually, it is not possible to dilate the cervix once it has started to close. Furthermore, an early decision to perform a cesarean section minimizes maternal and fetal mortality. A doe that has been actively straining for 1½ hours, has had active labor cease or has had more than 12 hours of restlessness and abdominal discomfort without active labor should be examined. Any obvious abnormal fetal presentations should be corrected as soon as they are detected.

The diagnosis of a dystocia is made by vaginal examination after cleaning the perineal region. Uterine torsion may be diagnosed by detecting vaginal folds or twists.

INCOMPLETE CERVICAL DILATION

Incomplete cervical dilation is a serious and common finding. The examiner will feel firm rings, usually 2 bands 0.5 to 1 cm wide. A well-dilated cervix, on the other hand, will be barely palpable at the neck of the uterus. Attempts at manual dilation of a cervix open 2 to 5 cm often tear the cervix and uterus. If a nondilated cervix is present in a doe that is also demonstrating cool skin and ears and muscle weakness, treatment for hypocalcemia should be initiated. The animal should be rechecked for dilation in 3 hours. A bovine milk fever solution (60 ml), such as Cal Dextro No. 2, may be given intravenously or subcutaneously. This hypertonic solution may be diluted in 200 ml of sterile water or saline for added safety and also to reduce the probability of subcutaneous abscess formation.

Incomplete cervical dilation is commonly a sign of prolonged dystocia, and cesarean section is indicated.

UTERINE TORSION

Torsions are uncommon, and the initial examination may be made too late to save the kids or doe. The examiner is at a further disadvantage because a rectal examination, to diagnose the direction of the twist, as in bovine dystocias, is not possible.

Prior to attempting correction of the torsion by rolling the doe, a vaginal examination with the doe on her side should be repeated. If the torsion is 180° or less, the vaginal twists will be more open when the doe is laid down on the same side as the direction of the twist. A plank pressed against the abdomen or a leg of the fetus grasped through the vagina may be used to hold the uterus stationary while the doe is rolled. After the torsion is corrected, several hours should be allowed for full dilation of the cervix to occur. Failure to untwist the uterus or inadequate cervical dilation after correction may necessitate a cesarean section. A doe with a friable, septic uterus containing an emphysematous fetus is a poor candidate for either manual correction or abdominal surgery.

FORCED EXTRACTION

If the cervix is well dilated and the fetal presentation can be corrected, forced extraction may be attempted. Manipulations must be clean, gentle and well lubricated, as it is very easy to rupture the uterus. A plastic garbage bag may be placed under the doe to keep bedding away from the perineal area.

When twins are presented simultaneously, attempts to repel one kid should be made. It is possible to pull a kid if the head is free and one forelimb is extended; the other forelimb will flatten along the thorax. Correction of an anterior presentation with the head retained toward the doe's right hip may be facilitated by laying the doe on her left side. A head snare or loop of stiff nylon cord may be necessary to retrieve the head.

EPIDURAL ANESTHESIA

Epidural anesthesia may facilitate manipulation, but experience is necessary for satisfactory results. Two per cent lidocaine (2 to 5 ml) is deposited between the sacrum and first coccygeal vertebra with an 18- or 20-gauge 1 inch needle.

FETOTOMY

When a dead kid presents head first with forelimbs retained, decapitation should be considered rather than repulsion of the head to correct the position. If the kid has started to swell, there may not be enough room for the head and limbs in the birth canal. A subcutaneous embryotomy may be necessary on oversized, malformed or emphysematous kids. Fetomony equipment designed for cattle is too large to be useful in goats, and unguarded obstetric wire will damage the uterus.

Removal of a forelimb or head may permit forced extraction. A finger knife or scalpel blade may be used to incise the skin. The incision should encircle the proximal carpus and then continue along the medial side of the limb to the axilla. Blunt finger dissection will allow the scapula to be pulled free. Amputation of the head is best performed externally. Repelling the forelimbs and applying traction to the head should allow the fetal head to protrude far enough from the vagina to be cut off without injury to the doe.

Occasionally, a more complete fetotomy is necessary. After the forelimbs are removed, the skin can be stripped away from the thorax, the ribs fractured, and the spinal column twisted to remove the anterior half of the fetus.

GENERAL CARE AFTER INTERNAL MANIPULATIONS

Oxytocin (10 to 20 units intravenously) may be used to control postextraction uterine and cervical bleeding. The owner can repeat the same dose subcutaneously in 2 hours. Goats are also susceptible to tetanus. Vaccinated animals should be given a booster injection of toxoid. If the animal has not been vaccinated, 1500 IU of tetanus antitoxin should be administered.

Systemic antibiotics should be given 5 days postpartum. Penicillin G procaine (22,000 IU/kg BID, IM or SQ) or oxytetracycline (11 mg/kg BID, IV, IM or SQ) may be used. While many newer antibiotics are effective, very few are approved for goats, so dosage and withdrawal recommendations are the practitioner's responsibility. Subcutaneous injections will be easiest and safest for the owner to administer.

If the uterus is contaminated during manipulation or if an embryotomy is performed, the uterus should be rinsed with warm fluid. Two commonly used solutions are dilute chlorhexidine and tamed iodine. A disinfected calf esophageal feeder holds 3.5 liters of solution. It is more sanitary than stomach tubes and pumps and is much quicker and more economical than prepared IV fluids, bottles and tubing.

Bolus or fluid antibiotics may be placed in the uterus after manipulations. Usually, it is not possible to insert boluses by hand more than 24 hours postpartum.

Kids delivered by extraction need to be stimulated

to breathe, perhaps through vigorous rubbing or by placing straw in the nose. Fluids should be drained by gravity. Colostrum (50 ml/kg) should be fed by stomach tube if the kids are too lethargic to nurse.

Reference

1. Bowen JS: Pregnancy toxemia, milk fever and kidding difficulties. Dairy Goat J 56:20, 1978.

Cesarean Section in Goats

Sally Vivrette, D.V.M.
Cornell University, Ithaca, New York

Cesarean section is usually performed to relieve dystocia, to obtain gnotobiotic kids for research or to obtain caprine arthritis-encephalitis (CAE)–free kids.

PREOPERATIVE CONSIDERATIONS

The doe should be given a careful physical evaluation before surgery. A vaginal examination will ensure that a cesarean section is indicated. If signs of shock, such as hypovolemia and cardiovascular collapse, are evident, intravenous fluid therapy and other supportive treatment should be given. Tetanus prophylaxis should be given if the doe has not been vaccinated in the past year.

RESTRAINT AND ANESTHESIA

The operation can be performed via a right flank or ventral midline incision but is most easily accomplished by left flank celiotomy with the doe in right lateral recumbency. With this approach, the rumen prevents the small intestines from entering the surgical field.[1] If the doe is profoundly depressed, she may require only leg restraint and local anesthesia at the incision site using approximately 30 ml of 1 per cent lidocaine. The regional therapy of choice is epidural analgesia using 0.5 per cent bupivacaine (Marcaine) at 1 ml per 7 kg (7 to 8 ml for an average-sized doe) at the lumbosacral junction. Bupivacaine has limited penetration across the placenta, minimizing fetal depression. If sedation is required, diazepam (Valium) (0.1 to 0.2 mg/kg IV) or xylazine (Rompun) (0.02 to 0.04 mg/kg IV) may be used. Concurrent sedation with butorphanol (Stadol) (0.01 to 0.03 mg/kg IM) will lessen the amount of diazepam or xylazine needed and minimize depression of the fetus.[2] If further immobilization is necessary, ketamine hydrochloride (Veta-

lar) (5.0 mg/kg IV) may be given following diazepam or xylazine administration. General anesthesia with halothane or isofluran can also be employed.

SURGICAL PROCEDURE

The left paralumbar fossa is clipped, prepared, and draped for aseptic surgery. A 15-cm incision, centered in the left paralumbar fossa, is made beginning approximately 4 cm ventral to the lumbar transverse processes. The skin, external abdominal oblique, internal abdominal oblique and transverse muscles of abdomen and peritoneum are incised or split separately. The gravid uterus is located and gently delivered to the incision. It is often possible to completely exteriorize the gravid horn. The uterus is incised along the greater curvature, preferably between rows of placentomes. This incision should be of sufficient length to avoid tearing the uterus. The fetal membranes are incised, and the fetus is extracted. Contamination of the abdomen with uterine fluids should be prevented. The umbilical cord is stretched and broken near the body wall. Excessive hemorrhage can be controlled with a simple ligature. The uterus should be evaluated closely for additional kids. These may be delivered through the original incision or, if necessary, a second incision may be made along the greater curvature of the other uterine horn. The uterus is closed after the practitioner has assured that there are no additional kids. The placenta may be partially resected to facilitate uterine closure. If the fetus is dead or emphysematous or if there is evidence of metritis, antibiotic or antiseptic boluses may be placed in the uterus.

The uterus is closed with 0 or 1 chromic catgut in 2 inverting layers, such as a Connell followed by a Lembert pattern. Alternatively, the Utrecht suture pattern may be used. This is a continuous inverting pattern inserted using oblique bites and buried knots.[3] The uterus is copiously lavaged with sterile saline and is returned to the abdomen. It is palpated to ensure that it is in normal position. The peritoneum and muscle layers are closed with 0 or 1 chromic catgut in a simple continuous pattern. The skin is closed with a nonabsorbable suture material.

Following surgery, the doe may be given 5 units of oxytocin intravenously or intramuscularly to aid in involution of the uterus. Within 24 to 48 hours the cervix will usually dilate and the placenta will be passed. Systemic antibiotic therapy, such as penicillin G procaine at 20,000 to 40,000 units/kg intramuscularly, twice a day for 3 to 5 days is advisable. Analgesics, such as flunixin meglumine (Banamine) (1.1 mg/kg IM or IV), may help relieve postoperative pain. The doe should be kept in a warm, clean pen until the skin sutures are removed 10 to 14 days after surgery.

PROGNOSIS

The prognosis for the doe's life and fertility after cesarean section is good if the surgery was performed electively. A guarded prognosis for life and fertility should be given if the fetus was emphysematous or macerated or if the doe was seriously ill prior to the operation.

CARE OF THE KID

The head and mouth of the kids should be cleared of fluid and mucus. If respiratory efforts appear depressed, doxapram hydrochloride (Dopram) (2 mg/kg) may be given intravenously using the jugular, lingual or umbilical vein. Doxapram hydrochloride may also be injected under the mucosa of the tongue, or a drop or two may be placed on the underside of the tongue. The navel should be dipped with 2 to 7 per cent iodine soon after birth. If the doe is depressed or recumbent or if the kids are too weak to nurse, 2 oz/kg of colostrum should be given via a nasogastric tube and repeated in 4 to 6 hours. Sedation of the doe with xylazine may cause depression of the kids for 4 to 8 hours. These kids will need to be kept warm and tube fed until a good sucking reflex is present.

References

1. Hudson RS: Surgical procedures on the reproductive system of the cow. In Morrow DA (ed): Current Therapy in Theriogeniology. Philadelphia, WB Saunders Co, 1980.
2. Hildebrand SV: University of California, Davis, Department of Veterinary Anesthesia, personal communication, 1984.
3. Turner AS, McIlwraith CW: Techniques in Large Animal Surgery. Philadelphia, Lea & Febiger, 1982, pp 278–283.

Uterine and Vaginal Prolapse in Goats

Jessica S. Franklin, D.V.M.
Dundee Veterinary Clinic, Dundee, Michigan

Uterine and vaginal prolapses are two distinct problems. Prepartum vaginal prolapses rarely cause postpartum uterine prolapses. The inexperienced goat owner may confuse a vaginal prolapse with the protruding amnionic sac, or may confuse a prolapsed uterus with a retained placenta. If these descriptions are to be relayed accurately by phone, one may contrast the pink or red firm swelling of a vaginal prolapse with the white, slippery, fluid-filled sac of an amnion. A prolapsed uterus will be a large mass, greater than 10 cm across, hanging to the animal's hocks; the owner can easily encircle the retained placenta with his thumb and forefinger at the vulvar lips. Furthermore, the surface of the prolapsed uterus will be dark red or blackened, and the bright red caruncles may have strands of placenta attached. In contrast to the protruding uterus placental membranes are stringy gray-tan, with pale pink cotyledons.

VAGINAL PROLAPSE

Although the protrusion of vaginal tissue through the vulvar lips is not as common as in pregnant sheep, it does occur occasionally during the last 5 weeks of caprine pregnancy.[1] Causes are similar to those for sheep and cattle. These include excess abdominal fill because of maternal fat or fetal mass, lax perineal tissues due to confinement, excess estrogen in forage, previous dystocia or hereditary factors.

Vaginal prolapses tend to recur on subsequent pregnancies.[2] The exposed tissues may be torn or infected, causing illness to the doe or dystocia. In addition, correction by retaining sutures will interfere with normal kidding.

A mild or incomplete vaginal prolapse can be recognized by a pink, peach-sized mass that is visible when the doe lies down but returns to its normal position in the standing animal. A complete vaginal prolapse on the other hand does not spontaneously correct itself upon standing and is larger and reddened because of trauma. It may contain the bladder or other abdominal organs. Frequently, the cervix can be detected as a hard bump in the center.

Treatment. An incomplete prolapse may be treated by increasing daytime exercise and by having the animal confined to a stall, with its hindquarters elevated at night. The owner can apply a lubricating antibiotic ointment to the exposed portion of the prolapse to keep it moist.

A complete vaginal prolapse should be corrected surgically. Epidural anesthesia (see the article Dystocia and Obstetrics in Goats) may help replacement and delay postoperative tenesmus for several hours. After cleaning and lubricating the mass, the tissue may be elevated to help the animal urinate and reduce the size of the prolapse. Holding the goat on her back on a slanted board, or having an assistant raise her hind legs will help ease replacement. After replacement, the vulva should be sutured to maintain the vaginal position. If 4 small loops of umbilical tape are placed in the skin lateral to each side of the vulva, a longer piece of umbilical tape can be used to shoelace the area. The owner can release the shoelace for parturition and replace it after a false alarm. Since prolapses rarely recur after parturition, the anchor sutures can be removed after the placenta has passed. Vaginal retainers designed for ewes may be used with a twine harness.

Persistent tenesmus will breakdown many prolapse sutures. Nonsteroidal analgesics such as aspirin (100 mg/kg BID oral) or flunixin meglumine (Banamine) (1.1 mg/kg BID subcutaneously) should be considered. After 140 days gestation, prostaglandin may be used to induce the birth of viable kids.

Prevention. The best preventive measure for vaginal prolapse is culling. Reoccurence of the prolapse on subsequent pregnancy is common. If the animal is to be kept, increase exercise, avoid obesity and allow a long open period to ensure that the stretched perineal tissues will heal. Lush clover or alfalfa roughage during pregnancy should be avoided, but an adequate diet should be provided.

UTERINE PROLAPSE

Uterine prolapse is the eversion of the postpartum uterus and cervix through the vulva. Dystocia, hypocalcemia and confinement without exercise during gestation all can increase the risk of this relatively uncommon problem.

Prognosis for recovery with breeding soundness is good if the tissue damage is minimal, the uterus has been everted less than 24 hours and the animal is still able to stand. Torn or badly soiled uterine tissue will increase the risk of metritis, peritonitis, and/or death.

Treatment. After cleaning and disinfecting the uterus and hindquarters, the remaining attached placenta should be removed. The hindquarters should be elevated as in the treatment of a vaginal prolapse. The uterus should be replaced with firm, gentle hand pressure, and epidural anesthesia may be necessary with severe straining. If the uterus is difficult to replace and epidural anesthesia has not reduced tenesmus, 2 mg IV or 3 to 5 mg IM of xylazine (Rompun) will sedate the doe and decrease straining. The horns should be everted and liquid or bolus antibiotics placed in the uterus. The vulva should be sutured with 2 mattress sutures or a purse string suture, which may be removed in 3 to 7 days. Postoperative care should include tetanus prophylaxis, oxytocin and systemic antibiotics and, if indicated, subcutaneous or intravenous calcium fluid therapy. Appropriate dosage schedules are listed in the article Dystocia and Obstetrics in the Goat.

The animal should be evaluated for shock. Unless sedated it should be able to stand once the prolapse is corrected. Weak, depressed does may respond to IV steroids and fluids. Three liters of lactated Ringer's provides 50 ml/kg to a milking doe weighing 60 kg.

References

1. Baker JS: Vaginal prolapse correction during cesarean section in the ewe. Bovine Pract 1:43, 1980.
2. Bowen JS: "Doc, my doe just kidded and . . ." Dairy Goat J 59:243, 1981.

Retained Placenta, Metritis and Pyometra

Jessica S. Franklin, D.V.M.
Dundee Veterinary Clinic, Dundee, Michigan

RETAINED PLACENTA

The afterbirth is considered retained if it is not passed within 12 hours of delivery of the last kid. Sixty-five herd owners who answered a nationwide survey in 1982 reported 3500 freshenings, with approximately a 6.4 per cent incidence of retained placenta. Herd problems caused by retained placenta may be attributed to a number of factors, including a selenium deficiency.[1, 2] Inadequate dietary selenium should be suspected when 20 per cent or more of the herd is affected. Dystocia and abortion may also increase the frequency of retained placenta.

Diagnosis of a retained placenta is complicated by the common habit of the doe ingesting the placenta and the difficulty of manually examining the narrow vagina even 24 hours after kidding. Therefore, diagnosis is based on the presence of hanging fetal membranes or straining the day after kidding. Often, the failure to clean may be attributed to an incomplete delivery; that is, a kid is still present in the uterus. A gloved vaginal examination should be performed after cleaning the perineum. If only the placenta is present, the uterus should be treated with antibiotics. Manual removal of the placenta should not be attempted, but administration of oxytocin (10 to 20 units subcutaneously at 12-hour intervals) until placental expulsion occurs is recommended. Systemic antibiotic therapy should continue for 2 to 5 days after the fetal membranes are passed. Furthermore, tetanus prophylaxis should be initiated.

Retained placenta may be prevented by adequate exercise and nutrition during the dry period. Selenium injections at 60 and 14 days prepartum may be used when oral intake is inadequate. Subcutaneous injection of 3 to 5 ml BO-SE provides about 0.05 mg of selenium per kilogram. If a placenta is not found, but a retained placenta is suspected, one dose of oxytocin may be administered.

METRITIS

Metritis or inflammation of the endometrium may be an important cause of infertility. Contamination of the uterus following dystocia or a retained placenta at kidding are common causes of postpartum metritis. Postbreeding metritis may cause a return to estrus within 10 days after breeding, with or without an increased vaginal discharge.

Clinical signs of acute metritis include a rectal temperature above 40°C, a dark red malodorous uterine discharge and anorexia. In chronic metritis the animal may be eating and afebrile, but a purulent vaginal discharge may persist and/or the animal may fail to conceive. This purulent discharge is more copious than the normally thick, scant white vaginal discharge of late estrus.

Systemic antibiotic therapy is the treatment for acute metritis. If the cervix is open, the uterus may be treated directly with a vaginal speculum and infusion pipette technique similar to that used in artificial insemination.

Chronic metritis will benefit from a prostaglandin regimen of 2.5 to 5 mg of dinoprost tromethamine (Lutalyse) injected subcutaneously. Estrus will return in 2 days if a corpus luteum is present. Systemic antibiotics are also used.

PYOMETRA

The classical pyometra, consisting of an enlarged, pus-filled uterus and persistent corpus luteum, is difficult to diagnose without laparotomy or paracentesis. Two more common causes of anestrus and abdominal distension should be considered before diagnosing pyometra: pregnancy and hydrometra. Pyometra is suspected in an anestrus animal discharging large amounts of pus. Treatment as with chronic metritis is recommended.

References

1. Cochran DE: Clinical selenium tocopherol deficiency in dairy goats. Dairy Goat J 58:48, 1980.
2. Guss SB: Management and Diseases of Dairy Goats. Scottsdale, Dairy Goat Journal Publishing Corporation, 1977, p 44.

Caprine Intersexes and Freemartins

Parvathi K. Basrur
A. O. McKinnon, B.V.Sc., M.Sc., A.B.V.P.
Ontario Veterinary College, Guelph, Ontario, Canada

Anomalous sex differentiation leading to the intersex condition is relatively common in goats. It is more prevalent in dairy goats of the Saanen, Toggenburg and Alpine breeds than in any other species of domestic animals.

APPEARANCE

Intersexes exhibit phenotypic variation ranging from nearly normal females to nearly normal males. They are generally femalelike at birth, but as they reach the age of sexual maturity, they become bigger than normal females, with a masculine head and erect hair on their neck. They carry small teats and a bulbus clitoris or a shortened penis. At puberty the clitoris becomes enlarged enough to be externally visible. Hypospadias may or may not be present, and one or two small lumps may be present in scrotal sacs or in the inguinal area (Fig. 1).

BEHAVIOR

The behavior of the intersexes varies greatly. Again, they are generally femalelike at birth, but at puberty they start to butt like a buck and act aggressively towards goats and people. Some dribble their urine or stretch out with a concave back and urinate forward between the legs. At about 5 months they develop the odor characteristic of the buck. A majority of the intersexes show pronounced male libido in the presence of a normal female goat in estrus. Some of the more femalelike intersexes lactate.

GONADS

Intersexes are named with reference to the gonads they carry. The term "true hermaphrodite" is used to distinguish the animal that carries both types of gonads from those that carry either one or the other type of gonads (pseudohermaphrodites). The term "male pseudohermaphrodite" is used to describe an intersex with testes, and the term "female pseudo-hermaphrodite" is used to indicate an intersex that carries ovaries.

With a few notable exceptions the gonads of intersex goats are testes. On this basis most caprine intersexes belong to the male pseudohermaphroditic category. The testes are generally intra-abdominal in the normal location of ovaries, or they may be partially or totally descended. The partially descended testes located in the inguinal region sometimes can be mistaken for udders especially when they begin to enlarge during puberty. In adults the seminiferous tubules are often atrophic, with abundant interstitium. The interstitium consists of mature and immature Leydig cells and small cells resembling fibroblasts. In general, the seminiferous tubules of the older animals are narrow or irregular in outline. The tubules, lined by Sertoli cells lack a lumen and are often hyalinized with thick basement membranes. Germ cells, seen occasionally in young animals, are almost always absent in the adult testes.[6]

Occasionally, a true hermaphrodite carrying ovotestes on both sides, or with an ovotestis on one side and a testis on the other side, occurs. Follicles at various stages of development are seen within these ovotestes (Fig. 2). Adult intersexes with abdominal ovotestes or ovaries often show gonadal hyperplasia and/or gonadal tumors.

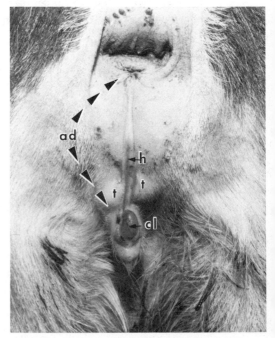

Figure 1. External genitalia of a 5-month-old polled intersex goat exhibiting female chromosome make-up in blood and skin. Note the enlarged clitoris (cl), increased anogenital distance (ad), hypospadias (h) and descended testes (t) in small scrotal sacs on both sides.

the intersexes showing short anogenital distances have intra-abdominal gonads, poorly developed wolffian ducts and well-developed müllerian ducts, whereas those with greater anogenital distance show a greater degree of masculinization of the external and internal genitalia. The gonads are generally intra-abdominal in intersex goats, with an anogenital distance ranging from 3 to 6 cm. This type of animal usually exhibits an enlarged clitoris, well-developed oviduct, uterine horns and cervix along with epididymis and vas deferens, while the accessory sex glands (seminal vesicles) may or may not be present.

Scrotal or inguinal gonads are present in intersexes that display an anogenital distance greater than 6 cm. These animals show extreme enlargement of the clitoris or an almost normal penis with sheath. This type of intersex shows both male and female duct systems including well-developed body and horns of the uterus.[6]

PREVALENCE IN BREEDS

The frequency with which intersexes are noted varies in different breeds of dairy goats. Among the goats raised in the United States, the incidence of intersexes in the Saanen and Toggenburg breeds used to be as high as 11 and 6 per cent, respectively. The overall frequency rises to 20.4 to 22.1 per cent among the progeny of the bucks and does of these breeds that have produced intersex kids previously, suggesting a strong familial tendency for caprine intersexuality.[3,4]

ETIOLOGY

Intersexes are more frequently seen in dairy goats that are polled (hornless). Various hypotheses have been offered for the prevalence of intersexuality in polled goats. The earlier hypothesis was that intersexuality (hermaphroditism) and horn traits are controlled by recessive genes and that these two loci are close to each other on the same chromosome (linked). Hornlessness (polled condition) is the result of a mutation at the horn locus. The polled trait (P), which is dominant to the horned trait (p), appears together with intersexuality (hermaphroditism—h) in PPhh or Pphh goats because the two loci are linked.[1] Thus, intersexes will be seen mainly among polled goats and only rarely among horned animals (pp) because of the occasional crossing over between the two loci, resulting in a pphh genotype. The second genetic explanation is that intersexuality is a pleiotropic effect of the gene for polled trait.[5] On this basis the major trait produced by the P gene is hornlessness, and all the phenotypic modifications noted in caprine intersexes are the minor (pleiotropic) effects of the polled gene, which may not always cause intersexuality.[3,4] This theory fails to account for the occurrence of intersexuality in some horned animals.

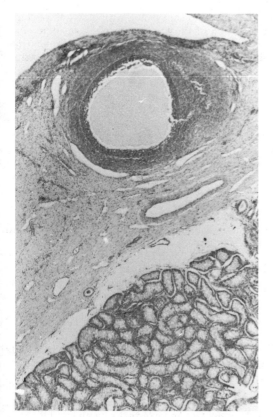

Figure 2. Abdominal ovotestis of a 5-month-old horned intersex showing "active" follicle in the cortex and seminiferous tubules in the medulla (H & E × 50).

STEROIDS

The principal steroid produced by the gonads in caprine intersexes is generally testosterone. Since the intersex testes are generally smaller than normal testes, the plasma testosterone levels tend to be lower than those of their normal male counterparts. The testosterone response to human chorionic gonadotropin (hCG) stimulation is lower in some of the intersexes even though the concentrations of testosterone in plasma may be similar to those of normal bucks.

DUCT SYSTEM

Intersexes exhibit an admixture of the derivatives of the mesonephric (wolffian) and the paramesonephric (müllerian) duct systems. The extent of ductal differentiation varies greatly. A criterion that generally serves as an indicator of the extent of masculinization is the anogenital distance. In a normal adult female this distance is close to 2 cm, and in a normal male it varies from 30 to 40 cm. In intersex goats the anogenital distance varies between 3 and 33 cm and shows a relationship to the type of gonads and gonaducts they carry. As a rule,

Cytogenetic evaluations of caprine intersexes clearly show that most polled intersexes are karyotypically female (XX), and the breeding histories of the parents indicate that the intersexes are homozygous for the polled trait.[6] The presence of male gonads in these homozygous polled (PP) intersexes of XX make-up suggests that they are sex-reversed females. In a female caprine fetus, which is homozygous for the polled gene, two doses of the P gene divert the process of sex differentiation in the male direction despite the presence of two X chromosomes.[2]

The association of the sex-reversed gonads (testes) with varying combinations of müllerian and wolffian duct derivative gonaducts suggests that the testes of the intersexes are not capable of exerting a total masculinizing effect on the duct system or on the external genitalia, even though the levels of testosterone detected in the testes of some adult intersexes are nearly normal for adult bucks of corresponding age.[10] The impact of the fetal steroids may not be sufficient to cause the virilization of the duct system even on the ipsilateral side in some cases. It would appear that the nonsteroidal hormone that inhibits the müllerian duct system (müllerian duct inhibiting factor) is also produced in insufficient amounts, or out of step with gonaduct differentiation, by the fetal testes, since müllerian duct derivatives are generally retained in caprine intersexes. Thus, the polled gene in the homozygous state simulates the Y chromosome in its impact on sex differentiation but succeeds only partially because of the presence of two X chromosomes. It is to be emphasized that this type of intersexuality occurs only in a genotype in which the P gene is in the homozygous state and the sex chromosome make-up is XX. The corollary to this is that all polled does that are fertile are heterozygous for the polled gene.

Another feature of the polled gene (P) is that it has a strong influence on fertility. The frequency of twins and triplets is higher among the progeny of polled (heterozygote, Pp) goats than those of horned goats. Polled does are significantly more prolific than horned does.[8]

The polled gene also has an effect on the sex ratio (the percentage of kids born that are male) in that it shifts the ratio in favor of males. In a polled-polled mating, if the buck is a homozygote for the polled gene (PP), the sex ratio is elevated to 61.4 even when the intersexes are included among the females. If the polled bucks are heterozygotes the ratio drops to 52.1, and when the buck is horned (and lacks the P gene) it is normal (50.7).

In matings of horned does to bucks with decreasing doses of the P gene, the sex ratio remains closer to the expected one, but the advantage shifts away from the male when the dose of P gene decreases. Thus, the sex ratios decrease from 48.6 to 47.5 to 46.3 when the buck's genotype consists of 2, 1 or no P genes (PP, Pp and pp bucks). In other words the trend is to have more females among the progeny if at least one of the parents, preferably the female is horned.[12]

The sex ratio shift is not attributable to selective destruction of the female conceptus in utero since frequencies of stillbirths and abortions remain unaltered in polled to polled matings.[3-5] It is possible that the Y-bearing spermatozoa from Pp bucks have a selective advantage over those carrying the X, or they reach the egg faster especially in those cases in which the Pp does shed multiple ova.

The gene for the polled trait also has an impact on the reproductive performance of the bucks. The bucks that are homozygous for the polled gene tend to become sterile. Testes in these bucks are of normal size (Fig. 3) and the seminiferous tubules display active and often precocious spermatogenesis. However, spermatozoa are not detected in the ejaculates because of a blockage in the caput epididymis. The trapped spermatozoa form hard masses of varying size that are palpable in the caput region of the epididymis.[6,13] In older bucks the seminiferous tubules close to the rete testes degenerate or rupture, causing the release of spermatozoa in the interstitium (extravasation), which often leads to sperm granuloma formation. This type of epididymal stenosis leading to sterility is detected in 10 to 30 per cent of polled bucks.

Thus, it would appear that the homozygous state for the polled gene is disadvantageous to both sexes. In the male it causes poor differentiation of the duct system, causing sterility, and in the genetic female it causes gonadal reversal leading to masculinization of the gonaduct and external genitalia.

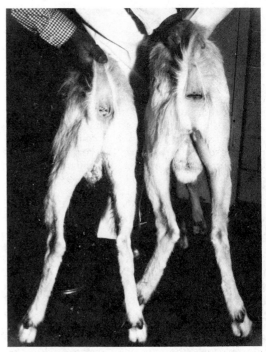

Figure 3. A hindview of a 6-month-old polled sterile buck (right) and his polled intersex sibling (left). Note the adult size scrotal testes in the buck and the poorly developed scrotal sacs of the intersex.

TWINNING AND FREEMARTINISM

The incidence of twinning is as high or higher than that of single births in goats. The birth weight of the kids in twin births is similar to that of single-born normal kids and perinatal mortality is the lowest in twins compared with that in single births and triplets. However, the incidence of intersexes is higher in twins and triplets than in singles.

It was once thought that all intersex goats might be the caprine counterparts of freemartins. Freemartinism is caused by the fusion of fetal membranes and the subsequent vascular anastomosis that allows the passage of cells and hormones from the male fetus to the female fetus. However, earlier observations showed no evidence of placental anastomosis between co-twin caprine fetuses, and on this basis, twinning as a cause of caprine intersexuality was generally rejected. Since the introduction of the leukocyte culture technique for the chromosomal confirmation of chimerism, freemartins have been frequently detected among the caprine intersexes.[7,11] A prerequisite for caprine freemartinism, as in other domestic animals, is birth as a twin to a male kid or as one of heterosexual multiplets. Sometimes birth as a twin may not be recognized as such if one of the twins had died in utero. In these cases the confirmation of freemartinism can be obtained from chromosome analysis, which would reveal the coexistence of male and female cells in blood and other hemapoietic tissues. In caprine freemartins the proportion of male cells in leukocyte cultures could be as low as 1 per cent, which necessitates careful examination of a large number of cells for an accurate diagnosis of freemartinism. Since twinning occurs in horned and polled goats, the freemartin-type intersexes can be seen among both types of goats. Various studies indicate that approximately 6 per cent of the intersexes may be expected to be freemartins. It is believed that in a majority of twin pregnancies in goats, vascular anastomosis either does not occur at all or occurs after the critical period in gonadal differentiation. The external and internal genitalia of caprine freemartins are similar to those of the polled intersexes. However, the masculine features are generally more exaggerated, and the gonads are partially descended testes devoid of germ cells.

TOTAL CHIMERAS

Intersexes that are chimeras are not always male pseudohermaphrodites or invariably a co-twin to a buck. Some of these are true hermaphrodites with a nearly normal ovary on one side and a testis or ovotestis on the other (Fig. 2). The testes are always inactive, and these animals generally resemble females more closely in their external genitalia and the gonaduct system. Karyotypic analysis shows that they are whole-body chimeras. Chimerism in these cases results from the fusion or cellular admixture of male and female embryos at an early stage in embryogenesis or from fertilization of the second polar body and ootid by X- and Y-bearing spermatozoa prior to the fusion of the polar body with the ootid.

The occurrence of this type of intersex is rare in goats, although approximately 1 per cent of all the caprine intersexes may belong to this category. Whole-body chimeras, like freemartins and the polled intersexes, are sterile.

MECHANISMS LEADING TO INTERSEXUALITY

In freemartins the ovary of the female co-twin is virilized to resemble a poorly developed testis, which generally remains abdominal or descends partially. Germ cells are detected up to 18 weeks of gestation, but they generally degenerate by the time the intersex is born.[6] Although testosterone from the male fetus can reach the female fetus through the shared placental vascular channel, the conversion of fetal ovary into testes is not likely to be brought about by testosterone from the male co-twin. Since chimerism has been detected in the gonads of co-twins in cattle, it is believed that the XY cells from the male co-twin entering the ovary may be responsible for the abnormal differentiation of the freemartin gonad. This assumption is supported by the detection of H-Y antigen in the fetal ovary of the freemartin.[14] It would appear that the H-Y antigen disseminated by the XY cells entices the sex cords to differentiate as seminiferous tubules, the cortex as the thick tunica albuginea and the mesonephric blastema cells as the Leydig cells. The H-Y antigen from each XY cell might be sufficient to organize a group of neighboring XX cells into programmed effector cells, or it might instruct a succession of XX cells to engage in the formation of seminiferous tubules without transferring the H-Y antigen to XX cells.[9] The XX germ cells of the ovary coated with H-Y antigen degenerate during the process of gonadal organization. This mechanism[9] will operate in caprine freemartins as well as in the true hermaphrodites with XX/XY whole-body chimerism. In the case of polled intersexes the P locus acts as a Y chromosome segment[15] and generates H-Y antigen to transform the fetal ovary into the testis. All three types of intersexes are therefore H-Y antigen positive.

References

1. Asdell SA: The genetic sex of intersexual goats and a probable linkage with the gene for hornlessness. Science 99:124, 1944.
2. Basrur PK, Coubrough RI: Anatomical and cytological sex of a Saanen goat. Cytogenetics 3:414, 1964.
3. Eaton ON: An anatomical study of hermaphrodism in goats. Am J Vet Res 4:333, 1943.
4. Eaton ON: The relation between polled and hermaphroditic characters in dairy goats. Genetics 30:51, 1945.
5. Eaton ON, Simmons VL: Hermaphrodism in milk goats. J Hered 30:261, 1939.
6. Hammerton JL, Dickson JM, Pollard CE, et al.: Genetic intersexuality in goats. J Reprod Fert Suppl 7:25, 1969.
7. Ilbery PLT, Williams D: Evidence of the freemartin condition in the goat. Cytogenetics 6:276, 1967.

8. Laor M, Barnea R, Angel H, Soller M: Polledness and hermaphroditism in Saanen goats. Israel J Agric Res 12:83, 1962.
9. Ohno S, Wachtel SS: Hormone-like role of H-Y antigen in bovine freemartin gonad. Nature 261:597, 1976.
10. Short RV, Hamerton JL, Grieves SA, Pollard CE: An intersex goat with a bilaterally asymmetrical reproductive tract. J Reprod Fert 16:283, 1968.
11. Smith MC, Dunn HO: Freemartin condition in a goat. JAVMA 178:735, 1981.
12. Soller M, Angel H: Polledness and abnormal sex ratios in Saanen goats. J Hered 55:139, 1964.
13. Soller M, Padeh B, Wysoki M, Ayalon N: Cytogenetics of Saanen goats showing abnormal development of the reproductive tract associated with the dominant gene for polledness. Cytogenetics 8:51, 1969.
14. Wachtel SS, Hall JL, Muller U, Chaganti R: Serum borne H-Y antigen in the fetal bovine freemartin. Cell 21:917, 1980.
15. Wachtel SS, Basrur PK, Koo GC: Recessive male determining genes. Cell 15:279, 1978.

Causes and Diagnosis of Abortion in Goats

Mary C. Smith, D.V.M.
Cornell University, Ithaca, New York

The female goat that is not an intersex is normally a very fertile animal. There are, however, numerous known reasons for failure of gestation.[1,7] These are listed in Table 1.

MEDICATIONS

A number of anthelmintics, including phenothiazine and carbon tetrachloride, should not be given to pregnant goats. Tetramisole has been reported by practitioners as causing abortion when administered in late gestation. Thiabendazole and fenbendazole can be safely used at this time. Undoubtedly, even safe drugs can develop a bad reputation if they are administered in a stressful way or if the herd is on the verge of an infectious abortion storm.

NUTRITION

A chronic (6-months duration) and severe vitamin A deficiency has caused epizootic abortions in adult goats; kids in the same herd showed diarrhea, lacrimation and corneal opacities. Such a deficiency is caused by a diet limited to dry feed, by severe infestation with liver flukes or by coccidiosis. When parasitism is involved, general unthriftiness is evident. It should be noted that impending starvation due to malnutrition, parasitism, exposure or a combination of these problems will often induce abortion a few days before the doe herself dies.

Manganese deficiency causes abortion at 80 to 105 days of gestation as well as low birth weights and paralyzed or deformed kids. Iodine deficiency is associated with stillbirths or weak and hairless kids. Sometimes the female kids are born dead and the males are born alive, suggesting that there is a sex difference in iodine requirements. Once identified, abortions caused by nutritional deficiencies can be easily prevented by appropriate dietary supplementation.

Although few reports are available, it is presumed that numerous poisonous plants can induce abortion in goats (see Table 1).

INFECTIOUS DISEASES

Many infectious diseases may cause failure of gestation. Some of these (chlamydiosis, campylobacteriosis, toxoplasmosis, Q fever and mycoplasmosis) are described in detail in other articles in this section.

Brucellosis. Brucellosis is currently not a very important disease in goats in the United States, although it is highly significant in Mediterranean countries and in Central and South America. Sporadic outbreaks have been observed in the southwestern United States, with documented reports from Texas[8] and Colorado.

Brucella melitensis is the principal cause of brucellosis in goats. *B. abortus* has occasionally been isolated from goats.[4] There do not appear to be any published reports of *B. ovis* infections as a cause of abortion in goats.

The organism enters through mucous membranes and may be found in any organ but tends to localize in the lymph nodes, udder and testes. Clinical signs include abortion, lameness, mastitis and orchitis. The first introduction of the disease on the farm will usually be accompanied by an abortion storm, with abortions being most frequent in the fourth month. On gross examination, the placenta is normal. Few abortions will occur in later years, but some of the goats may have chronic uterine lesions and remain sterile. Many infected goats will be symptomless, and abortion does not occur under endemic conditions if the environment and management are good.

Usually, infection of adults is lifelong, but some goats can recover from brucellosis. Apparently

Table 1. Reported Causes of Abortion, Stillbirth or Weak Newborns in Goats*

United States	Exotic
Anaphylaxis	Akabane disease
Anaplasmosis	Babesiasis
Anthrax, acute	Besnoitiosis, globidiosis
Blue tongue virus	Foot and mouth
Border disease	disease
Broomweed (*Gutierrezia*	Heartwater
sp.) poisoning	Nairobi sheep disease
Brucellosis	Peste des petits
Campylobacteriosis	ruminants
Caprine herpesvirus	Rift valley fever
infection	Theileriasis, East Coast
Chlamydiosis, enzootic	fever
abortion	Tick borne fever
Chromosomal defects	Wesselsbron disease
Copper deficiency	
Coxiella burnetii, Q fever	
Drug induced through	
estrogen, glucocorticoid,	
prostaglandin	
Goiter, iodine deficiency	
Japanese pieris poisoning	
Johne's disease,	
paratuberculosis	
Lathyrism	
Leptospirosis	
Levamisole toxicity	
Listeria abortion	
Liver fluke disease	
Locoweed (*Astragalus* and	
Oxytropis sp.) poisoning	
Manganese deficiency	
Malnutrition, protein-	
calorie starvation	
Mycoplasmosis	
Nitrate poisoning	
Phenothiazine	
Pregnancy toxemia	
Prolonged labor	
Salmonellosis	
Sarcocystosis	
Sheep X goat hybrids	
Slaframine toxicity	
Stress abortion	
Toxoplasmosis	
Uterine torsion	
Vitamin A deficiency	
Warfarin toxicity	
White muscle disease	

*From White ME, Lewkowicz J, Powers MS: Consultant Diagnosis/Sign Search Package. Version 1.1. Ithaca, New York State College of Veterinary Medicine, Cornell University, 1984.

healthy kids from brucellosis-positive mothers are often infected, and normal newborn kids rapidly become infected if they drink infected milk. Often these very young infected kids will have negative serologic tests. Opinions vary as to whether these kids will generally eliminate the infection before they are 4 months of age. Goats excrete the *Brucella* organisms intermittently in their milk even if they have not recently kidded. Brucellae may be excreted from the vagina of goats that have never kidded or aborted, and excretion continues for more than 3 weeks after parturition. Dust and soil are readily contaminated. Good data are not available on the probability of excretion in urine or feces.

Several diagnostic tests are available. Tube agglutination titers of 1:25 or higher are usually considered positive, while recently infected does may give negative reactions. Occasional false-positive reactions occur. The brucella card test has been used as a herd screening test. Whey agglutination tests are not sufficiently sensitive to detect infected goats. In one study only 24 of 174 infected goats gave positive whey test results. A stained antigen test similar to the milk ring test has been successfully used; after overnight incubation, a radiated deposit of agglutinated antigen is visible on the bottom of the tube. True rings are rarely seen.

Cultures of milk, vaginal swabs, necropsy specimens and fetal tissues such as abomasal contents, spleen and placenta are routinely processed aerobically at 37°C. Higher CO_2 tension is needed for *B. abortus*.

Vaccination of goats is neither needed nor permitted in the United States. If one animal in the herd is proved to be infected, the entire goat herd should be destroyed. If the owner refuses to permit elimination of the herd, testing and slaughter of all reactors should continue for several years before the herd is presumed clean. All new animals imported to an area or farm should have blood tests, and bucks should be tested before they are used for service. In parts of the country in which caprine brucellosis is essentially unknown, testing every 3 years is adequate. States adjacent to Mexico may find 6- to 12-month testing intervals to be more appropriate. Often, the first indication of brucellosis in goats is the occurrence of undulant fever in humans consuming unpasteurized milk or cheese.

Leptospirosis. Epizootics of leptospirosis occasionally occur in goat herds. *Leptospira grippotyphosa* is the most frequently reported strain.[6] A diagnosis based on clinical signs alone is often difficult. Icterus is not always present, and most animals are afebrile. In the hyperacute form the goats die of septicemia within 12 to 24 hours after the illness is first noticed. They stop feeding and may hold their heads low. Necropsy findings include anemia, an enlarged liver and enlarged, swollen kidneys. Goats with acute illnesses are sick from 1 to 3 days and show listlessness, inappetence and vague nervous signs before they die. The urine is often dark-red or brown, and abortions may occur. Goats with chronic illnesses are sick for about 1 week before they recover clinically without any treatment. The mucous membranes in these animals tend to be pale and icteric. The majority of infected goats become carriers without ever showing any signs and leptospiruria may last for at least 1 month.

Positive diagnosis can be made based on seroagglutination tests, dark field examination of the urine and culture procedures. Cultures of the liver and kidney are most apt to give positive results; blood, urine and milk may be injected intraperitoneally into white mice or guinea pigs, and the liver and kidney of the laboratory animals can then be cultured.

In species other than the goat treatment with 11 mg/kg of streptomycin intramuscularly twice a day for 3 days is usually effective in controlling the septicemia and preventing the carrier state. Vaccination every 6 to 12 months with the appropriate strain (based on serologic testing) should soon control the outbreak and prevent recurrences.

Listeriosis. Listeriosis is a common disease of goats. Signs vary from peracute deaths, to brainstem central nervous system (CNS) disorders lasting several days to undetected carriers. A carrier or recovering animal may shed the organism in urine, milk or semen as well as in nasal, ocular or vaginal discharges. Spoiled silage is another possible, though less common, source of infection. Oral dosing of pregnant goats with *Listeria monocytogenes* causes abortion or stillbirth. There are no diagnostic fetal lesions, and maceration is often well advanced by the time expulsion of the fetus occurs. In natural herd outbreaks abortion frequently occurs in the last month of gestation. The doe usually shows no illness prior to aborting but may develop a necrotic metritis and die soon afterward. Sometimes, the organism localizes in microabscesses in the endometrium; the aborting doe aborts again if rebred soon after the initial infection.

Antibiotic therapy using high doses of penicillin or tetracycline is often of no avail if advanced encephalitic signs are evident. The intracellular location of the organism protects it from antibiotic action. Prophylactic treatment of the remainder of the herd has been recommended to prevent new cases of either encephalitis or abortion. One such regimen involves administration of intramuscular tetracycline (3 mg/kg) for 3 days, followed by a week of oral tetracycline therapy. Dosages for prolonged tetracycline feedings are discussed under chlamydiosis.

Miscellaneous Bacterial Causes of Abortion. *Salmonella* infections have caused outbreaks of abortion in some goat herds. Details of the clinical findings are not available.

Johne's disease, or paratuberculosis, in goats is a chronic condition characterized by unthriftiness, weight loss and parasitism. Diarrhea may occur terminally. Ante mortem diagnosis may be based on an agar gel immunodiffusion test (AGID). Johnin tests are not very accurate, and fecal cultures for *Mycobacterium paratuberculosis* require several months. Fecal smears are rarely positive. The complement fixation test is negative until late in the course of the disease. At necropsy, the intestinal mucosa is thickened but generally is less rugose than the mucosa in cattle affected by Johne's disease. Mesenteric lymph nodes may be edematous, caseated or calcified. Microscopic examination of biopsy specimens from the ileal mucosa and ileocecal lymph node for acid-fast bacteria will confirm the diagnosis. Reproduction is generally poor when

animals are noticeably affected. Failure of conception, abortions and weak kids have all been reported. There is no effective treatment; animals with positive AGID tests or fecal cultures should be culled.

Viral Causes of Abortion. A syndrome of arthrogryposis and hydranencephaly has been reported in goats as well as in other domestic ruminants. The etiologic agent is the Akabane virus, which is thought to be an arbovirus. The syndrome has been recognized in Japan, Israel and Australia. Some deformed kids are aborted, while others go to term.

Experimental inoculation of does in the second month of pregnancy with the agent of border disease sometimes causes abortion or ataxic and shaker kids. Placentitis occurs in the doe. Hypomyelinogenesis and hypergliosis of the CNS are present in the kids, but hair coat defects have not been observed.

Abortions due to blue tongue virus in goats have been reported but are not well documented.[1]

Although goats have been experimentally infected with the infectious bovine rhinotracheitis (IBR) virus, they are not considered a natural host. Their response is generally limited to pyrexia and mild clinical illness. To date, there is no evidence that the IBR virus has any effect on reproduction in goats.[3] Instead, a serologically distinct herpesvirus has been shown to produce abortion in does and enteritis in kids.[5]

DIAGNOSIS OF CAPRINE ABORTION

A systematic approach is imperative for the diagnosis of abortions in goats. Many different etiologies need to be considered and each requires special tests. Be sure the pathologist is aware of which infectious agents are most likely to be present. The standard protocols for diagnosing bovine abortions due to brucellosis, leptospirosis, IBR, bovine virus diarrhea and campylobacteriosis will rarely solve a goat herd problem. Neither is mycotic abortion common in goats. Instead, the practitioner must obtain a good nutritional and clinical history, including possible exposure to carrier animals. When samples are submitted to a diagnostic laboratory, it is extremely important that placenta be included with the fetus. Without the placenta, identification of chlamydiosis and toxoplasmosis will be unlikely. Owners should be aware of the gross appearance of a mummy: a brownish, hairless fetus with an elongated muzzle and sunken eye sockets. All too often the owner learns that a mummy is unsuitable for either culture of histologic examination only after rushing it long distances to the laboratory. Whenever possible, fetuses and placentae from several aborting does should be submitted. Autolysis commonly obscures diagnostic changes, and in addition, more than one etiologic agent may be active in the herd.[2] The first abortion in the herd may be the most important, but many owners do not become seriously concerned until an abortion storm is evident. The owner should be instructed to freeze any fetuses and placentae, no matter how certain he or she might be that the abortion was caused by fighting or a fall. Does aborting later may eat their placentae. Acute serum samples should also be saved frozen from all aborting does. Paired serology may be required to confirm a suspicion of toxoplasmosis or chlamydiosis. In the meantime, if a positive diagnosis is not reached rapidly, the owner may choose to treat remaining pregnant does with tetracycline as described under chlamydiosis. Aborting does should be isolated from the remainder of the herd.

Most of the infectious diseases that cause abortion in goats are zoonotic, including chlamydiosis, Q fever, toxoplasmosis, campylobacteriosis, listeriosis and salmonellosis. The owner should be instructed to wear gloves when handling aborted fetuses and to burn or bury any placentae and fetuses not needed for diagnostic efforts. In addition, pasteur-

ization of goat milk for human consumption should be stressed.

References

1. East NE: Pregnancy toxemia, abortions, and periparturient diseases. Vet Clin North Am: Large Anim Pract 5:601, 1983.
2. Gunson DE, et al.: Abortion and stillbirth associated with *Chlamydia psittaci* var *ovis* in dairy goats with high titers to *Toxoplasma gondii*. JAVMA 183:1447, 1983.
3. Mohanty SB, et al.: Natural infection with infectious bovine rhinotracheitis virus in goats. JAVMA 160:879, 1972.
4. Renoux G: Brucellosis in goats and sheep. In Brandly CA, Jungherr EL (eds): Advances in Veterinary Science. Vol 3. New York, Academic Press, 1957.
5. Saito JK, et al.: A new herpesvirus isolate from goats: Preliminary report. Am J Vet Res 35:847, 1974.
6. Van der Hoeden J: Leptospirosis among goats in Israel. J Comp Pathol 63:101, 1953.
7. White ME, Lewkowicz J, Powers MS: Consultant Diagnosis/Sign Search Package. Version 1.1. Ithaca, New York State College of Veterinary Medicine, Cornell University, 1984.
8. Whiting RD, White BM, Stiles FC, Jr: An epizootic of *Brucella melitensis* infection in Texas. JAVMA 157:1860, 1970.

Chlamydiosis

N. E. East, M.S., D.V.M., M.P.V.M.
University of California, Davis, California

Chlamydia psittaci (enzootic abortion) appears to be the most common cause of infectious abortion in goats in the United States. Studies of *Chlamydia psittaci* have demonstrated species-specific antigens and have also shown that antigenic types are distinct and disease specific and that cross protection does not occur. The antigenic strains found in goats appear to be closely related to those in sheep; antigenic type 1 is implicated in abortions and the birth of stillborn and weak kids and in neonatal chlamydial pneumonia. Conjunctivitis and polyarthritis of growing and adult goats are caused by antigenic type 2.[5]

Enzootic abortion is of such serious economic consideration in some countries that compulsory government vaccination programs have been implemented.[4] In the United States in endemically infected herds 25 to 60 per cent of does kidding for the first time abort. Natural immunity is about 3 years, and in one herd observed, 24 per cent of the 4-year-old does (third kidding) aborted compared with 48 per cent of does aborting that kidded for the first time. Figures for losses due to weak kids are not known. Estimates for baseline pregnancy wastage are 2 to 8 per cent in the goat.

The epidemiology of *Chlamydia psittaci* is poorly understood. Intestinal shedding is common in endemically infected herds, and aborting does shed large numbers of the organism from the uterine fluids, fetus and placenta, particularly in the first 3 weeks following abortion, with complete elimination of *Chlamydia* from the uterus within 3 months.[2, 6] The route of infection is likely by ingestion. Does exposed for the first time to *Chlamydia psittaci* in the first half of gestation will abort that pregnancy. Does boarded for breeding may acquire the infection in endemically infected herds and abort, but several weeks of exposure appear to be required. Susceptible does exposed for the first time in the last half of pregnancy usually abort in the subsequent gestation. Newborn females in endemic herds may acquire the infection at or near birth, the infection is latent until their first pregnancy, which ends in abortion.[3] In experimental infections, abortion occurs about 4 weeks postinfection, but the fetus is not susceptible to infection until the last trimester of pregnancy.[3]

Abortion due to *Chlamydia psittaci* usually occurs in the last 4 weeks of gestation, but it can occur as early as day 100 of gestation.[2, 6, 7] Does are not normally ill but may separate from the herd, show slight depression and have a serosanguineous vaginal discharge 2 to 3 days prior to aborting. The fetus may be autolyzed or fresh; fresh full-term stillborns are commonly found in herd outbreaks. Some weak newborns may be expected, and a few does may retain the placenta.

Pathologic changes in the fetus due to enzootic abortion are nonspecific.[2, 8] The appearance depends on the amount of time that passes after the death of the fetus and subsequent expulsion from the uterus. A fetus aborted early in the last trimester is usually autolyzed, a condition characterized by thick sanguineous subcutaneous edema, excess serosanguineous peritoneal and pleural fluids, and soft internal organs. Sometimes dehydration occurs in utero, and the fetus appears mummified. Kids aborted near term are fresh; many have excess pleural and pericardial fluid, and some have subcutaneous petechiae on the skin of the limbs, neck and hips. Grossly, the placenta shows regional to generalized placentitis (white to yellow necrotic areas) involving the cotyledons and intercotyledonary areas.

Diagnosis is based on the demonstration of chlamydial elementary bodies (small, dark red, spherical, 200-nm diameter intracytoplasmic bodies) in the cotyledon using various stains but Giemsa stain is preferred.[8] Oil immersion with a light microscope is used to examine stained smears of the cut surface of cotyledons. An indirect fluorescent antibody technique is available in some areas. Serology is of little value. Isolation of *Chlamydia* in embryonated chicken eggs or in tissue culture is possible but is too expensive and time-consuming for diagnostic purposes. Differential diagnosis should include vibriosis (*Campylobacter fetus*), toxoplasmosis and Q fever.

Treatment in the case of outbreaks is twofold. First, does aborting should be removed from the herd for at least 3 weeks, and the fetus and placenta should be burned or buried in quicklime. Care should be taken not to contaminate buckets, feeders and implements. No feed should be offered on the ground, and feeders designed so that goats cannot get into them should be used. Second, antibiotics are given to all pregnant does. Tetracyclines are usually used with dosages of 80 to 450 mg per head per day continuously in feed or water, or injectable slow-release base tetracyclines* (9 mg/lb subcutaneously) are used twice a week until the last 4 weeks of gestation. Variable results have been obtained using antibiotics in outbreaks.[2,7] Does in the first half of gestation are most likely to benefit from antibiotic treatment.[7]

---

*Liquamycin LA 200, Pfizer

Prevention of chlamydial abortion is by far the best approach. Killed vaccines† for sheep are available in a number of states; in one study, a decrease in abortions by 50 per cent was seen, and other workers have reported a decrease of 70 per cent.[1,4,7] Timing of vaccination is important, the optimum time being 4 to 6 weeks prior to breeding. A loss of efficacy occurs if vaccination is done after breeding. The probable difference in the antigenic type of goat and sheep enzootic abortion agents may lead to lower efficacy when using sheep vaccines in the goat. Nevertheless, sheep vaccine has been fairly effective when used in the field. Vaccine trials in sheep have shown that protection from abortion lasts for about 3 years with one vaccination 4 to 6 weeks prior to the first breeding. Chlortetracycline fed at 80 mg per head per day from 10 days prior to exposure through gestation or at the rate of 150 mg per head per day 2 to 3 weeks prior to breeding has prevented chlamydial abortion under laboratory conditions.[7] Results in the field using antibiotics as a preventative are unknown, but the expense is greater than that associated with use of vaccine.

---

†Enzootic abortion vaccine (Ovine), Colorado Serum Company

References

1. Foggie A: Preparation of vaccines against enzootic abortion of ewes. A review of the research work at the Moredun Institute. Vet Bull 43:587, 1973.
2. Hall RF: Infectious abortions in ewes. Compend Cont Ed Vet 4:S216, 1982.
3. Munro R, Hunter AR: Infection of lambs by orally administered ovine abortion strain of *Chlamydia psittaci*. Vet Rec 109:562, 1981.
4. Polydorou K: The control of enzootic abortion in sheep and goats in Cyprus. Br Vet J 137, 4:411, 1981.
5. Schachter J, Banks J, Sugg N, et al.: Serotyping of *Chlamydia* isolates of ovine origin. Infect Immun 9:92, 1974.
6. Stortz J: *Chlamydia and Chlamydia Induced Diseases.* Springfield, Ill, Charles C Thomas, 1971.
7. Watson WA: The prevention and control of infectious ovine abortion. Br Vet J 129, 4:309, 1973.
8. Waldhalm DG, DeLong WJ: Laboratory diagnosis of ovine abortion. 23rd Annual Proceedings American Association of Veterinary Laboratory Diagnosticians: 1980, pp 183-185.

Campylobacteriosis (formerly Vibriosis)

K. L. Anderson, D.V.M., M.S.
University of Illinois, Urbana, Illinois

Campylobacter (vibrionic) abortion has been rarely documented as a cause of infectious abortion in goats. There are only three reports in the United States literature that implicate *Campylobacter* spp. in caprine abortions. Organisms implicated include *C. jejuni* in one report and *C. fetus* (subspecies unidentified) and a "vibriolike" organism similar to *C. fetus* in the others.

CLINICAL FINDINGS

Based on the descriptions from the limited number of cases of caprine *Campylobacter* abortion, *Campylobacter* spp. should be considered in the differential diagnosis of late gestation abortions in does and of weak and/or stillborn kids. Aborting does may or may not show signs of systemic illness. In one report, two of five aborting does had signs of systemic illness, including fever, depression and toxemia.[1] A mucopurulent or sanguinopurulent vaginal discharge was noted in all aborting does, either pre- or postexpulsion of the dead fetuses. A mild, pasty diarrhea was also noted in does in this herd, in which *C. jejuni* was isolated.

Characteristic fetal lesions in aborted fetuses cannot be accurately described from the limited number of cases. However, fetuses expelled following intrauterine death may exhibit subcutaneous edema and excess fluid in body cavities. In one report, multiple necrotic foci 2 mm in diameter were observed in the liver.

In a limited experimental study of caprine *C. jejuni*, two late gestation does were administered 3×10^9 viable *C. jejuni* orally in 10 ml of culture media while a late gestation (control) doe was administered 10 ml of culture media. Both *C. jejuni*-inoculated does developed fever, depression and mild fecal pastiness, and *C. jejuni* was reisolated from feces. One inoculated doe and the control doe kidded normally. The other *C. jejuni*-inoculated doe aborted triplets 8 days postinoculation. *C. jejuni* was reisolated in pure culture from several tissues of all three kids. At necropsy, *C. jejuni* was reisolated from the gallbladder and small intestines of both inoculated does. Prior to abortion, blood was culture-positive for *C. jejuni* in the aborting doe.

Mild intercotyledonary placentitis was observed in the aborting doe. Caution must be used in drawing conclusions based on such small numbers, but it appears that (1) *C. jejuni* (3×10^9 organisms) can cause abortion following oral inoculation of late gestation does; and (2) *C. jejuni* can colonize the small intestine of the goat.

DIAGNOSIS

Definitive diagnosis of *Campylobacter* abortion is accomplished by isolation of the organism from aborted fetuses.[1] This is most properly conducted by laboratories experienced in the procedure. Gram stains of fetal stomach contents may reveal gram-negative, S-shaped organisms. The organism can be cultured on 5 per cent bovine blood agar incubated at 37°C in 10 per cent carbon dioxide.

Serologic tests and tests for serotyping and phage-typing *Campylobacter* spp. isolates are available at a few specialized laboratories.[1-3]*

TREATMENT AND PREVENTION

Because of the apparent rarity of the disease, recommendations for treatment and prevention are empirical. However, because this disease may be similar to ovine *Campylobacter* abortion, it can be similarly treated. Recommended doses of penicillin-dihydrostreptomycin (10,000 IU/lb of procaine penicillin G and 5 to 10 mg/lb of dihydrostreptomycin) may be administered intramuscularly daily, and oxytetracycline (75 mg/head/day) may be administered orally in the feed.

Because of the probable oral route of infection, sanitary conditions, avoidance of fecal contamination of feedstuffs and isolation of aborting does are recommended.

PUBLIC HEALTH SIGNIFICANCE

C. jejuni has been recognized as a cause of a mild and self-limiting gastroenteritis in man, with more severe complications in some cases.[1-3] Domestic animals and unpasteurized milk are thought to be the source of *C. jejuni* infection in some human cases.[1-3] In Scotland, shepherds giving artificial resuscitation to *C. jejuni*-infected lambs have acquired *Campylobacter* gastroenteritis. Aborted fetuses infected with *C. jejuni* should be considered a potential source of *C. jejuni* infection in man and should be handled accordingly.

---

*The Vibriosis Research Laboratory, National Animal Disease Center, Ames, Iowa 50010.

References

1. Anderson KL, Hamoud MM, Urbance JW, et al.: Isolation of *Campylobacter jejuni* from an aborted caprine fetus. J Am Vet Med Assoc 183:90, 1983.

2. Blaser MJ, Reller LR: Campylobacter enteritis. New Engl J Med 305:1444, 1981.
3. Prescott JF, Munroe DL: *Campylobacter jejuni* enteritis in man and domestic animals. J Am Vet Med Assoc 181:1524, 1981.

Transplacental Toxoplasmosis in Goats

J. P. Dubey, M.V.Sc., Ph.D.

Animal Pathology Institute
V.S.D.A., A.R.S., Barc-East,
Beltsville, Maryland

Definition. Toxoplasmosis, caused by a protozoan, *Toxoplasma gondii,* is a common infection in goats, other livestock and people worldwide.

Infection in the Doe. Does become infected by ingesting food or water contaminated with oocysts from feces of infected cats. Following ingestion, motile one-celled organisms are liberated from oocysts in the small intestine. They invade and grow in cells of the intestine and associated lymph nodes. They enter the bloodstream and spread to other tissues of the doe within 2 weeks of ingestion of oocysts. The parasite then forms cysts in muscles, brain, liver and other tissues and may remain there for many months or for the life of the host. In the pregnant doe, *Toxoplasma* can invade and multiply in the placenta; it can also spread to the fetus. In either case it may cause abortion. If it spreads to the fetus, it can cause birth defects or illness in newborn kids.

Clinical Signs. Clinical signs vary with dose and the strain of *T. gondii*. Within 1 to 3 weeks of infection goats develop fever, anorexia, generalized muscle weakness, dyspnea and diarrhea, and some die. Goats that survive become clinically normal, although pregnant does may abort.

Effects on the Fetus. *Toxoplasma* infection may result in fetal death, resorption of the fetus, stillbirth, birth of a live but weak kid, or the birth of a normal kid, depending on the stage of pregnancy and the strain of the parasite.[1-5] Effects on the fetus are most severe when infection occurs in the first 3 months of pregnancy.[3]

Diagnosis. Does that abort because of toxoplasmosis are unlikely to be clinically ill at the time of parturition. Therefore, diagnosis is generally made

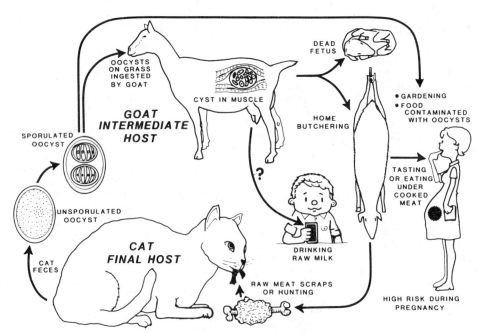

Figure 1. Toxoplasma in goats.

by examination of the fetal membranes and other fetal tissues. *Toxoplasma* produces characteristic necrotic lesions in the placenta. Color photographs of placental lesions have been published.[1] These lesions consist of microscopic to macroscopic, white to yellow foci of necrosis and calcification in the cotyledons; intercotyledonary areas are unaffected. Lesions are seen more easily if the placenta is thoroughly washed and then examined while submerged in isotonic solution so that villi float, untangle, and spread, exposing the deeper parts of the cotyledon. There are usually no specific gross lesions in fetal tissues. For confirmation, placentae and fetal membranes should be submitted to diagnostic laboratories. For shipment, they should be cooled, placed in a plastic bag and kept cold (but not frozen) during transit. *Toxoplasma* may be occasionally recognized in sections of placenta or fetal tissues, but in most instances, organisms are too few to be detected microscopically. Inoculation of tissues in mice can reveal even light infections but is time consuming and expensive. Serologic examination of the doe for antibodies to *T. gondii* may also aid in the diagnosis. An indirect fluorescent antibody test can detect *T. gondii* antigen in frozen sections and is also useful in making a rapid diagnosis.

Epidemiology and Prevention. At present, there is no vaccine to prevent toxoplasmosis. *Toxoplasma* infection prior to pregnancy generally results in protective immunity; therefore, does that have aborted should be retained for breeding in subsequent seasons. Cats are the key in the spread of toxoplasmosis because oocysts excreted by them can survive in soil for many months. Most cats become infected in nature by ingesting meat infected with *T. gondii* or by hunting (Fig. 1). Therefore, felines should not be fed uncooked meat or allowed to hunt. Grain containers should be kept covered to prevent cats from defecating in the grain. Placentae and fetal tissues should be burnt or buried because they may be infectious to people and animals. Tissues of goats butchered at home or bought from the store should be cooked well before consumption, and hands should be washed with soap and water after handling goat tissues or placentae.

References

1. Dubey JP: Epizootic toxoplasmosis associated with abortion in dairy goats in Montana. J Am Vet Med Assoc 178:661, 1981.
2. Dubey JP: Repeat transplacental transfer of *Toxoplasma gondii* in goats. J Am Vet Med Assoc 180:1220, 1981.
3. Dubey JP: *Toxoplasma*-induced abortion in dairy goats. J Am Vet Med Assoc 178:671, 1981.
4. Dubey JP, Sharma SP, Lopes CWG, et al.: Caprine toxoplasmosis: Abortion, clinical signs, and distribution of *Toxoplasma* in tissues of goats fed *Toxoplasma gondii* oocysts. Am J Vet Res 41:1072, 1980.
5. Munday BL, Mason RW: Toxoplasmosis as a cause of perinatal death in goats. Aust Vet J 55:485, 1979.

Coxiella burnetii Infection in Goats

R. B. Miller, B.Sc., D.V.M., Ph.D.
University of Guelph, Guelph, Ontario

N. C. Palmer, D.V.M., M.Sc., Ph.D.
Ontario Ministry of Agriculture and Food, Guelph, Ontario

M. Kierstad
Ontario Ministry of Agriculture and Food, Guelph, Ontario

DISTRIBUTION AND DISEASES PRODUCED

The causative agent of Q fever (Query fever) has been assigned to the genus *Coxiella* in the family Rickettsiaceae. The organism is an obligate intracellular parasite. *Coxiella burnetii* occurs in man, cattle, sheep, goats and many forms of wildlife throughout the world. In many countries, including the United States and Canada, the organism is associated with abortion in goats and sheep. Epidemiologic studies indicate that there may be strain differences in virulence. *Coxiella burnetii* may frequently be isolated from the placentae of sheep giving birth to normal lambs. Many workers suggest that uncomplicated infections with *C. burnetii* will not result in abortions and that additional factors must operate before abortion or stillbirth occurs. Other workers report that high exposures to *C. burnetii* alone may cause abortion.

TRANSMISSION

Large numbers of organisms are expelled into the environment via placental tissues, birth fluids, colostrum and milk. Birds may spread the organism, and some forms of wildlife may carry it. The prevalence of detectable antibodies in wildlife appears to be related to their association with infected livestock rather than the reverse. The organism is also carried by *Dermacentor* and *Ixodes* ticks; however, usual increases in antibody titers in livestock do not coincide with the high tick population season, so this may be a relatively unimportant source of infection. Because the organism is resistant to drying, dust in pens and holding yards may be an important means of transmission for animals and man.

Cattle frequently carry the organism for long periods and large numbers of organisms are excreted in placental tissues and birth fluids of cows. Thus, cows may be a source of infection for goats when they share pasture.

Initial transmission of the organism into a clean herd may be by ticks. Following abortions or normal parturition by infected animals, massive contamination of pastures occurs, permitting oral transmission to the remainder of the herd. Abortion or stillbirth with this agent usually occurs late in gestation. This may be because the extensive multiplication of *C. burnetii* that causes the severe damage to the placenta is delayed until the end of pregnancy.

USUAL HERD HISTORY

Some does abort without apparent clinical signs, while others are anorexic and depressed 1 to 2 days before aborting. The placenta may rarely be retained, and some does may not have milk. The abortion rate may reach 93 per cent but is more commonly 5 to 50 per cent.

DIAGNOSIS

In order to implicate *C. burnetii* as the causative agent of abortion or stillbirth, large numbers of organisms and severe, typical placental lesions must be demonstrated. At the same time, a rise in serum titer to *C. burnetii* and failure to isolate other causes of abortion including *Chlamydia* or *Campylobacter* are strongly supportive.

The organism and lesions are most abundant in the placenta, but the organism may be present in low numbers in abomasal contents, spleen, kidney, liver and lung. The organism is easily demonstrated in air-dried, heat-fixed impression smears of placenta using a modified Koster's stain. Stamps-modified Ziehl-Neelsen stain or a Gimenez stain may also be utilized. Immense numbers of pleomorphic acid-fast organisms with coccoid or filamentous forms are seen. The organism may also be demonstrated by the direct fluorescent antibody test. Ground tissue may be inoculated into guinea pigs or mice, and a rise in titer can be demonstrated by 14 days. In addition, the organism may be isolated by inoculation of embryonated hens' eggs.

Placental lesions are most conspicuous in the intercotyledonary zone, where there is abundant inspissated or fluid, white to red, exudate. The placenta underneath the exudate is thickened and may be diffusely red to brown with multifocal to confluent areas of mineralization appearing chalky white (Fig. 1 and 2). There is extensive necrosis of the cotyledonary villi and the intercotyledonary

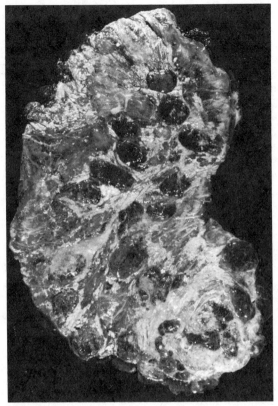

Figure 1. Chorioallantoic placenta of goat. This illustrates the thickening of the intercotyledonary placenta with suppurative exudate and mineralization. Macroscopically, there appears to be relative sparing of the cotyledons.

epithelium. A heavy neutrophilic infiltrate is present. The organism is conspicuous in trophoblastic cells of the chorion. The severe vasculitis commonly observed with chlamydial infection is not present. Gross lesions are not observed in the usually autolyzed fetus, but on microscopic examination, lymphoid accumulations may be observed around bronchioles.

For serology, acute and convalescent specimens (paired samples) should be assayed at the same lab. Complement fixation titers of greater than or equal to 1:8 are usually considered positive. Comparison of results from different laboratories is probably invalid because of the differences in assay techniques.

CARRIER STATE

Once infection is established, the organism is carried by the does indefinitely and is shed in the milk and at parturition. Repeated abortions are possible but unusual in the same animal.

PREVENTION AND CONTROL

A formalin-inactivated Phase I *C. burnetii* vaccine has been developed for use in calves and has also

of the organism at parturition. In one outbreak of abortion in goats, cessation of abortions followed feeding of chlortetracycline (200 mg/animal/day) for 19 days. The efficacy of antibiotic feeding in goats, however, has not been reported for controlled experiments.

ZOONOTIC IMPLICATIONS

While nearly all reports of Q fever infection in man indicate a benign self-limited infection, occasionally severe disease with endocarditis and atypical pneumonia may occur. The organism is killed by pasteurization but is readily transmitted by non-pasteurized milk. The usual source of infection for man may be milk, dust from contaminated pens or the handling of contaminated tissues. Veterinarians and livestock attendants should be aware of this danger, and precautionary measures should be taken.

Suggested Readings

1. Biberstein EL, Riemann HP, Behymer DE, et al: Vaccination of dairy cattle against Q fever *(Coxiella burnetii)*. Results of field trials. Am J Vet Res 38:189, 1977.
2. Crowther RW, Spicer AJ: Abortion in sheep and goats in Cyprus caused by *Coxiella burnetii*. Vet Rec 99:29, 1976.
3. McCaul TF, Williams JC: Developmental cycle of *Coxiella burnetii:* Structure and morphogenesis of vegetative and spo-rogenic differentiations. J Bacteriol 147:1063, 1981.
4. Palmer NC, Kierstead M, Key DW, et al.: Placentitis and abortion in goats and sheep in Ontario caused by *Coxiella burnetii*. Can Vet J 24:60, 1983.
5. Polydorou K: Q fever in Cypress: A short review. Br Vet J 137:470, 1981.
6. Ruppanner R, Riemann HP, Farver TB, et al.: Prevalence of *Coxiella burnetii* (Q fever) and *Toxoplasma gondii* among dairy goats in California. Am J Vet Res 39:867, 1978.
7. Waldhalm DG, Stoenner HG, Simmons RE, Thomas LA: Abortion associated with *Coxiella burnetii* infection in dairy goats. J Am Vet Med Assoc 173:1580, 1978.

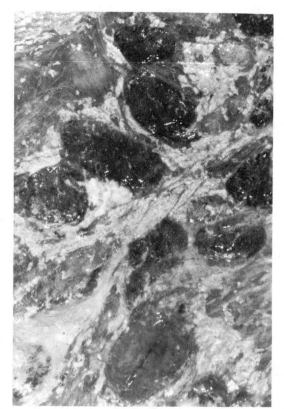

Figure 2. Chorioallantoic placenta of goat. Higher magnification of Figure 1. Acute suppurative intercotyledonary placentitis.

been used in cattle to reduce or eliminate passage of the organism in milk. The use of this vaccine in goats has not been reported.

Tetracycline therapy for a period of 2 weeks in cattle has been shown to reduce or prevent excretion

Mycoplasmosis

N. E. East, M.S., D.V.M, M.P.V.M
University of California, Davis, California

Mycoplasma spp. are of importance worldwide as pathogens of the goat.[1,2] Many outbreaks have been described in which the species of *Mycoplasma* has not been identified, and the clinical signs are similar for many species. Mycoplasemia (septicemia), fibri-nopurulent polyarthritis, pneumonia, agalactia, mastitis and conjunctivitis are often reported in varying degrees and combinations. Mortality rates are high, with reports of 10 to 100 per cent. Abortion due to *Mycoplasma* spp. is not the dominant clinical finding in outbreaks, but two species have been shown to cause abortion: *Mycoplasma mycoides* ss. *mycoides* (large colony type), and *Mycoplasma agalactiae*. In the United States, *M. mycoides* ss. *mycoides* is commonly isolated but only a few isolates of *M. agalactiae* have been made in recent years. *M. agalactiae* is common in parts of Europe, Africa and Asia and causes mastitis, conjunctivitis, polyarthritis, abortions and granular vulvovaginitis.[3] The disease is often chronic with shedding of the organism for months in milk, tears, urine, feces and uterine discharges. Initial exposure can result in mycoplasemia, and does in the last trimester of gestation may abort. Transmission of the disease to susceptible individuals is thought to occur through exposure to chronically infected animals.

Mycoplasma mycoides ss. *mycoides* primarily causes fibrinopurulent polyarthritis and pneumonia in nursing kids and mastitis with agalactia in adult does. Does can be chronic carriers of the organism, with first exposure occurring as kids from drinking infected milk or as adults, during milking. The organism is shed in the milk in very large numbers. Chronic carriers under stress may develop mycoplasemia and, if they are pregnant, abortion can occur. Does with mycoplasemia are very ill with pyrexia ($\geq 40.5°C$), agalactia, depression, and diarrhea; death may occur in 1 to 3 days. Does that abort from *M. mycoides* ss. *mycoides* infection will probably have the organism present in their milk, liver, kidney, spleen, amnionic fluids and placentomes, and it may also be found in the cotyledons, liver and spleen of the fetus.

Diagnosis of abortion due to *Mycoplasma* spp. is by culture (usually in special media) and serotyping of the isolate (USDA Plum Island).

Mycoplasma mycoides ss. *mycoides* and *Mycoplasma agalactiae* may be sensitive to tylosin or tetracyclines, but treated animals are likely to remain carriers. In other countries, treatment may be preferred for economic reasons, but in the United States slaughter is recommended. If slaughter is not possible, identification by milk cultures and strict isolation of infected animals is required.

References

1. Bar-Moshe B, Rappaport E: Contagious agalactia like disease in goats caused by *Mycoplasma mycoides* subsp. *mycoides* (ovine/caprine) serogroup 8. Refuah Vet 35 (2):75, 1978.
2. Cottew GS: Caprine-ovine mycoplasmas. In Barile MF, Razin S: The Mycoplasmas. Vol. 2. New York, Academic Press, 1979, pp 103-132.
3. Jensen R, Swift BL: Diseases of Sheep, 2nd ed. Philadelphia, Lea & Febiger, 1982, pp 25-27.

Abortion in Angora Goats

Maurice Shelton, Ph.D.
Texas Agricultural Experiment Station, San Angelo, Texas

Abortion has long been recognized as a major problem with Angora goats.[2, 5, 6] It is generally recognized that this problem is often of a type known as noninfectious abortion.[10] Heavy losses in non-Angoras, usually meat-type goats kept under poor feed conditions, have only recently come to the author's attention. It is not entirely clear why the goat is susceptible to noninfectious abortion, but at least two possible explanations can be suggested. In contrast to other domestic ruminants such as cattle or sheep, the goat is a corpus luteum–dependent species and any condition that causes a premature regression of the corpus luteum will result in abortion. Second, the goat does not fatten as readily as other species and is more dependent on a continuously available feed supply. The blood sugar level in goats seems to be more influenced by short-term variations in feed intake.[2, 9]

The high metabolic priority for fiber production in the Angora predisposes this breed to nutritional and other forms of stress to a greater degree than non-Angora goats. Most of the definitive research on noninfectious abortion has been done with Angora goats, and it is the writer's opinion that the basic underlying cause is the same among all breeds. Therefore, a discussion of the work completed with Angoras follows.

Definitive quantitative measures of the level of abortion under production conditions are difficult to obtain because the act of abortion or the abortus is only infrequently observed. However, in Angoras it is possible to determine the level of loss with reasonable accuracy. When an abortion occurs there is almost invariably some blood loss, which will stain the mohair on the tail and around the vagina. Blood stain is much darker in appearance than urine or fecal stain. In most flocks there are a number of does without blood staining that fail to kid. In these cases, it is not possible to distinguish between an early gestational abortion and fetal resorption.

In the United States, instances of recorded abortion in flocks with which the author has been associated have not exceeded 16 per cent.[1] However, oral reports of losses several times this level have occurred, and the writer has no difficulty accepting their validity. In South Africa instances of much higher losses have also been reported by Van Heerden,[5] who suggested premature regression of the corpus luteum as the cause of abortion.[4] More recent studies[6] suggest that this is an artifact, because corpus luteum regression occurs normally in conjunction with parturition without involving a direct cause and effect relationship with abortion.

It is generally accepted that in the United States most abortions occur in the range of 90 to 120 days of gestation and that they tend to occur more frequently in smaller does. Losses are also most frequently observed as "abortion storms" 1 or 2 days after a stress on the flock. Examples of stress may be changes in the weather or transport or similar events. Some outbreaks occur when the operator is unable to identify a specific stress but cannot be sure that some type of stress did not occur. In connection with the concentration of abortions in the 90- to 120-day period, it should be recognized that losses prior to this date may be largely unobserved and that losses occurring past 120 days may not be readily distinguishable from normal parturition.

The most definitive studies relating to abortion in Angora goats have been done in South Africa. For a period of time this work appeared to be contradictory to observations in Texas flocks. These differences have now been resolved with the realization that there are two types of abortion. One type is generally observed in younger, underdeveloped does that are subject to abortion storms resulting from stress ("stress aborters"). In these cases, the abortus is usually fresh and is often alive at expulsion. This is the major type of loss in production operations. In attempting to perform definitive studies on abortion, South African workers accumulated an experimental flock of does that had previously aborted.[6] These does were often larger, and the abortus was most often dead and edematous at expulsion. It is now realized that this type of abortion occurs in does known as "habitual aborters," which may abort in the absence of stress. A few habitual aborters (usually 0 to 5 per cent) may be present in most flocks unless they have been culled. The prevalence increases with age, and as a result of not raising kids, habitual aborters may become some of the larger does in the flock. The solution to this problem is simply to identify these individuals and remove them. The physiological mechanism by which they become habitual aborters is not known but is thought to result from an altered adrenal status (hyperadrenalism). It is known that these does are often the heaviest mohair producers early in life but may not be so in later life. It is not known if some of the initial stress aborters later become habitual aborters as a result of some altered endocrine status.

Because stress aborters constitute the primary problem, it is important to understand this phenomenon as well as possible. A recent series of studies by South African workers appears to provide an explanation for the concentration of losses between 90 and 120 days of gestation. Under normal conditions it is thought that the fetus is responsible for initiating parturition. The mechanism is apparently associated with the maturation of the fetal adrenal, and the time at which this occurs is species, and in some cases, breed dependent. The 90- to 120-day period coincides with a rapid increase in fetal nutritional demands, and it has been reasonably well established that a low blood glucose level is the triggering mechanism for abortion. It is postulated by Wentzel and associates[7, 8] that the hypoglycemic condition in the maternal organism results in a similar situation in the fetal circulation. This in turn activates the fetal hypothalamic-adrenal axis, resulting in an elevated output of steroids. Due to the immature state of the fetal adrenal, these steroids are thought to be estrogen precursors that result in excessive placental secretion of estrogens into the maternal circulation. Because estrogen is a relatively potent abortifacient, a number of abortions (abortion storms) may occur following any type of stress that results in maternal hypoglycemia. Abortions less concentrated in a particular time period may result from general undernutrition or inadequate size and development of the pregnant doe. The reduction in the level of abortion or at least the absence of abortion storms after 120 days is explained by the increasing maturity of the fetal adrenal, which has a more normal output and does not trigger excessive estrogen release.

Habitual aborters are thought to result from hyperfunction of the maternal adrenals. This condition tends to be chronic, although does with a history of abortion occasionally deliver a live kid. With advanced age, the habitually aborting doe tends to develop distinctive phenotypic features, including abdominal distention and finer mohair.

DEALING WITH ABORTION

The preceding explanation provides a basis for establishing guidelines for preventing abortion. The simplest recommendation is to deal with the habitual aborters. These animals should be identified and removed from the flock. Since the condition is by definition highly repeatable, the effect in subsequent seasons will be directly related to their proportion in the total flock. In theory, removing habitual aborters would have no effect because they would not have left offspring in the flock anyway. In fact, the elevated abortion problem in Angoras, in contrast to other types of goats, stems from their high metabolic tendency toward fiber production. A reduced emphasis on fiber production could be accomplished relatively easily, but this would be contraindicated by the demands of the industry. In theory, the goal should probably be an animal that has a high genetic potential for fiber production but can allow certain demands for reproduction to take precedence over fiber production at critical times. This goal is possible but would be difficult or slow to develop.

Management practices to prevent stress abortion appear to be more important and also are reasonably clear. These can be discussed under three headings:

1. Does should be physically mature prior to mating. At least with Angoras, there is clear-cut evidence that the small doe, even though reproductively mature, is more likely to abort. It may be desirable to delay breeding does that are not adequately developed to another season. Mating fol-

lowed by early abortion is not particularly damaging to the doe. The critical question is, does this establish a precedent in which this doe may become a habitual aborter, or do the conditions, such as small size and a very high level of fiber production, that trigger abortion in one year remain constant in the subsequent year?

2. An adequate ration should be provided to pregnant does to allow maintenance of normal blood glucose values. Angora goats have a high protein requirement due to their high level of fiber production, and, as a result, protein tends to be emphasized in supplemental feeding programs. However, for the pregnant doe there is reason to believe that energy should receive more emphasis. Under Texas range conditions, animals often feed infrequently and hence have inadequate energy intake compared with daily feeding. This practice of infrequent feeding is no doubt less acceptable with pregnant Angora does than with other classes of livestock.

3. Any form of stress that might trigger abortion storms should be avoided. For example, prolonged exposure to inclement weather results in a disruption of feeding and causes the animals to become chilled. Driving pregnant does for long distances during critical stages is another avoidable situation. Frozen water or a ground cover of ice or snow that prevents feeding has been observed to cause losses. Furthermore, abortion storms have been observed to occur when predisposing factors are not immediately apparent or explainable.

USE OF PROGESTERONE

In any technical discussion of abortion, the possibility of using progesterone or progestins is likely to arise. Crystalline progesterone would probably require daily or frequent injections, which seems impractical. Long-acting depot or oral progestins may be considered as alternative treatment strategies. However, it has been shown that these preparations in the ration or as injectables can cause difficulties at parturition. Thus, they should be removed prior to expected parturition, but few producers know the expected parturition date and understand the importance of treating each doe as an individual. Thus, the only treatment regime that appears to be feasible is the use of oral progestins during the critical period (90 to 120 days) that would be discontinued well in advance of expected parturition. However, it remains to be determined if this regime would be beneficial in reducing abortions. In one study involving small numbers, no adverse effects of short-term exposure to oral progestins was noted from this practice.[3]

References

1. Shelton M, Groff J: Reproductive efficiency in Angora goats. Tex Agric Expt Sta BU 1136, 1974.
2. Shelton M, Snowder G, Amoss M, Huston JE: The relation of certain blood parameters to abortion in Angora goats. Tex Agric Expt Sta PR 3896, 1981.
3. Shelton M, Amoss M, Lewis R: Influence of exogenous progestins on endogenous progesterone production in Angora goats. Tex Agric Expt Sta CPR 4026, 1982, p 40.
4. Van Heerden KM: Luteal failure as a cause of abortion in Angora goats in South Africa. Proceedings Fourth International Congress Animal Reproduction, The Hague, 1961.
5. Van Heerden KM: Investigations into the cause of abortions in Angora goats in South Africa. Onderstepoort J Vet Res 30:23, 1963.
6. Van Rensburg SJ: Reproductive physiology and endocrinology of normal and habitually aborting Angora goats, Thesis. DVM's University of Pretoria, Pretoria, South Africa, 1970.
7. Wentzel D, Morgenthal JC, Van Niekerk CH, Roelofse CS: The habitually aborting Angora doe: II. The effect of energy deficiency on the incidence of abortion. Agro Animalia 6:129, 1974.
8. Wentzel D, Morgenthal JC, Van Niekerk CH: The habitually aborting Angora doe. V. Plasma estrogen concentration in normal and aborter does with special reference to the effect of energy deficiency. Agro Animalia 7:35, 1975.
9. Wentzel D, Le Roux MM, Botha LJJ: Effect of the level of nutrition on blood glucose concentration and reproductive performance of pregnant Angora goats. Agro Animalia 8:59, 1976.
10. Wentzel D: Non-infectious abortion in Angora goats. Proceedings of Third International Goat Conference, 1982, pp 155–161.

Goat-Sheep Hybrids

Parvathi K. Basrur
Ontario Veterinary College, Guelph, Ontario

Breeders have attempted to cross domestic goats (*Capra hircus*) with their close relative, domestic sheep (*Ovis aris*), for centuries in the hope of developing a flock or herd that would provide milk, meat and wool as well as thrive well in hilly areas with poor grazing facilities. During the first half of this century, Warwick and Berry[3, 12, 13] observed that the fetuses from such matings did not survive and were generally aborted by the eighth week. Since then, other scientists have repeated their experiments using various breeds of goats and sheep, and these attempts are still being continued with a view to identifying the etiologic basis of hybrid fetal mortality.

MATING GOAT AND SHEEP

Rams and bucks often exhibit indiscriminate mating habits with ewes and does if both are present. Ewes will permit mounting by bucks, and rams enthusiastically mount does in season. However, fertilization of sheep eggs with goat spermatozoa occurs only rarely, and if fertilization is accomplished, the zygote never continues beyond the first few cleavage divisions. On the other hand, does mated to rams or inseminated with ram semen readily conceive. For these reasons, hybridization attempts are generally carried out using caprine females and ovine males.

FETAL MORTALITY

Goat-sheep hybrid fetuses conceived by does mated to rams die shortly after 30 days postconception, or they are aborted within 60 days of gestation. Fetuses aborted at 2 months are phenotypically indistinguishable from sheep or goat fetuses of corresponding age except in the nature of the tail. However, all hybrids show jaundice and hepatomegaly. The fetal abdomen is distended, and the peritoneum contains blood-stained fluid. The size of the recovered live hybrid fetus is smaller than an ovine fetus of corresponding age, and in some cases the size indicates an age 4 to 5 days less than that expected at the actual gestation period. The placental cotyledons are normal in size, shape and arrangement, although the fetal surface is irregular with small elevations and depressions. The fetal membranes are generally edematous. The allantoic fluid in some cases is yellow, and the volume is abnormally high, reaching a liter or more compared to the 200 ml or less obtained from the allantoic cavity of normal sheep or goats of similar gestational age. The amniotic fluid is normal and approximates 200 ml in volume, as in the normal doe with a goat fetus.[1, 7, 8]

The size of nonliving, unaborted fetuses recovered at laparotomy indicates that the death of these hybrids generally occurs between 30 and 50 days of gestation. The dead fetuses are brown or purplish-red with a gelatinous cover. Between 60 and 80 days after mating there is generally no evidence of a conceptus, suggesting that resorption is complete.

The reason for the death of the hybrid fetus is not known, although cytogenetic, immunologic and hormonal disparities between the two parental species have been considered as possible causes of fetal mortality.

CYTOGENETIC FEATURES OF GOAT-SHEEP HYBRIDS

The failure of hybridization is generally considered a reflection of the phylogenetic distance between the species mated. As a rule, different species of animals of the same genus interbreed and produce viable progeny if they are karyotypically identical. Viable but sterile hybrid progeny are obtained if the species mated are similar in the total number of chromosome arms, often referred to as the fundamental number (Nombre Fondamental, NF). Total failure to accomplish fertilization or to complete early embryonic development is a common feature of hybrid progeny of karyotypically dissimilar parents. Goats and sheep are different genera and carry a dissimilar chromosome make-up; the goat carries 60 single-armed (acrocentric) chromosomes, and the sheep carries 54, including 3 bi-armed (metacentric) chromosomes.

One of the causes of fetal loss in mammals is chromosome alteration in one or both of the parents leading to an absence or excess of chromosomes in the conceptus. The cytogenetic features of goat-sheep hybrids were among the first to receive attention in the search for an etiologic basis for failure of hybridization.

The first cytogenetic study was carried out on amniotic cells of goat-sheep hybrids by Berry,[3] who noted 57 chromosomes, including 3 metacentrics, in a majority of dividing cells in 30-day-old hybrid fetuses. Berry noted no evidence of mitotic aberrations leading to chromosome loss in the hybrids and concluded that the fetal mortality in these hybrids is not attributable to gross chromosome deficiencies. These studies were repeated using more refined methods including long-term fetal cell cultures and direct cell preparations from whole embryos.[6, 9, 10] Studies on cell suspensions from the embryos showed that the predominant cell type of the hybrids (92.7 per cent) carries 57 chromosomes and that the fetuses recovered between 24 and 31 days of gestation consist of more females than males (7 to 3). No consistent chromosome loss or gain (aneuploidy) or congenital malformation similar to those elicited by chromosome aberrations was detected.

IMMUNOLOGIC PROBLEMS

Immunologic differences between parents have a major impact on the survival of the conceptus. Fetal death may be precipitated by the immunologic incompatibility between the ram and the doe.[1, 11] The sera of pregnant does generally show hemolytic antibodies against the mated ram's blood cells, and the gross appearance of the hybrid fetus is reminiscent of children involved in Rh isoimmunization in man. These observations strongly suggest that hemolysins of maternal origin may be responsible for fetal death.[1] Further support for this hypothesis is that the time at which the trophoblast invades the cotyledons in goats and sheep (about the thirtieth day of gestation) and the appearance of hemolysins in maternal circulation (between days 35 and 50) coincide with the gestational stage at which the hybrid fetuses generally die. Maternal antibodies, however, do not reach a normal fetus in ungulates except when the placenta is defective. In the goat-sheep hybrid fetus, gross and histologic abnormalities are detected in the placenta. The maternal crypts and fetal villi are shallow, although the trophoblast is firmly attached to the uterine epithelium. The hybrid placentomes show platelet aggregation, lobular swelling of the vascular endothelium and other degenerative changes of the uterine epithelium reminiscent of injury related to antigen-antibody complexes. Furthermore, antigen-antibody complexes cannot be attributed to the reaction of the hybrid fetus against maternal antigens because the life of the hybrid fetus is generally shortened in does that had previously borne hybrid fetuses or had received the sire's skin graft or leukocyte injections.[11]

If an immunologic conflict is the basis of goat-sheep hybrid mortality, it should be possible to overcome this problem by immunization of the mother against the sire's red cell antigens. Scientists in Bulgaria[4] claim to have prolonged the pregnancy and obtained live goat-sheep hybrids at term after the does had been subjected to frequent intramuscular injections of the sire's blood prior to mating and during pregnancy. These investigators injected 10 to 15 ml of whole blood twice weekly from 3 months prior to mating and throughout pregnancy and claimed a 17.7 per cent hybrid embryo survival to term. They also reported that a hybrid fetus survives in a doe much better as a twin to the doe's own fetus than by itself. However, attempts to repeat this method not only failed to promote survival of the fetus, but in some cases, death occurred earlier in the pregnancy.[11]

In contrast, production of a low level of passive immunity in pregnant goats, either through a skin graft or through the injection of small amounts of antisera to suppress antibodies to antisheep hemolysins, prolongs the survival of the hybrid fetus.[1] However, eventually all hybrid fetuses die. Similarly, experiments in which hybrid embryos are transferred to does previously mated to bucks to produce twins, and in which does were injected with ram semen homogenate prior to mating to rams, show no detectable improvement in conception rate or hybrid embryo survival. Furthermore, immunologic incompatibility between the two species does not fully explain the death of some of the hybrid embryos prior to cotyledonary attachments.

HORMONAL PROBLEMS

Another possible contributing factor to hybrid fetal mortality is the difference between the two species in the hormonal concentrations and the pregestational fine-tuning of steroids. The progesterone levels in pregnant does are below those of sheep in similar stages of gestation, suggesting that progesterone deficiency may be causally related to the failure of hybrid pregnancy in does. The hybrid pregnancy resembles the progesterone deficiency syndrome in sheep. In both conditions there is a massive accumulation of allantoic fluid, and the fetus is aborted at about the same time. However, when goat-sheep hybrid embryos are transferred to synchronized ewes or does they undergo early embryonic development equally well in either species but fail to live beyond 60 days of gestation.

VIABLE GOAT-SHEEP HYBRIDS

Reports of living goat-sheep hybrids appear periodically in the news media. In most cases, these hybrids are kids resembling lambs or lambs resembling kids. The only reliable method of verifying the true identity of the animal is a chromosome examination that allows the visualization of sheep and goat chromosomes in the alleged hybrid. More recently, a hybridization venture that resulted in a fertile female goat-sheep hybrid has been reported from Logan, Utah.[5] The doe belonged to the "Spanish goat" breed (2n = 60), and the ram was of the "Barbados sheep" breed (2n = 54). Natural mating of these two animals produced a heterosexual twin set each carrying 57 chromosomes, including 3 metacentric autosomes. The female twin, backcrossed to a Barbados ram, also produced a set of heterosexual twins, thereby proving not only that the hybrids of this intergeneric cross are viable but also that the female hybrids are fertile. The chromosome number in the backcrosses was 55 including 5 metacentrics.[5]

In another study using a pure Saanen doe and a Barbary ram for hybridization, Bain,[2] in Cambridge, England, was able to obtain a set of stillborn twins showing no overt malformations. The Barbary sheep (aoudad) of North Africa is closer to a goat in some respects and is considered a "sheep goat." Natural mating frequently occurs between males of this species and female goats. The hybrids rarely go to term, although viable male and female hybrids are born occasionally.

INTERRELATIONSHIP OF GOATS AND SHEEP

It is believed that sheep and goats evolved from a common rupicaprid ancestor that carried 60 chromosomes, as in the present-day goat. The genus *Capra,* representing such species as *Capra ibex, Capra falconeri* and the domestic goat (*Capra hircus*), maintained the original chromosome number and remained chromosomally stable. The sheep line, represented by the Barbary sheep (aoudad), the Afghan wild sheep (*Ammon*) and the domestic sheep, underwent a series of translocations in their acrocentric autosomes resulting in a progressive reduction in the number from 60 to 54. Domestic sheep and their close relatives, the bighorns and mouflons (*Ovis canadensis* and *Ovis orientalis*), carry 54 chromosomes including three pairs of metacentric chromosomes. In all these ovine species the number of chromosome arms (the fundamental number) remains the same as in the caprine species despite the reduction in total number. It appears that the first of the series of translocations in the ovine line is that seen in the Barbary sheep (aoudad). The aoudad (*Ammotragus lervi*) carries 58 chromosomes including one pair of metacentrics. The next in this line of ovine evolution is the Afghan wild sheep *Ovis ammon* with 56 chromosomes including two pairs of metacentrics. These ovine species interbreed and produce fertile progeny.[5] The segmental details of the chromosome arms reveal homology, suggesting that the different species of the two genera differ only in the number of translocations sustained. The distinctive morphologic, physiological and behavioral features between members of these two lines are attributable to the accumulation of gene mutations beneficial to the ecologic niche in which they evolved. The specific gene mutations accumulated over the years by goats and sheep are bound to be different, and these differences cause a disharmonious combination at the gene level in their hybrids, forming an effective reproductive barrier between some members of these two genera. It is possible that some of the more primitive types of sheep are capable of successful hybridization with goats because they still retain similarity with goats in the gene loci controlling fetal growth and development.

References

1. Alexander G, Williams D, Bailey L: Natural immunization in pregnant goats against red blood cells of their sheep-goat hybrid features. Aust J Biol Sci 20:1217, 1967.
2. Bain AR: A cytogenetic study of a Barbary sheep *(Ammotragus lervia)* × domestic goat *(Capra hircus)* hybrid. Experientia 36:1358, 1980.
3. Berry RO: Comparative studies on the chromosome numbers in sheep, goats and sheep-goat hybrids. J Hered 29:343, 1938.
4. Bratanov C, Dikov V: Fecondation entre les especes brebis et chevres et obtention d'hybrides inter-especes. Proc 4th Int Cong Anim Reprod. The Hague, 4:744, 1961.
5. Bunch TD, Foote WC, Spillett JJ: Sheep-goat hybrid karyotypes. Theriogenology 6:379, 1976.
6. Buttle HL, Hancock JL: The chromosomes of goats, sheep and their hybrids. Res Vet Sci 7:230, 1966.
7. Dent J, McGovern PT, Hancock JL: Immunological implications of ultrastructural studies of goat × sheep hybrid placentae. Nature (Lond) 23:116, 1971.
8. Hancock JL: Attempted hybridization of sheep and goats. Proc 5th Int Cong Anim Reprod, Vol. 3, Toronto, 1964, pp 445–450.
9. Hancock JL, Jacobs PA: The chromosomes of sheep × goat hybrids. J Reprod Fert 12:591, 1966.
10. Ilberry PLT, Alexander G, Williams D: The chromosomes of sheep × goat hybrids. Aust J Biol Sci 20:1245, 1967.
11. McGovern PT: The effect of maternal immunity on the survival of goat × sheep hybrid embryos. J Reprod Fert 34:215, 1973.
12. Warwick BL, Berry RO, Horlacher WR: Results of mating rams to Angora female goats. Proc Am Soc Anim Prod 27:225, 1935.
13. Warwick BL, Berry RO: Intergeneric and interspecific embryo transfers in sheep and goats. J Hered 40:297, 1949.

The Reproductive Anatomy and Physiology of the Male Goat

Mary C. Smith, D.V.M.
Cornell University, Ithaca, New York

ANATOMY

The testes are normally present in the scrotum at birth and are positioned with the long axis vertical. The mature testes are quite large in proportion to the body weight compared with the testes of bulls. Approximately 15 to 20 efferent tubules collect spermatozoa from the rete tubules of the testis and join the head of the epididymis, which is located on the dorsolateral aspect of the testis. The body of the epididymis is located on the caudal aspect of the testis and slightly medial to it. Semen is stored prior to ejaculation in the tail of the epididymis, which is ventrally positioned.

The ductus deferens continues upward medial to the epididymis and passes through the abdominal inguinal ring as part of the spermatic cord. Blood vessels and nerves are also included in the cord and surrounded by tunics. The testicular artery is greatly convoluted; its close proximity to the pampiniform venous plexus serves to precool the blood going to the testis. The ductus deferens continues from the vaginal ring via the genital fold to the caudal part of the bladder. The terminal part of the ductus widens into the ampulla, passes under the body of the prostate and ends as a slitlike opening on the side of the seminal colliculus.

The vesicular glands (seminal vesicles) are compact glandular organs with a lobulated surface whose paired excretory ducts open at the seminal colliculus just lateral to each ductus deferens.

The prostate is entirely disseminated and completely surrounds the urethra. It has multiple ducts that open into the urethra in rows proceeding caudally from the seminal colliculus. The bulbourethral glands (Cowper's glands) are relatively large but are covered by dense fibrous tissue and partly by the bulbospongiosus muscle. They open under a fold of mucous membrane that forms a blind pouch in the urethra. It is currently believed that the secretions of the bulbourethral glands are involved in deterioration of fertilizing capability of spermatozoa used for artificial insemination. Washing the sperm to remove these secretions improves post-thaw fertility of frozen semen.[3]

The penis has a pronounced S-shaped sigmoid flexure except when it is fully extended at the time of ejaculation. A very thick tunica albuginea encloses highly developed erectile tissue. The terminal portion of the urethra lies in a groove on the ventral surface of the corpus cavernosum penis. Here, a slightly twisted urethral process extends 3 to 4 cm beyond the glans penis (Fig. 1).

CLINICAL EXAMINATION

Only the scrotal contents and the penis can be conveniently examined on the live buck.[6] Evaluation of the semen is discussed later. The examiner should position himself behind the buck with a hand on each side of the scrotum. Any dermatitis or skin wounds should be noted. The testes and epididymides are carefully palpated and compared. Cryptorchidism is easily recognized. Each testis should be large, slightly egg-shaped and mobile within the scrotum. Its consistency should be firm, similar to contracted muscle. Measurement of the circumference of each testis or of the entire scrotum and comparison with a normal goat of the same age and weight will permit identification of hypoplastic testes even if the examiner lacks previous experience with this diagnostic procedure. Normal scrotal circumference increases with both age and body weight, although charts have not yet been developed for bucks of dairy breeds. Scrotal circumference is also larger during the breeding season than in the spring. The normal epididymis is softer than the testis. The knotlike tail is the firmest part of the epididymis. Sperm granulomas are most commonly palpated in the head of the epididymis but should not be confused with normal lobulations. They are hard lumps of variable size and may be bilateral or unilateral. If the granulomas are large enough to completely obstruct the epididymis, sperm stasis and a tense, fluid feeling will be initially present in the testis. The testis will then degenerate and become softer and smaller. In some cases of testicular degeneration, the testicular tissue becomes mineralized and thus feels gritty. The value or safety of testicular biopsy as a diagnostic procedure for evaluating bucks with fertility problems has not yet been reported. Infarction of the testis can be expected if large blood vessels in the tunica albuginea are injured during the surgical procedure.

The buck's rudimentary teats should be examined for evidence of gynecomastia. Fused teats and other structural malformations are not desirable in the breeding buck because of the possibility that extra teats may be hereditary. The prepuce and penis are examined for wounds, strictures and congenital abnormalities such as hypospadias (suggestive of the intersex condition). While the buck is set up on his

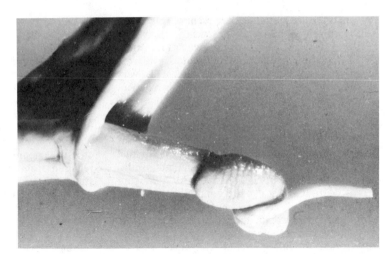

Figure 1. Normal buck's penis showing urethral process.

rump, the examiner grasps the shaft of the penis through the skin anterior to the scrotum with one hand and forces it upwards while working the prepuce posteriorly with the other hand. If protrusion of the penis is not achieved the buck may be sedated with 0.05 mg/kg of xylazine, but great care should be taken when using this unapproved drug on valuable bucks. Special attention should be given to the urethral process in which urethral calculi commonly lodge. Removal of the process does not interfere with breeding.

If the buck is large and the examiner's hand is very small, rectal examination of the internal genital organs may be possible, but this procedure has not been reported in the literature.

PUBERTY

The rate of male sexual development seems to vary with breed, birth weight and nutrition. The initial growth of the sex organs is gradual for the first 3 months of life. Then, with the onset of spermatogenesis, the weight of the testes, epididymides and seminal vesicles increases rapidly.[7] The spermatogenic cycle has been estimated to be 22 days in the buck kid, and mature spermatozoa are present in the epididymis by 3½ months.[8] Libido, it should be remembered, appears much earlier. The spermatogenic cycle of the adult buck has apparently not been studied.

The urethral process is initially located in a groove on the head of the glans penis. Separation from the glans and from the ventral wall of the prepuce begins at the distal tip of the process and proceeds toward the base, being complete by 4 months (Fig. 2). Separation of the penis from the remainder of the prepuce is usually not complete until after 5 months. These approximate times refer to dairy breeds under conditions of good nutrition; in these animals, fertile matings are easily possible by 5½ months. Buck and doe kids should be routinely separated before 5 months of age to prevent early breeding. Very large and fast-growing buck kids

may mature earlier and should be separated by 80 days of age for maximum safety.[8]

MALE SEXUAL BEHAVIOR

Bucks show very obvious courtship behavior when in contact with estrous does. They nose the female's perineum and udder as well as the ground where she has recently urinated. The urine odors elicit the flehmen reflex, in which the male extends his head and neck while retracting his upper lip. The buck also flicks out his tongue, strikes with a forelimb and makes low-pitched bleating sounds. He may butt the female's hindquarters or push them with his shoulders as a means of testing for heat. The female in standing estrus will remain still when urged to go forward. The buck then briskly assumes a position in direct line with and behind

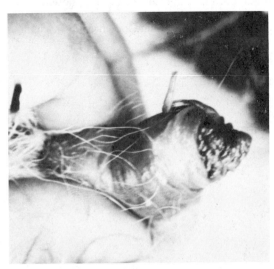

Figure 2. Partial separation of the urethral process and glans from the prepuce in a 3-month-old kid. Note the irregular surface of the glans.

the female. False mounting may occur during courtship. Frequently the male spills urine on his own head and forelegs or licks at the stream of his urine.

The reaction time, from first contact with the teaser or estrous doe to coitus, is normally very short—less than 5 minutes—if the animals have not been together continuously. During the nonbreeding season, bucks may refuse service. Often this is associated with misalignment, in which the buck puts his head on the doe's hindquarters, but his body is not in direct line with the doe's longitudinal axis.[4] The partially impotent buck maintains this improper position for a long time. As libido improves with resolution of a temporary problem, passing of the seasons, or administration of human chorionic gonadotropin, the axis will gradually be corrected until the potent buck is once more properly aligned. Mounting is rapid. The buck clasps the doe's body with his forelimbs and rapidly searches out and enters the vagina with his penis. An abrupt backward jerk of the head signals ejaculation. Coitus lasts a few seconds only, and the dismount follows immediately. Copulation can be repeated 20 times in a day.

The normal patterns of male sexual behavior are well established in kids housed in groups by the time they are 1 month old. Flehmen, perineal nuzzling and mounting occur, although the kid cannot extend his penis for several more months. If a male kid is raised in isolation, the animal may become imprinted on humans and mount the caretaker in preference to an estrous doe.

The male's typical and powerful odor, thought to be due in part to 6-trans nonenal from sebaceous glands caudomedial to the horns or bosses, stimulates a doe to show stronger heat than she would in the absence of a buck. Also, older and ranker males have a more positive effect than do young or descented bucks, and they will be sought out in preference by the average female. The buck whose scent, outside the breeding season, is more than his owner can tolerate can be made more presentable by trimming the beard and long facial hair, clipping the hair over the scent glands and wiping the crown of the head daily with a towel dampened with a mild disinfectant.

ENDOCRINOLOGY

The hormone patterns of the buck have not received as much attention as those of the ram. Under the influence of decreasing day length, increased amounts of luteinizing hormone (LH) are released from the anterior pituitary. LH in turn stimulates increased testosterone production by the testis.[2, 5] By September, the testes are enlarged and the buck's odor is pronounced. His libido increases, as does the frequency with which he urinates on his beard and forelegs. Libido and testosterone concentrations abate rapidly after the days begin to lengthen in the winter.[2] Spermatogenesis continues year round, because it requires a lower level of androgens than does maximum function of the accessory sexual glands.[5]

References

1. Bongso TA, Jainudeen MR, Zahrah AS: Relationship of scrotal circumference to age, body weight and onset of spermatogenesis in goats. Theriogenology 18:513, 1982.
2. Corteel JM: l'insémination artificielle caprine: Bases physiologiques, état actuel et perspectives d'avenir. World Rev Anim Prod 9:73, 1973.
3. Corteel JM, Paquignon M: Preservation of the male gamete (ram, buck, boar). Proc 10th Int Congr Anim Reprod AI, Illinois, June 10–14, 1984, pp II–20.
4. Fraser AF: Observations on the pre-coital behaviour of the male goat. Anim Behav 12:31, 1964.
5. Leidl W, Hoffmann B, Karg H: Endokrine Regulation und jahreszeitlicher Rhythmus der Fortpflanzung beim Ziegenbock. Zbl Vet Med Reihe A, 17:623, 1970.
6. Memon MA: Male infertility. Vet Clin North Am (Large Anim Pract) 5(3):619, 1983.
7. Skinner JD: Post-natal development of the reproductive tract of the male Boer goat. Agroanimalia 2:177, 1970.
8. Yao TS, Eaton ON: Postnatal growth and histological development of reproductive organs in male goats. Am J Anat 95:401, 1954.

Collection and Evaluation of Caprine Semen

Kent R. Refsal, D.V.M., M.S.
Michigan State University, East Lansing, Michigan

There has been considerable interest in progeny testing and artificial insemination of dairy goats in recent years. Also, the purchase of genetically superior bucks is becoming a substantial investment for breeders. Because of these factors, it is anticipated that there will be an increased demand for expertise in breeding soundness examination principles as applied to the buck. The purpose of this section is to describe methods of caprine semen collection and provide guidelines for evaluation of the ejaculate.

SEMEN COLLECTION

Use of an artificial vagina is the preferred method of semen collection, since the techniques are successful in a high percentage of bucks and a representative ejaculate is obtained. An artificial vagina is easily constructed with inexpensive components (Fig. 1). Support is provided by a stiff rubber tube (radiator hose, for example) 13 to 16 cm long and 5 to 8 cm in diameter with a combination air and water-filling valve placed in its wall. A cylindrical rubber liner, 23 to 25 cm long by 4 to 5 cm wide, is positioned inside the tube, and both ends of the liner are folded over the ends of the tube and secured with rubber bands (Fig. 2). The space between the tube and the liner is filled with 55°C water. The inner wall of the liner is lightly lubricated with sterile lubricating jelly that is not toxic to sperm cells. The space between tube and liner is further inflated with air via the valve until the inner lumen of the artificial vagina is occluded to the point where one finger can be easily inserted. A rubber cone with attached glass collection vessel is placed over the lesser-lubricated end of the artificial vagina. The collection vessel should be insulated to prevent cold shock of the spermatozoa. This can be accomplished by covering the cone and vessel in a padded insulation bag or suspending the vessel in warm water contained in a plastic bag that encloses the cone and is fastened to the stiff tube. The optimal temperature in the inner lumen of the artificial vagina is 40° to 45°C.

Unless a buck has been trained to mount an inanimate object, semen collection with the artificial vagina will be made during attempts to breed a mount doe. An estrual doe is the most optimal mount animal. Many bucks, especially if used in a hand-breeding management program, will readily attempt to serve a nonestrual doe that is sufficiently restrained to limit both lateral movement and rearing on the hind limbs. This author has failed to collect semen when excessive movement in a large nonestrual doe intimidated a yearling buck, or when a nonestrual doe would not support the weight of an older, experienced breeding male.

The collection site should have good footing and provide sufficient room for freedom of movement for the buck and handlers. Dirt and debris should be gently removed from the buck's preputial orifice.

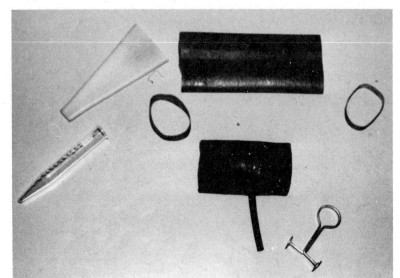

Figure 1. Components of a homemade artificial vagina, prior to assembly.

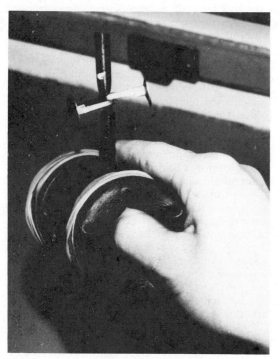

Figure 2. Testing pressure of the artificial vagina by thumb insertion.

After the artificial vagina is prepared, the collector should kneel laterally to the doe's hindquarters, on the same side of the doe as the hand used to hold the artificial vagina, i.e., if the artificial vagina is held in the left hand, the collector should be on the doe's left side. The buck is slowly led to the doe's hindquarters. His first response will be to sniff at the doe's perineal region and begin to protrude his penis. When mounting is initiated, the buck will grasp the doe's hindquarters and begin short pelvic thrusts to bring the extended penis into contact with the vulva. At this time, the collector should gently grasp the prepuce and divert the tip of the penis into contact with the artificial vagina opening, which is held at the level of and behind the doe's hip (Fig. 3). A pronounced pelvic thrust usually accompanies ejaculation, and the collector should hold the artificial vagina at the preputial orifice as the buck dismounts. Sometimes a buck will repeatedly dismount when the prepuce is grasped and diverted to the artificial vagina. Increasing the artificial vagina temperature may result in successful collection. The collector could allow more time for searching movement before grasping the prepuce, but this may result in an undesired mating if the mount doe is in estrus. Fortunately, 2.5 to 5 mg of prostaglandin $F_{2\alpha}$ is a very effective abortifacient in the goat 5 days or more after breeding. After an ejaculate is collected, the buck and doe should be separated because breeding attempts may be quickly reinitiated.

Semen samples may also be collected by electroejaculation, using an ejaculator that provides variable control of intensity and duration of current. The buck's rectum should be emptied by a warm-water enema. The buck is held in either a standing or a lateral recumbent position, and a ram probe is inserted with electrodes positioned toward the pelvic floor. A rhythmic and increasingly intensified application of electronic current is administered, with the current on for 2 to 5 seconds and off for 2 to 3 seconds. The desired response is penile extension followed by ejaculation. The sample is collected into a rubber cone with attached collection vessel.

The primary advantage of electroejaculation is that samples may be obtained when there is no mount doe available or when the buck is unwilling or unable to mount. There are several disadvantages of this method. First, the sample collected may not provide a true representation of the buck's ejaculate, especially for semen volume and concentration. Second, bucks tend to respond more vigorously to stimulation than rams and often elicit a loud vocal response that may be disturbing to owners or other observers. Lastly, many bucks less than a year old are too small for commercial ram probes.

SEMEN EVALUATION

At present data on minimal acceptable values for semen quality in bucks are limited. Most bucks breed a relatively small number of does each season, with most does bred more than once per estrus. These factors may result in good fertility records for bucks with questionable semen quality.

The buck's previous breeding schedule and the season at the time of examination may affect the results of semen evaluation. Males that have not been sexually active for several weeks prior to examination may have decreased motility and increased numbers of secondary sperm abnormalities due to epididymal sperm stasis. If this is the case, motility and sperm morphology should improve on successive samples collected 15 to 30 minutes after the first. There is a seasonal effect on sperm production, with decreased motility, reduced volume and decreased sperm cell numbers seen during the nonbreeding season in bucks maintained on a twice weekly artificial vagina collection schedule.

The semen sample must be kept warm (35° to 38°C), and motility should be assessed immediately after collection. A drop of raw semen is placed on a warmed slide and examined under the 10 × objective. Wave motion is categorized as rapid swirling, slow swirling, general oscillation or no oscillation. Another semen drop is mixed with warmed physiological saline, and a warmed coverslip is applied. The percentage of progressively motile spermatozoa is estimated by rapid observation of 8 to 10 low-power microscope fields. A stained smear, using eosin and nigrosin, for example, is made, and at least 100 spermatozoa are classified as being normal or having primary (major) or secondary (minor) defects. The incidence of specific abnormalities is recorded if they are com-

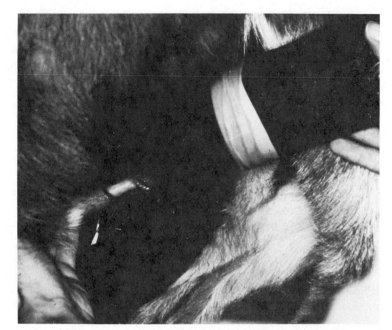

Figure 3. Semen collected via artificial vagina in the goat. The buck's partially extended penis is diverted toward the artificial vagina.

monly encountered. For example, high percentages of detached heads may indicate the presence of testicular degeneration. Another smear should be stained with new methylene blue or Wright's stain if there is suspicion that leukocytes or germ cells are present in the ejaculate.

Spermatocyte concentration can be quantified with red blood cell hemocytometer dilution or optical density comparison to known controls, or with automated cell-counting instrumentation. The number of sperm per ejaculate is calculated by multiplying spermatocyte concentration by ejaculate volume.

Based on previously reported guidelines and this author's clinical observations, the following values may be used as guidelines for assessing semen quality. Most ejaculates should range in volume from 0.5 to 2.0 ml and have 1.5 to 4.0 billion spermatozoa/ml. Bucks less than 1 year of age will have values near the lower end of these ranges.

An optimal semen sample should have rapidly swirling waves, and individual progressive motility should be greater than 75 per cent. At least 75 per cent of the spermatozoa should be morphologically normal.

There is great variability among bucks in regard to the time of puberty and the rate of sexual maturation. Some young bucks have good fertility at 5 to 6 months of age while others do not. There may be a considerable increase in sperm cell numbers per ejaculate between 5 and 8 months of age in a fast-growing buck. This period of maturation may be delayed if a young buck has had severe systemic disease (for example, coccidiosis or pneumonia) as a kid. Repeat examinations at 1- to 2-month intervals may be necessary to establish fertility potential.

References

1. Corteel JM: Collection, processing and artificial insemination of goat semen. *In* Gall C (ed): Goat Production. New York, Academic Press, 1981, pp 171–179.
2. Hayes B: Pre-breeding examination of the buck. Dairy Goat J 60:609, 1982.
3. Refsal KR, Simpson DA, Gunther JD: Testicular degeneration in the goat. A case report. Theriogenology 19:685, 1983.
4. Smith MC: Caprine reproduction. *In* Morrow DA (ed): Current Therapy in Theriogenology. Philadelphia, PA, WB Saunders, 1980, pp 992–994.

Infertility in the Buck

Mary C. Smith, D.V.M.
Cornell University, Ithaca, New York

Infectious causes of buck infertility are rare, but, significant problems do result from genetically determined intersexuality, testicular hypoplasia, cryptorchidism, sperm granulomas and testicular degeneration.

EPIDIDYMITIS AND ORCHITIS

Infections of the scrotal contents occasionally occur owing to penetrating wounds, hematogenous spread or possibly, organisms that ascend the urethra. Painful enlargement and abscessation of the epididymis or testis may occur. Unilateral castration is often attempted because the increased temperature of the inflamed organ adversely affects spermatogenesis in the remaining testis. Isolated organisms include *Staphylococcus pyogenes*, *Actinobacillus seminis* and *Brucella melitensis*. Experimental infections of male goats with *Brucella ovis* produced only transient epididymitis.

INTERSEXES AND TESTICULAR HYPOPLASIA

Caprine intersexes, or pseudohermaphrodites, are common. The problem has been discussed in a separate article in this text. It is important to realize that some intersexes are so masculine in both external appearance and behavior that karyotyping and semen evaluation are required to distinguish the XX intersex from a normal buck. The XX testes do not produce sperm cells. Almost all intersexes are polled. Unilateral and bilateral testicular hypoplasia have also been reported in male (XY) goats.

SPERM GRANULOMAS

Sperm granulomas are a common cause of sterility in the buck. If one or more of the efferent tubules in the head of the epididymis ends blindly, spermatozoa will migrate into the blind segments, undergo degeneration and release mycolic acid. While the initial lesion is merely that of sperm stasis and spermatocele formation, more advanced lesions have masses of spermatozoa in the interstitial tissue that are surrounded by histiocytes, lymphocytes, and plasma cell and Langhans' type giant cells.

Sperm stasis with testicular edema is followed by degeneration and calcification of the testis.

Careful examination by palpation or diagnostic castration of affected goats will reveal firm granulomas in the head, body or tail of the epididymis. These vary in size from a pinhead to several centimeters in diameter and are usually but not always bilateral. Some of the granulomas escape detection by being located deep in the parenchyma of the epididymis. Typically, the history reveals that the buck was once fertile but later became completely sterile, often quite suddenly. In these cases, spermatozoa will be absent from the ejaculate.

As with intersexuality, sperm granulomas are frequently associated with the polled condition. One study reports that approximately 50 per cent of homozygous (PP) polled males are completely sterile because of sperm granulomas. At least in the Alpine breed, the homozygous buck has a smooth head without scurs. The heterozygous buck has bean-shaped bony protuberances that often are surmounted by small, unsightly scurs.[4] In the past, breeders have unintentionally selected for the homozygous condition while attempting to achieve a smooth head on a polled buck.

Control of spermatic granulomas as a cause of infertility in the buck should include selection of horned, or at least heterozygous, bucks and careful palpation of all bucks before they are used for breeding. Affected animals should be eliminated from the herd or castrated.

CRYPTORCHIDISM

Not all cryptorchid goats are XX intersexes and therefore infertile. A form of cryptorchidism with possible recessive inheritance has been well documented in Angora goats, in which intersexes are very rare. These animals are known as ridglings. In studies conducted in Texas, the right testis always failed to descend, whereas studies in South Africa indicated that the left testis was invariably retained.[6] Sometimes the opposite testis was also retained. Frequently, thin but strong membranous attachments, in addition to the gubernaculum, connect the small, degenerate internal testis to the internal body wall near the ilium and to loops of intestine. It has been postulated that these adhesions, which interfere with descent, are inherited rather than cryptorchidism per se.

A unilateral cryptorchid buck should never be used for breeding, even if the condition may not always be hereditary. (Bilaterally affected animals are sterile.) Siblings and dams should also be discarded from the breeding herd. In one experimental herd, strong selection pressure over the course of 20 years reduced the prevalence of cryptorchidism from 50 per cent to 0.8 per cent.[7] The possible inheritance of the cryptorchid condition in breeds other than the Angora needs further study.

TESTICULAR DEGENERATION

Testicular degeneration is an important reason for loss of fertility in the buck. Not all cases are related to sperm granulomas. Typically, the testes are reduced in size by as much as one half. Shape also changes, so that the affected testes become small and spheroidal or have a smaller horizontal circumference and an elongated appearance. The consistency may become either soft, with extensive tubular degeneration, or excessively firm, with testicular calcinosis. In some advanced cases, the head of the epididymis loses its normal lobulations. Semen density and motility are decreased. An increased prevalence of sperm abnormalities such as separated heads, twisted midpieces and coiled tails will be found.[3] Occasionally, testicular degeneration is preceded by a period of gynecomastia with milk production in 3- to 4-year-old bucks.

There is no evidence that testicular degeneration is reversible or that treatment is possible. The buck should be replaced when his fertility is no longer acceptable. One study reports testicular degeneration induced by experimental *Trypanosoma vivax* infection; therefore, tsetse fly control may prevent some cases in tropical countries. Selection of horned bucks is also indicated to decrease the probability of sperm granulomas as a cause of testicular degeneration.

NUTRITIONAL INFLUENCES ON FERTILITY OF THE BUCK

A diet adequate for normal growth and maintenance of general health is usually also satisfactory for reproduction. Overfeeding of energy may result in an obese, lethargic goat with poor libido. If the animal is kept on an energy-deficient diet, the volume of the testes will decrease, but libido will usually remain until starvation is imminent. A severe protein deficiency will delay maturation of the testes and penis in young kids. In adults, sperm production will be adversely affected because spermatozoa are high in protein content.

The effect of trace mineral and vitamin deficiencies on male fertility in goats is largely conjectural. Presumably, iodine deficiency leading to goiter formation and poor body growth may be accompanied by decreased fertility. Likewise, a severe vitamin A deficiency may be expected to cause reversible atrophy of the testes and loss of libido. Testicular degeneration has been reported with vitamin E deficiency in goats, but details are not available. Finally, experimental zinc deficiency in goats causes listless, weak, unthrifty animals with dry hair coat, alopecia and very small testes. In addition, many seminiferous tubules are lined only by spermatogonia.

Posthitis

Posthitis (sheath rot or pizzle rot) due to a *Corynebacterium* infection is a problem when cas-

trated goats are kept on a leguminous or high nitrogen diet.[5] Angoras are most commonly affected, probably because the castrates are kept for years for mohair production. Wethers tend to urinate within the sheath. The urea-hydrolyzing corynebacteria produce degradation products that are more irritating to the mucous membranes than is normal urine. Affected goats have an ulcerated or scabby prepuce. When the orifice becomes distorted or covered by scabs, urination is accompanied by excessive straining.

Treatment with germicides is usually not effective. Prevention includes decreasing the protein in the feed and keeping males intact whenever practical. Testosterone implants have been used to prevent the problem in sheep in Australia, but these are not available in the United States.

Urolithiasis

Obstruction of the urethra by calculi is a common problem in castrated goats but also occurs occasionally in intact males. Any male goat of any age that is off feed or straining should be examined immediately to verify its ability to pass urine freely. Goats that are neglected for only a few days will progress to rupture of the bladder or urethra, uremia and death. If the buck is not observed to pass urine and the prepuce is not wet, a blood sample should be obtained to determine the creatinine level. The blood urea nitrogen (BUN) determination is not a dependable test in the goat, because animals may be completely obstructed and still have normal BUN values. Often the unobstructed goat will urinate promptly after being released from the restraint necessary to procure a blood sample.

Some cases of urinary obstruction may be easily diagnosed and treated because the calculus has lodged in the urethral process where it can be visualized. The buck should be positioned sitting on its rump and lightly tranquilized if necessary to facilitate exteriorization of the penis. The urethral process is snipped off with scissors. Subsequent breeding is usually unimpaired. Unfortunately, many bucks have additional calculi in the bladder or are already obstructed proximally in the penis, often in the region of the sigmoid flexure. The dilated urethra on the midline of the perineum may be turgid, painful and pulsating. It may be impossible to exteriorize the penis of a wether that was castrated before the breakdown of preputial adhesions. The urethral process must be amputated (or incised longitudinally if still adhered) to permit passage of a size 4 to 7 French urinary catheter. The catheter usually becomes lodged in the normal urethral diverticulum at the ischial arch; thus failure to reach the bladder is no proof that an obstruction remains.[1]

A wether with an obstruction proximal to the urethral process may be treated with a penectomy or urethrostomy performed under general or epidural anesthesia. If it is hoped to save an obstructed buck for later breeding, all calculi must be flushed out of the distal urethra via a cystotomy or urethrostomy and any urethrostomy incision closed. The prognosis is, at best, guarded.

If the animal has a distended abdomen, rupture of the bladder should be suspected. Palpation for a fluid wave and paracentesis 2 to 5 cm lateral to the prepuce will aid in the diagnosis. Abdominal surgery is indicated in these animals for repair of the bladder wall and for elimination of the inciting obstruction by cleaning sand from the bladder mucosa and backflushing the urethra. A distended but intact bladder can be detected by amplitude-depth ultrasound.

The cause of urolithiasis in goats has received little study. Presumably, information gained from sheep is applicable. Thus, high phosphorus diets (much grain accompanied by grass hay) are expected to be calculogenic in the goat. The author suspects that many cases are related to feeding male goats a ration that is designed for milking animals and is therefore excessive in both calcium (Ca) and phosphorus (P). Calcium-phosphorus ratios between 1:1 and 2:1 should be fed, but the total calcium requirement of the mature buck is only about 0.15 per cent of the diet on a dry weight basis. Thus, alfalfa hay and dicalcium phosphate supplements should be avoided in the feeding of the adult male goat. Excess magnesium (above 0.3 per cent) may be important in calculi formation.[2]

Prevention of calculi involves more than adjusting the mineral content of the ration. Clean water and salt must be continuously available. If a few fecal pellets fall into the water, the buck will drink very little. A heating element in the water container is valuable in cold climates to prevent freezing. Addition of salt (1 to 4 per cent) or ammonium chloride (2 per cent) to the concentrate is also helpful. Individual adult bucks, especially those that have become obstructed previously, can be given 1 tablespoon of ammonium chloride orally twice a day for several days after an episode of obstruction to dissolve remaining calculi by acidification of urine. One teaspoon of ammonium chloride three times a week is then given for maintenance. Supplementing the diet with 1 per cent sulfur has also been suggested for prevention of calculi on a ration that is otherwise calculogenic.

References

1. Hinkle RF, Howard JL, Stowater JL: An anatomic barrier to urethral catheterization in the male goat. J Am Vet Med Assoc 173:1584, 1978.
2. James CS, Chandran K: Enquiry into the role of minerals in experimental urolithiasis in goats. Indian Vet J 52:251, 1975.
3. Refsal KR, Simpson DA, Gunther JD: Testicular degeneration in a male goat. A case report. Theriogenology, 19(5):685, 1983.
4. Ricordeau G, Bouillon J, Hulot F: Pénétrance de l'effet de stérilité totale lié au gène sans cornes P, chez les boucs. Ann Génét Sél Anim 4:537, 1972.
5. Shelton M, Livingston CW Jr: Posthitis in Angora wethers. J Am Vet Med Assoc 167:154, 1975.
6. Skinner JD, VanHeerden JAH, Geres EJ: A note on cryptorchidism in Angora goats. S Afr J Anim Sci 2:93, 1972.
7. Warwick BL: Selection against cryptorchidism in Angora goats. J Anim Sci 20:10, 1961.

Semen Freezing and Artificial Insemination

George K. Haibel, D.V.M.
Ohio State University, Columbus, Ohio

FREEZING BUCK SEMEN

Although health requirements for AI sires have not been established for the goat, common sense dictates evaluation of the health of the individual as well as the herd of origin. The emergence of AI centers where semen is professionally processed from bucks not used for natural service awaits the demand for such quality.

Semen collection and evaluation are covered elsewhere in this section. Ejaculates accepted for processing should be of appropriate volume and concentration for the age of the buck and season of collection and should be free of inflammatory cells and gross debris. Higher quality samples are obtained using an artificial vagina rather than electroejaculation. Labeled ejaculates are placed in a waterbath at 35°C pending evaluation. An immediate 1:1 extension of each sample provides energy and buffer. Two or three ejaculates from the same buck obtained 20 minutes apart may be pooled for processing after total cell numbers are determined.

Many types of extenders have proved acceptable. Skim milk from powder remains a readily available and popular extender. Fresh milk must be heated to 95°C for 10 minutes to inactivate enzymes. If egg yolk is used in the extender, enzymes in seminal plasma may react with the yolk to form spermacidal breakdown products. This can be largely circumvented by washing and centrifugation of sperm in isotonic physiological solutions.

A requirement for the number of cells per breeding unit based on conception rate data does not exist. French workers suggest that two inseminations with 125×10^6 motile cells post-thaw ensure maximum fertility following induced heats. In the interest of processing a reasonable number of breeding units per collection, 100×10^6 motile cells per unit pre-freeze is convenient and results in good conception rates.

A two-step procedure with glycerol added after cooling to 5°C is standard. Desired volume after extension is computed from the total cells and the volume and numbers of cells in the inseminating dose. An initial half-final volume dilution is made, and the extended ejaculate is cooled to 5°C over a 2-hour period to avoid cold shock. A convenient system involves placing tubes of extended semen in a 250-ml beaker of 35°C water and then placing the beaker in the 5°C cold room or refrigerator. An equal volume dilution is then made by slowly adding precooled extender with 14 per cent glycerol (v/v) to obtain a final glycerol concentration of 7 per cent. An equilibration period of 2 hours appears to be necessary prior to freezing, during which time loading and sealing into ampules or straws can take place.

Freezing techniques vary with the packaging system. Glass ampules, by virtue of their slower conduction properties, require a more carefully controlled environment to achieve freezing rates of -0.5°C per minute from 5°C to -15°C. Plastic straws can be frozen with less sophisticated equipment by rack suspension in the vapor above liquid nitrogen in a closed insulated container. If pellets are to be used, they are frozen in premade wells in dry ice. An auto-pipetter facilitates achieving the desired 0.1 ml volume. Batches of frozen pellets are then dumped in liquid nitrogen prior to packaging in labeled bulk containers.

A sample breeding unit should be thawed and examined from each freezing sequence to verify the quality of each batch of semen. Post-thaw motility can vary from animal to animal and may provide a basis for correction factors in determining prefreeze sperm numbers per breeding unit. A useful range for expected post-thaw motility is 20 to 40 per cent.

ARTIFICIAL INSEMINATION OF THE DOE

Does selected for AI breeding should be healthy and in sound reproductive condition. Experience is best gained on multiparous does during the active breeding season due to the larger size of the cervix and vagina, greater ovulation rate, and more predictable estrous period. Semen should be secured well in advance of the breeding season to avoid delivery problems from small suppliers.

The primary difference in goat AI technique from that employed in the cow is the lack of cervical stabilization per rectum. The external os of the cervix is visualized with the aid of a speculum and light, and the inseminating instrument is directly manipulated past the well-aligned cervical rings (Fig. 1).

Equipment used is identical to that employed in bovine AI. Shortened goat-inseminating syringes and sheaths are available for straw-packaged semen but are not essential. Insemination pipettes for ampule-packaged and pelleted semen can be easily broken to a shorter length if desired.

Several speculum types are suitable for use in goat AI. Glass specula are easy to sanitize and can be made from 25×200 mm Pyrex test tubes or from straight glass tubing of a similar diameter and length. The end modified for entrance into the doe's vagina should be cut on a 45° angle and fire polished (Fig. 2). Nulliparous does may need a smaller diameter (20×175 mm) speculum.

Timing of insemination is only as good as the accuracy of heat detection and knowledge of the idiosyncrasies of particular does. Insemination is best accomplished in late standing heat. This is

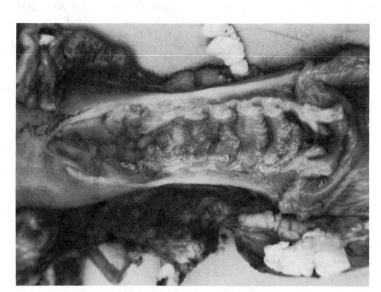

Figure 1. Goat cervix. Note regularity of cervical rings.

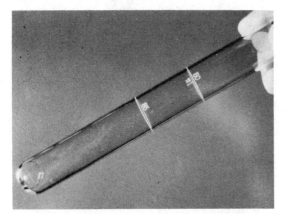

Figure 2. Test tube speculum.

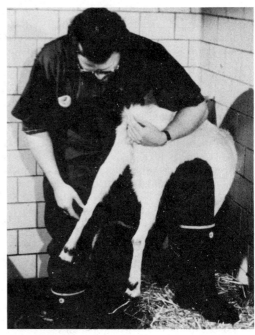

Figure 3. Restraint of the doe for artificial insemination.

close to the time of ovulation in the doe, yet the cervix is still relaxed for easy passage of the pipette. Earlier insemination is possible but requires confidence in the quality of the breeding unit to ensure post-thaw sperm longevity. Most does exhibiting a 24-hour estrus can be inseminated once at approximately 12 to 18 hours.

Restraint of the doe is essential for passage of the vaginal speculum and inseminating instrument. Calmer, more mature animals may be restrained by collar and crowded against a wall with the operator kneeling next to the doe. More nervous does are best restrained in a milking stanchion designed for goats. The operator faces to the rear of the doe, places the near foot on the milking platform and drapes the hindquarters of the doe over the thigh (Fig. 3).

The vulva and perineum are cleaned with a paper towel and water. A lightly lubricated speculum is passed through the vulva, directed over the ischial arch, past the vestibulovaginal sphincter and into the vagina. The oblique hole in the end of the speculum is directed to best expose the cranial vaginal floor. The cervix is located with the aid of a penlight. Cervical mucus may be present in such quantity that it needs to be removed by tipping down on the speculum or aspirated with the aid of a small suction apparatus fitted to a pipette. Cervical mucus provides a valuable aid in determining timing of insemination because it becomes progressively cloudier during estrus. Crystal-clear mucus thus indicates a doe that is not yet ready to be bred.

If timing is correct based on visual appraisal of the external os and cervical mucus, semen is thawed in accordance with the recommendations of the processor. In the absence of processor guidelines, ampules are best thawed in ice water for 10 minutes and straws are thawed in 35°C water for 10 to 20 seconds.

The vaginal speculum is reintroduced into the doe, and the loaded insemination instrument is visually guided through the external os and to the first cervical ring. By maintaining gentle but firm forward pressure the AI syringe or pipette tip can then be forced past successive cervical rings. Often a distinct "blip" can be felt or even heard as each ring is passed. Complete passage through the cervix is frequently not possible. Deep cervical insemination is thought to be as effective as intrauterine deposition, which can inadvertently result in placement of semen in a single uterine horn. Many operators routinely deposit a portion of the breeding unit during withdrawal if the cervix has been completely penetrated. The speculum is withdrawn following semen deposition and prior to removal of the breeding instrument. This is thought to prevent backflow of semen away from the external os.

Conception results vary with timing, quality of semen and skill of the technician but are thought to approach 60 per cent for a single AI breeding. Data on AI kidding rates compared with natural service kidding rates are not available, although some detrimental effect of AI would seem reasonable.

References

1. Corteel JM: Production, storage and insemination of goat semen. Symposium on Management of Reproduction in Sheep and Goats, Madison, Wisconsin, 1977, pp 41–57.
2. Drobnis EZ, Nelson EA, Burrill MJ: Effect of several processing variables on motility and GOT levels for frozen goat semen. *In* Proceedings, Western Section, American Society of Animal Science, Vol. 31, 1980. J Anim Sci 51 (Suppl 1):439, 1980.
3. Fraser AF: A technique for freezing goat semen and results of a small breeding trial. Can Vet J 3:133, 1962.
4. Purcella AW: A.I. (artificial insemination) of dairy goats. Dairy Goat J 52:3, 1974.

Castration and Preparation of Teasers

Mary C. Smith, D.V.M.
Cornell University, Ithaca, New York

CASTRATION

Goats are castrated for a variety of reasons. A male kid that is being raised for meat or mohair production or as a pet can be kept with the rest of the herd without fear of undesired matings. Also, the characteristic buck aroma is greatly subdued after castration and the meat is free of buck flavor. Goats that are castrated as adults retain their ability to ejaculate, often for a year or more, but the frequency of ejaculation decreases. The flehmen response to female urine also decreases somewhat, and the wether becomes less attractive to females.

Several techniques are commonly used. Tetanus prophylaxis is advisable with any method; the doe is vaccinated during the dry period to supply colostral antibodies, or 200 units of antitoxin is administered to the kid. Large bucks are given 500 units of antitoxin if they have not been previously vaccinated. Laymen sometimes castrate young kids with elastic castration bands, but the method is inhumane. A bloodless Venezuelan technique consists of twisting the testis around the spermatic cord and pushing it back into the inguinal canal, where it atrophies.[2] The use of a small Burdizzo emasculatome should be limited to young kids; after just a few months, the testes become too large to be completely resorbed. Each spermatic cord should be crushed twice, while minimizing the injury to the width of the scrotum. The end of the scrotum may be cut off with a scissors or a scalpel and the testes stripped out. An emasculator is necessary for hemostasis in all but the smallest kids. For adult bucks, separate U-shaped incisions may be made over the ventral aspect of each side of the scrotum. A final technique of castration, not yet evaluated in goat kids, is intratesticular injection of lactic acid.

A small kid may be restrained for castration by holding it upside down with all four limbs held together. A standing position may also be used, with the tail pulled upward. Larger animals may be given xylazine at a dose of 0.1 mg/kg intramuscularly. A local block may be performed by injecting 0.5 per cent lidocaine into the cord or testis and into the skin where the initial incision is to be made.

Care should be taken not to exceed 0.45 to 0.9 mg/kg of lidocaine, because toxicity, including opisthotonos and death, may result from higher doses. (Xylazine and lidocaine are both unapproved.) A fly repellent wound spray may be indicated but should be avoided in young nursing kids because any abnormal smell may cause the rejection of the kids by the mother.

TEASERS

When artificial insemination or planned mating is practiced, it is often convenient to have a teaser male in the herd that is able to stimulate and detect heat but that cannot successfully impregnate the doe.

A normal buck may be used temporarily as a teaser by simply fitting him with an apron. If a marking harness is also used, the owner can identify those does in heat with less frequent observations of the herd.

Several surgical procedures can be used to create permanent teasers while maintaining libido in the buck. Bilateral vasectomy can be performed, as is done with bulls or rams. A possibly simpler procedure involves removal of the tail of the epididymis.[3] Thirty days should elapse before the new teaser is used; this will allow for degeneration of sperm already in the tract beyond the epididymis, although most of the sperm will die sooner.

Because seminal fluids are resorbed in the head of the epididymis, obstruction or removal of the tail will not cause back pressure and testicular degeneration to the extent that libido is impaired. A spermatocele will form where the tail of the epididymis has been removed if ligation or cautery is not practiced. If the swelling later subsides, recanalization should be suspected. This may occur a year or more later.

Surgical deviation of the penis to the right flank hinders but does not prevent copulation;[1] the buck should be aproned if allowed to run with does. Libido may be decreased, but semen collection with an artificial vagina is simplified.

Male goats may be sterilized by injecting 200 µg/kg of cadmium chloride into each testis. This is reported to cause total destruction of the germinal cells, although the interstitium eventually regenerates. Leydig cell tumors have been reported in other species. The cadmium or some other sclerosing agent, such as 10 per cent calcium chloride, may be injected into the tail of the epididymis. A dose of 1 ml per epididymis is suggested.

Probably the simplest and most reliable teaser is the intersex goat. Many of these, although genetically female, develop marked masculine odors and behavior. If an intersex goat with female or intermediate external genitalia is used, copulation and any concomitant spread of disease will be impossible. Yet another alternative is intramuscular administration of 50 mg of testosterone propionate per day or 100 mg every 3 days to a normal female. The doe can be bred the same season with a minimal decrease in fertility, and the cost of maintaining a sterile animal is avoided.

References

1. Barker CAV: Penile deviation teaser bucks—A new development for dairy goat A/I. Dairy Goat J 55:67, 1977.
2. Gall C: Husbandry. *In* Gall C (ed): Goat Production. Academic Press, New York, 1981.
3. Shelton M, Klindt JM: A simple method of male sterilization for use with sheep and goats. Texas Agric Expt Sta Res Report, PR-3286, 1974.

Neoplasms of the Goat's Reproductive Tract

Mary C. Smith, D.V.M.
Cornell University, Ithaca, New York

NEOPLASMS OF THE FEMALE REPRODUCTIVE TRACT

Information concerning the prevalence of neoplasms of the doe's reproductive organs is scarce. One large granulosa cell tumor has been reported, and the author has personally seen a 1450-gm dysgerminoma in an aged doe.[3] Uterine adenocarcinomas, leiomyomas and fibromas as well as adenomas and fibromas of the vagina and vulva are infrequently seen. Numerous cases of lymphosarcoma have been reported in the goat, but there is no apparent predilection for the uterus.

Squamous cell carcinoma of the perineum is relatively common in animals with white or gray haircoats. These tumors are rounded, lobulated or ulcerated and may yield a foul exudate or become fly-blown. The squamous cell carcinoma must not be confused with the benign condition of ectopic mammary tissue in the vulva (Fig. 1). The animals with the latter anomaly show marked swelling and firmness of the vulvar lips just prior to each parturition; the swelling tends to regress completely in 60 to 70 days.[2] Milky fluid containing fat globules can be aspirated from nodules that are within the vulvar lips but are unattached to either skin or mucosa. If desired, a biopsy is easily accomplished through the vaginal mucosa. Occasionally, the vulvar swelling is large enough to interfere with defecation and urination.

Warts and melanomas of the perineum may also occur in the goat.

NEOPLASMS OF THE MALE REPRODUCTIVE TRACT

Information concerning the prevalence of neoplasms of the male reproductive tract is unavailable,

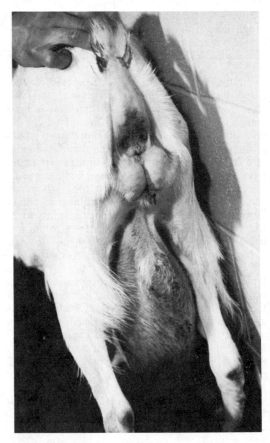

Figure 1. Postparturient vulvar enlargement due to ectopic mammary tissue.

with one exception. Adenomas of the adrenal cortex seem to be common in castrated male goats, especially in older Angoras.[1] Metastases and clinical signs are not reported. However, adrenal cortical inclusions have frequently been seen in the head of the epididymis, between the pampiniform plexus and the vasa efferentia of both male and intersex goats. It is postulated that the castrated male goat lacks sufficient endogenous testosterone to inhibit pituitary gonadotropins that mediate adrenal proliferation.

References

1. Altman NH, Streett CS, Terner JY: Castration and its relationship to tumors of the adrenal gland in the goat. Am J Vet Res 30:583, 1969.
2. Ramadan RO, El Hassan AM: Leiomyoma in the cervix and hyperplastic ectopic mammary tissue in a goat. Aust Vet J 51:362, 1975.
3. Smith MC: Caprine reproduction. In Morrow DA (ed): Current Therapy in Theriogenology. Philadelphia, WB Saunders Co, 1980.

Reproductive Health Programs and Records

Mary C. Smith, D.V.M.
Cornell University, Ithaca, New York

All livestock operations need good records, and goat herds are no exception. Because the proportion of novice goat owners in an area is often large, requests for assistance in setting up a preventive health program may be frequent. The records needed are determined by the procedures carried out on the animals and the purpose for which the herd is kept. Both individual lifetime records and herd summaries are needed. Goats have a propensity to destroy any valuable piece of paper in the barn. Therefore, permanent records (loose leaf, with holes reinforced) should be stored in the house, barn sheets should be hung high, and data should be transferred regularly to the permanent forms. Owners of commercial herds producing cheese or fluid milk should consider subscribing to a Dairy Goat Herd Improvement Association program if one is available in the area. Owners of purebred herds can also benefit from documentation of production capabilities of the animals they sell.

Treatments such as vaccinations, vitamin E/selenium injections, foot trimming and worming should be scheduled at appropriate times in the annual cycle of the herd. First, a plan is developed for the model goat from birth until maturity and through a year's lactation. Figure 1 shows a possible schedule for the first year of a goat's life, whereas Figure 2 applies to any doe in production. The back of the page can be used for health notations. If the kids are listed in order of birth and the does in order of kidding, similar work sheets for the year

can be constructed to serve as a reminder of tasks to be performed.

Care of the newborn kid involves a number of standard procedures not mentioned on the record sheet illustrated in Figure 1.[3] These include drying the kid (especially in cold weather when frost bite of the ears is likely) and dipping the navel in 7 per cent tincture of iodine. A careful examination should be made for congenital defects such as double teats, cleft palate or the intersex condition. Affected but viable kids are often raised for meat. If the kid does not receive colostrum from does given enterotoxemia and tetanus vaccination boosters in late pregnancy, then at least 150 to 200 units of tetanus antitoxin should be administered at the time of disbudding. The kid's own permanent vaccination series might also be begun earlier than 1 month of age.

The records for the lactating doe vary according to the intensiveness of the operation. Some full-time goat owners perform a California mastitis test and trim or at least check the feet once a month. Some record the milk production every day of the year. Others hardly ever find time to trim feet, or they milk into a pipeline so that no production records are available without special weigh days. Herds with mastitis problems need dry treatment, whereas many hand-milked animals never require such treatment. When a constant milk supply is desired, a portion of the herd may be housed under 16 to 20 hours of light a day in the winter for spring breeding after the lights have been turned off. Owners of show herds commonly clip all the does before the show season begins.

As a veterinarian develops experience with goat herds in a given area, the program should be modified. For instance, Figures 1 and 2 represent current needs of herds in the Northeast. In areas where selenium deficiency is not a problem or where additional selenium can be added to the diet by prescription, the emphasis on vitamin E/selenium injections would be dropped. Similarly, if a certain infectious disease has been identified in the area as a cause of abortion, prophylactic measures would be built into the program. An example would be the use of a chlamydial vaccine before breeding to

Dam_____ Breed_____ Tattoo LE_____

Name_____ Color_____ RE_____

Sire_____ Reg. No._____

Birth date_____ Number in litter_____

Horned or polled_____

Date disbudded and tattooed (1 week)_____

Date 1st E/SE (birth)_____

Date 2nd E/SE (1 month)_____

Date 1st CD/tetanus (1 month)_____

Date 2nd CD/tetanus (6 weeks)_____

Coccidiostats used _____ _____ _____ _____

Dates _____ _____ _____ _____

Dewormed with _____ _____ _____ _____

Dates _____ _____ _____ _____

Foot trim dates _____ _____ _____ _____

Comments

Weight at 7 months (goal-65% of adult weight)_____

Prebreeding E/SE date_____ Date lights on_____ Lights off_____

Heats, not bred _____ _____ _____ _____

Bred to buck _____ _____ _____ _____

Dates _____ _____ _____ _____

Date due _____

Date prekidding E/SE (-30 days)_____

Date prekidding CD/tetanus booster (-30 days)_____

Date kidded_____ Sire of kids_____ Number of kids_____

Figure 1. Health program for kids.

Name_____   Breed_____   Tattoo _____

Reg. No._____   Color_____   Class. Score_____

Date Kidded_____ Placenta passed_____ Weight after kidding_____

Kids born: sex   _____ _____ _____ _____

      disposal or tattoo   _____ _____ _____ _____

Dewormed with   _____ _____ _____ _____

          Dates _____ _____ _____ _____

Monthly operations: <u>Date</u>   <u># Milk</u>   <u>CMT</u>   <u>Feet</u>   <u>Comments</u>

    1.
    2.
    3.
    4.
    5.
    6.
    7.
    8.
    9.
  10.
  11.
  12.

305 day production: # Milk_____   # Fat_____   # Protein_____

Date dried off_____   Dry treated with_____

Lights on_____   Lights off_____

Heats, not bred   _____ _____ _____ _____

Bred to buck   _____ _____ _____ _____

          Dates _____ _____ _____ _____

Checked pregnant   _____   Date due_____

Date prekidding E/SE (-30 days)_____ Date CD/tetanus booster (-30 days)_____

Date kidded_____   Sire of kids_____   Number of kids_____

Figure 2. Health program for does.

prevent chlamydial abortion. In herds that show extensively the manager may wish to use sore mouth vaccine 6 weeks before the show season begins.

The parasite control program has been left intentionally vague in these figures. It will vary tremendously from herd to herd depending on the success of management techniques designed to control parasitism. Worming a lactating doe in a commercial herd is very expensive due to the need to discard milk after treatment. Hence, anthelmintics are avoided when possible, but they become more and more necessary as herd size and crowding increase.

An alternative record system, or one that can replace the cumbersome barn sheets, is a 3- by 5-inch file card for each goat each year.[4] The months of the year are listed across the card while vaccinations, worming, heats, breedings, fresh date, body weight and foot care are noted vertically. Appropriate dates are filled in on the grid. The back of the card is used for health notations and details concerning breeding or freshening.

The health program for the buck is often slighted because of the pervasiveness of his aroma. Yet his feet, his vaccinations, his parasite status cannot be ignored. In addition, a record should be kept of all does bred and the breeding dates each season.

These lists should be tallied to determine the conception rate for the buck. If does are returning to heat after breeding, part of the evaluation of the problem should be a breeding soundness examination of the buck.[1] Semen evaluation, as discussed previously in this volume, would complement a thorough physical examination of the animal.

Angora goats represent a very different type of livestock operation from a dairy herd. Herd health programs will probably need to concentrate on parasite control.[2] Because of the high proportion of wethers in a herd, dietary management to prevent urolithiasis is important. Production records are greatly simplified because the mohair is generally clipped only twice a year.

References

1. Ott RS, Memon MA: Breeding soundness examinations of rams and bucks. A review. Theriogenology 13(2):155, 1980.
2. Ross JD: Herd health program for Angora goats. *In* Howard J (ed): Current Veterinary Therapy Food Animal Practice. Philadelphia, WB Saunders Co, 1981, pp 203–204.
3. Williams CSF: Herd health program for dairy goats. *In* Howard J (ed): Current Veterinary Therapy Food Animal Practice. Philadelphia, WB Saunders Co, 1981, pp 199–203.
4. Wortham A: Records, anyone? Dairy Goat J 61(7):630, 1983.

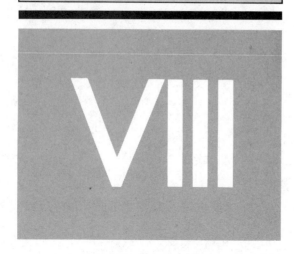
***Additional Pertinent Information Found in the First
Edition of Current Therapy in Theriogenology:***

Schryver HF, Hintz HF: Nutrition and Reproduction in the Horse,
p 768.

Management of the Breeding Stallion

J. M. Bowen, F.R.C.V.S.

Texas A & M University, College Station, Texas

STALLION SELECTION

It is commonly assumed that the selection of a stallion should be done purely on the basis of pedigree and little else. Often this is the case, particularly in thoroughbreds in which race performance is most important. In other breeds other factors such as the stallion's temperament and his eligibility as a representative of the breed as a whole should be taken into account. Full attention to the breed requirements and popular type is of paramount importance. The markings and colors of the horse should also be considered, especially in those breeds in which color is important, as this can greatly affect the demand for a sire. Consideration should also be given to preventing the possibility of propagating certain hereditary defects. Monorchism is a congenital defect that should be included in this category; in potential sires both testes should have descended and be within the scrotum.

Some countries have regulations concerning the registration and licensing of stallions and list the conditions that they consider to be hereditary, including navicular disease, ring-bone, cataracts and laryngeal hemiplegia. In the United States no such government regulations exist, and it is up to the individual owners and breed societies to encourage the castration of all males that do not meet breed specifications.

The Society for Theriogenology's manual for clinical evaluation of a stallion lists the following conditions considered to be genetically controlled: cryptorchism, combined immunodeficiency, parrot mouth, hemophilia, cataracts, aniridia, multiple exostoses and the wobbler syndrome.[11] Any stallion found to have any of these conditions should be considered ineligible as a sire.

MARE NUMBERS

The number of mares that should be covered by one stallion in a breeding season has been the subject of much debate. The traditional number has been about 40 mares for a stallion used in natural service. From a genetic point of view, taking into account the population of each breed, the number of mares put to each stallion should probably not exceed 55.[12] The more a single stallion is used, the narrower the genetic base of the breed becomes, increasing the risk of propagating genetic defects. Unfortunately, few owners take an altruistic view of their breed, and it is not uncommon for a stallion used in an artificial insemination program to have to cover 150 to 200 mares in a season, with the more popular stallions booked to 250 to 400 mares. Increased numbers of mares booked to any one stallion increase the owner's risk of having infertile and inferior mares sent to their stallion. Excessive numbers of mares result in increased demands for labor and decreased conception rates, reflecting poorly on the fertility of the horse and increasing the number of mares to be rebred the following season. In addition, unsuccessful progeny at the racetrack will devaluate the stallion and his offspring.

One criterion for judging a horse's fertility is the daily sperm output, which is very important when using a horse in an artificial insemination program. It has been postulated that the minimal insemination dose for each mare bred is 500 million motile spermatozoa,[13] although other authors have suggested that as few as 100 million live spermatozoa is commensurate with good fertility.[21] Thus, the average stallion in an artificial insemination program that produces 7 billion live spermatozoa at every collection would be able to cover 14 to 70 mares per ejaculate, depending upon the sperm dose chosen. Not all stallions will achieve their greatest fertility at the level of 100 million spermatozoa; thus, it should not be assumed that all stallions are capable of having their semen diluted to this extent.

In natural cover stallions are usually booked to about 40 mares, although this number is rising. It is not unusual to find that some popular stallions are booked to 50 or more mares in a season. In Australia it is common for a stallion to cover between 80 and 120 mares per season, while one stallion in Ireland has been reported to have covered in excess of 200 mares per season for several seasons with good fertility.

A rough guide to the numbers of mares a stallion should be able to cover, depending upon his age and maturity, is shown in Table 1.

Table 1. Number of Mares a Stallion Can Cover Based on Age and Number of Mares

Age of Stallion	Number of Mares
3 years	20 to 25
4 years	25 to 30
7 years	45 to 55
Mature	55 to 70
20 years	20 to 25

EXERCISE

Stallions need daily exercise and should be allowed to exercise freely when possible. Ideally, they should be turned into a small pasture or enclosure where they are safely contained to move about as they please. When this is impossible, it is necessary to ride or lead the stallion in some daily exercise routine. In many cases, this is performed by a mechanical walker. While it is more time-consuming, riding is a much better way of keeping a stallion fit but does require experienced personnel. Stallions that are confined to a box stall without exercise become difficult to handle and will often bite the handler and act boisterously when taken to the breeding shed. It has been our experience at Texas A & M University that a stallion with one or two older pregnant mares as company in a small paddock becomes more docile and better suited to conditions in which not all personnel who wish to handle a stallion are experienced.

FOOT CARE

The stallion's feet should be checked regularly by the farrier. Usually, shoes are removed when the stallion arrives at the stud farm. Unless the stallion has some problem, such as a sandcrack in the forefoot, shoes are not applied. The farrier should be instructed not to rasp the sole excessively, as this may cause the feet to become tender. White feet are more prone to drying and cracking than are dark-walled feet. Excessive trimming is deleterious, as this causes the horn to dry more rapidly and to be predisposed to cracking. If a horse is walked over a rough surface, the feet will tend to wear, reducing the need for trimming. Gelatin added to the diet may aid in hoof wall growth, and water will tend to retain the flexibility of the outer wall.

HOUSING

Housing plays an important part in the attitude of the stallion toward his handlers. Many believe that the stallion should be within sight of his mares. To achieve this, the stallion is placed in a box stall (usually a corner box), from which he can see and call to the passing mares. The stallion box should be at least 5 m square, lined with boards to withstand his kicking, with an anticasting groove cut into the wood 1.25 m (4 feet) above the floor. This groove allows a cast horse to get a foothold so he can right himself. The box stall should have adequate ventilation. In tropical areas buildings with high ceilings and open sides are more comfortable. Even in temperate climates, the lack of adequate ventilation can lead to an increase in respiratory diseases among stabled horses.

HANDLING THE STALLION

It is ideal for one person to handle the stallion so he or she may establish the rapport necessary for a successful working relationship. The handler should also be the person who grooms and feeds the stallion. This contact will tend to counteract the effect of isolating the stallion from the rest of the herd. The person handling the stallion should be of calm disposition and have a quiet demeanor with horses. Shouting allied with rapid movements will increase the nervousness of the animal. The handler should move slowly and deliberately and talk constantly to the horse, so the stallion knows where the handler is located at all times. Talking calms the stallion, as he can recognize the tranquility of the handler's voice. The stallion must also learn that his handler will reprimand him if he misbehaves. Failure to correct a horse when required is foolish and potentially dangerous. Punishment should be fair, consistent and prompt. The stallion must never sense that those who approach him are afraid, as he will then be unwilling to respect their commands.

Many horses that come into the breeding shed have had a career in the show ring, the racetrack or some other competitive event and have been chastised (sometimes severely) for showing interest in a mare or filly. Patience is required in encouraging a young stallion to approach and cover a mare. New owners frequently inherit the problems created by previous handlers. The excessive use of restraint is discouraged, and success is based on having the necessary controlling mechanisms in place when needed. It is common in the United States for handlers to try to control a stallion with only a lead shank. When the horse starts to misbehave, they severely jerk on the shank. It is actually better to use a bit in the mouth of the horse to give the necessary control (Fig. 1). Horses must be handled with firmness and in such a way as not to discourage them from their tasks. Also, the stallion should be restrained lightly before he begins to behave in an overly exuberant manner. The handler must be alert to the needs and reactions of the stallion, but control can only be achieved by the cooperation of the stallion. If the stallion has a particularly difficult disposition, two people (one on either side) may be required to lead him. A bit and bridle rather than a halter and lead should be used to control the animal without resorting to physical violence. There is no need to employ a severe bit, as a plain snaffle or vulcanite bit will suffice. In special cases a Chifney bit may be used (Fig. 2). A stallion that is nervous or likes to play with a chain in his mouth is best fitted with a mouthing bit with keys. The handler should be in contact with the bit at all times, so the stallion is aware that he is under control. It is incorrect to let the horse have a slack rein and then jerk at it when he starts to become unruly. Harsh shouting, threatening behavior and the use of the whip will do little to gain the horse's confidence. Such behavior will only tend to rein-

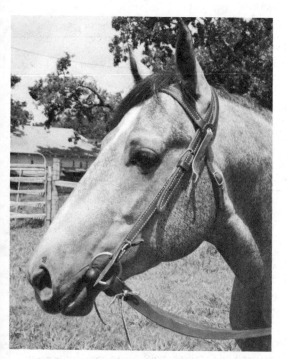

Figure 1. Stallion with a straight vulcanite bit.

force previous chastisement and will likely create a difficult stallion who is always in a state of apprehension and fear.

Occasionally, a vicious stallion will need to be managed. Such animals must be treated with the utmost of care. Preferably, there should always be two people to work with such a horse. Stallions of uncertain temperament and vicious horses need firm, skillful handling and rigid control at all times. Such animals are best left to the most experienced horse handler available.

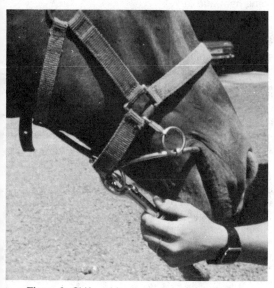

Figure 2. Chifney bit attached to a nylon halter.

MATING

The mating of stallions can be divided into three sections; pasture breeding, hand breeding and artificial insemination. Artificial insemination can further be divided into three subdivisions:

1. On-farm insemination using fresh raw or extended semen, with both the mare and stallion on the same premises.

2. Extended and cooled semen transported to the mare, which is on a farm different than the stallion's.

3. Semen previously collected and frozen in ampules or straws and stored in liquid nitrogen until the mare is scheduled to be inseminated.

A partial summary of the techniques that the breed registries will accept is listed in Table 2.

Pasture Breeding

With pasture breeding there is little the owner can or should do other than keep the fences in good repair and be sure that the stallion and mares will not be too close to any other group of horses. Preferably, the stallion should be experienced at pasture breeding. Young stallions should be hand mated several times to introduce them to their task. Shoes should be removed from horses run at pasture, with the exception that the front shoes may be left on some individual mares under special circumstances.

The stallion should be first introduced to a small band of older docile mares. After the stallion becomes accustomed to herding the mares together and controlling the herd, younger mares that might provoke or injure the stallion may be introduced. The breeding pasture should be of adequate size and clear of debris and wire. The horses should be checked for injuries twice daily. The daily feeding period allows an opportunity for closer examination of the animals. Mares should be examined for pregnancy at 2-week intervals beginning 1 month after introduction of the stallion. In the event that a stallion must be removed from the breeding pasture, 45 days should be allowed to elapse before a new stallion is introduced. The Quarter Horse Association allows the stallion to be replaced after 30 days, but this would seem to be inadequate for absolute certainty of parentage.

Care should be taken in approaching a stallion with a band of mares, as he may become protective of his herd. If stallions at pasture are approached slowly and deliberately, they are usually more tractable than stallions that are housed continuously. As with all methods of management, there are advantages and disadvantages in pasture breeding.

Advantages of Pasture Breeding. The greatest advantage of putting a stallion to pasture with a group of mares is that all work is done by the stallion, and the owner needs only to supervise the herd. The stallion is much better than his human companion at heat detection; thus, it is not unusual

Table 2. Regulations Concerning Artificial Insemination and Embryo Transfer

Breed Society	Artificial Insemination			Embryo Transfer
	On-Farm	Transported	Frozen	
Appaloosa	Yes	No	No	No
Arabian	Yes	No	No	Yes
Hanoverian	Yes	Yes	Yes	No
Holstein	Yes	Yes	?	?
American Paint	Yes	No	No	Yes
Quarter Horse	Yes	No	No	Yes
Standardbred	Yes	No	No	No
Thoroughbred	No	No	No	No
Trakehner	Yes	Yes	Yes	Yes

that a stallion bred at pasture will have a better conception rate than one that is hand bred. Bristol has recently reported that stallions breeding at pasture with a group of mares can obtain conception rates higher than 80 per cent in only one estrous period.[8] The other advantage, especially to those who wish to have early foals, is that regular ovulation and conception occur earlier in mares in contact with a stallion.[7] This male effect has been known in sheep for some time but has only recently been reported in the horse. This effect is not seen in mares kept with a stallion throughout the entire year but only when the stallion is introduced into the herd.

Disadvantages of Pasture Breeding. The greatest disadvantage of pasture breeding is the loss of supervision. When valuable animals are involved, it is impractical to consider pasture breeding, as the risk of injury is great. Horses are both gregarious and querulous by nature and quickly establish a social hierarchy that changes with each mare that moves into or out of the herd. There is much interplay among mares at feeding. Not only are there normal injuries from communal living, but the stallion is especially at risk, particularly if he is inexperienced. Injuries of the penis and prepuce are not uncommon. Not all mares are willing to be covered even when they are in estrus. An experienced stallion is necessary to cover these difficult mares. Young stallions will often find that the "boss" mare will try to prevent other mares from being covered when she is in estrus.

Recent observations of feral horses have shown that there is a danger to young foals when they are turned out with a stallion that is not their sire.[2] It has been postulated that when a new stallion takes over a band of mares for any reason, the new stallion will attack the foals that are not his. Young foals should only be put out with docile stallions, if at all.

In the event that a mare with venereal disease enters the herd, there is little chance of early observation of the problem or of preventing spread of the disease. Only during regular examination of the mares for pregnancy would such a problem come to light.

Hand Breeding

Breeding in hand is probably the most popular method of mating mares at the present time. The registry authorities who control thoroughbred breeding throughout the world do not permit the use of artificial insemination, and pasture breeding is considered too dangerous for valuable stallions. These restrictions leave hand breeding as the only alternative. When only a few mares are to be covered by a stallion, covering in hand is the method of choice.

The stallion is brought to the mare and mating takes place under restraint. Grass is an ideal surface for the stallion's footing and can act as a cushion if the stallion falls from the mare. In colder climates the need for protection (mostly for humans) has led to the development of the covering shed. Frequently, this is an oblong building open at both ends, with an area in which the mare can be prepared prior to mating. Octagonal breeding sheds are preferable, as they afford more room in which to work and are safer for the staff should an altercation occur between the mare and stallion. Octagonal buildings have the further advantage of being light and airy.

The floor of the covering area is an important feature. It should allow the stallion maximum grip when mounting the mare and should be a safe surface if the mare or stallion falls. The ideal surface is loose and dust free. Such things as tannin bark, pea gravel, and flint chips have all been utilized, as have artificial surfaces such as tarmacadam, Astroturf and Tartan. Sand and peat moss are too dirty (though adequate for grip and safety) and should not be used unless there is no alternative. Wood shavings can be used but should not be allowed to become damp, as the growth of bacteria, especially *Klebsiella,* will be promoted. The inside of the covering area should be clear of all obstructions, with the exception of a protective rail for spectators. A small pen should be available to contain the foal during the time of covering. It should be close enough for the mare and foal to communicate but not so close as to distract the mare.

The act of covering the mare is usually uneventful, especially if the mare is in strong heat. The mare should be brought to the covering area and her perineal region washed of any fecal material. After washing, the skin around the vulva is dried and the tail wrapped with a clean gauze bandage. The mare is led to the center of the area, where she is restrained prior to the act of covering. Hobbles may be used on quiet mares but can be dangerous if used on a high-spirited thoroughbred, since hobbles restrict the mare's ability to walk. Under these circumstances it is better to twitch the mare and hold one foreleg up with a leather strap until the stallion has mounted. In addition, felt boots can be put on the hindlegs of the mare to protect the stallion. Felt boots are difficult to place on some mares, and they may resent having to walk in them. If the mare is in strong heat, there is probably little need to restrain her unless the stallion is particularly boisterous in his approach to the mare.

Some owners prefer to tease the mares to be mated with the covering stallion. This allows the breeding shed manager to be sure that the mare is in heat prior to the time of mating and allows the stallion some stimulation. A teasing bar is installed in the covering shed that can be swung from the wall while the mare is teased and then returned to its original position along the wall during the act of covering. A teasing bar is particularly useful in the case of a mare that has a foal at her side and is slow to "break down" when teased. This bar may also afford protection for the stallion. Mares that do not show good signs of heat can constitute a hazard in the breeding shed. They must be fully restrained, and an experienced staff is necessary to cope with this type of mare. Such mares must be twitched, and a leg strap must be maintained in position throughout the act of mating.

The act of covering is straightforward when an experienced stallion is used. After teasing the mare, the stallion is moved to the side of the shed while the mare is restrained. The stallion, with penis in full erection, is led toward one side of the mare to make contact with her flank. From that position he is allowed to move around to mount from behind. By approaching in this manner, the stallion can test the way in which the mare will react to his presence and determine the best approach for covering the mare. Maiden mares are often frightened and are likely to bolt if alarmed and are best covered by an experienced stallion. It is sometimes recommended that the stallion's penis be grasped and guided into the vagina of the mare. Most stallions used in natural cover resent this attempt to aid them, and the procedure may be counterproductive. It is more useful to place the flat of the hand at the dorsal commissure of the vulva, preventing the penis from entering the rectum of the mare. Stallions that are particularly vigorous in thrusting may need the use of a breeding roll, which is a large padded roll placed under the tail of the mare and held on each side. The breeding roll prevents the stallion's penis from penetrating too deeply and injuring the mare's vagina and cervix. A breeding roll should also be used on mares that have had reconstructive surgery of the perineum. When the horse ejaculates, the tail moves up and down ("flags") with each ejaculatory pulse. Young stallions should be mated to older mares at the beginning of their breeding careers. Care must be taken to prevent the young stallion from charging nervously at the mare. This habit, once developed, can be quite unsettling in the breeding shed. The young stallion should be handled as calmly as possible and made to approach the mare directly from the rear rather than from the side, as would a more experienced stallion. This approach allows the stallion a better chance of mounting the mare correctly—from the rear, not from the side.

Particular care must be taken when the stallion dismounts, as mares will often kick at the male. In order to prevent kicking the mare should be turned toward the handler as the stallion dismounts. Turning the mare will unbalance her and reduce the chances of kicking. Some stallions (both young and old) will bite viciously—a difficult problem to overcome. In some cases it may be sufficient to lift the stallion's head with the bit as he tries to bite the mare's neck. The force should not be such that it causes the stallion to loose his concentration and dismount. If the stallion cannot be managed by lifting his head, it may be necessary to use a muzzle. The act of biting and nipping the mare is a stimulus to the young stallion and may be needed until he becomes accustomed to his role. Another method that may be used to prevent damage to the mare's neck is a leather drape that has a hard ridge across it. This is often a satisfactory way of controlling the problem while permitting the stallion to maintain his balance by gripping the drape with his teeth. A fourth method is to place a draft horse collar on the mare, which can be gripped by the stallion while covering.

When a young horse mounts incorrectly, it is necessary to make him dismount as quickly as possible. Care must be taken not to pull him over backwards. The pull on the bridle must be downwards and backwards. If the bridle is pulled backwards only, the stallion can be easily flipped over.[9]

When using a stallion in natural service, it is best to cover one mare per day. While it is possible to cover up to four or five mares per day, it is better to conserve the stallion as much as possible. If there is a need to cover more than one mare per day, these covers should be spaced as evenly as possible over the day.

Advantages of Hand Breeding. Hand breeding has some advantages over pasture breeding, particularly in the care of valuable animals. When the stallion and mares are kept separately from each other, there is little chance of an accident occurring. Supervision is optimal and this system is particularly suitable for owners who have a few mares to breed and whose stock is too valuable to turn out in a pasture. This system requires little equipment but does require considerable investment in housing facilities for the stallion and mares.

Disadvantages of Hand Breeding. The capital cost of housing could be considered a disadvantage, though this varies with location. The foaling rate from hand mating is lower than either pasture breeding or artificial insemination. This is probably due to two factors: the better heat detection rate of the stallion in pasture breeding and the greater sperm quality and disease control afforded by artificial insemination. Finally, the mares and stallion meet in the breeding shed, where the greatest possibility of injury occurs.

Artificial Insemination

When artificial insemination (AI) is practiced, the design of the facilities may be different from those needed for hand breeding. The collection area may be considerably smaller, as it is customary to collect the semen by allowing the stallion to mount a "jump mare" or phantom (also known as a dummy). The jump mare should be a small stocky mare, well able to bear the weight of the stallions. The jump mare should be ovariectomized, as such mares will allow covering at will and may show some slight signs of estrus because of a rise in the production of adrenal estrogens.[1] This rise of adrenal estrogen production is caused by the removal of the normal negative feedback effect of the intact ovaries, resulting in the release of high levels of follicle-stimulating hormone (FSH), the so-called "castration effect".[10] Jump mares will lose their acquiescence for a few days if given a therapeutic dose of dexamethasone.

The jump mare is usually hobbled, with the most convenient type of hobble being the California hobble, which allows the mare to walk while hobbled. It can be rapidly dismantled by quick release catches in the event of an entanglement. Hobbles are intrinsically dangerous and even the best-trained stallion can get caught in the ropes. It is essential that the cords be tied with quick release knots and that the quick release catches on the hock straps be fitted correctly.

Some breeders prefer to build a phantom on which they can collect their stallions. In Texas these are often made of two oil drums welded together and mounted on steel pipe. The phantom is set at about the height of the average mare. It is padded with several layers of plastic foam and covered with reinforced plastic or canvas. A leather cover, while expensive, is very durable, acceptable to the stallion and easy to clean. Many phantoms are too high and can cause physical discomfort or cause a fall when the stallion tries to thrust. There is no need to make the phantom as tall or as wide as a mare. Narrower dummies are more convenient.

As in natural service, the character of the flooring is important and should provide the stallion a good grip while thrusting. Some stallion owners use very confined quarters when collecting their stallions, especially if the stallion has problems in staying on the phantom. Many thoroughbreds are particularly unstable when serving a mare or a phantom.

Semen Collection. Semen for use in an AI program is usually collected into an artificial vagina (AV). There are several types of AVs available commercially. The more popular are the Colorado model, the Missouri model, the F.H.K. from Japan and the Goetze from Germany. They all consist of a hollow tube lined with rubber that can be filled with hot water. Some type of cup into which semen can be collected is attached to the distal end. Each type of AV is prepared differently and must suit the preferences of individual stallions. Some stallions prefer to work into a tight AV while others require a slack one. The temperature of the AV is also variable. Artificial vaginas such as the Colorado model with a double thickness of rubber liner are filled with water of a higher temperature than is the self-contained Missouri model. Air can be used in some AVs to augment the pressure and reduce the weight, an important factor when collecting a vigorous stallion. The preferences of the stallion should be noted for use at subsequent collections.

Preparation of the Stallion. The stallion should be brought from his stall to the breeding shed under full control of the handler. He should be allowed to see that he is about to enter the covering area and should be held back until he shows some degree of interest. If the stallion is slow to show interest, he should be allowed to enter the arena and see the jump mare or phantom. The stallion should be restrained until an erection is sustained. At this point, many stud managers wash the penis of their stallions. While the penis is erect, it is easy to hold and to wash the penis and sheath free of smegma and accumulated debris. Most stallions permit this procedure once they are accustomed to it and find it stimulating. Many owners and managers feel that washing is an essential part of the preparatory phase, as it delays the sexual act in the presence of the female, makes the stallion more eager and increases the chances of collecting a semen sample during the first mount.

Washing the stallion's penis has a long tradition in horse breeding. At first it was a somewhat desultory splash of cold water aimed somewhere in the vicinity of the penis as the stallion dismounted. With the advent of AI, a more thorough cleansing was implemented using soap. It was not until the diagnosis of contagious equine metritis (CEM) that serious methods of cleaning the penes of stallions used in natural service were considered. The use of a surgical scrub preparation seemed to be the most certain way of removing the offending organism from the penes. Little thought was given to the other effects of this procedure until overgrowth of *Pseudomonas aeruginosa* was found to be a problem subsequent to this washing routine.[3] Investigation showed that the use of effective antiseptic agents such as povidone-iodine surgical scrub and chlorhexidine gluconate surgical scrub could eliminate most of the bacteria, with the exception of the more resistant varieties. Such elimination of the normal bacterial flora of the skin of the penis allowed recolonization of the site with those pathogens that could best survive the strong antiseptics used in the washing procedure. Most of these organisms are also capable of causing disease in the uterus of the mare.

Swerczek reported in 1979 that the possibility of CEM transmission was increased by washing the penes of pony stallions with chlorhexidine surgical scrub.[20] Work at Texas A & M University showed the disruptive effects of different cleansing agents. In that experiment water, soap (Ivory) and povidone-iodine surgical scrub (Betadine) were compared. Seven stallions were washed daily for 2 weeks with each preparation. Two weeks rest was allowed between each treatment. The results are shown in Figure 3. It was demonstrated that water alone could disrupt the bacterial flora of the penis. Washing with soap tends to favor the establishment of coliform organisms, while washing with povidone-iodine surgical scrub, the most potent of the washing agents, produced an overgrowth of *P. aeruginosa* in all stallions used in the experiment.

In contrast, the bacterial flora of the penis of a control stallion left unwashed during the breeding season showed little variety in the types of bacteria isolated throughout the experiment. The bacteria isolated were mostly the normal species found on the penes of stallions. Pathogens appeared occasionally, but the conditions on the penis were not disrupted to encourage their establishment, as was

the case when stallions were subjected to the regular washing regimen. The conclusion drawn from this experiment is that the penes of stallions should not be washed regularily but only occasionally if the amount of smegma and keratinous debris demands removal.

An experienced stallion should be restrained for a short period of time prior to mounting the jump mare. After he attains a full erection, the stallion is allowed to approach the mare from behind and slightly to one side. He is allowed to mount and is quickly collected. Young stallions should be allowed to approach the jump mare and nuzzle her gently just behind the shoulder. They are then allowed to move back towards the mare's tail and smell under the tail. This will probably elicit a "flehmen" response from the stallion. Young stallions may also nibble at the hocks of the jump mare and care must be taken to prevent the stallion from biting the mare. Some young horses are initially slow to respond to the mare but when aroused react over exuberantly towards the mare, charging her and pushing her roughly. They will often mount from the side or over the withers and unsettle the mare. To prevent improper mounting, the immature stallion should be led back once a full erection is attained and made to approach the mare directly from behind rather than the usual side approach. In this way, they have a better chance of mounting

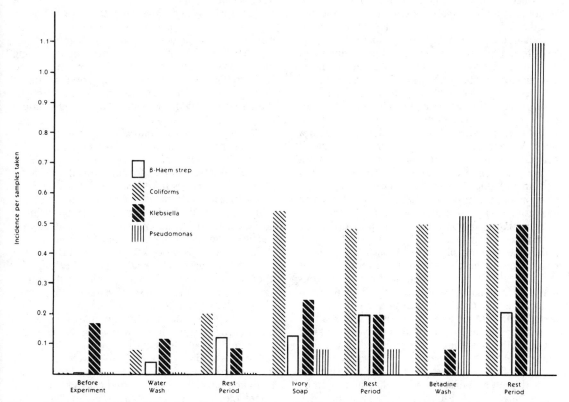

Figure 3. Incidence of bacterial isolates from the genitals of stallions washed with water, soap and povidone iodine surgical scrub.

correctly with one leg on each side of the mare, allowing them to remain on the mare during the collection. Some stallion managers prefer that a young stallion have the experience of covering one or two mares naturally before attempting to collect semen with the AV.

The following personnel are required for semen collection: a mare handler, stallion handler (or two) and a semen collector. The stallion is usually approached from the near or left side but it may become crowded on the near side of the mare and it is often easier to collect from the off or right side of the horse. Shy stallions, seeing several people congregating on the left side, may slide up the right side of the mare. If the collector is located on the right side, collection may be easier.

When collecting semen with an AV, it is best to divert the penis toward the AV and place the AV onto the penis. The stallion should not be expected to find the opening of the AV. The penis of young stallions should not be grasped firmly as they seem to resent this stimulus and may dismount. It may be necessary not to touch the penis after having placed the AV, although the urethral pulses occurring as the stallion ejaculates are an indication to the collector that the horse has ejaculated. After intromission, the AV is held with the distal end slightly elevated, approximating the normal plane of the mare's vagina. When ejaculation commences, the AV is lowered to allow the semen to flow into the collection bottle. Upon completion of the collection, the air and water are emptied from the AV and the collection bottle is taken to the laboratory.

Should the stallion fail to ejaculate, he is led away from the mare immediately after dismounting, as frustration may induce him to kick at the mare. The stallion is then encouraged to again attain a full erection and allowed to approach the mare and another collection is attempted. If the second attempt fails, the temperature and pressure of the AV should be checked. It is usual to start with a slack AV and increase the pressure with a hand-held bicycle pump. Several mounts may be required before the stallion ejaculates. If a stallion has not performed within 1 hour, the procedure should be postponed, as a frustrated stallion tends to become increasingly aggressive towards the jump mare.

Collecting a stallion on a phantom or dummy is by far the safest method. Stallions can be easily trained to mount a phantom by placing a mare in heat alongside the phantom or by covering the rear end of the phantom with urine from an estrous mare. Occasionally, a stallion will benefit from watching another stallion mount the phantom. This method can also be used with young stallions that seem to be particularly inept about covering mares.

Originally, phantoms were mounted in the covering arena, but now they are deliberately built in rather confined quarters, permitting the stallion to support himself against the side walls while mounted on the phantom. The only opening is on one side where the collector stands to manipulate the AV.

When the number of mares booked to the stallion exceeds the number of sperm doses obtained in one collection, it is necessary to obtain a second collection. Most stallions require some time to recover from a collection, and usually one must wait 1 hour before attempting a second collection.

The management of a stallion in the breeding shed requires a combination of patience and common sense along with a sound feeding and exercise routine—a contented stallion is easy to manage. If due regard is given to the social needs of stallions rather than to organizational conveniences, problems tend to resolve by themselves. A calm approach and quiet demeanor will gain the confidence of all horses, regardless of age, sex and temperament.

BREEDING PROBLEMS

Accidents and Injuries

In spite of precautions accidents do occur in the breeding shed, although the chances of injury to the stallion or mare running at pasture are greater. Kicks occur frequently, both between mares and between stallion and mare. Mares will always try to establish a social hierarchy, and the introduction of new mares will rearrange the social order. Stallions, on the other hand, are almost an appendage to the herd. The controlling influence is the "boss mare," who decides what the herd will do at any given time. It is she who decides when the herd will move from one place to another in the pasture. Stallions will herd their band of mares and group them together, especially if they feel threatened. Feeding time allows for great rivalry among the mares and leads to fighting over the amount of feed to be shared. To avoid trouble, several feeding troughs should be provided for mares. The troughs should be spaced well apart and placed some distance from the fence. Horses can and will trap rivals or their foals against the fence or in a corner. The water trough should be circular and centrally placed to allow greater freedom of movement in all directions. Provided that shoes have been removed, the damage sustained by the adult population from fighting injuries is usually slight, although fractured limbs do occur. In foals, the injuries can be severe, with fractured limbs and ribs being most common.

The stallion is also subject to injuries when around his mares. The stallion's liability depends upon his age, experience at running with mares, aggressiveness towards the mares and innate canniness. Many young stallions will be intimidated by the herd and will not cover many mares when first introduced. Others will be overly aggressive to the mares and savage to them at covering. Still other stallions will disregard their own well-being and may be severely punished by the mare band, losing teeth and developing bruises and exostoses in areas where they are kicked. Occasionally, stallions will be kicked by a mare in the act of covering or during attempts at mounting. Damage to the penis, scrotum, testes or sheath may occur. Such damage usually requires removal from the herd for at least 6 weeks.

Stallions have also been implicated in injuring foals when they are at pasture, especially those that are progeny of another sire. Highly virile stallions should be carefully monitored, as they are the most likely candidates for this antisocial behavior.

When hand breeding is practiced, there is a reduction in the number of injuries to horses but an increase in the danger to handlers and staff of the breeding farm. Often, the stallion is much less tractable and can be difficult to handle in the presence of a mare in heat. Sometimes his exuberance will frighten a nervous mare causing her to reject him, whereas he might have otherwise covered the mare had his approach been less aggressive.

Injuries incurred in hand breeding are similar to those encountered in pasture mating. The most serious problems are those that involve the prepuce, testes or penis. Hematomas are the most significant problem and require extensive hydrotherapy, with frequent applications of cold water. Hydrotherapy is most effective if applied for at least 1 hour at a time. It is preferable to treat a preputial hematoma with cold water for 1 hour once daily than to treat it for 20 minutes 6 times daily. About 20 minutes of therapy are required for a hematoma to begin to reduce in size; thus, short periods are less useful than long periods. When the penis is trapped by a hematoma, it is necessary to splint the penis with a rigid structure such as a plastic bottle, which has had the bottom removed. The end of the bottle is carefully padded to reduce chafing of the tissues.[18] The penis is placed within the bottle, and the entire support apparatus is pushed back into the sheath as far as possible. The splint is kept in place by four ties, two on either side of the flanks in front of the pin bones and two laid alongside the scrotum and run either side of the tail. All of the ties meet over the sacrum, where they are tied together. The support must be changed once or twice each day. This method may also be used in cases in which there is considerable edema of the sheath leading to paraphimosis. Sexual activity must be restricted following a hematoma of the penis or sheath. The length of time will depend upon the rate of recovery but should be a minimum of 3 weeks and may be up to 6 weeks or more.

Penile paralysis or priapism may follow the administration of drugs such as acepromazine and/or etorphine or as a result of debility or cold weather injury. If such cases are presented immediately, the condition is treated with benztropine mesylate at a dose of 8 mg by slow intravenous injection.[16] Support of the penis should not be necessary after the stallion can retract the penis. The use of the splint should be discontinued as soon as possible as it will excoriate the skin of the prepuce, penis and flank. Liberal application of petroleum jelly or lanolin ointment will reduce the chafing to a minimum. The prognosis for cases of penile paralysis should always be guarded, as stallions rarely regain the ability to

retract the penis. If the penis cannot be retracted, treatment consists of castration followed by either a "reefing" operation or amputation of the penis.

Occasionally, a mare may kick the distal end of the penis, resulting in a small cut on the glans penis. Such lacerations bleed profusely, causing the stallion to be withdrawn from the breeding program. The blood pressure within the erect penis of the stallion is approximately 7000 mmHg. As the corpus cavernosum and corpus spongiosum dilate, and blood pressure increases, the dorsal artery of the penis may spontaneously rupture allowing blood to rapidly fill the subcutaneous spaces. Such an injury must be treated as a traumatic hematoma, with the penis returned to the sheath and supported, as needed.

Trauma to the scrotum requires prompt treatment, as temperature regulation is important to spermatogenesis. It is essential that cold water therapy be instituted immediately to reduce the edema and hemorrhage, thereby preventing overheating of the testes. If the temperature of the testes is elevated for a period of time, the stallion can be rendered infertile temporarily or permanently.

Infections

Bacterial. Bacterial infections are of most concern in pasture breeding or hand breeding situations. There is considerable evidence that bacterial endometritis reduces fertility in the horse. Contagious equine metritis (CEM) is the only bacterial venereal disease of the horse. The proposed name of the causative organism of CEM is *Taylorella equigenitalis,* a small delicate microaerophilic micrococcus.[14] This organism can be found in the uteri of infected mares long after the initial infectious phase has passed and will be harbored by the stallion in the fossa glandis of the penis. *H. equigenitalis* has been recovered from colts born to mares infected with CEM. Perinatal infections have been reported to result in transmission to mares that were covered by carrier stallions.[19]

Other bacteria can also be spread by venereal transfer. These include *Klebsiella, Pseudomonas* and other ubiquitous organisms such as *Streptococci* and *Escherichia coli.* As mentioned previously, veterinarians and stud staff are much to blame for having instigated precopulatory washing as a routine, as this encourages the growth of resistant organisms and depletes the normal innocuous flora of the penes of horses. There is no evidence to date that anaerobic bacteria cause endometritis in mares, although these organisms have been found to affect fertility in cattle. Similarly, Ureaplasmas (*T. mycoplasma*) have not been isolated from equine reproductive tracts to date.

Treatment of bacterial venereal disease depends upon the sensitivity of the organisms involved. Prevention is best acheived by use of AI in place of hand breeding. When AI is not permitted, efforts must be made to eliminate the disease from the mare population to reduce the risk of spreading the infection.

Protozoa. Dourine is a venereal disease of Equidae rarely seen in North America. The disease occurs in Central and South America, North Africa and the Middle East. Dourine is caused by the trypanosome *Trypanosoma equiperdum* and is transmitted by coitus. If other modes of transmission are possible, they are of little importance. The disease is slow in onset, with an incubation period of up to 20 weeks. Initial clinical signs include a vaginal or urethral discharge, low recurrent fever and edema and ulceration of the external genitalia. Affected horses lose their conditioning and develop plaques on the flanks, which may persist for a few hours or days. These lesions are considered pathognomonic. Weakness is progressive, and nervous signs may develop, including incoordination, ataxia and paralysis. Those animals that have only mild signs will usually become carriers of dourine.[15]

Viruses. The viruses associated with the reproductive tract of the horse are both herpesviruses. Equine herpesvirus type I (equine viral rhinopneumonitis) causes abortion in mares but is not known to be transmitted venereally. Equine herpesvirus type III is transmitted by venereal contact and is known as coital exanthema. The disease is characterized by the formation of blisters on the penis of the stallion and around the vulva of the mare. While the lesions regress spontaneously, it is usual to withdraw an infected stallion from stud service for about 3 weeks in order to prevent further spread. Endometrial smears containing a high number of lymphocytes, suggestive of a viral stimulus, have been noted, but no correlation with either equine herpesvirus has been demonstrated.[4]

Other Infections. Orchitis is rare in the stallion but can originate from an ascending infection or localization of some systemic disease. *Klebsiella* is an organism that can cause an ascending orchitis in stallions, while *Streptococcus zooepidemicus* is an example of a systemic infection that can localize in the testes. Treatment of orchitis includes systemic antibiotics and hydrotherapy to cool the inflamed testes.

Urethritis is usually caused by the combination of trauma and an ascending infection and is often diagnosed because of its association with hemospermia. Diagnosis requires the use of a fiberoptoscope that allows examination of the entire urethra. Care must be taken to move the instrument gently, as iatrogenic irritation may lead to a misdiagnosis of urethritis. Urethritis is treated with highly soluble sulfonamides and antibiotics. In addition, stallion rings that may have been responsible for the condition are removed.

Hemospermia is thought by some to be of traumatic origin,[20] but it is more likely caused by secondary bacterial infection following trauma.

Hemospermia can occur without visible urethritis and is often seen as a mild condition characterized by a faint pink discoloration of the semen. In these mild cases little or no treatment is required, as it

Table 3. Tumors of the Equine Genital Tract

Tumor	Site	Treatment
Squamous cell carcinoma	Penis Prepuce	Cryotherapy Surgery
Granulomas (Habronema)	Penis Prepuce	Trichlorfon Ivermectin
Interstitial cell tumor	Testes	Surgery
Sertoli's cell tumor	Retained testes	Surgery
Seminoma	Testes (aged stallions)	Surgery
Teratoma	Retained testes	Surgery

does not interfere with motility or fertility of the spermatozoa. While it has been shown that considerable quantities of blood are deleterious to fertility,[22] the stallion, rather like man, appears to be able to tolerate a small amount of blood in his semen with no effect. Experience at Texas A & M University has suggested a strong correlation between hemospermia and *Klebsiella* present on the stallion's penis and in the bedding of his stall. Cases have been encountered in which the wood shaving bedding has been allowed to become and remain moist, encouraging the growth of *Klebsiella*. While this positive correlation has been noted, it has not been possible to isolate *Klebsiella* from the urethra in every case. *Klebsiella* has also been associated with cases of seminal vesiculitis, although this condition is less frequently seen in stallions than in bulls. The lesion is not palpable on rectal examination in the horse, as is vesiculitis in the bull. If structures similar to the seminal vesicles of the bull are palpated in the stallion, it is likely that the ampullae have been identified. The ampullae can become blocked in old stallions, rendering them infertile. The only clinical sign of seminal vesicle involvement in stallions is the presence of blood in the semen or of blood-tinged gel. It is frequently impossible to determine the cause of hemospermia in the horse, since a small lesion that is not obvious when searched for under tranquilization or anesthesia will become a gaping tear when subjected to the sudden increase in blood pressure produced by an erection.

Strangles can involve the testes and scrotum of the stallion, particularly if the stallion develops purpura hemorrhagica. In addition to orchitis, the skin of the scrotum can become necrotic, and the resulting edema and inflammation can affect the stallion's fertility.

Neoplasia

The most common tumor of the genitalia of the stallion is squamous cell carcinoma of the penis. This tumor can be slow in onset and insidious in its development. It is often mistaken for depigmentation of the penis rather than recognized as a tumor because it is not always raised from the skin surface. Diffuse circular lesions may be mistaken for healing vesicles that might follow coital exanthema. Diagnosis of squamous cell carcinoma is by biopsy of the lesion. The remaining tumors of the genital tract are listed in Table 3.

Behavioral Conditions

Impotence in the covering shed is not uncommon in the stallion. It may be due to inadequate or oppressive training or premature use of a stallion. Usually, it is possible to return the horse to normalcy with time, patience and kindness. Each case must be treated individually, but the primary ingredients for success are perseverance and calm handling. Some stallions will show little interest in the mare to be covered. In such cases an attempt may be made to increase the stallion's circulating testosterone level by the intravenous injection of 3000 to 5000 IU of human chorionic gonadotropin (hCG), which acts to stimulate the interstitial cells, resulting in an elevation of endogenous testosterone. Under no circumstances should repeated doses of testosterone be given to a stallion, as the stallion's endogenous levels of testosterone will be reduced.

Failure to ejaculate is another frequent problem in young stallions and in those that are not accustomed to the AV. It has been reported that stallions that persistently fail to ejaculate respond to treatment with 10 mg of the beta-blocker bunitrolol. The author has utilized propranolol hydrochloride, which is more easily available in the United States. The effect is transient and lasts for 7 to 10 days. Disinterest in the mare is also manifest as a failure to gain a complete erection of the penis. This condition is often seen in young immature stallions at the beginning of the breeding season. Treatment with 5 to 10 mg prostaglandin $F_{2\alpha}$ 20 to 30 minutes before attempting collection of semen is alleged to stimulate a more complete erection.

A few older stallions tend to urinate into the semen at the time of collection. This is presumably caused by the bladder sphincter's loss of ability to close when stretched during an erection. Urination during ejaculation is often a persistent problem, and some cases can be controlled by not allowing the stallion to tease prior to collection of semen. Treatment of persistent cases may be attempted by administering flavoxate hydrochloride.[5] On the day of collection 1 gm of flavoxate is given at 6:00 AM followed by a second 1 gm dose at 12:00 PM. The stallion is then collected 2 to 4 hours later (2:00 to 4:00 PM).

References

1. Asa CS, Ginther OJ: Glucocorticoid suppression of oestrus, follicles, LH and ovulation in the mare. J Reprod Fertil (Suppl) 32:247, 1982.
2. Berger J: Induced abortion and social factors in wild horses. Nature 303:59, 1982.
3. Bowen JM: Problems that can affect some stallions in the breeding season, and their management. Proc 18th Conv Equine Vet Assoc, Exeter, 1979.
4. Bowen JM, Bergeron H: Unpublished data.
5. Bowen JM, Martin MT, Bird EH: Unpublished data.
6. Bowen JM, Tobin N, Simpson RB, et al.: Effects of washing on the bacterial flora of the stallion's penis. J Reprod Fertil (Suppl) 32:41, 1982.
7. Bowen JM, Wiggington S, Bergeron H: Advancing the equine breeding season naturally. Proc 8th Equine Nutr Physiol Symp, Lexington, 1983, pp 90–95, 1983.
8. Bristol F: Breeding behaviour of a stallion at pasture with twenty mares in synchronized oestrus. J Reprod Fertil (Suppl) 32:71, 1982.
9. Dougall N: Stallions, Their Management and Handling. London, J. A. Allen, 1976.
10. Ganong WF: Role of the nervous system in reproductive processes. In Cole HH, Cupps PT (eds): Reproduction in Domestic Animals. New York, Academic Press, 1977, p 58.
11. Kenney RM (Ed): Theriogenology and the Equine. Part II. Hastings, Society for Theriogenology, 1983, pp 29–31.
12. Leighton-Hardman AC: Stallion Management. London, Pelham Books, 1974.
13. Pickett BW, Back DG: Procedures for preparation, collection, evaluation, and insemination of stallion semen. Colorado State University Experiment Station and Animal Reproduction Laboratory General Series 935, 1973.
14. Powell DG: Contagious equine metritis. Equine Vet J 10:1, 1978.
15. Robertson A (Ed): Handbook on animal diseases in the tropics. London, British Veterinary Association, 1976, pp 207–209.
16. Sharrock AG: Reversal of drug-induced priapism in a gelding by medication. Aust Vet J 58:39, 1982.
17. Swerczek TW: Aggravation of strangles, equine clostridial typhocolitis (colitis X) and bacterial venereal diseases in the horse by antibacterial drugs. Proc 25th Ann Conv Am Assoc Equine Pract, Miami Beach, 1979, pp 305–311.
18. Taylor T: Personal communication.
19. Timoney PJ, Powell DG: Isolation of the contagious equine metritis organism from colts and fillies in the United Kingdom and Ireland. Vet Rec 111:478, 1982.
20. Voss JL, Pickett BW: Diagnosis and treatment of hemospermia in the stallion. J Reprod Fertil (Suppl) 23:171, 1975.
21. Voss JL, Pickett BW: Reproductive management of the broodmare. Colorado State University Experiment Station and Animal Reproduction Laboratory General Series 961, 1976.
22. Voss JL, Pickett BW, Shideler RK: The effect of hemospermia on fertility in horses. Proc 8th Int Congr Anim Reprod AI, Krakow, 4:1093, 1976.

Physical Examination and Genital Diseases of the Stallion

William F. Braun, Jr., D.V.M.
University of Missouri, Columbia, Missouri

A breeding soundness examination of the stallion includes not only examination of various seminal characteristics but also evaluation of the stallion's physical condition and his ability to perform the arduous tasks involved in equine reproduction. The stallion must have the desire and ability to deliver fertile sperm into the reproductive tract of the mare or into an artificial vagina. In addition to the examination of the reproductive organs, a complete physical examination should be performed to evaluate the locomotor systems, including muscular, skeletal and neurologic components, and the visual function of the stallion.

The most reliable measure of fertility in an individual stallion is the pregnancy rate obtained when bred to mares of normal fertility and under ideal management. No single seminal parameter or physical characteristic of the stallion is highly correlated with fertility. Measurements of these characteristics and comparison of these to stallions of known fertility are sufficient to predict the potential potency of a given stallion. Stallions selected for evaluation include those about to be or recently purchased as a breeding animal, those about to enter the breeding season, those suspected of reduced fertility and young stallions being considered for their first breeding season.

The evaluation of the stallion for potential breeding soundness consists of five basic parts: (1) history, (2) general physical examination, (3) examination of the external genitalia, (4) examination of the internal genitalia and (5) collection and evaluation of a semen sample or samples.

HISTORY

The establishment of proper identification should include name, registration number, breed, color and identifying marks and tattoo number. Some authorities also recommend that photographs of the stallion be taken from each side and from the front to be included in the record. This identification is obviously important in cases in which the stallion has or is about to be purchased or in cases in which the stallion will be reevaluated at a future date.

A complete history should be obtained, but previous reproductive history may not be easily available. Previous usage, such as show, performance or breeding, past illness and past or present treatment information should be included as well as any behavioral difficulties. Vaccination history and negative serologic evidence of equine infectious anemia are also noted.

Previous reproductive history may be lacking in stallions used for the first time and in some purchased stallions whose past performance may not have been ideal. In breeding stallions, prior conception rates, frequency of ejaculation, problems related to breeding ability and handling techniques should be noted. Management as it relates to breeding behavior or performance may also influence libido and conception rates.

GENERAL PHYSICAL EXAMINATION

When evaluating the general physical status of the stallion, close attention should be paid to his physical ability to cover a mare in estrus. First, the general body condition of the stallion is noted. A stallion in poor condition may indicate inadequate nutrition, improper management or chronic, debilitating disease. In that these conditions may detrimentally affect semen quality, correction of these problems is needed before evaluation of the stallion's breeding soundness. These conditions should be corrected at least 60 days in advance of further evaluation so that spermatogenesis and sperm transport may reflect the stallion's improved condition.

The conformation of the stallion is assessed, and any conformational defects are noted. Inherited defects that should be considered include cryptorchidism, umbilical hernia, undershot and overshot jaws, wobbler syndrome and others. Because of polygenic transmittance and lack of controlled studies, it is difficult not to pass a stallion on the basis of these possible inherited defects, except perhaps in the case of cryptorchidism.

Of prime importance in evaluating the stallion's physical condition is his ability to approach and to mount the mare successfully. Any condition that adversely affects his mounting ability should be noted. Most of these conditions involve the musculoskeletal system of the back and hindlimbs. Chronic conditions such as osteoarthritis of any of the hindlimb joints, spondylosis of the vertebrae, chronic laminitis and bursitis may hinder his ability to approach and mount the mare for natural service. More acute problems may elicit enough pain that he is temporarily uninterested in performing. Acute problems are alleviated by the use of anti-inflammatory medication and correction of the basic problem, while the chronic conditions are accommodated by the use of pain relievers or change in management to counter the situation effectively, such as the use of a short phantom for the collection of semen.

An ophthalmologic examination should be included as part of the physical examination. A blind stallion or one in which blindness is developing will have difficulty in finding, approaching and mounting the mare. The satisfactory potential breeder must be willing and able to deliver a normal ejaculate to the proper place at the proper time. The stallion should not be blind or severely lame or have faulty conformation or disease conditions that interfere with foreplay, mounting, intromission or thrusting. Any unsoundness should be noted, and its degree of severity should be considered when evaluated.

Psychological as well as physical problems may adversely affect the stallion. Close observation of the handling of a stallion may be necessary to differentiate between decreased libido associated with physical problems and that associated with improper handling or mistreatment.

EXTERNAL GENITALIA

The penis and prepuce of the stallion are most conveniently examined at the time of washing. Examination of the scrotum and its contents is most readily performed after ejaculation, as the horse is more tractable at that time.

Penis and Prepuce

Anatomy and Examination. The penis of the stallion is of the musculocavernous type and encloses the extrapelvic portion of the urethra. It consists of three parts: the root or bulb that is attached at the ischial arch by two crura, the body or shaft that is the main part and extends from the crura to the glans and the glans that is the enlarged free end of the penis. When not erect the penis is approximately 50 cm long and 2.5 to 6 cm in diameter, with the distal 15 to 20 cm free in the prepuce. When erect, the penis doubles in length and thickness and the corona glandis increases three to four times in size. The urethra extends distally from the surrounding fossa glandis as the urethral process. A dorsal extension of the fossa becomes the urethral sinus, a bilocular diverticulum lined by thin skin.

The prepuce or sheath is a double invagination of the skin that covers the distal portion of the penis when not erect. It consists of an external and an internal part. The external sheath extends from the scrotum forward to within 5 to 10 cm of the umbilicus, where it reflects dorsally and caudally, forming the preputial orifice. The dorsal portion is continuous with the integument of the abdominal wall. The internal portion passes caudally from the orifice for 15 to 20 cm and then reflects cranially until it approaches the orifice and is again reflected caudally. The second reflection creates the internal preputial ring and forms the prepuce proper of the penis.

Examination of the stallion's penis and prepuce is conducted concurrently at the time of washing. The stallion is allowed to approach an estral mare until he is stimulated to let down, at which time the penis extends from the prepuce. Some stallions may be reluctant to be examined and cow kick at the examiner or kick out backwards. Care must be taken to prevent injury to the examiner or to the stallion.

The penis and prepuce are examined by manual and visual inspection. The penile shaft is grasped just proximal to the glans, and a careful examination is made of the glans and associated structures. Particular attention is given to the urethral process, where vesicular, neoplastic or parasitic lesions may be noticed. The urethral diverticulum is examined for the presence of partially inspissated smegma or the "bean". The examination is continued up the shaft of the penis, where any injuries, scars or other lesions are noted. With the extension of the penis, both the internal and external portion of the prepuce can be examined. An accumulation of greasy smegma is normally found at the base of the penis involving the preputial area.

Disease and Abnormalities. The penis and prepuce are common sites of traumatic injuries that may cause physical as well as psychological damage to the stallion. This is particularly true if the stallion is kicked by the mare during attempts at intromission. Other forms of trauma include lacerations from breeding sutures in mares, improperly fitted or cared for stallion rings and physical injuries unassociated with intromission. Hematoma of the penis is often the result of trauma associated with breeding, either from kicks or improperly handled artificial vaginas. Hemorrhage comes from vessels outside the tunica albuginea, unlike the bull, in which there is a rupture of the tunica.

Regardless of the cause, the severely traumatized penis rapidly enlarges because of inflammatory edema and extends beyond the protective confines of the prepuce, where it may become subject to further trauma. The epithelial covering may become excoriated, with some oozing of serum onto the surface. Minor trauma or lacerations may only involve local irritation and not present much of a problem.

Therapy is directed at reduction of edema and the prevention of further excoriation. Edema may be reduced by hydrotherapy, massage, pressure wraps and the judicious use of diuretics. During treatment the penis should be suspended close to the abdominal wall to prevent further accumulation of edema. Once reduced in size, the penis may be returned to the prepuce and retained by a purse-string suture in the preputial orifice. Injuries to the superficial epithelium may be treated with protective emollients or antibiotic ointments. Lacerations may be allowed to heal via granulation, or if severe, they may be properly sutured. Sexual rest is of prime importance because erection may further aggravate some injuries. This sexual rest should be maintained until full recovery has been achieved.

Paralysis of the penis results in the flaccid penis

extending from the prepuce. Causes associated or implicated with paralysis include spinal trauma, injury or lesions of the sympathetic function of the sacral nerves, infectious diseases (such as rhinopneumonitis, rabies or dourine), direct trauma to the penis, starvation and use of some phenothiazine tranquilizers. The paralyzed penis will undergo edema development and excoriation. Treatment is the same as that previously described. These stallions, however, usually fail to retract the penis and either a penile amputation or retraction surgery are often necessary. Stallions with penile paralysis will often retain their libido and mount estral mares but fail to achieve erection. It has been reported that by altering the temperature and pressure of the artificial vagina these stallions can still be collected.

Lesions of the penis and prepuce may be the result of neoplasms, parasites or viral infection. By far the most common neoplastic lesion of the penis and prepuce is squamous cell carcinoma. These carcinomas occur mostly in adult horses, and 45 per cent of all equine squamous cell carcinomas occur on the penis or prepuce. They begin as small, keratinized plaques that are slow to invade and considered to be of low malignancy. Cryosurgery on early lesions and surgical excision of more involved lesions are recommended. Other neoplastic lesions found are melanomas in old gray-colored horses, sarcoids and hemangiomas.

The most common parasitic lesions of the penis and prepuce are caused by the larvae of *Habronema muscae*. These larval lesions, summer sores or cutaneous habronemiasis, occur around the preputial ring or on the urethral process. The larvae initiate a granulomatous reaction that contains characteristic small yellow caseous granules in the invaded tissue. Large lesions on the urethral process may cause dysuria, and on the prepuce may leave scars that interfere with movement of the penis. Organophosphates are used as larvicidal drugs. Lesions may spontaneously disappear during the winter, with complete healing, but most must be surgically removed. Corticosteroid therapy is beneficial in the regression of most lesions. Edematous enlargement of the prepuce and scrotum have been associated with early cases of dourine caused by the parasite *Trypanosoma equiperdum*.

Equine coital exanthema or genital horsepox is caused by equine herpesvirus III, which creates numerous small, vesicular lesions on the prepuce and along the shaft of the penis. These vesicles develop into purulent papules and, finally, encrusted lesions. When the scabs are removed, a purulent ulcer is revealed. The disease is usually self-limiting, and sexual rest for at least 3 weeks is recommended. Transmission occurs during coitus, and the lesions cause mild pain. Uncomplicated cases do not decrease fertility, but libido will be reduced during the stage associated with painful lesions. Treatment consists of cleaning the penis and prepuce, reducing any inflammation and prevention of secondary bacterial infection.

Scrotum

Anatomy and Examination. The scrotum is an outpouching of skin in the inguinal area that encloses the testes. It is globular in form with a distinct longitudinal raphe on the midline, where the two sacs are fused. The scrotum may appear to be asymmetrical if one testis is larger than the other. The scrotum and its contents may be examined along with the penis and prepuce at the time of washing or after ejaculation when the stallion is more tractable and the scrotum and contents are more relaxed. The equine scrotum is not as pendulous as that of the bull but is held closer to the abdominal wall. Its skin is soft and pliable with a greasy feeling as a result of the sebaceous and sweat glands. The testicles should be freely movable within the scrotal sac, as the scrotum is important in thermo-regulation.

Disease and Abnormalities. Scrotal disease is rare and usually of traumatic origin. It may be in the form of lacerations or hematoceles induced by blunt trauma. Secondary inflammation causes a rise in temperature and may interfere with thermoregulation. Blood or serum will collect between the tunics in hematocele formation and may cause adhesions to form that will not allow free testicular movement. Cold water hydrotherapy will help reduce inflammation and antibiotic ointments or therapy may be necessary for laceration and abrasion therapy.

Scrotal edema may be the result of systemic illness, such as equine infectious anemia or equine viral arteritis, application of irritating substances like insecticide sprays or secondary to scrotal trauma. Edema may also be the result of scrotal dermatitis, which is a rare occurrence in the stallion. The edema will often subside with hydrotherapy, exercise or diuretic treatment. If the edema persists, it may interfere with thermoregulation or may cause testicular atrophy. Neoplasms rarely affect the scrotum.

Testicles and Epididymides

Anatomy and Examination. The testes are ovoid structures, compressed slightly from side to side, measuring 8 to 12 cm long by 6 to 7 cm high by 5 cm wide. Their long axis is horizontal, but when retracted, it becomes almost vertical. The visceral vaginal tunic surrounds each testis and is tightly adhered to the testicular tunica albuginea. The testis is retained in the parietal vaginal tunic by the mesorchium and proper ligament of the testis, which attaches the testis to the tail of the epididymis. The testicular parenchyma consists of the seminiferous tubules, in which spermatogenesis takes place, and the interstitial tissues, of which the Leydig's cells that produce androgens are the major component.

The epididymides are divided into three parts: head, body and tail. The head of the epididymis is closely attached to the anterior, dorsal aspect of the testicle where it passes from medial to lateral around the attachment of the spermatic cord. The epididymis then continues posteriorly along the dorsolateral surface of the testicle as the narrow, cylindrical body of the epididymis. The epididymis terminates as the rather large (2 to 3 cm diameter) tail of the epididymis that is loosely attached to the caudal pole of the testicle. A remnant of the gubernaculum, the scrotal ligament, attaches the tail of the epididymis to the scrotum.

The testicles and epididymides are palpated through the scrotal wall to determine their presence, size, symmetry and consistency. The normal stallion has two scrotal testicles that lie with their longitudinal axis horizontal. The testes should be freely movable within the scrotal sac. Digital palpation should show them to be of the same consistency and should reveal no abnormalities of shape or texture. The right testis is normally slightly smaller than the left.

Testicular size is determined by the measurement of the scrotal width of both testicles. Scrotal width may be measured by calipers and should be determined at the point of greatest lateral width in a stallion with a nonerect penis. Scrotal width is positively correlated with daily sperm production and daily sperm output. Normal scrotal widths range from 9 to 13 cm. Stallions older than 7 years of age tend to have greater scrotal widths than younger stallions. Training, racing and certain medications, particularly androgens, adversely effect testicular size.

The epididymides are palpable throughout their length. The head of the epididymis may be difficult to palpate because of the attachment of the cremaster muscle and spermatic vessels. The body may be difficult to palpate in older stallions. The tail of the epididymis is prominently displayed and, along with the scrotal ligament, serves as a landmark for identifying testicular torsion. The scrotal ligament is palpable as a small (5 to 10 mm) firm nodule at the dorsal posterior aspect of the tail of the epididymis.

Diseases and Abnormalities. Orchitis may be of traumatic or infectious origin but is usually rare in the stallion. Blunt trauma from kicks or invasion by infectious organisms either through penetrating wounds or hematogenous spread will cause acute inflammation. The testicle will be hot, sensitive and very tense, owing to swelling that is confined by the tunics. Spermatozoa concentration will be decreased, and abundant leukocytes will be present in the semen. Orchitis may extend to cause epididymitis or may progress to abscess formation. Beta-hemolytic streptococcus is commonly found on culture, but other organisms have also been reported. Treatment consists of hydrotherapy, high levels of antibiotics and anti-inflammatory therapy. Unilateral castration should be considered when only one testis is involved, to decrease the possibility of testicular degeneration in the remaining testis because of the associated confined swelling. Adhesions

of the testes to the scrotum may be a sequela of orchitis, hematocele or migration of strongyle larvae.

Testicular hypoplasia and degenerative atrophy both result in small testicles, usually uniform in shape and texture. Hypoplastic testicles fail to undergo normal development, and degenerative atrophy occurs in normally developed testicles that subsequently atrophy. The two conditions are difficult to differentiate and are usually differentiated on the basis of historical evidence. Both result in decreased sperm production. Chromosomal abnormalities have been detected in some cases of testicular hypoplasia. Testicular atrophy is the final step of many processes, and it is seldom easy to determine the precise cause.

Cryptorchidism is common in stallions. The genetic control is not fully known. The left testicle is most commonly retained. Congenital cryptorchid stallions are unsatisfactory breeders and should be castrated.

Neoplasia of the testes is rare. Any irregularity in form and texture of the testes should be considered abnormal. Seminomas, teratomas, and lipomas have been reported. Teratomas usually occur only in the retained testicle of the cryptorchid stallion.

Testicular torsion occurs as two different syndromes in the stallion. True torsion is rare but when it occurs causes a very acute, painful condition, and the stallion exhibits signs of severe colic. Examination shows that the testis has rotated at least 360° within the scrotum, causing occlusion of the spermatic vessels. Removal of the affected testicle is the treatment of choice. This condition should be differentiated from scrotal hernia, with the strangulated entrapment of intestines in the scrotum. The more common syndrome is the partial torsion of the testis. The testis lies in 180° rotation within the scrotum, with the tail of the epididymis identified on the anterior aspect of the testis. This condition seems to be a developmental defect in the descent of the testes and does not affect fertility.

Epididymal disease is rare in the stallion. No causative agent is associated with equine epididymitis, which is most often an extension of orchitis when it occurs. Occasional reports of sperm granulomas from blocked epididymal tubules have been recorded. Sperm stasis has been more frequently reported in stallions of low fertility. This condition is related to a defect in sperm transport through the epididymis and results in dead, nonmotile sperm, many of which have separated heads. Frequent ejaculation is necessary to maintain normal motile spermatozoa in the ejaculate.

Spermatic Cords

The spermatic cord extends from the abdominal inguinal ring to its attachment on the testis. It contains the convoluted testicular artery, network of small veins known as the pampiniform plexus, the ductus deferens and nerves. The external cremaster muscle is an integral part of the cord, running as an extension of the abdominal muscles to attach to the parietal vaginal tunic near the head of the epididymis. It acts to temporarily raise the testicle.

The cords should be palpated along their entire length. They should be of equal length and uniform diameter. The ductus deferens is surrounded by the cremaster muscle and cannot be delineated. Occasionally, varicoceles occur in the spermatic veins, some larger ones being a cause of scrotal edema.

INTERNAL GENITALIA

The ductus deferens is the continuation of the epididymis and runs from the tail of the epididymis, through the inguinal canal, to the area of the neck of the bladder. The duct is approximately 6 mm in diameter until it enlarges at the level of the bladder into the fusiform ampulla, which is 10 to 20 mm in diameter and 15 to 20 cm long, terminating at the colliculus seminalis of the pelvic urethra. With its crypts and main duct, the ampulla acts as a sperm storage organ.

The paired vesicular glands lie lateral and caudal to the ampullae and dorsal to the neck of the bladder. Both the ampullae and the anterior portion of the vesicular glands lie in the thin fascial sheet of the genital fold. The vesicular glands are 5 cm in diameter and 15 to 20 cm long in the stallion. These glands produce the gel fraction of the ejaculate. Each gland has a singular duct that joins with the ipsilateral ampullar duct to form a short ejaculatory duct in the colliculus seminalis.

The equine prostate gland is a single nodular gland consisting of two small lobes connected by a thin transverse isthmus over the dorsal aspect of the urethralis muscle, just caudal to the vesicular glands. The prostate empties its secretion into the pelvic urethra by a series of 15 to 20 small ducts from each lobe.

The paired bulbourethral glands lie on either side of the pelvic urethra at the ischial arch. They are covered by a dense fibrous capsule and the bulbospongiosus and bulboglandularis muscles. A series of 5 to 10 ducts lead from each gland and empty into the pelvic urethra just distal to the openings from the ducts of the prostate gland.

The vesicular glands, prostate gland, and bulbourethral glands are collectively known as the accessory sex glands. They all provide a portion of the seminal fluid but are not necessary for fertility.

These glands are normally examined by palpation per rectum. The prostate is located about wrist deep anterior to the anal sphincter on the floor of the pelvis. Craniolateral to the prostate are the vesicular glands. The vesicular glands are difficult to palpate, being essentially collapsed, empty saclike structures. After vigorous teasing, the vesicles enlarge, swollen by accumulation of the gel fraction, and are thus easier to palpate. The ampullae lie medial and anterior to the vesicular glands. Normally, the bulbourethral glands cannot be palpated.

The time for rectal examination is at the discretion of the examiner. The vesicular glands are more readily palpable after teasing. Most stallions are more tractable subsequent to ejaculation, but at this time palpation of the vesicular glands is more difficult. Pathology or disease processes of the equine accessory glands are quite rare, although vesiculitis has been reported. Acute vesiculitis would be accompanied by increased numbers of leukocytes in the ejaculate and pain on palpation.

The internal inguinal rings are located about 10 cm cranioventral to the pelvic brim and just lateral to midline. They are slitlike openings some 5 cm in length. The rings are evaluated rectally by sliding the fingers down the internal abdominal wall from the pelvic brim. They may be identified and evaluated by the insertion of one or two fingers and by the palpation of the ductus deferens and the pulsation of the spermatic artery. Adhesions and inguinal hernias are checked for, with enlarged rings suggesting a susceptibility to herniation.

The urethra is a long tube originating at the bladder and terminating at the distal tip of the urethral process. The pelvic portion is surrounded by the urethralis muscle that contracts vigorously during ejaculation. The colliculus seminalis is a prominence medially on the dorsum of the pelvic urethra about 5 cm distal from the bladder. The ejaculatory ducts open on either side of the colliculus, with the prostatic duct orifices arranged in two groups of openings lateral to the ejaculatory openings. Another 2.5 cm distally the ducts of the bulbourethral glands open in two small series close to the dorsal midline.

Fiberscopic examination of the penile and pelvic urethra is a very useful technique to further evaluate the penis and accessory sex glands. It is performed in the presence of an estral mare with the stallion lightly tranquilized. The penis is washed, and the sterilized scope is passed up the urethra aseptically by an assistant. The urethra may be evaluated for ulcers and erosions in cases of hemiospermia and an evaluation of the accessory gland openings may also be made.

GENITAL INFECTION

Diagnosis of genital infection in the stallion is contingent upon repeated isolations of a pathogen together with reduced semen quality. Healthy stallions harbor many kinds of nonpathogenic and potentially pathogenic microorganisms on their external genitalia. These organisms include environmental contaminants, hemolytic and nonhemolytic *Streptococcus* spp., *Staphylococcus* spp., *Escherichia coli*, *Klebsiella* spp., *Pseudomonas* spp. and contagious equine metritis organism (*Haemophilus equigenitalis* or the newly proposed name, *Taylorella equigenitalis*).

The distal portion of the penis and urethra harbor many types of bacteria, but the interpretation of their significance must be done with great care. Cultures of urethral swabs taken before ejaculation should have a great many mixed microbes, whereas swabs taken after ejaculation should have reduced numbers and types because of the flushing effect of ejaculation. If these cultures show no decrease, or even an increase, in numbers or if a pure culture of a potential pathogen is obtained, an attempt may be made to locate the source of bacteria.

External surface infections cause no observable irritation to the penis, and there is no build up of an inflammatory exudate. Separate swabs should be taken from the fossa glandis, penile surface, prepuce and distal urethra. Isolates found on repeat cultures are more significant than those found on only one attempt. *Pseudomonas* organisms that colonize the penile surface will fluoresce a bright blue green when examined by an ultraviolet lamp.

The internal genitalia of the normal stallion are free of bacteria and have no normal flora. Culture of semen collected by an artificial vagina will reflect organisms on the penis and not represent infection from the accessory glands. Semen collection with an open-ended artificial vagina is more reliable in reflecting bacteria from the urethra or internal genitalia. By a process of elimination, secretions may be collected separately from each of the accessory glands in order to evaluate the possible source of infection. Infections of the vesicular glands, prostate, bulbourethral glands and ampulla are extremely rare in the stallion.

Fluid from the bulbourethral glands can be collected by briskly massaging the glans of the erect penis. Upon release of the glans the stallion will emit preejaculatory fluid originating from the bulbourethral glands. The presence of large numbers of bacteria or inflammatory cells would indicate an infection of urethral origin or one of the bulbourethral glands.

After vigorous teasing, the vesicular glands will expand with a gel-like fluid and be easily palpable. A balloon-tipped catheter can be passed up the urethra to the level of the colliculus seminalis, and vesicular fluid can be collected by expression of the gland by rectal massage. The fluid from each vesicle may be collected separately by selective massage and by the use of separate sterile catheters.

The fluid from the glands of the ampulla and ductus are included in the first sperm-rich fraction of the ejaculate. An open-ended artificial vagina is used to collect this fraction. Infections higher in the tract, such as in epididymitis or orchitis, usually cause changes palpable through the scrotal wall.

Antibiotic treatment of the genital organs of an infected stallion is difficult at best. Systemic treatment with gentamycin with a regimen of 4.4 mg/kg twice a day for 34 days has been reported to be effective in treating infections caused by *Pseudomonas* and *Klebsiella* organisms. Systemic antibiotics may not penetrate the accessory glands sufficiently well to combat infection. Treatment of infections of the penile and preputial surface includes local cleansing with an antibacterial soap followed by the application of an antibiotic ointment. This may, however, lead to the reduction in the numbers of normal bacteria and the proliferation of more resistant species. Also, removal of natural smegma and oils by local treatment may cause some physical trauma to the penis such as soreness, cracking of the penile integument and hemorrhage.

Most stallions only harbor microorganisms on their genital organs or act as mechanical transmittors from one mare to the next. No stallion should be condemned on the basis of positive cultures. The one exception would be the removal from service of a stallion shown to be harboring the contagious equine metritis organism *Taylorella equigenitalis*. Those stallions found shedding other organisms may be utilized for breeding by the use of antibiotic-treated semen extenders.

Suggested Readings

1. Amann RP: A review of anatomy and physiology of the stallion. Equine Vet Sci 1:83, 1981.
2. Braun WF: The infected stallion. Equine Vet Data 3:54, 1982.
3. Pickett BW, Voss JL, Squires EL: Fertility evaluation of the stallion. Comp Cont Ed 5:S194, 1983.
4. Kenney RM, Hurtgen J, Pierson R, Witherspoon D, Simons J (eds): Society for Theriogenology Manual for Clinical Fertility Evaluation of the Stallion. Society for Theriogenology, 1983.
5. Thompson, DL, Pickett, DW, Squires EL, Amann RP: Testicular measurements and reproductive characteristics in stallions. J Reprod Fert Suppl 27:13, 1979.

Artificial Insemination and Semen Handling

Ted F. Lock, D.V.M., M.S.
University of Illinois, Urbana, Illinois

Artificial insemination is a management tool that can be very advantageous in an equine breeding program. Among its advantages are (1) more efficient use of stallions, (2) decreased risk of injury to horses and people, (3) opportunity to evaluate semen quality at each collection and (4) reduced risk of spreading infections by coitus. In order to achieve maximum fertility, excellent management is important in semen collection and handling as well as in estrus detection and timing of breeding.

SEMEN COLLECTION

Semen can be collected from stallions by using a jump mare exhibiting estrus or a phantom mare. Most stallions can be trained to mount a phantom mare, which makes the process safer and more consistent. The phantom should be designed so it is comfortable for the stallion to mount. It can be made with a variable height if more than one stallion will be using it.

If an estrous mare is used, her tail should be wrapped, and the perineal area should be cleaned well. Adequate restraint of the mare is important to prevent injury to the stallion or personnel involved. Restraint methods vary from a twitch to a breeding harness or breeding chute. The operator should determine the restraint methods required in each situation.

The ideal method for collection of stallion semen is an artificial vagina (AV). There are several models available, e.g., Colorado model, Missouri model and Japanese model (see the Appendix). Selection of the artificial vagina may depend on the stallion, as some stallions tend to prefer one model over another.

The artificial vagina is prepared by filling it with water to obtain the proper pressure and temperature. Due to the variations in penis size, the amount of water required to obtain proper pressure varies; however, a stallion should be able to penetrate an adequately lubricated artificial vagina without excessive resistance. The recommended internal temperature of the artificial vagina is between 45 and 48°C. Higher temperatures should be avoided in order to prevent irritation to the stallion's penis and damage to sperm.

The inside of the artificial vagina is lubricated with sterile nonspermicidal lubricant just before use. Products that contain disinfectants or other spermicidal substances should be avoided.

The collection bottle is warmed to body temperature and attached to the AV just before collection. Care should be taken to protect this receptacle from excessive temperature changes in order to prevent damage to sperm cells.

Polyester filters, which are designed to remove the gel portion from the semen, are also reported to retain sperm cells, thus reducing the number available for insemination. Removal of the gel by careful aspiration with a syringe or use of a nylon filter may help to reduce this loss.

PREPARATION OF THE STALLION

The stallion is exposed to an estrous mare until an erection is attained. The penis is washed with cotton or paper towels using warm water alone or with a mild, nonirritating soap. If soap is used, adequate rinsing is important to remove any soap residue, which may be detrimental to sperm.

The collection area should be large enough for the procedure to be carried out safely, and the floor should be designed to provide good footing for horses and handlers.

The stallion is allowed to mount the phantom or properly restrained mare only after he has a full erection. The stallion handler and collector should work from the left side. The stallion's penis is directed to the left side of the mare's buttocks and into the artificial vagina. Once this has occurred and once the pelvic thrusting begins, the ventral base of the penis can be palpated to detect the urethral pulsations that occur at ejaculation. During ejaculation the end of the AV should be lowered to allow semen to enter the collection bottle and to prevent loss from the open end. To ensure collection of the complete ejaculate, the AV should be kept in place until the stallion dismounts. The water is immediately drained from the AV to allow any remaining semen to flow into the collection bottle. When the stallion dismounts, the penis is rinsed again with warm water to remove any remaining lubricant. If a filter is used, it is removed to prevent the gel fraction from entering the semen. With unfiltered semen, the gel is aspirated from the semen at this time. Care should be taken to maintain the temperature of the receptacle and semen. The semen is then evaluated.

SEMEN EVALUATION

All supplies used in the semen evaluation should be maintained at approximately 37°C and should be free of any agent that may affect semen quality. Each ejaculate should be evaluated to assure that an adequate number of normal, progressively motile spermatozoa are used for insemination. The following evaluations are used to determine total sperm output and to calculate the insemination dose: volume, concentration, motility and morphology.

Volume. Total volume of gel-free semen should be recorded.

Concentration. Concentration can be determined by use of a hemacytometer or a spectrophotometer that has been properly calibrated.

Motility. Motility should be determined soon after collection. This is done by placing a drop of semen on a warm slide, covering it with a warm cover slip and estimating the per cent of progressively motile spermatozoa under a microscope. Highly concentrated samples may have to be diluted with warm saline or extender to obtain an accurate evaluation.

Morphology. Sperm morphology can be determined by microscopic evaluation of stained smears or, preferably, by phase-contrast microscopy of semen fixed in buffered formal saline. This eliminates artifacts seen in stained smears.

Total sperm output is calculated by multiplying volume and concentration. Total number of progressively motile sperm can be calculated by multiplying the product of volume and concentration by the percentage of progressive motility.

SEMEN EXTENDER

Several semen extenders have been evaluated for use in horses. The addition of extenders to stallion semen has not been shown to improve fertility in controlled studies. However, because stallion semen is contaminated with bacteria, the use of an antibiotic-treated extender is recommended. The following extender has been widely used for several years with good results:

Powdered milk (Sanalac)	2.4 gm
Glucose	4.9 gm
Sodium bicarbonate (7.5%)	2 ml
Gentamycin sulfate	100 mg
Distilled or deionized water	qs to 100 ml

After preparation, the extender is maintained at approximately 37°C, and the semen is added using a semen-to-extender ratio of 1:1 to 1:3.

INSEMINATION

Mares should be inseminated with a minimum of 100 million progressively motile, morphologically normal spermatozoa. Recommendations range up to 500 million normal motile sperm. Optimum fertility of individual stallions should be achieved by using insemination doses in this range. Insemination of mares is accomplished by depositing the semen into the body of the uterus using a clean plastic insemination pipette. Use of disposable equipment is recommended to prevent contamination during the insemination process. Sperm cells can be expected to remain viable in the mare's reproductive tract for at least 48 hours. Mares should be inseminated beginning on day 2 or 3 of estrus and every other day until ovulation occurs.

Most breed registration authorities require use of freshly collected semen for artificial insemination. Transport of equine semen is, therefore, limited. However, there is a trend toward acceptance of the use of transported semen by a few breed associations, provided requirements such as blood typing are met. Equipment for transporting fresh equine semen is commercially available (see the Appendix). Although its use has been limited, good fertility rates have been attained using fresh transported semen.

The use of frozen equine semen is also limited because of breed association restrictions. Although fertility with frozen semen is reportedly lower than with fresh semen, good conception rates have been reported.

Suggested Readings

1. Cooper WL: Artificial breeding of horses. Vet Clin North Am: Large Anim Pract 2:267, 1980.
2. Nishikawa Y: Studies on the preservation of raw and frozen horse semen. J Reprod Fertil Suppl 23:99, 1975.
3. Pickett BW: Use of artificial insemination in stallion management. In Morrow DA (ed): Current Therapy in Theriogenology 1st ed. Philadelphia, WB Saunders Co, 1980, pp 688–693.
4. Pickett BW, Gebauer MR, Seidel GE Jr, Voss JL: Reproductive physiology of the stallion: Spermatozoal losses in the collection equipment and gel. JAVMA 165:708, 1974.
5. Rossdale PD, Ricketts SW: The stallion. In Equine Stud Farm Medicine: 2nd ed. London, Bailliere Tindall, 1980, pp 158–161.

Breeding Soundness Examination of the Mare and Common Genital Abnormalities Encountered

Steven D. Van Camp, D.V.M.
North Carolina State University, Raleigh, North Carolina

A breeding soundness evaluation (BSE) should be conducted prior to purchasing a mare for breeding purposes or prior to each breeding season. However, frequently the veterinarian is not asked to examine a mare until after the purchase or when a problem is suspected. The complete BSE includes more than just evaluation of the reproductive tract. It includes evaluation of the entire animal and its previous history.

HISTORY

In order to evaluate a mare properly for breeding soundness it is important to know her general medical, environmental and utilitarian history plus a detailed reproductive history. A general history should include age, serologic tests, purchase date, vaccination history, animal contacts, boarding facilities, feed, previous use, intended use, medical problems, surgical problems, weight loss or gain and disease problems present on the farm.

The reproductive history should not only include foaling, heat and breeding dates but also age at first heat, age first bred, number of pregnancies, date of last foaling, abnormal foalings, interval between heats, length of heats, abnormal pregnancies, previous years breeding cycle pattern, number of breedings required at previous breeding for conception, foaling problems, evidence of discharges and problems with the foal. The methods used to tease and to breed the mare (pasture, natural hand breeding or artificial insemination) are also important. A brief history of the stallions used should also include the following: the number of mares bred, the number that conceived and foaled and historical evidence of infection in mares covered by the stallion. If possible, a breeding record from the previous season should be examined.

An in-depth history often reveals a breeding management problem that may have resulted in the mare's apparent infertility. This is often the situation when dealing with novice breeders. Indication of a breeding management problem will often be substantiated by normal reproductive physical examination and tests.

PHYSICAL EXAMINATION

General Physical

This is an essential, yet often overlooked, aspect of a breeding soundness examination. Hoof and leg infirmities such as a rotated third phalanx following acute laminitis may make a mare reluctant to stand for breeding or may make her unfit to carry a pregnancy to term. Pelvic injuries or abnormalities may predispose a mare to dystocia. Small stature, in some cases, has been related to certain chromosomal abnormalities. Hirsutism associated with a pituitary tumor may be the cause of a mare's unseasonal anestrus. Hypertrophic pulmonary osteopathy has been associated with certain types of ovarian tumors in mares. Thus, seemingly unrelated physical signs may have a direct bearing on a mare's soundness for breeding.

Reproductive Examination

Since most mares are seasonally polyestrous and demonstrate erratic cycles during the transition from anestrous to the breeding season and vice versa, the reproductive tract condition and structures identified on the ovaries must be evaluated in relation to the stage of the breeding season.

Seasonal Changes. During anestrus, the uterus is flaccid, thin walled and quiescent. The ovaries are small and firm (2 to 4 cm long and 2 to 3 cm wide). The vagina is pale and dry. The cervix (cx) is usually in the upper one third of the vaginal vault, pale and dry and tight (Cx 1 = high, dry, tight). Passage of a finger through the Cx 1 is difficult, and some time should be spent allowing it to soften and to dilate. In some cases the cervix may be very flaccid and even stand open during the anestrus period.

During the transition from anestrus to the normal breeding season or from the normal breeding season to anestrus the reproductive tract reflects the condition of the ovaries and the predominant hormones being produced by them. However, during the transitional periods an additional complication must be considered when evaluating the reproductive tract because in some cases the condition of the tract does not agree with the ovarian findings nor with the mare's behavior. This early season asynchrony between the ovaries and the uterus or cervix is thought to be caused by the ovaries' activity prior to the uterus' ability to respond to the hormones being produced. This may be a result of lack of hormone receptor induction within the uterus. Late in the year it may be due to reduced activity of the pituitary and diminished production of gonadotrophins or to a lack of responsiveness of the ovaries to the pituitary hormones.

Unfortunately, the early transitional period occurs in early spring, which is when breeders try to have the majority of the mares impregnated. This is done to take advantage of breed organization rules, which have indirectly defined this unseasonal breeding season. Artificial lighting may be used to obtain early pregnancies by stimulating cyclic ovarian activity during the winter anestrus and thus producing transitional periods and regular seasonal estrous cycles earlier in the year. Furthermore, boarding a cyclic mare in a dark, poorly lighted stall may precipitate early return to transitional period cycles. Owners of show animals who keep their mares under lights to maintain them in a "shed-out," sleek-hair coat condition must realize that this treatment will also alter the mare's reproductive cycles and may precipitate persistent irregular cycles at the same time that shows are planned. During these transitional periods mares may experience prolonged estrus, estrus without ovulation, ovulation without estrus, split estrus, persistent follicles, and asynchrony of ovaries and reproductive tract. During the physiological breeding season, the condition of the reproductive tract varies with the stage of the estrous cycle and the endocrine activity of the ovary.

Cyclic Changes. In general, estrogens from the follicles cause the uterus to become more edematous, congested and heavier. The cervix changes from a Cx 1 (high, dry and tight) to a Cx 2 (dropping), in which case the cervix is pinkish, softer, moister and lower in the vaginal vault. Also, the cervix develops folds of tissue extending from the external os toward the vaginal floor. It will readily admit one to two fingers. As the estrogen levels continue to rise, the cervix changes to a Cx 3 (hanging).

In this case the Cx 3 is very soft and pink. It is usually located in the lower third of the anterior vaginal wall, is very edematous, and glistens with moisture. The edematous folds of the external os actually touch the floor of the vagina, yet the cervix is still recognizable. Two to three fingers may easily be introduced through the Cx 3.

Near the time of ovulation, when estrogen levels have peaked, the cervix is at its softest and is designated a Cx 4 (laying). It is salmon pink in color, very moist and edematous and often appears as a mass of edematous folds on the floor of the vagina. Occasionally, a small pool of clear, serous mucus may be seen just caudal to the external os of the cervix. At this time, with stimulation, the cervix may dilate completely and readily allow the passage of the entire hand into the uterus.

An additional normal cervical condition that may be encountered is that of a "capped" cervix. This type of cervical appearance is similar to a Cx 1 (high, dry, tight and pale), but in this case the external os is not visible because of a cervical plug and the appearance that one of the cervical folds has covered and sealed off the end of the cervix. The "capped" cervix is often indicative of pregnancy. The reader is referred to Dr. Lieux's photographs in *Equine Medicine and Surgery* for examples of the changes that a cervix undergoes throughout the cycle.

The uterus of the normal cyclic mare after ovulation and during diestrus becomes less edematous, less congested and more tonic. It is easily identifiable as a firm tubular structure. The early pregnant uterus is also tonic and can be differentiated from the diestrus uterus by an amniotic vesicle bulge after about 20 to 25 days of pregnancy. The reader is referred to other sections of this text for a discussion of the palpable signs of pregnancy in the mare's reproductive tract.

EXAMINATION OF THE GENITALIA

After a general physical exam has been conducted, a detailed evaluation of the reproductive organs should be undertaken with the tail wrapped in gauze and tied out of the way. The mammary glands should be examined and palpated for evidence of mastitis, abscessation, neoplasia or injury. The *vulva* should be examined for conformation, apposition, tone and evidence of discharges. Malapposition of the vulvar lips or poor vulvar conformation (dorsal-cranial sloping with the anus several inches cranial to the vulva) may be signs of predisposition to pneumovagina and fecal contamination of the vaginal vault. Gentle separation of the vulvar lips and listening for aspiration of air can be used to diagnose pneumovagina in some cases. When examining a vulva that has a normal anal-vulvar relationship, the floor of the pelvis should be identified. Mares that have less than 70 per cent of the vulvar opening below the pelvic floor are also predisposed to pneumovagina in later life. The examination of the vulvar area continues with the examination of the clitoral fossa and clitoris. The cranial surface of the clitoris has three small sinuses located in it. These sinuses have been shown to harbor the contagious equine metritis (CEM) organism *Hemophilus equigenitalis.* If this disease is a concern, the sinuses should be expressed and cultured with the aid of a mini-swab and transported to the laboratory in Amie's plus charcoal medium. The examination then continues with either rectal or vaginal palpation.

Rectal Examination

Continuing with the *rectal examination* allows for the possibility of pregnancy to be ruled out. Before conducting a rectal exam it is advisable to "calibrate one's hand"; that is, identify certain measures such as joints, knuckles, or a thumb nail that can be used as size and diameter references when evaluating the tract. If the mare is pregnant, the procedures that follow will be altered. The mare's rectum is much more friable than a cow's, and therefore the examiner must take special precautions when conducting a rectal exam. The examiner's well-lubricated, gloved arm and hand should be introduced one finger at a time through the anal sphincter into the rectum. With the fingers held together, the cupped hand should clean out the feces as far cranial as possible prior to searching for the reproductive tract.

Some palpators locate one ovary first by reaching up into the sublumbar area ventral to the fourth or fifth lumbar vertebrae. However, if one identifies the uterus first and pregnancy is detected, there is no real need to examine the ovaries, which often have several large follicles in addition to corpora lutea on them. Therefore, it may be advisable to locate the uterus first.

The nonpregnant mare's *uterus* is T-shaped, with two short horns that extend upward toward the kidney-bean–shaped ovaries that must be differentiated from fecal balls in the small colon. The uterus can be located by inserting the arm approximately 45 to 50 cm into the rectum at a 20 to 30° downward slope in order to get under the fold of the mesorectum, which may interfere with grasping and identification of structures. Then, the closely opposed fingers are flexed slightly, and the arm is withdrawn approximately 10 cm. Usually, a band of tissue can be felt running through the palm of the hand from left to right. This is either the body of the uterus or the small colon with fecal balls in it. If it is the small colon, allow this band to slide out of the hand and withdraw the arm a little further and identify the next caudal band. This should be the uterus. If it is the uterus, it will curve upward toward the ovaries. The anterior ventral aspects of the uterus should be examined for evidence of a bulging or thinning, which may be an early pregnancy. If the mare is not pregnant, the uterus can be palpated more thoroughly, including slipping the folds of the endometrium through the uterine wall. Following examination of the uterine body, the horns should be followed to the left and right as they curve up to the ovaries.

The *ovaries* are suspended in the abdomen by a part of the broad ligament called the mesovarium, which attaches in the sublumbar region. They can usually be located just anterior to the ilium adjacent to the lateral abdominal wall and may have to be teased out from behind the mesovarium. The size of the ovaries varies with the season and the structures on them. Anestrus ovaries are small and firm, about 2 to 4 cm long and 2 to 3 cm wide and 3 cm thick. During the breeding season these dimensions may double, but in any case the normal ovary should fit into the palm of the hand. The ovary is cupped in the palm of the hand and examined with the tips of the thumb and fingers. Normally developing follicles in the mare ovary range between 2 and 6 cm and should not be confused with cystic structures. The mare ovulates through the ovulation fossa, which is the indentation in the ovary. The

corpus luteum forms within the structure of the ovary and does not protrude from the surface of the ovary. Corpora lutea are very difficult to palpate except by experienced examiners who have followed the development and ovulation of the follicles. The ovulation fossa is located ventrally and faces medially as the ovary hangs in the abdomen. This relationship helps identify cranial and caudal poles of the ovary for location of follicles on it. The uterine tube of the mare is short and not easily identified unless abnormal. The fimbria of the uterine tubes are closely apposed to the ovulation fossa. Occasionally, small cystic structures can be identified in the fimbria. After completing the examination of the ovaries and the uterus, the rectal examination is completed by evaluation of the bony pelvis for abnormalities that might interfere with breeding or parturition.

The *cervix* can be located by sweeping the hand across the floor of the pelvis and by identifying a cylindrical structure about 5 to 8 cm long and 2.5 to 5 cm wide. The nature of the cervix changes with the stage of the cycle. The firm Cx 1 is more easily identified than the soft Cx 4.

Vaginoscopic Examination

Preparation for a *vaginoscopic examination* involves a thorough cleansing of the vulva and perineum. After the tail has been wrapped and tied out of the way, a mild surgical scrub solution is used to disinfect the area. Caution must be used to prevent forcing fluid through the vulvar cleft into the vagina. The solution must be rinsed off completely to prevent irritation. After drying the area, the vulvar lips are separated and a sterile vaginal speculum, either tubular or the three-pronged Caslick speculum, is introduced into the vestibular area. The initial angle of introduction is dorso-cranial in order to pass above the ischium of the pelvis. Some resistance will be met as the transverse fold of the vestibulo-vaginal ring is met. This ring, which is a remnant of the hymen, will expand with moderate constant pressure and allow the speculum to pass into the cranial vagina.

Once fully introduced, and with the aid of a light, the speculum should be used to examine the cervical os for color and tone as soon as possible, since changes occur as cool air enters through the speculum. The vaginal wall should be examined for color, evidence of congestion or inflammation, tumors, lacerations and scars. The vaginal floor should be examined for evidence of exudate or fluid accumulation or injury. The dorsum of the vagina should be evaluated for evidence of injury or fistulation into the rectum. After the vagina is evaluated, the speculum should be slowly withdrawn and the vestibular area evaluated.

Some veterinarians prefer to obtain endometrial *cultures* through the vaginal speculum using a guarded uterine swab. Others prefer to introduce the swab manually using a sterile sleeve and sterile, nonbacteriostatic lubricant. In either case, the most valuable culture will be obtained if it is taken from the uterus while the mare is in heat. At other stages of the cycle one is more likely to culture a confusing array of nonpathogenic contaminants. The cultures should be submitted for identification of the organism and antibiotic sensitivity testing to allow for a rational choice of therapeutic agents, if treatment is necessary. The use of the manual technique allows for evaluation of the uterus by the bimanual technique after the swab is removed.

Bimanual Technique

The *bimanual technique* is practiced by some as an additional evaluation of the uterus. One gloved hand is introduced through the cervix into the uterus, while the other arm is introduced into the rectum. The walls and lumen of the uterus are examined between the hands. This technique can only be used when the mare is in estrus. After the uterine culture and/or bimanual palpation, endometrial biopsy is usually necessary in order to evaluate a mare's breeding soundness.

Endometrial Biopsy

The *endometrial biopsy* can reveal problems with the uterus that may not be revealed by palpation or culture of the uterus or examination of the vagina. Furthermore, it can be used in conjunction with the culture to decide when therapy is indicated. The biopsy can be taken at any stage of the cycle; however, penetration of the cervix is easiest during estrus. This is also the period when the uterus is most resistant to any infectious agents that might be introduced during the procedure. Furthermore, the effect of the biopsy procedure on altering the estrous cycle is minimal at this time. Evaluating the tissue sample for fibrosis and glandular nests is facilitated by taking the biopsy while the mare is in estrus, but some pathologists would rather evaluate a sample taken during diestrus because it gives a better indication of the glands, which are significant in maintaining pregnancy.

The preparation for biopsy is similar to that for vaginoscopy. The recommended biopsy punch is greater than 50 cm (20 inches) long and has alligator-type jaws with a basket that measures 20 mm long and 4 mm wide and 4 mm deep. The sterile biopsy punch is introduced into the uterus manually with the aid of a sterile-sleeved hand and arm. Once within the uterus, the jaws of the punch are opened, the arm is withdrawn and reintroduced into the rectum. The opened jaws are identified through the rectal and uterine walls. The uterine wall is pressed into the sides of the punch with the flat of the finger, the jaws are closed and the punch and arm are then withdrawn. The biopsy specimen should be fixed in 10 per cent formaldehyde (Formalin) or Bouin's solution. The mare usually shows very little discomfort from this procedure except when the punch is pressed under the arm against the pelvis while being introduced or when the cervix is dilated,

if necessary, for introducing the punch. Bleeding from the site should be minimal but occasionally a slight bloody discharge may be noted in the vagina or on the vulva the next day. The sites to be biopsied include any areas where abnormalities were previously noted/and or the junction of the body and horn of the uterus. Unless abnormalities are noted it is usually considered sufficient for evaluation to take one biopsy at the body-horn junction. The reader is referred to other sections of this text for an in-depth discussion of endometrial biopsies.

Some authors propose the use of *endometrial cytology* instead of biopsy to evaluate the endometrium of the mare. This procedure has not received as widespread acceptance as biopsy for evaluation of the endometrium and for prediction of or prognosis for fertility. The endometrium is swabbed with a sterile swab similar to the culturing technique, and the swab is then rolled on a slide that is fixed and stained. The cells on the slide are evaluated for white blood cells, neoplastic cells and bacteria. Evidence of neutrophils on the slide indicates inflammation of the uterus. Polymorphonuclear cells indicate acute inflammation, whereas mononuclear cells indicate a more chronic inflammation.

In some cases it is advisable to conduct a *fiberoptic examination* of the mare's uterus. This technique is especially valuable for evaluating abnormalities noted on rectal or bimanual examination. The mare is prepared as for endometrial biopsy, and the fiberoptiscope is passed into the uterus with the aid of a sterile sleeved arm. The uterine lumen is inflated to allow inspection. This technique may identify intraluminal adhesions, discharges, inflammation and tumors; however, these can often also be identified by the previous procedures.

Ultrasonography

Ultrasonographic equipment for use in the rectum of the mare is available. This equipment produces images from high frequency sound waves that have been reflected from different tissue layers. The probe is introduced with the hand into the rectum and held over the structure to be examined. With this equipment it is possible to identify the amniotic vesicle as early as day 15 of gestation. This instrument is valuable in predicting the presence of twins early enough in gestation to correct the problem without danger to the mare. In addition to pregnancy diagnosis, ultrasound is helpful in producing an image of various vaginal, uterine and ovarian masses to determine if they are solid or fluid filled.

These are the main procedures involved in the breeding soundness examination of the mare. There are, however, several ancillary laboratory tests that may be valuable in specific instances for arriving at a diagnosis of a mare's reproductive problem or status.

Hormonal Analysis

Hormone analysis for progesterone, estrogen and/or testosterone may be of value in differentiating the several causes of enlarged ovaries. Detection of pregnancy with pregnant mare serum gonadotropin (PMSG) requires a blood test. It is known to produce false-positive results if the mare loses the fetus after the endometrial cups are stimulated to produce PMSG. Therefore, this test can be used to differentiate a conception failure from early embryonic death after about 35 days of pregnancy. *Chromosomal analysis* may be of value in ruling out specific cases of persistent anestrus in mares.

Obviously, not all of these procedures will be applied in each case. The type and number of procedures will depend on the reason for the examination, the stage of the cycle, the status of the reproductive tract and the identification of specific abnormalities encountered. These abnormalities can be categorized according to the reproductive organ involved and whether it is smaller than normal, is enlarged or has evidence of abnormal structures associated with it.

COMMON GENITAL ABNORMALITIES ENCOUNTERED

Ovarian Abnormalities

Ovarian abnormalities identified on physical examination can be divided into small ovaries and large ovaries.

Small Ovaries. These may be either normal or abnormal. Prepubertal or juvenile ovaries are small; therefore, the age and previous cyclic history of the mare is important. During the anestrus season the ovaries are inactive and one half the size they will attain during the breeding season. In some small, docile, chronically anestrus mares a chromosomal anomaly called *XO gonadal dysgenesis* may be the cause of small ovaries. An endometrial biopsy from these mares often demonstrates glandular insufficiency. A karyotype is the only reliable means of diagnosing this condition, and there is no treatment. Unseasonally small ovaries may also be the result of other physical abnormalities. Mares that have experienced a severe weight loss may have small inactive ovaries. Mares with *pituitary tumors* have suppressed ovarian activity either because of their weight loss or from a lack of gonadotropin secretion from the pituitary. If only one ovary is small, firm and inactive, it is possibly being suppressed by an abnormality of the other ovary. This is often the case with a granulosa cell tumor on the opposite ovary. Suppressed activity of one ovary may be important for differentiating the several causes of enlarged ovaries. Additionally, there is another clinical situation in which unseasonally small ovaries occur. This is the case of the *"true" nymphomaniac mare*. These mares act as if they are in persistent estrus, yet often they will not allow mounting; some of these mares will demonstrate malelike behavior. Other than small, firm ovaries, no other abnormalities of the genital tract are noted in the nymphomaniac mare. The cause of nymphomania is

unknown and attempts to treat it are usually unsuccessful. Ovariectomy may or may not stop this behavior. In some cases the behavioral aberration can be controlled with exogenous progesterone.

Enlarged Ovaries. These may be a seasonal phenomenon. During the transitional periods, follicles may grow to abnormally large sizes and persist for various lengths of time before ovulating or regressing. These *persistent follicles* should be followed for several examinations over a period of time. They usually do not suppress activity in the other ovary and resolve themselves and cause no permanent problem. In the early transition period they can be treated with 1000 to 5000 IU of human chorionic gonadotropin (hCG), but results are variable. During the autumn transition period it is best to allow them to regress during the anestrus period. These persistent follicles are often diagnosed as cystic ovaries by practitioners unaccustomed to palpating the mare's ovaries. Cystic ovaries, such as those that occur in cows, do not occur in mares. The biggest problem in dealing with persistent follicles in mares is differentiating them from certain types of ovarian tumors.

Ovarian Tumors. In the mare ovarian tumors are usually classified according to the main type of cell making up the tumor. Most of these tumors are unilateral and rarely malignant. The *cystadenoma* must be differentiated from persistent follicles. These usually enlarge over a period of time, unlike the persistent follicle that remains the same or regresses. They probably arise from the surface epithelium of the ovary or the rete ovarii and have one or several large fluid-filled cavities within them. The ultrasound machine can be used to differentiate these from some of the more solid structures mentioned in the following discussion. Hormonal analysis or stimulation tests may be unrewarding when used to differentiate cystadenomas from other ovarian tumors. The only treatment is ovariectomy, and prognosis for fertility after removal is fair to good.

Granulosa-theca Cell Tumors. These are the most common ovarian tumor in the mare. Although they may grow to very large sizes if undetected, they are usually unilateral and benign. They produce a variety of hormones and usually suppress activity of the opposite ovary. Differences in ovarian size may be of diagnostic importance when trying to rule out other nontumorous causes of ovarian enlargement. Hormonal analysis before and after stimulation with hCG may help differentiate these tumors from ovarian abscesses or hematomas. They may be solid, single or multilocular in nature. An endometrial biopsy may also be helpful in diagnosing this tumor. Glandular hyperplasia of the endometrium has been reported to occur with progesterone-secreting granulosa cell tumors. The mare's behavior manifestation can range from states of anestrus to nymphomania and even to virility, depending on the predominant hormone produced by these tumors. Treatment is removal of the affected ovary, and the prognosis for fertility is fair to good, depending on the length of time that the tumor has existed and the degree of suppression of the opposite ovary. Mares will usually begin to cycle 1 to 4 months after the tumor is removed. Much less common ovarian tumors are teratoma and the dysgerminoma. The *teratoma* is a multiple tissue type tumor that usually has epithelial structures including cartilage, bone, hair and glandular epithelium. They are usually benign and produce no hormones, so the contralateral ovary usually remains functional, and the mare may continue to cycle. As in the other ovarian tumors, ovariectomy is indicated.

Unlike the previously discussed ovarian tumors, the *dysgerminoma* can be malignant. It arises from the germinal epithelium of the ovary and can become very large. Dysgerminomas have been reported to produce a type of hypertrophic pulmonary osteopathy condition in the mare similar to that which occurs in women. The tumors may be solid or contain fluid-filled multiple cysts. Ovariectomy is the treatment of choice.

Non-neoplastic Ovarian Enlargements. The other causes of ovarian enlargement are non-neoplastic. *Ovarian abscesses* and hematoma are not uncommon and are difficult to differentiate. The mare's temperature and white blood cell count may help identify the ovarian abscess, yet these abscesses are often encapsulated within the ovary and do not produce a systemic reaction after they become chronic. *Ovarian hematomas* often feel similar to ovarian abscesses. In both cases the opposite ovary usually remains functional and the mare continues to cycle. Ovarian hematomas usually regress over a period of time and cause no fertility problems. Hormone stimulation tests may differentiate these from ovarian tumors. An ultrasound examination may be of some help in differentiating them. Some authors report that the presence of an ovulation fossa in the enlarged ovary suggests an ovarian hematoma, but this author has not found that to be a reliable method of differentiating them.

The last cause of ovarian enlargement that should not be overlooked is the unusually large, normal cyclic follicle. Most cyclic follicles range in size from 2.5 to 6 cm in diameter prior to ovulation. Occasionally, one or several large follicles grow to 10 cm or more before ovulation. In this and all cases of ovarian enlargement, several examinations over a 15- to 30-day (or more) period are a valuable means of differentiating these ovarian abnormalities.

Uterine Tube Abnormalities

Abnormalities of the uterine tubes are difficult to identify in the mare. The incidence of *salpingitis* and *hydrosalpinx* seems to be very low when compared with cattle. European workers have reported observing a significant number of uterine tube lesions when the tracts of older mares were examined at slaughter. *Fimbrial cysts* are not a rare finding in the mare. These are usually small and inconsequential. Occasionally, they may grow large enough to interfere with the collection of the ovum by the fimbria. The primary concern with fimbrial cysts is

to differentiate them from other abnormalities of the ovary.

Uterine Abnormalities

Uterine abnormalities can be subdivided into (1) those associated with a uniformly enlarged uterus, (2) those associated with discrete abnormalities within the uterus and (3) parauterine abnormalities.

Uniformly Enlarged Uterus. This must be differentiated from *pregnancy* and a *postpartum uterus*. The mare's uterus usually involutes very rapidly after foaling in comparison to the cow's. By the beginning of foal heat, it should be no more than two to three times its normal size.

The other two major causes of a uniformly enlarged uterus are pyometra and pneumouterus. Unlike pyometra in the cow, mares with pyometra often cycle and intermittently discharge purulent exudate. The pathogenesis of pyometra in the mare usually involves an obstruction of outflow of the uterine secretions. These may include intraluminal adhesions, occlusion of the cervix or intra-abdominal adhesions of the uterine horns that hold them below the floor of the pelvis. If the damage to the endometrium is severe, the mare may remain anestrous, with a persistent corpus luteum caused by a lack of prostaglandin release from the damaged endometrium. Exogenous prostaglandins may evacuate the uterus of pyometritic mares unless an intraluminal occlusion is present. Evacuation of the uterus by lavage and siphoning may be helpful. The fluid should be cultured, and treatment should be instituted according to the sensitivity of the organisms identified. The chance of success is increased if one is able to break down the occlusion. Pyometra in the mare has a much poorer prognosis than in the cow and often recurs.

Pneumouterus is an occasional finding in the mare that has a pneumovagina or following a vaginoscopic examination when the mare is in heat. Correcting the pneumovagina will usually result in resolution of the pneumouterus. Tumors of the uterus are rare in the mare. The most common type of uterine neoplasia is leiomyoma, although fibroma, fibroadenoma and adenosarcoma have been reported.

Discrete Uterine Enlargements. These must be differentiated from *early pregnancy* by identifying the embryo as a discrete bulge in the uterine horn. Other enlargements include *endometrial cysts*, which result from blocked and dilated endometrial glands, *lymphatic lacunae*, which result from blocked lymph channels, *abscesses* in the uterine wall and *cornual dilatation* subsequent to atrophy of the uterine mucosa in older mares.

With the exception of cornual dilatation, the treatment for these enlargements is either drainage into the lumen or surgical removal followed by local and systemic antibiotics. Cornual dilatation is a degenerative condition that usually occurs at the junction of the body and horn near the implantation site. Treatment of these dilatations is usually unsuccessful, although infusion of hot saline may be beneficial in increasing the tone of the uterus in these areas.

Other discrete uterine abnormalities that can be diagnosed on physical examination include *luminal channels and tunnels* and *luminal adhesions*. These may be caused by endometrial injury or chronic endometrial inflammation. They are usually identified by either bimanual or fiberoptic examination techniques. They may interfere with placentation and/or possibly the delivery of the fetus. When recognized, they should be removed surgically.

Endometrial fold atrophy can be diagnosed by slipping the folds per rectum and by bimanual or fiberoptic techniques. Endometrial biopsy may be a valuable aid in making this diagnosis. These are degenerative changes and therapy is usually unrewarding.

Parauterine Abnormalities. Parauterine abnormalities diagnosed during the breeding soundness examination are mainly restricted to hematomas in the broad ligament of the uterus. These are not rare and are usually associated with parturition. A fresh hematoma should not be disturbed, and the mare should be treated with systemic antibotics to prevent abscessation. A chronic hematoma rarely causes a fertility problem and usually regresses over time.

Cervical Abnormalities

When evaluating the cervix, the normal variations during the estrous cycle and pregnancy must be kept in mind. The pinkness of estrus must be differentiated from the redness of inflammation. Cervicitis may be caused by contagious equine metritis (CEM), endometritis or vaginitis or may be secondary to pneumovagina or rectovaginal fistula. The most common noninfectious abnormalities noted are cervical adhesions and scars secondary to foaling or breeding problems. These abnormalities may prevent the cervix from opening and/or closing properly. A cervix that does not dilate fully prevents the stallion from ejaculating into the uterus and may make delivery of a foal difficult. A cervix that does not fully close predisposes the mare to endometritis and may prevent her from carrying a foal to term. Attempts to remove the cervical scars surgically are frustrating because the cervix adhesions readily reform adhesions.

Vaginal Abnormalities

Scars, adhesions and *lacerations* are some of the more common vaginal abnormalities. Vaginal abnormalities are often associated with foaling and breeding. Lacerations subsequent to breeding often occur in the fornix of the vagina. They are usually retroperitoneal and heal well. Occasionally, however, there may be an extension of a cervical tear, which results in cervical stenosis or insufficiency. Additionally, the rectovaginal fistula, which is a foaling accident, is not rare in the mare. Rectovaginal fistulas are usually caused by the foal sticking a foot through the dorsal wall of the vagina and through the ventral floor of the rectum. If the foot is not withdrawn into the vagina, the entire perineal body between the rectum and vagina may be torn, producing a *third degree perineal laceration*. Unless one is present and equipped to close these injuries immediately after they occur, it is best to allow 1 to 2 months rest before attempting to repair them surgically. In the meantime, the mare should be put on a laxative diet.

Undoubtedly the most common vaginal problem in mares is *pneumovagina* secondary to vulvar lip insufficiency. Pneumovagina can lead to vaginitis, cervicitis, and endometritis. It can be corrected easily by suturing the lips of the vulva together to the level of the pelvis (Caslick's operation). Care must be taken not to interfere with urination. Caslick's operation is performed routinely on many farms and may be one of the best management aids to overcome the problem of the barren mare. *Urine pooling* may be associated with pneumovagina or may be unrelated. The vaginal floor normally slopes anteriorly and ventrally. However, in the aged, heavily pregnant or postpartum mare, this slope may become exaggerated and prevent complete evacuation of urine from the vestibule. Urovagina may be temporary in the pregnant or postpartum mare and, therefore, not require repair. However, when urine pooling exists in other mares, attempts should be made to correct it prior to breeding. Mares with urovagina are usually infertile because of the spermicidal properties of urine. Several surgical procedures have been described for correction of this condition. Some surgeons attempt to form a dam with the transverse fold, while others prefer urethral extension. Urine pooling must be differentiated from the serous mucus that occasionally collects posterior to the cervix during estrus.

Vaginal abscesses occasionally occur subsequent to a vaginal laceration. They should be drained into the vagina, with care taken to avoid the large perivaginal blood vessels. Systemic and local antibiotics should be used to speed healing. The vaginal abscess must be differentiated from the *perivaginal hematomas* and vaginal cysts, such as *Gartner's cysts*. Hematomas should be allowed to resolve with time, and cysts usually do not cause a problem, but they may be drained if large. Occasionally, a complete or partial *persistence of the hymen* may occur in maiden mares. Very often a dark, thick fluid accumulates behind the hymen and may be discharged intermittently. If the hymen is completely imperforate, sufficient fluid may collect behind it to cause protrusion through the vulvar lips, and this may be confused with a vaginal prolapse. The persistent hymen can be identified by vaginoscopy. Correction involves manually or surgically dilating the hymen. Prepartum *vaginal prolapse* is rare in the mare. Occasionally, a persistent hymen, perivaginal abscess or hematoma may be mistaken for a vaginal prolapse.

Vulvar Abnormalities

The most common abnormality of the vulva is dorsocranial slope associated with pneumovagina. At least 70 per cent of the vulvar cleft should be below the brim of the pelvis. *Abnormal labial approximation* can result in the same problems as abnormal slope and should be corrected by Caslick's operation. Occasionally, a mare will be encountered that has suffered a severe vulvar laceration because an episiotomy was not performed on a mare that has had Caslick's operation. As mentioned previously, third degree perineal lacerations involve the vulva. Reconstructive surgery should be attempted. *Clitoral hypertrophy* is occasionally seen in fillies. This is usually a manifestation of pseudohermaphroditism. Clitorectomy is possible, but frequently the urethra opens through the clitoris and reconstructive surgery is necessary.

Neoplasia of the vulva is frequently identified, ranging from innocuous tumors, as in the case of fibromas or fibropapillomas, to proliferative malignancies, as in malignant melanomas common in grey mares to erosive, as in squamous cell carcinomas. Correction varies with the location and severity of the condition.

Suggested Readings

1. Baker CB, Kenney RM: 1st ed.: Systemic approach to the diagnosis of the infertile and subfertile mare. In Current Therapy in Theriogenology. Philadelphia, WB Saunders Co, 1980, Morrow DA (ed): pp 721–735.
2. Greenhoff SR, Kenney RM: Evaluation of the reproductive status of nonpregnant mares. JAVMA 167:449, 1975.
3. Hughes JP: Clinical Examination and Abnormalities in the Mare. In Morrow DA (ed): Current Therapy in Theriogenology. 1st ed. Philadelphia, WB Saunders Co, 1980, pp 706–721.
4. Hughes JP, Stahenfeldt GH, Kennedy PC: Estrous cycle and selected functional and pathological ovarian abnormalities in the mare. Vet Clin North Am: Large Anim Pract 2:225, 1980.
5. Lieux P: Reproduction and genital diseases. In Catcott EJ, Smithcors JF (eds): Equine Medicine and Surgery. 2nd ed. Wheaton, American Veterinary Publications, 1972, pp 597–622.

Estrous Synchronization in Mares

F. Bristol, B.V.Sc., M.Sc.

University of Saskatchewan, Saskatoon, Saskatchewan, Canada

The relatively long and variable length of estrus and the variation in the time ovulation occurs during estrus in the mare makes breeding management of mares very labor intensive. Estrus detection is tedious and time consuming, and failure to detect estrus is a major cause of infertility. Synchronization of estrus and ovulation would allow mares to be bred or artificially inseminated at a predetermined time, with or without estrus detection, thus simplifying breeding management and making more efficient use of stallions. When teasing is used for estrus detection, it can be done during a predetermined period of time, thus also reducing the amount of time spent teasing mares. Although synchronization of estrus in large groups of mares will probably not be used except on pregnant mare urine farms, it would be a useful technique for scheduling estrus in mares for heavily booked stallions. The major application, in the near future, will most likely be for synchronization of estrus and ovulation in donor and recipient mares destined for embryo transfer.

METHODS

Basically, three methods have been used to synchronize estrus in cycling mares, namely the following: (1) termination of the luteal phase of the estrus cycle with prostaglandin $F_{2\alpha}$ or a prostaglandin analog, (2) long- or short-term progesterone or progestogen treatment together with a luteolytic agent and (3) delay of foal estrus with short-term progesterone or progestogen treatment.

CYCLING MARES

Prostaglandins. Prostaglandin $F_{2\alpha}$ and its analogs have been shown to be very effective luteolytic

Figure 1. Procedure for synchronization of estrus in mares using two injections of prostaglandin.

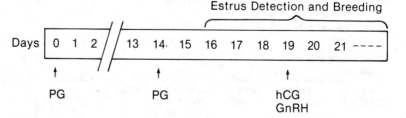

Table 1. Effect of hCG Given 5 Days after Second Prostaglandin (PG) Treatment and Insemination on Pregnancy Rate of Mares after Synchronization of Estrus

	Single Insemination (6 Days after 2nd PG Treatment)	Two Inseminations (6 and 8 Days after 2nd PG Treatment)	Inseminated on Alternate Days during Estrus
No. of mares	30	32	54
No. pregnant (per cent)	17 (56.6)	19 (59.4)	38 (71.7)

(Adapted from Hyland JH, Bristol F: J Reprod Fert Suppl 27:251, 1979.)

agents in mares; however, the corpus luteum is refractory to these agents until approximately 5 days after ovulation. Therefore, to synchronize estrus in large groups of cycling mares, at all stages of the estrous cycle, the double prostaglandin treatment originally developed for cattle has been adapted for mares. The regimen is illustrated in Figure 1. The interval between the two prostaglandin treatments has varied between 14 and 18 days.[1, 3, 4, 7, 8, 11] The onset of estrus was relatively well synchronized by the double prostaglandin regimen, and it has been shown that approximately 60 per cent of mares had begun estrus 4 days after the second prostaglandin treatment,[7] and between 75 and 90 per cent had shown estrus in 6 days.[2, 4, 7, 11] However, the interval from prostaglandin treatment to ovulation is very variable. Ovulations occurred from 2 to 12 days after prostaglandin treatment during the luteal phase.[3, 7, 12] Much of this variability depended on the size of the largest follicle at the time of prostaglandin administration. The greatest variation in response was observed in mares with follicles > 40 mm in diameter. Most of these ovulated shortly (5.1 ± 0.3 days) after treatment, while in some mares the follicles regressed and were replaced by another follicle, which ovulated 9.0 ± 0.7 days after treatment.[5]

Human chorionic gonadotropin (hCG) has been used in conjunction with the double injection of prostaglandin to hasten ovulation and to reduce the variability in the duration of estrus (Fig. 1).[3, 4, 7, 8, 11] Intramuscular doses of 1500 to 3300 IU hCG have been given 5 or 6 days after the second prostaglandin treatment or on the first or second day of estrus.

The use of hCG reduced some of the variability; however, some variation still existed.[7, 11]

Synchronized mares have been bred by artificial insemination with estrus detection and on predetermined days without estrus detection. When estrus detection was used, mares were inseminated on alternate days[1, 4, 12] or daily[12] during estrus, while those bred by appointment were inseminated once 6 days after the second prostaglandin treatment[4, 11, 12] or a number of times between 4 and 10 days after the prostaglandin injection (Tables 1 and 2). Fertility was normal in mares inseminated during estrus and in those mares inseminated four times without estrus detection; however, a single insemination cannot be recommended until ovulation can be more accurately controlled.

A synthetic gonadotropin-releasing hormone (GnRH)[12] and a GnRH analog[11] have also been given 5 days after prostaglandin treatment. This treatment did not hasten ovulation or shorten the duration of estrus.

Progesterone and Progestogens. Various regimens for synchronizing estrus using progesterone and progestogens have been developed: (1) long-term treatment (18 days) using either progesterone[3] or progestogen,[1, 3] (2) short-term (8 days) progestogen treatment with a prostaglandin injection on the last day of treatment[8, 9] and (3) short-term progesterone and 17-β estradiol treatment with prostaglandin. Because of the reduction in labor, the short-term treatments are more applicable for breeding management of mares.

The synthetic progestogen, altrenogest, has been used successfully for estrous synchronization. It has

Table 2. Synchronization of Estrus and Timed Insemination in Mares

	AI on Alternate Days During Estrus	AI on Alternate Days without Estrus Detection	AI Every Day without Estrus Detection
No. of mares	48	42	38
No. of mares showing estrus (per cent)	44 (91.6)	—	—
No. of inseminations per mare	3.49	4	8
No. of mares pregnant (per cent)*	25 (52.1)	27 (64.3)	24 (63.2)

*Pregnancy rates were not statistically different ($\times^2$, P > 0.05).
(Adapted from Bristol, F, unpublished data, 1983.)

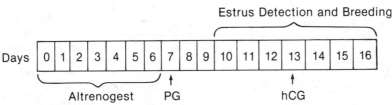

Figure 2. Procedure for synchronization of estrus in mares using altrenogest and prostaglandin. (Adapted from Palmer E: Proc 28th Int Congr Anim Reprod & AI, Krakow, pp 495–498, 1976.)

been administered for 8 to 12 days at a dose of 27 to 44 mg per day in the feed or by insertion of an intravaginal sponge impregnated with 0.5 gm of altrenogest.[8, 9] Because of the short duration of treatment it is necessary to give an injection of prostaglandin on the last day of progestogen therapy to remove any sources of endogenous progesterone production (Fig. 2).

Most mares began to show estrus 2 to 5 days after withdrawal of the progestogen treatment; however, synchronization of ovulation was not successful with ovulation occurring 8 to 15 days after withdrawal.[9] Most mares ovulated in a 4-day period if 2500 IU hCG was given 5 or 7 days after altrenogest withdrawal.[8, 9] As with prostaglandin synchronization, fertility was good (71 per cent pregnancy rate) when mares were bred every second day during estrus; however, when mares were inseminated at a predetermined time, the pregnancy rate was somewhat lower.[10]

Recently, short-term treatment using 10 daily intramuscular injections of 150 mg of progesterone and 10 mg of 17-β estradiol combined with prostaglandin $F_2\alpha$ on the last day of the regimen has been shown to be highly effective in the synchronization of both estrus and ovulation. Most mares (18 of 20) ovulated between 10 and 12 days after the last day of treatment.[6] This method appears to provide the best synchronization of ovulation; however, it is the most time consuming, as mares have to be injected on a daily basis.

EARLY POSTPARTUM MARES

Prostaglandins are not applicable for estrous synchronization in early postpartum mares. Although some mares ovulate as early as 6 days after partu-

rition, the majority of mares do not have a mature corpus luteum until approximately 18 days after parturition. Progesterone and progestogens have been used to delay foal estrus; however, they do not consistently prevent ovulation, resulting in poor synchronization of ovulation.[6] Injections of 200 mg progesterone and 10 mg 17-β estradiol given daily for 5 days beginning on the day of parturition were effective in delaying the onset of foal estrus and the first postpartum ovulation.[6] Delay of the first postpartum estrus for 1 to 10 days was used to synchronize estrus in postpartum mares. The mares were given a varying number of daily injections of progesterone and 17-β estradiol beginning on the day of parturition. Treatment for all mares ceased on the same day.[2] This regimen resulted in good synchronization of estrus, but there was greater variation in the distribution of ovulations following treatment in these mares (Table 3).

ANESTRUS MARES

The breeding season can be advanced by exposing mares to a daily regimen of 16 hours of light during the winter months. Estrus has been synchronized in anestrus mares using photoperiodic stimulation in conjunction with altrenogest, prostaglandin and hCG treatment.[9] (Fig. 3). Mares require at least 60 days of photoperiod stimulation before beginning the progestogen treatment.

SUMMARY

Estrus can be synchronized in mares using a double prostaglandin treatment and short-term pro-

Table 3. Effect of Progesterone and 17-β Estradiol on Control of Estrus and Ovulation in 36 Postpartum Mares

	Onset of Estrus (Days Post-treatment)			Ovulation (Days Post-treatment)			Number Pregnant
	n	Mean	Range	n	Mean	Range	
Mares treated 1 to 10 days postpartum	36	9.39	7–14	33	13.06	10–16	29

Note: Mares were inseminated every second day during estrus.
(Adapted from Bristol F, Jacobs KA, Pawlyshyn V: Theriogenology 19:779, 1983.)

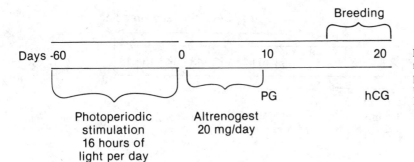

Figure 3. Procedure for synchronization of estrus in mares using photoperiodic stimulation and altrenogest. (Adapted from Palmer E: J Reprod Fert Suppl. 27:263, 1979.)

gestogen or progesterone and 17-β estradiol treatment with an injection on the last day of progestogen treatment. However, ovulations are not as well synchronized; some of the variability can be reduced if hCG is given 4 to 5 days after the second prostaglandin treatment or 10 days after the progestogen treatment. At present, the progesterone/estradiol treatment appears to be the most effective method of synchronizing ovulation in cycling mares.

References

1. Bristol F: Studies on estrus synchronization in mares. Proc Ann Mtg Soc Theriogenol. 1981, pp 258–264.
2. Bristol F, Jacobs KA, Pawlyshyn V: Synchronization of estrus in post partum mares with progesterone and estradiol 17B. Theriogenology 19:779, 1983.
3. Houltan DW, Douglas RH, Ginther OJ: Estrus, ovulation and conception following synchronization with progesterone, prostaglandin $F_2\alpha$ and human chorionic gonadotrophin in pony mares. J Anim Sci 44:431, 1977.
4. Hyland JH, Bristol F: Synchronization of oestrus and timed insemination of mares. J Reprod Fert Suppl 27:251, 1979.
5. Loy RG, Buell JR, Stevenson W, Hamm D: Sources of variation in response intervals after prostaglandin treatment in mares with functional corpora lutea. J Reprod Fert Suppl 27:229, 1979.
6. Loy RG, Pemstein R, O'Canna D, Douglas RH: Control of ovulation in cycling mares with ovarian steroids and prostaglandin. Theriogenology 15:191, 1981.
7. Palmer E, Jousset B: Synchronization of oestrus in mares with a prostaglandin analogue and hCG. J Reprod Fert Suppl 23:269, 1975.
8. Palmer E: Different techniques for synchronization of ovulation in the mare. Proc 8th Int Congr Anim Reprod AI, Krakow, 1976, pp 495–498.
9. Palmer E: Reproductive management of mares without detection of oestrus. J Reprod Fert Suppl 27:263, 1979.
10. Squires EL, Stevens WB, McGlothlin DE, Pickett BW: Effect of an oral progestin on the estrous cycle and fertility of mares. J Anim Sci 49:729, 1979.
11. Squires EL, Wallace RA, Voss JL, et al: The effectiveness of $PGF_2\alpha$, hCG and GnRH for appointment breeding of mares. J Eq Vet Sci 1:5, 1981.
12. Voss JL, Wallace RA, Squires EL, et al: Effects of synchronization and frequency of insemination on fertility. J Reprod Fert Suppl 27:257, 1979.

The Effects of Photoperiod on Reproduction in the Mare and Methods of Artificial Control

Dan C. Sharp, Ph.D.
University of Florida, Gainesville, Florida

SEASONAL REPRODUCTIVE PATTERNS

The annual reproductive cycle of the mare can basically be divided into a period of sexual competence (breeding season) and sexual incompetence (anestrus). The former is associated with spring and summer, thus relegating the mare to the category of "long-day breeders." The breeding season is characterized by repeated episodes of sexual receptivity (estrus) associated with follicular development and ovulation alternating with sexual nonreceptivity (diestrus) associated with corpus luteum function. The anestrous period is characterized by a relative lack of sexual receptivity and by gonadal regression and inactivity. However, this partitioning overlooks two periods of major interest from the standpoint of gaining a physiological understanding. These are the two transition periods, from anestrus to the breeding season, and from the breeding season into anestrus. Since the latter occurs in the fall when most breeders are not concerned with breeding, little more will be said about it here.

On the other hand, considerable attention has been given to the period of transition into the breeding season. This reflects the magnitude of the problem, since economic pressures compel breeders to strive for earlier foalings than is compatible with the mare's natural physiology. The lengthy transition period (30 to 60 days) is characterized by a complex chain of events that includes reinitiation of estrous behavior and ovarian follicular development. During this time follicle-stimulating hormone (FSH) is elevated,[2] which likely accounts for the sigmoid-shaped curve of follicle growth[18] (Fig. 1). However, luteinizing hormone (LH) remains basal throughout the transition period.[2, 16] Presumably, as a result of the basal LH secretion, ovulation does not take place throughout the transition period, even though many large (> 30 mm) follicles de-

velop. Finally, for reasons not yet understood, an LH surge occurs, and ovulation takes place, which by definition terminates the transitory period and begins the breeding season. As will be discussed later, this lengthy transition appears to be obligatory for most mares, and even if the timing of the first ovulation is somehow altered, the mare still undergoes a transition characterized by events previously described.[15] It is easy to understand why the transition period may be confusing and frustrating to breeders and practitioners, since mares may be sexually receptive and may have large follicles that feel preovulatory upon rectal examination, but since ovulation does not occur, breeding is futile until the transition is complete. Although there is much research still needed, results from our laboratory have indicated that because of their steroidogenic properties follicles from the early transition period behave differently than follicles from the late transition period. When tissues from the early or late transition follicles were incubated in vitro and examined for their steroid-producing ability, it was observed that the estrone-to-estradiol ratio changed markedly, favoring estrone in late transition and cycling mares.[13] Furthermore, the poor responsiveness of the early follicles to exogenous human chorionic gonadotropin (hCG) raises the question of whether or not the early follicles have a well-developed gonadotropin receptor system. This question stems from a preliminary experiment in which hCG (10,000 units) was administered (IV) to nine mares in transition at the time of detection of their first large follicle ($\geq$ 30 mm). A similar number of control mares received an injection of saline at the time of detection of their first follicle measuring 30 mm. Experience in this laboratory has indicated that the time from detection of the first 30 mm follicle to the time of the first ovulation of the year is approximately 25.6 ± 2.1 days. In theory the administration of hCG might cause ovulation of this first large follicle, which normally does not ovulate, thus advancing the onset of the breeding season. Two of nine control mares (11.1 per cent) ovulated within 4 days of detection of the first 30 mm follicles whereas the remaining seven mares did not ovulate for 25.7 ± 7.2 ($\bar{x}$ ± SEM) days. Only four of nine mares (44.4 per cent) receiving hCG at first detection of a follicle 30 mm or greater ovulated within 4 days of receiving the hCG, whereas the remaining five mares did not ovulate for 19.8 ± 5.7 ($\bar{x}$ + SEM) days. These results, while preliminary in nature, do not confidently show that ovulation can be induced effectively in mares during the early follicular development phase of the transition and raise the question of whether the early follicles are fully competent with respect to gonadotropin receptors. Whatever the mechanisms involved, it is clear that a better understanding of the transition events is necessary in order to develop rational methods for advancing the onset of the breeding season.

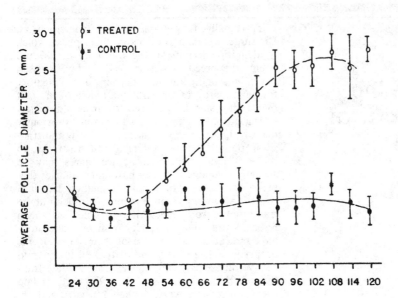

Figure 1. Changes in the average follicle diameter during the transition from anestrus to the breeding season. The open circles represent mares undergoing this transition; the closed circles represent mares still in anestrus (From Sharp DC, et al.: J Anim Sci 41:1368, 1975.)

The precision of the mechanisms involved in bringing about the change from anestrus to full reproductive competence is remarkable. Figure 2 illustrates the average date of first ovulation (Julian Calendar Date ± SEM) of ponies from a variety of experiments conducted at Florida over the years.

The vertical line represents the overall mean ± SEM of all experiments. Visual inspection of this graph reveals extremely good agreement in time of first ovulation among different experiments (conducted in different years with different environmental conditions), with the exception of groups labeled

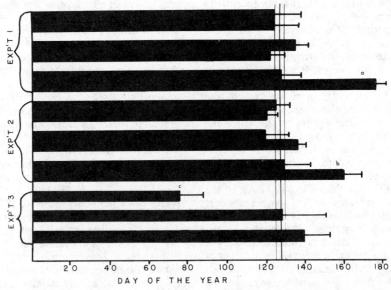

Figure 2. Date of first ovulation of mares from a variety of experiments from 1976–1980. The horizontal bars represent different groups of pony mares and the right hand edge of the bar represents the mean (± SEM) date of the first ovulation. The verticle lines represent the overall mean (± SEM) date of first ovulation of all experiments. Note that groups marked a, b, and c are the only experiments that markedly altered the onset of the breeding season. They were superior cervical ganglionectomy, pinealectomy and artificial photoperiod (2½ hours at sunset) for a, b and c, respectively. Note also the unmarked bar below c in experiment 3. These mares were exposed to the same light treatment as the mares in c but were also pinealectomized and did not respond.

a, b and c. This precise beginning of the breeding season appears to hold for a range of latitudes including about 43° N[2a] to about 15° N latitude,[12] which emphasizes the remarkable consistency of the mechanisms behind the breeding season.

INFLUENCE OF LIGHT

The consistency in timing of onset of the breeding season over a wide range of latitudes and range of environmental conditions within given latitudes offers a clue to the driving force behind the breeding season. The only environmental condition that is precise enough to serve as a cue for such consistent timing is photoperiod. The daily changes in daylength are precise and dependable; factors that surely would have been important to any species developing a time-keeping system for the purpose of perpetuating their species. Dependence on temperature, rainfall, nutrition or other factors for timing of the breeding season would be fraught with error, since the capriciousness of these factors in the environment is a common occurrence. Furthermore, even if such factors play a role in regulating the timing of the breeding season, they are driven themselves by changes in photoperiods. Therefore, it seems certain that changing photoperiod is the major impellor of seasonal reproductive rhythms.

Moreover, it is well known that artificial manipulation of the photoperiod can alter the timing of the breeding season. Burkhardt[1] demonstrated that artificially increasing the length of day at a rate twice that of the natural increase resulted in an earlier onset of the breeding season in mares. Nishikawa[8] and Oxender, Noden and Hafs[9] demonstrated an advance of the breeding season following exposure of mares to long photoperiods (> 14 hours of light) applied instantly (in contrast to a gradual increase). Finally, Sharp and Ginther[18] also advanced the onset of the breeding season by gradually increasing the length of day at the same rate as the natural increase but beginning much earlier (October). Thus, the onset of the breeding season can be advanced by artificially lengthening the day in a variety of ways, although a critical study has not been done to test the efficacy of one method over the other.

More will be said about use of artificial light for control of the breeding season in the last section of this article. The preceding discussion merely serves to illustrate the effectiveness of light in altering the natural timing of the breeding season.

POSSIBLE MECHANISMS AND PATHWAYS OF LIGHT

From the foregoing discussion it is apparent that the natural photoperiod is the likely signal for timing of the breeding season and that an artificially altered photoperiod leads to altered (usually advanced) entrance into the breeding season. The mechanisms by which mares utilize photoperiod in their time-keeping are not known, but some clues are available. It is known, for example, that the pineal gland is somehow involved. The pineal is a single unpaired organ located on the roof of the diencephalon. In lower animals (amphibia, reptilia) the pineal is directly photoreceptive, but in birds and mammals, the eye is the primary photoreceptor, and a complex neural pathway transmits the photic information to the pineal. Interruption of this nerve pathway (or surgical removal of the pineal itself) results in altered seasonal breeding patterns[4] (Fig. 2). When the photic pathway to the pineal is interrupted, or the pineal itself is removed, mares still undergo alternating periods of anestrus and sexual competence, but the onset of the breeding season is delayed 40 to 60 days. It is important, for practical reasons, to note that the pattern of changes from anestrus to the breeding season was similar to intact mares in appearance and length but was simply delayed.[4, 16] This suggests that the transition events may be obligatory in the renewal of sexual competence. The involvement of the pineal gland was further implicated in another study in which pinealectomized and pineal-intact mares were exposed to artificially lengthened days in order to accelerate the onset of the breeding season. The pineal-intact mares were significantly accelerated, but the pinealectomized mares were not[4] (Fig. 2). This indicates that the pineal is necessary in order to advance the onset of the breeding season and implies a role in the regulation of photic timing. These observations are important in that they indicate a mediatory role of the pineal in timing of seasonal reproductive events, but do not suggest that the pineal exerts control over these events.

The nature of the pineal's involvement remains to be elucidated. It is known, however, that the pineal's secretory function varies with photoperiod. Using measurements of peripherally circulating melatonin (a pineal hormone) as an index of pineal response to photoperiod, we have reported[4, 7] that in horses pineal secretion of melatonin is elevated during darkness and reduced during the day. The nighttime rise in melatonin is, in fact, closely coordinated with the time of sunset, and the daytime reduction occurs at about sunrise. Pinealectomy, which affects seasonal breeding rhythms, abolishes this day-night rhythm[4] (Fig. 3). Thus, it is clear that the pineal responds to photoperiodic stimuli by enhanced or reduced secretion of at least one of its hormones. Whether melatonin plays a direct role in regulating reproductive rhythms remains to be tested. Melatonin treatment (via chronic release mechanisms) of anestrous hamsters results in sexual recrudescence,[3, 11, 22] but the only report of melatonin treatment in horses of which this author is aware[21] showed no effect of melatonin on stimulation of early sexual recrudescence. Perhaps chronic administration of the hormone is inappropriate, however, since it is secreted in a rhythmic fashion by the pineal. This important concept deserves further testing.

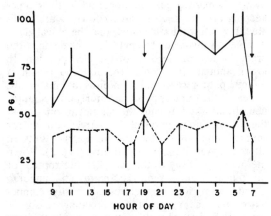

Figure 3. Effects of pinealectomy on melatonin secretion throughout 24 hours. The solid line represents melatonin secretion in intact mares; the dotted line represents melatonin in pinealectomized mares. The two vertical arrows represent sunset and sunrise. Note that pinealectomy completely abolished the day-night rhythm.

USE OF ARTIFICIAL LIGHTING

Because of the economic pressures and traditional beliefs, early-born foals are generally considered to be more desirable than late-born foals, although this depends somewhat on the breed. This need for early-born foals may be met by stimulating an early onset of the breeding season with artificial lights.

The question usually encountered in setting up a program of photostimulation is "How much light to use?" Unfortunately, it is not yet known what minimal amount of light is required to stimulate early sexual recrudescence. However, some guidelines can be drawn from the literature. First, it must be realized that at least three factors may be at play: (1) spectral wavelength, (2) light intensity and (3) duration and/or relative time of exposure to light. In the first category there is little or no research done. However, if the eye is the primary photoreceptor, then one can assume that activation of the retina would be maximal at wavelengths corresponding to activation of the photochemical rhodopsin. It is known that rhodopsin is maximally sensitive to light in the wavelength range of 550 nm (midrange), so it seems reasonable to utilize lighting systems that produce light near this optimum wavelength. Fluorescent bulbs, for example, generally favor lower wavelength emissions (yellow-green area, 500 to 600 nm), while incandescent and mercury vapor bulbs generally favor higher wavelength emissions (orange-red area, 550 to 650 nm and higher). As mentioned, it is not known how important spectral wavelength of light is for photostimulation of reproduction. Research using either fluorescent or incandescent bulbs has suggested, however, that either type bulb will work. A combination of fluorescent and incandescent bulbs will give a broad spectrum of wavelengths and cover all bases. Alternately, metal halide bulbs offer a broad spectrum of wavelengths, although they are more

expensive. In all, most types of bulbs appear to work, but more research is needed in order to comment on the relative effectiveness of one type compared with others.

The minimum intensity of light required to stimulate the onset of the breeding season also needs to be determined. Much research has been done with a variety of light intensities down to a minimum of 2 foot-candles (most studies used 10 foot-candles or brighter). In our lab we are conducting studies in an attempt to determine the minimum amount of light required for stimulation of reproduction in mares. Preliminary results of measurement of the retinal electrical response to light (electroretinogram—ERG) suggest that the threshold to light may be in the neighborhood of 1.0 to 1.5 log lux (less than 1 foot-candle).[5] It remains to be seen, however, whether the retinal response threshold is the same as the threshold for reproductive stimulation.

With the high cost of labor, breeders may wish to consider exposing mares to artificial photoperiod in a paddock situation instead of individual stalls. The same guidelines would likely apply. That is, a light source with broad spectral emission, such as metal halide, seems most appropriate, considering the current state of the art. Likewise, enough bulbs and fixtures should be utilized to achieve an average intensity of probably 5 to 10 foot-candles. Since the area of coverage is a function of type of fixture, shape and size of paddock, height of fixture and angle of the fixture to the ground as well as the number of fixtures and energy (wattage) of bulbs, some thought and expert lighting advice is highly recommended. An example of such a paddock lighting area employed at the Horse Research Center of the University of Florida is shown in Figure 4 for the reader's consideration. The lights were placed to provide an average minimum of 23.8 foot-candles, and the design was calculated through the courtesy of G.E. Sylvania Company (Danvers, Massachusetts). The paddock area (84 × 66 feet) required eight light fixtures (1000 W metal halide flood light) at a height of 20 feet in order to achieve the desired illumination. The circuitry design is such that only half of the bulbs can be turned on, so that in subsequent experiments, the light intensity can be reduced in order to study the minimum requirements. However, the results of the first year in paddock lighting were highly rewarding. In practice, mares assigned to the paddock group were permitted to graze during the day with control and other mares. At the late afternoon feeding, however, (4:00 to 4:30 PM) the paddock mares were led into the paddock where hay was available. Control mares returned to pastures distant from the paddock. At the time of sunset, the lights were automatically turned on and remained on for 2½ hours. At the time of lights off, the gate was opened and mares were permitted to graze in nearby pastures for the remainder of the night. Table 1 shows the date of the first ovulation of the year for paddock versus control mares. It is important to note that

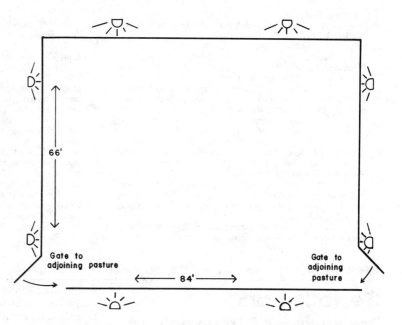

Figure 4. The paddock lighting system at the Horse Research Center, University of Florida. Dimensions of the paddock are 84 × 66 feet. The lights, Sylvania Model M/1000/CBD, 1000 W heavy duty, phosphor-coated lens metal halide flood lights, were distributed as shown. The lights were placed at a height of 20 feet and positioned at approximately 35 to 40°. Note the adjacent pastures to which the mares had access after lights out.

the highly significant advance of the breeding season (first ovulation) was achieved with a minimum of labor input. This is an important economic consideration. The other important consideration is that the acceleration of the onset of the breeding season was accomplished with only 2½ hours of additional light.

Previous studies from our lab have shown that such a short extension of the natural length of day is highly effective in advancing the breeding season if it is appropriately timed.[19] If, for example, the artificial light were applied 2½ hours prior to sunrise, it was totally ineffective. Therefore, it is our current recommendation that the artificial light be added beginning at the time of sunset and continuing for a short time only (2½ to 3 hours). These data, along with other recent publications,[6, 10] suggest that the mare has a unique period of time in her 24-hour rhythm in which she is uniquely or exquisitely sensitive to light. Such a period is well recognized in other mammals and is referred to as the "photosensitive period." It seems certain that with the high cost of labor and electricity, management systems, such as the paddock lighting system described here, that take advantage of the presumed

photosensitive period will need to be employed to a greater and greater extent.

In closing, it should be added that although we have acquired a great deal of knowledge about the effects and use of artificial light in equine reproduction, there is much to be learned. All the evidence to date favors the interpretation that the annual breeding cycle of the mare is internal in origin and is only modified by the environment, chiefly the photoperiod, to a rigid 12-month schedule. Continued research is necessary to understand the system completely, and therefore, deal with artificial adjustment of the breeding season rationally.

References

1. Burkhardt J: Transition from anestrus in the mare and the effects of artificial lighting. Agric Sci 37:64, 1947.
2. Freedman LM, Garcia MC, Ginther OJ: Influence of ovaries and photoperiod on reproductive function in the mare. J Reprod Fert Suppl 27:79, 1979.
3. Goldman B, Hall V, Hollister C, et al: Effects of melatonin on the reproductive system in intact and pinealectomized male hamsters maintained under various photoperiods. Endocrinology 104:82, 1979.
4. Grubaugh WR, Sharp DC, Berglund LH, et al: Effects of pinealectomy in pony mares. J Reprod Fert Suppl 32:293, 1982.
5. Gum GG, Sharp DC: Threshold of light intensity for electroretinogram response in anesthetized mares. (Unpublished results, 1983).
6. Johnson AL, Malinowski K: Influence of photoperiod on the daily rhythm of plasma cortisol in the mare. Proc 75th Ann Mtg Am Soc Anim Sci. Pullman, 1983.
7. Kilmer DM, Sharp DC, Berglund LA, et al: Melatonin rhythms in pony mares and foals. J Reprod Fertil Suppl 32:303, 1982.
8. Nishikawa Y: Studies on reproduction in horses. Japan Racing Assoc. Tokyo, 1959.
9. Oxender WD, Noden PA, Hafs HD: Estrus, ovulation and serum progesterone, estradiol, and LH concentrations in

Table 1. Use of a Paddock Lighting System to Accelerate the Onset of the Breeding Season in Mares

	Day of First Ovulation	Calendar Date
Paddock Group (n = 8)	33.4 ± 9.3	Feb 2*
Control Group (n = 6)	82.8 ± 14.2	March 24

* = P ≲0.01

mares after an increased photoperiod during winter. Am J Vet Res 38:203, 1977.

10. Palmer E, Driancourt MA: Photoperiodic stimulation of the winter anaestrus mare: What is a long day? In Ortavant R, Pelletier J, Ravault JP (eds): Photoperiodism and Reproduction. Nouzilly, INRA Publ, 1981, pp 67–82.

11. Reiter RJ, Vaughan MK, Balsk DE, Johnson LY: Melatonin: Its inhibition of pineal antigonadotropic activity in male hamsters. Science 185:482, 1974.

12. Saltiel A, Calderon A, Garcia N, Hurley DP: Ovarian activity in the mare between 15° and 22°N. Reprod Fertil Suppl 32:261, 1982.

13. Seamans KW, Sharp DC: Changes in equine follicular aromatase activity during transition from winter anaestrus. J Reprod Fertil Suppl 32:225, 1982.

14. Seamans KW, Sharp DC: Peripheral plasma androstenedione and testosterone concentrations during the transition from winter anestrus in pony mares. Proc 75th Ann Mtg Am Soc Anim Sci, Pullman, 1983.

15. Sharp DC: Environmental influences on reproduction in horses. Vet Clin North Am: Large Anim Pract 2:207, 1980.

16. Sharp DC, Garcia MC, Ginther OJ: Luteinizing hormone during sexual maturation in pony mares. Am J Vet Res 40:584, 1979.

17. Sharp DC, Kooistra L, Ginther OJ: Effects of artificial light on the oestrous cycle of the mare. J Reprod Fertil Suppl 23:241, 1973.

18. Sharp DC, Ginther OJ: Stimulation of follicular activity and estrous behavior in anestrous mares with light and temperature. J Anim Sci 41:1368, 1975.

19. Sharp DC, Seamans KW: Effect of time of day on photostimulation of the breeding season in mares. 72nd Ann Mtg Am Soc Anim Sci Ithaca, 1980.

20. Sharp DC, Vernon MW, Zavy MT: Alteration of seasonal reproductive patterns in mares following superior cervical ganglionectomy. J Reprod Fertil Suppl 27:87, 1979.

21. Thompson DL, Godke RA, Nett TM: Effects of melatonin and thyrotropin releasing hormone on mares during the nonbreeding season. J Anim Sci 56:668, 1983.

22. Turek F, Desjardin C, Menaker M: Melatonin: Antigonadal and progonadal effects in male golden hamsters. Science 190:280, 1975.

Gestation and Pregnancy Diagnosis in the Mare

S. J. Roberts, D.V.M., M.S.
Woodstock, Vermont

Equine theriogenology has rapidly advanced in the past 30 years with many significant reports being published on ovulation, fertilization, embryology, fetal and placental physiology and disease, endocrine studies, methods of pregnancy diagnosis, abortion and other diseases associated with pregnancy.

OVULATION, FERTILIZATION, EMBRYOLOGY, FETAL AND PLACENTAL DEVELOPMENT

Ovulation in mares requires a healthy, well-nourished mare and occurs naturally during seasons with increasing or long periods of daylight, such as late spring through early fall, or by artificial lighting in late fall through the early spring months. The transition period between anestrus and the normal breeding season in the early spring and late fall is characterized by irregular estrous cycles, abnormal estrous behavior and failure of ovulation. Maturing graafian or ovarian follicles grow rapidly during estrus and reach 1 to 3 or more inches (2.5 to 7.5 cm) in diameter before ovulation. Just prior to ovulation, which occurs in the ovulation fossa or concave aspect of the ovary, the follicle wall becomes softer and less tense. Once estrous cycles in mares have commenced in the breeding season, ovulation can usually be induced within 24 to 48 hours during estrus after intramuscular or subcutaneous injection of 2500 to 4000 IU of human chorionic gonadotropin (hCG). Repeated injections at subsequent estrous periods during the same breeding season have not been as effective in inducing early ovulations, possibly because of the production of antibodies to hCG. Gonadotropin-releasing hormone (GnRH) and pregnant mare serum (PMSG) have very limited value in inducing follicle formation and ovulation in the mare.

Most ovulations in the mare occur toward the end of estrus or within 24 to 48 hours before signs of estrus cease. Only occasionally do ovulations occur prior to 48 hours before the end of estrus or after estrus terminates. Following ovulation, the follicle fills with a large, soft blood clot, the corpus hemorrhagicum, that on rectal palpation may be mistaken for a follicle just prior to ovulation. The corpus luteum develops rapidly in the ovarian substance but is seldom palpable 4 or 5 days after ovulation because of the thick ovarian tunic. Various studies have reported that 15 to 30 per cent of equine estrous periods are characterized by twin or double ovulations. Ovulations during diestrus or during the first 120 days of gestation are not uncommon.

Since sperm capacitation time is short, and normal spermatozoa survive 2 to 4 or more days in the mare's genital tract during estrus, most mares are bred, and fertile sperm are present in the uterine tube, at the time of ovulation.

Equine ova are probably ovulated as primary oocytes that mature and are capable of being fertilized within a few hours after entering the uterine tube. Fertilization occurs soon afterward, with the first cell cleavage within 24 hours after ovulation. The fertilized, dividing ovum enters the uterus about 5 to 6 days after ovulation. Unfertilized ova ovulated during estrus, diestrus or pregnancy frequently remain in the uterine tubes for weeks or months. Recently ovulated ova die or lose their ability to be fertilized within a short period after ovulation, probably within 2 to 12 hours.

The gestation period, or pregnancy, extends from fertilization to parturition and has been divided into two periods.

In the mare the period of the embryo extends from conception to about 55 to 60 days of gestation, during which time the fertilized ovum, usually in the morula stage, enters the uterus from the oviduct. The zona pellucida fragments and the blastula, or blastocyst, develop and inhibit the release of the luteolytic substance, probably prostaglandin, from the endometrium. This occurs after about 12 to 15 days of gestation with the "maternal recognition of pregnancy." This prevents the normal involution of the corpus luteum, which is secreting progesterone necessary for endometrial development and release of uterine glandular secretions to nourish the blastocyst and early embryo.

During this period, especially the first half, rapid growth and differentiation of the tissues and the organs of the major body systems occur. By 38 days of gestation the embryo is recognizable as a horse. The embryonic (chorionic) vesicle, which is round in shape until about 25 to 30 days of gestation, increases in size from 2.5 cm at day 18 to 6 cm at day 38 of gestation. After day 30, the embryonic vesicle becomes more oval in shape. The chorionic girdle of the embryonic vesicle develops rapidly between days 25 and 36, when it is about 5 mm in width. Between days 36 and 38 the girdle separates from the fetal membranes, and its cells invade the endometrium to form the endometrial cups that by day 40 of gestation are producing large amounts of equine gonadotropin (ECG). By day 45 of gestation, the chorioallantois has extended beneath and replaced the entire surface of the chorioamniotic vesicle. It is probable that firm attachment of the placental villi to the endometrial sulci occurs between 50 and 70 days of gestation. Before 15 days of gestation there is definite evidence of transuterine migration of the conceptus between the right and left uterine horns and body in all pregnant mares.[2]

The period of the fetus extends from 55 to 60 days of gestation to parturition. During this period minor details in the differentiation of tissues, organs and systems occur, along with the growth and maturation of the fetus (Table 1). The increase in the size of the fetus during gestation is a geometric-like curve, with the weight increasing very rapidly during the last 2 to 3 months of pregnancy. For this reason, special attention to the level and quality of nutritive intake should be considered during the latter third of gestation. The equine fetal gonads reach a total weight of 50 gm or more at about 250 days of gestation because of a marked increase in the interstitial cells that secrete estrogens. This results in a marked rise in the concentration of that hormone in the dam's plasma. By 300 days the fetal gonads have begun their regression in size, with degenerative changes being apparent. The cause of this great increase in size of the equine fetal gonads between 120 to 280 days of gestation is not known.

Evidence indicates that fetal gonadal growth occurs concurrently, possibly coincidentally, with the involution of the endometrial cups.

Prior to the development of the chorioallantois, the nutritive needs of the developing embryo are absorbed from endometrial secretions through the blastodermic vesicle, the yolk sac and the amniotic chorion, respectively. At 20 to 30 days the yolk sac has largely regressed and the chorioallantois is nearly completely formed. By 90 days the chorioallantoic villi attached in the endometrial crypts provide for nutrients to and waste removal from the fetus via their respective circulatory vessels in the diffuse placenta characteristic of Equidae.

Toward the end of gestation the amount of amniotic fluid surrounding the equine fetus is 3000 to 7000 ml, and the amount of allantoic fluid is 8000 to 18,000 ml.[1] Amorphous, semisolid, amber-colored, soft, pliable, rubberlike, irregular-shaped, flattened masses or bodies with thin edges 2.5 to 15 cm in diameter and 0.3 to 3.8 cm in thickness are commonly found floating in fluids in the allantoic cavity. These are called hippomanes or "colts' tongues." In mares, the fetus is surrounded by the viscous amniotic fluid derived from the skin, amniotic epithelium, fetal urine, saliva and secretions of the nasopharynx of the fetus. The volume of amniotic fluid is somewhat regulated by ingestion of the fluid by the fetus. The fetus and the amniotic membranes in the mare float freely in the allantoic cavity, which is filled with watery allantoic fluid primarily from the excretion of the fetal kidneys. The equine fetus is attached to the amniotic and chorioallantoic membranes only by the long, 40- to 80-cm umbilical cord, which is usually moderately twisted.

The fetal membranes and fetus develop mainly in the body and one horn of the uterus, with a small extension of the membranes into the nongravid horn. Villi are present on the entire surface of the chorioallantois except in the region of the internal os of the cervix, the cervical "star" region. During the first half of gestation the equine fetus, which is small, can lie in any direction, but after the seventh month the fetus is longer than the diameter of the gravid uterine horn and body and is located longitudinally in these structures. Very rarely, 1 in 1000 gestations, single equine fetuses may develop in both horns as bicornual or transverse pregnancies. These usually result in severe dystocia at the time of parturition. During late equine pregnancy it is generally agreed that the fetus rests with its back on the ventrolateral abdominal wall in the dorsoilial or dorsopubic position. More than 99 per cent of equine fetuses are in anterior presentation with the fetal head toward the cervix by the eighth or ninth month of gestation.

TWINNING IN THE MARE

Twin births occur rarely, about 0.5 per cent, in the equine species. If observed abortions of twins

Table 1. Size and Characteristics of the Equine Fetus and Uterus During Pregnancy*

Day of Gestation	Size and Shape of Chorionic Vesicle	Amount of Fetal Fluids (ml)	Weight of Fetus	Diameter of Horn Containing Fetus	Length of Fetus (Crown-Rump)	Fetal and Placental Characteristics
16	5.2 cm Pigeon's egg (round)				0.32 cm	
20	6.0 cm Bantam's egg (round)				0.66 cm	
25	6.8 cm Pullet's egg (slightly oval)	30–40			0.6–0.85 cm	
30	7.5 cm Small hen's egg (oval)	40–50	0.2 gm	4.5–5 cm	0.9–1.0 cm	Eyes, mouth and limb buds visible, chorionic vesicle present only in the uterine horn
35	8.5 cm Large hen's egg (oval)	60–90		4.5–6.5 cm	1.5 cm	
40	10.0 cm Turkey's egg (oval)	100–150		7–8.5 cm	1.8–2.2 cm	Eyelids and pinnae have appeared
45	10.5 cm Goose's egg (oval)	150–200		7.5–9 cm	2.0–3.0 cm	
50	11.5 cm Orange (oval)	200–350		8.3–9.5 cm	3.0–3.5 cm	
60	13.3 × 8.9 cm Small melon (oval)	300–500	10–20 gm	8.9–10 cm	4–7.5 cm	Lips, nostrils and development of feet observed; eyelids partially closed; placenta not attached but beginning to go into the body of uterus
90	23 × 14 cm Small football (oval)	1200–3000	100–180 gm	12.5–15 cm	10–14 cm	Villi of placenta present but without firm attachment, mammary nipples and hooves visible, body and horn of uterus both involved and enlarged
120		3000–4000	700–1000 gm		15–20 cm	External genitalia formed but scrotum is empty; placenta attached, ergots and orbital areas prominent
150		5000–8000	1500–3000 gm		25–37 cm	May or may not have fine hair on orbital arch and tip of tail, prepuce not yet developed
180		6000–10,000	3–5 kg		35–60 cm	Hair on lips, orbital arch, nose and eyelashes and fine hair on mane
210		6000–10,000	7–10 kg		55–70 cm	Hair on lips, nose, eyelids, edge of ears, tip of tail, back and mane
240		6000–12,000	12–18 kg		60–80 cm	Hair on mane and tail, back and distal portion of extremities
270		8000–12,000	20–27 kg		80–90 cm	Short, fine hair over entire body
300		10,000–20,000	25–40 kg		70–130 cm	Body completely covered with short hair, prepuce developed, hair on mane and tail increased
330		10,000–20,000	30–50 kg		100–150 cm	Complete hair coat and hair coat gets its final color, testes descend

*Modified from Roberts SJ: Veterinary Obstetrics and Genital Diseases. 3rd ed. Ann Arbor, Edwards Bros Inc, 1986.

are included, this figure increases to about 1.5 per cent. Double ovulations occur in 4 to 44 (average 16) per cent of equine estrous periods and especially in certain "twin-prone" mares. There is presently a lack of published data to link twinning in mares with heredity, as occurs in other species. Double ovulations may be synchronous, occurring within several to 48 hours of each other, or asynchronous, occurring several days or more apart. Recent evidence indicates that twin pregnancy is usually associated with asynchronous ovulations rather than synchronous ovulations because of a well-developed "mechanism" in mares that eliminates one or both twin embryos resulting from synchronous ovulations. Nearly all equine twin pregnancies are of the fraternal or dizygotic type. Monozytotic twin pregnancies are rare. The incidence of triplets in mares is extremely rare, possibly 1 in 300,000 births. Evidence would indicate that in 95 per cent of mares with twin ovulations one or both ova or embryos are lost early in the gestation period. This could be a common cause of equine infertility. The surviving twin embryos are usually bicornual in location. Between 6 and 9 months of gestation one or both fetuses may die, and abortion of both fetuses is common. Even in twin pregnancies proceeding to term both twins are seldom born in a viable state. Usually, one is expelled dead or as a mummified fetus, together with a live but frequently small or weak twin. This high death rate, greater than 90 per cent, in twin pregnancies surviving beyond 120 to 150 days of gestation is apparently caused by a competition between twin fetuses for placental area. Although the chorions may fuse, anastomosis of blood vessels between the two placentae does not occur. One chorion invaginates into the other, and the smaller, growth-retarded fetus with the smaller placental area dies because of a lack of nutrients and is expelled prematurely along with the larger fetus. Alternatively, it may mummify and remain in the uterus to be expelled at parturition with the live fetus that had the larger placental area.

Various procedures have been tried in mares to avoid or prevent twin pregnancies.

These have included the following:

1. Monitoring ovulations by repeated rectal examinations of the "twin-prone" mare's ovaries and breeding only when one follicle matures.

2. If two large, mature follicles are found on rectal palpation do one of the following: (1) don't breed the mare until possibly the next estrus; (2) tap one follicle per vaginam with an ovarian needle; or (3) wait until one follicle ovulates and then breed 12 to 18 hours later, after the first unfertilized ovum has died.

3. If twin pregnancy is diagnosed early in pregnancy (20 to 35 days) by rectal palpation or ultrasound techniques, then abortion may be induced by one of the following methods: (1) attempt to crush one embryonic vesicle manually or destroy one embryo by inserting a needle or trocar into the embryonic vesicle after a laparotomy operation, which usually results in abortion of both embryos;

(2) dilate the cervix and douche the uterus to cause abortion and then rebreed at the next estrus; (3) inject the mare intramuscularly with prostaglandin $F_{2\alpha}$ ($PGF_{2\alpha}$) or a prostaglandin analog to produce luteolysis and abortion and then rebreed at the next estrus or (4) allow the twin pregnancy to proceed to term, with the hope that twin abortion will not occur and that one or both fetuses will be born alive.

4. Embryo transfer might be considered in the "twin-prone" mare.

None of these procedures used to prevent or to "treat" equine twin pregnancies is highly satisfactory in the control of this common condition.

Recent field studies have indicated that attempting to crush one embryonic vesicle manually may be a practical procedure if performed by a skilled veterinarian before 30 days of gestation and if the twin embryos are located separately, one in each horn. The use of a prostaglandin antagonist such as phenylbutazone (Butazolidin) or flunixin meglumine may be of value in this procedure. Further controlled studies are indicated. If mares with twin pregnancies are aborted after 35 to 40 days of gestation when the endometrial cups are formed and producing ECG, normal estrous cycling and ovulation usually do not occur until the endometrial cups have involuted several months later. Exogenous supplemental progesterone administered to mares with twin pregnancies may prevent impending abortion in the latter half of gestation and result in the birth of a live normal fetus and a mummified fetus at term. Pregnant mares in mid- to late gestation that suddenly show mammary development and leak milk and show marked relaxation of the perineum and vulva should be given 250 to 500 mg of progesterone in oil daily or 500 to 1000 mg of repositol progesterone every 2 to 4 days for several weeks until these signs recede. Some veterinarians continue supplementation with 1000 to 2000 mg of repositol progesterone every 4 to 7 days until 2 weeks before expected foaling. Injections of prostaglandin antagonists during signs of impending abortion may be desirable. Further studies are indicated.

HORMONAL CONTROL OF EQUINE GESTATION

After ovulation, the corpus luteum develops in the ruptured follicle and produces progesterone, which reaches a significant blood plasma concentration of 6 to 15 ng/ml by day 5. This production rate continues in the pregnant mare until about day 150 of gestation, after which progesterone levels markedly decline. PMSG or ECG is produced by the endometrial cups. The endometrial cups originating from the chorionic girdle of the embryonic vesicle produce PMSG levels detectable as early as 32 to 36 days of gestation. However, high or diagnostic levels of 40 to 80 IU/ml are not reached until 40 days of gestation and then persist at a high level until 90 days, after which the serum levels of PMSG decline rapidly. Mares carrying mule conceptuses have greatly reduced (one tenth) production of PMSG, while donkeys carrying hinny (horse-ass hybrids) conceptuses show greatly increased PMSG levels. It is now generally accepted that PMSG or ECG has no effect on the dam's ovaries. However, high levels of FSH and LH from the dam's pituitary gland cause follicle formation, ovulation and formation of secondary or accessory corpora lutea from days 30 or 40 to 120 of gestation. These corpora lutea regress or involute after 150 days of gestation.

Placental progestogen, especially the 5-pregnanes, production probably begins at approximately days 50 to 70 of gestation and supplements the progesterone produced by the primary and secondary corpora lutea until about midpregnancy, when the corpora lutea regress. Ovariectomy can be performed in the mare after 120 to 150 days of gestation without causing abortion. Progestogen plasma levels gradually rise in the latter half of pregnancy to 8 to 16 ng/ml until the end of gestation. Estrogen levels in the plasma of pregnant mares rise from 10 to 20 pg/ml before 120 days to a peak of 800 pg/ml between 180 to 270 days of gestation and then decline to about 150 pg/ml at parturition. Both estrogens and progestogens produced by the fetoplacental unit fall rapidly to very low levels after foaling.

Follicular development in ovaries of pregnant mares increases from 10 to 20 days of gestation to a peak in size and number at 50 to 60 days of pregnancy, probably under the influence of pituitary gonadotropins. Then follicular activity decreases, and by day 220 the ovaries contain no large follicles and are small, hard and inactive.[2]

The initiation of parturition or the termination of gestation in the mare is probably brought about by the presence of relatively high levels of estrogens, a modest increase in fetal glucocorticoids, an increase in prostaglandins and, terminally, an increase in levels of oxytocin. Other hormones such as relaxin may also play a role. Mares apparently can control the actual onset of labor by a number of hours, since 80 to 85 per cent of parturitions occur at night, with most occurring within 2 hours of midnight.

DURATION OF THE EQUINE GESTATION PERIOD

The duration of the gestation period of the mare varies from 327 to 357 days, with an average duration of 340 to 342 days. Draft mares may foal after a slightly shorter gestation period of 330 to 340 days. Ass-horse hybrids have a longer gestation of 350 to 355 days, approaching that of asses (356 to 375 days). Male fetuses usually have a gestation period that is 1 to 2 days longer than female fetuses. In the Northern Hemisphere foals born from January through April have gestation periods about 10 days longer than foals born from May through September. Short gestation periods in conjunction with abortions or premature births may be associated with twinning. Prolonged equine gestation periods of up to 375 days and even longer, with the delivery of a live foal, have rarely been reported. The duration of gestation in the mare may be shortened slightly by injections of prostaglandins, glucocorticoids, estrogens and oxytocin given late in gestation. The practical induction of parturition will be discussed in a subsequent article.

EQUINE TERATOLOGY OR INHERITED DEVELOPMENTAL ANOMALIES

Inherited or genetic lethal or semilethal defects reported in horses include atresia coli in Percherons, hemophilia, sterility (Fredricksborg lethal) in white horses, epitheliogenesis imperfecta of the lower limb (sex-linked lethal), hereditary ataxia in the Oldenburg breed and "wobbles" or incoordination seen in all breeds, especially in Thoroughbreds, Standardbreds and the American Saddle Horse. The latter is most common in male animals, and the inherited form of the disease results in a compression of the spinal cord in the cervical region caused by defective development of the cervical vertebrae. In recent years four or five other causes of incoordination or symptoms of "wobbles" have been described in horses. Other lethal defects include cerebellar hypoplasia in Arabian horses, absence of a retina, combined immunodeficiency in Arabian foals, hemophilia, hyperelastosis cutis, iliocolonic aganglionosis in white foals of Overo breeding and hydrocephalus.

Inherited nonlethal defects in horses include congenital blindness, aniridia with cataracts in Belgium horses, umbilical hernia, cryptorchidism, brachygnathia, subluxation of the patella (especially in ponies), multiple exostoses in Quarterhorses and Thoroughbreds, heaves or pulmonary emphysema, laryngeal hemiplegia (roaring) and hip dysplasia in Dole horses. Other possible nonlethal inherited defects include scrotal hernia, side bone, hypotrichosis congenita, nyctalopia (night blindness), osteochondrosis dissecans and sterility in mules and hinnies.

Congenital defects or anomalies of a nonhereditary nature are not uncommon in horses and may arise from ingested teratogens (including drugs or chemicals), radiation, endocrine disturbances, possibly nutritional deficiencies and possibly viral infections during the first third or half of gestation or from chromosomal anomalies caused by aging of the gametes in the uterine tube before fertilization, which is quite possible in horses. These congenital developmental errors include arthrogryposis, hydrocephalus, pharyngeal anomalies, cyclopia, polydactyly, polydontia, teratomas, hermaphrodites or intersexes, cardiac anomalies, cleft palate, ectopic urethra, persistent urachus, anomalies or failure in development of the gonads or genital tract, entropion, cataracts, optic nerve hypoplasia, ectopia o the patella, dentigerous cysts, dermoid cysts and others. Conjoined twin fetuses are extremely rare in horses.[3]

PREGNANCY DIAGNOSIS IN THE MARE

Indicative or subjective history and signs of pregnancy in a mare include the following:

1. Services by a stallion
2. Cessation of estrous periods as determined by regular teasing at 1- to 2-day intervals through 45 days after service
3. Increased gentleness and docility by the third month of gestation
4. Enlargement of the abdomen, especially the ventral portion (pear-shaped abdomen), by the fifth month of gestation
5. Observation of fetal movements, especially after drinking cold water, by the seventh to eight month of gestation
6. Enlargement of the udder
7. Relaxation of the pelvic ligaments by the tenth month.

"Spurious" conception because of persistence of the corpus luteum, which is common in mares, may follow a normal service in a healthy cycling mare, in which further estrous cycles apparently cease and rectal examinations at a later date reveal that the mare is not pregnant. However, these signs, especially the early ones, may be misleading. The breeding history of the mare in previous years is helpful. Others may conceive but abort or absorb an early embryo prior to 90 days of gestation and not exhibit estrus. Furthermore, some mares (up to 10 per cent) may show signs of estrus for a short period during early gestation or be indifferent to a teaser stallion and yet be pregnant. Thus, a broodmare may exhibit widely contradictory behavior in respect to her true state of pregnancy. Ballottement of the fetus during late gestation in the mare is difficult because of the thick abdominal wall and the tensing of the abdominal muscles by the mare during this maneuver.

Internal Examination for Detecting Pregnancy in the Mare

Before the internal examination for detection of pregnancy in the mare is performed, a good clinical breeding history should be obtained, if possible. The foaling and breeding dates, dates of estrus, frequency and efficiency of teasing before and after breeding and knowledge of the regularity of the mare in her estrous cycles and past foalings are helpful.

The rectal diagnosis of pregnancy in the mare by an experienced veterinarian, next to a skilled examination utilizing a good ultrasound machine, is the earliest and most accurate method available. In performing a rectal examination in a mare, the same equipment, dress and mode of procedure are generally used as for examination in the cow. Restraint is more essential in mares. Many mares require the application of a nose twitch to control and make them stand quietly and prevent them from kicking the operator. Some veterinarians have the mare's tail forced firmly dorsally and cranially over the sacrum as a form of restraint. Certain excitable mares that object to restraint must be handled gently and quietly if a rectal examination is to be performed. Often these mares may be examined only by having a foreleg elevated. In rare cases tranquilization or even sedation with acepromazine or xylazine (Rompun) in addition to using a twitch may be required. If breeding hobbles are used to restrain a mare, kicking is prevented but the hocks may be raised suddenly and injure the operator if he is standing too close to the rear quarters. A mare can be examined in stocks, over or around a stall partition or by being backed up to a manger or to several bales of hay or straw. If a mare is in stocks, the rear rope or board should be low so that if the mare drops her hindquarters suddenly the examiner's arm will not be injured. It is best to bandage the mare's tail or have it held upward and to one side by an assistant so that the long tail hair does not irritate the anus and rectum at the time the examiner's arm is inserted and so that the tail does not become soiled.

A bland, nonirritating lubricant should be used on the arm. The rectum of the mare is drier than that of the cow, and the operator's arm requires frequent, liberal lubrication. The author favors a bucket of soapy water made with a bland soap and applied with a sponge to the arm and anus during the rectal examination without causing irritation of the rectum. Commercial lubricants such as K-Y jelly are also helpful. The peristaltic waves in the mare are stronger than in the cow. The hand and arm should be withdrawn from the rectum when a peristaltic contraction occurs. Trauma to the rectum of the mare is more easily produced than in the cow and has more serious and sometimes fatal results because of the mare's increased susceptibility to peritonitis. In the last 15 years over 10 per cent of the total equine malpractice suits in the United States were caused by rectal lacerations. Rectal examinations should therefore be made with quiet restraint, care and gentleness. Withholding feed, especially roughage, for 12 to 24 hours aids the examination.

After entering the rectum of the mare and locating the bony pelvis, it is easier to first locate one of the ovaries until, with more experience, the uterus can be readily found. The distinct, fibrous, bean-shaped ovary, 4 to 8 cm long and 3 to 5 cm thick, is located about 10 to 20 cm cranial to the shaft of the ilium and about 5 to 10 cm below the lumbar vertebrae in the nonpregnant mare or the mare in early pregnancy. The operator who uses his right hand can more readily locate the left ovary of the mare and vice versa. After locating one ovary, the hand is passed down the utero-ovarian ligament to the uterus. The uterus is cupped in the hand between the fingers and thumb, and palpation of the cranial border and ventral and dorsal portions of the nonpregnant or early pregnant uterine horns, the opposite ligament and the opposite ovary is performed. The nonpregnant, completely involuted uterus is pliable, soft, flat and rather flaccid and measures 4 to 7 cm wide and 2 to 5 cm thick. In the maiden or young mare the nonpregnant uterus is suspended above the floor of the pelvis and abdomen. In older mares, especially the first month after foaling, the uterus may be located more ventrally and may be hanging cranial to the floor of the pelvis in the abdominal cavity.[3]

Uterine Changes During Pregnancy

In most mares rectal palpation of the uterus to diagnose pregnancy can be performed by an experienced operator with great accuracy from 30 to 40 days of gestation. Diagnosis is usually easier for the less experienced veterinarian from 40 to 50 days of pregnancy. Pregnancy diagnosis is easier in maiden mares or primigravidae and in barren, nonfoaling mares than in mares conceiving during foal estrus when the uterus has not completely involuted. Zemjanis[5] and others have described their apparently skilled, careful techniques for diagnosing equine pregnancy manually from 17 to 30 days of gestation. Great care must be taken not to injure the embryo or the chorionic or embryonic vesicle. It is often desirable to reexamine the mare once or twice at bimonthly intervals to make certain that embryonic or fetal death and resorption or abortion has not occurred. In the mare, as in the cow, early embryonic deaths are not uncommon, with an incidence of 2 to 10 per cent or greater between early pregnancy diagnosis and 110 days of gestation.

The thickness of the uterine wall increases slightly in both pregnant and nonpregnant mares from days 10 to 16 after the onset of estrus. From day 16 to 21 there is a threefold increase in thickness in the uterine wall in pregnant mares, while in nonpregnant mares the thickness of the uterine wall declines to a low point at the onset of the next estrus. The tone of the uterine wall follows the same pattern, showing a definite increase in the tone of the uterine wall of both pregnant and nonpregnant mares to day 16, followed by a decline in tone in nonpregnant mares to a soft, flaccid state about 1 day before the next estrus. In pregnant mares the uterine tone continues to increase after day 16, with the uterine horn becoming round and tubular about 5 days later.

Thus, a careful examination of a mare 18 to 20 days after service may provide a presumptive diagnosis of pregnancy if the mare's uterus and cervix are tonic and contracted, if the vaginal examination reveals no hyperemia, edema or estrual mucus secretion in the anterior vagina or relaxation of the caudal cervical os and if the mare rejects the advances of the stallion. Determination of the mare's plasma or milk progesterone level would be indicative of pregnancy if the values were high. The accuracy of these signs is probably about 75 to 80 per cent because of possible embryonic deaths, persistence of a corpus luteum and other factors.

Palpation of the Chorionic or Embryonic Vesicle

During pregnancy the uterine horns enlarge (Table 1). The earliest that this can ordinarily be detected is 20 to 30 days of gestation. This enlargement is characterized by a circumscribed ventral bulge or distention of the uterine horn, usually just to the right or left of the bifurcation of the horns. A dorsal bulging of the horn is not observed until after 40 days of gestation and then is not marked. Rarely, the embryo and its membranes may develop more laterally in either horn or in the body of the uterus. The spherical bulge or swelling is caused by the chorionic or embryonic vesicle during early gestation and later by the oval chorioallantoic vesicle containing the enclosed amniotic sac and embryo, the vitelline or yolk sac and the allantoic fluid. From 3 to 6 weeks the vitelline or yolk sac is large, and the amniotic cavity around the embryo is small. The allantoic cavity grows rapidly and fills with fluid from 5 to 7 weeks of gestation. This embryonic vesicle at first is round or slightly oval and then, as it enlarges, assumes a more ovoid, tubular or sausage-shaped outline and extends into the body of the uterus after about 60 to 90 days of gestation. The uterine wall during this early stage of pregnancy is more tubular in shape, has a more tonic feel and is thinner over the ventral bulge. As in the cow, these changes are primarily caused by filling of the uterine horn and body with fetal membranes and fluid, imparting the feel of a heavy, water-filled rubber balloon. By 60 to 70 days the chorioallantoic vesicle is so large that it is difficult to delineate its extent, and the early tonus is less evident.

Manual slipping of fetal membranes, as in the cow, is not done in the mare because the discrete, localized oval area of the uterus occupied by the conceptus in early pregnancy readily differentiates pregnancy from pyometra or mucometra. The diffuse attachment of the equine chorion to the endometrium and the anatomic arrangement of the equine allantoic vessels militate against the slipping of the fetal membranes in the mare, as can be performed in the cow. The thicker, more tonic equine rectal wall makes this technique hazardous. Furthermore, such vigorous handling of the vesicle in very early pregnancy might cause embryonic death.

Palpation of the changes in the size of the horn and body containing the fetus has been outlined in Table 1. Since the size of the round, and later oval, chorionic and chorioallantoic vesicle is closely correlated with the diameter of the apposed uterine horn, the diagnosis and duration of early pregnancy may be ascertained.

The pregnant uterus in the mare is usually suspended above or on the level of the floor of the pelvis until the third to fourth month of gestation, when it drops enough to rest on the abdominal floor, at which time the ventral surface of the uterus cannot be palpated. In older mares the uterus may rest on the abdominal floor by the third month. When the uterus lies deep in the abdominal cavity, it can be drawn caudally by retraction on the cranial border of the broad ligament. If the mare is more than 3 months pregnant, it will be difficult or impossible to pull back the uterus, owing to its weight; whereas if the mare is not pregnant, the uterus can be drawn back and palpated. By the fifth to sixth month of pregnancy the uterus is well forward in the abdominal cavity, and the broad ligament is under definite tension. The ovary may be 20 to 25 cm below the lumbar vertebrae and is moved with difficulty because of the tense mesovarium.

Palpation of the fetus through the rectal wall can usually be performed by 90 to 120 days of gestation, at which time the fetus feels like a small, heavy, submerged but floating object as the hand contacts it. In most mares it is usually possible to palpate the fetus per rectum from the third month throughout the rest of the gestation period. The size and weight of the equine fetus during the various stages of pregnancy are noted in Table 1. In a few deep-bodied mares palpation of the fetus may be difficult from the fifth to seventh months of gestation. In these mares the location of the uterus, the position of the ovaries and the palpation of the enlarged, "whirring" uterine artery will aid or confirm a diagnosis of pregnancy.

Unlike the cow, palpation of the ovaries of the mare during early pregnancy is of no value in determining which uterine horn contains the fetus. A portion of the corpus luteum is palpable for only a few days after ovulation in the region of the ovulation fossa before it is covered by the dense, fibrous ovarian tunic. Furthermore, although ovulation occurs more commonly (52 to 63 per cent) in the left ovary, up to 60 per cent of the fetuses develop in the right horn. The fertilized embryo can undergo intrauterine migration in both directions; thus, the percentage of pregnancies in each horn is about equal or is a few percentage points higher in the right horn.

Investigators have reported some interesting findings concerning the ovaries of mares during pregnancy. They divided the gestation period into four periods in relation to the changes that occur in the ovaries. The first period, from ovulation to 40 days, was characterized by the presence of a single corpus luteum of pregnancy. A number of various-sized follicles up to 5 cm in diameter were usually present in pregnant mares from 10 to 40 days of gestation on both ovaries. The second period, from 40 to 150 days, was characterized by marked ovarian activity with as many as 10 to 15 follicles over 1 cm in diameter and the formation of accessory or secondary corpora lutea. Ovulation occurred during this period. Usually three to five or more accessory

corpora lutea were present in each ovary. The diameters of the largest follicles were greatest about 50 to 60 days of gestation. This ovarian activity, with follicle and corpora lutea formation, was probably produced by the high level of gonadotropic hormones, especially FSH, secreted by the anterior pituitary gland. The third period, from 150 to 210 days, was characterized by a regression of the corpora lutea. Large follicles were absent. During the fourth period, from 210 days to foaling, no corpora lutea or follicles were present. Throughout these latter two periods gestation was maintained by steroid hormones produced in the placenta.[4]

The vaginal examination as an aid to pregnancy diagnosis may be helpful, especially about 18 to 20 days after service, as described previously. It is not as accurate as the rectal examination of the uterus. By 30 days of pregnancy the normal equine vagina and cervix are very white and pale on examination with a speculum. In fact, they are more white and pale than at any time during the estrous cycle and resemble a mare's vagina in anestrus during the winter months. By 60 to 90 days of pregnancy the mucous membrane is usually very dry, sticky and gummy. There is less tendency for the vagina to balloon when the speculum is inserted than there is during the estrous cycle. More of this gummy mucus is present on the mucous membrane of the vagina during pregnancy than during the anestrous period. About 75 per cent of pregnant mares show these characteristic vaginal changes. The other pregnant mares may show a more hyperemic or congested mucous membrane with less mucus. In rare cases a vaginitis with a mucopurulent exudate may be seen. The cervix in pregnant mares is usually tightly closed and small with a puckered external os. It is usually pulled downward and to one side. The external os of the cervix usually becomes covered with gummy, sticky mucus. In advanced pregnancy it may be easier to palpate the fetus through the vagina than through the rectum, as the mare objects less to the vaginal examination.

Differential Diagnosis

Differential diagnosis as part of pregnancy examinations should be considered by the inexperienced examiner. From 70 to 110 days a distended bladder may be confused with pregnancy. Pneumovagina, or a uterus filled with air, might be mistaken for pregnancy. From 90 to 120 days an enlarged or distended right colon or pelvic flexure of the colon might rarely be confused with a pregnant uterus. Pyometra and mucometra associated with focal cystic degeneration of the endometrium are occasionally found in the mare. In this condition the uterine wall may be thick and heavy, and the fluid contents of the uterus are sluggish. Tumors, usually leiomyomas, are rare in the mare. Mummification of a single fetus has not been observed in the mare. Fetal maceration is uncommon.

Double ovulation occurs in 16 to 20 (range 4 to

44), per cent of mares, and twin pregnancies are quite commonly diagnosed. But the incidence of twin births is low (0.5 per cent) because of embryonic or fetal death and abortion of possibly one or, more often, of both fetuses. Twin embryos may be detected from 20 to 60 days of gestation by the palpation of two chorioallantoic vesicle or ventral bulges, often with one vesicle in each horn. Occasionally, both vesicles are in one horn and result in a uterine enlargement that is up to twice as large as would be expected for a normal single vesicle at that stage of gestation. Later, twin fetuses might be palpated and both uterine arteries might be enlarged. Embryonic deaths in mares may be diagnosed at 30 to 45 days by a loss of fluid and tone in the chorioallantoic vesicle. The uterine wall, however, may remain tonic and thick for a considerable period, even though the size of the ventral bulge regresses. These mares may not return to estrus for 40 to 80 days, possibly because of the "persistence of the corpus luteum." Douching the uterus with 500 ml of warm saline, if performed before 35 to 38 days of gestation, or the injection of 10 mg of $PGF_{2\alpha}$ usually results in a return to estrus within a few days in these mares. If these treatments are instituted after 40 days of gestation when the endometrial cups are present, normal estrous cycling and ovulation does not usually occur for 2 or more months. If early embryonic death is suspected, repeated examinations per rectum may be necessary for confirmation.

Other abnormalities of the mare's uterus that might be confused with early pregnancy include large endometrial cysts up to 5 cm or more in diameter; a doughy, flaccid myometrial lymphatic lacuna and a focal atony of the myometrium and endometrium in the region to the right and left of the uterine bifurcation that may cause ventral bulges of the uterine horn. However, careful palpation will usually reveal that these pathologic structures are thicker walled and lack the fluid feel of an embryonic vesicle and that the uterine wall lacks the characteristic marked tonicity noted in pregnant uteri. These findings are usually seen in older mares.

Biologic and Other Tests for Pregnancy in the Mare

The biologic tests for pregnancy in the mare are based on the presence of high levels of certain hormones at various stages of pregnancy. Some of these tests are highly accurate and useful in very nervous or vicious mares and small ponies, in which rectal examinations are dangerous or impossible, and also when the veterinarian is not experienced in manual examination for pregnancy.

The most practical biologic tests for pregnancy in the mare determine the presence of PMSG or ECG between 40 and 120 days of gestation. This hormone is produced by the endometrial cups. Tests commonly used for detecting PMSG in mare's serum are the Aschheim-Zondek (A-Z) rat test, or rabbit test and the mare immunologic pregnancy (MIP) test. The former A-Z immature rat test, or its modification, is still commonly used in many laboratories having a ready supply of young rats. The MIP test is presently the most widely used test in the United States because it can easily be performed in the field or office, is over 90 per cent accurate and results can be obtained within a few hours.

The MIP test is a hemagglutination inhibition test utilizing the principle that PMSG inhibits the agglutination of sheep erythrocytes coated with PMSG in the presence of PMSG antiserum from rabbits. Recent studies have shown that between 40 and 120 days of gestation the MIP test and the A-Z test are more reliable than the rectal palpation method for diagnosing pregnancy, unless the palpation is performed by a highly experienced diagnostician. Early embryonic or fetal death loss from 45 to 90 days of gestation is fairly common in mares. If PMSG levels become elevated before the death of the conceptus, these levels will remain high and give a false-positive test. The incidence of false-negative MIP tests is generally low, unless blood is drawn from mares before 40 days or after 120 days of gestation, the mare is carrying a mule fetus or the serum is overheated.[3]

Other less practical and less accurate mare biologic pregnancy tests include the Cuboni method for detecting high levels of estrogen in the urine between 120 and 290 days of gestation. This chemical test is most accurate from 150 to 250 days.

Tests such as radioimmunoassay (RIA) or competitive protein binding for determining levels of progestogens or estrogens in blood serum can be used about 17 to 21 days after service and ovulation to determine whether conception possibly occurred. However, when mares are teased regularly, less than 7 per cent of the nonpregnant mares have not returned to estrus by 24 days.

References

1. Arthur GH: Veterinary Reproduction and Obstetrics. 4th ed, London, Bailliere and Tindall, 1975.
2. Ginther OJ: Reproductive Biology of the Mare. Cross Plaines, Wisconsin, 1979.
3. Roberts SJ: Veterinary Obstetrics and Genital Diseases. 3rd ed, Woodstock, Vermont, 1986.
4. Rossdale PD, Ricketts SW: Equine Stud Farm Medicine. 2nd ed, Philadephia, Lea & Febiger, 1980.
5. Zemjanis R: Diagnostic and Therapeutic Techniques in Animal Reproduction. Baltimore, The Williams & Wilkins Co, 1970.

Ultrasound: An Aid for Pregnancy Detection in the Mare

S. J. Burns, D.V.M., M.S.
G. E. Layton, D.V.M.
Paris, Kentucky

Ultrasound examination in human reproduction has become commonplace, although the objective is primarily to examine a fetus for abnormalities rather than to diagnose pregnancy. The procedure is utilized well after the completion of organogenesis, with the scanning head applied over the abdominal wall. This scanning method has been attempted in domestic animals in an effort to establish an early diagnosis of pregnancy. The method has not been satisfactory for mares, producing an accurate diagnosis in only 59 per cent of examinations performed at less than 18 days; 86 per cent of examinations performed at 18 to 60 days; 77 per cent of those performed at 61 to 90 days and 52 per cent of those performed at 121 to 260 days.[14] The major obstacles to success using this method include the large abdominal size of the mare, the distance between the soundwave source and the target and the presence of gas-filled bowel between the sound source and the uterus. The primary objective for the use of ultrasound examination in animal reproduction is to assist in the early, accurate detection of pregnancy, so the technique is employed much earlier in the animal's gestation than in the human patient.

The probe that emits the sound waves is inserted into the rectum, allowing much closer approximation to the target organs being examined. The first serious effort to apply this concept to examination of the mare was reported by Fraser and colleagues,[4] who used a doppler ultrasound transducer in the rectum to detect a fetal pulse—occasionally as early as day 42 and consistently after day 90. Palmer and Draincourt[9] were the first to use a real-time multi-crystal probe to observe the equine conceptus in 1979. The clinical application of ultrasound as an aid for pregnancy detection in mares is still very recent, so there are many questions regarding its use that remain unresolved. A more complete understanding of the events of early pregnancy in mares shall emerge as experience and acceptance of the technique increases.

PHYSICS OF ULTRASOUND

It is worthwhile to eliminate some of the mystery of ultrasound physics before exploring clinical applications. Sound waves produce echoes that vary in intensity depending on the density of the reflecting surface. The echoes produced as one walks down a tile-lined hallway are more pronounced than those produced if the corridor is lined with less dense acoustic tile. Almost no echo would be produced if the hall were lined with an even less dense material, such as cotton. These physical laws remain unchanged when passing ultrasound waves through tissues of varying densities.

Sound waves, as we hear them, are actually alterations in compression of air molecules that travel in a straight line. They are longitudinal waves with repetitive patterns of compressed air (compression) followed by areas of decreased density (rarefaction). These wave lengths can be measured in the number of cycles per second, referred to as hertz. The upper limit of human hearing is about 20,000 cycles/second (hertz). Most units used for diagnostic ultrasound operate at a frequency of 2 to 5 million cycles/second; 1 million cycles/second is called a megahertz, hence the term "ultrasound," meaning sound waves well beyond the range of human hearing. As these sound waves are produced and pass through tissue, the echo reflected by the tissue will vary with the density of the tissue or acoustical impedance. The greater the density, the stronger the echo it will return.

The sound produced by a vibrating object is determined by its size, which controls its resonant frequency. A large bell produces longer sound waves of a lower tone than a small bell. To make ultrasound, it is necessary to make a very small object vibrate. This is accomplished by electrical stimulation of a piezoelectric crystal. The molecular arrangement of these crystals is very rigid. Rather than being deformed by the energy of an electrical impulse, the whole crystal will vibrate. This vibration produces the waves that are directed at the target tissue for reflection. The transformation from electrical to mechanical energy is called transduction. The source of the ultrasound waves in the rectal probe is therefore called a transducer. The crystal is subjected to high frequency bursts of electricity and it will return to its resting state between stimulations. While in its resting state, we can "listen" for any returning echoes from the tissues penetrated by the ultrasound beam. The crystal may be pulsed 1,000 to 2,000 times each second and the crystal will vibrate at a rate of 2 to 5 million times per second during each individual pulse.[10]

Having gone to all this trouble to produce an ultrasound echo that cannot be heard, we must convert this energy to something we can sense for interpretive evaluation. We can make visual appraisal of this information by using a cathode ray tube to trace the amplitude (hence the term A-mode) of the echoes produced as a function of time or distance. This mode will measure echoes as waves but will not easily portray anatomic information. A second method of evaluation converts the echo to various intensities of brightness on a series of spots on the face of the cathode ray tube, hence the term B-mode for brightness. When enough of these dots are present and there are adequate differences in brightness, an image can be formed on a display screen that allows a two-dimensional view of the tissue directly under the transducer. The combination of a transducer coupled with a B-mode display produces the B-scan commonly used in clinical practice. If the B-mode display is moved over a recording device at a constant rate, it will record any motion of the tissue reflecting the echo, hence the term M-mode.[11]

The brightness of the dots on the cathode ray tube is projected in various shades of gray much like a black and white photograph. Echoes of many amplitudes will be produced, but the display system will group them into 10 to 64 different shades of gray. The human eye can only detect about 10 different shades of gray if there is no contrast with which to compare them. A greater range of gray level above 10 will increase contrast and shading, thereby producing a more blended image. If these images are produced and erased in rapid sequence, they will reveal any motion in the tissue being imaged. This is the basis of "real-time" scanning. The rapid scanning and erasing can be accomplished in two ways. The transducer can be made to rock back and forth on its long axis producing a pie shaped image referred to as a sector scan. A second system involves electrical stimulation of many small transducers lined up side by side. These produce a rectangular display called a linear scan. We will now comment on the mechanical techniques used in the examination of mares with this greatly simplified explanation of ultrasound wave propagation as a foundation.

EXAMINATION TECHNIQUE

Ultrasound examinations should be unhurried and methodical. It is difficult to examine more than six to eight mares an hour unless the mares are concentrated in one area and presented for examination in rotation in two or more stocks. It is quite possible to overlook features or misinterpret images if the operator is too hasty. Ultrasound machines are relatively expensive, so it is best to leave the unit outside the stall during the course of the examination. This can be accomplished if the mare is placed in stocks or is placed with her hind quarters halfway out of the stall door. The examination area should be fairly dark as images are very difficult to see and follow if the display screen is in excessive light. Most mares will tolerate examination with only the usual amount of restraint employed during rectal-digital examination. The feces are removed from the rectum, and the reproductive tract is

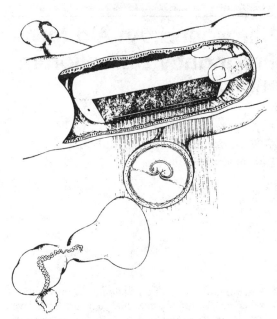

Figure 1. The scanner probe in a mare's rectum, with the verticle linear array beam giving a cross-sectional or "bacon slice" image of the conceptus in the pregnant uterine horn.

palpated to determine its location, size and targets of interest. The examiner will make mental note of the distance of the tract from the anal sphincter, for this will assist in placing the transducer in the proper position over the uterus. The transducer emitting surface is coated with a lubricant so that no air pockets will occur between the transducer and the tissues being examined. The transducer is inserted into the rectum and advanced with the emitting surface beamed ventrally toward the uterus. The transducer is placed in the rectum parallel to its long axis and thus at nearly a right angle to the long axis of the uterus. It is quite surprising how frequently the first identifiable structure observed will be the pregnancy. This, however, does not signal the conclusion of the examination. The uterus will appear gray while fluid-filled structures such as the vesicle or an endometrial cyst will appear dark or black. The image on the display is presented as if the viewer is looking down the long axis of the uterus and examining the cross section of each of the slices. The uterus will appear as a reasonably circular structure with a granular gray center. The surrounding tissue will appear a more dense, lighter gray. The uterus will appear larger and darker during estrus due to its increased lumenal fluid content and endometrial edema. The probe is moved laterally in both directions to examine both uterine horns. The circular image of the uterus is maintained on the center of the display by moving the transducer cranially or caudally as necessary. The termination of the uterine horn may be noted by visualization of the ovary identifiable by the appearance of several small spherical "cysts," which are follicles. The ovary may be very difficult to visualize if there are no follicles on it. Each uterine horn should be examined at least twice to reduce the possibility of overlooking a pregnancy.

Normal Observations

An embryonic vesicle can be observed with ultrasound 14 days after ovulation. From 15 to 20 days the pregnancy will appear as a black circular structure that may have an echogenic spot at its dorsal or ventral limits. The embryo is probably not visible at this time. From days 20 to 25 the shape of the vesicle may appear irregular or triangular, as its fluid pressure is not great enough to overcome pressure from the uterine walls. The embryo appears as a small flat disc on the border of the vesicle, which gradually becomes circular and approaches the center of the vesicle. A fetal heartbeat may be detected as early as 24 days. From day 25 to 30 the vesicle develops sufficient fluid pressure that it is once again nearly circular. The fetal heartbeat should be reasonably evident if the conceptus is normal and the lighting and adjustments on the display screen are properly set. From days 30 to 50 the vesicle increases in size rapidly, and the embryo is readily apparent. The size of the vesicle increases with the days of pregnancy and is influenced by the type and breed of mare. Draft mares seem to average larger vesicles, while vesicles in mares carrying their first foals seem to be smaller than average. There is great variation in size within vesicles of the same age. Standard deviations resulting from examination of 1075 vesicles were so wide that it is evident that size alone is a very unreliable indicator of the age of the vesicle.[2]

Ultrasound is highly accurate in detecting pregnancy. Chevalier and Palmer[2] were able to confirm a pregnancy in 95 per cent of subsequent examinations (n = 453). This percentage may actually be low, for all failures were assumed to be diagnostic error with no allowance for early fetal loss. In this same study there were 62 mares that did not return to estrus after a negative diagnosis by ultrasound. Reexamination found 10 (16 per cent) of these mares to be pregnant, and the remaining 84 per cent were confirmed as nonpregnant. This normal rate of false-negatives must be considered when applying ultrasound as an aid to detect twin conceptions and may be an expected rate of error.

Abnormal Observations

A large number of examinations (n = 2135) made by Chevalier and Palmer[2] on trotter, draft and pony mares revealed some abnormal observations. While different from a Thoroughbred population, the outcome of these abnormalities is worthy of review. A diagnosis of an abnormality was accepted as valid only if it was detected on two separate examinations.

1. Single vesicles that appeared too large (larger than the mean plus the standard deviation) were confirmed in 24 cases. Seventy per cent proved to be single pregnancies, 13 per cent were confirmed as twins and 17 per cent became nonpregnant.

2. Vesicles that appeared too small (smaller than the mean minus the standard deviation) were confirmed in 123 cases. Twenty-one per cent resulted in a single pregnancy, 1 per cent resulted in twins and 78 per cent became nonpregnant.

3. Abnormal shape or echoes within the vesicle were confirmed in 48 cases. Seventy-seven per cent were single pregnancies, 2 per cent were twins and 21 per cent became nonpregnant.

4. A "divided" vesicle was confirmed in 12 cases. Sixty-seven per cent proved to be single pregnancies, 25 per cent were twins and 8 per cent became nonpregnant.

The pregnancy may be found in unexpected places in early examination and often in a more normal position on a subsequent examination.

1. Location in the body of the uterus was confirmed in 11 cases. Sixty-four per cent continued a normal pregnancy, while 36 per cent became nonpregnant.

2. Location high in one uterine horn was confirmed in nine cases. Thirty-three per cent remained pregnant, and 66 per cent became nonpregnant.

It is evident that when an abnormality is suspected, particularly on an early examination, confirmation on a second examination should be considered before corrective action is undertaken by the clinician.

CLINICAL APPLICATION OF ULTRASOUND

Maximum benefits from diagnostic information provided by ultrasound examination require an adequate understanding of equine reproductive physiology. A very brief review will assist in demonstrating that there is a very narrow time period in the pregnancy during which an accurate ultrasound examination can assist any corrective measures contemplated.

The normal interovulatory period for the mare is 21 to 22 days. Following ovulation, the lifespan of the resulting corpus luteum is normally 13 to 14 days if no pregnancy is established. There is a marked increase of plasma progesterone during the function of the corpus luteum (diestrous phase of cycle), which makes the mare unreceptive to the male. The interovulatory period includes two follicle-stimulating hormone (FSH) surges that are about 10 days apart. The first is present in conjunction with ovulation, and the second occurs about 10 days later in diestrus.[3] Follicular activity and even ovulation may be observed in diestrus because of this second FSH surge. These diestrous ovulations can be fertile if viable spermatozoa are present in the oviducts. Multiple ovulations in the same interovulatory period may be separated by minutes or up to 10 days. This ability for multiple and/or diestrous ovulations, while normal, complicates management efforts to avoid twins.

Pregnant mares form structures called endometrial cups at 36 to 38 days gestation. These cups are of fetal origin, coming from chorionic girdle cells. These cells invade the endometrium and produce a chorionic gonadotropin, or pregnant mare serum gonadotropin (PMSG). This substance may assist in the maintenance of the pregnancy,[13] and cup failure in early pregnancy may result in fetal loss. Normal endometrial cups will continue to function for 90 to 120 days once imbedded in the lining of the uterus, even though the pregnancy may be lost to other causes. A positive mare immunopregnancy (MIP) test assures only that the mare was pregnant at day 36 to 38 and that she did form endometrial cups. Should the pregnancy be lost after the cups have formed, most mares will not cycle as expected until cup function ceases 90 to 120 days later, which greatly reduces the possibility of establishing another pregnancy. The following three key figures should be considered:

1. About 14 days is the earliest that a vesicle is visible on ultrasound examination.

2. There may be as much as 10 days difference in the ages of two vesicles occurring during one estrous cycle.

3. All observations must be made and confirmed, corrective action must be taken and the results of that action must be known prior to the formation of endometrial cups at day 36 to 38.

The critical period for examination is then between days 24 and 36. Examinations on day 24 should allow for the opportunity to find both members of a pair of twins, even if 10 days apart in age, and day 36 should allow for termination of an abnormal pregnancy with a reasonably good expectation of resumption of normal cyclic activity. Without considering economic factors, there are specific times in the pregnancy that ultrasound examinations can provide useful information for improved reproductive performance. There are specific objectives for each examination time:

Examinations on days 19 to 21 following ovulation.

1. Determine that the failure to return to estrus is because of the establishment of pregnancy and not because of prolonged luteal function.

2. Screen for the appearance of two vesicles with the understanding that "visualization of two dark circular areas is not proof of two conceptuses."[2] A younger vesicle more than 7 days apart from the first may not be detected.

Examination on days 25 to 30 following ovulation.

1. Visualize the second vesicle that may have been too young to detect at days 19 to 21 or confirm a single pregnancy.

2. Examine suspected twins found on the first exam for continued enlargement, each dark circular area now containing a visible embryo with a heartbeat.

3. Eliminate one vesicle by crushing and evaluate the success of the vesicle rupture.

Examination on days 35 to 36 after ovulation.

1. Clarify any unusual observations made on the first two examinations.

2. Demonstrate the maintenance of a single viable embryo with a heartbeat following vesicle rupture of its twin prior to day 30.

3. Determine that both pregnancies have been lost and administer prostaglandin $F_{2\alpha}$ to resume normal cyclic activity.

ULTRASOUND AS AN AID IN THE MANAGEMENT OF TWIN PREGNANCY

Detection and control of twinning is currently a motivation for the clinical use of ultrasound in mares. Ultrasound is a diagnostic aid to complement and to confirm diagnoses made by rectal palpation. Palpation alone has not proved to be an adequate diagnostic aid to prevent twin conception in mares, and the frequency of twin births as recorded in stud books has not declined with its use. This unfortunate state of affairs can be explained by the observation that multiple ovulations are frequently undetected. The second follicle may be deep in the ovarian stroma and thus not palpable, or it may be adjacent to the primary follicle and appear to be part of it. The second ovulation may occur after the mare has gone out of estrus and examinations have ceased. It is accepted that twins in mares are almost always dizygotic,[7] so that two conceptuses confirm that two ovulations occurred. Failure to detect these ovulations by palpation alone is reflected in one report that 76 per cent of 107 mares pregnant with twins conceived on a "single" ovulation.[5] This observation is confirmed by Allen,[1] who noted that 70 per cent of 51 cases of twins were conceived on "single" ovulations.

The frequency of multiple ovulations appears to be influenced by breed, being much higher in Thoroughbreds and much lower in ponies. Multiple ovulations were reported in 19 per cent (n = 347) of Thoroughbred mares by Ginther[5] and 15.6 per cent (n = 2646) by Allen[1] compared with 9 per cent in light horses such as Appaloosas and Quarter horses (n = 2597) and 2 to 3 per cent for ponies.[5] The breeding status of the mare also affects the frequency of multiple ovulations, as foaling mares have a lower frequency than do nonfoaling mares, regardless of breed. Ginther[5] reported that 6.6 per cent (n = 1492) of foaling mares had multiple ovulations compared with 16.1 per cent (n = 1244) of nonfoaling mares, while Allen[1] indicated that 13 per cent (n = 1589) of foaling Thoroughbred mares had multiple ovulations, while 19.5 per cent (n = 1057) of barren or maiden Thoroughbred mares had multiple ovulations. These figures are very interesting, but they do not reveal that multiple ovulation is highly probable in repeated cycles in some mares and very unlikely in other members of the same breed.

It is evident that the Thoroughbred mare has a greater frequency of multiple ovulations and is at higher risk to conceive twins. It is a common practice with Thoroughbred mares to either not breed when two follicles are present or to wait for one follicle to ovulate and then mate the mare in hopes of producing a pregnancy from the second ovulation. This has resulted in lost cycles, lost time, fewer pregnancies and increased costs—all preferable to a mare pregnant with twins.

There is reasonable evidence to suggest that mares mated on synchronous (within 48 hours) ovulations have a higher fertility rate than single ovulators. Fifty to 54 per cent of normal single ovulating mares will become pregnant on any given estrous cycle.[5] If we accept that fertilization and survival of each resulting embryo is independent of the other, we can consider that the double ovulation is equal to two cycles superimposed on each other. In a single cycle with a single ovulation, 54 per cent of the mares should become pregnant, leaving 46 per cent for the next cycle. Fifty-four per cent of this population will become pregnant for an added 25 per cent ($0.54 \times 0.46 = 0.248$). One would expect 79 per cent of normal mares to become pregnant with a single foal when given two opportunities for conception, be it two cycles of single ovulation or one cycle with two ovulations. Such appears to be the case, for Ginther[5] reported that 39 of 47 (83 per cent) mares with double ovulations became pregnant with a single foal.

There is a risk of twinning when a mare is mated accompanied by multiple ovulation. Ginther[5] has suggested that twin conceptions come only from asynchronous ovulations (greater than 48 hours apart), based on a study of broodfarm records that reveal 9 out of 57 mares with asynchronous ovulations conceived twins, while 0 out of 39 mares with synchronous ovulations conceived twins. These figures were obtained from a population of mares (n = 1396) with an overall twinning rate of 4 per cent (n = 61), much lower than the rate in a Thoroughbred population.

Ultrasound examination in 3699 cases showed that two vesicles of equal respective diameter gave the highest rate of twins, confirmed on two separate examinations. Sixty per cent remained with twins when the vesicles were separated, and 50 per cent remained with twins when the vesicles were adjacent.[2] This suggests that synchronous or nearly synchronous ovulations were more successful in resulting in twin conceptions. When two vesicles of unequal size (asynchronous ovulations?) were present, the smaller vesicle developed in only 2 out of 25 cases.[2]

Reports of ovulatory patterns compared with abortion or foaling of twins indicate that 76 per cent (n = 107) of twins result from mating to a "single" ovulation.[5] Since the second ovulation necessary to produce twins was undetected, it remains unknown if the ovulation was synchronous or asynchronous. When two follicles were known to be present, 10 per cent conceived twins when there was one ovulation plus a large follicle present, and 14 per cent conceived twins on an asynchronous ovulation for a total of 24 per cent. This is what would be expected if the probability of fertilization of ovum was only 50 per cent and independent of each other in a population of double ovulations. One would expect that in one fourth of the cases both ova would become fertilized; in one half of the cases one or the other would become fertilized, and in one fourth of the cases neither would become fertilized. One can conclude that there is an increased probability of pregnancy with double ovulation and one would expect about a 25 per cent chance of twin conceptions. This is confirmed by Allen and Simpson,[1] who reported on 51 cases of twins, 30 per cent of which became pregnant on known double ovulations.

Ultrasound examination with palpation allows for an earlier and more accurate diagnosis of pregnancy than does palpation alone. Palpation very early in pregnancy may provide observations that are highly suggestive of pregnancy, such as increased uterine tone, tubularity, contortion of the uterine horns and a tightly closed cervix. There is a very wide range in the size of the normal vesicle, and its size is influenced by the uterus. The conceptus size increases from days 15 to 18 and tends to stop at a diameter of about 27 mm until day 28, when it continues to grow.[2] The accurate detection of twins by palpation alone is often difficult before day 30 because of this delay in size increase. "Although rectal palpation is highly accurate beyond day 25 after ovulation when performed by experienced equine clinicians, it is nevertheless difficult to be certain that a mare which is in prolonged diestrus is not, in fact, pregnant before about day 40 after mating. Furthermore, it is often not possible to diagnose twins positively when one conceptus is in each uterine horn until after day 35, and it is impossible to detect twins per rectum at any time if both fetal sacs are lying adjacent in the same uterine horn."[12]

Once twins have been diagnosed, there are three possible outcomes, of which only one is desirable. The mare may deliver a single live foal, abort or deliver twins or cease to be pregnant. The relatively high frequency of multiple ovulations compared with the low incidence of twin births suggests that twinning may be the leading cause of noninfectious fetal loss and barren mares or that there may be some method of embryoreduction in mares pregnant with twins. Ginther[5] proposed that embryoreduction operates after the embryos enter the uterus on day 6 and before twin embryos are detectable by palpation. A report on 30 pairs of twins diagnosed by palpation on days 28 to 30 indicated that 43 per cent terminated in a single pregnancy, while 17 per cent delivered twins and 40 per cent ceased to be pregnant. When twins were diagnosed at 40 to 42 days (n = 16), only 6 per cent had a single foal, 31 per cent had twins and 63 per cent lost both fetuses. "The data were likely influenced to an unknown extent by palpation errors."[5]

There are three options available once twins have been confirmed. One can abort both and start anew, attempt selective destruction of one by crushing or elect nonintervention. Crushing of one of the vesicles has been attempted with some success. Vesicle rupture was performed on 23 mares pregnant with twins of less than 30 days. Two mares remained pregnant with twins, 13 continued with a single pregnancy and eight became nonpregnant for a success rate of 57 per cent. Seventeen other mares were left without intervention from which 11 aborted or delivered twins, two delivered a single foal and four became nonpregnant for a success rate of 12 per cent.[2] Allen and Simpson[1] reported on 24 cases of twins in separate horns. Attempts to crush one vesicle prior to day 45 resulted in 72 per cent single pregnancies and 8 per cent becoming nonpregnant. Nearly all the losses were incurred when the attempt was made beyond day 30. Each day after day 30 increases the probability of failure until days 36 to 38, at which time the mare forms endometrial cups. After this time, intervention is of value mainly to allow an early start at the next breeding season. Intervention by crushing from days 24 to 30 appears to be the most favorable management option. Should both conceptuses be lost following the attempt, the mare can be expected to return to normal estrus. When nonintervention is practiced beyond days 30 to 35, one can expect either a barren mare or twins for the coming season.

Management practices suggested with the utilization of ultrasound as a diagnostic aid include the following:

1. Breeding on cycles involving multiple ovulations to take advantage of higher fertility, accepting the risk of possible twin pregnancy.

2. Practice nonintervention from ovulation to day 20.

3. Confirm twins on days 24 to 30 and attempt to crush one vesicle followed by IV injection of 500 mg flunixin meglumine.

4. Confirm ongoing pregnancy 7 to 10 days later and observe fetal heartbeat. If both are lost, administer prostaglandin.

The use of ultrasound appears to be quite safe, as there has been no increase in fetal loss following its clinical application. The rate of loss of single pregnancies reported by Chevalier and Palmer[2] was 11 per cent (n = 1000) when the diagnosis was made before 25 days, 11 per cent when the mare was examined between days 25 and 35 and 7 per cent when she examined beyond 35 days giving an overall loss rate of 9 per cent. Allen and Simpson,[1] observed that pregnancy loss under 100 days following examination was 2.5 per cent (n = 16) in maidens, 7.2 per cent (n = 335) in nonfoaling mares and 7.9 per cent (n = 856) in foaling mares.

Layton[8] reported a 7.5 per cent (n = 295) fetal loss prior to 45 days of pregnancy.

CONCLUSION

Ultrasound is a valuable aid to confirm rectal palpation diagnoses and to allow for more confidence in early pregnancy detection. As such, it offers new hope for the evolution of more satisfactory management options than those afforded by palpation examination alone. The technique is not infallible. Chevalier and Palmer[2] reported a false-negative diagnosis in 16 per cent (n = 62) of mares not returning to estrus. A negative diagnosis is never positive! If the survival and detection of each embryo in a pair of twins is independent of the survival and detection of the other, failure to find 16 per cent of mares pregnant with twins may be anticipated in mares examined with ultrasound only once. Even so, it remains a dramatic improvement in our diagnostic skill when compared with palpation alone.

References

1. Allen WR, Simpson PJ: Personal Communication. Equine Fertility Unit, Animal Research Station, 307 Huntingdon Road, Cambridge CB3 OJQ, UK, 1982.
2. Chevalier F, Palmer E: Ultrasound echography in the mare. J Reprod Fert Suppl 32:423, 1982.
3. Evans MJ, Irving CHG: The serum concentrations of FSH, LH and progesterone in the oestrous cycle and early pregnancy in the mare. J Reprod Fert Suppl 23:193, 1975.
4. Fraser AF, Keith NW, Hastie H: Summarized observations on the ultrasonic detection of pregnancy and foetal life in the mare. Vet Rec 92:20, 1973.
5. Ginther OJ: Twinning in mares: A review of recent studies. Eq Vet Sci 2:127, 1982.
6. Ginther OJ, Douglas RH, Woods GL: A biological embryo-reduction mechanism for the elimination of excess embryos in mares. Theriogenol 18:475, 1982.
7. Jeffcott LB, Whitwell KE: Twinning as a cause of foetal and neonatal loss in Thoroughbred mares. J Comp Pathol 83:91, 1973.
8. Layton GE: Personal communication. P.O. Box 31, Paris, Kentucky 40361, 1982.
9. Palmer E, Draincourt MA: Use of ultrasonic echography in equine gynecology. Theriogenol 13:203.
10. Powis R: A Thinkers Guide to Ultrasonic Imaging. Baltimore, U. Schwarzenberg, 1982.
11. Rantanen NW, Torbeck RL, DuMond SS: Early pregnancy diagnosis in the mare using transrectal ultrasound scanning techniques: A preliminary report. Eq Vet Sci 2:27, 1982.
12. Simpson PJ, Greenwood RES, Ricketts SW, et al: Use of ultrasound echography for early diagnosis of single and twin pregnancy in the mare. J Reprod Fert Suppl 32:431, 1982.
13. Urwin VE, Allen WR: Pituitary and chorionic gonadotrophic control of ovarian function during early pregnancy in equids. J Reprod Fert, Suppl 32:371, 1982.
14. Wallace AK, Voelkel SA, Thompson DL, Godke RA: Evaluation of ultrasonic pregnancy detection in Thoroughbred and Quarter Horse mares. Baton Rouge, Louisiana State University. Livestock Producers Day Report 21:211, 1981.

Delayed Embryonic Development and Prolonged Pregnancy in Mares

Marcel M. Vandeplassche
State University, Ghent, Belgium

Two well-controlled and interesting clinical observations at this clinic have initiated a more detailed study of delayed embryonic development and prolonged pregnancy in the mare.

First, on a number of occasions we have been consulted about mares in prolonged pregnancy because the owner was concerned about the risk of dystocia and the survival of an oversized and overmature foal. However, the majority of such mares in advanced pregnancy prove to be less heavy than normal, and the owner sometimes doubts that the mare is pregnant. Preparatory symptoms for parturition occur at about 12 months of gestation instead of 11 months and result in spontaneous foaling and delivery of a normal mature foal (Fig. 1).

A second interesting clinical observation has been the fact that in mares presented for diagnosis of pregnancy by rectal palpation between 30 and 50 days of gestation the uterine enlargement was quite variable, and some mares were found with a marked underdevelopment of the pregnant horn. For example, a mare presented 50 days after the last breeding had a firm, tightly closed cervix, the uterine horns contracted when palpated, but the distention of the pregnant horn was similar to that of a 30-day pregnancy.

The objective of this study was to define these two clinical observations in order to institute appropriate treatment without disturbing the normal course of gestation and parturition.

MATERIALS AND METHODS

For the past 6-year period all cases of excessively prolonged pregnancy for which veterinary practitioners and owners sought advice were studied. An attempt was made to gather accurate information about the date of the last breeding, the course of gestation and parturition, the size, maturity and vitality of the foals and expulsion and structure of the placenta.

Since 1978 special attention has been given to mares with a gravid uterus obviously smaller than expected for the time since the last breeding. These mares have been reexamined by rectal palpation as gestation advanced in order to assess uterine enlargement. In addition to rectal palpation, a blood sample was taken whenever possible for detection of pregnant mare serum gonadotropin (PMSG) in mares more than 40 days after breeding in order to estimate the stage of development of the conceptus more accurately. These mares were observed until foaling to determine the exact length of gestation, the type of parturition and the characteristics of the foal. Every attempt was made to obtain accurate information regarding the exact dates of estrus, last breeding and parturition.

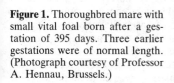

Figure 1. Thoroughbred mare with small vital foal born after a gestation of 395 days. Three earlier gestations were of normal length. (Photograph courtesy of Professor A. Hennau, Brussels.)

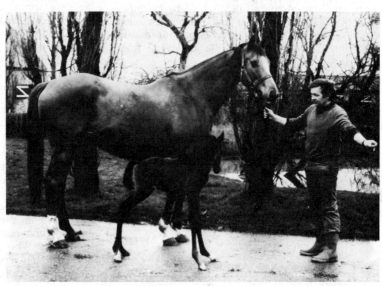

Table 1. Length of Pregnancy in Days (Viable Foal) in the Mare (Based on Review of Literature)

Average: 336
Physiological variation: 320 to 350 (93%)
Variation between extremes: 309 to 370
310 to 370
310 to 374
315 to 387
Prolonged gestation: over 360 (4.4%)
over 365 (0.34%)
over 370 (1.3%)

OBSERVATIONS AND DISCUSSION

Prolonged Gestation

The literature was reviewed to obtain data about the length of gestation in mares that deliver a normal foal. This information from a number of publications is summarized in Table 1. Most authors attribute the diversity in gestation lengths of 320 to 350 days to "physiological variations." In this study, emphasis was placed on the excessively prolonged gestations, which are reported to be from 370 to 387 days. The incidence of extremely prolonged pregnancies varies from one report to another but is probably about 1 per cent.

The literature was also reviewed to determine the factors that influence gestation length in mares. This information is presented in Table 2. When the nine factors reported to influence gestation length are considered, it may be concluded that they could be responsible for prolonging gestation by a few days but it is unlikely that gestation would be prolonged by 30 to 63 days.

To date, 21 mares with excessively prolonged gestation periods have been studied. Detailed data concerning these pregnancies are shown in Table 3. Five of these mares delivered twins after a mean gestation length of 384 days compared with a mean of 375 days for 16 single pregnancies. The twin foals were small but mature as determined by examination of the teeth, haircoat and hooves. Detailed characteristics of the five cases of prolonged twin gestation are presented in Table 4. Several foals

Table 2. Factors Influencing the Length of Gestation in Mares (Based on Review of Literature)

1. Breed: ± 1.5 days
2. Sex of foals: colts 2 days longer than fillies
3. Age of mare: no influence
4. Stallion: + −
5. Dam: + −
6. Month of conception: spring, longer than autumn
7. Daylight: over 80 per cent of mares foal by night (between 6:00 PM and 6:00 AM stimulated foaling)
8. Severe undernutrition: in second half of gestation +4 to +10 days
9. Overfeeding in second half of gestation: − a few days
10. Stress: delayed foaling for 1 to 2 days

from the single pregnancies were judged by the owners to be undersized or typical of twin foals. The fact that most of these breeders had expected an oversized foal probably made it more difficult for them to be objective.

A thorough macroscopic examination of the placentae from 12 single and four twin pregnancies was made, and no differences between these and those from gestations of normal length were observed.

Delayed Embryonic Development

In Mares. Under the conditions of field practice it is difficult to obtain complete histories in cases of delayed embryonic development diagnosed by rectal palpation. The case histories of 12 mares with markedly retarded embryonic development are presented in Table 5.

Upon initial examination such mares might be considered nonpregnant, but none had been in estrus for 3 to 6 weeks following the last service, and no mature graafian follicles were palpated. The cervix was firm, and the uterine horns were slightly asymmetric and, most importantly, uterine contractions were obvious during palpation. Equipment for echographic examination was not available. Distention of the pregnant horn, permitting the diagnosis of pregnancy, was obvious when these mares were reexamined about 3 weeks subsequent to the initial examination. During the second half of gestation, the owner may question the normalcy of the pregnancy because the abdominal distention of the mare and movements of the fetus may be delayed. Ten of these 12 mares in which delayed embryonic development was diagnosed had a prolonged or excessively prolonged gestation period. While the mechanism by which pregnancy is terminated in the mare is not as well defined as that in ruminants, it is apparent that maturity of the fetoplacental unit probably plays an important role in the initiation of parturition in mares. Thus, it is reasonable that following an embryonic diapause of 3 to 5 weeks, the fetoplacental unit needs the normal gestation length plus an additional 3 to 5 weeks in order to reach maturity.

Serum samples from five of these 12 mares were assayed for the presence of PMSG two or three times at intervals varying from 11 to 35 days. The tests used (bioassay in female rats and hemagglutination inhibition) reliably detect the presence of PMSG from day 43 of pregnancy onward. It is apparent in these five cases that the development of the endometrial cups and the appearance of PMSG in the blood was delayed for 20 to 25 days, while the delay of embryonic development, as detected by rectal palpation, was 20 to 30 days (Table 5).

From these observations we have concluded that in some equine pregnancies the early embryo enters an embryonic rest or diapause of approximately 3 to 4 weeks. When this period of time is added to a normal gestation period, a markedly prolonged gestation occurs. It is also possible that an embryonic

Table 3. Prolonged Gestation in Mares Carrying Single and Twin Conceptuses

Animal Number	Breed	Gestation Length (Days)	Parturition (Normal = N; Difficult = D)	Status of Foals at Birth (Live = +; Dead = −; Mature = M; Dysmature = A)
Single Conceptus				
1	HB	385	N	+M
2	WB	382	D	+M
3	BHD	378	N	+M
4	HB	370	N	+M
5	WB	374	N	+M
6	BHD	372	N	+M
7	BHD	370	N	+M
8	HB	382	N	+M
9	WB	375	N	+M
10	BHD	385	N	+M
11	HB	385	N	+M
12	WB	381	D	−A
13	BHD	382	D	+M
14	WB	379	N	+M
15	TB	345	N	+M
16	TB	362	N	+M
		(mean 375)		
Twin Conceptuses				
17	BHD	399	N	+M
18	BHD	382	N	+M
19	HB	385	N	+M
20	WB	382	N	−M
21	BHD	370	N	+M
		(mean 384)		−M
				+M
				−M
				−M
				−M

BHD = Belgian Draught Horse; WB = Warmblood; HB = Halfblood; TB = Thoroughbred

rest of a few days is a common occurrence during early gestation in mares.

The period during which delayed embryonic development occurs is not well defined. Direct examination of the embryo is not possible because of the sporadic incidence of the phenomenon. It is postulated that the rest period must start after the embryonic signal has been given at days 15 to 16 after fertilization[2] to prevent regression of the corpus luteum of pregnancy. Development of the endo-

Table 4. Characteristics of Five Cases of Prolonged Twin Gestation

1. Type of parturition
     spontaneous: 5/5
2. Vitality of foals
     1 vital foal and 1 mummy: 3/5
     2 vital foals: 1/5
     2 dead foals: 1/5
3. Maturity of foals
     Vital foals: 5/5 normal
     Dead foals: 2/2 normal
     Mummy: ± 7 months development
4. Expulsion of placenta
     Normal: 4/5
     Retained: 1/5 (2 vital foals)

metrial cups and PMSG production begin around day 35 of pregnancy. In all five mares with embryonic rest the secretion of PMSG was delayed for at least 20 to 25 days (Table 5). It is concluded, therefore, that the slowed or arrested development of the embryo starts before day 35 of pregnancy and can continue for up to 30 days. Embryonic rest occurs before the attachment of the embryonic villi to the endometrial crypts during which time the conceptus depends upon the absorption of histotrophe for nourishment. Thus, the phenomenon of embryonic rest could be defined as delayed implantation.

In Other Mammals. Embryonic rest is a common occurrence in several species of mammals and is caused by factors such as season, stress and hibernation in minks, badgers and weasels and lactation and suckling stimulus in marsupials, rats, mice and rabbits.[3] Embryonic dormancy resulting in "split parturition" has been described in the sow.[6]

The experimental induction of embryonic rest and subsequent reactivation of the dormant blastocyst has been attempted with various exogenous hormones, primarily estrogens and progesterone. Early pregnancy in the mare is characterized by a rapid increase in circulating progesterone, with a

Table 5. Delayed Embryonic Development

Animal Number	Breed of Horse	Day Since Ovulation	Estimate (Per Rectum) Stage of Development of Conceptus (Days)*	Presence of PMSG in Blood (+ or −)	Gestation Length (Days)	Parturition (Normal = N)
1	WB	55	32	−	389	N
		75	55	+		
2	HB	48	−	−	336	N
		59	+	+		
3	WB	51	28	−	365	N
		79		+		
4	WB	41	28	−	384	N
		66	35	−		
		76	60	+		
5	HB	53	−		374	N
		58	−	+		
		63	45			
6	HB	63	30	+	362	N
7	WB	43	−	43: −	392	N
		62	+	62: +		
8	HB	28	−		379	N
		42	+			
9	WB	35	−		345	N
		53	+			
10	WB	40	−		362	N
		54	+			
11	BHD	42	−		367	N
12	TB	40	−		395	N

WB = Warmblood; HB = Trotter; + = normal size for stage; − = smaller than normal; TB = Thoroughbred.

maximum of 8 ng/ml at day 16, followed by a decline to 5 ng/ml until day 40 of pregnancy when accessory corpora lutea develop and peripheral progesterone concentrations rise to 15 ng/ml (Fig. 2). The period of low peripheral progesterone levels corresponds

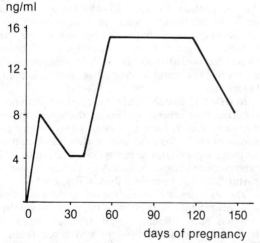

Figure 2. Mean circulating concentrations of progesterone in mares (3).

well to the phase of embryonic rest. Since peripheral levels of progesterone vary considerably from one mare to another, it is hypothesized that exceptionally low levels of progesterone under certain circumstances could induce a retardation of embryonic growth by suppressing the synthesis of ribonucleic acids in the blastocyst. Further, increased progesterone at about day 40 of pregnancy could reactivate the metabolism of the embryo.

A similar hormonal mechanism has been documented in marsupials. The single corpus luteum following the postpartum ovulation remains small for the 7-month period that the pouch-young is suckling in continuous attachment to the nipple. During lactation, the intrauterine blastocyst remains in a state of metabolic rest. Most reports indicate that the most probable factors that maintain the blastocyst in diapause are a lack in quality or quantity of specific endometrial proteins and vital amino acids.[4] During the first 4 days after the pouch-young stops suckling and leaves the pouch, a marked growth of the corpus luteum occurs that is characterized by hypertrophy and hyperplasia of luteal cells. This renewed luteal development probably results in increased levels of progesterone, which induces the secretory activity of the endometrium responsible for the resumption of metabolic activity and growth of the blastocyst.[1]

PRACTICAL IMPORTANCE OF THE OBSERVATIONS

Delayed Embryonic Development

Practicing veterinarians should be aware of the occurrence of delayed embryonic development when examining mares for pregnancy by rectal palpation, particularly during the period of 40 to 60 days after the last breeding. A smaller than expected pregnant uterine horn and even a negative test for PMSG do not exclude the possibility of pregnancy, especially when slight uterine asymmetry and uterine contractions are present. The blastocyst might be detected by echographic examination if the growth block did not start too early. Plasma progesterone levels would be useful in identifying nonpregnant mares only if concentrations were less than 1 ng/ml. Since the induction of luteolysis with prostaglandin or intrauterine infusion of saline will terminate pregnancy in most cases, treatment should be delayed until the pregnancy status of the mare is accurately determined by reexamination in 2 to 3 weeks. In pregnant mares the uterine contents will have developed sufficiently to enable an accurate diagnosis of pregnancy.

Excessively Prolonged Pregnancy

Veterinarians are frequently consulted by the anxious owner of a mare in which the gestation period appears to have exceeded 1 year. In such cases the breeding records should be critically reviewed, since it is not unusual to find errors in the breeding date or calculation of gestation length. When the breeding information appears to be correct and the mare is in good health with normal development of the abdomen and visible movements of the fetus but lacks relaxation of the vulva and pelvic ligaments and development of the udder, the possibility of embryonic rest should be considered. Artificial induction of parturition is contraindicated, since spontaneous delivery can be expected in almost all of these mares. When the mare shows excessive development of the abdomen, has lost condition or has suffered bouts of colic, rectal examination is indicated to determine the size and viability of the fetus. Uterine torsion and dorsoflexion of the uterus should be differentiated from prolonged gestation and treated as indicated.[5]

SUMMARY

Embryonic rest of a few days may be a common occurrence in mares. A diapause of 3 to 5 weeks is rare but has been observed between days 16 and 35 of gestation, a period during which peripheral progesterone levels are low. A long block of embryonic growth is suggestive of nonpregnancy, but the immediate induction of luteolysis could provoke abortion. A long period of embryonic rest usually results in a markedly prolonged gestation period and spontaneous delivery of a normal-sized vital foal. Consequently, most gestation periods longer than 1 year do not need any special treatment.

References

1. Anonymous: What maintains an embryo in diapause? Res Reprod 6:4, 1974.
2. Douglas RH: Effects of the blastocyst on the maternal recognition of pregnancy in the equine. Newsletter Am Assoc Equine Pract 1:58, 1980.
3. Enders AC (ed): Delayed Implantation. Chicago, University of Chicago Press, 1963.
4. Mead RA, Rourke AW, Swannack A: Changes in uterine protein synthesis during delayed implantation in the western spotted skunk and its regulation by hormones. Biol Reprod 21:39, 1979.
5. Muylle E, Vandeplassche M, Nuytten J, et al: Dorsoflexo uteri tijdens de dracht bij de merrie. Vlams Diergeneesk Tijdschr 50:155, 1981.
6. Vandeplassche M: The physiological explanation of double parturition in the pig and other mammalian species. Ann d'Endocrinologie 30:328, 1969.

Induction of Parturition in the Mare

Carla L. Carleton, D.V.M., M.S.
Michigan State University, East Lansing, Michigan

Walter R. Threlfall, D.V.M., Ph.D.
Ohio State University, Columbus, Ohio

Induction of parturition in the mare is primarily a method to permit convenient observation and professional assistance at foaling. It is most often used with valuable or problem mares but is becoming an established, accepted procedure of convenience. It is a commonly accepted practice on many large breeding farms to hire attendants to provide 24-hour a day observation of near-term mares. The relative costs of intensive labor can be negligible compared with the value of a lost foal and/or mare if unobserved dystocia occurs and no assistance is available. Apart from the conservation of farm labor, there are clinical situations in which induced parturition can be recommended, such as prolonged gestation, uterine atony, preparturient colic or impending rupture of the prepubic tendon.[8]

Induction is also warranted when mares have suffered physical damage in accidents or at a prior parturition. If the healing process following a pelvic fracture has reduced adequate pelvic space for fetal passage, the need for manual assistance at foaling may be required. In the case of soft tissue trauma the reduction in elasticity in the vulvar lips must be considered, with perhaps an episiotomy being necessary. If the mare has undergone surgery to repair foaling lacerations of the perineal body or cervix, observation and assistance at subsequent foalings may serve to eliminate a recurrence or damage to the repaired site. There are, in addition, other justifications for inducing a mare at term, including preparturient loss of colostrum, the teaching value of an observed parturition, research investigations involving parturition or neonatal physiology and induction to permit use of a mare as a nurse mare for a valuable orphan foal.[11]

EVALUATION OF CANDIDATES FOR INDUCED PARTURITION

Prior to parturition induction a physical examination of the mare should be performed, including determination of the presentation, position and posture of the foal. The practitioner should be aware that the fetus may normally lie in a dorsopubic or dorsolateral position, with flexed posture turning to a dorsosacral position and extended posture only during the first and early second stages of labor.[13] The basic criteria for induced parturition, in addition to a normal physical examination, include a gestation of not less than 320 days (calculated by a *known* breeding date) if a live foal is the goal, mammary development present with colostrum available and some relaxation of the cervix to permit a more rapid delivery.[8]

If a mare has a history of 330- or 340-day gestations, arrangements can be made to wait longer to initiate treatment, since optimum survival is achieved when the fetus is induced within 10 to 14 days of term. Udder size can vary, depending on size, age, breed and parity of the mare. The major changes occur within two weeks of foaling. To allow the mare to approach term as closely as possible, owners should be instructed to observe for the changes in udder size, consistency and the presence of colostrum. Owners should be capable of evaluating the character of the secretion daily or more frequently as the mare approaches term. Beginning a few weeks before term, the secretion will appear cloudy and straw colored and be quite viscous. Closer to the natural foaling date, the secretion will become more fluid and the udder will become larger and firmer. Distinctive color changes of the milk have been reported as progressing from clear to a smokey-gray color, and finally, a few hours to a few days before parturition, the color becomes opaque-white.[8, 12] Owners should be instructed to contact a veterinarian when the smokey-gray color appears. Waxing may or may not become apparent on the teat ends the week prior to natural foaling. The daily manipulation of the teat ends has been an added benefit in maiden mares in that they become accustomed to the teats being handled.

At the time the mammary gland is developing, the cervix will be relaxing. If the breeding date is confirmed and the mammary gland is showing development, induction can be safely practiced even if the cervix is closed. Many veterinarians prefer not to induce a mare with less than a 3- to 4-cm cervical dilation.[12] The relaxation of the pelvic ligaments is more subtle in the mare than in the cow, and this should not be relied upon as a major parameter to gauge the time of parturition.[9] Vaginal and cervical examination should be conducted with proper technique. With a tail wrap on the mare and the perineum thoroughly cleaned with a gentle soap, the cervical softening (becoming more compressible and dilated) can be evaluated by vaginal speculum or by palpation.

Not to be overlooked are the circumstances in which parturition should not be induced. For example, induction should not be considered if signs of impending abortion are present, if foul-smelling, cloudy or red-colored vaginal discharge is noted, if the mare is febrile or if on rectal palpation the status of fetal viability is in question. If such a situation is present, the veterinarian and the procedure may be held responsible for the dead and/or weak foal and any postpartum sequelae (retained placenta, metritis, laminitis) that the mare may experience. If the mare is systemically ill or abnormal vaginal and cervical discharges are noted, it would be better to delay induction and treat the primary illness first. In cases in which the value of the mare exceeds that of the foal, and the owner is alerted to the situation prior to treatment of a toxic mare, induction may still be considered a viable option if foal survivability is irrelevant.

PREPARATION OF MARE

If possible, a mare for which induced parturition is planned should be introduced to the foaling environment 2 to 4 weeks before the actual foaling. Vaccination of the mare will vary with farm management. Prior to treatment, the mare should be placed in a quiet stall that is clean and bedded with straw and preferably removed from other farm activities. Rectal examination of the mare at this time will usually permit evaluation of fetal presentation, position and posture as well as the viability status of the fetus. A tail wrap should be placed on the mare and her perineum thoroughly washed.

METHOD OF INDUCTION

Oxytocin Administration

The most frequent induction hormone employed is intravenous or intramuscular oxytocin.[6, 7, 8, 11, 12] Once the mare preparation has been completed, a vaginal examination should be performed to evaluate cervical dilation. The dosage administered varies with the degree of cervical relaxation. If the cervix is relaxed at least 2 cm internal diameter, 40 to 60 units of oxytocin are administered as an intravenous bolus. Delivery of the fetus should occur within 90 minutes. If the cervix is closed or relaxed less than 2 cm diameter, oxytocin can be administered in 10-unit increments as intravenous boluses at 15- to 30-minute intervals. Cervical relaxation can be evaluated prior to each additional increment. Birth is usually induced by the time four to five of the 10-unit doses have been given. If the cervix dilates, but the mare shows no labor, additional oxytocin can be given (40 to 60 units). Checking the dilation of the cervix and examining fetal progress allows evaluation of fetal presentation, position and posture and correction of it prior to the development of a severe dystocia.

The stages and signs to be anticipated following a single 40- to 60-unit dose are presented in Table 1 with the approximate time sequence.

In a pluriparous mare the sequence may be more rapid, with stage II completed within 30 minutes from the time of oxytocin administration. In many practices oxytocin has been traditionally administered by the intramuscular[5, 6, 7, 11, 12] or intravenous (IV drip and/or bolus) routes.[1, 8] Much of the recent literature has reiterated the observation that the mare's response (both in speed and violence) is proportional to the dose of oxytocin given.

Other Induction Treatments

Other treatment regimens have been utilized but with less reliability than oxytocin. Estradiol cypionate (4 to 6 mg) and diethylstilbestrol have been used as aids for cervical dilation when given 12 to 24 hours before the administration of oxytocin.[6, 11] Corticosteroids such as dexamethasone have been given (100 mg at 24-hour intervals), until parturition occurs. The average induction time is 4 ± 1.6 days.[2] Although most investigations have reported satisfactory foal survival following induction by dexamethasone, repeated steroid treatments create the potential for lowered resistance (increased disease

susceptibility) in the foal.[2, 3, 8] Because of this as well as the long delay and unreliable response between treatment and delivery steroids are not recommended. Prostaglandin $F_{2\alpha}$ ($PGF_{2\alpha}$) causes the strongest smooth muscle contractions of all of these alternative drugs. Foal survival with $PGF_{2\alpha}$ is compromised because of the strong myometrial contractions, which lead to early placental separation and increased fetal weakness and mortality.[3, 4, 5, 15] Prostaglandin analogs, such as fluprostenol (Equimate), have less smooth muscle activity and therefore can be successfully used for induction. Mares can be induced, including those with a closed cervix and no milk (if the intent is to save the mare), with a dose of 1 μg/lb. The delivery should occur in approximately 4 hours.[1, 14] Because of the disadvantages of other methods of induction, oxytocin has remained the most commonly used and possibly the most efficacious choice because of its safety and rapid action.

None of the mentioned treatment regimens have been associated with an increased incidence of placental retention.

AFTERCARE

If the amnionic membrane has not ruptured during delivery, it should be removed from the foal's head immediately after expulsion to prevent asphyxiation. This should be performed in such a way as to minimize disturbance to the mare.

When the mare is adapted to a clean environment, umbilical treatment is optional. If the foaling area is less than ideal, the abdomen (umbilicus) can be wrapped with a clean or sterile towel, taped in place and left on for 1 to 1½ hours. The usefulness of preparing the umbilicus with iodine is questionable.

Ten per cent of the foal's body weight in colostrum should be fed within the first 24 hours of life. A maximum of 1 liter should be given within the first hour, with at least five additional feedings occurring thereafter. Foal vaccination against var-

Table 1. Stages and Signs of Parturition Following Oxytocin Administration*

Stage	Time (Minutes)	Remarks
I	5–10	Restlessness, anorexia, colicky pains (looking at the flanks), minor tail movements
	15–20	Stall walking, frequent defecation, getting up and down, elevation of the tail, repeated stretching, sweat on shoulders and neck and behind the elbows
	20–25	Restlessness, tail switching, sweat on ribs and flanks
II	25–30	Acceleration of respiratory and pulse rates, with rupture of the chorioallantoic membrane and beginning of the abdominal press
	35–40	Amnionic membrane at vulvar lips
	45–50	Stage II completed with passage of foal
III	30	Initial phase completed with passage of placenta

*Single 40- to 60-unit dose

ious diseases is dependent on the mare's vaccination status.

Careful examination of the placenta to determine whether it is intact is imperative in the possible prevention of metritis and laminitis, which may occur if fragments remain in the uterus. Any placental abnormalities should be recorded. A positive correlation between the foal's health and placental abnormalities has been recognized.[13]

The mare's vaccination history should be obtained when possible. If any doubt exists, a tetanus toxoid booster should be administered. Examination of the mare's reproductive tract for a second fetus, lacerations and uterine tone should be performed, as is indicated with any assisted delivery. The uterus, cervix, vagina, vestibule and vulva should be included in the examination. Placental passage usually occurs within 3 hours following the induced parturition.

It is critical to keep in mind that the period from induction to foaling in a mare is extremely brief. Once the induction has been initiated, the attending veterinarian should remain on the farm until stage II of parturition is completed. The major advantages of being present are to permit successive vaginal examinations, if indicated, and to assist, if necessary, in the delivery process. If a postural defect exists, it can be corrected by manually extending and drawing the extremities into the cervical lumen. This is less difficult to accomplish early in the delivery process compared with later on when the uterine contractions have made fetal repulsion impossible. The amnionic membrane may or may not rupture during the early stages of labor. If the amnion has not ruptured and assistance is necessary, the membrane may be incised with a finger knife. If the normal progress of parturition is delayed, examination of the fetus should be performed to reevaluate presentation, position and posture. Observed parturition also permits foal examination after parturition. Mares with a history of foals suffering neonatal isoerythrolysis may have their foals removed and colostrum supplied from a compatible mare.

Before utilizing any hormone or hormone-like substance to induce parturition, the veterinarian is responsible for determining adequate fetal gestational age and adequate mare lactational capability. If there is any doubt, gestation should be allowed to continue, with regular evaluations performed.

As discussed earlier, any mare approaching term should have her udder and milk secretion evaluated once or twice a day. This procedure allows the veterinarian to choose the most convenient and safe time for induction. Additionally, there is no association of induction with impaired future reproductive efficiency.[13]

References

1. Allen WR, Pashen RL: The role of prostaglandins during parturition in the mare. Acta Vet Scand Suppl 77:279, 1981.
2. Alm CC, Sullivan JJ, First NL: Induction of premature parturition by parenteral administration of dexamethasone in the mare. JAVMA 165:721, 1974.
3. Alm CC, Sullivan JJ, First NL: The effect of a corticosteroid (dexamethasone), progesterone, oestrogen and prostaglandin $F_{2\alpha}$ on gestation length in normal and ovariectomized mares. J Reprod Fert Suppl 23:637, 1982.
4. Bristol F: Induction of parturition in near-term mares by prostaglandin $F_{2\alpha}$. J Reprod Fert Suppl 32:644, 1982.
5. Hillman RB: Induction of parturition in the mare. In Morrow DA (ed): Current Therapy in Theriogenology. 1st ed. Philadelphia, WB Saunders Co, 1980, pp 753–755.
6. Hillman RB: Induction of parturition in mares. J Reprod Fert Suppl 23:641, 1975.
7. Hillman RB, Ganjam VK: Hormonal changes in the mare and foal associated with oxytocin induction of parturition. J Reprod Fert Suppl 27:541, 1979.
8. Jeffcott LB, Rossdale PD: A critical review of current methods for induction of parturition in the mare. Equine Vet J 4:208, 1977.
9. Neely DP, Liu IKM, Hillman RB: Equine reproduction. Belvidere, Hoffman-LaRoche Inc, 1983, p 80.
10. Pashen RL: Oxytocin—the induction agent of choice in the mare? J Reprod Fert Suppl 32:645, 1982.
11. Puvis AD: Elective induction of labor and parturition in the mare. Proc AAEP, 1972, pp 113–118.
12. Puvis AD: The induction of labor in mares as a routine breeding farm procedure. Proc AAEP, 1977, pp 145–160.
13. Roberts SJ: Veterinary obstetrics and genital diseases. Ann Arbor, Edwards Bro 1971, pp 46, 204–205.
14. Rossdale PD, Jeffcott LB, Allen WR: Foaling induced by a synthetic prostaglandin analogue (fluprostenol). Vet Rec 99:26, 1976.
15. Townsend HGG, Tabel H, Bristol FM: Induction of parturition in mares: Effect on passive transfer of immunity to foals. JAVMA 182:255, 1983.

Equine Obstetrics

R. S. Youngquist, D.V.M.
University of Missouri—Columbia, Columbia, Missouri

Parturition in the mare is a rapid and violent process. Fortunately, the incidence of dystocia in horses, reported at about 4 per cent, is low when compared with the incidence in cattle. However, when dystocia exists, the life of the foal is usually in jeopardy, and the health and future reproductive performance of the mare are often compromised.

GESTATION AND PARTURITION

The normal gestation period of the mare is usually stated as 340 days, but it may vary considerably from this average. Foals are not capable of extra-uterine survival before day 300 and are premature if born before day 320. Vandeplassche[7] reported that delayed embryonic development may account for prolonged gestation periods, resulting in the spontaneous delivery of normal foals after gestation periods of up to 385 days. The mare appears to have the ability to exercise some control over the onset of labor, and most foals are born at night when stable activity is at a minimum.

The signs of impending parturition vary from mare to mare and are generally not as dramatic as those in the cow. In late gestation slight relaxation of the sacrosciatic ligaments occurs but may not be obvious because of the heavy croup muscles of the mare. The vulva becomes slightly edematous, and the vulvar cleft lengthens during the last few weeks prior to parturition. Udder development occurs during the last 1 to 1½ months of gestation, and leakage of colostrum or "waxing" may be seen 24 to 48 hours before foaling in most, but not all, mares.

The presentation, position and posture of the fetus as it approaches the maternal pelvis are used to describe both normal and abnormal birth. The presentation of the fetus refers to the orientation of the spinal axis of the fetus in relationship to that of the dam and the portion of the fetus approaching the dam's pelvis. If the spine of the fetus is parallel to that of the dam, the presentation is longitudinal and may be either anterior or posterior, depending upon whether the head or tail is approaching the pelvis. When the spine of the fetus is perpendicular to that of the dam, the presentation is described as transverse and may be either dorsal or ventral, depending upon which body surface of the fetus is presented to the maternal pelvis. The position of the fetus refers to the relationship of the dorsum of the fetus to the four quadrants of the maternal pelvis—sacrum, left and right ilium and pubis. The fetal posture is defined as the relationship of the extremities of the fetus to its body. The foal is normally delivered in anterior presentation, dorso-sacral position, with the head and neck and forelimbs extended. Approximately 50 per cent of equine fetuses are in posterior presentation in early gestation, but by 6½ months most have rotated to anterior presentation. One in 500 equine fetuses are reported to be in posterior presentation at the time of delivery. During the last half of gestation the fetus is in the dorsopubic position, with the head and forelimbs flexed.

Delivery of the foal is a continuous process and includes active participation by both the dam and the fetus. For purposes of description, it is convenient to divide the normal events of labor into three stages.

First Stage of Labor. During the first, or preparatory, stage of labor the fetus extends its head and forelimbs and rotates to dorsosacral position, probably because of a combination of its own reflex action and myometrial contractions. Mares vary in their display of clinical signs during the first stage of labor. Some show minimal signs of discomfort, while others may perspire or show more marked signs of colic. Two to four hours are required for cervical dilation and completion of the first stage of labor. In some mares the first stage of labor may not be followed by the second stage. Delivery of the foal may be delayed for several hours or days. A normal delivery may be preceded by several bouts of false labor.

Second Stage of Labor. The second stage of labor, or delivery of the fetus, is initiated by rupture of the chorioallantois and by release of the watery allantoic fluid. The fetus enters the birth canal in a slight dorsoilial position to take maximum advantage of the oval pelvis of the mare. The shoulders enter the pelvis successively, thus the hoof of one forelimb rests at the level of the fetlock of the other. The head lies between the carpal joints. The amnionic membrane is forced through the cervix and should protrude between the vulvar lips within 5 minutes of the rupture of the chorioallantois. Abdominal straining begins shortly after the onset of the second stage of labor. While some mares begin the expulsive stage while standing, most assume lateral recumbency for delivery of the fetus. The second stage of labor is normally short in the mare, usually being completed in 20 to 30 minutes. The equine placenta separates from the endometrium rapidly, and fetuses not delivered within a relatively short period of time after the onset of the second stage of labor are deprived of their oxygen supply.

Third Stage of Labor. Following delivery of the fetus the myometrium continues to contract, aiding in expulsion of the placenta and involution of the uterus. Expulsion of the equine placenta usually occurs within 30 minutes to 3 hours after delivery of the foal.

Dystocia or difficult birth exists when either of the first two stages of labor is prolonged or not progressive, and examination of the birth canal and fetus is indicated to determine the cause of the impediment. Foaling attendants should be instructed to seek veterinary assistance as soon as any abnormality is detected in the foaling process. Early and proper intervention may allow the delivery of a living foal and reduce the damage to the mare's reproductive tract caused by prolonged labor.

EXAMINATION OF THE PARTURIENT MARE

The amount of restraint necessary for examination will vary depending upon the temperament of the mare, the manipulations required to relieve the dystocia and the preference of the operator. The first requisite for examination is to place the mare in a clean environment with good footing and away from obstructions that might cause injury to the mare and/or the obstetrician should the mare assume recumbency. Mechanical restraint in the form of a twitch, a sideline or breeding hobbles may be useful. Stocks are not desirable for obstetric operations because of the tendency of mares to attempt to lie down during expulsive efforts stimulated by manipulations within the genital tract.

Chemical restraint may be necessary in some cases to allow for examination of the mare in dystocia. A number of sedatives, analgesics and anesthetics are useful in the mare. In cases in which the fetus is still alive, care should be taken not to cause unnecessary depression of the fetus. Acepromazine maleate (0.04 to 0.08 mg/kg) administered intravenously reduces spontaneous activity. Xylazine, while inducing profound sedation, may not diminish the defense reactions of the mare, and some individuals respond adversely, especially to operations involving the hindquarters. A combination of xylazine (1.0 mg/kg intravenously) followed by ketamine (2.0 mg/kg intravenously) induces muscular relaxation and analgesia for short periods (10 to 15 minutes) allowing examination and short obstetric procedures. For procedures requiring more extensive manipulation, intravenous or volatile general anesthetics are indicated.

Epidural anesthesia is indicated in many cases of dystocia to relieve pain and abolish abdominal straining, facilitating a thorough examination and repulsion and mutation of the fetus. An 18 gauge, 3 inch disposable spinal needle with a stylette has been found to be useful in entering the epidural space between the first and second coccygeal vertebrae. The dose of 2 per cent lidocaine will vary with the size of the mare. An initial dose of 6 to 8 ml is adequate to relieve straining in a 450 kg mare without causing loss of motor function in the hind legs.

After the mare has been restrained and sedated, if necessary, the mare's tail should be bandaged in a manner suitable to control the tail hairs and to be held out of the way. The tail should be tied to the halter to prevent injury to it if the mare lies down. All procedures involving invasion of the genital canal must be completed with strict attention to sanitation. The perineal region and buttocks of the mare should be cleaned with a surgical scrub. The hands and arms of the operator should be similarly cleaned.

Adequate and effective lubricants are indispensable for examination of the genital tract and obstetric manipulations. Sterile, water-soluble lubricants such as methylcellulose are adequate in many cases for the initial examination but are quickly diluted and washed away by the fetal fluids. Petrolatum is preferred as a lubricant for mutation and fetotomy. Adequate amounts should be applied to the genital tract of the mare, the fetus, obstetric instruments and the hands and arms of the operator. Frequent reapplication of lubricant is necessary to protect the genital tissues of the mare.

A thorough examination of the birth canal should be conducted, with inspection for evidence of previous trauma and adequacy of relaxation and size. The presentation, position and posture of the fetus must be accurately determined and a plan for delivery should be formulated. An attempt should be made to determine whether or not the fetus is living.

OBSTETRIC OPERATIONS

Four basic procedures are available to the practicing theriogenologist for the resolution of an equine dystocia. They are mutation of abnormal posture, position or presentation; forced extraction; fetotomy (partial or complete) and cesarean section.

Mutation. Delivery of the equine fetus can proceed normally when it is in anterior presentation, dorsosacral (or partial dorsoilial) position, with the head, neck and forelimbs extended. When dystocia is caused by fetal abnormalities, mutation followed by extraction is usually attempted. Repulsion of the fetus out of the maternal pelvis into the uterine cavity where more space is available for correction is the first step in mutation. The fetus and birth canal must be well lubricated, and abdominal straining must be abolished by epidural anesthesia of the dam. It is preferable in most cases to have the dam standing prior to attempting repulsion of the fetus. Extreme care should be used when repelling a fetus, as uterine rupture may result from excessive pressure. Various instruments have been advocated for repulsion of the fetus, but none are superior to the hands and arms of the obstetrician. In protracted cases the uterine wall is tightly contracted around the fetus and repulsion should not be attempted.

If the fetus is not in dorsosacral position, an attempt should be made to rotate the fetus into normal position. Prior to attempting rotation, the fetus and birth canal should be lubricated and the fetus repelled as far cranially as possible. Version is defined as rotation of a transversely presented fetus into either anterior or posterior longitudinal presentation.

Malposture of the fetal extremities is the most common cause of dystocia in the mare. The extremities must be extended to allow passage through the birth canal unless the fetus is smaller than normal or the dam's pelvis is larger than normal. In most cases the fetus must be repelled deeply into the uterine cavity to gain sufficient space for mutation of malpostures. In order to correct flexion of an extremity, the proximal end must be repelled, the middle portion rotated laterally and traction applied to the distal end. Repelling and rotating forces are best applied by the operator's hand and arm. Traction may be applied by the operator if sufficient space is available to permit introduction of both arms into the birth canal or by an assistant using an obstetric chain or snare. At all times the birth canal of the mare must be protected from trauma caused by instruments or fetal parts. When mutation involves a leg, the fetal hoof should be covered by the operator's hand. If mutation cannot be completed in a relatively short period of time (< 15 minutes), an alternate form of delivery should be adopted.

Forced Extraction. An absolutely or relatively oversized fetus is not commonly encountered as a cause of dystocia in the mare. Forced extraction is usually attempted after fetal malposture has been corrected. Traction snares or chains are placed around the fetal pasterns, with the eye of the snare on the dorsal aspect of the limb. Traction devices should be used with caution on the fetal head and should be used only to direct the head, not as a point of extractive force. The bones of the skull of the foal are not as well developed as those of the calf; thus, eye hooks are relatively more dangerous to use in equine dystocia.

The oval shape of the pelvis of the mare and the long, slender body of the foal provide favorable conditions for extraction; obstruction by the fetal head, thorax or pelvis is less common in the mare than in the cow. Only moderate amounts of traction should be applied to the equine fetus. As a general rule, the efforts of two or three persons should be sufficient to deliver a foal. Mechanical aids for applying traction are easily misused and have little, if any, place in equine obstetrics. Traction should be applied smoothly and simultaneously with the abdominal press of the mare. Obstruction by the fetal hindparts ("hip-lock") is uncommon in the mare due to the shape of the maternal pelvis; thus, rotation of the fetus from dorsosacral to dorsoilial position is not necessary in the mare, as it is in the cow. If delivery does not progress rapidly after the application of traction, the fetus should be reexamined, and the cause of the impediment should be determined and corrected.

Fetotomy. Reduction of fetal size or amputation of an extremity in malposture can be quickly and easily accomplished with a fetatome properly designed by an obstetrician familiar with the techniques described for fetotomy.[2] In most cases of equine dystocia a partial fetotomy will allow removal of the impediment to delivery followed by extraction of the remainder of the fetus. Only rarely is a complete fetotomy required to deliver an oversized fetus. Restraint of the mare for fetotomy will vary with the demeanor of the mare and the projected length of time of the fetotomy operation. Epidural anesthesia and sedation are indicated in almost all cases to minimize straining of the mare. General anesthesia should be used in mares that are uneasy or prone to sudden movements and in cases in which more than one or two cuts with the fetatome are anticipated. Repeated applications of non-water soluble, nonirritating lubricant are required to protect the genital canal and endometrium of the mare. Sequellae to fetotomy in the mare include retained placenta, metritis, peritonitis, laminitis, vaginal and cervical lacerations, delayed uterine involution and nerve paralysis (radial and facial). The severity of sequellae is related to the number of cuts required to relieve the dystocia and the duration of labor prior to presentation. In cases requiring partial fetotomy and presenting within 12 hours of the onset of labor, the prognosis for the mare's survival is good.

Cesarean Section. Delivery of a foal by laparohysterotomy is indicated in cases of transverse presentation, uterine torsion, malposture of the living fetus that cannot be corrected rapidly, an oversized fetus and maternal pelvic deformities. Restraint and anesthesia will vary with the preference of the operator, the temperament of the mare and facilities available. The operation has been reported to have been successfully performed in the standing mare under sedation and local anesthesia and in the recumbent mare using various general anesthetics. When the fetus is living, general anesthesia should be maintained at a light plane until the fetus is removed from the uterus, to avoid respiratory depression. Several sites for the abdominal incision have been described, including the paralumbar fossa, the ventral midline and the paramedian area; however, several authors report a preference for the lower left flank because less restraint of the mare is required. The uterus is incised along its greater curvature, avoiding large blood vessels. Hemorrhage from the large subendometrial veins must be controlled prior to closure of the uterine incision. A hemostatic suture is placed around the margins of the incision to clamp the three layers of the uterine wall together, thus, preventing intraluminal hemorrhage. Both a simple continuous and a continuous interlocking suture pattern are reported to have been successfully used. Following the hemostatic suture, the uterus is closed with an infolding suture pattern. Aftercare should be provided as indicated, with attention given to preventing or to controlling postsurgical infections, laminitis and retained placenta.

Vandeplassche[9] has compared the results of fetotomy and cesarean section in the mare and has reported several observations which are listed in Table 1.

Table 1. Results of Fetotomy and Cesarean Section

	Fetotomy (Per Cent)	Cesarean Section (Per Cent)
Mare Mortality	10	20
Retained Placenta	28	50
Fertility		
Pregnancy	42	50
Abortion	10	30
Foal Mortality	100	70
Impossible Delivery	10	0

DYSTOCIA

Dystocia may be caused by an abnormality of the fetus and is thus defined as fetal dystocia or by an abnormality of the dam, which is defined as maternal dystocia.

Fetal Dystocia in Anterior Presentation

Carpal Flexion Posture. Dystocia may be caused by uni- or bilateral carpal flexion. The condition is described as "engaged carpal flexion" when the limb, along with the head, is impacted in the maternal pelvis and is described as "disengaged carpal flexion" when the limb lies in front of the maternal pelvis. Correction of the malposture requires repulsion of the affected limb along with the fetus into the uterine cavity for manipulation of the long limb of the equine fetus. The hand corresponding to the side of the displacement is introduced into the birth canal, and the metacarpus is grasped immediately above the fetlock. The limb is lifted dorsally, flexing the shoulder and elbow joints. When the fetlock joint is above the pubis, the hoof, cupped in the operator's hand, is brought into the pelvic inlet. Traction applied with a snare fixed at the fetlock is useful in correcting cases of carpal flexion. While the carpus is lifted and repelled with one hand, gentle traction is applied to the snare with the other hand.

In some cases of engaged carpal flexion, delivery without correction may be possible if sufficient space in the maternal pelvis is available. Traction is applied to the extended limb, the fetal head and the carpus of the affected limb. Extension of the shoulder joint of the affected limb by application of repelling pressure to the shoulder and extractive force to the flexed carpus may aid in overcoming obstruction to delivery in uncorrected cases.

In cases in which the fetus is not living, carpal flexion posture is easily corrected by partial percutaneous fetotomy. The affected limb is amputated by placing the saw wire around the limb immediately distal to the carpal joint. The carpal joint is left intact to provide a point to anchor an obstetric chain.

If the malposture cannot be corrected rapidly and the fetus is living, cesarean section is indicated.

Shoulder Flexion Posture. In this malposture the forelimb lies alongside or under the fetal abdomen. The condition may be uni- or bilateral and may be engaged or disengaged. When attempting correction with the hand and arm, the hand corresponding to the side of the displacement is introduced into the birth canal, and the radius is grasped and pulled upward toward the pelvis, converting shoulder flexion into carpal flexion, which is further mutated. Mutation of shoulder flexion is difficult because of the long limbs of the equine fetus. A traction snare placed below the carpus with the aid of a snare introducer may be useful but is often difficult to apply because the carpus is situated deeply within the uterus. Extractive force is applied with the snare while the hand within the uterus is used to repel the shoulder, mutating the limb into a state of carpal flexion.

Forced extraction of the fetus without correction of unilateral shoulder flexion should be considered only if attempts at correction fail and the maternal pelvis is large and/or the fetus is small. The fetus must be well lubricated prior to the application of traction to the head and extended limb. Severe trauma to the fetus is likely if this procedure is attempted.

Relief of dystocia caused by shoulder flexion posture by percutaneous fetotomy is facilitated by amputation of the head, which allows access to the limb. The limb is amputated by first making an incision in the fetal skin over the dorsal border of the scapula. As the saw wire is positioned between the fetal scapula and the thorax, it is placed in the incision to prevent it from slipping down the limb. In bilateral cases, it may be necessary to remove only one limb prior to delivery of the remainder of the fetus.

Foot-Nape Posture. In this malposture, one or both forelimbs are displaced upward and lie on top of the fetal head. Common sequellae to foot-nape posture are rupture of the vagina, rectovaginal fistula and third degree perineal laceration. Immediate correction is necessary to prevent or minimize trauma to the birth canal. The fetal head must be lifted and repelled while assistants apply traction in a downward and lateral direction with snares attached to the fetlocks until the digits lie in a normal position.

If the hooves have penetrated the vaginal and rectal walls, an attempt may be made to replace them within the vagina prior to correction of the malposture. When the case has progressed to the point at which a rectovaginal fistula has been created, incision of the mare's perineum and conversion to a third degree perineal laceration may be indicated.

Percutaneous fetotomy procedures used to relieve foot-nape posture include amputation of the displaced limb or limbs within the vagina or within the rectum, if necessary. If the head prevents access to the limbs, it should be amputated and removed prior to amputation of the limbs.

Shoulder-Elbow Flexion Posture. In this relatively rare type of malposture the progress of the limbs is retarded, and the fetal muzzle lies in the area of the fetlocks rather than in the carpal joints. The elbows are impacted on the pubis, and the humerus lies in a vertical plane rather than the normal horizontal plane. This condition can be corrected by repelling the fetal head while simultaneous extractive force is applied to the limbs. Fetotomy is rarely needed to correct this type of malposture, but amputation of the head or one of the forelimbs may be considered.

Ventrovertical Presentation ("Dog-Sitting"). In this type of fetal malpresentation, delivery is impeded by the hind limbs, which are flexed at the hip joints. The digits of the posterior limbs may be impacted against the pubis or may lie in the vagina alongside the fetus. The anterior portion of the fetus is delivered normally, but delivery is impeded as the thorax emerges from the vulva. Delivery does not progress when extractive force is applied. Continued or forceful attempts at extraction may drive the fetal digits through the uterine wall. Attempts to deliver the fetus with the malpresentation uncorrected are not likely to be successful. Correction of ventrovertical presentation into normal anterior presentation may be attempted by rotation of the fetus to dislodge the digits. If the operator's arm is of sufficient length, an attempt to repel the hindlimbs by grasping the fetlocks, flexing the limb, and repelling the hindlimbs deeply into the uterine cavity should be considered.

Dystocia due to ventrovertical posture may be relieved by transverse division of the fetal trunk posterior to the last rib. After the forepart of the fetus is removed, an attempt may be made to deliver the hindquarters intact or the fetal pelvis longitudinally divided by directing the saw wire over the dorsum of the pelvis and between the hindlimbs.

Lateral Head Posture. Malposture of the fetal head and neck is a common cause of dystocia in the mare. The relatively long neck of the fetus makes manual correction extremely difficult. Congenital curvature of the cervical vertebrae ("wry-neck") cannot be corrected and must be differentiated from lateral deviation. In cases in which the fetus is exceptionally small delivery may proceed with the head deviated laterally, but most must be corrected.

If the head is within reach, the operator may attempt correction with the hand and arm. After abdominal straining has been relieved with epidural anesthesia, the mare is placed in lateral recumbency with the fetal head uppermost. The operator's hand corresponding to the side of the displacement is introduced deeply enough to grasp the fetal mouth. Pressure is exerted to move the head toward the midline of the dam, and the fetal head is brought into the pelvic inlet by grasping the muzzle with the fingers while maintaining pressure against the side of the fetal head with the palm of the hand. Traction for correcting malposture of the head and neck may also be applied by grasping the orbital grooves with the thumb and middle finger or by grasping the

lower jaw. A mandibular snare made of soft rope is useful in applying traction for correction of lateral head posture. The snare is placed around the lower jaw, and traction is exerted by the operator while maintaining repelling pressure against the fetal face with the opposite hand within the birth canal. Only moderate traction should be used when redirecting the head with a mandibular snare.

Partial percutaneous fetotomy is indicated when the fetal head is beyond reach, the malposture cannot be rapidly corrected or "wry-neck" is suspected. The head and neck are amputated at the point of deviation and removed from the birth canal, then the remainder of the fetal body is delivered. When sufficient space is not available within the maternal pelvis for amputation of the neck, the forelimb on the side opposite the displacement is amputated and delivered, allowing easier access to the flexed neck.

Cesarean section is indicated if the fetus is living and the malposture cannot be easily corrected.

Breast-Head Posture. Various degrees of breast-head posture have been described. *Vertex posture* is defined as the fetal head resting with the bridge of the muzzle against the maternal pubis and the poll directed into the pelvic inlet. Cases in which the head is displaced still further and the nape of the fetal neck is presented to the pelvic inlet are described as *nape posture*. True *breast-head posture* occurs when the fetal head is displaced still further between the forelimbs, and the jaw of the fetus rests against the sternum.

A mandibular snare is useful in attempting to correct breast-head posture. One of the operator's hands is used to apply repelling pressure to the poll while the other hand is used to apply traction with the snare, displacing the fetal head upward and forward. After it is sufficiently displaced, the fetal head is guided into the pelvic inlet.

Spontaneous delivery or delivery by extraction may be possible in some cases of nape posture if the maternal pelvis is of normal or larger size.

Percutaneous amputation of the displaced head is indicated if the fetus is dead; cesarean section should be considered if the fetus is living and the malposture cannot be rapidly corrected.

Hydrocephalus. Dystocia due to fetal monsters is not common in the mare. Hydrocephalus of the fetus is encountered occasionally. The cranium of the affected fetus will vary in size and degree of bone development. Some cases may be relieved by incising the soft portion of the skull, releasing the accumulated fluid and collapsing the skull sufficiently to allow for a safe delivery. Small instruments should not be introduced into the uterus without first attaching them to a long (100 cm) piece of umbilical tape held externally so they may be retrieved should they slip from the operator's hand. When bone development is more extensive, it may be necessary to reduce the size of the head by percutaneous fetotomy. The saw wire is placed around the indented portion of the cranium near its base, and the enlarged portion is amputated, collapsed and delivered. The body of the hydrocephalic fetus is usually smaller than normal and presents no further impediment to delivery.

Fetal Dystocia in Posterior Presentation

Posterior presentation of the fetus as a cause of dystocia is exceptional in the mare. When malposture of the hindlimbs occurs, mutation is difficult because of the extreme length of the fetal limbs and the limited space available.

Hock-Flexion Posture. Dystocia is caused when the fetus is presented posteriorly with the hindlimb flexed at the tarsal joint. The malposture may be uni- or bilateral and engaged or disengaged. When attempting to correct the malposture with the hand and arm, the operator grasps the lateral aspect of the metatarsus and displaces the hock upward and forward until the hoof can be directed into the pelvic inlet. Opposing forces may be applied, with the hand of the operator repelling and lifting the hock while traction is applied with a snare placed distal to the fetlock.

Percutaneous amputation of the affected limb or limbs immediately distal to the hock is indicated if the malposture cannot be corrected. The hock is left intact for application of a traction snare.

Hip-Flexion Posture. Delivery in posterior presentation may be impeded by complete flexion of one or both hip joints, resulting in displacement of the limbs under the fetal body. Correction of this malposture is difficult but may be attempted by placing the mare in lateral recumbency, with the affected limb uppermost. An attempt is made to mutate hip-flexion posture to hock-flexion, which is further mutated. Uncorrected delivery using a snare or anal hook has been described but is likely to be neither successful nor safe.

Dystocia due to hip-flexion posture can be relieved by percutaneous amputation of the affected limb or limbs followed by delivery of the remainder of the fetal body.

Fetal Dystocia in Abnormal Position and Presentation

Dorsoilial or Dorsopubic Position. Abnormal position resulting in dystocia occurs when the fetus fails to rotate to the normal dorsosacral position during the early phases of labor. When the fetus lies with its spine directed towards the maternal pubis or abdominal floor, the position is defined as dorsopubic. Partial rotation of the fetus with the fetal spine directed toward the left or right maternal ilium is described as dorsoilial position. Unless the fetus is small the malposition must be corrected before the fetus can be delivered. The condition must be differentiated from uterine torsion.

Obstetric chains are fixed to both fetal limbs, and

the head is secured by blunt eye-hooks or a mandibular snare. The operator's hand is introduced and placed below the ventral fetal limb, and the humerus is grasped near the shoulder joint. While an assistant applies traction to the dorsal limb in a downward and medial direction, the operator lifts the fetus upward until rotation into dorsosacral position is complete. The fetus must be freely moveable within the uterus prior to attempting rotation, or uterine torsion may be produced.

Fetal Dystocia in Transverse Presentation

Dystocia due to transverse presentation occurs following a gestation in which the fetus develops to a greater or lesser extent in both uterine horns and the body (bicornual pregnancy). This condition is fortunately rare and has been estimated to occur in less than 0.1 per cent of deliveries.

Ventral Transverse Presentation. This form is more commonly encountered in the mare. The fetus lies with its longitudinal axis oblique or perpendicular to that of the mare, with its limbs and abdominal surface presented to the pelvic inlet. The condition must be differentiated from twin pregnancy by determining that all limbs belong to the same fetus. Mutation of the transversely presented fetus is difficult, and cesarean section should be considered. If delivery by mutation is attempted, the fetus should be converted to posterior longitudinal presentation, dorsosacral position by repulsion and rotation. The forelimbs of the fetus are amputated prior to attempting version. It may be necessary to amputate the hindlimbs at the tarsal joints to gain access to the forelimbs. The forepart of the fetus is then repelled deeply into the uterine cavity while traction and rotation are applied to the hindlimbs.

Ventral transverse presentation may be complicated by rotation of the uterus. During late gestation the fetus and uterus rotate 90 to 180 degrees and lie beneath the uterine body and vagina, with the limbs of the fetus directed towards the dam's head. Stretching of the vagina results in an extremely long and narrow birth canal. Delivery by mutation or fetotomy is not likely to be successful because the fetus is out of reach; thus, delivery by cesarean section is indicated.

Dorsal Transverse Presentation. This form is less common than ventral transverse presentation. The fetus lies horizontally in front of the pelvis with the limbs directed towards the dam's head. Delivery by mutation requires that the forepart of the fetus be repelled while the hindpart is extracted and rotated, bringing the fetus into posterior presentation and dorsosacral position. If a saw wire can be passed around the lumbar area of the fetus, transverse division may allow delivery of the anterior and posterior portions of the fetus separately. Mutation and fetotomy are likely to be difficult, and delivery by cesarean section should be considered.

Maternal Dystocia

Difficulty in delivery of the fetus caused by an abnormality of the dam is less frequently encountered in the mare than is fetal dystocia.

Uterine Torsion. Torsion of the uterus in the mare is usually accompanied by signs of severe abdominal discomfort. Diagnosis is based on palpation of displacement of the broad ligaments. The broad ligament on the side to which the uterus is twisted is pulled tightly under the uterus while the one on the opposite side is stretched over the top of the uterus. In contrast to the cow, uterine torsion in the mare does not usually involve the anterior vagina or cervix. Torsion may be in either direction but is most commonly toward the left.

Several methods are described to correct uterine torsion in the mare. Rolling the anesthetized mare rapidly in the direction of the torsion has been reported to be successful but may be complicated by uterine rupture or abortion. Uterine torsion may also be corrected by abdominal surgery. The standing position is preferred. A laparotomy incision is made in the flank on the side of the torsion, and the uterus is repositioned by lifting the lower portion and repelling the upper portion. If the fetus is dead, it is removed by hysterotomy. Live fetuses are left in place, with most expected to continue to term.

Abdominal Hernia. Rupture of the prepubic tendon is seen more commonly in draft mares than other types. It usually occurs in the last 2 months of gestation and may or may not be associated with a history of trauma. The prognosis in all cases is poor because the mare cannot effectively apply abdominal pressure during the second stage of labor. Several methods have been advocated for the management of rupture of the prepubic tendon, including elective cesarean section near term, repeated vaginal examinations followed by extraction of the fetus when the cervix dilates and induced parturition accompanied by extraction. Euthanasia of the mare following delivery of the foal is indicated in many cases.

Abnormal Pelvis. Fractures or exostoses of the pelvis that result in stenosis of the birth canal are rarely encountered in the mare. Management of these cases will depend upon the degree of stenosis. Elective cesarean section should be considered if such cases are identified prior to the onset of labor.

Vaginal Cystocele. The urinary bladder of the mare may interfere with delivery if it enters the vagina either by eversion through the urethra or prolapse through a rupture in the vagina. In either case the bladder must be replaced after first abolishing abdominal straining and repelling the fetus. The everted bladder must be massaged and inverted through the urethra. In the case of a prolapsed bladder accumulated urine may be removed by catheterization of the urethra or by cystocentesis. The bladder is replaced and the vaginal wound sutured. The fetus is then delivered by traction.

References

1. Benesch F, Wright JG: Veterinary Obstetrics. Baltimore, Williams & Wilkins Co, 1951, pp 156–259.
2. Bierschwal CJ, deBois CHW: The Technique of Fetotomy in Large Animals. Bonner Springs, VM Publishing Co, 1972, pp 9–50.
3. Blanchard TL, Bierschwal CJ, Youngquist RS, Elmore RG: Sequellae to percutaneous fetotomy in the mare. JAVMA 182:1127, 1983.
4. Edwards GB, Allan WE, Newcombe JR: Elective cesarean section in the mare for the production of gnotobiotic foals. Equine Vet J 6:122, 1974.
5. Pascoe JR, Meagher DM, Wheat, JD: Surgical management of uterine torsion in the mare: A review of 26 cases. JAVMA 179:351, 1981.
6. Roberts SJ: Veterinary Obstetrics and Genital Diseases. 2nd ed. Ithaca, SJ Roberts, 1971, pp 274–299.
7. Vandeplassche M: Obstetrician's view of the physiology of equine parturition and dystocia. Equine Vet J 12:45, 1980.
8. Vandeplassche M: The normal and abnormal presentation, position and posture of the foal-fetus during gestation and at parturition. Mededelingen der Veeartsenijschool van de Rijksuniversiteit te Gent, nr. 1, 1957, pp 3–36.
9. Vandeplassche M, Spincemaille J, Bouters R, Bonte P: Some aspects of equine obstetrics. Equine Vet J 4:105, 1972.

Equine Fetal Diseases

T. W. Swerczek, D.V.M., Ph.D.
University of Kentucky, Lexington, Kentucky

The reproductive efficiency of the domesticated mare is poor compared with other farm animals. Among the factors that cause a lowering of the foaling rate, fetal wastage is of paramount importance. This is compounded in some cases because the cause of the abortion may have a lasting effect on the reproductive tract of the mare. Frequently, in some mares there is a vicious cycle of abortion, infection and nonproduction. The increased number of barren mares in recent years is of considerable economic importance to the horse breeding industry.

This article will discuss the common causes of fetal wastage, as recorded in the necropsy examination of fetuses submitted to the University of Kentucky from area horse farms. Hundreds of fetuses not found but aborted early in gestation are never recorded or submitted. It is this category of aborted fetuses that account for the greatest percentage of fetal wastage, from 5 to 15 per cent as

Table 1. Causes of Equine Fetal Loss in 935 Aborted Fetuses (Recorded at the University of Kentucky from 1973 to 1975)

Cause	Percentage of Aborted Fetuses
Placental Disease	29.8
Twins	19.1
Herpesvirus 1	14.7
Neonatal Asphyxia	11.7
Noninfectious disease (placental edema, fescue)	10.0
Congenital anomalies	9.7
Bacteremia	2.5
Miscellaneous	2.6

(From the proceedings of the annual meeting of The Society for Theriogenology, September 15–17, 1976, Lexington, Kentucky.)

compared with 2 to 5 per cent of the fetal wastage in which the fetuses are found and examined. Unfortunately, more attention is focused on the lesser important causes of wastage because these fetuses are aborted later in pregnancy and are submitted for necropsy. A survey of the causes of 935 aborted fetuses during a 3-year period from 1973 to 1975 (Table 1) was recorded in 1976.[10] The cause of fetal wastage has remained the same in recent years, with the exception of one disease category—herpes virus 1 abortion, in which there has been a significant decrease in the number of cases. This is because the planned herpes virus 1 infection is no longer practiced. Its use caused a small percentage of abortion on most farms where it was administered, especially in the maiden mares, but large abortion storms were prevented on a single farm. The planned infection program has been replaced by vaccination programs that do not cause abortions; they maintain immunity in a herd, which also prevents large-scale abortion storms. As a result, the incidence of virus abortion has dropped significantly. Other necropsy surveys have been reported earlier from Kentucky[1] and from England.[7, 13]

EARLY FETAL LOSS

There are a variety of causes of early embryonic or early fetal loss. These are related to infections of the uterus, venereal diseases, hormonal dysfunction, genetic abnormalities, cervical lesions, uterine lesions, urine pooling, poor conformation of the vulva, vagina and cervix, pneumovagina and others. In these cases, however, conditions generally affect the mare individually, and most can be identified; a few can be corrected. More often the end result is a problem mare, usually an older mare, that is a habitual aborter either early or late.

Another cause of early embryonic and early fetal loss in otherwise normal healthy mares is related to nutrition or nonseasonal breeding and nutrition.[11] This form of early embryonic and fetal loss affects the healthy mare and occasionally multiple mares of all ages in an otherwise normal, healthy herd. Mares that are bred before the natural breeding season, which starts in late April in the Northern Hemisphere, seem to have a higher incidence of early embryonic and fetal loss if they are exposed to a drastic change in nutrition from a dry winter ration to lush spring grass while they are pregnant. These mares have excessive ovarian follicular development and a more relaxed cervix when compared with control mares in a dry lot not receiving fresh green grass. The sudden increase in the plane of nutrition, a result of the green grass, seems to flush the mare. A similar flushing phenomenon, even in nonpregnant mares, occurs when there is a seasonal change from dormant, dry summer pastures to lush green fall pastures. This fall flushing causes a dramatic increase in fetal losses; the mare may be 6 to 7 months pregnant, and the aborted fetus is found to have an ascending bacterial and/or mycotic placentitis secondary to cervical relaxation. A similar ascending placentitis is seen when mares are "conditioned" for shows or for the fall and winter horse sales. The sudden change and/or elevated plane of nutrition produces a flush similar, but less significant, to the one produced by the lush spring or fall grass. The best conditioned mares seem to have the highest incidence of this type of ascending placentitis.

Any condition that encourages the onset of estrus in the mare contributes to cervical relaxation. Another important cause is transporting mares for long distances. Nonpregnant mares have a tendency to come into estrus or to show signs of estrus activity a few days after hauling. The same phenomenon has also been observed in mares early in pregnancy, with the loss of the fetus a few days to a few weeks after hauling. Mares are stressed from hauling and are exposed to a new environment, new horses and a different type of ration on the new farm. The combination of these factors is very conducive to early fetal loss and infectious placentitis.

BACTERIAL AND MYCOTIC DISEASES

The common bacterial organisms found in aborted fetuses are coliforms, *Escherichia coli*, *Pseudomonas aeruginosa*, *Klebsiella pneumonia*, *Streptococcus zooepidemicus*, *Staphylococcus aureus*, and *Actinobacillus equuli*. Other bacteria occasionally found include *Salmonella* spp., *Brucella abortus*, *Leptospira* spp. and *Listeria* spp. Frequently, bacteria that normally are thought of as nonpathogenic are found in the fetus, and in some cases these nonpathogens are the likely cause of abortion, especially in early embryonic and fetal development.

The fungus most often associated with abortion is *Aspergillus fumigatus*, but *Mucor* spp., *Allescheria boydii*[5] and *Coccidioides immitis*[4] also have been reported as causing mycotic abortion in mares.

It is difficult in many cases to determine if the pathway of infection is hematogenously spread from the maternal side or if it ascends from the cervix and vagina. It appears that the majority of cases result from an ascending infection secondary to cervical relaxation and from organisms that are commonly found in the vaginal tract. It is obvious in cases of *Streptococcus zooepidemicus* and fungal infections that the infection is ascending secondary to cervical relaxation. In other cases, in which cervical relaxation and an ascending infection with coliform organisms are likely, the placental lesions indicating contamination are not as obvious because these organisms rapidly spread throughout the placenta, and the fetus dies before placental lesions have time to develop. The cause of abortion in most instances is placentitis and, in some cases, a secondary fetal septicemia.

BACTERIAL PLACENTITIS

Bacterial placentitis is by far the most common cause of fetal wastage in the mare. Placental infection from an ascending pathway occurs throughout pregnancy. The greatest loss occurs early in pregnancy, and many of these fetuses are not found. It is reasonable to assume then that this type of fetal wastage is responsible for the majority of abortions in mares. The placental lesions seen in bacterial placentitis vary with the type of causative bacteria.[8] *Streptococcus zooepidemicus* produces a chronic placentitis, with necrosis and chronic inflammation around the cervical star and extending up into the body. The fetus has slight growth retardation, and the organs are slightly autolytic. In contrast, bacteria such as *E. coli, Pseudomonas* spp., *Klebsiella* spp. and coliforms produce acute infection. The placental lesions are acute, the inflammatory response is minimal and numerous bacteria can be seen in the chorionic villi. The fetus is usually very autolytic, and the body cavities contain blood-tinged fluid. The fetal organs contain the causative organism.

Another very common form of apparent bacterial placentitis appears to be related to bacteria normally considered nonpathogenic, such as microaerophilic streptococci or *Acinetobacter* spp. The placenta in this case has a chronic inflammation, with focal areas of necrosis, bacteria scattered throughout the villi and frequently foci of dystrophic calcification. The fetus is autolytic and either is free of bacteria or contains the "nonpathogenic" bacteria.

MYCOTIC PLACENTITIS

The two most common fungi causing mycotic placentitis are *Aspergillus fumigatus* and *Mucor* spp. The infection is ascending, apparently secondary to a relaxed cervix, and leads to contamination of the chorioallantois around the cervical star, with progression up in the body. Typically, the mare shows signs of heat earlier in pregnancy, then several months later the mare aborts with an ascending mycotic placentitis. As discussed earlier, the incidence of mycotic placentitis seems to be higher when flushing conditions prevail, that is, a wet fall and abundant pasture.

Fetuses that abort from a mycotic placentitis are usually fresh. Frequently, foals are born prematurely and have marked growth retardation resembling a twin. If they are near term, the chances for survival are similar to those of a twin born alive near term.

The chorioallantois from a mycotic placentitis is characterized by evidence of an ascending infection from the cervical star area. The chorioallantois is thickened and leathery and usually contains a thick tenacious mucoid exudate, which will vary with the causative agent. There is a sharp line of demarcation between the infected and the normal chorioallantois. Histologically, there is a marked metaplasia of the chorion to squamous type epithelium, necrosis and inflammation, with the necrotic tissue laden with mycotic hyphae. In cases of infection by *Aspergillus* spp. there are occasionally metaplastic, cystlike nodules on the allantoic surface. The fetal organs are usually fresh, with the most dramatic lesions found in the liver, which on gross examination is pale, enlarged and mottled. Histologically, the liver is fatty, with portal hepatitis and bile ductule proliferation. The changes in the liver are likely caused by a combination of fetal starvation and toxic fungal products from the placental lesions because mycotic organisms are rarely found in the liver. Occasionally, mycotic hyphae are found in the lungs, and in these cases there is a focal to diffuse chronic pneumonia.

BODY PREGNANCY

This condition is caused by the failure of the horns of the uterus to expand, and the chorioallantoic horns are underdeveloped. The fetus develops in the body of the uterus and is usually very retarded in growth. Abortion occurs from 7 to 10 months of gestation. The placenta is commonly thickened because of a chronic inflammation, and the fetus has no characteristic lesions other than those associated with placental insufficiency. The cause of this condition is unknown. It seems reasonable to assume that the cause may be nonspecific and related to pathologic lesions in either the uterus or the placenta or both.

PLACENTAL INSUFFICIENCY

Fetuses aborted with this condition have growth retardation caused by a variety of pre-existing pathologic lesions in the uterus. These may be chronic metritis with fibrosis of the endometrium, multiple cysts in the uterine mucosa and general atrophy of the uterine mucosa. The end result is a malnourished fetus that is aborted or a term foal that is underdeveloped and weak at birth. Because of the uterine lesions, the chorionic villi are irregular, atrophied and poorly developed. Often, there is a chronic placentitis with dystrophic calcification of the chorionic villi.

PREMATURE PLACENTAL SEPARATION

When the placenta prematurely separates at parturition, the fetus frequently dies perinatally. In these cases, the entire chorioallantois is thicker than normal, but the area at the cervical star is very thick, red and edematous. The edema gradually lessens in the body, and the chorioallantois becomes thinner. This placental area, but not the cervical star, ruptures at parturition.

The cause of premature placental separation and placental edema may be multifactorial. There are two common causes of placental edema: fescue grass toxicity and stress in combination with excessive nutrition. In the case of fescue grass toxicity, there is a history of fescue grass exposure either through the pasture, hay or bedding. Typically, prolonged gestation, agalactia characterized by the absence of mammary gland development or occasionally mammary gland development with little or no milk secretion indicates the toxicity. The entire chorioallantois and amnion are edematous, thick and heavy. If foals do not suffocate at birth, they may be weak at birth and frequently die from a variety of neonatal diseases, since they are compromised from the fescue toxicity and, on occasion, from the lack of colostrum.

The second cause of premature placental separation and placental edema is associated with stress to the mare late in gestation. The stress may be from drastic changes in weather, hauling, changing of pastures, anthelmintic treatment, medication, vaccination or illness. In addition to the stress, there is a history of an excessively nutritious diet either in the form of lush pastures, legume hay, and/or excessive protein and carbohydrate rations. This combination seems to trigger the phenomenon of premature placental separation, but unlike fescue toxicity, the foals are usually born prematurely, mammary gland development is present if near term and milk may be secreted if near term. There may or may not be evidence of a bacterial or mycotic infection at the cervical star. In these cases it appears that the cause of the placental edema around the cervical star and into the body is related to cervical relaxation. Possibly, as the cervix and the body of the uterus near the cervix relax, there is a gradual detachment of the chorion from the uterus. As this occurs, fluid accumulates in the chorioallantois because of continuous circulation from the fetus but no corresponding circulatory contact from the maternal side, resulting in edema between the chorion and allantois. The process is not spontaneous, as there is fibrin formation between the chorion and allantois and around major vessels. The result is a very thick, edematous and tough chorioallantois that is difficult to tear. In these cases the cervical portion of the chorioallantois may separate at the body, and the foal suffocates from premature placental separation. The cause of this lesion is unknown, but frequently there is a coincidental history of stress from many conditions and/or excessive nutrition in many forms. Mares maintained in a dry lot and not excessively fed usually have very thin placentas that are in sharp contrast to mares with the placental edema syndrome.[12] The condition is an important cause of fetal loss and seems to be on the increase in recent years. Also, the condition varies from year to year, possibly owing to grass-growing conditions and weather conditions that are closely related.

CONGENITAL MALFORMATIONS

Congenital anomalies occur in approximately 1 per cent of the foals that are born each year. Many of these are minor, allowing the birth of live foals. There seems to be an unending list of developmental malformations that occur in fetuses and foals with new variations appearing each year. One cannot help from speculating that the recent avalanche of new drugs given to pregnant mares may be responsible for many of these anomalies. Unfortunately, we have been unable to determine the etiology of any of the field cases, but experimentally an anthelmintic was shown to cause limb abnormalities in pony foals.[3]

The most common form of developmental malformation is contracted forelimbs and occasionally contracted hind legs. A more severe form may be related to this and includes varying degrees of cranial-facial deformities, torticollis and scoliosis. These malformations are important because they are usually responsible for dystocia and the occasional death of the mare. There are numerous other malformations that occur in fetuses and foals that are reported elsewhere.

Abnormalities of the umbilical cord frequently occur, but often it is difficult to determine the significance of these changes, as similar lesions are seen on the umbilical cords of apparently normal term foals. The most common forms of abnormal umbilical cords are sacculations filled with fluid and calcified cysts. There are cases in which the umbilical cord is excessively twisted, causing edema and hemorrhage and an obvious fatal circulatory disturbance to the fetus. Fetuses that die of umbilical cord obstruction usually have subcutaneous edema and hemorrhage of the ventral abdomen around the navel and excess blood in the body cavities. In other cases there may be an elongated navel stalk, an umbilical hernia and an enlarged dilated urachus and urinary bladder.

FETAL DIARRHEA

As the name indicates, fetuses with this condition defecate a large amount of usually soft liquid meconium in the later stages of fetal development. This meconium is frequently aspirated into the lungs. Depending on the degree of fetal defecation, abortion may occur late in gestation or foals may be born weak, with a poor prognosis.

The aborted fetuses and term foals are stained by the meconium, thus appearing jaundiced. The lesions seen at necropsy will vary in severity, but the typical cases will have hyperplasia of the adrenal glands and marked lymphoid depletion in the thymus and splenic follicles. The kidneys occasionally are swollen and inflamed with an interstitial nephritis with dystrophic focal calcification. The lungs contain meconium in the bronchiolar tree and alveoli. Often, fetal diarrhea occurs with other primary lesions such as placental infarction and congenital anomalies. The etiology is unknown, but the cause appears to be related to fetal and/or maternal stress. The syndrome possibly has multiple causes, and fetal diarrhea may be a reaction to fetal stress.

VIRAL DISEASES

Herpesvirus 1

Equine herpesvirus 1 is a respiratory virus of young and adult horses. Often, the virus is inapparent in adults, but if pregnant mares are exposed to the virus after 7 months of gestation, they may abort. In the majority of cases herpesvirus 1 abortion occurs sporadically in a herd, with the maiden mares most often affected. Multiple abortions of all age groups usually indicate a lack of immunity in a herd that was recently exposed to the virus. Usually, in these circumstances a new horse has recently been added to the herd, which was kept in isolation for several months or years. Virus abortion is rare in mares that are kept in a group with no addition of new mares to the herd after the first trimester of pregnancy. Mares usually abort suddenly, with no mammary gland development, and the fresh fetus is still attached to the placenta. The placenta may be heavier than normal due to congestion and edema and is usually stained with meconium, giving it a jaundiced appearance. Foals that are born near term may have severe respiratory signs and very low white blood cell counts.

The pathologic lesions produced in cases of herpesvirus 1 abortion vary greatly and generally depend on the stage of gestation. Fetuses affected at 7 to 10 months of gestation have widespread lesions in the liver, lungs, thymus, lymph nodes, adrenals and subcutaneous tissues. As the fetus nears term, the lesions are most severe in the lungs, with a gradual decrease in severity of lesions elsewhere. In general, most fetuses will have the following lesions in varying degrees and areas: (1) hyperemic and hemorrhagic mucous membranes of the eyes and mouth, (2) varying degrees of jaundice in the subcutaneous tissues, placenta and hooves, (3) subcutaneous edema, especially along the forehead and neck, (4) occasional severe edema of the upper neck and around the larynx and anterior trachea, (5) excessive clear yellow fluid in body cavities, (6) varying degrees of consolidation, with focal hemorrhage and interlobular edema in the lungs, (7) few to many minute foci of necrosis on the surface and throughout the liver, (8) perirenal edema, (9) hemorrhagic adrenal glands, (10) hyperplastic spleen with prominent splenic follicles and (11) necrotic thymus, as seen on the cut surface.

Histologically, the lesions are characteristic, and viral intranuclear inclusion bodies can be demonstrated in necrotic tissues of the liver, lung, thymus, adrenals and lymph nodes. In the liver in addition to focal necrosis, there is often a reactive portal hepatitis with variable proliferation of reticulum cells, round cells and bile ductules. The adrenals have foci of necrosis with hemorrhage. Necrosis of lymphocytes also occurs in the thymus, splenic follicles and lymph nodes, especially nodes near the lung, liver and intestine. Lastly, a necrotizing bronchiolitis and a focal pneumonitis are found in aborted fetuses, with a diffuse pneumonitis generally present in term foals.

Equine Viral Arteritis

The equine arteritis virus is also a cause of abortion. This disease does not show any characteristic lesions, but the virus can be isolated from affected fetuses. The only known cases of abortion have occurred when the very virulent form of the virus existed.[2] Currently, the virus is so avirulent that either obvious clinical signs are not observed or very mild clinical signs are seen when sporadic outbreaks occur.[6] The virus seems to be endemic in Standardbreds in a subclinical form, but in April 1984 it was diagnosed in Thoroughbred stallions and mares on a Kentucky stud farm. The virus has spread to mares bred to affected stallions and then to other mares and foals.

Equine Infectious Anemia

Pregnant mares infected with equine infectious anemia (EIA) may have virus-infected foals. The virus is transmitted by intrauterine passage or through the milk.[9] We have not recorded any cases of abortion that were attributed directly to the EIA virus. However, it is possible that mares acutely affected with EIA may abort at the height of the febrile reaction, as is the case with other infectious diseases of the mare. If EIA does cause abortion, the incidence is very low.

TWINS

Twinning is a common cause of abortion, especially in Thoroughbreds, in which the incidence is 1 to 2 per cent. It appears that the highest incidence of twins occurs when mares conceive during the natural breeding season. In this season the plane of nutrition from spring and early summer grass is the highest, and the photoperiod is the longest; therefore, it is reasonable to expect multiple ovulations during this season in comparison to the usual nonbreeding season. It is common for the mare to have multiple follicles and multiple ovulations. Many twins are conceived but few are carried to late gestation or to term. It is not unusual to find evidence of mummified remains of a twin in the placenta of a single foal of normal size. With the use of ultrasound in diagnosing early pregnancy, it has been observed that mares conceiving twins commonly *absorb* one fetus during the first month of development. In these cases there is no evidence of fetal remnants left in the placenta of the other twin at foaling. It would be of interest and of considerable importance to determine which factors are involved in this phenomenon of multiple ovulation, twin conception and absorption of one twin in the majority of cases. It is likely that nutrition plays a role. Also, certain mares have a tendency to conceive twins, indicating a genetic influence.

When both twins survive the early part of gestation, they are usually aborted, or occasionally underdeveloped weak foals are born at or near term. In these cases one foal is usually larger and may survive. The fetal loss appears to be caused by lack of nutrition from competition with the other twin. This obviously occurs to a certain extent because of the inadequate placental space. However, it does not explain why one fetus dies early in development when space is not as critical. It is not unusual for the fetus with the largest placental space to die first. Possibly such mechanisms as interfetal incompatibility, immunologic reactions as well as nutrition are responsible for early twin absorption as well as late fetal death. When mares are carrying twins, the mammary glands commonly develop prematurely and secrete milk. This apparently occurs when one fetus dies.

When twins are aborted late in pregnancy, one fetus is usually alive and the other is mummified and in various stages of autolysis from a fetal death of a few hours to several months. The fetus is underdeveloped, and the liver is mottled, pale and enlarged. Histologically, the liver is fatty and has a mild portal triad hepatitis with histiocytes and plasma cells. The changes in the liver appear to be related to the placental insufficiency and possibly an immunologic response from the other twin. The placentae from twins can be readily identified as a twin placentation by a sharp line of demarcation where the chorioallantois of the two fetuses come in contact with each other. The chorionic villi are lacking where the chorion of each twin contacts each other. There are many variations in the size and shape of the placenta of each fetus and this may play a role in the length of time the mare carries the twins. Generally, if the placentae are nearly equal in size, the twins are more likely to be carried to term.

STILLBIRTHS AND NEONATAL ASPHYXIA

Foal death at birth or perinatally is frequently caused by dystocia. Other causes are premature placental separation, placental edema, obstruction of the nose with the fetal membranes and premature rupture of the umbilical cord. Other cases have no apparent reason, but in the majority there is a history of abnormal foaling, usually a prolonged foaling time.

References

1. Dimock WW, Edwards PR, Bruner DW: Infections observed in equine fetuses and foals. Cornell Vet 37:89, 1947.
2. Doll ER, Bryans JT, McCollum WH, Crowe MEW: Isolation of a filterable agent causing arteritis of horses and abortion by mares. Cornell Vet 47:3, 1957.
3. Drudge JH, Lyons ET, Swerczek TW, Tolliver SC: Cambendazole for strongyle control in a pony band: Selection of a drug-resistant population of small strongyles and teratologic implications. AJVR 44:110, 1983.
4. Langham F, Beneke ES, Whitenack DL: Abortion in a mare due to coccidiodomycosis. JAVMA 170:178, 1977.
5. Mahaffey LW, Rossdale PB: An abortion due to *Allescheria boydii* and general observations concerning mycotic abortions in mares. Vet Rec 77:541, 1965.
6. McCollum WH, Bryans JT: Serological identification of infection by Equine Arteritis Virus in horses of several countries. Paris, Proc 3rd Int Conf Equine Infect Dis, 1972, pp 256–263.
7. Platt H: Infections of the horse fetus. J Reprod Fert Suppl 23:605, 1973.
8. Prickett ME: Abortion and placental lesions in the mare. JAVMA 157:1465, 1970.
9. Stein CD, Mott LO: Studies on congenital transmission of Equine Infectious Anemia. Vet Med 37:370, 1942.
10. Swerczek TW: Pathology and pathogenesis of equine fetal diseases. Lexington, Proc Soc Theriogenology, 1976.
11. Swerczek TW: Early fetal death and infectious placental disease in the mare. Proc 26th Ann Conv AAEP, 1985, pp 173–179.
12. Swerczek TW: Unpublished data, 1985.
13. Whitwell KE: Investigations into fetal and neonatal losses in the horse. Symposium on equine reproduction, Vet Clin North Am: Large Anim Pract 2:313, 1980.

Abortion and Other Gestational Diseases in Mares

S. J. Roberts, D.V.M., M.S.
Woodstock, Vermont

Abortion is the expulsion of a nonviable or dead fetus. Expulsion of the embryo or fetus following death between 20 and 90 days of pregnancy is rarely observed. Most abortions, even on a well-supervised breeding farm, are usually not observed until after 4 or 5 months of gestation. For this reason most early embryonic and fetal deaths, which are common from 20 to 90 days of gestation, are considered to be a form of infertility. Early death of the embryo is usually associated with a regular or slightly delayed estrous cycle. The incidence of early fetal death in mares between 30 and 90 days of gestation is reported as ranging from 7 to 30 per cent, with the average being 8 to 15 per cent (see Table 1, Size and Characteristics of the Equine Fetus and Uterus During Pregnancy, page 672). An increase in early pregnancy losses has been associated with the following: (1) use of certain stallions; (2) short postpartum intervals of less than 20 days before service; (3) mares over 18 years of age; (4) infertile mares or those that aborted at the previous breeding season; (5) injudicious, rough manual examination of mares in early pregnancy, i.e., before 40 days; (6) poorly managed breeding, in which excessive aging of spermatozoa or ova occurred in the uterine tubes prior to fertilization, resulting in chromosomal abnormalities; (7) malnourished mares between 25 and 31 days of pregnancy; (8) uterine infections; (9) an abnormal endometrium with fibrotic, atrophied endometrial glands and (10) excessive stress due to overheating, trucking and working.

The incidence of observed equine abortions after the fourth month of gestation usually constitutes only a small percentage of total pregnancy wastage (about 2 to 12 per cent of all pregnancies). Abortions may be caused by either infectious or noninfectious agents that affect the normal function and development of the fetus, fetal membranes and genital tract. Given an accurate and complete history and prompt delivery of a blood sample and the chilled, aborted fetus with placental membranes to a competent diagnostic laboratory, the cause of the

abortion can usually be ascertained in about 50 to 60 per cent of the submitted cases. Frequently, the fetus dies in the uterus and is not expelled for 2 to 3 days, with resultant autolytic changes that make a definitive diagnosis very difficult. Autolysis of the equine fetus is characterized by opacity of the cornea, soft, mushy internal organs and gelatinous, blood-tinged subcutaneous and placental tissues.

INFECTIOUS CAUSES OF EQUINE ABORTION

Bacteria

Bacterial causes of equine abortion include *Streptococcus zooepidemicus, Salmonella abortus equi, Leptospira pomona* and possibly other *Leptospira* organisms, *Escherichia coli, Staphylococcus aureus, Corynebacterium equi, Pseudomonas aeruginosa, Brucella abortus* and other *Brucella* organisms. *Klebsiella pneumoniae var. genitalium, Actinobacillus, Streptococcus equi* and other streptococci and staphylococci.

Most of these organisms gain entrance to the uterus through the cervix, invade the cervical portion of the placenta and spread to the allantoic and amniotic cavities and the fetus. They are often found in the stomach or lungs of the fetus as a result of its swallowing or inhaling infected amniotic fluid. Some of these bacterial organisms, such as salmonella and leptospira, can enter the uterus from the bloodstream and pass to the fetus through the placenta. Most of these organisms cause abortion during the last trimester of gestation or are present in the newborn foal at parturition.

Streptococcus zooepidemicus, a β-hemolytic streptococcus, is the most common bacterial cause of abortion at any stage of gestation. This organism is commonly found on the external genital organs of mares and stallions. It may be recovered by culture of the genital tract from more than 90 per cent of foaling mares for several days after parturition and is the most common organism associated with vaginitis, cervicitis and metritis secondary to pneumovagina. These "strep" abortions occur most commonly on poorly managed farms where proper breeding hygiene, including prebreeding examination and culture of mares, and proper washing of the external genitalia of the mare and stallion before and after breeding, is not followed. In addition, such abortions are common on farms where frequent services at "foal" heat, excessive frequent breeding of older mares and unsanitary foaling procedures occur.

The normal, healthy genital tract in mares not prone to infection is quite resistant to small numbers of *S. zooepidemicus* or other organisms introduced at parturition or breeding. Abortions caused by this organism are sporadic because infection is limited to the genital tract and is not spread by ingestion or by other means. The organism is usually readily recovered from the infected fetus, infected fetal membranes and genital discharges after abortion. Infected mares may require local antibiotic therapy of the genital tract, preferably at estrus; vulvar suturing, if the mare has pneumovagina; limited services performed in a careful, hygienic manner or artificial insemination with semen treated with antibiotics and possible douching of the uterus with antibiotics 12 to 24 hours after service. Older, chronically infected mares can be a serious problem and require a guarded prognosis.

Salmonella abortus equi as a cause of contagious equine abortion was first described in the United States in the late nineteenth century and was a common cause of outbreaks of abortion in Kentucky in the early twentieth century. Abortions caused by this agent have been reported in many states as well as worldwide. Except for two small, isolated outbreaks, salmonella abortion in mares has not been reported in the United States since 1932. The reason for the near disappearance of this previously common disease is not known.

The salmonella organism is spread by ingestion of feed and water contaminated by fecal or genital wastes. The incubation period is 10 to 28 days, and the incidence of abortion in a group of infected mares may reach 50 to 90 per cent. The fetus is usually autolyzed, and the placenta is edematous, necrotic and hemorrhagic. The organism can be readily recovered by culture, and the agglutination test performed on the mare's serum will demonstrate antibodies with a titer of 1:500 to 1:5000. The use of bacterins as a prophylactic measure has been highly effective in the past in preventing outbreaks of salmonella abortions.

Leptospira pomona and other leptospirae have occasionally been reported as a cause of abortion in mares. Abortions may occur without any history of prior disease but often occur 1 to 3 weeks after a mild illness that is characterized by a moderately elevated body temperature, anorexia, slight depression and icterus. Usually, the fetus shows autolysis, and demonstration of the leptospiral agent is unsuccessful by culture, staining or fluorescent antibody techniques; however, the aborting mare will frequently show a rising antibody titer.

The other bacterial agents usually cause only sporadic abortions and are associated with conditions and disease factors similar to those associated with *S. zooepidemicus*. Preventive measures and appropriate local treatment of the genital tract with antibiotics are indicated.

Viruses

Viral causes of equine abortion include rhinopneumonitis or equine herpesvirus 1, equine arteritis virus and equine infectious anemia.

Equine herpesvirus 1 (rhinopneumonitis virus) is widespread in the United States, Canada, Japan and European countries. It commonly affects foals in the fall of the year at weaning time and produces a mild, febrile (102 to 104°F or 38.8 to 40.0°C) respiratory disease, with coughing, nasal discharge ("snots"), inappetence and depression. Occasionally, ataxia, paresis, prostration and death may occur in horses when the virus invades the central nervous system. The incubation period of the respiratory disease is 2 to 3 days in foals. The signs of the disease may linger in foals for 2 to 6 weeks. Spread of the disease is mainly by inhalation or droplet infection or occasionally by ingestion. The disease is highly contagious and infectious, and animals may experience several attacks at 6-month to 2-year intervals. The respiratory disease in older horses that have previously been infected is very mild, with few or no clinical signs. The incubation period for abortion in natural cases averages 20 to 30 days, but it may extend up to 90 days. This long incubation period may be caused by the persistence of the virus in the leukocytes of the mare and in the chorion of the placenta before it finally invades the susceptible fetus, causing its death and expulsion.

Fetal death and abortion due to this virus rarely occur before the fifth month of gestation, and 90 per cent of cases occur from 8 months to term. Infected foals may be born at term but die within 2 to 9 hours of birth. The incidence of abortion in a group of mares varies from 1 to 90 per cent, depending on factors such as the degree of immunity, virulence of the virus and numbers of mares in advanced pregnancy. Abortions may occur over a period of 2 weeks to 3 months, with 90 per cent of abortions occurring within 60 days. Fetuses usually die and are expelled promptly in a fresh state. Some infected fetuses show no significant lesions, but many have edema and petechial hemorrhages in the lung or small whitish-yellow foci of necrosis in the liver. Intranuclear inclusion bodies are frequently found in the bronchial epithelium and the liver cells. Virus abortion due to equine herpesvirus 1 is probably the most common single cause of abortions in the last trimester of pregnancy. Permanent immunity, as with other herpesviruses, does not occur, and carriers of the virus are common. The prophylactic use of vaccine is discussed elsewhere.

Equine arteritis virus will produce rare outbreaks of a severe general systemic and respiratory disease, with abortion as a complication. This virus was found to cause abortion about 15 to 20 years ago soon after the occurrence of severe "shipping-fever-like" disease outbreaks, which were characterized by elevation of the body temperature (103 to 106°F or 39.4 to 41.1°C), conjunctivitis, lacrimation, photophobia, palpebral edema (pink eye), severe depression, rapid respirations, weakness, stiffness, anorexia, rapid loss of weight and sometimes edema of the lungs and abdominal wall. Deaths occasionally occurred in old or young horses. The course of the disease was 2 to 15 days, with abortion usually occurring 1 to 14 days after the onset of illness. The incidence of abortion ranged from 1 to 50 per cent. Most abortions occurred between 5 and 10 months of gestation, and as they did not occur promptly after fetal death, the fetuses underwent autolytic changes prior to expulsion. No inclusion bodies were present, but the virus could be recovered from fetal tissues such as the liver and lung. Horses that recovered had a prolonged immunity to reinfection. Although an effective vaccine has been developed and has been commercially produced, its use is closely regulated.

Equine infectious anemia in pregnant mares is occasionally characterized by early fetal death or abortion. Abortion may be caused by the virus invading the fetus during the last half of pregnancy, or it may be associated with the stress produced in the mare by an acute febrile episode of the disease. Further study is needed to elucidate the mechanism of abortion in equine infectious anemia.

Fungi

Mycotic or fungal causes of equine abortion include *Aspergillus fumigatus, Mucor* spp. and *Allescheria boydii,* with *A. fumigatus* being by far the most common. Mycotic abortions in mares, like abortions from miscellaneous bacterial causes, are sporadic. The fungus probably invades the fetus through the cervix and placenta or possibly through the bloodstream directly to the placenta. In most mycotic abortions the placenta, especially the chorioallantois, is extensively and diffusely involved. Mycosis may be responsible for 5 to 30 per cent of all infectious abortions. Most mycotic abortions occur late in gestation after the placenta has been infected for many weeks. Fetuses are usually small because of growth retardation caused by chronic placental disease. Some of these infected fetuses may be expelled alive. Infection, especially with *Mucor* sp., may cause a mycotic pneumonia in the fetus. Skin lesions rarely occur. The causal organism may readily be cultured from the placenta and occasionally from the fetal organs. The chorioallantois is usually extensively diseased, edematous, thickened and necrotic. Rarely, abortions due to *Histoplasma, Coccidioides immitis* and the yeasts *Candida* and *Cryptococcus* have been reported.

Protozoal Causes

Protozoal causes of equine abortion include *Trypanosoma equiperdum* and *Babesia equi* or *B. caballi,* which cause dourine and piroplasmosis, respectively. Abortion due to these agents is rare in horses. It is not certain whether the fetus and placenta are invaded by *T. equiperdum.* If invasion does not occur, abortion is probably caused by the stress produced by the disease in the mare. Dourine is present only in tropical countries and has been eradicated from North America. It is transmitted primarily by sexual contact.

Babesiasis or piroplasmosis may result in abortion in severely affected mares, possibly because of the stress produced by the disease. Signs of the acute disease resemble those of equine infectious anemia, except that icterus and hemoglobinuria may also be present. Presently this disease is largely limited to the state of Florida in the United States but is endemic in many tropical countries. The fluorescent antibody technique is applied to red blood cells from infected fetuses, foals or dams to determine the presence of the parasite. This, together with the complement fixation test, is highly efficient for diagnosing babesiasis and for differentiating it from equine infectious anemia, leptospirosis, equine herpesvirus 1 and neonatal isoerythrolysis. Therapy for mares affected with piroplasmosis is available and is generally effective.

NONINFECTIOUS CAUSES OF EQUINE ABORTION

These may include twinning, drugs or chemicals, hormones, chromosomal abnormalities and physical causes.

Twinning

Twinning is the cause of 20 to 30 per cent of all observed equine abortions. About 60 to 80 per cent of twin fetuses that survive through the fourth month of gestation are aborted. These abortions are usually caused by fetal death from a lack of placental area. (See the previous discussion on equine twinning.)

Chemicals, Drugs and Poisonous Plants

Phenothiazines and thiabendazole, purgatives such as arecoline and aloes, sudan grass or sorghum pastures, sodium iodide, organophosphate anthelmintics, ergot and others have occasionally been reported as causing equine abortions. However, the evidence or scientific basis for incriminating these chemicals, drugs or agents as causes of abortion has not been adequately determined.

Hormones

Hormonal causes of equine abortion have included estrogens, glucocorticoids, oxytocin, prostaglandins and possibly a progesterone deficiency.

Estrogens in large doses induce abortion or parturition in cows and ewes. There is some reported evidence that large, repeated doses of estrogen may cause abortion in ponies. Further studies are needed to prove that estrogen can be abortifacient in the mare.

Glucocorticoids, such as dexamethasone, at doses of 100 mg/day for 4 days given during the tenth month of gestation will hasten or induce parturition. The author's experience and that of others working with pregnant mares have shown that the stresses of transport, close housing after pasture, sudden reduction and changes in feed and water intake, debilitating conditions or diseases and other stresses, especially from 3 to 5 months of gestation when progesterone levels from the corpora lutea are declining, will cause abortions. Mitchell[4] reported that about 50 per cent of pregnant yearling mares aborted between 30 and 160 days of gestation, probably because of stress factors. Certain mares are definitely more easily stressed than others. Mares that conceive promptly but have a history of abortion should be managed so as to avoid stress throughout gestation, especially after 60 days.

Oxytocin, 20 to 100 IU intramuscularly, is highly effective for inducing parturition in mares in an average of 50 to 60 minutes during late gestation, near term, or during moderately prolonged gestations.

Prostaglandins in single or multiple doses, 2.5 mg of prostaglandin $F_{2\alpha}$ ($PGF_{2\alpha}$) every 12 hours, will cause abortion in pony mares between 80 and 300 days of gestation. An average of 3.7 injections were given with a mean interval from first injection to abortion of 36.6 hours.[1, 4]

Progesterone deficiency has been incriminated as a cause of abortion in mares and other animals. Ganjam and co-workers[2] have shown that the half-life of progesterone in the mare is extremely short. Giving 150 to 300 mg of progesterone daily maintains normal blood levels (6 to 8 ng/ml) of this hormone in ovariectomized mares or those in deep anestrus. Therapy consisting of 500 mg of repositol progesterone every 6, 10 or 30 days is presently being used as an aid in preventing equine abortion supposedly caused by progesterone deficiency. However, this is obviously a very low dose in light of the report just cited. It is possible that a sudden decline in progestogens may precipitate twin abortion late in the gestation period when one of two fetuses dies because of a lack of placental area.

Chromosomal Abnormalities

Chromosomal anomalies are seldom a cause of abortion from 3 months to term. However, as mentioned earlier, death of the early embryo or fetus, especially before 90 days, might be caused by chromosomal anomalies, as has been reported in other mammalian species.

Physical Causes

Physical causes are seldom responsible for abortions in mares (other than those abortions deliberately performed). These causes include abnormalities of the umbilical cord, trauma or severe injury to the mare or to the embryonic vesicle, natural service during pregnancy and manual dilatation and douching of the pregnant uterus.

Abnormalities of the umbilical cord that are potentially lethal to the fetus are caused by excessive length of the cord and result in the following:

1. Strangulation of the amniotic portion of the cord around portions of the fetus, resulting in deep grooves and local edema in the head, neck, legs, back and thorax.

2. Excessive torsion of the amniotic part of the cord with urachal obstruction and vascular occlusion. Urachal obstruction can cause excessive distention of the fetal bladder and rupture of the bladder prior to or during birth or can even cause dystocia. Rupture of the urachus with urine passing into the amniotic cavity has also been described by Whitwell.[5] Vascular occlusion of the umbilical cord is a major cause of death and the subsequent abortion of an autolyzed fetus. In these cases the amniotic portion of the umbilical cord is markedly twisted and is associated with hematomas, aneurysms, thromboses, ecchymoses and edema. Usually, a distended bladder and a dilated urachus are also present. Torsion or strangulation of the umbilical cord is responsible for about 1 per cent of fetal deaths and abortions and occurs most commonly between 5½ and 7½ months of gestation.

3. Whitwell[5] described 11 abortions in conjunction with long umbilical cords associated with ischemic necrosis of the cervical pole of the chorioallantois that was distinct from infectious cervical placentitis.

Trauma or injury resulting in severe stress to a pregnant mare, such as in prolonged difficult transport, hard sustained work, difficult long surgical operations and vigorous struggling and trauma in a "cast" mare may cause abortion. This is probably caused by stress and the production of glucocorticoids that initiate abortion, as previously described. Rough, traumatic manipulation of the embryonic vesicle during manual pregnancy diagnosis, especially from 16 to 40 days of gestation, should be avoided. Evidence would indicate that this could cause the death of the early embryo in horses as well as in cattle. Conversely, if this examination is done gently and skillfully by a highly experienced diagnostician, apparently few deaths are produced.

Natural service during the first 3 months of gestation occurs occasionally, possibly because of the increased estrogen levels associated with follicular ovarian activity during this period. Abortions following natural matings during pregnancy are rare because of the constricted cervix.

Manual dilatation of the cervix and the introduction of several hundred milliliters of physiological saline, dilute Lugol's solution or iodized oil in a clean, sanitary manner readily produce abortion within 3 to 10 days in most mares. A second treatment may occasionally be necessary. Aborting mares after 3 or 4 months of gestation is usually not recommended because complications may arise as a result of the large size of the fetus.

Induction of abortion or prevention of conception is occasionally performed when mismating has occurred or when an owner has purchased a pregnant mare with an undesired pregnancy or has decided after breeding a mare to terminate the pregnancy. If the mismated mare is still in estrus or was bred only 12 to 72 hours previously, a large, single injection of 100 to 200 mg of repositol diethylstilbestrol or several injections of 10 to 20 mg of estradiol given every 36 to 48 hours would probably prevent pregnancy, much as such therapy does in other domestic animals. If the bred mare fails to show heat signs at the next expected estrous period or if she is diagnosed pregnant, then at subsequent examination, she may be given an intrauterine douche, as previously described, or one or multiple injections of 2.5 to 5.0 mg of $PGF_{2\alpha}$ or a suitable prostaglandin analog, at 12-hour intervals to cause abortion.[3] The use of large dosages of estrogens or glucocorticoids or both to produce abortion in mares requires further study.

MISCELLANEOUS DISEASES AND ACCIDENTS OF THE EQUINE GESTATION PERIOD

Fetal Mummification

Fetal death in horses that occurs from the third to tenth month of gestation and does not result in abortion or maceration is followed by autolytic changes in the fetus and placenta, absorption of the placental and fetal fluids and mummification of the fetus. In the horse fetal mummification is uncommon and has only been reported as occurring in one of twin fetuses that has died during pregnancy, possibly because of placental insufficiency. In twin equine fetuses the smaller twin usually dies, and both twins are aborted, but if one twin mummifies and remains in the uterus for several months, it and its fetal membranes will be expelled with the viable fetus when the latter is aborted or delivered at term. The great discrepancy in size between the mummified fetus and the viable twin fetus may lead to an erroneous diagnosis of superfetation. The mummified fetus with its membranes may not be observed because of its small size. Single mummified fetuses have never been reported in the mare.

Fetal Maceration

Maceration of the equine fetus is rare but may occur at any stage of gestation from 2 months to term. Fetal death may be due to any of the various causes of abortion, but if the cervix fails to dilate sufficiently and the fetus remains in the uterus, autolysis proceeds to emphysema and maceration, metritis and pyometra and, in some cases, a fetid vulvar discharge. The diagnosis of fetal maceration can usually be determined from the breeding history and an evaluation, following vaginal and rectal examination, of the uterus and its contents. The cervix of the mare should be gently dilated manually with frequent lubrication, and the fetus and placental remnants should be carefully removed. In rare cases fetal emphysema and maceration in late gestation may require a partial fetotomy or even cesarean section if the cervix cannot be well dilated. The uterus and cervix should then be treated as for metritis and cervicitis with broad-spectrum antibiotics in an oily base. Aftercare may also require systemic antibiotic therapy and treatment to prevent acute laminitis.

Hydrops Amnii and Hydrops Allantois, Edema of the Chorioallantois and Fetal Dropsy

These conditions are extremely rare in the equine species. Hydrops amnii has not been reported in mares. The author has observed mild-to-moderate cases of edema of the chorioallantois, no cases of fetal anasarca or dropsy or excessive fetal ascites. Hydrops allantois is also rare. In the latter case rupture of the prepubic tendon and ensuing shock may result in the mare's death. Induced abortion, with slow IV infusion of oxytocin, possibly preceded by a large dose of estradiol, or surgical intervention through laparotomy or dilatation of the cervix and rupture of the membranes with very slow removal of allantoic fluid to prevent shock, may be necessary if spontaneous abortion does not occur.

Extensive Unilateral Ventral Hernias

Extensive unilateral ventral hernias occurring in mares during late gestation are rare. These may be associated with excessive uterine weight in cases of twinning or of hydrops allantois. Affected mares may be treated in a manner similar to that used for rupture of the prepubic tendon and should be given prompt assistance at foaling to avoid the delivery of a dead foal because of the inability of the abdominal muscles to assist adequately in its expulsion. Repair of these extensive hernias is impossible, and the breeding life of the mare is usually terminated.

Rupture of the Prepubic Tendon

Rupture of the prepubic tendon (prepubic desmorrhexis) is a rare occurrence in light mares in advanced pregnancy but is more common in draft mares. Usually, this condition is preceded by an area of marked, tense, painful edema, 4 to 6 inches thick on the abdominal wall, extending from the udder to the xiphoid process. Affected mares move very slowly and cautiously and refuse to lie down. In a few cases rupture of the prepubic tendon may occur suddenly because of trauma or violence without the usual development of severe edema. When rupture does occur, it is associated with severe distress, pain, sweating, rapid respiration, fast and weak pulse and possible internal hemorrhage and shock. Collapse and death usually follow within a few minutes or hours. Even in the few animals that survive, the mare's usefulness is so severely limited that she is usually humanely destroyed. Mares that develop a severe ventral edema and a stiff, cautious gait indicative of a possible impending rupture of the prepubic tendon should be confined and have exercise limited; large, bulky feeds should be avoided and a light, laxative concentrate ration should be fed. A wide, heavy canvas girdle, with straps that can be tightened, should be placed around the mare's abdomen for support. Heavy padding should be placed over the spine to prevent pressure necrosis. Affected mares should be watched closely for the initiation of parturition, so that assistance can be given promptly, since abdominal contractions are weak. Induction of parturition late in gestation with oxytocin should be seriously considered.

Extrauterine Pregnancy

True extrauterine pregnancy in the mare in which the embryo or conceptus establishes nutritive relationships with tissues other than the endometrium has never been described. False or secondary uterine pregnancy in which the fetus develops normally but escapes into the abdominal cavity through a uterine wall rupture, usually late in gestation, is very rare and generally follows trauma or violence to the mare. The fetus dies promptly, often followed by the death of the dam because of abdominal complications. In the mare the uncommon rotated or compound bicornual pregnancy may be mistaken for an extrauterine fetus because the birth canal is very long and the fetus, which is located in both uterine horns, may be palpated beneath the stretched vagina and uterine body.

Torsion of the Uterus

Torsion of the uterus occurs in the later stages of gestation, possibly associated with the mare's rolling or falling or with excessive activity of the fetus. Differing from the cow, equine uterine torsion is seldom associated with parturition. This condition is rare in the mare because of the dorsally attached broad ligaments, and many cases are limited to about a 180° twist. Signs of uterine torsion are restlessness, anorexia, abdominal pain or colic and frequent attempts at urination. These prolonged signs resemble those seen in the early stages of parturition, and when these are observed in advanced pregnancy, usually with a tightly closed cervix, the anterior vagina should be examined for the twisting or folding of the wall, indicative of torsion. A rectal examination should also be performed to determine the direction of the torsion and the degree of tension on the broad ligaments. In many equine uterine torsions the twisted portion of the genital tract only involves the body of the uterus cranial to the cervix and not the anterior vagina. If the condition is diagnosed early and fetal death and rupture of a large blood vessel have not occurred, the prognosis is usually guarded to favorable. The torsion may be relieved by sedating or anesthetizing the mare and by rolling her in the direction of the torsion, preferably by using Schaffer's method, which utilizes a plank placed on the abdomen to hold the fetus in place while the mare is slowly rolled in the direction of the torsion.[1, 2] If these conservative methods fail, a laparotomy through the left flank of the standing or recumbent mare may be performed, with the torsion corrected manually.

Hemorrhage of Pregnancy

Occasionally, violence or trauma, especially to an older mare in late gestation, may cause rupture of a large uterine blood vessel that results in a fatal intra-abdominal hemorrhage or a large hematoma in the broad ligament. Signs of excessive hemorrhage include markedly increased respiration and heart rate, weakness, staggering, sweating, pale mucous membranes and the rapid onset of prostration, shock and death. Treatment with large quantities of blood or blood substitutes is indicated in severe cases, but this is difficult to implement within a short period.

Older mares in advanced pregnancy may rarely show occasional, slight, recurrent bleeding from the vulva. This is of concern to the owner but usually is not serious and often does not require treatment. This bleeding does not usually come from the uterine cavity but from a ruptured "varicose" or surface vein in the vaginal or hymenal region. Such lesions usually heal spontaneously after foaling, but ligation or cautery of the lesion may be indicated. Rarely, bleeding from the vulva may be due to a traumatic lesion of the vulva, hymen or vagina or to a tumor involving those structures.

References

1. Douglas RH and Ginther OJ: J Reprod Fert Suppl 23:257, 1975.
2. Ganjam VK and Keaney RM: Proc 21st Ann Conv AAEP, 1975, pp 263–275.
3. Mitchell D and Allen WR: J Reprod Fert Suppl 23:531, 1975.
4. Roberts SJ: Veterinary Obstetrics and Genital Diseases. 3rd ed. Woodstock, Vermont, 1986.
5. Whitwell KE: J Reprod Fert Suppl 23:599, 1975.

Control of Abortigenic Herpesviral Infections*

John T. Bryans
George P. Allen
University of Kentucky, Lexington, Kentucky

THE VIRUS

The predominant cause of abortigenic viral disease of Equidae is a typical member of the Herpetoviridae known as equine herpesvirus 1 (EHV-1).† The disease is worldwide in distribution. Infection by EHV-1 may result in respiratory and neurologic disease, but abortion is, economically, the most important disease produced by the virus. Equine herpesvirus 1 exists as two antigenically distinguishable subtypes. These are called EHV-1[1] and EHV-1[2]. Both subtypes cause respiratory disease, which is most severe in immunologically naive young horses. However, EHV-1[1] causes the great majority of abortigenic infections and neurologic disease, while EHV-1[2] appears to be responsible for most epizootic herpesviral respiratory disease in young horses. The viral subtypes are identifiable by several methods of antigenic analysis, by their ability to infect productively specific cell types in culture and by differences in the structure of their genomes (DNA), detectable by restriction endonuclease "fingerprinting" techniques. Genetic variation in both subtypes has been discovered, but neither the immunologic nor the epidemiologic significance of such variation has yet been fully defined.

DIAGNOSIS

Abortion resulting from infection of the fetus by EHV-1 is a sudden event. Mares exhibit no signs of disease and usually no premonitory signs of abortion. The placenta is grossly normal in appearance and is usually delivered with the fetus. Almost all (96 per cent) infected fetuses are aborted in the last 4 months of pregnancy. The damage done to the fetus from the time it is infected until abortion occurs does not kill it. It dies as a result of suffocation, first as a result of separation of the placenta early in the sequence of events that lead to abortion, and second as a result of pulmonary edema that impairs respiratory function. It therefore presents without evidence of postmortem decomposition. Its footpads are commonly stained by meconium, and petechial and ecchymotic hemorrhages may be visible on the mucous and serous membranes. Some fetuses may be delivered alive, but most succumb within minutes or hours as a result of pulmonary insufficiency. The lungs are heavy with fluid, and the interlobular septa are distended. The thoracic cavity usually contains excessive clear, straw-colored transudate, which may amount to a liter or more. Small, gray necrotic foci may be seen under the capsule of the liver, and focal hemorrhage may be observed in the adrenal cortices. The thymus is commonly necrotic and therefore abnormally friable.

Confirmation of the results of gross necropsy examination may be accomplished by histologic and virologic examination of fetal tissues. Veterinarians unable to obtain necropsy diagnostic services should submit formalin-fixed specimens of lung, liver and thymus to a diagnostic laboratory for histologic examination along with frozen specimens of the same tissues for virologic examination. Because the majority of mares of breeding age normally carry some humoral antibodies specific for EHV-1 and because abortions occur after the mare has mounted a secondary antibody response to infection, the results of serologic diagnostic tests are often uninterpretable.

Although a thorough discussion of EHV-1 neurologic disease is beyond the scope of this article, such disease may occur concomitantly with abortions caused by the virus. This form of disease occurs about a week to 10 days after the mare is infected. It presents as a proprioceptive defect, which may be quadrilateral but which usually affects only the pelvic limbs. Usually the earliest signs of such disease in pregnant mares are dependent edema of the pelvic limbs and a reluctance to move. Paralysis of the bladder and tail and signs of central nervous system involvement may appear during the first day after the initial signs are noted. The severity of the clinical signs depends on the extent and location of damage to nerve tracts; signs are established during a short period of time and are generally not progressive. Affected mares may not abort, and their foals may be born uninfected by the virus. The pathogenesis of EHV-1 neurologic disease has not been fully defined, but it appears that the lesion is produced by an immunologic (Arthus-like) reaction to virus-infected endothelial cells in many organs that, in the central nervous system, leads to ischemic damage to nerve tracts. In many cases, the virus is coincidentally demonstrable in the buffy

*The investigation reported in this article (No. 84-4-90) has been done in connection with a project of the Kentucky Agricultural Experiment Station and is published with approval of the Director.
†Equine rhinopneumonitis and equine viral abortion are synonyms for the disease.

coat of the blood of acutely affected animals. Veterinarians wishing to submit samples to a diagnostic laboratory for virus isolation should obtain 20 ml of sterile citrated blood and deliver it refrigerated (not frozen) without delay.

Diagnosis of acute herpesviral respiratory disease may be obtained by isolation of virus from the nasopharynx of infected horses or by serologic methods. Samples for virus isolation should be taken by swabbing the nasopharynx with a small surgical sponge attached to a suitable sampling instrument. Although the virus may be isolated for a week or more after clinical signs become apparent, samples are best obtained during the acute febrile stage of disease. Such samples should be soaked in about 3 to 5 ml of a simple sterile virus fluid transport medium, refrigerated and then transported to a laboratory without delay. Serologic diagnosis requires both acute and convalescent serum samples. Several serologic tests, complement fixation, serum neutralization and ELISA (enzyme-linked immunosorbent assay) tests are available for the purpose.

EPIDEMIOLOGY

Herpesviruses survive by virtue of their ability to produce a carrier state in the host. The biologic mechanisms that condition establishment of the carrier state in the horse have not been defined, but there is sufficient epidemiologic evidence for its existence. Recurrent lesions of herpesviral disease and an infectious process productive of new virus are known to be induced in herpesviral carriers by various forms of stress. Management practices contrived to avoid as much stress as possible can therefore influence the occurrence of herpesviral disease in horses and other species. Immunity to infection by EHV-1 is comparatively short-lived. Horses that have experienced infection may become reinfected repeatedly. The initial infection results in severe respiratory disease and an immune response that protects for only a few months. Second infections produce less severe disease, and subsequent infections may produce no clinically defineable signs. Horses contracting such infections amplify the amount of virus in the environment, and pregnant mares may abort. Both subtypes of the virus are transmitted by the respiratory route.

Prior to the recognition of the existence of subtypes of EHV-1, epidemiologic information obtained by serologic methods that did not distinguish viral subtypes, suggested that outbreaks of herpesviral respiratory disease among weanlings were of singular importance in the genesis of abortigenic infections of broodmares. It is now appreciated that most such occurrences of respiratory disease among weanlings are caused by EHV-1[2], a virus that is rarely the cause of abortion. Nevertheless, because EHV-1[1] can cause clinically indistinguishable outbreaks of respiratory disease among weanlings, management practices that serve to separate bands of weanlings from pregnant broodmares are important in the control of abortigenic disease.

Most occurrences of herpesviral abortion (70 per cent) involve only one or two mares in a herd. Multiple abortions may occur in both closed herds with little or no horse traffic as well as in herds that are subject to a high level of new additions or transients introduced from other farms or racetracks. Outbreaks of viral abortion that result in multiple fetal losses are, however, most common in herds in which the population is crowded and in which there are additions to the herd during the final months of the foaling season. Such circumstances produce stress and condition the occurrence of epidemic spread of the virus. The incidence of herpesviral abortion is significantly higher in mares that have been transported in late pregnancy and in mares that have gone through sales. Other stress factors such as severe weather, especially extreme variations in temperature during the spring, may contribute to the incidence of the disease.

Because, under natural circumstances, the majority of mares of breeding age are clinically immune to respiratory disease but not to abortigenic infection, spread of EHV-1 infection through a herd occurs commonly without clinically noticeable signs. Although incubation periods of 60 days or more from the time of intranasal inoculation of pregnant mares with virulent virus to abortion have been recorded, most mares inoculated by this natural route abort within a month. The spread of infection within a population of pregnant mares that have been exposed to a mare that has experienced abortigenic disease depends on the immune resistance of individuals to infection of the respiratory tract. Evidence from serologic testing of mares in contact with a mare that has aborted has shown that all mares in some herds became infected at about the same time as the mare that aborted. In other herds, similar evidence shows that the infection was limited to only the mare that aborted or one or two of its cohorts. Serologic or virologic evidence of infection of cohorts is not predictive of ensuing abortigenic disease. It is therefore advisable not to remove pregnant mares from a group in which one mare has aborted unless these mares can be placed in a location where they will not come into contact with unexposed pregnant mares. The most dangerous source of infection for the cohorts of mares that have aborted is the infected fetus, which is a rich source of infectious virus. The mare itself does not shed virus from either the respiratory or the reproductive tract at the time of abortion.

TREATMENT

Although certain antiviral drugs have been shown to be more or less effective for treatment of specific herpesviral diseases of other species, these have not been critically evaluated in horses. Barring complications not connected with viral infection of the fetus, abortigenic infection by EHV-1 does no apparent damage to the reproductive tract. Mares recover as if they had experienced normal parturition. Such mares are no more susceptible to postparturient bacterial infections than are normal foaling mares. Veterinarians may, therefore, considering the individual's reproductive history, follow the same procedures of postparturient reproductive management that they apply to normal mares in their practice.

Foals that suffer herpesviral respiratory disease may experience severe secondary infections, evident as purulent rhinitis, pharyngitis and pneumonia. Antibiotic therapy applied during the acute and convalescent stages of EHV-1 respiratory disease may serve to prevent or modify complicating infections.

Foals infected by EHV-1 may be born alive if they are aborted during the terminal days of a normal gestational period. In addition to pulmonary damage, necrosis of lung parenchyma and edema, such foals have hepatic, adrenal and extensive lymphoreticular damage. They are extremely susceptible to secondary bacterial infection. There are no reports of successful attempts to preserve the life of such foals.

IMMUNITY AND PROPHYLAXIS

The characteristics of their behavior as pathogens suggest that herpesviruses have evolved with the hosts they infect. Although these viruses produce formidable diseases, these occur most frequently in immunocompromised individuals, in newborn and infant animals or, in the case of certain viruses such as simian B and pseudorabies, in species other than the natural host. Herpesviruses are among the more efficient parasites; they have apparently "learned" to integrate their genetic information with that of their hosts as well as to compromise certain functions of the immune system, thereby influencing favorably their ability to exist latently.

The approaches to development of a successful method for prophylactic immunization against a virus with these characteristics are somewhat obfuscated by an inadequate understanding of the function of those immune factors that protect the host from infection. We know that horses respond to infection by EHV-1 in several classic ways: they develop cellular immune responses, interferons, and specific immunoglobulins that neutralize viral infectivity, and they exhibit immunopathologic reactions such as delayed hypersensitivity and Arthus reactions. Because the role of these responses, singly or in combination, is incompletely understood, it is difficult to define, with a reasonable degree of confidence, the relationships between information from in vitro tests and resistance.

Although sophisticated techniques for preparation of candidate vaccines and for in vitro measurement of their comparative ability to stimulate immune responses are available, it remains the present "state of the art" that vaccine efficacy, safety and strategies are most reliably evaluated by vaccination and controlled challenge of the natural host.

Approaches to vaccination of mares against abortigenic disease caused by EHV-1 have employed a variety of immunogenic preparations of varying potency; both infectious-attenuated and inactivated virus vaccines have been used. One vaccine is presently licensed as an aid in protection of mares against such disease—an inactivated, adjuvant EHV-1[1] preparation manufactured in the United States.* This vaccine has been widely employed by veterinarians in the United States and several foreign countries since 1980. Several million injections have been administered, providing a reasonable basis for assessment of both its safety and its efficacy in practice. The strategy for employment of the vaccine is based on results of vaccination and challenge experiments in horses and on knowledge of the epidemiology of the disease. It is recommended that pregnant mares receive vaccine during the fifth, seventh and ninth months of gestation. This strategy is contrived to maintain immunity to infection by EHV-1 at the highest achievable level during the period when mares are at maximum risk for abortigenic infection.

The effects of application of this vaccination protocol on the incidence of EHV-1 abortions have been closely monitored in the highly concentrated broodmare population of central Kentucky since the vaccine became routinely available. Approximately 65 per cent of the pregnant mares in that area have been vaccinated each year since 1980. During the 4 years immediately prior to use of the inactivated vaccine, 9.8 per cent of 1568 aborted equine fetuses were found to be infected by EHV-1. During the period 1980–1983, 4.5 per cent of 1566 aborted fetuses were found to be infected. The average number of EHV-1 abortions per year during the 23-year period prior to use of this vaccine was 7.4 per 1000 pregnant mares. The EHV-1 abortion rate for the whole population, both vaccinated and unvaccinated during the period 1980–1983, was 2.9 per 1000, which is approximately 70 per cent of the lowest annual incidence ever observed among Kentucky mares prior to use of the inactivated vaccine. The abortion rate for the vaccinated sector of the population during this period was 1.7 per 1000, which is less than half the lowest annual incidence ever recorded in this area. The decrease in incidence of EHV-1 abortion is coincident with a greater than 50 per cent increase in the number of pregnant mares at putative risk to the disease in the test population.

Neither this vaccine nor any other vaccine that has been developed will immunize pregnant mares against EHV-1 infection with an absolute degree of reliability. The pathogenesis of abortigenic infection by EHV-1 involves transport of virus from the circulation of the pregnant mare transplacentally by an immunologically privileged mechanism that pre-

---

*Pneumabort-K; Fort Dodge Laboratories, Fort Dodge, Iowa.

sumably involves a leukocyte capable of transplacental migration. Whether the cell that harbors and conveys the virus to the susceptible fetus is productively infected by the virus or whether it carries the virus latently is not known. Viremia occurs following infection of the respiratory tract of the mare. Prevention of such infection is the key to prevention of abortigenic disease. Immunity to overt disease of the respiratory tract is a product of repeated infection or contrived immunization. Such a quality of immunity is not difficult to achieve by either means. However, immunity to infection productive of new virus, when achieved, persists for a period of only a few months. When reinfection occurs, viremia may follow, placing pregnant mares at risk of aborting. Epidemiologic observations suggest that individual latently infected mares may abort as a result of recrudescence of latent virus precipitated by stress, a situation that vastly complicates any approach to prevention by vaccination. The inactivated vaccine, on the record of its performance, is the best that can be recommended.

In advising their clients, veterinarians should be mindful of the fact that management practices such as crowding of pregnant mares, casual horse traffic in broodmare bands, indiscriminate mingling of horses of various age groups, the environment of sales and other factors that produce stress can significantly influence the occurrence of EHV-1 disease. Observance of sound management practices in conjunction with implementation of a complete vaccination program offers the best means available for prevention and control.

The most efficacious use of the inactivated vaccine in providing a period of immunity to EHV-1 respiratory infection has been obtained in adult populations that are immunologically conditioned by the experiences of repeated vaccinations and perhaps by one or more prior natural infections by the virus. Comparable levels of immunity to respiratory challenge of young, immunologically naive foals with either of the subtypes of EHV-1 has not yet been achieved by a primary series of two injections of the inactivated virus vaccine. In vaccination and challenge trials conducted on weanling foals, the vaccine was not effective in preventing infection or the development of clinically recognizable disease.

Neither the inactivated virus vaccine nor a modified live virus vaccine* advertised for control of herpesviral respiratory disease contains the subtype of EHV-1 responsible for causing the majority of herpesviral respiratory disease in young horses. Because the subtypes are antigenically related, however, repeated vaccination of foals with these subtype 1 vaccines produces a quality of immunity to the subtype 2 virus that modifies both the severity and the duration of the disease. The use of such vaccines timed to give maximal protection during periods of greatest susceptibility to infection (weaning, sales), along with management practices designed to minimize the stress of weaning and to limit exposure of foals to the stressful environments of sales, trafficking, and new horse populations, offers the best currently available approach to prevention of EHV-1 respiratory disease in young horses.

---

*Rhinomune; Norden Laboratories; Lincoln, Nebraska

References

1. Allen GP, Turtinen L: Assessment of the genetic relatedness between the two subtypes of equine herpesvirus 1. J Virology 44:249, 1982.
2. Allen GP, Yeargan MR, Turtinen LW et al.: Molecular epizootiologic studies of equine herpesvirus 1 infections by restriction endonuclease fingerprinting of viral DNA. Am J Vet Res 44:263, 1983.
3. Bryans JT: On immunity to disease caused by equine herpesvirus 1. J Am Vet Med Assoc 155:294, 1969.
4. Bryans JT: Serological responses of thoroughbred mares to vaccination with an inactivated equine herpesvirus 1 vaccine. Am J Vet Res 41:1743, 1980.
5. Bryans JT: Application of management procedures and prophylactic immunization to the control of equine rhinopneumonitis. Proceedings 26th Annual Convention, American Association of Equine Practice, 1980, p 259.
6. Doll ER, Bryans JT: Epizootiology of equine viral rhinopneumonitis. J Am Vet Med Assoc 142:31, 1963.
7. Doll ER, Crowe MEW, Bryans JT, McCollum WH: Infection immunity in equine virus abortion. Cornell Vet 45:387, 1955.
8. Turtinen LW, Allen GP, Darlington RW, Bryans JT: Serologic and molecular comparisons of several equine herpesvirus type 1 strains. Am J Vet Res 42:2099, 1981.
9. Turtinen L, Allen G: Identification of the glycoproteins of equine herpesvirus 1. J Gen Virology 63:481, 1982.

Termination of Unwanted Pregnancy in the Mare

R. M. Lofstedt, B.V.Sc., M.S.
Tufts University School of Veterinary Medicine, North Grafton, Massachusetts

Occasionally it may become necessary to terminate pregnancy in a mare. Reasons for abortion might include unintentional service of a mount mare during semen collection, other cases of mismating, diagnosis of twin pregnancy, undesirable gravity stress on an orthopedic injury, changes of ownership with consequent change of function of the mare (i.e., broodmare to show mare), teaching and research.

For the convenience of the reader, the subject of terminating pregnancy has been divided into several sections, each relating to a particular stage in gestation during which different physiology is operative and different therapy applies.

ABORTION BEFORE THE STAGE OF MATERNAL RECOGNITION OF PREGNANCY

The corpus luteum is maintained by a uterine signal of pregnancy received approximately 10 to 11 days after ovulation. It is usually a simple matter to terminate pregnancy prior to the twelfth day of gestation. During this period, pregnancy can be terminated by any common method of luteolysis—i.e., either prostaglandin administration or uterine infusion with approximately 400 to 1000 ml (depending on the size of the mare) of sterile saline to cause the release of endogenous prostaglandins. Prostaglandin therapy is probably preferable because it is very effective and does not require invasion of the genital tract with the attendant threat of endometritis. It is also more rapid and occasionally more cost-effective—i.e., a farm call is not necessary because the client can be given the drug and told to administer it intramuscularly.

Most research has been conducted on the use of prostaglandin $F_{2\alpha}$ and one of its potent analogs, fluoprostenol. However, it is highly probable that a luteolytic dose of any prostaglandin would work well. Effective doses for these drugs in a 500-kg mare are: 5 mg prostaglandin $F_{2\alpha}$ intramuscularly; 2 mg prostalene intramuscularly or 250 μg fluoprostenol intramuscularly. The cloprostenol analog of prostaglandin is not approved for use in mares, but this author and others have routinely used it at a dose of 100 μg intramuscularly to cause luteolysis. At this dose, therapy was very inexpensive and no side effects were noticed in treated mares. However, the author emphasizes that the veterinarian employs this drug in the mare on his own recognizance.

The veterinarian must recognize the fact that the mare is generally refractory to luteolytic treatments before the fifth day postovulation, and therefore abortifacient treatment is most effective after day 7 or 8 postestrus. The mare can be expected to return to estrus within 5 days (usually 3 to 4) and to experience an estrous period of normal length. The mare should be teased and monitored per rectum and per vagina to ensure that abortion has occurred.

The fertility of estrous periods following early abortion has not been well studied, but a consensus of opinion suggests that it should be normal.

ABORTION AFTER MATERNAL RECOGNITION OF PREGNANCY

Once pregnancy has been recognized, the corpus luteum is endowed with a longevity that may interfere with the return of the mare to functional estrus. One may abort the mare at this stage of pregnancy by crushing the fetoplacental unit through rectal palpation, by using prostaglandins, or by flushing the uterus as described above.

To crush the fetoplacental unit, excitable mares may need tranquilization. The author prefers to employ tranquilization for this purpose in all mares because it increases relaxation of the rectal wall. The fetoplacental unit usually bursts with moderate pressure, and the conceptus is passed within 96 hours. Occasionally it may be impossible to crush the conceptus despite two or three attempts on successive days. In these cases, rupturing of the placental unit is not obvious, and the allantochorion merely appears to flatten and stretch out. Tone is recovered within several days, and pregnancy progresses to term. For this reason, it is suggested that prostaglandin be used (see below) to induce abortion when rupture is not evident. Fetoplacental crushing has not been associated with decreased future fertility or significant rectal damage.

If the equine embryo is crushed or removed by physical means even shortly after the mare has received the signal to maintain the corpus luteum for pregnancy, the corpus luteum will often be retained for periods of 10 to 90 days (usually 20 to 30 days), causing a delayed return to estrus. It should also be noted that the uterine tone that is typical for pregnancy is usually maintained until the primary corpus luteum of pregnancy eventually undergoes luteolysis. One may expect that flushing the uterus with saline or crushing the fetoplacental unit would release sufficient endogenous prostaglandin to cause luteolysis and a rapid return to estrus. However, this effect is inconsistent, and return to estrus is unreliable. For this reason, it is preferable to use prostaglandin to terminate gestation after the tenth to the twelfth day of gestation.

Normal luteolytic doses of prostaglandins given once will usually terminate pregnancies between the twelfth and thirty-fifth day and cause the onset of estrus within 4 to 5 days of treatment. However, there is some suggestion that prostaglandin dosage should be moderately increased (± 20 to 30 per cent) after the recognition of pregnancy. The fertility of estrous periods following abortion at this length of gestation has not been well documented. Therefore, it may be prudent to "short cycle" the mare using prostaglandin to ensure that the uterus has involuted fully before rebreeding is contemplated.

Human chorionic gonadotropin (hCG) therapy may occasionally cause abortion prior to 35 days. This effect is poorly documented and even more poorly understood. Abortion in these cases may result from increased circulating estradiol levels following follicle maturation due to hCG therapy. In this regard, estrogens in high doses are believed to cause placental villous degeneration in horses and cattle. Parenteral estrogen therapy has also been used as an abortifacient in horses, but its effect is unpredictable.

ABORTING THE MARE WHEN THE ENDOMETRIAL CUPS ARE FUNCTIONAL

It is difficult to abort a mare with a single luteolytic injection of prostaglandin while the endometrial cups are functional—i.e., between 35 and 120 days of gestation. It appears that pregnant mare serum gonadotropin (PMSG) or other factors coincident with its production have a protective effect on the accessory corpora lutea of pregnancy. One may also speculate that the accessory corpora lutea have different or fewer binding sites for the prostaglandin molecule. Nevertheless, three to five daily injections of prostaglandin at luteolytic doses usually cause luteolysis with subsequent abortion. Abortion usually occurs before the fifth day of therapy, and it is seldom necessary to employ more than four to five prostaglandin treatments.

When the endometrial cups are functional, abortion is not generally followed by the onset of estrus, and therefore the mechanism of fetal expulsion is poorly understood. In fact, in some studies estrus and ovulation were delayed until day 100 or 120, when the endometrial cups regressed. Occasionally, however, estrus with ovulation may follow 2 to 3 days postabortion, but the fertility of these estrous periods has not been well documented. Anovulatory estrus with substantial follicular development may also occasionally occur before the endometrial cups have ceased to function.

Prostaglandin therapy appears to have no effect on the function of the endometrial cups, and mares remain positive to tests for PMSG even after abortion has occurred. An identical situation occurs in the case of spontaneous abortion at this stage of gestation (see Fig. 1). Due to the fact that PMSG appears to suppress cyclicity in the postabortion mare, it is essential to terminate pregnancy before 35 days of gestation if the mare is expected to be rebred in the same breeding season. Mares with a history of twinning should be examined for twin pregnancies at 18 to 19 days of gestation by ultrasound or at 28 to 33 days by rectal palpation for the same reason (see the section later in this article, Elective Abortion of Twin Pregnancies).

During the period when the endometrial cups are functional, pregnancy may also be terminated by intrauterine infusions of larger volumes of saline than those used in earlier pregnancies. Volumes of 500 to 2000 ml have been used depending on the duration of pregnancy. If one intends to invade the uterus, it is probably prudent to add antibiotics to the flushing medium. This author suggests that a solution of 2 million IU of sodium penicillin G added to 1 liter of saline be used for the initial flushing. This medium should be infused into the uterus using a sterile intravenous set and a 22-inch uterine infusion tube. The infusion rate should be slow to avoid endometrial splitting and excessive backflow. Pretreatment with 10 mg of estradiol 24 hours before flushing may facilitate and hasten abortion by causing cervical relaxation. However, estradiol treatment is not essential because the cervix usually relaxes spontaneously within 3 or 4 hours of infusion.

The time of expulsion of the fetoplacental unit after flushing is rather variable. It may occur almost immediately or it may be delayed for more than a day. However, it usually occurs within 24 hours. If it has not occurred by 24 hours, the flush should be repeated. It may be necessary to repeat the flush two or three times at 24-hour intervals.

It should be remembered that flushing does not interfere significantly with the production of PMSG. Therefore, the time needed for return of estrus may be as prolonged as that when prostaglandin is used for abortion. It is possible that irritating media such as 0.5 per cent iodine or tetracyclines in propylene glycol may cause decreased endometrial cup function, but this has not been studied. Caution should be exercised in this regard because the irritating effect of these substances on the rest of the endometrium may compromise future fertility.

Flushing techniques are best reserved for mares that are less than 80 days pregnant. In these mares, the allantochorion does not abut firmly on the cervix, and fluid infused through the cervix flushes around the conceptus rather than entering the fetoplacental unit itself. Fluid flushed around the conceptus probably separates the microvilli from the endometrium with greater ease than if the punctured allantois is overfilled with fluid.

After 80 days, pregnancy can be terminated by

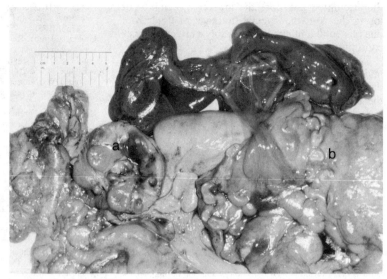

Figure 1. A 2-month-old equine conceptus that is in the process of undergoing spontaneous abortion. In spontaneous and induced abortion after day 35, the corpora lutea (a) undergo luteolysis, but the endometrial cups (b) remain viable. The endometrial cups produce PMSG up to 120 days of gestation, usually preventing the mare from returning to estrus.

penetrating the cervical seal with a finger and gently dilating the cervix over a period of 10 to 20 minutes. The allantochorion is ruptured, and the fetus is gently removed by traction on its limbs. The placenta will usually follow readily because placental attachment is not well developed at this stage. Pretreatment with 10 mg of estradiol the day before abortion will cause cervical relaxation and may facilitate this procedure. If the allantochorion is merely ruptured and the fetus is not withdrawn, abortion usually occurs in 2 to 7 days. However, the reliability of this latter method is poorly documented.

If mares are ovariectomized at less than 4 months of gestation, they will usually abort within 4 to 6 days.

TERMINATION OF PREGNANCY AFTER 4 MONTHS OF GESTATION

It has been shown that prostaglandin $F_{2\alpha}$ will terminate pregnancy after 4 months when it is administered repeatedly at daily doses of 1 mg per 45 kg—i.e., approximately 2 times the normal luteolytic dose. Approximately 70 per cent of mares so treated can be expected to abort during the first week of treatment and the remainder within the next 21 days. The optimal number of prostaglandin treatments has not yet been determined. Apparently the stage of gestation does not affect the time lapse to the onset of abortion. However, a stage of pregnancy must be reached when the interval to abortion decreases remarkably because it is known that prostaglandin is capable of inducing foaling within 2 hours of treatment after the tenth month of gestation.

The use of uterine infusions after 120 days of gestation is often ineffective. If abortion occurs in these cases, it usually does so only if the fetal membranes are ruptured or if very large volumes

(>3 liters) of fluid are used to flush the uterus. If physical means are to be employed, the method of cervical dilation and withdrawal of the fetoplacental unit may be preferable. The latter method has been used in pregnancies as advanced as 150 days.

ELECTIVE ABORTION OF TWIN PREGNANCIES

Mares that have twin pregnancies should be aborted as early as possible in pregnancy so that the breeding season can be salvaged. Although real-time ultrasonic examination can reveal pregnancies reliably as early as 15 days of gestation, it is prudent not to examine mares for twin pregnancy as early as this because there is often a 4- to 5-day age difference between twins. This small difference in age may cause the younger twin to be invisible during an examination at 15 days.

If the pregnancy has been diagnosed by ultrasound at 18 to 19 days, the pregnancy can be terminated with prostaglandin and the mare will return to estrus within 3 to 4 days. However, if the twin pregnancy is diagnosed after the endometrial cups have been formed—i.e., after 35 to 40 days—selective abortion of one twin should be attempted. Unfortunately, this often results in the abortion of both twins, but because there is a good chance that the breeding season will be lost anyway (see previous discussion), the attempt at selective abortion is usually justified. Some owners will not request treatment but may elect to wait and see if spontaneous abortion of a co-twin occurs. In practice, this abortion frequently occurs. Therefore, each case of twinning may be treated differently.

Unfortunately, there is no reliable method available that will abort one twin and allow maintenance of the other. Despite the use of progesterone and prostaglandin synthetase inhibitors, rupture of one of the placental units appears to result in abortion of the twin in 50 to 90 per cent of cases. The later the attempted abortion, the greater the chance of losing the co-twin. Vaginal drainage of fluid from one placental unit almost invariably causes the other conceptus to be aborted.

Care should be taken to examine the mare for maintenance of the remaining co-twin at least 10 days after the first twin has been destroyed because the remaining pregnancy may appear to be maintained for the first 4 to 7 days after crushing or drainage has taken place. Abortion may occur as late as 3 weeks after one twin has been crushed.

There is some evidence that twin pregnancies may be reduced to single pregnancies by decreasing the mare's food intake to hay alone for 2 to 4 weeks or until one twin has died. However, this method requires further study.

Suggested Readings

Bosu WTK, McKinnon AO: Induction of abortion during midgestation in mares. Can Vet J 23 (12):358, 1982.

Douglas RH, Ginther OJ: Effects of prostaglandin $F_{2\alpha}$ on the oestrous cycle and pregnancy in mares. J Reprod Fert Suppl 23:257, 1975.

Ginther OJ (ed): Reproductive biology of the mare. In Endocrinology of Pregnancy. Ann Arbor, McNaughton and Gunn, 1979.

Ginther, OJ: Twinning in mares: A review of recent studies. Equine Vet Sc 2(4):127, 1982.

Holtan DW, Squires EL, Lopin DR, Ginther OJ: Effect of ovariectomy on pregnancy in mares. J Reprod Fert Suppl 27:457, 1979.

Kooiska LH, Ginther OJ: Termination of pseudopregnancy by administration of prostaglandin $F_{2\alpha}$ and termination of early pregnancy by administration of prostaglandin $F_{2\alpha}$ or colchicine or by removal of embryo in mares. Am J Vet Res 37:35, 1976.

Merkt H, Jungnickel S, Klug E: Reduction of early twin pregnancy to single pregnancy in the mare by dietetic means. J Reprod Fert Suppl 32:451, 1982.

Pascoe RR: A possible new treatment for twin pregnancy in the mare. Equine Vet J 11:64, 1979.

Pascoe RR: Methods for the treatment of twin pregnancy in the mare. Equine Vet J 15:40, 1983.

Roberts CJ: Termination of twin gestation by blastocyst crush in the broodmare. J Reprod Fert Suppl 32:447, 1982.

Squires EC, Hillman RB, Pickett BN, Nett TM: Induction of abortion in mares with Equimate: Effect on secretion of progesterone, PMSG and reproductive performance. J Anim Sci 50:490, 1980.

Endometritis in the Mare

A. C. Asbury, D.V.M.

University of Florida, Gainesville, Florida

It is surprising, in this age of sophisticated antimicrobial drugs, that a disorder of apparently simple bacterial etiology has stubbornly refused to disappear. In fact, bacterial infections of the mare's uterus seem to have the same incidence as they had before penicillin was discovered. The economic impact on the horse-breeding industry due to infertility caused by endometritis is actually increasing as the value of horses rises. This situation suggests that the real cause of infectious infertility is not yet properly defined and that adequate control of the problem will not be achieved until the pathogenesis is better understood.

Research into the complexities of equine uterine defense mechanisms is underway at a number of institutions around the world. The resulting information should produce better understanding and hence better management of endometritis. It is conceivable that by the time this book is revised again, antibiotic therapy for bacterial infections of the mare's uterus will be relegated to a secondary role, yielding to management of the immune aspects of the disease.

PATHOGENESIS

In fertile mares, the tremendous contamination of the reproductive tract that is an inevitable part of breeding and foaling is dealt with promptly and efficiently. Microorganisms and inflammatory by-products are cleared from the uterus within days to allow the embryo to survive. The valvelike action of the cervix, vestibular sphincter and vulva promotes removal of foreign material during estrus. Mucus, exudates and transudates flow to the outside while air and surface contaminants are excluded.

Neutrophils migrate rapidly from the circulation to the uterine lumen where they ingest and kill contaminating organisms. These cells are then promptly eliminated mechanically. The efficiency of the entire defense system is best appreciated when considering the responses of fertile mares in the early postpartum period. The bacteria that gain access to the uterus during parturition and those deposited during breeding within the first 2 weeks are eliminated by 5 days after ovulation to allow pregnancy to become established. The demands on the system are even greater when mares are bred by natural service. It is not unusual on the best-managed farms to achieve a 50 per cent conception rate following natural service during the foal heat.

Aging, repeated foaling, anatomic breakdown and slowing of the cellular immune mechanisms eventually decrease the efficiency of bacterial clearance. If the uterine environment suffers from a prolonged inflammatory process, embryos die and mares recycle.

In its most extreme form, loss of uterine resistance will allow establishment of endometritis merely from the irritation of pneumovagina. Breeding these mares, even artificially, inevitably results in prolonged purulent exudation. Antibiotic therapy, either local or systemic, may help in reducing the bacterial population but will not alter the underlying failure that precipitated the infection.

The causal organisms of endometritis are common surface, fecal and soil bacteria. Streptococci, *Pseudomonas* and enteric genera are easily transferred to the mare's uterus during breeding, foaling or examination. The severity of the contamination is unimportant in healthy mares. Stallion semen is normally contaminated with billions of bacteria from the penis, prepuce and the urethra. Vulvar contaminants are added during natural service, and the entire ejaculate is usually deposited directly into the uterine lumen. Those bacteria that have antibiotic resistance, such as *Pseudomonas aeruginosa,* are important only if they become established in a prolonged inflammatory process. Finding such bacteria in stallion semen is not an automatic signal of impending infertility.

Failure of uterine defenses may occur abruptly following serious trauma to the reproductive tract, or gradually. Repeated parturition tends to stretch and remodel the pelvic and perineal anatomy. Changes in perineal conformation and integrity of the function of the vulvar, vestibular and cervical sphincters results in greater irritation and contamination from the outside. Uterine susceptibility may occur, however, without noticeable anatomic change. In these cases, defects in the phagocytic function of neutrophils is a real possibility.

Recently reported studies indicate that phagocytic failure may relate to a defect in opsonization of bacteria in the uterine lumen. Lack of efficient adherence of bacterial cells to each other and to the cell membranes of neutrophils can result in slower clearance of organisms. In this work, complement appeared to be a more important opsonin than antibody.[1, 2]

Undoubtedly the entire immune process, which is important in the pathogenesis of endometritis, is complex. Interactions between various defense mechanisms and differences in dealing with various specific organisms must be defined to understand the cause of this important aspect of mare infertility.

DIAGNOSIS

Intrauterine or systemic treatment for endometritis is time consuming, costly and potentially complicating. It is imperative, therefore, that only infected mares be treated. Accuracy in diagnosis will reduce the chances of mistakenly treating the noninflamed mare or, conversely, failing to recognize the low-grade inflammation that needs therapy. History, physical examination and laboratory aids are all part of the diagnostic regimen.

Endometritis is an inflammation of the uterus. Diagnostic procedures should, therefore, be targeted at detecting the signs of inflammatory change. Recovery of bacteria by itself is not an adequate criterion for making the diagnosis because the organisms involved are mostly commensals and can easily contaminate the culture.

The physical examination should have the highest priority in the diagnostic workup. Changes in the tubular tract that are evident on rectal or vaginal examinations often provide immediate evidence for or against the presence of inflammation. Examination of the vaginal tract and cervix through a speculum is an absolute necessity. Changes in color of the mucosa, presence of exudate originating beyond the cervix or pooling in the vagina, traumatic lesions and conformational faults may all be detected through the speculum. Rectal palpation of the uterus and cervix is less rewarding but may on occasion suggest fluid accumulations in the uterus or local lesions in the tract. The rectal examination alone is not enough to give reliable diagnostic information on the presence or absence of inflammation. Changes in size, tone and texture of the uterus are too often related to stage of cycle, time since parturition, age, and other factors unrelated to endometritis.

Support for the provisional diagnosis of inflammation may come from examining uterine cytology or endometrial histology. The detection of significant numbers of neutrophils on endometrial smears is virtual assurance that inflammation exists in the mare's uterus. Simple staining procedures are adequate and may be done at the site of examination to provide immediate evidence. Since there is no "normal" neutrophilic migration in the equine uterus, their presence must relate to some antigenic stimulus. Of course, because not all endometritis is of bacterial origin, factors such as urine pooling, pneumovagina or treatment with irritant drugs must all be considered in evaluating neutrophil numbers.

Examination of the endometrial changes via uterine biopsy is another valid supportive procedure when significant inflammatory changes are evaluated. The established inflammation produces a superficial lymphocyte and plasma cell infiltration. Neutrophils are fairly transient in the tissue but may be evident when the process is still active. Caution in interpretation of mild inflammatory changes is indicated, since no clear dividing line exists between "normal" degrees of cellular infiltration and those that are associated with clinical inflammation.

The uterine culture is not an aid in confirming or ruling out endometritis. The presence or absence of bacteria on the culture plate is poorly correlated with the degree of inflammation. The culture is therefore used to suggest the etiology of an already confirmed inflammatory process. Culture techniques should ensure that the results are indicative of uterine bacterial populations. Some method of guarding the culture swab until it is in the uterine lumen is an essential requirement in taking valid cultures.[4]

The culture should yield information on numbers

as well as types of bacteria grown. Direct plating on media, without intermediate holding in nutrient media, is necessary to obtain both qualitative and quantitative information.

The principal bacterial pathogens involved in endometritis are *Streptococcus zooepidemicus, Escherichia coli, Pseudomonas aeruginosa,* and *Klebsiella pneumoniae.* These organisms are recovered in the great majority of confirmed cases of uterine infection. In the presence of documented inflammation, *Corynebacterium* spp., *Proteus* spp., and *Staphylococcus* spp. should be considered as pathogens. Most isolates of alpha-hemolytic streptococci, *Enterobacter* spp. and *Staphylococcus epidermidis* are rarely if ever correlated with inflammation and are viewed as contaminants.

Yeasts from the *Candida* spp. and fungi such as *Aspergillus* may be isolated from mares with concurrent signs of inflammation. Repeated recovery is necessary to confirm their role in the disease. Often yeasts and fungi develop secondarily to antibiotic therapy for bacterial endometritis. When established in the reproductive tract, they have the potential for producing severe and irreversible tissue damage.

As long as culture results are viewed in perspective, as suggestions for the etiology of a known inflammation, the integrity of the diagnostic regimen is ensured. Treatment based purely on cultural findings is not without risk. Negative cultures in mares with proven inflammatory signs are always perplexing. Chronicity, low bacterial numbers and improper culture techniques are possibilities in these situations. One should always consider that a causal agent may be involved that will not be recovered by conventional means. The emergence of contagious equine metritis in the United Kingdom and Europe in the late 1970s provides a strong reminder of the value of negative cultures.

THERAPY

The principles of management of mares with endometritis must include (1) correction of anatomic defects when indicated, (2) reduction of the inflammation and bacterial numbers in the uterus and (3) prevention of recurrence of the disorder.

In some mares with poor vulvar conformation, all three objectives can be achieved with a Caslick's operation. This simple procedure for excluding air and contaminants from the vaginal tract is probably still the most effective therapeutic procedure in the management of infected mares. Anatomic defects of a more serious nature will need more complex reconstructive surgery of the perineal area.

The second objective, reduction of inflammation and associated organisms, is currently best accomplished with antimicrobial therapy. Newer concepts in stimulating the natural defense mechanisms are promising but have not yet been critically tested. The current status of this treatment concept will be presented with cautions appropriate to new therapeutic ideas.

Antimicrobial therapy includes both antibiotics administered locally (intrauterine) or by systemic routes and antiseptic therapy administered locally. Little precise information is available to guide the practitioner in the selection of drugs, routes of administration, dosage and treatment schedule when antibiotic therapy is undertaken. Most guidelines are based on experience, anecdotal information and the innate creativity of the practicing veterinarian.

ANTIBIOTIC THERAPY

Critical investigations on tissue levels of various drugs in the endometrium are beginning to produce useful data on systemic dosing schedules. The advantages of systemic antibiotic therapy for endometritis are largely related to elimination of the need for invading the vaginal canal to infuse materials through the cervix. An additional advantage is that treatment is easily continued through the diestrous phase of the cycle, and in fact, tissue levels of some antibiotics are higher during diestrus. Inhibitory concentrations of drugs in endometrial tissue may not totally correlate with efficacy of treatment; however, antibiotic concentrations in the uterine lumen may be of greater consequence in reversing the inflammatory processes. It will be difficult to compare systemic with local therapy objectively until a predictable model is developed.

Nevertheless, increasing reports of success in treating endometritis by systemic means are emerging. In particular, several refractory cases of streptococcal infection have been treated with trimethoprim in combination with sulfamethoxazole.*† The treatment schedule was 3 mg/kg trimethoprim and 15 mg/kg sulfamethoxazole, by mouth twice a day for 10 days.

The majority of equine practitioners continue to favor the intrauterine approach to treatment of uterine infections. That feeling is shared by the author, and the following guidelines are based on personal opinion. (1) Select as specific an antibiotic as possible, based on culture results and in vitro antibiotic sensitivity testing. (2) Select both drugs and vehicles that are known to be nonirritating to the endometrium. (3) Administer by intrauterine infusion, using aseptic technique. Treat daily, during estrus, for at least 3 days and longer when time and economic circumstances permit. (4) Infuse a total volume of at least 200 ml per treatment, promoting dispersal of the infusion throughout the uterine lumen.

Some notable variations from these guidelines should be observed. Antibiotic sensitivity testing does not always correlate with in vivo efficacy when applied to the equine uterus. For example, poly-

---

*Bactrim, Roche Laboratories, Nutley, NJ 07110.
†Moore, B., personal communication.

myxin B, which is invariably effective on sensitivity plates against *Pseudomonas* and *Klebsiella*, is seldom of value in the treatment of endometritis caused by these bacteria. Nitrofurazone, although widely used, is similarly unimpressive as an intrauterine medication. Drugs from the tetracycline family should never be placed in the mare's uterus because of potential irritation. Antibiotics with a primary antibacterial spectrum should never be used when yeasts or fungi are the cause of the disorder.

Table 1 lists antibiotics that have been used successfully for intrauterine infusion in the mare. Not all of these drugs are officially approved for this purpose, and appropriate discretion is advised.

A particularly perplexing problem encountered in managing specific bacterial infections is the so-called superinfection. In these cases the primary organism is eliminated from cultural findings, but another, usually more stubborn one takes over. This situation may be noted when treatment for streptococci results in a pure recovery of *Pseudomonas* at the next estrus. Occasionally *Pseudomonas* and *Klebsiella* are involved in the same interaction. The phenomenon of superinfection has been noted to occur spontaneously in experimentally infected mares in which no antibiotic therapy has been employed. This observation suggests that both organisms are involved initially, but one is masked by the other. Changes in the uterine environment may predispose the reduction in numbers of one agent and favor multiplication of the other. Superinfection, if noted often, may be an indication for use of broad-spectrum antibiotics or combinations of narrower spectrum drugs.

ANTISEPTIC THERAPY

Many cases of endometritis, particularly the more chronic cases, do not yield specific bacteria on culture, yet the tissues are known to be inflamed.

A decision must be made in these instances whether to use antibiotic therapy without knowledge of the etiologic agent involved or to use a less specific, nonantibiotic approach. Previous cultural history may aid in the decision.

The use of irritating disinfectant solutions in the mare's uterus should be approached cautiously. The mare is extremely sensitive to irritant substances introduced into the reproductive tract and may respond with necrosis and subsequent fibrotic changes of the endometrium, cervix and vagina. Strong iodine solutions and chlorhexidine diacetate* are contraindicated.

One nonantibiotic regimen that has been used with some success in chronic and culturally negative cases is infusions with dilute povidone iodine solutions. A variety of these compounds are marketed, and the available or titratable iodine content of each should be noted to calculate the appropriate dilution. The maximum strength of the infused solution should not exceed one part of a stock solution containing 1 per cent available iodine in 10 parts of final solution.

Even at these concentrations the solutions are irritating to some mares. Discomfort and straining following infusion may be noted. Prior to each subsequent treatment, evaluation of the degree of irritation caused by the previous infusion should be made. Any cervical or vaginal edema or hyperemia indicates discontinuation of therapy. Failure to monitor the irritation carefully may result in severe and rarely permanent changes in the reproductive tract. A few cases have been seen by the author in which sensitivity to povidone iodine was so severe that small, dilute residues on examination equipment produced severe vaginitis.

Ideally, the povidone iodine infusions, using 250 to 500 ml of solution, should continue for 5 or 6 days. Histologic evidence of an improvement in the

*Nolvasan, Fort Dodge Laboratories, Fort Dodge, IA.

Table 1. Suggested Antibiotics for Uterine Infusion

Drug	Dose (per infusion)	Comments*
Amikacin	2 gm	Gram-negative spectrum
Ampicillin	3 gm	Use only soluble products
Carbenicillin	6 gm	At this dose this drug is effective in some *Pseudomonas* cases
Chloramphenicol	2–3 gm	If oral solution used, may precipitate in saline
Gentamicin sulfate	2 gm	Buffer with NaHCO$_3$ when using small volumes (less than 200 ml)
Kanamycin sulfate	1–2 gm	Most *E. coli* are sensitive
Neomycin sulfate	4 gm	*E. coli*, some *Klebsiella* but seldom *Pseudomonas*
Potassium penicillin G	5 ml units	Preferred for streptococci
Ticarcillin	3–6 gm	Most endometritis pathogens are susceptible. High dose recommended for *Pseudomonas*
Amphotericin B	50 mg	Use the IV preparation. Dilute in water, *not* saline. For *Candida* spp and fungi

*Except where indicated, sterile saline is the appropriate vehicle.

endometrium has been observed with this treatment, and fertility has been restored in a number of difficult mares.

TREATMENT TO ENHANCE THE NATURAL UTERINE DEFENSE MECHANISMS

The possibility that a defect in opsonization of bacteria in the uterus of susceptible mares is responsible for inefficient phagocytosis has been suggested.[2] Since the principal opsonins in serum or plasma are IgG and complement, intrauterine plasma has been investigated as replacement therapy for deficient opsonins.[1] Whether or not the concept will withstand critical evaluation, there appears to be a beneficial effect from infusing the uterus with plasma.

Since 1982, researchers at the University of Florida have documented 44 cases of persistent endometritis, 50 per cent of which have been resolved, with the mare delivering live foals subsequent to the following treatment scheme:

1. Plasma is harvested from the affected mare by aseptic collection of blood, to which 10 units of heparin per ml of blood are added. Plasma is separated by centrifugation and either infused within an hour of collection or frozen for later use.

2. During estrus, the mare's uterus is lavaged with large volumes of sterile saline, which is infused and collected through a large-bore Foley catheter. Three separate 1-liter flushes are made in a manner similar to that of an embryo flush. The clarity or cloudiness of the recovered flush is noted. Cloudy recoveries indicate a need for repeating the flush 2 days later.

3. A volume of 100 ml of plasma is infused into the uterus after the saline is completely evacuated. The plasma infusion is repeated daily, irrespective of flushing, for 5 days during estrus.

4. The mare is evaluated during a subsequent estrous period and, if found clinically normal, is bred. Plasma is infused for 1 to 2 days after breeding.

Additional numbers of mares have been treated with either plasma alone or plasma in combination with saline flushes purely on a postbreeding basis. Large-volume flushes can be used for as long as 3 to 4 days after ovulation without compromising conception.[3] Plasma infusions may also be combined with certain antibiotics after breeding.

Currently, only the mare's own plasma has been evaluated by the University of Florida group. Various practitioners report success using plasma from other donors.

These treatments are neither suggested as primary courses of therapy nor as panaceas. Most of the cases have been unsuccessfully treated with antibodies before the plasma regimen was tried, suggesting that more unconventional approaches offered little downside risk.

EVALUATION OF THERAPY AND MANAGEMENT TO PREVENT RECURRENCE

No matter what therapy is used to control endometritis in mares, evaluation is based on disappearance of clinical signs of inflammation. The same diagnostic criteria are employed. Physical changes should regress, neutrophils should be notably absent from cytologic specimens and endometrial inflammation should improve. Cultures, again, are only part of the story. A negative culture, post-treatment, is unreliable if inflammation is persisting.

Once the uterus has been returned to an acceptable state, careful management is indicated to prevent recurrence of the infection because the uterine defense mechanisms are as important as the initial therapy. Indiscriminate breeding or failure to maintain anatomic integrity will usually cause an immediate recurrence of the problem.

Artificial insemination using antibiotic extenders is the best management tool for these susceptible mares. When AI is not permitted, mares should be managed for minimum contamination at breeding. The infusion of antibiotic semen extenders into the uterus just prior to natural service is helpful. Limitation of the numbers of natural breedings is also indicated. Post-breeding infusion with antibiotics may be used for 48 hours after ovulation without compromising embryo survival.

References

1. Asbury AC: Uterine defense mechanisms in the mare: The use of intrauterine plasma in the management of endometritis. Theriogenology 21:387, 1984.
2. Asbury AC, Gorman NT, Foster GW: Uterine defense mechanisms in the mare: Serum opsonins affecting phagocytosis of *Streptococcus zooepidemicus* by equine neutrophils. Theriogenology 21:375, 1984.
3. Asbury AC: Post-breeding treatment of mares utilizing techniques that improve uterine defenses against bacteria. In Proc 13th Ann Con AAEP, Dallas, 1984, pp 349–356.
4. Blanchard TL, et al.: Comparison of two techniques for obtaining endometrial bacteriologic cultures in the mare. Theriogenology 16:85, 1981.

Supplemental Readings

1. Baker CV, Kenney RM: Systematic approach to the diagnosis of the infertile or subfertile mare. *In* Morrow DA (ed): Current Therapy in Theriogenology. Philadelphia, WB Saunders, 1980.
2. Conboy HC: Diagnosis and therapy of equine endometritis. *In* Proceedings of the Twenty-Fourth Annual Convention of the AAEP. St. Louis, Missouri, 1978, pp. 165–171.
3. Garg RC, Powers TE: Some interactions, incompatibilities and adverse effects of antimicrobial drugs. *In* Morrow DA (ed): Current Therapy in Theriogenology. Philadelphia, WB Saunders, 1980.
4. Hughes JP: Clinical examination and abnormalities in the mare. *In* Morrow DA (ed): Current Therapy in Theriogenology. Philadelphia, WB Saunders, 1980.
5. Kenney RM: Cyclic and pathologic changes of the mare endometrium as detected by biopsy, with a note on early embryonic death. J Am Vet Med Assoc 172:241, 1978.
6. Woodcock JB: Equine endometritis: Diagnosis, interpretation and treatment. Vet Clin North Am, Large Anim Pract 2(2):241, 1980.

Equine Endometrial Biopsy

R. M. Kenney, D.V.M., Ph.D.
University of Pennsylvania,
Kennett Square, Pennsylvania

Paul A. Doig, D.V.M., M.Sc.
Syntex Agribusiness,
Mississauga, Ontario

Endometrial biopsy is evolving as a useful technique for aiding in the diagnosis and prognosis of the endometrium's ability to carry a foal to term. The ability to carry a foal to term was chosen as the prognostic end point[14] rather than pregnancy because it was found that pregnant mares often lost the conceptus as a result of microscopic pathologic changes in the endometrium. In view of the fact that so many organs and events are involved in producing a live foal, it is surprising that there is such a strong[7, 8, 19] yet imprecise relationship between the histologic examination of 0.1 per cent of the endometrium (the percentage of endometrium represented by a biopsy) and the foaling rate. While this correlation probably points to the central role of the endometrium in the process of producing a foal, the impreciseness of the relationship no doubt reflects the fact that this is not a definitive test for fertility because a multitude of factors are involved, including the stallion and overall management.

Endometrial biopsy is a relatively easy and safe technique that can be performed with a minimum of equipment. The biopsy should never be used alone but in conjunction with a detailed history, visual examination of the external genital organs, manual examination of the internal genital organs, uterine swab culture and vaginoscopy. When used properly, the technique can provide valuable information needed by the clinician to evaluate accurately the reproductive capability of the mare.

The technique is particularly useful in detecting causes of reduced fertility that are not diagnosable in any other way. In addition, the results of biopsy can often provide a basis for therapy as well as a means of evaluating its efficacy. Taken together with the other findings, the biopsy can provide a major component for predicting the future ability of the uterus to carry a foal to term, but it must be kept in perspective. It is neither foolproof nor the final answer to fertility prognostication. It does help to increase the accuracy of prognoses. When normal, it points away from the endometrium and toward other areas.

INDICATIONS

Endometrial biopsy has been shown to be of diagnostic value with a number of types of subfertile mares. These include mares found barren after the previous breeding season, "repeat breeder" mares during the breeding season, mares with a history of early embryonic death and mares with clinical endometritis or pyometra. In addition, the biopsy may be valuable as a prognostic aid prior to surgical correction of genital abnormalities such as urovagina, cervical adhesions or lacerations, and genital tract neoplasms. It may also be used as an adjunct to fertility evaluation.[14]

TECHNIQUE

A number of biopsy instruments*† have been used to obtain acceptable endometrial samples. The tissue sample obtained should be a minimum of 10 to 20 × 3 × 3 mm in size for proper histologic interpretation. It would be ideal to sample the roof and floor of each uterine horn and body, but because of the need for hygienic preparation and procedure for each sampling, routinely taking six samples is impractical. It has been shown that one sample is essentially representative of the endometrium as a whole.[2] To maximize the usefulness of one sample, it is essential to ascertain that the size, shape and texture of the uterus and endometrial folds are uniform throughout with no focal abnormalities.[16] When palpably variable areas are detected, a sample should be taken from each as well as a sample from a uniform area. In spite of these necessary precautions and the remarkable uniformity of changes, the changes may be incompletely uniform on occasion.[11] Proper instrumentation and handling of the specimen are important to minimize the development of artifacts that make interpretation difficult.

Because of the ease of dilating the equine cervix, the procedure may be performed during any stage of the estrous cycle. It is important, however, to be aware of the changes that occur in the endometrial architecture due to ovarian steroids that vary with the season of the year and the stage of each estrous cycle.[6, 14] To minimize this variability and avoid misinterpretation, the inexperienced practitioner may prefer to obtain the biopsies only during diestrus when the endometrium is under maximum luteal influence.[18] Regardless of the timing, the person evaluating the biopsy should be informed of the stage of the cycle and the physical findings at the time the sample was obtained.[17]

Since the most common pathologic endometrial changes are inflammatory, it is important to obtain

---

*In USA, Pilliag Surgical Instrument Co, Fort Washington, PA 19034.

†In Canada, Dr. JCL Harris, RR1, Campbellville, Ontario, Canada, LOP 1BO.

a valid endometrial swab for culture. The results of the biopsy and the culture are used for their mutual interpretation.[4, 5] Because the swab must be passed through areas that are apt to be contaminated, it is essential that the swab be guarded, preferably doubly guarded, and have a removable distal occlusion,* both features designed to avoid contamination.[3] If a serious effort is not made to avoid contaminants from the equipment, air, vulva, vagina and cervix, the results of endometrial swabbing are of no consequence. It is essential to take the swab before the biopsy to further minimize contamination.

In preparation for sampling, the rectum is emptied, and a detailed palpation of the internal genital tract through the rectum is performed.[10] A tail bandage is then applied, and the vulva and perineum are thoroughly washed and dried. In order to avoid contamination of the area, the endometrial swab is taken with a sterile gloved hand rather than opening the vagina to the environment with a speculum. A sterile gloved hand, lubricated with sterile surgical jelly and without bacteriostatic chemicals, is used to carry the protected swab through the vagina to the cervix. The tip of the guarded swab is passed by the index finger, inserted through the cervix and into the body of the uterus where the swab is exposed to the endometrium for 2 to 3 minutes. The swab is withdrawn into its guard and then withdrawn from the mare. The process is repeated with the biopsy punch, being careful to avoid carrying contamination into the uterus. With the punch in the uterus, the gloved hand is then withdrawn from the vagina and inserted into the rectum. This hand is used to relieve any pneumovagina by exerting ventral pressure on the vagina. Next, using the same hand, the tip of the punch is located and directed to a point just inside either the left or right uterine horn. The punch is then rotated in order to approach the endometrium on its side. The jaws are opened, and the endometrium is pushed between the jaws and pinched off. A sharp pull completes the taking of the sample. If indicated, an appropriate antibiotic may be infused into the uterus to complete the procedure.

TISSUE PREPARATION

The biopsy specimen is carefully dislodged from the jaws of the punch with a fine hypodermic needle and dropped in Bouin's solution. Great care must be exercised to avoid squashing or other mishandling that produces artifacts. Bouin's solution tends to produce a firmer specimen than formalin with less tissue distortion on sectioning. Following 2 to 24 hours in Bouin's solution, at a ratio of 1 part tissue to 10 parts fixative, the specimen is placed in 70 per cent ethyl alcohol or 10 per cent formalin, either of which may be used as the transport me-

---

*Harford Veterinary Supply, 9100 Persimmon Tree Road, Potomac, MD 20854

dium to the laboratory. Routine histopathologic procedures follow, and the sections are stained with hematoxylin-eosin.

INTERPRETATION

Histopathologic assessment of endometrial samples and development of an epicrisis should be done by a person who is knowledgeable in both the clinical aspects of horse reproduction and the reproductive physiology and pathology of the mare.[11, 18] Normal variations in endometrial architecture that occur during the estrous cycle, transitional stages and anestrus have been well documented and should be appreciated prior to interpreting the biopsy specimen.[11, 14]

Evaluation of an endometrial sample should include four components: (1) making certain that there is sufficient tissue (i.e., ≥ 1 linear cm of tissue), (2) assessing the histologic stage of the cycle, (3) assessing any inflammatory (cellular) response, and (4) assessing the degree and extent of endometrial degenerative changes such as fibrosis, lymphatic lacunae, and cystic glands.

Histologic Variation Between Seasons of the Year

Although endometrial histologic features vary predictably with the season of the year, they actually result from changes in ovarian steroidal levels. The physiological "seasons" of the mare year are imprecisely divided periods in which ovarian activity is characteristic for the mare population in the hemisphere in which they reside.[10]

In the northern hemisphere, the physiological breeding season starts in the spring and extends into the summer, with the peak centering around the summer solstice in June. The histologic features of this season are those associated with changes in stage of the estrous cycle (see next section).

The nonbreeding season begins during late fall and winter when the ovaries are inactive and the endometrium is in atrophy. The endometrium in atrophy is characterized by cuboidal luminal and glandular epithelia and straight rather than tortuous glands. Inspissated secretions also tend to accumulate. Since mares in deep anestrus are without ovarian steroids, these are also the features of endometria in such gonadectomized states as the surgically ovariectomized mare and mares with gonadal dysgenesis resulting from chromosomal abnormalities.[14]

Between the period of winter endometrial atrophy and the cyclic endometrium of the physiological breeding season, the endometrium goes through a transition period from complete inactivity (atrophy) to full activity. There is also a reverse transition period in the fall. The length of the transition period may be very short because some mares conceive on the first estrus of the year with an endometrium found to be atrophic within the 2 weeks prior to ovulation. It is probably more common for the transition period to be considerably longer. The time required for reactivation of the endometrium varies among individuals but tends to lag behind the recommencement of ovarian and behavioral estrous cycles.[14] For this reason it is possible in the early spring to find various degrees of residual endometrial atrophy in mares that have had one or more ovulatory cycles. Mares with this type of endometrium appear to undergo repeat breeding, which may result in the submission of a biopsy for evaluation. It should be recognized with this type of endometrium that normal fertility for that individual returns when the endometrium recovers from atrophy. However, the criteria for predicting the individual versus the population time lag required have not been developed (see below).

In a recent retrospective study (P. A. Doig and J. D. McKnight, unpublished data), 87 standardbred mares were sampled in the months of February through April and placed in one of two seasonal stages based on the degree of residual endometrial atrophy (glands atrophic or active). All mares had either a category I (see later section, A Proposed Standard Classification System of Histologic Changes) or category IIA endometrium,[9] had been in estrus, and were inseminated when ovulation was impending and the cervix relaxed. The length of time for mares in each stage of endometrial atrophy to be bred and become pregnant was determined (Table 1).

In the first 30 days, only 2 of 37 mares (5 per cent), in which initially there was predominant residual gland atrophy (early to mid-transition stage), were judged to be ready to be bred on the basis of the follicle and cervix. One mare was bred on day 12 after the biopsy and the other on day 22, and both became pregnant. By 60 days, less than half (46 per cent) of these mares had been bred, but again there was a high pregnancy rate among those bred. In contrast, during the same period, in the second group of mares (which had been judged initially to have recovered from seasonal endometrial atrophy) 54 per cent were inseminated within 30 days and 92 per cent by 60 days.

These findings indicate that among mares determined to have substantial endometrial atrophy despite the presence of one or more behavioral estruses, only 5 per cent met criteria for breeding and had been inseminated in the first 30 days and only 50 per cent by 60 days. In contrast, in mares whose endometria were initially substantially out of atrophy, about 50 per cent were pregnant in the first 30 days and over 90 per cent had been inseminated by 60 days. When either class of mare had an ovulating follicle and relaxed cervix, they were fertile regardless of the state of the initial biopsy. However, most of those whose endometria are substantially out of atrophy will be breedable within 60 days. When either class of mare has an ovulating follicle and relaxed cervix, they will be highly fertile regardless of the state of the initial biopsy.

Histologic Variations Related to Stages of the Estrous Cycle Within the Physiological Breeding Season

The histologic features of the endometrium during the physiological breeding season more or less reflect the relative levels of the ovarian steriods[14] in several ways. More edema tends to be evident during proestrus, but this is difficult to evaluate since edema is produced in a surgically derived specimen. The most reliable feature of spontaneous edema is the "proestral nest" created by differential distribution of tissue fluid. Such nests occur in 15 to 20 per cent of cases at this stage.[14]

The luminal and ductular epithelia appear to respond more quickly to changing steroid levels than either the mid or basal gland epithelia. They are the first to become active when the endometrium emerges from atrophy and the last to undergo atrophy when the endometrium enters atrophy. The luminal epithelium appears to vary in height in concert with the ovarian cycle. It reaches a peak height of 30 to 40 μm during early estrus, drops to 15 to 20 μm in late estrus or early diestrus and then increases in height through diestrus and proestrus.[14] Luminal epithelial cell height often varies within a section, so estimation should be based on the predominant type.

Margination is the phenomenon in which polymorphonuclear (PMN) leukocytes become closely associated with the endothelium of capillaries, venules and veins. This occurs during estrus and in inflammation. In estrus, the PMNs marginate but do not migrate through the stroma, although small numbers do migrate through the luminal epithelium and into the uterine lumen (margination without migration). In inflammation, they both marginate in the vessels and migrate through the stroma.

Glandular tortuosity can be helpful in estimating

Table 1. Relationship Between Residual Endometrial Atrophy as Assessed by Biopsy During the Transition Period (February–April) and Pregnancy Rates Obtained During the Next 60-Day Period

		30 Days					60 Days			
		Insem.		Preg./ Insem.		% of Total	Insem.		Preg./ Insem.		% of Total
Endometrial Glands	No.	No.	(%)	No.	(%)	Preg.	No.	(%)	No.	(%)	Preg.
Majority atrophic	37	2	(5)	2/2	(100)	5	19	(51)	17/19	(89)	46
Majority active	50	27	(54)	23/27	(85)	46	46	(92)	42/46	(91)	84

the stage of cycle. The more tortuous the glands, as indicated by a series of glandular cross sections or a very scalloped outline, the higher the progesterone/estrogen ratio.[14] That is, tortuosity indicates luteal dominance.

Assessment of Inflammatory (Cellular) Response

The inflammatory response may be acute or chronic or occasionally may consist of a chronic response on which an acute reaction is superimposed. In acute reactions, polymorphonuclear leukocytes (PMNs) predominate, usually in the stratum compactum or luminal epithelium as well as in the capillaries and venules of the stratum compactum. Only infrequently are PMNs found in the uterine lumen, presumably because they were lost during processing. Rarely, PMNs may be present deeper within the lumen of dilated glands. Since chronic reactions usually have PMNs passing through them, it is common to find PMNs in the lumen overlying a chronic reaction in the stroma.

Chronic inflammation is characterized by infiltrations of lymphocytes and less commonly by plasma cells, siderophages, eosinophils and mast cells. Chronic reactions usually involve the stratum compactum but can involve the deeper stratum spongiosum as well, usually in the form of discrete foci that have either a scattered or widespread distribution.

The presence of moderate to severe chronic reactions, especially if plasma cells are present, is indicative of continuing antigenic stimulation. This should alert the clinician to the possibility of an infectious etiology and the need for appropriate diagnostic or therapeutic procedures.

Siderophages are macrophages that have phagocytosed blood and converted it to hemosiderin. Thus they represent previous hemorrhage and can be a sign of trauma, although more often they indicate parturition, abortion or early fetal death.

Eosinophils are occasionally observed as discrete or diffuse foci, usually more frequently in inflamed uteri during estrus.[14] Eosinophils are inconsistently frequent in fungal endometritis,[13] whereas they characterize the acute inflammation of pneumouterus.[20] These are two conditions partially related to conformational defects, a point the clinician should be alerted to in the epicrisis.

Increasing severity of endometrial fibrosis appears to be associated with a corresponding increase in the incidence of inflammatory cell infiltrations.[9] Moderate to severe inflammatory responses should be resolved before breeding is attempted. These mares should also be protected from further bacterial exposure at the time of breeding through the use of a minimum contamination technique.[15] As with other pathologic changes, a key point is that the more widespread the inflammation, the greater the reduction in the endometrium's ability to carry to term.

Both the cause of inflammation and its role in reducing the endometrium's ability to support pregnancy are proper areas of concern. Traditionally, there has been little association between the incidence of inflammation and recovery of aerobic bacteria. However, as improved cultural techniques have reduced contamination, the discrepancy has increased,[3, 4, 5] so that it is now more common than not to obtain a "no growth swab" in the presence of inflammation. This raises the question of involvement of other types of organisms and noninfectious mechanisms in the genesis of inflammations.

A category II level of inflammation has been shown by Asbury[1] to reduce the pregnancy rate by 40 per cent compared with category I and to have a 37 per cent loss of those pregnancies while category I endometria lost only 2 per cent. These observations confirm that category II inflammations lead to reduced pregnancy rates and reduced ability to carry to term unless they are treated and the affected mares bred with a minimum contamination technique.[9]

Assessment of Endometrial Fibrosis

An evaluation of the degree of endometrial fibrosis is a very important assessment of a biopsy sample because endometrial fibrosis, in contrast to inflammatory changes, is permanent and, when widespread, becomes one of the main limiting factors in subsequent reproductive performance of the mare.

The deposition of collagen most commonly occurs around glands or in association with the basement membrane of the luminal epithelium. The first evidence of impending deposition of collagen is the loss of randomization of stromal cells (and their nuclei) of the stratum compactum or stratum spongiosum, particularly around glands. Periglandular fibrosis may involve isolated, individual gland branches, or a number of branches can be ensheathed to form a nest.[14] The severity of fibrosis can be rated as to degree (number of periglandular layers) and frequency (number of fibrotic foci per linear field). The finding that the more widespread the fibrosis, regardless of the degree of severity, the lower the ability of the uterus to carry a foal to term (just as in the case of inflammation and lymphatic lacunae) led to its inclusion in the development of classification systems for assessment of equine endometrial biopsies.[9, 14]

Nonfibrotic nests, clusters of gland branches tightly coiled together and distinctly separated from other glands by stroma, are distinguished from fibrotic nests by the lack of nonrandom, circumferential stromal nuclei as well as lack of deposition of collagen. In addition, they occur most commonly during seasonal anestrus and the transitional periods.[11]

It has recently been shown that 12 biopsies in the same area did not increase the incidence of fibrosis.[11]

Assessment of Lymphatic Lacunae

Lymphatic lacunae are derived from dilated lymphatic vessels and can occur in the lamina propria or core of endometrial folds singly or in clusters and can be focal or diffuse. When individual lacunae coalesce and enlarge they become endometrial cysts.[14, 16] Histologically, they should be differentiated from surgically induced edema.[16] Their precise role in reducing the ability to carry to term is not clear, but when widespread and detectable by palpation of thickened endometrial folds, they appear to greatly reduce the ability to carry a foal to term. When present in association with lymphatic cysts, their detrimental effect appears to be cumulative. They must be differentiated from the condition known as severe, widespread edema.[12]

Assessment of Endometrial Cysts

Endometrial cysts are derived from lymphatic vessels and vary in size from microscopic to $\simeq 12$ cm in diameter. They can originate in the lamina propria or in the connective tissue core of folds. Only the smaller ones will be detected on biopsy, where they appear as exaggerated lacunae. The large ones are far too large to be seen in biopsy samples. However, the biopsy punch can be used to remove a portion of the larger ones to enable them to drain, thereby aiding therapy.

Embryonic death associated with cysts has been observed. The connection is not clear, because afflicted endometria usually have concurrent problems.

Assessment of Cystic Glands

Cystic distention of glands is common in fibrotic nests. Distention with inspissated secretion is common in seasonal atrophy. Cystic distention without fibrosis and without inspissation can occur during the physiological breeding season.[14] This change does appear to be associated with repeat breeding when widespread.

Effects of Barrenness

The number of years that a mare has been barren under good breeding management appears to influence the foaling prognoses significantly within fibrosis categories. Mares with moderate endometrial fibrosis but barren only 1 year were found to have foaling rates that were twice those of similar mares barren 2 years or more (62 per cent versus 28 per cent).[9] The adverse effect from "years barren" was also apparent in the mild fibrosis group.[9] The reason for the apparent difference in foaling rates for mares in the same fibrosis category is not entirely clear but is partially related to susceptibility to bacterial exposure because the effect is reduced through treatment of inflammation and use of minimum contamination breeding.[9]

Effects of Minimum Contamination Breeding

Minimizing bacterial contamination of the uterus at the time of breeding through a minimal contamination technique can be a critical determinant in improving foaling rates.[15] It is recommended for endometria with category II inflammatory changes or with any endometrium recovered from inflammatory changes. In endometria with moderate fibrosis coupled with inflammation, treatment of the inflammation and breeding with a minimum contamination technique has virtually doubled the foaling rate.[9]

CLASSIFICATION SYSTEMS OF HISTOLOGIC CHANGES

The initial classification system[13] of histologic changes employed three categories: an essentially normal group (category I) with a foaling rate reflecting the overall management scheme, a severely affected group (category III), whose foaling rate reflected severe changes in the endometrium, and an in-between group (category II), whose foaling rate reflected endometrial changes plus management factors including veterinary care. It was anticipated that category II and possibly category III could eventually be subdivided as criteria for more accurately predicting foaling rate were developed. It was also recognized that endometria in categories II and III could be moved up in a category when one or more of the pathologic changes (widespread diffuse inflammation or widespread lymphatic lacunae) were reduced or eliminated, with the qualification that after improvement of the inflammation, they should not be exposed to raw semen but should be bred with one of the minimum contamination techniques.[15] The process of subdivision was initiated when it was found that the extent of fibrosis could be further subdivided[9] in a way that reflected differing degrees of ability to carry to term. In addition, a nonhistologic feature, the number of years barren, was found to influence the foaling rate within categories. For example, a mare with a category IIA endometrium that had been barren only 1 year would have an 80 per cent prospect of foaling, but this would be only 50 per cent if barren for 2 years or more. Dividing the extent of fibrosis into four categories—namely, absent, mild, moderate and severe—resulted in a more precise prediction of foaling probability than the three-category system. Both rating systems, however, used the same criteria for the most severe group to identify those endometria with extremely poor ability to carry to term. This is a critical feature for any rating system—that is, a well-defined group of endometria that have an extremely poor potential for carrying a foal to term—since mares with these uteri represent a large burden on the owner. Mares with such endometria are not sterile, but they are very poor producers, and their identification is a major objective of the procedure.

A PROPOSED STANDARD CLASSIFICATION SYSTEM OF HISTOLOGIC CHANGES

Owing to the widespread use and acceptance of the three-category system, it is proposed that until the basis for the subdivisions is fully documented, any modification should retain the original numerical designations.

An understanding of several terms used to describe the pattern of distribution of lesions in biopsy samples is very important. The overall distribution of a type of lesion is designated as widespread or scattered. *Widespread* lesions are numerous and appear widely throughout the sections, whereas *scattered* ones are few and irregularly distributed. The more widespread a lesion, the more likely it will lower the ability to carry to term.

In addition, there are two particularly important terms for pathologic foci. Discrete foci have concentrated changes with rather sharp, well-defined margins, whereas the contents of diffuse foci are spread out with indefinite margins. The more diffuse a lesion the greater its depressing effect on the ability to carry to term. For instance, widespread, diffuse lesions of any degree of severity appear to be more serious than scattered, focal severe lesions.

In this modified system, category I and category III endometria remain as previously defined while the broad category II is divided into two groups designated as IIA and IIB. Others have used this technique successfully to divide group II endometria into two categories termed II high and II low.[18] Using the modified criteria, the following classifications can be made:

Category I. The endometrium is neither hypoplastic nor atrophic, and either there are no pathologic changes or any existing changes (such as inflammation or fibrosis) are slight and sparsely scattered.

Category IIA. Inflammatory changes that qualify an endometrium for inclusion here include slight to moderate, diffuse infiltrations of the stratum compactum or scattered but frequent foci in the stratum compactum and stratum spongiosum. Qualifying fibrotic changes include frequent scattered involvement of individual gland branches of any degree of severity (but usually one to three layers) or fibrotic nests of gland branches averaging less than two per 5.5-mm linear field in an average of four or more fields.

Lymphatic lacunae that become sufficiently extensive to produce palpable changes in the endometrial folds are also grounds for placing this type of endometrium in category IIA. If the lacunae are lost either spontaneously or through therapy, the endometrium reverts to category I providing it qualifies otherwise.

Partial endometrial atrophy late in the physiological breeding season, in contrast to atrophy before the physiological breeding season, with behavioral and ovarian cycling, is a fourth basis for classifying an endometrium as category IIA until the cause of the atrophy is determined and corrected. During the transitional seasons, atrophy has an additive transitory effect on the three other types of changes in depressing ability to become pregnant and carry to term.

Endometria with these criteria from mares that have been barren two or more years are put in category IIB.

The inflammatory, fibrotic, lymphatic and atrophic changes are additive, so when more than one change is present, the category is lowered stepwise. For instance, if both inflammatory and fibrotic changes are present, each of which qualifies the endometrium for category IIA, the endometrium is categorized as IIB. If the inflammatory changes are corrected, the endometrium may be recategorized as IIA providing the mare is bred with minimum contamination technique.[14]

Category IIB. Qualifying inflammatory changes are widespread, diffuse and moderately severe foci. The fibrotic changes are also more severe and extensive than those found in category IIA. The fibrotic involvement of individual gland branches in this category is very widespread and of uniform distribution, usually with up to four or more layers, or there are an average of two to four fibrotic nests of glands per 5.5 mm of linear fields in an average of four or more fields.

If qualifying inflammatory changes are present in combination with qualifying fibrotic or lymphatic changes, the endometrium is placed in category III. Elimination of the inflammatory or lymphatic changes allows upward reclassification to category IIA or even higher,[9] providing a minimum contamination technique of breeding is used after reduction or elimination of inflammation.

Category III. The criteria for the four changes that qualify an endometrium for category III are as follows: Widespread, diffuse, severe inflammatory changes are one of the qualifying criteria for placing an endometrium in this category. Uniformly widespread fibrosis of gland branches of five or more fibrotic nests per 5.5 mm of linear fields and lymphatic lacunae so severe that they produce a "jelly-like" feel of the endometrial folds or uterine wall are also qualifying changes. If a mare has an endometrium in deep atrophy in the physiological breeding season, the endometrium is categorized as III until the cause of the atrophy is removed. If two or more of the four types of changes are present at one time, the situation is that much worse. Because such types of endometria are not totally incapable of carrying a foal to term, such mares are not sterile.

If endometria have qualifying levels of fibrotic

Table 2. Expected Foaling Rates of Mares According to Categorization of Endometrium

Category	Degree of Endometrial Change	Expected Foaling Rate (Per Cent)
I	Absent	80–90
IIA	Mild	50–80
IIB	Moderate	10–50
III	Severe	10

changes as well as one or more of the other changes, therapy for the inflammatory or lymphatic changes can be helpful, but because the fibrotic changes are widespread the chance for upward reclassification is very slim.

A mare should never be condemned on the basis of one biopsy sample for several reasons, although it has been repeatedly shown that such endometria are of considerably reduced ability to sustain a foal to term.

1. First, mares with these endometria are not sterile. Thus a mare's offspring may be worth the cost of sustaining and breeding the mare over several years. Mares with such endometria produce an average of one foal every 10 years.

2. Although the pathologic changes are surprisingly uniform throughout the endometrium,[2] they are sometimes incompletely uniform,[11] and therefore confirmation of the changes by biopsy at a different site is in order.

3. Unless one considers the effect of season, the results can be misleading.

FOALING PROGNOSTICATION

Because of the previously outlined factors, any "probable foaling rate" index for the various categories must utilize a range to allow for the influence of those variables (Table 2).[17, 18]

EPICRISES

If the person reading the biopsy is not the clinician for the case, that person should write an epicrisis of the case. This means that the histologic findings, both normal and pathologic, should be interpreted by taking into consideration the history, physical, behavioral, and microbiologic findings. When possible, the epicrisis can include recommendations for therapy and prognosis for alternative approaches to the case including additional diagnostic tests.

References

1. Asbury AC: Some observations on the relationship of histologic inflammation in the endometrium of the mare to fertility. Proceedings of the 28th Annual Convention of the American Association of Equine Practitioners 1982, pp 401–404.
2. Bergman RV, Kenney RM: Representativeness of a uterine biopsy in the mare. Proceedings of the 21st Annual Convention of the American Association of Equine Practitioners, Boston, Dec., 1975, pp 355–361.
3. Blanchard TL, Garcia MC, Hurtgen JP, Kenney RM: Comparison of two techniques for obtaining endometrial bacteriologic culture in the mare. Theriogenology 16(1):85, 1981.
4. Blanchard TL, Cummings MR, Garcia MC, et al.: Comparison between two techniques for endometrial swab culture and between biopsy and culture in barren mares. Theriogenology (16)5:541, 1981.
5. Blanchard TL: Erroneous diagnosis of endometritis in the mare. Theriogenology Proceedings, Spokane, Wash., Sept. 23–25, 1981, pp 247–255.
6. Britton BA: Endometrial change in the annual reproductive cycle of the mare. J Reprod Fert Suppl 32:175, 1982.
7. Carroll CL, Mitchell G: The role of endometrial biopsy. J Reprod Fert Suppl 32:639, 1982 (abstract).
8. de la Concha-Bermejillo A, Kennedy PC: Prognostic value of endometrial biopsy in the mare: A retrospective analysis. J Am Vet Med Assoc 181(7):680, 1982.
9. Doig PA, McKnight JD, Miller RB: The use of endometrial biopsy in the infertile mare. Can Vet J 22:72, 1981.
10. Greenhoff GR, Kenney RM: Evaluation of reproductive status of nonpregnant mares. J Am Vet Med Assoc 167(6):449, 1975.
11. Gross TL, LaBlanc MM: Seasonal variation of histomorphologic features of equine endometrium. JAVMA 184:1372, 1984.
12. Henry G, Vandeplassche G, Coryn M, et al.: Excessive oedema of the genital tract of the mare. Zbl Vet Med A 28:390, 1981.
13. Hurtgen JP, Cummings MR: Diagnosis and treatment of fungal endometritis in mares. Proceedings Annual Meeting of the Society for Theriogenology, 1982, pp 18–22.
14. Kenney RM: Cyclic and pathologic changes of the mare endometrium as detected by biopsy with a note on early embryonic death. J Am Vet Med Assoc 172:241, 1978.
15. Kenney RM, Bergman RV, Cooper WL, Morse GW: Minimal contamination techniques for breeding mares: Technique and preliminary findings. Proceedings 21st Annual Convention American Association Equine Practitioners, Boston, Dec., 1975, pp 327–336.
16. Kenney RM: Clinical aspects of endometrial biopsy in fertility evaluation of the mare. Proceedings, 23rd Annual Convention of American Association of Equine Practitioners, Vancouver, Dec., 1977, pp 105–122.
17. Kenney RM: The role of endometrial biopsy in fertility evaluation of the mare. Proceedings 24th Annual Convention of American Association of Equine Practitioners, St. Louis, 1978, pp 177–184.
18. Neely DP: Evaluation and therapy of genital disease in the mare. *In* Equine Reproduction. Veterinary Learning Systems Co., Inc., 1983.
19. Shideler RK, McChesney AE, Voss JL, Squires EL: Relationship of endometrial biopsy and other management factors to fertility of broodmares. J Eq Vet Sci 2(1):5, 1982.
20. Slusher SH, Freeman KP, Roszel JF: Eosinophils in equine uterine cytology and histology specimens. J Am Vet Med Assoc 184:665, 1984.

Treatment of Uterine Infections in the Mare

Walter R. Threlfall, D.V.M., M.S., Ph.D.
The Ohio State University, Columbus, Ohio

Carla L. Carleton, D.V.M., M.S.
Michigan State University, East Lansing, Michigan

In the past, uterine treatments have been evaluated primarily by the response of clinical cases following therapy. However, one of the problems often associated with this type of study is the lack of a definitive diagnosis. Another major drawback of the "clinical impression" evaluation is the *absence* of controls, since known infected mares are seldom left untreated. In addition, the lack of clinical records to substantiate the clinical impression reduces credibility. This summary of the treatments available in the literature is designed to credit those completed research efforts and to point out the vast number of unknown, unsubstantiated therapies that need to be investigated to determine their efficacy and lack of associated detrimental side effects.

To permit uniform understanding and evaluation of infertility, it is necessary to define the severity of the condition, both infectious and inflammatory. *Endometritis* is an infection or inflammation of the endometrium. The most common causes of endometritis have been reported to be insemination at the wrong stage of the estrous cycle and breeding too often. It is also a common sequel to abnormal parturition or to metritis and lacerations of the uterus. Uterine contamination and inflammation are normal occurrences at the time of parturition and should be distinguished from clinically significant endometritis. The inflammation or contamination that occurs at parturition can progress to a clinically significant condition, but generally the normal involutionary process of the uterus is responsible for eliminating contaminating organisms and reducing inflammation.

The diagnosis of endometritis may involve endometrial culture or endometrial biopsy or may be based merely on observation of purulent exudate from the cervix with substantial proof that a cervicitis is not present. It is imperative to obtain a culture of the lumen of the uterus and not of the vagina or cervix. The lack of correlation between various culture sites has been demonstrated.[32] Uterine cultures can be taken during any stage of the estrous cycle because the cervix is easily dilated.[43]

Although many clinicians at present disregard the significance of uterine cultures in the absence of other clinical signs of infection, the work demonstrating the major differences in conception rates between clinically normal uninfected mares and clinically normal streptococcal infected mares should be noted.[31] The conception rates for these two groups were 80 per cent and 52 per cent, respectively, based on a total of 225 Thoroughbred mares. The classification of a clinically normal infected mare utilized culture and thorough vaginal and cervical examinations but did not involve endometrial biopsies. Rectal examination may not disclose any abnormality of the uterus because by definition only the lining of the uterus is involved. Estrous cycles are usually normal in length but may be altered due to modifications in the release of endogenous luteolytic factor.

Metritis is an extension of the condition involving the endometrium into the deeper layers of the uterus. The uterus may have a tendency to increase in size and decrease in tone. There may be an accumulation of fluid in the lumen of the uterus. The endometrial folds may become less defined on palpation or fiberoptic examination.

Acute toxic metritis is seen less frequently in the mare than in the cow and is characterized by signs of metritis plus systemic involvement, which can include signs of increased temperature, depression, loss of appetite, laminitis and other signs representative of a toxemia or septicemia. This may lead to *perimetritis* or *parametritis,* which indicates that the infection or inflammation has progressed to the peritoneal surface of the uterus and the peritoneal cavity.

Pyometra is characterized by an accumulation of pus within the lumen of the uterus in addition to the persistence of a corpus luteum beyond its normal life span. Pyometra in the mare results in the expected increased and sustained level of progesterone. The failure of estrus may be due to an altered capability of the endometrium to produce the luteolytic factor.[20] Mares with pyometra do not exhibit systemic clinical signs, and the volume of fluid retained in the uterus varies greatly.[21] Although uterine cultures usually reveal mixed organisms or sometimes no bacterial growth, the most common organism isolated is *Streptococcus zooepidemicus.*

A uterus distended with purulent material and incapable of drainage due to cervical adhesions has also been referred to as pyometra. However, if the corpus luteum is not maintained, it may be correctly defined as a metritis, which has cervical adhesions. The presence of a retained corpus luteum is an important distinction between metritis with fluid and pyometra. A mare with metritis may eventually develop a pyometra, but as long as she continues to cycle she stands a much better chance of self-recovery than would a mare with pyometra. Due to the absence of systemic involvement, this condition may go undetected for years in nonbroodmares, and owners seek veterinary assistance only when they note the copious intermittent vulvar discharge.

It should be recognized that the lumen of the normal nonpregnant uterus is bacteriologically sterile.[27] Also, if the mare is similar to the cow, bacteria do appear during pregnancy, and the type or numbers of bacteria may account for whether the pregnancy is maintained or terminated.[37] Many mares may not warrant treatment for an infection if their uterine biopsy results indicate an extremely poor reproductive prognosis. Furthermore, it should be stated that prevention of uterine infection with proper foaling and breeding practices should supersede any consideration regarding therapy. Once uterine disease has occurred, early detection and immediate treatment of infertility are recommended.[44]

Assuming that the severity of the condition and the etiologic agent have been determined, therapy to correct the cause of the infertility can be instituted. Uterine therapy can be accomplished by several different routes. The first and most commonly used approach is the local instillation of antibiotics, antiseptics, immunoglobulins or other substances directly into the uterus. Another approach is systemic antibiotic treatment. Hormones and hormone-like products can be administered locally or systemically for "desired effects." Vitamins, minerals and other dietary supplements do not appear to be of benefit when mares are already receiving an adequately balanced diet. Surgical correction of problems such as pneumovagina should always precede any other form of therapy since the abnormal conformation is often responsible for the uterine infection.

The primary reason for treating uterine disease should be to save reproductive time by assisting the mare in the bacterial elimination process. It is reported that normal mares artificially exposed to large numbers of pathogenic organisms have returned to a noncontaminated, noninfected state within a few days. However, the mare that is not normal may require longer to eliminate the bacterial organisms or may not be able to do so without assistance. Therapy, therefore, is of value in reducing lost reproductive time and in assisting the abnormal mare. Some authors have recommended sexual rest as a treatment for metritis (Skewes, personal communication). The resistance of the reproductive tract is highest during estrus, and mares that cycle normally have repeated periods of high resistance. It must be emphasized that extreme caution should be directed at local uterine therapy, so that the treatment selected does not pose a greater danger to reproductive health than the disease itself. Extra-label use of numerous products as intrauterine medications in mares is common in spite of the lack of information about their potentially damaging properties.

Mares that appear *more* susceptible to endometritis must be handled with greater care than normal mares. Recommendations for these problem mares, including intrauterine infusions of semen extender containing an antibiotic before breeding and the day after breeding may appear justified.

Opinions relating to treatment objectives and anticipated responses are widely varied and stimulate much controversy. Most veterinarians agree that elimination of infectious organisms, reduction in uterine size, improvement of uterine tone and elimination of uterine fluid are all desirable in a treatment program. Divergent opinions arise concerning the method and means used to obtain these objectives.

The first consideration regarding intrauterine infusion is the choice of the most effective antibiotic. With regard to the use of antibiotics to eliminate bacterial infections, one should remember that bacterial cultures and antibiotic susceptibilities are the best way to approach the problem of selecting an efficacious antibiotic. Combinations of antibiotics should be avoided with uterine therapy because they are often of little value due to drug incompatibility. The same can be said for antibiotic and antiseptic combinations or of these combinations plus hormonal or other "preparations" to be used intrauterine. The organisms most commonly present within the infected uterus are *Streptococcus* spp., *Klebsiella* spp., *Staphylococcus* spp., *Proteus* spp., *Pseudomonas* spp. and *Corynebacterium* spp. Beta-hemolytic streptococcal organisms account for an estimated 65 per cent of all equine uterine infections. *Proteus* spp., *Pseudomonas* spp., and *Klebsiella* spp. account for an additional 30 per cent.

The antibiotics most commonly utilized for intrauterine infusion are penicillin, tetracycline, gentamicin, ampicillin, streptomycin, chloramphenicol, nitrofurazone, polymyxin B, neomycin and the sulfonamides. The antibiotics effective against the majority of pathogenic organisms generally are ticarcillin, ampicillin and chloramphenicol.

The majority of reports of equine uterine infections have dealt with how and when infections occur and the organisms responsible. Evaluation of the intrauterine medications has been determined by production of a foal the following year, conception rates, elimination of the organism from the uterus, or improvement in uterine size and tone.

More common risks associated with local antibiotic therapy in the uterus are changes in the pathogenic flora and development of resistant strains of microorganisms due to "indiscriminate" use of antibiotics. One observation reported in the literature and made by this author is that some mares treated successfully for a streptococcal infection with various local antibiotics will re-culture a growth of *Pseudomonas* spp.

A report on gentamicin stated that of the following organisms isolated from 120 mares, the percentage of those sensitive to the antibiotic were *Staphylococcus* spp., 100 per cent, *Streptococcus* spp., 97 per cent, *Micrococcus* spp., 100 per cent, *Bacillus* spp., 100 per cent, *Pseudomonas* spp., 100 per cent, *Enterobacter*, 100 per cent, *Alcaligenes* spp., 100 per cent.[19] Conception and foaling data were obtained on 98 of the mares, with 69 conceiving and 18 of 25 pregnant mares followed to foaling at term. In another study involving 60 mares with endometritis treated with 1.0 to 2.5 gm of gentamicin daily for 3 to 5 days, 86 per cent of these mares had "no growth" cultures following treatment and 74 per cent produced foals.[22] The antibacterial results of the total of 185 cultures indicated that 100 per cent of the *Staphylococcus* spp., 97 per cent of the *Streptococcus* spp., 100 per cent of the *Pseudomonas* spp. and 100 per cent of the enterobacteria were sensitive to gentamicin. It has been suggested that *Klebsiella* uterine infections can be successfully treated by using 800 mg of gentamicin twice daily intramuscularly for 8 days[9] or 2 to 2.5 gm gentamicin plus 250 ml of saline infused into the uterus once daily for 3 days.

Chloramphenicol is commonly utilized as a treatment for uterine infection because of its effectiveness, economic feasibility and availability. Chloramphenicol is reported to be effective against *Staphylococcus* spp., *Streptococcus* spp., *E. coli*, *Proteus vulgaris*, *Corynebacterium* spp., *Pseudomonas* spp. and *Shigella* spp.[19]

Results of uterine cultures and antibiotic sensitivities at The Ohio State University Veterinary Hospital[45, 46] indicated that 10 per cent of the *Pseudomonas* isolates were sensitive to chloramphenicol. Sixty-six per cent of the *Klebsiella* isolates, 75 per cent of the *Proteus* isolates, 98 per cent of the *Streptococcus* isolates, 99 per cent of the *E. coli* isolates and 100 per cent of the *Staphylococcus* isolates were sensitive to this antibiotic.

The stage of the estrous cycle influences the pharmacokinetic variables in cattle, and if this is true in the mare, the dosage of the antibiotic may need to be altered depending on estrous activity. In the mare, chloramphenicol was rapidly absorbed after infusion, with peak serum levels occurring within 1 hour.[42] There were no detectable serum levels present within 12 hours of infusion.

Penicillin has been reported to be effective against *Streptococcus* species; however, it is rapidly absorbed from the uterus. The therapeutic blood levels are short, indicating that treatment may need to be repeated four or five times per day. Allen (1978)[21] reported that intrauterine administration of penicillin should be repeated at 5-hour intervals in pony mares in order to maintain therapeutic levels of this antibiotic. This recommendation was based on the disappearance of penicillin from the serum. Other investigators have shown in the cow that oxytetracycline is absent from the serum within 12 hours postinfusion, sulfamethazine by 12 hours, penicillin by 12 hours and dihydrostreptomycin by 48 hours. Serum levels are probably significant, especially when the majority of antibiotic is absorbed. Absorption of sodium benzylpenicillin following intrauterine administration is 1/10 of that following intramuscular injection. The stage of estrous cycle does not appear to affect the absorption of this antibiotic, but endometrial irritation such as swabbing did result in a higher percentage absorbed. Intramuscular administration of penicillin produced levels in the endometrium equal to 50 to 75 per cent of those found in the serum. Intravenous administration produced similar results except that tissue levels were not maintained longer than 8 hours, whereas with intramuscular administration, levels lasted 24 hours. The recommended dosage from this study was 13,000 to 26,000 IU per kg.

It has been reported for penicillin that plasma concentrations can be increased by decreasing the volume infused, expelling air from the vagina after infusion and by infusing 10 per cent Lugol's solution into the uterus before the penicillin.[9] Penicillin is thought to be one of the most effective antibiotics available, and this can be understood when examining the organisms responsible for equine uterine infection. It was recommended that intrauterine treatments be administered "at 24 hour intervals in order to maintain a therapeutic level."[23]

Ampicillin at systemic dosages of 11 to 16 mg per kg has been successful in maintaining endometrial concentrations for 8 hours. It was therefore recommended that three to five injections per day could be successful in maintaining antibiotic tissue levels and eliminating uterine infections.

Ampicillin, when infused into the lumen of the mare's uterus, was found to result in "a white, chalky material resembling ampicillin suspension" that covered the endometrial surface 3 days after infusion.[30] The substance was still present at 7 and 14 days but appeared to be green in color.

One study on the absorption of ticarcillin sodium* from the mare's uterus indicates that little if any of this antibiotic appears in serum, in contrast to high peak serum levels occurring 20 to 45 minutes following intramuscular administration.[47] The intrauterine doses were 1 and 3 grams. Ticarcillin is reported to be active against penicillin-susceptible strains of *Staphylococcus aureus*, *Streptococcus pyogenes* and *Streptococcus pneumonia* but is slightly less active than ampicillin against these organisms. Ticarcillin is more active than ampicillin against penicillinase-producing strains of *Staphylococcus aureus* and many strains of *Enterobacter aerogenes*, *Escherichia coli* and indole-positive *Proteus* species.[18, 41]

Ticarcillin is also reported to have an in vitro activity at least twofold greater than carbenicillin against *Pseudomonas* spp. Local intrauterine administration of ticarcillin in mares resulted in higher levels in the uterus and cervix than did intramuscular administration, although therapeutic levels were still achieved by the systemic route.

Although oxytetracycline is not routinely the antibiotic of choice in the mare because of the bacteria implicated in equine infertility, it has been shown that absorption of this substance from the uterus appears to be slow in estrous mares.[29] It was also reported that one mare had what appeared to be a foreign body present within the uterus that was thought to be the result of intrauterine infusion of oxytetracycline.[30] Oxytetracycline at 20 times the penicillin concentration has been shown to be effective in treating some uterine infections.[23]

---

*Beecham Laboratory, Bristol, TN.

Dihydrostreptomycin was ineffective against any organisms found in the uterus.[23] This re-emphasizes its limited usefulness. Nitrofurazone was stated to be effective against some uterine pathogens.[23] Some investigators have had excellent success using nitrofurazone solutions to treat uterine infections,[33] but these authors have not had satisfactory results.

One major problem with many sulfa preparations is that they are insoluble and remain in localized areas of the uterine lumen for long periods of time.[37] Sulfamethazine is absorbed from the uterus of normal diestral cows, reaching peak levels in the blood within 2 hours following administration.[6] Therapeutic levels were maintained for up to 12 hours. This duration of therapeutic blood levels was later found to last up to 24 hours.[36]

It requires approximately 60 ml of fluid to cover the endometrial surface of a normal mare's uterus.[33] Most veterinarians, however, report using quantities of from 100 to 500 ml for the abnormal uterus. The primary objective is to infuse sufficient volume to obtain complete endometrial contact by the substance in use. Up until the mid to late 1960's uterine treatment as well as cultures were performed only while the mare was in heat. A slow transition away from that practice has occurred with no attributable damage to the mare.[33]

The frequency of antibiotic infusion into the uterus in the past has probably been determined on a "convenience" basis rather than on sound medical judgment. The most popular treatments clinically have included recommended or larger than systemic doses infused daily for 3 to 5 days,[7, 51] or every other day infusions for two to five treatments. It is generally not practical to infuse mares more frequently than once per day. Frequency of treatment, however, should probably be based on the length of time the antibiotic is active in the uterus. Davis and Abbitt suggested that "correct usage" of antibiotics was essential if treatment was to be successful and resistance avoided. Placement of an Indwelling Uterine Infusor* in mares to facilitate more frequent treatments has been described.

Some investigators have argued that local antibiotic therapy is a technique held over from the days of local antiseptic therapy; they compare the uterus to the udder with regard to the presence of higher tissue levels in the udder following systemic therapy than with local treatment.[17] It has also been noted in favor of systemic therapy that intrauterine infused antibiotics are rapidly absorbed from normal animals. However, in cows with endometritis, absorption other than to the endometrium is reduced.

In cattle, support for systemic versus local therapy has been found in one report in which the intramuscular route of oxytetracycline administration resulted in substantial concentrations in other tissues of the genital tract such as the oviduct and ovaries, whereas local administration resulted in no detectable levels in these tissues at 24 hours following treatment. The intrauterine route, however, had

very high luminal and endometrial concentrations for 72 hours following treatment.[17] This has also been found to be true for ticarcillin.[28]

The basic question to be addressed is what tissues are involved in the uterine infection being treated. If the infection involves deeper layers of the uterus and other genital tissues, systemic therapy would be necessary. If, however, the infection is limited to the endometrium, then local therapy is probably warranted due to very high sustained levels of antibiotic in the lumen and endometrium. It has been suggested that in the case of severe endometritis antibiotics may be retained and degraded in the uterine lumen.[17] The fact that antibiotics are not absorbed into the circulation does not, however, indicate that they are degraded nor that they are not as beneficial or are more beneficial locally than systemically administered antibacterial agents. It is questionable whether local therapy for endometritis would be less successful than systemic therapy. More severe conditions such as metritis, pyometra or perimetritis may, however, deserve systemic therapy if antibiotics alone are to be used in treatment.

It has been suggested that the majority of uterine infections are the result of contamination by organisms from the mare's intestinal tract. In light of this, it has been recommended that mares be placed on sulfonamides. Ninety-five per cent of sulfonamides are excreted in the feces. These drugs are "minimally" nontoxic in addition to their effectiveness against coliforms in reducing this contamination and infection.

Antiseptics are used mainly to reduce the size and increase the tone of the uterus by direct irritation. These agents have also been used to decrease the viscosity of uterine fluid to aid in its expulsion. Furthermore, in conditions of chronic inflammation without infection, they are capable of changing the inflammatory status to that of an acute one. Antibiotics are of no value in this situation unless they are irritating. Antiseptic preparations are also generally, as the name implies, antibacterial and possibly antifungal.

A partial list of antiseptic agents used in the past includes acriflavin, bismuth subnitrite, boric acid, charcoal, chlorine, iodine and iodine solutions, iodoform, perborate and silver oxide. Lugol's infusion (10 per cent solution) of three mares resulted in an endometrium that was "virtually altered" and contained blood, serosanguineous fluid and fibrin strands. Furthermore, although the epithelial surface "regained a normal appearance," there were areas of ulceration present 21 days after the infusion. This, however, is in contrast to the author's clinical case reports (unpublished) and research data completed to date regarding Lugol's. In the bovine, the infusion of dilute Lugol's solution (2 per cent) has been shown to be capable of chemically irritating the uterus enough to cause regression of the corpus luteum, depending on the stage of the estrous cycle, and regeneration of the endometrium 5 days later.[38] Whenever chemical curettage is used

---

*Fort Dodge Laboratories, Fort Dodge, IA.

as an intrauterine treatment, one must remember not to inflict further damage by too harsh or too concentrated a treatment solution.

Chlorhexidine* suspension is available for intrauterine infusion of mares and is in common use. Chlorhexidine solution, however, should not be used, or *if necessary,* should be used with extreme caution. The most serious abnormality observed on reproductive tracts of mares presented to The Ohio State University has occurred in mares with a history of treatment with chlorhexidine solution. This also has been reported by Voss.[22]

Mares that are prone to uterine infection at breeding should be bred as few times as necessary to obtain conception. Palpation of these mares and breeding one time close to but before ovulation is recommended.[3] Daily intrauterine infusions following breeding until the cervix closes have been recommended for mares that become infected following natural service. However, the routine use of postbreeding infusions on all mares (normal and abnormal) may decrease foaling rates in the normal mare. Mares with chronic or recurring uterine infections should be bred only by utilizing antibiotic-treated semen extender or by the minimum contamination technique.[25]

Prostaglandins are commonly used in cows with pyometra to evacuate the uterus and to reestablish cycling activity.[16] They are also gaining acceptance as a treatment for metritis and endometritis in the mare. Prostaglandins will short-cycle a mare with a corpus luteum. The subsequent estrus will increase her resistance to infection by the influence of estrogen. Prostaglandins may also have a direct beneficial effect on the myometrium by their activity on smooth muscle fiber.

Estrogen has been recommended as a means of enhancing uterine involution.[3] It has been suggested that estrogen, when administered to the mare systemically and followed 48 hours later with oxytocin, would exogenously produce a situation similar to estrus.

Enzyme preparations used locally to enhance recovery from pyometra have also been reported. Products such as pepsin, papain, urea and yeast have been utilized in the uterus because of their possible effect on tissue debris. However, the ability of these products to enhance recovery is doubtful.

Intrauterine dimethylsulfoxide (DMSO) has been used for a number of different purposes. Studies as to its beneficial or harmful effects are lacking. When 120 ml of DMSO was applied cutaneously twice daily for 10 days, the systemic changes noted included hemoglobin depression, platelet number reduction and decreased sedimentation rate but no change in prothrombin clotting time.[13] Marked "alterations" occurred in sorbitol dehydrogenase and serum glutamic oxalacetic transaminase levels. There were no local changes. DMSO has been shown to be "mildly" antifungal and antibacterial.[26] This same report noted that skin exposed to once daily treatments with DMSO "rapidly became tolerant" to the irritating properties of this product.

Fungal infections of the uterus usually become established following long-standing chronic contamination, such as with pneumovagina, or following prolonged antibiotic therapy used to eliminate a bacterial infection.[12] Most treatments have consisted of eliminating the initial cause and then allowing the mare to self-correct or of infusing iodine solutions, nystatin or amphotericin B. *Candida* spp. appear to be the most common organisms associated with fungal uterine infection.[39] The success of treatment with Lugol's solution and mycostatin* is represented by a report in which 6 of 13 infected mares receiving either or both conceived when bred on the heat following treatment.[53] Of the nontreated controls, one of three conceived after 3 months of repeated breedings.

Mycostatin was reportedly used on one mare for the treatment of a *Candida rugosa* infection that had followed successful treatment of a *Pseudomonas aeruginosa* infection with carbenicillin.†[1] However, the discharge continued and the organism was still present. The mare was then treated with 0.3 per cent iodine solution, but the discharge continued for an additional 6 weeks. Four months later the mare underwent culture and sensitivity tests, and no bacterial or fungal organisms were present. She was bred and conceived.

Amphotericin B has been used to treat successfully *Monosporium apiospermum*[35] and clinically used for *Candida* sp. Another report suggested using 200 mg of amphotericin B or 2.4 million units of intrauterine mycostatin daily for 4 days.[14] Gentian violet has also been used successfully on two mares with a mold infection.

Uterine flushes have proved to be of value in the elimination of fluid, stimulating blood flow, improving tone and decreasing size.[3] Hot saline (40° to 45°C) has been used successfully for treatment of myometrial atony and endometrial atrophy to enhance myometrial tone.[24] The response was rapid but transient. Also, saline flushes at day 6 of the cycle[15] have been shown to induce luteal regression, whereas this did not occur at day 1 or day 11 of the cycle. Uterine flushes on alternate days for 9 days with warm and cold salt solutions have been reported to be successful as a therapy for uterine infection.

Another successful method of handling uterine infection that has been recommended is the use of a "pressure-infusion treatment."[50] This report was based on the conventional treatment of 16 mares with uterine infections using gravity infusion of the uterus, which resulted in only three conceptions. However, when the remaining 13 mares were

---

*Nolvasan, Fort Dodge, IA.

*Nystatin, Squibb.
†Geopen, Roerig, New York, NY.

treated with pressure-infusion, nine conceived and the other four had no-growth cultures following therapy. This technique employed a Denta Porta-Pac* as the pressure source and controls.

The Caslick's surgical procedure, named after its describer, is recommended whenever mares have faulty vulvar conformation that leads to pneumo-vagina.[8] This procedure, which is used routinely, has greatly improved fertility by elimination of chronic contamination, especially in Thorough-breds. Many infected mares become free of infection within 2 to 3 months following this procedure without any other therapy.

Any abnormality that can be eliminated by surgery should be corrected to improve the probability for breeding success. Conditions such as third degree perineal lacerations, rectovaginal fistulas, cervical lacerations, and urine pooling are examples. One report of uterine curettage involved 17 infertile mares. Following curetting, 16 of the mares conceived, and eight of these produced live foals.

Reexamination of infected mares following therapy is as important as the original diagnosis of a problem. Therapy of any type is rarely 100 per cent effective, and therefore reevaluation is necessary to ascertain success.

The length of time recommended between uterine therapy and subsequent culture is 30 days.[7] The authors have used 14 days following the last treatment with excellent results.

Probably the most important and most promising aspect of uterine infection prevention and treatment—local immune responses and natural local defense mechanisms—has received the least amount of attention and research. This could be and probably is the reason why some mares become infected following bacterial contamination of the uterus and others do not. These natural uterine mechanisms have been separated into cellular and noncellular.[34] Cellular mechanisms involve the phagocytes. Non-cellular factors include opsonins, thermal-stable factors and the leukocytic tide. The opsonins *prepare* bacteria for phagocytosis, the thermal-stable factors *have the ability* to kill bacteria, and the leukocytes move into the uterus and engulf the bacteria.

Immunoglobulins within the uterine luminal fluid of normal and abnormal mares have been reported to include what the report authors describe as IgA, IgG, IgG(T), and IgM.[4] Comparison indicated that mares with reduced fertility (lowered resistance) had increased amounts of IgA, IgG and IgG(T). Insufficient data was obtained to determine a difference for IgM. Earlier work had failed to demonstrate the presence of IgT and IgM, but did report the presence of IgG(a), IgG(b) and IgG(c).[25] A more recent report indicated that although IgA was increased, IgG and IgG(T) were not elevated in infected mares.[49] The differences may be due in part to the differences in abnormal animals selected in each study.

Uterine antibody response may be related to ovarian hormones. In cattle and mice an increased responsiveness of immunoglobulins was detected when the animals were under the influence of estrogen in contrast to progesterone. Studies in ovariectomized mares indicated that estrogen did hasten the elimination of bacteria from the uterus compared with mares receiving no estrogen.

It has been reported that the infected uterus of a mare has lost its ability to eliminate contaminating organisms and overcome infections.[20, 34] The mechanisms involved are not understood. This loss of ability is possibly related to failures in the immune system. The uterus of a normal maiden mare responds rapidly to experimental inoculation of *Streptococcus zooepidemicus* organisms. In contrast, the older, chronically infected mare may show little or no response.

Mares resistant to uterine infection have substances in the uterine fluid that are capable of opsonizing bacteria, thereby enhancing phagocytosis. However, mares that are susceptible to uterine infection do not have this opsonization capability. Furthermore, the addition of serum to uterine washings of both groups of mares enhances opsonization of bacteria.

It has been suggested that a practical method of overcoming inadequate immune defense mechanisms of the uterus is to place substances, such as colostrum or plasma already containing these antibodies, in the uterine lumen. In a group of 20 infertile mares, colostrum was infused into the uterus in an attempt to improve uterine resistance to infection.[11] During the mating estrus, 120 ml of colostrum and 380 ml of normal saline were infused into each mare. Of these 20 mares, 15 were diagnosed as pregnant at 40 days following the last breeding date. Four of six mares diagnosed as pregnant and followed to term had normal foals.

The reduction of uterine size, elimination of fluid and improved tone should be accomplished before antibiotic therapy commences. This can be accomplished with flushes, hormones, antiseptics or combinations of these. Antibiotic treatment guidelines should be based on culture and sensitivity results on all mares treated. General or routine treatment of all problem mares with the same antibiotic will not ensure the best treatment results. To obtain maximal treatment efficacy, mares must be handled as individuals. Guidelines recommended by these authors include using antibiotics indicated by sensitivity tests. The antibiotics most commonly used are chloramphenicol, ampicillin and ticarcillin. These are administered by intrauterine instillation according to systemic dose recommendations of the pharmaceutical company. Daily infusions are administered with a volume sufficient to obtain complete endometrial contact with the infused material. This generally ranges from 100 to 500 ml. The infusion is performed after the mare's tail is wrapped and held or tied to one side and the perineal area has been thoroughly cleansed. A sterile sleeve, treatment rod and lubricant are used

---

*Model 3412, Kentucky Dental Supply Company, Inc., Lexington, KY.

for the infusion. Medication is placed in the uterus by gravity flow by connecting the free end of the rod to the inverted bottle via a sterile simplex.

Uterine therapy, like uterine biopsy and culture, can be performed at any time during the estrous cycle or during anestrus. Two weeks following therapy, the uterus is re-cultured to determine effectiveness of treatment.

Most, if not all, of the preceding techniques have been applied to the treatment of infertility. The only summary one can make of this vast amount of information is that at present there is no single treatment that can be used for all uterine disease. To ensure the best results from our therapy, each mare must be treated as an individual.

One of the most important challenges that must be met is not simply to treat the infection successfully but to manage mares subsequently so that they will not become re-infected.

References

1. Abou-Gabal M, Hogle RM, West JK: Pyometra in a mare caused by *Candida rugosa*. J Am Vet Med Assoc 170(2):177, 1977.
2. Allen WE: Plasma concentrations of sodium benzylpenicillin after intrauterine infusion in pony mares. Equine Vet J 10(3):171, 1978.
3. Arthur GH: Veterinary Reproduction and Obstetrics, 4th ed. London, Bailliere-Tindall Co, 1975, pp 467–487.
4. Asbury AC, Halliwell REW, Foster GW, et al.: Immunoglobulins in uterine secretions of mares with differing resistance to endometritis. Theriogenology 14(4):299, 1980.
5. Bain AM: The role of infection in infertility in the Thoroughbred mare. Vet Rec 78:168, 1966.
6. Bierschwal CJ, Dale HE, Uren AW: The absorption of sulfamethazine by the bovine uterus. J Am Vet Med Assoc 126:373, 1956.
7. Blanchard TL, Woods GL: Reproductive management of the barren mare. The Compendium on Continuing Education for the Practicing Veterinarian II(9):S141, 1980.
8. Caslick EA: The vulva and the vulvo-vaginal orifice and its relation to genital health of the Thoroughbred mare. Corn Vet 27(2):172, 1937.
9. Crouch JRF: Klebsiella infections in mares. Vet Rec 105(4):335, 1979.
10. Davis LE, Abbitt B: Clinical pharmacology of antibacterial drugs in the uterus of the mare. J Am Vet Med Assoc 170(2):204, 1977.
11. Dewes HF: Preliminary observations on the use of colostrum as a uterine infusion in Thoroughbred mares. NZ Vet J 28:7, 1980.
12. Doyle AW, O'Brien HV: Genital tract infection with *Candida albicans (Monilia)* in a Thoroughbred mare. Irish Vet J 23:90, 1969.
13. Edds GT, Kirkham WW: Dimethylsulfoxide: Tests for safety in horses. J Am Vet Med Assoc 150(11):1305, 1967.
14. Ellsworth KS: A practical approach to the treatment of endometritis. Proc Am Assoc Equine Pract 18:490, 1972.
15. Ginther OJ, Meckley PE: Effect of intrauterine infusion on length of diestrus in cows and mares. Vet Med/Sm Anim Clin 67:751, 1972.
16. Gustafsson B, Backstrom G, Edquist LE: Treatment of bovine pyometra with prostaglandin F_2: An evaluation of a field study. Theriogenology 6:45, 1976.
17. Gustafsson BK, Ott RS: Current trends in the treatment of genital infections in large animals. The Compendium on Continuing Education for the Practicing Veterinarian 3:147, 1981.
18. Hoffler D, Dalhoff A, Koeppe P: Pharmacokinetics of ticarcillin in patients with normal and impaired renal function. Dtsch Med Wschr 103:931, 1978.
19. Houdeshell JW, Hennessey PW: Gentamicin in the treatment of equine metritis. Vet Med/Sm Anim Clin 67(12):1348, 1972.
20. Hughes JP, Loy RG: The relation of infection to infertility in the mare and the stallion. Equine Vet J 7(3):155, 1975.
21. Hughes JP, Stabenfeldt GH, Kindahl H, et al.: Pyometra in the mare. J Reprod Fert Suppl 27:321, 1979.
22. Jackson RS, Skewes AR, Voss JL, et al.: Equine Infertility—Doctor to Doctor Seminar. Kenilworth, NJ, Schering Corporation, 1972, pp 4–53.
23. Kendrick JW: Report on dairy cattle fertility: Cause, prevention, and treatment of uterine disease. Kansas Vet 31:16, 1978.
24. Kenney RM, Ganjam VK: Selected pathological changes of the mare's uterus and ovary. J Reprod Fert Suppl 23:335, 1975.
25. Kenney RM, Khaleel SA: Bacteriostatic activity of the mare's uterus: A progress report on immunoglobulins. J Reprod Fert Suppl 23:357, 1975.
26. Kligman AM: Dimethyl sulfoxide studies in man. JAMA 193(10):796; 193(11):923, 1965.
27. Knudsen O: Endometrial cytology as a diagnostic aid in mares. Corn Vet 54(3):415, 1964.
28. Lock TF, DiPietro JA, Ott RS, et al.: Distribution of ticarcillin in the reproductive tract of pony mares following parenteral and intrauterine administration. Proceedings 61st Annual Meeting Research Work in Animal Disease, Chicago, December 1980, p 16.
29. Lock TF, Memon MA, Bevill RF, et al.: Oxytetracycline concentration in plasma after intravenous and intrauterine administration in mares. Ninth International Congress on Animal Reproduction, Madrid, Spain, 1980.
30. Mather EC, Refsal KR, Gustafsson BK, et al.: The use of fibre-optic techniques in clinical diagnosis and visual assessment of experimental intrauterine therapy in mares. J Reprod Fert Suppl 27:293, 1979.
31. Millar R, Francis J: The relationship of clinical and bacteriological findings to fertility in Thoroughbred mares. Aust Vet J 50:351, 1974.
32. Newcombe JR: Comparison of the bacterial flora of three sites in the genital tract of the mare. Vet Rec 102:169, 1978.
33. Northway RB: A treatment regimen for equine cervicitis and metritis. Vet Med/Sm Anim Clin 68(3):269, 1973.
34. Peterson FB, McFeely RA, David JSE: Studies on the pathogenesis of endometritis in the mare. Proceedings 12th Annual Convention American Association Equine Practitioners, Houston, Texas, 1969, pp 279–287.
35. Reid MM, Frock IW, Jeffrey DR, et al.: Successful treatment of a maduromycotic fungal infection of the equine with amphotericin B. Vet Med/Sm Anim Clin 72:1194, 1977.
36. Righter HF, Mercer HD, Kline DA, et al.: Absorption of antibacterial agents by the bovine involuting uterus. Can Vet J 16:10, 1975.
37. Roberts SJ: Veterinary Obstetrics and Genital Diseases, 2nd ed. Ithaca, author, 1971.
38. Sequin BE, Morrow DA, Louis TM: Luteolysis, luteostasis, and the effect of prostaglandin F_2 in cows after endometrial irritation. Am J Vet Res 35:57, 1974.
39. Sonnenschein B, Weiss R, Bringewatt W: Über Vorkommen und Bedeutung von Sprosspilzen auf equinen Genitalschleimhauten. Dtsche Tierzarztl Wschr 85:389, 1978.
40. Stabenfeldt GH, Hughes JP, Kindahl H, et al.: The influence of chronic uterine infection on luteal activity in the mare. Proceedings, VIII International Congress on Animal Reproduction and Artificial Insemination, Cracow 1976, pp 645–648.
41. Sutherland R, Burnett J, Rolinson GN: Carboxy-3-thienylmethyl-penicillin (BRL 2288), a new semi-synthetic penicillin: In vitro evaluation. Proceedings Tenth Interscience Conference on Antimicrobial Agents and Chemotherapy, Chicago, October 1970, pp 390–395.
42. Threlfall WR: Antibiotic infusion of the uterus of the mare. Proceedings, Society for Theriogenology Meeting, Mobile, Alabama 1979, pp 45–47.
43. Threlfall WR: Broodmare uterine therapy. The Compendium on Continuing Education for the Practicing Veterinarian II(11):246, 1980.
44. Threlfall WR: Diagnosis and treatment of infertility in the mare. Vet Med/Sm Anim Clin 75:483, 1980.
45. Threlfall WR: Unpublished update (1976–1978) of bacterial

organisms isolated from the equine uterus and susceptibilities of those organisms to antibiotics. Presented to the Ohio Equine Practitioners Workshop, Columbus, Ohio, January 1979.

46. Threlfall WR: Uterine therapy in the broodmare. Proceedings, Society for the Study of Breeding Soundness Meeting, Lexington, Kentucky 1976, pp 1–7.
47. Threlfall WR, Keefe TJ: Ticarcillin administration to the equine: intrauterine and intramuscular. Theriogenology 19(2):169, 1983.
48. Wearly WK, Murdick PW, Hensel JD: A five year study of the use of post-breeding treatment in mares in a Standardbred stud. Proc Am Assoc Equine Pract 17:89, 1971.
49. Williamson P, Dunning A, O'Connor J, et al.: Immunoglobulin levels, protein concentrations and alkaline phosphatase activity in uterine flushings from mares with endometritis. Theriogenology 19(3):441, 1983.
50. Wilson GL: A modified treatment of the equine uterus. Vet Med/Sm Anim Clin 76:493, 1981.
51. Woolcock JB: Equine bacterial endometritis—diagnosis, interpretation and treatment. Symposium on Equine Reproduction. Vet Clin N Am/Large An Pract 2(2):241, 1980.
52. Varadin M: Endometritis: a common cause of infertility in mares. J Reprod Fert Suppl 23:353, 1975.
53. Zafracas AM: Candida infection of the genital tract in Thoroughbred mares. J Reprod Fert Suppl 23:349, 1975.

Management Factors Affecting Equine Fertility

Peter G. Honey, B.V.Sc., M.S.
Orbost, Victoria, Australia

Average foaling rates in mares that are hand bred approach 60 per cent while foaling rates among pasture-bred horses are often around 90 per cent.[2, 7, 20] Little advancement has been made over the years toward improved foaling rates under intensive management.[9] Management factors, therefore, appear to play a major role in equine fertility.

THE BREEDING SEASON

Most breed societies impose an arbitrary breeding season that starts February 15th in the northern hemisphere and continues through the first week of July. In the southern hemisphere the breeding season starts in August and proceeds through December. Owners attempt to breed their mares as early as possible, with the conviction that earlier foals become larger and more marketable as yearlings than late-born foals. Unfortunately, the operational breeding season does not correlate with the true physiological breeding season.

The arbitrary breeding season begins when only 25 to 33 per cent of mares are cycling and ovulating, but ends when the number of mares capable of producing ova available for fertilization approaches 100 per cent.[22, 30] As mares emerge from winter anestrus they pass through a transitional period in which psychic heat may be displayed without ovulation.[30] In addition, mares with palpable and psychic evidence of cycling do not necessarily show histologic evidence of cyclic endometrial glandular function.[19] Thus the uterus may be unprepared to nurture a zygote early in the operational breeding season. Breeding mares during such periods of receptivity results in wasted services and increases the opportunity for genital tract infection.

Semen production by the stallion is lowest in the period coinciding with the mare's transitional period.[24] In contrast, the physiological breeding season is at its peak in midsummer, when sperm output is at its highest in the stallion and when mares have their highest incidence of ovulation and shortest estrous period.[22, 24, 30] The net result of breeding horses early in the arbitrary breeding season is a low conception-to-service ratio.

Studies have shown that foals born early in the year are smaller and lighter than foals born late in the year and that differences persist at 18 months of age.[14] The objective of breeding bigger foals, therefore, does not justify the reproductive inefficiency caused by breeding early in the operational breeding season.

TEASING PROGRAM

A well-run teasing program is essential to sound broodmare management. The management objective is to allow the stallion to elicit a response in the mare that will indicate her cycle status. Mares are generally bred on the second day of standing heat and every 48 hours thereafter until ovulation is detected or estrous behaviour ceases. This is sound practice because spermatozoa can be expected to survive in the female tract and be capable of satisfactory fertilization for at least 36 to 48 hours.[8, 16]

However, teasing programs do have their limitations. In the wild state, a stallion is in attendance of a harem group of mares continuously throughout the day.[10] In the artificial domestic situation, many mares are exposed fleetingly to a stallion that is kept in isolation with little or no social contact. In addition, the task of supervising teasing is often relegated to persons low in the management hierarchy who have little interest in interpreting the complex physiological events that are occurring.

Teasing should be conducted with a view to thoroughness and safety. When both the mare and the stallion are restrained for the encounter, rhythmic exposure of the clitoris (winking) and a squatting stance best indicate estrus and kicking best indicates diestrus.[34] While several nonlactating mares can effectively be teased simultaneously in a properly constructed chute, lactating mares, because of anxiety for their foals, need to be individually exposed to the stallion.

Unfortunately, there is often a disparity between the behavioral and physiological status of mares.[13, 31] This, combined with other intrinsic weaknesses in teasing programs, makes the use of other complementary management aids necessary.

PALPATION PER RECTUM

Palpation per rectum gives the skilled operator an excellent indication of the status of the reproductive tract. However, palpation, like the other management aids, has its flaws and must serve as an adjunct to other procedures rather than as a substitute for good management. Some studies have suggested that palpation of the tract per rectum may cause longer heat periods and reduce conception rates.[34] Also, it seems to be difficult to interpret palpation findings, and premature prediction of ovulation may result in a cessation of breeding with resultant infertility. Similarly, a failure to detect ovulation may result in continuing unnecessary services, with the risk of infecting the mare. Without the assistance of other management aids, the palpation of a mid-diestrous follicle could be a cause of mismanagement in the mare. Because a mare is likely to be again in diestrus 18 days after breeding on a mid-diestrous follicle, she could be mistakenly palpated as pregnant because of the tone of the tract. Tone and tubularity of the tract play a major part in interpreting palpation findings.[27]

RECORDS

Effective records help in analyzing the progress of the breeding season. A color-coded wall chart of the whole herd can indicate at a glance how many mares are cycling normally and the number of pregnancies per cycle. Extra attention can be paid to evaluating certain mares if events can be anticipated from the chart. In addition, individual mare records should be kept with a page for each mare containing teasing, palpation and breeding data as well as other relevant information on foaling date, treatments, history and identification.

As essential as they are, records are only as good as the objective information they contain. Usually they do not contain enough information early in the operational breeding season to contribute to improved efficiency at this difficult time.

BREEDING AT THE OPTIMUM TIME

The effect of season has been discussed. The ideal situation is to breed mares in the true physiological breeding season. However, manipulation of photoperiod, careful management of nutrition

and judicious use of hormone therapy can help to reduce some of the difficulties of breeding mares at a less than optimal time of year.

A 200-watt incandescent bulb placed in each stall can be used to increase daylength in a step-wise manner to 15 to 16 hours. The program is usually begun about 3 months before the beginning of the operational breeding season so that mares will be under the full light regime by the time breeding begins.[5] Other methods of achieving a 16-hour daylength have also been effective in bringing about an improved wintertime breeding program.

Provided the mares are either showing estrous activity or have some palpable follicular activity, therapeutic stabilization of erratic cycles with resultant fertile breedings is possible. For example, progesterone in oil at 100 mg a day can be administered for 7 days, and ovulatory heat often occurs 2 to 3 days following withdrawal.[32] Allyl trenbolone, an oral progestin, appears to have similar success when administered for 14 days.[28]

Mares that are gaining weight at the beginning of the breeding season have an earlier onset of ovarian cyclic activity than mares not gaining weight.[11] For this reason, management programs are designed to restrict nutrition in barren mares until prior to the commencement of the operational breeding season and then to feed for weight gain as the season approaches.

Ideally, mares should be bred within 48 hours of ovulation. Fertility falls off rapidly in mares bred more than 12 hours after ovulation.[16] Breeding mares every 48 hours until ovulation is detected should maximize chances of conception. However, one study[15] in which ovulation was detected by a subsequent rise in progesterone showed that detection of the actual event of ovulation by palpation can be difficult. Mistakes in interpretation of palpation can lead to either a premature cessation of breeding or a continuation of breeding after ovulation. The first leads to infertility, the second increases the opportunity for contamination of the reproductive tract with pathogens. Of 15 mares bred in this study, 11 became pregnant. Of the four that were open, three were bred more than 48 hours out of synchrony with ovulation. All pregnant mares had been bred within 48 hours of ovulation. Palpation results had been confirmed among three operators.

Breeding at the optimum time improves probability of conception and therefore reduces the number of services and decreases chances of infection.[33]

PREPARATION OF MARES FOR THE BREEDING SEASON

Barren mares need to be evaluated for reproductive soundness at the end of their unsuccessful operational breeding season. Most mares will be still actively cycling at this time, and a true estimation of future breeding potential is possible. Seasonal variation in uterine morphology early in the operational breeding season could result in an inaccurate evaluation.[19] Later histopathologic evaluation of uterine biopsy specimens allows one to make a prognosis of breeding potential and also gives an index of success of intrauterine therapy.

Apart from breeding, the most serious cause of genital tract contamination in the mare is pneumovagina due to conformational faults or persistent relaxation of the vulva.[4] An index has been devised whereby the effective length of the vulva (length in centimeters of the vulval opening between the dorsal commissure and the brim of the pelvis) is multiplied by the angle of declination of the vulva from the vertical. By performing Caslick's procedure on all mares with an index greater than 150, an overall increase in fertility can be expected.[23] Pregnant mares needing Caslick's surgery should be sutured as soon as pregnancy is confirmed. Open mares should have the surgery performed in late summer or early fall so that further contamination of the tract is curtailed while the mare is still cycling and the natural defenses that operate during estrus[18] can combat existing infection. Each mare should be reappraised seasonally because the index varies with age and nutritional status.

USE OF ARTIFICIAL INSEMINATION

Where breeding societies allow its use, artificial insemination helps to control infection within the herd because contamination of the mare's tract by natural breeding is avoided. Although most mares in good reproductive health can mount a transient inflammatory response and eliminate bacteria following breeding, infection and disease can become established if natural defense mechanisms are inadequate.[17] Additional protection is provided by the use of semen extenders containing antibiotics. In one study, semen diluted with extender containing sodium penicillin and gentamicin sulfate showed an average 91 per cent reduction of bacteria within 15 minutes after collection.[26]

Artificial insemination also contributes to fertility management by facilitating continuous evaluation of the stallion's semen quality.

A RATIONAL APPROACH TO HYGIENE

Measures should be aimed at preventing the transmission of potentially pathogenic organisms. However, many hygiene programs seem to be aimed more at rendering each individual horse bacteriologically sterile. Outbreaks of contagious equine metritis (CEM) have borne this out. Normal nonpathogenic bacterial flora of the reproductive tract have been shown to inhibit the growth of the CEM organism.[29] The practice of extensive washing of both the mare and the stallion with antibacterial agents may therefore be contributing to the growth of pathogens by removing normal flora. Similarly,

indiscriminate use of antibiotics in the mare's reproductive tract may be contraindicated.

Objectively designed hygiene programs stress the use of disposable gloves and bucket liners, running water and sterile speculae and instruments. Training of stud farm personnel in basic epidemiology of infection is also emphasized.[6] Bland soaps rather than antiseptics[25] are recommended for washing.

Although infection is a major cause of female infertility,[3, 21] arbitrary treatment regimes cannot be relied upon to improve fertility in a mare band.[33] In fact, an ill-conceived therapeutic approach may lead to selection of resident flora of a more pathogenic nature[1] and the establishment of a chronic endometritis that is very difficult to treat. Excessive use of intrauterine antibiotics may be followed by the establishment of fungi and yeasts and a poor prognosis for fertility.[36]

Mares suspected of having endometritis should be subjected to a thorough evaluation including culture and sensitivity tests, endometrial biopsy, palpation and visual examination of the external genital organs, vagina and cervix. The history and general condition of the mare should be taken into consideration.[12] Before treatment is undertaken, the appropriate antibiotic should be selected and steps taken to remove predisposing factors.

CONCLUSION

Improving fertility in a brood mare operation involves improved general management techniques. Mares should be bred when they are cycling normally. Steps should be taken to synchronize breeding as closely as possible to ovulation and to avoid unnecessary services to the stallion. An epidemiologically sound program of infection control should be instituted.

References

1. Ashbury AC, Held JP: Interpretation of cultural findings in the diagnosis of endometritis in mares. Proceedings Annual Conference of the Society of Theriogenology, Mobile, 1979, pp 41–47.
2. Bain AM: Problems associated with infertility in the brood mare. Aust Vet J 24:152, 1948.
3. Bain AM: The role of infection in infertility in the Thoroughbred mare. Vet Rec 78:168, 1966.
4. Caslick EA: The vulva and the vulvo-vaginal orifice and its relation to genital health of the Thoroughbred mare. Cornell Vet 27:178, 1937.
5. Cooper WL, Wert NE: Wintertime breeding of mare using artificial light and insemination: Six years' experience. Proceedings 21st Annual Meeting American Association of Equine Practitioners, 1975, pp 245–253.
6. David JSE, Frank CJ: Contagious metritis 1977. Vet Rec 101:189, 1977.
7. Day FT: Some observations on the causes of infertility in horse breeding. Vet Rec 51:581, 1948.
8. Day FT: Survival of spermatozoa in the genital tract of the mare. J Agric Sci 32:108, 1942.
9. Dimock WW: Equine breeding hygiene. J Am Vet Med Assoc 94:469, 1939.
10. Feist JD, McCullough DR: Behaviour patterns and communication in feral horses. Z Tierpsychol 41:337, 1976.

11. Ginther OJ: Occurrence of anestrus, estrus, diestrus and ovulation over a 12-month period in mares. Am J Vet Res 35:1172, 1974.
12. Greenhoff GR, Kenney RM: Evaluation of reproduction status of non-pregnant mares. J Am Vet Med Assoc 167:449, 1975.
13. Hancock JL: Notes on oestrus, ovulation and pregnancy in the mare. Vet Rec 60:679, 1948.
14. Hintz HF: A review of recent studies on the growth of horses. Calif Vet 33:17, 1979.
15. Honey PG: The use of milk progesterone assay as an aid to broodmare management. Thesis, Texas A & M University, 1980.
16. Hughes JP, Loy RG: Artificial insemination in the equine. A comparison of natural breeding and artificial insemination of mares using semen from six stallions. Cornell Vet 60:463, 1970.
17. Hughes JP, Loy RG: The relation of infection to infertility in the mare and stallion. Equine Vet J 7:155, 1975.
18. Kenney RM, Whaleel SA: Bacteriostatic activity of the mare uterus: A progress report on immunoglobulins. J Reprod Fert Suppl 23:357, 1975.
19. LeBlanc MM: Seasonal variation in uterine morphology of mares: A clinical and histopathologic study. Proceedings of the Annual Meeting Society of Theriogenology, Milwaukee, 1982, pp 168–175.
20. Mahaffey LM: Studies of fertility in the Thoroughbred mare. Aust Vet J 26:267, 1950.
21. Millar R, Francis J: The relation of clinical and bacteriological findings to fertility in Thoroughbred mares. Aust Vet J 50:351, 1974.
22. Osborne VE: An analysis of the pattern of ovulation as it occurs in the annual reproductive cycle of the mare in Australia. Aust Vet J 42:149, 1966.
23. Pascoe RR: Observations on the length of declination of the vulva and its relation to fertility in the mare. J Reprod Fert Suppl 27:299, 1979.
24. Pickett BW: The effect of season, sexual stimulation, frequency of ejaculation and testicular size on spermatozoal output. Proceedings 31, University of Sydney Post Graduate Committee in Veterinary Science, Semen Refresher Course, 1977, pp 16–37.
25. Pickett BW: Horse artificial insemination. Proceedings 31, University of Sydney Post Graduate Committee in Veterinary Science, Semen Refresher Course, 1977, pp 49–59.
26. Simpson RB, Burns SJ: Microflora in stallion semen and their control with a semen extender. Proceedings of the 21st Annual Meeting of the American Association of Equine Practitioners 1975, pp 255–261.
27. Solomon WJ: Rectal examination of the cervix and its significance in early pregnancy evaluation of the mare. Proceedings of the 17th Annual Meeting of the American Association of Equine Practitioners, 1971, pp 73–80.
28. Squires EL, Stevens WB, McGathlin DE, Pickett BW: Effect of an oral progestin in the estrous cycle and fertility of mares. J Anim Sci 49:799, 1979.
29. Swerczek TW: Contagious equine metritis—Clinical signs, diagnosis, treatment, and current status of the disease. Proceedings of the Annual Meeting of the Society of Theriogenology, Oklahoma City, 1978, pp 26–31.
30. Trum BF: The estrous cycle of the mare. Cornell Vet 40:17, 1950.
31. Vandeplassche M, Henry M, Caryn M: The mature and midcycle follicle in the mare. J Reprod Fert Suppl 27:157, 1979.
32. Van Niekerk CH, Coubrough RI, Doms HWH: Progesterone treatment of mares with abnormal oestrous cycles early in the breeding season. J S Afr Vet Med Assoc 44:37, 1973.
33. Varadin M: Endometritis, a common cause of infertility in mares. J Reprod Fert Suppl 23:353, 1975.
34. Voss JL, Pickett BW: Reproductive management of the broodmare. Colorado State Univ Bull, Gen Series 961, 1976, pp 9–12.
35. Wearly WK, Murdick PW, Hensel JD: A five year study of post-breeding treatment in mares in a standardbred stud. Proceedings 17th Annual Meeting of the American Association of Equine Practitioners, 1971, pp 89–95.
36. Zafracas AM: Candida infection of the genital tract in Thoroughbred mares. J Reprod Fert Suppl 23:349, 1975.

Surgery of the Male Equine Reproductive System*

J. T. Vaughan, D.V.M.

Surgery of the reproductive system of the male horse is classified according to anatomy and etiology. Anatomically, the penis, prepuce, scrotum and testes constitute the organs important to a discussion of surgery. Since it is difficult to separate certain maladies, such as diseases of the penis from disorders of the urinary system or cryptorchidism from invasion of the peritoneal cavity, there are instances in which the discussion may border on other systems or disciplines. Etiologically, the principal concerns involve injuries, infections (including parasitisms), neoplasms, hernias, congenital anomalies and surgical complications.

PENIS AND PREPUCE

Injuries

Injuries occur during breeding, fighting with other stallions, falling on fences and stall partitions and in various other ways. One of the most serious injuries to the breeding stallion is a kick to the erect penis by a poorly restrained mare. Severe contusions cause hemorrhage and intense inflammatory edema of both penis and prepuce. In contrast to the internal hematoma due to rupture of the corpus cavernosum penis in the bull, the parallel injury in the horse usually produces hemorrhage originating external to the tunica albuginea.

The immediate result of the rapid congestion and edema of the injured part is acute paraphimosis, characterized by an inability to retract the turgid (vis à vis tumescent) organ into the prepuce. In fact, the obstacle to retraction may be the inflammatory swelling (posthitis) in the preputial laminae even more than the inflammation of the penis proper (balanitis). Inflammatory swelling and hem-

*Revised from the original, which appeared in Jennings PB Jr (ed): The Practice of Large Animal Surgery. Philadelphia, WB Saunders Co, 1984, pp 1083–1105.

orrhage are complicated further by the edema of stasis and gravitation caused by the restricted venous and lymphatic drainage in the pendulous state. Also, it seems likely that stagnation of blood in the sinusoidal spaces of the corpus cavernosum penis and corpus spongiosum urethrae is as aggravating a factor in traumatic balanoposthitis as it is in the flaccid paralysis associated with adverse reactions to the phenothiazine-derivative tranquilizers.

Delay in reestablishment of circulation allows for clotting and organization of humoral elements of inflammation, leading quickly to chronic prolapse and either a protracted course of recovery or a refractory condition that may require preputial reefing, surgical retraction (the Bolz technique) or even amputation of the penis.

To mark the progression from acute to chronic paraphimosis, the doughy character of the pitting edema undergoes gradual induration. The thin, glossy skin of the swollen part becomes dry and inelastic, and patchy excoriations develop into indolent ulcers. In this irritated state, the ability to retract the penis may return before the desire to do so. Recovery is predicated in terms of weeks and usually proceeds apace with epithelialization and reduction of scarring.

Recovery may be interrupted at any point by pathologic changes that prevent the normal telescoping of the prepuce and penis. If the problem is focal, a simple elliptical excision of the scar and closure of the wound under suture may be all that is required. If the problem is circumferential and limited to the dermis, a preputial reefing operation is indicated, but this still falls within the classification of revisional skin surgery. If the problem is generalized and involves the penis as well as the prepuce, the two surgical options (after conservative care has been exhausted) are the penis retraction operation (Bolz technique) and the penis amputation. In both instances, the patient is a gelding or a candidate for gelding in that the subsequent use of the horse as a stallion has been, of necessity, relinquished.

Abrasions of the penis result from exposed breeding sutures used to protect the Caslick closure of the vulva in mares that have been operated on for pneumovagina. Strangulation of the collum glandis may occur with an ill-fitting stallion ring. Obstruction of the urethra may stem from a dissecting hematoma of the sinusoidal tissues of the penis. Rupture of the bladder and urine peritonitis may be further complications. Disruption of the urethra may produce regional urine cellulitis. Chronic irritation, with or without infection, may result in varices, ulcers and granulomas of the urethra that are manifested as dysuria and hemorrhage on ejaculation (hemospermia). Lacerations and puncture wounds of the penis may also compromise the course of the urethra. Misdirected castration surgery and/or postoperative infections not infrequently cause paraphimosis and other injuries, however unintentional, to the penis and prepuce.[25, 50, 57]

Nonoperative Management

Treatment of contusions should commence when the injury occurs with the application of ice packs to the site of the injury in an effort to prevent edema. Afterward, treatment of acute paraphimosis is directed at early reduction of the edema by promoting improved circulation by massage, hydrotherapy, and suspension of the prolapse to relieve the pendulousness. The skin should be protected against maceration with emollients, and overuse of water sprays should be avoided in consideration of this fact. Pre-existing infections, such as in castration wounds, should be treated vigorously. As soon as physically possible, the penis and internal laminae of the prepuce should be manually returned to their normal retracted position and retained there by a stallion supporter or an improvised nylon mesh bag. This material permits uninhibited urination and is easily cleaned. Alternative methods, although less desirable, include the use of a cylindrical pessary and retention sutures in the external orifice of the prepuce. Systemic antibiotics, anti-inflammatory drugs and diuretic agents (to reduce edema) are discretionary. Tranquilizers are specifically contraindicated. Stallions should be isolated from mares, preferably out of sight and sound. Exercise ad libitum or regulated at the halter is helpful to reduce edema and prevent its return.

Conservative treatment of chronic paraphimosis follows the general guidelines for the acute form, except that greater effort must be directed toward keratolysis of dry, thickened skin; gradual healing of ulcers and excoriations; and resolution of indurated subcutaneous tissues. Retention of the penis in suspension should be encouraged and daily care conscientiously maintained until function is restored, bearing in mind that, if nonoperative methods fail, surgery is the alternative. Salvage of a useful stallion is the incentive for much nursing care.

It should be emphasized that free urine output should be confirmed if necessary by catheterization and that, until the horse is observed in the natural act of urination, this function should never be taken for granted. The stallion should also be studied carefully upon his first return to the breeding shed. Hemospermia may be inapparent at all other times than on intromission and ejaculation. Prior history of this disorder requires urethroscopy and contrast radiography. Chronic, bleeding lesions of the urethra require special attention for diagnosis as well as treatment. Ascending tract infections must be cultured and urethral mucosal scrapings examined for cytologic findings. Granulomas, varices, and ulcers can be treated by debridement, curettage or cautery either transurethrally or by urethrotomy. Retrograde medication with infusions or suppositories may be used in conjunction with systemic treatments, such as urinary antiseptics and pH alterants (which are ordinarily acidifiers in herbivores). Ammonium chloride by mouth or administered in the feed can be used to reduce the pH below 7 and to maintain acidity for the several weeks of methenamine therapy necessary to render the environment of the urinary tract inhospitable to pathogens. Sexual rest is mandatory.

Management of sharp wounds of the penis and prepuce should follow the principles that apply to injuries of the hollow organs in general, i.e., provide decompression to areas of occlusion, relieve obstructions (such as encroaching hematomas, abscesses, granulomas), prevent ascending tract infections (especially when the external sphincter has become incompetent), and prevent cicatricial strictures upon healing. Surgical reconstruction should be as prompt, anatomically accurate and secure as wound characteristics permit. Drainage catheters should be used with scrupulous regard for asepsis. If a catheter is left indwelling, it is imperative that a one-way (exit) valve be used to prevent aspiration of air and the attendant contaminants. Even so, it is good practice to change catheters every 24 to 48 hours to avoid accumulation of urine salts. If the catheter is used for bougienage, care should be taken to avoid provoking fresh hemorrhage from the site of stricture (the wound site). However, if hemorrhage does occur, the catheter should be left in place and sterile irrigations administered until bleeding is controlled so that blood clots are not retained in the bladder and urethra. Even with relatively little special attention, the urethra shows a remarkable capacity for healing if physiologic rest and daily hygienic wound care are provided.

Neoplasms and Parasitisms

Neoplasms and parasitisms are discussed in the same section because of gross similarities that require differential diagnosis. Neoplasms may be organized as epithelial or mesenchymal lesions. Epithelial tumors of the hair-bearing skin surface of the external prepuce reflect the same distribution as tumors of the skin anywhere else on the body, such as sarcoids, melanoma, mastocytoma, hemangioma and squamous cell carcinoma. However, the most common tumor of the penis and internal laminae of the prepuce of the horse is the squamous cell carcinoma, which seems to show a predilection for this site.[71] Typical lesions are sessile, cauliflower-like growths, often multifocal, with a gross appearance that may be confused with sarcoid or the benign squamous papilloma of the equine genitalia. Squamous cell carcinoma of the penis and prepuce is slow growing at the outset, and circumscribed lesions can usually be successfully removed surgically by local excision or cryotherapy. Later, invasion of the deeper layers of the penis with the possibility of metastasis to the superficial inguinal lymphatics and the lungs makes radical excision necessary. There is, in addition, the tendency for the lesion to recur.[11, 32, 45]

Representative of the mesenchymal tumors of the prepuce and penis is the rare fibrosarcoma. This is not an important group from the standpoint of incidence.[32]

The most significant of the tumorlike lesions is the chronic granuloma caused by the larval migrations of the *Habronema* species. This form of granulomatous habronemiasis must be differentiated from squamous cell carcinoma, squamous papilloma and sarcoid to establish a rational basis for treatment. Although each type bears identifying features and much could be said to support the gross morphologic diagnosis, a final decision should always depend on the biopsy made in the histopathology laboratory. This may be made on a sample or on the lesion in toto, in which case the completeness of the excision can be assessed.

Habronemiasis lesions show a propensity for the urethral process and the preputial ring. The surface of the granuloma may be an ulcerated, red proliferation. Numerous caseous, mulberry-shaped masses, which are indistinguishable from the Bollinger's granules seen in botryomycosis, are found on the cut surface. These are surrounded by eosinophilic, histiocytic and lymphocytic infiltrations. The parasite itself may occasionally be demonstrated in the cut paraffin section.

The diagnosis of space-occupying lesions of the penis and prepuce is also confused by the misleading appearances of carcinoma and the occasional occurrence of other diseases. Once it starts to spread, squamous cell carcinoma can cause fixation of the penis within the prepuce (phallocrypsis). It can result in deep-seated abscesses that fistulate to the outside and mimic the inguinal abscess of strangles or other varied causes. Of course, the familiar surface ulcerations and raw, red granulations of superficial carcinoma may closely resemble the *Habronema* granuloma.

Representative of less common diseases of this anatomic region is the microfilariasis attributed to *Onchocerca* and *Setaria* species that causes swollen genitals and "erysipelatoid" lesions of the prepuce with dry, crusted, and fissured skin and firm, pendulous swellings of the prepuce.[75] Another example that has been described was a spirochete infection of the prepuce and penis, suspected of being caused by the genus *Treponema*. This infection was characterized by multiple circumscribed gummatous lesions and irregular shallow ulcers through the external and internal folds of the prepuce and extending onto the free body of the penis. Spirochetes were found in the semen, and the left testis was observed to be slightly indurated, both findings reminiscent of syphilis in man.[53] *Hyphomyces destruens* was recovered from an enlarged inguinal lymph node apparently related to a refractory lesion of chronic phycomycosis in the hindleg of a thoroughbred filly.[47]

Nonoperative Management

Common lesions frequently treated by means in addition to or other than surgery are sarcoids, *Habronema* granuloma and squamous cell carcinoma. Sarcoids possibly have the greatest diversity of treatments, including the induction of immune response by initial sensitizing injections followed at weekly intervals by repeated infiltrations around the tumor base with bacillus Calmette-Guérin (BCG), tuberculin, or bovine transfer factor, with anticipated regression or remission of the lesion during the ensuing weeks. Escharotic therapy has been used with Tn. podophyllin 25 per cent in pine tar applied topically once daily until the lesion gradually sloughed or regressed under eschar. Topical 5-fluorouracil in propylene glycol has been applied daily to the open site of surgical excision as an antimetabolite to reduce the incidence of recurrence. Electrofulguration is an older modality of treatment that has met with varying success. Cryotherapy is a somewhat more recent method that has been widely used in the 1970's, with enthusiastic acceptance by many, for the reasons that local immunity to the viral agent of sarcoid was thought to be enhanced while, at the same time, the frozen lesion was undergoing a slough.

Habronema granulomas, once treated by either thermocautery or surgical excision, are now recognized to be vulnerable to organophosphate medication. It is common practice to treat small lesions topically and large ones both topically and systemically with trichlorfon. The topical form can be prepared by mixing 4.5 gm of trichlorfon in 4 oz of nitrofurazone cream. This is applied once daily if the lesion is left open and every several days if the granuloma is placed under bandage. In the context of this discussion, the first method would have more frequent applications. The topical use of fenthion offers another possibility. Systemic medication can be given by mouth as a calculated anthelmintic dose of trichlorfon or by vein at the dosage rate of 22 mg/kg of body weight diluted in 1 to 2 liters of sterile physiologic saline solution and administered by slow intravenous drip. Atropine and pralidoxime chloride should be on hand in the event that adverse reactions due to organophosphate toxicity require an antidote. Introduction of the avermectin group of systemic anthelmintics provides a potentially fruitful avenue of investigation. Efficacy and safety are the objectives of newer treatments.

Nonoperative treatment of squamous cell carcinoma of the penis and prepuce may include radiation therapy by gamma sources such as radon implants placed in the tumor bed following surgical excision. However, this form of treatment is not ordinarily used. By the same token, it would not be inappropriate to use conventional radiotherapy on sites of deeper invasion or on lymphatic metastases, but such instances are thought to be infrequent. Cryotherapy has been reported as successful in treating localized lesions.[69]

Operative Surgery of the Penis and Prepuce

Surgical procedures involving the incised approach include the total or partial circumcision of the prepuce (known as the reefing operation), the surgical retraction and fixation of the penis and the amputation of the penis.

Reefing Operation (Posthioplasty)

Although posthioplasty is commonly used to refer to total circumcision, it is correct to include partial posthetomy in this discussion. Indications are extirpation of the circumscribed neoplasms that are confined to the dermis, revision of chronic scarring of the prepuce that has resulted from repeated *Habronema* parasitisms, extensive removal of the prepuce necessitated by chronic intractable posthitis and, in rare instances, posthioplasty for congenital anomalies of the prepuce and penis.

Although for different reasons, the objective of both procedures is restoration of the telescoping function of the concentric elastic sleeves that facilitate extension and retraction of the penis. The prepuce is divided into internal and external reflections that are readily opposed by scars, granulomas, neoplasms and other such space-occupying lesions. The surgery consists of the removal of the obstruction and the apposition under suture of the neighboring normal prepuce. Excision may be in the form of an ellipse for circumscribed lesions or a ring in the case of circumferential lesions, e.g., an extensive granuloma scar of the preputial ring. Limited reefing will salvage the use of a breeding stallion. Extensive reefing places such future service in doubt. There are no established safe minimums to use as guides; therefore, discretion of the surgeon must be exercised in each case.

Success depends on optimum healing with minimal scarring and early return to function. These are ensured by control of sepsis and hemorrhage and by accurate reconstruction under suture. The patient is restrained under general anesthesia in dorsal recumbency and prepared for aseptic technique. The urethra is catheterized, and the penis is fixed in forward extension by a traction tape secured around the collum glandis. Surface ulcerations or other breaks in the skin should be disinfected. Use of a tourniquet is optional but advantageous in the face of chronic inflammatory engorgement. Gum-rubber tubing secured proximal to the site is satisfactory. The lesion is bracketed by skin incision. The dissection plane is the loose subcutaneous fascia external to the tunica albuginea of the penis. Scissor dissection is helpful. Bleeders should be controlled as identified, loosening the tourniquet periodically for this purpose. The lesion should be isolated from the dissection to prevent contamination by microorganisms, tumor cells or the like and removed from the field as soon as possible. Suture reconstruction is done in two layers. The subcutaneous fascia is approximated by multiple simple interrupted sutures of 0 medium chromic surgical gut or the equivalent. No attempt is made to quilt fixation points to the underlying tunica albuginea. The skin is closed with interrupted mattress sutures (vertical or oblique) taken with 00 polypropylene. If the suture line is long, it may be permissible, in the interest of time, to close the skin with a continuous vertical mattress suture pattern that is cut and tied at each quadrant. This minimizes the constricting effect of an uninterrupted circular suture line.

Postoperative care should include daily wound hygiene and topical medication as needed and systemic antibiotics for prophylaxis, since it is impossible to render the surgical site free of contaminants. Stallions should be isolated. Skin sutures are left in for 10 to 14 days.

Surgical Retraction of the Penis (Phallopexy)

When conservative care has not resulted in recovery of spontaneous retraction and when posthioplasty is not the answer, phallopexy offers an alternative to amputation. The advantages are a simpler procedure with less chance of postoperative complications such as hemorrhage, dehiscence, delayed healing, and urethral constriction. The candidate should be a gelding with complete healing of the castration wound. Premature phallopexy in the incompletely healed castration site is inadvisable. All nonoperative efforts to reduce the morbid swelling of the penis should have been exhausted. Infection should be controlled, and physical placement of the penis into the prepuce should be possible. Surgical revision of scar tissue may be done in advance or at the same time, although the former is preferred. Epithelialization of ulcerated skin should be essentially complete.

The patient is restrained in dorsal recumbency under general anesthesia with the hind legs in passive abduction. Strained positions caused by forced abduction predispose to obturator nerve injury and complicated recovery from anesthesia. The penis is catheterized but is neither fixed in traction nor placed in a tourniquet. The field is prepared for aseptic technique. A skin incision 10 cm long is made on the median raphe just behind the castration scar. The loose, subcutaneous fascia is separated by blunt dissection to expose the penis, which is pulled up into the incision sufficiently to expose the annular thickening at the point of attachment of the internal lamina of the prepuce to the free body of the penis. This lies at the forwardmost extent of the plane of dissection. The procedure should be done without unduly disrupting the loose tissue bed of the penis so that vascular and lymphatic pathways remain as undisturbed as possible. The retraction required causes slight sigmoidation of the penis, but dysuria has not been a reported problem. A traction suture of noncapillary synthetic material is placed in the annular thickening on each side of the urethra (identified by catheter location), avoiding entry of the preputial cavity. The suture ends are brought through the skin alongside the incision with eyed needles and then are retained by passing them through a short length of polyvinyl laboratory tubing used as a suture splint. The suture ends on each side can then be pulled in sufficient tension to retract the glans penis into the external preputial orifice.

The ends are tied in a bow knot or can be held together by a small clamp to permit adjustment of tension and, thus, extent of retraction after the horse regains his feet. It is important to be able to regulate the position of the glans so that it is concealed but not so deeply retracted as to cause urine scald inside the prepuce. This adjustment is difficult to estimate when the patient is lying on his back. After placement of the traction sutures, the loose adventitia is closed with interrupted sutures of fine surgical gut. A Penrose drain is optional. The skin incision is closed with interrupted vertical mattress sutures of polypropylene or other suitable skin suture.

Postoperative care consists of providing daily local wound hygiene and discretionary antibiotic therapy. The site can be kept clean more easily if the patient is restrained, standing by crossties and given regular exercise at the halter. The use of fly repellents will reduce any self-irritation that might be caused by much switching of the tail between the legs. The traction sutures can be removed after 14 days. Recently gelded horses and those that retain some stallion behavior should be separated from both mares and stallions during the first 2 to 4 weeks. Evaluation should be made after this time to allow for recession of swelling and soreness.

Amputation of the Penis (Phallectomy)

The common indications for amputation are squamous cell carcinoma of the glans or free body of the penis and intractable paralytic paraphimosis. In the circumscribed carcinoma in situ, limited excision may be successful; however, once the lesion has invaded the tunical layer, amputation is necessary. If there is palpable or visible evidence of lymphatic spread or of phallocrypsis, en bloc resection offers an alternative to euthanasia. Radiation therapy may also be tried.

The preferred method of management of unresponsive paraphimosis is phallopexy; however, if morbid swelling of the penis (phalloncus) or other changes are so extensive as to prevent mechanical retraction, the last resort must be amputation.

The patient is restrained in dorsal recumbency under general anesthesia. The penis is catheterized, pulled into forward traction, and tourniqueted. The field is prepared for aseptic technique. Using the method described by Williams,[18] a site is chosen well above the pathologic process, and a triangular section of skin, subcutaneous fascia, retractor penis and bulbospongiosus muscle, and corpus spongiosum overlying the urethra is carefully dissected away from the urethra. The base of the triangle (3 cm) corresponds to the cross-sectional plane of amputation. The two sides of the triangle (4 cm) represent the bilateral reflections of the urethra as the incised edges are spatulated over the cut surfaces of the corpus spongiosum. The apex of the triangle points backward. After the urethra has been exposed, the ventral wall is split and sutured to the skin sides of the triangle with multiple simple interrupted sutures of 00 polypropylene or synthetic surgical gut (polyglycolic acid), which seems to hold up well in the presence of moisture. Closely spaced sutures are necessary to prevent worrisome hemorrhages from the corpus spongiosum, particularly during the immediate postoperative time. The V-shaped spatulation is a safeguard against cicatricial stricture of the urethra after healing.

Once the sides of the urethra are sutured, the remainder of the penis is amputated at the line established by the base of the triangle. The plane of transection is directed slightly craniad from ventral to dorsal so that urine flow will be diverted downward during the natural act. Before the urethra is sutured in this plane, the individual bleeders must be identified and ligated. Owing to chronic hyperemia of the pathologic process, some of the vessels are greatly engorged and may require transfixation ligatures. Small vessels may be safely cauterized by electrofulguration. The cut surface of the corpus cavernosum penis can be closed by placement of sutures in the tunica albuginea. The cut edge of the urethra is included in this layer. Interrupted sutures are preplaced to ensure even spacing and to avoid puckering the closure. The first suture bisects the circular cross-section of the penis, passing through the urethra and the tunica albuginea at the center of the urethral groove, up over the corpus cavernosum, down through the dorsalmost centerpoint of the tunica albuginea, and thence through the skin. The suture ends are held together with small hemostatic forceps while succeeding sutures are placed. The second and third sutures divide the halves into quarters. The next four sutures divide the quarters into eighths, and so on. When enough sutures are preplaced, they are tied in the same sequence. When done properly, the skin is evenly apposed to the urethra, and hemorrhage upon release of the tourniquet is negligible. Nevertheless, it is not unusual for some minor bleeding to occur for the first few postoperative days, particularly during the act of urination. Indwelling catheters are unnecessary. Prophylactic antibiotics are discretionary but usually advisable. If still exhibiting stallion behavior, the patient should be isolated from mares. Healing should be complete in 14 to 21 days.

Complications of phallectomy include hematoma of the suture line, which causes partial or complete dehiscence, and resultant healing by granulation, which may or may not be further complicated by exuberant granulation. This may necessitate debridement or reamputation. Wound infection and urethral stricture are the other important complications.

En Bloc Resection

If invasive or metastatic carcinoma is evident, radical inguinal dissection is sometimes considered as an alternative to euthanasia. Preparation is the same as for simple amputation, except for the tourniquet. The penis may or may not be fixated in retraction (phallocrypsis). Radical dissection differs from the simple form in that the entire prepuce and free body of the penis are removed together with the superficial inguinal lymph glands on both sides— all in one mass. In keeping with good technique of tumor dissection, skin incisions and dissection planes should be located well into normal neighboring tissue, and venous and lymphatic drainage pathways should be controlled and mobilized early in the dissection to prevent further spread at the time of surgery. The surgical specimen should be draped and isolated from accidental contact with normal host tissues, and changes of gloves, linens, and instruments should be made as indicated to minimize the chance of spread. Amputation of the penis in the perineal region necessitates a urethrostomy, done in much the same way as the operation in the male of the bovine and ovine species. The stump of the penis is sutured into the skin incision to permit spatulation of the urethra to the skin. Owing to the extensive dissection and unavoidable areas of dead space, Penrose drains are required. For the same reasons, wound hygiene, a clean stable, prophylactic antibiotics, and regulated exercise are necessary. All tissues, both preoperative specimens and the surgical specimens, should be submitted for biopsy. Consideration should be given to the feasibility of radiation therapy with the understanding that only in selected cases with access to appropriate clinical facilities would such management be proposed.

SCROTUM AND TESTES

Castration of the normal and the cryptorchid horse and surgical management of complications of castration account for most surgical procedures in this region. Correction of hernias, revision of anomalies and production of teasers round out the list.

Castration (Orchiectomy)

Candidates for elective castration are selected on the basis of disposition, trainability and breed characteristics. The operation can be done at any age, although there are advantages for deferment to postpuberty so that the gelding displays masculinity. Selection of bloodstock should depend on performance testing as well as conformation, and this cannot be well determined until maturity in most cases. For these reasons, a case is made for elective castration no earlier than 2 years of age, although it is conceded that there may be perfectly valid reasons for earlier castration in the individual horse.

An infrequent, but not rare, argument for castration has been autocannibalism, flank-biting or self-mutilation. One source attributed this problem to chronic unilateral purulent seminal vesiculitis due to a β-hemolytic streptococcus. The behavior disappeared following resection of the affected seminal vesicle through an eccentric perineal (pararectal) approach.[19]

In the temperate as well as in the subtropical zones, castration by the open method is best done during the cooler months of the year because there is less aggravation by insects and a somewhat reduced incidence of wound infection during these seasons. In much of the southern border of the United States and in the nations to the south, screw worms continue to be a problem, necessitating special aftercare of all surgical wounds.

Castration of horses is well established as a field procedure, i.e., one that does not require the use of an operating room or a period of hospitalization. Even when performed at a clinic, the horse is usually treated as an outpatient. This is basically a matter of economics, and the current safety record for general anesthesia of horses has not changed this fact. As long as this remains the case, the great majority of horses will be operated on by the open wound method, with certain complications such as eventration, wound infection and hemorrhage accepted as calculated risks.

Anesthesia

The great change that the procedure has undergone in the past 20 years is the widespread acceptance of humane technique, using either local or general anesthesia. Even the advantages of succinylcholine chloride in speed and physical restraint have not obscured the central fact that its use does not abolish pain. Hence, neuromuscular blockade does not have universal approval, and those who follow this practice continue to find it necessary to justify its existence. There are, of course, other risks associated with suppression of respiration and plasma cholinesterase levels.

Whether the patient is restrained in a standing or recumbent position is a matter of choice by the owner or veterinarian. The use of the double-sideline casting harness has been virtually abandoned in light of advanced anesthetic pharmacology. It is debatable whether standing castration is much faster than that using the ultrashort general anesthetics such as thiamylal sodium. The objectional foundering during induction and recovery is less of a problem with the use of combinations of tranquilizers and muscle relaxants for preanesthetic and anesthetic medication. Certainly, cryptorchidectomy and management of hernias, hemorrhages and the like are sufficient reasons for having the capability to do castrations under general anesthesia. The defensible arguments for standing castration include the controllable patient with bilateral testicular descent and no evidence or history of scrotal hernia. Lack of needed assistance and use of facilities unsuitable for safe induction of general anesthesia may have an added bearing on the choice. Perhaps the only justification for the use of succinylcholine chloride in castration is for management of the uncontrollable horse, in which case attempts to anesthetize the animal by slower intravenous infusion or by local infiltration would place the personnel at unnecessarily high risk of injury.

Examples of acceptable local anesthetics are mepivacaine hydrochloride and lidocaine hydrochloride 2 per cent solution (with epinephrine). There are at least three methods of infiltration: direct infiltration of the spermatic cords at the superficial inguinal ring, infiltration by long needle (15 cm) of the spermatic cords and infiltration of the testicular parenchyma. In the last-named method, anesthesia of the cord occurs by diffusion. Profound skin anesthesia at the sites of scrotal incision usually requires direct subcutaneous infiltration except in the first-named technique, in which scrotal anesthesia may result if enough anesthetic is distributed. Needle sizes vary from 18 to 23 gauge according to the preference of the operator and the sensitivity of the patient. The amount of anesthetic varies from 10 to 30 ml per side, depending on the size of the testis and cord and the technique of the operator.

What has come to be known as chemical restraint for standing castration can be provided by a variety of agents used singly or in combination. The simplest is a tranquilizer such as acepromazine (IV) with the small risk of chemically induced priapism or penile paralysis (terms used are not to imply synonymity). Other agents include xylazine or pentazocine, usually with acetylpromazine. Intravenous chloral hydrate ± magnesium sulfate has been valued for years. Xylazine (0.3 mg pound or 0.66 mg/kg IV) with the same dose of morphine is ascribed superior efficacy.

General anesthetic, tranquilizer and muscle relaxant combinations are subject to even wider variation. These include acetylpromazine, promazine, xylazine and diazepam (tranquilizers); pentazocine (analgesic); glyceryl guaiacolate (muscle relaxant); sodium thiopental and thiamylal sodium (barbiturate anesthetics); ketamine hydrochloride (nonbarbiturate anesthetic); halothane and methoxyflurane (inhalant anesthetics); and meperidine hydrochloride (narcotic analgesic).

An example of a combination anesthetic for a 454-kg horse would be 30 to 40 mg of acetylpromazine IV followed in 20 minutes by 2 gm of thiamylal sodium and 50 gm of glyceryl guaiacolate in 1 liter of 5 per cent dextrose solution given rapidly (12- to 14-gauge needle) by gravity flow IV injection. The animal's fall should be controlled by snubbing a strong halter rope to a wall ring or equivalent with a dally (as opposed to a knot) so that tension can be tightened or loosened according to need. The hind quarters can be directed by holding the tail during the casting. If the calculated dose is given and the injection is arrested at that point, surgical anesthesia is provided for 15 to 20 minutes, with a struggle-free recovery. If, on the other hand, the unexpected occurs, such as scrotal eventration, the IV infusion can be resumed by slow drip and the patient maintained under surgical anesthesia for up to an hour or so with little problem. If complications require general anesthesia much beyond an hour, considerable advantage is gained with halothane anesthesia and the capability to give mechanical assistance to ventilation.

Other combinations that have been reported are as follows.[44]

1. Acetylpromazine (0.04 mg/kg) IV followed by glyceryl guaiacolate (100 mg/kg) and thiopental (4 mg/kg) IV.

2. Xylazine (1 mg/kg) IV followed by same as above.

3. Xylazine (1 mg/kg) IV followed by thiopental alone (same dosage).

4. Xylazine (1 mg/kg) IV followed by ketamine (2.2 mg/kg) IV.

5. Diazepam (0.2 mg/kg) IM and xylazine (1 mg/kg) IV followed by ketamine (2.2 mg/kg) IV.

Operative Technique

Despite many variations, all orchiectomies follow a common technique. First, the procedure should take advantage of anesthesia. Second, it should be done with a scrupulous regard for asepsis. The surgical field may be only a halo of cleanliness in a generally germy environment, and field procedures cannot duplicate the controlled conditions of the operating room. Nevertheless, it should be assumed that all castrations benefit from a surgical scrub of both the site and the surgeon and that aseptic technique is practiced in every way possible.

In the open wound method, orchiectomy is done through the ventral scrotum, and the most common approach is made through two parallel skin incisions lengthwise over the two testes. The incisions should be equidistant from the median raphe and should extend the full length of each testis, through the dartos, and to the scrotal fascia. Care should be exercised to avoid opening the parietal tunic (tunica vaginalis parietalis) until after the testis has been freed from the scrotum to midway up the extra-abdominal spermatic cord. The dissection plane is the scrotal fascia. Then, an incision is made through the parietal tunic over the cranial pole of the testis and extended upward along the exposed spermatic cord. The testis is prolapsed from the vaginal cavity through this incision, at the same time everting the caudal sac of the parietal tunic with the fingertips to provide a handle on the tunic to oppose the retractile action of the external cremaster muscle. The testis now hangs suspended by the mesorchium and visceral pedicle composed of the testicular artery, veins, lymphatics, nerves and ductus deferens. In preparation for amputation, the mesorchium is perforated by the fingertip, and the opening is enlarged sufficiently to admit the jaw of the emasculator. The visceral (or vascular) pedicle is divided separately and apart from the musculofibrous component of the spermatic cord, which prevents stretching the testicular artery at the time of emasculation and minimizes serious hemorrhage (all other things being equal). After the musculofibrous cord is divided with the emasculator, the remaining loose tags of scrotal fascia are trimmed to prevent interference with drainage.

Minor hemorrhage stops spontaneously if the wound is undisturbed and the horse is kept quiet for a few minutes. If hemorrhage continues, the wound should be explored for the source, most often the testicular artery. If this is the case, the artery should be ligated immediately by slipping a snare ligature of No. 2 chromic gut over kidney forceps (Stille vessel clamps or the equivalent) used to cross-clamp the arterial stump. If circumstances do not permit ligation, the alternative is sterile gauze packing retained with sutures or clips in the scrotal incision. The adjunctive use of systemic exogenous clotting factors such as conjugated mare estrogens has been thought to be of value in selected clinical cases.

Postoperative care includes tetanus immunization, wound hygiene and regulated exercise to facilitate drainage from the open wound. Insect irritation can be controlled by use of topical insect repellents over the entire horse as well as around the wound. The use of topical and systemic antibiotics is optional, depending on the cleanliness of the environment and the reliability of the attendants. Given an either/or choice, liberal exercise in a clean surrounding would be of greater benefit than antibiotics and no exercise. Usually one is faced with a compromise.

Observation during the healing period is emphasized. The greatest risk is during the initial 24-hour postoperative period. In one series of 371 cases, small intestinal eventration occurred in 11 horses. Seven eventrations happened within 2 hours, one in 4 hours, two in 24 hours, and one 6 days later. Although this accounts for only a small number of the total cases, it must be remembered that 11 elective procedures turned into emergencies with an ominous mortality rate of 63.6 per cent.[34]

In addition, hemorrhage of consequence can take place during the first postoperative day, and there are unusual instances of late-occurring hemorrhages after the first day. One case of hemorrhage followed heavy exercise that was allowed prematurely in the first convalescent week.

Penile paralysis from adverse reaction to the use of a phenothiazine tranquilizer (promazine, acetylpromazine) becomes a major problem if unattended for even 12 hours. In fact, if recovery of retractility of the penis fails to occur within 4 to 8 hours, the use of a suspensory should be considered without further delay. Comparing the problem to "drug-induced priapism" in the human, a 3-year-old thoroughbred gelding so affected after receiving 30 mg acetylpromazine IV was treated successfully with benztropine mesylate 8 mg IV, given 2½ hours after the acetylpromazine injection. The priapism was reversed in 30 minutes.[62]

Unusual edema of the scrotum and prepuce, with or without paraphimosis, may herald wound infection and should receive early attention. A sudden fever rise may indicate wound infection, or it may mean putrefaction of a retained blood clot in a poorly drained wound. Such infections can lead to chronic complications, namely, champignon (a streptococcosis of the spermatic cord stump), botryomycosis (a staphylococcosis of the cord), and aggravated paraphimosis, even penile paralysis. Septicemia, peritonitis and urinary obstruction are representative of acute complications. Survivors of either group must be subjected to further surgery upon localization of the wound infection for incision and drainage of the inguinal abscess and debridement of the purulent sinuses and chronic inflammatory granulomas of the cord stumps.[37, 50]

Primary closure castration by aseptic technique is done with the patient restrained in dorsal recumbency under general anesthesia. The skin incision is oriented with the spermatic cord extending upward to the proximity of the superficial inguinal ring. The incision is deepened through the parietal tunic into the vaginal cavity, exposing the visceral components of the cord. The incision is extended sufficiently to permit exteriorization of the testis and adnexa (after cutting the gubernacular ligament). The visceral cord is then ligated and amputated, and the stump is returned to the vaginal cavity. The parietal tunic is closed with gut sutures, then the fascia is closed, and finally the skin. Operative time for both sides is about 30 minutes. Aftercare includes moderate regular exercise, tetanus prophylaxis and discretionary use of antibiotics.[33, 38]

Cryptorchidism

The transabdominal migration of the fetal testis during the first 9 months of gestation may be attributed to both testicular migration and differential growth of the fetus. An example is the testicular hypertrophy due to increasing numbers of interstitial cells up to about 7½ months of gestation, after which regression occurs (to a greater degree in the right testis than in the left). Distally, the testis is attached to the inguinal region by a column of mesenchyme known as gubernaculum, divided into intra-abdominal and extra-abdominal parts as it descends into the peritoneal eversion forming the vaginal process. For the first 8½ months, these structures grow at nearly the same rate, except that the caudal gonadal ligament (forerunner of the proper ligament of the testis) lengthens more rapidly than the gubernaculum (future ligament of the tail of the epididymis), which causes a wide separation between the caudal pole of the testis and the cauda epididymidis. This accounts for the fact that the cauda epididymis may occupy the vaginal process inside the inguinal canal as early as the fifth month of gestation. Owing to the length of the caudal gonadal ligament, hypertrophy of the fetal testis, small diameter of the vaginal ring and lack of tension on the gubernaculum, descent of the testis through the inguinal canal does not occur until the eleventh month, by which time testicular regression and differential development of the vaginal process (producing increased tension on the gubernaculum) combine to usher the testis into the inguinal canal, where it resides until after birth. This is in contrast to the human, in whom the testes reach the scrotum by the end of the eighth month of gestation.[29, 49, 61, 65]

A somewhat dissimilar account credits the final stages of descent as being principally due to continuous pressure of peritoneal fluids causing expansion of the vaginal process around the gubernaculum, drawing the testis to the internal ring. Further, the oft-repeated anecdotal reports of the testes that are palpated in the scrotum of the newborn only to be found retained later on are explained as the greatly enlarged gubernaculum that undergoes a 10-fold increase in size before the 300th day of gestation and can be palpated at birth as soft, ovoid masses in the scrotum indistinguishable from testes. The truly cryptorchid testis never descends, owing to a failure to enter the internal inguinal ring prior to closure, which occurs near or shortly after birth.[7]

The cause of maldescent remains unresolved and, indeed, may be due to several factors. Studies in the human have proposed (1) defective hypothalamic-pituitary axis and deficiency of luteinizing hormone, which fails to explain the more commonplace (three to five times) unilateral cryptorchidism; (2) mechanical defect, i.e., gubernacular abnormality, inadequate abdominal pressure for proper expansion of the vaginal process, inadequate growth of the post-testicular mass that precedes the testis through the inguinal canal, or displacement and incarceration of the testis in the pelvic cavity; (3) genetic factor, based on familial and inherited tendencies; (4) defect in the testis itself, resulting in a deficiency of the testicular production of androgens, which influence the ductus deferens, epididymis and gubernaculum during descent (or a defect in the end-organs themselves, resulting in a different response to testicular androgens), which may offer the best answer for unilateral cryptorchidism; and (5) testicular dysgenesis based on abnormal testicular chromosomes.[7, 61]

In the horse, abdominal cryptorchidism shows an interruption of development at the 5-month fetal stage, with or without descent of the cauda epididymidis.[65] Despite the effectiveness of human chorionic gonadotropin (HCG) in the treatment of undescended testes in man,[61] use of HCG for treating abdominal cryptorchidism in the horse is considered unjustified by some.[65] Clinical impressions tend to support this claim and increase the dependence on surgery for rectifying the problem.

Prevention, on the other hand, appears to rest on the public conscience, which shows an amazing disregard or ignorance of the fact that equine cryptorchidism is considered an inherited abnormality. Although in other species it is classified as a recessive trait, the disorder in horses is reputedly of dominant inheritance.[35, 58] Interestingly, of 29 equine breed associations reporting to the AVMA Council on Veterinary Service (published in 1976)[4] on unacceptable surgical procedures for eligibility and qualification for registration with the respective breed association, only one, the Appaloosa Horse Club, Inc., specified "surgical correction of cryptorchidism or monorchidism." Only two, the Spanish-Barb Breeders Association and the American

Suffolk Horse Assocation, specified surgical correction of hereditary defects or procedures that mask hereditary defects. The National Trotting and Pacing Association, Inc. and the United States Trotting Association specified "surgical correction of inguinal or umbilical hernia, without castration."[4] In a retrospective study of 350 cases of cryptorchidism seen over a 14-year period at a large midwestern United States university clinic, 49 per cent of the cases were observed in quarter horses, as compared with 4 per cent for American saddle horses, 3.7 per cent Arabians, 3.1 per cent standardbreds, and 1.4 per cent thoroughbreds.[70] Unacceptable surgical procedures reported by the American Quarter Horse Association were "removal of white spots, cosmetic ear surgery, and tail surgery."[4]

Analysis of cases has revealed the probabilities of distribution. Of a series of 350 cases, 59.4 per cent of the cryptorchid testes were abdominal,[70] which compares favorably with another series of 417 cases in which 60.2 per cent were abdominal.[39] Unilateral cryptorchidism in the two series ranged from 86 per cent of 350 cases to 93 per cent of 417 cases, 7 to 14 times the incidence of bilateralism, an even higher statistic than for humans. Unilateralism favored the left side from 53 per cent of 350 cases to 65 per cent of 417 cases, except for the fact that in position, the inguinal retention occurred more commonly on the right side (58 per cent of 350 cases). Conversely, 75 per cent of the abdominal retentions occurred on the left side, reminding us of Smith's observation that the regression of the hypertrophied fetal testis appeared to be slower on the left side.[39, 65, 70]

Cryptorchidism is often associated with congenital anomalies such as pseudohermaphroditism. True hermaphroditism has been observed in rare instances.[22, 41]

Diagnosis

Diagnosis of cryptorchidism has long been a source of speculation and much discussion. Since known castrates may exhibit stallion behavior,[9, 12] and since many candidates for cryptorchidectomy have histories of previous (unsuccessful) surgery, the patient is not infrequently presented as a diagnostic problem. Short of exploratory surgery, the common diagnostic approaches include (1) external palpation of the scrotum and superficial inguinal rings, (2) pelvic palpation per rectum and (3) laboratory testing for plasma androgen concentrations. A new modality that is finding increasing acceptance in various diagnostic applications is ultrasonography.[56]

External palpation is done to detect the retractile testis lying just outside the superficial inguinal ring, the inguinal testis that is occasionally palpable through the ring or the scarred stump of the spermatic cord. The horse must be controllable, and relaxation of both horse and examiner is necessary. The examination may be facilitated by prior tranquilization or sedation of the patient.

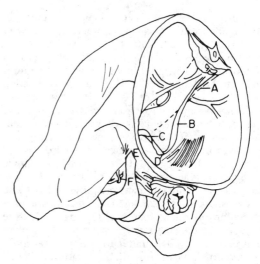

Figure 1. Anatomy of the inguinal region. Route of the left ureter (dotted line) (A); mesorchium (B); ductus deferens (C); vaginal ring (D); superficial inguinal ring (E); and spermatic cord within tunica vaginalis parietalis (F). (After Nickel R, et al.: The Viscera of the Domestic Mammals. New York, Springer-Verlag, 1973, pp 351–392.)

Palpation per rectum places the same premium on cooperation. Correct diagnosis on the basis of this method has been reported in as many as 88 per cent of 350 cases that were confirmed at the time of surgery.[70] Objectives are palpating the testis per se or the ductus deferens entering the vaginal ring or noting the absence of the same. It is not difficult to trap the cryptorchid testis against the wall of the caudal abdomen by carefully sweeping the region of the deep inguinal ring with the hand in the relaxed rectum. The soft, hypoplastic testis can be felt to slip under the fingertips or the edge of the hand as it passes from the linea alba upward toward the vaginal ring. A full bladder will interfere with the procedure and may necessitate catheterization or voluntary urination before the examination can be completed. Palpation of the vaginal ring just cranial to the pelvic inlet is done most easily by feeling the caudal abdominal wall from the midlateral region downward to detect the slitlike opening in the parietal peritoneum. If the epididymis has descended into the vaginal process, the ductus can be felt entering the ring. Absence of pulsations differentiates it from the external pudendal artery. Of course, this does not obviate the possibility that the testis may still reside in the abdomen, but it does at least ensure the chances of retrieval by a noninvasive procedure (in the sense of peritoneal cavity)[1, 3, 52, 70] (Fig. 1).

Laboratory assay of androgen levels in the plasma has become a useful way to detect the presence of testicular tissue in questionable animals, particularly those not yielding easily to physical examination and those with a history of previous surgery. The test is based on the Leydig cell elaboration of testosterone in increased amounts in response to the injection of human chorionic gonadotropin (HCG); hence, the frequent reference to the HCG test. The procedure calls for the comparison of testosterone levels in paired plasma samples harvested from heparinized blood drawn at 0 minutes and 30 to 120 minutes after the intravenous injection of 6000 to 12,000 IU of HCG.[12, 13, 15] Testosterone and other plasma androgens are measured by either competitive protein-binding assay (CPBA) or radioimmunoassay (RIA).[1] Basal concentrations of testosterone in the stallion range widely from <100 pg/ml to >1500 pg/ml. In one study of known geldings, the values averaged 15.3 pg/ml. In previously castrated animals that were presented as "false rigs" (ostensible cryptorchids), the mean basal concentration of testosterone was 17.7 pg/ml. In true cryptorchids the comparative mean was 423 pg/ml. Between 0 and 120 minutes following intravenous injection of 12,000 IU of HCG, testosterone levels in the plasma of the stallion experienced a 4- to 30-fold increase. In geldings, the highest concentrations were from about a 1.5- to 3-fold increase above the average. The comparative figures for "false rigs" did not differ significantly from that for geldings. This has also been shown to be true for castrates with intact epididymides ("proud cut").[15, 16] In contrast, HCG response in cryptorchids demonstrated greater than a threefold increase of the mean within 30 minutes postinjection.[15] The technique varies somewhat in human testing, in which the child is given HCG, 2000 IU daily for 4 days, and plasma assay is run on the fifth day. If normally responsive gonads are present, there may be as much as a 10-fold increase over baseline. The point is made, however, that any rise in the testosterone level after HCG treatment is evidence of functioning testicular tissue until proved otherwise.[61] It has also been observed that individual cryptorchid horses with low initial testosterone concentrations show a tendency to respond more to HCG than those with higher initial concentrations.[15]

Other work has sought to compare the total estrogen levels in plasma of male horses; levels were significantly higher in the bilaterally cryptorchid animal and higher in the animal with a cryptorchid testis than in one with a scrotal testis in unilaterally cryptorchid animals. The lowest levels were in the gelding. Thus, it was hypothesized that simultaneous measurement of total estrogen and androgen levels in horses may be a more useful method to determine the presence of viable testicular tissue than the HCG test.[28]

Operative Technique

The undescended testis can be approached through (1) the inguinal canal, (2) the ventral abdominal wall (paramedian) or (3) the lateral abdominal wall (flank). Experienced and ardent advocates can be found to support the advantages of each. It may be safe to say that if sufficient numbers of patients are presented under varied circumstances, one might justify the use of all three.

Inguinal Approach. With the patient restrained under general anesthesia in dorsal recumbency and prepared for aseptic surgery, a skin incision approximately 10 cm long is made over and aligned with the superficial inguinal ring. Accidental injury to the large subcutaneous branches of the external pudendal vein can be avoided by limiting sharp dissection with the scalpel to the skin incision. The inguinal fascia is separated with the fingertips, and the inguinal canal is explored for the vaginal process and contents or for the scarified stump of spermatic cord of the castrate. Notation of skin scar and inguinal fibrosis raises expectation of the latter, but only the demonstration of all the components of the spermatic cord, including ductus deferens, vessels, tunica vaginalis and external cremaster muscle, should serve to cancel the further search for the retained testis. In not a few instances, the epididymis is amputated in the mistaken belief that it is a hypoplastic inguinal testis. In such cases, the testis is retained in the abdomen and usually requires invasion of the peritoneal cavity.

If the vaginal process is encountered, it should be grasped by forceps and retracted to permit incision, revealing the gubernaculum, epididymis and ductus deferens. The incision can be lengthened by either scissor or fingertip toward the vaginal ring, and gentle traction on the epididymis will produce the small, soft testis most often found.[1, 77] A characteristic feature is the increased length of the caudal gonadal ligament (proper ligament of the testis) separating the caudal aspects of the testis and epididymis.

If the search fails to yield the vaginal process or if it is thought to be inverted, the forceps technique of Adams can be employed to grasp the gubernaculum through the rudimentary vaginal process (presumed to exist). Curved 10-inch Foerster sponge forceps are manually guided into the deep (internal) inguinal ring to the peritoneal covering of the vaginal ring. The partially opened jaws are pressed carefully into the vaginal process and closed to grasp a small fold of the process. Care must be taken not to tear the peritoneum. The inverted process is retracted into the canal until it can be seen. Palpation through the process will reveal the cordlike gubernaculum. A small incision in the process can be made safely with Mayo dissecting scissors, and the access is thus provided for grasping the gubernaculum, retraction of which produces the epididymis and, finally, the testis.[1]

Alternatively, the index and middle fingers can be introduced through the vaginal ring to grasp the gubernaculum, epididymis or ductus deferens.[42, 66] Retrieval of the testis follows retraction of these structures. The procedure is facilitated by dietary reduction of colon bulk and by elevation of the hind quarters (using differential padding or an inclined plane). A variation of this technique is to perforate the medial muscular wall of the inguinal canal just inside or just outside the superficial inguinal ring. In the latter case, the aponeurosis of the external oblique muscle must also be perforated. In all three instances, the search is conducted in much the same way. In the event the limited exploration is unsuccessful, the coned fingers are used to enlarge the opening to admit the hand. The pelvic inlet is explored for the respective ductus, leading from the ampulla in the genital fold above the urinary bladder, over the lateral ligament of the bladder, to the epididymis of the retained testis. It is advantageous to use the right hand to explore the left canal and the left hand to explore the right canal so that the palm and flexor surfaces of the fingers face medially and backward.[66] If it is necessary to introduce the hand in small subjects, it is better to use the paramedian or flank approach to avoid unnecessary disruption of the inguinal canal. This is also advisable if the testis is tumorous and too large to deliver through the canal.[14, 39]

The exteriorized testis and epididymis can be amputated with angiotribe forceps and ligature or simply with an emasculator. If the funiculus is too short to permit exteriorization, a chain écraseur can be used. Lacking that, a snare ligature can be slipped over the retracting forceps and tightened around the funiculus inside the abdomen. Blunt-pointed scissors can be manually guided into the abdomen to make the amputation a safe distance from the ligature. On other occasions, an emasculator has been manually introduced inside the abdomen, but great caution must be exercised to avoid accidental injury to the bowel or mesentery.

Following orchiectomy, the wound is closed under suture in three layers. The superficial inguinal ring, which is a slit in the aponeurosis of the external abdominal oblique muscle, is closed with either surgical gut or polyglycolic acid (PGA) synthetic No. 2 gut double-strand in a simple continuous pattern. The secret in the strength of the repair is to initiate the row beyond the cranial end of the ring and terminate it beyond the caudal end to avoid unnecessary distraction and tension on the end knots. A flat hernia needle is used to facilitate manual placement without breaking asepsis, which occurs inevitably when sharp-pointed needles are so used. The distance from needle hole to ring margin is staggered to avoid common stress lines. The pattern is vertical, i.e., perpendicular to the principal direction of aponeurotic fibers. Approximately six bites are necessary to close the ring. Slight adduction of the corresponding thigh during the closure reduces the distraction of the ring margins.

The second suture layer consists of interrupted gut or PGA sutures in the inguinal fascia, and the third layer is a row of interrupted mattress sutures of noncapillary nylon or polypropylene in the skin incision. Primary closure of cryptorchidectomy incisions is axiomatic if aseptic procedure has been followed. The only excuse for packing such wounds today is the presence of gross contamination, which may occur in the field procedure but should never be accepted as a part of the surgical plan. If the primary closure is done as described, herniation, eventration and abscess are not anticipated sequelae.

Postoperative care is the same as that provided for any such procedure that involves the abdominal wall and peritoneal cavity, whether invasive or not. The horse should be allowed the use of a private box stall with clean bedding, fresh water and light hay. Hand walking can be started the first 24 hours after surgery and gradually increased as soreness subsides. Paddock exercise ad libitum may be permitted by the second or third day if the horse is confined to a private paddock. Skin healing should allow suture removal in 10 days. Tetanus immunization is mandatory and use of prophylactic antibiotics is discretionary.

Paramedian Approach. Preparation and restraint parallel those described for the inguinal approach. A 10-cm longitudinal skin incision is made 6 to 8 cm off the midline and alongside the external preputial orifice. Because it is extensile, the incision can be readily lengthened caudad for easier access to the region of the deep inguinal ring. Parenthetically, this is much the same approach as that used for access to surgery of the urinary bladder in the male. This plane of dissection is deepened progressively through the superficial and deep abdominal fascia, the conjoined aponeuroses of the external and internal abdominal oblique muscles (superficial sheath of the rectus), and the longitudinal fibers of the rectus abdominis muscle. The aponeurosis of the transversus abdominis muscle (deep sheath) can be incised in the same longitudinal plane, which transects its fibers, or it can be split transversely along its fibers, employing the principle of a grid incision. The fatty layer of fascia transversalis lies just underneath and covers the final layer, the peritoneum, which is perforated to admit the hand. Again, exploration is facilitated by reduced bulk in the colon and the elevation of the hind quarters. The wound margins can be retracted manually or mechanically, according to the surgeon's preference. The retrieval of the testis follows the same procedure as that described previously. An advantage of this method is that bilateral abdominal testes can be removed through the one incision, with some slight preference expressed for the left paramedian incision in such cases. An écraseur may be required for access to the contralateral testis. A disadvantage is that its use is confined to the abdominal cryptorchid, necessitating accurate preoperative diagnosis.[14, 39]

Closure of the incision is subject to some variation. Peritoneal suture is optional. The deep sheath of the rectus should be closed with gut or PGA sutures. However, this layer will support very little tension, and continuous sutures must be preplaced, pulling up slack on several bites at once to avoid tearing the thin aponeurosis. Whether suturing peritoneum or the deep sheath, tension should be taken synchronous with the patient's inspirations to take advantage of the greater degree of relaxation of the abdominal musculature at this time. This phased tightening of several bites at once avoids the undesirable tearing and fenestration of thin tissue planes. The main purpose of this layer is to keep the retroperitoneal fat out of the ensuing closure. The next layer of sutures is taken in the superficial sheath and provides the major support. Gut has been used successfully in simple interrupted pattern, as have nonabsorbable synthetics (nylon, Dacron or polypropylene) in a continuous, imbricating mattress pattern (modified Mayo), starting and finishing beyond the ends of the incision to eliminate the weak point of knot-break strength. Care should be taken to exclude fat and muscle from the overlapped interface of aponeurosis. The edge is sutured down with a continuous row of the same material. The superficial abdominal fascia is closed with interrupted sutures of gut placed in reverse to invert the knots. The skin is closed with interrupted mattress sutures of a noncapillary synthetic. Synthetic absorbable sutures have enjoyed increasing popularity because of their early strength and prolonged dependability as well as the absence of suture sinus seen occasionally with nonabsorbable sutures. Aftercare is the same as that previously described.

Flank Approach. This method is performed as a field procedure on the standing horse under sedation and local anesthesia. As with the paramedian approach, its use is confined to the abdominal cryptorchid, and the location of the testis must be known beforehand. The flank site also offers an alternative approach for access to the unilateral testicular tumor (commonly teratoma). In this case, surgery is usually done on the patient restrained in lateral recumbency under general anesthesia because of the obvious benefits afforded by relaxed abdominal musculature. Inasmuch as only grid incisions are made in the lateral abdominal wall, delivery of large masses through such incisions is mechanically impractical, if not impossible, in the standing patient.

The practicality of the standing operation, however, is that both in the horse undergoing surgery for abdominal cryptorchidism and in the mare for ovariectomy the procedure can be performed satisfactorily in the field without the facilities or assistance required for responsible administration of general anesthesia. It has been adopted as a routine approach by many practitioners who prefer this method, especially for the retention of a unilateral abdominal testis. Therefore, any balanced discussion of the subject requires its inclusion.

Sedation is provided by tranquilization (see Castration) with or without sedation by intravenous chloral hydrate, 7 per cent solution or stronger concentrations, combined with magnesium sulfate. Local anesthesia is by line infiltration or inverted L field block of the incision site with 2 per cent lidocaine or mepivacaine. Preoperative medication with intravenous hydrocortisone sodium succinate suppresses the noxious effects on the circulation when the peritoneal cavity is invaded in the conscious horse.

A 15- to 20-cm transverse skin incision is made in the midflank, equidistant from the last rib and the tensor fasciae latae. The superficial fascia is divided in the same plane. The external oblique muscle is divided in the direction of its fibers running caudoventrad from the rib. The internal oblique muscle is divided in the cranioventral direction. The transversus abdominis muscle is divided in the plane of the skin incision, and the peritoneum is perforated with the fingertips. At this point, additional local anesthetic can be used topically to provide better anesthesia of the peritoneum. The left hand, with the palm upward and backward, is used to explore the left side; the right hand, the right side. Upon entering the peritoneal cavity, the palm of the hand, turned upward to locate the kidney, is passed caudally to identify the mesorchium, which extends from the region behind the kidney caudoventrad toward the inguinal canal. This leads directly to the testis. If a visceral mass makes this difficult, the pelvic inlet can be explored for the ductus deferens (see earlier discussion). When located, the testis is exteriorized for emasculation. Again, in the case of the short funiculus, écrasement or blind emasculation may be required. If the testis is inguinal in location, successful removal may require a second approach through the inguinal canal under general anesthesia. In the bilateral abdominal cryptorchid, it is possible, but difficult, to remove both testes through the one side, and the procedure does require a remote amputation.[73]

The flank wound is closed easily with individual layers of simple interrupted gut sutures to appose the separated planes of muscle and to obliterate dead space. The peritoneum is not sutured. The superficial abdominal fascia should be closed carefully with No. 2 gut interrupted sutures. The skin incision is apposed with interrupted mattress sutures of noncapillary synthetic material. Aftercare parallels that of the other laparotomy approaches.

Scrotal Hernia

Inguinal hernia occurs in both sexes and may be congenital or acquired, emergency or elective, reducible or strangulated, or correctable or irreparable (Fig. 2). Heritability[58] remains somewhat of a moot issue in some cases, such as whether the mature stallion that herniated while breeding a mare may have had a predisposing weakness since birth. Direct hernias (versus indirect) occur through a rent in the fascia alongside the canal, usually as a result of trauma.[78] Although some surgeons have performed scrotal herniorrhaphy without castration,[8] this borders on malpractice and is expressly in violation of the rules of several breed associations.[4] The lay public should be able to look to the profession for guidance in such matters, and if we vacillate on the issues, the layman can scarcely be expected to do better. Herniorrhaphy without castration is certainly no technical feat and nothing to brag about; rather it is something to explain and show

Figure 2. Scrotal hernias. The internal pathology is transposed from left to right in the external manifestation for the sake of illustration. A knuckle of bowel entrapped in the vaginal ring and proximal inguinal canal (A). No outward signs apparent. A limb of bowel is incarcerated in the vaginal cavity of the spermatic cord (B). This is visible and palpable in the external inguinal region. A limb of bowel has herniated into the vaginal cavity of the scrotum, distorting the architecture, and is grossly visible (C). Torsion of the spermatic cord (D) causing painful swelling and mimicking the hernia in B. (After Nickel R, et al.: The Viscera of the Domestic Mammals. New York, Springer-Verlag, 1973, pp 351–392.)

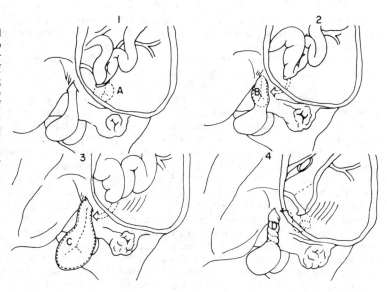

cause for. In such instances as the breeding stallion, if there has been no evidence of scrotal hernia as a familial problem, correction with retention of the testes may be justified, but the records should clearly show the conditions that dictated such a decision.

Hernia may first appear in the newborn in which there is defective development of the inguinal canal. The hernial ring is large, and the contents can be easily reduced with very little concern for strangulation. In fact, if the foal strains at the bowel movement, e.g., meconial obstipation, the worry is that the hernia will enlarge. Surprisingly, if there is no such complication, some of these hernias will correct themselves spontaneously. This does not reduce the need for vigilance against strangulation but does argue the case for watchful waiting. Meanwhile, in the absence of other problems, the foal grows stronger, muscles gain tone, anesthetic risk diminishes and tissues will provide better support for sutures if surgery is necessary. Such individuals should be marked for castration whenever the proper time arrives. The only justification for delaying castration is to allow for development of masculine traits.

The visible and reducible hernia is a known entity, and treatment is elective. There should be little problem in dealing with these. It is the obscure hernia, recurrent or not, that causes problems either as a complication of castration (eventration)[34] or as a strangulation. Although inguinal or scrotal swelling is not a consistent feature of scrotal hernia, if there is a history of such signs (characterized by occurrence and disappearance) in the candidate for castration, time should be taken to palpate per rectum for enlargement of the vaginal rings prior to surgery. If this is suspected, primary closure of the castration wound is warranted.

The strangulated hernia is presented as an acute colic, characteristically of small intestinal locus. It

need not be in a breeding stallion, although if such signs occur directly after breeding, strangulated hernia should be assumed until proved otherwise. Some cases are difficult to diagnose because there may be no externally visible or palpable evidence of the hernia. The entrapped limb of small intestine (usually the case) may be confined to the inguinal canal. Even on palpation per rectum, it can be misdiagnosed as torsion of the spermatic cord. However, this does not alter the course of action, which is surgical invasion of the inguinal canal. One instance of this diagnosis is recalled with some embarrassment, as it was made at the time of an exploratory laparotomy through the linea alba. This serves to underscore the importance of a searching palpation per rectum on every case when possible.

Herniorrhaphy Procedure

The preoperative preparations will range across the spectrum of possibilities; therefore, the discussion simply addresses the mechanics that are common to all.

The patient is restrained under general anesthesia in dorsal recumbency and prepared for aseptic surgery. The skin incision is made over the superficial inguinal ring and extended downward over the scrotum for a distance required by the size of the hernia. Adhesions necessitate more dissection. The tunica vaginalis parietalis is freed from the scrotal fascia by blunt dissection, and the hernial contents are "milked" back into the peritoneal cavity. A time-honored method of doing this on reducible hernias, which simultaneously retains the reduction until ligated, is to twist the tunica (with the testis in the fundus of the sac) on itself, winding up the cord as it were, to obliterate the vaginal cavity and force the intestines out. Then, the cord is ligated with transfixation at the level of the superficial ring. The cord is transected, and the stump is allowed to retract into the inguinal canal. The closure of the ring and other layers parallels that described for inguinal cryptorchidectomy.

If the hernia is irreducible, the parietal tunic must be opened, incarcerated intestines freed of adhesions and decompressed of gas or fluids, and the hernial ring enlarged if necessary to permit return of the hernial contents to the abdomen. If the hernia is strangulated, the preferred course is decompression of the intestine (if required) and return to the abdomen. If viability of the gut has been compromised, resection is necessary. It may be possible to extend the contents sufficiently to provide room for this. The alternative is to reduce and return the devitalized bowel to the abdomen and exteriorize it through a ventral laparotomy. The justification is that the architecture of the inguinal canal is preserved, undesirable traction on bowel and mesentery is avoided, and resection and anastomosis can be done without tension. In such cases, the inguinal canal and abdomen must be treated as contaminated, and appropriate safeguards such as drains and prophylactic antibiotics should be used.

Reconstruction of the canal has been described previously.

Space-Occupying Lesions of the Scrotum and Testes

A differential diagnosis should consider the major possibilities: (1) orchitis, which in turn may be sterile and possibly accompanied by seroma or hematoma, or septic with abscess; (2) cyst of the testis, e.g., hematocyst; (3) effusion of the vaginal cavity, e.g., hydrocele and hematocele; and (4) neoplasm.

Orchitis may result from trauma, such as a kick, or from infection, although the latter is somewhat less frequent a cause in the horse than in other domestic species.[58] Fluctuation is not a reliable diagnostic feature in such cases because of the tension under the tunica albuginea as well as the plaque of scrotal edema that so often overlies the testis. Therefore, differentiation of seroma, hematoma and abscess will likely depend on needle aspirates and signs of leukocytosis, fever and pain or possibly on surgical incision for drainage.

The cystic testis may present a problem in the abdominal cryptorchid as well as in the horse with a scrotal testis. In the former case, much of the parenchyma has been displaced by serous fluid, which may account for an increase in size by several times that of the normal gonad. Paracentesis may be effective in reducing it sufficiently so that it can be removed through an inguinal approach. In the animal with a scrotal testis, a hematocyst is usually the result of trauma, and the physical findings are those of orchitis.

Serous effusion of the vaginal cavity or hydrocele in the horse is more common following castration and is characterized by a painless, noninflammatory, fluctuant swelling that gives the appearance of a scrotal testis. Paracentesis yields clear peritoneal fluid. Hematocele is the presence of whole blood, usually clotted, in the same space and is thought to be caused by trauma.[31]

Neoplasms of the equine testis are uncommon but do occur with sufficient frequency to be a diagnostic consideration. Teratoma is the most important testicular tumor in the horse, and the equine accounts for the greatest incidence of this tumor type among the domestic animals. Teratomas are composed of multiple tissues foreign to the part in which they arise, e.g., bone, cartilage, skin, hair, epithelial ducts, dentigerous cyst formation, mammary tissue, and nerves. They may be bilateral, may occur during the first five years of life and may affect the cryptorchid testis in as many as 25 per cent of cases.[11, 45] The large size of some lesions necessitates laparotomy for successful removal.[20]

Other neoplasms of the equine testis include seminoma, Sertoli cell tumor and interstitial cell adenoma, all rare but reported, usually in the older stallion.[45, 55] Unilateral lesions may be removed and the fertility of the horse salvaged if the opposite testis is normal;[31] however, the prognosis of breeding soundness may be clouded by the suppressant effect of hemicastration.[27]

Surgical management of these masses is by incision and drainage or resection. Techniques employed are those used for castration and cryptorchidectomy.

Vasectomy and Epididymectomy

Teasers for the breeding industry have been produced with various methods including penile deviation (retroversion),[5] epididymectomy,[21] and vasectomy.[60] The advantage of retroversion is that accidental intromission is prevented; however, the method has not been adopted for general use since its description over 25 years ago.[5] The epididymectomy has stimulated some interest, but there is concern about the likelihood of sperm granuloma. A technique of vasectomy that can be performed as field surgery has been proposed more recently.[60]

The patient is restrained in lateral or dorsal recumbency under intravenous general anesthesia and prepared for aseptic surgery. A skin incision is made over the caudomedial aspect of one testis near the median raphe of the scrotum and is aligned with the oblique course of the ductus deferens in its ascent from the cauda epididymidis to the spermatic cord. The incision is deepened through the dartos, fascia, and parietal tunica vaginalis to open the vaginal cavity. The ductus is exteriorized and a 2-cm section excised, double-ligating the cut ends with 00 silk to prevent sperm granuloma. The tunic is closed under fine gut suture, and through the same skin incision the scrotal septum is opened along the medial side of the opposite testis for access to the other ductus deferens. The vasectomy is repeated on the second side, and the tunic, septum, fascia, and skin are closed in separate layers. Sequential semen evaluations have shown the disappearance of all viable spermatozoa by the sixth postoperative week.

A related subject with different indications is the chemical suppression of spermatogenesis by intramuscular injection of a repositol form of microencapsulated testosterone propionate, which causes depressed output of pituitary gonadotropins LH and FSH. The effects of the injection last 3 to 6 months and are reversible. There is no effect on libido. Field trials on feral stallions reduced foal counts by 5 times.[36]

References

1. Adams OR: An improved method of diagnosis and castration of cryptorchid horses. J Am Vet Med Assoc 145:439, 1963.
2. Amann RP: A review of anatomy and physiology of the stallion. J Equine Vet Sci 1:83, 1981.
3. Ashdown RR: The anatomy of the inguinal canal in domesticated mammals. Vet Rec 75:1345, 1963.
4. AVMA Council on Veterinary Services: Council report—Unacceptable surgical procedures applicable to domestic animals. J Am Vet Med Assoc 168:947, 1976.
5. Belonje CWA: The operation for retroversion of the penis in the stallion. J South Afr Vet Med Assoc 27:53, 1956.
6. Bergevin JD, Merritt FD, Schoenberg RA: Field-adapted equine castration technique with ligation of spermatic vessels and vaginal tunics left in place. Proceedings of the 23rd Annual Convention of American Association of Equine Practitioners, 1977, pp 193–195.
7. Bergin WC, Gier HT, Marion GB, Coffman JR: A developmental concept of equine cryptorchidism. Biol Reprod 3:82, 1970.
8. Bignozzi L: Surgical treatment of scrotal hernia in foals and yearlings, without orchectomy. Tijdschr Diergeneeskd 98:1025, 1973.
9. Bishop MWH, David JSE, Messervy A: Some observations on cryptorchidism in the horse. Vet Rec 76:1041, 1964.
10. Bracken FK, Wagner PC: Cosmetic surgery for equine pseudohermaphroditism. Vet Med/Small Anim Clin 78(6), 879, 1983.
11. Cotchin E: A general survey of tumours in the horse. Equine Vet J 9:16, 1977.
12. Cox JE: Surgery of the Male Reproductive Tract in Large Animals. Published by the author, University of Liverpool Veterinary Field Station, Leahurst: Neston, WIRRAL, L64 7TE, Merseyside, England, 1977.
13. Cox JE, Williams JH: Some aspects of the reproductive endocrinology of the stallion and cryptorchid. J Reprod Fertil 23 (Suppl): 75, 1975.
14. Cox JE, Edwards GB, Neal PA: Suprapubic paramedian laparotomy for equine abdominal cryptorchidism. Vet Rec 97:428, 1975.
15. Cox JE, Williams JH, Rowe PH, Smith JII: Testosterone in normal, cryptorchid and castrated male horses. Equine Vet J 5:85, 1973.
16. Crowe CW, Gardner RE, Humburg JM, et al.: Plasma testosterone and behavioral characteristics in geldings with intact epididymides. J Equine Med Surg 1:387, 1977.
17. Damodaran S, Ramachandran PV: A survey of neoplasms of equidae. Indian Vet J 52:531, 1975.
18. Danks AG: Williams' Surgical Operations. Published by the author, Ithaca, 1945, pp 84–87.
19. Deegen E, et al.: Surgical treatment of a chronic purulent seminal vesiculitis in a stallion. Dtsch Tieraerztl Wschr 86:140, 1979.
20. DeMoor A, Verschooten F: Paramedian incision for the removal of abdominal testicles in the horse. Vet Med/Small Anim Clin 62:1083, 1967.
21. Dietz O, Gangel H, Richter W: Die Sterilisation des Ebers und des Hengstes. Mhefte Vet Med Leipzig 29:906, 1974.
22. Dunn HO, et al.: Two equine true hermaphrodites, with 64,XX/64XY and 63,XO/64,XY chimerism. Cornell Vet 71: 123, 1981.
23. Easley KJ, Genetzky R, Schneider EJ: Management of a deep penis laceration in the horse: A case report. Calif Vet 35 (10): 14, 1981.
24. Finocchio EJ, Merriam JE: Surgical correction of myiasitic urethritis granulosa in the horse. Vet Med/Small Anim Clin 71:1629, 1976.
25. Firth EC: Dissecting hematoma of corpus spongiosum and urinary bladder rupture in a stallion. J Am Vet Med Assoc 169(8):800, 1976.
26. Frank ER: Veterinary Surgery, 7th ed. Minneapolis, Burgess Publishing, 1964, pp 292–294.
27. Frerichs WM: Effect of imidocarb ipropionate and hemicastration on spermatogenesis in pony stallions. Am J Vet Res 38:139, 1977.
28. Ganjam VK, Kenney RM: Androgens and oestrogens in normal and cryptorchid stallions. J Reprod Fertil 23 (Suppl): 67, 1975.
29. Getty R: Sisson and Grossman's Anatomy of the Domestic Animals, 5th ed. Vol. 1. Philadelphia, WB Saunders, 1975, pp 531–541.
30. Goetz TE, Boulton CH, Coffman JR: Inguinal and scrotal hernias in colts and stallions. Comp Continuing Ed 3:S272, 1981.
31. Gygax AP, Donawick WJ, Gledhill BL: Hematocoele in a stallion and recovery of fertility following unilateral castration. Equine Vet J 5:128, 1973.
32. Hall WC, Nielson SW, McEntee K: Tumours of the prostate and penis. Bull WHO 53:247, 1976.
33. Hoffman PE: Castration of normal and cryptorchid horses by a primary closure method. In Proceedings of the Nineteenth American Association of Equine Practitioners, Atlanta, 1973, pp 219–223.
34. Hutchings DR, Rawlinson RJ: Eventration as a sequel to castration of the horse. Aust Vet J 48:288, 1972.
35. Jones WE, Bogart R: Genetics of the horse. East Lansing, Michigan, Caballus Publishers, 1971, pp 241–278.
36. Kirkpatrick J, Turner JW, Perkins A: Reversible chemical fertility control in feral horses. J Equine Vet Sci 2:114, 1982.
37. Lindley WH: Some complications in a series of equine castrations. Mod Vet Pract 63:728, 1982.
38. Lowe JE, Dougherty R: Castration of horses and ponies by a primary closure method. J Am Vet Med Assoc 160:183, 1972.
39. Lowe JE, Higginbotham R: Castration of abdominal cryptorchid horses by a paramedian laparotomy approach. Cornell Vet 59:121, 1969.
40. Lundall RL: The urinary system. In Oehme V, Prier JE (eds): Textbook of Large Animal Surgery. Baltimore, Williams & Wilkins, 1974, p 459.
41. McIlwraith CW, Owen R, Basrur PK: An equine cryptorchid with testicular and ovarian tissue. Equine Vet J 8(4):156, 1976.
42. Merriam JG: Inguinal approach to equine cryptorchidectomy. Vet Med/Small Anim Clin 67:187, 1972.
43. Moore JN, Johnson JH, Garner HE, Traver DS: A case report of inguinal herniorraphy in a stallion. J Equine Med Surg 1:391, 1977.
44. Moore JN, Johnson JH, Tritschler LG, Garner HE: Equine cryptorchidism: Presurgical considerations and surgical management. Vet Surg 7:43, 1978.
45. Moulton JE: Tumors in Domestic Animals, 2nd ed. Berkeley, University of California Press, 1978, Chaps. 10 and 11.
46. Munger RJ, Meagher DM: Surgical repair of a fistula of the urethral diverticulum in a horse. Vet Med/Small Anim Clin 71:96, 1976.
47. Murray DR, Ladds PW, Johnson RH, Pott BW: Metastatic phycomycosis in a horse. J Am Vet Med Assoc 172(7):834, 1978.
48. Nash JG, Voss JL, Squires EL: Urination during ejaculation in a stallion. J Am Vet Med Assoc 176:224, 1980.
49. Nickel R, Schummer A, Seiferle E, Sack WO: The Viscera of the Domestic Mammals. New York, Springer-Verlag, 1973, pp 351–392.
50. Nickels FA: Complications of urogenital surgery. Proceedings of the Annual Convention of the American Association of Equine Practitioners, 1976, pp 261–265.
51. Nyack, Buxton, et al.: Castration of mules by unskilled laymen—Surgical correction of traumatic results.

52. O'Connor JP: Rectal examination of the cryptorchid horse. Irish Vet J 25:129, 1971.
53. Osborne VE: Genital infection of a horse with spirochaetes. Aust Vet J 37:190, 1961.
54. Pascoe JR, Ellenburg TV, Culbertson MR, Jr, Meagher DM: Torsion of the spermatic cord in a horse. J Am Vet Med Assoc 178:242, 1981.
55. Peterson DE: Equine testicular tumors. Equine Vet Sci, 4:25, 1984.
56. Rantanen N: Conditions diagnosed with ultrasound. Equine Vet Sci 4(1):17, 1984.
57. Roberts MC: Ascending urinary tract infection in ponies. Aust Vet J 55:191, 1979.
58. Roberts SJ: Veterinary Obstetrics and Genital Diseases (Theriogenology). Ithaca, NY, published by the author, distributed by Edwards Brothers, Ann Arbor, 1971.
59. Scott EA: A technique for amputation of the equine penis. J Am Vet Med Assoc 168(11):1047, 1976.
60. Selway SJ, Kenney RM, Bergman RV, et al.: Field technique for vasectomy. In Proceedings of 23rd Annual Convention of the American Association of Equine Practitioners, Vancouver, 1977, pp 355–361.
61. Shapiro SR, Balaza IB: Current concepts of the undescended testis. Surg Gynecol Obstet 147:617, 1978.
62. Sharrock AG: Reversal of drug-induced priapism in a gelding by medication. Aust Vet J 58:39, 1982.
63. Shira MJ, Genetzky RM: Equine cryptorchidism. Iowa State Vet 44(2):77, 1982.
64. Sisson S, Grossman JD: Anatomy of the Domestic Animals, 3rd ed. Philadelphia, WB Saunders, 1938.
65. Smith JA: The development and descent of the testis in the horse. Vet Ann 15:156, 1975.
66. Stannic MN: Castration of cryptorchids. Mod Vet Pract 41:30, 1960.
67. Stick JA: Teratoma and cyst formation of the equine cryptorchid testicle. J Am Vet Med Assoc 176:211, 1980.
68. Stick JA: Surgical management of genital habronemiasis in a horse. Vet Med/Small Anim Clin 76:410, 1981.
69. Stick JA, Hoffer RE: Results of cryosurgical treatment of equine penile neoplasms. J Equine Med Surg 2:505, 1978.
70. Stickle RL, Fessler JF: Retrospective study of 350 cases of equine cryptorchidism. J Am Vet Med Assoc 172:343, 1978.
71. Strafuss AC: Squamous cell carcinoma in horses. J Am Vet Med Assoc, 168(1):61, 1976.
72. Sundberg JP, Burnstein T, Page EH, et al.: Neoplasms of Equidae. J Am Vet Med Assoc 170:150, 1977.
73. Swift PN: Castration of a stallion with bilateral abdominal cryptorchidism by flank laparotomy. Aust Vet J 48:472, 1972.
74. Taylor NR: Traumatic balanoposthitis in a yearling Appaloosa colt. Vet Rec 197:154, 1980.
75. Thomas AD: Microfilariasis in the horse. J South Afr Vet Med Assoc 34:17, 1963.
76. Trotter GW, Aanes WA: A complication of cryptorchid castration in three horses. J Am Vet Med Assoc 178:246, 1981.
77. Valdez H, Taylor TS, McLaughlin A, Martin MT: Abdominal cryptorchidectomy in the horse using inguinal extension of the gubernaculum testis. J Am Vet Med Assoc 174:1110, 1979.
78. Vasey JR: Simultaneous presence of a direct and an indirect hernia in a stallion. Aust Vet J 57:418, 1981.
79. Williams PFB: Removal of a urinary calculus from a gelding. NZ Vet J, 27:223, 1979.

Equine Urogenital Systems*

J. T. Vaughan, D.V.M.

Surgery of the reproductive system of the female horse is classified by anatomy and etiology. According to surgical access, the female reproductive system can be divided into the cranial tract, including uterus and ovaries, and caudal tract, composed of the vulva, vagina and cervix. Other systems are involved secondarily. The rectum and colon may be sites of injury or prolapse. The urinary system is subject to obstruction, disruption and malposition. Iliac and uterine arteries may be the source of spontaneous hemorrhage associated with advanced pregnancy. Any component of the system may be affected by neoplasia, surgical infections and congenital anomalies.

*Revised from the original, which appeared in Jennings PB Jr (ed): The Practice of Large Animal Surgery. Philadelphia, WB Saunders Co, 1984, pp 1122–1150.

INJURIES

The caudal tract, including the rectum, vagina and intervening perineum, is more vulnerable to injuries, especially those due to foaling, than is the cranial tract (Fig. 1). Other causes are accidental injury to the rectum during manual examinations of the pelvic and abdominal viscera or accidental injury to either the rectum or the vagina by the stallion (misdirected intromission or mismatched size) by overly forceful correction of dystocias and malicious acts of sadism. These injuries may be retroperitoneal and confined to the pelvic space, or they may extend by perforation into the peritoneal cavity. A second consideration is the transmural migration of infection in the pelvis into the peritoneal cavity. Therefore, a pelvic abscess that results from a retroperitoneal injury of the rectum or vagina may extend with little opposition into the peritoneal cavity and result in a localized pubic or inguinal abscess or a generalized peritonitis.

Injuries to the cervix and uterus are almost invariably dystocial, whether delivery is natural or assisted. The cervix is either stretched or torn, and, as with any sphincter injury, valvular function is compromised. The divided circular muscle fibers retract, and the injured surfaces heal by epithelialization without reunion. The result can be permanent incompetence of the sphincter.

The uterine injury takes the form of rupture or hemorrhage. Somewhat different from hemorrhage following the other injuries, consequential hemorrhage from uterine vessels (intra- or extramural) is usually spontaneous and preparturient. Owing to

Figure 1. Anatomy of the caudal tract. *Left,* Rectum (A), cervix (B), anus (C), vagina (D), perineal body (E), urinary bladder (F), urethral orifice (G), vestibule (H), vulva (I), clitoris in fossa clitoridis (J), fossa clitoridis (K), fossa glandis (L). (After Nickel R, et al.: The Viscera of the Domestic Mammals. New York, Springer-Verlag, 1973, pp 351–392.) *Right,* Uterus (A), cervix (B), mesometrium (C), urinary bladder (D), transverse fold (E), external urethral orifice (F), clitoris (G), fossa clitoridis (H), vulva (I). (After Sisson S, Grossman JD: The Anatomy of the Domestic Animals. 3rd ed. Philadelphia, WB Saunders Co, 1983.)

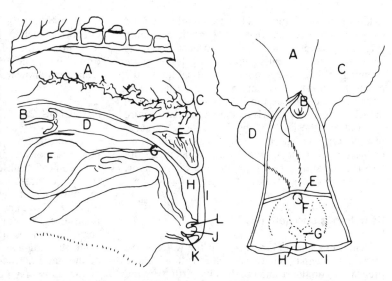

the diffuse placentation, this is more of a problem in mares than in cows.

DISPLACEMENTS

Complications of pregnancy and parturition are uterine torsions, rectal and uterine prolapses, eversions of the urinary bladder, and eventrations through ruptures in the rectal prolapse or through vaginal tears. All except uterine torsion are associated with tenesmus. Of course, rectal prolapse can occur in either sex and from causes other than parturition.

A more insidious displacement is that of splanchnoptosis in the older pluriparous mare, in which the normal caudoventrad slope of the vagina changes to horizontal or cranioventrad. This reverses the gradient of urine flow and results in vesicovaginal reflux with retention of voided urine in the vaginal fornix. Selected cases may respond to urethroplasty, which creates an extension of the urethra beyond the dividing line of outflow versus inflow.

SPACE-OCCUPYING LESIONS

Neoplasms, cysts, abscesses, hematomas, granulomas and seromas account for the majority of these lesions. Diagnosis is established on the basis of paracentesis and biopsy as well as physical characteristics and location.

Neoplasms

Neoplasms are divided into those of the female tubular genital tract, the ovaries, the cutaneous perineum, and the mammary gland. Tumors (neoplasms and cysts) described in the mare have included adenoma of the uterine tube (oviduct); paramesonephric (Müllerian) duct cysts of the fimbria; fibrosarcoma, leiomyosarcoma, and lymphosarcoma

of the uterus and cervix; cystic hyperplasia of the endometrium; lymphangiectasia in the ventral part of the body of the uterus in aged mares; mesonephric duct cysts of the mesometrium and myometrium; squamous metaplasia of the surface endometrium in pyometra; squamous cell carcinoma, malignant melanoma, fibrosarcoma, hemangioma and hemangiosarcoma of the vagina and vulva; and carcinoma of the mammary gland.[60, 68]

Tumors of the ovary of the mare receive the most attention owing to their relatively greater incidence and their effects on fertility and psychological behavior. The most common by far is the granulosa cell tumor of sex cord–stromal origin.[29, 62, 68, 71] This tumor is typically unilateral and may be diagnosed fortuitously or upon examination because of infertility or abnormal behavior, as might be characterized by hypersecretion of estrogen and/or androgen.[56, 68] Teratoma is the second most common tumor and can be presumptively diagnosed on palpation per rectum by its hardness and irregular surface (having points and edges). Malignant tumors are represented by cystadenocarcinomas and secondary (metastatic) lymphosarcomas. The only common ovarian cysts in the mare are the subsurface epithelial (germinal) cysts and parovarian cysts of the mesovarium and mesosalpinx. Graafian follicle cysts are of clinical importance in the cow and sow, but not in the mare, and are frequently misdiagnosed.[71]

Focal lesions of the uterus are occasionally confused with early pregnancy on palpation per rectum. Examples are muscular atrophy, focal myometrial atonia, myometrial lymphatic lacunae and endometrial cysts. These are mainly diagnostic problems and fall more in the province of theriogenology than surgery; however, reference to surgical removal of endometrial cysts has been made.[56]

Abscesses

The abscess of greatest clinical importance is the pelvic abscess, which usually originates from injury to the vagina or rectum and less frequently is caused by wounds to the base of the tail or the perineum (Fig. 2). Abscesses are usually suspected on the basis of a stormy course marked by fever, pain, straining, pelvic phlegmon (often apparent in the perineal region), constipation and dysuria. Additionally, there may be the history of a penetrating or lacerating injury. Pelvic examination may require epidural anesthesia and general sedation. Paracentesis is confirmatory. One case revealed adhesions of the colon to the vagina around a necrotic core and a fecal fistula perforating into the vaginal floor. The mare had recently been delivered of a dystocia.

Hematomas and Seromas

Hematoma and seroma occur in the walls of the uterus and vagina and are associated with advanced pregnancy and the trauma of difficult birth. Circumscribed hematoma of the vaginal wall may be confused with vascular tumors and varices. Hematocyst has been diagnosed in the ovary, but great care must be exercised to avoid mistaking this for the unilocular cystic granulosa cell tumor. Pelvic hematoma has been seen in the barren mare. This is due to spontaneous rupture of vessels and also to laceration or rupture of the pelvic vasculature, e.g., the obturator artery by sharp bone splinters and pelvic fracture. The significance of hematomas extends the full range of the spectrum from incidental findings to life-threatening events.

Granulomas

Granulomas of a chronic, inflammatory nature may arise from external parasitisms, such as cutaneous habronemiasis of the vulva, or from internal infections, such as staphylococcal botryomycosis of the cervix. Identification requires differentiation from the common neoplasms of the region, notably melanoma and carcinoma.

PHYSIOLOGICAL SURGERY

Not fitting any pathologic classification of diagnoses but constituting important categories of what has been called physiologic surgery are the cesarean section (cesarotomy) and the bilateral ovariectomy for purposes of neutering. Indications for cesarotomy are the immutable dystocias that do not lend themselves to fetotomy. These include the transverse lie or presentation of the fetus during labor when the long axis of its body crosses the long axis of the maternal body and cases in which the ends of the fetus may occupy both horns of the uterus. Certain fetal monsters may pose problems for nonoperative means of delivery, such as the hydrocephalus, in which a greatly enlarged calvarium may resist the most strenuous efforts to reduce the size to one compatible with the pelvic diameter. Perosomus and multiple arthrogryposis are examples of other monsters.[81] An occasional indication for cesarotomy is delivery of a live foal when normal birth is prevented by pelvic deformity, uterine torsion or other mechanical obstacles or in emergency delivery from a mare that has just died.

Bilateral ovariectomy is performed to neuter the mare valued only for work to eliminate the undesirable periods of estrus and also to correct the ungovernable behavior of the chronic nymphomaniac. It is important to the prognosis to understand that although bilateral ovariectomy assures sterility, it does not promise altered behavior. The prospects

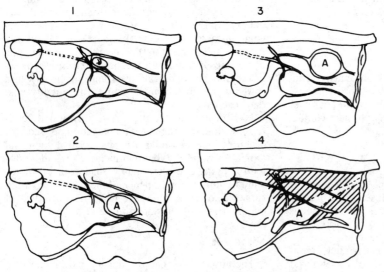

Figure 2. Pelvic abscess. *1,* The pelvic viscera in normal relationships. *2A,* A pelvic abscess in the vesicogenital pouch, partially obstructing the urethra and causing distention of the urinary bladder. *3A,* A pelvic abscess in the rectogenital pouch, partially obstructing the rectum and interfering with defecation, owing to pain as well as space occupied. *4A,* A pelvic abscess originating from a perineal wound and migrating forward to the pubic region. Access for drainage would be in the pubic or inguinal regions. Shaded zone represents widespread pelvic cellulitis. Urination and defecation compromised.

are favorable in the normal mare and in the mare with a mild type of chronic nymphomania. In the severe type, viciousness and other unacceptable behaviors are apt to be so ingrained as to make the mare incorrigible even after surgery. The risk of injury to life and limb of personnel and the undesirable influence on other livestock may dictate euthanasia as the practical alternative. Recovery of desirable traits in nymphomaniac mares has been quoted as 60 per cent successful after spaying. Interestingly, the ovaries recovered from such mares may display no abnormalities or may be small and atretic, as opposed to the enlarged follicular cysts that often attend nymphomania in cows.[81]

Surgery of the Caudal Tract

Procedures fall into two categories: (1) revision or reconstruction of structural defects (lacerations, sphincteric incompetence, fistulae, splanchnoptosis, adhesions, displacements and anomalies) and (2) extirpation and drainage of space-occupying lesions (neoplasms, cysts, abscesses and hematomas). The vulvovaginal procedures account for the majority of such operations. These include (1) episioplasty (Caslick operation) for faulty conformation and first and second degree injuries to the dorsal commissure of the vulva and the perineal body and (2) reconstruction of third-degree perineal lacerations and rectovaginal fistulae.

Foaling injuries to the caudal tract are graded first, second or third degree in order of increasing severity. First-degree injuries involve the mucosa of the ceiling of the vestibule and the dorsal commissure of the vulva, including the skin. Disruption of underlying muscle bundles is minimal. Second-degree injuries involve stretching or disruption of the vulvovestibular musculature, especially in the perineal body but sparing the rectal floor and anal sphincter. Third-degree injuries occur usually in the primipara when hard labor contractions force the foal's foot upward at such an angle as to catch in the dorsal transverse membranous fold of the vaginovestibular junction. If the foot is retrieved and the malposition is corrected in time, only a fistula results. If not, the foot (feet) extends through the rectovaginal septum into the rectal lumen and in the ensuing course of labor traumatically divides the perineal body, anus, vulva and cutaneous perineum.

Episioplasty

The Caslick operation was initially introduced as a means of reducing the size of the mucocutaneous cleft of the vulva to prevent aspiration of air associated with ascending tract infections. However, the concept of this operation has since been expanded to include repair of the compromised function of the constrictor muscles of the vulva and vestibule, which serve, together with the labia, as the first line

of defense against the environment, especially around the perineum. One has only to compare the vulvovestibular characteristics of the normal tract with those of the chronic windsucker to appreciate the functional deficit in the latter case. When the labia of the normal tract are parted (overriding the constrictor vulvae muscle), the constrictor vestibulae still provides closure of the vestibule. This is especially apparent by the closure effected at the vaginovestibular junction just craniad to the urethral orifice and at the site of the hymen. The efficacy of this function of the hymenal ring in the young, healthy mare has been demonstrated time and time again by the ability of some animals to be bred successfully despite third-degree perineal lacerations or rectovaginal fistulae that were located caudad to the vaginovestibular junction. In the chronic windsucker, however, the vulva may stand open; or if closed, the simple act of parting the labia will usually provoke aspiration of air, as no effective valvular action remains in the vestibule.

One of the common causes of pneumovagina is the injury to the perineal body sustained at parturition, particularly the dystocia that produces a first- or second-degree laceration. The circular muscles forming the sphincters of the anus, vulva and vestibule cross each other in the rectovaginal septum, and the primary intersection of these decussating bundles of smooth muscle is the perineal body. On sagittal section, the cut surface has roughly the shape of a right-angle triangle, with the base being the cutaneous perineum, the hypotenuse the ceiling of the vestibule, and the perpendicular the floor of the rectum.[69] When these muscle fibers are disrupted ("lacerated"), they retract on themselves. Despite the rapid healing that results from granulation and epithelialization, spontaneous reunion of sphincters does not occur, and the function is either diminished or lost altogether. The first line of defense to the outside environment has been violated, and restoration usually requires reconstructive surgery.

Successive parturitions may be expected to add to problems that were minimal at the outset; therefore, pneumovagina is a greater problem in the aging mare than in the young animal. Not infrequently, the sagging viscera (splanchnoptosis) associated with gradual stretching of mesometrium and enlargement of the abdominal cavity is an attendant feature that may necessitate urethroplasty concurrently with episioplasty. Other contributing factors include malnutrition, parasitism, dysmasesis and other chronic problems that cause a deterioration in the constitution, resulting in weight loss and generalized atony of smooth and skeletal musculature. The desired outcome from reconstructive surgery is partially dependent on the successful management of the constitutional disease.

The complexity of surgical repair somewhat parallels the grade of injury or conformational defect. The conventional Caslick operation suffices for the majority of juvenile windsuckers (racing fillies) and mares with comparatively minor malconformation of the vulva, e.g., inversion of one labium, separation of labia, or sloping perineum. Using local anesthesia, the edges of the labia are infiltrated with 2 per cent lidocaine hydrochloride. A narrow (6 to 8 mm) strip of mucous membrane is removed with scissors from the mucocutaneous junction at the edges of both labia from the dorsal commissure down to a level just below the bony floor of the pelvis. The raw margins are apposed with a single row of simple continuous suture using 00 polypropylene monofilament swaged on a general closure needle (or the equivalent).

The repair will approximate a fraction of the vulvar cleft and is subject to the degree of correction required by the individual animal. Closure should not be so extensive, however, as to cause dysuria. Also, if breed association regulations require a natural cover, the opening must be sufficient to allow for intromission. It is customary to culture or biopsy the uterus and to treat for existing infections prior to doing the Caslick operation, although treatment by intrauterine infusions through a vaginal cylinder can be done after the surgery. In this case, as in breeding, the repair can be protected from accidental dehiscence with a single mattress tension suture (breeder's stitch) of 0.6-mm Vetafil suture (or equivalent) taken at the lowest point of the closure, exercising caution against tying it too tightly, causing a stitch abscess, or so loosely that the exposed limb of suture abrades the dorsal surface of the penis during breeding. A breeding roll is used to limit the depth of intromission, protecting both the mare and the stallion. Skin sutures are removed upon healing in about 10 days. The breeder's stitch is removed when treatments are discontinued or upon termination of breeding. The closure line should be opened, usually with scissors or a blunt-pointed bistoury, just prior to foaling. If the mare foals through the unopened Caslick closure, irregular tears may result, and the repair is unnecessarily complicated.

Episioplasty for second-degree injuries and more extensive defects requires special dissection and reconstruction of the perineal body and ceiling of the vestibule as well as the dorsal commissure of the vulva. The operation is done on the standing patient, tranquilized and restrained in stocks. Local anesthesia of the cutaneous perineum and vestibule up to the depth of the hymenal ring is provided by epidural injection of approximately 6 to 7 ml of 2 per cent lidocaine or mepivacaine hydrochloride in mares weighing approximately 450 kg. If additional anesthesia is required, local infiltration (field block) of the ischiorectal region will usually suffice. No change in feeding routine is necessary since the rectum is not involved; therefore, this repair can be scheduled at the convenience of the surgeon, paying attention to the condition of the specific tissues and the total patient.

The objective of the dissection is to expose a triangular area of the dorsal aspect of the defect to conform to the sagittal sectional area of the perineal body or to the amount that has been disrupted in the estimation of the surgeon. Exposure for the submucous resection requires dorsal retraction of the tail and dorsal commissure and bilateral retraction of the labia. The lines of incision through the mucous membrane can be drawn with the scalpel in the shape of the right-angle triangle previously described. The mucous membrane is elevated by tissue forceps and scissor or scalpel dissection for a distance of about 10 cm craniad from the edge of the labium. This should approximate the length of the vestibule and reach the vicinity of the vaginovestibular junction. Suture closure of the triangulated field starts in the forwardmost depths of the wound with interrupted bites of 0 or 00 surgical gut or polyglycolic acid (PGA) placed in a quilting pattern out to the line of mucosal incision.

A variation is described by Gadd[41] in which the submucous resection is done in a continuous field, finally removing a V-shaped gore to create the desired area for apposition (Fig. 3). The cut edges of mucosa are closed in the initial line of sutures, and the exposed face of the perineal body is approximated with successive rows of buried interrupted sutures using 0 or 00 PGA sutures or equivalent.

Skin closure for reconstruction of the commissure defect is made with 00 polypropylene in an interrupted vertical mattress pattern. Aftercare consists of tetanus immunization, systemic antibiotic therapy for 72 hours, maintenance of wound hygiene and removal of skin sutures in about 10 days. Natural breeding can resume when uterine cultures are negative.

Repair of Third-Degree Perineal Lacerations

Surgery involving the rectum requires adjustment of the diet so that the bowel movement becomes soft and reduced in volume. Painful or difficult defecation (dyschezia) is as responsible as errors of technique for surgical failure. Straining on defecation subjects the wound repair to excessive tension, and dehiscence results. Crash diets and laxatives are used to soften the feces but are less preferred than natural means, notably pelleted feeds, which have a tendency to produce a softer bowel movement, and bran mashes, long used for this effect. The advantage of pelleted feeds is that they furnish a balanced ration. On the other hand, if the mare is in constitutionally good health when placed on a diet, no adverse effects will result from feeding bran mashes for the 3 weeks usually required. It is also recommended that the change from the regular feed to pelleted feed or bran mash be done gradually over at least a period of 1 week to prevent any digestive disturbance that might otherwise occur. The day of surgery is scheduled at the discretion of the surgeon when the bowel movement is judged to be sufficiently soft and reduced in volume for the procedure. It must be kept this way for at least 2 weeks postoperatively, accounting for a total time of about 3 weeks on a restricted diet. Twenty-four

Figure 3. The Gadd modification episioplasty. *1,* Anus (A), dorsal commissure of vulva (B), line of incision of submucous resection (C), dissected flap of vulval mucosa reflected ventrally (D), vaginovestibular junction (orifice) (E), urethral orifice (F), floor of vestibule (G), fossa clitoridis (H), ventral commissure of vulva (I). *2D,* Redundant flap resected. *3C,* Cut edges of resected mucous flap apposed by first row of deep sutures. *4E,* Cut surfaces of perineal body exposed by submucous resection and apposed by second row of deep sutures. *5E,* Episioplasty completed by apposing incised margins of labia with third row of sutures. (After Gadd JW: Proc 21st Ann Con Am Assn Equine Prac, Boston, 1975, pp 362–368.)

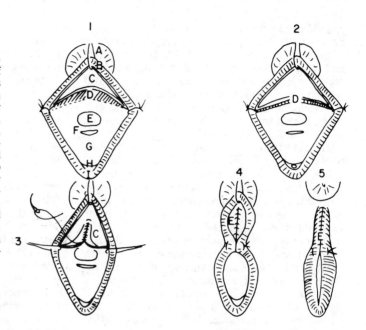

hours prior to surgery, the mare is given a 1-gallon mineral oil gavage, and feed is withheld for the last 12 hours. It is misinformed to suggest that mineral oil is contraindicated because of possible interference with healing. This is no more true than the suggestion that intestinal resection and anastomosis are precluded in animals with intestinal obstruction that have been treated for colic with mineral oil. Nevertheless, the idea crops up from time to time, usually to support the argument for saline cathartics or for dihydroxyanthraquinone. It is enough to say that the argument strains the evidence.

The second requirement for successful surgery is the health of the tissues at the wound site. At the time of initial injury, the tissues are somewhat atonic and edematous in preparation for parturition. Although commonly referred to as a laceration, the tissues are not sharply divided but are literally torn apart, often in eccentric planes. If there is a delay of as long as 4 to 6 hours between the time of injury and the repair, the tissues become even more edematous and desiccated on the surface. Irregular tags of tissue become devitalized, and the superficial layers become infected. Repairs attempted at this time will not be very successful. Careful observations of both natural and experimental wounds show that 3 to 4 weeks are required for the host's natural defense and repair mechanisms to return the tissues to a degree of health to support primary healing of an elective surgical procedure. Therefore, if circumstances do not favor reconstruction at the time of injury, the next opportunity occurs about 1 month later. Then, if the foal survived the delivery, there is the choice as to whether or not to subject the youngster to the enforced confinement necessitated by the strict diet imposed on the mare as well as to the hazards, noxious influences and nosocomial infections to which foals are so susceptible. Sound

judgment opposes this option in favor of postponing the surgery until the foal is weaned, which may be done as early as 3 to 4 months of age with the help of milk formula and dietary supplements for the suckling. By waiting an additional 6 to 8 weeks beyond the earliest advisable date, the wound will have undergone further healing by contraction and differentiation. The defect at 12 weeks is significantly smaller than at 4 weeks, and the tissues are better able to respond to surgery. The same thing is true of rectovaginal fistulae, which may reduce in diameter to a surprising degree in even 1 month, improving the chances for successful repair. In fact, some fistulae may heal spontaneously during the waiting period.

A note of precaution: a small percentage of foaling injuries may cause sufficient pelvic irritability that resultant straining predisposes to complications such as prolapse of pelvic viscera and even rupture with eventration or hemorrhage. For this reason, the mare should be kept under close observation and given daily care for the first week or so after injury, even if she is turned out to pasture thereafter. This can avert the occasional statistic of a mare that is sent home to wait for 6 weeks for elective surgery only to become the victim of major complications a day or two later. Referral clinics should have good communications and clear understanding with both practitioner and owner as to what is involved in postponement of surgery.

The surgery is done with the animal standing, preferably using restraint provided by stocks. The rectum is emptied by hand and cleansed with a mild antiseptic wash that is safe for use on mucous surfaces. A low enema can be used but should precede the epidural block. Local anesthesia is by epidural injection as previously described under Episioplasty. One injection usually suffices for the one to one and one-half hours required for surgery. Some like to leave a spinal needle indwelling for additional anesthetic, if needed. The tail is wrapped and reflected dorsally. The defect is retracted laterally by tension sutures placed in the margins of the old wound and anchored in the hairline over the ischiatic area on either side. The kickboard, sides of the stocks, and the hind quarters peripheral to the field should be draped.

The defect extends caudally from the vaginovestibular junction in the ceiling of the vestibule in almost every case. The field should be well-lighted to facilitate dissection and suturing. The dissection is made in a frontal plane starting in the shelf, which is the remains of the rectovaginal septum in the forwardmost part of the defect. The shelf should be split from side to side, leaving the rectal floor as thick as possible to support suture closure. Dissection by both scissors and scalpel is aided by placing the tissues in tension with forceps. The plane started in the shelf is continued around on either side at the line of junction of healing of the rectal and vaginal mucosa, recognizable by the slight difference in color of the two mucous membranes. This junctional incision is deepened into the sides of the defect sufficiently to free rectal and vaginal (vestibular) flaps on each side that can be brought together in the middle without tension. Inattention to this most important step is thought to be a common cause of failure. The bilateral dissection is extended to the cutaneous perineum with a modification in the posterior half, consisting of a triangulated submucous resection over the cut face of the perineal body as described under the repair of second-degree perineal lacerations in the section on Episioplasty. This part of the dissection can be deferred until the anterior half of the wound has been reconstructed under suture. This ensures a fresher and less contaminated tissue surface for suture closure.

The suture pattern in the cranial part of the dissection is the modified Goetze pattern, after Straub and Fowler (1961).[92] All these sutures are interrupted, nonabsorbable, noncapillary synthetic sutures placed no more than 1 to 1.5 cm apart with a curved needle. The first two sutures are placed as vertical mattress bites ahead of the defect, so as to create a fold in the margins of the defect that will merge smoothly into the apposed surfaces. Closure of the defect is made with a six-bite vertical suture that starts in the left vaginal flap at least 3 cm from the margin; goes directly upward into the left rectal flap, emerging at the submucosal margin *without* perforating the mucosa; reenters the right rectal flap at the same spot, emerging at least 3 cm from the margin; goes directly downward through the right vaginal flap, 3 cm from the margin; and then turns medially to pass through the near margins of the vaginal flaps to be tied by hand (not instrument) on the left side of the now apposed vaginal defect. The suture material should have tensile strength sufficient to permit ties snug enough to effect intimate apposition of the rectal margins with *no* exposed suture, either visible or palpable. Failure to do this may cause fistulization or total dehiscence of the repair. The principle of repair is much the same as that required by a milk fistula or laceration through the teat canal of a dairy cow.

Repair of the perineal body, exposed by the triangular submucous resection, is the same as that described for the second-degree laceration except that the wound in the rectum and anus must be closed. The use of Ob-Gyn gut or PGA gut in this area gives a stronger, longer-lasting closure; however, others report the successful use of buried polypropylene sutures.[91] The cutaneous perineum is repaired as described under Episioplasty. The skin sutures and the nonabsorbable synthetic sutures tied inside the vagina (vestibule) are removed in 11 to 14 days. No anesthetic is required for the usual case. The reconstruction is completed in one operation. Despite variations in wound characteristics,[45] it has not been necessary to resort to the phased procedures[1, 2] to achieve primary healing.

Postoperative care consists of the use of prophylactic antibiotics for 5 to 7 days, mainly to guard against stitch abscesses that might predispose to fistulae. Pelvic phlegmon and fascial abscess have not been common problems. Dyschezia is an occasional problem in the mare that may have been operated on for the second or third time, but this complication can usually be averted by reducing the colon content and maintaining a laxative bowel movement during the 2 weeks after surgery. This is not an inconvenience to either the mare or the manager.

Splanchnoptosis and urine reflux are unusual in the primipara; therefore, it is anticipated that the majority of such cases that benefit from primary healing on the first try can be returned to breeding. It is a consideration, however, to provide attendance on successive parturitions.

Repair of Rectovaginal Fistula

Preparation parallels that for repair of the third-degree laceration. The dissection is made in the frontal plane in its entirety. The skin incision extends from side to side between the buttocks and midway between the anus and the vulva. Thereafter the perineal body and rectovaginal septum are split sideways in the same fashion, so as to separate the rectum from the vagina (vestibule) to a point 2 to 3 cm beyond the fistula. The thickness of the rectal floor is maintained at the expense of the vaginal roof. The rectal fistula is closed transversely, i.e., at right angles to the long axis of the rectum, which is in alignment with the principal lines of stress when the rectum contracts in peristalsis. This is done in essentially the same way as the Heineke-Mikulicz operation for pyloroplasty by preplacing a series of interrupted Lembert sutures (0 or 1 surgical gut or PGA). The first suture bisects the fistula, the next two divide the halves into quarters, and the next four divide the quarters into eighths until intimate closure has been effected. The sutures are tied in the same sequence. This is repeated on the vaginal fistula except that the closure is oriented on the longitudinal rather than the transverse plane. After both fistulae have been closed, the divided septum and perineum are reunited with a series of interrupted fine gut sutures placed out to the cutaneous perineum, which is closed with mattress skin sutures. There is little tension on this part of the reconstruction, and high tensile strength sutures are not required. Postoperative care is the same as for the third-degree laceration.

There are occasional references made to conversion of fistulae to third-degree lacerations for use of repair techniques adapted to the latter injury. This is justified if the fistula has healed (see earlier description) and still remains so large as to impose an unusual tax on the conventional fistula repair. In such cases, the perineum that remains intact may be a narrow isthmus of tissue, which makes the wound a fistula only in a technical sense. Often this is the result of previous unsuccessful attempts to reconstruct a third-degree laceration. Therefore, in these instances, conversion to a full-fledged third-degree laceration is merely a technicality. However, if the characteristics of the fistula do not conform to these exceptions, the defect should be operated as a fistula in accordance with the principles of Forssell described more than 50 years ago.

Urethroplasty

For relief of splanchnoptosis and urine reflux, two surgical procedures are currently favored—the episioplasty and the urethroplasty. The first operation was introduced more than 40 years ago,[37] the second a little more than 10 years ago.[65] Since then, both procedures have been adopted by the profession and have undergone some modifications.

The urethroplasty is a revisionary technique for caudal extension of the urethra[22] in the mare that has been rendered infertile at least partially because of vesicovaginal reflux with retention of voided urine in the vaginal fornix. Chronic cervicitis and endometritis are the expected consequences. Understandably, the competence of the vulvovestibular closure and the morphologic condition of the endometrium must be carefully assessed[55] before predicting the benefits of urethroplasty. This done, the mare is prepared and anesthetized for pelvic surgery in the standing position as described in the previous section. The labia are retracted by stay sutures or self-retaining retractors. Two procedures have been described.

The Monin technique[65] fixes the transverse membranous fold overlying the external urethral orifice in a posterior position by denuding the lateral edges of the retracted fold and suturing these edges to similarly denuded recipient sites along the sides of the floor of the vestibule. Caution is observed to provide a channel large enough to prevent dysuria. Intimate apposition of tissue avoids fistula formation. A continuous suture pattern with 00 polypro-

pylene, Ob-Gyn gut, or PGA material is satisfactory. Prophylactic antibiotics are recommended. A healing time of about 2 weeks is required. Success is based on the disappearance of urine pooling in the cranial vagina. Treatment of endometritis and correction of vulvovestibular incompetence must be managed separately, often concurrently for return of breeding soundness.

The Brown technique[22] may be likened to the surgical separation of the rectum from the vagina in the reconstruction of the third-degree perineal laceration (Fig. 4). The shelf is the membranous fold overlying the urethra. This is split from side to side, extending the incision bilaterally along the sides of the vestibular floor backward to about 3 cm from the labial margins. The plane of dissection is deepened to free flaps, dorsal and ventral, of mucous membrane. These flaps are then brought together in the middle by two or three layers of sutures to construct a membranous extension of the urethra back to the vulvar cleft. Number 00 polypropylene or PGA suture material in continuous, mattress patterns is used to appose the cut mucous edges in eversion. The third (optional) layer can be used in the submucosa between the two mucosal layers for added support in case there is tension on the suture line. Postoperative procedures are the same as for the Monin technique. Breeding thereafter has been accomplished by both natural and artificial means.

Pouret (1982)[77] advanced a technique for correction of pneumo- and urovagina that employs a frontal plane of dissection originating midway between the anus and vulva and extending craniad 8 to 12 cm after the fashion of the Forssell approach to correction of rectovaginal fistula. Presumably, this plane of dissection undergoes cicatricial contraction upon healing, taking up some of the slack, as it were, in the vestibule and vulva.

Repair of Vaginal Adhesions and Anomalies

Partitioning defects of the vagina occur as congenital anomalies as well as traumatic adhesions (Fig. 5). They may be two-dimensional or three-dimensional, longitudinal or transverse. They cause diagnostic problems and may or may not be surgically remediable.

Longitudinal bands in the sagittal plane are usually identified as persistent median walls of the embryonic Müllerian duct system. They may be discovered fortuitously upon a routine examination, and since they may present a mechanical obstacle to breeding or foaling, these bands should be excised. This is done most simply under local or no anesthesia (craniad to the hymenal ring) with long-handled dissecting scissors to sever the band at its junctions with the vaginal floor and ceiling. Hemorrhage is negligible, and healing occurs by second intention.

Transverse, two-dimensional partitions may be

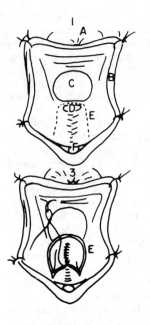

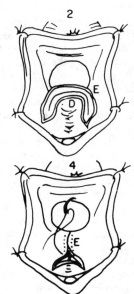

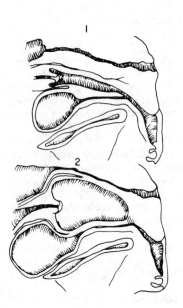

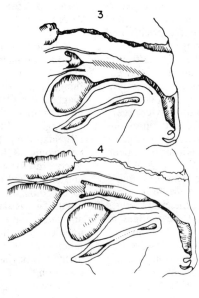

Figure 4. Urethroplasty according to Brown and colleagues. *1,* Anus (A), labium of vulva (B), vaginovestibular junction (C), urethral orifice (D), line of proposed incision in mucosa of floor of vestibule (E), clitoris (F). *2,* Urethral orifice (under reflected edge of mucosa) (D). Line of incision completed (E). *3,* Inner (inferior) edge of mucosa apposed with first row of sutures to create urethral extension (E). *4,* Outer (superior) edge of mucosa apposed with second row of sutures to complete urethral extension (E). (After Brown MP, Colahan PT, Hawkins DG: JAVMA 173:1005, 1978.)

congenital or acquired. The persistent hymen is the congenital form, usually broken by the first breeding or speculum examination and rarely requiring surgery. The imperforate hymen is uncommon, may be attended by mucometra or at least some accumulation of mucous secretions and detritus, and, in such cases, requires surgery. Traumatic adhesions may mimic imperforate hymen in every respect, with the possible exception of bacteria in the trapped secretions. This may justify the designation in some cases of pyometra, although the typical example of pyometra includes adhesions of the cervix rather than of the vagina.

Demonstration of the two-dimensional characteristics may be done by palpation per rectum and per

vaginam as well as by needle test puncture and aspiration. Under local anesthesia and suitable preoperative preparation, the partition is incised from quadrant to quadrant, and the four flaps of redundant tissue created by the cruciate incision are excised by scissors, scalpel, or electric scalpel. Retraction of the labia and illumination of the field are essential. If a large volume of mucus and/or exudate has been trapped in the uterus and vagina, tenesmus may be a prominent clinical sign, and heavy sedation as well as epidural anesthesia may be required to facilitate surgery. Also, it may be advisable to drain such accumulations by indwelling catheter or release incisions as part of the preparations for surgery. This, in itself, may suffice to

Figure 5. Adhesions of the caudal tract. *1,* Sagittal section of the normal tract. *2,* Two-dimensional adhesion of the vaginovestibular junction (diagonal lined area), with distention of vagina and uterus by entrapped fluids and detritus. Evacuation of rectum and urinary bladder is also compromised as depicted by distention. *3,* Three-dimensional adhesion of the vagina (diagonal lined area). *4,* Adhesion of cervix with pyometra or mucometra.

control the violent straining. If dysuria is an attendant problem, an indwelling balloon catheter may also be desirable. If the urinary catheter is to remain postoperatively, it should be fitted with a one-way valve (such as a split latex glove finger) to prevent aspiration of air and contaminants into the bladder—the unavoidable cause of ascending infection if this feature is overlooked.

Three-dimensional adhesions must be distinguished by medical history from the segmental aplasia of the tubular tract that is seen occasionally. Since neither problem is common, diagnosis may be confusing unless it is established that the patient is or is not a maiden mare. The only likely explanation for an acquired defect other than injury by dystocia would be by breeding or a malicious act (sadism).

Correction is accomplished either by restoration of the preexisting lumen or, when this is not possible, by ovariohysterectomy. Mechanical breakdown of adhesions must be done under local anesthesia on the standing patient with the organs suspended in situ and free of the intraabdominal pressures present in the recumbent position that displace and compress the pelvic viscera. Alternatively, recumbent positioning would require cranioventral tilt to displace the abdominal viscera forward. Fibrolysis is done primarily by scissor dissection, spreading, and cutting, as adhesions are distinguished from the vaginal wall. The urethra should be identified by catheter and the bladder evacuated to avoid accidental injury. The rectum should be emptied and cleansed to permit periodic palpation per rectum. The dissection must be followed closely by manual palpation to maintain proper orientation with the cervix, which is, of course, obscured from view in such cases. The tract should be reentered manually at regular intervals during the convalescence to prevent cicatricial constriction and recurrence of adhesions before epithelialization is complete. Hysterectomy for segmental aplasia with mucometra is discussed under the surgery of the cranial tract.

Repair of Prolapses

Prolapses of the caudal tract can be ranked in order of importance as rectal, uterine and vesical. Rectal prolapse may or may not occur as complications of urogenital disease but usually results from some cause of straining, such as dystocia or pelvic irritability, e.g., an inflammatory or space-occupying lesion. Initially, rectal prolapse may be described as a proctitis complicated by edema of the rectal mucosa that bulges and protrudes through the anus. If treatment is prompt and the cause, such as dyschezia, corrected, the problem responds to conservative care. If neglected, the problem can lead to prolapse of the small colon. Turner and Fessler classified four types of prolapse: (1) mucosal prolapse, (2) complete prolapse, (3) complete prolapse with invagination of the colon, and (4) intussusception of the peritoneal rectum or colon through

the anus. The segmental blood supply to the terminal small colon and rectum resembles that of the esophagus in that collateral circulation is comparatively poor, and if the tissue bed and terminal mesocolon are sufficiently disrupted so as to compromise the blood supply, infarction results unless the involved bowel is resected. For this reason, replacement of sizable rectal prolapses and pursestring suture of the anus are not high on the list of successful treatment modalities in the horse. Certainly, if this "conservative" course of management is elected, the condition of the rectum and of the total patient should be carefully monitored for at least the postoperative week. A more cautious course in such cases would be intraoperative evaluation of the small colon by laparotomy, with colostomy a consideration if the viability of the colon was in question.[20]

Fortunately, the majority of cases requiring surgery can be handled by submucosal resection. Done under epidural anesthesia, a ring of the prolapsed and edematous mucosa and submucosa is dissected free from the underlying tissue. The healthy margins of anus and rectum are joined first with a row of interrupted horizontal mattress sutures of No. 2 medium chromic surgical gut. Then the mucosal edges are apposed with a second row of No. 3–0 PGA suture in a simple continuous pattern interrupted at the quadrants. Tension on the dissection and reconstruction is relieved by skewering the prolapsed portion with two 6-inch, 18-gauge spinal needles passed through the base from 12 to 6 o'clock and from 9 to 3 o'clock. After suture closure is complete, the needles are removed and the repaired anatomy allowed to return inside the anus. Pursestring suture of 0.6- to 0.8-mm Vetafil or equivalent can be used with caution, understanding that such sutures meet with somewhat less success in horses than in cattle. Straining must be controlled with maintenance of a laxative bowel movement (mineral oil) and tranquilizers, sedatives, analgesics and nonsteroidal anti-inflammatories PRN for up to 1 week after surgery. Systemic antibiotics and tetanus immunization are also mandatory.[96]

When amputation is required, the technique should closely follow the principles of intestinal resection and anastomosis. The procedure is performed under epidural anesthesia if possible, and the site of anastomosis is near the cutaneous anus. Stay sutures of umbilical tape or the needle skewers are used to cross the diameter of the bowel at the four quadrants. These serve to stabilize the tissues for further dissection and to orient even suture placement. It may be necessary to open the prolapse lengthwise for a distance to provide access to the interior wall for accurate suturing. An interrupted mattress pattern is used circumferentially, with enough sutures to prevent constriction of the lumen. Although 00 to 0 gut or PGA suture can be used, a technique used in cattle has been tried successfully in horses. This employs a 0.4- to 0.6-mm synthetic nonabsorbable suture tied tightly so as to create a slough of the diaphragm of tissue at the site of amputation 10 to 14 days postoperatively. Alternatively, a cylindrical plastic prolapse ring, drilled with a series of holes around its circumference, is introduced into the prolapse and sutured in place with the same type of sutures designed to slough by 14 days. The sutures pass through the holes in the cylinder in a mattress pattern and are tied on the outside. The prolapse is amputated just beyond the sutures. The plastic cylinder maintains patency of the rectum during the healing time and then is voided upon sloughing of the sutured diaphragm of tissue. Prophylactic antibiotics, laxatives by gavage (mineral oil and dioctyl sodium sulfosuccinate) and dietary changes are required during convalescence.

Uterine Prolapse

Advice on the management of this relatively infrequent problem parallels that given for rectal prolapse in that much advantage is gained by early attention. Once again, the controversy regarding epidural anesthesia in the mare should be laid aside, since its use is very beneficial to suppress straining, particularly in the hot-blooded breeds. The concurrent use of tranquilizers, sedatives, and narcotics is certainly indicated to quell sensitivity, but nothing controls pelvic-origin tenesmus so effectively as epidural anesthesia.

Scrupulous toilet of all exposed surfaces should also consider the limitations of time and irritation factors. The race is against development of thrombosis of the engorged and stagnated uterine vasculature, after which replacement of the organ is a somewhat futile effort since infarction and death are the likely sequelae. Amputation of the gangrenous uterus in the mare should be done when the need is evident, but it ranks among the truly heroic procedures, with opportunity for success slight. Treatment of shock is the major factor. In the replacement procedure in the mare, as in any species, care should be taken to ensure that the retroverted tips of the horns are repositioned completely and that thought is given to mural as well as intraluminal hemorrhage. The conjugated estrogen products of equine origin were developed for control of just such hemorrhage in the human female and, barring a major arterial injury, are indicated for such need in the mare.

Recurrence of prolapse following replacement seems not to be the problem in the mare that it is in cattle; however, the continuation of tranquilization for a time thereafter is indicated with the proviso that it be in agreement with blood pressure and any premonitory signs of shock.

Vesical Prolapse

Displacement of the urinary bladder takes two forms—extrusion through a break in the floor of the vagina and prolapse (eversion) through the urethra. The latter is more frequent in the mare, although both are uncommon. As with other prolapses, the principal causes are increase in intra-abdominal pressure, primarily during terminal gestation and parturition, and straining, usually precipitated by the presence of a mass in the pelvis or by pelvic irritability. For these reasons and because of the short and distensible urethra of the female, vesical prolapse is a gynecological problem, most often associated with pregnancy.[39, 58] Other causes include acute distention of the bowel from intestinal obstruction due to mechanical or paralytic ileus[36] and pelvic irritation associated with third-degree perineal lacerations. Haynes and McClure (1980)[44] described two cases, one 6 weeks postpartum and one 5 months postpartum. In both cases, the everted urinary bladder was occupied by a herniation of the pelvic flexure of the left colon, necessitating reduction per laparotomy. Both cases were attended by severe straining somewhat refractory to epidural anesthesia and attempted reduction by manipulation.

Diagnosis is based upon recognition of the retroverted or everted bladder lying in the floor of the vestibule and protruding through the vulva. In the rare retroversion, the urethra is blocked and urine flow prevented. The distention must be evacuated by paracentesis before the bladder can be returned. If the peritoneal reflection in the pelvic cul de sac is broken, the principal risk is pelvic abscess. The defect in the vaginal floor should be freshened and repaired under suture if feasible in consideration of the duration and nature of the injury. An indwelling urinary catheter with a one-way valve would be a further consideration. Antibiotics that reach effective levels in the urine would also be indicated.

The true prolapse, commonly referred to as an eversion, is recognizable by its mucous surface and the two elevated openings of the ureters that appear on the dorsal surface of the organ near its neck. Inflammatory swelling in the bladder wall may cause some retardation of urine flow from the ureters and perhaps even some ureteral distention, but no obstruction exists beyond that. For this reason, a chronic form of vesical prolapse has been described in which the bladder could not be returned and amputation of the corpus vesicae beyond the ureteral orifices was successfully accomplished. The healed stump returned to the vestibule, and the ureters discharged directly thereinto.[39]

In the more typical case, the acute prolapse that occurs around the time of parturition should receive immediate care while it is still possible to reduce the edema in the bladder wall sufficiently to return the everted organ through the urethra. This requires patient manipulation and gentle massage under epidural anesthesia to suppress straining. If replacement is difficult and the bladder wall is friable, urethral sphincterotomy may be helpful. After replacement, prevention of recurrence is the problem, suggesting the need for an inflatable, indwelling balloon catheter of a capacity of 100 ml or more (such as a human rectal retention catheter). Also, chronic cystitis requires long-term urinary antibiotic therapy. Control of straining by use of tranquilizers, sedatives, and narcotics is necessary.

Repair of Cervical Lesions

Lesions of the cervix include (1) injuries sustained during foaling (rupture of muscle fibers and tearing of the mucosa), (2) consequences of chronic inflammation (cervicitis with adhesions or chronic granuloma due to persistent bacterial infection), and (3) congenital anomalies (e.g., segmental aplasia or incomplete development). When dystocial injuries of the cervix impair its function as a valve to close the tube between the vagina and uterus, the disorder is referred to as an incompetent cervix and may constitute a cause of infertility. The condition may be remediable if healing is attended by recovery of muscle tone or if discrete tears ("lacerations") can be freshened and reconstructed under suture. The latter may be done through a metal speculum (bivalve or trivalve) in some mares or without speculum in others. Knowles cervical forceps can be used as effectively for retraction of the cervix into the reach of conventional instruments for dissection and suturing. Alternatively, traction sutures can be used. Without this, the structure is all but inaccessible. Even so, suturing is difficult and often is done blindly. Old defects that encompass no more than one-quarter of the circumference can be freshened with a long-handled scalpel, exerting forceps traction on the cervix to facilitate more accurate dissection. Interrupted sutures of 0 or 1 Ob Gyn gut or PGA material must be placed with circular, cutting edge, or trocar point needles. If retraction of the cervix is inadequate for the length of conventional needle holders, the Knowles forceps can be used for this purpose as well as for a tissue forceps. If the defect is more extensive than 45°, the chances of successful surgical reconstruction are greatly reduced. Also, the interior lumen of the cervix does not lend itself so well to such external methods of repair. However, the external os for a variable distance inward (depending upon the architecture and temperament of the individual mare and the dexterity of the surgeon) is accessible for such procedures.

Evans and associates (1980)[38] emphasize the importance of a three-layer closure on full thickness tears. A continuous horizontal mattress suture is placed in the cervical mucosa-submucosa to evert the mucosa into the cervical lumen. A simple continuous pattern is used to appose the muscularis. Finally, a second mattress suture layer is placed in the vaginal mucosa-submucosa to evert that layer of tissue into the vaginal lumen. Evans and coworkers also advocate the placement of two indwelling traction sutures to lift the cervix off the vaginal floor for the first week of healing to prevent adhesions. These sutures pull the cervix outward and upward by passing the suture limbs through a ring of suture fixed in the vaginal roof and on backward to be tied in the hymenal remnant.

Correction of cervical incompetence due to atony or defects not amenable to debridement and reconstruction may be achieved by any of several variations of purse-string or retention sutures placed in the base of the cervix at its junction with the vaginal fornix, in fact, near the internal os in the retracted state. Wheeless (1981)[105] described the Shirodkar technique using a fascia lata strap buried submucosally and the McDonald operation using a quadrantally placed purse-string suture of large, monofilament polypropylene or nylon. Evans and colleagues used a 5-mm ribbon suture of Mersilene or two strands of No. 2 Mersilene lubricated with antibiotic surgical ointment and placed around the cervix through two short incisions made at 6 and 12 o'clock. After the circle of suture was pulled tight and knotted, the mucosal incision was sutured over the knot. The surgery is performed during the first 48 hours following breeding and ovulation, and, like the Caslick suture, the suture must be removed prior to foaling.

Sometimes the cervix is badly stretched with no apparent surface disruption, and the mare may appear unresponsive to treatment. These animals should be examined and treated as required for endometritis, pneumovagina and urine pooling and then turned out to pasture or returned to physical work with the best general health maintenance possible. In some animals in which local treatment of the organ system is to no avail, the recovery of overall muscle tone will be attended by recovery of cervical function.

When chronic cervicitis results in adhesions, pyometra may be the ensuing complication. To treat or to prevent this may require the use of an indwelling cannula to maintain cervical patency and to provide continuous drainage of the uterus when needed. An acceptable item in standard supply is the inert plastic cannula and inflatable cuff used for barium enema in the human to perform contrast radiography of the rectum. The rectal retention cannula is self-retaining in the mare's cervix when the cuff is inflated inside the body of the uterus. The cannula can be fitted with flexible plastic laboratory tubing to provide the length necessary to drain outside the vulva. The exit end is covered with a glove fingertip valve to prevent aspiration of air and reflux of exudate. If fitted with a sealable second-lumen infusion tube, the uterus and cervix can be irrigated or infused PRN without disturbing the drainage tube. However, it is advisable to change drainage tubes at least once every 48 to 72 hours. Latex or red rubber tubes should be changed more frequently, partly because of the tendency to build up crystals of urine salts and adherent deposits of exudate.

An alternative is to drain the uterus daily without an indwelling tube, infusing the cervix with a combination triamcinolone-antibiotic ointment to prevent reformation of cervical adhesions.

Chronic granuloma of the cervix is an infrequent lesion and, based on very limited experience, is regarded as resistant to treatment. It is a space-occupying lesion palpable per rectum and should be viewed with concern as far as future breeding soundness. Diagnosis is based upon biopsy. When due to *Staphylococcus*, it has been assigned the name botryomycosis of the cervix, after the comparable condition seen in postcastration infection of the stump of the spermatic cord.

Of the several types of congenital anomalies seen in the cervix of the domestic animals, two have been observed in the mare—complete aplasia with no lumen whatsoever and incomplete development of the muscular walls with a lumen but no effective sphincter. As mentioned earlier in this section, segmental interruption of the tubular tract predisposes to either mucometra or pyometra, necessitating hysterectomy if luminal patency cannot be established. Both degrees of aplasia are permanent conditions of unsoundness to be regarded more as diagnostic than therapeutic problems.

Surgical Management of Space-Occupying Lesions

Neoplasms of the caudal tract are most often the malignant melanoma in the gray horse and squamous cell carcinoma in horses with white skin areas. Both types metastasize by blood and lymph, although metastasis is slow at first, and cutaneous as well as mucosal sites may provide the origin for the primary tumor. Complete surgical excision with a generous margin of normal tissue remains the most reliable and most practiced modality for the circumscribed lesion with no known metastasis. Evidence of regional or remote spread is usually regarded as a contraindication for surgery. When radiation therapy is used for such surface lesions, it is in conjunction with surgical excision. No special surgical techniques have been developed as standardized approaches to such lesions in the mare.

Cysts are usually of the mucous retention type. They are due to displaced embryonal remnants in the walls of the tubular tract and are rarely of clinical importance. When drainage is required, liberal excision is done to evacuate the contents and to permit cauterization or dissection of the lining.

Hematoma of the vaginal wall must be differentiated from hemangioma, and if not enlarging or associated with varicosities, it may be managed simply by incision and evacuation or, if small, left undisturbed. If continued hemorrhage is anticipated, particularly of a major artery in an undisclosed location, the best course may be one of watchful waiting. Conjugated estrogens may be given. Opinion is divided as to the value of parenteral fluids in cases of truly consequential hemorrhage in the parturient or preparturient mare. Absolute quiet and judicious use of sedatives are advised. Unless the exact source of the hemorrhage is known (and is surgically accessible), much dependence is still placed on spontaneous arrest, as in the case of uterine arterial hemorrhage into the mesometrium or uterine wall.

Abscesses involving the caudal tract are, in the majority of cases, pelvic in location. Frequently originating through wounds in the vaginal wall, the lesion ranges from a small, focal abscess to a dan-gerous pelvic phlegmon, not only causing dyschezia and dysuria but also threatening peritonitis and septicemia. Tenesmus is a prominent clinical sign, and if the vaginal wall is broken, eventration may even result. It should be remembered that the pelvic fascia is confluent with the fascia transversalis of the abdominal wall, and there is no barrier to extension of infection other than the humorocellular host defenses. Transmural migration of infection to the peritoneal cavity occurs freely. Therefore, pelvic cellulitis of an infectious nature should be treated as a systemic problem as well as a local one.

Once the process has localized and an abscess has formed, an attempt is made to locate the most direct and the most benign drainage route. Pelvic examination per rectum and per vaginam requires epidural anesthesia to control staining. Confirmation of the abscess and identification of contents are made by paracentesis and examination of the aspirate. The three avenues most often employed for drainage are the vaginal, perineal and abdominal routes. The superficial abscesses located on the floor or sides of the pelvic canal can be drained through incisions made in the perineum or vaginal wall. Deep-seated abscesses that extend to or beyond the pubic brim may require drainage through an incision in the caudal abdominal wall in the inguinal or pubic regions. In this case, an exploratory laparotomy can be done concurrently to determine the best location. The drainage path is made through the retroperitoneal fascia so as to avoid direct soilage of the peritoneal cavity. It may be possible to place a through-and-through drain (fenestrated tube or Penrose drain), exiting at a remote point such as the perineum, to allow irrigation of the abscess. Antibiotic therapy is based on the infectious organism and whether the process is contained within the region or not. As with any acute and consequential pelvic disease, maintenance of normal urination and defecation is a primary consideration.

EXTIRPATION OF THE CLITORAL SINUSES

The accidental introduction of contagious equine metritis (*Haemophilus equigenitalis*) into the United States in 1977 led to a new surgical procedure: extirpation of the clitoral sinuses. As described by Zent (1980),[110] the fossa clitoridis and fossa glandis are excised by scissor dissection under local infiltration anesthesia. The plane of dissection is the submucosa-subcutis. The clitoris is left partially intact; only the external mass is removed. Hemorrhage is no problem, and the wound is allowed to heal by second intention by preference. Daily wound toilet with a mild solution of chlorhexidine is recommended for the first five days or until healed.

OPERATIVE SURGERY OF THE CRANIAL TRACT

Surgical procedures commonly performed on the cranial reproductive tract of the mare are the ovariectomy, detorsion of the uterus, and cesarean section. Much less often done is the ovariohysterectomy for pyometra, neoplasia, or anomaly. All these share the involvement of the peritoneal cavity, whether by colpotomy for the vaginal spay or by laparotomy in the flank or ventral body wall. Otherwise, the techniques vary widely, even those with the same objective.

Ovariectomy per Colpotomy

The patient is restrained in stocks and prepared for pelvic surgery as previously described. The classic vaginal spay, as it has been practiced for many years, involves a stab incision through the vaginal fornix performed under epidural anesthesia on the standing mare. In order to do this safely, it is imperative that the bladder and rectum be empty, the colon contents reduced, and the vagina free of infection. Also, the mare must stand quietly without straining. The mare is stimulated to balloon the vagina by infusing 1 liter of warm saline solution. A knife (scalpel or bistoury) is carried into the ballooned vagina, and an incision is made through the vaginal wall in the upper right hand quarter of the fornix at the 1:30 o'clock position. The knife is removed, and Mayo dissecting scissors are carried in to make a stab through the vaginal incision so as to perforate the peritoneum in the cul-de-sac. The scissors are removed, and the gloved hand is introduced by deliberately stretching the incision one finger at a time until the coned hand is admitted to the peritoneal cavity. A gauze sponge, attached to long strands of umbilical tape to ensure safe retrieval, is saturated with lidocaine and carried in the palm to wrap around the ovarian pedicle for local anesthesia. The sponge is removed, and the chain loop of the écraseur is carried in. The ovaries are resected one at a time with the chain loop, removing each ovary into the vagina as amputated.

The greatest caution should be taken to ensure that only the ovary passes through the loop—not mesentery or intestine. At the moment of écrasement, the mare must not be allowed to make sudden movements lest the pedicle be torn, causing severe hemorrhage. Before leaving the site, the cut stump should be palpated gently to detect arterial hemorrhage. If all goes well, the mare is removed from the stocks after a few minutes and is placed standing in cross-ties in an individual stall. She should be monitored for signs of shock or straining, since the two major concerns during the first postoperative hours are hemorrhage and eventration. The preoperative fast can be broken and the mare allowed to eat light hay and bran mash or pelleted feed. Prophylactic antibiotics should be continued for 5 days as a safeguard against peritonitis. The mare should be hand-walked at the halter at regular intervals during the day but should be restrained standing in cross-ties otherwise for the first 5 days until all risk of eventration is past. The vaginal

wound may be expected to heal by second intention in 2 weeks.

Ovariectomy per Laparotomy— Grid Flank Technique

This approach is most often used for removal of a single diseased ovary too big to be removed per vaginam. The procedure can be done under local anesthesia on the standing patient if the ovary is not too large or under general anesthesia with the patient in lateral recumbency if the patient is difficult to manage or if problems are anticipated with exteriorization and hemostasis.

The technique for grid flank laparotomy is essentially the same as that described in Cryptorchidectomy, with the exception that incision dimensions may be somewhat greater. The lower flank permits more flexibility of tissue planes and can be used for access and delivery of the large tumors while retaining the advantages of a grid approach. This recommendation is emphasized by the fact that one of the sites of choice for the cesarean section is the Marcenac incision, which is a grid approach through the low flank.

Upon entry into the abdomen, the ovary is easily located in proximity to the respective flank, especially if tumefied. To aid exteriorization, cystic tumefactions of the ovary can be aspirated. Solid ones can be elevated to the abdominal incision to permit the placement of vulsellum forceps and/or heavy gauge guy sutures (e.g., umbilical tape) in the tough fibrous cortex of the ovary. This allows the surgeon to use external traction on the enlarged ovary while manually retracting the separated muscle planes. Delivery of the ovary to the outside puts considerable tension on its attachments, and caution must be taken to avoid accidental rupture of the blood vessels, which are often engorged owing to the chronicity of such lesions. In the process of dissecting the mesovarium and associated structures, it is important to control the ovarian arteries and veins by double transfixing ligatures before dividing the proper ligament of the ovary. This acts as a safeguard against abrupt or inadvertent stretching of the vasculature. Attempts to ligate all structures indiscriminately in one loop may work where engorgement due to ovarian pathology is absent. However, when this is not the case, the same reasoning applies for differential ligation of the vascular components of the ovarian pedicle as for selective emasculation of the visceral (versus the musculofibrous) part of the spermatic cord in castration of mature and well-developed stallions. Once the vessels are safely ligated and the mesovarium, uterine tube (oviduct) and ligament are transected, the stump of the pedicle is examined carefully for hemorrhage before returning it to the abdomen. If the opposite ovary is to be removed from the same side, there should be provision for intra-abdominal écrasement if the ovary is small. If it is pathologic, and the blood supply is therefore increased, remote écrasement without ligation is inadvisable. An important point to remember, especially when securing a remote ligature by hand, is that the cross-sectional shape of a pedicle changes with tension as opposed to relaxation. Thus, a ligature that may seem to be snug and secure on a stretched pedicle prior to écrasement may loosen and slip or, if transfixed, simply fail to constrict bleeders once the tension is released. This offers one explanation why the occasional patient will hemorrhage consequentially albeit unseen after an otherwise routine and presumably careful ovariectomy. The problem can be avoided by always remembering to relax the traction on a vascular pedicle at the moment the ligature is tightened. If this is not possible, then the need to ligate each vessel individually before dividing the proper ligament of the ovary is even greater. The closure and aftercare of the abdomen parallel that of the flank cryptorchidectomy incision.

Ovariectomy per Laparotomy— Ventral Abdomen Technique

Approach through the ventral paramedian or midline incision requires general anesthesia and dorsal recumbency. It is justified on the basis of preference or in the case of a very large tumor that would tax the limits of a grid incision. The ventral incision is extensile and can be started small for exploration and lengthened as needed.

The midline incision is made on the linea alba and gives maximum exposure and access to either side. The tissue planes incised are skin, superficial abdominal fascia, linea alba, the fatty fascia transversalis and peritoneum. Upon entry into the abdomen, the tumor is handled in the same way as described in the flank approach. Suture closure of the peritoneum is optional, and opinion is somewhat divided as to its desirability. If done, the peritoneum can be effectively closed with a continuous suture of No. 0 or 1 gut placed in bootlace fashion and tensed during the patient's inspiration. The incision in the conjoined aponeuroses at the midline is closed by preference with a continuous oblique modified Mayo imbricating mattress suture pattern taken with doubled strands of a high tensile-strength nonabsorbable synthetic suture material. The overlapping margin is fixed securely to the superficial sheath of the rectus muscle with a second row of continuous suture taken with a single strand of the same material. The superficial abdominal fascia is closed with a third row of No. 2 chromic gut placed in an interrupted mattress pattern and tied with inverted knots. The skin is closed with a fourth row of interrupted horizontal or oblique mattress sutures of any acceptable noncapillary, nonabsorbable material. A stent bandage is oversewn and, if desired, a protective support bandage (corset) is applied

over that. Healing allows removal of the skin sutures in 14 days.

It is freely acknowledged that alternative techniques make satisfactory use of two- or three-layer closures of aponeurosis and musculature with interrupted sutures of No. 2 medium chromic gut, polyglycolic acid suture material, or the equivalent. Skin should be closed with a noncapillary, nonabsorbable material placed in either a horizontal or vertical interrupted mattress pattern.

The *paramedian incision* is usually made 4 to 8 cm lateral and parallel to the midline over the respective ovary. The tissue planes incised are the skin, superficial abdominal fascia, superficial sheath of the rectus abdominis (composed of the deep abdominal fascia and the conjoined aponeuroses of the external and internal abdominal oblique muscles), the musculature of the rectus abdominis (with intersecting tendinous inscriptions), the deep sheath of the rectus abdominis (aponeurosis of the transversus abdominis muscle), the fatty retroperitoneal fascia transversalis and the peritoneum. The superficial sheath and muscle belly of the rectus are always opened longitudinally and coincident with the skin incision. The fibers of the deep sheath run transversely and are cut by a longitudinal incision. For this reason, some prefer separating the fibers of the deep sheath transversely, in the manner of a grid incision, continuing then with a longitudinal incision of the peritoneum. This is an acceptable alternative; however, the argument strains the evidence. The deep sheath is a very thin, weak layer that contributes little to the strength of the closure of the ventral laparotomy while restricting exposure and limiting access. Also, the grid defeats the purpose of using an approach through the ventral abdomen to take advantage of the extensile feature of ventral longitudinal incisions. Therefore, it seems more practical to use the through-and-through paramedian incision made in the same sagittal plane. Ovariectomy is routine.

Closure of the paramedian incision approximates that of the linea alba except for the muscle mass. Closure of the peritoneum is as previously described. The deep sheath is closed with horizontal mattress bites if incised (longitudinally) and with vertical sutures if separated (transversely). No sutures are placed in the muscle fibers of the rectus abdominis muscle. The superficial sheath provides the major support and is closed by preference according to the technique described for the linea alba with a two-layer overlapping mattress suture. Because of the close attachment of the underlying muscle, however, it is necessary to free the undersurface of the superficial sheath on the overlapping side so that a fascia-to-fascia healing interface is created. Muscle or fat interposed between the fascial overlap will weaken the eventual union and predispose to dehiscence and herniation. Some care should be taken when reflecting the muscle from the rectus sheath to avoid unnecessary hemorrhage from the multiple vascular branches of the superficial abdominal arteries that perforate the rectus sheath. Once the incision in the sheath is repaired, the superficial abdominal fascia and skin are closed according to the previous description. Aftercare is also the same.

Detorsion of the Uterus per Laparotomy

Torsion of the uterus occurs less frequently in the mare than in the cow, but it is a more serious problem in the mare owing to the relatively greater difficulty in correction and the lower survival rate. In one compilation of more than 50 cases in the mare and more than 400 cases in the cow, the mortality rate in the mare was greater than three times that in the cow.[81, 86, 104] This may be due partly to the high percentage of success with the nonoperative technique of reduction by rolling the cow with a torsion versus the much more frequent need in the mare for surgical reduction per laparotomy. Physical problems of restraint and patient safety cannot be compared when one considers the basic difference in casting a cow with a rope squeeze, rolling her over in fully conscious recumbency, and allowing her to jump up to her feet, as opposed to casting a mature mare, which, in this modern age, means either general anesthesia or the use of some profound muscle relaxant or neuroleptic that may last for at least 15 to 20 minutes before the mare is able to regain her feet, somewhat unsteadily. Add to this the vulnerability of the uterus of the mare to rupture as a result of such manipulations or to break and hemorrhage spontaneously to a consequential degree, and it is understandable why uterine torsion is regarded with more gravity in the mare than in the cow. Be that as it may, Bowen and coworkers and Guthrie join the ranks of those who believe that selected cases of torsion can be safely reduced by rolling, modifying the procedure somewhat to fit the peculiarities of the mare.[18, 19, 43]

Diagnosis is based on careful examination of every case of colic or malaise seen in the pregnant mare, especially during the last 4 months of gestation. Labor contractions are usually absent because the fetus cannot be presented into the pelvis so long as the torsion exists. On manual examination of the pelvic canal per rectum, the torsion can be palpated as either a clockwise (more prevalent) or a counterclockwise rotation by feeling the broad ligaments (mesometrium) of the uterus pulled into tense bands crossing the uterus dorsally from right to left or left to right. The actual twist of the uterine body may be less readily detected. The common dorsosacral position of the term fetus may have assumed a dorsopubic posture, unless of course the torsion has increased from 180° to 360° or greater. On examination per vaginam, contorted folds may or may not be apparent or palpable in the fornix. Pascoe, Meagher, and Wheat (1981)[76] emphasized the un-

reliability of vaginal examination for diagnosis in the mare versus the cow. Maxwell (1979)[59] cited a case in which vaginal examination was diagnostic.

It is possible that the cervix may have dilated and that the torsion is not great enough to prevent introduction of the hand. Herein lies a hazard. In such cases, the torsion may go unrecognized, and the temptation is to provide an assisted delivery by external traction. If this is attempted in a torsion of 180°, for example, the odds are great that the uterus will be ruptured by the effort and that the mare will die early from hemorrhage or later from peritonitis. Therefore, be on guard against hasty conclusions at the time of such pelvic examinations, and if torsion is present, do whatever is necessary to correct it.

Although no great confidence has been placed in rolling the mare, there will be some cases in which the method is justified. The mare is cast on the side toward which the torsion is directed and then turned rather quickly in the direction of the twist, with the objective of turning the body around the uterine axis, counting on inertia in the gravid uterus to keep the fetal position constant while the maternal position changes. The surgeon may elect to follow the course of events with one hand in the vagina, holding onto a part of the fetal anatomy if the cervix is open. Rolling may need to be repeated several times. Guthrie (1982)[43] described rocking the mare back and forth in dorsal recumbency to dislodge a somewhat static torsion before it finally slipped loose. Bowen and associates have found it valuable to use the plank method commonly employed in the cow.[18, 19] The plank consists of a long, 2×8 inch (or wider) wooden board, one end of which is placed on the mare's abdomen prior to turning. The other end is placed on the ground some distance away in the same direction as the legs. One or two assistants then stand in the middle of the plank as the patient is turned over on its back to the other side in the same direction as the torsion. This may be repeated several times before the torsion is reduced. The major contraindication would be an edematous and friable uterus or one suspected of thrombosis due to a 360° torsion, especially if of long duration. If it is unsuccessful or if this method is not used, the alternative is manipulation through a grid flank laparotomy in the standing mare, done under local anesthesia as described for the flank cryptorchidectomy.

Although both sides have been used successfully, there seems to be some reason for approaching the torsion from the side toward which the twist is directed. One paramount consideration is that correction is best accomplished by pushing rather than pulling. Therefore, if the uterus is twisted to the right, entry through the right flank would permit pushing the gravid horn back over the uterine (or somatic) axis. This is facilitated by elevation of the gravid horn from underneath by manually lifting with one arm while pushing with the other to cause the displaced horn to roll back over. Great care should be exercised to avoid perforating or tearing the uterine wall by overzealous efforts, remembering that the tissues may have been rendered somewhat friable.

Once the torsion has been corrected, there is still concern for the blood supply, which may have been strangulated long enough to cause thrombosis, which will result in infarction of the gravid horn and very probably death of the mare. In torsions that approximate parturition, it must be determined whether labor will be affected. If the mare has gone full term, has come to milk, and is dilated, the decision may be to assist delivery, either by induction of labor with oxytocin or by more direct manually assisted delivery.

In the event the torsion cannot be corrected per flank laparotomy or if that alternative is not appropriate to the circumstances, the last resort is cesarean section, and incorrectable uterine torsion is a justifiable indication for this procedure.

Cesarean Section

Proper emphasis dictates that cesarean sections should be done only when the fetus cannot be delivered by either mutation of malposition or fetotomy or when the latter technique would be unduly injurious to the mare or would unnecessarily sacrifice a live fetus. These considerations stress the importance of prompt assessment and quick action while the fetus is still alive or before the dam develops further complications. Treatment for shock should be presumptive and, regardless of clinical signs, administration of parenteral fluids and prophylactic antibiotics should commence with preparations for surgery. The use of adrenocortical steroids and antihistamines is discretionary but should be considered in light of the frequency of shock and laminitis in such cases. If a mechanical respirator and oxygen are available, they should be readied for use.

Hypotensive tranquilizers and barbiturate anesthetics are generally contraindicated if the fetus is alive or if the mare has been greatly stressed. Vandeplassche recommended the combination of epidural anesthesia to suppress tenesmus and relax the abdominal wall, intravenous glyceryl guaiacolate to induce relaxation of skeletal muscle necessary for recumbent positioning, and local infiltration or incisional anesthesia.[98-101] Low-level halothane by inhalation is also well tolerated and eliminates the need for continuous drip glyceryl guaiacolate, which tends to retard recovery owing to its calcium-binding action. The use of inhalation anesthesia also makes possible simultaneous mechanically assisted ventilation. The principal advantage of the glyceryl guaiacolate method is that it is readily available for use in the field for emergency purposes, and if inhalation equipment must be dismantled and transported for such use, the time lost in the process may be the margin between fetal life and death. Therefore, it is necessary that the alternative

method be available and familiar to the surgeon. The calcium-binding effect of intravenous glyceryl guaiacolate can be countered by the cautious infusion of 10 to 20 per cent solution of calcium borogluconate during the postanesthetic recovery period, being careful to monitor heart action all the while.

The choice of incisions for cesarean section is somewhat a matter of preference between the low flank grid through an oblique incision and the ventral midline incision. Both have been used widely and should provide alternative methods. The chief criticisms of the ventral technique are vulnerability of the incision to disruption, greater compromise of the pleural space, and interference with respiration due to the intra-abdominal pressure on the diaphragm and the occasional inadvertent production of obturator paralysis by failure to support or suspend the weight of the hind legs hanging in abduction. The major criticism of the grid technique is comparatively smaller exposure, requiring greater retraction, and perhaps some risk of radial nerve paralysis in the dependent foreleg. To stretch a point, the anesthesiologist argues the case of the congested downside lung and the poorly perfused upside lung caused by protracted lateral recumbency. Needless to say, these disadvantages can be met and minimized by use of precautionary methods and competent technique.

The low flank oblique incision, often referred to as the Marcenac approach, is directed caudoventrad from a point midway down the costal arch along a line extending backward and downward to a point inside the fold of the flank. The left side is usually preferred owing to the mobility of the bowel on that side, as opposed to the capacious cecum and fixed limbs of the colon on the right side. The superficial abdominal fascia is incised in the same plane. The deep abdominal fascia, recognizable by its yellow, elastic fibers, runs at a right angle to the incision and must be incised or separated. The fibers of the external abdominal oblique muscle and aponeurosis are separated in the direction of the incision, and the underlying aponeurosis of the internal oblique muscle is separated as it runs at a right angle to the incision. The transversus abdominis muscle runs in a transverse direction that splits the right angle between the oblique muscles and is also separated in the direction of its fibers. The upper edge of the rectus abdominis muscle is encountered in the lower extremity of the incision and must be retracted downward. The fatty fascia transversalis and peritoneum are incised in agreement with the skin incision, and all the muscles are retracted sufficiently to permit the elevation of the tip of the gravid horn of the uterus into the incision.

Manipulation of the uterus follows the methods advocated in detorsion of the uterus. Undue pulling and tugging on one part may cause a weakening or rupture of the uterine wall. If edema and friability of uterine wall pose grave threats to attempted exteriorization of the gravid horn, the decision to incise the uterus in situ may be justified. Vigorous suction and liberal use of lap drapes and absorbent pads will greatly minimize contamination of the peritoneal cavity with fetal fluids. This risk is a tradeoff to prevent rupture of the uterus and possible major hemorrhage. Posterior presentations place the fetal head and forelegs in the uterine tip and require proportionately longer incisions for delivery than when the feet and hocks of the hind legs are encountered in the anterior presentation.

Incision of the uterus should be on the greater curvature and should avoid the tip near the junction with the uterine tube (oviduct). The contents should be handled as contaminated and carefully drained to the outside. The use of plastic laparotomy drapes placed so as to protect the laparotomy wound margins from contamination will reduce the number of postoperative wound infections and ensure stronger repairs. This becomes of special importance in ventral midline incisions.

The live foal should be laid alongside the mare with the umbilical cord left intact until the foal is breathing normally and pulsations in the umbilical vessels have stopped. Then, the cord should be broken or severed at the slight constriction a few centimeters away from the cutaneous navel. This should be done without tugging roughly on the site of attachment to the foal, which may predispose to umbilical hernia. If the foal is alive, the placenta may be difficult to remove and should be left inside the uterus. If the foal is dead, the membranes should be removed if possible. The cavity of the uterus should be medicated with an antibiotic compatible with that used systemically.

Closure of the uterus should take account of the problem in achieving adequate hemostasis along the cut margins of the uterine incision. Because of the diffuse placentation in the mare, ligation of discrete bleeders in a few locations is inadequate to control mural hemorrhage, which continues to cause bleeding into the lumen of the uterus after a conventional closure. This has been recognized as a significant cause of maternal mortality. The use of a continuous interlocking suture, through all layers of the uterine wall and around the entire margin of the incision, has been recommended for control of this problem and has been credited with much of the reduction of mortality rate in one series of 71 cases.[99-101] After placement of this row, the uterus is closed with inverting rows of Lembert or Cushing suture pattern of No. 1 chromic gut or PGA swaged on a curved atraumatic needle. Care is taken to exclude any remaining placenta from the suture lines. The uterus is cleansed and returned to the abdomen.

Closure of the grid incision is effected by placement of simple interrupted or continuous sutures in each plane of muscle or fascia independently. The superficial abdominal fascia and skin are closed as previously described. Upon completion, oxytocin, 20 IU, is given intravenously to aid in expulsion of the remaining placenta, fluids, and detritus. If the membranes are retained beyond the fourth postpartum hour, 50 IU of oxytocin diluted in 1 liter of physiologic saline solution is given intravenously by continuous drip over 30 to 60 minutes.[98-101]

Thereafter, the treatments already initiated for complications described should be maintained as needed until the mare's condition is rated safe. This may include manual disruption of early adhesions by palpation of the uterus per rectum on the fourth day, lavage and siphonage of the uterus if an unusual accumulation of lochia occurs, administration of small doses of oxytocin if involution is slow, maintenance of a laxative diet for constipation, continuation of antibiotics for infection, attention to the wound, and constant alertness for signs of peritonitis, hemorrhagic shock, laminitis and metritis.[98-101]

OVARIOHYSTERECTOMY

If chronic pyometra has made the mare permanently barren, if the uterus is the site of localized neoplasia, or if there is segmental aplasia of the cervix with mucometra, and if the mare is otherwise sound for work, ovariohysterectomy is justified.

The procedure is done through the ventral midline with the patient under general anesthesia in dorsal recumbency. The hind legs should be supported by side cushions or suspended in semiflexion from above to prevent the obturator paralysis that will result from unsupported hind legs hanging too long in passive abduction. Preoperative antibiotics are advisable. The approach is the same as that described for cesarean section. The ovarian and cranial uterine blood supply is controlled by double ligation as the mesovarium and mesometrium are dissected. This allows both ovaries and uterine horns to be resected en bloc. At this point, they are exteriorized and packed off to guard against accidental contamination of the peritoneal cavity during the subsequent amputation. The uterus is retracted sufficiently to expose the uterine body, which is tourniquetted (with gum rubber tubing or equivalent) as close as possible to the cervix. A second tourniquet is placed near the bifurcation, leaving at least an 8-cm space between the two tourniquets. The uterine body is transected within this space, closing the stump with double-layer inverting sutures according to Parker-Kerr technique and oversewing to ensure seal against contamination. The surgical specimen (uterus and ovaries) is removed from the field along with any soiled drapes. As the remaining tourniquet is loosened, care is taken to ligate any bleeders originating from the bilateral urogenital arteries that supply the caudal uterus. Once hemostasis and asepsis are secured, the field is cleansed and undraped, and the abdominal incision is closed as described under cesarean section. Aftercare is routine. If the procedure has gone according to plan, recovery should be relatively uneventful, but prudence dictates that the mare's condition be monitored carefully for the first 2 postoperative weeks.

References

1. Aanes WA: Progress in rectovaginal surgery. Proceedings of the 19th Annual Convention of the American Association of Equine Practitioners, 1973, pp 225–240.
2. Aanes WA: Surgical repair of third degree perineal laceration and rectovaginal fistula in the mare. J Am Vet Med Assoc 144:485, 1964.
3. Adams SB: Oophoritis in a horse. Vet Surg 10:67, 1981.
4. American Veterinary Medical Association Council on Veterinary Services: Council report—Unacceptable surgical procedures applicable to domestic animals. J Am Vet Med Assoc 169:947, 1976.
5. Ansari M, Matros LE: Surgical repair of rectovestibular lacerations in mares. Compend Continuing Educ 5:129, 1983.
6. Azzie MAJ: Temporary colostomy in the management of rectal tears in the horse. J S Afr Vet Assoc 46:121, 1975.
7. Baker CB, Newton DI, Mather EC, Oxender WD: Luteolysis in mares after endometrial biopsy. Am J Vet Res 42:1816, 1981.
8. Barber SM: Torsion of the uterus—A cause of colic in the mare (case report). Can Vet J 20:165, 1979.
9. Basv WTK, et al.: Ovarian disorders: Clinical and morphological observations in 30 mares, Can Vet J 23:6, 1982.
10. Becht JL, McIlwraith CW: Jejunal displacement through the mesometrium in a pregnant mare. J Am Vet Med Assoc 177:436, 1980.
11. Belling TH Jr.: Surgery of the vulva: Modifications of the traditional Caslick operation. Vet Med/Small Anim Clin 78:870, 1983.
12. Bergeron H: Granulosa theca cell tumor in a mare. Compend Continuing Educ 5:141, 1983.
13. Blanchard TL, Bierschwal CJ, Youngquist RS, Elmore RG: Sequelae to percutaneous fetotomy in the mare. J Am Vet Med Assoc 182:1127, 1983.
14. Blanchard TL, Cummings MR, Garcia MC, et al.: Comparison between two techniques for endometrial swab culture and between biopsy and culture in barren mares. Theriogenology 16:541, 1981.
15. Blanchard TL, Evans LH: Congenitally incompetent cervix in a mare. J Am Vet Med Assoc 181:266, 1982.
16. Blue MG, Bruere AN, Dewes HF: The significance of the XO syndrome in infertility of the mare. N Am Vet J 26:137, 1978.
17. Blue MG, Oriol JG: Conception in mares following intrauterine therapy with amikacin. J Equine Vet Sci 2:200, 1982.
18. Bowen JM, Gabowry C, Bousquet D: Nonsurgical correction of a uterine torsion in the mare. Vet Rec 99:495, 1976.
19. Bowen JM, Taylor TS: Personal communication on nonsurgical correction of uterine torsion in the mare, 1983.
20. Brown MP: Conditions of the rectum. Vet Clin North Am Anim Pract 4:185, 1982.
21. Brown MP: Modified treatment for uterine pooling. J Am Vet Med Assoc 174:458, 1978.
22. Brown MP, Colahan PT, Hawkins DL: Urethral extension for treatment of urine pooling mares. J Am Vet Med Assoc 173:1005, 1978.
23. Bruere NA, Blue MG, Jaine PM, et al.: Preliminary observations on the occurrence of the equine XO syndrome. N Z Vet J 26:145, 1978.
24. Buoen LC, et al.: Sterility associated with an XO karyotype in a Belgian mare. J Am Vet Med Assoc 182:1120, 1983.
25. Caslick EA: The vulva and vulvovaginal orifice and its relation to genital health of the thoroughbred mare. Cornell Vet 27:178, 1937.
26. Caudle AB, Purswell B, Williams DJ, Brooks P: Skin staples for nonscarified Caslick procedures. Vet Med/Small Anim Clin 78:782, 1983.
27. Caudle AB, Purswell BJ, Williams DJ et al.: Endometrial levels of amikacin in the mare after intrauterine infusion of amikacin sulfate. Theriogenology 19:433, 1983.
28. Chisholm FR: Uterine prolapse in the mare. Can Vet J 12:267, 1981.
29. Clark TL: Clinical management of equine ovarian neoplasms. J Reprod Fertil (Suppl) 23:331, 1975.
30. Concha-Bermejillo Andrés de la, Kennedy PC: Prognostic value of E.B. in the mare. J Am Vet Med Assoc 181:680, 1982.
31. Cotchin E: A general survey of tumours in the horse. Equine Vet J 9:16, 1977.
32. Danks AG: Williams' Surgical Operation, Ithaca, NY, published by the author, 1945, pp 84–87.
33. Davis LE, Abbitt B: Clinical pharmacology of antibacterial drugs in the uterus of the mare. J Am Vet Med Assoc 170:204, 1977.
34. Dawson FLM: Recent advances in equine reproduction. Equine J 9:4, 1977.
35. Doig PA, McKnight JD, Miller RB: The use of endometrial biopsy in the infertile mare. Can Vet J 22:72, 1981.
36. Donaldson RS: Eversion of the bladder in the mare. Vet Rec 92:409, 1973.
37. Engle MJ, Black T: Urine pooling in the mare (in the vagina). Iowa State Univ Vet 42:5, 1980.
38. Evans LH, Tate LP, Jr, Cooper WL, Robertson JT: Surgical repair of cervical lacerations and the incompetent cervix. Proceedings of the 25th Annual Convention of the American Association of Equine Practitioners, 1980, p. 483.
39. Frank ER: Veterinary Surgery, 7th ed. Minneapolis, Burgess Publishing Co, 1964, pp 292–294.
40. Gabal MA, Hogel RM, West JK: Pyometra in a mare caused by Candida rugosa. J Am Vet Med Assoc 170:177, 1977.
41. Gadd JW: The relationship of bacterial cultures, microscopic smear examination and medical treatment to surgical correction of barren mares. Proceedings of the 20th Annual Convention of the American Association of Equine Practitioners, 1975, pp 362–368.
42. Getty R: Sisson and Grossman's Anatomy of the Domestic Animals, Vol. 1, 5th ed. Philadelphia, WB Saunders, 1975, pp 531–541.
43. Guthrie RG: Rolling for correction of uterine torsion in a mare. Clinical Report. J Am Vet Med Assoc 181:66, 1982.
44. Haynes PF, McClure JR: Eversion of the urinary bladder: A sequel to third-degree perineal laceration in the mare. Vet Surg 9:66, 1980.
45. Heinze CD, Allen AR: Repair of third-degree perineal lacerations in the mare. Vet Scope 11:12, 1966.
46. Held JP, Buergelt C, Colahan P: Serous cystadenoma in a mare. JAVMA 181:496, 1982.
47. Held JP, et al.: Serous cystadenoma in a mare. JAVMA 181:496, 1982.
48. Howlett JR: Complete uterine prolapse in a mare. Vet Med/Small Anim Clin 76:655, 1981.
49. Hughes JP, Trommershausen-Smith A: Infertility in the horse associated with chromosomal abnormality. Aust Vet J 53:253, 1977.
50. Hurtgen JP, Whitmore HL: Induction of estrus and ovulation by endometrial biopsy in mares with prolonged diestrus. J Am Vet Med Assoc 175:1196, 1979.
51. Hurtgen JP, Whitmore HL: Effects of endometrial biopsy, uterine culture, and cervical dilatation on the equine estrous cycle. J Am Vet Med Assoc 173:97, 1978.
52. Jackson PGG: Rupture of the prepubic tendon in a Shire mare. Vet Rec 111:38, 1982.
53. Jones RD: Diagnosis of uterine torsion in a mare and correction by standing flank laparotomy. Can Vet J 17:111, 1976.
54. Jones WE, Bogart R: Genetics of the Horse. East Lansing, Caballus Publishers, 1971, pp 241–278.
55. Kenney RM: Cyclic and pathologic changes of the mare endometrium as detected by biopsy, with a note on early embryonic death. J Am Vet Med Assoc 172:241, 1978.
56. Kenney RM, Ganjam VK: Selected pathological changes if the mare uterus and ovary. J Reprod Fertil (Suppl) 23:335, 1975.
57. Lock TF, Macy DW: Equine ovarian lymphosarcoma. J Am Vet Med Assoc 175:72, 1979.
58. Lundall RL: The urinary system. In Oehme FW, Prier JE (eds.): Textbook of Large Animal Surgery. Baltimore, Williams & Wilkins, 1974, p 459.
59. Maxwell JAL: The correction of uterine torsion in a mare by caesarean section. Aust Vet J 55:33, 1979.

60. McEntee K, Nielsen SW: Tumours of the female genital tract. Bull WHO 53:217, 1976.

61. McLennan MW, Kelly WR: Hypertrophic, osteopathy and dysgerminoma in a mare. Aust Vet J 53:144, 1977.

62. Meagher DM, Wheat JD, Hughes JP, et al.: Granulosa cell tumors in mares—a review of 78 cases. Proceedings of the 22nd Annual Convention of the American Association of Equine Practitioners, 1977, pp 133–145.

63. Meek DG, DeGrofft DL, Schneider EE: Surgical repair of similar parturition-induced ventral hernias in two mares: A comparison of results. Vet Med/Small Anim Clin 72:1066, 1977.

64. Mills JHL, Fratz PB, Clark EG, Ganjam VK: Arrhenoblastoma in a mare. J Am Vet Med Assoc 171:754, 1977.

65. Monin T: Vaginoplasty: A surgical treatment for urine pooling in the mare. Proceedings of the 17th Annual Convention of the American Association of Equine Practitioners, 1972, pp 99–102.

66. Moore JN, Johnson JH, Tritschler LG, Garner HE: Equine cryptorchidism: Pre-surgical considerations and surgical management. Vet Surg. 7:43, 1978.

67. Moorthy ARS, Spradbrow PB, Eisler MED: Isolation of mycoplasmas from the genital tract of horses. Aust Vet J 53:167, 1977.

68. Moulton JE: Tumors in Domestic Animals, 2nd ed. Berkeley, University of California Press, 1978, Chaps 10 and 11.

69. Nickel R, Schummer A, Seiferle E, Sack WO: The Viscera of the Domestic Mammals. New York, Springer-Verlag, 1973, pp 351–392.

70. Nickels FA: Complications of urogenital surgery. Proceedings of the 23rd Annual Convention of the American Association of Equine Practitioners, 1978, pp 261–265.

71. Nielsen SW, Misdorp W, McEntee K: Tumours of the ovary. Bull WHO 53:203, 1976.

72. Nyack B, Johnson AD: A mammoth granulosa cell tumor in a mare. Vet Med/Small Anim Clin 78:218, 1983.

73. Osborne VE: Genital infection of a horse with spirochaetes. Aust Vet J 37:190, 1961.

74. Pascoe RR: Observations on the length and angle of declination of the vulva and its relation to fertility in mares. J. Reprod Fertil (Suppl) 27:299, 1979.

75. Pascoe RR: Caslick's operation and its relation to fertility in mares. In Australian Advances in Veterinary Science, Australian Veterinary Association, Artarmon, Australia, 1979, pp 25–26.

76. Pascoe JR, Meager DM, Wheat JD: Surgical management of uterine torsion in the mare: A review of 26 cases. J Am Vet Med Assoc 179:351, 1981.

77. Pouret EJM: Surgical technique for the correction of pneumo- and urovagina. Equine Vet J 14:249, 1982.

78. Reid MM, Frock IW, Jeffrey DR, Kaiser GE: Successful treatment of a madurmycotic fungal infestion of the equine uterus with amphotericin B. Vet Med/Small Anim Clin 72:1194, 1977.

79. Richardson GF, Honey PG, Karns PA, et al.: Vet Med/Small Anim Clin 78:398, 1983.

80. Roberts SJ: Twin pregnancy in mare: A live foal and a mummified fetus. Cornell Vet 68:196, 1978.

81. Roberts SJ: Veterinary Obstetrics and Genital Diseases (Theriogenology). Ithaca, NY, Published by the author, distributed by Edwards Brothers, Ann Arbor, 1971.

82. Schmidt GR, Cowles RR, Jr, Flynn DV: Granulosa cell tumor in a broodmare. J Am Vet Med Assoc 169:635, 1976.

83. Schneider JE, Leipold HW, White SL, Korsgaard E: Repair of congenital atresia of the colon in a foal. J Equine Vet Sci 1:121, 1981.

84. Shideler RK, McChesney AE, Voss JL, Squires EL: Relationship of endometrial biopsy and other management factors on fertility of broodmares. J Equine Vet Sci, 2:5, 1982.

85. Sisson W, Grossman JD: The Anatomy of the Domestic Animals, 3rd ed. Philadelphia, WB Saunders, 1938.

86. Skjerven O: Correction of uterine torsion by laparotomy. Nord Vet Med 17:377, 1965.

87. Slone D: Personal communication on use of triamcinolone-antibiotic infusions to prevent cervical adhesions in chronic pyometra, 1982.

88. Smith JM: Hydrallantois in the mare. Mod Equine Med, 1983.

89. Stabenfeldt GH, Hughes JP, Kennedy PC: Clinical findings, pathological changes, and endocrinology secretory patterns in mares with ovarian tumors J Reprod Fertil (Suppl) 27:277, 1979.

90. Stashak TS, Knight AP: Temporary diverting colostomy for the management of small colon tears in the horse: A case report. J Equine Med Surg 2:196, 1978.

91. Stickle RL, Fessler FJ, Adams SB: A single stage technique for repair for rectovestibular lacerations in the mare. Vet Surg 8:25, 1979.

92. Straub OC, Fowler ME: Repair of perineal lacerations in the mare and cow. J Am Vet Med Assoc 138:659, 1961.

93. Sundberg JP, Burnstein T, Page EH, et al.: Neoplasms of Equidae. J Am Vet Med Assoc 170:150, 1977.

94. Swerczek TW: Elimination of CEM organism from mares by excision of clitoral sinuses (letter). Vet Rec 105:131, 1979.

95. Torbeck RL, Kittleson SL, Leathers CW: Botryoid rhabdomyosarcoma of the uterus of a filly. J Am Vet Med Assoc 176:914, 1980.

96. Turner TA, Fessler JF: Rectal prolapse in the horse. J Am Vet Med Assoc 170:1028, 1980.

97. Turner TA, Manno M: Bilateral granulosa cell tumor in a mare. J Am Vet Med Assoc 182:713, 1983.

98. Vandeplassche M: Caesarean section in the mare. Vet Rec 96:412, 1975.

99. Vandeplassche M: Embryotomy and cesarotomy. In Oehme FW, Prier JE (eds): Textbook of Large Animal Surgery. Baltimore, Williams & Wilkins, 1974, pp 521–537.

100. Vandeplassche M: Caesarean section in the horse. In Grunsell CSG, Hill FWG (eds): The Veterinary Annual. Bristol, John Wright, 1978, pp 73–78.

101. Vandeplassche M, Bouters R, Spincemaille J, Bote P: Caesarean section in the mare. Proceedings of the 22nd Annual Convention of the American Association of Equine Practitioners, 1977, pp 75–80.

102. VanDyk E, Immelman A, VanHeerden JS: The use of amikacin in the treatment of endometritis caused by Pseudomonas aeruginosa in the mare. J S. Afr Vet Med Assoc 53:124, 1982.

103. Washburn SM, Klesius PH, Ganjam VK, Brown BG: Effect of estrogen and progesterone on the phagocyte response of ovariectomized mares infected in utero with β-hemolytic streptococci. Am J Vet Res 43:1367, 1982.

104. Wheat JD, Meagher DV: Uterine torsion and rupture in mares. J Am Vet Med Assoc 160:881, 1972.

105. Wheeless CR: Atlas of Pelvic Surgery. Philadelphia, Lea & Febiger, 1981, pp 166–169.

106. Wilson GL: Hysteroscopic examination of mares. Vet Med/Small Anim Clin 78:568, 1983.

107. Wilson GL, Arnold JF: Uterine torsion. Mod Vet Pract 58:265, 1977.

108. Wingfield-Digby NJ, Ricketts SW: A method for clitoral sinusectomy in mares. Equine Pract 4:145, 1982.

109. Witherspoon D: Personal communication on treatment of CEM by extirpation of the clitoral sinuses, 1982.

110. Zent WW: Surgical removal of the clitoral sinus(es) for elimination of the contagious equine metritis carrier state in mares. International Symposium on Equine Venereal Diseases, September 1979. Newmarket, England, Animal Health Trust, 1980, pp 43–45.

Clinical Experience with Equine Hysteroscopy

Gary L. Wilson, D.V.M., M.S.
Equine Reproductive Clinic, Lexington, Kentucky

As a result of technological advances, methods for visual examination of the uterine lumen have progressed rapidly in recent years. Notable among these advances were the introduction of fiberoptics, which made possible the use of high-intensity proximal light sources, and the development of new methods for the distention of the uterine lumen. Along with the development of new instruments there has been increasing interest among veterinarians in hysteroscopy as a diagnostic and therapeutic tool in equine theriogenology. The development of reliable hysteroscopic procedures should improve the diagnostic accuracy of equine clinicians, enabling them to treat uterine abnormalities more effectively.

The visual examination of the mare's endometrial cavity by means of a flexible optic instrument has been attempted infrequently by veterinarians. The clinical application of fiberoptics has been delayed because of inadequate visualization as a consequence of insufficient illumination and inadequate distention of the cavity. If equine hysteroscopy is to become a routine procedure in the evaluation of reproductive soundness, these problems must be consistently overcome. Recent mechanical and optical innovations give the equine practitioner this capability. Continued developments in photography and video recording produce reliable documentation of hysteroscopic observations.

INSTRUMENTS

Hysteroscope

A hysteroscope with a sheath designed specifically for use in the mare has not been manufactured. Human endoscopes have been adapted for use in mares.

Our initial experience was obtained in using a flexible bronchoscope attached to a 150-W halogen cold light supply. The optical information obtained with that instrument was insufficient due to inadequate illumination. Most recently, we have used a GIF type 2T flexible esophagealscope. The instrument has an outside diameter of 12.6 mm and a

working length of 1100 mm. Foreoblique optics are adjustable by hand control knobs. Located at the proximal end of the instrument are the eyepiece, focusing rim, controls for regulation of vacuum, and air flow and fluid inflow and outflow valves. The distal end of the instrument contains the lens system vacuum channel orifices for air, irrigating fluid and surgical instruments.

Under normal conditions, the uterine cavity is collapsed and must be distended with some medium to permit visual examination. After trying several types of fluid, we have adopted sterile water as a distention medium for the production of transient hydrometra during examination.

Ancillary Equipment

Fluid or air for irrigating or distending the endometrial cavity may be injected through stop-cocks on the proximal end of the instrument. Operating channels of 1.2 or 2.3 mm (7 Fr) in the fiberoptiscope accommodate ancillary instruments such as flexible biopsy forceps or scissors, calibrated probes, small tissue forceps and small suction tubes. Rubber nipples seal the channel when catheters or biopsy forceps are in place. Using these instruments, intraluminal adhesions, cysts or polyps can be incised and removed.

Photography

Endoscopic photography enables the operator to record observations, a capability that is useful in client education and in the documentation of the results of the examination and treatment. Photographic equipment should be available at all times during the endoscopic examination. Records are kept of each exposure including the signalment, date, endoscopic results and exposure settings of the camera.

Proximal flash or "exoflash" generators are available and vary widely in design, price and performance. The endoscopic light source and camera must be compatible and optically synchronized for best results. Photographs made through sterile water or high-viscosity fluid are clear and have good resolution. The authors have used cinematography to record the technique of hysteroscopy and its diagnostic applications.

Personnel

Equipment maintenance and the skill of the assistant and operator are important factors in an efficient endoscopic exam. Responsibility for maintenance of the instruments and provision of supplies should be specifically delegated. Manipulation of photographic and videorecording equipment and record-keeping must be coordinated to facilitate the procedure.

Discussions with the owner, which include informational videotapes prior to the examination and demonstration of the findings after the examination, improve owner acceptance of the procedure.

Maintenance

Maintenance of the hysteroscope and accessory instruments is similar to the care given to all endoscopic equipment. After each use, the channels are irrigated and the lens and probes cleaned. If high-viscosity solutions are used to distend the endometrial cavity, the instruments must be soaked in hot water immediately after completion of the procedure. Hot water, not force, should be used in attempting to free obstructions of forceps jaws or stop-cocks. The fiberoptiscope and accessory instruments can be adequately disinfected by soaking them for 20 minutes in any of a variety of disinfectant solutions. Fiberoptic instruments cannot be safely autoclaved and frequent gas sterilization is impractical.

TECHNIQUE

Prior to hysteroscopy, mares are sedated with xylazine (150 mg per 450 kg) and morphine sulfate (300 mg per 450 kg) given intravenously. Additional doses of ataractics may be necessary during the procedure. Chemical restraint reduces movement of the mare, permitting a more complete examination, and reduces the possibility of damage to the instruments.

Preparation

The mare is restrained in padded stocks and the tail wrapped. The perineal region is scrubbed with bactericidal soap, rinsed with tamed iodine solution, and dried with disposable towels.

A pipette is passed through the cervical canal through which 3 to 4 liters of sterile water are infused by gravity flow to establish transient hydrometra. The pipette is then withdrawn, and the flexible endoscope is introduced into the endometrial cavity. The flow of irrigating fluid into the uterus is controlled by means of a stop-cock. Vacuum controls permit the aspiration of fluid and intrauterine debris.

Postoperative Patient Care

After the diagnostic procedure is completed, the fiberoptiscope is withdrawn and the mare is given a narcotic antagonist before being returned to a bedded stall.

ENDOSCOPIC FINDINGS

Normal Variations

Although it is easy and safe to insert a flexible endoscope, interpretations of the findings and procedures can be difficult for the inexperienced operator. Common technical problems are inability to maintain sharpness of the image and sufficient separation of the uterine walls. Purulent exudate can interfere with the hysteroscopic examination. The presence of blood causes a diffuse red image. Water that may condense on the eyepiece obsures vision.

The endoscope is inserted just beyond the internal os of the cervix. The flow of sterile water into the uterine lumen is controlled with the stop-cock on the fiberoptiscope. If resistance to flushing is encountered, the instrument is too close to the endometrial surface.

The initial hazy red view seen occasionally through the fiberoptiscope disappears soon after the introduction of the fluid medium. If the field does not clear following the infusion of additional media, the endoscope should be withdrawn and focused on the cervix. A persistently obscured view may indicate mucus or blood adhering to the lens, and the instrument must be removed and the lens cleaned.

The normal endometrial cavity is slitlike, and the walls are in apposition, preventing adequate inspection without prior distention of the uterus. The endometrial folds are arranged longitudinally. The bifurcation of the uterine body and horns is readily identified and serves as a landmark. The uterotubal junction is located by gently passing the instrument craniad until the uterine horn comes into view with the tubal papilla at its apex. Tubal papillae may be round, oval or stellate and vary in size. The tubal papilla can accommodate a 1-mm cannula. Occasional contractions cause changes in the size of the papilla during the examination.

During diestrus, the endometrium is thin, yellow and smooth. Occasional blood vessels are visible. In the estrous phase of the cycle, the endometrium is thickened, undulating and pink or tan in color, and small submucosal blood vessels are obvious. The ends of accessory instruments sink into the velvety surface.

The endometrial folds are visualized by aspiration of the distending medium, which permits collapse of the endometrial cavity. As contraction of the uterus occurs, the endometrial folds come into view and resume their normal position. Folds are evaluated for size, contour, color and consistency. Abnormalities such as cysts, atrophy, ulcers and plaques are noted.

The cervical canal is usually examined at the conclusion of the procedure as the instrument is withdrawn. Normally the cervical canal is circular with a smooth mucosal membrane that is white in color, distinctly different from the lining of the uterine lumen. The length of the cervical canal varies with cervical relaxation.

At the conclusion of the examination, observations are recorded on the form shown in Figure 1.

Pathologic Conditions

Fiberoptiscopic examination of the uterine lumen for diagnostic and therapeutic procedures has been performed on 100 infertile mares with histories or clinical findings suggestive of intrauterine pathology. Abnormalities that can be identified include adhesions, polyps, ulcers and cysts. Purulent exudate that was not previously diagnosed by rectal palpation is found frequently. Atrophic endometria resemble those seen during the diestrous phase of the cycle and the endometrial cavity is shrunken and uniformly smooth.

The results of the examinations of 100 mares are as follows: endometritis, with or without exudate, 51 mares; normal endometrial cavity, 16 mares; fibrosis, 12 mares; endometrial cysts, 8 mares; intraluminal adhesions, 5 mares; endometrial polyps, 3 mares; endometrial atrophy, 3 mares; uterine sacculation, 1 mare; and intraluminal foreign body (detached culture swab), 1 mare.

Intrauterine adhesions can develop following the infusion of irritating solutions into the uterus, dystocia or abortion. Transverse luminal adhesions appear as bridgelike tags connecting one endometrial surface across the lumen to the opposite surface. Marginal luminal adhesions seem to project inward from the endometrium in the distended uterus. In the five mares cited above with intraluminal adhesions, all of the transverse adhesions and most of the marginal adhesions were removed by pushing with the tip of the fiberoptiscope under visual control. Two of the five mares in which adhesiotomy was performed conceived during the subsequent breeding season.

CLINICAL USES OF HYSTEROSCOPY

A history of infertility is the most frequent indication for hysteroscopic examination. It provides a method of assessing endometrial vascularization and health. Samples of endometrial fluids for microbiologic culture can be obtained by inserting a cannula through the operating channel and aspirating the fluid. Lavage and aspiration of purulent exudate can be performed with the fiberoptiscope, allowing the clinician to visualize the uterine lumen to ensure complete removal of the debris. Endometrial cysts, polyps and adhesions can be diagnosed and removed, although further studies are needed to determine the role of these abnormalities in equine infertility. Hysteroscopy also is beneficial in evaluating the results of endometritis therapy.

Date _____

Owner _____ Mare's Name _____

Breeding History _____

_____

Operative Procedures:

☐ Flexible Hysteroscopy   ☐ Photography   ☐ Adhesiotomy, Cautery
☐ Rigid Hysteroscopy   ☐ Polaroid   ☐ Polypectomy, Cautery
☐ Biopsy   ☐ Slides   ☐ Cystoectomy, Cautery
☐ Cytology   ☐ Videotape   ☐ Culture Swab/Fluid
                   ☐ D & C

Endoscopic Findings _____

_____

_____

_____

_____

_____

_____

_____

Biopsy/Specimens/to Pathology _____

Postoperative Dx _____ Signature _____ D.V.M.

Figure 1. Hysteroscopy worksheet.

SUMMARY

Hysteroscopy adds a new dimension to the management of mares with common reproductive problems. Its use increases the accuracy of diagnosis and serves as an adjunct to treatment of uterine abnormalities. Hysteroscopy is a safe, simple and economical procedure. The authors have been using hysteroscopy for examination of the uterine lumen for 2 years and have adopted a liquid medium for uterine distention.

Suggested Readings

1. Edstrom K, Fernstrom I: The diagnostic possibilities of a modified hysteroscopic technique. Acta Obstet Gynec Scand 49:327, 1970.

2. Kevine RV: A symposium on advances in fiberoptic hysteroscopy. Contemp Obstet Gynec 3:115, 1974.
3. Lindeman HJ: A symposium on advances in fiberoptic hysteroscopy. Contemp Obstet Gynec 3:115, 1974.
4. Mather EC, et al.: The use of fiber-optic techniques in clinical diagnosis and visual assessment of experimental intrauterine therapy in mares. J Reprod Fert Suppl 27:293, 1979.
5. Wilson GL: Hysteroscopic Examination of Mares. Vet Med/Small Anim Clin, April 1983, 568–578.
6. Wilson GL: Equine Hysteroscopy: A Window to the Internal Reproductive Tract. Vet Med/Small Anim Clin, September 1983, 1455–1459; 1462–1466.
7. Wilson GL: Equine Hysteroscopy: Normal Intrauterine Anatomy. Vet Med/Small Anim Clin, November 1984, 1388–1393.
8. Wilson GL: Equine Hysteroscopy: Diagnostic Endoscopic and Photographic Equipment. Vet Med, April 1985, 76–88.
9. Wilson GL: Recognition & Treatment of Recurrent Equine Intrauterine Hemorrhage. Vet Med, September 1985, 76.
10. Wilson GL: Diagnostic and Therapeutic Hysteroscopy for Endometrial Cysts in the Mare. Vet Med, October 1985, 59–63.

Laparoscopic Examination of the Reproductive Tract of the Mare

Gary L. Wilson, D.V.M., M.S.
Equine Reproductive Clinic, Lexington, Kentucky

Laparoscopy, also called peritoneoscopy and pelvioscopy, is one of the more commonly used endoscopic techniques in human gynecology. Techniques for visualization of the tubular genitalia have progressed rapidly in recent years in human medicine but have not gained wide acceptance in veterinary medicine. Notable among these advances has been the introduction of fiberoptics, which make possible the use of high-intensity proximal light sources.

Veterinarians involved in equine practice are aware of the limitations of examination of the mare's reproductive tract by rectal palpation and vaginal speculum examination. Accurate diagnoses of lesions of the vulva, vagina, cervix and uterine body are made by augmenting palpation and visual inspection with special procedures such as microbiologic cultures, cytologic examinations and endometrial biopsies. The internal genitalia beyond the level of the uterus have been inaccessible to these direct procedures. Because of the uncertainties of exploratory abdominal surgery, this method has not been widely used in the field of veterinary gynecology. Surgical intervention may be an excessive act and is rarely justified.

Methods of examination similar to those used to examine the vagina and cervix may be applied to the internal pelvic organs without resorting to abdominal surgery. Laparoscopy may be used to inspect the pelvic reproductive organs and obtain tissue samples for biopsy as well as samples for microbiologic and cytologic examination. The information obtained is similar to that obtained by exploratory laparotomy, but laparoscopy is simpler and less traumatic and can be performed with minimal risk. Laparoscopy offers the theriogenologist the advantage of visual examination of the abdomen without the necessity for a large incision. The postoperative period is short and the cosmetic results are acceptable, thus making laparoscopy an attractive procedure.

EQUIPMENT

The instruments necessary for laparoscopy include a laparoscope, a trocar with sheath to permit introduction of the instrument through the abdominal wall, a Verres needle and pneumoperitoneum control system, a light source with a fiberoptic conduction system and various ancillary instruments.

The laparoscope is a fiberoptiscope with an illuminated optical system that does not require a mechanism for focusing. The standard instrument has a direct or 180° view and foreoblique view (145° to 165°) and right angle or 90° view. In addition to the lens and prisms, the laparoscope contains the fiberoptic bundles that transmit cold light to the distal end of the instrument.

A remote source of light is condensed and transmitted through the fiberoptic conduction system of the laparoscope. The light is then projected onto the field to be examined by the objective lens. The intensity of the cold light can be varied depending on the source. A 150-watt light source is sufficient to examine the internal genital organs of a mare, but cinematography and videorecording require 500 watts of power. For still photography, an adjustable external electronic flash and a reflex camera are recommended.

The Verres needle is a small trocar that is introduced into the peritoneal cavity through which nitrous oxide is transmitted for the purpose of displacing the organs from the abdominal wall. The pneumoperitoneum control system delivers the gas at a rate of 1 liter per minute at a pressure of less than 20 mm Hg. The flow is decreased when the intra-abdominal pressure increases and is interrupted at a pressure of 40 mm Hg.

A surgical laparoscope will permit passage of a biopsy forceps, which can be utilized to obtain samples from the ovary and other pelvic organs. Other instruments that may be introduced through the laparoscope include probes for manipulation, swabs for obtaining samples from the infundibulum for microbiologic cultures and suction equipment for obtaining ovarian fluid.

TECHNIQUE

Laparoscopy is a surgical procedure to be performed under strict aseptic conditions with the mare properly restrained in padded stocks. A 24-hour fast is required to reduce the volume and motility of the intestines.

Chemical restraint for laparoscopy include sedation with xylazine (150 mg intravenously) and morphine sulfate (300 mg intravenously). The abdominal wall at the incision site is desensitized with a local anesthetic. Additional sedation may be necessary during the procedure. Proper sedation eliminates the mare's anxiety and induces relaxation during introduction and manipulation of the instruments.

The optimal site for penetration of the abdominal wall is immediately caudal to the last rib at the insertion of the dorsal crus of the internal abdominal oblique muscle. After a 1-cm incision is made in the skin, subcutaneous tissue and fascia, the sharp-pointed Verres needle is gently inserted. The needle can be felt to penetrate the fascia, and penetration into the abdominal cavity is completed by advancing and directing the needle toward the axis of the pelvic inlet. The operator must rely on a sense of touch to complete this phase. Care is taken to ensure that the needle penetrates the peritoneum to avoid retroperitoneal introduction of gas. The correct placement of the needle may be determined by attaching a syringe to the needle to detect the aspiration of air into the abdominal cavity. One or two drops of sterile saline may be placed in the needle, creating a suckinglike sound when the needle penetrates the abdominal cavity. Free movement of the needle also signifies proper placement.

Table 1. Indications for Diagnostic Laparoscopy

1. Infertility
2. Ovarian biopsy
3. Biopsy of pelvic masses
4. Microbiologic culture of the infundibulum
5. Examination of tubal patency
6. Aspiration of cysts

If the position of the needle is in doubt, it should be reinserted.

The nitrous oxide tubing is then connected to the needle. After gas flow has been initiated, the operator must monitor the intra-abdominal pressure gauge throughout the introduction of gas. As the intra-abdominal pressure increases, the flow rate of gas decreases and is interrupted at a pressure of 40 mm Hg. The initial insufflation rate should be no greater than 1 liter per minute. After 2 to 4 liters of nitrous oxide have been introduced, the gas valves are closed and the needle is withdrawn.

After the operator inspects the instrument for proper function, a truncated cone trocar within the sheath is cautiously advanced through the muscle and fat layers with a rotary pushing motion. After the peritoneum has been penetrated, the sharp instrument is withdrawn approximately 3 cm into the sheath, and the sheath is advanced approximately 2 cm. If the sheath can be easily advanced, the trocar is removed. A gush of escaping gas indicates that the previously inflated abdominal cavity has been penetrated.

The laparoscope with the light source attached is then inserted through the sheath. Fogging of the lens of the laparoscope is prevented by immersion of the instrument in 37°C saline. The nitrous oxide tube is then connected to the sheath for automatic or intermittent insufflation.

Initially, the abdominal organs are identified and inspected for evidence of hemorrhage, perforation or other abnormalities. The ovaries may be more easily inspected if an assistant holds them per rectum. The operating laparoscope allows the introduction of instruments that may be used to obtain ovarian biopsy or drain a cyst without damage to vessels on the surface of the ovary.

After the procedure is completed, all instruments except the laparoscope sheath are removed. The sheath is maintained in position and the intra-abdominal gas allowed to escape. The skin is closed with one or two sutures. A narcotic antagonist (0.4 mg naloxone hydrochloride) is administered intravenously. The mare is removed from the padded stocks, allowed to stand in the recovery room for 5 minutes and returned to a bedded stall.

INDICATIONS

There are several indications for laparoscopy in the field of equine reproduction (Table 1). Laparoscopy may be indicated in the evaluation of infertile mares. Direct inspection of the internal genitalia in conjunction with ovarian biopsies and microbiologic cultures provides the veterinarian with more information on which to base a diagnosis, formulate a plan for therapy and offer a prognosis.

The possibility of performing repeated laparoscopic examinations offers the veterinarian the opportunity to observe and study ovarian and uterine tubal function. Areas of needed research that may benefit from the use of laparoscopy include the study of stimulation and suppression of ovulation, ovum transport and uterine tubal motility and secretions.

CONCLUSION

Laparoscopy provides the veterinarian specializing in equine reproduction a diagnostic and thera-peutic technique useful in evaluating the upper portion of the reproductive tract. This instrument spans the void between rectal palpation and exploratory laparotomy and will aid in the study and understanding of equine infertility.

References

1. Heinze H: Pelviscopy in the mare. J Reprod Fert Suppl 23:319, 1975.
2. Steptoe PC: Laparoscopy in Gynecology. Edinburgh and London, E and S Livingston, 1967, p. 18.
3. Witherspoon DM, McQueen RD: Development of equine peritoneal fistula device. Am J Vet Res 31:387, 1970.
4. Wilson GL: Laparoscopic Examination of Mares. Vet Med/Small Anim Clin, October 1983, 1629–1633.

Equine Neonatal Respiratory Distress and Resuscitation

John W. Ludders, D.V.M.
David B. Brunson, D.V.M., M.S.
University of Wisconsin, Madison, Wisconsin

The transition from fetus to neonate involves a multitude of interrelated anatomic, physiologic and behavioral processes. If the transition from fetal to neonatal status is delayed, severe neonatal stress can occur and may result in the death of the foal or render it susceptible to secondary complications. In the equine species, this condition has been referred to as the "neonatal maladjustment syndrome."[1] A major factor in this condition is asphyxia and hypoxia at or shortly after birth. It may be due to a variety of factors including partial or premature placental separation, compression, damage or knotting of the umbilical cord, impairment of the maternal cardiopulmonary system as may occur during cesarean section, dystocia, pharmacologic agents such as anesthetics, trauma or septicemia.[7, 9, 12]

This chapter will describe normal fetal development characteristic of the equine, normal postnatal behavior of the foal, and treatment regimens that the veterinarian may use to enhance the survival of a term but weak newborn foal. This section is not concerned with resuscitation of the foal born prematurely or with congenital defects. For a more detailed discussion of fetal and neonatal anatomy and physiology, the reader is referred to the section in this text entitled Resuscitation and Intensive Care of the Newborn Calf.

FETAL DEVELOPMENT

The placenta serves as the gas and metabolite exchange structure between the dam and the fetus. In the equine species, the placenta is a highly efficient structure for oxygen and carbon dioxide exchange because of the microcotyledonary circulation, the small intercapillary distances between maternal and fetal vessels, and the fairly high rate of uterine blood flow relative to umbilical blood flow.[14] For these reasons, the oxygen and carbon dioxide gradients across the placenta are minimal, especially when compared with those in other species such as sheep, cows and pigs. In comparison with other species, changes in the arterial Po_2 of the mare are immediately reflected in the umbilical venous blood as evidenced by a fall in the umbilical venous Po_2.[14]

In many species (man, monkey, ruminant), the affinity of fetal blood for oxygen is increased when compared with adult blood due to the physicochemical difference in fetal hemoglobin. This increase in affinity of fetal hemoglobin for oxygen facilitates the transport of oxygen across the placenta. In contrast, the equine fetus does not have fetal hemoglobin. The hemoglobin in the fetus is identical to that of the adult horse. The slight increase in affinity for oxygen of equine fetal red blood cells compared with the adult is due to decreased amounts of 2,3-diphosphoglycerate (2,3-DPG). The 2,3-DPG binds to hemoglobin, thus decreasing the affinity of hemoglobin for oxygen. The concentration of 2,3-DPG increases immediately after birth of the foal and approaches the concentration observed in the adult horse within 3 days.[6] Acidosis of any origin can inhibit the formation of 2,3-DPG.

Although the fetal lungs are mechanically inactive and receive only 25 per cent of the fetal cardiac output, the respiratory system does become primed in several ways for functioning at birth. Lung liquid is formed by the lungs and leaves via the trachea to be swallowed or added to the amniotic fluid, which serves as a protective cushion for the fetus. Near term, this volume of lung liquid is similar to the functional residual capacity of the neonatal lung. At birth, the lung liquid is primarily removed via absorption into the lymphatic system. With the onset of breathing and inflation of the lungs, radial traction is created within the lung parenchyma, expanding the lymphatic plexuses in the peribronchial and periarterial connective tissues. This results in an increase in the hydraulic conductivity of the pulmonary epithelium, thus facilitating absorption of the lung liquid.[15] Without this change, absorption would be very slow.

Cells within the lung tissue produce surfactant, which lowers surface tension and reduces the tendency of alveoli to collapse. In the equine fetus, surfactant is present in the lumina of alveoli at 200 days of gestation, but it is not fully developed until about 300 days of gestation or later.[8] A lack of surfactant can be due to a primary defect in the production of surfactant or it may be secondary to other causative factors.

Finally, there are respiratory movements in the fetus that are not due to asphyxia.[15] The fetal breathing movements indicate that the respiratory centers and other neuromuscular mechanisms necessary for breathing are present and capable of functioning at an early stage of development.

INITIATION OF RESPIRATION

At birth, many factors interact to initiate neonatal breathing. The factors include a low Pao_2 and an elevated $Paco_2$, tactile stimulation, lowered temperature and gravity. The onset of breathing and placental separation initiate profound and immediate changes in the circulatory system of the neonate. With the reduction of placental blood flow, there is an increase in vascular resistance for the left side of the heart. Concurrently, as the lungs expand with the first breaths there is a reduction in pulmonary vascular resistance. This causes a lowering of blood pressure on the right side of the heart. These changes in direction of the pressure gradients between the right and left sides of the heart cause functional closure of the foramen ovale. With the onset of breathing, the Pao_2 increases from fetal levels and causes the ductus arteriosus to constrict, thus restricting the flow of blood from the pulmonary vein through the shunt to the aorta. In the foal, a murmur can normally be auscultated over the region of the ductus arteriosus for up to 3 weeks.[5]

NORMAL NEONATAL BEHAVIOR IN THE FOAL

The behavior pattern of the mare during parturition and of the foal following birth are character-istic. If the behavior of either the dam or the foal is abnormal, it may indicate that there are problems with the foaling. In the thoroughbred, the following are considered to be important normal events at the time of parturition following an average gestation period of 340 days. First, the onset of stage II labor is marked by rupture of the chorioallantoic membrane, with full delivery of the foal within 30 minutes of this event.[10, 11] In most cases, the mare delivers the foal while in the recumbent position, which may allow for transfer of a significant amount of blood from the placenta to the foal.[10, 13] The umbilical cord ruptures when the mare stands following delivery. Within seconds of delivery, the normal foal establishes a respiratory rhythm, and within a few minutes its ability to right itself becomes obvious. Furthermore, within 100 minutes of birth the foal is able to stand and nurse. Variation from this behavior pattern may indicate that the foal is not normal or needs assistance if it is to survive. A key step in this cascade of events is the ability of the foal to initiate respiration and take its first breaths.

RESUSCITATION PROCEDURES FOR THE NEONATAL FOAL

As soon as the foal is delivered, it must be observed to determined whether it can successfully make the transition from fetal to neonatal status. Once the face, nares and oral pharynx are cleared of mucous and fetal membranes the heart rate, color of the mucous membranes and respiratory efforts should be evaluated. This establishes a baseline for future evaluations. If the heart rate is slow, the mucous membranes are pale, and the foal appears unable to initiate or maintain ventilation, resuscitation procedures should be started immediately. Since inflation of the lungs is essential in the transition from fetal to neonatal status, the initial steps in resuscitation are oriented toward inflating and ventilating the lungs. The resuscitation procedure involves intubation of the foal, positive pressure inflation and ventilation of the lungs, nursing care and use of pharmacologic agents if needed.

Intubation of the depressed foal with a normal upper airway is easy to perform and requires a minimum of equipment. The head of the foal should be extended on its neck so that the orotracheal axis approaches a straight line. A 10- to 12-mm (inside diameter) endotracheal tube can be used in thoroughbred foals. To facilitate intubation, a full roll of 1-inch tape can be used as a mouth gag. The tube is passed through the roll of tape, over the tongue and back into the pharynx. Because of the narrow, small mouth of the foal the tube is passed into the larynx and trachea without direct visualization. The tube is passed into the larynx using firm but gentle movements. If resistance is met, the tube should not be forced, but withdrawn, slightly rotated and advanced again. When the tube enters the larynx and trachea, the tip of the tube can be felt to slide past the tracheal rings. If the tube is in the esophagus, there is a feeling of smooth resistance. To ensure proper placement, the neck can be gently palpated to ascertain the presence of the tube in the trachea and not in the esophagus.

Very negative intrathoracic pressures are generated when a neonate takes its first breaths of air. Pressures as low as -80 cm H_2O have been recorded,[2] indicating the tremendous effort required of the neonate to inflate the lungs. Weak foals may not be able to generate the muscular effort required to inflate the lungs. In these cases, positive pressure ventilation is required.

A variety of devices for positive pressure ventilation are readily available for use in the field or clinical situation. The Hudson demand valve* is one example. It uses oxygen that can be supplied from an easily portable E cylinder equipped with a two-stage regulator that should permit regulation of line pressure. When connected to an endotracheal tube, the Hudson demand valve provides positive pressure ventilation when a button on the valve is depressed. If the button is held down the valve will continue to deliver oxygen until the pressure within the airway reaches approximately 54 cm H_2O. In the neonatal foal that is unable to fully inflate its lungs, the initial two or three positive pressure lung inflations with airway pressures of up to 54 cm H_2O may be appropriate. Thereafter, pressures up to 25 to 30 cm H_2O should be sufficient to inflate the lungs. Without a pressure gauge to measure pressure in the airway the adequacy of ventilation can be approximated by watching for normal chest wall excursions during positive pressure inflation. The Hudson demand valve will also deliver oxygen to a spontaneously breathing animal.

The Vetaspirator† is another portable device that can be used for positive pressure ventilation. In addition, it has a feature that allows operator-controlled aspiration. However, as mentioned earlier, the normal primary route for removal of lung liquid is through absorption, not drainage or aspiration.

Hand-operated mechanical inflation devices, such as the Ambu-bag, can also be used to inflate the lungs. However, lacking any of this equipment, the veterinarian can use his or her own lung volume and blow through the endotracheal tube to inflate the lungs of the neonatal foal.

Once the foal is able to maintain ventilation the veterinarian must provide adequate and proper nursing care. Although the foal can maintain its deep body temperature over a wide range of ambient temperatures within a few hours of birth, the potential for hypothermia is present. The foal should be dried and kept in a clean, draft-free environment.

Fluid therapy may be indicated in foals with a low intravascular volume and inadequate perfusion of tissues as determined by capillary refill time (CRT). Digital pressure on the gums causes blanching of the tissues. If perfusion is adequate the gums will regain their pink color within 1 to 2 seconds. A CRT greater than 2 seconds indicates inadquate perfusion. In addition, if metabolic reserves are depleted glucose should be given intravenously.

Alkali therapy may be of benefit in foals with severe acidosis that is slow to respond to the therapy detailed above. However, sodium bicarbonate therapy is not without hazards. It is usually administered as a hypertonic solution and has been associated with intracranial hemorrhage. In addition, bicarbonate dissociates into carbon dioxide and water. If the foal cannot ventilate adequately, the carbon dioxide will accumulate and a "paradoxical" worsening of the acidosis will occur.[3]

Neonatal animals display characteristic behavior patterns when they are anoxic.[9] Initially there is struggling, gasping, hypertension and bradycardia. This is followed by a short period of apnea, and then by a period of more regular and deeper gasping with a slight increase in heart rate. Following this is a second period of apnea that is often fatal, resulting in cardiovascular failure. Stimulatory drugs such as doxapram have been used in apneic animals in an attempt to stimulate ventilation. In low doses, doxapram stimulates respiration by stimulating carotid chemoreceptors, but in higher doses it stimulates both respiratory and nonrespiratory centers in the medulla.[4] Doxapram and other stimulatory drugs are not effective if used during the second period of apnea since the chemoreceptors are already maximally stimulated. These drugs may be of some benefit if used in the initial period of apnea. However, the key to resuscitation of the neonate in the latter stages of anoxia is full inflation of the lungs with air or oxygen by positive pressure ventilation.

In summary, resuscitation of the term but weak neonatal foal involves intubation, positive pressure ventilation, and nursing care that may include fluids and glucose given intravenously. Pharmaceutical agents such as respiratory stimulants or alkalinizing agents may be beneficial in some severe cases.

References

1. Arvidson G, Astedt B, Ekelund L, et al.: Surfactant studies in the fetal and neonatal foal. J Reprod Fertil Suppl 23:663, 1975.
2. Dejours P: Principles of Comparative Respiratory Physiology, 2nd ed. Amsterdam, Elsevier/North/Holland Biomedical Press, 1981, p 170.
3. Eidelman, AI Hobbs JF: Bicarbonate therapy revisited. Am J Dis Child 132:847, 1978.
4. Franz DN: Central nervous system stimulants. *In* Gilman AG, Goodman LS, Gilman A (eds): The Pharmacologic Basis of Therapeutics, 6th ed. New York, Macmillan, 1980, pp 585–591.
5. King AS: A Guide to the Physiological and Clinical Anatomy of the Thorax, 3rd ed. Liverpool, University of Liverpool Press, 1974, Chap. 10.
6. Kitchen H, Bunn HF: Oxygen transport and adaptation in the

---

*Model 5040, Hudson Oxygen Therapy Sales Co., Wadsworth, Ohio.

†Vetaspirator, Veterinarian's Specialities, Cedar Rapids, Iowa.

fetus and newborn foal. Proc Am Assoc Equine Pract 17:81, 1971.

7. Martens RJ: Perinatal physiology and pathobiology of the foal. Proc Am Assoc Equine Pract 24:411, 1978.

8. Pattle RE, Rossdale PD, Schock C, et al.: The development of the lung and its surfactant in the foal and in other species. J Reprod Fertil Suppl 23:651, 1975.

9. Randall GCB: Perinatal mortality: Some problems of adaptation at birth. Adv Vet Sci Comp Med 22:53, 1978.

10. Rossdale PD: Clinical studies on the newborn Thoroughbred foal: (I) Perinatal behavior. Br Vet J 123:470, 1967.

11. Rossdale PD: Clinical studies on the newborn Thoroughbred

foal: (II) Heart rate, auscultation and electrocardiogram. Br Vet J 123:521, 1967.

12. Rossdale PD, Leadon D: Equine neonatal disease: A review. J Reprod Fertil Suppl 23:685, 1975.

13. Rossdale PD, Mahaffey LW: Parturition in the Thoroughbred mare with particular reference to blood deprivation in the new-born. Vet Rec 70:142, 1959.

14. Silver M, Comline RS: Transfer of gases and metabolites in the equine placenta: A comparison with other species. J Reprod Fertil Suppl 23:589, 1975.

15. Strang LB: Growth and development of the lung: Fetal and postnatal. Ann Rev Physiol 39:253, 1977.

Neonatal Isoerythrolysis in the Foal

Michelle M. LeBlanc
University of Florida, Gainesville, Florida

Neonatal isoerythrolysis, a hemolytic disease of foals, is due to an incompatible blood group reaction between serum antibodies of the dam (concentrated in colostrum) and erythrocytes of the neonate. Hemolytic crisis occurs when a mare that is negative for the antigen inherited by the fetus from the stallion is isoimmunized.

ISOIMMUNIZATION AND PATHOGENESIS

Isoimmunization of the dam may occur naturally or iatrogenically, although the actual mechanism has not yet been demonstrated. In natural isoimmunization, it is thought that sensitizing amounts of fetal antigen (paternal in origin) gain access to maternal circulation as a result of placental hemorrhage. Leakage of blood may occur late in gestation or during labor and may be enhanced by cesarean section, vaginal delivery, manual separation of the placenta or placental dysfunction. Resulting isoantibodies are selectively concentrated in colostrum prior to parturition.[3] These antibodies are ingested and absorbed by the intestine and pass into the systemic circulation where they destroy erythrocytes of the foal. The severity of hemolysis depends on the quantity and nature of the antibodies absorbed. In foals, clinical symptoms occur only after ingestion of colostrum, in contrast to the human fetus, in which the antibodies pass the placental barrier before birth.

During the last month of pregnancy, a sensitized mare will show a rise in the level of circulating antibody to the offending fetal antigen. It is possible, therefore, to identify potential cases of neonatal isoerythrolysis by screening mares prior to foaling and thus prevent the condition from occurring by withholding colostrum. The degree of maternal sensitization is relatively weak following the first pregnancy. Exposure to the same antigen in subsequent pregnancies stimulates an anamnestic response, which produces sufficient antibodies to cause hemolytic disease. The majority of cases are seen between the fourth and seventh pregnancies.

Iatrogenic isoimmunization of the dam has also been reported. Incompatible blood transfusions, injections of pregnant mare serum gonadotropin, pituitary luteinizing hormone, homologous blood vaccines (tetanus antitoxin) and tissue vaccines—namely, the intranasal vaccine of rhinopneumonitis (equine origin)—have all been incriminated as causes of hemolytic disease. Isoerythrolysis has also been reported in the cow and the sow, the majority of cases appearing to be associated with vaccination (anaplasmosis and babesiosis vaccine in the cow, hog cholera vaccine in the sow).[4] These vaccines, produced by pooling blood or blood-containing tissues from two or more sensitized animals, are ideal for production of isoantibodies.

BLOOD GROUPS

Eight blood groups (i.e., antigens on the surface of the erythrocyte) containing various blood factors are presently recognized in the horse (A, C, D, K, P, Q, T, U).[3, 4, 5] Neonatal isoerythrolysis occurs owing to differences among individual blood groups. Each group is completely independent and is inherited in a direct manner, one phenogroup arising from the dam and the other from the sire. Blood factor A of group A and Q of group Q account for the majority of hemolytic cases in the horse.[5] Both are highly antigenic and act primarily as hemolysins in the presence of fresh rabbit complement. Brood mares possessing both A and Q are at low risk of having foals that develop neonatal isoerythrolysis. Those lacking one or both, and with a titer of anti-A or anti-Q of $\geq$ 1:8 within a week or two of parturition are at a high risk. The most severe and peracute hemolytic crises occur with anti-A titers. Maternal isoantibodies formed against factor Q are less antigenic and have a slower disease onset. A high incidence of blood factor A is observed in thoroughbreds and Arabians. A 30 per cent lower frequency of both factors is present in Shetland ponies, making them good candidates for blood donors.

Of the remaining blood factors, blood group D, which functions primarily as an agglutinin, and factors RS of group Q (found together) also cause hemolytic disease. Neither is as antigenic as factors A or Q. The only reliable test for their detection in vitro is the antiglobulin test (direct Coombs').[3, 7]

CLINICAL SIGNS

The clinical picture observed in foals can vary with the type of antibody in colostrum, the amount ingested and the antigenic composition of erythrocytes of the foal. At birth all foals are normal because there is no transfer of passive immunity in utero. In most instances, the first signs of weakness and dullness are seen by 24 to 36 hours. The foal is reluctant to suckle for long and may become easily exhausted just by following his dam in the paddock. Breathing is rapid and shallow and the foal may repeatedly yawn. Heart rate is markedly increased and easily palpable through the chest wall.[2] Progressive lethargy and weakness follow until the foal is unable to stand.

Depending on acuteness, icteric mucous membranes may or may not be present. Acutely affected foals (within 12 to 14 hours of birth) may not develop jaundice until 1 to 2 days after the massive loss of circulating erythrocytes. Hemoglobinuria may occur prior to icterus. Foals afflicted within 12 hours of parturition have rapid circulatory collapse and dark red to muddy brown mucous membranes. These foals die within 12 to 36 hours, apparently as a result of anaphylactic shock, mediated by an antigen-antibody reaction.[1] Primary lesions observed on necropsy are pulmonary edema, icterus and splenomegaly due to sequestration of abnormal erythrocytes, and hemoglobinuria.

DIAGNOSIS

A fairly reliable diagnosis can be based on clinical signs. Few other diseases of the newborn present a similar picture. The hemogram reflects the severity of hemolytic crisis and is very important in the decision for treatment. Packed cell volume (PCV) and hemoglobin are usually low (PCV < 20 per cent). In peracute cases, PCV may be high due to hemoconcentration. The erythrocyte count drops below 3 million per cubic millimeter. White cell count will be normal unless an ongoing septicemia is present. Clinically inapparent hemolytic disease may be more common than is generally realized. It increases susceptibility of the foal to secondary pathogens by decreasing stress tolerance. When hemograms are performed on these subclinically affected foals, erythrocyte counts will be well below normal.

The definitive diagnosis is made serologically by demonstrating maternal isoantibodies present on the erythrocytes of the foal. The use of the Coombs' direct antiglobulin test will detect agglutination.[2] To detect hemolysins "coating" the erythrocytes of the foal, complement obtained from absorbed rabbit serum is added to the erythrocytes. Testing erythrocytes of the foal prior to nursing against colostrum of the mare to identify sensitization is of limited usefulness. Colostrum tends to induce marked rouleaux formation, which mimics agglutination. Due to false positive results, many foals will be denied the needed colostral protection from their dam. Unfortunately, most field tests are simple agglutination tests and are not adequate for detecting incompatibilities due to hemolysis.[1]

Detection of antigenic sensitization in the mare is based on abbreviated blood typing. This is the preferred technique for prevention of neonatal isoerythrolysis. Hemolysins are tested for by using absorbed rabbit or guinea pig serum as a source of complement.[6] Mares should be screened for the presence of anti-A or anti-Q titers 2 to 3 weeks prior to foaling. If a titer is greater than 1:8, colostrum of the dam is withheld from the foal following birth. When lower titers are present, the mare is rebled in 10 to 14 days to identify a possible rise in titer.[5]

Blood from mares needing to be typed may be sent to a commercial laboratory.* Two 10-ml blood samples, a serum tube and an ACD tube need to be drawn. Following 1 hour of refrigeration, samples may be mailed in a Styrofoam shipper.[6]

TREATMENT

Treatment needs to be directed toward maintenance of hemostasis. In very acute cases, transfusion is essential or the foal will quickly die from hemolytic anemia. Blood transfusion is also necessary when the total erythrocyte count is less than 3 million per cubic millimeter and PCV is less than 12 to 14 per cent. One large exchange of 4 to 6 liters administered slowly is more helpful than several small transfusions. One of the best sources of erythrocytes is the dam. Her erythrocytes will not be lysed by her own colostral antibodies. Cells must, of course, be free of serum from the mare and be checked against serum from the foal for the possibility of naturally occurring lysins. Four to six liters of blood should be collected from the dam in transfusion bottles containing acid citrate and spun in a centrifuge to remove plasma. Cells are washed three times in sterile normal saline to remove the majority of remaining plasma. A 50 per cent suspension of the washed erythrocytes is made with lactated Ringer's solution. This solution is administered slowly at the rate of 1 liter per hour and can be repeated in 24 to 48 hours if necessary. In an emergency, blood can be collected from the mare and left to stand for an hour. Once most of the cells have settled out, the majority of the plasma can be

---

*Stormont Laboratories, Woodland California.

aspirated. Some plasma will remain trapped within the cells, but the effect of this will be far outweighed by the beneficial effect of intact and compatible donor erythrocytes.[3]

If there is a massive acute intravascular hemolysis with severe icterus, an exchange transfusion with whole blood is indicated. A healthy donor, particularly an unrelated male or a Shetland pony whose washed red cells are compatible with the serum of the dam, can be used. If possible, select for the absence of A and Q blood factors. The sire is not an acceptable donor because his erythrocytes will react with passively acquired circulating antibody.

Support therapy is critical. Fluids (a balanced multiple-electrolyte solution) are necessary to maintain circulating blood volume, replace metabolic deficits and stimulate renal function.[1] Glucose should be administered to severely affected foals to compensate for hypoglycemia, a common sequela. To prevent additional anaerobic glycolysis in the peripheral tissues (due to reduced oxygen-carrying capacity of the blood), foals must be kept *quiet*. Antibiotics may be administered to prevent secondary bacterial infections. Corticosteroids, if given, will stimulate erythropoiesis and attempt to stabilize "coated" erythrocytes of the foal both directly and by interference in antibody-antigen complexes.

MANAGEMENT

The foal must be prevented from nursing and should be muzzled with a soft leather cloth or nylon stocking. Colostrum from an unrelated source or an artificial milk replacer should be fed. The mare will need to be milked for the first 36 hours following parturition. Titers should drop in 8 to 16 hours. The foal may be allowed to nurse its dam after 36 hours because he usually is unable to absorb immunoglobulins after 24 to 36 hours. A low percentage of foals will have an acute hemolytic crisis when allowed to nurse after several days. Separation of the mare and foal should be avoided because this added stress will compound problems.

PREVENTION

When a mare is being immunized by her own fetus, it is possible to detect the presence of antibodies in her circulation. Screening mares 2 to 3 weeks prior to foaling for anti-A, anti-Q and anti-RS titers incorporating the abbreviated blood typing is the preferred method. Other tests include the indirect antiglobulin test (examining serum and precolostrum of the mare for antibody production against erythrocytes of the stallion) and comparison of stallion and mare blood types prior to breeding. Since neonatal isoerythrolysis is a relatively uncommon disease, it is impractical to sceen all pregnant mares. It is reasonable to screen pregnant A-negative mares because anti-A titers produce the most serious clinical effects. If a mare has had a hemolytic foal, there is no reason for her to lose another foal with this condition. These mares should be tested for rising isoantibody titers in the last few weeks of subsequent pregnancies. A good prognosis may be given if the condition is diagnosed sufficiently early and appropriate treatment is instituted promptly.

References

1. Martens RJ: Neonatal isoerythrolysis. *In* Mansmann RA, McAllister ES (eds): Equine Medicine and Surgery, Vol I, 3rd ed. Santa Barbara, American Veterinary Publishers, 1982, pp 352–355.
2. Rossdale PD, Ricketts SW: Equine Stud Farm Medicine, 2nd ed. Philadelphia, Lea & Febiger, 1980, pp 345–349.
3. Scott AM, Jeffcott LB: Hemolytic disease of the newborn foal. Vet Rec 103:71, 1978.
4. Stormont CJ: Neonatal isoerythrolysis in domestic animals. A comparative review. Adv Vet Sci Comp Med 19:23, 1975.
5. Stormont CJ: Blood groups in animals. J Am Vet Med Assoc 181:1120, 1982.
6. Stormont C: Personal communication, 1983.
7. Tizard I: An Introduction to Veterinary Immunology, 2nd ed. Philadelphia, WB Saunders, 1982, pp 281–283.

Contagious Equine Metritis

David G. Powell
University of Kentucky, Lexington, Kentucky

Following the first reported outbreak of contagious equine metritis on stud farms in the Newmarket area of England during 1977, the disease has been diagnosed among equine populations in many parts of the world. Contagious equine metritis is caused by a previously unrecognized gram-negative coccobacillus and can persist in the genital tract of mares and stallions for an indefinite period. Several reviews of the disease have been published in many languages, and recent reviews in the English language have been published by Platt and Taylor[8] and Brewer.[2]

BRIEF HISTORY OF THE DISEASE

During April, 1977, a large public stud farm in the Newmarket area, housing mares from many parts of the world, reported that an unusually large proportion of bred mares were returning to estrus after a shortened diestrous period. This was associated, in some mares, with varying amounts of a mucopurulent uterine discharge that developed 48 hours after covering. In some cases this was copious, causing a vulval discharge coating the hindquarters and tail. The majority of affected mares did not conceive, but the stallions that had covered the mares appeared healthy. Extensive laboratory studies failed initially to identify the causal agent, but eventually a gram-negative coccobacillus was isolated from endometrial swabs cultured on chocolate (heated) blood agar. The plates had been incubated at 37°C in an atmosphere containing 5 to 10 per cent carbon dioxide following 48 hours incubation. Transmission studies undertaken in ponies confirmed the organism as the causal agent. Similar results were obtained at the same time in Ireland, where the disease was also under investigation. Sensitivity tests indicated that the organism was sensitive to a wide range of antibiotics including penicillin but was resistant to streptomycin. Initially, difficulties were encountered in isolating the organism from the genital tract of stallions that had covered affected mares. These were due to heavy contamination of culture plates by commensal and environmental bacteria and were overcome with the aid of a selective medium containing streptomycin.

Because of the disease outbreak, breeding on a number of stud farms in the Newmarket area was suspended, and by the end of the season it was estimated that approximately 200 mares and 23 stallions on 29 stud farms had contracted the disease. The outbreak received widespread publicity and a ban on the movement of horses from France, Ireland and the United Kingdom was imposed by a number of countries including the United States, Canada, Australia and New Zealand. Despite these precautions contagious equine metritis was confirmed in Australia later in 1977 and in the United States during the spring of 1978. A feature of the U.S. outbreak, which occurred among Thoroughbred horses in Kentucky, was the isolation of two strains of the organism, one sensitive and the other resistant to streptomycin. During the autumn of 1977 a code of practice to control the disease was published in the United Kingdom by a scientific committee convened by the Horserace Betting Levy Board, and similar codes were published in Ireland and France.

DISTRIBUTION

Knowledge of the geographic distribution of contagious equine metritis is still incomplete because in many countries the appropriate bacteriologic methods have not been included in routine laboratory procedures. In Europe the disease has been reported in the United Kingdom, Ireland, France, Germany, Belgium, Italy, Yugoslavia and Austria, and in Scandinavia from Denmark and Sweden. It is also present in the United States, Australia and Japan (see Table 1). Among several European

countries the disease has been diagnosed among Thoroughbred and nonthoroughbred animals, especially standardbred or trotting mares and stallions.

ETIOLOGY

Considerable detail regarding the characteristics of the causal organism has been published by Platt and Taylor[8] and Brewer.[2] Two strains of the contagious equine metritis organism are currently recognized—a streptomycin-resistant strain first isolated by Taylor and colleagues[20] in 1977 and deposited in the U.K. National Collection of Type Cultures (type strain NCTC 11184), and a streptomycin-sensitive strain initially isolated by Swerczek[15] in the United States (type strain NCTC 11225). The organism is a nonmotile, gram-negative, non–acid-fast coccobacillus with a mean diameter of 0.8 μm (range 0.7 to 1.0 μm) with occasional filaments 5 to 6 μm in length. The morphology is influenced by the culture medium, the conditions of incubation and the age of the culture with the proportion of coccal and bacillary forms varying considerably. The ultrastructure of the organism has been studied by Swaney and Breese,[14] who suggested the presence of a capsule.

The media most readily supporting growth in the laboratory is chocolate (heated) blood agar incubated at 37°C in an atmosphere containing 5 to 10 per cent carbon dioxide. Small opalescent glistening colonies less than 0.5 mm in diameter appear within 48 hours, but on further incubation for 3 to 4 days, these reach a maximum 1 to 2 mm in diameter. Other agar media that support growth include heated blood agar prepared from tryptose or Eugon agar. On these media there is a greater tendency for variation in colony size and morphology that is not always maintained on subculture. For this reason, the use of Eugon agar for primary isolation is not recommended. The contagious equine metritis organism grows under a variety of atmospheric conditions, indicating that it is not truly microaerophilic.

The organism is asaccharolytic but is catalase, cytochrome oxidase and phosphatase positive and is unreactive to other conventional biochemical tests. The DNA composition is 36.1 per cent guanine-cytosine. Serologic studies using antisera to the contagious equine metritis organism prepared in rabbits have not indicated any close relationship with any other bacterial genus. On the basis of their initial studies Taylor and colleagues[20] proposed that the organism should be named *Haemophilus equigenitalis*. However, it does not possess certain properties associated with the genus *Haemophilus* and the possibility that it should be placed in a genus of its own has been considered. Sugimoto and co-workers[13] have recently suggested that it should be reclassified in a new genus *Taylorella* as *T. equigenitalis*.

Table 1. Geographic Distribution of Contagious Equine Metritis

Region	Country	Type of Horse	Streptomycin	
			Sensitive	*Resistant*
Europe	United Kingdom	TB + nonTB		+
	Ireland	TB		+
	France	TB + nonTB	+	+
	Italy	TB		+
	Germany	TB + nonTB	+	+
	Belgium	nonTB	+	
	Yugoslavia	not known	+	
	Austria	nonTB		+
North America	United States	TB + nonTB	+	+
Asia	Japan	TB		+
Australasia	Australia	TB		+
Scandinavia	Denmark	nonTB	+	
	Sweden	TB + nonTB	+	+

TB, thoroughbred, nonTB, nonthoroughbred

TRANSMISSION

Contagious equine metritis is disseminated primarily by venereal transmission, although during the early outbreaks it was recognized that the handling of the genital tract of mares and stallions by stud farm personnel and the use of contaminated veterinary instruments to examine mares also contributed to the spread of the disease. The ability of the contagious equine metritis organism to persist indefinitely in the genital tract of mares and stallions is well recognized. It is readily isolated from the clitoral sinus of the "carrier" mare and from the urethral fossa of positive stallions. The organism has been isolated from the placentae of positive mares[9] and from the genital tracts of several colts and fillies.[24] An investigation of the history of the colts and fillies suggested that in some cases the organism was acquired in utero or following transmission at the time of parturition. In other cases the probability was that the genital tract of the foal became contaminated with vaginal discharge from mares showing clinical signs of contagious equine metritis during the nursing period. There was also the possibility that transmission occurred in the training stable during the practice of washing the external genitalia of colts prior to a racing engagement.

PATHOLOGY

Because contagious equine metritis is not a fatal disease a study of its pathology has been restricted to observations following the autopsy of pony and crossbred mares experimentally infected with the contagious equine metritis organism and to endometrial biopsies obtained from field cases of the disease. The most recent experimental study, published by Acland and Kenney,[1] reported the findings from 23 mares that had been challenged by intra-uterine inoculation and had undergone necropsy after intervals of 2 to 115 days. Up to 14 days after the mares were inoculated the organism was readily isolated from the lumen of the uterus and the cervix. It was isolated less frequently from the vagina, vestibule, clitoral fossa and sinus, and uterine tube. After 21 to 116 days the organism was occasionally found on the ovarian surface, the uterine tubes, uterus, cervix and vagina but more frequently in the clitoral sinuses and fossa. The pathologic changes observed were those of a severe endometritis with extensive cellular infiltration and edema. This caused a severe necrosis and shedding of the endometrial epithelium into the lumen of the uterus, contributing to the profuse discharge that emanated from the cervix. The changes were most obvious during the first 14 days but decreased thereafter to a mild or multifocal lymphocytic endometritis. After 14 days large numbers of plasma cells accumulated in the stratum campactum of the uterus. It was considered that they may well have contributed to local antibody production, accounting for the inability to isolate the contagious equine metritis organism from the uterus and cervix after 14 days. The authors concluded that lesions caused by other pathogenic bacteria were similar to those observed with contagious equine metritis and that there were no characteristic histologic lesions that might be diagnostic of the disease. In mares that became carriers histologic examination of the clitoris revealed some infiltration of macrophages and plasma cells into the epithelium, but the specificity and significance of these changes was considered doubtful. No lesions have been reported in the stallion.

DIAGNOSIS

Currently, the diagnosis of contagious equine metritis is confirmed by isolation of the gram-negative coccobacillus from the genital tract of a mare or stallion. To reduce the possibility of obtaining a false-negative result it is imperative that samples be obtained from the appropriate sites in the correct manner, placed immediately in transport medium and cultured as quickly as possible in a laboratory that is familiar with the fastidious nature of the organism.

Sites to Swab in the Mare

Swabs should be taken from the lining of the endometrium or cervix during early estrus and from the clitoris including the clitoral sinuses. The sinuses are found on the dorsal aspect of the clitoris and are usually three in number. They have narrow openings that are not readily observed until the clitoris is partially extruded and held downward. Each sinus contains varying amounts of smegma, which may be extruded from the central sinus as a small hard pea. Some mares resent having a swab placed in the sinus, so adequate restraint is necessary. A small swab moistened in sterile water should be inserted in the sinuses and then placed in transport medium. An endometrial swab should always be taken from a subject with a suspected case of contagious equine metritis, but for routine screening the clitoral swab has the advantage that it may be taken from the nonpregnant mare at any stage of the cycle and from the in-foal mare at any stage during pregnancy.

Sites to Swab in the Stallion

The stallion or colt should always be sampled with the penis in the extruded position. Swabs should be taken on at least three occasions before the stallion can be considered free of the disease. Samples should be obtained from the urethral fossa, the urethra, the folds of the sheath and skin of the penis and, if possible, the pre-ejaculatory fluid. It may be necessary to moisten the swab in sterile water. On occasion, swabs may be heavily contaminated with other organisms such as *Proteus* and *Pseudomonas*, which tend to overgrow in the culture plates and inhibit the growth of the contagious equine metritis organism. This may be partially overcome by the use of selective media, although following the treatment of a positive stallion, it may be necessary to breed the stallion to a test mare. The test mare may then be screened bacteriologically and serologically to determine if transmission of the organism has occurred. In the absence of test breeding, the stallion should be swabbed on three occasions with negative results, the first sample not to be taken until 7 days after treatment has ceased.

Transport Media

All swabs should be placed in a transport medium, preferably Amies with charcoal, and kept at 4°C or on ice and delivered to the laboratory within 24 hours. Inhibitors or antibiotics should not be added to the transport medium.

Isolation and Confirmation

Details of the bacteriologic techniques for the isolation of equine genital infections have been published by Mackintosh.[5] Swabs taken for possible contagious equine metritis isolation should be plated onto a rich peptone-based agar medium to which L-cystine (300 mg per liter) or the soluble L-cystine hydrochloride (100 mg per liter), sodium sulfite (200 mg per liter), and 2 to 5 per cent heated horse or sheep blood have been added. The addition of 5 mg per liter of amphotericin and 1 mg per liter of crystal violet helps reduce fungal contamination. One plate should contain streptomycin sulfate, 200 mg per liter, and each swab should be inoculated onto two plates, one with streptomycin and one without. The blood agar plates should be incubated at 37°C in 5 to 10 per cent carbon dixoide. The contagious equine metritis organism usually grows within 24 to 48 hours, although plates should not be discarded until after 6 days incubation. A subculture should be made from a single colony onto a nonselective medium, which allows confirmatory tests to be performed on a pure culture. Suspect colonies should be tested for oxidase, catalase and phosphatase activity; if positive and if they reveal gram-negative coccobacilli on Gram stain, such colonies should be submitted to a series of sugar tests. If the organism is unreactive to these tests and does not grow aerobically on blood agar and gives a positive agglutination reaction with specific rabbit antisera, then contagious equine metritis organism is confirmed.

Serology

A variety of serologic tests including serum plate and tube agglutination, complement fixation, passive hemagglutination, enzyme-linked immunosorbent assay (ELISA) and immunodiffusion have been developed to detect antibody to the contagious equine metritis organism in serum. A comparison of the various tests undertaken by Sahu and colleagues[11] indicated that the ELISA and passive hemagglutination tests were superior to other serologic methods in detecting infected mares. Field application of the various serologic tests has demonstrated that they are a useful adjunct to isolation in identifying positive mares during an outbreak of contagious equine metritis. Mares with an endometritis following contagious equine metritis develop a humoral response that can be measured within 40 days of challenge. The present serologic tests appear to be of little value as a screening procedure to identify chronically infected or carrier mares. Antibody levels in these mares have waned and the contagious equine metritis organism has localized in the clitoral sinuses, where it does not appear to stimulate a detectable humoral response. There have been no reports of finding humoral antibody to contagious equine metritis in the stallion. Both field and experimental studies have demonstrated considerable individual mare variation in immune response to infection, and there is an apparent difference in response between breeds of horses.

Alternative Methods of Diagnosis

Gram-stained smears of cervical and vaginal exudate provided the first clues to the etiology of contagious equine metritis in 1977. In acute cases a presumptive diagnosis can be made from the microscopic examination of Gram- or Giemsa-stained smears taken from the endometrium. They reveal large numbers of inflammatory cells, predominantly polymorphonuclear leukocytes and numerous small gram-negative coccobacilli, located free or phagocytosed within the cytoplasm of neutrophils. Smears prepared from chronically infected or carrier mares are of little value. When there is strong circumstantial evidence to suggest that a stallion or mare has transmitted contagious equine metritis but it has proved impossible to isolate the organism, a procedure of inoculation of test mares using smegma from the subject animal has been recommended.[18] In the laboratory a variety of methods have been attempted to improve the isolation and identification of the contagious equine metritis organism. These include development of a selective medium[25] and the use of gas liquid chromatography to identify the organism.[6]

TREATMENT

Mares recovering from contagious equine metritis infection may be considered under three categories: the majority, which recover spontaneously and from which the organism can no longer be isolated; cases that recover following treatment; and cases from which the organism continues to be isolated despite treatment. The latter constitute a very small proportion of affected animals but have proved to be the focus from which fresh outbreaks of the disease have occurred.

Experience has shown that topical treatment is the most efficacious, although a single course of treatment does not necessarily eliminate the organism in every case. Uterine infusions given daily for 5 to 7 days have included benzyl penicillin, ampicillin, neomycin and nitrofurazone given either alone or in various pharmaceutical combinations. Daily infusions of 5 to 10 mega units of penicillin in 100 ml of water have been successful. Problems associated with the persistence of the organism in individual mares following a single course of treatment may be attributable to an insufficient dose rate or inadequate duration of treatment.

Special attention must be given to the clitoris and sinuses, which should be thoroughly cleansed with a 4 per cent solution of chlorhexidine using an intramammary syringe. They should then be packed with nitrofurazone, penicillin or chlorhexidine oint-ment. The procedure should be repeated daily on five occasions. Mares with a known history of contagious equine metritis may have their clitoris and sinuses cleansed with chlorhexidine on each of two or three days in early estrus prior to being covered.

Swerczek[16] has suggested that antibiotic therapy prolonged the course of the disease and promoted persistence of the organism in the genital tract. He observed that certain bacteria inhibited the growth of the contagious equine metritis organism in utero and suggested that a similar situation might exist in vivo where the normal flora of the reproductive tract inhibited the growth of pathogenic bacteria including the contagious equine metritis organism.

The topical treatment of stallions with chlorhexidine and nitrofurazone has proved highly successful. The external genital organs should be thoroughly cleaned with the penis in the extruded position, using a solution of not less than 2 per cent chlorhexidine, and then dressed with nitrofurazone ointment. This should be repeated for 5 days, paying particular attention to the cavities of the urethral fossa, the folds of the sheath and the skin of the penis. There have been no reports of impaired fertility in mares or stallions following successful treatment.

EPIDEMIOLOGY

Although contagious equine metritis was first recognized in 1977, it is probable that the causal agent was present in the equine population prior to that period. O'Driscoll and colleagues[7] described an outbreak of genital infection among Thoroughbred horses in 1976 that was clinically and epidemiologically similar to contagious equine metritis. The isolation of the organism from 2-, 3- and 4-year old Thoroughbred horses during 1978 and 1979 with no history of sexual experience further supports their view. Prior to 1977 swabs taken from the genital tract of mares and stallions were cultured only aerobically allowing the organism to remain undetected.

To date all strains of the contagious equine metritis organism recovered in the United Kingdom, Ireland and Australia are streptomycin-resistant. Assuming that the resistant strain evolved from the sensitive strain, it is likely that contagious equine metritis was introduced into the equine population of these countries following the importation of a carrier animal. This has been established for the origin of the outbreaks in the United States, the first outbreak in Kentucky originating from the importation of two Thoroughbred stallions from France in 1977, and the second in Missouri from the importation of a Trakehner stallion from Germany during the same year.

The isolation of the sensitive strain from several horse breeds, especially trotting or standardbred horses, in several European countries suggests that the disease may have been circulating in the horse population for some time. Nonthoroughbred horses receive less veterinary attention than Thoroughbred horses, so cases of genital disease would not have been investigated, thus allowing contagious equine metritis to become more widely distributed.

The origin of the contagious equine metritis bacteria is still a matter of speculation. It may have been present in other animal species as a pathogenic or commensal organism, although studies indicate it has a limited host range. The disease has been reproduced in donkeys,[22] but not in cattle, sheep or pigs,[23] although laboratory animals appear to be more susceptible.[21] Alternatively, it may have evolved as a mutant of another bacterial species because there are reports that it does cross-react to some degree with several other gram-negative bacteria including *Moraxella, Acinetobacter* and *Haemophilus*.[12] Seroepidemiologic studies in the human[19] and bovine[3] have demonstrated antibody to contagious equine metritis antigen in these species. It is therefore possible that a similar or related organism may be present in other domestic animals and man that may or may not be a cause of genital disease.

CONTROL

The control of contagious equine metritis is dependent on the ability to reduce the incidence of the disease within the equine population by identifying and successfully treating positive mares and stallions. Considerable success has been achieved since 1977 in reducing the incidence of the disease in countries where it has been reported. This was brought about by the implementation of the codes of practice, the first of which was introduced in the United Kingdom prior to the 1978 breeding season. The codes emphasized the significance of the prompt diagnosis of contagious equine metritis and the standards of hygiene necessary on the stud farm to prevent the spread of the disease. An extensive bacteriologic screening program of mares and stallions was recommended to identify the clinical or carrier case. Only after positive mares and stallions had been treated and found not to harbor the contagious equine metritis organism were they allowed to participate in the breeding program. In Europe, a common code has been in operation for several years to control the disease among Thoroughbreds in France, Ireland and the United Kingdom, and similar codes have been introduced in Italy, Sweden and Germany. Outbreaks of the disease that have occurred since the codes were introduced have been few, involving only a small number of animals. The origin of these outbreaks has invariably been traced to the introduction of a carrier mare. As a consequence, mares with a known history of contagious equine metritis infection have been placed in the "high risk" category and must be swabbed from the endometrium and the clitoris including the clitoral sinuses with negative results, on at least three occasions. Even so, a number of mares have given false-negative results,

and consequently prophylactic treatment of the clitoris prior to mating and surgical removal of the clitoral sinuses has been advocated.[17] This latter procedure has been incorporated in the requirements for importation of mares into the United States from countries in which the disease has been reported.

The available evidence suggests that the prevalence of contagious equine metritis is low, although as the techniques for isolation of the organism become more widely used, it is likely that the reported distribution of the disease will increase.

The possibility of developing a vaccine against contagious equine metritis was investigated by Fernie and colleagues[4] and Sahu.[10] In both studies, although vaccinated ponies developed a high level of circulating antibody, the antibody did not protect against subsequent challenge. Vaccinated animals that were challenged showed less severe clinical signs and harbored the organism for a shorter period compared with control animals, suggesting that some degree of immunity, possibly local, did exert a protective effect.

The antiseptic precautions undertaken on stud farms prior to 1977 were not effective in preventing the spread of contagious equine metritis. The codes of practice recommended the introduction of procedures involving greater use of disposable and sterile equipment, which has proved to be extremely effective in helping to eliminate the spread of contagious equine metritis and other genital infections.

References

1. Acland HM, Kenney RM: Lesions of contagious equine metritis in mares. Vet Pathol 20:330, 1983.
2. Brewer RA: Contagious equine metritis: A review/summary. Vet Bull 53:881, 1983.
3. Corbel MJ, Brewer RA: Antibodies to *Haemophilus equigenitalis* in bovine sera. Vet Rec 106, 35, 1980.
4. Fernie DS, Batty I, Walker PD, et al.: Observations on vaccine and post infection immunity in contagious equine metritis. Res Vet Sci 28:362, 1980.
5. Mackintosh ME: Bacteriological techniques in the diagnosis of equine genital infections. Vet Rec 108:52, 1981.
6. Neill SD, O'Brien JJ, McMurray CH, Blanchflower WJ: Contagious equine metritis—use of gas liquid chromatography in identifying the causal agent. Equine Vet J 16:430, 1984.
7. O'Driscoll J, Troy PT, Geoghegan FJ: An epidemic of venereal infection in thoroughbreds. Vet Rec 101:359, 1977.
8. Platt H, Taylor CED: Conagious equine metritis. *In* Easmon CSF, Jeljaszewicz J (eds): Medical Microbiology, Vol. I. New York, Academic Press, 1983, pp 149–196.
9. Powell DG, Whitwell K: The epidemiology of contagious equine metritis (CEM) in England 1977–1978. J Reprod Fertil Suppl 27:331, 1979.
10. Sahu SP: Contagious equine metritis: Effect of vaccination on control of the disease. Am J Vet Res 42:45, 1981.
11. Sahu SP, Rommel FA, Fales WH, et al.: Evaluation of various serotests to detect antibodies in ponies and horses infected with contagious equine metritis bacteria. Am J Vet Res 44:1405, 1983.
12. Smith JE, Young CR: Agglutinins to causative organism of contagious equine metritis 1977 in human serum. Lancet 1:1266, 1978.
13. Sugimoto C, Isayama Y, Sakazaki R, Kuramochi S: Transfer of *Haemophilus equigenitalis* Taylor et al 1978 to the genus *Taylorella* gen. nov. as *Taylorella equigenitalis* comb. nov. Curr Microbiol 9:155, 1983.

14. Swaney LM, Breese SS: Ultrastructure of *Haemophilus equigenitalis*, causative agent of contagious equine metritis. Am J Vet Res 41:127, 1980.

15. Swerczek TW: Contagious equine metritis in the U.S.A. Vet Rec 102:512, 1978a.

16. Swerczek TW: Inhibition of the CEM organism by the normal flora of the reproductive tract. Vet Rec 103:125, 1978b.

17. Swerczek TW: Elimination of CEM organism from mares by excision of clitoral sinuses. Vet Rec 105:131, 1979.

18. Swerczek TW: Contagious equine metritis: Test for suspect carriers. Vet Rec 108:420, 1981.

19. Taylor CED, Rosenthal RO: Agglutinins to the causative organism of contagious equine metritis 1977 in human serum. Lancet 1:1038, 1978.

20. Taylor CED, Rosenthal RO, Brown DFJ, et al.: The causative organism of contagious equine metritis 1977: Proposal for a new species to be known as *Haemophilus equigenitalis*. Equine Vet J 10:136, 1978.

21. Timoney PJ, Geraghty VP, Dillon PB, McArdle JF: Susceptibility of laboratory animals to infection with *Haemophilus equigenitalis*. Vet Rec 103:563, 1978b.

22. Timoney PJ, McArdle JF, O'Reilly PJ, et al.: Successful transmission of CEM to the donkey. Vet Rec 104:84, 1979.

23. Timoney PJ, O'Reilly PJ, McArdle J, Ward J: Attempted transmission of contagious equine metritis 1977 to other domestic animal species. Vet Rec 102:152, 1978a.

24. Timoney PJ, Powell DG: Isolation of the contagious equine metritis organism from colts and fillies in the United Kingdom and Ireland. Vet Rec 111:478, 1982.

25. Timoney PJ, Shin SJ, Jacobson RH: Improved selective medium for isolation of the contagious equine metritis organism. Vet Rec 111:107, 1982.

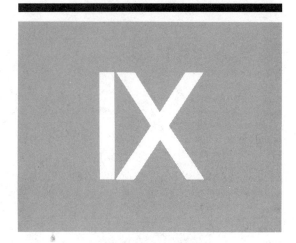

Physiology and Endocrinology of the Feline Estrous Cycle

Donelle R. Banks, Ph.D.

California State University, Sacramento, California

SEASONALITY-PHOTOPERIODISM

The reproductive cycle of the domestic cat has some unique features that are often overlooked. Unfortunately, it is convenient to lump dogs and cats together as "small animals." Cats, however, are induced, or reflex, ovulators and do not spontaneously ovulate during estrus. Thus, cats are reproductively more similar to rabbits (or ferrets and voles) than they are to dogs. In addition, dogs have an anestrous period unrelated to season, whereas the anestrus of cats is determined by the seasonal change in length of day (photoperiodism).

In the absence of mating queens will usually be in estrus every 2 to 3 weeks throughout the reproductive season. In the Northern Hemisphere this season generally begins in January as the day lengthens and continues until September. The duration and frequency of estrus throughout this period are variable among individuals.

In queens allowed to breed there will often be just two estrous periods (and two subsequent litters) per season. A January estrus with a litter born in March and a second estrus in May or June with a subsequent litter in July or August is a typical pattern. It is possible to have a third fertile estrus before the onset of the seasonal anestrous period in September.

The age at the first estrus (puberty) is dependent not only on physical maturation but also on the season. Kittens born in June, for example, may be sexually mature the following January and thus have their first estrus at 6 months of age—if they have attained a body weight of 2.3 to 2.5 kg.[15] Kittens born early in the year (e.g., March) would attain pubertal weight and age during anestrus and would not commence estrous cycles until the following January or February. The range of ages at puberty, therefore, is generally from 6 to 10 months.

Since the seasonal anestrus is a result of decreasing photoperiod, it can be modified by changing the natural light conditions. Cats exposed to artificial lighting in homes may continue to have estrous cycles in the months of October and November. Under laboratory conditions of 12 to 14 hours of artificial light per day, queens will cycle year-round. Additionally, the breed of the cat may influence seasonality. In one study 90 per cent of the long-haired cats exhibited seasonal anestrus, whereas only 40 per cent of the short-haired cats became anestrous.[8]

Recent studies have been designed to investigate the mechanism of the onset of ovarian inactivity during anestrus. The two hormones prolactin and melatonin are known to change in response to light-dark cues in many species. Prolactin is secreted from the anterior pituitary, which is under control of the hypothalamus. Melatonin is secreted by the pineal gland in the absence of light. In the cat, as in many other species, prolactin concentrations are higher during the dark hours; this results in a diurnal rhythm of prolactin secretion.[3] Melatonin secretion also increases during the dark period.[10] Melatonin is even more sensitive to changes in photoperiod than prolactin, so that with the seasonal decrease in light, melatonin levels are elevated for an increased number of hours. During seasonal anestrus, follicular growth in the ovaries is suppressed while these two hormones are elevated. Laboratory studies have shown that exogenous melatonin administration suppresses ovarian activity but not quite to the same degree as a short photoperiod.[11] It is still not known, however, whether changes in prolactin and/or melatonin concentrations are the cause or effect of photoperiod-induced anestrus.

THE ESTROUS CYCLE

The stages of the feline estrous cycle are usually described as proestrus, estrus, metestrus and anestrus. Metestrus is actually an "interestrous" period between two estrous periods if breeding does not occur. Anestrus in the cat is the seasonal period of ovarian inactivity, as previously described. Therefore, the cycles during the breeding season are composed of alternating estrus, interestrus and so on until the onset of the seasonal anestrus. If a sterile mating occurs during estrus, ovulation and corpora lutea formation are induced. This luteal phase can be termed diestrus. Therefore, there are three possibilities for a feline estrous cycle:

1. Proestrus, estrus (nonbred), interestrus
2. Proestrus, estrus (sterile mating), diestrus, interestrus
3. Proestrus, estrus (fertile mating), pregnancy

Vaginal Cytology

The stages of the estrous cycle correlate with changes in the vaginal epithelium, since both are caused by the changing levels of estrogen. Unfortunately, vaginal cytology cannot be used to predict the onset of estrus in the cat. This is because the behavioral signs of estrus often coincide with the increased vaginal cornification. In one study one third of the queens showed signs of estrus *before* the vaginal smear contained clearly detectable cornification.[19] The information obtained from vaginal cytology is primarily used, therefore, for following the stages of the estrous cycle or for verifying estrus.

The ease with which vaginal smears are obtained depends largely upon the personality of the cat, its familiarity with the handler and the stage of the estrous cycle. It is recommended that the sample be taken as quickly as possible, and it is usually desirable to have the cat restrained by a second person unless the queen is sexually receptive. In this case she may assume mating posture for the vaginal swabbing. Care must be taken not to stimulate the cervix with the swab, as ovulation may then be induced.

The technique involves gently swabbing the vaginal wall approximately 1 to 1½ cm inside the vaginal orifice with a sterile cotton swab. The swab should be premoistened with distilled water or saline to prevent irritation. After one full rotation, the swab is withdrawn and rolled on a slide to make one or two rows. The slide is then immediately immersed in 90 per cent methanol for not less than 1 minute. Air-dried slides can be stained immediately with a stain such as Giemsa or Wright's stain. When using the Giemsa stain (Azure II Eosin), it should be freshly prepared. The slides are stained for 20 minutes followed by a 5-second rinse in distilled water and air drying. An alternate stain useful in clinical situations is the Dif-Quick system, which has the advantage of being rapid (5-second dip in each of three solutions—fixative, eosin, counterstain) and of giving reliable color even after long storage of the stain.

When observed under the microscope, most slides will contain several cell types. By counting 100 cells, the per cent of each of the four different cell types can be determined. The four kinds of cells are parabasal, intermediate, superficial and anuclear. There are usually two or more cell types seen in a smear but the predominant type of cell (Fig. 1) indicates the stage of the estrous cycle as follows:

1. Anestrus—parabasal (small basophilic cells)
2. Interestrus—intermediate (large cells with distinct nuclei)
3. Proestrus—superficial (large cells with small, pyknotic nuclei)
4. Estrus—superficial and anuclear (cornified)

In addition to the changes in the predominant cell types during the estrous cycle, there is also a change in the background appearance of the slide because of increased mucous secretion during estrus. The smear shows a noticeable absence of noncellular debris at this time, resulting in a clear background. This "clearing" of the vaginal smear usually occurs before the onset of estrus.[19]

Behavior

Proestrus is characterized by an increase in the rubbing activity of the queen's head on inanimate or animate objects (including the owner and handler), often interpreted as affection. This behavior

may continue for 1 or 2 days before the queen is sexually receptive. On the other hand, proestrus may be unnoticed before estrus.

During estrus the queen will often vocalize and frequently assume a posturing position with the pelvis elevated, especially in the presence of a tom. While the queen is exhibiting lordosis, her tail is laterally deviated and the hind limbs tread actively. The male mounts by grasping the back of the queen's neck with his teeth and then begins a series of pelvic thrusts. Intromission and ejaculation occur after ½ to 7 minutes from the time of mounting.[19] At this time the queen emits a loud cry, which is presumed to occur when the cervix and vaginal wall are stimulated by the "spines" on the penis (or by a glass rod or cotton swab if mechanical stimulation by a person is used). Inexperienced cat owners may not realize that this piercing cry indicates that a successful mating has occurred. Immediately following this cry the queen actively rejects the male by hissing and striking or spitting at him. She then grooms her vulva and rolls around, sometimes quite violently. This behavior is known as the "after reaction." After approximately 5 to 20 minutes, the queen will usually posture again and allow the male to remount. There may be as many as 5 to 7 matings within 1 or 2 hours if the pair is not disturbed (Fig. 2).

A queen in estrus does not always mate even when this is desired by the owner. There are a number of factors that may prevent mating, such as the following:

1. Size incompatibility: A small male may have difficulty mating a large female unless his neck grasp is farther back on the neck region.

2. Unfamiliar surroundings: A tom brought to a new area may be more interested in "marking" the territory and investigating new smells than in breeding. Likewise, an estrous female may becomes less receptive when placed in an unfamiliar area, though generally, it is more important for the male to be in familiar surroundings than the female.

3. Personality: Shy or timid females may reject an aggressive male. If this occurs, the owner can pet the queen and stimulate her to posture for the male. Occasionally, a queen will reject one male but accept another. In most cases, a fully receptive female will allow more than one male to mount her during the estrous period. Thus, if it is the desire to have only one male be the father of an entire litter, the queen should be kept isolated from other males every day that she is sexually receptive.

The length of estrus among queens varies considerably but is usually from 5 to 8 days. In some studies mating seemed to shorten the length of estrus slightly.[12, 16] Other investigators have shown no significant differences in length of estrus between nonbred and bred queens.[26] In one study bred animals were in estrus longer (8.4 days) than animals that were not allowed to mate (6.2 days) but were still exposed to males.[19]

Continuous estrus of 3 or more weeks occasionally occurs even though there is regular cyclic ovar-

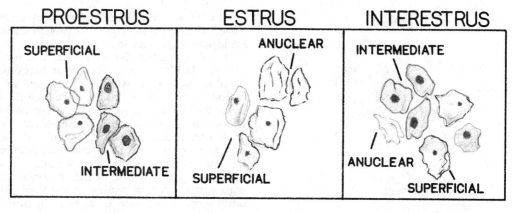

Figure 1. Vaginal cytology of the cat. Predominant cell types seen during three stages of the estrous cycle.

ian function. In this situation hormone analysis indicates that there have been separate waves of follicular growth and regression even though the queen exhibited continuous sexual receptivity. At the other extreme some queens do not exhibit estrus behavior even when vaginal cytology and estrogen levels indicate the estrous stage of the reproductive cycle. An example of this situation may occur when a timid queen is placed in new surroundings. Also, there are a few queens that exhibit overt estrous behavior only in the presence of a male. Therefore, an isolated queen may go through estrus unnoticed.

With so many deviations from average estrous behavior, it is apparent that the duration of nonestrous behavior between any two estrous periods can be very short (1 to 2 days) or very long (months). The average interestrous period is usually described as 8 to 9 days for nonbred animals. When a female is bred and becomes pregnant, the next estrus is delayed until 1 to 2 weeks after weaning (about 4 months total time from the last estrus). When a cat is mated with a vasectomized or sterile male, ovulation is induced and the follicles transform into corpora lutea. The next estrus is delayed until after the corpora lutea regress. This interestrous period is variable, ranging from 30 to 73 days but most commonly between 45 and 50 days.[14, 18, 26] This long luteal phase is sometimes called pseudopregnancy, as it is in the dog, but signs of lactation are infrequently present in the cat. If kittens from another queen are allowed to suckle a pseudopregnant cat, milk production may occur, presumably as a result of prolactin release in response to the suckling stimulus.

ENDOCRINOLOGY

In recent years the results of several studies have given a fairly complete picture of the hormonal events associated with the feline estrous cycle, ovulation and pregnancy. Hormones assayed in feline plasma include 17-β estradiol, estrone, progesterone, luteinizing hormone (LH), prolactin and relaxin. In addition to giving a graphic description of pituitary and ovarian activity, hormone analysis can be useful in verifying estrus, ovulation, pseudopregnancy and pregnancy.

In anovulatory estrous cycles, the waves of follicular development can be detected by a rise and fall of 17-β estradiol in the peripheral blood. The frequency and duration of consecutive follicular phases can thus be determined. In Figure 3 the first two cycles show a typical pattern for one cat. Levels of 17-β estradiol above 20 pg/ml indicate the days of the follicular phase.[19] Estrous behavior usually commences within 1 or 2 days following the initial rise of estradiol above 20 pg/ml. There may be a 1- or 2-day proestrus; however, many cats do not exhibit noticeable proestrous behavior. The average length of the follicular phase is 7.4 ± 2.3 days, with a range of 3 to 16 days.[19] The interval between follicular phases (that period when estradiol levels are less than 20 pg/ml) is generally 1 to 2 weeks.[19, 23]

Progesterone, another ovarian hormone, remains at basal levels (<1 ng/ml) during anovulatory estrous cycles, since no corpora lutea are formed.

Pituitary LH secretion, in the absence of coitus or mechanical stimulation of the cervix, remains at basal levels during estrus.[5, 21, 26] Pituitary follicle-stimulating hormone (FSH) secretion patterns in the cat have not, as yet, been reported.

As was previously mentioned, ovulation requires cervical stimulation by coitus or artificial means. These actions evoke pituitary LH release, presumably through a neurohormonal mechanism involving LH-releasing hormone (LHRH) from the hypothalamus. Pituitary LH release can also be evoked by injection of synthetic LHRH.[4, 9, 21]

When the queen breeds during estrus, the pitui-

POSTURING

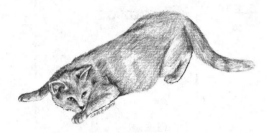

MATING

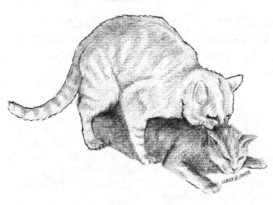

AFTER REACTION

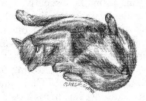

Figure 2. The posturing position of an estrous female (upper). Mating position; male grasping neck of female (middle). "After reaction" of queen; rolling and twisting (lower).

tary secretes LH into the bloodstream within 10 minutes after coitus. The amount of LH released in response to coitus varies with (1) the day of the follicular phase on which coitus occurs, (2) the number of coital contacts and (3) the frequency of coital contacts.

Cats mated two or three times on the first day of estrus do not always respond with an ovulatory LH surge. The amount of LH released by the pituitary may be insufficient to cause ovulation.[1, 26] Queens that are allowed to mate only once on the third day of estrus ovulate only about 50 per cent of the time. However, with four or more copulations on the third day of estrus, LH release is generally adequate to induce ovulation.[5, 25] It has not yet been determined whether there is an optimum frequency of coital contacts to ensure ovulation.

There is considerable variation in the pattern of postcoital LH surges. Some LH profiles show an immediate surge with short duration while others show a long, sustained release. This is caused in part by a lack of complete correlation between the onset of estrous behavior and the stage of the follicular phase. Some cats are in heat on the first day of the follicular phase, while others do not show estrus until the second, third or even fourth day of the follicular phase. It has been found that if a cat shows estrus early in the follicular phase, the pituitary may not be capable of responding to coitus with an ovulatory release of LH. A typical endocrine pattern of a cat mating on the third day of estrus is shown in Figure 3. The resulting ovulation may occur as early as 25 hours after coitus when the coital contacts occur within a 1 hour period,[19] or ovulation may occur later when there are fewer coital contacts, which are spaced over a period of hours.[26]

In addition to inducing ovulation, the pituitary LH release stimulates corpora lutea formation and the secretion of progesterone. A sustained, elevated progesterone concentration by the fifth or sixth day following coitus indicates that ovulation has previously occurred.

The mechanism by which LH causes the follicle to rupture seems to be different than the mechanism by which LH causes luteinization and progesterone secretion. Studies on rabbits have shown that prostaglandin synthesis within the follicle is necessary for the eventual follicular rupture but not necessary for progesterone secretion.[7] An attempt has been made to block ovulation after coitus in the cat by the administration of the drug indomethacin. This drug blocks prostaglandin synthesis and was found to be 100 per cent effective in blocking ovulation in rabbits.[13] In cats indomethacin administration is only partially effective in blocking ovulation even when two or three injections are administered over an 18-hour period (Banks, unpublished observations, 1979). There have been no other known reports regarding pharmacologic methods of successfully blocking ovulation in the cat.

It was previously mentioned that a definitive luteal phase (a period of elevated progesterone concentrations) occurs in the cat only when ovulation is induced without subsequent pregnancy. The ova in this case are not fertilized either because coitus occurred with a sterile (e.g., vasectomized or infertile) male or ovulation was induced artificially by stimulation with a glass rod or by injection of LH or human chorionic gonadotropin (hCG). The resulting luteal phase (or pseudopregnancy or pseudocyesis) is that period when progesterone levels are maintained at >1 ng/ml, usually peaking at >20 ng/ml in about 3 weeks. Progesterone levels during this time are similar to those during pregnancy but begin to decline after about 3 weeks to <1 ng/ml at about 35 to 40 days.

During the luteal phase queens do not usually exhibit estrus. Some animals may gain weight and have an enlarged uterus. The ovaries continue to

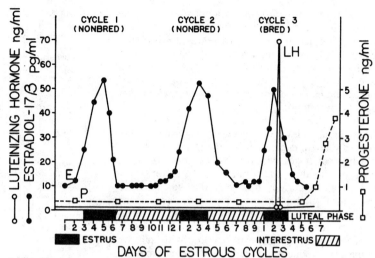

Figure 3. Composite of the hormonal events of the cat during three estrous cycles. Cycles one and two are anovulatory (nonbred) cycles. Cycle three shows a coitus-induced LH surge with subsequent corpora lutea formation, as indicated by the rise of progesterone concentrations.

have waves of follicular growth, although the number of follicles is fewer than during estrus.[26] Following the decline in progesterone to <1 ng/ml, there is a period of 7 to 10 days before the next estrus. This results in an overall interestrous period of 45 to 60 days.

Pharmacologic methods have been employed to shorten the luteal phase, although it is not generally recommended. Repositol progesterone or repositol diethylstilbestrol may be given. The use of prostaglandin $F_{2\alpha}$ or a methylester analog depresses progesterone levels somewhat but neither significantly shortens the luteal phase [18, 24] (Banks, unpublished observations, 1980).

PREGNANCY AND LACTATION

The gestation period in cats is approximately 65 days. The average litter size is dependent upon the

age and breed of the queen as well as her state of nutrition. Litter mates may have different male parentage (superfecundation) if the female is allowed to mate with more than one male.

The endocrinology of pregnancy has recently been investigated in the cat.[3, 17, 23] During the first half of pregnancy 17-β estradiol, LH and progesterone patterns are similar to those of the nonpregnant luteal phase. During the second half of pregnancy progesterone continues to be elevated until approximately 3 weeks before parturition, at which time progesterone concentrations begin a gradual decline.[2, 17] Concomitant with the progesterone decline is a rise in plasma prolactin, which peaks 2 to 3 days before parturition. The initial rise in prolactin occurs at about the sixth week of pregnancy.[2] Another hormone usually associated with parturition, relaxin, has been measured in the cat[22] and is included in the composite of pregnancy hormone relationships shown in Figure 4.

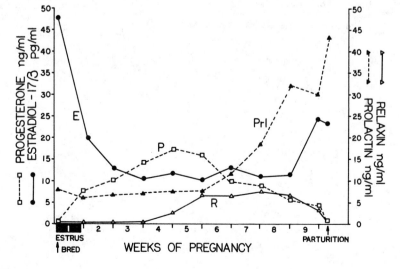

Figure 4. Composite of the hormonal events of the cat during pregnancy.

Concentrations of 17-β estradiol often fluctuate during the second half of pregnancy, indicating that waves of follicular growth and regression probably occur. Many cats exhibit peak 17-β estradiol levels during the last week of pregnancy.[17] An occasional queen will exhibit estrous behavior during pregnancy and can be bred, resulting in a litter of mixed ages (superfetation).

During the lactation period prolactin concentrations remain elevated for the first 4 weeks, then show a gradual decline during the next 2 weeks and reach basal levels within 2 weeks after weaning.[3] Most queens do not exhibit estrous behavior during the lactation period; however, this has been reported.[16] Usually, the first postpartum estrus occurs from 1 to 3 weeks following weaning and can result in pregnancy.[2, 17]

With increasing age, estrous periods usually become less frequent but do not cease completely. The number of ovulations decreases, resulting in smaller litters being born to queens over approximately 8 years of age.

References

1. Banks DR, Stabenfeldt GH: Luteinizing hormone release in the cat in response to coitus on consecutive days of estrus. Biol Reprod 26:603, 1982.
2. Banks DR, Paape SR, Stabenfeldt GH: Prolactin in the cat. I. Pseudopregnancy, pregnancy and lactation. Biol Reprod 28:923, 1983.
3. Banks DR, Stabenfeldt GH: Prolactin in the cat. II. Diurnal patterns and photoperiodic effects. Biol Reprod 28:933, 1983.
4. Chakraborty PK, Wildt DE, Seager SWJ: Serum luteinizing hormone and ovulatory response to luteinizing hormone-releasing hormone in the estrous and anestrous domestic cat. Lab Anim Sci 29:338, 1979.
5. Concannon P, Hodgson B, Lein D: Reflex LH release in estrous cats following single and multiple copulations. Biol Reprod 23:111, 1980.
6. Colby ED, Stein BS: The reproductive system. In Pratt PW (ed): Feline Medicine. Santa Barbara, American Veterinary Publications, Inc, 1983, pp 511–554.
7. Grinwich DL, Kennedy TG, Armstrong DT: Dissociation of ovulatory and steroidogenic actions of luteinizing hormone in rabbits with indomethacin, an inhibitor of prostaglandin biosynthesis. Prostaglandins 1:89, 1972.
8. Jemmett JE, Evans JM: A survey of sexual behaviour and reproduction of female cats. J Small Anim Pract 18:31, 1977.
9. Johnson LM, Gay VL: Luteinizing hormone in the cat. II. Mating-induced secretion. Endocrinology 109:247, 1981.
10. Leyva H, Addiego L, Stabenfeldt G: The effect of different photoperiods on plasma concentrations of melatonin, prolactin and cortisol in the domestic cat. Endocrinology 115:1729, 1984.
11. Leyva H, Stabenfeldt G: Effect of different photoperiods and chronic melatonin administration on estrous cycle activity of the domestic cat (In press).
12. Liche H: Oestrous cycle in the cat. Nature 143:100, 1939.
13. O'Grady JP, Caldwell BV, Auletta FJ, Speroff L: The effects of an inhibitor of prostaglandin synthesis (indomethacin) on ovulation, pregnancy and pseudopregnancy in the rabbit. Prostaglandins 1:97, 1972.
14. Paape SR, Shille VM, Seto H, Stabenfeldt GH: Luteal activity in the pseudopregnant cat. Biol Reprod 13:470, 1975.
15. Scott PP: Cats. In Halez ESE (ed): Reproduction and Breeding Techniques for Laboratory Animals. Philadelphia, Lea & Febiger, 1970, pp 192–208.
16. Scott PP, Lloyd-Jacob MA: Some interesting features in the reproductive cycle of the cat. Stud Fertil 7:123, 1955.
17. Schmidt PM, Chakraborty PK, Wildt DE: Ovarian activity, circulating hormones and sexual behavior in the cat. II. Relationships during pregnancy, parturition, lactation and the postpartum estrus. Biol Reprod 28:657, 1983.
18. Shille VM, Stabenfeldt GH: Luteal function in the domestic cat during pseudopregnancy and after treatment with prostaglandin $F_2\alpha$. Biol Reprod 21:1217, 1979.
19. Shille VM, Lundstrom KE, Stabenfeldt GH: Follicular function in the domestic cat as determined by estradiol-17β concentrations in plasma: Relation to estrous behavior and cornification of exfoliated vaginal epithelium. Biol Reprod 21:953, 1979.
20. Shille VM, Stabenfeldt GH: Current concepts in reproduction of the dog and cat. In Bradley CA, Cornelius CE (eds): Advances in Veterinary Science and Comparative Medicine. New York, Academic Press Vol. 24, pp 211–243.
21. Shille VM, Munro C, Farmer SW, et al.: Ovarian and endocrine responses in the cat after coitus. J Reprod Fert 68:29, 1983.
22. Stewart DL, Stabenfeldt GH: Relaxin activity in the pregnant cat. Biol Reprod 32:848, 1985.
23. Verhage HG, Beamer NB, Brenner RM: Plasma levels of estradiol and progesterone in the cat during polyestrus, pregnancy and pseudopregnancy. Biol Reprod 14:579, 1976.
24. Wildt DE, Panko WB, Seager SWJ: Effect of prostaglandin $F_2\alpha$ on endocrine-ovarian function in the domestic cat. Prostaglandins 18:883, 1979.
25. Wildt DE, Seager SWJ, Chakraborty PK: Effect of copulatory stimuli on incidence of ovulation and on serum luteinizing hormone in the cat. Endocrinology 107:1212, 1980.
26. Wildt DE, Chan SYW, Seager SWJ, Chakraborty PK: Ovarian activity, circulating hormones, and sexual behavior in the cat. I. Relationships during the coitus-induced luteal phase and the estrous period without mating. Biol Reprod 25:15, 1981.

Fetal and Neonatal Growth and Development

Ezra Berman, D.V.M.

MD-74C Environmental Protection Agency,
Research Triangle Park, North Carolina

The complicated and usually coordinated process of growth begins shortly after fertilization of the ovum and, in the strictest sense, does not end until death. Growth can be expressed in terms of changes in morphologic units, e.g., body weight or linear measurements, or in the incidence of appearance of structures or behavior. There are a variety of physiologic, behavioral and functional alterations that are part of this grand process. Growth is looked upon as normal maturation. However, the clinician should be aware of pathologic states in which or from which growth is abnormal or detrimental.

PRENATAL GROWTH

The clinician is sometimes called upon to make value judgements about the degree of maturity of a fetus. If the fetus has normal morphologic findings, and has little post-mortem change if dead, the weekly age can be accurately estimated by measurements of the crown-rump length and by observation of external characteristics. Table 1 contains data from observed breedings that occurred within 3-hour periods with known sires in a scientific production colony. The crown-rump length values are from Nelson and Cooper.[6] The external characteristics are personal observations by the author

on fetuses collected similarly from a different group of breedings. Of the three criteria in Table 1, the external characteristics will prove most useful as a clinical estimator of age.

The bony skeleton begins its appearance in the fetus as early as the fifth week of gestation, but these small depositions of bone may not be visualized on radiographic examination. By 6 weeks of age the fetus has sufficient bone to ensure that individuals are discernible in the uterus. The five bones of the appendicular skeleton of the cat fetus listed in Table 2 have a steady rate of growth, doubling in length in approximately 14 days. Even when these bones can be seen in a radiograph of the queen, measurements for age are not practical in the clinic because of unknown magnification and distortion factors in such radiographs.

The clinician is sometimes presented with a case of suspected superfetation in which a single fetus of a litter appears relatively immature but normal in all other respects. Superfetation has been reported in case histories,[4, 5] but the sexual lives of the involved queens were not fully controlled. In the scientific production colony previously noted fetuses that might ordinarily be considered superfetations were found in pregnancies from single breedings. The characteristics of the pregnancies detailed in the case histories and the singly bred pregnancies were similar: a relatively immature but normal live fetus among littermates seemingly 2 or 3 weeks older. Both the physiologic improbability of superfetation and the comparison of reported cases of superfetation with normal gestational variability lead us to believe that feline superfetation will remain theoretical.

POSTNATAL GROWTH

From birth the kitten's growth is dependent upon the amount and quality of available nutrition (milk supply), the presence of transmissible diseases in littermates, environmental conditions and a host of other influences. Because of its convenience as a measurement, body weight is a successful and conventional criterion of growth. Periodic weighing is

Table 1. Weight, Length and General External Characteristics of Aged Feline Fetuses*

Fetal Age (days)	Weight (gm)†	Crown-Rump Length (cm)†	N†	Characteristics
21	0.16 ± 0.09	1.48 ± 0.32	18	—
28	0.89 ± 0.2	2.43 ± 0.46	17	Opened eyes and ears; digits without claws
35	4.98 ± 1.2	4.73 ± 0.90	19	Closed eyes and ears; claws
42	17.8 ± 5.6	7.24 ± 1.07	21	Vibrissae follicles
49	40.7 ± 6.5	9.54 ± 0.90	18	Fine body hair without pattern or color
56	75.6 ± 15.0	11.7 ± 0.80	21	Full body hair with color and pattern
63	102 ± 24.6	13.8 ± 1.03	18	—
65 (birth)	97.1 ± 23.1	13.7 ± 0.92	78	—

*Values are mean and standard deviation. N = number of fetuses.
†Data from Nelson NS, Cooper J: Growth 39:435, 1975.

Table 2. Mean Lengths (cm) of Appendicular Bones in Fetal Cats (N = 9 to 14)

Bone	Week of Gestation			
	6	7	8	9
Humerus	0.73	1.17	1.49	1.87
Radius	0.68	1.08	1.36	1.70
Ulna	0.70	1.20	1.53	1.85
Femur	0.62	1.00	1.32	1.82
Tibia	0.58	1.06	1.41	1.80

the most common assay for continuing health and growth. A number of references contain growth tables using the body weight of the cat. These are not included here because of the difficulties associated with any attempt to compare weight curves among a feline production colony and a commercial cattery, pet environment or clinical situation. In absence of any chart, three rules may be applied:

1. A nursing kitten gains 7 to 10 gm or more per day.

2. Any loss of weight is a detrimental sign.

3. Birth weight (male or female) is approximately 100 ± 10 gm.

The pattern of eruption of teeth reflects age, and examination of the mouth for estimation of age is as accurate in the cat as in other species. Recogni-

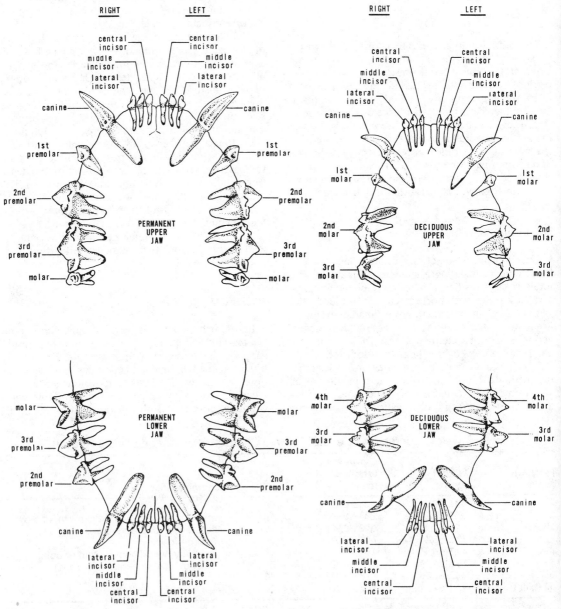

Figure 1. The deciduous and permanent teeth of the domestic cat. (From Berman E, et al.: Lab Anim Care 17:511, 1967.)

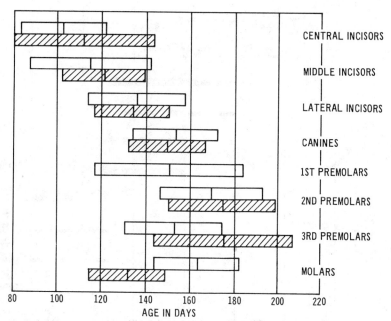

Figure 2. Age of eruption of the permanent teeth of the domestic cat. Upper teeth are represented by the clear bars, lower teeth by the cross-hatched bars. Values are mean ± 95 per cent CL. (From Berman E, et al.: Lab Anim Care 24:929, 1974.)

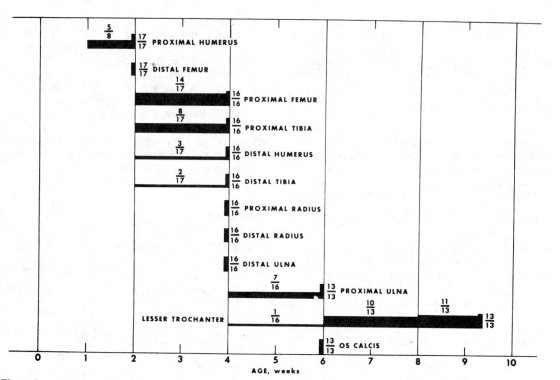

Figure 3. Appearance of ossification centers in the cat. Fractions are number of individuals with the ossification center on radiographs over total number examined.

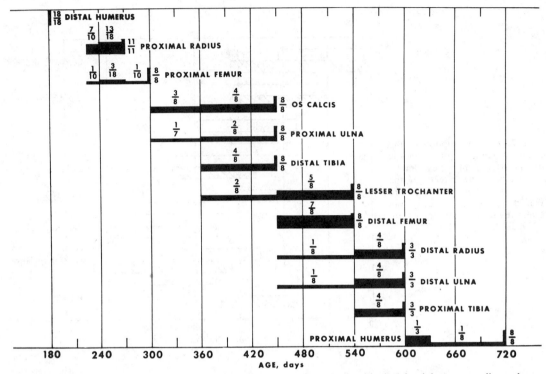

Figure 4. Epiphyseal closure in the cat. Fractions are number of individuals with closed epiphyses on radiographs over total number examined.

tion and identification of individual deciduous and permanent teeth can be made more accurately using dental charts such as the one in Figure 1.[2] Relatively unskilled personnel can use dental charts to collect data like those in Figure 2,[1] which shows the ages at which the permanent teeth of the upper and lower jaws emerge. The incisors, for example, normally erupt at 100 to 120 days of age but may appear as early as 80 days. The latest that teeth may erupt can be after 6 months of age. Generally, teeth of both sexes on both sides of the mouth and upper and lower jaws erupt at similar times, and the progression of emergence is to the rear of the mouth. Jayne[3] has made a thoroughly detailed examination of cats' teeth after birth.

Jayne[3] has also studied the growth of bones in the cat as they develop after birth. More recently Smith[7, 8] has clearly described the developing skeleton of the cat, giving extensive charts and data derived from radiographs. Figure 3 contains previously unpublished data of the initial appearance on radiographs of ossification centers of cats of known age. These cats were from the production colony previously noted, and no more than one male and one female from the same litter were used in the compilation of data. Because ossification centers make a stepwise appearance with age, radiographic examination of the skeleton can be a useful tool for estimating the age of a cat that does not yet have a fully developed skeleton. Other examinations of the

skeleton, such as bone length and epiphyseal closure, require more exacting skill than most practitioners possess. Epiphyseal closure measurements (Fig. 4) require skillful radiographic technique to visualize the epiphyseal line correctly and may need a time-series of radiographs to ensure that the line is not developing further. The measurement of length of a bone shaft affords a more exact value but is confounded when the diaphysis is not clearly separable on a radiograph. Length and closure measurements also require consideration of magnification factors inherent in any radiographic image.

References

1. Berman E: The time and pattern of eruption of the permanent teeth of the cat. Lab Anim Sci 24:929, 1974.
2. Berman E, Davis J, Stara JF: A dental chart of the domestic cat (Felis catus L.). Lab Anim Care 17:511, 1967.
3. Jayne H: Mammalian Anatomy. London, J. B. Lippincott Co., 1898.
4. Jepson SL: A case of superfetation in the cat. Am J Obstet 16:1056, 1883.
5. Markee JE, Hinsley JC: A case of probable superfetation in the cat. Anat Rec 61:241, 1935.
6. Nelson NS, Cooper J: The growing conceptus of the cat. Growth 39:435, 1975.
7. Smith RN: The developing skeleton. J Am Vet Radiol Soc 9:30, 1968.
8. Smith RN: Appearance of ossification centres in the kitten. J Small Anim Pract 9:497, 1968.

Management of Artificial Breeding in Cats

Nickolas J. Sojka, D.V.M., M.S.
University of Virginia Medical Center, Charlottesville, Virginia

SEMEN COLLECTION AND STORAGE

Reasons for Semen Collection

There are at least three generally recognized uses of collected semen: artificial insemination, diagnostic purposes and use in research. Semen may be used for artificial insemination in the form of a fresh, whole ejaculate, a "pooled" sample from several ejaculates, an extended (diluted) product that can be deposited in total or divided between recipients or a previously frozen sample. Conditions that suggest the collection and use of fresh or extended semen, as opposed to natural breeding, include disease control such as ringworm or respiratory infections and male or female breeding problems, which may be either psychological or physical, e.g., intensively aggressive, combative or other antisocial behavior, abnormal external reproductive anatomy or a physical handicap or injury that adversely affects the ability of the animals to assume an effective breeding position.

The decision to use fresh or extended samples implies a prior determination of semen normality. However, not all single ejaculates are large enough in volume or concentrated enough in total viable sperm to be sufficient to ensure pregnancy either by natural breeding or by artificial insemination. One answer to this difficulty is the pooling of several samples from the same donor. The desirability of perpetuating such defects is not under consideration here but should be a part of the decision-making process in all cases of assisted breeding.

The use of previously frozen semen can be said to have all the potential advantages of other methods as well as at least three additional ones. It abrogates distance: Animals widely separated geographically may be bred without either one suffering the stress of travel. It enables breeders to maintain a favored line in spite of debilitating injury or death. And, it provides sufficient material for repetitive experimental manipulations.

Collected semen can also be used as a diagnostic tool. Investigation of suspected abnormalities of the reproductive and endocrine systems that result in azoospermia, oligospermia or excessive percentages of immature, abnormal, dead or immotile sperm is the most obviously advantageous use. The extent to which certain drugs are affecting the donor may also be indicated by the manner or degree of their effect on spermatogenesis and/or semen characteristics. Unfortunately, due to the extremely small volume of the feline ejaculate, some of the diagnostic procedures available for use with larger volume ejaculates are difficult to duplicate outside the research laboratory.

Feline semen collection for use in biomedical investigations has been limited primarily to purposes associated with feline reproduction, i.e., to gain a more thorough understanding of feline reproductive physiology, to compare characteristics with those of other species and to contribute to, on a limited basis, in vitro fertilization and embryo culture studies. Considering the tractability of many toms in training to the artificial vagina, they have been underused in drug studies evaluating short- and long-term gonadal toxicity.

Techniques for Collection

The two most common methods of feline semen collection are the artificial vagina (AV) and electroejaculation. An effective, inexpensive artificial vagina can be assembled using a rubber aspiration bulb, a 4-cm tube and a small plastic container, which serves as a warm water jacket (44 to 46°C) to control temperature (Fig. 1).[5] The primary advantages of an artificial vagina, in addition to its low cost, are its humaneness (neither chemical nor physical restraints are needed) and the fact that a single technician can perform the entire procedure without assistance (Fig. 2). Its principal disadvan-

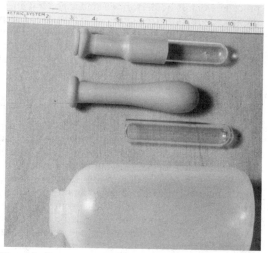

Figure 1. Components for an artificial vagina for tomcats. From top are pictured an assembled collection tube, a pasteur pipette bulb, the 6 × 50 mm glass test tube and the 100 ml polyethylene bottle, which serves as a warm water jacket (44–46°C) to control temperature.

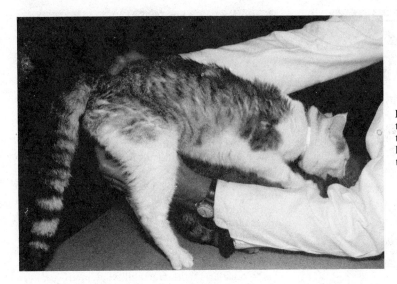

Figure 2. Collection of semen from a trained male. The collection apparatus is out of site between the male's hind legs; the male is holding the teaser queen by the neck.

tages result from the necessity, in most cases, of providing a "teaser" queen (either a female in heat or a spayed female treated with estrogen) and from the 2- to 3-week training period necessary for accustoming the toms to the device. Even with this time period, not all toms can be trained.

Electroejaculation is accomplished with the use of an electric stimulator and a rectal probe. Its principal advantages are that it can be performed on any tom that can be safely anesthetized, and it provides a "split" ejaculate (one sperm-free and one sperm-rich fraction) if this is desired. A more detailed discussion of exact methodology is presented elsewhere.

For specific needs, sperm may also be collected by lavage from the vagina, using buffered saline in a 1-ml syringe with a smooth tip or collected directly from the uterus or oviducts. The direct collection procedures must be performed under general anesthesia and are more frequently used for the research rabbit. All three methods can provide an excellent indication of the behavior and viability of samples after exposure to female tract secretions, should problems in that area be suspected.

Semen Handling and Dilution

Semen collected by AV or electroejaculation can be diluted with 0.1 ml saline (0.9 per cent sodium chloride) for determination of sperm concentration and examination for the per cent of abnormal forms and estimation of overall motility. Further dilution with saline will provide several samples for direct artificial insemination. As with the semen of other species, samples should be "handled" as little as possible. Critical conditions include temperature, light, pH and degree of dilution. Samples should be held at 25 to 37°C, preferably in the dark or in shielded containers. If the extended semen is to be held without freezing for several hours before insemination, containers should be stoppered or covered to prevent pH changes resulting from pro-

longed exposure to air. Excessive dilution is detrimental to the fertilizing capacity of feline sperm; and, care should be taken to avoid direct contact with preservatives and metal ions, as these are generally toxic to sperm.

Storage

While motility can be maintained in saline-extended samples left in a water bath and shielded from light for up to 8 hours, the best method of maintaining the fertilizing capacity of feline sperm over extended periods of time is by freezing. Normal pregnancies have been reported using extenders similar to those successfully employed for other species.[2] Samples may be preserved as either pellets prepared on dry ice or as a liquid in vials; both are placed in liquid nitrogen for long-term storage. In either case insemination should take place immediately upon thawing to ensure maximum fertilizing capacity. Samples frozen in defined media of the type used to support frozen storage of fetal kidney cell lines maintain excellent post-thaw motility but have, so far, failed to produce successful pregnancies (E. M. Cline, personal communication).

SEMEN EVALUATION

The mean volume of feline semen collected using an artificial vagina has been observed to be 0.04 ml (range 0.03 to 0.12 ml) containing 56.5×10^6 sperm (range 0.96 to 51.01×10^8/ml), while electroejaculation produced a mean volume of 0.23 ml (range 0.08 to 0.74 ml), with 28×10^6 sperm (range 0.10 to 1.53×10^8/ml)[3]; motility averaged 78 per cent (35 to 100 per cent) and 60 per cent (47 to 81 per cent), respectively. Abnormal forms occurred with a 1 to 10 per cent frequency and all the common anomalies have been observed: bicephalic, biflagellate, abnormal shapes and sizes of heads and acrosomes, club tails, separation of head and tail and immature forms. Abnormal motility can result from conformational anomalies or from cold shock. Sperm concentration, per cent motility and type motility can be determined using a Fuchs-Rosenthal hemocytometer and a microscope; live-dead analysis and morphologic abnormality can be observed using eosin aniline blue and Giemsa staining.[4]

Feline semen is usually milky white in appearance unless contaminated with urine or blood (rare). The mean pH is reported to be 7.4 (range 7.0 to 8.2). A whole ejaculate will contain varying amounts of exfoliated epithelial cells, cytoplasmic droplets, bacteria and cellular debris.

Any evaluation should include determinations of semen volume, per cent rapid, progressive motility, sperm concentration and per cent abnormal forms. Semen characteristics will vary widely among males and can vary just as widely among several collections from the same male. Judgments about the potential fertilizing capacity of a male must never be based on a single evaluation.

ARTIFICIAL INSEMINATION

Full details of the queen's estrous cycle are presented elsewhere in this text. However, for the purposes of artificial insemination it is important that the proestrous phase of the vaginal epithelial cycle be clearly identified. During late proestrus the vaginal epithelial cells reach maximal hypertrophy; they appear as large, round cells with clearly defined cell membranes and round or ovoid nuclei; few, if any, leukocytes should be present at this stage. Proestrous epithelial cells are readily identifiable on wet mount slides (using Wright's stain or toluidine blue) prepared from either vaginal lavage using distilled water in a pipette or from a cotton swab inserted gently into the vagina and then rolled across the glass slide.

Ideally, a first insemination is performed when the vaginal epithelial cells have reached their maximum size, the nuclei have begun to shrink and the queen is showing that she is ready to breed by her restlessness, calling and willingness to assume a breeding stance. Typically, she will yowl and move quickly away from the inseminating device once it has come into contact with the cervix, after which she will vigorously wash the perineal area. Immediately following insemination, administer 50 to 75 IU human chorionic gonadotropin (hCG) intramuscularly to induce ovulation. The insemination process (including hCG injection) should be repeated after 24 hours, at which time many of the vaginal epithelial cells should be anuclear with irregular, crumpled membranes; they frequently appear as sheets of cells at this point.

Concentrations of 5×10^6 to 3×10^8 sperm in 0.1 to 0.2 ml of diluted semen have produced successful pregnancies; therefore, 50×10^6/ml has been suggested for routine use in artificial insemination. This sperm suspension may be deposited in either the anterior vagina or posterior cervix using a 0.25-ml syringe with a 20-gauge needle bulbed at the tip or shielded at the tip with a 1-cm piece of polyethylene tubing. Easy entry into the cervical os should be suspect, as this opening is tightly closed except during pregnancy or in the presence of uterine infection.

ELECTROEJACULATION OF THE CAT

The reasons for employing semen collection procedures as opposed to natural mating have already been presented. However, the specific conditions indicating use of electroejaculation as the method of first choice may need further elucidation. For either physical or psychological reasons, some males may not be usable for natural breeding or collection of semen via artificial vagina. Additionally, electroejaculation is unique in the cat, generally resulting in a far larger ejaculate because of a significant increase in the amount of seminal plasma; the sources of this excess fluid are probably the prostate and bulbourethral glands, which are apparently overstimulated by electroejaculation.[2] The seminal plasma, largely sperm-free, is thus readily available for use in diagnosis or for research purposes.

Platz and colleagues[2] published full details of both the materials and methods essential for feline electroejaculation. Basically, the necessary equipment includes an electric stimulator,[1] a rectal probe, wire leads, 110 volt AC current and a vessel to receive the ejaculate.

Male subjects are anesthetized with ketamine hydrochloride (33 mg/kg), administered intramuscularly, then placed on their sides before insertion of the lubricated probe into the rectum (approximately 9 cm). If necessary, the probe is removed for cleaning off of fecal material and then reinserted so that the electrodes are directed ventrally. The collection tube is applied to the penis in such a way as to expose the penis before stimulation begins. A series of three sets of electrical stimulations (of gradually increasing voltage), with rest periods between each, is used to induce ejaculation. Care should be taken to avoid interference with the response caused by fecal material.

All materials that come into contact with the semen should be maintained at 25 to 37°C to avoid cold shock. Semen quality is apparently unaffected by routine once-a-week electroejaculation. Although males have shown no ill effects with regard to weight, activity or behavior, care should be taken to ensure that due consideration is given to humane concerns in the use of this equipment.

References

1. Lang CM: A technique for the collection of semen from the squirrel monkey (*Saimini scuirens*) by electroejaculation. Lab Anim Care 17:218, 1967.
2. Platz CC, Wildt D, Seager SWJ: Pregnancies in the domestic cat using artificial insemination with previously frozen spermatozoa. J Reprod Fertil 52:279, 1978.

3. Platz CC, Seager SWJ: Semen collection by electroejaculation in the domestic cat. J Am Vet Med Assoc 173:1353, 1978.

4. Saacke RG: Morphology of the sperm and its relationship to fertility, animal reproduction and artificial insemination. Proc

3rd Tech Conf, Chicago, National Association of Animal Breeders, 1970, pp 17–29.

5. Sojka NJ, Jennings LL, Hamner CE: Artificial insemination in the cat *(Felix catus L.).* Lab Anim Care 20:198, 1970.

Estrous Cycle Control—Induction and Prevention in Cats

David E. Wildt, Ph.D.
National Zoological Park, Smithsonian Institution, Washington, D.C.

No pharmacologic therapies are formally approved in the United States for stimulating or inhibiting reproductive function in the female cat (queen). Reasons for the lack of previous efforts are numerous. Public demand for manipulating reproductive activity in the cat traditionally has been less intensive than for the dog.[1] Escalating research costs and strict federal requirements for new drug development have compromised initiative and severely limited new advances. Much of this concern resulted from early studies showing that cats treated with gonadal steroids are predisposed to the development of cystic endometrial hyperplasia (CEH).[21] It is also likely that a major factor slowing this field has been, until recently, a surprisingly weak informational base on the physiology of reproduction for the species.

It is evident that perhaps the difficulties associated with manipulating reproductive activity in the queen are related, at least in part, to the unique reproductive style of the species which is described elsewhere in this section. It is likely that the complications and variations reported in pharmacologic manipulation of reproduction in the cat are caused in part by a rather continuous and dynamic flux in reproductive-endocrine function within individual females. Consequently, it is imperative that a complete and accurate reproductive status be established prior to any attempt to stimulate or suppress reproductive activity.

ESTRUS AND OVULATION INDUCTION

The interest in estrus and ovulation induction in the queen is principally related to the seasonal nature and unpredictable onset of sexual activity.

Certain queens often exhibit irregular estrous cycles, abbreviated or lengthy estrous periods or no sexual behavior at all. Methods for inducing estrus and ovulation may be particularly important to the breeder of valuable purebred queens, which display prolonged periods of sexual inactivity or fail to conceive following ovulation. For breeders this causes frustrating delays, demonstrating the need for therapeutic intervention. Similar concerns may be evident in commercial catteries or laboratories employing cats as biomedical research models.

Sexual activity in the cat is responsive to environmental factors. Queens maintained indoors will frequently initiate cyclic behavior within several weeks of being exposed to a 12/12 hour light/dark cycle. In such conditions housing females in groups or in close approximation to a male will sometimes facilitate onset of estrus. Occasionally, introducing a highly demonstrative estrous female to anestrous queens will stimulate sexual behavior. As with certain farm animals, transport of queens will both induce and synchronize estrous activity. Of 21 laboratory cats translocated, 16 exhibited onset of estrus within 18 to 31 days of transport.[18]

Exogenous hormones may be used to stimulate reproductive activity in the queen. The objective of hormonal therapy is to induce both sexual behavior and ovulation. Frequently, a major misconception and error in stimulating estrous cyclicity in the queen concerns the function of exogenous estrogens. Estrogens or estrogenic compounds cause intense sexual behavioral displays. However, such steroid therapy actually inhibits ovarian activity and prevents ovulation. Therefore, administration of estrogen to an anestrous female for the ultimate goal of achieving pregnancy is useless. For induction of estrous behavior alone, estradiol benzoate (50 μg/animal) or 17-β estradiol cypionate (Estracyp-V or ECP; 0.25 mg/animal) injected intramuscularly is effective.[7] Onset of estrus after treatment is variable (2 to 7 days) and may last 2 to 4 weeks. It is recommended that no more than 8 mg of estrogens be given in any one 4-month period because of the chronic toxicity of these compounds.[17]

The events leading to ovulation in mammalian species have two distinct components: the development and maturation of ovarian follicles and subsequent ovulation and formation of corpora lutea. Follicular maturation is primarily under the stimulus of pituitary release of the gonadotropin follicle-stimulating hormone (FSH). The release of luteinizing hormone (LH) gonadotropin, also from the pituitary and as a result of copulation, is responsible for eliciting ovulation. Sexual receptivity or estrus is a direct consequence of elevated estrogens produced by maturing follicles. Several hormonal preparations have been used and are commercially available for producing FSH/LH-like responses in the cat.

FSH-P (follicle stimulating hormone-pituitary) is a highly purified, lyophilized hormone obtained from selected pituitary glands of domestic animals. The action of this pharmaceutical is primarily like that of FSH. Pregnant mare serum gonadotropin (PMSG) is a highly potent compound obtained from the serum of pregnant mares and is commercially sold in the lyophilized form. Although PMSG principally exerts an FSH-like influence, it also has inherent LH-like activity. Human chorionic gonadotropin (hCG) is purified from the urine of pregnant women and acts in an LH-like mode by inducing rupture of mature follicles. Gonadotropin-releasing hormone (GnRH) is a synthetic hypothalamic hormone that acts by stimulating endogenous discharge of FSH and LH from the pituitary.

Both PMSG and FSH-P have been used successfully to induce overt sexual behavior and ovarian follicle development in cats. Initial research efforts were conducted with PMSG employed in a specific dose schedule.[10] During seasonal anestrus (September–June), PMSG was given intramuscularly as follows: on the first day 100 IU and 50 IU each day thereafter for 5 to 6 days. During the natural breeding season (February–August), the PMSG dosage was reduced to 25 IU, depending on the degree and rapidity of behavioral response. Estrous behavior was frequently induced, and mating and conceptions occurred, resulting in a birth rate of 4 kittens/litter. More recent studies have suggested that multiple doses of pregnant mare serum gonadotropin (PMSG) at the previously recommended levels are too severe. One investigation reported a conception rate of only 18 per cent in queens treated subcutaneously with 100 IU PMSG on day 1 and 50 IU of PMSG on each subsequent day for 4 or 5 days.[5] The latter study achieved more success using a conservative approach involving one subcutaneous injection of 100 IU PMSG followed by one intramuscular injection of 50 IU of human chorionic gonadotropin (hCG) 6 days later. Duration of estrus was not different from natural estrus controls and all queens accepted mating attempts by the male. Fourteen of fourteen control queens conceived versus seven of nine PMSG-treated females. Although ovulation rates were not reported, an average litter size of 4.5 kittens was produced in the latter group. Further evaluations of PMSG, particularly its effectiveness compared with follicle-stimulating hormone-pituitary (FSH-P), have also confirmed that the feline ovary appears to be highly sensitive to overdosing with either hormone.[22] Multiple injections of low-dose PMSG resulted in an excessive number of ovulations, cystic follicle production and prolonged periods of estrus. Because PMSG also exerts luteinizing hormone (LH)-like effects, premature luteinization of early developing follicles can occur. Another major problem is that potency estimates of PMSG preparations can vary considerably from one commercial lot to another. Addi-

tionally, PMSG physically is a large glycoprotein and has been suspected of causing an immunologic response with repeated injections. No data are available on subsequent reproductive capabilities of queens previously treated with single or multiple dosages of PMSG. Although it has been suggested that the CEH-pyometra complex may be associated with excessive PMSG therapy, no specific clinical data are available.[7]

FSH-P is highly effective in stimulating follicle maturation and estrous behavior in the cat.[22] Because of its relatively short half-life, multiple injections of FSH-P are required. However, this characteristic lessens the incidence of a hyperstimulative effect. A dosage of 2 mg given intramuscularly and daily for 5 days is effective; however, recent data indicate that reducing the FSH-P dosage to 1.0 or even to 0.5 mg on the second through fifth day may be equally efficacious. Prolonged use beyond 5 days should be avoided, as eventually cystic follicles can develop even in the absence of overt sexual behavior. FSH-P treatment should be discontinued as soon as the female is sexually receptive and mates. If the queen fails to display estrual behavior within 7 days following the last (fifth) FSH-P injection, the treatment regimen can be repeated in 5 to 6 weeks.

As with all gonadotropic therapy, there is interest in whether the ova matured and released as a result of hormonal treatment are normal and capable of fertilization and development. Recent studies by Goodrowe and Wildt (unpublished data) involving embryo recovery from FSH-P–treated, naturally mated queens indicate that these embryos appear morphologically normal. FSH-P has also been used safely on repeated occasions in the same female without eliciting a refractory response. Usually, FSH-P–injected queens are in estrus within 5 to 6 days after the onset of treatment and remain sexually receptive for about 6 days. Although ovulation number is generally greater in these queens (8 to 10 corpora lutea) than in naturally mated controls (3 to 6 corpora lutea), conception rates and litter size are comparable. Furthermore, normal offspring result from FSH-P–treated females artificially inseminated with fresh or frozen-thawed spermatozoa.[14]

A major key to successful ovulation induction with FSH-P is adequate handling and management of the breeding pair before, during and following hormonal treatment.[22] Young (less than 1 year), sexually naive, timid or extremely aggressive females do not respond well to therapy. Although ovarian activity is stimulated, these cats usually fail to display the classic symptoms of sexual receptivity. Similar results have been observed in PMSG-treated queens.[7] It is critical that the treated female be familiar and compatible with the male designated as the mating partner. Even queens exhibiting intense and natural behavioral estrus will sometimes refuse the copulatory attempts of strange males. Therefore, it is unreasonable to expect hormonally stimulated females to openly solicit and copulate freely upon abrupt exposure to an unfamiliar male.

Queens should be handled frequently and monitored both before and during FSH-P treatment. In our facilities queens are conditioned prior to treatment to ensure that each animal will allow physical contact, particularly to monitor the onset of sexual receptivity. This is accomplished by the handler gently stroking the perineal region in the vulvar area while observing for signs of lordosis, tail adjustment and treading movement of the hind limbs. Any queen that ferociously reacts to such testing is not likely to show normal sexual behavior after gonadotropin therapy. A second indication of the candidate's suitability is its pretreatment reaction to the chosen male partner. A female that aggressively attacks the male will not likely be responsive to copulation after hormonal treatment.

Socially well-adjusted queens 1 to 6 years of age are the optimal candidates for therapy. Each female should be taken to the male's quarters and the pair allowed to interact for 15 to 30 minutes, beginning 3 to 5 days before treatment and continuing daily through at least 1 week after therapy. Sexual behavior and the mating attempts can often be facilitated by the handler's gentle restraint of the queen and the initiation of the sexual display by stroking the perineal region. Aggressive handling, noise and other distractions should be strictly avoided. Repeated matings should be encouraged since copulatory frequency in the cat is necessary to ensure LH release and thus ovulation. If possible, ad libitum mating should be allowed. However, in facilities in which males are used frequently and sexual exhaustion is a concern, conception rates are normal in queens mated three times/day at 3- or 4-hour intervals during the first 3 days of estrus.[15]

Both hCG and gonadotropin-releasing hormone (GnRH) will cause rupture of vesicular follicles developed as a result of natural estrus or treatment with FSH-P. Neither of these two pharmaceuticals probably is necessary or facilitate ovulation or improve conception rates in estrual queens receiving adequate mating stimuli. Additionally, the injections of hCG normally prolongs the behavioral estrus interval by several days.[20] The primary usefulness of hCG and GnRH is the hormonal induction of ovulation in queens failing to mate and designated for artificial insemination. The number of follicles ovulating has been shown to increase with the dose of hCG. Over 90 per cent of all mature follicles ovulate at dosages of 250 or 500 IU of hCG.[20] A dose of 250 IU hCG injected intramuscularly on the first 2 days of estrus is recommended. Similarly, a high percentage of naturally estrous queens ovulate when 25 µg of GnRH is injected intramuscularly on the first 2 days of estrus.[4] Although specific data are unavailable, GnRH likely results in endogenous FSH release and, therefore, theoretically could have follicle-developing properties. However, unpublished work from our laboratory indicates that twice daily intramuscular injections (10 µg) of GnRH for as long as 5 days are generally ineffective in stimulating either follicle development or estrus.

INHIBITION OF ESTRUS AND OVULATION

Practical methods of suppressing or inhibiting reproductive function can generally be classified into surgical or pharmacologic approaches.

Surgical sterilization (ovariohysterectomy) is the most effective and low-risk method for sterilizing the queen.[21] While controlling reproduction and eliminating the nuisances associated with estrus, this method also affords a health advantage by virtually eliminating common intrauterine diseases such as mucometra and pyometra. Because of pet owners' resistance—due to psychological and economic factors—ovariohysterectomy has not been the answer in controlling animal overpopulation. Emotional considerations of owners for their pets often result in opposition to irreversible surgical sterilization. Surgical procedures are not inexpensive, and the adequate facilities required for proper procedures are costly to construct and maintain. Few efforts have been made to examine other surgical techniques for sterilizing the female cat. Tubal ligation or cauterization has been suggested as one possible alternative.[1, 19] This procedure can be performed using minimally invasive, rapid techniques such as laparoscopy.[1, 19, 21] Although the behavioral annoyances associated with intact gonadal systems are not alleviated, tubal ligation may have practical application for mass sterilization in clinics[19] that carry out neutering.

Because of the irreversibility and cost of surgery, considerable interest has been generated in pharmacologic methods of suppressing or prohibiting reproduction. Although fertility can be controlled in the queen by administering various steroid compounds or their derivatives, often pathologic changes in the uterus are induced, necessitating mandatory ovariohysterectomy. These agents generally are progestational in nature and exert a highly potent negative feedback effect on the hypothalamus and pituitary. It should be emphasized that indiscriminate use of all known exogenous progestogens can cause CEH, mucometra and endometritis and other complications including obesity, mammary hyperplasia, neoplasms, diabetes mellitus and various metabolic disorders.[1, 2, 21] The incidence of these negative side effects is less in queens than in similarly treated bitches.

Progesterone in a repository type base (Reprogest) prolongs absorption and action for up to 14 days. In the cat estrus can be effectively delayed by intramuscular injections of 2.2 to 4.4 mg/kg of body weight (BW) of Reprogest at 5- to 10-day intervals, as required. Several other progesterone-like compounds have also been investigated. Medroxyprogesterone acetate (MAP or Depo-Provera) given orally at a dose of 5 mg/day will alleviate behavioral signs of estrus and mating activity within 24 hours.[7] To continue the delay, four additional daily doses of MAP are recommended. Alternatively, 25 to 100 mg of MAP can be injected. The interval of estrus inhibition is variable, usually lasting 2 to 4 months. The compound delmadinone acetate (DMA) is also a systemically active progestin that additionally exerts antiestrogenic and antiandrogenic effects. For prolonged prevention of estrus, the adult queen receives 0.25 to 5 mg/kg BW subcutaneously twice/year.[9] For suppression of clinical manifestations of estrus, DMA is given orally and daily for 6 days at a dosage of 0.5 to 1 mg/kg BW or subcutaneously in 1 or 2 injections in 24 hours at a rate of 2.5 to 6.75 mg/kg BW. The effect lasts an average of 2 to 4 months after oral medication and 6 to 9 months after injection. At the dose levels used and over the time employed DMA has been safe and efficacious.

Probably the most extensively used progestin is orally active megestrol acetate (Ovaban).[2, 12] This product also has marked antiestrogenic properties and no anabolic or androgenic activity and is rapidly metabolized and rated as palatable. To suppress estrus, megestrol acetate is given at a dosage of 5 mg/animal for 3 consecutive days. During this period the female should be isolated from the male. Anestrus can be maintained by a dose of 2.5 to 5 mg once/week. Treatment should not be extended for more than 10 weeks. Estrus is delayed as long as the maintenance dose is continued. To postpone estrus, queens can be given 2.5 mg/day for up to 60 days. When discontinued, onset of estrus can occur from 2 to more than 24 weeks later, the variations due primarily to seasonality. Temporary minor side effects include increased appetite, diarrhea, decreased activity and weight gain. It is recommended that cats treated with either of the long-term regimens have an untreated estrus before further therapy. Extended administration of Ovaban should also be avoided, as recent observations indicate occasional instances of pyometra and diabetes mellitus in chronically treated females.

Mibolerone (dimethyl-nortestosterone or Cheque) is an androgenic, anabolic steroid devoid of progestational or estrogenic activity.[2, 3] This compound is effective in inhibiting estrus only when treatment is initiated prior to the onset of estrus. Daily oral administration of 50 μg/animal of mibolerone to adult queens for 6 months prevented estrus. There was no post-treatment effect on subsequent estrus, mating, pregnancy rates or litter size. Because mibolerone has severe toxic potential if misused or given in gross overdoses, this product is currently not recommended for control of estrus in the cat. The major concerns are increased thyroid-parathyroid weights, time-related changes in serum cholestrol concentrations, pancreatic dysfunction and liver toxicity. Additionally, mibolerone can cause slight masculinization in queens, including thickening of the cervical dermis, clitoral hypertrophy and slight erythema in the clitoral fossa.

MISMATING (POSTCOITAL OR INTERCEPTIVE) TREATMENT

Various hormones are used to terminate early pregnancy following mismating. 17-β estradiol cypionate (Estracyp-V or ECP) can be injected intramuscularly 40 hours after copulation or up to 5 days after coitus at a dosage of 125 to 250 μg/animal.[7, 11] This steroid is considered to retard oviductal transport of the fertilized ovum, block the embryo from entering the uterus and/or interfere with the normal development of the uterine endometrium. The chronic effects of 17-β estradiol cypionate in the cat have not been studied intensively and, therefore, extreme caution should accompany its use. 17-β estradiol cypionate may prolong estrus, produce genital irritation and result in follicular cysts, endometritis or even CEH-pyometra. A similar abortifacient effect can be achieved in the cat with diethylstilbestrol (DES).[10, 17] Following an unwanted series of copulations, DES can be given intramuscularly 24 to 48 hours later at a dosage of 1 to 2 mg/animal. Treatment should be repeated 8 days later. DES is highly toxic to cats[8] and daily administration can result in hepatic, pancreatic and cardiac lesions. Pyometra and aplastic anemia are also not uncommon in DES-treated queens. Because of these severe and variable side effects, neither 17-β estradiol cypionate nor diethylstilbestrol can be highly recommended as reliably safe practices to eliminate an undesirable pregnancy. The most suitable alternative is ovariohysterectomy of the queen during the first month of pregnancy.

Prostaglandin $F_{2\alpha}$ ($PGF_{2\alpha}$) has been considered as an abortifacient compound in cats. In one study intramuscular injection of $PGF_{2\alpha}$ at doses of 0.5 to 1 mg/kg BW was reported to induce abortion in the queen after day 40 of gestation.[13] This result was never repeated and a later investigation demonstrated that $PGF_{2\alpha}$ alone failed to stimulate complete luteolysis and abortion in the cat during late pregnancy.[24] Two independent studies more recently demonstrated that $PGF_{2\alpha}$ given during the early luteal phase at doses of 0.5 to 5 mg/kg BW is ineffective in prematurely terminating corpus luteum function.[16, 23] It is evident that this compound at the tested doses is not luteolytic in the queen and, therefore, currently is not recommended for interceptive treatment of an unwanted pregnancy.

References

1. Burke TJ: Fertility control in the cat. Vet Clin North Am 7:699, 1977.
2. Burke TJ: Pharmacologic control of estrus in the bitch and queen. Vet Clin North Am 12:79, 1982.
3. Burke TJ, Reynolds HA, Sokolowski JH: A 180-day tolerance-efficacy study with mibolerone for suppression of estrus in the cat. Am J Vet Res 38:469, 1977.
4. Chakraborty PK, Wildt DE, Seager SWJ: Serum luteinizing hormone and ovulatory response to luteinizing hormone-releasing hormone in the estrous and anestrous domestic cat. Lab Anim Sci 29:338, 1979.
5. Cline EM, Jennings LL, Sojka NJ: Breeding laboratory cats during artificially induced estrus. Lab Anim Sci 30:1003, 1980.
6. Colby ED: Induced estrus and timed pregnancies in cats. Lab Anim Care 20:1075, 1970.
7. Colby ED: Suppression/induction of estrus in cats. In Morrow DA (ed): Current Therapy in Theriogenology. 1st ed. Philadelphia, WB Saunders Co, 1980, pp 861–865.

8. Dow C: The pathology of stilbestrol poisoning in the domestic cat. J Pathol Bacti 75:151, 1958.
9. Gerber HA, Jochle W, Sulman FG: Control of reproduction and of undesirable social and sexual behaviour in dogs and cats. J Small Anim Pract 14:151, 1973.
10. Herron MA: Feline reproduction. Vet Clin North Am 7:715, 1977.
11. Herron MA, Sis RF: Ovum transport in the cat and the effect of estrogen administration. Am J Vet Res 35:1277, 1974.
12. Houdeshell JW, Hennessey PW: Megestrol acetate for control of estrus in the cat. Vet Med Small Anim Clin 72:1013, 1977.
13. Nachreiner RF, Marple DN: Termination of pregnancy in cats with prostaglandin $F_2\alpha$. Prostaglandins 7:303, 1974.
14. Platz CC, Wildt DE, Seager SWJ: Pregnancy in the domestic cat after artificial insemination with fresh or frozen spermatozoa. J Reprod Fertil 62:279, 1978.
15. Schmidt PM, Chakraborty PK, Wildt DE: Ovarian activity, circulating hormones and sexual behavior in the cat. II. Relationships during pregnancy, parturition, lactation and the postpartum estrus. Biol Reprod 28:657, 1983.
16. Shille VM, Stabenfeldt GH: Luteal function in the domestic cat during pseudopregnancy and after treatment with prostaglandin $F_2\alpha$. Biol Reprod 21:1217, 1979.
17. Stein BS: The genital system. In Catcott EJ (ed): Feline Medicine and Surgery. 2nd ed. Santa Barbara, American Veterinary Publications, 1974, pp 303–354.
18. Wildt DE: Effect of transportation on sexual behavior of cats. Lab Anim Sci 30:910, 1980.
19. Wildt DE: Laparoscopy in the dog and cat. In Harrison RM, Wildt DE (eds): Animal Laparoscopy. Baltimore, Williams & Wilkins, 1980, pp 31–72.
20. Wildt DE, Seager SWJ: Ovarian response in the estrual cat receiving varying dosages of HCG. Horm Res 9:144, 1978.
21. Wildt DE, Kinney GM, Seager SWJ: Reproduction control in the dog and cat: An examination and evaluation of current and proposed methods. J Am Anim Hosp Assoc 13:223, 1977.
22. Wildt DE, Kinney GM, Seager SWJ: Gonadotropin induced reproductive cyclicity in the domestic cat. Lab Anim Sci 28:301, 1978.
23. Wildt DE, Panko WB, Seager SWJ: Effect of prostaglandin $F_2\alpha$ on endocrine-ovarian function in the domestic cat. Prostaglandins 18:883, 1979.
24. Wyckoff JT, Ganjam VK: Successful termination of pregnancy in cats by the administration of a combination of adrenocorticotrophic hormone and prostaglandin $F_2\alpha$-Tris (hydroxymethal) amino-methane salt. Fed Proc 38:1189, 1979.

Pregnancy, Obstetrics and Postpartum Management of the Queen

Louise Laliberté, D.V.M., M.Sc.
Hôpital Vétérinaire Vimont,
Auteuil-Laval, Québec, Canada

PREBREEDING CONSIDERATIONS

Prebreeding Examination

Both prospective parents should be presented for a complete prebreeding examination, during which the previous medical history is reviewed, and general health is evaluated. The examination should take place early enough before breeding to allow for time to complete laboratory tests, vaccinations and deworming and for detection of congenital or acquired abnormalities. All cats must be tested for feline leukemia virus (FELV) infection. Tests for antibody to feline coronavirus (FIP) are often requested by breeders, although the interpretation of the results is controversial; it may be important, however, to know the coronavirus antibody titer of a cat when it is to be introduced into a coronavirus antibody-negative cattery.

An exhaustive review of congenital defects in cats, with a complete bibliography, has been published by Saperstein, Harris and Leipold.[12] Hip dysplasia and chronic patellar luxation are becoming more prominent in certain breeds, and both conditions are suspected to be congenital. Affected cats should not be allowed to breed. Inverted nipples are not uncommon in cats and should be detected early, so that problems with lactation may be avoided by daily extracting of the nipple and massaging during pregnancy. Pelvic deformities are common sequelae of injuries and might compromise normal delivery.

During the prebreeding visit clients should be instructed about care and possible complications during pregnancy and parturition. A time for a prepartum examination should be arranged. The method for estimating the delivery date should be explained in order to allow for clients to plan their schedule and to be available at parturition.

General Recommendations about Breeding and Gestation

The queen is presented to the stud on the second or third day of estrus and may stay for 1 to 2 days. It is advisable to prepare the long-haired queen for breeding by shortening the perineal fur. A good meal given before mating also seems to calm the cats and to encourage a favorable disposition. It is customary that the female visits the male, since the male seems to feel more secure on his own ground. The breeding area should not be cluttered with unnecessary furniture and should not be brightly lit, as cats feel safer under low lighting. Partners are to be presented to each other gradually to avoid fights and possible injuries. It is recommended that they be isolated at first, but with the possibility of seeing and smelling each other, by placing them in adjacent cages. Even after some time in separate but adjacent enclosures, it is not unusual for the female to reject the male temporarily. Once compatibility is established, some males and females go through a courtship ritual with coitus occurring up to six times hourly, as long as the pair is left together.

Owners should be advised to isolate the dam from other males after mating during the remainder of estrus in order to prevent superfecundation: fertilization of separate ova by sperm cells from different males is commonly observed in cats.

Since females that live together tend to cycle at similar intervals, breeding two females at the same time is a good management practice, which makes a foster mother available if problems occur. Lactating queens rarely reject other kittens if a few precautions are taken (see the article Neonatal and Orphan Kitten Care).

PREGNANCY

Duration

Gestation periods of 56 to 71 days have been reported, but average feline gestation is between 63 and 65 days. The mortality of kittens born after a gestation of fewer than 61 or 62 days appears greater than that of kittens born 63 to 66 days after mating. There seems to be no increased risk of mortality for kittens born after a gestation of 67 to 69 days.

Breed differences with regard to gestation length have been occasionally reported but are far from being well documented. Environmental factors such as moving the mother, hospitalization or boarding may delay onset of parturition and appear to increase the length of gestation. Maternal weight and age, size and number of fetuses, level of nutrition and exercise during pregnancy as well as the number of previous pregnancies are other factors that may account for variations in length of gestation in cats. In obese queens parturition may be delayed and significantly prolonged. Early parturition of large litters is commonly observed.

Finally, because of repeated coitus, the time of conception may be difficult to establish, and the exact due date may not be easy to predict. Since ovulation takes place between 24 and 48 hours following coitus, fecundation will not occur for at least 24 hours postcoitum. It may be safe to expect birth any time within the period from 63 days (plus 24 hours) after the first mating to 63 days (plus 24 to 48 hours) after the last mating.

Pregnancy Diagnosis

There are no chemical pregnancy tests available for the cat. Some queens show behavioral changes very early in pregnancy and become quieter, devoting more time to eating and sleeping and adopting a more subdued lifestyle while seeking more human contact. Some females may be partially anorexic, while others may display a sudden increase of appetite. Occasional vomiting may be noticed. Breeders often depend upon a change of appearance of the queen's nipples, which become bigger and rosier during the second and third weeks of pregnancy. A sudden weight gain is not a reliable sign, nor is it any more normal for the queen than for the human female to double her weight during the

first phase of gestation. It is only after 1 month of gestation that one may note a slight enlargement of the abdomen; by the sixth week, abdominal distention is obvious.

Abdominal palpation is the easiest method of diagnosing pregnancy. Individual rounded uterine swellings measuring about 1.5 to 2 cm in diameter can be accurately felt and counted between the third and fourth weeks of pregnancy. Palpation is best achieved by having the cat stand on its four limbs with the tail toward the practitioner. With one hand placed on the lumbar vertebrae, the abdomen is cupped with the other hand, and the bladder is identified; starting just behind and above the bladder, the practitioner moves fingers cranially along the uterine horns and counts the discrete swellings. After 4 weeks, palpation becomes unreliable, as uterine masses become confluent.

Although fetuses can be counted by palpation, radiography remains the only method for determining the precise number of fetuses prepartum; this method is most successful after 50 days. Uterine embryonic swellings have been visualized as early as 17 days. Ossification begins in the embryo at day 25,[4, 15] and the skeleton becomes radiographically visible between days 36 and 38 of gestation.

Ultrasonic scanning techniques used in human obstetrics have been tried in veterinary medicine, but their application in cats has not been practical. The Doppler instrument can detect heart beat and placental blood circulation only after the fourth week of gestation,[5] thus providing no distinct advantages over skilled abdominal palpation. This method also gives a high percentage of false-negative results, even in late pregnancies.[9] Echography has also been tried in cats.[9] It allows accurate visualization and measurement of the fetal ampulla after the third week of pregnancy. Some difficulties in adapting the ultrasonic probe to the focal distance needed for small animals have been encountered, and the instrument has not been properly adapted for use in cats. The Doppler and Echosonograph instruments are costly, and their use is still considered to be experimental and limited to veterinary teaching hospitals.

Care of Dam During Pregnancy

It is important to disturb the queen as little as possible during pregnancy. The pregnant queen should receive good nutrition, have adequate exercise, live in a clean environment and be protected from undue stress. However, since pregnancy is a physiological condition, the queen should continue her usual lifestyle, and owners should not exaggerate their concern. Although total isolation is unnecessary, the pregnant queen should be kept away from males, since approximately 10 per cent of the pregnant queens may display typical estrous behaviour and copulate between the third and sixth weeks of gestation.

Normal exercise should never be restricted during pregnancy, as it is probably one of the most important single factors in a successful delivery. During the last 4 weeks of pregnancy, when the abdomen becomes considerably enlarged, the female should be protected from other cats or dogs, as she will be less agile. Vigorous exercise should be minimized in order to reduce the risk of abdominal injuries.

The dam should not be allowed to become overweight during pregnancy: obesity may lead to difficult parturition because of a narrowed birth canal and poor muscle tone. Food should not be increased before midgestation. Active adult cats require 80 Kcal/kg body weight, requirements for the pregnant cat are about one third more. A 7-lb pregnant female (3.5 kg) does not need more than 250-300 gm of good moist food daily throughout gestation. The daily ration should be given in three to four small portions rather than in one or two large meals. There is no need to supplement the diet of a pregnant female fed a good commercial cat food; however, special needs during pregnancy should be supplemented when mixed or when poor diets are fed. Protein requirements are unique in the cat and are much higher than in other animals of the same size. Not less than 30 per cent protein of high biologic value should be the basis of the pregnant cat's diet. The cat also has a high demand for vitamin A; deficient mothers either fail to implant or produce a high proportion of kittens with malformations. Considerable quantities of folates are transferred across the placenta during the last third of pregnancy; to meet this need, organ meats and green leafy vegetables should be provided if the diet is of doubtful quality. A minimum of 200 mg/day calcium should be given to the pregnant cat with a Ca:P ratio of from 0.9 to 1.1 parts calcium to 1 part phosphorus in order to promote sound growth in the fetus.[3]

Medications, particularly steroids and griseofulvin, should be avoided, as should any elective surgical procedures. However, there is no need to postpone urgent surgery, since no abortion or inhibition of implantation have resulted from repeated laparotomies performed on laboratory cats to study fetal development.[6]

If the cat is used to being bathed, there are no contraindications to regularly bathing the pregnant queen, as long as the owner is careful to avoid chilling her. During the last week before parturition, the queen is often so heavy that she is unable to groom herself, particularly her perineal area. Gentle bathing must be done by the owner. Her nipples should be massaged and cleaned in the same way. The need for trimming the hair around genital and abdominal areas in long-haired cats is debatable, but this practice will certainly ease the postpartum cleaning.

Abnormal Pregnancy

Extrauterine Pregnancy (Ectopic). The cat has been described as being relatively resistant to uterine rupture, and extrauterine pregnancy is considered to be rare; however, the few reports that have been described may not accurately reflect the true incidence of this condition,[1] and they have been later questioned. Primary ectopic pregnancy involves fertilization and development of an ovum in the abdominal cavity. Nidation can take place on various abdominal structures, and development of the fetus continues until placental insufficiency related to the abnormal locus and inadequate blood supply occurs. Death of the fetus follows with maceration and mummification.

Most reported cases of extrauterine fetuses have been associated with a rupture of the uterus as a result of abdominal trauma, with subsequent passage of the fetus into the abdominal cavity. The diagnosis of secondary extrauterine pregnancy occasionally can be substantiated at surgery by finding a uterine rupture or cicatrix on the uterus; in most cases, however, this is impossible to locate on the fully involuted uterine horn. In these cases the ectopic pregnancy may mistakenly be considered as primary, but if the owners are questioned, they will often remember that the cat had been injured during the pregnancy.

Herniated Gravid Uterus. Herniated gravid uterus has been reported as a possibility but is a rarity in the cat. Trauma or injury are generally the cause. Radiography and palpation will confirm the diagnosis.

Pseudocyesis. Since the cat is an induced ovulator, pseudopregnancy is observed following a nonfertile ovulation brought on by mating with a sterile or vasectomized male, mechanical stimulation of the cervix or exogenous hormonal treatment. Pseudopregnancy usually lasts from 30 to 45 days. Changes observed in the uterus and mammary gland are similar to those occurring in gestation, but it is unusual that lactation will ensue. Intervention is rarely necessary in cats, and signs of estrus will often be evident within 1 to 2 weeks after the end of pseudopregnancy. If the manifestations are severe, mild tranquilization or hormonal therapy such as repositol progesterone (1 mg/lb of body weight) may be indicated. A second treatment may be necessary on rare occasions and should be repeated after 1 week.[14]

Uterine Torsion. Although uterine torsion is considered rare in cats, a surprisingly high number of cases have been reported,[7] probably because of the catastrophic aspect of the condition. This condition is serious, especially when it occurs in late pregnancy or during parturition. Onset is sudden, characterized by collapse and abdominal pain, subnormal temperature and pale mucosal membranes—all clinical signs consistent with severe shock. Abdominal palpation is greatly resented because of pain. Some light sanguineous vaginal discharge is usually observed. In most cases a single horn is partially or completely rotated on its longitudinal axis. In some cases the extent of the torsion can be up to two and one half complete turns.

Once uterine torsion is suspected, immediate abdominal exploration must be carried out. The exteriorized uterus appears reddish and engorged, and in most cases a complete hysterectomy is necessary. Despite intensive and prompt treatment, prognosis is grave, since severe shock or massive hemorrhage from the engorged placenta may cause death. The exact cause of uterine torsion is unknown.

PARTURITION

Prepartum Examination

The pregnant female is examined at the end of the eighth week of gestation. It is good practice to obtain lateral and ventrodorsal radiographs of the abdomen to determine the number of fetuses, thus preventing an unnecessary emergency call from the clients who suspect the presence of another fetus in utero.

During the prepartum visit the clients are instructed about parturition. They are advised how to select a suitable place for delivery and how to prepare themselves psychologically for the event. They are encouraged to read about the topic, as it will certainly help them feel more secure and stay calm during parturition. The owners should be instructed to warn the clinician that parturition is impending and then to call at the onset of contractions. They should report complications by telephone and avoid bringing the queen to the hospital unless so instructed, since moving the queen unnecessarily may stop or delay labor.

Prior to parturition the clients should prepare a kittening box, bedding replacement, hot water bottles and a suitable disinfectant for the umbilical cord. The kittening box may consist of a simple cardboard box lined with a flannel sheet. Terry cloth rags or towels should be avoided as kittens have well-developed claws that can get caught, leading to subsequent injuries or strangulation of kittens. The chosen kittening area should be quiet, darkened, clean, draft-free with an environmental temperature around 30°C (85°F) and isolated from other cats or dogs. If the queen does not seem to like the selected area, there is no need to worry, as the family can be moved to the chosen place a few hours after parturition is completed.

At the onset of the first signs of parturition, the clients should observe the female and take note of the following: time of first bed scratching, first contraction and onset of vaginal discharge, if any, and amount of food consumed during the last few days.

Signs of Parturition

A decrease in rectal temperature during the preceding 12 hours or in the first stage of labor may be noted, although this sign is not as reliable as in the bitch. Presence of milk in the engorged mammary glands is also not a precise sign of approaching parturition. In primiparous females, lactation may be established less than 24 hours before parturition, while after several pregnancies, colostrum can be detected as early as 1 week prepartum.

Changes of behavior are more often reliable but these can vary enormously from one female to the next and can be highly subjective. During the ninth week, the queen is generally less active and is obviously heavy with kittens. The queen, and especially the primiparous queen, becomes more nervous and apprehensive in the last 2 days, searching for a place in which to deliver.

It is believed that most cats retreat to secluded, sometimes even inaccessible places to deliver litters. While this may be true for feral cats, most pet cats will follow the owner and may refuse to stay alone in the kittening room. Owners should try to reassure the queen and stay with her only until she agrees to lie in the box. Some queens will refuse all food from 12 to 24 hours before delivery, while others will not become anorexic at all and will even eat between kittens.[14]

Normal Parturition, or Eutocia

Normal parturition will take place only if the following conditions are met: (1) the fetus is normal in size and conformation; (2) the pelvic canal is large enough to allow passage of fetuses, and the cervix, vagina and vulva are properly relaxed and dilated; (3) uterine contractions are normal, with proper duration, strength and frequency and (4) there are no environmental disturbances.

It is customary to divide parturition into three stages, but in multiparous species, the second and third stages are difficult to separate. The first stage corresponds to the preparation of parturition, while the latter stages involve the expulsion of the fetus and the passage of placental membranes, respectively.

Stage 1. From 2 to 12 hours before queening, vocalization, tachypnea and pacing may be observed. The queen may tear up and rearrange the bedding, turn around in circles and wash herself constantly. As labor approaches, the queen will lie in the kittening box, purring loudly and continuously. Initial uterine contractions are intermittent and difficult to detect. Discharge of clear fluid may be noted, and the vulva and perineum become more flaccid.

Stages 2 and 3. The second stage corresponds to the active expulsion of the fetus. Irregular contractions may be seen and felt while the female remains on her side. As contractions become more vigorous, she may get up and occasionally lower her hind quarters into a semisquatting position, standing on her phalanges with the calcaneous bones pointed almost straight up and wide apart. More intense contractions will correspond to the entry of the fetus into the pelvic canal, and the cat may groan or cry.

Regular uterine contractions accompanied by stronger abdominal contractions will result in delivery of the first kitten between 3 to 5 and 30 to 60 minutes after onset of the second stage. The birth of the first kitten is usually the longest (Fig. 1A). Unexperienced females may turn vigorously, groan and try to bite at the fetus. The owner should not be overly concerned but should only reassure the female without interfering because cannibalism of normal kittens is extremely rare in cats.

On expulsion, the kittens are enveloped in the thin amniotic sac, which usually ruptures during progression within the pelvic canal; if the sac does not rupture, it will be torn by the dam (Fig. 1B). Some queens are more busy with cleaning and licking their wet perineal area than with caring for the kitten. If the queen does not tear the membranous sac and it is intact on delivery, the membrane should be ruptured at once by the owner. Normal newborn kittens are strong, can cry and immediately search for a nipple.

Within 5 to 15 minutes and following mild, short contractions, the brownish-pink placenta will be expelled. The dam will not generally sever the umbilical cord until the placenta is extruded, although an actively licking female may do so. The placenta is usually consumed by the dam as she proceeds to bite through the umbilical cord. If the dam does not cut the cord, the owner should take over and sever it by simple stretching: the cord is grasped about 4 to 5 cm from the kitten and firmly held by the right-hand fingers well wrapped in a clean cloth. The fingers of the left hand pull away the cord attached to the placenta, stretching it until it breaks. Extreme care must be taken not to exert any traction on the newborn's umbilicus (Figs. 1C to F).

If a large litter is born, the dam should not be allowed to eat all the placental membranes, since this may cause digestive problems. After a rest of 10 to 60 minutes, the second stage will resume, followed again by the third stage, until all the kittens are born. Placental delivery should be carefully supervised, and all placentae should be counted, since retention may result in uterine infection. Occasionally, two kittens from alternate horns may be born within a few minutes of each other, with both placentae being delivered only after the second kitten. The same number of placental sacs as the number of kittens should be expelled, but if monozygous twins occur, two fetuses may have shared the same placenta. It may be difficult to recognize twins especially in solid-colored kittens, but in colored or marked kittens the patterns will appear as mirror images.

Queening is usually completed in 2 to 6 hours, but normal parturition may also last up to 10 to 12 hours, particularly in older females. Litter size varies between one and nine kittens, with an average size litter being 3.5 to 4.6 kittens. Seventy per cent of the litters consist of four, five or six kittens. For primiparous females, it has been shown that litter size may be smaller, with an average of 2.8 kittens. In small surveys, Siamese and other Oriental breeds with an elongated body were found to be more prolific than long-haired and cobby-type breeds such as Persian or Himalayan.[10, 13] Larger cats tend to have larger litters, but the birth weight of kittens born of smaller mothers is proportionately greater than that of kittens born of larger mothers. Older females tend to have smaller litters. Overall, there are no significant differences in sex ratio for any breeds of cats.

Dystocia, Signs and Management

It is generally believed that cats rarely experience problems with parturition. Feline practitioners are well aware, however, that dystocia is far from uncommon; in some practices, especially in those dealing with numerous purebred catteries, Cesarian sections are considered routine surgeries.

Classification of Dystocia. Dystocia is usually classified as either of maternal or of fetal origin. From a clinical point of view, however, an etiological classification of dystocia due to obstruction or functional deficiency is more logical.

Obstructive dystocia always involves a disproportion between the pelvic canal diameter and fetal volume. A small pelvic diameter due to immaturity, congenital malformation or deformity following healed fractures will prevent the passage of the fetus. Insufficiently dilated soft tissue in the birth canal, a congenitally malformed uterus (uterus unicornis) or benign uterine torsion may also result in dystocia. In multiparous cats, or in cats with a history of previous dystocias, the birth canal may be narrowed by fibrosis of the uterus, the cervix, the vagina or the vulva. A uterine prolapse occurring before the expulsion of the last kitten may also cause obstructive dystocia.

Dystocia due to obstruction may also be related to fetal malposition, although this problem does not commonly occur in the cat. Posterior presentation is considered normal in cats and occurs in approximately two out of five births. Posterior presentations have, however, been related to predisposition to dystocia, as mechanical dilation of cervical uteri may be inadequate. Transverse presentation and simultaneous presentation of two fetuses are other possible causes of obstruction. Fetal posture errors in cats are infrequent compared with other species, but head or limb flexion still may prevent normal expulsion of the fetus, since flexion increases overall fetal dimensions.

Obstructive dystocia is most commonly caused by fetal oversize, especially following prolonged gestation or abnormal fetal development, such as congenital hydrocephalus or partial duplication of the body, resulting in dipygus (double pelvis) or diprosopus (double head).[14] Genetic selection for a large flat head such as it occurs in the Persian or Himalayan breeds may predispose the queen to obstructive dystocia.

Uterine inertia is the main cause of dystocia in cats. Primary inertia, for which a hereditary tendency has been suggested, is characterized by the failure of the myometrium to expel a normally sized fetus through an intact birth canal. Contractions are weak, infrequent and nonproductive. Environmen-

All photographs courtesy of the author.

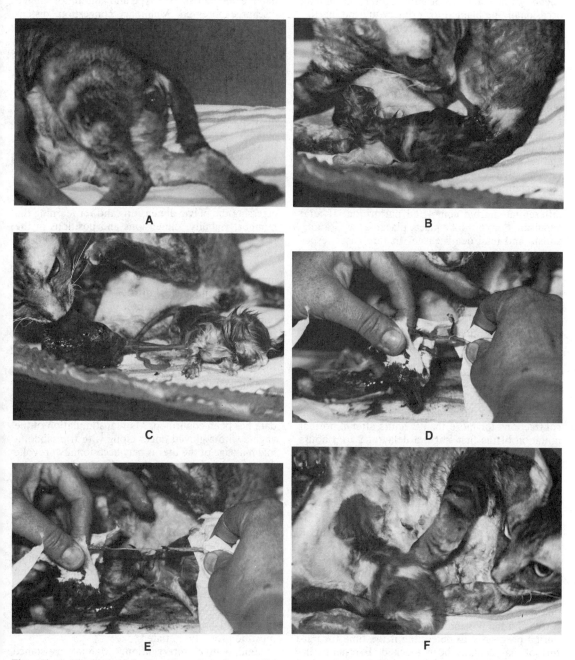

Figure 1. *A,* The birth of the first kitten is the longest. In some cases, an evaginated portion of the amnion may be seen at the vulva for 60 minutes and more. *B,* Posterior presentation is considered normal in cats and occurs in approximately two out of five births. In those cases, the tail may often appear at the vulva. The owner should not be overly concerned, as the feet of the kitten will appear shortly. *C,* The dam consuming the placenta as she proceeds to bite through the umbilical cord. *D* and *E,* If the dam fails to cut the umbilical cord, the owner should take over and sever it by simple stretching. The cord is grasped about 4 to 5 cm from the kitten and firmly held by the right-hand fingers well wrapped in a dry and clean cloth. The fingers of the left hand pull the cord attached to the placenta, stretching it until it breaks. Extreme care must be taken not to exert any traction on the newborn's umbilicus. *F,* Normal newborn kittens are strong and immediately search for a nipple.

tal stress such as unnecessary hospitalization, introduction of new animals or human intervention may occasionally be blamed for primary uterine inertia. Uterine inertia is also seen frequently in older or obese females and in females affected with debilitating diseases as well as in females with extreme uterine distension when very large litters are carried.

Secondary uterine inertia occurs after prolonged uterine contractions and following obstructive dystocia. Extreme pain experienced during a difficult expulsion also may cause secondary uterine inertia. In some cases the queen begins a normal parturition and delivers one or more fetuses but subsequently (and mostly because of muscle fatigue) fails to expel the remaining fetuses, although the birth canal is unobstructed. Secondary uterine inertia must be differentiated from completed parturition. If fetal expulsion does not take place, placental separation, anoxia and fetal death ensue. In rare cases, especially in the absence of infection, the queen may tolerate the presence of dead fetuses to term without any clinical signs. These kittens are mummified or macerated. In cases of uterine infection fetuses will become emphysematous; within 24 hours severe clinical signs will be noted. The female becomes depressed, hypothermic, toxemic and rapidly dehydrates; a brownish and malodorous vaginal discharge is usually present.

Recognizing Dystocia. Dystocia should be suspected if the owner reports any of the following: a true delay in parturition (2 days or more past the latest expected due date), strong and ineffective contractions for more than 2 hours after a normal initiation of the first stage, a delay of 2 to 3 hours following the uneventful birth of a first kitten, weak and unproductive contractions that are diminishing in frequency, green vaginal discharge in absence of contractions or a partially presented kitten.

Examination of the Parturient Queen. When a kitten is partially presented, simple assistance is within the capability of the instructed owner. In all other cases a complete examination should be carried out on the parturient cat.

Special attention should be given to the case history, especially when a delay in parturition is suspected. The practitioner should recalculate the due date with the owner by reviewing the time of estrus and the possibility of an occurrence of estrus during pregnancy to determine if the time for parturition has actually been reached. Erroneous information provided by insistent breeders often has led to an unnecessary cesarean section, which ended with the extraction of immature fetuses. Alternately, the queen simply may not be pregnant or may be experiencing a pseudopregnancy. Questioning the owner about presence of straining or behavioral changes may also be useful, as he may not be aware that in his absence parturition has been initiated and subsequently stopped because of outside stress or other causes.

Evaluation of the female's general health status should be made. The nature and frequency of contractions should be noted, the vulva and perineum examined and the type and amount of vaginal discharge observed. Mammary congestion, distension and size of the glands should be evaluated while verifying the presence of milk. Abdominal palpation will reveal the presence of fetuses, but their number and size may be difficult to evaluate. Fetal movements may or may not be detected, since fetuses tend to be less active toward the end of gestation. Digital exploration may help to appraise dilation of the cervix and vagina, detect obstructions and determine the presence and presentation of the fetus in the pelvic canal. The examination should be carried out with care because of the potential for initiating an ascending infection. Ultrasound, if available, is especially useful for determining fetal viability. Radiography is a valuable method for assessing the pelvic dimensions and for learning the number, viability, dimensions and positions of the fetuses. Accumulation of gas within or around the fetuses as seen on radiographs suggests that they are dead and decomposing; other signs of death may be alteration in the fetal skeleton, such as overlap of skull bones, dissociation of limb bones in the case of mummification or grouping of fetal bones with high contrast following the resorption of fetal fluids.

Therapeutic Approach to Dystocia

Medical Treatment. Medical management should be tried first in primary uterine inertia, provided there is no obstruction and that the correct delivery date has been confirmed. Manual stimulation of the vagina with a gloved finger along with transabdominal massage of the uterus may occasionally provoke onset of contractions and expulsive efforts. Drugs should be used with great discretion, and owners should never be allowed to use any unless closely supervised. Posterior pituitary hormone (oxytocin) is administered subcutaneously or intramuscularly (2 to 5 units USP) to stimulate uterine contraction. If the hormone is ineffective after 45 minutes, a second dose is given. Slow intravenous injection of 1 to 3 ml of 10 per cent calcium gluconate solution is often helpful in sensitizing the uterus. Close supervision of the treated female is necessary. If contractions are not initiated 30 to 45 minutes after the second hormonal injection, surgical treatment must be promptly initiated.

Manipulative Intervention. Manual assistance with delivery is only indicated when the female is actively contracting, the disproportion between fetal and pelvic size is slight, only one or two fetuses that are of little value to the owner are retained, a kitten already has entered the birth canal and its expulsion is likely to allow normal expulsion of the remaining kittens, a dead fetus is within reach or a kitten is partially presented at the vulva; in the last case simple assistance by the owner is usually sufficient.

Manual assistance must be carried out aseptically. The genital area is washed with organic iodine, and all maneuvers are carried out by a sterile gloved hand. It is essential to lubricate the vaginal vestibule and fetus with a sterile water-soluble lubricant instilled as far as possible into the anterior portion of the vagina.

Partial retention of a kitten at the vulva may be managed by telephone instructions to the owner, since waiting for arrival of the veterinarian may result in death of the kitten.

The client should be instructed as follows: In an anterior presentation with the tip of the nose visible the first priority is to tear away the amnion so that respiration can start, since the maternal blood supply may be cut off by compression of the cord. The lips of the vulva may be pushed up to improve access to the fetus. A clean, dry cloth is helpful, as fetal fluids tend to make the fetus slippery. The fetus is grasped as far as possible behind the head by one hand while the other hand is holding and pushing upwards on the abdomen of the dam. The mother's forelegs may be elevated. Traction must be gentle and limited to easing out only, taking advantage of the mother's contraction efforts. Traction must be directed caudally and then ventrally and slightly to each side to allow alternate passage of the fetal shoulders. Uncontrolled vigorous traction may easily result in dislocation of the fetal spine. Once the shoulders are free, delivery should be easy. A posterior presentation is indicated by appearance of hind feet or the tail at the vulva. The appearance of a tail should not call for immediate assistance as the author has often witnessed a tip of the tail protruding from the vulva for more than half an hour, with the subsequent birth of a healthy kitten. If one or both feet are present and a true obstruction is suspected, the maternal vulva should be pushed up and a good grip obtained as far proximal as possible on the legs or on the fetal pelvis in front of the ileum. At this moment the occiput may impede further delivery; it can be freed by rotating the fetus slightly into an oblique position on its side to facilitate delivery of the head. Prompt clearing of membranes and fluid from the fetal nose and throat is again very important. Fluid may be removed from the mouth and pharynx by suction or by holding the kitten head-down and swinging it vigorously.

Although instrument-assisted delivery is theoretically possible, it is not recommended, since the risk of injury to both the queen and fetus is high because of the small size of the cat's pelvic canal. The use of obstetrical forceps is virtually impossible, while the use of an ovariectomy hook to assist with delivery (as described for the dog) although less traumatic, is still impractical in cats.

An episiotomy may be indicated in rare cases in which insufficient dilation of the vulva is observed, but a cesarean section is preferred.

Cesarean Section. A timely cesarean section involves minimal risk for the queen and her kittens. The female normally recuperates very rapidly, readily accepting her kittens. If the history and examination have revealed a full-term pregnancy, a cesarean section should be considered in the following situations: (1) in a 70-day pregnancy when medical induction has not been possible, (2) in unresponsive primary or secondary uterine inertia, (3) in irreducible obstructive dystocia, (4) when kittens are valuable and it is believed that other manipulations may damage kittens or the dam's genital system (especially if two or more fetuses are retained), (5) when a heavy discharge is present and uterine infection is suspected and (6) in a female with a history of recurrent cesarean sections. Surgery should be considered in females with elevated or subnormal temperatures, since operation may be less stressing than prolonged labor.

POSTPARTUM CARE OF THE DAM

Immediate Postpartum Examination

Routine postpartum examination of the dam and litter is not recommended. If delivery is considered to have progressed normally and the dam and kittens appear content, there is no need to move the litter from its home environment, since this move may result in needless stress and compromise normal lactation. Owners should, however, be instructed to bring the queen and kittens for examination if the kittens cry or show any inability to nurse, the queen is reluctant to care for the kittens, she is anorexic for more than 24 hours or her body temperature rises over 39.5° C (103° F).

Care and Management of the Newborn Litter

Chilling accounts for a high proportion of kitten deaths that cannot be attributed to other specific causes.[11] A heated floor or pad, or hot water bottles frequently replenished are helpful in keeping a 30° C (85 to 86° F) environment. The close proximity of the mother, whether she is long haired or short haired, is usually sufficient to avoid chilling. The queen will appreciate calm surroundings, and visitors should not be allowed near the newborn litter. Lactating queens require two to three times more food than usual, depending on the number of kittens, and their size and age. Fresh water always should be available, and a diet high in protein should be fed. In order for bones to develop, protein, calcium and phosphorus are needed, and kittens obtain these from the mother's milk. Lactating queens require about 600 mg of calcium daily.[3] Multivitamin supplementation should be prescribed if the nutritional balance and quality of the diet are questionable.

Normal kittens will attempt to nurse immediately or within 1 to 2 hours of birth. An experienced and calm queen will usually allow and encourage kittens to nurse as soon as they are born, even while experiencing labor with another kitten. The owner should not be alarmed, however, if she refuses to nurse until all kittens are born. In the latter situation kittens should be closely watched or even temporarily separated from the dam and placed on heated pads or in a box lined with hot water bottles.

During 12 to 24 hours following parturition the queen normally remains continuously with the kittens, leaving the nest only to feed and to eliminate. Her appetite may be decreased during this period, which is considered normal, especially if she has ingested all placental membranes. During the first week, the dam may spend up to 90 per cent of her time with the kittens.[2]

Postpartum Uterine Diseases

Uterine Prolapse. Uterine prolapse is infrequently seen in practice and only sporadic cases are reported in the literature. A prolapse generally occurs in queens over 2 years of age and after one or more uneventful litters. The uterus prolapses almost immediately or within a few hours following the delivery of the last kitten. The prolapse can be complete with both horns protruding from the vulva or limited to the body and one horn. Although causes are difficult to establish, lack of exercise during pregnancy, weakness of uterine ligaments because of overbreeding, prolonged second-stage labor, incomplete placental separation or relative oversize of a kitten may all be factors responsible for uterine prolapse. If veterinary intervention is not immediately available, the everted uterus quickly becomes engorged and edematous, and the animal's condition will severely deteriorate. In a few cases the cat appears to suffer no ill effects for up to 2 hours after the prolapse; however, the sooner the cat is treated, the more successful the treatment and the more favorable the prognosis.[14] Depending on the severity of the prolapse, its duration and the condition of the mucosa, several approaches may be taken. In some instances replacement of the prolapsed horn and its proper reposition in the abdomen can be achieved by digital manipulation, assisted by a thick-walled glass test tube or a plunger from a syringe and by irrigation of the everted uterus with cold 50 per cent dextrose solution to reduce the edema. In most cases, however, amputation of the everted uterus is necessary, followed by ovariectomy. In all cases, intensive antibiotic therapy is required. If treatment is prompt, the recovery is uncomplicated and the queen can be allowed to resume the care of her kittens.

Postpartum Acute Metritis. Acute metritis is a serious condition affecting queens within 12 to 48 hours following parturition. Postpartum acute metritis is usually related to the presence of a retained fetus or placental membrane but also may result from unclean obstetric manipulation or surroundings. The common presenting complaint is that the queen neglects the kittens and is depressed, febrile and polypneic. She may also be dehydrated and have vomiting and diarrhea. In the majority of cases the vaginal discharge is copious, malodorous and dark. The presence of a retained fetus is easily confirmed by plain abdominal radiographs, but retained placental membranes are seldom demonstrable on radiographs and will be found by palpation of a local enlargement of the uterus accompanied by green lochia 24 hours postpartum.

If a retained fetus is found, surgical removal is recommended, as the fetus rarely will be evacuated by medical treatment. Intensive supportive care is necessary with intravenous administration of fluids and electrolytes. Ovariohysterectomy is the treatment of choice but is rarely acceptable to the owner when dealing with a highly valued breeding queen. As an alternative, the use of prostaglandin F_{2a} given subcutaneously at a dose of 0.1 mg/lb daily until all discharge stops (an average of 3 to 8 days) will cause dilation of the cervix and evacuation of uterine contents. Antibiotics should be continued for 10 to 12 days. Even after successful evacuation of the uterus by prostaglandin, future fertility is often jeopardized. Untreated acute metritis will usually degenerate into pyometra, uterine rupture and peritonitis.

Uterine Rupture. Uterine rupture associated with parturition is seen less frequently in cats than in other species, probably because of the relatively low weight carried by the gravid uterus. The condition may, however, occur spontaneously during unattended obstructive dystocia or as a result of injury occurring in late pregnancy.[14]

Lactational Disorders

Agalactia. Starvation of kittens is frequently reported by owners but total lack of milk supply is rare in the cat. True agalactia may be observed in premature parturition or in early cesarean section. However, a tendency toward poor milk production is definitely associated with heredity and possibly augmented by stress. Primiparous, nervous or confused queens often will experience temporary agalactia. Reassurance by the owner and occasionally a mild sedative (acepromazine maleate at low dosage) may help the nervous queen become calmer and subsequently accept the kittens. In some instances older, stronger and more determined kittens from another litter may force the queen to relax and once lactation is initiated, she will accept her own kittens. If all else fails, kittens should be hand fed but not necessarily separated from the dam, as she may still demonstrate other maternal behavior, such as licking and cleaning. When agalactia is suspected, the queen should be examined for presence of other disorders.

Galactostasis. Milk production may be adequate, but milk may be unobtainable because of delayed or insufficient nursing, abnormal nipples or edema of the gland.[14] The condition is usually seen after death of a litter or after early weaning. Occasionally, galactostasis occurs without an obvious cause a few hours after parturition. Massage and warm-water compresses along with a mild diuretic will reduce the edema and allow milk to flow. The best stimulation is often achieved by stronger, older and aggressively nursing kittens.

Acute Mastitis. Mastitis is relatively infrequent in cats and generally is first recognized by illness or sudden death of the nursing kittens. Upon presentation, one or more mammary glands appear hot, enlarged and painful. The queen is anorexic, febrile, dehydrated and depressed, and the milk is purulent and yellowish. Culture of the milk most often reveals staphylococci and streptococci organisms. The most probable route of infection is through the teat orifice or damaged overlying skin of the mammary gland following trauma caused by the sharp nails of kittens; hematogenous spread of organisms has also been suggested.[14] In all cases kittens should be immediately separated from the queen and hand fed. Systemic antibiotics given for 10 days with warm-water compresses and topical antimicrobial ointment massage is the recommended treatment. Surgical débridement and drainage is required when abscessation occurs. Untreated acute mastitis generally degenerates into gangrenous mastitis.[8]

Lactational Tetany. Feline lactational tetany has sporadically been reported in the literature.[14] Affected queens were nursing 2- to 5-week old litters of four to six kittens. Ataxia was first noticed, followed by tonic spasms of limb muscles and polypnea. The condition is generally associated with a calcium-deficient diet during lactation.

Treatment consists of slow intravenous administration of 2- to 5-ml doses of 10 per cent calcium gluconate solution repeated to effect. As hypoglycemia may follow hypocalcemia, the intravenous administration of 10 per cent dextrose solution has been recommended.[14] Calcium supplement should be prescribed, and the diet should be completely reevaluated. Kittens should be prevented from nursing but allowed to stay with the queen in order to avoid the risk of behavioral abnormalities in the kittens.

References

1. Bark H, Sekeles E, Marcus R: Extrauterine mummified fetus in the cat. Fel Pract 10:44, 1980.
2. Beaver B: Veterinary Aspects of Feline Behaviour. St. Louis, CV Mosby Company, 1980.
3. Brewer NR: Nutrition of the cat. JAVMA 180:1179, 1982.
4. Boyd JS: The radiographic identification of the various stages of pregnancy in the domestic cat. J Small Anim Pract 12:501, 1971.
5. Burke TJ: Feline reproduction. Vet Clin North Am 6:317, 1976.
6. Colby ED: Induced estrus and timed pregnancies in cats. Lab Anim Care 20:1075, 1970.
7. Groulade P: Anomalies de la parturition chez la chatte. Anim Compagnie 1:83, 1976.
8. Gruffydd-Jones TJ: Acute mastitis in a cat. Fel Pract 10:41, 1980.
9. Mailhac JM, Chaffaux ST, Legrand JJ, et al.: Diagnostic de la gestation chez la chatte: utilisation de l'échographie. Rec Méd Vét 156:899, 1980.
10. Povey RC: Reproduction in the pedigreed female cat. A survey of breeders. Can Vet J 19:207, 1978.
11. Prescott CW: Neonatal diseases in dogs and cats. Aust Vet J 48:611, 1972.
12. Saperstein G, Harris S, Leipold HW: Congenital defects in domestic cats. Fel Pract 6:18, 1976.
13. Scott FW, Geissinger C, Pletz R: Kitten mortality survey. Fel Pract 8:31, 1978.
14. Stein BS: The Genital System. In Catcott EJ (ed): Feline Medicine and Surgery. 2nd ed. Santa Barbara, American Veterinary Publications, 1973.
15. Tiedermann K, Henschel E: Early radiographic diagnosis of pregnancy in the cat. Fel Pract 10:18, 1980.

Neonatal and Orphan Kitten Care

Louise Laliberté, D.V.M., M.Sc.

Hôpital Vétérinaire Vimont,
Auteuil-Laval, Québec, Canada

CARE FOR THE HEALTHY NEONATE AFTER NORMAL DELIVERY

A healthy and contented kitten is quiet and spends its life either feeding (up to 8 to 10 hours per day) or sleeping. Careful handling of newborn kittens is not detrimental and, on the contrary, may stimulate their development and sociability, provided that human intrusion does not upset the queen.

The owner is well advised to disinfect the umbilical cord with weak iodine soon after it has been cut as a preventive measure against omphalitis caused by environmental contamination or overzealous licking from the dam. At the same time gentle examination of each kitten for congenital defects should be carried out with special attention given to detection of umbilical hernia and cleft palate, probably two of the most frequently encountered congenital anomalies in cats. The sex of the newborn can also be determined at this point.

It is good practice to weigh the kittens at birth and to note daily gain thereafter. On the average, a newborn kitten weighs between 75 and 150 gm at birth, with mean birth weight around 105 to 110 gm. Kittens may lose a few grams or may not gain any weight during the first 24 hours. They should gain approximately 15 gm daily during the first week, so that the birth weight generally doubles after 7 days. Owners are instructed to keep a chart for each kitten and to report any drop in weight. The growth rate may decrease during the following weeks, but a normal kitten should weigh close to 400 to 450 gm at 1 month of age.

Newborn kittens spend most of their time nursing. Feeding sessions that can occur almost hourly during the first day or two are in most cases initiated by the dam. The suckling reflex is present at birth and is very strong in the healthy neonate. By 2 to 3 days of age the kittens should be skilled at suckling without any help from the queen or the owner. While nursing, kittens usually tread or knead, pressing their forepaws alternately against the mammary gland. (This behavior may stimulate milk flow.) Teat preferences have been observed in approximately 80 per cent of kittens.[1]

The kitten's eyes remain closed until 5 to 12 days after birth. Full visual acuity is not achieved before 2 months of age. Pupillary response generally appears within 24 hours after the eyes open, taking 2 to 3 days to develop normal speed. Until this time, the kitten will usually turn its head away from the light source. It is also during this critical period that most mothers will begin to move the litter into a darker place.

Development of hearing in the kitten is not complete at birth: the totally closed external auditory canal will begin to open between 6 and 14 days of age.

The sense of smell is highly developed at birth. Within the first two days, the kitten can show a strong avoidance reaction to offensive odors. It is not unusual that a 2-day-old kitten will hiss when picked up by unfamiliar hands. Olfaction is well developed at this early age because of its importance in guiding the young animal to the mammary gland for nursing. Because the smell of the nest gives security to the kitten, bedding should not be changed too often, unless it is essential for hygienic purposes. Like olfaction, the sense of touch is fairly well developed at birth, probably because it also plays a role in orientation of the neonate. Tactile response is present at birth and cutaneous pain is felt within the first 4 days after birth. Kittens will cry if accidentally stepped on by the dam. Their cries are strong stimuli to the mother and make accidental crushing of kittens very unlikely. If a kitten is found dead under the mother, chances are that the kitten was already dead or too weak to cry.

Kittens are born with a well-developed coat but with very few fat reserves. At birth the homeostatic mechanisms are not functioning completely, and kittens normally tend to huddle together or in the fur of the queen to maintain their body temperature.

The neonate cannot voluntarily urinate and defecate, since both functions are under the control of the urogenital reflex. This reflex is stimulated by the mother's licking the kittens' anogenital area. Excrement and urine will be ingested by the dam. Spontaneous elimination begins at 3 weeks of age.

The environment of the newborn should be quiet and comfortable. The litter should be isolated from dogs and other cats until 3 to 4 days after the kittens receive their first vaccination. This isolation not only will avoid undue stress but also will prevent infection from potential disease carriers. The area should be draft-free and dimly lit, at least for the first week and until 2 days after the eyes are completely opened. The ideal temperature is around 30°C (85°F) for the first 2 weeks, decreasing to 25°C (80°F) until 4 weeks of age.

INTENSIVE CARE OF THE NEONATE AFTER DYSTOCIA OR CESAREAN SECTION

When the kitten is being delivered by cesarean section, the head must be immediately freed from the amniotic sac, and the umbilical cord must be clamped by a hemostat and cut. The kitten is then rubbed briskly with a towel so that circulation and breathing are initiated. The mouth is gently wiped to remove any mucus and the kitten is held upside down in order to drain the mucus from the nose and throat. If further stimulation of the kitten is required, it is firmly held on its back in the palm of the hand, with the head supported by the fingers and its face and abdomen covered with the other hand. The kitten is then swung sharply up and down. The pressure difference caused by the swing will stimulate respiration. Respiratory and cardiac stimulants such as doxapram hydrochloride may be dropped on the tongue or given intravenously through the umbilical or the sublingual vein.

Once the kitten is breathing and showing some strength, it is placed in a small box containing a heating pad or hot water bottles while the mother is recovering from anesthesia. Care should be taken to prevent burning of the kitten by the heating pad. There is no need to feed newborn kittens until the awakened dam is ready to accept them, since glycogen reserves in the liver can maintain kittens for several hours. They should be fed by 12 hours after birth, however, because hypoglycemia and hypothermia may develop at that time. The author has noticed that bottle-feeding the kittens within 1 to 2 hours of delivery will help maintain their suckling reflex. It may help to present the kittens to the dam's nipples as soon as surgery is over, inviting them to nurse while the dam is still recovering from anesthesia. If later rejection of the kittens occurs, they will have at least received some colostrum.

As soon as the dam is awakened, the kittens are presented to her one at a time while her reactions are carefully supervised. Some queens will accept the kittens within 4 to 6 hours after the surgery while others will reject them for up to 24 hours. If the kittens are still not accepted by the dam after 6 to 8 hours, hand feeding should be initiated.

ORPHAN OR REJECTED KITTEN CARE

Using a foster mother with kittens is the ideal way to care for orphaned or rejected kittens, as this method will not only provide maternal care but also allow for interaction with peers, which is essential for the development of normal adult behavior. Most breeders will help each other and will willingly agree to put the orphans with one of their nursing queens if they feel she can raise a larger family. The prospective foster mother should have a litter that is similar in age to the fosterlings. Most nursing queens will promptly adopt additional kittens. If difficulties are expected, the dam should be temporarily removed from her kittens while fosterlings are introduced to the nest and made to mix with the other kittens so that all smells are alike. Direct introduction of the orphans may also be successful if their genital area is first presented to the dam. Once the fosterlings have been fed and licked, they can be considered as definitely accepted.

If a foster mother is unavailable, the owner must prepare to hand-raise the kittens. In some instances an animal with strong maternal instincts will be willing to care for the kittens; female dogs and even neutered toms have been reported to accept such tasks. This is to be encouraged, as the orphan will not only find warmth and cleaning care, but the owner's chore will also be reduced.

Hand raising includes feeding, ensuring elimination, handling and providing a warm, clean and stable environment. The first 48 hours are critical for survival of the orphan kittens that have never nursed. If they are alive after that period of adjustment, they are likely to survive. Hand raising healthy neonates is to be encouraged and can be highly rewarding but a runt or malformed kitten should be euthanatized, since its adult life may be compromised.

Orphan kittens should be kept in an environment with a constant temperature of 30°C (85°F). A heating pad, regularly replenished hot water bottles or heat lamps are successful kitten warmers. The box should be small and lined with a flannel sheet. This sheet should not be changed too often, as the smell of the nest will be the only security provided to the orphans. With adequate cleaning and elimination induced by the owner, the nest will stay reasonably clean.

During the first week of life feeding sessions must occur every 2 to 3 hours, including throughout the night. The milk formula fed must be as similar to cat's milk as possible. A newborn weighing 125 gm requires 380 kcal/kg and a daily ration of approximately 30 gm, which ideally should consist of 72 per cent water, 9.5 per cent protein, 6.8 per cent fat, 10 per cent carbohydrates, 0.7 per cent ash and 0.035 per cent calcium; this ration provides 142 kcal/100 gm.[3] Cow's milk is unsuitable, as it is lower in protein than cat's milk. Several homemade milk formulas have been suggested: They usually consist of canned evaporated milk diluted with an equal part of water and mixed with one tablespoon of corn syrup, one egg yolk, liquid vitamins or liquid proteins such as Diamino 4x. The easiest method for ensuring proper nutrition of orphan kittens is to use commercial milk replacements such as KMR: these are also the best milk substitutes. The milk substitute should be given at the cat's body temperature (38 to 38.5°C). All equipment should be washed promptly after each use, thoroughly rinsed

and sterilized. The same equipment should be used each time, as familiar odors and shapes will stimulate the kittens to feed. Tube feeding has been recommended for speed and efficiency, but the author feels that tube feeding, in addition to the risk of pharyngeal and gastric lesions, causes kittens to lose their suckling reflex. Only in cases in which the kittens are weak and unable to suckle should tube feeding be encouraged. A 3-ml syringe (which has the added advantage of allowing easy measurement), a doll bottle or a curved glass feeding bottle (Catac Foster feeding bottle) is recommended.

When bottle fed, a kitten should never lie on its back but should be held in a position similar to the one used while nursing the dam. The kitten should be approximately at a 45° angle, resting on a towel arranged on the lap of the owner. Normal intake averages have been determined, but it is better to rely on the kitten's behavior. If it is eagerly suckling and suddenly turns its head away from the nipple, it is likely to be satisfied. During the first week, 2 to 3 ml/feeding (10 to 12 feeds/day) should be sufficient. Afterward, the number of daily feedings can be reduced to six or seven; the kitten should be taking 5 to 7 ml/feeding. By keeping a daily weight-gain chart, the owner is able to evaluate whether the intake is satisfactory.

Semisolid food can be added to the milk formula after 2 weeks of age, but larger holes should be pierced in the nipple. At 3 weeks of age orphan kittens are introduced to solid food by letting them lick baby food off the fingers; most of them will quickly start licking the finger, which is then directed to the bowl. The kitten will follow and start licking directly from the bowl within 1 or 2 days.

After each feeding, the anogenital area of the kitten must be gently wiped with cotton balls dampened in warm water to provoke urination and defecation. By 3 weeks of age, voluntary urination and defecation are possible. A shallow pastry pan or a small box with a little litter or torn newspapers placed near the kitten's sleeping areas should ensure successful training. Queens are normally very meticulous about the cleanliness of their kittens and long grooming sessions usually take place in the nest. The hand-raised orphan also should receive such care once or twice daily. A soft fingernail brush or a face cloth very slightly moistened are good grooming aids. The coat should always be perfectly dry.

In order for their sociability to develop, orphan kittens should be handled as much as possible but not at the expense of their sleeping time. Supervised contact with other healthy cats as well as the family dog is also to be encouraged but preferably after the orphans have been vaccinated.

For orphans that have never nursed the dam and have apparently received no colostrum, an early vaccination program is highly recommended, since kittens receive 75 to 80 per cent of the maternally derived antibodies through the colostrum within 48 hours of birth. If there are some doubts about the quantity and specificity of maternal antibodies or if the dam has not been vaccinated against the common viral infections, thus suggesting a low titer of maternal antibodies at birth, kittens should be fully vaccinated around their third week of age, with revaccination every 2 to 3 weeks thereafter.

NEONATAL DISEASES

A high incidence of preweaning mortality has repeatedly been reported in feline reproduction surveys.[5, 6, 8] Mortality rates of up to 30 per cent have been recorded in breeding colonies, while it was shown that barrier-maintained cat colonies also experienced preweaning losses of up to 13 per cent.[2, 7] Losses are particularly high during the first week of life. Breed predisposition to morbidity and mortality have been reported, but important differences have also been observed between individual catteries even when the same cat breed was involved.[4]

Neonatal diseases are often fatal even when diagnosis and intensive therapy are quickly instituted. The following neonatal conditions typically affect kittens less than 1 week old.

Starvation and Maternal Neglect. Maternal neglect or agalactia resulting in starvation may account for 10 to 20 per cent of neonatal mortality during the first week of life. Finding such early deaths should always indicate necropsy of the kitten and examination of the queen. The starved or neglected kitten will usually have an empty stomach and a full bladder, suggesting that it had not eaten and that urination had not been stimulated. The remaining kittens must be hand raised.

Cannibalism. Cannibalism as well as accidental trauma of the kitten occurs rarely. An overzealous queen may accidentally injure or kill the kitten while eating the placental membranes, but other cases of cannibalism should be suspect, since the consumed kitten may have been malformed and dying if not already dead. Repeated disturbance of the queen and her litter or other stress such as loud construction noise have been associated with cases of cannibalism.

Bacterial Infections. Sudden death of the kitten within the first week of life is typical of septicemia or bacterial pneumonia. *Escherichia coli*, staphylococci and streptococci are commonly associated with bacteremia in newborns. Infections may originate in utero, while traversing the vagina, or through contaminated milk from infected mammary glands.

Acute and usually fatal gastroenteritis of neonatal kittens is characterized by foamy vomitus and liquid feces. These neonates cry continuously, have abdominal pain, rapidly dehydrate and die within 24 hours after onset of the condition. Rehydration and oral antibiotics (ampicillin) may save a few kittens, but most treatment is usually futile. The dam should be examined for mastitis or metritis.

Omphalitis is often found in 1-week-old kittens and is usually associated with lack of hygiene. This disorder is manifested by persistence of a soft umbilical cord and redness in the umbilical region. The kitten should be treated at once with systemic antibiotics (ampicillin), since omphalitis may lead to fatal septicemia. Local disinfection is also essential. On necropsy kittens with omphalitis-caused septicemia will have abscesses distributed throughout the abdominal cavity, particularly on the liver and mesentery.

Bacterial conjunctivitis is commonly observed in kittens and should be treated with local ophthalmic antibacterial ointment. Systemic antibiotherapy is seldom indicated.

In all cases of recurrent bacterial diseases in neonates, the queen should be examined, and in future gestations antibiotics may be given to her from 1 week prior to parturition until 2 weeks postpartum.

Fading Kitten Syndrome. This syndrome occurs with kittens that are from several days old to 2 to 3 weeks old. Kittens that are apparently born healthy become less active, stop nursing, become hypothermic and show no interest in their surroundings. This syndrome has been referred to as the "fading kitten syndrome."[4] After exhibiting these symptoms, kittens may survive for up to several days. The condition has been associated with various bacterial and viral infections and metabolic diseases. A fading kitten could be born from a leukemic dam: one of the effects of feline leukemia virus infections is the atrophy of the kitten's thymus gland. The thymus is intimately involved in the development of the immune system, and the destruction of this gland makes these kittens highly susceptible to septicemia.[4]

Another possible cause of the fading kitten syndrome may be thyroid malfunction. Although the exact etiology and pathogenesis are unknown, affected kittens were shown to have lower levels of circulating thyroxine (T_4) than age-matched normal kittens. Empirical treatment consisting of 3 to 5 μg of levothyroxine given per os daily has given dramatic results: Fading kittens resume normal activity and normal growth rates, often as soon as 2 days after beginning of treatment. In at least two cases thyroid hypoplasia was detected microscopically (Johnson and Laliberté, unpublished data, 1981).

In all cases of fatal neonatal diseases necropsy should be performed with particular attention to thymus and thyroid development. Bacterial and viral cultures should be done, and the dam should be tested for leukemia virus infection.

References

1. Beaver B: Veterinary Aspects of Feline Behavior. St. Louis, CV Mosby Company, 1980.
2. Festing MFW, Bleby J: Breeding performance and growth of SPF cats (Felix catus). J Small Anim Pract 11:533, 1970.
3. National Academy of Sciences: Nutrient Requirements of Cats. Number 13 of Nutrient Requirements of Domestic Animals. Washington, D.C., 1978.
4. Povey RC: Reproductive problems. In Grunsell CSG, Hill FWG: (eds): The Veterinary Annual. 18th Issue. England, John Wright, 1978.

5. Povey RC: Reproduction in the pedigree female cat. A survey of breeders. Can Vet J 19:207, 1978.
6. Prescott CW: Reproduction patterns in the domestic cat. Aust Vet J 49:126, 1971.
7. Robinson R, Cox HW: Reproductive performance in a cat colony over a 10-year period. Lab Anim 4:99, 1970.
8. Scott FW, Geissinger C, Peltz R: Kitten mortality survey. Fel Pract 8:31, 1978.

Cattery Management and Health

Joan M. Arnoldi, D.V.M., M.S.
Wisconsin Department of Agriculture, Madison, Wisconsin

Veterinary medicine has, until very recent times, tended to treat small animals rather than individual species. The cat, because it has been treated like a small dog, has suffered from such a lumping of species. In fact, the cat has many unique characteristics that distinguish it from other small animals.

Veterinary care of the cattery differs from that of the kennel and most certainly differs from treating the individual pet or even pets in the multicat household. Like any other animal-raising enterprise, economics plays a very definite role in treatment, which the practitioner should appreciate. The sentimental value given a household pet is not the factor that determines the degree of treatment in a cattery any more than it is in the production of rabbits, goats or beef cattle.

If the challenge of aiding a breeder to produce a healthy product and to improve a breed, as evidenced by show wins, is meaningful, then working with cattery owners can be most satisfying.

The average feline breeder usually has a history of no planning. Few have made a conscious decision to enter into the hobby or the business of breeding cats. The greatest percentage of those involved purchased their first purebred animal as a pet and eventually became fascinated with some aspect of breeding—perhaps raising kittens or showing their animal. A few breeders have entered the field from other animal enterprises, usually with dogs or horses. These breeders consistently enter with a great deal more knowledge of genetics, reproduction and showing.

Because cattery owners have received little attention by veterinarians, many have obtained in desperation what knowledge they could find and, right or wrong, have begun diagnosing and treating. Some of these habits may be self-destructive and difficult to change. The veterinarian must essentially sell the breeder on what he or she has to offer and not be offended by the client's slow acceptance.

Even new breeders will be subjected to the peer pressure of older breeders to do it "our" way.

Breeders having the feline fancy accept a degree of reproductive failures and kitten mortality that would be unacceptable in any other animal production unit. Usually, these problems arise from a few basic and poorly understood management mistakes.

First, a solitary or loner animal is subjected to close confinement. Second, the reproduction of this species is poorly understood by both veterinarians and breeders. Only very recently have some research groups begun to explore myths surrounding feline reproduction—the tom and queen are unique in their sexual and reproductive habits.

Because of these factors the cattery presents the veterinarian with a variety of problems. This article will discuss several aspects of cattery management, the effect of catteries on reproduction and disease prevention.

CATTERY CONSTRUCTION

The existing catteries are as variable as the breeds themselves. As stated earlier, very little, if any, planning goes into the decision to breed cats and thus, the facilities for their care are haphazard. One may find 10 breeding animals stacked in carriers in a closet with little or no light or ventilation or a large well-planned and constructed facility that rivals the finest research colony. Unfortunately, the former situation is more common. If the veterinarian can influence the construction of a new facility, many future problems can be prevented; however, very little factual information is available on construction.

The two most prevalent problems are overcrowding and lack of ventilation, with poor sanitation running a close third. Under ideal conditions ventilation should include six air changes per hour without creating a constant draft that affects any one cage or animal.

If the importance of controlled lighting in a breeding facility is understood by the breeder, it becomes easy to convince him or her of the need for a timer on the cattery lights, so that at least in an indoor cattery the estrous cycles of the queens can be somewhat controlled.

With an understanding of feline territorial mating behaviors in both sexes, it soon becomes obvious to the novice that impervious surfaces are a must both for sanitation and odor control. Although there are breed variations, most breeding toms spray urine consistently, and when overcrowded or in heat, many females will also spray. Therefore, the surfaces with which each animal has any contact, up to spraying height (18 to 24 inches), must be impervious and readily accessible for regular cleaning. In addition, all cracks between wall and floor surfaces must be adequately sealed to prevent urine from soaking into underlying materials.

Novice breeders should understand that keeping an intact male is a commitment on their part to confine the animal for the remainder of its life. They should be encouraged, therefore, to keep only those males that have special breed attributes and to understand that these animals will be used for breeding purposes. If such decisions cannot readily be made, neutering should be encouraged at the proper age or when the show career has been completed. Only exceptional males should be retained for breeding.

Animals that are constantly confined must have adequate space for exercise. For the cat this includes space for jumping or climbing. The walk-in run with spaced resting shelves and possibly a climbing post is most satisfactory. The walk-in run also makes cleaning and sanitation easier. For prevention of aerosol transmissions, it is best to have impervious dividers between adjacent cages or runs.

Ideally, there should be a separate queening area. The queen should be moved to a cage in this area about 3 weeks prior to queening and should be provided with an adequately sized queening box in her cage so that she can lie on her side and nurse a litter comfortably. The box should offer the queen a feeling of security but should have an opening large enough for her to be observed.

A separate nursery for queens and their offspring over 3 weeks of age should provide adequate exercise space for the growing, active kittens. Enclosures in this area must be larger than ones in the queening area.

A food preparation area with refrigeration and running water is desirable, as is a treatment area with good light and a table on which to perform such routine tasks as nail trimming or examining and medicating.

The importance of an isolation area with separate ventilation and sink should be stressed especially to the breeders who have a constant flow of animals through the cattery: cats going to and from shows, queens arriving for breeding and new purchases. The space itself is not beneficial unless the person caring for the cats on a day-to-day basis understands the principles of isolation. While true isolation may not be possible, efforts toward that goal are essential.

The outdoor cattery has advantages over indoor catteries because ventilation and constant odor control are not major problems. However, in place of those problems one must be concerned about security, fly control, rodents and parasites such as fleas. The animals must be provided with adequate protection from both sun and precipitation. If cats are allowed on the ground, litter pans must be provided to discourage the use of natural surfaces.

EFFECTS OF CATTERY LIFE ON REPRODUCTION AND POSTNATAL DEVELOPMENT

The life of a cat in the average cattery differs substantially from that of a cat born and raised in a colony. Typically, in a cattery a kitten is selected from a litter at a rather early age as a potential show animal. If more than one kitten in the litter shows this promise, they are sold as either "show quality" or "breeder stock." The remainder of the litter is sold as pets.

The selected showable kittens must be routinely handled and introduced to grooming procedures at an early age if they are to be amenable to showing as adolescents or young adults. Some are shown as kittens (4 to 8 months), others are not "taken out" until after 8 months. Maturity for show purposes varies greatly with various breeds. The selected kitten may thus become a pampered pet for the first year or two of its life—allowed to run free "on the floor" rather than being routinely caged. Eventually, the cat may not live up to its anticipated show potential, may be shown successfully for as long as it is competitive or may begin to show undesirable sexual characteristics such as coming into heat and/or spraying behavior. At this time the pampered pet is thrust into a caged existence and expected to reproduce. A few purebred animals never seem to recover from this abrupt change in life-style. A year or two of frustrated attempts to breed this animal may follow, and there may be nonacceptance of the opposite sex, failure to conceive or resorptions. Eventually, the animal is neutered and sold as a pet. Thus, the necessary adaptation to cattery life may not be possible in a few of these highly inbred animals.

The larger percentage of animals do, of course, adapt to living in the cattery. The toms, if introduced properly to an experienced queen in the first few breedings, become adept at breeding strange queens. A mistake often made by the novice breeder is to introduce the virgin queen to a novice tom. The results will often produce a shy male who thereafter has difficulty breeding queens. In their haste for the perfect mating, these novice breeders do not take the time to first train the young male and give him a few positive experiences with experienced queens.

The virgin queen has an even more difficult role to fulfill. She is having her first or second estrus, which is quite upsetting to her both physically and psychologically. She is often shipped some distance, perhaps via airplane halfway across the country, arrives in strange surroundings with strange cats and is immediately tossed into the cage with an eager tom. It is a small wonder that any of these breedings are successful. The first reaction of a young queen is to "go out of heat." She then may be shipped back home to try again at a later date or, with hope, held in her new surroundings until she begins to cycle again. Some queens never do start cycling and after a considerable period of time, 10 months or even a year, are sent back home, where they may soon resume cycling.

If the young queen is successfully bred either in the home cattery or elsewhere, she must now be able to adapt to being pregnant in the crowded cattery. If she were able to select her own environment at this time, she would prefer to be off by herself—especially toward the last half of her gestational period. Some queens adapt to crowding at this time; others do not. Many of the queens who cannot adapt, do not go to term.

When a queen successfully produces a litter of kittens, she is subjected to the stress of protecting a litter from her immediate threatening environment that is full of cats. Her personality undergoes an immediate change within a few hours after delivery from acceptance of her surroundings to apprehension and the desire for seclusion. Experienced breeders will attempt to give her some form of seclusion—a covered cardboard box in her cage or a blanket over her cage. If she cannot find seclusion to her satisfaction at this time, she may cannibalize her young, partially or entirely. Suddenly, an entire kitten may be missing, with no evidence of the queen's actions. She may pick up a kitten and carry it in her mouth, pacing incessantly, paying no attention to the littermates. Eventually, the skin on the nape of the neck of this kitten may necrose. The mother may not lie down long enough for the kittens to nurse; after about 12 hours, the hungry kittens will begin to cry, and this adds to the mother's frenzy. She may refuse all nourishment, causing her milk production to fall off in 3 to 4 days, or she may not "let her milk down." She may show aberrant behavior, treating the kittens as prey—such as pouncing on them each time they move or cry or tossing them in the air. Queens that are able to react positively to their surroundings will successfully raise healthy litters.

After raising three or four litters for a breeder, the queen may be sold or traded to another cattery so that another breeder may use her bloodlines. A few queens do not make this adjustment in middle age and will not reproduce in the new surroundings.

Once again, we have taken an animal that prefers solitude, especially in reproduction except for the actual mating, and have forced it to adapt to the environment of an overcrowded cattery. We have taken a pampered pet and attempted to make it into a breeding animal, and we have taken a highly inbred animal with personality variables and have expected it to perform in a standardized manner. It is therefore not surprising that reproductive problems plague cattery owners even more than problems of disease, nutrition or genetics.

In a cattery the kitten's postnatal development is relatively uneventful during the first 3 weeks of life, providing the queen is a good mother. The kittens respond only to the queen, providing the temperature is adequate and food from the queen is suffi-

cient. Such kittens should be handled on a daily basis; those handled in this way develop earlier and appear to be less fearful of humans during their entire life span.

At 3 to 4 weeks of age the kittens respond to each other and begin to take some notice of their surroundings. If entirely cage-raised until sold or sent to new surroundings at 8 to 16 weeks of age, they may never be able to adapt to a new home complete with children, dogs or other cats. It becomes most important that they are given some socialization "on the floor" from about 6 weeks of age until a permanent home is provided for them. This is even more important if the kitten is expected to adapt to showing. Although this may be in direct conflict with disease control procedures, a trade-off may be necessary.

Socialization should include new, but not frightening experiences, such as introduction to strangers, being handled by children or experiences with friendly dogs. This will produce an emotionally stable animal for its entire life, in contrast to the caged, nonsocialized animal that will never be able to adapt to a new environment and may become a "behavior problem" either in the show ring or in its new home. There are breed differences as well as individual differences in the amount or degree of socialization necessary to produce this sound animal. Experienced breeders, while aware of breed differences, may fail to consider those of the individual.

CLEANLINESS AND SANITATION

In working with a new breeder one of the most important concepts to communicate is the necessity for cleanliness and sanitation procedures. If proper decontamination procedures are followed religiously, all other health management efforts, such as immunization, will be much more effective. It is much more difficult to break a pattern of poor management practices in an established cattery. The tendency is to give more and more "shots" to prevent or to cure severe disease problems than routinely to expend efforts in thoroughly cleaning and disinfecting the cattery. The importance of sanitation cannot be overemphasized to either the novice or the experienced breeder even at the risk of causing antagonism.

Breeders have a tendency to purchase a large variety of deodorizers and disinfectants. These solutions are used in copious quantities, often undiluted and in violation of directions, with the idea that large quantities of strong disinfectants replace a good soap and water scrub. The cattery owner must be encouraged to establish a set routine for maintaining the cattery in a spotless condition. A vacuum with disposable filters is helpful in removing hair; this should be followed by washing all surfaces with a detergent, followed by a disinfectant rinse. It is important that the disinfectant be viricidal;

recent research has shown that the most effective viricidal agent for common cat viruses is household bleach diluted with water (4 oz/gal). It is important to emphasize that all organic debris must be removed before any disinfectant becomes effective.

Special attention must be given to cleaning the floors in the cattery. This area is often neglected because the animals are not usually running on the floor; however, viral and bacterial agents may drop to the floor, making it a highly contaminated area through which there is usually traffic to all areas of the cattery. Regular scrubbing and disinfecting of the floor are therefore just as important as scrubbing areas that are in direct contact with the cats. Litter pans should be soaked in the bleach solution for 10 minutes whenever litter is changed. Solids should be removed at least once or preferably twice daily and litter changed completely when spent, or every 3 to 4 days, depending on usage. Water and food dishes, if disposable, should be discarded daily. If nondisposables are used, they should be washed daily in soap and water, then soaked 10 minutes in the bleach solution and dried on a rack.

If there are sick cats, it is important to emphasize that the healthy cats should be cared for first, before the sick animals. Protective clothing and shoe covers are necessary when caring for the sick animals and should be removed before entering the rest of the cattery.

PREVENTIVE MEDICINE: DISEASE PREVENTION PROGRAM

A program for disease prevention in any species makes the following basic assumptions: (1) the level of nutrition is adequate for the age and productivity of the animal in question, (2) a reasonable level of cleanliness is routinely maintained, (3) there is shelter from all types of environmental stress and (4) the animals in question are in good health to begin the disease prevention program. If any of these conditions are not being met, steps should be taken to correct any problems before the success of a disease prevention program can be predicted.

The most readily salable program to the breeder is a vaccination program for the prevention of feline viral diseases. Inoculating kittens at 7 to 9 weeks, with reinoculation at 12 to 14 weeks, is highly protective against feline panleukopenia. Annual boosters for adults are necessary to ensure their continued protection. Some breeders neglect boosters after several years of freedom from "feline distemper." This should be discouraged, as viral infections can surface at any time in a cattery.

More than any other health advance in recent times, the advent of the feline respiratory disease vaccine allowed successful breeding and showing of cats. Prior to this, respiratory disease was rampant in many catteries and made showing purebred animals a serious risk. Although the vaccines available do protect cats quite well against feline viral rhinotracheitis (FVR), feline calicivirus (FCV) and feline

pneumonitis, chronic upper respiratory infections of unknown etiology continue to exist in some catteries because of presence of carrier states and varying strains of FVR and FCV. Carrier queens may transfer viruses to their kittens when maternal immunity wanes. Some catteries have succeeded in breaking the infection cycle by weaning kittens at an early age from the carrier queens. Other catteries use intranasal vaccines in kittens starting at 3 weeks of age and repeat the procedure every 2 weeks until injectable vaccines may be given (14 weeks). This method, though somewhat controversial, has been successful when other means have failed.

Kittens should be vaccinated for FVR and FCV as well as for pneumonitis at 7 to 9 weeks of age and again at 12 to 14 weeks. These vaccines may be combined with panleukopenia vaccine. Breeding queens should receive boosters at least 2 weeks prior to breeding.

Although vaccination for these diseases is highly successful, overwhelming infections in the cattery will still produce disease. Cats returning from shows or after breeding in other catteries as well as newly purchased animals should be isolated for 10 to 14 days. Known carriers should be eliminated when possible.

To date, a commercial vaccine for feline leukemia virus is not available. Initiation of a health program in any cattery should include testing for feline leukemia of all cats but not young kittens. Once the base line information is established, yearly sampling of 10 per cent of the animals as well as of any sick animals should be satisfactory. Written proof of a negative feline leukemia test during the past 3 months is essential for all purchased animals and/or any animals incoming for breeding.

Currently, there is no successful vaccine for feline infectious peritonitis (FIP) available, and there are no meaningful serologic test procedures. The breeder should be as knowledgeable as possible about the diseases so that he will not unknowingly pick up "bargain" breeders from a cattery that is going out of business or suddenly is "reducing breeding stock."

Removal of cats that are not clinically diseased because they have an FIP antibody titer is completely unwarranted. In catteries and some research colonies, 80 to 90 per cent of the cats have been found to have an antibody titer to FIP. Test and removal of titered cats is ineffective, since sources of negative cats are not available or perhaps not even desirable. Prevention of the disease other than by good management procedures, which have already been discussed, is not possible with presently known methods. When breeders are encouraged to routinely run FIP antibody titers, either a false sense of security results if titers are low or healthy cats with high titers are eliminated from the colony. Neither of these methods is known to prevent or control the disease.

Parasite control depends upon whether the animals are housed indoors or outdoors. Consistent surveillance for evidence of external parasites, such as fleas, and evidence of ringworm lesions is essential. This requires at least a weekly examination and handling of each animal by the caretaker. Control of internal parasites by sanitation, daily litter cleaning, emptying litter completely and regular disinfection of litter pans are invaluable aids. Newly purchased cats, breeding queens and composite samples from litters of kittens should be tested for parasites by fecal examination.

RECORDS

The importance of record keeping must be emphasized and may have to be proved to the breeder. The novice with one or two animals sees no need for record keeping, but 3 to 5 years of breeding may result in 30 or more animals and recollection of individual performances becomes impossible. Usually, breeders keep vaccination and show-win records, or a more knowledgeable person may also keep records of kittens produced. However, once a kitten has been sold there is usually no attempt made to follow up on the production or performance of those animals.

The veterinarian can be of service by providing the breeder with guidance about the value of specific records as well as by establishing a valuable diagnostic aid. Busy practitioners seldom keep sufficient individual animal records to provide the information needed when problems develop within the cattery. These records should be kept by the owner, as is the case in most other animal production units. Such records are best kept in a loose-leaf notebook and should be shown to the veterinarian each time an animal is presented for examination.

Individual animal records should include at a minimum identification of the animal, vaccination records, diagnostic test procedures (both dates and results), illnesses including a date, diagnosis, symptoms, and treatment as well as a record of any surgery performed.

To be of further value, a reproductive record should be kept and show dates of estrus, breedings, confirmed pregnancies, any treatments given and a record of numbers of progeny delivered, including sex, color, size, stillbirths and congenital anomalies or inherited defects. Breeders should be encouraged to set goals for individual animals as well as for the cattery. When breeding performance is evident from available records and the breeding potential of an individual animal is determined, intelligent culling can be encouraged.

A further record-keeping step that will enable the veterinarian and breeder to evaluate the operation is a cattery breeding record. This record will quickly enable the veterinarian and the breeder to determine if previous breeding goals have been met. Breeding performance of individuals is evident as compared with others in the cattery. Significant trends in reproductive problems that are affecting the entire unit are more evident from the cattery record than from examination of individual records. A review of overall health problems, nutritional levels and cats' ages will pinpoint a possible cause for problems in these areas.

Suggested Readings

1. Beaver B: Veterinary Aspects of Feline Behavior. 1st ed. St. Louis, CV Mosby Company, 1980, chapters 5 and 6.
2. Cornell Feline Health Center: *Felis domesticus*: A Manual of Feline Health. 1982–83, pp 114–121, 161–168.
3. Houpt KA, Wolski, TR: Domestic Animal Behavior for Veterinarians and Animal Scientists. Cedar Rapids, The Iowa State University Press, 1982, chapters 4–6.
4. Morrow DA: Current Therapy in Theriogenology. 1st ed. Philadelphia, WB Saunders Co, 1980, pp 552–563, 832–845.
5. Pratt PW: Feline Medicine. 1st ed. Santa Barbara, American Veterinary Publications, Inc, 1983, chapters 4, 15, 19.

Infertility from Noninfectious Causes

Mary A. Herron, D.V.M., Ph.D.
Texas A&M University, College Station, Texas

Noninfectious causes of infertility may be grouped under five broad categories: endocrine disorders, congenital/genetic causes, nutrition, behavior and environment and neoplasia. Infertility arising from these causes presents a diagnostic challenge, since detailed research and case reports concerning these causes are not abundant. Recent advances in defining feline hormone levels and feline karyotyping are a part of the pioneering efforts to provide the basis for understanding, diagnosing and treating some of these noninfectious causes of infertility.

ENDOCRINE DISORDERS

Anestrus, cystic endometrial hyperplasia (CEH), cystic follicles and hypoluteoidism resulting in infertility are thought to be hormonal in origin. This is suggested by clinical and pathologic signs rather than by documented alteration of hormone levels or receptor sites. These conditions are diagnosed by interpreting clinical signs and eliminating other probable causes. Serum hormone levels for the cat are now being studied. Establishment of a range of levels in endocrine disorders would assist diagnosis by fact rather than by elimination.

Failure to cycle, anestrus, may result from inadequate hormonal stimulation of the ovary. Impatience to breed specific individuals may prompt clients to request hormone treatment for animals they believe to be anestrous. Hormone therapy should not be instituted until ordinary causes of anestrus and uterine disease are eliminated and the risks of treatment are thoroughly explained to the owner. It must be kept in mind that some young females, particularly Persians, may not have initial estrus until 1 year of age. In other instances the first estrus may be accompanied by mild or brief signs that the owner fails to recognize. In all cases in which anestrus is the complaint, the history and examination should eliminate the possibilities that the female has been neutered or that the female has not had sufficient exposure to light to stimulate estrus. A thorough investigation of medications presently or recently given should be made, since progesterone-containing medications given for dermatologic or behavioral problems can suppress estrus.

Pregnant mare serum gonadotropin (PMSG) and follicle-stimulating hormone (FSH) have been used to stimulate estrus in research colony queens.[4, 5, 23] One hundred IU of PMSG followed in 7 days by an intramuscular injection of 50 IU human chorionic gonadotropin (hCG) has produced results comparable with natural mating.[4] Two milligrams of FSH were administered intramuscularly each day for not more than 5 days. If estrus was stimulated, 250 IU of hCG were administered intramuscularly.[23] Breeding was begun on the day of hCG administration. Vaginal smears and daily observation during either treatment would be a useful aid in detecting the onset and progression of estrus. Superovulation, induction of cystic ovaries and CEH are possible side effects of treatment.

CEH-pyometra complex is less common in cats than in dogs, but the clinical effects and pathologic signs are similar. CEH is a progressive progesterone-dependent uterine disease of the older female, usually over 5 years of age. Dow describes four histologic subdivisions.[8] In the initial phase the endometrium is lined with small or large translucent cysts. The cysts may be distributed in patches or diffusely over the endometrium. The last three phases represent progressive inflammatory changes of acute, subacute and chronic endometritis. The affected uteri are generally enlarged and have thickened walls if the cervix is open. Variable amounts of exudate, depending on the patency of the cervix, are retained in the uterine lumen. The color and consistency range from thick yellow or green to watery brown or red. In most cases corpora lutea are present on the ovaries. In initial stages the clinical signs may be simply nonconception. As inflammatory changes progress, intermittent vaginal discharge, abdominal enlargement and periods of dullness, depression and inappetence may be reported. Some stability in condition may be attained if the cervix is patent and drainage occurs; however, if drainage cannot occur, rapid deterioration of body condition is seen. Total white blood cell counts are elevated, with the most dramatic elevations occurring in queens with a nonpatent cervix. Ovariohysterectomy is curative, but animals in the later stages of the disease are poor surgical risks and require intensive monitoring before, during and after surgery. A few pregnancies have followed treatment by laparotomy and uterine lavage along with corpora lutea removal.[12] Prostaglandin $F_{2\alpha}$ and antibiotics have been administered to cats for successful treatment of pyometra. Dosages of 0.2 to 0.5 mg/kg SQ have stimulated uterine contraction and concomitant emptying of uterine content within a few hours; the cats eventually became pregnant.[21, 22]

The treatment may be repeated daily until there is no discharge. At the higher dosage levels side effects include restlessness, increased heart rate, increased respiratory rate, vomiting and diarrhea.[22] No commercial prostaglandin $F_{2\alpha}$ product is approved for use in the cat. Refinement of dosage and evaluation of efficacy in true cases of cystic endometrial hyperplasia await further reports and research. Treatments other than ovariohysterectomy require an appraisal of the individual case. Frequently, in chronic cases there is extensive uterine degeneration that cannot be restored to reproductive function.

Follicular cysts produce signs of hyperestrogenism, primarily expressed as intense estrous behavior. The cysts may be multiple or single. Not all cysts of the ovary are follicular cysts. Cysts arising from remnants of the mesonephric tubules and the rete tubules and cystadenomas are commonly observed in the cat during necropsy or ovariohysterectomy. Successful medical treatment of feline follicular cysts is not reported; ovariohysterectomy is the treatment of choice. If the cyst is singular or the cysts are few in number and the diagnosis is made before severe uterine changes, laparotomy and cyst rupture might be attempted.[11] If the surgical treatment appears successful, breeding should take place at the first opportunity, since recurrence of the cystic condition is likely.

Repeated abortions in the latter half of pregnancy in the absence of infection seems to suggest that a progesterone deficiency (hypoluteoidism) could exist. The logic of this assumption is not yet supported by information on serum progesterone levels. If low levels of progesterone can be documented, supplemental oral or injectable progesterone could be given to maintain the pregnancy. Careful monitoring and withdrawal of treatment before expected parturition would be necessary, since progesterone inhibits relaxation of the cervix, and an extended pregnancy could be produced. Bacterial and viral causes of endometritis and abortion should be thoroughly investigated before hypoluteoidism is considered and progesterone levels should be determined for diagnosis and to assist treatment.

CONGENITAL/GENETIC CAUSES

Genital anomalies are rare in the cat but must be included in the differential diagnosis of infertility, particularly in the young cat. Vulval and vaginal atresia may occur simultaneously or separately. Small labia with or without stenosis of the vestibule are observed in the former, while stenosis of the vaginal canal is observed in the latter.[18]

Uterine anomalies include uterus unicornis and segmental aplasia. Uterus unicornis, the absence of one horn, is usually an incidental finding at necropsy or ovariohysterectomy, since normal pregnancies are carried in the existing horn. However, litter sizes may be small. The absence of the ovary, kidney and ureter ipsilateral to the absent horn is frequently associated with the condition. If segmental aplasia exists, portions of one or both horns are represented by a fibrous, nonpatent cord. Clinical signs vary with the position of the aplastic tissue. If the aplasia involves the anterior portion of one horn, pregnancies in the remainder of that horn or in the contralateral horn are possible. Pregnancies are not possible if the aplasia obliterates the connection of both horns to the uterine body. Mucometra may result in normal portions of horns that are isolated from the cervix by aplastic tissue. These portions of the horn become distended with uterine secretions and are palpable. The distended segments may be surgically removed, or ovariohysterectomy may be performed.

Ovarian hypoplasia and ovarian agenesis are rare, and both result in anestrus and sterility. The diagnosis is confirmed by observing small fibrotic ovaries and histopathologic examination of the gonadal tissue. Karyotyping and G-banding are useful diagnostic tests that may help to identify a genetic basis for some gonadal anomalies. A monosomy (37, XO) was recently documented in an adult Burmese cat.[13] Associated clinical signs were small body size and anestrus that was resistant to gonadotropin treatment. Existing evidence suggests that the condition is ovarian dysgenesis rather than hypoplasia or agenesis.

The most common genital anomaly of the male is cryptorchidism. Cryptorchidism may be bilateral or unilateral in the cat. Bilaterally cryptorchid males are sterile. Unilaterally cryptorchid males are fertile but should not be used for breeding, since the condition is probably heritable. The incidence of cryptorchidism in a breeding population may be reduced in a few generations by removing both parents of affected males from the breeding pool. Monorchidism, or unilateral testicular agenesis, and testicular hypoplasia are also reported in the male cat.[8]

Sterility in the male cat with a tricolor coat is known to be genetic in origin. The XXY condition in the male cat results in a phenotypic male, with testicular hypoplasia and lack of spermatogenesis. Since the X chromosomes carry the alleles for coat color, X^0 (orange) and X^{0+} (nonorange), the presence of the alleles in the XXY male will produce the calico or tortoiseshell coat pattern typically associated with females. Those males with the XXY genotype that do not carry the alleles are also sterile but are not distinguished by coat color. The condition may arise from nondysjunction of the sex chromosome during meiosis. The tortoiseshell pattern may also arise through chimerism. In these males two genotypic cell populations exist; one population must contain a Y for maleness, and two X chromosomes carrying the alleles for coat color must be present. A few of these males may be fertile.[16] Sexual behavior varies in these animals from absent to normal.[15]

Two intersex conditions, hermaphroditism and male pseudohermaphroditism, have been reported in cats.[9, 11] Hermaphroditism is characterized by the presence of ovarian and testicular tissues as separate gonads or ovotestes. The external genitalia are immature or sexually intermediate. Male pseudohermaphrodites have only testicular tissue. The gonads are located intra-abdominally, and the external genitalia are basically female in appearance although immature or misplaced. Clitoral enlargement as documented in the canine male pseudohermaphrodite is not yet documented in the cat. The genotypes of feline intersexes have not been studied; nor have sex steroid levels been reported.

NUTRITION

Specific cases of nutritionally induced infertility are not reported, and in most cases it is unlikely that reproductive signs would be the only signs that accompany a dietary deficiency. However, the role of nutrition should not be disregarded as a cause or a contributing factor to infertility.

Anamnesis should include information on the quality of cat food, its quantity, acceptability and storage method. Commercial cat foods (dry, semimoist or wet) may provide adequate nutrition for reproduction. The label "complete and balanced nutrition" authorized by the American Association of Feed Control Officials (AAFCO) ensures that the food product will support reproduction.[14] Homemade diets should be viewed with suspicion, particularly if one food ingredient, such as heart or milk, is used. Heart has a high phosphorus content and will produce calcium deficiency and resultant skeletal problems. Milk is deficient in niacin, which may result in diarrhea. Diets composed only of meat may be deficient in iodine. The cat requires an unusually high level of dietary iodine (400 μg/day).[2] Reported reproduction-related signs of iodine deficiency (anestrus, dystocia and congenital deformities) are accompanied by signs of thyroid hypertrophy.[25] Dog foods are unsuitable for cats. The cat is more strictly a carnivore while the dog can easily utilize nutrients of vegetable origin. Dog foods are deficient in both fat and protein. A diet containing 9 per cent fat (dry weight basis) is recommended for cats; 5.5 per cent is recommended for dogs.[6, 7] The fat content of the feline diet is needed to provide energy and improve palatability. Experimentally produced essential fatty acid deficiency in cats has resulted in loss of libido, anestrus and male hypogonadism as well as listlessness, dry hair coat and increased susceptibility to infection.[6, 25] Adult feline dietary protein requirements are five times greater than canine requirements.[25] In addition, taurine, a beta amino acid required by the cat, is usually deficient in dog foods formulated from vegetable products and bovine milk. Taurine deficiency leads to degeneration of retinal photoreceptor cells and to blindness in the cat.[2]

The history should determine the quantity of food consumed and more importantly the palatability. A nutritionally sound diet is useless if not eaten. Cats are selective eaters and are sensitive to odors and taste. Their eating habits or food consumption may also be influenced by stress.

Food storage should be appraised. Long storage times should be discouraged even though purchasing food in quantity affords a better price. Moisture, heat and infestation with insects or rodents can alter the quality and acceptability. Vitamin A content may deteriorate during storage. Cats require preformed vitamin A and cannot convert beta carotene into retinol. In addition to the classical signs of vitamin A deficiency (hair loss, weight loss, night blindness), reproduction-related signs of anestrus (conception and implantation failures, abortion, congenital defects) are seen. Males show depressed libido and spermatogenesis.

Hypervitaminosis A does occur naturally in cats that are fed primarily raw liver. The principal reported lesion is exostoses of the cervical vertebrae accompanied by pain and reluctance to move.[3] Reproduction might be secondarily affected by reluctance to copulate.

Pregnant and lactating queens require special attention. Naturally, a highly palatable, nutritionally balanced diet should be fed. The National Research Council suggests caloric intake of 100 kcal/kg body weight during gestation and up to 250 kcal/kg during lactation. Food may be given freely to allow the queen the opportunity to consume the additional calories and nutrients. High quality protein supplements and calcium supplements may be added to commercial diets. Calcium requirements increase dramatically during gestation and lactation. The normal 200 mg/day calcium requirement increases during gestation and lactation to 600 mg/day during peak lactation periods.[25] The supplemental calcium should be balanced with the dietary phosphorus. The Ca:P ratio for the cat is 1.2:1, and bone meal is a good balanced calcium source.

BEHAVIOR AND ENVIRONMENT

Abnormal breeding behavior and environmental conditions can lead to copulatory inadequacy or failure, which may be perceived as infertility. Diagnosis is usually made by careful observation or detailed history of breeding performance. Patience and good breeding management will correct most of the problems. Copulatory failure or inadequacy is more likely to arise in individuals from single-cat households than in those from catteries. Sheltered household pets with low exposure to other cats may not breed readily. A female in estrus that experiences a radical environmental change, such as transport to a breeding facility, may cease estrous behavior. Estrous behavior may resume if she is simply left in the tom's environment for several hours or days. An alternative solution is to place these queens in the new environment several days before estrus to allow for time to adjust to the environment. Occasionally, a queen rejects specific males for unknown reasons. Alternative partners should be made available. Ovulation failure may be responsible for infertility. Queens are induced ovulators, but the degree of stimulus required to induce ovulation in individuals varies. The stimulus of a single coitus may be insufficient to induce ovulation in some queens. Multiple matings are suggested if anovulation is suspected.[24] Serum LH or progesterone levels following breeding would help in the detection of anovulation. These tests are not now in routine use.

It is customary to bring the female to the male's environment for breeding. Although some males will mate anywhere, most prefer a familiar area or room. In a foreign environment the male may spend hours inspecting and marking the environment before copulating. Mounting behavior may also affect breeding. Males should grasp the skin over the female's lower cervical vertebrae before mounting. This grasp helps to control the female and positions the male genitalia over the vulva. If the male grasps the skin over the thoracic area, malpositioning results. Malpositioning may also result from pairing a long-bodied female with a short-bodied male. If the short-bodied tom grasps the proper neck area, the genitalia are placed over the sacrum. Position adjustments are usually corrected by the pair, or some assistance may be necessary. However, human intervention or even activity around the breeding area may inhibit or delay copulation.

The initial breeding of an individual may proceed slowly. Breeding two novices will compound the inexperience; therefore, it may be preferable to pair a novice with an experienced breeder. Selection of the mate for the initial breeding experience should be made with care. Overly aggressive mates may create a bad experience that could inhibit future performance of the novice.

A lack of libido, particularly in older males, may account for breeding failures. Testosterone injections (0.25 to 0.5 mg/kg) may improve their response. Chronic use of testosterone is not encouraged, since long-term use could depress spermatogenesis, and no studies are available to guide dosage levels. Libido could also be affected by thyroid function. Hypothyroidism is not documented in the cat but should not be discounted as a possibility. Libido may also be inhibited by the urethral irritation associated with the feline urologic syndrome. Treatment of the syndrome followed by 1 or 2 months of sexual rest is suggested.[12]

Oligospermia and azoospermia may account for some cases of male infertility. A semen sample may be collected for evaluation by electroejaculation, if equipment is available, or samples may be collected from the vagina following a breeding. The latter collection samples will allow detection of azoospermia, but the degree of oligospermia would be difficult to ascertain. Ejaculates collected by artificial vaginas are reported to contain a mean spermatozoa count of 56 million,[19] while samples collected by electroejaculation contain fewer spermatozoa. Although the insemination of as few as 5 million sperm may result in pregnancy,[19] no firm minimum number of sperm for fertilization has been established.

Three causes of low sperm concentration are sexual over-use, elevated testicular temperatures and age. Mature cats bred three times per week maintained sperm concentration with no increase in abnormal forms or decrease in motility.[19] Daily collections for 4 consecutive days will reduce the concentration by half. Therefore, under normal circumstances a tom may be allowed to breed routinely three times a week. Daily use for short periods of time is also acceptable.

Testicular temperature may increase in the presence of an inguinal hernia or lacerations on or close to the scrotum and in febrile animals. Normal sperm production returns after correction of the initiating factor.

Although males are usually fertile by 10 months of age, sperm maturity (evaluated by observation of the presence of protoplasmic droplets) and concentration may be inadequate to support a breeding program. Breeding programs are usually initiated after the male is 1 year of age. Old age, no doubt, results in declining sperm concentrations, but no data is available to relate concentrations, breeding effectiveness and age.

NEOPLASIA

Neoplasia in the feline genital tract is not a major consideration in infertility because feline genital tumors are extremely rare and most of those that are reported occur in cats over 8 years of age, past the prime breeding age.

Unlike the canine male the feline male has no reported neoplasia of the prostate, and testicular tumors are rarely reported. Sertoli's cell tumors of the testicles have been reported in aged males. Descended or undescended testicles may be involved, and the condition may be bilateral or unilateral. Clinical signs are related to the increased size of the gonad. Abdominal enlargement, abdominal discomfort and scrotal enlargement may be seen; however, no feminization signs have been reported.[20] Castration is the treatment of choice. Metastasis does occur, but radiation treatment and chemotherapy have not been reported.

In general, ovarian tumors are unilateral, not highly metastatic and attain a large size before discovery. Most clinical signs are related to the compromised abdominal viscera. Signs include abdominal distention and discomfort, ascites, vomiting, anorexia, intermittent intestinal obstruction and weight loss. Half of the reported feline ovarian tumors are granulosa-theca cell tumors. Persistent estrus, bilaterally symmetrical alopecia and cystic endometrial hyperplasia are frequently associated with these ovarian masses and suggest steroid production by these tumors.[1]

Dysgerminomas, the next most common feline ovarian tumor, arise from germ cells. Hormone-related signs of persistent heat and masculinization may occasionally occur. Ovarian teratomas may contain tissue arising from all three embryonic germ layers. Epithelium, bone, hair and other tissues may be identified in the excised tumor. Since this tumor frequently mineralizes, radiography is a useful diagnostic tool.

Other ovarian tumors include cystadenoma, cystadenocarcinoma, adenocarcinoma, leiomyoma and metastatic tumors.[1]

The highly malignant endometrial adenocarcinoma accounts for most reported cases of feline uterine neoplasia, but leiomyosarcoma, fibroma, lipoma and leiomyoma are also reported. Most clinical signs—straining, anorexia, constipation, abdominal enlargement—result from the size and position of the tumor. However, vaginal discharge and estrous irregularity may be reported.

Clinical signs and physical examination may suggest genital tract tumors, but definitive diagnosis requires histopathologic examination of extirpated masses or biopsy specimens. Treatment for all ovarian and uterine tumors is ovariohysterectomy. Prognosis is good for nonmetastasized neoplasia.

Pedunculated fibroma and leiomyoma of the feline vagina are reported. The most common clinical sign is constipation from pressure of the mass on the rectum. Breeding could also be inhibited by the masses. Surgical removal of the tumors combined with ovariohysterectomy is suggested, since a hormonal etiology is possible.[20]

Benign and malignant mammary tumors do occur in cats, but most are diagnosed in females over 7 years old, which is after the prime breeding age. All mammary masses deserve immediate attention, since carcinoma with metastasis is common. Unlike mammary tumors, mammary hypertrophy occurs in young, sexually intact females. Feline fibroadenomatosis, fibroadenoma and fibroepithelial hyperplasia are all terms that have been applied to the condition. This progesterone-dependent dysplasia frequently follows an estrus, and the female may or may not be pregnant.[10] When the condition is diagnosed in spayed females and males, it is usually associated with preceding progestin therapy.[10] In affected individuals one or more of the glands enlarges. The swelling may be mild or dramatic, with accompanying pain and necrosis. Proliferation of duct epithelium and stroma is seen microscopically. The swelling may regress and affected females may become pregnant, but the condition often recurs in the next postestrous period, and the female's acceptability as a breeder is reduced. Ovariohysterectomy is curative.

References

1. Barrett RE, Theilen GH: Neoplasms of the canine and feline reproductive tracts. In Kirk RW (ed): Current Veterinary Therapy VI. Philadelphia, WB Saunders Co, 1977, p 1263.
2. Brewer NR: Nutrition of the cat. JAVMA 180:1179, 1982.
3. Clark L: Hypervitaminosis A: A review. Aust Vet J 47:568, 1971.
4. Cline EM, Jennings LL, Sojka NJ: Breeding laboratory cats during artificially induced estrus. Lab Anim Sci 30:1003, 1980.
5. Colby ED: Induced estrus and timed pregnancies in cats. Lab Anim Care 20:1075, 1970.
6. Committee on Animal Nutrition, National Research Council: Nutrient Requirements of Cats. Washington, D.C., National Academy of Sciences, 1978, p 25.
7. Committee on Animal Nutrition, National Research Council: Nutrient Requirements of Dogs. Washington, D.C., National Academy of Sciences, 1972, p 26.
8. Dow C: The cystic hyperplasia-pyometra complex in the cat. Vet Rec 74:141, 1962.
9. Felts J: Hermaphroditism in the cat. JAVMA 181:925, 1982.
10. Hayden DW, Johnston SD, Taing DT, et al.: Feline mammary hypertrophy/fibroadenoma complex: Clinical and hormonal aspects. Am J Vet Res 42:1699, 1981.
11. Herron MA, Boehringer BT: Male pseudohermaphroditism in the cat. Fel Pract 5:30, 1975.
12. Herron MA, Stein B: Prognosis and management of feline infertility. In Kirk RW (ed): Current Veterinary Therapy VII. Philadelphia, WB Saunders Co, 1980.
13. Johnston SD, Buoen DC, Madl JE, et al.: X-chromosone monosomy (37, XO) in a Burmese cat with gonadal dysgenesis. JAVMA 182:986, 1983.
14. Kealy RD: Feline nutrition. In Morrow DA (ed): Current Therapy in Theriogenology. 1st ed. Philadelphia, WB Saunders Co, 1980.
15. Lang SE, Gruffy DD, Jones DM: Male tortoiseshell cats: An examination of testicular histology and chromosome complement. Res Vet Sci 30:274, 1980.
16. Patterson DF: Disorders of Sexual Development. AAHA's 50th Annual Meeting Proceedings, 1983, pp 453–457.
17. Platz CC, Wildt DE, Seager SWJ: Pregnancy in the domestic cat after artificial insemination with previously frozen spermatozoa. J Reprod Fert 52:279, 1978.
18. Saperstein G, Harris S, Leipold HW: Congenital defects in domestic cats. Fel Pract 6:18, 1976.
19. Sojka NJ, Jennings LL, Hamner CE: Artificial insemination in the cat (Felis catus). Lab Anim Care 20:198, 1970.
20. Stein BS: Tumors of the feline genital tract. J Am Anim Hosp Assoc 17:1022, 1981.
21. Tadashi A, Yoshio K: Treatment of feline pyometra with prostaglandin F$_2\alpha$. J Japan Vet Med Assoc 33:115, 1980.
22. Wiessing J, Thompson KS: Treatment of feline pyometra with dinoprost. N Z Vet J 26:112, 1980.
23. Wildt DE, Kinney GM, Seager SWJ: Gonadotropin-induced reproductive cyclicity in domestic cat. Lab Anim Sci 28:301, 1978.
24. Wildt DE, Seager SWJ, Chakraborty PK: Effect of copulatory stimulus on incidence of ovulation and on serum LH in the cat. Endocrinology 107:1212, 1980.
25. Wilkinson GT: Nutritional deficiencies in the cat. Vet Ann 21:183, 1981.

Infectious Causes of Infertility, Abortion and Stillbirths in Cats

Gregory C. Troy, D.V.M., M.S.
Mary A. Herron, D.V.M., Ph.D.
Texas A&M University, College Station, Texas

Infertility, abortions, stillbirths and neonatal mortality in the cat may result from a variety of environmental, behavioral, nutritional, hormonal, genetic and infectious factors. Infectious agents are perhaps the most commonly incriminated cause of these reproductive disorders in cats. Although documentation of abortion rates is lacking, stillbirth rates in the cat have been reported to range from 6 to 12 per cent. Certain catteries have reported preweaning death rates as high as 50 per cent. Because of the potential for spread of infectious agents and the subsequent high losses that may result, the veterinarian should have a good working knowledge of the common infectious agents that are observed in clinical practice (Table 1). Routes of transmission, carrier states and sanitation practices are particularly important in relation to the infectious diseases.

The diagnosis of infertility, abortions, stillbirths and neonatal mortality should begin with a complete history and physical examination. Histories of both the individual animal and the cattery should be included. Particular emphasis should be placed on the following items:

1. Housing (type of cages—individual or group cages—isolation facilities and practices, sanitation procedures)

2. Nutrition (type of food, sanitation of feeding utensils)

3. Vaccination program (vaccination schedules and products used)

4. Past disease-related problems (feline leukemia, feline infectious peritonitis, panleukopenia, upper respiratory infections, toxoplasmosis)

5. Past reproductive history of the cattery and individual animals

The current medical history should be dealt with last. The veterinarian can establish a good working foundation by outlining clinical signs observed, progression of the disease process, number and age and sex of the affected animal, immediate past breeding histories of toms and queens, recent animal acquisitions and treatment protocols used.

Once an adequate history is obtained, the physical examination should be performed. Particular attention should be paid to the genital tract of both

Table 1. Infectious Agents Incriminated in Reproductive Disorders in Cats

Bacterial Agents
Escherichia coli
Streptococcus sp.
Staphylococcus sp.
Salmonella sp.
Mycobacterium sp.

Viral Agents
Feline herpesvirus I
Feline panleukopenia virus
Feline infectious peritonitis virus
Feline leukemia virus

Protozoan Agent
Toxoplasma gondii

males and females. Genital discharges should be cultured and evaluated cytologically. Specimens should be collected for hemograms, biochemical profiles, urinalyses, tests for feline leukemia virus, feline infectious peritonitis and toxoplasmosis titers. Whenever possible, affected kittens, aborted fetuses or stillborn kittens should be histopathologically examined.

BACTERIAL AGENTS

Bacterial organisms most commonly enter the uterus when the cervix is dilated, i.e., during breeding and parturition. They enter the uterus from the vagina, by way of the male genital tract or from the environment. Bacteria entering at the time of breeding are more likely to cause fetal deaths or abortion than those entering at parturition, which may result in acute or chronic endometritis. Bacterial growth is enhanced when the uterus is under the influence of progesterone. Commonly isolated organisms from clinical cases are *Escherichia coli*, *Staphylococcus* sp. and *Streptococcus* sp. *Salmonella* sp. and *Mycobacterium* sp. have also been reported.

Clinical signs of bacterial abortion include anorexia, pyrexia, malaise, depression, abdominal discomfort, straining and vaginal discharge. Vaginal discharge usually precedes abortion and is fetid and yellow to brownish red. In the advanced stages of pregnancy fetuses or portions of fetuses may be recognized in various stages of decomposition. Unless cattery management is substandard, bacterial abortion is uncommon.

Bacterial endometritis in cats is not as common as in dogs. Both acute and chronic forms are diagnosed. Acute cases are marked by fever and systemic illness, while infertility and failure to conceive are observed in chronic cases. Vaginal discharges are scant and may not be recognized by the owner because of the cleaning habits of the feline species. Clinical signs are frequently mild and go unnoticed.

Treatment of bacterial infections is twofold: (1) eliminate the infection and (2) evacuate the uterus.

Antibiotic therapy should be dictated by culture and sensitivity tests and initially should be given for 2 to 3 weeks. Follow-up cervical swabs should be performed during the subsequent heat cycle to detect any residual infection. Evacuation of the uterus is helpful when there is palpable or radiographic evidence of uterine enlargement. Ergonovine maleate (Ergonil, 0.05 mg BID for 2 to 5 days) and recently prostaglandin $F_{2\alpha}$ (Lutalyse, 25 to 50 µg/kg BID for 3 to 5 days) have been used to evacuate the uterus.[7] Prostaglandins are not approved for use in cats.

VIRAL AGENTS

Feline herpesvirus I is a DNA virus that plays a major role in diseases of the feline upper respiratory tract. This agent is particularly important in catteries where the respiratory complex is prevalent. The major routes of infection are intranasal, oral or conjunctival, and as many as 80 per cent of infected animals may remain chronic carriers. Carrier animals may shed the virus spontaneously and intermittently after periods of stress.

In most instances of feline herpesvirus-induced reproductive problems, clinical signs are mainly related to the respiratory system. Anorexia, depression, fever, coughing, ocular and nasal discharges and keratitis are frequently observed in affected animals with respiratory disease. Abortions that result from feline herpesvirus I occur during the fifth or sixth week of gestation. Virus and viral antigen cannot be demonstrated in the placenta, uterus or fetuses of animals infected via the intranasal route. Experimentally, intravenously administered virus produces lesions within the placental vasculature.[5] Abortions that are the result of naturally occurring disease are thought to be a nonspecific reaction to the respiratory infection.

Devastating losses of neonatal kittens may also result from feline herpesvirus I infection. Shedding of the virus from carrier adults may result in respiratory infection in kittens in the early neonatal period. Rhinitis, tracheitis, bronchopneumonia, keratitis and focal hepatic necrosis are characteristic pathologic lesions observed in neonates.

Definitive diagnosis of feline herpesvirus I is based on clinical signs and virus isolation. Because of the high incidence of feline herpesvirus I infections in catteries, viral isolation studies are the most advantageous test for detection of infection and carrier animals. Serum neutralization titers and direct immunofluorescence testing on ocular and nasal discharges may be useful diagnostic aids in isolated instances of infection.

Prevention of feline herpesvirus I infection is best accomplished by vaccination and strict management procedures. Parenteral and intranasal vaccines are available. A commercially available intranasal vaccine shows promise because of more rapid and complete protection. Chronic carrier states may also be prevented by this intranasal product; however, at present this protection seems to be of short duration. Isolation of affected animals, good disinfecting procedures and early and frequent vaccination of kittens will help to prevent dissemination.

Feline panleukopenia is caused by a small, single-stranded DNA virus. Viral transmission occurs by direct contact of susceptible animals with saliva, feces, urine or vomit from infected cats. The virus is highly resistant to heat, drying and most disinfectants. Infected animals may shed the virus for up to 1 year in their urine, thereby providing a continued source of infection for susceptible animals.

Infection of pregnant queens may produce abortions, stillbirths and teratogenic effects (cerebellar hypoplasia). These signs may be observed without the classical gastrointestinal signs (fever, vomiting, diarrhea and dehydration) in the queen. Vaccination of pregnant queens with modified live vaccines may also produce these clinical signs. With natural infections, viral replication can be demonstrated within placental cells; however, histopathologic lesions are not evident. Transplacental passage of the virus does not necessarily result in infection of all fetuses in a litter.

Diagnosis of panleukopenia is confirmed by history, clinical signs, laboratory findings, histopathology and virus isolation. Urine and feces are good sources of virus for use in isolation studies.

Treatment of animals with panleukopenia depends upon the clinical signs. If gastrointestinal disease is present, fluids, antiemetics, antibiotics and general supportive care are indicated. There is no treatment for neonates with cerebellar hypoplasia; however, the neurologic dysfunction in range, rate and force of locomotion is nonprogressive, and moderately affected kittens may learn to adapt and become functional pets.

Strict sanitation practices and vaccination prevent panleukopenia. Parenteral products provide adequate protection against the disease. Three vaccinations administered 1 month apart starting at 8 weeks of age and yearly booster vaccinations should be given. Vaccination of pregnant queens should not be done, except in extreme circumstances. If vaccination is warranted in a pregnant queen, killed vaccines should be used. Sanitation procedures should be strictly followed in outbreaks of panleukopenia. Sodium hypochlorite (1:32 dilution) has been found to be a satisfactory disinfectant.

The feline infectious peritonitis virus (FIPV) is a member of the genus *Coronavirus*. This was the first coronavirus isolated in cats. Recently, another feline coronavirus, which causes enteritis and is antigenically similar to the FIPV, has been identified.

The FIPV has been implicated as a cause of infertility, repeat breeding, stillbirths, endometritis, abortion, chronic upper respiratory disease, fetal resorption, "fading" kitten syndrome and cardiovascular disease. This group of reproductive disorders has been called the "kitten mortality complex"

by some authors. Whether or not other infectious agents or factors are also responsible for this complex has yet to be determined. Several excellent reports have been written about the kitten mortality complex involving catteries and breeding colonies.[8, 9] These affected catteries and breeding colonies have been found to be relatively free of other infectious agents (feline leukemia virus, toxoplasmosis, panleukopenia and upper respiratory viruses). FIPV was the only agent or factor that could be identified.

Clinical signs in affected queens are usually mild. Abortions occur late in gestation, with the majority occuring during the last several weeks of gestation. In some instances, vaginal bleeding may be prolonged after abortion.

Endometritis is also observed in affected queens. Purulent or sanguineous vaginal discharges are evident; this is occasionally accompanied by mild systemic signs (anorexia, depression and fever). These animals frequently require "repeat breeding" if normal estrous cycles are present.

Stillbirths and high kitten mortality rates are frequently reported in catteries or colonies of cats with FIPV. A high incidence of "fading" kittens is observed. Failure to gain weight, anorexia and emaciation are characteristic of animals that die within the first weeks of life.

Diagnosis of FIPV is based on clinical signs, appropriate clinical pathologic tests and histopathologic and serologic test results. Serologic testing is presently the best method of detecting FIPV infection. Serologic tests should always be correlated with the signs, clinical pathologic tests and histopathologic lesions. The recent identification of the enteric coronavirus places some confusion upon past FIPV serologic surveys. Because these viruses are antigenically similar, they may be difficult to distinguish from one another by current serologic tests. High antibody titers (greater than 1:1600) are uncommon in cats infected with the enteric coronavirus. Fourfold increases (greater than 1:1600) in antibody titer may help in identification of active infections with FIPV.

Prevention of FIPV is through isolation of affected animals and serologic screening of new animals. The virus is readily destroyed by most disinfectants (sodium hypochlorite, quaternary ammonium compounds). At present there is no vaccine available for prevention of the disease.

The feline leukemia virus is a member of the family Retroviridae, genus *Oncovirus*. This virus has been implicated in a variety of different clinical manifestations and syndromes. Lymphosarcoma, leukemia, aplastic anemia, glomerulonephritis, fetal thymic atrophy, infertility, abortion and fetal resorption have all been reported to be associated with feline leukemia virus (FELV) infections.[3]

Abortions and fetal resorption may occur from the third week of gestation until term. Surveys of cats presented for these reproductive disorders have shown positive test results in as many as 92 per cent of affected cats. Abortion is spontaneous without preceding systemic signs in the queen. Damages to the maternal-fetal attachments are thought to induce the fetal loss.

Clinical signs are not usually observed in queens with FELV-induced reproductive disorders. Absence of estrus or repeat breeding should suggest the possibility of FELV infection.[1]

The fetal thymic atrophy syndrome results in weak, immunologically deficient kittens that fail to gain weight and die in the early neonatal period. Secondary bacterial and viral infections, especially upper respiratory and enteric infections, commonly lead to death of affected animals.

Diagnosis of FELV-associated abortions or fetal resorption should be based on the use of the direct immunofluorescent antibody (IFA) test or the enzyme-linked immunosorbent assay (ELISA) test. In cattery situations it is essential that all animals be tested for FELV. Only negative animals should be added to the colony and yearly testing should be done to keep a "closed," noninfected colony. At present there are no vaccines available; however, experimental work has been encouraging.*

PROTOZOAN AGENT

Toxoplasmosis is caused by the protozoan parasite *Toxoplasma gondii*. The cat is the only definitive host for this parasite. Serologic surveys indicate that most infections in the cat are subclinical. Infections have also been reported in most domestic species and in man.

Toxoplasmosis has long been incriminated as a cause for abortions and congenital infections in cats; however, documentation is lacking. Transmission of toxoplasmosis, both naturally and experimentally, has been shown to occur transplacentally and through ingestion of intermediate hosts infected with oocysts. Transplacental transmission is more common in sheep and man.

Congenital infections in neonatal cats are characterized by anorexia, depression, dyspnea, ocular discharges, incoordination and death.[2] Queens do not appear to have clinical signs related to the infection. These congenital infections are thought to occur in the last third of gestation. It should be noted that toxoplasmosis is an uncommon cause of abortion and neonatal infection in cats. Therefore, until further documentation is presented, it should not be considered in the differential diagnosis unless all other known infectious diseases and factors are eliminated.

Serologic testing has been used in the diagnosis of toxoplasmosis in cats. Complement fixation, indirect hemagglutination, indirect immunofluores-

ence, Sabin-Feldman dye test and enzyme-linked immunosorbent assays have all proved reliable in clinical situations. A fourfold increase in antibody titers indicates a recent infection. In cattery situations serologic testing can help to identify active infections when they occur; however, animals with stable antibody titers may be immune to infection and therefore do not need to be removed from the cattery.

Prevention of toxoplasmosis is by strict sanitation practices and dietary management. Litter pans should not be interchanged between animals, and feces should be removed daily to prevent exposure to sporulated oocysts. Cats should not be fed raw meat and should be prevented from hunting and consuming intermediate hosts, which carry toxoplasmosis.

SUMMARY

Infectious agents are only one of many causes for infertility, abortion and neonatal deaths in cats. Accurate and rapid diagnosis is needed to help prevent spread of infectious agents among animals. Particular attention should be paid to the history-taking part of the examination. Past and present medical problems of individual animals and catteries should be included in the examination. Management practices should also be considered in reference to general procedures.

Specimen collection should include cytologic, bacteriologic (aerobic and anaerobic), hematologic and serologic tests. Histopathologic examination of aborted fetuses, stillborn kittens or neonatal deaths is helpful in diagnosis of some infectious agents.

Prevention of infertility, abortion and stillbirths is best accomplished by strict management practices, isolation of affected animals, vaccination and maintenance of a "closed" colony when possible.

References

1. Colby ED: Infertility and disease problems. In Morrow DA (ed): Current Therapy in Theriogenology. 1st ed. Philadelphia, WB Saunders Company, 1980, pp 869–874.
2. Dubey JP, Johnstone I: Fatal neonatal toxoplasmosis in cats. J Am Anim Hosp Assoc 18:461, 1982.
3. Hardy WD: Feline leukemia virus non-neoplastic diseases. J Am Anim Hosp Assoc 17:941, 1981.
4. Herron MA, Stein B: Prognosis and management of feline infertility. In Kirk RW (ed): Current Veterinary Therapy VII. Philadelphia, WB Saunders Co, 1980, pp 1231–1237.
5. Hoover EA, Griesemer RA: Experimental feline herpesvirus infection in the pregnant cat. Am J Pathol 65:172, 1971.
6. Huxable CR, Duff BC, Bennett AM, et al.: Placental lesions in habitually aborting cats. Vet Pathol 16:283, 1979.
7. Lein DH: Pyometritis in the bitch and queen. In Kirk RW (ed): Current Veterinary Therapy VIII. Philadelphia, WB Saunders Co, 1983, pp 942–944.
8. Norsworthy GD: Kitten mortality complex. Fel Pract 9:57, 1979.
9. Scott FW, Weiss RC, Post JE, et al.: Kitten mortality complex (neonatal FIP?). Fel Pract 9:44, 1979.

---

*Since this article was submitted for publication, a commercially available feline leukemia vaccine has been introduced by Norden Laboratories, Lincoln, Nebraska.

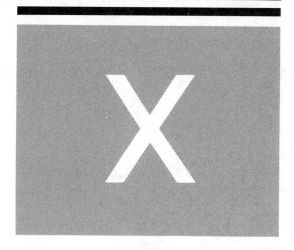

SECTION X

OVINE

E. D. Fielden

Consulting Editor

Selection for Reproductive Performance and Hereditary Aspects of Sheep Reproduction

A. L. Rae, M.Agr., Ph.D.

Massey University, Palmerston North, New Zealand

Improvement in the reproductive performance of the ewe is a major requirement in a wide variety of sheep enterprises. Except under harsh environmental conditions in which multiple births may lead to high lamb mortality or place the life of the ewe at risk, increased litter size will contribute substantially to the efficiency and profitability of sheep production. Indeed, the continuing existence of sheep farming in many countries is now dependent on producing sheep with a substantially increased reproductive rate. Furthermore, a higher reproductive rate is important because it results in a larger number of young sheep being available for selection and thus leads to accelerated genetic gain in other productive traits.

The limited information available on genetic correlations between reproduction rate and other traits indicates a positive relationship to yearling body weight and probably a near-zero relationship to fleece weight.

MEASUREMENT OF REPRODUCTIVE PERFORMANCE IN THE EWE

Reproductive performance may be measured in many ways. Because the emphasis is on selection for reproductive performance, the measures used have to be made on the individual ewe under near-normal conditions of flock management. For this purpose the usual measure is reproduction rate, which is defined as the number of lambs weaned per ewe per year. It is a function of fertility (whether or not the ewe lambs), fecundity (the number of lambs per pregnancy) and survival (the ability of the lamb to survive to weaning). Reproductive rate is thus a complex trait, with its variation resulting from effects contributed by the ewe, the ram and the lamb and the interactions among them.

GENETIC AND PHENOTYPIC PARAMETERS OF REPRODUCTION RATE IN THE EWE

Although a major gene, which in the heterozygous state increases mean litter size by one lamb, has been identified in the Booroola Merino, the reproduction rate is usually found to be controlled by many genes. In Table 1 the range of estimates for the repeatability of reproduction rate and its components—fertility, fecundity and survival—is summarized. From the table one may conclude that (1) both heritability and repeatability are generally low for all traits, (2) the number of lambs born per ewe has a slightly higher heritability factor than the number of lambs weaned per ewe and (3) fecundity has, in most cases, higher repeatability and heritability factors than fertility, i.e., selection for lambs born is likely to be more effective than selection *against* barrenness.

The reproduction rate and all its components are markedly influenced by the age of the ewe and by differences in environmental conditions from year to year. It is desirable that these nongenetic factors should be eliminated when making comparisons between the performances of different sheep within the flock for selection purposes. This is achieved by expressing each ewe's annual record as a deviation from the average reproduction rate of her contemporaries (i.e., the ewes in the flock of the same age and in the same year). Thus, if a ewe in her 3-year-old lambing weans two lambs and all 3-year-old ewes in the flock in the same year averaged 1.3 lambs weaned, her record would be $(2 - 1.3) = + 0.7$ lamb.

DIRECT SELECTION FOR REPRODUCTION RATE

In selecting for improved reproductive performance, it is necessary to assess the breeding value of the young ewes and rams for reproduction rate in order to choose those that will enter the flock. In this context the breeding value of an individual is an estimate of the average reproduction rate of the daughters of that individual. Since reproduction rate can be measured only in the ewe, the records for predicting the breeding value of the young rams and ewes (if they have not yet had a lambing) must

Table 1. Range of Estimates of Genetic Parameters for Reproduction Rate and Its Components

Trait	Repeatability	Heritability
Lambs weaned per ewe	0.03–0.25	0.03–0.22
Lambs born per ewe	0.05–0.30	0.03–0.35
Fertility	0.08–0.18	0.03–0.12
Fecundity	0.04–0.30	0.04–0.26
Survival	0.03–0.15	0.02–0.10

come from female relatives such as the dam, grandams, half-sisters and daughters.

Records of the Dam. The dams of the young rams and ewes born in a particular year will differ in age, in the years over which they have had lambing records and in the number of such records. The first two effects are eliminated, as shown earlier, by expressing each record as a deviation from the average performance of the contemporaries. These deviations are then averaged. The breeding value of the son or daughter is thus predicted.

$$BV = \frac{\frac{1}{2}kh^2}{1 + (k - 1)t} \text{ (average deviation)}$$

In this equation, h^2 is the heritability, t is the repeatability of reproduction rate and k is the number of records included in the average deviation. The breeding value (BV) is expressed in terms of the number of lambs born or weaned (as the case may be). Its mean over the flock is expected to be zero.

Records of the Grandams. The records of the paternal grandam are easily included in the prediction of breeding value along with those of the dam, the coefficient in the prediction being one-half that just given for the dam. Use of the records of the maternal grandam is more complicated because some of the information that these supply is already contributed by those of the dam.

Records of Half-Sisters. Some of the young rams will have half-sisters that have had lambing records in the flock. The prediction of breeding value from this source is the following:

$$BV = \frac{\frac{1}{4}nh^2}{1 + (n - 1)\frac{1}{4}h^2} \text{ (half sister's average deviation)}$$

Here, n is the number of half-sisters in the average deviation. This information will usually be added to the estimate of breeding value obtained from the dam's records to give a useful increase in the accuracy of prediction.

Records of Daughters. With a sex-limited trait of low heritability, one would expect the average records of the daughters of a sire to be a valuable estimator of his breeding value. The progeny test is certainly the most accurate assessment of the breeding value of a ram. However, it substantially increases the generation interval on the sire side (in most cases from about 2½ to about 4½ to 5½ years) because of the time required to get the daughters' records. Thus, progeny testing is likely to be worthwhile only when progeny-tested rams can be used widely by artificial insemination.

Relative Accuracy of the Various Methods. The accuracy of the various methods of selection can be compared by using the correlation between the records used and the true breeding value. Using a heritability of 0.10 and a repeatability of 0.15, the following correlations are found:

One record of dam	0.16
Average of three records of dam	0.24
Average of four records of dam	0.26
Average of five records of dam	0.28
Average of three records of dam plus average of three records of paternal grandam	0.27
Average of three records of dam plus average of three records of maternal grandam	0.26
Average of three records of dam plus average of 20 half-sisters	0.38

With the possible exception of the last method, the generation interval is unaffected.

INDIRECT SELECTION

Because improvement of reproduction rate by direct selection is often slow and costly and sometimes difficult to measure, the study of more easily measured traits that are related to reproduction is of interest.

Although there is evidence of a phenotypic correlation between face cover and reproduction rate, the genetic correlation is small and of little value for indirect selection. The same is true of the degree of skin fold in Australian Merino sheep. The genetic correlation between yearling body weight and reproduction rate is being used in combination with the lambing records of the dam in New Zealand, but the genetic relationship appears to vary from breed to breed and needs more investigation. Resistance to facial eczema is highly heritable, and the selection for it that is being undertaken in New Zealand will increase reproduction rate through reducing the incidence of this disease.

Several promising possibilities are being investigated at present. They are (1) determining the ovulation rate by endoscopy (results to date suggest that ovulation rate not only controls much of the variation in reproduction rate but has a higher heritability), (2) measuring the number of estrous cycles before the first mating, (3) measuring luteinizing hormone (LH) and follicle-stimulating hormone (FSH) levels and (4) assessing testis growth.

CONCLUSION

When records of the lambing performance of the dam are available and all selection is devoted to reproduction rate, selection experiments have shown rates of gain in the number of lambs born per ewe to be of the order of 0.01 to 0.02 per year. Thus, heritability and the size of the selection differentials that can be achieved are sufficiently large to allow for a useful selection response.

Under conditions of extensive husbandry in which no records of relatives are kept, choosing twin-born rams and ewes is a possible approach in selecting for reproductive rate. This method is equal in accuracy to the use of one record of the dam.

Usually, the objectives in breed improvement will include other traits in addition to reproduction rate. In these circumstances selection index procedures to give suitable weighting to the traits included in the objective will commonly be used.

References

1. Bradford GE: Genetic control of litter size in sheep. J Reprod Fertil (Suppl) 15:23, 1972.
2. Land RB: Physiological criteria and genetic selection. Livestock Prod Sci 8:203, 1981.
3. Rae AL: National sheep breeding programmes—New Zealand. Proc 1976 Int Cong Sheep Breeding. Perth, Western Australian Institute Technology, 1976, pp 33–39.
4. Piper LR: Selection for increased reproduction rate. Madrid, Proc 2nd World Cong Gen Applied Livestock Prod 5:271, 1982.

Mating Management and Health Programs

A. Neil Bruere, B.V.Sc., Ph.D., M.R.C.V.S., F.H.C.V.Sc.

Massey University, Palmerston North, New Zealand

Sheep are found in the most diverse climates. They are husbanded at latitudes relatively near to the North and South Poles, where the breeding season is short and only the hardy breeds survive, and in semidesert areas where the breeding season is longer but survival is also difficult during prolonged drought periods. In some countries housing and hand feeding are practiced; while in others, greatly improved pastures, which are available to sheep the year round, have produced animals of exceptionally high productivity.

It is difficult, therefore, to give a precise account of management for so diverse a geographical range to which a wide variety of breeds have been adapted. However, it is possible to give general advice on sheep management, some of which will apply to one area more than to another. The annual pattern of sheep husbandry is shown in Table 1. The seasons are referred to in a general way, and the approximate months of the year are given for the Southern and Northern Hemispheres, respectively. Obviously, the nearer one goes to the equator, the less demarcated are the seasons, the longer the possible breeding season and the less it may be necessary to provide special feeding conditions.

Some countries have diseases that do not occur in others, so that any references to vaccinations and medication are to cover what may be considered the major international aspects of sheep health. This includes the prevention of trace element diseases, clostridial diseases, principal viral diseases, foot diseases and endo- and ectoparasitism.

Ewes are usually shorn prior to or soon after weaning, and the plane of nutrition is reduced temporarily to cause a rapid cessation of lactation.

However, it is prudent to soon improve the level of feed to ensure that ewes are at acceptable body weights for mating, since there is a high correlation between ovulation rates and body weight at tupping. Body weight will vary according to breed and from country to country, but for the heavier British breeds, e.g., Suffolks and Border Leicesters, body weights at mating are frequently over 65 kg and up to 80 kg. The wooled breeds such as the NZ Romney are usually tupped at about 55 kg. Ewes are now selected for their mating flocks and are mated on a flock basis with from 2 to 3 per cent of rams or less under some circumstances. However, in the case of pedigree animals, ewes are mated in smaller groups to individually selected rams.

It is now common practice in some countries to use vasectomized (teaser) rams to stimulate overt estrus. In addition, mating rams are frequently harnessed with tupping crayons that identify individual ewes as they are served by the ram.

The crayon color is usually changed every 14 to 15 days, just short of the average estrous period. Rams are usually mated to the ewes for four breeding cycles, and frequently in the case of wool breeds or dual-purpose breeds of sheep, a down ram is used for the final cycle so that late lambing ewes can be culled from the flock. In addition, the progeny of such ewes are slaughtered and are not kept for breeding.

Prior to mating, sensitizing vaccinations against enterotoxemia, tetanus and abortion (Chlamydia and Campylobacter) should be given. This is indicated for ewes that have not previously been vaccinated and when a long passive immunity is intended for the lambs. Also at this stage, trace elements such as selenium should be given to the ewe, and pretupping drenching, as practiced in some countries, should be carried out. Dipping and spraying for ectoparasites is usually undertaken before mating. In many countries this is compulsory.

Management during pregnancy is aimed at providing a lower plane of nutrition during the second and third months, followed by a steady increase for the final 2 months. In the last month of pregnancy, ewes may be given annual booster vaccinations against tetanus and enterotoxemia. Other clostridial diseases, namely black leg and malignant edema, should be covered at this period. Final doses of selenium and iodine should also be given to ewes within the last 2 months of pregnancy in areas where

Table 1. Calendar of Sheep Farm Events

Season	Northern Hemisphere	Southern Hemisphere	Operation
Midsummer	June July August	November December January	Ewe and ram shearing Weaning Ewes on lower plane of feed Attend to foot conditions (foot rot)
Late summer	August	March	Dipping Body weight check prior to mating Ring crutch prior to mating Chlamydial and Campylobacter vaccination (enzootic abortion)
	September	April	Drenching—dose selenium; sensitizing clostridial vaccinations Mating (tupping)
Autumn or fall	September October November	April April–May May	Reduce feed (mob stocking) Begin winter feeding Dose iodine (if endemic goiter area) or feed brassicas
Winter	November February	June July	Dose selenium, copper, iodine Vaccinate booster clostridial vaccines
Spring	March	August	Crutch, prelamb shearing Lambing, early lambing ewes segregated Docking (tailing, castration, ear marking)
	April	September	Vaccinate lambs if necessary for clostridial diseases, scabby mouth Where endemic—blue tongue
	May	October	Drench lambs (Nematodirus) Louping ill vaccination (ovine encephalomyelitis)

deficiency occurs (see the article Perinatal Lamb Mortality).

Before lambing, ewes are either crutched or pre-lamb shorn and sorted into early and late lambing flocks from either crayon color marks from tupping or from udder development. In some countries, lambing ewes are carefully shepherded either in small flocks or in enclosures where they are hand fed. Under these conditions, considerable attention is given to individual ewes, and all dystocia cases are treated. Alternatively, in many sheep areas where labor costs are high, "easy-care" sheep are being developed. Under the easy-care system, the labor input is reduced and lambing supervision is minimal. Easy-care sheep must have a reduced incidence of dystocia and are also selected for good mothering ability. They must be well exercised and their diet carefully regulated during late pregnancy to reduce the incidence of fetal dystocia.

When intensive and assisted lambing is carried out, lambing kits containing obstetrical jelly, antibiotics, nylon lambing cords, identification sprays and antiseptic are invaluable.

Tailing and castration of lambs (docking) usually takes place at 2 to 3 weeks of age, and in most areas lambs are weaned between 10 and 14 weeks of age. In some countries, creep feeding is practiced before weaning, and early weaning is carried out.

Development of the Female Reproductive Tract, Oogenesis and Puberty

W. R. Ward, Ph.D., B.V.Sc., M.R.C.V.S.
University of Liverpool, Leahurst, Neston,
South Wirral, England

The female reproductive tract develops in the sheep embryo in a fashion similar to that of other domestic species. There is little of special interest to the clinician; intersex conditions are far more common in goats and pigs, as are freemartins in cattle. Of interest in the sheep are the pigmented caruncles and fallopian tubes (oviducts) present in the embryo. The embryology of the Merino sheep has been documented by Cloete.[2]

OOGENESIS

Oogenesis, the formation and development of the egg, begins in the embryo and is completed when a spermatozoon penetrates the zona. As in most mammals, primitive germ cells become oogonia, which multiply by mitotic divisions to form oocytes (whose number cannot increase) in the embryonic ovary. The primary oocytes, with 54 chromosomes, begin meiosis in the embryo, and at the time of birth, most have reached diplotene—the fourth of the five stages of prophase, which is the first of the four stages of meiosis. When the sheep is in estrus, a small number of oocytes (one to three in most breeds) resume meiosis while the surrounding follicles (graafian follicles) enlarge. The dominant follicle is unique in its ability to synthesize estradiol under the influence of follicle-stimulating hormone (FSH) and luteinizing hormone (LH).[1] By the time the follicle has reached its maximum size of 10 mm, the oocyte has completed meiosis to produce a first polar body, which is discarded, and one secondary oocyte, with 27 chromosomes. A second meiotic division passes through a rapid prophase but is arrested in metaphase until fertilization, which in the oviduct stimulates resumption of meiosis to form the egg nucleus and the second polar body. Ovula-tion appears to require prostaglandins, since indo-methacin prevents its occurrence.[5] Laparoscopy shows that ovulation is not explosive but involves a slow trickle of fluid with some blood from the follicle.

The number of ova produced depends on an interaction between genotype, nutrition over a long period of time and a rise in plane of nutrition in the 3 or 4 weeks prior to mating (flushing).[6] Although very fat ewes, condition score 3.5, produce more ova than those with a score of 2.75, they have been found to produce fewer embryos.

PUBERTY

Puberty in the female sheep occurs in the first or second year of life. Suffolk lambs born early in the year reach puberty at the beginning of the breeding season; those born later reach puberty toward the middle of the season at 6 months of age; lambs born later still do not achieve puberty until their second year.[4] Merino ewes in Australia first dem-onstrate estrus in February or March, during declin-ing day length, at ages ranging from 5 to 9 months.

Lambs reared on a high plane of nutrition reach puberty earlier than those on a low plane. This is partly a reflection of the tendency to reach puberty only above a certain body weight and partly a direct effect of nutrition on the reproductive system.

In a small group of ewe lambs measurement of progesterone concentration in peripheral blood showed that there was no ovulation until the time of the first estrus detected by a ram. In another small group ewe lambs ovulated once or twice before demonstrating estrus.[3] The first ovulation commonly produces a corpus luteum that lasts only 1 to 4 days. Lambs at 8 weeks are able to ovulate when treated with pregnant mare serum gonadotro-pin (PMSG) and human chorionic gonadotropin (hCG). Spontaneous estrus and ovulation, however, appear to depend on the initiation of hypothalamic activity by estrogens.

References

1. Baird DT: Factors regulating the growth of the preovulatory follicle in the sheep and human. J Reprod Fert 69:343, 1983.
2. Cloete JHL: Prenatal growth in the Merino sheep. Onders J Vet Sci Anim Ind 13:417, 1939.
3. Hare L, Bryant MJ: Characteristics of oestrous cycles and plasma progesterone profiles of young female sheep during their first breeding season. Anim Prod 35:1, 1982.
4. Hammond J Jr: On the breeding season in sheep. J Agric Sci 34:97, 1944.
5. Murdoch WJ, Dunn TG: Luteal function after ovulation block-ade by intrafollicular injection of indomethacin in the ewe. J Reprod Fert 69:671, 1983.
6. Rattram PV, Jagusch KT, Smith JF, et al.: Flushing responses from heavy and light ewes. Proc NZ Soc Anim Prod 40:34, 1980.

The Breeding Season and the Estrous Cycle

W. R. Ward, Ph.D., B.V.Sc., M.R.C.V.S.
University of Liverpool, Leahurst, Neston,
South Wirral, England

(FSH) and luteinizing hormone (LH). The ovaries contain small numbers of large follicles, but corpora lutea (indicating ovulation) are found only at the end of the anestrous period. In the middle of the anestrous season, infusion of gonadotropin-releasing hormone (GnRH) induces ovulation, without overt estrus, and the resultant corpus luteum is short lived. Intermittent injections of GnRH or LH are followed by normal ovulation and luteal function. Seasonal anestrus may be caused by the greater reduction in the frequency of LH pulses, attributed to low concentrations of estradiol.

THE BREEDING SEASON

North of latitude 35°N and south of 34°S most breeds of sheep breed during a restricted time period during the year and are intermittently polyestrous. It is presumed that the young will be born at a time of year when they have the best chance of growing to maturity. Sheep begin to breed when the days are shortening and are sometimes classed as "short-day breeders" in contrast to "long-day breeders," such as the mare.

Movement of sheep between Northern and Southern Hemispheres is followed by adaptation to the appropriate breeding season. Regulation of artificial lighting in housed sheep[7] demonstrated that the length of daylight is an important factor in timing of the breeding season. Decreasing periods of light at a time of year when sheep were normally anestrous induced estrous cycles, and this remains a method of producing more than one crop of lambs a year in housed sheep. Yeates[10] found that the actual length of the daily light periods was not important, thus showing that breeding was not dependent upon a critical total amount of light. The annual breeding season is not controlled by an intrinsic rhythm.[6] Blinded sheep were able to respond to artificial changes in light periods only when housed with a sighted ram.[5]

The level of nutrition exerts some effect on the time of onset of breeding in sheep, as does environmental temperature. The effect can be measured when the differences in diet have ended almost 12 months earlier and when differences in body weight between experimental and control ewes have disappeared. Under laboratory conditions it was found that ewes maintained at 7°C began breeding 30 to 40 days earlier than ewes at normal ambient temperatures of 27 to 32°C.

The length of the breeding season clearly differs among breeds. In general breeds of mountain origin have short seasons, while lowland breeds have longer seasons. The season remains roughly symmetrical around the shortest day, however. The Merino and Dorset Horn breeds have very long breeding seasons. Treatment with melatonin can bring forward the beginning of the breeding season.[1]

During seasonal anestrus the pituitary contains large amounts of follicle-stimulating hormone

THE ESTROUS CYCLE

The estrous cycle lasts for 16 to 17 days during the middle of the breeding season but varies widely at the beginning and end of the season when longer cycles are common. Estrus lasts about 36 hours (Fig. 1).

On the day before estrus one or more follicles grow rapidly and the concentration of 17-β estradiol in the blood increases from about 10 to 20 pg/ml. The estrogen causes behavioral estrus. Other effects of the estrogen include stimulation of the production of a small amount of cervical mucus, erythema of the vulva and the growth of thick, stratified squamous epithelium in the vagina. These changes are of limited value to the clinician, and the usual indication of estrus is marking of the ewe by a harnessed ram.

Estradiol, along with hypothalamic GnRH, stimulates release of LH from the pituitary. The concentration of LH in the blood rises to a peak of about 80 ng/ml 10 hours after the beginning of estrus, and then both LH and estradiol concentrations fall rapidly. LH stimulates ovulation, which occurs about 14 hours after the LH peak, i.e., about 24 hours after the beginning of estrus. Throughout the rest of the estrous cycle, the LH concentration remains very low, 2 to 3 ng/ml.

At the same time as the LH peak, FSH reaches a maximum of about 170 ng/ml and then falls rapidly. Unlike LH, it rises to a second peak 24 hours after the first. After estrus, FSH concentration is elevated at day 3, and from days 8 to 12 it rises to about 80 ng/ml and then declines to about 40 ng/ml before the next estrus. The function of the rises in FSH concentration during the sheep's estrous cycle is not clear. It is usually stated that FSH stimulates growth of follicles. There is growth of follicles (which later undergo atresia) between 6 and 9 days and 13 and 15 days after estrus. The two obvious peaks of FSH are, however, ill-timed to be regarded as causing follicular growth.

Synthetic GnRH stimulates release of physiological amounts of LH and FSH. The separate release of FSH without LH at the end of estrus may be explained by the effect of the previous high concentration of estradiol; this sequence can cause release of FSH alone in anestrous ewes.[9]

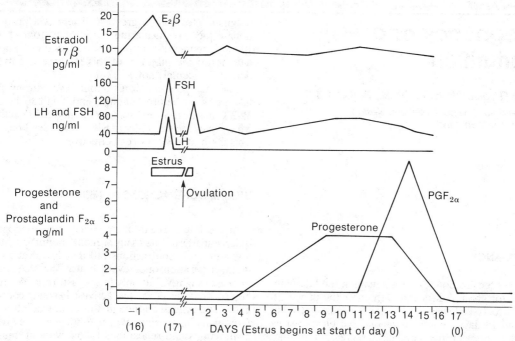

Figure 1. Diagram of hormone concentrations during estrous cycle of sheep. (Prostaglandin $F_{2\alpha}$ in uterine vein blood; other hormones in jugular vein blood.)

If no embryo is present in the uterus on the twelfth day, the corpus luteum later regresses, and estrus recurs. On the twelfth day in the nonpregnant (and pregnant) ewe, prostaglandin $F_{2\alpha}$ ($PGF_{2\alpha}$) increases in concentration. In the nonpregnant sheep $PGF_{2\alpha}$ reaches a peak on the fourteenth day at a concentration in the uterine vein of about 10 ng/ml. $PGF_{2\alpha}$ is established as the luteolysin in the sheep and reaches the corpus luteum by means of the close apposition of the uterine vein and ovarian artery. The release by the ovary of oxytocin, in amounts that are greatest at the time of luteal regression, suggests a role in luteolysis, but hysterectomy depletes the ovary of oxytocin without preventing luteolysis by cloprostenol.[8] The CL of the pregnant ewe requires more $PGF_{2\alpha}$ to cause luteolysis; this relative resistance might be produced by prostaglandin E from the uterus.[3]

The corpus luteum shows histologic evidence of regression on the fifteenth day. By day 16 the concentration of progesterone is basal (< 0.2 ng/ml). This fall in progesterone concentration stimulates estradiol secretion by the growing follicles, and the absence of progesterone permits stimulation of gonadotropin release by estradiol. Progesterone is also believed to be a necessary precursor for the production of estrous behavior by the estradiol.

A role for androstenedione in the control of gonadotropin release is indicated by the increase in ovulation rate following either passive or active immunization against a protein conjugate (now available commercially in some countries). Similar effects are shown by conjugates of estrone, estradiol

and testosterone.[4] Prolactin is released throughout the cycle but particularly at estrus. Prolactin and LH together are able to maintain the corpus luteum in ewes hypophysectomized just after ovulation.

References

1. Arendt J, Symons AM, Laud CA, Pryde SJ: Melatonin can induce early onset of the breeding season in ewes. J Endocrinol 97:395, 1983.
2. Goodman RL, Bittman EL, Foster DL, Karsch FJ: Alterations in the control of luteinizing hormone pulse frequency underlie the seasonal variation in estradiol negative feedback in the ewe. Biol Reprod 27:580, 1982.
3. Huie JM, Magness RR, Reynolds LP, et al.: Effect of chronic ipsilateral or contralateral intra-uterine infusion of prostaglandin E (PGE₁) on luteal function of unilaterally ovariectomised ewes. Prostaglandins 21:945, 1981.
4. Land RB, Morris BA, Baxter G, et al.: Improvement of sheep fecundity by treatment with antisera to gonadal steroids. J Reprod Fert 66:625, 1982.
5. Legan SJ, Karsch FJ: Importance of retinal photoreceptors to the photoperiodic control of seasonal breeding in the ewe. Biol Reprod 29:316, 1983.
6. Perry JS: The Ovarian Cycle of Mammals. Edinburgh, Oliver & Boyd, 1971.
7. Sadleir RMFS: The Ecology of Reproduction in Wild and Domestic Mammals. London, Methuen, 1969.
8. Sheldrick EL, Flint APF: Regression of the corpora lutea in sheep in response to cloprostenol is not affected by loss of luteal oxytocin after hysterectomy. J Reprod Fert 68:155, 1983.
9. Wheaton JE, Recabarren SE, Mullett MA: GnRH-FSH and LH dose-response relationships in anestrous sheep and effects of estradiol-17 and progesterone pretreatment. J Anim Sci 55:384, 1982.
10. Yeates NTM: The breeding season of sheep with particular reference to its modification by artificial means using light. J Agric Sci 39:1, 1949.

Pregnancy and Parturition

R. J. Fitzpatrick, B.Sc., Ph.D., M.R.C.V.S.
University of Liverpool, Leahurst, Neston,
South Wirral, England

PREGNANCY

After fertilization, the ova remain in the fallopian tubes for about 4 days and then enter the uterus at the 8- to 16-cell stage. Attachment occurs between 14 and 18 days, which means that the blastocyst is able to prevent the "cyclical" regression of the corpus luteum before being attached, possibly by day 12. This may be effected by inhibition of the release of uterine luteolysin ($PGF_{2\alpha}$), which occurs in nonpregnant ewes between days 12 and 19. The corpus luteum of pregnancy initially secretes progesterone, but the developing placenta assumes this function. After about the fiftieth day, pregnancy is not terminated by ovariectomy or by administration of luteolytic doses of prostaglandins.

In the first half of pregnancy there is rapid growth of membranes and accumulation of fluids. Ossification of the fetus has begun by day 50 but diagnosis of pregnancy by radiology of the fetal skeleton is unreliable before about the twelfth week. Fetal circulation may permit pregnancy diagnosis by ultrasound employing the Doppler effect, but this has been superceded recently by the use of ultrasound scanning and imaging; this is safer, cheaper and more convenient than radiography and is more accurate and more useful than the Doppler method. Ultrasound scanning gives 100 per cent diagnosis of pregnancy, distinguishes multiple fetuses from singletons with 98 per cent accuracy and gives the precise fetal number with 97 per cent accuracy. This is achieved between days 50 and 100 and permits matching maternal food intake to fetal growth requirements, resulting in profitable increases in fetal and maternal survival and well being. The method may be mastered in one week.[12]

During the second half of pregnancy growth of the fetus dominates, i.e., its weight doubles during the last month. It is toward the end of this phase of exponential fetal growth that the incidence of pregnancy toxemia is greatest. There is a proportionate increase in uterine blood flow from about 100 ml/minute before pregnancy to 1500 ml/minute near term; the majority of this increase is cotyledonary (placental) flow.

Body temperature drops about 0.5°C during the last 48 hours before lambing, and a fall to below 39.2°C has been proposed as a method for selecting which ewes are due to lamb within the next 2 days.[13] This method is 80 per cent effective.

UTERINE CONTRACTIONS AT TERM

In the last 2 weeks of pregnancy the previously quiescent uterus shows infrequent, nonpropagated low amplitude contractions (10 mmHg) of about 5 minutes duration once every hour. The frequency increases slightly, but only in the last 12 to 24 hours before delivery does this activity become coordinated and regular, although still of low amplitude. Eventually, approximately 2 to 8 hours before birth, contractions and relaxations follow without pause, the amplitude increases to 20 mmHg and the ewe is in advanced first-stage labor. In twin pregnancies, one horn, often the larger, is dominant in initiating contractions, and the fetus of this side first engages the cervix, which is now compliant, semirelaxed and yields to the pressure exerted by the distended membranes and fetus. Stretch receptors of the cervix and vagina are activated, and the expulsive pressure is increased by two reflexes: (1) the release of oxytocin, which augments myometrial contractility to pressures of 40 mmHg and (2) the contractions of abdominal muscles, which are thus precisely superimposed on uterine contractions. The ewe is now in second-stage labor, and birth follows in a few minutes. Immediately after delivery, separation of the placenta and uterus commences, and the placenta is delivered a few hours later. Powerful rhythmic contractions continue, probably under the influence of prostaglandins, during the third stage and for several days afterward to discharge the final necrotic placental shreds and the lochia.

The contractility of the myometrial cells, as with all muscle cells, is precipitated by a rise in intracellular free calcium ions, which activate the contractile protein. Although this is relevant to uterine inertia of the hypocalcemic ewe, hormones are the more interesting variables, affecting the contractile mechanism at a slightly earlier stage. Chief among these variables are progesterone, which inhibits this mechanism, and the prostaglandins, which stimulate it. Parturition effectively begins when the concentration of circulating progesterone falls and that of estrogens and prostaglandins rises.

THE ENDOCRINE CONTROL OF LABOR

The changes of hormone secretion before birth have been thoroughly studied in sheep,[3] and in this species it is now well established that the fetus influences its own birth.[9, 10] The sequence of events starts with activation of the hypothalamus and pituitary of the fetus by a mechanism as yet unknown. It is, however, certain that about 5 days before birth, adrenocorticotropic hormone (ACTH) is secreted and stimulates the fetal adrenal glands to liberate cortisol. Cortisol acts on the steroid-secreting cells of the fetal cotyledon, which for most of pregnancy have been actively secreting the progesterone essential for the maintenance of the pregnancy. Cortisol induces an enzyme, 17α-hydroxylase, which in effect switches steroid production from progesterone to estrogen.[1, 6] Fetal estrogen crosses the placenta, where it becomes unconjugated estradiol. At the same time the clearance rate of progesterone increases.

The change to estrogen dominance over progesterone is important in several respects but particularly in the production of prostaglandin $F_{2\alpha}$ ($PGF_{2\alpha}$) in the cells of the myometrium and maternal placenta. Unconjugated estrogens promote the synthesis of $PGF_{2\alpha}$ in sheep, whereas progesterone inhibits this; conversely, the enzymatic degradation of prostaglandins is enhanced by progesterone throughout pregnancy but is depressed by the dominance of estrogen during the last few days before birth. Thus, the endocrine changes promote the production of $PGF_{2\alpha}$ and also of PGE_2, both of which are powerful stimulants of uterine muscle. Uterine contractions themselves then facilitate the further release of the intracellular lysosomal enzymes that synthesize prostaglandins, and the whole process becomes self-perpetuating.

The ultimate effect of uterine contractions, in combination with cervical relaxation and other changes, is to advance the fetus into the cervix and anterior vagina, which will elicit the reflex release of oxytocin. This augments the myometrial contractions, with the liberation of even more prostaglandins, so that the whole sequence takes on a cascading effect. The significance of this and the reflex-synchronized abdominal effort is to increase the efficiency and decrease the duration of second-stage labor, when the risks of anoxia and other hazards are maximal. Each uterine contraction outlasts the accompanying abdominal spasms which is important in maintaining uterine "tone," without which a flaccid uterus could be damaged by compression against the fetus and could also be everted with the fetus at birth.

INDUCTION

Induction of parturition in sheep in the last few days of pregnancy can be achieved with glucocorticoids[2] or estrogens,[11] but not effectively with prostaglandins. In husbandry systems, where the date of mating and, hence, the date of full term, is known to within 1 week, estrogens and corticoids are equally reliable but exogenous estrogen prolongs the ewe-lamb bonding period, and this facilitates the fostering of surplus lambs. Earlier induction is possible with large doses of glucocorticoids, but if a substantial number of lambs are born before day 140, as would occur in flocks with imprecise mating dates, then there is an unacceptable lamb mortality due to prematurity.

SOFT TISSUE CHANGES AT BIRTH

Parturition is more than mere contraction of the uterus. The increase in expulsive force must be coincident with decrease in resistance, which, for practical purposes, means softening of the collagen of the cervix, uteri, vagina and pelvic ligaments. Recent studies on the sheep cervix have revealed that the dense connective tissue of the wall softens dramatically at the very end of pregnancy, ultimately becoming gel-like, so that the cervix is held together during the passage of the fetus by the external muscle layer and the mucosa only.[4, 5] Both the total amount of collagen and its concentration fall, and there is a marked increase in water. Histologically, the collagen bundles become disaggregated and the fibrils dispersed. This is associated with changes detectable in the proteoglycan constituents.[4, 5, 7] Together, these increase the compliance or distensibility of the cervix over a period of 12 to 18 hours under the influence of the decline in progesterone secretion and the increase in that of estrogens, prostaglandins and relaxin. Failure of the cervix to dilate (ringwomb) is almost certainly caused by failure of the endocrine control or of the tissue response to secretions. Although PGE_2[8] and estradiol[5] can elicit softening of the cervix experimentally, trials of these substances in ringwomb have proved them to be ineffective within an acceptable time period.

References

1. Anderson ABM, Flint APF, Turnbull AC: Mechanism of action of glucocorticoids in induction of ovine parturition: Effect on placental steroid metabolism. J Endocrinol 66:61, 1975.
2. Bosc MJ: The induction and synchronisation of lambing with the aid of dexamethasone. J Reprod Fert 28:347, 1972.
3. Chamley WA, Buckmaster JM, Cerini ME, et al.: Changes in the levels of progesterone, corticosteroids, estrone, estradiol-17β, luteinizing hormone and prolactin in the peripheral plasma of the ewe during late pregnancy and at parturition. Biol Reprod 9:30, 1973.
4. Fitzpatrick RJ, Dobson H: The cervix of the sheep and goat during parturition. Anim Reprod Sci 2:209, 1979.
5. Fitzpatrick RJ, Dobson H: Softening of the ovine cervix at parturition. In Ellwood DA, Anderson ABM (eds): The Cervix in Pregnancy and Labour. Edinburgh, Churchill-Livingstone, 1981, pp 40–56.
6. Flint APF, Goodson JD, Turnbull AC: Increased concentrations of 17,20-dihydroxy-pregn-4-en-3-one in maternal and fetal plasma near parturition in sheep. J Endocrinol 67:89, 1975.

7. Fosang AJ, Handley CJ, Santer V, et al.: Pregnancy related changes in the connective tissue of the ovine cervix. Biol Reprod 30:1223, 1984.
8. Ledger WL, Ellwood DA, Taylor MJ: Cervical softening in late pregnant sheep by infusion of prostaglandin E$_2$ into a cervical artery. J Reprod Fert 69:511, 1983.
9. Liggins GC, Fairclough RJ, Grieves SA, et al.: The mechanism of initiation of parturition in the ewe. Rec Prog Hormone Res 29:111, 1973.
10. Liggins GC: Parturition in sheep. In The Fetus and Birth. Ciba Symposium No. 47, Amsterdam, Elsevier, p 3, 1977.
11. Restall BJ, Herdegen J, Carberry P: Induction of parturition in sheep using oestradiol benzoate. Aust J Exp Agric Anim Husb 16:462, 1976.
12. White IR, Russel AJF, Fowler DG: Real time ultrasonic scanning in the diagnosis of pregnancy and the determination of fetal numbers in sheep. Vet Rec 115:140, 1984.
13. Winfield CG, Makin AW: Prediction of the onset of parturition in sheep from observations of rectal temperature changes. Livestock Prod Sci 2:393, 1975.

Pregnancy Diagnosis in the Ewe

D. M. West

Massey University, Palmerston North, New Zealand

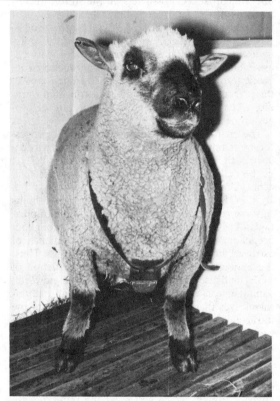

Figure 1. Ram with harness and crayon for marking ewes when serving.

The accurate prediction of pregnancy in ewes would greatly add to the efficiency of sheep farming. A reliable technique for the early detection of pregnancy and the diagnosis of multiple fetuses would enable the culling of barren ewes and the appropriate feeding of pregnant ewes for the remainder of gestation.

The useful techniques for pregnancy diagnosis can be grouped under two headings: (1) aids to diagnosis and (2) most reliable methods of diagnosis.

AIDS TO DIAGNOSIS

Use of a Harness and Crayon on the Ram. The use of a harness and colored crayon (Fig. 1) to detect mating patterns within a flock is now almost a standard technique. It is important to choose the crayon according to the weather conditions prevailing at the time of use, as sudden cold weather may prevent the crayon from leaving a mark. The harness must be carefully fitted to the ram, ensuring that it is comfortable and is positioned correctly to mark the ewe. Problems of the harness chafing or slipping should be checked regularly, but these will be minimized if the rams have a fleece length of 1 to 2 cm. At intervals of 14 to 16 days the color of the crayon should be changed so that ewes returning to the ram are marked with a different color. Care must be taken in interpreting the results of crayon marking, as very light marks may go undetected and not all ewes that are marked necessarily produce a lamb.

Ballottement and Subjective External Examination. Pregnancy diagnosis by external examination and abdominal palpation is a useful technique in late gestation. It has been shown to be 80 to 95 per cent accurate in Merino ewes that are 90 to 130 days pregnant, the accuracy increasing with increasing gestational age. It is advantageous to withhold feed and water for 12 to 24 hours before diagnosis, especially when the ewes are in better condition. The ewe is held in a sitting position approximately 2 feet above ground level by an assistant. With one hand pressed against the left side of the ewe's abdomen, the operator ballottes the lower abdominal area with the fingertips of the other hand. Although the technique is simple and relatively fast (up to 200 ewes per hour), the number of fetuses cannot be determined accurately, and this limits its usefulness.

MOST RELIABLE METHODS OF DIAGNOSIS

The most reliable methods of pregnancy diagnosis include (1) vaginal biopsy, (2) radiology, (3) laparotomy and peritoneoscopy, (4) ultrasonic techniques, (5) blood progesterone assay, (6) rectoabdominal palpation and (7) detection of pregnancy-specific antigens.

Vaginal Biopsy. The vaginal biopsy method was most favored by Richardson[4] in a review of pregnancy diagnosis in the ewe. Sections of vaginal mucosa taken from the wall of the vagina just anterior to the urethral orifice are examined histologically. The stratified squamous epithelium of the nonpregnant ewe is gradually replaced during early pregnancy by layers of cells that tend to be cuboidal in shape, with accompanying changes in the nuclei and cytoplasm. The method has been found to be approximately 93 to 97 per cent accurate after 40 days of gestation, rising to 100 per cent after 80 days. However, nonpregnant ewes are more difficult to detect. Of 204 of these ewes, only 167, or 81 per cent, were correctly diagnosed as being nonpregnant. Multiple pregnancies are not indicated by vaginal biopsy, and this factor, plus the time delay and laboratory expense in arriving at a diagnosis, precludes its use in the field.

Radiology. Most investigators agree that for accuracy, radiography is the best method of pregnancy diagnosis. By 80 days of gestation the fetal skeleton is well calcified, making the radiologic diagnosis of pregnancy and fetal numbers relatively simple and accurate. Mobile units have been developed using video fluoroscopy so that an enhanced image of the ewe's abdominal contents is instantly displayed on a screen. However, the capital cost of this equipment limits its application to experimental flocks.

Laparotomy and Peritoneoscopy. Lamond[3] demonstrated that pregnancy can be diagnosed in early gestation by the digital palpation of the uterus via a 5-cm paramedian laparotomy incision. At 4 weeks gestation the pregnant uterus is tense, thin walled and about 1 cm in diameter, extending beyond the pelvic brim. At 6 to 7 weeks the uterine horns are 5 to 10 cm in diameter, and cotyledons can be detected. It is apparent that for diagnosis of pregnancy alone, digital palpation or direct observation of the internal genitalia would be highly accurate, but this would be of limited value in predicting multiple fetuses.

Ultrasonic Techniques. Numerous ultrasonic devices are available to test sheep for pregnancy, ranging from simple pulse-echo devices to those that provide an instantaneous image of the tissue being scanned.

Early work with externally applied pulse-echo devices indicated an accuracy approaching 100 per cent after 60 to 70 days of pregnancy in sheep. Accuracy of identifying nonpregnant ewes is lower, averaging 80 to 90 per cent. Most observers record a rate of about 120 ewes/hour.[5]

Similar results have been achieved using the Doppler pregnancy testing instruments, in which pregnancy is diagnosed by detecting the change in frequency of an ultrasonic wave as it strikes moving objects (such as blood flow or a heart beating). These devices can be used either externally or intrarectally. However, attempts to diagnose multiple pregnancies and/or litter size have so far met with limited success.

Recently, ultrasonic devices have been improved to provide an instantaneous image, enabling the abdominal contents of the ewe to be visualized. This offers considerable advantages in accuracy of predicting litter size, but for satisfactory results, the operator must be skilled. Apart from the considerable cost of the equipment, other disadvantages of this technique include the need to examine sheep well restrained on their backs and the need to ensure adequate contact by removing wool from the lower abdomen.

Despite these improvements, the early hopes of the widespread use of ultrasonics in pregnancy detection in ewes have not been realized.

Blood Progesterone Assay. The development of rapid and sensitive assays of plasma progesterone in sheep has permitted the diagnosis of pregnancy with an accuracy of approximately 90 per cent by day 28 of gestation. Furthermore, a success rate of 65 per cent has been claimed in predicting litter size at 90 to 105 days gestation, although this was achieved under optimal conditions of standardization. A similar method, measuring progesterone levels in milk, has been adapted for pregnancy diagnosis in cattle. It must be remembered that with dairy cattle in particular, milk is readily available, and differentiation between single and multiple pregnancies is not required. Except for research purposes, progesterone assay for pregnancy diagnosis in sheep will be limited because of the cost, the time delay and the lack of sensitivity in differentiating singles from multiples.

Rectoabdominal Palpation. Pregnancy diagnosis by rectoabdominal palpation has been described by Hulet.[1, 2] It is recommended that the ewes be fasted overnight. The ewe is restrained on her back in a cradle, and a lubricated rod is inserted into the rectum a distance of about 30 cm. With one hand on the posterior abdomen, the other hand guides the rod so that the distal end palpates the region that should accommodate the fetus. In early pregnancy (before 70 days) it is advantageous to have the ewe tilted forward so that the gut falls forward, away from the genitalia, but this is not necessary in later pregnancy. Virtually 100 per cent accuracy at 70 to 110 days after mating can be obtained in differentiating nonpregnant from pregnant animals. However, the overall accuracy rate in differentiating between single and multiple pregnancies is only about 70 per cent.

Rectoabdominal palpation has the advantages of immediate results, speed (approximately 120 ewes per hour) and economy. The disadvantages include the necessity of fasting the ewes overnight and the danger of inflicting internal injuries with the rectal probe. Losses from ewe deaths and abortions have been reported following the use of this technique.

Detection of Pregnancy-Specific Antigens. Recently, a technique has been described in which antigens specific to pregnancy in the ewe can be detected using a hemagglutination test. Hemagglutination occurred when rabbit anti-sheep embryo serum was added to a few drops of blood from ewes between days 6 and 50 of pregnancy, but not when added to blood from nonpregnant ewes, rams or wethers. The test offers very early detection of pregnancy, but its usefulness is limited at present because (1) it cannot differentiate single from multiple fetuses and (2) the time delay of about 30 minutes necessary for hemagglutination to occur requires identification and a further gathering of ewes.

CONCLUSION

The economic justification for the diagnosis of pregnancy in ewes in commercial flocks lies in saving supplementary feed to nonpregnant sheep and efficient feeding of ewes carrying multiple lambs. However, for a technique to be acceptable certain criteria must be attained. Equipment and materials

should be inexpensive, and the diagnosis should be rapid, safe and accurate. After 100 days of gestation, an accuracy of almost 100 per cent in detecting pregnancy and 90 per cent in separating singles from multiples would appear to be reasonable goals. None of the techniques described can currently reach these criteria.

In contrast, there are very useful methods of pregnancy diagnosis for research purposes. These include vaginal biopsy, laparotomy peritonescopy, blood progesterone estimations and detection of pregnancy-specific antigens, all of which achieve accuracies approaching 100 per cent early in gestation. By 80 days gestation the number of fetuses can be accurately determined by the use of radiology.

References

1. Hulet CV: A rectal abdominal palpation technique for diagnosing pregnancy in the ewe. J Anim Sci 35:814, 1972.
2. Hulet CV: Determining fetal numbers in pregnant ewes. J Anim Sci 36:325, 1973.
3. Lamond DR: Diagnosis of early pregnancy in the ewe. Aust Vet J 39:192, 1963.
4. Richardson C: Pregnancy diagnosis in the ewe—a review. Vet Rec 90:264, 1972.
5. Thwaites CJ: Development of ultrasonic techniques for pregnancy diagnosis in the ewe. Anim Breed Abstr 49:427, 1981.
6. Turner CB, Hindson JC: An assessment of a method of manual pregnancy diagnosis in the ewe. Vet Rec 96:56, 1975.

Infectious Ovine Abortion

E. D. Fielden, B.Agr.Sc., B.V.Sc., F.R.C.V.S., F.A.C.V.S.

Massey University, Palmerston North, New Zealand

Although sporadic cases of abortion and fetal mummification are regularly observed on sheep farms, the major causes for concern are those enzootics that occur from time to time and that lead to substantial loss of potential progeny, not only from abortion but also from perinatal death of lambs. Some of the agents concerned directly attack the fetus or placenta or both, leading to what is often called a primary abortion. Others, because of the marked systemic disturbance caused to the ewe, result in secondary abortion. References are made to congenital infections and their relationship to perinatal lamb deaths in the article Perinatal Lamb Mortality.

Two major problems confront the veterinarian faced with one of these outbreaks: first, the need to establish a diagnosis and second, control of the disease. Diagnosis is not difficult if one is aware of the type of problem that exists in the area with which you are concerned. Careful gross examination is made of several dead or dying lambs and their placentae which contain many characteristic lesions associated with diseases causing ovine abortion. Care must be taken in selection and transport of specimens to a competent diagnostic laboratory. Control, both because of problems of cost and because of our limited knowledge of the epidemiology of many of these diseases, may be an entirely different matter. It would not be possible, within the limitations of this article, to deal comprehensively with all the infectious agents that may cause abortion and perinatal mortality in sheep. I have therefore selected and tabulated some of the more important conditions that have been described and have commented particularly on matters that are relevant to their diagnosis and control (Table 1). Further information concerning these diseases can be obtained from the references listed.

SELECTION AND TRANSPORT OF DIAGNOSTIC SPECIMENS

1. Reliable laboratory diagnosis depends on a correct selection of specimens that reach the labo-

Table 1. Infectious Diseases Causing Ovine Abortion and/or Perinatal Loss

Disease	Transmission	Clinical Features	Gross Pathology of Fetus and Placenta	Diagnostic Aids
Vibriosis				
Campylobacter fetus ss. *fetus* affects sheep. The same serotype occasionally affects cattle and man. Several biotypes occur. Vibriosis is widespread and is regarded as an important cause of ovine abortion in Britain, the United States and New Zealand.	Ingestion, especially during last 2 months of gestation. Rapid spread occurs during close confinement of ewes during lambing. Sheep are regarded as the primary source of infection; other animals and birds may act as secondary reservoirs of infection.	Abortions in late pregnancy, stillbirths and birth of weak infected progeny occur. The disease tends to occur in epidemic form every 4 to 5 years; seldom seen as cause of serious loss in same flock in successive years. Metritis may occur after abortion; other ewes die from peritonitis following retention of dead lambs. The incubation period from infection to abortion is 7 to 25 days.	Placentitis with edema and necrosis of cotyledons is present, with cotyledons sometimes diffusely pale. The placental lesions are usually not as severe as with brucellosis. Fetus shows usual signs of intrauterine death, with subcutaneous blood-stained edema and excess fluid in body cavities. In about 40 per cent of cases characteristic circumscribed necrotic foci 10 to 20 mm in diameter occur in the liver.	Culture and direct microscopy are used to identify organisms from placenta, fetal stomach contents and uterine discharge after abortion. Immunofluorescent techniques are used in some laboratories.

Control of Vibriosis

1. During an outbreak careful attention should be paid to hygiene if at all practical. Thus, affected ewes (and their surviving lambs) should be isolated until genital discharges cease; dead fetuses, lambs and placentae should be burnt or destroyed with quicklime; the pen area or lambing site should be disinfected. Spreading out the ewes in advanced pregnancy over a wide grazing area reduces contact with infective material.

2. The prophylactic use of an adjuvant vaccine containing killed organisms will protect ewes from challenge. The same biotypes as occur in the area should be included in the vaccines. If vaccination is not carried out, running ewes in early pregnancy, and those not yet bred, with aborting ewes helps spread natural immunity in the flock.

3. The use of vaccination during an outbreak is of questionable value unless lambing is spread over a long period of time. Intramuscular injection of in-contact ewes with combinations of penicillin and streptomycin has been suggested as a way of reducing losses, provided early diagnosis is made; the economic merit of such a procedure requires careful consideration. When evaluating potential control programs, the cyclical nature of this disease on a property should be kept in mind.

Disease	Transmission	Clinical Features	Gross Pathology of Fetus and Placenta	Diagnostic Aids
Brucellosis				
Brucellosis melitensis affects sheep, goats and other species including man. It is recorded in continental Europe, Mediterranean countries, Africa, Central America and rarely in the	Ingestion is the main method of transmission, especially during the lambing period. Droplet inhalation and entry both through the conjunctival membrane and broken skin occasionally occurs.	Abortions in late pregnancy, stillbirths and birth of weak infected progeny occur. Congenital infections may persist throughout life (especially *B. melitensis*). Systemic effects may be seen	The essential lesion is placentitis, with edema and necrosis of cotyledons. The intercotyledonary membrane may be thickened, yellow-brown and leathery; cotyledons show yellow-	Culture and direct microscopy are used to identify organisms that are plentiful in the placenta, fetal stomach and vaginal discharge of the ewe. Modified Ziehl-Neelsen technique is satisfactory

Table continued on next page

Table 1. Infectious Diseases Causing Ovine Abortion and/or Perinatal Loss *Continued*

Disease	Transmission	Clinical Features	Gross Pathology of Fetus and Placenta	Diagnostic Aids
Brucellosis *Continued* *B. abortus* only occasionally affects sheep. United States.	Venereal transmission following natural mating is rare.	in the dam with fever, lameness (associated with joint swellings), sometimes central nervous system (CNS) signs.	brown necrotic areas, often with adjacent hemorrhage. Mucopurulent material may be adherent to the allantochorion. Fetus shows usual signs of intrauterine death.	for staining for direct microscopy. Complement fixation (CF) test on sera of aborting ewes.
B. ovis affects sheep only and has been reported in central Europe, South Africa, the western United States, Australia and New Zealand.	Method of natural transmission in ewes is not known, although in the absence of the ram, spread from ewe to ewe is thought to be of little consequence.	Pathogenicity for the ewe is low and outbreaks of abortion are rare. *B. ovis* is much more important as a cause of ram wastage.	The same pathology is present when the ewe is affected.	As above (for diagnosis of the disease in rams see the Caprine section).

Control of Brucellosis

1. Test and slaughter policy can be used when the disease is under control and appropriate testing of replacement stock can be undertaken.
2. Otherwise, general hygiene at lambing and protection of ewes before first breeding using *B. melitensis* (Elberg Rev 1) or *B. abortus strain 19* vaccines.
3. For control of *B. ovis*, attention is focused on the ram.

Salmonellosis (Paratyphoid Abortion) *Salmonella abortus ovis*, which is host specific, is relatively uncommon but endemic in the south of England and in parts of Europe. Other salmonellae species, which are widespread throughout the world and affect many animals including man, may cause abortion in sheep, e.g., *S. dublin, S. typhimurium, S. montevideo*.	Ingestion of contaminated food and water usually from carrier animals. Ewes in late pregnancy appear more susceptible. Overcrowding and other forms of stress favor an outbreak. Unless the infecting dose is large or the strain exceptionally virulent, infection seldom causes clinical disease in the absence of some predisposing factor resulting in stress.	Abortions, stillbirths, birth of weak infected progeny that usually die within 7 days of birth. Ewes may show high fever before aborting; most recover, but some die from metritis and/or septicemia. Some ewes and newborn lambs show diarrhea; in the lamb this is usually fatal. When infection is endemic, abortions tend to be confined to the younger ewes.	No specific placental lesions have been reported. Aborted fetuses show usual signs of intrauterine death. Septicemia lesions may be seen in those lambs dying during or shortly after birth.	Culture of organisms from fetus, placenta and uterine discharge may be continuous. Serum agglutination tests, when available, may be useful on a flock basis for identifying presence of the particular organism.

Control of Salmonellosis

1. Maintenance of a closed flock, avoidance of overcrowding and other stress situations and rodent control when food contamination is a problem should be followed. During an outbreak normal hygienic precautions as described for vibriosis help reduce the rate of spread.
2. Mass treatment of exposed animals with drugs is generally disappointing and usually economically unjustified. Individual animals can be given trimethoprim plus sulfadiazine (fluid therapy in conjunction with, or even instead of, such treatment may be just as effective).
3. Autogenous vaccines given before unavoidable exposure of susceptible ewes to the disease have been suggested as being of value. Because of the natural immunity that develops following exposure to the disease, careful evaluation of the real merit of such vaccines is required.

Disease	Transmission	Clinical Features	Gross Pathology of Fetus and Placenta	Diagnostic Aids
Toxoplasmosis *Continued* *Toxoplasmosis gondii* affects a wide range of animals as well as man. It is widespread and has been reported in Australia, New Zealand, Britain, Turkey, USSR and North America. Cats and other Felidae are considered the primary host and excrete oocysts; species such as sheep and man are regarded as secondary hosts. In these species the organism is found in two forms: tachyzoites, which are actively multiplying, invasive and found in the acute state of the disease, and cysts containing bradyzoites found in the chronic phase of the disease.	Oocysts excreted in cat feces are thought to provide the major source of infection. Congenital transmission from ewe to lamb is established. Further epidemiologic knowledge is required to establish how the disease spreads during an epidemic.	Ewes infected in the earlier stages of pregnancy either resorb the embryo, or fetal death and mummification (often only one of a twin pair) may occur. Infection in late pregnancy leads to abortion and perinatal losses of lambs. Many congenitally affected lambs survive. Disease in the adult is generally asymptomatic, occasionally CNS signs develop. In endemic areas only younger ewes usually lose lambs.	Gross lesions of the cotyledons (numerous grey-white foci 1 to 3 mm in diameter) are indicative of the disease. Not all cotyledons are equally affected, and such lesions should be differentiated from nonspecific calcification. Focal leukoencephalomalacia in the CNS of stillborn lambs or lambs dying shortly after birth is a common finding—microscopy of brain sections is nearly always necessary to confirm this.	Histology of cotyledon to demonstrate focal areas of necrosis and organism; histology of fetal brain to demonstrate foci of glial cells and leukoencephalomalacia. A range of serologic tests has been developed by different laboratories to assist with diagnosis of this disease.

Control of Toxoplasmosis
Since the immunity that is induced following natural infection leads to a reduction in subsequent losses of lambs, a recommended practice is to run unbred flock replacements with aborting ewes to aid the development of natural immunity.

Disease	Transmission	Clinical Features	Gross Pathology of Fetus and Placenta	Diagnostic Aids
Border Disease (Hairy Shaker Disease) The cause is infection of the pregnant ewe with a pestivirus closely related to, if not identical with, bovine viral diarrhea (BVD) virus. The disease has been described in Britain, North America, New Zealand, Australia, Greece and Ireland. Several strains appear to be involved.	Vertical transmission from ewe to lamb during gestation is well established, and venereal spread of the disease seems likely. Surviving lambs can transmit the virus both vertically and laterally for years. Most of the more obvious clinical signs result from infection of pregnant ewes in the first half of gestation. Severe loss is likely if susceptible pregnant ewes are introduced to infected flocks or if infected ewes are mixed with resident ewes having no immunity to the disease.	Losses of potential progeny at any stage during pregnancy and in the postnatal period occurs. Infertility with a marked increase in barren ewes, fetal mummification and/or maceration, abortions, stillbirths and losses of lambs born alive are all features of the disease. When the fleece has developed, it tends to be hairy and may be pigmented. If born alive, lambs may show muscular tremors causing incoordination and difficulty in nursing.	Cotyledons tend to be small for fetal age; they occasionally show areas of focal necrosis (1 to 3 mm). Fetal mummification; hairy pigmented coats if the wool has developed; fetus small for gestational age; muscular tremors and incoordination if lambs are born alive When late gestation fetuses or young lambs encounter the disease, nodular periarteritis, which is slow to resolve, may occur.	CNS shows hypomyelino-genesis, and the skin shows characteristic skin lesions on histologic studies. BVD-neutralizing antibodies in the serum of dam or lamb may help to differentiate the disease from enzootic ataxia.

Table continued on following page

Table 1. Infectious Diseases Causing Ovine Abortion and/or Perinatal Loss *Continued*

Disease	Transmission	Clinical Features	Gross Pathology of Fetus and Placenta	Diagnostic Aids
Control of Border Disease 1. Eradication is probably only feasible by total depopulation and repopulation from virus-free sources. This is unlikely to be practicable in large flocks in which the disease is endemic. 2. Running of breeding stock with affected lambs during the nonpregnant period and well before mating begins helps spread resistance. Vaccines for controlling the disease, while possible experimentally, have yet to be shown to be of value in the field.				
Enzootic Abortion (EAE, Chlamydial Abortion) This is caused by a chlamydial agent that affects sheep, occasionally goats and cattle and rarely man. Abortion-producing strains differ antigenically from strains producing polyarthritis (sheep and cattle) and ovine conjunctivitis. The disease appears to be of greatest importance in Britain, Europe and the western United States.	Ingestion during the lambing period following contamination of food and surroundings by aborted fetuses, placentae and vaginal discharge are the routes of transmission. Spread is more rapid when ewes are confined.	Late abortion, stillbirths and birth of weak infected progeny are the main features. Fetal mummification is occasionally seen. Lambs with congenital infections usually abort during their first pregnancy; ewes infected in the last month of pregnancy may not abort until the next gestation period; i.e., latent infections occur. Ewes seldom abort more than once.	A chorionitis with chorionic epithelial cells packed with elementary bodies appears to be the essential lesion.	Placental smears and smears of vaginal discharge (but not fetal stomach) stained by the modified Ziehl-Neelsen technique should be done. Organisms can be cultured in yolk sac of embryonating chicken eggs. CF test may also be used.
Control of Enzootic Abortion 1. During an outbreak, all aborting ewes, weak lambs and their dams should be isolated until uterine discharges cease and surviving lambs are normal. Infected placentae, dead lambs and lambing areas should be handled as for vibriosis. 2. Although treatment of in-contact ewes with long-acting oxytetracycline has been reported to have value in field outbreaks, it is doubtful whether the return justifies the cost. At the time of impending abortion, irreversible damage may already have taken place. 3. Immunization of susceptible ewes before breeding with a commercial killed vaccine appears to offer reasonable protection in areas where the disease is endemic.				

ratory in a satisfactory condition for processing. A comprehensive case history concerning the problem under investigation should be submitted with the specimens (see previous comment on the value of gross examination of dead and dying lambs and placentae).

2. Remember the cardinal law of diagnosis is that you have every chance of not finding what you don't look for! It is therefore generally better to submit too many samples rather than too few.
3. You should consult with your own diagnostic servicing laboratory personnel concerning their requirements regarding selection of diagnostic material and method of packaging and transport in your own particular area. Submission of the following material will generally permit diagnosis to be made of known infectious diseases causing abortion in sheep:
   a. Placenta including placental cotyledon—fixed and fresh.
   b. Fresh fetuses—chilled if they can be delivered rapidly to the laboratory. Otherwise:
      (1) Fetal liver and lung—fresh and fixed.
      (2) Fetal abomasum and contents—fresh.
      (3) Fetal heart blood or exudate from body cavities, or both—fresh.
      (4) Fetal brain—fixed.
   c. Whole blood (only if specimen reaches the laboratory in 24 hours) or sera from affected ewes.

   d. Vaginal discharge from affected ewes—fresh.
4. Fresh material to be used for microbiological examination should be packaged individually in sterile containers to avoid cross contamination and should be chilled (use coolant packs and insulated containers). Deep frozen tissues are generally suitable for virologic and most bacteriologic examinations but not for histopathologic studies.
5. Material for histopathologic examinations should be fixed in neutral solutions of 10 per cent formalin (1 volume of commercial formalin with 9 volumes of water) as soon as possible after collection. Brains, cotyledon and placental tissue should be fixed whole. Several slices of lung and liver (about 5 mm thick, using boundary zones including normal and abnormal tissue when this can be seen) permit better fixation for these specimens.

References

1. Barlow RM, Patterson DSP: Border disease of sheep: A virus-induced teratogenic disorder. Adv Vet Med Suppl 36:90, 1982.
2. Garcia MM, Eaglesome MD, Rigby C: Campylobacters important in veterinary medicine. Vet Bull 53:793, 1983.
3. Martin WB (ed): Diseases of Sheep. Palo Alto, Blackwell, 1983.

Dystocia

K. G. Haughey, B.V.Sc., M.A.C.V.S.

The University of Sydney,
Camden, New South Wales, Australia

Dystocia is defined as parturition that results in hypoxic or traumatic injury to the fetus or traumatic injury to the ewe that is prejudicial to its survival. In addition to causing asphyxiation during birth, severe asphyxia also depresses the thermoregulatory and feeding activity of affected neonatal lambs, so that they are prone to hypothermia during cold weather. Neonatal survival is further prejudiced as maternal behavior of dystocic ewes is severely depressed.[1] Thus, dystocia is a major cause of perinatal mortality because it causes neonatal as well as parturient death.

OCCURRENCE AND PATHOGENESIS

The prevalence of dystocia is usually higher in meat breeds, e.g., Texel, Dorset Horn and Romney, than in wool breeds, e.g., Merino and Scottish Blackface, grazed under extensive management. Reasons for the increased susceptibility of meat breeds probably include their more favorable nutritional circumstances during pregnancy, different carcass and skeletal characteristics of both ewe and fetus and the effect of reduced natural selection against dystocia, resulting from intensive shepherding during lambing. Disproportion between the sizes of the fetus and that of the maternal birth canal, maldisposition of the fetus (involves deviation of the fetal axis and extremities from normal presentation, position or posture), uterine work load, i.e., the weight of fetal and placental tissues and fluids to be delivered, and uterine inertia, acting singly or in combination, are implicated in the pathogenesis. Maternofetal disproportion and maldisposition are the most prevalent causes. Maternal components of the disproportion include small pelvic inlet, failure of cervical ripening and dilatation ("ringwomb") and low distensibility of vaginal and vulval tissues. Large size of the usually single fetus is invariably the fetal component.

Small size of the pelvic inlet has been associated with a high prevalence of dystocia,[5, 7, 8] indicating a strong maternal influence. This is not invariably so, as dystocia, primarily of fetal origin, has been identified in one Merino strain because of a heritable postmaturity and resultant fetal oversize. Nutrition of young replacement breeding stock and genetic influences are likely determinants of mature pelvic size. Fetal size has a genetic as well as a nutritional basis. Within- and between-breed sire effects on birth weight have been demonstrated. The effects on birth weight of varying the level of nutrition in the last third of pregnancy have been extensively documented.

"Ringwomb" causes sporadic dystocia in mainly multiparous ewes showing otherwise normal parturition. The etiology is not understood. Because experiments suggest that one or more prostaglandins, probably in the presence of low progesterone-to-estrogen ratios, is necessary for normal cervical ripening,[4] pathogenesis is thought to involve hormonal imbalance or dysfunction. Treatment rests largely on cervicotomy or cesarean section, as prostaglandin therapy has been disappointing. The effect of uterine load on dystocia is reflected in the high positive correlation between the total weight of fetal and placental tissues and fluids expelled and the duration of second stage labor. The mean duration of second stage labor was significantly longer in multiple-bearing Merino ewes than in single-bearing ewes. To that extent, multiple-bearing ewes are often dystocic, causing increased fetal asphyxia. Dystocia characterized by uterine inertia and low distensibility of vaginal and vulval tissues is one manifestation of catastrophic reproductive failure caused by prolonged ingestion of estrogenic clover pastures in Australia. High mortality of ewes results from retention of fetuses.

Maldisposition is usually positively related to birth weight. Anterior presentation with flexion of the shoulder and flexion, or less frequently, extension, of the elbows is the most common maldisposition. Less prevalent maldispositions include anterior presentation with flexion of the neck and posterior presentation with flexion or extension of the hip joints and, to a lesser extent, flexion of the stifle and hock joints. The other permutations of presentation, position and posture occur sporadically. Mechanisms involved in maldisposition with anterior presentation include inability of the fetus because of lack of space to convert from a state of flexion during most of pregnancy to one of extension shortly before parturition, and impaction of the fetal chest and upper forelimbs in the pelvic inlet during second stage labor in cases of maternofetal disproportion. The reasons for posterior presentation are unknown. It is noteworthy that epidemics of arthrogryposis and hydranencephaly caused by fetal infection with Akabane virus are nearly always characterized by posterior presentation of the fetus.

TREATMENT

Obstetric intervention is facilitated by placing the ewe in a supine position with hindquarters raised in a special cradle, the placement of up to 0.5 liter of methyl cellulose obstetric gel (1.5 per cent) in the uterus with a large metal syringe prior to intervention, the use of a 10-cm gauze bandage as snares for the limbs and the use of blunt and sharp ovine obstetric hooks for traction on the eye socket or fetal trunk. The delivery of nearly all dystocias can be achieved by correction of maldisposition and standard obstetric procedures, including embryotomy. Anterior presentations with intrauterine retention of one forelimb can usually be delivered by judicious traction alone. The delivery of very large fetuses in normal anterior presentation can often be facilitated by repelling one forelimb back in the uterus and delivering the fetus as a head and one forelimb presentation. Retained forelimbs of a dead fetus, presenting only a large swollen head, are most easily retrieved by amputation of the head.

Episiotomy, cervicotomy and embryotomy greatly minimize the need for cesarean section in cases of "ringwomb" or low distensibility of vaginal and vulval tissues. Incision of the cervix, vagina or vulva enables the birth canal to be enlarged, at the same time giving some control over the site, direction and extent of tearing. For cervicotomy, grasp the partially dilated cervix dorsally, with two pairs of vulsellum forceps, one on either side of the midline, and draw it as far as possible towards the vulva. Slit the cervix in the dorsal midline with blunt scissors. For episiotomy of lowly distensible vaginal or vulval tissue, grasp the constricting tissues similarly and incise them dorsally with a scalpel. Careful traction on the fetal head and limbs will tear the birth canal to an appropriate size for delivery. Suturing of the torn tissues is optional. Aftercare includes prophylactic antibiotic therapy of the ewe and supportive nursing of ewe and any surviving progeny.

Dystocic ewes and their surviving progeny should be culled from purebred flocks because of the repeatable and heritable nature of rearing failure.

PREVENTION

Regular exercise of ewes in late pregnancy appears to reduce the prevalence of dystocia, as prevalence was 17 per cent in housed Dorset Horn ewes exercised on a treadmill for 20 minutes daily for 14 days prior to lambing compared with 50 per cent in their unexercised controls (JM George, personal communication, 1984). Because rearing failure, including dystocia, is repeatable and heritable, selection for rearing ability offers greatly improved prospects for reducing the prevalence of dystocia. A suitable selection program is outlined in the article Perinatal Lamb Mortality. Improved lamb survival, due in part to a reduction in the prevalence of dystocia, and less need for shepherding during lambing have been associated with the implementation of similar selection programs.[2, 3, 6, 9]

References

1. Alexander G: Maternal behaviour in the Merino ewe. Proc Aust Soc Anim Prod 3:105, 1960.
2. Atkins K: Selection for skin folds and fertility. Proc Aust Soc Anim Prod 13:176, 1980.
3. Donnelly FB: A practical attempt to breed for better lamb survival. Proc Aust Soc Anim Prod 14:30, 1982.
4. Fitzpatrick RJ, Dobson H: The cervix of the sheep and goat during parturition. Anim Reprod Sci 2:209, 1979.
5. Fogarty NM, Thompson JM: Relationship between pelvic dimensions, other body measurements and dystocia in Dorset Horn ewes. Aust Vet J 50:502, 1974.
6. McSporran KD, Buchanan R, Fielden ED: Observations on dystocia in a Romney flock. NZ Vet J 25:247, 1977.
7. McSporran KD, Fielden ED: Studies on dystocia in sheep. II. Pelvic measurements of ewes with dystocia and eutocia. NZ Vet J 27:75, 1979.
8. Quinlivan TD: Dystocia in sheep: Preliminary observations on within- and between-breed differences in various skeletal measurements. NZ Vet J 19:73, 1971.
9. Quinlivan TD: Cooperative ram breeding. Proceedings No. 58, Refresher Course on Sheep. Postgraduate Committee in Veterinary Science, University of Sydney, Australia, 1981, p 280.

Perinatal Lamb Mortality

K. G. Haughey, B.V.Sc., M.A.C.V.S.
The University of Sydney, Camden, New South Wales, Australia

Perinatal lamb mortality, defined as deaths occurring before, during or within 7 days of birth, is the major known source of wastage to the sheep industry. In Australia and New Zealand, for example, the respective losses average 25 per cent and 15 per cent of lambs born, rising to as high as 45 per cent in individual grazing breeding flocks. Nearly all deaths occur during or within 3 days of birth. The majority of losses result from repeated rearing failure by a minority of ewes. Losses vary greatly within and between flocks, districts and seasons.

ESTIMATION OF PERINATAL LOSS

Perinatal loss may be estimated directly or indirectly. Direct estimation involves counting the number of lambs born and expressing those dying as a percentage of the total born. This method is practical only in closely shepherded lambing flocks in areas free from predators and scavengers. Indirect estimation involves "wet-drying" the breeding flock after lambing, i.e., the identification and removal of all ewes not rearing a lamb or lambs. "Wet-drying" can be carried out any time up to weaning but is more reliable when undertaken within a few weeks of lambing, usually at the time of lamb marking. It is the most practical technique for estimating losses in large flocks that are not intensively shepherded during lambing. The flock is classified into dry (not lambed) ewes and lambed ewes. This latter group can be subdivided into those rearing a lamb, or lambs, and those losing all lambs.

The classification is based on the following: body condition and fleece quality of the ewe, presence of "lambing stain," i.e., contamination of the posterior surface of the udder and hocks with the discharges resulting from lambing, udder development and the nature of udder secretions. Dry ewes have neither udder development nor "lambing stain" and usually show better body condition and fleeces than lambed ewes. Lambed ewes have enlarged udders, usually show "lambing stain" and have poorer fleeces and body condition than dry ewes. Ewes rearing lambs have full, resilient udders containing milk. The teats and adjacent areas are clean, soft and pliable as a result of the lamb's sucking activity. Ewes that have lost all lambs have variably developed udders with a tendency for cleavage between the two glands. The teats are stiff and dirty, with udder secretions ranging from normal to thin, watery or honey-colored viscous material. The perinatal mortality rate is defined as the number of ewes losing all progeny, expressed as a percentage of the total number of ewes lambing. The estimate represents minimal loss because it does not take into account the extent of cross-mothering or situations in which one or both twins die. However, because about 90 per cent of mortality occurs during or within 3 days of parturition, the estimate is a reliable reflection of minimal perinatal lamb mortality. The minimal incidence of multiple births is expressed as the percentage of lambs marked over ewes lambing.

INVESTIGATION OF PERINATAL MORTALITY

Necropsy, supported by appropriate microbiologic and histopathologic examinations, is the simplest and most reliable method of determining causes of loss. The method is deficient in that it does not identify cases of neonatal starvation caused by aberrant maternal or neonatal behavior. An adequate sample (arbitrarily 50 carcasses that are representative of mortality throughout lambing) must be examined to arrive at a realistic assessment of the relative contributions that various entities make to total mortality. Table 1 lists the minimum number of carcasses required to detect a specific entity in at least one carcass with 95 per cent confidence, given a designated theoretical prevalence in the flock.

Table 1. Sample Size Required To Detect a Specific Pathologic Entity in at Least One Carcass Given a Specified Flock Prevalence*

	Flock Prevalence (%)																		
	5	10	15	20	25	30	35	40	45	50	55	60	65	70	75	80	85	90	95
Number of Carcasses To Be Examined	58	28	18	13	10	8	7	6	5	4	4	3	3	2	2	2	2	1	1

*$p = 0.95$

Fetal membranes should be collected with dead lambs when possible because they are invaluable in the diagnosis of congenital infections. A knowledge of weather conditions during the previous 24 hours (e.g., hot, warm or cold; wet or dry; calm or windy) and a determination of the dead weight of lambs allow more reliable interpretation of necropsy findings. Dead weight often represents birth weight or is a reflection of birth weight of lambs dying within a few days of birth. High proportions of small lambs (< 3 kg) succumb during cold or hot weather because of their relatively greater surface area, whereas large lambs (> 4.5 kg) are more prone to dystocia. Birth weight is influenced by single or multiple births, nutrition during late pregnancy and genetic factors.

A full necropsy, including examination of the central nervous system (CNS), is carried out using a systematic technique.[6] Using this method, which classifies the time that lambs die relative to birth, the following groups can be recognized:

1. Anteparturient deaths—dying before the commencement of birth.

2. Parturient deaths—dying during birth or within a few hours of birth.

3. Postparturient deaths—dying more than a few hours after birth.

Anteparturient deaths usually constitute an insignificant proportion (< 2 per cent) of losses, leaving parturient and postparturient deaths to account variably for 25 to 75 per cent of losses, depending on the flock, district and season. The classification is a valuable diagnostic aid, as specific entities are more likely to occur in specific time-of-death categories (Table 2).

GENERAL NATURE OF PERINATAL MORTALITY

Perinatal lamb mortality results from a variety of environmental and intrinsic maternal and fetal causes operating singly or together. In the past the importance of maternal and fetal factors has probably been underestimated. Rearing ability in a number of sheep breeds is now reported to have low levels of repeatability and heritability, variously estimated in the range of 0.1 to 0.2,[13] suggesting that significant improvement in lamb survival of current and subsequent generations may result from selection for rearing ability.

Table 2 summarizes the occurrence of common causes of perinatal loss among Australian and New Zealand grazing flocks relative to time-of-death classification. Usually, less than 20 per cent of losses are accounted for by lethal congenital malformations, deficiencies of essential trace elements, infections acquired during pregnancy and after birth and predation. Because these are mainly environmental influences they tend to occur randomly.

The majority of deaths fall into two categories:

1. Those animals dying during or shortly after (and presumably because of) birth, showing evidence of birth stress at necropsy.

2. Those animals constituting the starvation-mismothering-exposure (SME) complex, characterized by death 1 to 2 days after birth, evidence of starvation, severe depletion of brown fat reserves and other lesions of hypothermia at necropsy.

Nutritional Considerations

Nutrition during pregnancy exerts a powerful influence on birth weight and indirectly on lamb

Table 2. Cause of Death in Relation to Time of Death Relative to Birth

Cause of Death	Time of Death		
	Before	During	After
Incidence (%)	<2	75–25	25–75
Lethal congenital malformations	+	+	+
Congenital nutritional deficiencies	+	+	+
Congenital infections	+	+	+
Birth injury	−	+	+
Infections acquired after birth	−	−	+
Predation	−	−	+
Starvation			
Mismothering	−	−	+
Exposure			
Miscellaneous	−	−	+

survival.[12] This results from the combined effects of the amount of substrate available for placental growth during early pregnancy and for fetal growth during late pregnancy. Good feeding of single-bearing ewes in late pregnancy results in large lambs predisposed to dystocia.

Even moderate underfeeding of multiple-bearing ewes restricts placental and fetal growth, resulting in undersized lambs, particularly vulnerable to fatal hypothermia early in neonatal life. Underfeeding during pregnancy also depresses the level of milk production and may delay its onset. Placental weight accounts for most of the variance in birth weight, and nutrition of the ewe during the second and third month of pregnancy is one of the major determinants of placental weight. This suggests that improved nutrition in the second and third months should achieve improvement in placental growth in multiple-bearing ewes. The reliable detection of multiple pregnancies as early as 40 days after conception by ultrasonic imaging[5] should facilitate their improved nutritional management.

THE DIAGNOSIS AND CONTROL OF COMMON CAUSES OF PERINATAL MORTALITY

The complex nature of perinatal mortality is often manifest by carcasses showing lesions having more than one origin. The following are some of the commonly seen lesions.

Birth Injury to the Fetal Central Nervous System[6, 10]

A variety of subdural, subarachnoid and extra-dural hemorrhages at single or multiple sites in and around the cranial and spinal meninges are the most common lesions found at necropsy of parturient and postparturient deaths. Male and female and single and twin lambs are affected, and the lesions occur independently of assistance during delivery. In our investigations prevalence ranged from 56 to 86 per cent of deaths in individual flocks. The lesions were exclusive to lambs dying during or shortly after birth and to those classified as having the SME complex. Meningeal hemorrhage is present in virtually all parturient deaths and is often accompanied by other manifestations of trauma and asphyxia during birth. These include subcutaneous edema of the presenting portion of the fetus; abdominal hemorrhage caused by rupture of the liver or tearing of the liver capsule; subepicardial, subendocardial, subpleural and subcapsular thymic petechiae and ecchymoses. In those classified as having the SME complex prevalence ranged from 30 to 55 per cent, accompanied almost invariably by evidence of cold injury and starvation.

Meningeal hemorrhage has been interpreted as a manifestation of injury to basic neural elements of the fetal CNS, resulting from trauma and hypoxia during birth. Experimentally, the prevalence of meningeal hemorrhage rises with increasing levels of stressful birth. The variables implicated in pathogenesis include duration of second stage labor, vigor of tenesmus, fetopelvic proportions and fetal blood gas status. Severe injury causes death during or immediately after birth, whereas less severe injury, by markedly impairing sucking activity, leads to rapid exhaustion of fetal energy reserves and death within 1 to 2 days of birth from secondary hypothermia when ambient temperatures are less than thermoneutral or to dehydration and heat exhaustion when temperatures are hot ($> 28°C$).

Control. Predisposition to dystocia and birth injury is genetically based, as descendants of ewes with high lifetime rearing efficiency sustained fewer losses from dystocia and birth injury than descendants of ewes with low lifetime rearing efficiency.[8] See the section Selection for Improved Lamb Survival.

Hypothermia and the SME complex

The SME complex has a multiple etiology and may account for up to 65 per cent of perinatal losses in grazing flocks. At temperatures less than 28°C in "still" air and at higher temperatures during wet windy weather the newborn lamb maintains body temperature by shivering, catabolism of brown fat and peripheral vasoconstriction. Fatal hypothermia, which may be primary or secondary, occurs when heat loss exceeds heat production for more than a few hours. Primary hypothermia occurs during severely cold, wet, windy weather because heat loss outstrips heat production even in the presence of adequate energy reserves. Secondary hypothermia occurs during moderately cold, usually dry weather because of factors that prevent the lamb from feeding and replenishing depleted fetal energy reserves or that impair its thermogenic ability. Lambs less than 3 kg are particularly vulnerable to hypothermia because of immaturity, low fetal energy reserves and a wide surface area-to-body mass ratio, allowing more heat loss compared with heavier lambs. Heat loss is modified also by ambient temperature, wind velocity, thickness and dampness of the birth coat and genetically determined susceptibility to cold.[14] Heat production is modified by pre- and intrapartum hypoxia due to placental insufficiency or stressful birth[3] and by any postpartum factor that precludes replenishment of depleted energy reserves, including aberrant maternal and neonatal behavior,[15] hypothermia,[2] agalactia or abnormalities of the teats and udder.

The lesions of hypothermia include catabolism of brown fat, subcutaneous edema of the distal limbs and adrenocortical changes.[7] Brown fat at perirenal, pericardial and other sites is pinkish white at birth or in newborn lambs exposed to temperatures greater than 28°C. Below thermoneutral temperatures, brown fat depots are important sites of non-shivering thermogenesis. Fat depletion occurs during exposure to cold and independently of starvation. In the process the fat depots change to a red-brown color, the extent and duration of the rise in metabolism modifying the degree of color change. Varying degrees of yellow subcutaneous edema (up to 5 mm thick) invariably occur in the distal hind limbs and often at the base of the tail and the distal forelimbs. Changes in the adrenal cortex, including hypertrophy and focal hemorrhage, result from severe systemic stress. All these lesions occur to greater or lesser degrees in newborn lambs exposed to cold. They are more marked in lambs that died as a result of exposure to cold.

Treatment. Hypothermic lambs can be resuscitated by correcting hypoglycemia with an intraperitoneal injection of 20 per cent solution of glucose (10 ml/kg) and by rewarming them in air at 40°C in an enclosed chamber with a 3 kw domestic electric fan heater until the rectal temperature is 38°C.[4] Subsequent attention to nutrition, including administration of colostrum, and husbandry are critical to high rates of resuscitation.

Prevention. Losses from hypothermia can be reduced by adequate feeding during pregnancy to prevent small fetuses, provision of shelter for lambing ewes and selection to reduce the prevalence of heritable traits predisposing animals to hypothermia, notably susceptibility to cold, birth injury to the fetal CNS and probably aberrant maternal behavior. The expense usually precludes housing of lambing ewes. Prelamb shearing of grazing ewes, not more than one month prior to lambing, thereby inducing them to seek and lamb in natural or specially prepared, cheap, low-level shelter, has shown promising results.[1]

Hyperthermia

Lambs born in hot, semiarid environments, particularly if they are small, often die from hyperthermia and dehydration. Their necropsy is characterized by severe dehydration, an empty alimentary tract, no color change of fat depots and intense leptomeningeal congestion. Dehydration is often caused or exacerbated by depressed sucking activity due to the same factors contributing to secondary hypothermia.

Predation

Although primary predation is a constant source of low-level loss under the extensive grazing conditions experienced in Australia, in isolated instances losses may be heavy. However, predation by wild animals and occasionally by birds may be overrated as a cause of lamb loss because lambs of low viability killed before death (secondary predation) and carcasses mutilated post-mortem are included in the estimate. Death can be attributed to primary predation only when the carcass shows extensive and severe ante-mortem trauma and no other gross lesions. Fat depots will not be catabolized, and there will be evidence of milk absorption when the lamb has sucked. A substantial portion of the carcass should be skinned, as not only are external appearances misleading regarding the degree of mutilation, but the nature of the mutilation may also indicate the predator species involved.

Lethal Congenital Malformations

Lethal congenital malformations usually constitute about 1 per cent of losses. (See the article Congenital and Inherited Defects in Sheep.)

Deficiency of Essential Trace Elements

Swayback, cardiac myopathy and goiter, associated respectively with dietary deficiency of copper, selenium and iodine, occur congenitally and are usually endemic to certain districts where sporadic outbreaks may cause heavy losses. Dietary supplementation by top-dressing pasture or by parenteral administration of slow-release intraruminal devices effectively controls these mineral deficiencies (see the article Feeding Sheep for High Reproductive Performance).

Infections

Infections occur widely at low prevalence in Australia and New Zealand, occasionally causing heavy losses. (For a discussion of congenital infections see the article Infectious Ovine Abortion.)

A wide variety of bacterial infections have been associated with perinatal lamb loss.[11] The prevalence rises with high-grazing pressures and intensive husbandry systems such as shed-lambing. Most bacterial infections are acquired at or soon after birth, although their pathologic manifestations may extend beyond the defined perinatal period.

Common pathogens include the following:

1. *Clostridium septicum, C. chauvoei* and *C. novyi,* manifested by gangrene around the umbilical stump and localized or generalized serofibrinous peritonitis.

2. *Pasteurella haemolytica* causes localized or generalized serofibrinous peritonitis often accompanied by pneumonia.

3. Infection by *Staphylococcus aureus, Streptococcus* sp., *Corynebacterium* sp., *Fusobacterium necrophorum* and *Haemophilus somnus* are manifested by pyemia with multiple purulent foci in the liver, kidneys, heart, lungs, muscles and joints.

4. *Escherichia coli* causes a variety of syndromes characterized by enteritis, polysynovitis, septicemia or leptomeningitis.

5. *Erysipelothrix insidiosa* and *Chlamydia* sp. infections are manifested by polysynovitis.

Diagnosis is confirmed by microbiologic and histopathologic examinations of appropriate specimens or whole carcasses. Annual vaccination of ewes within 3 to 4 weeks of lambing effectively controls losses due to *Clostridium* sp. by providing the lamb with a colostral immunity.

Table 3. Program for Improving Lamb Survival by Selection for Rearing Ability

Rearing Performance at Lamb-Marking	Lambing Year				
	1	**2**	**3**	**4**	**5**
Dry (not lambed)	retain	cull	cull	cull	cull
Lambed, failed to rear	cull	cull	cull	cull	cull
Lambed, rearing at least one lamb	retain	retain	retain	retain	retain

SELECTION FOR IMPROVED LAMB SURVIVAL

Table 3 summarizes a selection program used increasingly in New Zealand and Australia for successfully improving lamb survival in grazing flocks. The program recognizes maternal and fetal defects contributing to the pathogenesis of perinatal loss, the repeatable and heritable nature of rearing ability and the fact that rearing performance at maiden lambing is indicative of subsequent performance.[9] The program also aims at developing flocks that require minimal care during lambing.

The program should begin with maiden ewe replacements so as to spread the cost of heavy culling over 4 to 5 years. Maiden ewes failing to rear their lambs should be culled, identifying them at lamb marking by the "wet-dry" technique. Maiden ewes losing their lambs have about an equal chance of failing to rear at least twice in a 4-year breeding life. That age group should similarly be culled in subsequent years. Do not assist dystocias except to salvage and cull ewes so affected; retention of such ewes and their progeny facilitates the perpetuation of genes for poor rearing ability. Mate the elite ewes to rams born of ewes with impeccable rearing ability. In New Zealand and Australia cooperative ram breeding schemes and progressive studs are making such rams increasingly available. Because small maternal pelvic size has been associated with repeated rearing failure in a number of breeds (see the article Dystocia), ensure good nutrition of young female stock to 2½ years of age, at which time the pelvic centers of ossification close. The potential for increasing rearing efficiency by selection can only be realized by adopting appropriate husbandry and disease control measures, excluding obstetric assistance to live dystocic births. The cost of the heavy culling required initially can also be offset by retaining dry (not lambed) maiden ewes for another year, as most lamb consistently in subsequent years, and their rearing ability can be extremely high.[9]

After 4 to 5 years, all ewes in the flock, except replacements, will always have reared at least one lamb, making for minimal care at lambing. Flock owners culling ruthlessly for rearing failure report significant improvement in lamb survival in the medium term.

CONCLUSIONS AND SUMMARY

Perinatal lamb mortality has a complex etiology involving the action and interaction of many causes, including weather conditions, genetic factors, deficiency of gross and specific nutrients during pregnancy and after birth, predators, infections, aberrant maternal and neonatal behavior and birth injury to the fetal CNS. Necropsy, accompanied by examination of specimens in the laboratory, will identify most of the causes of death. Until recently, measures aimed at increased lamb survival have concentrated on improving nutrition during pregnancy, the provision of shelter and supervision of lambing ewes and disease control. These measures are often labor-intensive and costly, and the results are frequently disappointing. The major role of maternal and fetal factors, indicated by the repeatable and heritable nature of rearing ability, on perinatal mortality has now been recognized.

Lamb survival to weaning has to be seen mainly in the perspective of a compatible partnership between mother and offspring throughout pregnancy, parturition and lactation. "Wet-drying" at lamb-marking is a critical test of the success of that partnership. Selection for rearing ability, backed by appropriate nutrition, disease control and husbandry, offers greatly improved prospects for increasing lamb survival. In addition, these measures develop flocks requiring minimal supervision during lambing.

References

1. Alexander G, Lynch JJ, Mottershead BE, Donnelly JB: Reduction in lamb mortality by means of grass wind-breaks. Proc Aust Soc Anim Prod 13:329, 1980.
2. Alexander G, Williams D: Teat-seeking activity in newborn lambs: The effects of cold. J Agric Sci Camb 67:181, 1966.
3. Eales FA, Gilmour JS, Barlow RM, Small J: Causes of hypothermia in 89 lambs. Vet Rec 110:118, 1982.
4. Eales FA, Small J, Gilmour JS: Resuscitation of hypothermic lambs. Vet Rec 110:121, 1982.
5. Fowler DG, Wilkins JF: The identification of single and multiple bearing ewes by ultrasonic imaging. Proc Aust Soc Anim Prod 14:492, 1982.
6. Haughey KG: Vascular abnormalities in the central nervous system associated with perinatal mortality. 1. Pathology. Aust Vet J 49:1, 1973.
7. Haughey KG: Cold injury in newborn lambs. Aust Vet J 49:555, 1973.
8. Haughey KG: Selective breeding for rearing ability as an aid to improving lamb survival. Aust Vet J 60:361, 1983.
9. Haughey KG, George JM: Lifetime rearing performance of Merino ewes and its relationship with pelvic size and early rearing status. Proc Aust Soc Anim Prod 14:26, 1982.
10. Haughey KG: New insights into rearing failure and perinatal mortality. Proceedings No. 67, Refresher Course, Sheep Production and Preventive Medicine. Post-Graduate Committee in Veterinary Science, University of Sydney, Australia, 1983, p 135.

11. Hughes KL, Haughey KG, Hartley WJ: Perinatal lamb mortality: Infections occurring among lambs dying after parturition. Aust Vet J 47:472, 1971.
12. Mellor DJ: Nutritional and placental determinants of foetal growth rate in sheep and consequences for the newborn lamb. Br Vet J 139:307, 1983.
13. Piper LR, Hanrahan JP, Evans R, Bindon BM: Genetic variation in individual and maternal components of lamb survival in Merinos. Proc Aust Soc Anim Prod 14:29, 1982.
14. Slee J: A review of genetic aspects of survival and resistance to cold in newborn lambs. Livest Prod Sci 8:419, 1981.
15. Stevens D, Alexander G, Lynch JJ: Lamb mortality due to inadequate care of twins by Merino ewes. Appl Anim Ethol 8:243, 1982.

Congenital and Inherited Defects in Sheep

Stanley M. Dennis, B.V.Sc., Ph.D., F.R.C.V.S., F.R.S.Path.
Horst W. Leipold, Ph.D., D.V.M.
Kansas State University, Manhattan, Kansas

A variety of structural and functional defects have been described in lambs.[2, 4, 5, 8–10] Sheep have the highest incidence of craniofacial defects in mammals, including man. Defective development may be manifested by embryonic mortality, fetal death, abortion, premature birth, full-term stillbirth, non-viable or viable neonates and dysmaturity. Defects are usually obvious at birth, but detection depends on the nature and extent of the defect. Only under unusual circumstances, such as a defect occurring repeatedly in the same flock or geographic area, is a defective lamb likely to come to the attention of veterinarians or scientists.[2, 7] Thus, most defective lambs go unrecorded. Only recently has there been a perceptible change in attitude toward the importance of congenital defects or diseases in sheep.[11]

NATURE OF CONGENITAL DEFECTS

Congenital defects may affect a single structure or function, involve several body systems or combine structural and functional alterations. Defects may be lethal, semilethal or compatible with life.

A defective lamb is an adapted survivor from a disruptive event at one or more stages in the complexly integrated process of embryonic or fetal development. Before attachment, the zygote is resistant to teratogens but susceptible to genetic mutations and chromosomal aberrations. During the embryonic period the embryo is highly susceptible to teratogens, but this decreases with age as the critical developmental periods of various organs are passed. Except for later-differentiating structures such as the cerebellum, palate and urogenital system, the fetus becomes increasingly resistant to teratogenic agents as it ages. The estimated ovine embryonic mortality of 20 per cent suggests unidentified lethal genes or chromosomal aberrations may be active during this critical period.[3]

FREQUENCY

The frequency of congenital defects in sheep is difficult to assess. Because they are caused by genetic and environmental factors, the frequency of individual defects varies with breed, breeding practices, location, year, level of nutrition, sex, parental age and other environmental factors. Based on studies in Australia, New Zealand and the United States, the incidence ranges from 0.2 to 2.0 per cent of all lambs born.[8]

Body systems principally involved in a large number of defective lambs studied at necropsy included musculoskeletal, 55.4 per cent; digestive, 12.7 per cent; cardiovascular, 9.7 per cent; urogenital, 8.0 per cent; central nervous, 6.0 per cent; special senses, 3.5 per cent; integument, 3.2 per cent and endocrine, 1.5 per cent. As determined by necropsy and survey findings in a large sheep population, the common congenital defects were (in alphabetical order) agnathia, arthrogryposis, atresia ani, bowed forelegs, brachygnathia, cleft palate, conjoined twinning, cryptorchidism, entropion, hernia, hypospadias, interventricular septal defect, limb defects, microtia, partially bifurcated scrotum, perosomus elumbis, polythelia, prognathia, tail defects and torticollis.[4, 5]

EPIZOOTIOLOGY

Congenital defects in sheep are probably more common than reports indicate. Many defective lambs are not observed because of common ovine husbandry practices, and of those defective lambs observed, many are not reported unless the number is high.[7] This means that many sporadic cases, which would include many genetic defects, are not reported. Unless the rancher routinely examines newborn dead lambs, most defects (i.e., semi- or non-lethal ones) will be observed during castration or other procedures, and most lethal defects will be unrecognized.

CAUSE

Congenital defects are caused by genetic or environmental factors or by their interaction. Some

Table 1. Ovine Defects Reported To Be Inherited

Defect	Mode of Transmission
Agnathia	Recessive
Alopecia	Recessive
Ancon dwarf sheep	Recessive
Anotia	Incomplete dominant
Atresia ani	Recessive
Arthrogryposis	Recessive
Blindness (microphthalmia to anophthalmia)	Recessive
Cataracts	Dominant
Cerebellar ataxia	Recessive
Collagen dysplasia	Recessive
Cryptorchidism	Recessive
Dwarfism	Recessive
Earless and cleft palate	Recessive
Goiter	Recessive
Hyperbilirubinemia	Recessive
Inguinal hernia	Recessive
Lethal gray	Incomplete dominant
Luster mutant	Dominant
Mammary hypoplasia	Dominant
Muscular dystrophy	Recessive
Neuroaxonal dystrophy	Recessive
Paralysis	Recessive
Photosensitivity	Recessive
Polythelia	Dominant
Rigid fetlocks	Recessive
Short ears	Recessive
"Wattles"	Dominant
Yellow fat	Recessive

defects are inherited, others are suspected to be, but the heritability of the majority is unknown (Tables 1 and 2).

Genetic defects are caused by mutant genes or chromosomal aberrations. Most known genetic defects in sheep are autosomal recessives that occur in any environment (Table 1). Except for chromosomal aberrations, genetic defects occur in intra- and intergenerational patterns. Several chromosomal aberrations have now been reported in sheep.[3]

All genetic defects have their counterpart in environmentally induced phenocopies. The problem is to recognize which defects are genetic and which are environmental; this may be difficult in sheep.

Teratogenic factors are difficult to identify but often follow seasonal patterns, known stressful conditions, medication and maternal disease. They do not follow a familial pattern, as do genetic causes. Only a few environmental factors have been incriminated as being teratogenic for sheep (Table 3). Border disease has been reported in Europe, Australia, New Zealand and the United States and is emerging as a serious cause of ovine reproductive failure.[1]

DIAGNOSIS

When a defective lamb is born, determining whether the cause is genetic or environmental is the problem. This is difficult because the etiologic agent exerted its effects approximately 4 months before the defect is recognized. Even with several defective lambs, it is not easy to eliminate the possibility of disease, teratogenic plants, drugs or nutritional deficiencies. When affected ewes are restricted to a single flock or area, environmental factors are usually investigated first. Spontaneous epizootics of congenital defects are unlikely to be genetically induced.

Factors hindering diagnosis of congenital defects in sheep include defects not being reported, inadequate history, inadequate records and lack of interest in teratology by some veterinarians and diagnosticians.[7]

History. A detailed history is necessary for diagnosing congenital defects and should include breed, geographic region, season, type of pasture and soil, exposure or suspected exposure to teratogenic plants or viruses or drugs, feeding and management practices, breeding records, health history of the flock, drugs used (routine or new) and congenital defects previously observed.

Diagnosing Genetic Defects. The basis for diagnosing genetic defects is the fact that they tend to run in families. Mutant genes become evident over two or more generations by one of four major breeding patterns: dominant, incompletely dominant, recessive and overdominant. The patterns involve certain characteristic ratios of normal to defective progeny that form the basis for genetic diagnosis. Several factors prevent accurate diagnosis of hereditary patterns and ratios in sheep: rarity of particular defects, phenocopies, wide genetic diversity, inadequate breeding records and nonreporting or reporting only extreme cases. It is nearly impossible to have enough cases of many ovine defects to identify the hereditary pattern; the pattern must be

Table 2. Ovine Congenital Defects Suspected To Be Hereditary

Adactyly
Anury
Brachygnathia
Cerebellar atrophy
Cyclopia
Epitheliogenesis imperfecta
Entropion
Hernia
Holoacardius acephalus
Hypotrichosis
Limb defects
Micrencephaly
Osteogenesis imperfecta
Palatoschisis
Partially bifurcated scrotum
Perosomus elumbis
Persistent umbilical hemorrhage
Prolonged gestation
Pseudohermaphroditism
Syndactyly
Testicular hypoplasia
Ventricular septal defect

Table 3. Agents Reported To Be Teratogenic for Sheep

Teratogenic Agent	Major Body System Affected
Viruses	
Akabane	CNS
Blue tongue	CNS
Border disease	CNS
Bovine virus diarrhea	CNS
Plants	
Veratrum californicum	CNS and skeletal
Astragalus sp.	Skeletal
Blue lupins	Skeletal
Oxytropis sp.	Skeletal
Swainsonia sp.	CNS
Trachymene sp.	Skeletal
Goitrogenic plants	Endocrine
Drugs	
Parbendazole	Skeletal
Aminopterin	Skeletal
Nutritional	
Iodine deficiency	Goiter
Copper deficiency	CNS and skeletal
Selenium deficiency	Muscular
Physical	
Hyperthermia	CNS and skeletal
Irradiation	Skeletal

(CNS = central nervous system)

repeated several times before it can be clearly identified. Genetic defects are differentiated from nongenetic defects by identifying supporting or contradictory evidence of a characteristic hereditary pattern or by establishing one or more nonhereditary patterns. Diagnosing a defect in a single lamb as genetically induced is impossible.

Most known genetic defects in sheep are caused by recessive genes. They are usually characterized by a small number of defective lambs from normal-appearing parents. Recessive genes are insidiously perpetuated from generation to generation by normal carriers or heterozygotes.

Test mating of sheep to confirm genetic defects is impractical in commercial flocks. It is simpler to detect recessive defects by having all defective lambs reported.

Recommended Diagnostic Procedures. The following procedures are recommended for diagnosing congenital defects in sheep: encourage reporting of defects; record all defective lambs; obtain an adequate history; perform a detailed necropsy; collect serums from affected and in-contact ewes and live defective lambs for viral serologic examination; check for possible exposure to teratogens, especially during mating and early pregnancy and examine chromosomes of live defective lambs and analyze records for genetic cause.[7]

PREVENTION

Determining whether the defect is genetically or environmentally induced is important, as proper identification indicates which control measures are applicable. It is essential to recognize inherited defects early to control their insidious spread. The difficulty of identifying normal carriers makes control of recessive defects virtually impossible.

To minimize the effects of congenital defects in sheep, the following measures are recommended:

1. If possible, establish an accurate diagnosis.

2. If not possible, regard all congenital defects as genetic until proved otherwise.

3. Do not breed defective sheep.

4. Eliminate defective lambs to keep the incidence of recessive defects low.

5. Seek help from the regional diagnostic laboratory.

6. Encourage ranchers to report all defective lambs.

7. If the defect is environmentally induced, adjust the management program.

8. Report all defective lambs, as they serve as biomedical indicators of environmental hazards that may have public health significance.

9. Finally, develop an interest in teratology.

References

1. Barlow RM, Patterson DS: Border disease of sheep: A virus-induced teratogenic disorder. Berlin, Paul Parey, 1982, pp 1–80.
2. Binns W, Keeler RF, Balls LD: Congenital deformities in lambs, calves and goats resulting from maternal ingestion of *Veratrum californicum:* Harelip, cleft palate, ataxia, and hypoplasia of metacarpal and metatarsal bones. *Clin Toxicol* 5:245, 1972.
3. Bruere AN: Application of cytogenetics to domestic animals. In Grunsell CSG, Hill FWG (eds): Veterinary Annual 20:29, 1980.
4. Dennis SM: A survey of congenital defects of sheep. Vet Rec 95:488, 1974.
5. Dennis SM: Perinatal lamb mortality in Western Australia. 7. Congenital defects. Aust Vet J 51:80, 1975.
6. Dennis SM, Leipold HW: Agnathia in sheep. External observations. Am J Vet Res 33:339, 1972.
7. Dennis SM, Leipold HW: Diagnosing congenital defects in sheep. Zuchthygiene, March 1976.
8. Dennis SM, Leipold HW: Ovine congenital defects. Vet Bull 49:233, 1979.
9. Ercanbrack SK, Price DA: Frequencies of various birth defects of Rambouillet sheep. J Hered 62:223, 1971.
10. Hughes KL, Haughey KG, Hartley WJ: Spontaneous congenital developmental abnormalities observed at necropsy in a large survey of newly born dead lambs. Teratology 5:5, 1972.
11. Pearson H: Changing attitudes to congenital and inherited diseases. Vet Rec 105:318, 1979.

Development of the Male Reproductive Tract, Spermatogenesis and Puberty

K. R. Lapwood, B.V.Sc., Ph.D.
Massey University, Palmerston North, New Zealand

EMBRYOLOGICAL DEVELOPMENT OF THE REPRODUCTIVE ORGANS

Gonadal Development. As in other species, the testes of rams are derived from undifferentiated gonads on the ventromedial surfaces of the embryonic urogenital ridges. The undifferentiated gonad is covered by two or three layers of epithelial cells from which groups or strands of epithelial cells extend into the underlying mesenchyme. Primordial germ cells, presumably derived from yolk sac endoderm, are present in sheep gonads as early as day 29 after conception. Histologic evidence of the differentiation of gonads to testes first becomes apparent at 34 to 35 days with the appearance of the tunica albuginea. By day 42 of development, testis cords containing gonocytes and indifferent or supporting cells are formed, while interstitial cells are prominent between the cords. At this stage the gonocytes are centrally located within the testis cords and are surrounded by indifferent cells.

Subsequent development of the sex cords involves a gradual increase in their diameter as a result of mitosis of both indifferent cells and gonocytes and an increase in the amount of indifferent cell cytoplasm. The indifferent cells have poorly defined cell membranes and tonguelike processes that extend into the center of the sex cords. While the sex cords enlarge, the interstitial cells increase in number and develop eosinophilic cytoplasmic granules; such granules are present in most interstitial cells by day 70 of fetal life.

Testicular descent into the scrotal pouches occurs as a result of traction exerted by the gubernaculum, which shortens slightly while the surrounding structures undergo substantial elongation. In rams testicular descent is completed by day 80 of fetal life.

Reproductive Tract Development. Detailed analyses of the course of embryologic development of the reproductive tract and accessory sex glands of rams do not appear to have been published. However, it is assumed that this course of development is unremarkable compared with development in other domestic species. One of the few points worthy of note is that the degree of ventral and anterior migration of the scrotum is extreme.

Regulation of Sexual Differentiation. Differentiation of the indifferent gonads and differential development of male, rather than female, reproductive tract primordia occur as a result of secretion of testosterone and androstenedione by the fetal gonads. In rams these two androgens can be detected in the testes from day 30 of fetal life, and probably it is their secretion before day 40 of fetal life that determines sexual differentiation. In the absence of fetal androgen, potentially female structures such as the müllerian ducts develop, rather than male precursors such as the wolffian ducts. Fetal gonadal androgen secretion up to 40 to 60 days after conception also determines the sexual differentiation of adult sexual behavioral patterns and the sexual dimorphism of hypothalamic secretion. Androgen exposure at this critical stage abolishes the female-type cyclic control potential of the preoptic hypothalamic area so that male-type tonic control influences from the mediobasal hypothalamus become dominant. Fetal testicular androgen secretion reaches peak levels at about day 70 and then falls with the approach of parturition.

SPERMATOGENESIS

The Immature Testis. At birth, the testicular sex cords contain peripherally situated supporting cells and centrally placed gonocytes. Fibrous connective tissue located between the sex cords contains blood vessels and interstitial cells arranged in clumps or cords or singly. Prior to puberty only minor changes occur. Both gonocytes and supporting cells continue to multiply, and the gonocytes are transformed into prospermatogonia. During this transformation the number of nucleoli is reduced from two to four original nucleoli to one nucleolus, and nuclear dimensions increase. At the same time there is a reduction in the proportion of interstitial cells containing eosinophilic granules.

Pubertal Changes. Pubertal development of ram testicular germinal elements follows a uniform pattern despite slight breed differences in the ages and body weights at which particular changes are observed. Data from Ile-de-France rams indicate that when the testis weighs 6 gm, prospermatogonia move to the basement membrane, transform into type A spermatogonia and then start multiplying rapidly. Primary spermatocytes are first seen in 12-gm testes (about 105 days of age), spermatids in 30-gm testes (120 to 125 days) and spermatozoa in 65-gm testes (140 to 150 days); full adult testicular weight is about 200 gm. At the same time as the gametogenic elements develop, the supporting cells transform into Sertoli cells. This transformation occurs just before the first appearance of spermatids and involves an increase in nuclear size as well as the extension of cytoplasmic processes between the germinal cells so as to provide points of attachment for spermatids. Seminiferous tubule lumen formation also occurs at about this time. During pubertal development the size of groups of interstitial cells is reduced.

Testicular growth curves are sigmoid in shape, growth being slow in the first 2 to 3 months after birth. It then becomes rapid between 2 to 3 and 5 months when spermatogenesis is being established, then subsequently slows. In fact, the time at which rapid testicular growth commences is better correlated with body weight than with age. Typically, prospermatogonia appear at a body weight of 15 kg, type A spermatogonia appear at 21 kg and all spermatogenic cell types are present at 27 kg. However, there are breed differences in the exact body weight at which each stage commences.

Maximal efficiency of spermatogenesis does not occur until several months after the first appearance of spermatozoa. This is partly due to the variability in the onset of spermatogenesis within the seminiferous tubules and partly due to an initial high rate of degeneration of spermatogenic cells. In rams this degeneration mostly affects intermediate spermatogonia and decreases with age. Adult spermatogenic production is not reached until testis weight is about 100 gm.

Spermatogenesis in Adult Rams. A detailed description of the histologic course of spermatogenesis in the ram is beyond the scope of this article.

Using nuclear staining methods such as the Feulgen-hematoxylin technique, it has been shown that the spermatogenic cycle of the ram's seminiferous tubules is divided into eight stages, each consisting of distinct associations or groupings of four to five generations of gametogenic cells. Generally, in rams a stage in the cycle occupies an entire cross section of the seminiferous tubule. The period between successive appearances of the same stage in the cycle at a particular point in a tubule is 10.4 days, while the total duration of spermatogenesis in rams is 49 days.

Estimates of the daily sperm output of rams have been highly variable, ranging from 5.5 to 13.9 $\times$ 10^9 sperm/day. This deviation has been attributed to technical variations in methods of estimating daily sperm output as well as to breed, age, and individual and seasonal effects. Daily sperm output varies with testis size, which in turn varies seasonally. Seasonal effects are compounded because sperm production per gram of testis weight varies seasonally and is about 20 per cent lower in the nonbreeding than in the breeding season. Seasonal effects on spermatogenesis primarily result from seasonal variations in the daily photoperiod. However, extreme elevation of environmental temperature can disrupt spermatogenesis (the susceptible stage in rams is the pachytene stage of meiosis), so that the number of primary spermatocytes is reduced.

After release from the seminiferous tubules and passage through the rete testis, ram sperm spend 10 to 14 days in the epididymis undergoing the final stages of maturation.

PUBERTY

Puberty in the male may be defined as the time at which reproduction is possible, i.e., when spermatozoa are released. The course of gonadal development through the period of puberty has already been discussed.

Reproductive Tract and Accessory Organ Development at Puberty. The development of the reproductive tract and accessory organs is more highly correlated with physiological growth and testicular growth than with age. These associations in rates of growth occur mainly as the result of increased androgen secretion before and during puberty. Thus, in ram lambs high correlations exist between the rates of growth of the testes and those of the epididymides, seminal vesicles, bulbourethral glands and ampullae and the concentration and total content of fructose and citric acid in ejaculates. Penile-urethral adhesions are broken down; adhesions first disappear from the urethral process, then from the glans penis and finally from the penile shaft. Failure of breakdown of penile adhesions may predispose to the development of ovine posthitis in wethers. Penile growth, particularly growth in circumference, occurs at or shortly after puberty. In horned breeds horn growth precedes penile growth. Testicular androgens can also influence the rate of body growth so that ram lambs grow 3 to 8 per cent more rapidly than wethers if nutrition is adequate.

Neuroendocrine Induction of Puberty. Postnatal reproductive hormone secretion patterns of rams are becoming established. Plasma luteinizing hormone (LH) levels increase from birth to a peak at about 70 days of age and then decline. On the other hand, plasma follicle-stimulating hormone (FSH) levels peak at about 5 weeks. During the prepubertal period both gonadotropins, particularly LH, are secreted in an episodic manner, and peak plasma LH levels are higher in rams of high fecundity breeds. However, because of the relatively low heritability of adult fecundity and because of low within-breed correlations between LH levels and fecundity potential of individual animals, measurement of prepubertal plasma gonadotropin levels is unlikely to assist in genetic selection for fecundity. Pituitary LH and FSH responses to exogenous gonadotropin-releasing hormone (GnRH) peak at approximately the same time as peak plasma levels are recorded.

Plasma testosterone levels are low after birth and then increase to peak levels at 5 to 9 months of age. Androstenedione is always secreted in low concentrations, and these levels decline during the first 2 months of age. Plasma prolactin concentrations are low in lambs born in autumn until a short sharp elevation occurs at 10 to 12 weeks of age; this peak coincides with the onset of spermatogenesis. In lambs born in spring the normal seasonal elevation of prolactin secretion obscures any such peak.

The precise nature of the neuroendocrine interactions that trigger puberty are unknown. It is presumed that maturation of hypothalamic androgen-sensitive tissues is involved. This maturation probably takes the form of a decrease in sensitivity to androgen-negative feedback, which allows increased gonadotropin secretion to occur. The time course of pubertal development and endocrine changes can be modified by factors such as nutrition and photoperiod. Undernutrition inhibits body growth and reproductive development because pituitary secretion of gonadotropins is inhibited; consequently, androgen secretion is retarded. A declining daily photoperiod stimulates reproductive hormone secretion and may advance the pubertal endocrine surge slightly.

Endocrinology of the Adult Ram. In adult rams LH and prolactin, but not FSH, are secreted in pulsatile patterns, while peaks of testosterone secretion follow within 30 minutes after each plasma LH peak. Under some conditions plasma prolactin levels are elevated nocturnally, but the other reproductive hormones are not secreted in a circadian pattern.

Marked seasonal fluctuations in mean plasma hormone concentrations are superimposed on these acute secretory patterns. Prolactin secretion shows the greatest seasonal variations, with peak levels occurring in midsummer and lowest levels occurring in winter. Subsequent to the peak of prolactin secretion, LH output is elevated in mid-to-late summer, while seasonal peaks of FSH and testosterone follow in early autumn, coincident with the increase in testis size and libido at the commencement of the breeding season. Seasonal changes in the length of daylight contribute most to regulating seasonality of reproductive hormone secretion, probably as a result of influencing a retinopineal-hypothalamohypophyseal-gonadal axis. Despite considerable between-breed differences in the extent of reproductive seasonality in ewes, breed appears to have little influence on the seasonality of hormone secretion in rams. Effects of factors such as temperature, nutrition and pheromones on hormone secretion patterns await more adequate investigation.

The functions of individual reproductive hormones have, in many cases, been difficult to elucidate. Testosterone regulates functions such as reproductive behavior as well as maintains anatomic and physiological integrity of the reproductive tract and accessory structures. LH controls testosterone secretion of the Leydig cells, and prolactin may function as a "permissive" or "conditioning" hormone that synergizes with the endocrine effects of LH and testosterone. The endocrine regulation of spermatogenesis in the ram is complicated and requires further study. Multiplication of gonocytes and supporting cells in the impuberal testes requires LH and FSH. Testosterone may also be involved in this control, as well as in regulating primitive type A spermatogonium production. This steroid also controls the meiotic divisions resulting in spermatid production, although the final stages of spermatid maturation probably require FSH secretion. LH affects spermatogenesis in postpubertal rams indirectly by its stimulation of androgen production.

Suggested Readings

1. Courot M: Semen quality and quantity in the ram. In Tomes GJ, Robertson DE, Lightfoot RJ (eds): Sheep Breeding: Proc Int Congr Muresk, W.A. Institute of Technology, 1976, p 276.
2. Dyrmundsson OR: Puberty and early reproductive performance in sheep. II. Ram lambs. Anim Breed Abstr 41:419, 1973.
3. Lincoln GA, Short RV: Seasonal breeding: Nature's contraceptive. Rec Prog Horm Res 36:1, 1980.

Sexual Behavior of Sheep

R. J. Holmes, B.V.M. & S.S., Ph.D., M.R.C.V.S.
Massey University, Palmerston North, New Zealand

MATING SEQUENCE

Since the first edition of this book, useful reviews have been published about behavior and reproduction by Wodzicka-Tomaszewska and colleagues[3,4] and Gonyou.[1] Normal mating behavior was also well described and illustrated in the first edition[2] of this book. Therefore, this article will concentrate on aspects of sexual behavior that will allow for accurate assessment and management of breeding flocks.

The order of ram behavior between nosing and mounting the female has been found to alter with experience in the early pubescent period. Variation has also been found in the age of occurrence of component behaviors, the number of components expressed and their repetition.

Ewe lambs (Perendale) in their first and second estrus failed to tail fan, head turn, exhibit lordosis, maintain proximity and overtly solicit rams. They did not tend to form groups around rams (harem formation) as do older ewes. Thus, mating management of ewe lambs requires greater confinement and ram attention for maximum conception rates.

Two-tooth ewes (about 1½ to 2 years old) were found less likely to approach tethered rams than were older ewes. This may partly account for the lower mating percentages of young ewes in paddocks.

Ovariectomized and androgenized adult ewes show the complete repertoire of male sex behavior, including ejaculatory thrust and subsequent quiescence, but at a quantitatively lower rate. Treated ewes can be used to induce early or out-of-season estrus.

RAM SHOCK

Joining ewes and rams early in the breeding season, after isolation since the last breeding season, is a routine management technique that causes a marked increase in incidence and synchrony of estrus.

Sudden exposure of anovular ewes (Merinos in Australia), which had been sexually isolated for at least 1 month, induced ovulation in a proportion of ewes 72 hours later and estrus 17 days after that. Ewes living in tropical areas cycle throughout the year and respond to introduction of rams with 25 per cent showing estrus the next day. In New Zealand (latitude 38°S) short exposure (48 hours) in small flat paddocks (0.1 ha) was found to be just as effective in stimulating estrus as longer periods (17 days) in larger paddocks (7 to 10 ha). Because little or no estrus is expected within the first 48 hours at the beginning of the sexual season, intact rams could be used for this purpose. In small areas one ram could be used for different groups for successive short periods.

Intact rams have been found to be more effective in producing the ram shock effect than vasectomized rams, and Dorset Horns are more effective than New Zealand Romneys.

The factor or factors involved in this phenomenon have not been determined, but evidence suggests that smell is involved. Ewes respond when penned close to but unable to see or touch rams. Ewes also respond to both androgenized ewes and wethers. It has also been suggested that rams walking past ewes, or ewes using yards previously used by rams, has an estrus-stimulating effect. Wool and wax from rams' sebaceous glands have been found effective when used alone.

Apart from olfactory stimulation the stress of the sudden change in sexual environment may be a contributing factor to the ram shock effect.

RAM'S SENSE OF SMELL

The ram's sense of smell is not essential for determining the female's sexual state, which he does by her response to his sexual challenge. Estrous females cooperate for mounting. It is possible that, as in other species, the male learns to associate odor and receptivity with estrus. Some sexually uninterested rams showed immediate withdrawal after genital sniffing of estrous ewes, as though they found the estrous smell aversive. The rams then went directly across to a tethered ram.

Anosmic adult rams required more time than smell-intact rams to detect estrous ewes but were eventually just as successful. Their courtship was unaltered. It would seem, therefore, that the sense of smell facilitates speed of estrus detection by mature rams.

DISTRIBUTION OF SEXUAL ATTENTION

Large variation has been observed between ewes in the number of services received per estrus, although there was no apparent difference in their receptivity. Ewes may vary in attractiveness to rams as well as competing between themselves for proximity to the ram.

When a number of females are simultaneously in estrus and there is only one ram present, they are unlikely to receive equal sexual attention. Rams exposed to eight estrous ewes per day for single-sire mating did not mate more than five ewes per day. Younger females (up to 2 years old) are usually subordinate to adult ewes, and this reduces the chances of being mated when run with older ewes. Experienced ewes seek the ram, whereas ewe lambs tend not to do so. Older estrous ewes gather around a ram, showing harem formation.

During an estrous period some ewes appear to be more attractive. The same ewes at one estrus received greater attention by different rams when a single-sire mating technique was used. However, when rams were paired, the dominant ram showed preference for some ewes and mated them more often, but the subordinate ram mated randomly. Therefore, multi-sire mating would be expected to result in a greater proportion of ewes being served.

Some experienced rams working within larger flocks have been seen serving ewes only once, giving mated ewes little more than a nosing before moving on to serve preferentially unmated females. Experimentally, rams have been seen to show sexual habituation, i.e., loss of sexual responsiveness, to the same estrous female.

Dispersion and increased grazing time by ewes on large paddocks, especially when markedly underfed (5 kg body weight loss in 60 days), has been found to reduce ram-ewe contact. Reduced ram-ewe contact leads to lower pregnancy rates in larger paddocks.

Rams show sex preference for ewes of their own breed or appearance. It has been estimated that on average ewes are served two to four times during an estrus. The greater the number of ejaculations the greater the probability of conception. When mated with continuously working rams, females may need to be inseminated several times to receive sufficient spermatozoa for fertilization. In fact, it has been estimated that conception rates of ewes in multi-sire mating systems increased with the number of rams by which they were served.

RAM BLOCKING

Rams, usually dominants, have been seen preventing heterosexual interactions by blocking, by either walking or pushing between the ewe and ram and then staying between them. Rams with either normal or low sexual responses to estrous females have shown blocking behavior. When done by rams with low libido, blocking may reduce conception rates. This supports the need for libido testing, especially before multi-sire mating.

DOMINANCE BETWEEN RAMS

Competition between rams for access to an estrous female results in one ram's subsequent priority in access, i.e., dominance. The rank order (or dominance hierarchy) from sexual competition for

a group of rams was found to be identical to the feeding competition order. If this observation is found to apply generally, the feeding order would be a convenient predictor of sexual rank order. However, different sexual rank orders for the same rams were found when they sexually competed in a pen and again in a paddock.

Subordinate rams working singly have shown decreased mounting and ejaculation frequency in the sight of dominants in nearby pens. This "psychological inhibition" has been called the "audience effect." The ejaculation frequency of a dominant ram, however, was unchanged when he was watched by subordinates, but he was more dexterous, i.e., showed less mounts per ejaculation.

Some authors have reported dominants mounting more frequently than subordinates in multi-sire mating. The difference between dominants and subordinates decreased with increasing dispersal in paddocks and sex ratio. Mounting by subordinates appears often to depend upon distance or visual isolation from the dominant.

Although sexual dominance may be exerted in pens and small paddocks, subordinate rams do successfully mate when outside the sphere of influence of the dominant. Subordinates have also been seen working within a harem surrounding the dominant ram.

The ejaculation rate was halved when a dominant and subordinate worked together in a small area (1.23 ha) compared with their rate when mated individually. When they worked together, the dominant served less ewes and the subordinate more, but the total number of ewes mated was greater than when each ram worked singly. In that study dominance was not related to serving capacity. There appears to be individual variation between the sexual responses of subordinates in proximity to dominants. One variable could be the libido of the competing rams.

Another study showed that higher-ranking rams ejaculate at an earlier age and more frequently, although they mounted less, i.e., had superior mating dexterity. Other studies have found that higher-ranking rams served more ewes.

When kept in groups in the nonbreeding season, rams, particularly dominants, will mount and ejaculate into the rectum of rams. This may result in ram-ram transmission of infectious agents such as *Brucella ovis*.

In conclusion it appears that dominance has an effect on ram sex behavior in some circumstances. This depends upon space available, visual isolation, libido of rams involved and position of a ram in the sexual rank order.

LIBIDO

Sex drive of rams has been measured in several ways, e.g., time taken before there is no sexual activity within a standard period (usually 20 to 30 minutes), number of ejaculations per unit time (varying from 20 minutes to 2 hours—serving capacity), time from introduction to ejaculation (reaction time), intervals between successive ejaculations and a scoring system for sexual vigor (libido score).

The serving capacity (SC) appears to be the most useful measure for predicting sexual performance of flock rams. Potential benefits from using high-SC rams are the following: fewer rams required, shorter mating, and hence lambing period, higher percentage of daughters getting pregnant as ewe lambs and greater proportion of high-SC sons.

The reliability of pen tests in predicting paddock performance has been questioned, and several reasons for failure have been suggested as follows. Rams less than 2 months old were found insufficiently developed to give useful predictions of post-puberal behavior; pen-reared rams may be disturbed by strange testing facilities and handling—they should be tested in the usual living area by the normal stockhandler; there should be sufficient number of animals to be mounted and sufficient time allowed for differences between rams to be fully expressed; distinction should be made between sex drive and ability to mate swiftly with minimum energy use. Performance of rams in larger paddocks can be expected to be affected by walking and foraging abilities.

Several ejaculations from a continuously working ram appear necessary for the achievement of sufficient sperm numbers for fertilization. In multi-sire paddock mating most rams (New Zealand Romneys and Merinos) were observed to ejaculate 10 times in 8 hours of daylight, with many rams serving 20 times in that period.

Australian research with Merinos has shown significant positive correlations between SC and the number of ewes inseminated in both single and multi-sire flock mating. A group of four mature rams with higher SC served a greater proportion of ewes during the first cycle (17 days) than a similar group with lower SC. However, there was no difference between proportions of ewes lambing in the two flocks. The female progeny of the high-SC group when mated at 8 months had a significantly higher lambing percentage than the equivalent low-SC progeny.

Other work showed some low-SC rams obtained pregnancy rates as high as medium- and high-SC rams. However, serving capacity generally gave a good indication of flock mating performance. High-SC rams may also improve the reproductive efficiency of maiden ewes.

Repeatability between SC tests was greater (0.8) when there was no visual contact between rams. It was found that many rams took at least one introductory 20-minute period to familiarize themselves with the pen.

The present recommended method of measuring SC is to calculate the mean of two 1-hour tests for a ram tested singly in a 6 m × 6 m pen with four estrous ewes. The SC test without competition would not be expected to predict reliably small paddock performance when competition could affect sexual success. Restrained anestrous ewes (× 10) with lubricated vaginas have also been used to test 12 rams at once. The rams were first allowed to watch other rams serve for 5 minutes before being allowed to serve for 20 minutes.

FACTORS AFFECTING LIBIDO

Genetic. High libido appears to be genetically inherited and positively correlated with prolificacy. Differences occur between breeds, e.g., Finn ram lambs reach puberty earlier and are more effective than Merinos, and between strains within breeds, e.g., the more prolific Merino strains show greater sexual activity. High correlations have been found between libido of sire and sons. High-SC sires tend to have a smaller proportion of low-SC male offspring.

Hormones and Photoperiod. Testosterone treatment of ram lambs between 5 and 8 weeks of age decreased the number of adult rams with low libido. Treatment with antitestosterone antiserum during that age decreased their libido as adults. Androgens naturally circulating at this time may affect the sensitivity of central nervous system (CNS) centers to sexual stimulation.

Libido of the adult ram requires a minimum level of circulating testosterone. Androstenedione and other hormones may also be involved. Libido declined slowly after postpuberal castration and was returned to 92 per cent of the original measurement level by injection of 15 μg testosterone. Higher doses increased aggression but not libido. Although testosterone has been found to return libido during the long photoperiod, it has had no effect on active or inactive rams during the breeding season.

Rams transported to a shorter photoperiod showed better libido than before. The sexual responsiveness of androgenized castrates was greater when days were getting shorter, and libido of entire rams has been found to be higher at this time.

Although there are seasonal variations in basal levels of testosterone, it is probable that seasonal variation of CNS centers is involved in sexual responsiveness. It may be that CNS function is more important than testosterone in producing seasonal variation in libido.

Weather. Libido reduces during a sudden cold snap and returns with warmer weather. Short periods of high temperature (41°C for 4 to 13½ hours) prolonged reaction time (RT). After 13½ hours, RT was significantly increased. It was most prolonged 3 weeks after the heat stress.

Rearing. Rearing of ram lambs in groups from weaning (3 months) to 16 months of age without exposure to females was associated with lack of sexual responsiveness to an estrous ewe by half the rams. These rams were the more dominant in their groups. Their inappropriate sex behavior may have reflected the association of mounting with dominance within all-male groups. Rams that showed low sexual response to an estrous female also showed most frequent mounting within their all-male group.

Rearing of ram lambs either in physical contact or in proximity without physical contact, resulted in a lower proportion of rams that would not mate. Another study reported rams kept in close proximity to ewes ejaculated more frequently than isolated rams. Repeated exposure (about 40 times) or time (9 days) with estrous ewes has increased the proportion of rams showing sexual interest in ewes.

It appears, therefore, that rearing of ram lambs without females may have temporary effects on heterosexual behavior. However, rearing with ewes or keeping ewes close to rams may increase the probability of rams mating at the first instance required.

Learning. Rams modify their sexual behavior with experience. After training for semen collection, an adult ram mounted and ejaculated within 2 seconds and without courtship. Rams have shown a decline in foot striking when tested with restrained ewes. Having been trained to mount a dummy for semen collection, rams became indifferent to it when repeated attempts to ejaculate were thwarted by barriers.

It is to be expected that searching and mounting will decline when it is associated with pain, e.g., foot abscess and arthritis.

Nutrition. For maximum libido, rams should be adequately fed and free of disease. Poor nutrition (below maintenance levels) of the ram for more than 5 weeks has been implicated in loss of libido. It has been suggested that underfeeding will adversely affect libido before spermatogenesis. There is often a loss of ram body condition during the breeding period, but the causes have not been determined. Obesity has been associated with increased reaction times and difficulty in mounting.

MATING RATIO

The optimal mating ratio will vary with age of females, SC of ram or rams, size and terrain of mating area, whether one or more rams are to be used per female group and weather.

For Australian conditions at least one ram per hundred ewes (1:100) has been recommended when rams and ewes are mature Merinos. For maiden ewes this should be decreased to 1:50. A ratio of 1:400 for mature sheep resulted in lowering of proportions of ewes mated and pregnant.

Under New Zealand conditions a 1:100 ratio has been found to be conservative when rams are fertile, healthy and working in small flat paddocks. No loss in reproductive performance of Merino and New Zealand Romney ewes more than 2 years of age (4-tooth and older) was found when intensively managed at grass for mating with mature rams at 1:200. Ratios of 1:350 and even 1:400 have been used satisfactorily with semen-tested high-SC mature rams in optimal conditions. Young rams, i.e., 2-tooths, are not necessarily as active as mature rams and, therefore, the ratio should be lowered. Young females (lambs or hoggets and 2-tooths) achieve better conception rates when mated separately from old ewes, especially when there are large numbers of females. With 2-tooths the percentage mated in the first cycle decreased with an increase in mating ratio. During all these New Zealand trials 80 to 95 per cent of females were mated in the first 17 days.

It appears that 1:100 is a reasonable ratio, which can be modified according to circumstances. Under optimum conditions, with mature animals and rams of high libido and good semen quality, the ratio can be raised for successful mating over two cycles.

References

1. Gonyou HW: The role of behavior in sheep production: A review of research. Appl Anim Ethol 11:341, 1984.
2. Holmes RJ: Normal mating behavior and its variations. In Morrow DA (ed): Current Therapy in Theriogenology. 1st ed. Philadelphia, WB Saunders Co, 1980, pp 931–936.
3. Wodzicka-Tomaszewska M, Kilgour R, Ryan M: "Libido" in the larger farm animals: A review. Appl Anim Ethol 7:203, 1981.
4. Wodzicka-Tomaszewska M, Edey TN, Lynch JJ (eds): Behavior in relation to reproduction, management and welfare of farm animals. Rev Rural Sci 4. Armidale (N.S.W., Australia), University of New England, 1980.

Examination of the Ram for Breeding Soundness

A. Neil Bruere, B.V.Sc., Ph.D., M.R.C.V.S., F.A.C.V.Sc.
Massey University, Palmerston North, New Zealand

The veterinary inspection of rams for breeding soundness prior to either sale or mating is now practiced in many sheep-raising countries. As a result, considerable information has been recorded, and the incidence of disease affecting the genitalia of rams has been reported to be as high as 10.7 per cent in rams of all ages in Australia, rising to 35 per cent in aged rams. In New Zealand up to 20 per cent of ram lambs in some flocks have been rejected for unsoundness of the genitalia. Also, as a result of these investigations, an extensive range of diseases and defects of the penis, prepuce, scrotum, testes and epididymides of rams has been documented. Many of these conditions affect the subsequent breeding performance and fertility of the ram either permanently or temporarily. The veterinarian involved in ram soundness examinations must have a wide knowledge of and experience with these diseases and must realize that in some instances their diagnosis, control, eradication and prevention are now possible, while in others we have a very poor understanding of either their etiology or transmission, let alone their control. The veterinarian should also recognize that he has an obligation to two different types of sheep farmer, the stud or pedigree breeder producing rams for sale to the commercial sheep farmer who, in turn, is aiming at maximum reproductive performance from his flock.

THE EXAMINATION

Whole-flock examination should be conducted with the rams in the standing position and should involve an examination of the scrotum and its contents and the prepuce. Rams that require more detailed examination should be tipped over.

Single-ram examination of pedigree and valuable animals should also include a general clinical examination. In either case a diagnosis of soundness or unsoundness may be supported by a semen test and other ancillary diagnostic aids.

Identification by either a wool or an ear tag of rams that have passed a veterinary examination may be useful for sheep that are destined for sale within a short time of examination. Technically, a ram can *only* be guaranteed sound on the day of examination.

If a certificate is issued following either a whole-flock or a single-ram examination, it should state clearly what was done, e.g., an examination of the scrotum and its contents and prepuce or a full clinical examination. The results of other tests, if conducted, should also be included.

The timing of the ram examination is very important. Rams should be inspected regularly and well before the start of the mating season. In general two situations must be considered. First, the owners of stud or pedigree ram flocks and commercial ram-producing flocks have a particular responsibility to the sheep industry because they must supply rams that are not only of sound genetic background but also of good fertility and free from the major defects to be outlined shortly. In order for information to be gathered on the overall incidence of genital disease in a given stud flock, the first veterinary inspection of rams should take place soon after weaning. At least two to three inspections of rams between weaning and the two-tooth stage (1 year and 1 year, 6 months) not only acquaints the flock owner with any problems but also enables control measures to be initiated if disease is detected. Regular examination and record-keeping also provide important local and national data from which priorities for research can be established.

Second, in the case of flock rams at least one annual examination per month prior to mating will ensure that animals are in rising health and free of known disease. Likewise, treatment and replacement of defective rams can take place in plenty of time to ensure enough sound rams for mating.

CATEGORIES OF SOUNDNESS

For clinical differentiation the following categories of soundness or unsoundness are suggested for general use. A *genitally sound ram* is one that has no congenital, physical or genital abnormalities or any condition that in its progression will cause a ram to become incapable of service. A *fertile ram* is one that is able to serve and is capable, in the opinion of the examining veterinarian, of impregnating the ewes mated to him. A *certifiable ram* must be one that is both genitally sound and fertile, but for practical purposes of inspection three separate degrees of breeding soundness are recognized:

1. The *full sound ram*, which is free from all defects of the genitalia and, as far as can be gauged by clinical examination, is sound for sale and mating.

2. The *temporarily unsound ram*, which has some defect that can be treated and the ram is restored to full soundness.

3. The *permanently unsound ram*, in which the defect or disease will permanently nullify or impair the performance of that ram.

SPECIFIC CONDITIONS CAUSING UNSOUNDNESS IN THE RAM

There are a number of conditions that contribute to genital unsoundness in the ram that for descriptive purposes are best dealt with in the order of the regions inspected. The inspection usually begins with the prepuce and penis, followed by the scrotum, and finally the testes and epididymides are palpated through the scrotum. A full examination of the penis is not carried out in large numbers of commercial rams but is essential in valuable animals or in those that are to be mated alone to selected ewes.

The Prepuce

Phimosis. Phimosis is recorded in some breeds of rams and may be detected either when the penis cannot be extruded or when ewes return to service or fail to produce lambs. It is generally accepted as a congenital condition causing permanent unsoundness.

Balanoposthitis or Pizzle Rot. The most common condition affecting the penis and prepuce of rams is balanoposthitis or pizzle rot. This disease is caused by a bacterium that grows profusely in the alkaline urine produced by sheep fed a protein-rich diet. It is seen very commonly in those countries in which such diets are produced by rapidly growing improved pasture. The causal bacterium produces ammonia from the urea excreted in the urine as a result of such a diet. The ammonia is the cytotoxic agent and has a direct scalding effect on the penis and prepuce, producing the characteristic signs of pizzle rot. The disease is venereal in nature and can be transmitted freely between ewes, rams, wethers and lambs. Cattle can also become affected and act as carriers.

This condition is easy to detect. The veterinarian should instruct the farmer about the nature of this disease and emphasize that it can be prevented. This can be done by ensuring that infected animals are isolated from other mating animals. Such animals should be treated and cured well before mating. It is also highly desirable to eliminate the conditions under which the causative bacterium flourishes. This can be done by keeping the male animals carefully shorn around the prepuce. Any stained wool from this area should be destroyed and not left to contaminate the environment. At certain times of the year it may be necessary to restrict the diet carefully of male animals in order to produce an acid urine, which will automatically clear minor external lesions of pizzle rot.

In the case of mild external lesions (posthitis), a few days of restricted diet with ad libitum water will usually effect a cure without the need for topical medication. With severe internal lesions as well (balanoposthitis), it may be necessary to dose the ram with ammonium chloride (1 to 3 gm, two to three times daily) and, in addition, to irrigate the prepuce with suitable antiseptic solutions. In severe cases it may be necessary to incise the prepuce to allow drainage of urine and pus. In such severe cases the urethral process and penis are frequently damaged, and the ram becomes permanently unsound.

The Penis

The examination of the penis of the ram requires the animal to be held in a sitting position with its forelegs held by an assistant. The examiner must then secure the penis near the sigmoid flexure with one hand and move it out of the prepuce, where it is held firmly by the other hand. The main defect of the penis is damage to the urethral process, which occurs frequently during shearing. Its subsequent effect on fertility is largely unknown. Nevertheless, it does represent a defect and should certainly be noted in pedigree and valuable rams. Blockage of the urethral process by calculi is very common in some countries. As a result, the process frequently becomes necrotic and sloughs off. The necrosis can, and often does, extend to involve the glans penis as well.

The Scrotum

Three important features should be noted in the examination of the scrotum: wool length, the presence or absence of scrotal abscesses and chorioptic mange.

Wool Length. It is important to see that rams with woolly scrota (e.g., Romney, Merino, Corriedale) do not carry excess wool during the mating season. (Note that this is not indicative of unsoundness as such.) Wool length can affect testis size, and an optimum wool length is about 0.5 to 1.0 cm at mating.

Scrotal Abscesses. These occur frequently in rams and are a common cause of both temporary and permanent unsoundness. They should be treated carefully, as they tend to extend to deeper structures and often permanently damage the genitalia (Fig. 1).

Chorioptic Mange. Chorioptic or scrotal mange is one of the primary diseases affecting the external genitalia of rams. The causative mites (*Chorioptes bovis*) live and feed on the skin of sheep, goats, cattle and horses. Their life cycle is about 3 weeks from the egg to the larval stage to the egg-laying female. The disease is not confined solely to the ram but is probably widespread in both sexes in most sheep flocks. The mites are usually found on the lower half of the body, particularly on the scrota of rams, around the dew claws and brisket and often on the poll. Many sheep have mites without mange, but when mange does occur, it is generally on those areas of the body on which the mites concentrate. Paradoxically, however, in individual sheep the extent of the mange is not necessarily related to

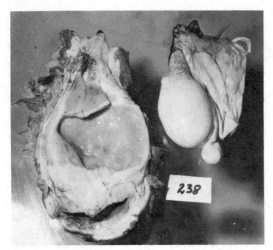

Figure 1. Penetrating scrotal abscess of the left testis. Note severe atrophy of right testis.

mite numbers. Mildly infested sheep may have the most severe mange. Rams without lesions of chorioptic mange are just as likely to be infected with mites as those with lesions. Furthermore, rams with old inactive lesions may be free of mites.

Severe mange in the scrotum will reduce fertility and may even cause temporary or permanent sterility. Outbreaks of scrotal mange can be quite explosive and unpredictable and under suitable conditions will persist over long periods of time. Its control is therefore of considerable importance to the ram breeder.

From this summary of scrotal mange, the following implications can be drawn when considering ram soundness: First, lesions of chorioptic mange must be diagnosed as either active or inactive. Active lesions when rubbed usually produce a marked nibbling or biting response by the ram. Active lesions when scraped or manipulated leave a bleeding area or at least a noticeable hyperemia. Such areas may be pinhead sized or larger. If such lesions are found, the ram is temporarily unsound and must be removed from the flock for treatment. Severe active or inactive lesions covering approximately more than half of the scrotum render animals totally unsuitable for mating during that season and may even render them permanently unsound. It is important to remember that all animals without lesions may carry mites, and this must be considered when advising the farmer on treatment and control.

Control and Treatment. Treatment can be applied either locally, i.e., to the affected scrotum, or generally, i.e., application by shower dip of a suitable parasiticide, of which the organophosphorous compound Diazinon is most widely used. Topical treatment is satisfactory for individual cases, but for flock treatment the use of shower dipping at the higher recommended concentrations of Diazinon is highly efficient for both treatment and prevention.

The Testes

Testis Size. As many examinations will be carried out on ram hoggets (4 months to 1 year of age) actually completing puberty, it is pertinent to remember the following points: There appears to be a closer relationship between testicular growth and body weight than between testicular weight and ram age. When body weight increases beyond 20 kg, testicular weight increases at a greater rate, maximum growth taking place between 23 and 27 kg. Puberty is reached at approximately 140 days of age and at 35 kg of body weight. However, there are wide between-breed differences (e.g., Suffolk, 112 days; Merino, 225 days). Increased testicular size implies increased spermatogenesis, and this is more so in younger than in older animals.

It must also be remembered that not uncommonly one testis in the ram descends before the other. Also, there is frequently a size differential between testes during puberty that becomes inapparent at maturity. This must be considered carefully when rejecting young rams because of either hypoplasia or atrophy of one testis.

In the examination of the testis of the mature ram, we must ensure that both size and tone are adequate. Testis size is related proportionately to the sperm output of the individual ram. The ram with large symmetrical testes that are free from defects is likely to produce semen of good quality. In fact, the manual examination of ram genitalia is now considered much more important and is generally more relevant to fertility prediction than a single semen examination. Semen examination, unless expertly executed, can lead to quite erroneous conclusions concerning the suitability of a particular ram for mating. Small testes are likely to produce semen of poor quality.

Hypo-orchidism. It is clinically difficult to differentiate testicular atrophy from testicular hypoplasia unless the former is associated with an obvious defect such as concurrent epididymitis. Also, the inexperienced veterinarian must acquaint himself or herself with the seasonal variation in testes size, particularly noticeable in such breeds as the Romney. A sound ram at the height of the breeding season should have large oval testes that are firm to the touch and of equal size. The thin nonresilient testis is usually seen out of the breeding season or may be associated with poor health. Note also that remarkable changes in size and form can take place in the testis of the ram once mated.

The term hypo-orchidism has been coined to include both testicular atrophy and testicular hypoplasia. Distinct forms of testicular hypoplasia (Figs. 2 to 5) include the following:

1. Unilateral testicular hypoplasia.

2. Testicular hypoplasia due to cryptorchidism and monorchidism.

3. Primary micro-orchidism (XXY chromosomal complement).

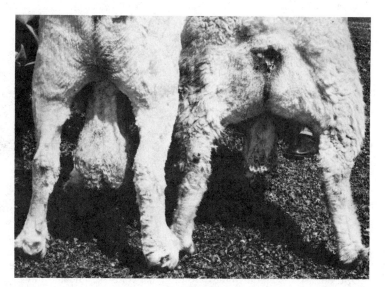

Figure 2. Scrotum and testes of a normal Romney ram (left) compared with those of a ram with severe testicular hypoplasia.

4. Micro-orchidism of unknown etiology.

5. Hypo-orchidism in association with segmental aplasia of the epididymis.

6. Bilateral epididymal spermiostasis and hypo-orchidism.

7. Hourglass testes and hypo-orchidism.

8. Hypo-orchidism and inguinal hernia.

9. Hypo-orchidism in association with varicocele.

Testicular atrophy can be seen in association with systemic disease and other physical and chemical factors. It can also be seen as a result of epididymitis and chorioptic mange. Therefore, extreme caution should be exercised when giving a decision on the soundness of a ram with hypo-orchidism. Many animals may have to be regarded as temporarily unsound and should be reexamined at a later date.

The many types of hypo-orchidism may need particular investigation to determine their etiology. For example, in valuable rams chromosome analysis may reveal individual cases of primary micro-orchidism in which rams have two X chromosomes as well as a Y chromosome.

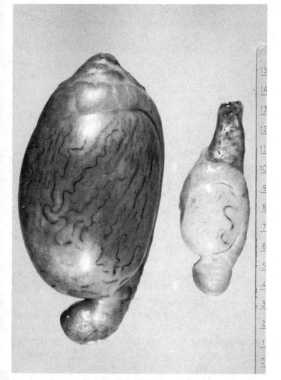

Figure 3. Testis of normal ram (left) and testis from ram of same age with primary micro-orchidism (right).

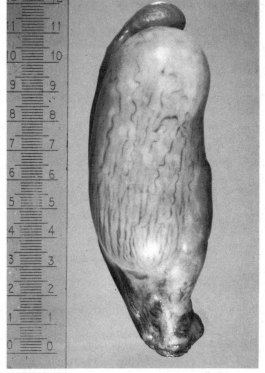

Figure 4. Hourglass testis caused by stricture of the tunica vaginalis testis.

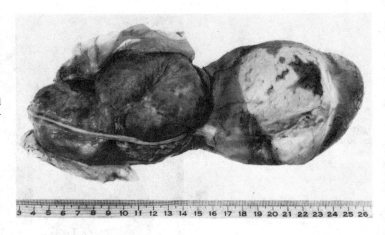

Figure 5. Testis of a ram and associated varicocele. The varicocele was intra-abdominal.

The Epididymides

Disorders of the epididymides are the most common cause of ram wastage, accounting for over half the rams rejected for genital unsoundness. There are several known bacterial etiologic agents, of which the most common are *Brucella ovis*, *Actinobacillus* sp., *Corynebacterium* sp. and *Pasteurella pseudotuberculosis*.

The detection of palpable lesions of epididymitis presents few problems to the experienced veterinarian. The important factor is the diagnosis of the cause.

Brucella Ovis. Brucellosis of rams has been recorded in many sheep-raising countries of the world and is a major cause of epididymitis. Under some circumstances the organism can cause a placentitis with subsequent abortion in ewes, but as a cause of abortion in sheep its role is probably overemphasized. In many flocks the incidence of brucellosis is low, and the effect of the few rams with reduced fertility caused by epididymitis is offset by overmating, i.e., using 2 to 3 per cent of rams. However, in flocks in which the incidence among mating rams is high, there is good clinical evidence to support the belief that low fertility may result and that the lambing will be spread over a longer period than normal. The detection of affected rams and the control of this disease are therefore of considerable importance to sheep production.

Transmission. *Brucella ovis* may be transmitted from sheep to sheep by a number of ways. However, it would appear that rectal transmission from ram to ram, particularly young rams following sodomy, is the main means of spread in affected flocks. Rams may also acquire infection following passive venereal transmission from ewes, and some ewes may carry infection from one lambing season to the next. There is also evidence that suggests that some ram lambs may be born infected with *B. ovis* and survive to infect other rams at puberty. *B. ovis* may also be recovered for up to 10 days from the vagina of some ewes that abort or expel infected placentae, so that the postabortion estrus that normally follows 6 months later may be an important avenue of spread of brucellosis. However, it is generally believed that the majority of ewes do not remain infected into the following mating season.

Diagnosis. Following active infection, palpable lesions of epididymitis can be detected within 5 weeks. At this stage the epididymis, usually the tail, will be hard and swollen, but as the lesions progress, the testis atrophies, and the lesions attain relatively enormous size and frequently appear larger than the atrophied testis itself. Lesions may be palpated in the body and the head of the epididymis as well as in the tail, and both testes are often affected. (Fig. 6).

A confirmed diagnosis of *B. ovis* may be made in several ways. First, it is possible to culture the organism from semen ejaculates obtained even from rams with nonpalpable lesions, since *B. ovis* resides in the secondary sex glands as well as in the epididymides. Semen culture is not absolutely reliable, and several ejaculates may need to be examined before either a positive or negative diagnosis may be made. The organism is acid-fast and stains readily by the Ziehl-Neelsen technique.

Second, autopsy of the affected ram and pathologic and histopathologic examination of the lesions will also be helpful but not completely diagnostic. Early lesions consist mainly of epithelial cysts with epithelial hyperplasia and fibrosis with lumen obstruction of the epididymides. The common lesion is a spermatic granuloma, with rupture of the epididymal tubule and extravasation of spermatozoa. Testicular degeneration fibrosis and calcification are the usual sequelae.

The third and main aid to diagnosis is the complement fixation (CF) test for *B. ovis*. This test is highly accurate in the hands of reliable operators. For the accurate diagnosis of infected rams, fresh serum samples need to be prepared and forwarded to a diagnostic laboratory as soon as possible, avoiding high temperatures. The CF test is, however, of no value in detecting affected animals if a vaccination policy of control has been introduced (see following paragraphs), since CF antibodies persist in vaccinated rams for several years.

Control. There is no known therapy for *B. ovis*

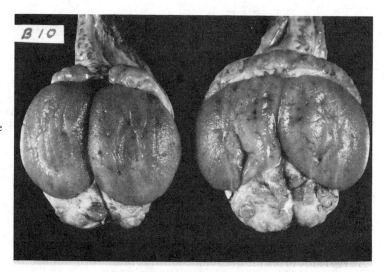

Figure 6. Acute epididymitis of the right testis caused by *Brucella ovis*.

in sheep; therefore, control either by detection and slaughter of affected animals or by vaccination is essential.

In pedigree and ram breeding flocks the regular inspection of all rams and sires for sale is essential. Once a diagnosis of brucellosis is confirmed, the regular use of the CF test for the detection of carrier animals is required for eradication. The use of this test will depend on the state of infection in the flock. Initially, it may be necessary to repeat the screening of all rams twice a year, but once the incidence has been reduced, the annual testing of ram hoggets at about 10 to 12 months of age and of breeding rams at least 1 month prior to mating is probably adequate.

All rams to be introduced into the flock should be isolated and tested via CF before contact with the main flock. A *B. ovis* eradication scheme based on the CF test has been successful in markedly reducing the incidence of this disease in Tasmania and New Zealand.

In commercial flocks, particularly those with large numbers of mating rams, protection against brucellosis may have to be given by vaccination, using an oil-based vaccine. The correct vaccination procedure is 2 doses of the oil-based vaccine at 6-week intervals. The alternative procedure involving the use of oil-based *B. ovis* vaccine together with *B. abortus* strain 19 is now not favored because of undesirable side effects produced by the strain 19 vaccine in some young rams. Before such a procedure is introduced all the rams to be vaccinated must be diagnosed as free from brucellosis by using the CF test. Vaccination usually gives good protection for the serviceable life of the ram.

Control by the segregation of the different age groups of rams has been practiced prior to the development of the CF test and a vaccine. This produced some degree of success but necessitated the mating of each age group of rams with their corresponding age group of ewes. The management problems are obvious.

Actinobacillosis. There are reports from several major sheep-raising countries, Australia, New Zealand, South Africa and the United States, of a specific epididymitis of young rams caused by the organism *Actinobacillus seminis*, of which there are apparently many antigenically different strains. The organism has also been associated with a suppurative polyarthritis and posthitis in sheep.

Infection with *A. seminis* is seen as either an acute or chronic orchitis, epididymo-orchitis or epididymitis. The disease is usually very acute and mainly seen in ram lambs at or soon after puberty. It is occasionally seen in older rams but usually in the chronic form. The lesions are characterized by intense swelling and pain of the scrotal contents accompanied by a severe systemic reaction. Frequently, lesions rupture to the exterior and discharge copious gray-to-yellow pus. Animals lose condition, and death has followed in some instances (Fig. 7).

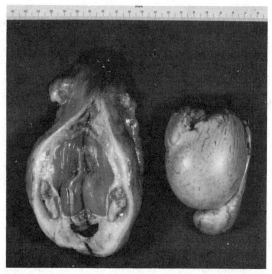

Figure 7. Chronic epididymitis and orchitis of left testis caused by *A. seminis*.

The chronic and more insidious epididymitis as seen in *B. ovis* disorders also frequently follows *A. seminis* infection. The lesions are permanent and are detected easily on palpation of the genitalia.

Transmission. The route of transmission has not been established. It is believed that between rams transmission may be by sodomy, but such venereal transmission is in doubt. It would appear that the organism may be transmitted by a variety of routes so that merely overcrowding young rams may be a major method of spreading the disease. In flocks with a high incidence of actinobacillosis, the carrier rate of infected rams increases rapidly from puberty to about 8 months of age. It then declines until about 1 year of age when only a few rams remain carriers of the disease. During the carrier phase the semen of such rams is of poorer quality and probably not suitable for mating.

Control. Control of actinobacillosis is difficult. Clinically affected animals should be removed from the flock and slaughtered. The detection of carrier animals is also difficult, but a CF test has been shown to be valuable in South Africa. It is emphasized, however, that a number of antigenic strains need to be included in the test.

At present there is no vaccine available for the prevention of this disease. It is probable that vaccine production will be difficult because of the pleomorphic state of the organism.

Other Causes of Epididymitis. Other organisms (as just named) have been isolated from instances of epididymitis in rams; they are, however, relatively unimportant and sporadic in occurrence. In summary it should be emphasized that in addition to the specific conditions described here, the general health and conformation of rams should be considered during a soundness examination. In some countries a full soundness examination includes evaluation of teeth, feet and other factors.

CONCLUSIONS

Genital disease of rams accounts for a high wastage in the sheep industry of most countries, so that the examination of rams for breeding soundness has become an accepted and highly economical veterinary procedure.

Three broad categories of breeding soundness are now recognized for the ram: sound, temporarily unsound and permanently unsound. The examination requires a highly skilled and informed approach with the use of a wide range of ancillary aids to diagnosis, including semen examination and serologic, microbiologic, pathologic and other special tests. There is an ever-increasing demand from the sheep industries for sound, disease-free rams. The veterinary profession should be aware of the many new advances in knowledge of genital disease of sheep in order to be able to deal with this demand.

Suggested Readings

1. Bruere AN: Some clinical aspects of hypo-orchidism (small testes) in the ram. NZ Vet J 18:189, 1970.
2. Gunn RMC, Sanders RN, Granger W: Studies in fertility in sheep. Bull Coun Scient Ind Res Melb No. 148, 1942.
3. Hughes KL: The epidemiology of *Br. ovis* infection. Proceedings of the New Zealand Veterinary Association Sheep Society. 2nd Seminar. Massey University, 1972, p 55.
4. Miller SJ, Moule GR: Clinical observations on the reproductive organs of Merino rams in pastoral Queensland. Aust Vet J 30:353, 1954.
5. Quinlivan TD: Breeding soundness in the ram: A review of the proceedings and resolutions from two seminars held in 1964 and 1969. NZ Vet J 18:233, 1970.
6. van Tander EM: *Actinobacillus seminis* infection in sheep in the Republic of South Africa. I. Identification of the problem. II. Incidence and geographical distribution. III. Growth and cultural characteristics of *A. seminis*. Anderstepoor J Vet Res 46:129, 135, 141, 1979.
7. Watt DA: Testicular abnormalities and spermatogenesis of the ovine and other species. Vet Bull 42(4):181, 1972.

Semen Collection and Evaluation

I. C. A. Martin, B.V.Sc., Ph.D., F.R.C.V.S.
The University of Sydney, Sydney, Australia

In most sheep breeding management systems as few rams as possible are introduced into the ewe flock without jeopardizing the target of maximum fertility and fecundity. In recognition of the risks to reproductive performance inherent in using rams of undefined fertility, techniques for the rapid assessment of the reproductive fitness have been developed by workers at many centers. The detail of the techniques employed for the ranking of rams, based on factors thought to be correlated with fertility, differs according to the intensity of selection desired or to what is practically possible. Examination of a sample (or samples) of semen from each apparently physically normal ram is an essential step in this diagnostic program.

Obviously, the selection pressure will be much greater when rams are being considered for use in artificial insemination programs, in which case factors such as libido (ejaculation frequency) and daily sperm output as well as semen quality become very important.

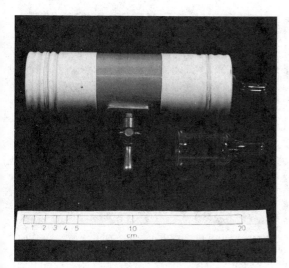

Figure 1. Artificial vagina for rams and a semen collection tube designed to fit inside the inner latex rubber liner.

SEMEN COLLECTION

Three methods of semen collection from the ram are practically relevant. These include the artificial vagina (AV), electroejaculation (EE) and aspiration of semen from the vagina of a ewe after service has been observed. Semen obtained using an AV is the best indicator of the ejaculate naturally produced by the ram. Recent research into the technique of EE has improved the reliability of this method of obtaining ejaculates whose characteristics are prognostic of the semen normally ejaculated by the ram.

Although time consuming and probably always demanding the availability of a number of ewes per ram tested, collection of ejaculates from the vagina has some value in assessing untrained, unrestrained rams. An adaptation of this method by Synnott and colleagues,[4] using a modified condom as a vaginal insert, is useful for the estimation of the sperm production rates of rams free to mate with small groups of estrous ewes.

The method of collection chosen for any project depends on the number of rams to be examined, their tractability, the emphasis placed on service behavior and ejaculatory frequency and the detail required in terms of total sperm produced and semen characteristics measured. When the semen is required for artificial insemination, only collection by AV and EE can be considered.

Artificial Vagina

The AV shown in Figure 1 is a development from that described by Emmens and Robinson[1] and is simple to construct, assemble, use and clean. When the AV is assembled for use, the collection tube is placed almost completely within the case and liner, serving the two purposes of keeping the tube warm and ensuring that ejaculation occurs into it with little or no semen deposited on the liner.

The AV should be between 41 and 44°C for collection, and its liner must be lightly coated with a germicide- and spermicide-free lubricant, such as a water-based (surgical) gel (KY Jelly-Ethnor) or petroleum jelly. Of course, care must be taken, particularly with water miscible gels, that minimal amounts of lubricant are used. Otherwise, the characteristics of the semen sample will be distorted by the presence of gel. It has been found that use of a water-miscible lubricant simplifies the cleaning after use of the liner.

Time must be allowed for training rams to serve an AV, and the amount of previous handling, e.g., penning and feeding, will influence how quickly rams can be trained for semen collection. In general, the training sequence should allow rams to serve estrous ewes in the collection area, with the semen collector present. Following that the rams should be progressively conditioned until they will serve the decoy ewe while simultaneously permitting the collector to touch them. Once this stage has been reached, training usually proceeds quickly, i.e., within a day, to the point at which rams regularly serve the AV and ejaculate.

AV collection is preferable to the other methods of collection if time can be afforded for the initial training period, which may occupy several weeks. However, a number of rams, for example, 30 per cent of flock rams having no early experience of close proximity with and handling by farm staff and collectors, cannot be trained for AV semen collection even though EE of these rams will usually indicate that they are producing normal semen.

Electroejaculation

Using currently available stimulators, which can incorporate timing circuits to give a preprogrammed pattern of stimuli, most rams will ejaculate within 30 seconds so that semen samples can be collected quickly without training rams for the AV. Figure 2 shows a stimulator and probe of this type that has been used to obtain semen from 100 to 150 rams in a working day. Most modern circuits operate at low voltages (approximately 10 V) and for reasons of electrical safety are powered by rechargeable batteries, so that while being used, the stimulator is completely isolated from a main source of electricity. The characteristics of the electrical stimuli most likely to produce ejaculation have been defined[3] and are sine- or square-wave pulses at 30 to 50 hz delivered through a bipolar rectal electrode in volleys of 3- to 5-second duration followed by a similar period of rest. Such a pattern of stimulation repeated for up to 1 minute will in most cases produce ejaculation. However, the ejaculatory response is significantly affected by the duration of the rest and stimulation periods. Fewer sperm are ejaculated following two cycles of "on" for 20 seconds and "off" for 40 seconds than to stimuli applied for 5 seconds with a 10-second rest repeated eight times.[3] Commonly used patterns of stimulation are 3- to 5-seconds "on" with a similar period of 3- to 5-second rest repeated nine or ten times.

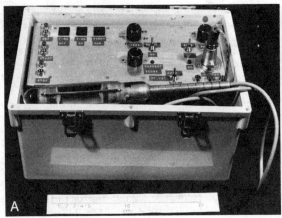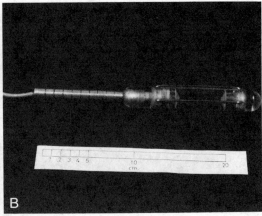

Figure 2. *A,* Stimulator developed for the electroejaculation of rams with options of sine or square wave, variable frequency and amplitude of stimulus. The stimulator is controlled by a preset timer for the delivery of volleys of stimuli of several seconds duration. The stage reached in the stimulation sequence is indicated by a digital display. *B,* A rectal probe for the electroejaculation of rams. It carries three longitudinal electrode strips set 60° apart, which are directed ventrally in the pelvic space.

Bipolar rectal electrodes deliver stimuli to the pelvic contents, and on most rectal probes the electrodes are arranged as longitudinal strips (Fig. 2) that span the pelvic space from the last lumbar vertebra to the third sacral foramen.

Rams are usually restrained in lateral recumbency, with hindlegs in moderate extension for EE. It is not a usual practice to clear the rectum mechanically or with an enema before inserting the probe. However, failure to ejaculate is often associated with fecal accumulation on the probe. This possibility should always be checked whenever stimulation has been unsuccessful; EE can then be repeated immediately after clearing feces from the rectum and probe.

For collection of semen the penis is manually extended and, while the shaft of the penis is held, the glans and urethral process are inserted into a dry, warm (37°C) graduated collection tube (a 12 or 15 ml graduated centrifuge tube is suitable).

SEMEN EVALUATION

Whether semen samples from large numbers of rams are examined in flock surveys or whether several ejaculates from each of a much smaller number of rams are assessed much more critically for suitability in an AI project, the principal objective is to assess the number of motile, morphologically normal spermatozoa in an ejaculate (or series of ejaculates in which the daily sperm output is being determined). Thus, volume of semen, sperm concentration, proportion of motile spermatozoa and spermatozoal morphology must be measured with the greatest possible accuracy under field conditions. Of these variables, sperm motility is the most difficult to assess repeatably unless the specimens are carefully protected against cold shock by using prewarmed glassware for collection, are col-

lected into clean specimen tubes and are examined soon after collection. The motility of sperm in normal ram semen diminishes rapidly if held at 35°C or higher after collection.

Although various sensors of the electrical and optical characteristics of ram semen have been tested for their value in semen appraisal, particularly with reference to rapid determination of spermatozoal concentration and to quantification of motility, no instrument has yet been developed that satisfies the requirements of portability, durability and speed and simplicity of operation. Advances in microcomputer design and transducer (sensor) technology have enhanced the prospects for the manufacture of such instruments, but currently, the light microscope is the central instrument for the evaluation of semen.

A good quality microscope, preferably equipped with phase-contrast illumination and objectives with $10\times$, $40\times$ and $100\times$ magnification, is needed for semen evaluation. If spermatozoal motility is to be observed consistently, the microscope should also be fitted with a warm stage so that specimens are always evaluated between 37 and 39°C. Intensity of wave motion (scored on a scale of 0 to 4, for example) within undiluted semen is the most usual record of motility, but the intensity of motility and the proportion (per cent) of spermatozoa progressing can be estimated from samples diluted into a suitable buffer. Standardized cells for scoring of motility can be built on ordinary microscope slides, or a hemocytometer may be used. The Makler Cell (Israel Electro-Optical, Rehovot) permits examination of a thin film (10 µm) against a ruled graticule of 1 mm² and is useful for determining both sperm concentration and motility. However, a hemocytometer is cheaper and nearly as satisfactory (Model 1475 produced by AO, Buffalo, NY, for phase-contrast studies is particularly useful).

If large numbers of ejaculates are to be studied,

sperm counts are best obtained photometrically by measuring the optical density of highly diluted (1/200 to 1/400) semen. The Bausch & Lomb Spectronic 20 has been widely used for this purpose. A subsample of semen is diluted in 154 mM NaCl containing 0.5 per cent formaldehyde to immobilize the spermatozoa. This method requires the calibration of the optical density readings of the photometer against counts of the diluted samples made with hemocytometers.

Microscopic examination of the diluted semen will quickly indicate whether sperm morphology is grossly abnormal. However, it is usual practice to make simple films of semen for later studies of morphology. Commonly, supravital stains employing eosin (or Congo red) and nigrosin (or fast green FCF)[2] will also be prepared, as these stains permit assessment of unstained (viable) spermatozoa as well as morphology. Rose bengal, modified Wright's stain, Giemsa or hematoxylin-eosin have all been suggested as stains useful for delineating sperm for morphologic examination. With any of these stains or, indeed, with formalin-fixed specimens (examined as wet mounts in phase-contrast illumination) aberrations in shape and size of sperm heads and defects in midpieces and tails are readily detected using the 100 × (oil immersion) objective. Watson[5] described a useful variant of the Giemsa stain that preferentially stains acrosomes and permits evaluation of abnormality in, or damage to, that organelle.

RELATIONSHIP OF SEMEN CHARACTERISTICS TO FERTILITY

When the techniques of scrotal palpation are applied together with semen examination of palpably normal rams, poorly fertile or infertile rams can be rapidly identified and eliminated from the flock. Then, if rams selected as satisfactory on these criteria are mated with large groups of ewes or if their semen is used extensively for AI, less than 20

per cent of differences in fertility among rams can be accounted for in the ranking of any of the preceding criteria of semen quality or in any indices of quality produced by combining several criteria together with data of longevity of sperm on incubation. Mating frequency tests and appraisal of the daily sperm output by repeated semen collection may enhance the accuracy of estimates of potential fertility, but these tests demand time and limit their use to relatively few rams.

As a general, practical guideline, a minimally acceptable semen sample will contain 1000 million spermatozoa, of which 60 per cent will show strong, progressive motility, and fewer than 30 per cent will have morphologic abnormalities.

Any prognostication on potential fertility must also take into account the lability of sperm output by rams in response to changes in environment or altered health status. Semen quality can change substantially in those breeds that show seasonality in reproduction, and in many farm production situations semen from rams can only be usefully evaluated 2 to 3 weeks before mating is due to start. Various stresses, e.g., high ambient temperature or shearing, are well known as causing a decline in semen quality. Various disease processes, e.g., foot rot, foot abscess or fly strike, though not involving any part of the reproductive tract, will have acute and adverse effects on semen quality.

References

1. Emmens CW, Robinson TJ: Artificial insemination in the sheep. *In* Maule JP (ed): The Semen of Animals and Artificial Insemination. Farnham Royal, C.A.B., 1962, pp 205–251.
2. Entwistle KW: Congo red-fast green FCF as a supra-vital stain for ram and bull spermatozoa. Aust Vet J 48:515, 1972.
3. Martin ICA: The principles and practice of electroejaculation of mammals. Symp Zool Soc Lond 43:127, 1978.
4. Synnott AL, Fulkerson WJ, Lindsay DR: Sperm output by rams and distribution amongst ewes under conditions of continual mating. J Reprod Fert 61:355, 1981.
5. Watson PF: Use of a Giemsa stain to detect changes in acrosomes of frozen ram spermatozoa. Vet Rec 97:12, 1975.

Artificial Breeding Techniques in Sheep

S. J. Miller, M.V.Sc., F.A.C.V.Sc.
Warwick, Queensland, Australia

Artificial breeding has been utilized in sheep to extend the use of superior sires or to spread a specific character, such as "polledness," rapidly through a population. It has also been used to help in the speedy elimination of undesirable characteristics.

The economic importance of artificial breeding depends largely on the anticipated monetary return from using known superior sires that provide more rapid genetic gains or from overcoming infertility arising from certain causes in difficult environments, especially in the tropics. The likely results will depend on the skill of the operation and the way it is incorporated into any system of sheep breeding.

Note that the techniques described in this article are those used basically in Australia—brief reference is made to some variations carried out in other countries.

SELECTION AND MANAGEMENT OF RAMS

Artificial breeding programs should be conducted when ewes are cycling, e.g., late summer, autumn or early winter. If inseminations are to be carried out in spring/early summer, the use of vasectomized rams can be considered. When ewes are induced to ovulate in spring by the sudden introduction of vasectomized rams, then ovulation occurs in about 48 hours without estrus. Some ewes will then have short cycles and reovulate in 5 to 6 days, and others will have a normal cycle in 17 days. The former group will exhibit first estrus 22 to 26 days after ram introduction. However, in some environments rams may be infertile when needed unless precautions are taken. Thus, the events that occur 2 months prior to a program largely influence the results. Eight to ten weeks prior to use, rams should be shorn, treated for internal and external parasites and wounds and have their feet trimmed. They should also be kept cool and should preferably be shed housed and adequately fed. (Rations containing 10 to 12 per cent crude protein and 55 per cent total digestible nutrients in a mixture containing 55 per cent roughage and 45 per cent concentrate are

satisfactory). Two-tooth (1½-year) rams should be segregated from older rams to avoid fighting and sodomy. Shed-housed rams become quiet and are easier to train to an artificial vagina (AV).

During use rams should be penned individually while waiting their turn as semen donors. This prevents their mounting one another or fighting, and they quickly become accustomed to walking from pen to serving bail and back, saving considerable time.

SEMEN COLLECTION, DILUTION AND STORAGE

An artificial vagina is used to collect the semen, as this gives a maximum output over a period of time. Semen can be collected from most rams at least three times per day over a 17-day insemination period without a drop in semen quality. During an artificial breeding program, semen is assessed rapidly after each collection for volume, color, density and motility, and a visual estimate is made of live-dead ratios.

Semen is mostly used undiluted in Australia but can be diluted up to fourfold, depending on the initial concentration. The most common diluents used are whole, skimmed and reconstituted cow's milk that has been heated to 90°C for 10 minutes. Ultra-high temperature (UHT) milk can be used without heating. Egg yolk, glucose citrate (15 per cent egg yolk; 0.8 per cent glucose anhydrous; 2.8 per cent sodium citrate dihydrate in glass-distilled water) has also been used successfully as a diluent. In practice dilution rates greater than 1:2 are seldom used. Dilutions are made with the diluting solution at 30 to 35°C.

If not used immediately, diluted semen is cooled to 2 to 5°C over a 2-hour period and held at this temperature. Although some motility is retained for 14 days at this temperature, the fertilizing capacity decreases rapidly after 24 hours of storage, and semen should be used within this period. In France[2] semen is stored at 15°C in milk diluent and gives good fertility after storage for 14 to 16 hours.

Preservation of semen by freezing has proved to be more difficult with rams than with bulls, and fertility rates comparable with those achieved by either natural mating or liquid semen techniques have still to be regularly achieved.

Salamon and Visser[8] have conducted experiments on the effect of diluents, glycerol concentration, dilution rate and egg yolk concentration on sperm survival after freezing spermatozoa by the pellet method and storing the pellets at −196°C in liquid nitrogen. Thawed pellets frozen with raffinose-citrate-yolk-glycerol and used after 3 years resulted in a 50 per cent lambing. Lambings of 55 per cent have been achieved using pellet-frozen semen in TRIS-glucose-yolk-glycerol diluent. The semen is

Table 1. Semen Dilution with a Tris-based Diluent

| | Dilution Rate (Semen/Diluent) | | | |
	1 + 1	1 + 2	1 + 3	1 + 4
Tris (gm)	5.814	4.361	3.876	3.634
Glucose (gm)	0.8	0.6	0.533	0.5
Citric acid (gm)	3.184	2.388	2.123	1.99
Egg yolk (ml)	24	18	16	15
Glycerol (ml)	8	6	5.3	5
Glass-distilled water to 100 ml				

The chemicals are first dissolved in approximately 60 ml of distilled water before adding the glycerol and egg yolk. The volume is then made up to 100 ml with water.

diluted at an appropriate rate (usually 1:2) with a tris-based diluent as shown in Table 1.

Dilution is carried out at 30°C. The diluted semen is cooled to 5°C over a 2-hour period before freezing in pellet form on dry ice that has had molded holes engraved on it for the purpose. Pellet size is usually about 0.1 to 0.2 ml, containing about 200 million spermatozoa. After freezing for 2 to 3 minutes, the pellets are transferred into liquid nitrogen. Pellets are thawed at 37°C and used as liquid semen.

Freezing in pellets is the system most commonly used when ewes are to be inseminated at a natural estrus. However, the system is tedious when ewes are inseminated at a synchronized estrus, and under these circumstances, as described in France, semen is frozen in straws, which gives acceptable fertility.

MANAGEMENT OF THE EWE FLOCK

Accurate and early detection of estrus is essential. Estrus in ewes is detected by vasectomized rams (teasers) wearing harnesses with crayons (see Fig. 1 in Pregnancy Diagnosis of the Ewe). Teasers should be young, healthy and free from disease. In Australia, 1 per cent of teasers are joined with the ewes the day before insemination commences, and marked ewes are removed (drafted) that afternoon. These ewes are either discarded (as precise onset

of estrus is not known) or else inseminated early the next morning to familiarize assistants with the task being undertaken and to test equipment. Only ewes with increased amounts of clear mucus are inseminated. Ewes are then drafted at 9 AM and 4 PM each day, the 9 AM draft selecting those ewes that came in estrus after the afternoon draft, and the 4 PM draft selecting those ewes that came into estrus during the day. Inseminations take place between 7 and 8 AM next morning for the 4 PM draft and between 10 AM and 3 PM the same day for the 9 AM draft. This ensures that most ewes are in their last 12 hours of estrus when inseminated, that the labor force is used efficiently and that semen collection can be satisfactorily spaced. Two teams of teasers are alternated every 3 days to ensure efficient teasing. Teasers become inefficient when an increasing number of ewes with creamy mucus are presented. This indicates that estrus has terminated and that the teasers may not have been marking ewes early in estrus.

In some countries (France and Norway) AI with frozen semen is usually conducted in conjunction with estrous synchronization. This involves the use of progestogen-impregnated intravaginal sponges plus pregnant mare serum gonadotropin (PMSG), with animals giving satisfactory pregnancy rates when inseminated 55 hours after the PMSG injection.

Ewes are normally held in a large yard with access to water between the morning and afternoon drafting to save remustering. This has no effect on fertility or body weights, provided ewes are released to good feed following the afternoon draft. When large numbers (4000 to 5000 ewes) are handled in a 17-day program, well-designed facilities are required.

INSEMINATING TECHNIQUE

Nonsurgical. The ewe is generally restrained with her hindquarters elevated. Special cradles have been devised in Australia for this purpose, although

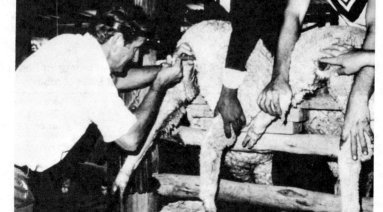

Figure 1. Method of positioning ewes for large-scale insemination program.

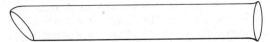

Figure 2. Diagram of Pyrex glass speculum made from a test tube (180 × 25 mm). Note lip at beveled end that is helpful in positioning entrance to cervix.

simpler facilities can usually be utilized in the normal shearing shed (Fig. 1). When large numbers have to be handled, some operators have the ewe backed up to a rail or strap, with the inseminator standing in a pit. Either way, using two catchers, ewes can be inseminated at the rate of 100 per hour.

The instruments required are simple: a speculum, a head lamp, a Pyrex inseminating tube about 6 inches long and a 1-ml syringe that is attached with a 2-inch rubber connector to the tube. Several types of speculums have been used, including the small duck bill type, a metal tube, a plastic speculum with a built in light source and a Pyrex test tube with the end cut off at an angle (Fig. 2). The latter instrument is preferred, as it can easily be cleaned, reflects light from the head lamp well, gives a good view of the cervix and allows the operator to position the entrance of the cervix with the lip of the speculum. Plastic instruments are rather more difficult to clean, whereas glassware can be boiled and oven dried. Detergents and disinfectants should be avoided unless thorough rinsing with glass-distilled water is undertaken following the initial disinfection.

The ewe is restrained to limit its movement. The speculum, lubricated with liquid paraffin, is inserted into the vagina by an assistant. The inseminator, using the 1-ml syringe, draws up 0.05 to 0.1 ml of semen into the inseminating tube, with a similar volume of air behind it. The tip of the inseminating tube is inserted into the cervical canal; this can usually be penetrated 1 to 3 cm if small-caliber nozzles are used. The long, tortuous canal and the firm cervical wall normally preclude deeper penetration. In old ewes either the annular fold of the canal may be prolapsed through the cervical opening or there may be tissue tags at the opening, making the actual entrance difficult to find. Once the nozzle

is in the canal, the plunger of the syringe is depressed, and the speculum withdrawn before the tip of the inseminating tube is removed from the cervical os. This procedure allows the walls of the vagina to collapse and the semen to be retained in the cervical canal. It is important to ensure that semen is deposited in the entrance of the cervical canal; if deposited only in the anterior vagina, larger volumes of semen and greater sperm numbers are needed to achieve comparable conception rates.

Laparotomy. High fertilization rates can be achieved when semen is deposited into the uterus, but fertility levels are disappointing as a result of high embryo mortality.[7]

The technique has found widespread use to inseminate ewes involved in embryo transfer programs.

Laparoscopy. Killeen and Caffery[4] described a technique for intrauterine insemination carried out with the aid of a laparoscope. Inseminations are carried out under local anesthesia, with the ewes restrained in a laparotomy cradle tilted to an angle of 30°. Satisfactory levels of fertility can be obtained with this method using frozen/thawed semen.[5] The problem of embryo mortality, which occurs with intrauterine insemination following laparotomy, seems to be greatly reduced. The sperm dose for intrauterine insemination is at least one third of the dose required for cervical insemination of frozen/thawed semen. Pregnancy rates over 65 per cent have been achieved with this technique using frozen/thawed semen.

TIMING OF INSEMINATIONS

It has been clearly demonstrated that ovulation occurs about 30 hours after the onset of estrus, which lasts approximately 20 to 24 hours in the ewe. Ova survive in the fallopian tube from 4 to 10 hours. Spermatozoa need several hours to capacitate in the genital tract of the ewe, but they may be recovered from the fallopian tube 5 minutes after insemination. Midestrus is therefore the optimum time for insemination, and in practical terms satisfactory results have been achieved when inseminations are performed 12 to 24 hours after the onset of estrus. If this procedure is followed, fertility levels will not be improved by reinseminating 12 hours later; a second insemination will improve conception rates

Table 2. Relationship between Types of Mucus at Time of Insemination and Percentage of Ewes Lambing

Stage of Cycle	Type of Mucus	Number of Ewes Inseminated	Ewes Lambing (Per Cent)
Early estrus	Clear and sparse	100	50
Midestrus	Clear and copious	200	68
	Cloudy and copious	103	65
Late estrus	Cloudy	108	55
	Creamy	90	32
Postestrus	"Cheeselike"	80	12

5 to 10 per cent when the first insemination is performed early in the estrous cycle.

The type of vaginal mucus present provides a good practical guide to the stage of the cycle at which insemination should be carried out (Table 2).

Ewes should be inseminated with a minimum of 50 million sperm in volumes of 0.05 to 0.1 ml of semen if satisfactory results are to be achieved (good quality ram semen should contain 150×10^6 sperm per 0.05 ml). Provided these standards are observed, good results can be achieved using diluted or undiluted semen.

Failures in sheep artificial insemination programs are mainly due to poor organization and technique. Thus, poor pretreatment of rams, failure to have adequate feed for ewes, inefficient teasing and unnecessary handling of ewes after insemination all lead to unsatisfactory results. Faults in technique commonly observed include lack of speed, failure to deposit semen in the cervical canal (particularly if too much air is used to expel the semen, since this tends to blow the semen back into the vagina) and not withdrawing the speculum before the semen is deposited.

References

1. Colas G: Fertility in the ewe after artificial insemination with fresh and frozen semen at the induced oestrus, and influence of the photoperiod on the semen quality of the ram. Live Prod Sci 6:153, 1979.
2. Colas G, Courot M: Storage of ram semen. Int Sheep Breed Cong, Muresk and Perth, 455, 1976.
3. Dunn RB: Artificial insemination of sheep. Aust Vet J 35:256, 1959.
4. Killeen ID, Caffery GJ: Uterine insemination of ewes with the aid of a laparoscope. Aust Vet J 59:95, 1982.
5. Killeen ID, Caffery GJ, Holt N: Fertility of ewes following intrauterine insemination with the aid of a laparoscope. Proc Aust Soc Reprod Biol Abstr no. 104, 1982.
6. Morrant AJ, Dun RB: Artificial insemination of sheep. Aust Vet J 36:1, 1960.
7. Salamon S, Maxwell WMC, Firth JH: Fertility of ram semen after storage at 50°C. Anim Reprod Sci 2:373, 1979.
8. Salamon S, Vissar D: Fertility of ram spermatozoa frozen and stored for five years. J Reprod Fertil 37:433, 1974.

Estrous Synchronization and Control of the Estrous Cycle

M. F. McDonald, M.Agr., Ph.D.
Massey University, Palmerston North, New Zealand

Procedures are available that will induce and synchronize estrus in young animals near puberty, in anestrous ewes during the nonbreeding season or during lactation or in cyclic ewes in the breeding season.[1,2,4] Control of breeding can also be linked with methods to increase ovulation rate and therefore alter litter size.[3] Hormonal techniques are the most widely used, but alteration of the photoperiod (by keeping animals in light-controlled rooms) or stimulating ewes by an exteroceptive factor ("social" effect of the ram; pheromone) will regulate or modify breeding activity. With housed sheep and selected breeds a combination of photoperiodic and hormonal control has allowed accelerated lambing programs to be successfully applied.

ESTROUS SYNCHRONIZATION

The number of ewes that show estrus on any one day is usually proportional to the length of the estrous cycle. Synchronization of cycles occurs when most ewes are in estrus during a restricted period, usually of 24 to 48 hours.

Successful synchronization implies a short mating period and also a high level of fertility at the synchronized ovulation. With natural mating, and depending upon flock size, additional rams will be necessary to provide a 1:10 ram-to-ewe ratio to "cover" the concentration of ewes in estrus. With artificial breeding, fertile insemination at a fixed time independent of estrus detection has practical advantages.

The main compounds used for estrous control are progestogens (progesterone, medroxyprogesterone acetate—MAP, Provera), flurogestone acetate (FGA, Cronolone), chlorgestone acetate (CAP, Chlormadinone), and prostaglandin $F_{2\alpha}$ and its synthetic analogs. The former are administered orally, by injection or subcutaneous implant or in an intravaginal device (impregnated polyurethane sponge or pessary or Silastic dispenser). The progestogens act as an artificial corpus luteum and either prolong an existing estrous cycle or are substitutes for a nonexisting one. Prostaglandins can be injected intramuscularly and will cause regression of the corpus luteum and thus shorten the existing cycle. They are ineffective in the nonbreeding season. Of all the systems available, the use of intravaginal sponges is probably most widespread.

INDUCTION OF ESTRUS IN YOUNG EWES

Puberty occurs in lambs or hoggets around 9 months of age. Breeding may be induced 2 to 3 months earlier by treatment with progestogen for 10 to 14 days and injection of 400 to 600 IU of pregnant mare serum gonadotropin (PMSG); 70 to 100 per cent of the animals will be in estrus and up to about one half will conceive. Earlier treatment may cause substantial follicular growth, but ovulation does not occur consistently. Lambs induced to ovulate may not necessarily continue cyclic activity, and this is related to the age of the hogget and the time within the year when treated.

The use of an intravaginal sponge to supply the progestogen can be used with hoggets, but this method is sometimes not as suitable as it is with mature ewes, owing to the difficulty of inserting and removing the device, especially with small-sized animals.

INDUCTION OF ESTRUS IN MATURE EWES IN THE NONBREEDING SEASON

Sheep that are seasonally anestrus will respond to progestogen given over 10 to 14 days and 500 to 800 IU of PMSG injected at the time of withdrawal of progestogen or within 24 hours. The dose of PMSG should be related to the time within the season when the treatment is given, the breed of ewe and the required ovulation rate. In commercial sheep practice when the ewe is expected to carry the pregnancy and rear her offspring, only low or moderate ovulation rates are required, with one to three lambs born as a result. Excessive PMSG stimulation can result in variable spread of ovulation, higher than desirable ovulation rates, large litters with low survival rates in the small lambs and, frequently, failure to conceive among many ewes.

Lactation anestrus will occur in ewes lambing at any time of the year. In ewes that normally lamb in the late winter or spring months lactation anestrus will merge with that caused by passage into the nonbreeding season. Out-of-season lambing is still followed by anestrus, but cyclic activity will resume while the ewe is still lactating and nursing its offspring. Progestogen and PMSG (600 to 800 IU) treatment, similar to that for the seasonally anestrous ewe, can be used, although conception rates are usually lower than in seasonally anestrous ewes and lower in spring-lambing than in autumn-lambing sheep.

The conception rate to the induced estrus increases with a lengthening interval between parturition and insemination but rarely exceeds 40 per cent until 6 weeks postpartum. It is also influenced by the ewe breed, number of lambs suckled, the level of lactation and whether or not a cycle of ovarian activity has occurred prior to insemination. These constraints to breeding the ewe early in lactation inhibit the development of accelerated lambing programs, so that lambing at 6-month intervals is impractical. Instead, the production of three crops of lambs every 2 years is feasible using suitable breeds with a short nonbreeding season and some hormonal treatment.

ADVANCEMENT OF THE BREEDING SEASON

Promoting an earlier start to the breeding season is often sought for reasons of management in relation to feed supply and for the marketing of lambs.

In the transition period from anestrus the ewe can be synchronized by progestogen with or without PMSG. The combined treatment will cause estrus in most ewes. With progestogen alone the response will be increased when rams are joined with the ewes at the end of treatment and will exert a stimulatory effect resulting in ovulation.

The sudden introduction of rams to a flock will frequently synchronize estrus in a high proportion of the ewes. The synchronization caused by the "ram effect" is less predictable than that achieved after hormone treatment, but the ram effect technique requires little cost or effort, and fertility rates at induced estrus are higher. Receptive ewes will ovulate without estrus within 3 to 4 days and will show estrus 17 to 24 days after joining. The synchronization is not tight, owing to premature regression of the corpora lutea in about 50 per cent of the ewes. This leads to another ovulation and a second peak of estrus 22 to 24 days after joining. Priming with progestogen before "teasing" ensures estrus, ovulation and a normal life span of all corpora lutea.

SYNCHRONIZATION OF ESTRUS WITHIN THE BREEDING SEASON

In the cyclic ewe estrus can be regulated after the ovary has been released from the suppressive influence of progestogen or following destruction of the corpus luteum by use of prostaglandin $F_{2\alpha}$. A major problem of either method is the low conception rate recorded at the estrus immediately after treatment. This is primarily caused by poor sperm transport and survival and is exacerbated by low sperm number and artificial insemination. It may be partly overcome by using a 200×10^6 dose of sperm in a dense inseminate. A more practical solution is to ensure mating at second estrus when synchronization is still adequate and conception rates are normal.

Use of Progestogen. This treatment needs to be given for at least 14 days to block the discharge of ovulatory luteinizing hormone (LH) effectively, and then synchronized estrus will occur within 2 to 3 days. Rams should be joined with ewes at withdrawal or preferably 24 hours later. A small dose of PMSG (500 IU) at the end of progestogen therapy will improve the precision of ovulation control. In the absence of estrus detection the ewes should be inseminated once at 54 hours or twice at 48 and 60 hours after the sponge is withdrawn. About 60 per cent of ewes inseminated once and 70 per cent inseminated twice will lamb as a result of the synchronized ovulation.

Use of Prostaglandins. These will not induce luteolysis prior to days 4 to 5 of the cycle. Thus, to ensure that all ewes are at a responsive stage, two injections spaced about 9 days apart are necessary. The ewes are in estrus about 2 to 4 days after the second injection, but fertility at this time is variable and often low. An increase in fertility is obtained at the subsequent estrus, which is still adequately synchronized. The use of double-injection therapy is more costly than progestogen sponge treatment and offers no real advantage, especially if ewes are not mated until the second estrus after treatment. A further method involves a combination of progestogen for 8 days and prostaglandin injected at withdrawal; this treatment will synchronize estrus and sometimes allow for a better conception rate than following a double-injection prostaglandin regimen.

INCREASE IN OVULATION RATE AND MULTIPLE BIRTHS

Multiple ovulations can be induced in the ewe through two methods—gonadotropin therapy and steroid hormone immunization. Both alter the level of follicular activity in the ovaries and modify the ovulation rate.[4]

Gonadotropin Therapy. PMSG and horse anterior pituitary (HAP) extract administered near the end of the cycle are effective in elevating the ovulation rate. Optimal results occur when PMSG is given on days 12 to 13 of the natural cycle. Pretreatment with progestogens for synchronization requires the PMSG to be given at the end of progestogen administration. Effective dose rates range from 600 to 1500 IU, mainly in relation to the size of the ovulatory response sought. High doses may cause excessive luteinization of follicles and inhibition of ovulation.

Treatment with HAP should be given over 3 days, commencing on day 12 of the cycle; the quantity to be injected should be assessed on the basis of a preliminary trial, as the potency of the material can vary markedly.

The superovulatory response of mature animals alters with breed, age, live weight, stage of estrous cycle, season of year, plane of nutrition and postpartum interval. Individual responses to standard doses of gonadotropin therefore will be variable, especially when more than 1000 IU of gonadotropin are given. Responses to repeated treatment will decline because of ovarian refractoriness. An in-

crease in complete failure of fertilization in some ewes following superovulation is a practical limitation to the use of high-dose rates.

Steroid Hormone Immunization. This technique relies on the production of antibodies, which temporarily inactivate some of the steroid hormone normally produced by the ovary. As a result, there is less feedback to the hypothalamus, and extra gonadotropin is produced, which causes additional ovulations and more multiple births (mostly twins). Commercially developed immunogens exert good control of the immune response. These cause a high proportion of the ewes to produce an extra ovulation, giving a lambing percentage increase of 20 to 30 per cent and also avoiding excessive antibody production that results in suppression of estrous behavior and even failure of ovulation and barren ewes.

Immunization can be induced following two injections 4 weeks apart and with a further 3 to 4 weeks to allow for development of the maximum ovulatory response when the ewes should be mated. Elevated ovulation rates persist for about 3 months. In subsequent years a single booster injection is required 1 month before mating occurs.

The effectiveness of immunization treatments needs to be examined for different breeds in a variety of environments and management systems. It appears that the responses of ovulation rate to immunization are additive to those effects caused by breed, level of nutrition and feed ingredient. Commercial immunogens should be sought that will provide moderate and consistent rises in ovulation rate.

References

1. Lamond DR: Animal Breeding Abstracts 32:269, 1964.
2. Robinson TJ: The Control of the Ovarian Cycle in the Sheep. Sydney, Sydney University Press, 1967.
3. Scaramuzzi RJ, Cox RI, Hoskinson RM: Proceedings World Congress on Sheep and Beef Cattle Breeding (New Zealand) 1:359, 1982.
4. Thimonier J: Proceedings World Congress on Sheep and Beef Cattle Breeding (New Zealand) 1:351, 1982.

Surgical Procedures of the Reproductive Tract of Sheep

M. D. Copland, B.V.Sc., M.A.C.V.Sc., M.R.C.V.S.

Department of Agriculture, Animal Health Laboratory, South Perth, Western Australia

CASTRATION

Most ram lambs not required for breeding are castrated to facilitate controlled breeding and to produce a more valuable carcass. The operation is usually performed at the time the tail is docked by using rubber rings, the Burdizzo instrument or a knife. In general, one specific technique is no more advantageous than any other. Partial methods of castration have been described but appear to offer little practical advantage.

The necessity for castrating ram lambs destined for the fat lamb market is questionable, since these lambs are slaughtered before puberty and, particularly if feed is not limiting, the intact lamb produces the heaviest and leanest carcass.

Castration of the Ram Lamb

Rubber Ring Method. Using an Elastrator, rubber rings are placed around the neck of the scrotum, dorsal to the testis. Avascular necrosis ensues, and the scrota and testes slough after 3 to 4 weeks. This method requires minimal preparation but incurs a greater risk of tetanus and the possibility of fly strike. Faulty technique may result in only partial castration. The older a lamb is when castrated with rubber rings, the greater is the risk of failure and the possibility of reduced growth rates.

Burdizzo Method. The Burdizzo instrument effectively deprives the testes of their blood supply by crushing the spermatic cords. Each cord is held in a lateral position and placed between the jaws of the instrument, which are then closed. Care should be taken not to include the median septum, as this may result in sloughing of the scrotum. Preferably each cord is crushed twice.

The method has the advantage that the skin remains unbroken and the procedure is bloodless. Failures may be common if the instrument is improperly adjusted or is in a state of disrepair.

Open Method. A sharp knife or scalpel is used to incise the scrotal sac and vaginal tunic along their posterior and ventral margins. Each testis is then extruded and removed, either by scraping and then severing the cord with the knife or by pulling.

Untoward sequelae that may follow this method include local infection, hemorrhage and possible fly strike. Such sequelae may be minimized by adopting sound hygiene procedures and by castrating only young lambs in clean temporary yards.

Castration of the Adult Ram

Adult rams may be castrated with the Burdizzo instrument in a manner similar to that described for the lamb or by the open method. When using the open method, local analgesia or general anesthesia may be used. General anesthesia may be obtained with pentobarbital, 20 mg/kg, or with the shorter-acting but more expensive steroid CT1341 (Saffan), 0.3 ml/kg. Hemostasis is essential because of the greater blood supply to the adult testis. This may be achieved either by using crushing emasculators or preferably by using a transfixing ligature around the spermatic vessels. The effect of either method on subsequent performance has not been evaluated.

VASECTOMY

Vasectomized rams are used to detect ewes in estrus and to provide ewes with a ram stimulus prior to the onset of the *physiological* breeding season.

To implement an artificial insemination program it is necessary to detect ewes in estrus. The number of vasectomized rams required is approximately 2 per cent of the ewes to be inseminated. After vasectomy, the rams are divided into two groups that are then used alternately every 3 days.

Many studies have shown that the practice of joining vasectomized rams with breeding ewes for 14 days prior to the joining with fertile rams leads to an early onset of the breeding season and to a degree of synchronization during the resultant lambing. The degree of synchronization may not always be predictable because of differences between years in the onset of physiological breeding activity. Claims have been advanced that vasectomized rams are not as effective as entire rams in producing this ram stimulus.

Even though sperm may be seen in the ejaculate of vasectomized rams for some months after the operation, the rams are rendered sterile within 2 weeks of surgery. Farmers should be advised not to use the rams during these 2 weeks and to identify them permanently to avoid any confusion between them and intact rams. The veterinarian should consider the possibility of subsequent litigation and, if

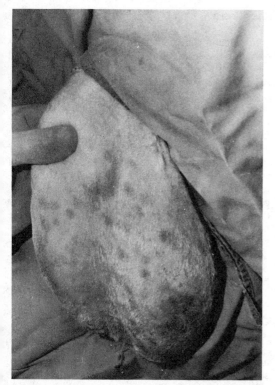

Figure 1. The posterior aspect of the testes, showing the left spermatic cord restrained by the operator's left hand prior to incising the skin.

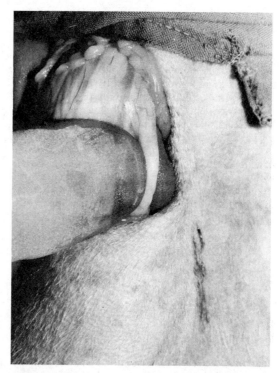

Figure 2. The vas deferens immobilized between the index finger and thumb prior to incising the vaginal tunic.

necessary, should take the precaution of obtaining histologic confirmation of the tissue removed during the operation.

The ease with which some rams may be sterilized by injecting sclerosing agents into the epididymis continues to attract attention. However, the reliability of the technique and the future welfare of the ram require further investigation before this technique can be recommended.

Operative Procedure

An assistant secures the ram in right lateral recumbency with the left hind leg extended and restrained anteriorly. After the usual skin preparation, local anesthesia is infiltrated into the spermatic cords and the skin over their caudal margins. The left side of the scrotal neck is then firmly grasped between the thumb and the fingers of the operator's left hand (Fig. 1). A 5-cm incision is made through the anesthetized skin, dartos muscle and fascia. Any loose fatty tissue present is bluntly dissected away from the cord, which is then exteriorized using the index finger of the operator's left hand. By rolling the cord between the thumb and index finger, the vas deferens will be felt as a thick-walled tube that can be isolated and immobilized beneath the vaginal tunic (Fig. 2). A small incision (1 cm) is made through the tunic over the vas deferens, and a loop

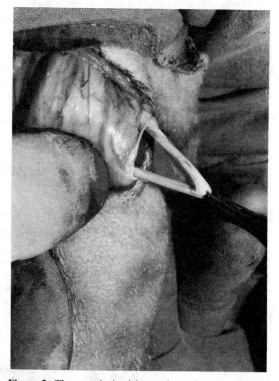

Figure 3. The exteriorized loop of vas deferens prior to ligation and removal.

of the duct is withdrawn (Fig. 3). Two ligatures approximately 3 cm apart are placed around the duct, and the segment in between is removed. After replacing the cord, the skin is sutured. Similarly, a section of the right deferent duct is removed by using the right hand to hold and immobilize the duct and the left hand to incise the tunic.

With experience this procedure may be expedited by locating and immobilizing the ducts externally by palpation through the scrotal skin. All tissues external to the duct are then excised over a distance of 1 to 2 cm and a loop of the duct is removed without having to exteriorize the spermatic cord from the incision (Fig. 4). A cranial midscrotal approach has been described, and it is claimed that such an approach simplifies this operation.

CESAREAN SECTION

The literature contains a number of references to the cesarean operation in the ewe. These show that in this species the operation was developed primarily for the relief of ewes suffering from partial dilation of the cervix (ringwomb) and less commonly for other obstetric complications that preclude successful delivery per vaginam. The latter include relative and absolute fetal oversize, emphysema, fetal monsters and hydrallantois.

In many cases, because of the high cost of the operation, the economic benefit to the farmer is only marginal. Indirectly, this may have the advantage that the veterinarian is more likely to be presented with the ewe at the clinic, where better facilities may exist, rather than having to carry out the procedure on the farm.

Vaginal prolapse and pregnancy toxemia have been listed as other possible indications for cesarean section; however, greater success and economic benefit may accompany the induction of parturition with glucocorticoids in these cases.

Anesthesia

In selecting an anesthetic technique the indications for the operation, the available facilities and the viability of the lambs need to be considered. All general anesthetic techniques incur some risk of regurgitation, and many depress the fetus. General anesthesia may, however, be the method of choice when obtaining gnotobiotic lambs by hysterectomy. In the author's experience the use of the steroidal anesthetic CT1341 (Saffan), 0.2 to 0.3 ml/kg, for the induction of anesthesia, together with minimal concentrations of halothane and oxygen for maintenance, is accompanied by little depression. In general, however, local analgesia is preferred, and the administration of a local anesthetic by any one of several techniques such as local infiltration, inverted L block, paravertebral injections and epidural injections have all proved satisfactory for this purpose. Should it be necessary, tranquilization may be achieved with diazepam (Valium) 0.2 mg/kg.

Operative Procedure

The available facilities and the viability, position and number of lambs present at the time of surgery should be considered when selecting the site for the abdominal incision. Most surgeons would probably utilize an approach through the left flank, although the midline, paramedian, right and left dorsoventral and oblique abdominal incisions have all been successfully used.

Adopting normal surgical procedures, an incision of approximately 15 cm is made through the abdominal wall and into the peritoneal cavity. The most accessible extremity (often the hind limb) or the head of the lamb is then palpated within the uterus and gently manipulated through the incision. The uterine wall is incised in a relatively avascular region, avoiding any cotyledons. The incision should be made over a sufficient length to enable easy manipulation and rapid delivery of the lamb. Pro-

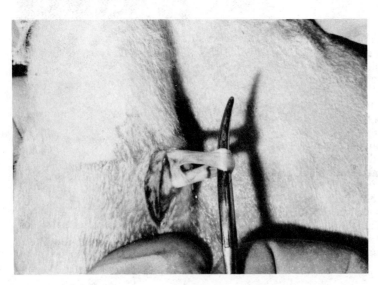

Figure 4. The posterior aspect of the testes, showing the small incision required to exteriorize a loop of the vas deferens by the alternative method.

longed manipulation of the lamb in utero should be avoided, as this may stimulate the lamb to breathe amniotic fluid, which is often contaminated with meconium. When more than one lamb is present, an attempt is made to deliver the remaining lambs through the same incision. If this proves difficult, the other uterine horn is incised. Unless readily removable, the fetal membranes are left in situ.

The uterine and abdominal incisions are then closed in accord with general surgical principles.

Lamb Resuscitation

After the lamb is delivered, amniotic fluid is "milked" from the muzzle, pressure is applied over the thorax and any fluid present in the pharyngeal region is aspirated. If the lamb does not breathe after 2 minutes, an endotracheal tube (4 mm diameter) is inserted, and intermittent positive ventilation is initiated. A severely depressed lamb is characterized by failure to breathe, a heart rate of less than 100/minute and poor withdrawal reflexes. These lambs are usually acidotic, and the intravenous administration of sodium bicarbonate (5 mEq) and glucose (5 ml of a 10 per cent solution) should be considered. Once breathing, the lamb is dried, placed in a warm environment (37°C) and allowed to suckle its mother or, if this is not possible, is fed colostrum.

Postoperative Sequelae

Included in the literature are reports of 191 ewes subjected to cesarean section because of obstetric complications. Seventy-six per cent of these ewes survived the operation, and 69 per cent of 85 lambs alive at delivery were successfully reared. It is likely that better results could be anticipated in ewes subjected to elective cesareans.

Post-mortem findings for 13 ewes that died after the operation showed severe endometritis in every case and delayed uterine involution in most cases. Other findings recorded were delayed uterine healing, retained placenta and septic peritonitis.

No records are available regarding the subsequent breeding performance of ewes after cesarean section although, as with cattle, some depression in fertility is to be anticipated.

Suggested Readings

1. Copland MD: The effects of CT1341, thiopentone and induction-delivery time on the blood-gas and acid-base status of lambs delivered by caesarean operation and on the onset of respiration. Aust Vet J 53:436, 1977.
2. Hopwood JB: Bacterial flora of the genital tract of ewes undergoing caesarean section. J Comp Path 66:187, 1956.
3. Lofstedt RM: Vasectomy in ruminants: A cranial midscrotal approach. JAVMA 181:373, 1982.
4. Louw BP, Marx FE, Yates GD: The influence of vasectomized rams on the lambing pattern of spring-mated Corriedale ewes. S Afr J Anim Sci 4:167, 1974.
5. Torell DT, Duelke BD, Bon Durant RH: Sterilising lambs by chemical sclerosing of epididymi. J Anim Sci 49: Suppl 1:204, 1979.
6. Trengrove RB: Vasectomy of rams under field conditions. J S Afr Vet Med Ass 36:119, 1965.

SECTION

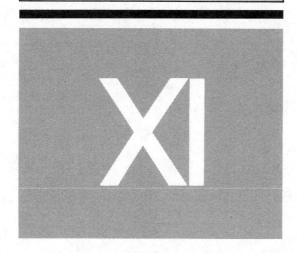

XI

PORCINE

John P. Hurtgen, D.V.M., Ph.D.

Consulting Editor

*Additional pertinent information found in the first
edition of Current Therapy in Theriogenology:*

Physical Examination of the Sow and Gilt

Wayne L. Singleton, Ph.D.
Purdue University, West Lafayette, Indiana

Careful physical examination of females is a useful tool in selecting potentially fertile breeding animals. Gilts with structural or genitalia abnormalities can be culled prior to breeding, thus eliminating costs associated with the development of these animals to breeding age. A physical examination along with a herd history derived from records of previous management, reproductive ability and health conditions are helpful in the diagnosis of reproductive failure in individual animals or in breeding groups within a herd. When indicated, internal reproductive organs should be recovered from slaughtered animals for a thorough examination. The clinician can often gain useful information from such an examination when other procedures fail.

EXTERNAL EXAMINATION

Structural Soundness. With the trend toward environmentally controlled rearing and breeding, structural soundness of females is becoming increasingly important. Soundness in replacement gilts is especially significant, since most structural faults and weaknesses are aggravated with age and confinement rearing. Special attention should be given to selecting gilts free from foot, leg and joint problems, which may impair their future reproductivity. A moderate slope to the pasterns provides the animal with a cushion to the foot and leg joints, enabling her to cope with solid surfaces in confinement.

Gilts and sows with hoof cracks, sole bruises or other foot problems should be culled because attempted treatments are often unsuccessful. Such problems may arise from abrasive or damp, slick flooring. These and other traits of unsoundness may have genetic implications, and certain genetic lines may be more predisposed to them than others.

Too much slope in the rump area tends to make the animal more prone to unsoundness as she matures. A steep rump also displaces the vulva to a low position and angle so that boars often experience difficulties in entering the sow during mating.

Extreme muscling has been implicated as a characteristic of some females with reproductive problems—mainly delayed puberty, low conception rate, farrowing difficulty and poor mothering ability. Again, the acceptable degree of muscling in females is difficult to define, but in general, females should be selected primarily for soundness and productivity.

External Genitalia. Observing the vulva of replacement gilts at 5½ to 6 months of age can help detect potentially sterile or slow-breeding females. The most commonly observed abnormality is the infantile vulva. The infantile vulva is usually accompanied by small, prepubertal ovaries and uterine horns. This condition is more frequently observed in gilts reared in confinement, but it occasionally occurs in females reared in pasture. The incidence of inactive ovaries varies within and between herds. For example, puberty occurs later for Yorkshire, Duroc and other meat-type breeds as compared with the Landrace and Large White breeds. Puberty is also delayed in gilts that reach 6 months of age during summer months as compared with winter months. Onset of puberty is hastened by exposure of gilts to boars, relocation to different pens or facilities, outside rearing and transport stress. However, gilts with delayed puberty seem to respond less well to these stimuli than expected.

Treatment of gilts with 500 to 1000 IU of pregnant mare serum gonadotropin (PMSG) has also shown success in some herds. Treatment with exogenous hormones is not encouraged because of the possible implications involved in propagating females predisposed to this problem.

The dorsally "tipped vulva" is another abnormality that is less frequently observed (Fig. 1). Its relationship to future reproductive potential is unknown. Boars may experience difficulty in servicing gilts having this trait. Such gilts should be eliminated as potential breeding herd replacements.

Injuries of the vulva may occur from fighting or at parturition. Unless they are severe, they generally do not contribute to future reproductive problems.

Atresia ani, or imperforate anus, is a congenital defect observed in all breeds. In gilts the rectum and vagina may be joined, forming a rectovaginal fistula just anterior to the vulva. Males die because they are unable to defecate. Gilts defecate via the vulva opening. This condition is easily detected in newborn pigs. Inheritance of atresia ani is thought to be controlled by two pairs of dominant genes.

Occasionally, an unusually large percentage of females within a group is observed to have red, swollen vulvas, typical of females in estrus. This observation, when coupled with mammary development in nonpregnant females and barrows, indicates the presence of exogenous estrogenic substances such as zearalonone in the feed. Diagnosis is often difficult because the feed source has been completely used before the effects are observed.

Mammary System. A sound underline is a fundamental characteristic to consider when selecting gilts as herd replacements. The underline should have at least six functional, well-developed and evenly spaced teats on each side, with three in front

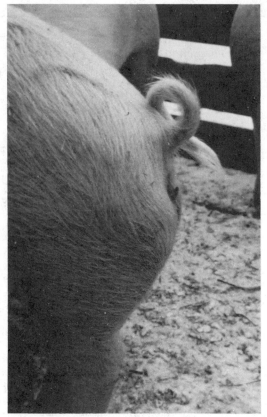

Figure 1. Tipped or "sky-hooked" vulva.

of the navel (Fig. 2). Gilts with a blind teat (one that does not fully develop), a pin nipple or an inverted nipple should not be considered as replacement animals (Fig. 3). Constant selection is required to maintain acceptable underlines in a breeding herd. Selection can be initiated soon after birth by observing underlines of gilt pigs. Gilts with sound underlines and adequate teat numbers farrowed from productive dams can be ear marked for consideration as potential replacements when final selections are made at 5 to 6 months of age. Although

not proved experimentally, abrasive concrete flooring in farrowing crates or pens has been implicated as a causative factor in herds experiencing a larger than normal incidence of underline problems in young gilts.

At the time of weaning the mammary system of lactating sows should also be evaluated for the presence of abscesses and teat occlusion caused by nursing or flooring injuries. Older sows should maintain 10 functional mammary glands; otherwise, piglet viability and growth rates during subsequent lactations will decrease.

INTERNAL EXAMINATION OF THE REPRODUCTIVE TRACT

Surveys conducted in the United States and Europe indicate that 5 to 10 per cent of all virgin gilts have abnormal reproductive tracts. Heritabilities of many abnormalities have not been estimated. Reproductive tracts from infertile animals or problem breeders are seldom recovered at slaughter. However, in herds with a high incidence of reproductive failure that are not diagnosed by other methods, examination at slaughter is recommended. Females should be tattooed prior to slaughter for identification so that the individual animal's reproductive history can be related to the observed reproductive tract disorder. The normal slaughter procedure is to sever the tract by a cut through the vagina. The abattoir personnel will usually remove the tract intact if requested. If pathologic study is indicated, a heavy string should be tied around the posterior end of the vagina to prevent contamination. The intact tract is then placed into a plastic bag with a numbered card corresponding to the tattoo identification. Specimens should then be packed in ice and transported to the laboratory for study.

The presence and size of follicles, corpora lutea and cysts should be noted and recorded for each ovary. Any adhesions surrounding the ovaries or within the ovarian bursa should be noted. The size of the uterine horns should be recorded. Externally,

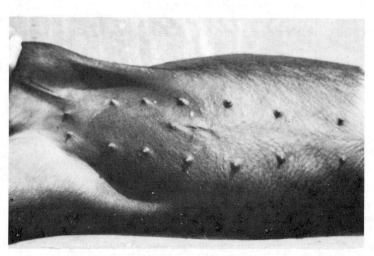

Figure 2. Four-month-old gilt with excellent teat placement. Note presence of three teats on each side in front of the navel.

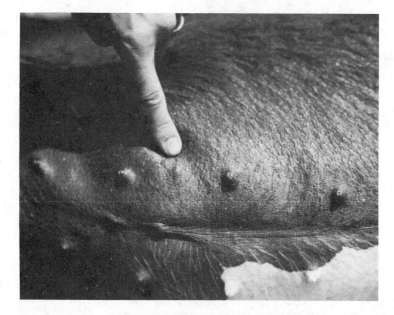

Figure 3. Pin nipple.

each oviduct and uterine horn to the vagina should be traced, with the practitioner looking for occlusions, missing parts or adhesions (Fig. 4). If pathologic study is not indicated, an insemination apparatus may be used to inject fluid into the tract to facilitate detection of occlusions. After gross examination has been completed, open the tract beginning at the vulva and continue through the cervix and each horn. Examine the uterine endometrium and note the presence and characteristics of fluid or embryonic tissue.

If bacteriologic status of the uterus is desired, the uterus must be opened in a sterile manner. Full-thickness (¼ inch) pieces of uterus or oviducts obtained at various sites should be fixed in Bouin's solution.

Occasionally, it is helpful to determine the serologic status of females at slaughter. Using a syringe and small-gauge needle, fluid can be aspirated from follicles on the ovaries. This fluid is then submitted for serologic analysis in the same manner as that for serum. In most cases, the follicular fluid would be tested for antibodies to pseudorabies virus, porcine parvovirus, enteroviruses, leptospirosis and brucellosis.

ANATOMIC AND HORMONAL ABNORMALITIES

Hydrosalpinx and Pyosalpinx. Hydrosalpinx and pyosalpinx refer to distention of oviducts with clear fluid and puslike material, respectively. These conditions occur more frequently in gilts than in sows and are caused by an occlusion or distention of the oviducts that blocks the passage of spermatozoa and ova. It is thought that these conditions, as well as most other defects, result from abnormal embryonic

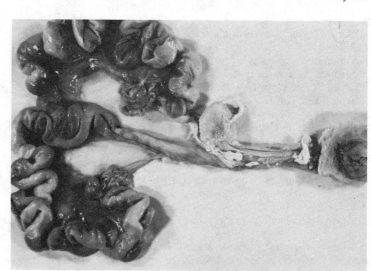

Figure 4. Intact reproductive organs from normal cycling gilt.

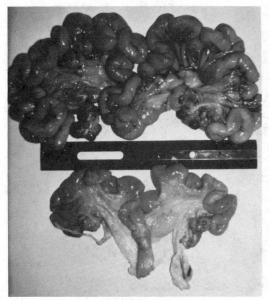

Figure 5. Reproductive tracts from two 8-month-old gilts of the same age and from identical management conditions. *Top,* Normally developed tract from gilt that experienced two previous estrous cycles.

development and may be hereditary. Affected females have regular estrous cycles but are prone to repeat breeding and reduced litter size. If lesions are bilateral, affected females are sterile. Recent reports on the reproductive pathology of repeat breeders suggest that occlusion of the oviducts is the most commonly observed abnormality. Patency of the oviducts should be tested by cannulating the infundibulum with the end of a plastic syringe and infusing water, saline or a dye.

Segmental Aplasia. Segmental aplasia may occur at any position along the uterine horn but most commonly occurs near the uterine body. Occasionally, an entire uterine horn may be absent. Afflicted females will cycle normally. It is possible to have pregnancy in the patent side, but litter size is usually reduced.

Blind, Double and Missing Cervix. These abnormalities occur infrequently. Females with either condition cycle normally. If part or all of the cervix is missing, the female is sterile. Pregnancy can be achieved in females with a double cervix.

Infantilism. This is a common abnormality and is generally but not always associated with confinement-reared gilts (Fig. 5). The presence of a very small vulva and the absence of estrus are suggestive of this condition. The infantile tract is approximately 30 per cent of the size of a tract from a normally cycling gilt. The ovaries are hypoplastic and nonfunctional, with numerous small follicles and no corpora lutea. This condition is common in gilts with delayed puberty or gilts less than 6 months of age.

Adhesions. Adhesions have been observed in all areas of the reproductive tract but more frequently in the oviduct and ovarian bursa. They are generally

associated with intraperitoneal injections given to baby pigs or improper injections at older ages. Cyclic activity is normal. Reduced litter size and infertility are frequently noted.

Intersexuality. Intersex pigs occur infrequently but are more predominant in the Yorkshire breed (Fig. 6). They are usually genetic females in which a portion of the reproductive tract has differentiated into its male homolog. A majority of these conditions are inherited, with the mode of inheritance thought to be autosomal recessive accompanied by modifier genes. Exact classification must be done by combined chromosomal and anatomic study. Some individuals can be distinguished by the presence of an ovotestis, which may be internal or external, whereas others may have a prominent clitoris and "sky hook" vulva. Some intersexes show male characteristics such as tusk development and mounting behavior. When possible, a pedigree study of such animals should be made and possible carriers removed from the breeding herd.

Cystic Ovaries. Much remains to be learned about cystic ovaries in swine. Cystic ovaries originate in a complete or partial failure of ovulation. Therefore, cystic follicles may appear on the same ovary as normal-appearing corpora lutea. Although sows may be pregnant when one or more follicles fail to ovulate, fertility is reduced. Luteinization of the

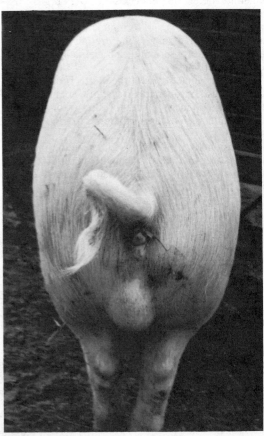

Figure 6. Intersex with descended ovotestis and "sky-hooked" vulva.

anovulatory follicle is common. Cysts may vary in size from 12 to 50 mm. Serum progesterone is usually lower than that of the mid-diestrous female. Affected females may be anestrous or exhibit near normal estrous cycle patterns. Under practical conditions, diagnosis in the living animal is difficult or impossible except by ovarian palpation per rectum. This procedure is difficult to perform in swine. Most attempts at treatment are ineffective.

SUMMARY

Systematic physical examination of the female and female reproductive tract and careful consideration of herd history records are useful when selecting potential breeding animals and when attempting to diagnose reproductive failures.

Clinical examination of the internal reproductive organs recovered from nonbreeders at slaughter is helpful in cases of anestrus, repeat breeding and

reduced litter size. Serum hormone analyses are a useful adjunct to slaughterhouse evaluations in problem herds.

Because of the apparent genetic basis for many of the structural and anatomic abnormalities that impair reproductivity, treatment is usually not attempted. The importance of this discussion is not only in the treatment of such problems but also in creating an awareness of them so that the veterinarian and swine producer can improve upon their ability to select potentially sound, productive females and to detect and to cull sterile or problem breeders.

Suggested Readings

1. Perry JS, Pomeroy RW: Abnormalities of the reproductive tract of the sow. J Agri Sci 47:238, 1956.
2. Rasbeck NO: A review of the causes of reproductive failure in swine. Br Vet J 125:599, 1969.
3. Wrathall AE: An approach to breeding problems in sows. Vet Rec 89:61, 1971.

Sexual Development and Initiation of Puberty in the Pig

G. D. Dial, D.V.M., Ph.D.
H. D. Hilley, D.V.M., Ph.D.
K. L. Esbenshade, Ph.D.
North Carolina State University, Raleigh, North Carolina

In the commercial swine industry herd replacements are reared solely for reproduction. Delays in the onset of puberty of replacement animals result in delays in the commencement of their productivity. Delayed puberty can potentially disrupt the breeding stock replacement schedule and thereby either cause less productive females to be retained in the herd longer than desirable or lead to less than optimal numbers of animals being bred and farrowed. Disruptions of the replacement schedule also cause an increased cost for maintaining nonproducing and poor-producing breeding stock in the herd. Because the offspring must bear the maintenance expenses of the breeding herd, production becomes less profitable. It is, thus, usually desirable to promote and, in some cases, to control the onset of puberty. This article will emphasize techniques for the practical management of the prepubertal gilt and boar for the optimization of reproductive potential.

THE GILT

Maturation of the Reproductive System

Although puberty is an abrupt process in the gilt, the pubertal commencement of ovarian and estrous activity is preceded by gradual maturational changes in each of the components of the hypothalamo-hypophyseal-ovarian axis. These maturational changes commence prior to birth, continue at differing rates and culminate in a series of endocrine events resulting in the onset of puberty.

Ovaries. At midgestation, all of the ova of the fetal gilt are concentrated in discreet areas of the ovaries, called egg nests. There is a progressive decrease in the percentage of egg nests as fetal age increases, until the nests are seldom observed after 20 days of postnatal age. Egg nests are replaced during mid to late gestation by undifferentiated primordial follicles. Primordial follicles begin differentiating into primary follicles (having a single layer of squamous epithelium around the oocyte) at approximately 70 days post coitum. Secondary follicles (with two layers of cuboidal cells around the oocyte) become differentiated at about the time of birth and increase steadily in number postnatally. Tertiary follicles (multilayered structures with antra) do not become evident until 40 to 60 days of age. Coincident with development of antral follicles is an abrupt increase in ovarian size. From about 70 to 110 days of age the ovaries of prepubertal gilts undergo a period of rapid follicular development and become able to respond to exogenous gonadotropins with increased steroidogenesis and with ovulation. The number of small antral follicles (1 to 3 mm in diameter) increases linearly between 70 and 110 days of age, after which time their numbers decrease. This decrease is accompanied by the rapid development of large, antral follicles (> 3 mm). These reach their highest number at approximately 140 days of age and then remain relatively constant until puberty.

Reproductive Tract. From birth to 70 days of age, there is a slow but linear increase in the weights and lengths of the uteri and oviducts that corresponds closely to the increase in body weight. During this period, the uterine wall and endometrium increase in thickness, and the uterine glands begin their differentiation. An accelerated rate of growth commences at approximately 70 to 80 days and continues until puberty. At puberty there is an abrupt increase in the size of the entire female reproductive tract. Additional increases in the size of the uterus occur at the subsequent estrous cycles and during gestation. Even though puberty seldom occurs prior to 150 days, the morphologic development of the uterine glands, endometrium and myometrium is completed by approximately 120 days of age. (The endocrine events associated with puberty are discussed in the article The Clinical Endocrinology of Reproduction in the Pig.)

Factors Affecting Onset of Puberty

Age, Weight and Growth Rate. The weight and growth rate of pigs are usually a reflection of age and are influenced largely by genotype and nutrition. Because age, weight and growth rate are intimately related, it is difficult to distinguish their relative contributions to the onset of puberty. Nonetheless, there appears to be a consensus among researchers that chronologic age is a more accurate indicator of sexual maturity than weight or growth rate. Although the results may be confounded by nutritional effects, one study has reported that when gilts were fed at rates that allowed them to reach the same weight at different ages, females of 135 days of age took substantially longer to reach puberty after boar exposure than gilts of 160 or 190 days.

Genetics. Breed and mating systems have long been recognized to influence the age of puberty. As shown in Figure 1, some breeds, such as the Landrace, consistently reach puberty at a younger age than other breeds. From study to study, however, there is a considerable variation in the relative rates at which the other breeds achieve puberty. The variability between genetic lines within a breed makes absolute ranking of the various breeds difficult. Because of heterosis, crossbred gilts generally reach puberty at an earlier age than their purebred counterparts. Since the heritability of age of puberty has been estimated to be approximately 0.30, there appears to be a genetic basis for selection for this trait.

Boar Exposure. The exposure of peripubertal gilts to boars can accelerate the maturational changes leading to the onset of puberty. When gilts are introduced to boars at about 160 days of age, the majority commence estrous activity within 2 to 3 weeks. The exposure of gilts to boars at less than 140 days results in an increased interval from first boar contact to puberty and no advancement of the age of puberty. The introduction of gilts to boars at greater than 170 days of age causes gilts to reach puberty at an older age relative to gilts of 140 to 170 days. It appears that boar introduction when gilts are approximately 160 days of age minimizes both the interval from first boar contact to puberty and the age at which gilts reach puberty.

The type of male exposure influences the age of onset of puberty in gilts. Females that are reared with intact boars reach puberty earlier than when raised with barrows. Daily boar exposure for 30 minutes appears to be just as effective and, in some cases, more effective than continuous exposure for the induction of puberty. Boars that are 11 months of age or older are more effective in inducing puberty in gilts than younger males.

Pheromones produced by the boar are potent sensory stimuli for the gilt. In fact, gilts that are unable to perceive pheromones because of olfactory bulbectomies commence puberty at a time coincident with intact gilts not exposed to boars but delayed relative to intact females introduced to the boar.

Management Stimuli. When gilts of about pubertal age are removed from familiar environments, moved to the breeding herd and exposed to boars, estrus often occurs within a few days. Typically, 20 to 60 per cent of the prepubertal gilts show synchronous estrus within 2 weeks of movement. As shown in Table 1, the highest percentage of gilts

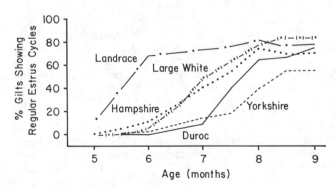

Figure 1. Influence of breed on the age of commencement of estrous activity in gilts reared in confinement. (Redrawn from Christenson RK, Ford JJ: J Anim Sci 52:821, 1981.)

Table 1. The Influence of Different Forms of Management Stimuli on the Initiation of Puberty in 165-Day-Old Gilts

No. of Gilts	Mixing	Management Stress Transport	Relocation	Boar Exposure	Percentage Reaching Puberty within 10 Days
25	+	−	−	−	7
25	+	+	−	−	8
25	+	+	+	−	28
25	+	+	+	+	87

From Zimmerman et al.: J Anim Sci 42:1362, 1976.

reach puberty when they are subjected to multiple management stimuli, such as mixing, transport, relocation and boar exposure. The most potent of these stimuli for facilitating the onset of estrus appears to be boar exposure.

Social Environment. The environment in which the gilt is reared can influence the age at which it commences estrous cyclicity. Rearing gilts in confinement can cause a retardation of the onset of puberty. The number of gilts per pen and stocking density may also influence the onset of puberty; however, results of scientific studies are controversial. Some studies have shown that crowding gilts stimulates early sexual maturation, while other investigations have demonstrated either no effect or a detrimental effect on the onset of puberty. Gilts reared individually show delays in the commencement of puberty. Table 2 lists the approximate floor space that should allow for prepubertal gilts to mature at a normal rate.

Climatic Environment. The domestic pig has been found in recent years to have pronounced seasonal breeding patterns. One manifestation of seasonality in swine may be the timing of the onset of puberty. Gilts that are farrowed in the fall have been found in some studies to reach puberty earlier than females born in the spring. The adult female shows a decrease in fertility and a diminished ability to return to estrus following weaning during the summer. One explanation for the delayed onset of puberty in spring-born gilts is that they reach a pubertal age during the "nonbreeding season" and are thus less

Table 2. Estimates of Floor Space that Will Allow for Normal Maturation of Replacement Gilts*

Average Weight (lb/pig)	Space† (ft²/pig)
45–75	3.6
75–105	4.5
105–135	5.5
135–165	6.4
165–195	7.3
195–225	8.2
> 225	4 ft²/100 lb

*Adapted from Ford JJ, Teague HS: J Animal Sci 47:828, 1978.
†Values given are only to be considered as guidelines for the *approximate* floor space that will allow prepubertal gilts to mature at a normal rate. Absolute, minimum space requirements (below which puberty is delayed) have not been established.

able to commence ovarian cyclicity during this summer anestrous period. Not all studies have observed seasonal changes in the onset of puberty.

The seasonal influences on the initiation of puberty could reflect circannual changes in temperature and photoperiod. In the adult female elevations in environmental temperature cause a decrease in estrous activity as well as decreased farrowing rates and embryonic survival. Although evidence is limited, the elevated temperatures that characterize the summer months may also adversely affect the initiation of puberty.

Several studies have shown that lighting regimens with 12 or more hours of daylight induce an earlier onset of puberty than occurs with daylight of 6 hours or less. Thus, long length of day would appear to be conducive to the early maturation of gilts. It might be noted that seasonal infertility in swine has its peak incidence after the summer solstice (maximum daylight hours) when photoperiod is decreasing. Although the optimal light-dark schedule for the advancement of puberty has not been elucidated, it appears that exposure to natural changes in photoperiod or to artificial photoperiods of at least 12 hours of light will allow for normal onset of puberty.

When considering the combined influences of photoperiod and temperature, it becomes apparent that spring-born gilts may be potentially stimulated by increasing photoperiod and inhibited by increasing environmental temperatures. In contrast, females born in the fall may be inhibited by decreasing photoperiod and stimulated (or left uninhibited) by decreasing temperatures. The seasonal influence on age of puberty of gilts in commercial herds may, therefore, be pronounced or absent, depending upon the environment within the building in which gilts are housed.

Nutrition. Since weight and growth rate appear to have very little influence on the onset of puberty, it might be expected that the nutrition of the gilt would similarly have an insignificant effect on the pubertal process. Depending upon the study, plane of feeding and composition of the diet, however, may or may not influence the age of puberty.

Numerous studies have compared the responses of the prepubertal gilt with full and limited feeding. Results are controversial. Some studies have observed that gilts fed a restricted diet have a delayed onset of puberty relative to their full-fed counterparts. Other studies have noted no influence of plane of feeding on puberty. Similarly, the restriction of energy in the diet was found to delay the onset of puberty in some studies, but in others it had no effect. Most studies agree that deficits in protein intake or amino acid imbalances can increase the age of puberty. The influence of vitamins and minerals on the onset of puberty has not been well documented.

The overall conclusion that can be made is that if a ration promotes adequate growth rates in a group of commercial replacement gilts, then it is unlikely that nutrition has a significant impact on the attainment of puberty.

THE BOAR

Maturation of the Reproductive System

While the onset of puberty is abrupt in the gilt, it is a more gradual process in the boar. Like that of the gilt, sexual maturation in the boar is a culmination of gradual maturational changes in each of the components of the hypothalamo-hypophyseal-gonadal axis.

Androgen-stimulated descent of the testes from the abdomen commences at about midgestation and is completed shortly after birth. During the last weeks of gestation and the initial few weeks following birth there is a rapid phase of testicular development that is attributable largely to Leydig cell proliferation. At about 1 month after farrowing the Leydig cells begin regressing and cause a decrease in testicular weight. The negative feedback control of gonadotropin secretion by testicular steroids appears to be established at about this age. During the perinatal period there is also increased lengthening and coiling of the seminiferous tubules. The Sertoli cells develop their morphologically distinct forms at about 40 days after birth and form the blood-testes barrier at 110 to 120 days. At about 100 days of age a period of rapid testicular growth commences. This is largely attributable to tubular development and a substantial increase in the number of germ cells. After approximately 110 days, spermatogenesis has been completed in many seminiferous tubules. By 120 to 150 days of age there are often sufficient spermatozoa in the epididymus to impregnate gilts. Testicular size increases throughout the prepubertal period and continues to increase following puberty (Fig. 2).

The actual age of puberty is usually defined as the time at which a maturing boar is able to produce sufficient sperm to impregnate a female. Boars typically have spermatozoa in their testes by about 4 to 5 months of age. Some males can ejaculate at 5 to 6 months; however, others are reluctant or unable to ejaculate until 8 to 9 months. Thus, there appears to be discrepancies in the ages of physiological and psychological maturity in some boars. The inability to collect semen from these boars precludes the accurate assessment of the age of puberty. Since most boars have reached puberty by

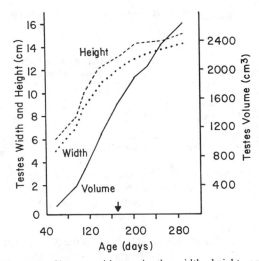

Figure 2. Changes with age in the width, height, and volume of the testes of the pre- and postpubertal boar. The age at which semen could first be collected from boars in this group is indicated by the verticle arrow. (Adapted from Esbenshade KL, et al.: J Anim Sci 48:246, 1979.)

8 to 9 months of age, young boars should not be judged as infertile until they are at least that age.

Factors Affecting Onset of Puberty

The influence of rearing conditions on the attainment of puberty by the boar has not been well studied. It appears that boars reared in groups reach puberty at an earlier age and demonstrate greater sexual aggressiveness as compared with boars raised individually. In addition, the exposure of prepubertal boars to mature sows and gilts during sexual maturation improves postpubertal sexual behavior. Both sexually receptive and nonreceptive females are able to promote the behavioral aspects of sexual development. The exposure to females appears to have a greater effect on mating behavior than exposure to other males. Prepubertal rearing experiences have no influence on the development of either the testes or the reproductive tract of boars. Contrary to what is commonly believed, rearing boars in confinement apparently has no effect on sexual development relative to boars maintained in pasture lots.

Suggested Readings

1. Christenson RK, Ford JJ: Puberty and estrus in confinement-reared gilts. J Anim Sci 49:743, 1979.
2. Dyck GW, Swierstra GW: Growth of the reproductive tract of the gilt from birth to puberty. Can J Anim Sci 63:81, 1983.
3. Esbenshade KL, Singleton WL, Clegg ED, Jones HW: Effect of housing management on reproductive development and performance of young boars. J Anim Sci 48:246, 1979.
4. Ford JJ, Teague HS: Effect of floor space restriction on age at puberty in gilts and on performance of barrows and gilts. J Anim Sci 47:828, 1978.

5. Kirkwood RN, Hughes PE: The influence of age at first boar contact on puberty attainment in the gilt. Anim Prod 29:231, 1979.

6. Zimmerman DR, Bourn P, Donovan D: Effect of "transport phenomenom" stimuli and boar exposure on puberty in gilts. J Anim Sci 42:1362, 1976.

The Clinical Endocrinology of Reproduction in the Pig

G. D. Dial, D.V.M., Ph.D.
J. H. Britt, Ph.D.
North Carolina State University, Raleigh, North Carolina

One of the leading problems in commercial swine production throughout the world is reproductive failure. Many of the common reproductive problems encountered in swine have been related to a dysfunction of the endocrine system. By understanding the reproductive endocrinology of the pig, the veterinary practitioner should be better able to understand the etiopathogenesis and thereby make diagnoses and formulate therapeutic strategies for some of the common reproductive disorders of swine.

HORMONAL CHANGES IN THE FEMALE

Fetal and Prepubertal Periods. There is a gradual maturation of ovarian follicles during the later stages of gestation and the first few postnatal months. Tertiary (antral) follicles capable of endocrine function do not develop until 60 to 90 days after birth. This is the approximate age at which the ovaries of prepubertal gilts are first able to respond to exogenous gonadotropins with increased steroidogenesis and with ovulation. Normal circulating concentrations of estradiol remain relatively low from the time of birth until 150 to 210 days of age. Thus, even though spontaneous steroidogenesis appears to be minimal until just before puberty, it appears that the porcine ovary is able to respond to gonadotropins, whether exogenous or endogenous, well in advance of puberty.

The maturation of the hypothalamo-hypophyseal axis is thought to regulate the rate of ovarian development through release of gonadotropins. Circulating levels of luteinizing hormone (LH) in the gilt are highest around the time of birth and then decrease gradually until midpuberty (Fig. 1). In contrast, concentrations of follicle-stimulating hormone (FSH) increase from the time of farrowing and remain elevated throughout the prepubertal period. As puberty approaches, there is an increased pulsatile release of gonadotropins that stimulates the progressive development of ovarian follicles. Both gonadotropins likely act in concert to promote follicular development and consequently steroidogenesis. Gonadotropin-stimulated increases in circulating levels of 17β-estradiol triggers the preovulatory release of LH that initiates ovulation at puberty.

Estrous Cycle. As the gilt commences estrous cyclicity at puberty, predictable hormonal profiles begin to occur. The pig typically has an estrous cycle of approximately 21 days duration, but it commonly varies from 17 to 25 days in length. The porcine estrous cycle can be divided into three distinct phases: diestrus (luteal phase), proestrus (follicular phase) and estrus (sexual receptivity).

Following ovulation of 6 to more than 20 follicles, luteinization of follicular remnants results in the formation of multiple corpora lutea (CL). A rise in circulating levels of progesterone is generally observed 2 to 4 days after estrus (day 0 being the first day of estrus). Concentrations increase in a near-linear fashion until a maximum is reached during mid to late diestrus (Fig. 2). After peaking, concentrations of progesterone may fluctuate dramatically in individual animals from day to day until they begin a decline coincident with luteolysis on days 13 to 15. Lysis of the CL is accompanied by increased circulating levels of the presumptive luteolysin, prostaglandin F_2 alpha ($PGF_{2\alpha}$) (Fig. 3). The decline in progesterone concentrations usually reaches a nadir between 14 and 18 days after estrus. In contrast to other species the CL of the pig appear to be essentially autonomous throughout diestrus and once formed do not require additional hypophyseal support. Porcine CL are not able to respond to increased $PGF_{2\alpha}$ concentrations with luteolysis until after day 12 of an estrous cycle.

As progesterone levels decline during late diestrus, the hypothalamo-hypophyseal axis is released from the inhibitory feedback effects of the steroid. Consequently, there is an increased frequency of episodic release of LH. This stimulates augmented development of follicular receptors for gonadotropins and increased maturation of antral follicles to preovulatory graafian follicles. Gonadotropin-stimulated steroidogenesis is thought to involve increased androgen production by thecal tissue followed by an increase in the aromatization of androgens to estrogen by the granulosa cells. The net effect of luteal demise is, thus, an increase in circulating levels of estrogen, primarily 17β-estradiol, between days 18 and 20 of the estrous cycle.

As follicles grow toward a preovulatory size of 5

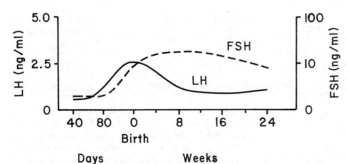

Figure 1. Circulating levels of luteinizing hormone (LH) and follicle-stimulating hormone (FSH) during the sexual maturation of the gilt. (Redrawn after Elsaesser F: In Cole DJA, Foxcroft GR (eds): Control of Pig Reproduction, Boston, Butterworth Scientific, 1982, p 93.)

to 12 mm during proestrus, a threshold level of estradiol is eventually reached that triggers the hypothalamo-hypophyseal release of LH (Fig. 2). The preovulatory discharge of gonadotropins has several effects. It induces luteinization of the theca granulosa tissue of follicles and thereby causes a rapid decline in estradiol production, with a concomitant gradual increase in progesterone release. It also stimulates resumption of oocyte maturation and ultimately ovulation.

In the immediate postovulatory period the abrupt decrease in circulating estradiol levels allows a marked increase in the release of FSH that continues for 2 to 3 days after estrus. This increased release has been suggested to be in response to removal of follicular sources of either estradiol or inhibin (folliculostatin). Inhibin apparently acts on the pituitary to inhibit FSH release. Estradiol feeds the hypothalamus and/or pituitary to inhibit gonadotropin release. In other species the postovulatory rise in FSH levels is thought to be associated with recruitment of the crop of follicles destined to ovulate at the subsequent estrus.

The onset of estrus in the pig typically follows the peak in proestrous concentrations of estradiol (Fig. 2). Depending upon age, females may be sexually receptive for 1 to 3 days. Onset of estrus

coincides ($\pm$ 12 hours) with the preovulatory LH surge. Ovulation occurs in most gilts during the latter part of the second day after the onset of estrus. As luteinization of the corpus hemorrhagicum occurs, new CL are formed, and the diestrous phase of the estrous cycle is recommenced.

The preovulatory rise in LH is coincident with increased circulating prolactin levels. The role of prolactin during the estrous cycle of swine remains uncertain.

Pregnancy and Parturition. When sows remain unmated or fail to conceive, the CL undergo a functional demise. In contrast to nonpregnant sows, females that conceive at their estrual matings show no decline in circulating concentrations of progesterone and maintain lower levels of $PGF_{2\alpha}$ (Fig. 3). It has been suggested that the preimplantation embryo provides luteotrophic support for the continued maintenance of the CL during pregnancy or alternatively causes $PGF_{2\alpha}$ produced in the endometrium to be secreted into the lumen of the uterus rather than into the uterine vein. Progesterone production by the CL appears to be required for the maintenance of pregnancy, since ovariectomy, corpus luteal enucleation or prostaglandin treatment after day 12 postcoitus causes abortion. Hypophyseal support of the CL is required throughout ges-

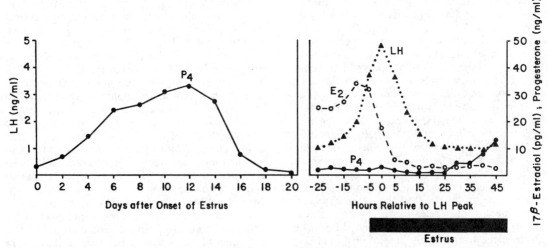

Figure 2. Mean circulating concentrations of progesterone (P_4) throughout the estrous cycle and levels of P_4, luteinizing hormone (LH) and estradiol-17β (E_2) around the time of estrus in the gilt. (Redrawn from Guthrie HD, et al.: Endocrinology 91:675, 1972; Van de Wiel DFM, et al.: Biol Reprod 24:223, 1981.)

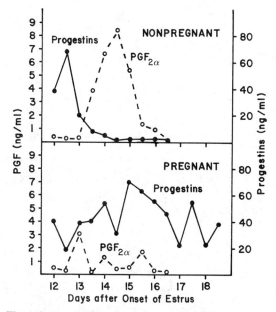

Figure 3. Levels of prostaglandin F (PGF$_{2\alpha}$) and progestins in the utero-ovarian vein of the nonpregnant (upper panel) and pregnant gilt (lower panel). Figure redrawn from Moeljono MPE, et al.: Prostaglandins 14:543, 1977.

tation in the pig. At least four embryos are required on day 12 after breeding to prevent luteolysis and ensure the maintenance of pregnancy.

During gestation, circulating concentrations of progesterone are elevated, and as a result, the uterine myometrium remains quiescent. As term approaches, a cascade of endocrine events is begun that terminates in parturition. As discussed in detail by First and Bosc,[3] it appears that the fetal pigs initiate the farrowing process. Presumably, near the time of parturition, fetal pituitary release of adrenocorticotropic hormone (ACTH) stimulates production of glucocorticoids by the fetal adrenal (Fig. 4). Cortisol, in turn, stimulates increased release of PGF$_{2\alpha}$ from the gravid uterus. Increasing maternal circulating concentrations of prostaglandins at term promote luteolysis and thereby cause decreased concentrations of progesterone. This facilitates an increased frequency of uterine contractions and the initiation of parturition. Elevated PGF$_{2\alpha}$ levels at term promote release of relaxin from the CL and oxytocin from the neurohypophysis. Relaxin allows a relaxation of the cervix and a widening of the birth canal. Oxytocin promotes myometrial activity of the estrogenized, prepartum uterus and causes reflex mammary myoepithelial contraction at suckling. Gestation in the pig usually lasts 114 to 116 days.

Lactation. The demise of the CL prior to parturition is associated with a sharp decrease in circulating levels of progesterone and a gradual increase in plasma concentrations of estrogen, which fall rapidly following farrowing. This periparturient increase in estrogen, presumably of fetoplacental or-

igin, may accompany an anovulatory estrus in some sows within the first few days after farrowing.

At parturition there is only modest follicular development, and the CL have regressed to their less functional remnants, corpora albacantia. As lactation progresses, the number of follicles as well as follicle size increases steadily from 7 to 10 days postpartum. Along with this follicular development is a gradual increase in circulating concentrations of estrogen (Fig. 5). While levels of gonadotropins are low during the first weeks of lactation, there is an increase in both LH and FSH during the latter weeks of a 4- to 5-week lactation. The increased follicular development as lactation progresses may reflect this increase in gonadotropin secretion. Progesterone levels remain low throughout lactation.

The endocrine mechanisms that inhibit follicular development and gonadotropin secretion during lactation are not completely understood. It appears that LH and FSH secretion during lactation may be inhibited by different mechanisms. Ovarian secretion of a nonsteroidal substance (folliculostatin) during lactation has been suggested as selectively inhibiting the release of FSH but not LH. The secretion of LH is presumably suppressed by neural afferents from the mammary gland that are stimulated at suckling.

Prolactin levels in sows are much higher during lactation than during the postweaning period. Removal of piglets causes a rapid decrease in circulating concentrations of prolactin. This suggests that suckling not only acts to inhibit LH release from the hypothalamo-hypophyseal axis, but it may also act to inhibit hypothalamic release of prolactin-inhibiting factor (PIF) and thereby cause increased prolactin levels. As in other species, prolactin is thought to facilitate lactogenesis in the pig. It does not appear to interfere with pituitary or ovarian function in the lactating sow, as has been proposed in other species.

Postweaning Period. While there is only modest follicular development prior to weaning, the removal of piglets from the sow at weaning causes an abrupt acceleration in follicular growth and a corresponding increased production of ovarian estrogens (Fig. 5). This appears to be a consequence of the increased pulsatile secretion of LH following weaning. As during the estrous cycle, the gradually increasing concentrations of estradiol prior to ovulation trigger a preovulatory discharge of LH that initiates the ovulatory process. Although the percentage varies with season, the majority of sows exhibit estrus from 3 to 7 days following weaning.

Anestrus. Not all sows return to estrus and ovulate following weaning. Sows that persistently remain in anestrus after weaning appear to be of two types: Those that are anestrous and have anovulatory, acyclical ovaries (anovulatory anestrus) and those that fail to show estrus but have active, cyclical ovaries (behavioral anestrus).

The majority of persistently anestrous sows are of the anovulatory, anestrous type. These sows show an absence of spontaneous, cyclical changes in cir-

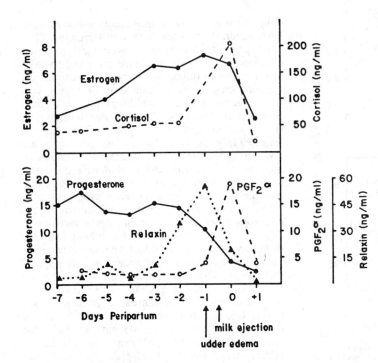

Figure 4. Circulating levels of progesterone, prostaglandin F_2 alpha ($PGF_{2\alpha}$), relaxin and total estrogens in the dam and cortisol in the fetus around the time of parturition. (Redrawn from First NL, Bosc MJ: J Anim Sci 48:1407, 1979.)

culating levels of steroid or gonadotropin hormones. The ovaries of these sows show varying degrees of follicular development, but follicles seldom reach preovulatory size during extended periods of time following weaning. Anovulatory, anestrous sows are able to respond to exogenous gonadotropins (e.g., pregnant mare serum gonadotropin, PMSG, or human chorionic gonadotropin, hCG) with increased follicular growth, increased steroidogenesis and ultimately ovulation.

Behaviorally anestrous sows show cyclical changes in progesterone levels that are similar to those occurring during the estrous cycle of the pig. Because these sows ovulate, they are assumed to have cyclical changes in circulating levels of LH and estradiol. It is not known if the behavioral centers in the hypothalami of these sows are unresponsive

to cyclic changes in estradiol or if the increases in estradiol levels prior to ovulation are insufficient to evoke estrous behavior. Behaviorally anestrous sows do not show estrus in response to exogenous gonadotropins or to exogenous estradiol.

Pathologic Conditions. The endocrine changes that occur during the reproductive diseases of swine have not been well studied.

Cystic ovarian disease is a common cause of reproductive failure in swine. Single, variable-sized cysts are frequently observed in sows having apparently normal estrous cycles and do not appear to influence fertility. Two other types of ovarian cysts, however, can cause ovarian dysfunction. Multiple small cysts are occasionally observed in anestrous sows. These cysts are typically slightly larger (10 to 15 mm) than normal follicles of ovulatory size and

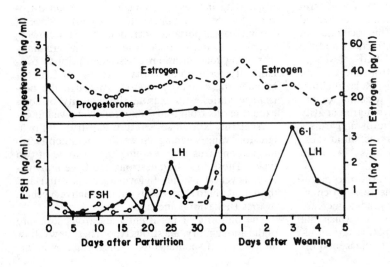

Figure 5. Mean concentrations of luteinizing hormone (LH), follicle-stimulating hormone (FSH), estrogen and progesterone in the peripheral circulation of sows during lactation and after weaning. (Redrawn from Stevenson JS, Britt JH: Theriogenology 14:453, 1980; Stevenson JS, et al.: Biol Reprod 24:341, 1981.)

are usually more abundant (> 15) than the normal number of preovulatory follicles present at proestrus. Small multiple cysts secrete high levels of estrogen. Multiple large cysts are relatively common in acyclic sows. These cysts are larger than preovulatory follicles (> 15 mm) and may reach enormous sizes (5 to 10 cm). The number of large cysts observed is usually similar to the number of follicles (6 to 20) that normally develop during proestrus. Large cysts can have completely luteinized walls or have only patches of luteinized tissue scattered throughout their walls. These cysts frequently release significant amounts of progesterone. When ovarian cysts are steroid-secreting cysts, they may interfere with cyclic reproductive activity by the feedback inhibition of gonadotropin release.

Mycotoxicoses commonly cause reproductive failure in swine throughout the world. The most common mycotoxin associated with dysfunction of the reproductive system is zearalenone (zearalenol, F-2 toxin, a metabolite of *Fusarium roseum*). Zearalenone has a potent estrogenic activity that is very obvious in prepubertal gilts. Even though vulvas are swollen and reddened, and mammary glands are frequently well developed, prepubertal gilts exposed to this mycotoxin commonly show ovarian atrophy, an absence of follicular development and low circulating levels of estradiol. Puberty, if it occurs, usually fails to commence at a normal time. Prepubertal boars fed contaminated diets have depressed testosterone levels, delayed sexual development, abnormally small testes and diminished libido. Cyclic gilts exposed to zearalenone often enter into a pseudopregnant status, with the prolonged maintenance of the corpora lutea and continued elevations in circulating levels of progesterone. Moldy feed in the diet of pregnant sows has been associated with decreased litter sizes and increased incidences of abortion, weak pigs, stillbirths and fetal mummification. Morphologic changes in the genital tract depend upon whether the CL are maintained, causing a progestational influence, or whether the estrogenizing effects of the mycotoxins are manifested. Zearalenone is thought to have potent negative feedback effects on hypothalamo-hypophyseal secretion of gonadotropins. Thus, gonadal production of steroid hormones is very low.

Replacement gilts commonly have delays in the onset of puberty. Frequently, gilts do not show estrus for months after their penmates have commenced pubertal cyclicity. As with the persistently anestrous weaned sows, gilts experiencing delayed puberty are of two types: those that fail to either show estrus or commence ovarian cyclicity (anovulatory, anestrous) and those that initiate ovarian activity but fail to exhibit estrus (behaviorally anestrous). The anovulatory, anestrous gilts show no cyclical changes in circulating concentrations of steroid hormones or gonadotropins. Behaviorally anestrous females have cyclical changes in levels of LH, progesterone and estradiol that are similar to those occurring in the normal cycling gilt.

The loss of an entire litter during mid to late gestation commonly leads to pseudopregnancy. The pseudopregnant sow fails to farrow at the anticipated time, never "bellys-down," or shows only a modest increase in abdominal girth, and does not return to estrus. Some degree of mammary development is occasionally observed. Progesterone levels remain elevated in these pseudopregnant sows, as the CL are maintained beyond the normal time of parturition. Presumably, the absence of living fetuses prevents the initiation of the endocrine cascade that culminates in parturition. The uterus of the pseudopregnant sow usually contains mummified fetal remnants, and the sow fails to recognize that the fetuses have died. Thus, production of prostaglandins by the uterus is prevented, and the CL of pregnancy are maintained.

ENDOCRINOLOGY OF THE BOAR

Prepubertal Boar. During the late fetal and early neonatal periods there is rapid differentiation of the Leydig, Sertoli, and germ cell components of the testes. This differentiation is accompanied by an increase in steroid production. Around the time of birth, circulating levels of testosterone, LH and FSH are elevated and reach a maximum at about the second week after farrowing. Following this peak, concentrations of steroids and gonadotropins decrease until a second rise in testosterone levels is observed between 40 and 220 days of age (Fig. 6). An increase in peripheral levels of estradiol lags behind but parallels the rise in testosterone concentrations. Estradiol is produced either by the Sertoli cells of the testes from steroid precursors synthesized in the Leydig cell or by the Leydig cell itself. Testosterone is produced within the Leydig cell. Estradiol is thought to act in concert with testosterone in the maturing boar to stimulate the development of the accessory sex glands and the onset of sexual behavior.

After their postnatal decline, circulating concentrations of LH and FSH remain relatively constant throughout the prepubertal period. As the boar matures, there is a curvilinear increase in testicular size and weight and presumably an increase in steroidogenic tissue. In addition, there also appears to be an increase in the sensitivity of the Leydig cells to gonadotropins during sexual maturation. Thus, circulating levels of testicular hormones increase during puberty even though mean serum LH concentrations do not change substantially as the boar matures.

Mature Boar. Androgens produced primarily in the Leydig cells play vital roles in sustaining spermatogenesis, in supporting development of the penis and accessory sex glands and in stimulating the development of the secondary sex characteristics. Even though functionally very important, testosterone becomes quantitatively less important as the boar matures. The principal steroids found in the peripheral circulation of older boars are the 16-androstenes (16-unsaturated C_{19} steroids). This class

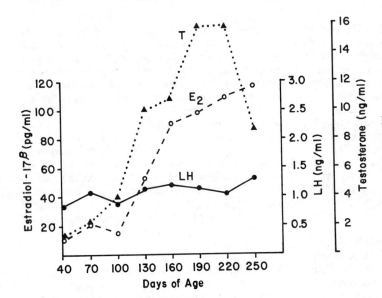

Figure 6. Circulating levels of estradiol-17β (E₂), luteinizing hormone (LH) and testosterone (T) during the sexual maturation of the boar. (Redrawn from Allrich RD, et al.: J Anim Sci 55:1139, 1982.)

of steroids is responsible for the "boar taint" or musk smell that characterizes the mature male. These compounds are the pheromones of the pig and can be used to facilitate the induction of estrous behavior when presented in aerosol form to the female. The 16-androstenes accumulate in the submaxillary salivary gland of the boar and are released into the saliva.

Like those of the stallion, the boar testes secrete substantial amounts of estrogens. In fact, levels of unconjugated estrogen in boar plasma are substantially higher than those in the plasma of estrous gilts. It is thought that the estrogens in boar plasma may originate from the aromatization of androgens. Estrogens have been shown to enhance the behavioral response of castrated boars to testosterone. The administration of estrogen alone, however, induces female sexual behavior in the barrow. In the growing boar estrogen appears to enhance the growth-promoting effects of androgens.

As in the female, LH secretion in the boar is pulsatile. Transient elevations in LH are followed within 60 minutes by large pulses of testosterone. Copulation, the presence of an estrous female or exposure to an aggressive boar causes abrupt increases in testosterone levels. Thus, the concentrations of testosterone in the peripheral circulation are highly variable between samples taken from the same boar and among blood samples taken from different boars.

The control of gonadotropin secretion in the boar has not been fully elucidated. However, it appears that the boar is similar to males of other species in that testicular steroids, especially estradiol and testosterone, feed back on the hypothalamo-hypophyseal axis to inhibit release of LH. Because of their potent feedback effects, the use of anabolic steroids as growth promotants have been suspected of interfering with the maturation of the boar and with sperm production.

DIAGNOSTIC ENDOCRINOLOGY

A rapidly growing area in veterinary diagnostic medicine is the use of hormonal measurements and endocrine challenges to diagnose reproductive diseases and to improve reproductive management in commercial herds.

Pregnancy Diagnosis. At least three endocrine tests have been evaluated for use in the early diagnosis of pregnancy in swine. The analysis of progesterone concentration in blood collected between 17 and 24 days after mating has been found to be an accurate means of diagnosing pregnancy. This test is based upon the fact that progesterone levels should be low (< 5 ng/ml) in sows that do not conceive and elevated in pregnant females that have maintained CL during this interval. The progesterone pregnancy test is higher than 90 per cent accurate in confirming pregnancy and is approximately 60 to 90 per cent correct in detecting nonpregnant sows. In the practical application of the test blood samples are collected 17 to 19 days after coitus, the results are analyzed within 1 day and the results are called back to the producer prior to day 21 when open sows would be expected to return to estrus. The accuracy of the test is limited by the occurrence of longer or shorter than normal estrous cycles. Fetal death after the day the blood is drawn also causes inaccurate results.

The measurement of blood and urinary estrogens has also been used as a basis for a pregnancy test. The technique is based upon the principle that the fetoplacental unit synthesizes large quantities of estrogens, causing increased maternal blood and urinary estrogen content. Concentrations of estrogen are increased in the maternal circulation 16 to 18 days after coitus, reach a maximum between days 24 and 30 and decline to a nadir by days 35 to 50. This peak is composed predominantly of a sulfated conjugate of estrogen (the water soluble form), estrone sulfate. With this test, blood samples are drawn between 22 and 32 days of gestation. Elevated levels imply pregnancy; low levels indicate a nonpregnant status. Extensive field trials are required before the accuracy of the test can be estimated. The advantage of the test is that there is a broad range of time (10 or more days) over which blood samples can be drawn. One disadvantage of the test is that it appears to be less accurate than the progesterone test when used on the days prior to anticipated return (< 21 days after mating). As with the progesterone test, late embryonic death can cause nonpregnant sows to be detected as pregnant. A promising aspect of the estrone sulfate pregnancy test is that maternal levels are correlated positively ($r = 0.5$ to 0.6) 20 to 26 days after coitus with the number of fetuses. Thus, in the future, levels may be used to estimate litter size or to predict which sows have experienced early fetal death.

After conception, the presence of viable conceptuses prevents the secretion of $PGF_{2\alpha}$ into the uterine vein between 11 and 16 days after breeding. Thus, low maternal circulating levels of prostaglandin (or prostaglandin metabolites) during this period should be an indication of pregnancy, and high levels should reflect ongoing luteolysis and nonpregnant status. The prostaglandin pregnancy test offers support of this hypothesis. The test was approximately 90 per cent accurate in determining that sows were pregnant and between 68 and 72 per cent accurate in uncovering nonpregnant females when blood samples were drawn between 13 and 15 days after mating.

Assessment of Ovulation. During the estrous cycle circulating levels of progesterone are elevated for 14 to 18 days of the 21-day cycle. Thus, progesterone is increased for approximately 75 per cent of the entire cycle. If a single blood sample is drawn from a cyclic gilt in which the date of the last estrus is not known, there is only a 75 per cent chance of observing an elevated progesterone level. By taking multiple samples throughout the 21-day estrous cycle, ovulatory status can be accurately assessed. Since this is usually clinically impractical, an alternative approach is to determine the progesterone levels in two samples of blood taken at 10-day intervals. Elevation in circulating levels of progesterone (> 3 ng/ml) in one or both of the samples confirms that luteal structures are present. By using this sampling interval, it is possible to determine the ovulatory status of an individual animal or the percentage of gilts in a group that are cycling. Females that are pseudopregnant or pregnant, have persistent CL or have luteinized ovarian cysts will also have elevations in progesterone levels.

Endocrine Challenge. In the future it is likely that there will be increased use of hormone preparations as endocrine probes to evaluate the individual components of the hypothalamo-hypophyseal-gonadal axis of problem animals. Although much additional research is needed, clinical techniques may be developed that use (1) exogenous gonadotropins (such as PMSG or hCG) to assess ovarian or testicular function of animals of unknown or suspect fertility, (2) exogenous estrogen to evaluate the activity of the hypothalamo-hypophyseal system of problem animals or (3) gonadotropin-releasing hormone (GnRH) to assess pituitary function.

References

1. Allrich RD, Christenson RK, Ford JJ, Zimmerman DR: Prepubertal development of the boar: Testosterone, estradiol-17β, cortisol and LH concentrations before and after castration at various ages. J Anim Sci 55:1139, 1982.
2. Elsaesser F: Endocrine control of sexual maturation in the female pig and sexual differentiation of the stimulatory oestrogen feedback mechanism. In Cole DJA, Foxcroft GR (eds): Control of Pig Reproduction. Boston, Buttersworth Scientific, 1982, p 93.
3. First NL, Bosc MJ: Proposed mechanisms controlling parturition and the induction of parturition in swine. J Anim Sci 48:1407, 1979.
4. Guthrie HD, Henricks DM, Handlin DL: Plasma estrogen, progesterone and luteinizing hormone prior to estrus and early pregnancy in pig. Endocrinology 91:675, 1972.
5. Moeljono MPE, Thatcher WW, Bazer FW, et al.: A study of prostaglandin $F_{2\alpha}$ as the luteolysin in swine II. Characterization and comparison of prostaglandin F, estrogens and progestin concentrations in utero-ovarian vein plasma of nonpregnant and pregnant gilts. Prostaglandins 14:543, 1977.
6. Stevenson JS, Britt JH: Luteinizing hormone, total estrogens and progesterone secretion during lactation and after weaning in sows. Theriogenology 14:453, 1980.
7. Stevenson JS, Cox NM, Britt JH: Role of the ovary in controlling luteinizing hormone, follicle stimulating hormone, and prolactin during and after lactation in pig. Biol Reprod 24:341, 1981.
8. Van de Wiel DFM, Erkens J, Koops W, et al.: Periestrous and midluteal time courses of circulating LH, FSH, prolactin, estradiol-17β and progesterone in the domestic pig. Biol Reprod 24:223, 1981.

Pharmacologic Control of Estrus and Ovulation in the Pig

G. D. Dial, D.V.M., Ph.D.
North Carolina State University, Raleigh, North Carolina

G. W. BeVier, D.V.M., M.S.
Pig Improvement Company, Franklin, Kentucky

Because of the intensive rearing conditions that typify modern swine production, it is usually essential that females are bred and farrowed in relative synchrony. When sows and gilts are bred over long periods of time, rather than within a few days of each other, the movement of the females as a group from one stage of production to another is disrupted. Consequently, farrowing rooms and nurseries cannot be used in an "all-in, all-out" manner. Since pigs of different ages must be mixed, disease control programs are compromised, and production becomes less efficient. The net effect of asynchronous breeding of females is inefficient pig flow throughout all stages of production and less than optimal utilization of both facilities and breeding stock. This article will emphasize practical techniques for synchronizing the times of onset of estrus and ovulation in groups of female swine. Only those treatments that have been proved effective with minimal adverse consequences and that could be practically applied by the veterinary practitioner will be discussed. It should be emphasized that even though commonly used in European countries, no drugs have been approved for use in American swine herds for the synchronization of estrus or for the induction of ovulation.

PRETREATMENT CONSIDERATIONS

Efforts to control the timing of ovulation and the onset of estrus have developed along two lines: the induction of ovulation in acyclic, anovulatory females and the regulation of the luteal phase of the estrous cycle of cyclic, ovulatory pigs. Because the treatments and the response to treatment differ between cyclic and acyclic females, it is important to establish ovarian status prior to attempts at synchronization. A history should be taken and should include the approximate ages of gilts and the most recent stage of production of sows. The percentage of females in the group that have shown signs of estrus or have had vulvar swelling during past weeks should be determined. In some herds it may be necessary to evaluate pregnancy status. If a laboratory with cooperative personnel is available, the endocrine evaluation of ovarian activity prior to treatment will help to maximize response to therapy. When reproductive status cannot be established, the veterinary practitioner should forewarn the producer that response to treatment will likely be less than optimal.

ACYCLIC FEMALE

During recent years numerous hormonal treatments have been evaluated for efficacy in the stimulation of ovarian activity in acyclic, anovulatory females. Hormones that have been used in attempts to promote follicular growth and induce ovulation in the pig include pregnant mare serum gonadotropin (PMSG), human chorionic gonadotropin (hCG), luteinizing hormone (LH), follicle-stimulating hormone (FSH), gonadotropin-releasing hormone (GnRH) and its synthetic analogs, prostaglandin F2 alpha ($PGF_{2\alpha}$) and the prostaglandin analogs and estrogen and its congeners.

To date, PMSG has been the most commonly used and the most effective therapy for the induction of follicular growth, ovulation and estrus in swine. In many countries of Europe PMSG is available commercially and is used therapeutically to induce fertile estrus in persistently anestrous sows and in gilts experiencing delayed puberty. PMSG is also used prophylactically to decrease the interval from weaning to estrus in the postlactational sow, to induce ovulation in the lactating female, to promote the onset of puberty in gilts and to induce supraovulation in the cyclic sow.

Other hormonal treatments besides PMSG are not as efficacious in the induction of both estrus and ovulation. By itself hCG will induce ovulation but is relatively ineffective in initiating estrus. Exogenous estrogens, such as estradiol benzoate (17β estradiol-3-benzoate), and estradiol cypionate (estradiol 17β-cyclopentylproprionate) will consistently induce estrus and a preovulatory-like discharge of LH in anovulatory females but will only sporadically induce ovulation, and then at rates less than normal. When females are treated with hCG plus estradiol, both estrus and ovulation occur, but litter size is usually reduced. Combinations of LH and FSH have been found to be effective in inducing ovulation in swine, but their short half-lives relative to PMSG (approximately ½ hour versus 36 hours) require that large doses or multiple injections be given. Thus, the practical use of the natural gonadotropins in the induction of ovulation in groups of females is limited. The administration of a single dose of GnRH will induce transient (< 3-hour duration) hypophyseal release of endogenous gonadotropins but will not induce estrus or ovulation. The pulsatile administration of GnRH (1 injection/hour until estrus) to anovulatory females will induce estrus and ovulation but is impractical for commercial application. Treatment with $PGF_{2\alpha}$ or one of its analogs will induce a return to estrous activity in sows that have persistent corpora lutea but will not promote ovulation in females that do not have responsive luteal tissue.

Since PMSG remains the treatment of choice for the induction of estrus and ovulation in the anovulatory female, special consideration of its effects are warranted. There is a linear relationship between dose of PMSG and number of induced ovulations. Although it is possible to induce a supraovulatory response with high doses of PMSG, litter size is not consistently increased above normal. The size of the litter following PMSG-stimulated supraovulation is limited by an increased ovulation of immature ova, an elevated rate of fertilization failures and an increased early embryonic mortality. Because of these adverse consequences, therapies utilizing PMSG should be directed toward achieving a physiologically normal ovulatory response.

Prepubertal Gilt. The gilt is first able to ovulate in response to exogenous gonadotropins at approximately 100 days of age. There is a gradually improved ovulatory response as puberty is approached, with optimal response occurring in gilts of 160 days of age or older. The most common regimens used to induce ovulation are the administration of 500 to 1000 IU PMSG followed in 48 to 96 hours by approximately 500 to 750 IU hCG and the injection of 400 IU PMSG in combination with 200 IU hCG. The split-dose and combination treatments appear to induce comparable rates of ovulation and estrus. When PMSG is given without hCG, ovulation rates and the per cent of gilts showing estrus are reduced relative to treatments utilizing hCG in conjunction with PMSG. Exogenous GnRH has been used in lieu of hCG at 48 to 60 hours after PMSG administration to induce synchronized ovulation; however, a more reliable response appears to occur when hCG is given after PMSG. The time of ovulation following treatment with the PMSG/hCG combination is approximately 110 to 120 hours. When either hCG or GnRH is given following PMSG, ovulation occurs at approximately 40 to 44 hours following the second injection.

Although conception rates of 40 to 90 per cent are common following gonadotropin-induced ovulation, less than 60 per cent of gonadotropin-induced gilts are typically able to maintain successful pregnancies. It is thought that in some gilts induced corpora lutea (CL) are not able to retain their viability 20 to 30 days after ovulation. If females are mated at the spontaneous estrus that occurs in some gilts at approximately 21 days following induced ovulation, farrowing rates are markedly improved. The presence of boars after induced ovulation enhances the ability of gilts to maintain cyclic, ovarian and estrous activities.

Delayed Puberty. Gilts reared in confinement commonly show an onset of puberty that is substantially delayed relative to penmates. As discussed in other articles, these anestrous females may have acyclic, anovulatory or cyclic, ovulatory ovaries. Most gilts that are anovulatory and anestrous are able to respond to exogenous gonadotropins with both estrus and ovulation. Prepubertal females that are anestrous and have cyclic ovaries (behaviorally anestrous) are not able to respond to increased circulating levels of estradiol and thus cannot respond to gonadotropin therapy with estrus. They are, however, able to ovulate and to form accessory CL in addition to their primary CL.

Lactating Sow. During lactation, the ovaries of sows show only modest follicular development. There is gradual but progressive development of follicles as lactation proceeds. Females are able to ovulate in response to exogenous gonadotropins as early as 15 days postpartum, but pregnancy rate is improved when treatment is initiated at 25 days or more following farrowing. The procedure found to be most effective for inducing ovulation in the lactating sow involves the administration of 1500 IU of PMSG followed after 96 hours by 1000 IU of hCG. Since estrus is not consistently observed, females should be artificially inseminated at 24 hours and again at 36 to 42 hours following hCG administration. The separation of the sow from her litter for one to three 12-hour periods prior to treatment appears to improve the response to gonadotropin.

Postweaning Sow. Following weaning, the majority of sows show signs of estrus within 3 to 7 days. Exogenous gonadotropins have been used to decrease the weaning-to-estrus interval and to improve the synchrony of the postweaning estrus. Gonadotropins have also been used prophylactically to decrease the incidence of sows that fail to return to estrus following weaning. PMSG can be used alone or in combination with hCG to promote earlier onset of the postweaning estrus. For maximum effectiveness, PMSG should be administered on the day following weaning.

Anestrous Sow. It is not uncommon in some herds for sows to fail to return to estrus for 30 or more days following weaning. As with delayed puberty, anestrous sows may have acyclic or cyclic ovarian activity. Females that have anovulatory ovaries are able to respond to PMSG with a fertile estrus. The combination of estrogen (1 mg of either estradiol benzoate or estradiol cypionate) and hCG (1000 IU) has been used to return anestrous sows to productivity. However, additional studies are warranted to establish the efficacy of this treatment. Because of its luteotrophic effects in the pig, exogenous estrogen may induce prolonged diestrus in anestrous sows with cyclical ovaries. Estrogens should be used with caution in the pig.

CYCLIC FEMALE

The estrous cycle of the pig can be altered by suppressing ovarian activity and thereby delaying the spontaneous demonstration of estrus. It can be modified by inducing premature regression of corpora lutea and thereby hastening the onset of estrus. It can also be altered by the artificial induction of premature follicular growth and ovulation. Therapeutic approaches for synchronizing the estrous cycles of pigs have been developed along these lines.

Suppression of Ovarian Activity. Progesterone and the synthetic progestins suppress follicular development in cyclic females. The parenteral administration of progesterone at doses of at least 100 mg/day for 14 consecutive days or more will delay the onset of estrus and allow estrous synchronization with normal fertility. Numerous orally active progestins have been used to synchronize the estrous cycles of swine. Most of these synthetic progestins have been found to have significant adverse effects, such as the production of cystic follicles, the failure to synchronize onset of estrus tightly, the reduction of litter size, the reduction of conception and farrowing rates or the induction of fetal teratology.

One synthetic progestin, allyl trenbolone (Regumate), has proved to be a very useful tool in the regulation of estrus and ovulation. Feeding cyclic gilts individually or in groups at a rate of 15 to 20 mg/day for 14 to 18 consecutive days produces a synchronous onset of estrus between 2 and 8 days after the last progestin feeding. Approximately 65 to 80 per cent of the treated gilts can be expected to be in estrus within 2 days of each other, and more than 90 per cent will be in heat within 4 days. Estrous synchronization with altrenogest allows for breeding to be planned in advance and facilitates the introduction of randomly cycling, replacement gilts into the breeding herd. Using altrenogest, the onset of estrus in gilts can be coordinated with that of weaned sows. In this manner less desirable, mature breeding stock can be efficiently replaced with young females. The day of the estrous cycle that gilts are initially treated with altrenogest does not influence the response to the progestin. Treatment with altrenogest does not appear to hinder fertility.

Induction of Luteolysis. The porcine CL remains unresponsive to the acute administration of $PGF_{2\alpha}$ or its analogs until days 12 to 14 after ovulation. Prior to this time, treatment with prostaglandins causes no decline or only a transient decline in circulating levels of progesterone. As the porcine CL typically commences its natural demise because of endogenously secreted prostaglandins 14 to 17 days after estrus, there is only a transient period during which exogenous prostaglandins are effective in initiating luteolysis in the pig.

ABORTION SYNCHRONIZATION

The porcine CL become responsive to the luteolytic effects of prostaglandins at about day 12 of the estrous cycle. CL that are maintained because of pregnancy are similarly sensitive to the lytic effects of prostaglandins. Females that are treated with prostaglandins at any stage of gestation undergo luteolysis, abort and subsequently return to fertile estrus. At least three regimens have been used to abort swine: 15 mg of $PGF_{2\alpha}$ followed in 12 hours by 10 mg of $PGF_{2\alpha}$, 1.0 mg of cloprostenol followed in 24 hours by 0.5 mg of cloprostenol, and a single injection of 0.5 mg of cloprostenol. The relative efficacies of these regimens and the minimum effective dose of prostaglandin that will induce abortion have not been determined. The time to onset of abortion varies with stage of gestation but usually occurs between 30 and 45 hours after prostaglandin administration. Aborted sows return to estrus 4 to 10 days following treatment. Conception rates at the first postabortion estrus are usually higher than 80 per cent. Because this procedure is commonly used, boars are added to a group of gilts, and random matings are allowed to occur for a period of at least 20 to 30 days. Two or more weeks following removal of the boars, gilts are treated with prostaglandins. Pregnant sows subsequently abort and return to estrus in synchrony.

Sexual Behavior Problems in the Male and Female Pig

P. H. Hemsworth, B.Agr.Sc., Ph.D.
C. G. Winfield, B.Sc., M.Sci.
Department of Agriculture, Werribee, Victoria, Australia

The sexual behavior of the pig has received little research attention in the past. Recently, however, this area has become recognized as having important practical implications. Although it is difficult to estimate the influence of low levels of sexual behavior on reproductive efficiency of the herd, it is obviously important that each breeding pig is able to develop fully and maintain its sexual behavior. Therefore, problems with the sexual behavior of both the male and female pig are discussed in this article.

LOW COPULATORY CAPACITY IN BOARS

Definition. While there is little documentation on boar wastage, experience from several artificial insemination centers and a few commercial piggeries indicates that 20 to 50 per cent of culled boars are unable to copulate or copulate at an insufficient frequency. This condition results from either low sexual motivation or low mating competency. Limited evidence suggests that this condition is more severe in intensive rather than extensive production systems, and its incidence may increase with age, perhaps because of the increased susceptibility to locomotor disturbances in such environments.

Diagnosis. The pertinent information for diagnosing the cause of low copulatory capacity includes past illness and injury, age, onset of condition and reproductive record, including frequency of copulation and frequency of refusal to copulate. Since the social, physical and climatic environments may be responsible for the condition,[1] information should be sought on these aspects. The boar's pen and mating pens should be inspected to assess the amount of female contact available to the boar, the pen size, the floor type and condition, obstructions in the pen and the possibility of prolonged elevated temperatures. Information on the social environment of the boar during rearing and around puberty should also be sought.

The clinical examination should focus on the behavioral response of the boar to a highly receptive female in the normal mating arena. The mobility of the boar should be observed to detect locomotor disturbances that may adversely affect the boar's mating competency or dexterity. These disturbances will be most apparent when the boar is attempting to mount or during mounting and thrusting.

After 24 hours of rest, a boar of adequate sexual motivation, when introduced to the female, should quickly engage in courtship and attempt to mount within 2 minutes. Once the boar mounts, the penis should be observed for problems such as attached frenulum, failure to attain satisfactory erection or protrusion, deviation of the penis and hemorrhage from lacerations or abrasions. The etiology of these functional failures is unknown in most cases. Some authors have suggested that the condition of an attached frenulum may have a hereditary basis. Since failure to ejaculate may progressively reduce sexual motivation, boars that will not mount should be examined under anesthesia if problems of the penis are suspected.

Penile problems may inhibit copulation because of pain, while injury sustained during copulation may carry a psychological effect for some time after physical recovery has occurred, again inhibiting copulation.

Poor orientation of the mounting response, such as head mounting, is often seen in the young boar. However, proper orientation is probably a learned response, and if the boar is of satisfactory sexual motivation, mating competency should improve with the positive reinforcement of copulation.

Once the boar copulates, he should be observed for evidence of discomfort, such as uneven or changing distribution of weight on the hindlegs, forelegs resting on the back of the female and straight joints of the hindlegs and arched back. With females that are highly receptive, ejaculation should last for 5 to 15 minutes.

If the boar is free of locomotor or penile disturbances but fails to copulate, then it is likely that the boar is of low sexual motivation. In the mature boar isolation from females causes a depression in the level of sexual behavior; however, this effect is reversible by housing female pigs nearby. In the young prepubertal boar social restriction, particularly lack of tactile contact with other pigs, causes a severe depression in the level of sexual behavior, which may be permanent. In contrast to the mature boar the adverse effects of isolating young postpubertal boars from females are longer lasting and may even be permanent.

Evidence from other species, together with breed comparisons of boars, suggests that the sexual behavior of the boar may have a heritable basis. Elevated environmental temperatures may reduce the sexual behavior of the boar, but this effect is generally only temporary.

Despite the fact that recommendations are often made, little is actually known of the effects of frequent mating. A high mating frequency (for example, up to 10 copulations per week) for either the young or mature boar does not appear to be detrimental to the subsequent long-term sexual behavior of the boar. Although unconfirmed, long periods of abstinence may depress sexual behavior for some time.

Prevention and Treatment. To prevent locomotor disturbances, postpubertal boars should be housed individually, and the boar pen should be large enough (greater than 10 sq m) to allow for exercise. Ideally, matings should take place in a separate pen specifically designed for mating. An octagonal- or hexagonal-shaped pen removes corners in which the female's rear quarters may be inaccessible to the boar, thus prompting interference by the attendant. The floor of the mating pen, as for the home pen, should be kept dry, and although it should not be slippery, it should not be abrasive to the animal's feet. The mating arena should be free of obstructions such as feeders or drinkers or other features such as damaged slats, damaged walls or wire-mesh walls, which may trap the leg of an unbalanced boar. If slats are used in the home pen, the slats should be well maintained, should be spaced close enough to provide stability for the boar and should have a good pencil-type edge.

The incidence of locomotor disturbances may be reduced by careful selection for desirable conformational traits of the feet and legs and by selection against undesirable traits such as uneven claw size.

A number of penile disturbances can be treated, such as persistent frenulum, balling of the penis in the diverticulum as well as some injuries to the penis. Again, prevention of penile injuries should include attention to the design and maintenance of the mating arena.

Boars that are sexually inexperienced or may have suffered a traumatic experience when copulating should be introduced to quiet, highly receptive females in familiar surroundings. It may be useful to stimulate the boar sexually by first allowing it to observe another boar courting and copulating. Another useful method is to make a series of short individual introductions to a number of females, removing each female as the boar starts to court. Once the boar has copulated, he should be regularly mated; for example, at least two copulations per week to develop its sexual behavior.

If the boar is suspected of having low sexual motivation, examine the social environment first. Pens for working boars should be located close to the female's pens (less than 15 m), as odor from the female appears to be the main stimulus. The detrimental effects of social deprivation during rearing and around puberty are difficult to overcome and may be permanent. Therefore, young boars selected for breeding should be kept in groups with other pigs during rearing for as long as practical. If it is necessary to measure individual feed intake, the use of individual feeding stalls in the group pens will ensure both feed intake monitoring and full development of sexual behavior. Alternatively, young boars could be housed in individual pens from 12 weeks of age; however, it is essential that they receive tactile contact with other pigs, such as the contact available with neighboring pigs through a wire mesh pen division. Young postpubertal boars should be housed near female pigs, and, therefore, quarantine procedures applied to newly introduced young boars should include contact with female pigs, perhaps culled females.

If elevated temperatures are suspected to be the cause of low sexual motivation, insulation, ventilation and cooling systems should be improved.

Finally, if hand and supervised matings are practiced, the behavior of the attendant toward the pigs should be observed. An attendant that uses fearful stimuli (for example, shouting and waving), punishes the animals, makes fast and unpredictable movements and is impatient will likely have a negative effect on a boar, particularly a young boar that lacks confidence. This negative effect may inhibit the boar's sexual response to a female when in close proximity to a human.

FAILURE TO DETECT OVULATING GILTS OR SOWS

Definition. Failure to detect ovulating females appears to be a significant problem in both the gilt and sow. Reports from commercial and experimental piggeries suggest that the incidence of this condition in the gilt is from 6 to 22 per cent of all gilts. In sows not mated within 3 weeks of weaning the percentage of ovulating sows not detected in estrus may vary from 19 to 83 per cent. Failure to detect an ovulating female results from either an unattentive herder, an inefficient estrous detection procedure or a reduced intensity in signs of estrus in the female. This condition may be revealed by a high percentage of gilts (more than 20 per cent) not mated by 240 days of age or a higher percentage of sows (more than 20 per cent) not mated by 21 days after weaning. Although only limited research has been conducted on this topic, a number of social factors have been implicated in the condition.[2-4] Some, although not all, of the research data indicate that the incidence of this condition is higher in intensive, rather than extensive, production systems.

Diagnosis. In a situation in which a high percentage of females remain unmated within the expected period, it is necessary to differentiate between those that have ovulated (but have not been detected) and those that have not ovulated. Plasma progesterone levels in two blood samples taken about 10 days apart or post mortem examination of ovaries of a sample of females will determine the ovarian status.

If the problem is a failure to detect ovulating females, pertinent information should be sought on (1) estrus detection procedures and (2) factors in the social environment likely to depress estrus expression. Relevant background information includes average age of mating of gilts, average weaning-to-mating interval for each parity group of sows, any evidence of an influence of season on these two parameters and the first occurrence of the problem.

If a boar is relied on to identify estrous females, the sexual behavior of the boar and the contact time allowed in relation to the size of the group of females should be assessed. However, research has shown that boars approach estrous and nonestrous females on a random basis, relying on the female's behavioral response to determine whether they are receptive or not. Boars used in this manner to identify estrous females can be very efficient, but there may be problems with the efficiency of this procedure if the boars are of low sexual motivation, the females to be tested are in large groups, there are a number of females in estrus at once or the boar is allowed insufficient time to test each female.

If the attendant is relied on to identify estrous females, the use of the "back-pressure test" or the "riding test" would appear to be the most efficient and practical estrus detection procedure. The efficiency of this test is greatly enhanced if females are tested adjacent to boars at the place where they receive intense boar stimulation. Separation from boars by as little as 1 m can reduce the efficiency of the test. Intense olfactory, auditory and visual stimuli from the boar facilitate the standing response of estrous females to pressure on their backs. Non-behavioral symptoms of estrus, such as appearance of external genitalia, are less reliable characteristics of estrus. In any procedure that depends on the attendant, it is obviously important that the animals are not fearful of the attendant and that the attendant is competent, thorough and observant.

The social environment around estrus influences the estrus detection rate. Cycling females kept very close to boars, separated by only a wire-mesh pen division, have been shown to have a lower estrus detection rate than those kept opposite boars across a 1-m wide corridor. (In both treatments the back-pressure test was used to detect estrous females while they were held adjacent to boars.) Females continuously housed adjacent to boars may receive such continuous and intense stimulation from the boars that they become refractory to those signals that enhance the standing response to the back-pressure test. It is not yet known whether a boar could have detected and mated these "over-stimulated" females.

Although research data are very limited, it appears that group size and space allowance for grouped females may influence their estrus detection rate. For example, cycling gilts housed in groups of six had a lower estrus detection rate when allowed 1.0 m² per gilt compared with either 2.0 or 3.0 m² per gilt. Also, a lower percentage of gilts was detected in estrus when in groups of 24 compared with groups of 8. (Both treatments had a space allowance of 0.9 m² per gilt.)

Other factors that appear to affect estrus detec-

tion rate are season (summer lower than other seasons), breed (purebred lower than crossbred, and Landrace, Hampshire and Yorkshire breeds lower than Large White and Duroc breeds) and sexual age (pubertal estrus lower than subsequent estruses).

PREVENTION AND TREATMENT

Proper control of boar contact and estrus detection procedures will prevent and treat the condition in most situations. The back-pressure test is probably the most efficient and practical procedure available, but it is important to ensure that the following measures are taken:

1. A boar (preferably an adult of high sexual motivation) is close to the female at the time of testing, for example only separated by a wire-mesh wall.

2. The attendant should quietly approach and apply hand or sitting pressure gently but firmly on the midregion of the back of the female. It may be useful to massage the flanks of the female manually prior to applying pressure to the back.

3. Records of other signs of estrus are kept (either in a notebook or with marks on the female's back), so that suspected females can be double checked with the back-pressure test. Other signs of estrus include swelling and reddening of the vulva for several days prior to estrus (the intensity of these signs may decline as estrus occurs), the presence of viscous mucus in the vulva, particularly in the second half of the estrous period, and behavioral symptoms such as an attraction to the boar, increased restlessness, attempts to court and mount pen-mates and a low-pitched growl.

The efficiency of the procedure will obviously be affected by the competency and attitude of the attendant. If the attendant is unsatisfactory in this regard, a procedure that relies on a boar should be adopted or the attendant should be replaced.

In procedures that rely on a boar to detect estrous females, it is important to remember that the boars are highly motivated, that the test females are in small groups (for example less than 10) and that there is sufficient time (5 minutes or more for a group of 10 females). It is preferable to remove each female as it is identified to allow the first boar or a fresh boar to test for further receptive females. It is a good idea to allow the boar to regularly mate some of the detected females in the detection arena in order to maintain its interest.

To ensure adequate expression of estrus, gilts and sows that are to be mated should be housed near, but not too close to, mature boars. Housing opposite to boars with a 1.0-m or more wide corridor between the two appears suitable. Small groups of females (less than 10) with adequate space (2.0 m² per animal) are preferable.

If seasonal, breed or sexual age problems are suspected, there is little that can be done without changing the management policies. Concentrating on the earlier discussed points may alleviate the extent of the problem.

References

1. Hemsworth PH: Social environment and reproduction. In Cole DJA, Foxcroft GR (eds): Control of Pig Reproduction. London, Butterworths, 1982, pp 585–601.

2. Hemsworth PH: Sexual behavior of gilts. J Anim Sci Suppl (in press).
3. Signoret JP: Reproductive behavior of pigs. J Reprod Fert Suppl 11:105, 1970.
4. Wrathall AE: Reproductive disorders in pigs. Commonwealth Agricultural Bureau, Review Series No. 11, Commonwealth Bureau of Animal Health, England, 1975.

Pregnancy Diagnosis in Swine

J. Ross Buddle, B.Sc., B.V.Sc., D.V.P.H., M.A.C.V.Sc.

Murdoch University, Western Australia

Veterinarians should be able to obtain highly accurate results with at least two methods of pregnancy diagnosis in sows. A single test that is appropriate for all situations is not currently available. Veterinarians are frequently asked to give advice to clients about the use and accuracy of various pregnancy tests, to help train farm staff in their use, to provide accurate pregnancy diagnoses to assist farmers in making management decisions and to obtain accurate pregnancy diagnoses when investigating reproductive disorders.

Four general points should be noted:

1. We do not have a highly accurate test for nonpregnancy; most of the tests are for pregnancy. Nonpregnancy is merely inferred when a test for pregnancy is negative.

2. The tests do not indicate the fate of the pregnancy.

3. The routinely available tests do not predict the number of fetuses.

4. There has been relatively little comparative evaluation of the tests. The oldest test (returns-to-service) is the least evaluated. Most assessments of tests have been done on a single test, with the presence or absence of a subsequent farrowing being the ultimate criterion as to whether the sow was pregnant or not. Because sows can lose a litter after being positive to a test, the tests have not been assessed as tests for pregnancy but rather as tests for the prediction of farrowing. This means the number of false-positives may have been overestimated in these assessments and therefore the specificity and diagnosability of the tests underestimated.

MEASUREMENTS OF ACCURACY

It is misleading to talk about the "accuracy" of a test without specifying which accuracy is meant. Four "accuracies" are used to measure the reliability of a diagnostic test.

1. "Sensitivity" is the probability of a diagnostic test correctly identifying as positive those animals that truly have the characteristic being tested. The result is often expressed as a percentage.

2. "Specificity" is the probability of a diagnostic test correctly identifying as negative those animals that truly lack the characteristic being tested.

3. "Diagnosability" is the percentage of test positives that truly have the characteristic being tested. Sensitivity and specificity are indicators of the ability of the test to reveal correctly the true situation in the animals. Diagnosability is an indicator of the truth of positive results. When assessing a test's accuracy, both sensitivity and specificity should be considered.

4. "Overall" accuracy is the total percentage of animals correctly identified.

REASONS FOR PREGNANCY DIAGNOSIS

Detection of Nonpregnant Sows. In this case one assumes that the test is negative for all the nonpregnant sows but not for any of the pregnant ones. If the test is not 100 per cent accurate, it can err in one of two ways. It might give negative results for all the nonpregnant plus a few pregnant (false-negatives) or give negative results for most of the nonpregnant but none of the pregnant. The worse error is for pregnant sows to be determined as nonpregnant, i.e., false-negatives. Therefore, a test for the detection of nonpregnant sows should give few false-negatives, i.e., have a high sensitivity.

Reasons for requiring the accurate detection of nonpregnant sows include: (1) monitoring herd reproductive performances to detect problems promptly, (2) investigating reproductive disorders, (3) detecting individual nonpregnant sows so they may be remated, treated or culled, (4) checking reputedly anestrous sows for nonpregnancy before they are treated or culled and (5) checking sows selected for culling for nonpregnancy.

Detection of Pregnant Sows. In this case one assumes the test is positive for all of the pregnant sows but not for any of the nonpregnant ones. If the test is not 100 per cent accurate, it might give positive results for all of the pregnant plus a few nonpregnant (false-positives) or most of the pregnant but none of the nonpregnant. The worse error is for nonpregnant sows to be determined as pregnant, i.e., false-positives. Therefore, a test for the detection of pregnant sows should give few false-positives, i.e., have a high specificity.

The reasons for requiring the accurate detection of pregnant sows include (1) aiding the decision of whether injured sows should be treated or culled, (2) detecting pregnant sows when matings have been unsupervised or mating records have been lost or sow identification is uncertain, (3) checking that sows being sold as pregnant are pregnant, (4) predicting production levels and (5) identifying sows to be transferred to gestation accommodation.

TESTS FOR PREGNANCY DIAGNOSIS

Returns-to-Service

Absence of estrus is equated with pregnancy and the presence of estrus with that of nonpregnancy. Accurate estrus detection is vital to the success of this test. Although reddening and swelling of the vulva and the behavior of the boar are helpful indications, behavioral changes in the sow are the most important. Sows in estrus are restless, have a capricious appetite and frequently grunt or squeal. They seek the company of a boar and will stand firmly to pressure applied over their loins by the stockman, i.e., the "back-pressure test." The accuracy of this test is higher in the presence of a boar. The conclusive sign is the sow's willingness to stand for mating. An instrument that measures the conductivity of the vaginal mucus has been developed to assist detection of estrus.

Costs. This test is generally regarded as the cheapest because there is no additional capital outlay, but labor costs can be high, particularly if sows beyond 18 to 24 days after mating are tested.

Advantages. It is easily performed by farmers. Of the currently available tests it provides the earliest confirmation of pregnancy (18 to 24 days), except for the vaginal biopsy test in some circumstances. It also tests for nonpregnancy, there is a minimal capital outlay and it requires no special equipment or laboratory tests.

Disadvantages. It can be deceptively time-consuming and therefore labor intensive. It is not applicable when the sow does not appear to be returning, nor is it useful for routine testing outside the 18- to 24-day period after mating or multiples of this period. False-positives (low specificity and diagnosability) are caused by barren sows (anestrous even though not pregnant), the inability of sows behaviorally to express their desire to seek a boar because of stalls, bullying, or husbandry, and delayed returns, which are unlikely to be detected unless the test is rigorously applied outside the 18-

to 24-day period. In some reproductive disorders delayed returns can be 60 per cent of the total returns-to-service. False-negatives are rare.

Usage. This test is the most appropriate for many farm situations as the earliest indication of non-pregnancy. It is of little use to veterinarians, although the results from the client's usage are most important. Its usefulness for the selection of pregnant sows (specificity) is markedly reduced in herds in which estrus is suppressed in nonpregnant sows.

Manual (per Rectum) Palpation

Manual (per rectum) palpation detects changes resulting from pregnancy in accessible pelvic organs. The criteria used (in descending order of usefulness) are the following: fremitus, the size and position of the middle uterine artery, the tone and tension of the cervix, the size, weight and contents of the uterus, and the corpora lutea. The sow should be restrained in a standing position. Adequate obstetric lubricant should be applied to the gloved hand and forearm. One or two fingers are inserted through the anus, and by holding the hand in the obstetric-cone shape, the entire hand enters the rectum. Remove all feces and allow peristaltic waves to pass over your hand rather than force your hand through them. Slide your hand gently forward to locate the pelvic brim with the tips of your fingers. Then rotate your hand through 90° and move it dorsally and laterally to locate the shaft of the ilium (the right ilium if using your left hand, the left if using your right). The external iliac artery (EIA) runs caudally and ventrally along the medial aspect of the shaft. It is attached to the bone and is about the diameter of a pen (8 to 10 mm). The middle uterine artery (MUA) branches from the aorta caudal to the origin of the EIA. Initially, it runs parallel to the EIA then curves cranially to cross it medially about half way down the shaft before going beyond reach into the abdomen. A smaller artery that supplies the bladder crosses the EIA below the MUA and can lead to a false-negative diagnosis if confused with the MUA.

Spontaneous fremitus can be felt in a few sows at about 4 weeks of gestation and its presence increases steadily to about 70 per cent of sows at full-term. Fremitus can be induced by slowly pushing the MUA against the bone dorsal to the cross-over point, then slowly releasing the pressure. Induced fremitus occurs in about 20 per cent of sows at 2 to 3 weeks of gestation and in almost 100 per cent from 4 weeks. Repeat twice on both MUA before diagnosing nonpregnancy. Avoid accidental occlusion of the EIA to avoid false-positives.

Locate the cross-over of the two vessels. In the nonpregnant sow the MUA is about the diameter of a piece of string (2 to 3 mm but up to 5 mm in multiparous sows), is loosely held against the bone and, particularly in multiparous sows, may be quite tortuous. As pregnancy advances, it increases in size, so that by 4 weeks gestation it is half the size of the EIA in 50 per cent of sows. If the MUA is smaller than the EIA, the arteries on the other side of the pelvis should be examined because occasionally with small litters the MUA on one side is small. During estrus the MUA may increase to about 4 mm in diameter, with a distinct but normal pulse. As the weight of the uterus increases, the D-shape between the EIA and the MUA becomes thinner. Occasionally, the MUA may lie cranial to the EIA for most of its length.

For about 6 days during estrus the cervix becomes hard, arched, tubular and about 40 to 50 mm in diameter, with the bifurcation of the uterus projecting horizontally forward into the abdominal cavity. During diestrus and pregnancy it becomes soft and pliable and feels about 25 mm wide. The uterine bifurcation becomes less distinct with advancing gestation. The weight of the uterus is detected by lifting the cervix with the tips of your fingers. In diestrus there is negligible tension on the cervix.

From about 3 weeks gestation the uterus begins to feel enlarged, with thin soft walls, and from about 4 weeks the bifurcation is indistinct, with the cranial cervix dilating into an ill-defined, thin-walled uterus that falls into the abdomen. Fetuses are palpable close to full-term only.

To palpate the ovaries, follow the cranial edge of the broad ligament from the flank down into the abdomen. Use your free hand to press against the ovaries from outside the flank. Corpora lutea can be detected on the ovaries as small, firm nodules 18 to 24 days after mating. With advancing pregnancy the ovaries are pulled cranially out of reach.

Advantages. This is the cheapest of the tests other than absence of return-to-service. The test requires no special equipment except obstetric lubricant and gloves. If the MUA only is examined, the test is very quickly done and averages about 1 minute per sow, depending on time taken for restraint. It may provide additional information about pathologic changes to the reproductive organs, e.g. large ovarian cysts.

Disadvantages. It is usually not applicable to nulliparous sows (the pelvic cavity is too small), may cause trauma to the sow (this is rare if performed carefully), may expose the veterinarian to injury if the sow suddenly changes position and requires some experience for accurate interpretation. False-positives may be caused by endometritis, a large MUA in multiparous sows or accidental occlusion of the EIA. False-negatives may be caused by only a small increase in the MUA or by mistaking the bladder artery for the MUA.

Usage. Manual palpation remains the basic test for veterinarians, as their responsibilities extend from pregnancy diagnosis for management decisions to solving reproductive problems. It is useful for the detection of both nonpregnant and pregnant sows.

A-Mode Ultrasonography (Amplitude Depth or Pulse Echo)

A-mode machines emit pulsed ultrasound energy from a transducer placed on the skin of the sow. Some ultrasound energy is reflected to the transducer and, depending on the type of machine, converted to electrical energy either in the form of audible or visual (oscilloscope or light-emitting diodes—LED) signals. The machines detect fluid-filled organs at a depth of 10 to 20 cm. Ultrasound energy is reflected from interfaces between different tissues, and some machines can also be used to measure back fat thickness.

The test is best performed with the sow standing, but it can be done with the animal in lateral recumbency. Restraint in a stall is preferable, although the testing may be done while sows are eating or standing still in a pen. Ultrasound transmission gel or vegetable oil (not as viscous as gel) is applied to the transducer, which is placed on the skin of the lower caudal abdomen, approximately above the second to last teat and in the center of the relatively hairless triangular area cranial and ventral to the stifle. The transducer is directed slightly cranially and dorsally toward the reproductive organs. If a signal indicating pregnancy is not present, the interior of the abdomen is searched by keeping the transducer in the same place but slowly moving the handle in an increasing spiral, so the ultrasound beam within the abdomen describes the side of an ever-increasing cone, the apex of which is at the transducer. With advancing pregnancy the weight of the contents pulls the uterus downward and forward into the abdomen, so the position of the transducer on the skin should be adjusted correspondingly. Always ensure that there is coupling medium between the transducer and the skin. Pregnancy is indicated by the relevant signal from the machine. Once familiar with the use of the machine, the operator can infer nonpregnancy when 2 minutes of searching fails to produce a positive signal.

Advantages. This test provides immediate results, usually taking only one half to 1 minute per sow. The machine is easy to use, and a training period is unnecessary. The cost is reasonable: Machines range from $500 to $1500. Those with oscilloscopes and back fat measuring capabilities are usually more expensive. They appear to be reasonably sturdy with a long life span and low service costs. The oscilloscope type is potentially more prone to damage. The machine can be used while sows are eating and on nulliparous sows, the results are easy to check (repeat the test), and it is not harmful to the sow or fetuses.

Disadvantages. The test requires a special machine, and the interpretation of signals in an unusual pattern (oscilloscope or rows of diodes) may be difficult. False-positives can be caused by urinary bladder, pyometra, or a dead litter. False-negatives may be caused by use before 30 or after 90 days gestation when a decrease in the ratio of fluid-to-fetal tissue in the pregnant uterus occurs, or missed or misinterpreted signals.

Usage. A-mode ultrasonography is probably the most frequently used method of pregnancy diagnosis by farmers after absence of returns-to-service. For veterinarians it is a useful adjunct to manual palpation. The test is more useful for the detection of nonpregnant rather than pregnant sows.

Doppler Ultrasonography

The Doppler phenomenon is the change in sound frequency of a moving object as perceived by a stationary observer. Doppler ultrasound machines detect frequency change and, therefore, movement, usually converting it to an audible signal via a loudspeaker or stethoscope. Movements indicative of pregnancy include blood flow in the middle uterine artery, blood flow in the umbilical arteries, the fetal heartbeat, and fetal movements.

The method used is basically the same as that for A-mode ultrasonography. However, sows should be restrained so that their movement is minimized. Feeding increases confusing intestinal sounds. The earliest sound heard is blood flow in the MUA. To detect this, the transducer is placed in the same position as for A-mode ultrasonography, but is initially pointed straight across the abdomen and slightly dorsally toward the flank on the opposite side. The direction is more caudal and dorsal than that for A-mode machines. A rectal probe has been used but has little advantage over external application of the transducer. Blood flow in the MUA produces a strong regular sound repeated at 60 to 80 beats/minute (the sow's pulse rate) and has a whistling or swishing quality. It can be heard as early as 21 days but is not reliably present until 30 days. Blood flow in the umbilical artery has a similar quality at a slightly higher pitch and has a pulse rate that decreases from about 240/minute at 45 days gestation to 160/minute at full-term. It can be heard from about 32 days gestation. The fetal heartbeat occurs at the same rate as umbilical artery sounds but has more of a clapping or galloping quality to its sound. Fetal movements are loud, strong, swishing and often irregular sounds.

Once familiar with the method, the operator can infer nonpregnancy when 2 to 3 minutes of searching fails to produce a sound consistent with pregnancy.

Advantages. The test produces an immediate result and is reasonably quick, averaging 2 minutes per sow, slower than that with the A-mode machine. It is easy to use once the technique is mastered. The machine is reasonably priced, $500 to $1000. It can be used on nulliparous sows, results are easy to check (repeat the test) and the test is not harmful to sow or fetuses. Fetal sounds are definite indications of live fetuses. Fetal heart rate may indicate the stage of pregnancy and, therefore, predict the farrowing date. The test can also check for fetal heartbeat at farrowing if fetuses are thought to remain in the uterus.

Disadvantages. The test requires a special machine and some experience to detect and to distinguish the sounds of pregnancy from other abdominal sounds. Sows must be less mobile than with the A-mode machines, and feed cannot be used to distract sows. False-positives may be caused by increased blood flow to the uterus, e.g., endometritis or an agitated sow. False-negatives may be caused by missed or misinterpreted sounds.

Usage. It takes longer to become experienced with interpretation of sounds and the method is more difficult and time consuming than that of the A-mode machines. Machines with padded headphones are more comfortable to wear and help eliminate extraneous piggery noise. False-positives tend to be fewer (specificity is higher) than with A-mode machines, although false-negatives tend to be higher (sensitivity is lower). Hence, Doppler ultrasound is particularly useful when it is necessary to know that specific sows are definitely pregnant, e.g., certification of pregnancy prior to sale.

Real Time Ultrasonography

Real time ultrasonographic machines scan a plane rather than the beam used by A-mode machines. The reflected signal is converted to a moving pictorial image on a cathode ray tube. Small portable machines (cost is about $20,000) have been developed for veterinary use, predominantly for horse stud work. Preliminary use with swine suggests that they should be at least as useful as in horses, but they have not yet been assessed as a diagnostic test. Although unlikely to be widely accepted for commercial use in the near future, they could become a useful research tool, as they have the potential to indicate pregnancy at an early stage, along with the number of embryos or fetuses present.

Vaginal Biopsy

The histologic appearance of the vaginal epithelium changes under the influence of the varying hormone levels during the estrous cycle and pregnancy.

Two main types of instruments have been used to obtain the sample: a general biopsy instrument (cost about $20), such as that used for human rectal biopsies or a specially designed instrument in which one tube rotates inside another, cutting off a small piece of mucosa through a slot in the outer tube. The vulva is cleaned and the lips are parted, and the sterile instrument, in the closed position, is inserted into the vagina. Initially, it is directed cranially and dorsally, so the tip slides along the roof of the vagina, thus avoiding the urethral opening. When the cervix is reached, the instrument is withdrawn 2 cm to avoid the cervix. The slot is pushed against the mucosa of the anterior vagina, and the inner tube is rotated through 360° to cut off a piece of mucosa and enclose it within the tube.

After withdrawing the instrument, the biopsy sample is carefully removed with a pair of fine forceps and placed in fixative for dispatch to a laboratory. The biopsy instrument is cleaned and disinfected prior to reuse. Hemorrhage from the biopsy site is rare and, if undisturbed, clots without complications.

Advantages. With adequate sow restraint, collection takes one half to 1 minute per sow, or 2 minutes per sow to collect and dispatch samples. Samples taken 18 to 19 days after mating can provide a result with a high sensitivity on days 19 or 20, i.e., earlier than any of the other currently available routine tests. The test can be used on nulliparous sows.

Disadvantages. It does not provide an immediate answer and may be expensive because laboratory processing and interpretation are required ($3 to $5 per biopsy), although this service may be free through a government diagnostic service. Mating dates should be known for maximum accuracy. The specificity is reduced in some reproductive disorders. False-positives may be caused by collection from a nonpregnant sow in the late luteal phase of the estrous cycle (hence avoid collection 30 to 35 days after mating), early fetal death, delayed returns-to-service, low-farrowing rate, cystic or quiescent ovaries, or a biopsy taken from the cervix. False-negatives may be caused by testing before 18 days after mating, biopsy from vaginal vestibule or oblique section of epithelium.

Usage. For routine testing, the vaginal biopsy has been superseded by ultrasonography, despite the greater capital outlay for the latter. It can provide a diagnosis earlier than ultrasonography and can also be useful as an ancillary test on the same day if an ultrasonographic test on a nulliparous sow is equivocal. The test is particularly useful for routine monitoring of pregnancy when samples can be obtained on days 18 or 19 after mating and the result is obtained within 1 or 2 days. Frozen tissue sections have been used, but fixed samples are likely to be more applicable in the field.

Plasma Estrone Sulfate Assay

Estrone sulfate is produced by the embryo, and plasma levels peak between days 23 and 30. Initial studies have indicated that the test can provide accurate results before 4 weeks and perhaps 3 weeks. False-negatives are very low. The 10 per cent false-positives (based on subsequent farrowing) in a large trial is unsatisfactory. Comparison of plasma levels from known pregnant and nonpregnant sows suggests that most of the false-positive sows were pregnant at the time of blood sampling. Hence, this test may become very useful for early pregnancy diagnosis.

Plasma Progesterone Assay

In nonpregnant sows plasma progesterone levels decline rapidly on days 17 to 19 of the estrous cycle.

High levels of plasma progesterone 18 days after mating are suggestive of pregnancy. This test has mainly been used experimentally, but in one commercial situation blood was collected on day 17, so results were available by the expected time of a normal estrus. A high sensitivity was obtained. In the presence of a reproductive failure problem, 21 per cent false-positives (based on subsequent farrowing) reduced the specificity to 60 per cent. Of the sows that did not farrow, none of those returning at a normal interval were incorrectly diagnosed as pregnant, but 46 per cent of those returning at a delayed interval were. If these "false-positives" were actually pregnant at the time of testing, this test, as with the plasma estrone sulfate test, is applicable for pregnancy diagnosis at about 3 weeks gestation in herds in which mating dates are accurately known, and blood samples can economically be collected within a narrow gestational range.

Laparoscopy

Laparoscopic examination of the reproductive tract has provided very early diagnosis of nonpregnancy, using luteal regression as early as day 12 and ovarian follicular development, hyperemia of the uterine horns and peristaltic contractions of the horns as early as day 15. A 100 per cent accuracy was reported, although only 15 sows were tested. This test is likely to remain a research technique only because of the necessity for anesthesia, surgery and the time to perform the test.

Blood Prostaglandin Assay

Estrone from embryos, by blocking prostaglandin synthesis, helps to maintain the corpora lutea during pregnancy. A normal blood prostaglandin level between days 11 and 16 indicates nonpregnancy. The radio-immunoassay test for blood prostaglandin has considerable potential because it is a test for nonpregnancy and is applicable very early in gestation. The reported accuracies indicate further research on the test is necessary before it is useful in the field.

COST/BENEFIT ANALYSIS

If pregnancy diagnosis is to be used routinely, its cost/benefit analysis must be compared with the situation in which no pregnancy diagnosis is performed. Hence, accurate records of the farrowing rate to first service should be known. Assuming this is 80 per cent in a 100-sow herd, the cost of not performing pregnancy testing is the maintenance cost for 20 sows for 16 weeks. However, pregnancy diagnosis would not prevent all of this loss. If we use a pregnancy test with a sensitivity of 95 per cent and a specificity of 90 per cent we will have 78 test positives (76 truly pregnant plus 2 false-positives) and 22 test negatives (18 truly nonpregnant and 4 false-negatives). Hence, to be beneficial, the cost of testing 100 sows, plus the maintenance cost of 2 false-positives and the loss of profit from 4 false-negatives, must be less than the maintenance cost of 18 sows from testing to expected farrowing.

SELECTION OF THE APPROPRIATE PREGNANCY TEST

On most farms the majority of sows are pregnant; therefore, a test of equal sensitivity and specificity will produce more false-negatives than false-positives. Hence, for general use a test with a very high sensitivity is preferable.

It is desirable that veterinarians in practice should be competent in the use of at least two tests. Currently, the three tests appropriate for most occasions are (1) manual palpation, (2) A-mode ultrasonography (high sensitivity and moderate specificity from 30 to 90 days), or (3) Doppler ultrasonography (moderate sensitivity, high specificity from 30 to 115 days).

The use of one or more tests on the same day reduces the number of false-positives, although it may not increase the number of correctly predicted farrowings. Repeat tests on sows previously tested as negative can eliminate false-negatives. Both can be performed with relatively little increase in cost of testing and thus markedly increase the cost/benefit analysis of pregnancy diagnosis.

Suggested Readings

1. Balke JME, Elmore RG: Pregnancy diagnosis in swine: A comparison of the technique of rectal palpation and ultrasound. Theriogenology 17:231, 1982.
2. Buddle JR: Pregnancy diagnosis in sows: A comparison of Doppler ultrasound, vaginal biopsy and manual (per rectum) techniques. Proc VIth Int Pig Vet Soc Congr, Copenhagen, p 30, 1980.
3. Cox RI, Pan YS, Wong MSF, Hoskinson RM: Differentiation of pregnancy and nonpregnancy in pigs from plasma oestrone sulphate levels. Proc 13th Ann Conf Aust Soc Reprod Biol, Christchurch, Abstr 98, 1981.
4. Diehl JR: Pregnancy diagnostic methods for the sow. In Morrow DA (ed): Current Therapy in Theriogenology. 1st ed. Philadelphia, WB Saunders Co, 1980, pp 1057–1064.
5. Fraser AF, Nagaratnam V, Callicot RB: The comprehensive use of Doppler ultrasound in farm animal reproduction. Vet Rec 88:202, 1971.
6. Meredith MJ: The detection of pregnancy in pigs: Parts 1 and 2. Unit for Veterinary Continuing Education, The Royal Veterinary College, London, 1980.

Physiology of Late Pregnancy and Parturition in Swine

Geoffrey C.B. Randall, Ph.D., B.V.Sc., M.R.C.V.S.

Animal Diseases Research Institute, Nepean, Ontario, Canada

THE FETUS DURING GESTATION

The duration of pregnancy in swine is normally 114 to 116 days, with variations occurring between both breeds and strains. Unfortunately, we still have very few details of the factors controlling growth and development during this period, which occupies almost 40 per cent of the life of commercially produced pigs.

While ovulation may be uneven, intra-uterine migration prior to implantation leads to a fairly even distribution of fetuses between horns, with the rapid elongation of the chorion establishing the uterine "territory" of each embryo. The subsequent fusion of the allantois with the chorion provides the diffuse allantochorionic placenta, although at the distal portions the chorion remains a discrete, relatively avascular zone of demarcation between fetuses.

The increase in fetal body weight follows a sigmoid pattern; a relatively slow increase in weight until day 50, steady growth between days 55 and 110 and slower growth during the last 5 days. While severe dietary protein or energy restrictions may lower birth weight, there is little evidence at present that it can be increased by overfeeding the sow. Although growth hormone (GH) is produced by the fetal pituitary, decapitation at 45 days gestation does not result in growth retardation for the trunk, although its maturation is disturbed. Chorionic somatomammotropin (placental lactogen), which can bind to GH receptors in some species, has not been identified in pigs, and the actions of other trophic hormones, such as insulin, are unclear.

At birth, hypothermia is a major hazard to the newborn pig, which has only a limited capacity for gluconeogenesis and very little fat to act as either insulation or energy reserves. The total fat content at birth is about 1 per cent, mostly of a structural nature, and there is no "brown fat," which acts as a heat and energy source in other neonates. During fetal life glucose is the main fetal source of energy, and although very high fructose levels are present in fetal blood, there is no evidence that fructose is a major source of energy. Carbohydrate stores, as liver and striated-muscle glycogen, are the major energy reserves at birth. Their deposition starts at about day 60 but is most rapid between days 100 and 107; the control mechanisms are not known,[8] but in other species, GH and glucocorticoids have been reported as stimulating liver glycogen deposition. Pronounced differences in liver and muscle glycogen content occur between individuals within litters, but their relationship to subsequent survival is not known. The ability to mobilize glycogen rapidly, which is essential after birth, is already present 15 to 20 days before birth and is probably under autonomic control, since fetal catecholamine infusions into the fetus induce glycogenolysis.[3] Whether this plays a role as a source of glucose during fetal life is not known.

During late gestation fetal PO_2, PCO_2, pH and per cent hematocrit remain remarkably stable,[6] although fetal arterial PO_2 (22 to 25 mm Hg) is considerably lower than that of the uterine vein. However, the fetal oxygen dissociation curve is displaced to the left of adult blood (P_{50} = 24 to 27 mm Hg versus P_{50} = 36 mm Hg), allowing higher saturation at lower PO_2 values. There is no distinct fetal hemoglobin in the pig during late pregnancy and the shift in P_{50} is caused by lower 2,3-diphosphoglycerate levels in the fetal red blood cells.[2] These differences permit a higher oxygen-carrying capacity for fetal blood and, together with increases in umbilical and uterine blood flow, enable fetal oxygen requirements to be met throughout pregnancy.

The initial crisis for the newborn is the establishment and maintenance of pulmonary respiration. This requires that the surfactant system be fully developed and that the respiratory muscles function without fatigue. Lamellated osmiophilic bodies, which are associated with surfactant production, first appear at about 90 days of gestation.[1] This coincides with declining lung glycogen reserves and the period when squamous epithelium replaces the cuboidal cells lining the alveoli. Whether surfactant is present in the lung fluid at this time is unknown. By 105 days the number of lamellar bodies has increased to the number seen postnatally, and this is compatible with casual observations that respiration can be established in fetuses removed at 105 to 107 days. There is little information on the control of lung maturation in the pig. Corticosteroids and other hormones, e.g., thyroid hormones, have been implicated in other species, but the data presented here suggest that in the pig maturation occurs at a time when concentrations of fetal corticosteroids are low, although there is clinical evidence in the pig linking low surfactant production with possible thyroid defects.[11] It is well established in many species that fetal respiratory movements occur long before birth and that fetuses spend a large proportion of their time "breathing," thus explaining why the respiratory muscles function without fatigue. In ovine fetuses long periods of rapid irregular breathing (RIB) are associated with rapid eye-movement sleep. Similar periods of RIB are seen in fetal pigs, but additional periods of slower regular breathing movements lasting up to 15 minutes are frequently seen. The stimuli to either type of fetal breathing is not known in the pig.

As with other species, the sow's uterus is not quiescent during gestation, and irregular episodes of prolonged electrical activity that are coincident with elevated intra-amniotic pressure occur. Such episodes have been related to transient disturbances of fetal PO_2, heart rate or "breathing" patterns in other species, but similar studies have not been carried out in pigs. Heart rate is extremely variable in cannulated pig fetuses and may vary from 135 to 225 beats/minute over a 60 minute period. Some of this variability may be associated with the marked fetal activity that can be seen on the sow's flanks, but other short-term variations are observed, and their association with either fetal breathing or uterine activity is not known at present.

PARTURITION

Successful parturition depends upon the rapid and efficient delivery of fetuses sufficiently mature to survive in an extrauterine environment. This must coincide with anatomic, physiological and behavioral changes in the sow that enable her to develop and to maintain a relationship with the litter during the nursing period. Delivery of the fetuses depends upon the synchronized contraction of the uterine smooth muscle, which is aided during the expulsive phase of birth by the striated muscles of the abdominal wall. This muscular activity must be preceded by structural changes in the connective tissue of the cervix, vagina, uterus and pelvic ligaments. The connective tissue of the human cervix during gestation is composed of densely packed collagen fibrils dispersed within a glycoprotein matrix. Shortly before labor both the quantity and chemical composition of the mucopolysaccharides are altered, allowing the connective tissue water content to increase, with resulting separation of the collagen fibers. Thus, the cervix becomes softer and distensible ("ripens"), permitting its easy dilatation. A similar increase in water content of the cervix is seen in the pig in response to injections of relaxin, a hormone whose plasma concentration increases dramatically during the last 3 to 4 days of gestation. Current opinion holds that cervical "ripening" in the sow is brought about by relaxin, but the possibility exists that other hormones, e.g., estrogens or prostaglandins, may also be involved. Changes occurring in the connective tissue of the pelvic ligaments, uterus and vagina are presumed to be similar to those seen in the cervix.

The changes in myometrial activity during parturition have been described by Taverne and co-workers.[10] Although progesterone concentrations may decrease 24 hours before delivery, the pattern of myometrial activity does not change until 9 to 4 hours before delivery of the first piglet. At this time uterine activity increases significantly and changes from the infrequent, long, synchronous periods of activity seen throughout late gestation to more frequent, shorter, propagated contractions, which result in more marked increases in intrauterine pressure. While these increases in activity are under the general control of endocrine changes, structural changes in the myometrial cells similar to those that have been described in other species may also occur in the pig. These include increased numbers of oxytocin receptors in response to rising estrogen levels and the formation of gap junctions between muscle cells in response to falling progesterone and rising estrogen levels, which may allow a more rapid and coordinated propagation of uterine contraction.

During delivery of the fetuses myometrial contractions may begin at either the cervical or the tubal end of the uterine horn and act either to propel fetuses toward the cervix or to shorten the horn. Following delivery of the last fetus from a horn, contractions generally begin at the tubal end only.

A number of external signs of impending delivery are coincident with these internal changes. During the last 3 to 4 days of gestation the vulval lips swell and may be slightly reddened. The udder enlarges more rapidly during the last week of pregnancy so that individual glands are delineated. Over the last 2 to 3 days small beads of secretion may be detectable in some, but not all of the glands, and its presence in any one gland is somewhat variable. Within 24 hours of delivery the glands become more turgid and tense (especially noticeable in the teats) and, at varying times, milk becomes progressively easier to obtain, although this is not a very reliable prognostic aid to the timing of delivery. In the last 24 hours the sow undergoes characteristic behavioral changes. Initially, there is an increased "alertness," which changes to restlessness with continuous alteration in position. Later (usually within 12 hours of delivery), the sow shows signs of "nest building," which include vigorous pawing movements with the forelegs, scraping bedding (or food) into a heap and chewing or rooting at bars or other objects in the pen or farrowing crate. Some authors have attributed onset of nest building to the beginning of labor pains, but recent evidence suggests that it may begin prior to increased uterine activity. Attempts to defecate or urinate are often more frequent during this period of intense activity. Finally, there is a period of relative quiescence (1 to 2 hours) when the sow settles, strains and draws the hind legs up to the abdomen. A small amount of blood- or meconium-stained fluid may escape during this period, indicating cervical patency. The passage of each pig through the pelvis is heralded by vigorous flailing of the tail.

Most sows deliver the litter in 3 to 4 hours, although some "normal" farrowings may take longer. Assessment of the need to assist in delivery must be made in terms of the absence of or the relative strength or productivity of contractions. In general, the mean interval between fetuses is 10 to 15 minutes, although it may be slightly longer between the first and second and before the last fetus.

The order of delivery from either horn is random, and there is evidence that fetuses may occasionally be delivered before litter-mates situated closer to the cervix. Between 25 and 45 per cent of piglets are born in posterior presentation, but there is little evidence that this increases morbidity. Most fetuses are in a dorsosacral position when delivered and, if presented anteriorly, the forelimbs lie alongside the chest wall. However, major deviations in limb position, including breech presentation, cause few problems in fetuses of normal size.

THE FETUS DURING DELIVERY

Until recently it was assumed that mild asphyxia was a normal part of delivery, since contractions interfere with uterine blood flow (and hence fetal oxygenation). Samples taken shortly after birth contained increased lactic acid concentrations and had a lowered pH. However, redistribution of fetal blood flow to increase placental flow allows the fetus to tolerate these transient periods of hypoxia without becoming asphyxiated. In fully viable fetuses mean PO_2, PCO_2 and pH values between contractions are relatively stable until the last hour before birth despite the presence of strong uterine contractions (during which fetal PO_2 may fall by 25 per cent) 8 to 9 hours before delivery.[5] Individual variation occurs, with no change seen in these parameters in some fetuses, while minor alterations occur during the last 2 to 3 hours of labor in others. Since this variation is not always associated with position in the farrowing order, it suggests that other factors, such as placental attachment or blood flow, may be involved. Fetal blood glucose and lactic acid concentrations and heart rate remain stable during delivery, although the latter increases transiently during the initial stage of uterine contractions.

Immediately after delivery, pronounced changes (which may be catecholamine induced) occur: Heart rate increases (by up to 100 per cent), hematocrit increases transiently and blood glucose rises. With the onset of breathing PO_2 increases rapidly, and PCO_2 falls. However, pH falls by 0.1 to 0.3 units during the first few minutes of life, and this is associated with increased blood lactic acid, resulting from a redistribution of blood flow to skeletal muscle. These changes occur so rapidly after birth that samples taken 2 minutes after delivery bear little association with intrauterine conditions.

Following birth there is a short period of apnea (< 10 seconds) followed by a short series of gasps and a period of panting prior to the onset of regular respiration. The gasping, which may be induced by the transient hypoxia experienced during the final stages of delivery, acts to facilitate aeration and removal of liquid from the lungs. The rapid increase in PO_2 that follows the onset of breathing may act to reset peripheral and central chemoreceptor thresholds from fetal to adult levels so that normal patterns can be established. Piglets attempt to stand within 1 or 2 minutes of birth and then move craniad on the sow, sucking at any protuberance until they encounter a teat.

MORTALITY DURING DELIVERY

Approximately 25 per cent of newborn piglets die before weaning, and one fourth of these losses have been loosely designated as stillborn. While "outbreaks" of stillbirths are associated with some infections or nutritional deficiencies, the most serious economic losses result from the deaths of one or two pigs in about one third of all litters. Stillborn piglets can be subdivided into those that died *prepartum* and those that died during labor (*intrapartum*), the larger group. Most piglets dying during birth are alive at delivery, although a slow heart beat may be the only evidence of life. When pH, blood gases and lactic acid levels are determined in such piglets, the severe respiratory and metabolic acidosis (pH 6.5 to 6.9; PCO_2 > 150 mm Hg; lactic acid > 150 mg/100 ml) suggests that the severe depression is a result of asphyxiation during delivery. Asphyxiation in utero may increase fetal peristalsis and relaxation of the anal sphincter, so that meconium is passed into the amniotic fluid. At the same time severe hypoxia stimulates deep fetal gasps so that amniotic fluid, and any debris in it, is drawn into the trachea. Meconium- or blood-stained fluid may be found in the respiratory tract in up to 85 per cent of *intrapartum* deaths, its presence generally being an indicator rather than a cause of asphyxia. Thus, asphyxia during delivery is a significant cause of losses and may account directly for 20 per cent of all preweaning losses. In addition, on the basis of a composite viability score, reduced viability in liveborn piglets can be correlated with acidemia, suggesting they have been subjected to less severe or shorter-lived periods of asphyxia. Such piglets, because of depressed functions and less activity, may be more susceptible to trauma and chilling during the immediate postparturient period and less competitive in nursing. Transient periods of hypoxia mobilize liver glycogen reserves, further reducing their chances of survival.

At term, fetal pigs have a short survival time when subjected to asphyxia. If the umbilical circulation is experimentally occluded in utero, the time to last gasp (TLG) is about 5 minutes, although the heart may continue to beat for 20 to 25 min.[7] It follows that if fetal oxygenation is completely blocked (e.g., premature rupture of the umbilical cord), delivery must occur within 5 minutes if the fetus is to survive without external resuscitation. However, a recent study of a naturally occurring case[9] suggested that a different pattern is seen when the hypoxia is less severe but more protracted, e.g., during premature placental separation. In this case periods of gasping and severe bradycardia occurred near the end of each uterine contraction but were absent between contractions. The period during which gasping was recorded lasted 35 minutes, but the heart ceased beating within 5 minutes of the last gasp. Clearly, more studies are needed to clarify relationships between etiology and the clinical state.

While *prepartum* deaths occur randomly, 70 to 80 per cent of *intrapartum* deaths occur in the last third of the litter to be born. Although prolonged deliveries result in a higher incidence of stillbirth, the majority of stillborn piglets occur in litters delivered in less than 4 hours, suggesting alternate causes. At present, there is no conclusive evidence that the stillbirth rate can be reduced by administration of oxytocin or other drugs to shorten the farrowing time. In most *intrapartum* deaths the umbilical cord has already ruptured at the moment of delivery. The proportion of all piglets (i.e., live and dead) in which the cord is broken at the time of birth increases later in the birth order, and it is probable that the distribution of stillbirths is associated with increased tension and rupture of the umbilical cord during the later stages of delivery. It is not known whether the incidence of premature rupture of the cord can be reduced. *Intrapartum* asphyxia may also result from premature placental separation, which may be more common late in farrowing, or from reduced oxygen carrying capacity of maternal or fetal blood, as in iron-deficiency anemia.

Synchronized batch-farrowing with prostaglandins may permit closer attention to piglets at birth; cleaning of the upper respiratory tract and drying and moving the depressed piglets to a warm environment will also reduce losses. Milosavlejević and coworkers[4] have reported that up to 30 per cent of *intrapartum* stillborns can be resuscitated using artificial ventilation, but our experience with small numbers using ventilation combined with bicarbonate (1 mEq IV) to counter acid-base disturbances has been less successful in achieving a fully viable piglet. This difference may be a result of the duration of asphyxiation and the degree of brain damage occurring prior to resuscitation.

References

1. Baskerville A: Histological and ultrastructural observations on the development of the lung of the fetal pig. Acta Anat 95:218, 1976.
2. Comline RS, Silver M: A comparative study of blood gas tensions, oxygen affinity and red cell 2,3 DPG concentrations in foetal and maternal blood in the mare, cow and sow. J Physiol 242:805, 1974.
3. Comline RS, Fowden AL, Silver M: Carbohydrate metabolism in the fetal pig during late gestation. Qly J Exp Physiol 64:277, 1979.
4. Milosavlejević S, Miljković V, Sôvljanski B, et al.: The revival of apparently stillborn piglets. Acta Vet (Belgrade) 22:71, 1972.
5. Randall GCB: Changes in fetal and maternal blood at the end of pregnancy and during parturition in the pig. Res Vet Sci 32:278, 1982.
6. Randall GCB: Daily changes in the blood of conscious pigs with catheters in foetal and uterine vessels during late gestation. J Physiol 270:719, 1977.

7. Randall GCB: Studies on the effect of acute asphyxia on the fetal pig *in utero*. Biol Neonate 36:63, 1979.
8. Randall GCB, L'Ecuyer C: Tissue glycogen and blood glucose and fructose levels in the pig fetus during the second half of gestation. Biol Neonate 28:74, 1976.
9. Taverne MAM, Randall GCB: Heart rate changes and gasping during intra-partum asphyxiation of a piglet. A case report. Theriogenology 19:797, 1983.
10. Taverne MAM, Naaktgeboren C, Elsaesser F, et al.: Myometrial electrical activity and plasma concentrations of progesterone, oestrogens and oxytocin during late pregnancy and parturition in the miniature pig. Biol Reprod 21:1125, 1979.
11. Wrathall AE, Bailey J, Wells DE, Hebert CN: Studies on the barker (neonatal respiratory distress) syndrome in the pig. Cornell Vet 67:543, 1977.

Induction of Parturition in Swine

John P. Hurtgen, D.V.M., Ph.D.
New Freedom, Pennsylvania

REASONS FOR INDUCTION

There are a number of factors affecting management and productivity that can be better controlled through induced parturition. For example:

1. The number of personnel and management efforts can be increased and planned if farrowings can be effectively induced during specific time periods. For example, weekend and night farrowings can be minimized.

2. Simultaneous farrowings aid in the cross fostering of pigs and the equalization of pig size within litters and pig numbers between litters. This practice may be particularly helpful when one or more sows with poor mammary systems or aggressive behavior are due to farrow.

3. The age differential of pigs within a farrowing group can be reduced. This factor has the potential of reducing disease and stress within the farrowing group and, subsequently, in the nursery.

4. The effective use of induction of parturition has the potential to increase sow productivity. Sow productivity should be increased because of these factors as well as the frequently reported reduction in the mastitis-endometritis-agalactia (MMA) syndrome in sows following prostaglandin induced farrowing.

PROCEDURE FOR INDUCTION

The most efficacious method for the induction of parturition in sows and gilts is injection of prostaglandin $F_{2\alpha}$ ($PGF_{2\alpha}$) or one of its analogs. Pregnant females should not be treated until day 111 or later in gestation to avoid compromising piglet birth weight and viability. In fact, under farm conditions, it is advised that sows be treated on or after day 112. The majority of sows farrow the first pig 24 to 30 hours after prostaglandin treatment. The duration of farrowing is comparable to spontaneous parturition, i.e., about 4 hours. Although other prostaglandin analogs may also be effective in the induction of farrowing, a dosage of 10 mg $PGF_{2\alpha}$, 175 µg of cloprostenol, or 1, 2, or 3 mg of alphaprostol is widely used.

Frequently, a prostaglandin product is administered in the morning so that most females will farrow during daylight working hours the following day. In order to decrease the interval and variability in the interval from treatment to onset of farrowing, 30 IU of oxytocin may be administered 20 to 24 hours after prostaglandin treatment.

The use of prostaglandin to induce farrowing does not compromise the onset of lactation or the availability of colostrum in treated females. Some research reports suggest that prostaglandin-treated sows have a decreased incidence of MMA.

The interval from prostaglandin treatment to onset of farrowing is dependent on length of gestation and the sow's readiness for farrowing. If colostrum can be expressed from the teat ends of the near term female, farrowing may commence in 2 to 6 hours as opposed to 24 to 30 hours after treatment.

Some sows exhibit an increased respiratory rate and anxiety following prostaglandin $F_{2\alpha}$ treatment. These side effects are rarely observed in sows treated with one of the prostaglandin analogs.

Although synthetic glucocorticoids administered to sows in late gestation will decrease the length of gestation, farrowings are not well synchronized, treatments need to be given repeatedly and piglet viability tends to be compromised.

SUMMARY

Prostaglandin is an effective agent for the induction of farrowing in swine. Females should be treated on or after day 112 of gestation. Farrowing usually occurs 24 to 30 hours following injection. When used in this manner, piglet birth weight and viability are not compromised. Induction of parturition may help to minimize MMA in herds with a high incidence of the syndrome.

Suggested Readings

1. Einarsson S, Fischier M, Karlberg K: Induction of parturition in sows using prostaglandin $F_{2\alpha}$ or the analogue cloprostenol. Nordisk Vet 33:354, 1981.
2. Holtz W, Hartmann FJ, Welp C: Induction of parturition in swine with prostaglandin analogs and oxytocin. Theriogenology 19:583, 1983.

Factors Influencing Live Litter Size

L. Kirk Clark, D.V.M.

University of Minnesota, St. Paul, Minnesota

There is little evidence that litter size at birth or weaning has improved in the past years despite the many management schemes that have been developed to improve swine reproductive efficiency. Improvements in the number of live pigs per sow year over the past 10 years have been the result of increasing litters per sow year, not live pigs per litter.[1] The number of pigs weaned per litter in the United States has varied little from 7.4 during the last 40 years. With preweaning mortality estimated to be approximately 17 per cent, the average live-born litter size in U.S. herds would be about 9.5 pigs. The genetic potential for liveborn litter size in swine is estimated to be 10.5 to 11 pigs. If this potential could be achieved through the implementation of management techniques, known to improve live-born litter size, weaned litter size should also improve.

Management of the breeding herd is tantamount to the improvement of litter size. Many causes of small litter size are responsive to management change. Unfortunately, their relative importance and interactions remain unknown. Except for those cases in which excessive numbers of stillborn and mummified fetuses are presented at farrowing, small litters are usually not caused by infectious reproductive diseases. Therefore, this article will emphasize the noninfectious factors and management techniques that affect litter size.

GENETICS

Historically, most breeds of swine were not developed and/or maintained for prolificacy. Although some breeds are more prolific than others, observations of data from several large swine herds show that litter size varies within breeds as much as among them. Attempts to improve litter size through direct genetic selection have not been promising. The low calculated heritability of reproductive traits is believed to be responsible for this lack of progress. In practice, the maintenance of prolific lines and the use of cross-breeding schemes to optimize heterosis should maximize potential litter size within a herd. To date, little evidence exists to show that genetic selection has overcome any of the limiting factors imposed upon the breeding herd by the following management variables affecting live litter size and reproductive efficiency.

PARITY

Ovulation rate increases with advancing age or parity. Live-born litter size reaches its maximum around the fourth parity and then slowly declines because of increasing percentages of stillborn pigs. The size of the first litter is influenced by the age of the gilt and the number of estrous cycles prior to mating. However, when measuring the average reproductive performance during the first four parities, early-bred females produce as well as those bred at later estrous cycles. Herd reproductive efficiency is usually not compromised by small litters from gilts bred during first estrus. However, if the cull rate and percentage of gilts is increased, herd reproductive efficiency could suffer. Analysis of records of several large confinement herds in the United States shows large numbers of first parity females (30 to 60 per cent) in herds producing small litters. Gilts are often unjustly culled because of small litter size. Average live-born litter size of second parity females rises less than one half pig above first parity females, and extensive culling is again instituted. The average parity of sows that have farrowed is reduced to about two, and live-born litter size becomes a limiting factor of reproductive performance.

After first parity gilts are weaned, nearly 40 per cent fail to return to estrus within 14 days. Less than 20 per cent of females in other parities fail to return to estrus within 14 days. The first parity females that do return to estrus within 14 days (60 per cent) have a marked reduction in litter size (nearly two pigs less than the herd average). However, if those that fail to return to estrus in 14 days are not culled and are rebred at their next estrus, they produce large litters (more pigs per litter than the herd average). Without considering cull rate or days from weaning to estrus, the second-parity litter size is generally equal to or slightly greater than the litter size of first-parity females.

Investigations of herds with low litter size should include a review of the management of first and second parity females and also an analysis of the herd's parity distribution. Close examination of culling procedures and time and rate of return to estrus is also important for improving litter size in early parity females.

PREVIOUS LENGTH OF LACTATION

Because of the advanced management techniques for raising very young pigs, early weaning has become increasingly popular. Consequently, producers are able to take advantage of increases in litters per sow year with early weaning programs (removing pigs from sows less than 28 days after farrowing). Early weaning has little effect on most parameters of the sow's subsequent reproductive performance unless average weaning age is less than 21 days. However, early weaning has been shown to reduce subsequent litter size. If early weaning is practiced, lower litter size through all parities will occur.[6]

To determine the effects of 21 ± 3-day (early weaning) versus 28 ± 3-day (late) weaning on subsequent live litter size and farrowing rate, a retrospective analysis of 6350 litters born over a period of 7 years in a large commercial herd in south central Minnesota was completed. The litters were categorized into early and late weaned groups only by the length of lactation of their previous litter. They were not continuously weaned early or late. To avoid the confounding influence of time between weaning and mating, all litters were removed from the litter size analysis that had wean-to-breed intervals longer than 14 days. Therefore, farrowing rates were calculated as the percentage of sows of a group that had mated within 14 days of weaning and farrowed a live litter. Early weaned sows (1768) farrowed 1433 litters and had a farrowing rate of 81 per cent as compared with late-weaned sows (5688) that farrowed 4749 litters with a farrowing rate of 83.5 per cent. The early weaned sows (mean weaning age 21.9 days) produced a mean of 9.55 live pigs per litter compared with late weaned sows (mean weaning age 27.5 days) that produced a mean of 10.12 live pigs per litter. The difference favored the late weaned sows by a 2.5 per cent increase in farrowing rate ($P < 0.025$) and by 0.57 live pigs per litter ($P < 0.001$). These data show that early weaning was associated with reduced litter size and farrowing rate in the subsequent litters in a commercial herd.

Reduction in live litter size because of early weaning occurs during implantation, 10 to 20 days after coitus.[4, 5] Whether the physiological changes that occur during implantation can be manipulated to reduce the losses observed after early weaning awaits future research. Unless it can be determined that early weaning does not affect subsequent litter size within a given herd, producers should view weaning earlier than 28 days with caution.

MATING MANAGEMENT

Mating management can affect reproductive performance with regard to normal and abnormal re-

turns to heat and variation in litter size. Fertility of the boar, timing of mating and the number of matings per estrus all influence the preceding parameters. Since boars of low fertility are often culled, most boars influence reproductive efficiency through variation in litter size of subsequent litters, reduced conception rate and low birth weights.

Many boars that have poor reproductive efficiency are hidden in herds in which two different boars are mated to the same female during a single estrus. Others with poor reproductive efficiency are kept in herds that do not keep production records on boars. Single-boar matings, when one boar is repeatedly mated to a female during the estrous period, allow for the assessment of individual boar fertility. Using multiple boars to mate a female has resulted in slightly higher conception rate and litter size, although subfertile boars will not be detected.

Litter size and conception rate can be adversely affected by the timing of mating and number of services per estrus.[3] Litter size and conception rate are maximized when mating occurs 6 to 10 hours prior to ovulation, which occurs approximately 38 to 42 hours after the onset of estrus. The enhanced conception rate and litter size observed after multiple matings, per estrus, is probably more a function of proper timing than the number of matings. Other factors can affect boar fertility, including high ambient temperatures, scrotal frostbite, lameness and overuse.

The technology of artificial insemination has not yet been developed to equal the reproductive efficiency of natural service. When compared with natural service, conception rate is often 5 to 15 per cent lower, and litter size is one half to two pigs less per litter. At this time, artificial insemination should be avoided if conception rate and live litter size are a problem within a herd.

SEASONAL EFFECTS

Although reproductive efficiency can be adversely affected by seasonal or climatic conditions, there is little evidence that live litter size is affected. A current study of a large Minnesota herd showed no significant live litter size variation when comparing mean litter size per month over a 7-year time period. However, there is a trend toward smaller live litter size born subsequent to breeding in late winter and the hot summer months. Recent analyses of other herds suggest similar trends. Although the cause is unknown, it is possible that environmental temperature prior to breeding may affect semen quality at the previously mentioned times. Proper housing and environmental management of the boar during extremely hot and cold weather are necessary to minimize seasonal influence on litter size.

EFFECTS OF INFECTIOUS DISEASES

Small litter size is usually not the only clinical sign observed with infectious reproductive failure.

Infections, such as parvovirus, enterovirus, leptospirosis and toxoplasmosis, may result in small liveborn litters in some females within the herd.[1] Other signs of reproductive failure observed during these infections include abortion, stillbirth, mummified fetus, normal and abnormal return to heat and sows found not-in-pig (NIP). When small liveborn litter size is observed, along with these signs, efforts to isolate causative agents and serologic studies should be instigated.

NUTRITION

The nutrition of the breeding herd has commanded considerable attention in the past 20 years, as evidenced by the volume of literature devoted to this topic. Nutritional effects on litter size are minimal unless diets that grossly deviate from National Research Council (NRC) requirements are fed for prolonged periods of time.

Using NRC recommendations, plus 15 per cent to provide a margin of safety, the breeding herd should be fed to condition on an individual animal basis. When considering long-term reproductive efficiency, emphasis should be given to maintaining good condition of first- and second-parity females. These females should not lose excessive weight during lactation. A rule of thumb to maximize reproductive efficiency is to full feed a high energy ration during the lactation and weaning-to-estrous period.

Changes in nutrition that might influence reproductive efficiency during the reproductive cycle include the following:

1. Increasing feed intake (flushing) in gilts 14 days prior to mating (positive).

2. Reducing feed consumption to 5 to 6 lb per head per day immediately following conception through the first 30 days of gestation (positive?).

3. Feeding limited quantities of feed during cold weather in thin sows (negative).

PARTURITION

Since evidence of infectious diseases has been found in only 30 per cent of stillborn pigs, the largest cause of stillbirth (a major cause of small liveborn litter size) appears to be from problems during parturition.[2] After the fourth parity, the per cent of stillborns increases with increasing parity, limiting optimum liveborn litter size. Studies have also shown stillborn rates to rise dramatically as total litter size increases above 12 pigs per litter. Proper farrowing house management, including induction and observation of parturition, particularly in older sows, will help reduce high stillborn rates.

HOUSING

Many changes in housing of sows have occurred in the past 20 years without documented evidence of a direct influence on live-born litter size. However, housing does affect management of nutrition, ambient temperature, photoperiod and social environment, which are all important for optimum reproductive efficiency.

SUMMARY

Live-born litter size is the net result of the genetic potential of the female to produce a litter minus those factors that influence litter size, acting independently or through interaction during the reproductive cycle of the sow. Veterinarians and swine producers must continuously assess and refine these factors to achieve maximum reproductive performance. This can best be accomplished through the use of adequate records and their timely analysis.

In general, the following techniques can be used to help maximize litter size:

1. Use prolific breeds and cross-breeding systems that maximize heterosis in those breeds.

2. Maintain average parity of sows that have farrowed as near to four as possible.

3. Use 4-week weaning systems unless the negative effects of earlier weaning have been assessed within the herd.

4. Mate sows twice at 24-hour intervals or three times at 12-hour intervals during estrus with a different boar each mating.

5. Do not expose boars to extreme temperatures prior to usage.

6. Vaccinate to prevent the effects of disease on reproductive efficiency.

7. Flush gilts (increased energy intake 14 days prior to mating).

8. Feed the herd individually and maintain good body condition throughout each reproductive cycle.

9. Attend the last one third of parturition, especially in sows of advanced parity that are known to produce large litters. Synchronize farrowing when necessary.

10. Use facilities that allow for easy implementation of these techniques.

References

1. Kingston HG: The problems of low litter size. Pig Vet Soc Proceed 8:54, 1981.
2. Randall GCB: Observations on parturition in the sow. II. Factors influencing stillbirth and perinatal mortality. Vet Res 90:183, 1972.
3. Tilton JE, Cole DJA: Effect of triple versus double mating on sow productivity. Anim Prod 34:179, 1982.
4. Varley MA, Cole DA: Studies on sow reproduction. 5. The effect of lactation length of the sow on the subsequent embryonic development. Anim Prod 22:79, 1976.
5. Varley MA, Cole DJA: Studies on sow reproduction. 6. The effect of lactation length on pre-implantation losses. Anim Prod 27:209, 1978.
6. Walker N, Watt D, MacLeod AS, et al.: The effect of weaning at 10, 25, or 40 days on the reproductive performance of sows from the first to the fifth parity. J Agric Sci Camb 42:449, 1979.

Management of the Farrowing and Lactating Sow

Marianne Ash, D.V.M.
Staff Veterinarian, Yeager & Sullivan, Inc., Camden, Indiana

It is the objective of farrowing and lactation management to wean the maximum number of strong and healthy piglets. To accomplish this goal, it is necessary to understand what is normal, so that the slightest deviations from this state will promptly be recognized. Thorough knowledge in this area is also required so that unnecessary interference will not occur during normal delivery and lactation.

PREDICTING PARTURITION

The gestation period of the sow is generally recognized as 114 ±2 days. However, individual sows may have normal gestation periods that vary over a wide range. Therefore, both good records and close observation are essential to ensure that the sow is in the right place at the right time for farrowing.

The sow demonstrates several signs of impending parturition. These include the following:

1. Changes in the texture of the mammary gland. The mammary gland changes from a soft flabby structure to one of increased firmness and turgidity as parturition nears. These changes usually become noticeable several days prior to delivery.

2. Availability of milk. A serous secretion may be expelled from the mammary glands of some sows as much as 48 hours prior to delivery. This secretion changes to a milky consistency near delivery. When milk becomes readily available, one can expect the first pig within 6 to 8 hours.

3. Bed making and restlessness. As parturition approaches, there is an overall increase in activity on the part of the sow. She gets up and down frequently and may attempt to collect things within her reach to make a nest. She may also paw at the floor, chew on anything available and become more vocal. Urination and defecation may increase in frequency.

4. Vulvar swelling and discharges. Swelling of the vulva becomes obvious 3 to 4 days prior to delivery. The vulva becomes moist, and blood-stained fluids may be observed within about 2 hours of farrowing in a majority of sows. Small amounts of meconium are often expelled prior to the first pig. When this is observed, the first pig will usually arrive within 30 minutes.

5. Respiration, pulse and rectal temperature all tend to increase as farrowing approaches and as general sow activity increases.

Although these factors have been discussed independently, predicting the time of farrowing is most reliable when all factors and observations are considered collectively.

FARROWING

The Sow. Baby pigs are usually delivered with the sow in lateral recumbency. The degree of restlessness exhibited by the sow will vary considerably. Sows tend to appear more nervous at the time of delivery of the early pigs. It is at this time that the greatest danger from crushing and mutilation exists. After the last pig has been born, a nervous sow will usually become relaxed and settle down to nurse her pigs.

Delivery time for individual sows may vary greatly. It has been reported to range from 30 minutes to over 10 hours, with the average observed time to be a little over 2½ hours. The interval between births may range from as little as a minute to more than 1 or 2 hours. However, the average interval between pigs is about 15 minutes.

In most cases all fetal membranes are passed after delivery of the last pig. This is not, however, always the case. Portions of placenta may be passed between pigs. Retained placenta is not common in the pig, and when present, usually indicates the presence of additional pigs in the reproductive tract.

The Pigs. Baby pigs may be delivered almost as frequently "hind feet first" as "nose first." Pigs delivered "nose first" should appear in a dorsoventral position with the front legs extended back along the chest. Pigs that are delivered "hind feet first" should also be in a dorsoventral position with the hind legs extended. Any deviation from either of these positions would be considered malpresentation.

In most instances the umbilical cord is still attached at birth but usually breaks within 5 minutes. Baby pigs are often seen nursing with the cord still attached. Pigs born with the cords already ruptured are most often those born latest in the litter.

Baby pigs are on their feet within minutes after birth. On the average they will have nursed successfully within 45 minutes following delivery. Occasionally, pigs may be born partially or completely enveloped in the afterbirth. The majority of these will struggle free with no negative aftereffects.

OBSTETRIC PROBLEMS

Various observers have noted that less than 1 per cent of sows or gilts farrowing require assistance with delivery. However, the following signs may be indicative of a problem:

1. Signs of farrowing without the onset of birth, e.g., abdominal straining and vulvar discharges without delivery of pigs.

2. Cessation of abdominal straining following delivery of only one or two pigs.

3. An interval of greater than 1 hour passing since the delivery of the previous pig, with continued abdominal straining on the part of the sow.

4. Presence of a foul smelling, colored vaginal discharge.

5. Anorectic, depressed, ill-appearing sow because of the farrow.

Difficulty with delivery of the pigs is referred to as dystocia and may be of maternal or fetal origin.

Maternal Faults. One of the more common causes of dystocia in the sow results from failure of the uterus to contract. This is referred to as uterine inertia. Primary uterine inertia refers to cases in which uterine contractions fail to begin, and the sow appears to never enter the second stage of labor. The exact mechanism of failure is not well defined but may result from interactions between several factors, such as hormone imbalances, nutrition, environment and disease. Secondary uterine inertia occurs when the uterus ceases contracting during a long and exhausting labor that may have been complicated by malpresentations, delivery of large piglets or delivery of an excessively large litter.

Treatment of uterine inertia usually begins with examination of the birth canal for evidence of obstruction followed by administration of oxytocin. Forcing the sow to rise and move about is often helpful in initiating parturition in cases of primary inertia. Manual removal of one or more pigs may also be beneficial. Cases of secondary inertia are usually relieved by manual delivery of the remaining pigs or by cesarean section.

Dystocia may occasionally occur in older sows with large litters because of deviation of the uterus. The weight of the litter pulls the uterus down over the brim of the pelvis, and when pressure is exerted during delivery, the uterus is projected caudally under the brim of the pelvis and delivery of the pigs is obstructed. Manual delivery of a few pigs will usually correct this problem.

Obstruction of the birth canal may also occur, resulting in difficulty in delivery of pigs. This obstruction may be caused by narrowing of the birth canal because of hematomas, a distended bladder, constipation, excessive fat, swelling and edema of soft tissues of the birth canal, previous pelvic fractures or the presence of a small immature pelvis. Rarely, a persistent hymen may be present, requiring rupture in order for birth to proceed. In cases in which the obstruction cannot be reduced nor the pigs delivered manually, cesarean section may be required.

Fetal Faults. A difficult birth is often a result of an oversized fetus, malpresentation of the fetus or malformation of the fetus. In most cases delivery can be accomplished with assistance. If not, a decision must be made as to whether a cesarean section is indicated.

LACTATION

The baby pig's ultimate well-being is largely dependent upon its ability successfully to attain adequate nutrition shortly after birth. The sow's antibodies do not cross the placenta to the unborn pig, making adequate colostral intake during the first few hours essential to the survival of the newborn pig. During the course of lactation many factors affect the baby pig's access to adequate nutrition. Identifying these factors and minimizing their effects must be a primary goal of management.

The Mammary Gland. To maximize the baby pig's opportunity for adequate nutrition it is desirable that 14 to 16 functional teats be present. Teat abnormalities such as blind and inverted teats should be avoided, and even spacing of the teats along the udder is desired. Adequate exposure of the lower row of teats during nursing is frequently a problem, especially because the rearmost teats in older sows have large pendulous udders. This must be recognized as effectively reducing the rearing capacity of the sow. Selection of gilts with underlines closer to the midline may be helpful. Since the problem is more common in older sows, timely culling will help. A comfortable floor surface is also felt to help encourage the sow to expose all teats adequately. Research has shown that certain mammary gland characteristics have a low heritability. There are times when selecting for them may result in selection against other desirable traits, such as growth rate or feed efficiency. These facts should be considered in decisions concerning gilt selection and sow culling.

Nursing. The normal nursing pattern consists of a uniform time interval of somewhat less than 1 hour between each feeding, and this pattern continues over a 24-hour period. The nursing period lasts for only a few minutes, with abundant milk flow for only about 20 seconds.

Teat Order. Immediately following birth, fierce competition occurs among pigs of a litter for the mother's available teats. Once the teat order is established, a given pig usually maintains his chosen teat until weaning. Pigs show a definite preference for certain teats, particularly the anterior teats. As fighting occurs for these teats at each milk letdown, some pigs lose, and because of the short period of milk flow, they may miss a feeding altogether. With each successive feeding missed, their chances for success during the next feeding are lessened, as are their chances for survival. In situations in which rear teats are being left vacant, an observant and patient manager can sometimes encourage apparently unsuccessful contenders for the front teats to take nutrition from teats more posterior. Since one pig claims one teat at each feeding, it is essential that any pigs in excess of the number of functional exposed teats be immediately recognized and alternative provisions be made for their rearing.

Crossfostering. As earlier mentioned, the sow frequently delivers more or less pigs than she is capable of rearing. For this reason crossfostering can be a very effective means of increasing pig survival, especially in large herds with batch farrowing. It is likely to be of greatest benefit in those herds having large litters with a lot of variability in birth weight. Extra pigs from one litter may usually be transferred successfully to a sow with surplus teats if done within 3 days of farrowing. After that time the surplus glands may have begun to dry up. Likewise, smaller pigs may be grouped and transferred to a foster mother to eliminate their need to compete with larger littermates and thus improve their opportunity for nutrition. For whatever reason, crossfostering will be most successful the sooner it is done after farrowing. To increase the opportunity for successful crossfostering, large operations may want to consider the use of hormones to induce parturition. This will allow most pig transfers to be done within 5 to 6 hours after birth.

MILK SUPPLY

The sow's ability to produce an adequate supply of milk requires sufficient genetic potential, access to adequate nutrition, healthy mammary glands and absence from disease in general. It is recognized that differences in milking capacity exist between breeds and individuals. Three-week litter weights are probably the best indicator of the sow's milk yield, as up to this time the amount of growth is almost entirely dependent upon the sow's milk supply. Some indication of milk yield should be considered as important to any sow evaluation system. Systems have been designed for adjusting weights at variable weaning ages back to a 3-week figure, so that varied weaning ages can be taken into consideration.

FARROWING QUARTERS

Adequate housing is fundamental to the success of any farrowing operation. There are many systems that will work, so long as certain basic requirements are met. It has been long recognized that to achieve optimum farrowing performance requires specialized facilities for the sow and pigs. The primary goals of this specialized housing have been (1) optimizing microenvironments for the pigs and sow through temperature control and good ventilation, (2) helping to ensure the baby pigs' access to adequate nutrition, (3) improving hygiene and reducing challenge from disease and (4) protecting the baby pigs from crushing and other sources of injury.

FACTORS TO CONSIDER IN HOUSING

The Crate. The crate should be designed to help control movements of the sow so that as she attempts to lie down she can do so in a controlled manner rather than falling suddenly onto her side. In addition, it is necessary that the design is such that the sow does not slide under the lower bars and become trapped. It is also important that the bars of the crate do not interfere with the baby pigs' access to the nipples of the udder. Traditionally, straight-sided crates with an internal width of approximately 22 inches have been used. To further control overlay, crates with an 18 inch internal width are considered by some to be most desirable. As crates have become narrower, they also have been modified over the years to include such options as lower bars that are adjustable in height, lower bars that bow outward, making the crate much wider at the base, or lower bars that have been raised from a height of about 10 inches above the floor to 13 to 15 inches, with downward pointing prongs attached at an outward angle. The latter option is becoming increasingly popular. In addition, various moveable attachments have been designed in the form of bars that in effect further narrow the crate and, therefore, slow the sow's descent but are hinged or counterbalanced in such a way that they move out of the way as the sow rises.

Tether versus Crate. In recent years there has been increasing interest in the use of tethers for restraint of sows in gestation and farrowing. Stated advantages of the tether system over the traditional crate systems include economy of construction, improved animal visibility and better access to pigs and sow. In general, the girth tether has been preferred to the neck tether. The girth tether appears more comfortable and is easier to adjust (Fig. 1).

Crate Orientation. To minimize cost of construction, many farrowing facilities are designed with either a rear access to the farrowing pens or a front access but not with both. The need at farrowing time for frequent observation of the rear of the sow in order to detect promptly the need for assistance to the sow or pigs makes the rear access very desirable. Likewise, the need to give such aid with minimal disturbance to the sow indicates preference for the rear passage.

Pen Size. The preferred farrowing pen size will depend on the age of weaning and to some extent on the floor material used. Floors with high voidage will stay fairly clean, and less space is required. The traditional 5 by 7 foot pen is, however, probably the minimum desired.

Flooring. The important considerations in selection of floor surface material include adequate traction for sow and pigs to minimize injury, degree of cleanliness and labor required for cleaning, overall comfort of sow and pigs, durability of materials chosen and initial cost. The final choice is influenced by such factors as age of weaning, size of operation, cost of labor and capital available. To help ensure

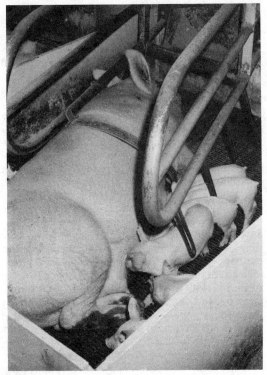

Figure 1. Sow during lactation. Sow is restrained by a girth tether and side partitions. Addition of prongs to the lower bar of the partition allows the piglets better access to the sow's udder. The flooring surface is woven wire.

maximum cleanliness at minimum cost, the trend in recent years has been toward the use of partial or totally perforated flooring in the farrowing crate. It has become generally recommended that in such cases, perforations or gaps in the floor should not exceed 10 mm in width.[5] Plastic-coated expanded metal flooring is one of the least traumatic materials available, but because it has less open space it does not clean as well as some other surfaces. Woven wire flooring has become quite popular and is considered by many producers to be a good compromise among cost, comfort, cleanliness and durability.

Room Size. In large continuous farrowing operations it is advantageous to keep the farrowing room size small. This makes all-in all-out scheduling practical and permits frequent and thorough cleaning of farrowing quarters between farrowings. It allows for placing in the rooms a group of sows that will all farrow within a few days. The result is minimal age variation within the group. The net result is better hygiene and reduced disease challenge.

Temperature Control. Heating of farrowing and lactation quarters becomes a compromise between the requirements of the sow and those of the baby pigs. The ideal temperature for the newborn pig is recognized to be 28 to 30°C. In contrast, the sow will farrow and lactate more readily in a cooler environment. Providing localized heat for the baby pigs is the most common approach to the problem. Numerous methods for supplying this heat are available. A suspended lamp or heater, underfloor heating or heating pads are most frequently used. It is recommended by some that when floor heating is used that a light be used during the first 48 hours to attract the pigs to the warmed area. Regardless of the system chosen, the important factor is close observation of the pigs. The best indicator of comfort is the pig itself, not the thermostat. Make such observations and adjust heat output accordingly.

Creep Location. The preferred location for the pigs' creep area is disputed. Creeps are usually located either at the side of the sow in close proximity to the udder or at the front of the crate near a front access passage. The stated advantages of the forward creep include best access to pigs, pigs are farthest away from danger, and pigs are easiest to lid and to box, if so desired. The major advantages of the side creep include nearness to the udder, which is the pigs' natural preference, and less distance to travel shortly after birth. Some people recommend that if forward creeps are used, supplementary heat lamps should be placed behind or at the side of the sow at farrowing. As a compromise, a triangular creep may be preferred. This is achieved by setting the crate at an angle across the pen. This provides a sensible zone in which the pigs may lie in reasonable safety and yet be near the udder. With rear access farrowing pens this configuration may somewhat limit access to the pigs.

Water. Nipples or bowls may be used to supply water to the sow. If a nipple is used, it is best mounted low and over the feed trough. If the nipple is mounted too high, water may run down the sow's neck and wet the crate floor, particularly when solid floors are used. If baby pigs are weaned onto nipples in the nursery, it is advantageous to use a nipple as the water source while the pigs are in the crate.

Lighting. It is generally recommended that lighting in the farrowing quarters be rather subdued. Excessive brightness is believed to contribute to increased restlessness of the sows. However, little scientific work has been done on the effect of photoperiod and light intensity on the sow during farrowing and lactation. Some limited studies suggest that low light intensity may have an unfavorable effect on the growth of baby pigs, and additional lighting during the night may possibly increase milk production and reduce mortality rate. This information may be important to consider in the management of facilities using equipment for creep heating that does not act as a continuous light source.

Agalactia in Sows

Stig Einarsson, Ph.D., D.V.M.
Swedish University of Agricultural Sciences, Uppsala,
Sweden

Agalactia is a common disorder in postpartum sows, resulting in serious economic losses. It has become more prevalent in recent years, especially in areas where swine production is intensive and confinement farrowing is practiced. More common than agalactia, which means no milk secretion, is hypogalactia (reduced milk secretion). The incidence of the disease varies very much from herd to herd and among countries. A recent study carried out in the United States revealed that about 13 per cent of sows were affected. The incidence of lactation failure has increased significantly in Sweden during the last two decades, with the incidence being higher in large breeding units. Several other factors, such as age of the sow, season of the year and the environment within the herd, influence the incidence of postpartum agalactia. Affected sows usually recover clinically, but the reduced milk production quickly leads to starvation, neonatal diseases associated with malnutrition or even death of the suckling piglets.

CLINICAL SIGNS

The main clinical symptom is a failure of the sow to nurse the piglets adequately. This failure appears within 1 to 3 days after parturition. However, even under normal conditions, the sow does not provide its piglets milk every time nursing appears to take place. Close observation of nursing behavior has shown that milk ejection fails in approximately 25 per cent of all nursings.

Except for a varying degree of lactation failure in diseased sows a number of other symptoms are often observed. Clinical observations and health status of sows affected with agalactia and of normal sows in the same herd are presented in Table 1. Vaginal discharge was recorded in normal and agalactic sows. The discharge of agalactic sows was somewhat more mucopurulent and of a larger quantity than that found among the healthy sows. Apparently, the occurrence of vaginal discharge in the postpartum sow is a normal condition. It is clear from several studies, including necropsy examinations, that metritis is rarely a significant component of the disease.

Macroscopic signs of mastitis were found in approximately 50 per cent of the diseased sows. Pure cultures of *Escherichia coli* are isolated from the majority of diseased sows simultaneously, with increased numbers of cells in the milk. Severe udder edema is often associated with the more severe cases of agalactia. Examination of milk samples from "healthy sows" revealed several sows with pure culture of *Escherichia coli* and high cell content without any clinical disease symptoms, so-called subclinical cases.

PATHOLOGY

Lesions are confined to the mammary glands. The subcutaneous tissue is edematous over affected parts of the udder. Histologic examination reveals several lesions in the udder that had not been recognized earlier. The noncoliforms are not associated with severe histologic lesions. It is not known how spontaneous invasion of the udder cistern of the sow takes place. American scientists demonstrated significant numbers of coliform bacteria in about one fourth of mammary gland samples prior to parturition. Serologic typing of isolates from sows with mastitis revealed an extreme multiplicity of serologic types not only within a herd but also within distinct glands of the sow.

Gross examination of the reproductive tract from euthanatized diseased sows have revealed no or very mild pathologic lesions. Neither retained placenta nor retained fetuses have been observed in these sows. Examination of the digestive tract showed that the colon was atonic.

Table 1. Clinical Observations and Health Status of Sows Affected with Postpartum Agalactia and of Normal Sows in the Same Herd (71 Pairs of Sows)

Observation	Affected Sows	Normal Sows
Rectal temperature (°C)	40.15 ± 0.09	38.93 ± 0.03
Mastitis*	49%	0%
Vaginal discharge	97%	88%
Standing up at examination	61%	100%
Temperament		
Apathetic	20%	0%
Depressed	68%	1%
Feed consumption (none)	50%	0%
Water consumption (none)	31%	0%
Constipation	22%	5%

*Swelling and hardening of one or more mammary glands.

ETIOLOGY

Several etiologies for lactation failure in the sow have been presented, but the primary cause of the disease is still unknown. An interaction among endotoxins of bacterial origin, altered endocrine functions and predisposing factors causing "stress" has been postulated to result in lactation failure. An increased incidence has been associated with an altered feeding program. However, intestinal infusion of *Escherichia coli* endotoxin did not result in lactation failure.

A number of similarities have been demonstrated between clinical agalactia and endotoxin-induced agalactia (site of administration is IV, intrammary or IU). *E. coli* endotoxin given to sows on day 2 of lactation caused a marked suppression of prolactin secretion. The other effects of endotoxin such as fever, leukopenia and increased plasma cortisol level were also observed in the sow. Nachreiner and coworkers have proposed that the toxins responsible for the disease originate in inflammatory foci such as mastitic mammary glands.

TREATMENT

The primary goal for treatment is to reestablish the milk flow in the sow as quickly as possible. Under normal conditions each milk ejection is characterized by a sudden and sharp increase in intramammary pressure, rapidly reaching 20 to 40 mm Hg, then gradually returning to base line levels. In contrast to some other species such as the cow, in which milk can be obtained in part by passive removal, there is a necessity of oxytocin release for milk let-down in the sow. Milk ejection during suckling is caused by the release of oxytocin after activation of oxytocin-secreting neurons in the hypothalamus.

Exogenous oxytocin is widely used as a part of the therapy of affected sows to enhance milk ejection. Oxytocin will also cause uterine contractions and an increased tonus and peristalsis in the intestines. The half-life of injected oxytocin is very short. Treatment with oxytocin has, therefore, only a temporary effect in agalactic sows. The hormone should be administered intramuscularly or intravenously (20 to 50 IU and 5 to 10 IU, respectively). An alternative for treatment with oxytocin might, in more severe cases of agalactia, be a long-acting analog of oxytocin, inducing several hours of pharmacologic activity on the mammary glands. The milk let-down effect of an analog called dCOMOT (Ferring Pharmaceuticals Ltd, Sweden) lasted 4 to 5 hours. Treating agalactic sows with this long-acting oxytocin analog (dose = 0.6 mg/sow IM) gave better results than treating with natural oxytocin, in terms of recovery rate of the sows and weight gain of the piglets.

Treatment with antibacterial drugs against gram-negative organisms is generally indicated (sulfonamides or dihydrostreptomycin). In problem herds culture and sensitivity testing of milk samples from untreated diseased sows is recommended. Different treatment regimens may be indicated in different herds. The duration of antibiotic treatment should be about 3 days. Treatment with broad-spectrum antibiotics is sometimes indicated (trimethoprim-sulfonamide combination).

Additional treatment with a glucocorticosteroid may result in a significant reduction of piglet mortality. Synthetic corticosteroids are considered more effective than natural ones. The reason for this may be that corticosteroid-binding globulin does not bind synthetic corticosteroids with the same affinity. Corticosteroid treatment is not indicated in mild cases of agalactia.

The use of uterine infusion has not been demonstrated to be of significant value in treatment of common cases of lactation failure. However, herds with severe cases of acute metritis may benefit from a combination of systemic and local treatment. Exercise and a laxative diet are indicated, especially in the treatment of very early stages of the disease.

PREVENTION

Herd-health management must be considered. Environmental changes should be avoided during the last 2 weeks of pregnancy. The sows should therefore be moved to the farrowing stall early enough (2 to 3 weeks before expected farrowing) for them to adjust to the new surroundings. Efforts to reduce stress, especially near parturition, are important preventative measures. In particular, optimal humidity in the farrowing house has been reported to be of importance.

The hygienic quality of the feed and drinking water should receive special attention. The diet should be well balanced. Restricted feeding during late pregnancy has been recommended. In herds with established agalactic problems, a severely restricted feed intake for individual sows (minerals and vitamins are supplemented) during the last 2 to 3 weeks of gestation has proved effective in some herds. The feed is gradually increased to full-feed after the first week postpartum. These sows have been given additional feed between 30 and 100 days of gestation to equalize the total amount of feed given. In these cases it is important that the sows have access to straw.

Exercising sows during the periparturient period is recommended but is sometimes impractical for sows in confinement. Lack of exercise will contribute to reduced intestinal peristalsis. This could sometimes be prevented with mild doses of an oral laxative or a laxative-farrowing ration.

The rectal temperature should be measured morning and evening 1 to 2 days before and 2 to 3 days after farrowing in herds with a high incidence of postparturient disorders. In this manner it is possible to detect disease symptoms very early and to treat the sow before milk production decreases.

Induction of parturition with prostaglandin $F_{2\alpha}$

(PGF$_{2\alpha}$) reduces the incidence of agalactia in some herds with high agalactia problems. The specific mechanism behind the improvement is unknown. Possible explanations might be a shortened gestation length and/or duration of farrowing. Administration of PGF$_{2\alpha}$ on day 110 of pregnancy immediately increased the plasma level of prolactin, which is important for normal milk secretion in the sow.

Care of the Neonatal Piglet

Stanley E. Curtis, Ph.D.
Keith W. Kelley, Ph.D.
University of Illinois, Urbana, Illinois

James E. Pettigrew, Jr., Ph.D.
University of Minnesota, St. Paul, Minnesota

Birth is an abrupt and profound environmental change for the neonatal pig. The critical sequence of postnatal tasks facing the piglet makes the fact that any survive to weaning more remarkable than the fact that many do not.

INTRAPARTAL STRESS

Prenatal asphyxia is normal in all species, but it is especially severe in swine. Premature umbilical cord rupture contributes to the severe prenatal asphyxiation that can lead to low neonatal viability or even stillbirth. The duration of farrowing and the between-piglet interval also tend to be directly related to low viability and stillbirth frequency.

NUTRITION

Piglets have certain nutrient stores at birth, and they obtain additional quantities from colostrum and milk. These sources are adequate for most nutrients, but a deficiency of iron occurs without additional supplementation.

Iron does not readily cross the placenta, so the piglet is born with only a small reserve (about 50 mg); sow's milk contains little iron. The neonatal piglet's rapid growth leads to a high iron requirement (about 7 mg daily). The surest method of supplementation is to inject each piglet intramuscularly with 150 mg of iron dextran. Alternatively, the piglets can be given access to a commercial oral iron supplement beginning the second or third day after birth. Symptoms of iron deficiency include anemia, slow growth and reduced disease resistance.

Many piglets die because of inadequate energy supplies. Anything that increases birth weight—and thus, presumably the energy reserves—of a piglet improves its potential for survival. The amount of energy a piglet obtains from colostrum and milk can be increased by adding supplemental fat to the sow's diet during late gestation and lactation, which increases the fat content of both colostrum and milk.

ENVIRONMENTAL TEMPERATURE

Many more neonatal piglets would survive if they had warmer environments at their disposal, especially during the first 72 hours after birth. Chilling is often the underlying factor in death from such causes as crushing, diarrhea and hypoglycemia. As environmental temperatures decrease, the faster body heat will flow from the warm piglet to the relatively cool environment. During the critical first few days after birth, piglets are more prone to lie near the sow's udder than in a heated nest area, regardless of temperature preference. Thus, the general environment must be kept warm at this time, but if general environmental temperature rises above 27°C, dysgalactia may develop in the sows.

Roughly 10 per cent of the neonatal piglet's body heat is lost during the normal evaporation of water from its upper respiratory tract and skin. Another 15 per cent flows to the floor by conduction when the piglet is lying down. The floor's temperature and other thermal characteristics affect the rate of heat loss by conduction.

At least 75 per cent of the baby pig's heat flows to the environment by radiation or convection. The ratio between these two depends on environmental conditions. Wall and ceiling temperatures are the main factors determining radiant heat loss. Air temperature and air speed primarily affect convective heat loss. Decreasing wall and ceiling temperatures—even when air temperature remains the same—greatly increase heat loss from piglets. Thus, farrowing houses should be well insulated to ensure warm walls and ceilings.

The major effect of air speed on heat loss by convection occurs at very small departures from stillness. If a small draft is present, the effect is almost as great as that of a large draft. The piglet is sensitive to drafts that the human hand can hardly feel.

Straw bedding is probably the most effective means of providing baby pigs with a comfortable thermal environment. Covering the floor with 10 cm of straw in a 10°C environment has the same effect as raising environmental temperature to

18.5°C. When a piglet burrows in straw, the straw serves as a radiant shield between the pig and the wall and ceiling, as well as giving protection against drafts.

The temperature measured by a standard thermometer incompletely assesses the environment that the piglet is experiencing. A thermometer fails to give information about air speed or wall and ceiling temperatures. Also, air temperature at piglet level may be as much as 8°C lower than at human eye level. The piglet, by its behavioral reactions to the thermal environment, is still the best thermometer. If a piglet lies in a tense position or is huddled, it is not as comfortable as it should be.

The newborn piglet is at an extreme disadvantage with regard to thermal insulation. It has neither much hair nor much subcutaneous fat. The piglet's critical temperature is 35°C. The neonatal piglet must increase its metabolic rate to offset heat loss any time environmental temperatures are below 35°C under draft-free conditions. Given a choice of effective environmental temperatures ranging from 24 to 36°C, piglets in groups choose to reside at about 29.5°C.

General air temperature should be held between 21 and 27°C at piglet level until weaning even when supplemental radiant heat is provided in special zones. Floor drafts should be prevented by the use of straw or solid partitions at least 30 cm high between farrowing stalls.

IMMUNITY

Piglets are born practically devoid of antibodies in their blood. Piglets in farm environments need colostral antibodies for survival. Within 12 hours after nursing blood levels of immunoglobulins rise to 25 to 30 mg/ml. This whole process involves the accumulation of immunoglobulin proteins in the sow's colostrum, ingestion of colostrum by the piglets and subsequent absorption of the immunoglobulins by the piglet's intestinal epithelial cells. The immunoglobulins are transported through these cells and reach the blood by lymphatic drainage. After 24 hours, "gut closure" occurs, i.e., the small intestine loses its ability to transport macromolecules in intact form.

Piglets that die before weaning have lower blood levels of colostral immunoglobulins than do those that survive. Higher blood concentrations of colostral immunoglobulins are found in heavier and earlier-born piglets and in those with shorter birth intervals. In one study piglets born in the last half of the litter (tending to have lower birth weights) had only half as much immunoglobulin in their blood as did littermates born earlier. It is important that all piglets are able to ingest an adequate amount of colostrum before gut closure occurs. Exposure to cold seems to reduce teat-seeking behavior, and thus nursing vigor and suckling time are reduced.

BEHAVIOR

Within a litter piglets born earlier in the birth order tend to have a greater chance for survival. Piglets that are heavier or less stressed at birth are generally more vigorous and more successful in competition for colostrum and milk. Carbon monoxide generated by fuel-fired heaters may rise to concentrations in the air greater than 200 ppm, which can cause neonatal piglets to have diminished vigor and even to die. Sources of carbon monoxide in farrowing houses ought to be identified and eliminated, and adequate ventilation rates should be maintained.

Crossfostering is the removal of one or more piglets from their dam soon after birth and placing them with a different sow. Crossfostering may be practiced routinely to achieve a uniform number of pigs per litter or a uniform body weight of piglets. Crossfostering should be practiced in cases of sow death, agalactia or inadequate number of functional mammary glands and teats for the number of pigs farrowed. It is important that crossfostering be done as soon after farrowing as possible.

ARTIFICIAL REARING

Orphan piglets can be reared artificially, but much care and a proper diet are essential to success. An extremely clean and warm environment is also very important. Some piglets survive when fed a diet of milk, cream and eggs or a calf milk replacer, but their health and growth are much more satisfactory when fed a high-quality commercial milk replacer designed specifically for piglets. Such a product should be made mostly of milk products and it should include dry skim milk in particular. The crude protein level should be at least 25 per cent, and the fat level should be 10 per cent or higher. The liquid diet created by mixing this product with water either can be provided to the piglets several times daily or made available at all times. The diet must be kept fresh and clean, as it is an excellent medium for microbial growth.

DAY-ONE PROCESSING

Certain tasks should be performed on the first day after the piglets are born. The umbilical cord, if still attached, should be cut 5 cm from the body and dipped in a disinfecting solution. The piglet's needle (canine) teeth can inflict injury to littermates or to the sow's udder. Therefore, they should be trimmed with side-cutting pliers, with care being taken not to cut so deeply as to damage the gums. Permanent identification should be achieved by appropriate notching of the piglet's ears, using an instrument designed for this purpose. The tail should be docked 2 cm from the body, using side-cutting pliers. All instruments should be disinfected after processing each pig. Castration should be performed before the piglet is 2 weeks of age. The herder should remember that all of these operations are traumatic for the piglets and should be accomplished with as much gentleness and empathy as possible.

SPATIAL AND STRUCTURAL ENVIRONMENT

The spatial environment influences piglet survival because crushing by the sow is a major cause of piglet death in all types of farrowing and lactation accommodations. Any such accommodation must have a sow zone that will permit the sow to make necessary movements; an interaction zone, in which sow and piglets are together for various purposes, especially nursing, and a piglet zone, a place attractive to the young where they can rest safely and comfortably.

Choice of flooring material is important in minimizing injuries and disease, discomfort (including chilling) and inconveniences associated with sanitation. Of the materials currently available, wire mesh, plastic-coated expanded metal and concrete slats seem to be most suitable.

References

1. Curtis SE: Responses of the piglet to perinatal stressors. J Anim Sci 38:1031, 1974.
2. England DC: Husbandry components in prenatal and perinatal development in swine. J Anim Sci 38:1045, 1974.
3. Hartsock TG, Graves HB: Neonatal behavior and nutrition-related mortality in domestic swine. J Anim Sci 42:235, 1976.
4. Lecce JG: Rearing piglets artificially in a farm environment: A promise unfulfilled. J Anim Sci 41:659, 1975.
5. LeDividich J, Noblet J: Colostrum intake and thermoregulation in the neonatal pig in relation to environmental temperature. Biol Neonate 40:167, 1981.
6. Wilson MR: Immunologic development of the neonatal pig. J Anim Sci 38:1018, 1974.

Reducing Perinatal Mortality in Pigs

Jørgen Svendsen, D.V.M., M.Sc., Ph.D.
Lorraine Steen Svendsen, M.Sc., Ph.D.
Anne-Charlotte Bengtsson, M.Sc.
Swedish University of Agricultural Sciences, Lund, Sweden

OCCURRENCE AND CLASSIFICATION OF PREWEANING MORTALITY

Structural changes within sow production and the application of new techniques may have increased the profitability of swine production but have not, in general, led to a decline in losses due to death during the suckling period. Available statistics from many countries show rather unanimously that 20 to 25 per cent of the total number of pigs born die before weaning, and this high mortality rate does not appear to have changed significantly during the past 20 years.[1]

Main categories of losses of pigs during the preweaning period are presented in Table 1. The data presented in this table are derived from a 4-year study involving 5578 litters that was conducted in Denmark.[4] The total preweaning mortality observed in this study was 22.3 per cent. It should be emphasized that serious infectious swine diseases, such as transmissible gastroenteritis (TGE), hog cholera, brucellosis, leptospirosis and salmonellosis do not occur in Denmark.

The total preweaning mortality in a herd will be influenced by the litter size at birth and by the age of the sow. Thus, it was observed that an average of 2.5 pigs, or 14.3 per cent, were lost before weaning in litters of 8 pigs,[5] while 4.8 pigs, or 32 per cent, were lost from litters of 14 pigs.

There is considerable herd-to-herd variation in the incidence of preweaning mortality. A consistently low level of preweaning losses in a herd over

Table 1. Classification of Death Losses Before Weaning

Cause	Per Cent of Total Number of Pigs Born	Herd Variation
Antepartal death	1.6	(0.5–5.6)
Intrapartal death	4.5	(3.0–6.4)
Starved/undersized	3.5	(0.6–5.0)
Trauma	4.0	(1.3–7.1)
Gastrointestinal diseases	2.0	(0.5–3.9)
Pneumonias	0.6	(0.0–1.3)
Acute generalized infections	0.9	(0.4–1.7)
Malformations	1.1	(0.4–2.1)
Arthritis/polyarthritis	1.1	(0.2–1.7)
Miscellaneous	2.4	(0.6–3.6)
No cause found	0.5	(0.0–1.2)
Total Preweaning Mortality	22.3	(15.2–26.9)

(From Nielsen NC et al.: Disease control in sow herds. Institute for Internal Medicine, Royal Veterinary and Agricultural University, Copenhagen, 1976.)

a longer period of time and a correspondingly higher average number of pigs per litter are, to a great extent, a reflection of superiority of management and husbandry in the herd and are also indications of what may be achieved in commercial hog operations.

Most of the death losses before weaning occur during parturition or in the early neonatal period. This is illustrated in Figure 1, which shows that almost 80 per cent of the total preweaning mortality occurs during parturition and within the first 3 to 4 days of life. Therefore, particular attention should be given to the *perinatal* period when attempts are made to reduce the preweaning mortality. The losses incurred during the first days of life, such as losses due to death before or during parturition, to starved or undersized and weak pigs and to trauma, contribute greatly to the total preweaning mortality. By and large these losses are from *noninfectious* causes, and many of these may be caused by problems of development and adaptation. Thus, noninfectious death losses account for a very significant proportion of the total preweaning mortality. *Infections* are also important, not only as primary or secondary causes of death but also as significant contributors to morbidity.

This article will describe and discuss some of the economically important categories of losses due to death that occur during parturition and the early neonatal period (the first 48 to 72 hours after birth) and factors influencing these losses, beginning with the special problems of the newborn pig.

ADAPTATION TO EXTRAUTERINE LIFE

Neurologically, the newborn pig is relatively well developed but physiologically is immature. At birth, it leaves the security of intrauterine life and enters an extremely different environment where it is required not only to withstand the harassment of this environment but also to continue its process of maturation and growth. It is born sterile and without antibody protection against infectious agents. The sparsely pelaged newborn pig only contains 1 to 2 per cent fat, most of which is structural. It also lacks brown fat, which supplies heat via nonshivering thermogenesis. Therefore, lipid stores cannot be used as a major metabolic fuel, although these pigs can mobilize free fatty acids during starvation and cold exposure. In addition, pigs less than 1 to 2 days of age have a low capacity for fatty acid synthesis.

The glycogen deposits in liver and muscle at birth are relatively large in the pig and only decrease slightly during the first day. However, the newborn pig has a limited capacity for gluconeogenesis, and unsuckled or starved piglets become hypoglycemic

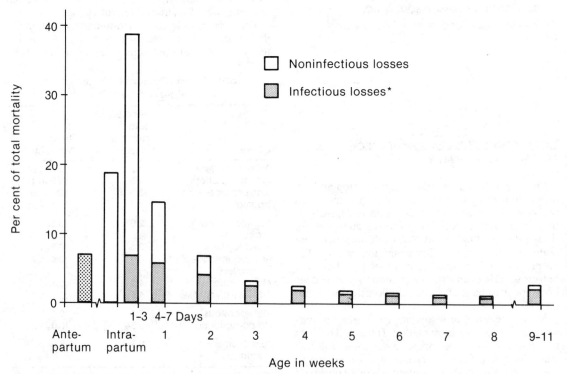

Figure 1. Per cent distribution of total preweaning mortality in pigs according to age. (Based on Nielson NC, et al.: Disease Control in Sow Herds. Copenhagen, Institute for Internal Medicine, Royal Veterinary and Agricultural University, 1976.)

*Infectious diseases such as transmissible gastroenteritis, hog cholera, brucellosis and leptospirosis do not occur in Denmark.

within 15 to 20 hours. Liver glycogen is an important energy source in the piglet; however, muscle glycogen must also be catabolized to provide the necessary glucose for metabolism, and this is accomplished by shivering.

Under commercial farrowing conditions, the newborn pig's only source of nutrition, besides the glycogen present in the liver and skeletal muscle, is in the colostrum and milk of the dam, which is essential not only for normal development and growth but also for passive protection against infections. Therefore, it is obvious that anything leading to a decrease in the production of the sow's milk, to a change in its composition or to a modification in the ability or the possibility of the pig to acquire and to utilize the colostrum and milk from the sow may also interfere with the health of the pig.

The ability of the newborn pig to regulate its body temperature is limited, especially in the smaller animals, which are born with a larger body surface and smaller energy reserves than larger animals. After birth, the body temperature of the pig decreases rapidly from approximately 39 to 37°C. In normal-sized pigs that start eating, the body temperature begins to rise again after 1 to 2 hours, but this recovery is somewhat delayed in smaller pigs. Body temperature in the newborn is maintained and regulated primarily by shivering. The "critical" temperature of the newborn pig is close to 35°C, and at least 75 per cent of the newborn pig's body heat flows to the environment via radiation or convection. During the first week of life, the thermoregulatory mechanisms of the pig improve, and the critical temperature falls to about 25°C. Thus, a 1-week-old pig is able to compensate relatively well for the changes in environment.

Post-mortem examination of pigs that died during the perinatal period show that several "mortality" groups can be identified.[1] Five mortality groups have been identified on the basis of clinical and post-mortem studies: stillborn intrapartum pigs, weak and/or undersized pigs, splayleg pigs, splayleg and weak pigs and traumatized pigs. Some basic characteristics of these groups will be described in the following sections, with the addition of the characteristics of stillborn antepartum pigs and pigs dying from umbilical cord bleeding.

MORTALITY IN RELATION TO PARTURITION

Stillborn Antepartum (stillborn a.p.). Such deaths occur at a certain low level in all herds and may show considerable herd-to-herd variation. They occur with approximately the same frequency in small litters as in large litters. Farrowing studies have shown that antepartum dead pigs are generally evenly distributed over the entire farrowing period (Fig. 2), and approximately 90 per cent are born in the fetal membranes or with a ruptured umbilical cord. The incidence of antepartal deaths among offspring from sows that have been strictly confined during the gestation period is the same as in litters from sows that have been maintained loose in pens. A multitude of factors may be involved, and it has been estimated that about 70 to 75 per cent of the antepartal mortality is because of noninfectious causes.

Stillborn Intrapartum (stillborn i.p.). Deaths during the intrapartal period account for a very significant proportion of the total preweaning mortality (Table 1). Most of these animals are normal sized, apparently normally developed pigs that are born to term.[1] Some of the pigs die during parturition, but approximately 70 per cent are born alive, although only the heart is beating, and these pigs die immediately after birth.[7] However, many of these pigs may be saved by using some form of resuscitation.

Studies of more than 700 litters showed that stillborn i.p. pigs occurred in 25 per cent of the litters, and 54 per cent of these pigs were born into litters having two or more stillborn i.p. pigs. The average weight of stillborn i.p. pigs was less than that of liveborn pigs from the same litters, and more males (57 per cent) died than females.[10]

Farrowing studies showed that the mean time for an individual pig to be born was 26 minutes. It took a significantly longer time for the birth of a stillborn i.p. pig than a liveborn and a significantly longer time for an intrapartum dead pig to be born than an antepartum dead pig. Generally, pigs born tail first took a longer time to be born than pigs born head first. Studies also showed that more than 70 per cent of the stillborn i.p. pigs were born with a ruptured umbilical cord or premature loosening of the fetal membranes, which was only seen among 13 and 2 per cent, respectively, of the unaffected liveborn pigs. The number of liveborn pigs with ruptured umbilical cords was generally evenly distributed over the entire farrowing period.[10]

These observations would indicate that the pig in some way is affecting the process of its birth and that one of the reasons apparently normal and well-developed pigs die during parturition is that there is some type of intrauterine "fight" or "battle" to be born, perhaps in combination with an abnormal position and/or a reduced ability to move. A pig that also lacks vitality or is deficient in a possible factor that accelerates the birth would slow down farrowing. The results can be, among others, an increased farrowing time and/or premature rupture of the umbilical cord, impeded blood flow, tenuous connections between the placenta and the uterus or other effects that result in asphyxiation because of a reduced or halted supply of blood from the mother to the fetus.[6]

Asphyxiation during parturition is normal in many species. However, species such as the pig, which are neurologically relatively mature at birth, are only able to withstand asphyxia and the resultant hypercapnia for a very short period of time. For this reason, intrapartal asphyxia may be associated not only with perinatal mortality but also with postnatal morbidity and mortality, and liveborn pigs that suffer asphyxia during delivery may often show

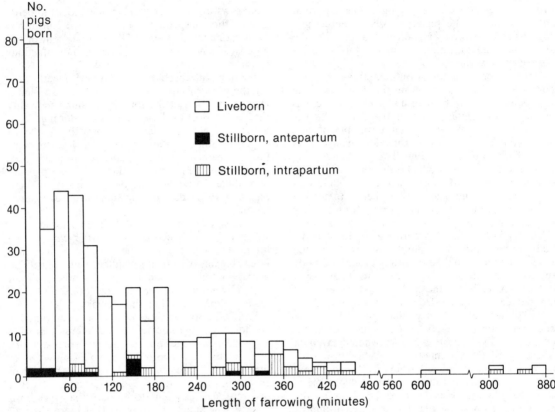

Figure 2. Distribution of liveborn and stillborn pigs over the farrowing period as determined by behavior studies at farrowing, 40 litters. (Based on Svendsen J, Bengtsson A-CH: Proc 14th Nordic Vet Congress, Copenhagen, 1982, pp 414–415.)

lower viability for several hours post partum, which endangers their ability to survive throughout the entire neonatal period.[7] Indeed, there may be a relationship between stillborn i.p. and the occurrence of weak pigs or splayleg pigs, since the number of weak pigs born was higher in litters with intrapartum dead pigs than in litters without them, whereas the number of splayleg pigs was lower in litters having one or more stillborn i.p. pigs.[10]

The number of stillborn i.p. pigs born increases greatly after a farrowing length of more than 4 to 5 hours[10] or after two thirds of the litter have been born.[7] The proportion of intrapartal dead pigs has been reported as the same in large litters as in smaller litters with the same parturition time. Increased parturition time increases the risk of prolonged asphyxia. A major proportion of the mortality due to stillbirth i.p. that exceeds 4 per cent may be explained by an increased length of parturition. Comparative studies of housing systems for sows in gestation have shown that sows confined in crates during gestation had a longer parturition time and, as a result, more intrapartal dead pigs than sows maintained loose in pens. After correcting for the linear effect of parturition time, the number of stillborn i.p. pigs born was independent of the type

of housing system for sows in gestation or for farrowing sows and of the age of the sow.

MORTALITY AFTER PARTURITION

Starved and Weak/Undersized (Weak) Pigs. *Starved* pigs are defined here as normal-sized pigs without apparent physical handicaps that have not received sufficient food because of the dam having agalactia, because the number of pigs in the litter is larger than the number of functional teats, or because of poor pen fittings. These pigs are a particular problem in herds having a high incidence of mastitis-endometritis-agalactia (MMA).

Weak pigs may be defined as liveborn pigs that at birth or during the first hours of life show signs of low viability or that because of their small size or locomotor disorders are judged unable to survive in an ordinary litter under standard husbandry conditions. Guidelines for this diagnosis may be a birth weight below 900 gm, a time-lapse of more than 20 minutes between birth and the first teat contact and/or apparent inability to obtain or to maintain a suckle even when helped. These pigs often have difficulty in orientation and in sensing their environment with regard to such items as the location and movements of the sow and the position of the heat lamp in the piglet area of the pen. Difficulties with locomotion appear as they become progressively weaker.

Detailed studies showed a morbidity of 5.3 per cent and a mortality of 2.8 per cent because of weak pigs, with a relatively even sex distribution. These pigs had a lower birth weight and a higher neonatal mortality, and a higher percentage were born in their fetal membranes or with a ruptured umbilical cord. Of the pigs in this group 91 per cent required more than 20 minutes to make the first teat contact, including 8 per cent that were unable to make teat contact. Body temperature studies of weak pigs showed that these pigs had a greater decrease in body temperature immediately after birth and a slower recovery than apparently normal littermates. The number of weakborn pigs increases with litter size and was higher among the offspring from older sows. No effect of sow housing in gestation or at farrowing was observed.

In general, weak pigs tend to be both weak and undersized, but normal-weight pigs may also be born weak. Many of the pigs in this group are viable, and approximately 50 per cent may survive the preweaning period under ordinary husbandry conditions. However, these pigs are *underpriviledged* in comparison to their littermates because they are unsuccessful in fighting for a teat and maintaining suckling during the crucial first 24 to 48 hours when the social order and suckling behavior of the litter is being established. Small pigs are also at a disadvantage in reaching teats that are placed too high or may be covered by the dam's body. Upon reaching a teat, these pigs may not be able to nurse vigorously and rapidly during the time that milk is available. Therefore, they have the problem of starvation to contend with in addition to whatever other physical difficulties they may have.

The pigs in this group quickly become weak and chilled because of starvation and because the smaller pigs have a relatively larger surface area than the heavier animals. Small pigs may need a relatively higher glycogen reserve than they have available in order to cope with this situation and, in addition, a weak pig may be unable to mobilize glycogen or may have a faulty glucose metabolism. Not receiving an adequate supply of colostrum, their own energy reserves quickly become exhausted, and they die as a result of hypoglycemia, trauma or infections. Occasional "helper" feedings by the stock person are undesirable for these pigs. If they are to survive they must have access to and help with receiving small amounts at frequent intervals. Intermittent feedings will only increase the metabolism of an already stressed animal, resulting in a more rapid reduction in the inadequate fuel supply of the body. This, together with an increase in the production of endogenous insulin, will further accentuate the hypoglycemic state.

Splayleg and Splayleg and Weak (Splayweak) Pigs. Splayleg is a "clinical" disease of newborn pigs that is characterized by a temporary functional disorder in which there is a reduced ability to adduct the limbs. The disease has been reported in several countries, and it appears to be particularly important within certain improved breeds, such as the Landrace, Large White and Pietrain[7] breeds. Detailed studies showed that two variants of this functional disorder could be clinically distinguished, the vital splayleg pig and the weak splayleg pig:

Splayleg Pigs. These pigs displayed signs of disease within the first 12 hours of life. Usually, only the hind legs are affected, and the piglets appear to be otherwise normal. When they attempt to stand, their hind legs extend sideways. Typically, the hind legs are bilaterally and equally affected, but in a few cases, both hind legs extend to one side, or one leg extends backwards. The disease appears to be most severe within the first 24 to 36 hours after birth. Although these pigs have difficulties in moving, they are still strong enough to compete for a teat and obtain a suckle.

Production data showed that the total mortality caused by splayleg was 1.9 per cent and the morbidity was 6.3 per cent. The pigs weighed only slightly less than unaffected littermates. Splayleg occurred much more frequently among males than females. Farrowing studies showed that these pigs had the same mean time for first teat contact (8.7 minutes) as did the unaffected pigs, but 21 per cent had ruptured umbilical cords at birth.

Splayleg appears to be a congenital, hereditary (the incidence varied from 0.8 to 11.7 per cent in offspring from different boars) disease with a significantly higher incidence in litters with 113 days or less gestation period. The occurrence of splayleg in a herd is apparently not influenced by litter size, parturition length, sow parity or housing systems for sows in gestation or at farrowing. In addition, the type of flooring in the pen apparently does not affect the incidence.

Apart from their locomotor handicap, the splayleg pigs appear strong and vital. Under normal husbandry conditions, and by taping the hind legs together to provide support, most of these pigs recover. Of the splayleg pigs that die, most die within 48 to 72 hours after birth, generally from trauma and starvation. Significantly, more males succumb. A distinct pattern of usually bilateral abrasions and injuries on the accessory digits, hocks and tail can be seen, and subcutaneous edema along the hind legs is a common feature.

Splayweak Pigs. These pigs show signs of splayleg very soon after birth while also appearing to be rather weak. Usually, both the forelegs and the hind legs extend to the sides, and the legs are bilaterally and equally affected. The condition of the pig rapidly deteriorates. The recumbent pig frequently lies with the hind legs extended along the body and the forelegs spread to each side.

Production data showed that most of the pigs with these clinical signs died after birth, accounting for 1.4 per cent of the herd mortality. The disease is apparently not influenced by gestation length, boar or sex. It is, however, a congenital disease syndrome that is diagnosed more often in litters also having splayleg pigs. Whereas the occurrence of weak pigs increased with the age of the sow and with litter size, no influence of parity on the occurrence of splayweak pigs was seen, and only a slight increase in the number of splayleg pigs with litter size was observed. More than 90 per cent of the splayweak pigs died and most died within the first 48 hours of birth, primarily from starvation. There was an equal sex distribution. At post-mortem examination a rather typical pattern of injuries and abrasions can be seen on the accessory digits, hocks, sternum, axillary and mandible.

Traumatized (Trauma) Pigs. Death losses caused by crushing of the piglet by the dam and other fatal traumatic lesions constitute the highest mortality group among liveborn pigs and contribute significantly to preweaning mortality. Detailed studies (Fig. 3) showed that most losses from trauma occur within the first 36 to 48 hours after birth and that the traumatized pigs weighed more than the other pigs that died during the neonatal period. More males than females died. Losses from trauma are greater in sow litters than in gilt litters, even after the litters are standardized, and greater in litters containing more than 11 pigs. There is no effect of gestation length.[9] Although postparturient diseases of the sow (such as MMA) have been implicated in the occurrence of trauma,[2] no such effect was seen.[9]

Most traumatizations occurred when the sow moved—upon standing up or laying down and when standing or walking. Most injuries were caused by the hindquarters and hind legs of the sow, irrespective of the arrangements of the creep area and of the sow being loose in a pen or fixed in a farrowing crate. About 30 per cent of all the traumas occurred around sow feeding times. Many traumatic injuries may be avoided by attendance around sow feeding times during the first day post partum.[9] About 25 per cent of the pigs in this group had a ruptured umbilical cord. However, the mean time required for first teat contact was the same as for the unaffected pigs. It was observed that 9.7 per cent of the normal weight, apparently normal pigs born had

been kicked or crushed severely and, in many cases, repeatedly. This implied that traumatic injuries occurred much more frequently than the production data indicated and that the repeated and/or severe traumatizations that did not lead immediately to death may result in the pig being noted as "weak" or being predisposed to infections, which subsequently are noted as the primary cause of death.

There is considerable herd-to-herd variation in the incidence of fatal traumatic injuries. In particular this is a result of differences in farrowing accommodations and management procedures. Comparative studies showed that losses from trauma were fewer in farrowing boxes that had a relatively high degree of fixation of the sow during the farrowing and subsequent neonatal period and in which the farrowing crates were provided with special fittings that "directed" the movements of the sow when she lay down. The occurrence of injuries was further reduced by improving the microenvironment of the newborn pig in the farrowing box. This was done by having a draught-free creep area close to, but outside of, the "danger zone" of the sow and a moveable heat lamp to direct the piglets away from the sow after birth. This provided a "local" temperature that approximated the critical temperature of the young pig. The fewest losses caused by trauma were observed in a special unit for farrowing and neonatal pigs that had a room temperature of 22°C and in cases in which the sow, maintained fixed in a farrowing crate as previously described, was kept on a totally perforated floor without straw bedding. The farrowing boxes had well-insulated, clean, draught-free creep areas parallel to the udder of the sow and moveable heat lamps and were constructed so that the stock person had easy access to the piglets.[9]

Umbilical Cord Bleeding. Over a period of time, bleeding from the umbilical cord may be a very important cause of perinatal mortality in certain herds. In general, the mortality due to umbilical cord bleeding is less than 0.1 per cent of all the pigs born and does not occur in all herds. However, in some herds mortality rates of more than 2 per cent of the pigs born have been recorded. The etiology is by and large unknown. However, it appears that

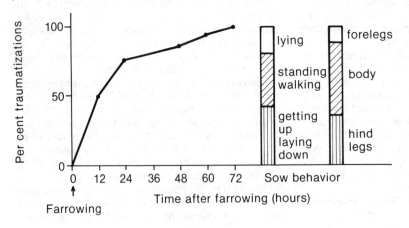

Figure 3. Causes of traumatic injuries in piglets. (Based on Svendsen J: Konsulentavdelningens rapporter, Allmänt 33, p 20:1, Uppsala, 1982.)

the condition may be related to the use of wood shavings as bedding in the farrowing box. Further investigations are needed to determine if a specific type of wood is implicated or if chemical compounds, such as wood preservatives, may cause the bleeding. Pigs having umbilical bleeding apparently do not show other bleeding abnormalities.

PRACTICAL PROCEDURES AND MANAGEMENT FOR REDUCING PERINATAL MORTALITY

The following text summarizes precautions that can be taken to reduce the losses that occur during parturition and the neonatal period.

Sows in Gestation. The housing and management of sows in gestation has a direct impact on the survival and vitality of their offspring. Besides receiving adequate nutrition, pregnant sows should be housed loose in pens in relatively small groups so that they have some access to exercise, are able to freely choose their location in the pen and lying positions and can keep themselves clean. It must be easy to supervise the animals and to give individual care and feeding when required. This will reduce losses from antepartal and intrapartal death, reduce the neonatal mortality and also decrease piglet losses due to infectious diseases.

Sows at Farrowing. In order to minimize the losses from trauma and low vitality at birth, sows should farrow in crates with fenders that can direct the movements of the sow when she lies down. The farrowing accommodations should be located in small, well-insulated farrowing units with relatively high room temperatures. Sows that show signs of prolonged parturition time should be treated properly and promptly to reduce the losses from intrapartal deaths and the number of liveborn hypoxic pigs. In addition, emphasis should be placed on the prevention or immediate treatment of diseases of the sow that cause agalactia, thus reducing losses from death caused by starvation and chilling.

The majority of farrowing boxes are designed for the maintenance of piglets until they are at least 3 weeks of age and represent a compromise between an adequate environment for the piglet and for the sow. These boxes also tend to be designed with the strongest of the litter in mind. We advocate the use of a special farrowing and neonatal care unit, in which a high level of hygiene can be maintained and the farrowing boxes and general environment are designed with emphasis on the special requirements of the newborn pig. Under these conditions the sow must remain fixed. After approximately 1 week when the piglets have doubled their body weight and are "swimming" in maternal antibodies, the sow and her litter may be moved to housing systems having less stringent requirements for equipment and optimal climate for the piglet and having more regard for the needs of the sow. It is hoped that future developments will lead to improvements in the farrowing conditions for both the piglets and the sow.

Newborn Pigs. The newborn pig should be kept warm at birth. The creep area should be clean, draught-free, close to but sheltered from the sow and warm. Using moveable heat lamps will ensure that the pigs will be maintained near their critical temperature and can be directed away from the sow after birth, toward the creep area. The piglets should be easily accessible to the stock person. Easily accessible, clean, fresh drinking water or other suitable liquids should be available for the newborn pig, thus reducing losses that are a result of underprivileged pigs.

Farrowings should be attended, making it possible to limit the death losses by instituting some form of resuscitation caused by asphyxiation, applying a ligature or clamp to the umbilical cord immediately after birth to reduce losses from umbilical cord bleeding in affected herds, giving proper care (warmth) to liveborn but hypoxic pigs in the first period of extrauterine life when they are still very weak, securing colostrum for each pig, making certain that each pig can obtain a functional teat, helping weaker pigs to suckle, removing or separating pigs from the sow just before and during sow feeding times the first two to three feedings after farrowing to reduce losses from trauma, forming litters containing pigs of similar size to reduce losses from starvation and providing special care for the weak and undersized pigs, including feeding them using a stomach tube with colostrum and milk from their dam.

Attempts to reduce neonatal mortality prove economically advantageous in a production program in which sows farrow in batches. This will make it possible to form uniform litters in which there is one functional teat available per pig, to secure an adequate supply of colostrum and milk for each animal and to reduce investment costs by requiring only a limited number of specially equipped farrowing boxes suitable for the newborn pig in the farrowing unit.

RECORD KEEPING AND BREEDING

A sow producing a large litter in which there is no perinatal morbidity or mortality obviously has the uterine capacity to retain and to nourish that number of pigs. Therefore, it appears sensible to select offspring from sows that produce large litters with little or no perinatal morbidity or mortality. This requires a well-adapted record keeping system that includes information on heredity, breeding, farrowing and litter size at birth and contains information on the type and nature of perinatal losses. When perinatal morbidity or mortality increases, diagnostic efforts should be implemented. The benefits of a carefully kept, up-to-date record system will rapidly exceed any initial difficulty in setting up and maintaining such a system.

References

1. Bille N, Nielsen NC, Larsen JL, Svendsen J: Preweaning mortality in pigs. II. The perinatal period. Nord Vet Med 26:294, 1974.
2. Bille N, Nielsen NC, Svendsen J: Preweaning mortality in pigs. III. Traumatic injuries. Nord Vet Med 26:617, 1974.
3. England DC: Husbandry components in prenatal and perinatal development in swine. J Anim Sci 38:1045, 1974.
4. Nielsen NC, Bille N, Svendsen J and Riising, H-J: Sygdoms-bekaempelse i svinebesaetninger (Disease control in sow herds). Institute for Internal Medicine, Royal Veterinary and Agricultural University, Copenhagen, 1976.
5. Nielsen NC, Christensen K, Bille N and Larsen JL: Preweaning mortality in pigs. I. Herd investigations. Nord Vet Med, 26:137, 1974.
6. Randall GCB: Observations on parturition on the sow. II. Factors influencing stillbirth and perinatal mortality. Vet Rec 90:183, 1972.
7. Randall GCB: Perinatal mortality: Some problems of adaption at birth. Adv Vet Sci Comp Med 22:53, 1978.
8. Stanton HC, Carroll JK: Potential mechanisms responsible for prenatal and perinatal mortality or low viability of swine. J Anim Sci 38:1037, 1974.
9. Svendsen J, Bengtsson A-Ch: Production systems for raising piglets: Methods of reducing the number of traumatized and crushed pigs. Konsulentavdelningens rapporter, Allmänt 33 20:1, Uppsala, 1982.
10. Svendsen J, Bengtsson A-Ch: Perinatal mortality in pigs. I. Effect of litter factors and herd factors on the occurrence of intra partum dead pigs. II. Behaviour studies of sows at farrowing to study the occurrence of intra partum dead pigs. Proc 14th Nordic Vet Cong Copenhagen, 1982, pp 414–415.

Artificial Insemination of Swine

L. E. Evans, D.V.M., Ph.D.
Iowa State University, Ames, Iowa

D. J. McKenna, D.V.M., M.S.
University of Illinois, Urbana, Illinois

Artificial insemination (AI) of swine has been successfully performed for several decades in many countries. In the last decade significant progress has been made in the development of extenders and equipment. Unfortunately, AI in swine has not been as widely accepted as AI in cattle for several reasons. First, the development and efficacy of cryopreservation of swine semen has not equaled that of bovine semen. Second, the methods for identification of superior boars are less clearly defined, and there is a potential for such boars to be rapidly displaced by their progeny because of the prolificacy of the species. Finally, fertility rates and litter sizes have often been below those expected for natural breedings.

There are several advantages to the use of AI in swine. Most important are its potential contributions to disease control and genetic improvement in the herd. AI makes it possible to introduce new genetic stock into the herd with a minimum risk of introducing disease organisms. It is possible to impregnate a minimum of 15 to 20 sows over a 2-day period with the single collection of a boar. Thus, the best sows can be mated to the best boars, and a 300-sow herd could require only three boars. Breeding boars can be given optimal housing and handling to avoid injury or environmental stress while genetically inferior boars can be utilized as teasers for the AI program. Under some circumstances it is more convenient to use AI at the second mating, without moving the females from their pens or gestation crates.

A disadvantage of AI in swine is the need for higher levels of management and increased labor demands. However, this may be offset by the resulting better record-keeping and the greater awareness of the reproductive performance of the herd.

BOAR TRAINING

Young boars with good libido are readily trained to semen collection on a dummy by observing the sexual activity of other boars on the dummy. Boars respond better to boar scent on the dummy than to female secretions. Reticent boars, particularly experienced boars, may require several collections on a sow in the same location before accepting the dummy.

SEMEN COLLECTION AND EVALUATION

The primary method of semen collection is the gloved hand technique, which elicits ejaculation by digital pressure on the spiral end of the boar's penis. Preparation of the boar before collection includes emptying the preputial sacs to reduce contamination at collection and clipping the long sheath hairs that may interfere with grasping the penis. A detailed description of the hand collection method can be found in this text in the article Semen Collection from the Boar.

Sperm cell motility should be estimated for each ejaculate to ensure sperm viability. If semen is extended, it is wise to recheck sperm motility. Samples with less than 70 per cent motility usually are discarded in an AI program. Sperm cell concentration may be approximated by color: creamy = 0.8 to 1 billion cells/ml, milky = 0.4 to 0.8 billion cells/ml and milky water = 0.2 to 0.4 billion cells/ml. Opaque samples may or may not have spermatozoa, since most of the color is from accessory secretion. Concentration can be estimated by hemocytometer units or by absorptiometers. Recently, a spectrophotometer has been developed for estimating semen concentration and breeding doses for equine AI. This instrument has potential for similar use in swine AI. Sperm cell morphology should be checked weekly with the light microscope for evidence of abnormalities. Samples with more than 10 per cent primary and 20 per cent secondary sperm abnormalities should be discarded or used with caution.

Under field usage a normal boar can be collected two to three times weekly at 48- to 72-hour intervals without reducing sperm output or semen volume. Daily sperm output for a mature boar is estimated to be 12 to 20 billion spermatozoa. This production is cumulative over a 2- to 3-day interval of collection.

SEMEN EXTENDERS

Semen extenders provide protection against temperature and changes in pH, increase semen volume, provide a source of nutrition for the spermatozoa and inhibit bacterial growth. Most extenders are formulated with glucose, electrolytes, buffers and antibiotics (Table 1). Sodium bicarbonate and sodium citrate are common buffers used in swine semen extenders. Penicillin G streptomycin, lincospectin and gentamicin are antibiotics that can be used in swine semen extenders.

The simplest extender to obtain is skim milk, which can be used for short-term storage of 24 hours or less. Skim milk should be heated to 90°C (195°F) for 10 minutes to inactivate enzymes that are detrimental to spermatozoa. When the milk has cooled, antibiotics are added, and sometimes a large egg yolk without the membrane or egg white is added to each liter of milk. The lipoproteins in egg yolk or milk afford protection to the spermatozoa down to a temperature of 5°C.

Semen diluted in glucose-citrate extenders without a lipoprotein source should not be cooled below 15°C (59°F). The Kiev, BL (Beltsville-1) and Modena are examples of this type of extender. They can be stored in dry form, with distilled water added before use, or they may be stored frozen until used.

Semen of good quality can be stored for 3 to 5 days in an Illinois Variable Temperature (IVT) that has been saturated with CO_2, sealed and held at 18 to 22°C. Several patented diluents, utilized by certain AI centers, are reported to protect spermatozoa effectively for 5 to 7 days.

Semen intended for immediate use is extended to the proper volume (number of sows to breed × 100 ml). Semen intended for storage is diluted at a ratio of one part semen to four to five parts extender. It is stored at the appropriate temperature in fully filled, sealed bottles. Sealing the bottle is particularly important in CO_2 saturated extenders. Before use, the stored semen is diluted to the desired insemination volume. Semen is mixed with extender by adding the extender slowly to the semen after the extender is within one to two degrees of the semen's temperature.

INSEMINATION DOSE

The insemination dose for sows is based upon two factors: number of sperm and volume of fluid. A minimum breeding dose of 1 billion progressively motile spermatozoa in 50 ml of volume is required to obtain adequate conception rates and litter sizes. For safety measures, a dose of 2 billion progressively motile sperm and 100 ml of volume is recommended at each breeding. Sperm cell viability and fertilizing ability are influenced by storage time. There is a need to increase the spermatozoa dosage in proportion to storage time. With most extenders litter size and conception rates fall gradually as the interval of storage exceeds 48 hours. Conversely, studies done with fresh semen collected, extended and used immediately at a breeding dose of 250 million spermatozoa resulted in normal conception rates and litter sizes. With this reduced dose, second

Table 1. Swine Semen Extenders

Component	BL₁	Kiev	Modena	IVT Mod.	Egg Yolk
Glucose (gm)	27.0	60.0	25.0	3.0	30.00
Na₃ citrate (gm)	10.0	3.75	6.9	20.0	
Citric acid (gm)			2.0		
Tris (gm)			5.65		
Cysteine (gm)			0.05		
BSA (Cohn Fr. V) (gm)*			3.0		
Sodium bicarbonate (gm)	2.0	1.20	1.0	2.1	1.5
Potassium chloride (gm)	0.3			0.4	
EDTA (gm)†		3.70	2.25		
Distilled water (ml)	1000.0	1000.0		1000.0	700.0
Potassium penicillin G (million unit)‡	1.0	1.0	1.0	1.0	1.0
Streptomycin sulfate (gm)‡	1.0	1.0	1.0	1.0	1.0
Egg yolk (ml)					300.0

*BSA = Bovine serum albumin
†EDTA = ethylenediaminetetraacetic acid
‡Lincospectin (6 ml/L) or gentamicin (100 mg) may be substituted

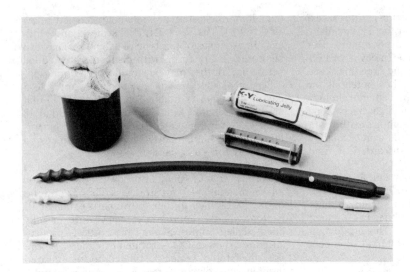

Figure 1. Equipment for artificial insemination of swine.

mating at a 12- to 18-hour interval was necessary for good fertility.

DETECTION OF ESTRUS

Perhaps the most critical factor in the success of swine AI is to ensure that the sows are bred at the proper time. The duration of estrus averages 60 hours in the sow and 44 hours in the gilt, with a variance of a few hours to several days. Determining the proper time to breed is based upon the time the female first shows estrus. The more frequently heat detection is attempted the more likely that proper breeding times will be achieved.

As estrus approaches, sows and gilts show increased sexual activity and some vulvar swelling. They may mount other animals and actively seek out boars. In true estrus the female will assume the mating stance in response to the boar, i.e., standing for manual back pressure and showing ear "propping" (an upward tilting of the erect ears). Generally, gilts or sows respond better to a mature male. Boars alone are often poor detectors of estrus because they randomly test females until one responds and then will neglect the other females. It is often better to move the boar among the females or leave him outside their pen and observe the females for interest in the boar. In some instances it is more convenient to move the gilts or sows past the boar pens and test the females that show interest. It is also possible to simulate the boar smell with an androgenic substance in an aerosol spray can (Boar Mate).

Best fertility occurs if the sow is mated 10 to 12 hours prior to ovulation and decreases rapidly if she is bred after ovulation. Ovulation occurs approximately 36 to 40 hours after estrus begins. Sows and gilts should be inseminated 24 to 30 hours after estrus begins and again 12 hours later. This practice reportedly increases conception rates by 10 to 20 per cent and litter size by one to two pigs.

SYNCHRONIZATION OF ESTRUS

Synchronization of estrus allows for efficient use of AI, since a number of females can be bred with a single collection. Weaning sows together will effectively synchronize 85 per cent of the animals over a 4-day period if the sows have been well fed and are weaned after 4 weeks lactation. Timed matings can be achieved with exogenous hormones given at weaning. This procedure should be used with caution in seed stock herds because it supersedes natural selection for fertility. (See other articles in this section on hormonal regulation of estrus and ovulation.)

INSEMINATION

Insemination equipment is designed to facilitate deposition of the semen into the uterus. Several catheters are available for this purpose (Fig. 1). These include a rubber (Melrose) spirette and several versions of disposable plastic pipettes. The rubber spirette is equipped with a soft corkscrew tip that is similar to the spiral end of the boar's penis. Counterclockwise rotation locks the spirette into the cervix. The spirettes must be thoroughly cleaned after each day's use. Flushing with distilled water or saline provides adequate cleansing between sows. Plastic pipettes fitted with a spiral tip or flange are available. Other pipettes have the anterior half inch bent at a 20° angle. These disposable pipettes are frequently cleansed between sows but discarded each day. The spirettes are preferred for inexperienced inseminators because they are more flexible and less likely to injure the sow. They provide the inseminator with a feel for cervical dilatation and usually result in less backflow of semen. Semen should be deposited in the uterus. Fertility is very poor if semen is deposited in the vagina.

Females selected for breeding may be bred in pens or crates affording minimal animal movement. Females will stand better if a boar is nearby or if stimulated with Boar Mate. The vulva is wiped with a clean paper towel, and the catheter, which is lightly lubricated with mineral oil, vegetable oil or KY jelly, is inserted along the dorsal wall of the vulva and vagina. It is important to miss the urethral opening, which is located ventrally in the posterior part of the vagina.

Once resistance is met, the spirette is rotated counterclockwise to lock into the cervix. Other catheters are manipulated accordingly to achieve intracervical location of the tip.

Semen is transferred through the catheter by connecting a syringe or plastic squeeze bottle. If backflow is observed, reset the catheter. Cervical stimulation with the catheter is sufficient to release oxytocin for uterine contractions and semen movement through the uterus. There appears to be no need of additional stimulation of the female.

Nondisposable equipment used for AI should be cleansed with warm tap water and a brush. It is advisable not to use detergents because of residues harmful to spermatozoa. After washing, rinse the equipment in distilled water and then boil it in distilled water for 15 to 20 minutes. A temporary sanitizing method is rinsing equipment in 70 per cent alcohol and allowing the alcohol to evaporate. Boiling or autoclaving is preferred to sanitization with alcohol because yeast and some bacteria are not adequately controlled by sanitizing the equipment.

It is advisable to examine the processed semen periodically for viability at each step of the breeding program. Semen may be inadvertently exposed to spermacidal substances during handling. Residual-cleansing agents, certain latex products (rubber gloves) and rubber plungers from resterilized syringes are sometimes spermicidal.

FROZEN SEMEN

The availability of frozen semen has become a reality in most countries, including the United States. Cryopreservation allows for long-term preservation and shipment of semen. Federal and state laws should be investigated before semen is shipped.

Most commercial companies freeze boar semen in plastic tubes in liquid nitrogen vapor or as small pellets on dry ice. These are stored in liquid nitrogen.

There is a great deal of variability in the fertility of boar semen once it is frozen. It is advisable to select semen from boars with known fertility after freezing. Special handling is required for use of frozen semen. This information is provided by the owner of the boar stud. Questions of fertility are best directed to the semen processor. In general, frozen-thawed semen results in lower conception rates and smaller litter sizes, but this may be minimized by carefully timing the matings.

CONCLUSION

Artificial insemination offers the producer an opportunity to introduce new genetic material into the herd or to utilize a desirable boar to breed more females in the herd. AI should not be regarded as a labor saving technique or as a method to overcome infertility in the herd. With good management, AI can equal conception rates and litter sizes obtained with natural service.

Viral Reproductive Failure

William L. Mengeling, D.V.M., Ph.D.
National Animal Disease Center, Ames, Iowa

Although numerous viruses have been reported as possible causes of reproductive failure of swine, only a few are known or believed to be of major clinical and economic importance. These are porcine parvovirus (PPV), porcine enterovirus (PEV), pseudorabies virus (PRV), hog cholera virus (HCV) and Japanese B encephalitis virus (JEV). Both PPV and PEV are found worldwide, whereas PRV, HCV and JEV are limited either by disease control or eradication programs (PRV, HCV) or by geographic distribution of a needed biologic vector (JEV). Neither HCV nor JEV is present among swine in the United States.

All of the aforementioned viruses can cross the maternal placenta to infect and kill the conceptus. However, the ultimate consequences of infection will depend largely on the stage of gestation and the particular virus involved. Dead embryos are usually resorbed without a trace, whereas fetuses, i.e., the conceptus after about 30 days of gestational age when skeletal development begins, will either become dehydrated (mummified) or be aborted. Moreover, some viruses, e.g., PRV, can kill fetuses at any gestational age, while others, e.g., PPV, are relatively innocuous during late gestation. A further variable is the effect of less than an entire litter being infected transplacentally. When this happens, littermates may be exposed by intrauterine spread of virus, and a variety of pathologic sequelae may be found in the same litter. This observation is of some general diagnostic significance because it strongly suggests the involvement of an infectious agent.

Maternal clinical signs, or the absence thereof, and other features of the disease associated with each of these viruses allow a tentative differential diagnosis, but whenever possible, appropriate samples should be tested in a diagnostic laboratory for corroboration. Although little can be done to alter the course of an epizootic of reproductive disease, correct diagnosis is emphasized by the availability of vaccines to prevent recurrence of the same problem among susceptible swine at subsequent intervals.

In general, male reproductive performance is at most only temporarily affected by the same viruses, and as a consequence, the following discussion focuses primarily on maternal infection and its sequelae.

TYPES OF VIRUS

Porcine Parvovirus. Porcine parvovirus[4] is distributed worldwide, and the incidence of infection approaches 100 per cent among older breeding stock in areas of intensive swine production. Swine are the only known hosts. Virus may be disseminated by clinically normal swine carriers—although this possibility has not been established unequivocally. During acute infection, PPV is shed in both secretions and excretions, and because of the extreme resistance of PPV to inactivation, a contaminated premise may remain infectious for months unless it is thoroughly cleaned and disinfected. Most swine are infected oronasally; however, the finding of PPV in boar semen suggests that in some cases apparent maternal infertility is caused by infection with PPV at the time of copulation. On the other hand, there is no evidence that infection affects the fertility of the boar. Most cases of PPV-induced reproductive failure are the result of maternal infection any time during about the first half of gestation. The interval between maternal and transplacental infection varies, but the mean is probably about 10 to 14 days. Within a few days after maternal exposure, virus and viral antigen are found in many maternal tissues, and a viremia can usually be demonstrated. Despite extensive viral replication, the dam is usually clinically unaffected, although a mild fever and leukopenia may develop. Early in gestation the immunologically incompetent embryos or fetuses succumb to infection, whereas fetuses of about 70 or more days of gestational age usually survive because, at least in part, of the production of antibody and the consequent suppression of viral replication. Nevertheless, the virus may persist, replicate at a low level and be further disseminated at the time of parturition. No developmental anomalies of the fetus have been reported. Abortion is uncommon, and if there is an increased incidence of stillbirth, it is probably because of the effect of

littermates that died during gestation and caused either a prolonged gestation or a prolonged farrowing interval or both. Note that in such cases one would expect to find a large number of mummified fetuses in addition to stillborn pigs.

Virus can frequently be isolated from affected fetuses even if the fetus is mummified. However, direct examination of fetal tissues by immunofluorescence microscopy is the diagnostic method of choice, since viral antigen persists after virus inactivation. In fact, viral antigen is so stable in mummified fetal tissues that failure to identify such antigen in any of several fetuses from an epizootic of reproductive failure would almost unequivocally eliminate PPV as a possible cause. The virus produces cytopathic changes in cell culture, but several serial passages in mitotically active cells are often necessary before such changes are easily detected.

Both modified-live-virus and inactivated-virus vaccines have been developed experimentally, and there are currently three federally licensed inactivated PPV vaccines commercially available in the United States.

Porcine Enteroviruses. Porcine enteroviruses[1] are distributed worldwide. The incidence of infection is known to be high; however, comprehensive serologic surveys are difficult to perform because at least eight serotypes exist. Swine are the only known host, and the virus is maintained by subclinically affected swine carriers. Porcine enteroviruses have been isolated from boar semen and may be the cause of apparent maternal infertility when introduced into the female genital tract at the time of copulation. Moreover, infection of the boar has been shown to affect semen quality adversely. The pathogenetic mechanism for enterovirus-induced reproductive failure is similar to that of PPV. Although microscopic developmental anomalies have been reported, they are not a cardinal feature of the disease. Occasionally, PEV can be isolated at term from tissues of affected pigs. The virus produces cytopathic changes in cell culture, and such changes are often obvious on initial inoculation of suspect material. Since four of the eight serotypes of PEV have already been incriminated in reproductive failure, an effective vaccine would have to be multivalent. A vaccine is not currently available.

Japanese B Encephalitis Virus. Japanese B encephalitis[5] virus has been identified in numerous Asian countries. In the United States a few cases of encephalitis due to JEV have been recognized in persons who have returned from Asia. However, the virus has not become established in the United States. Subclinical epizootics occur among swine and other animal species, sometimes coincidentally with clinical epidemics of encephalitis in man and horses. A single serotype has been described. The virus is maintained by subclinical infections and is transmitted by mosquitoes. In temperate climates the virus overwinters in the mosquito. Infection has not been reported to affect the boar or to be directly transmitted by the boar.

The pathogenetic mechanism of JEV-induced reproductive failure is similar to that of PPV and PEV except that fetal developmental anomalies, e.g., hydrocephalus, are a common feature of the disease. Moreover, JEV can also clinically affect fetuses later in gestation than either PPV or PEV. The sequelae of late infection are stillborn pigs and weak pigs that die shortly after birth with lesions of nonsuppurative encephalitis. Tissues from such pigs to be tested for virus should be kept cold to minimize decomposition. A tentative clinical diagnosis can be confirmed by virus isolation in mice (which develop encephalitis) or in cell culture.

Prevention can be accomplished by vaccination of breeding stock with modified-live-virus before gestation, by keeping stock away from the mosquito vector or by breeding so that gestation occurs during vector-free seasons.

Pseudorabies Virus. Pseudorabies virus[3] is widely distributed in swine throughout the world, but there are a few countries with significant swine populations, such as Canada and Australia, that are apparently free of the virus. Subclinical infection is common; however, unlike PPV, JEV and most strains of PEV, PRV also frequently causes severe and sometimes fatal disease of postnatal swine. Other domesticated and feral animals are also susceptible to PRV, and among these, infection is almost always fatal. The virus is believed to be maintained between epizootics by swine that are inapparent carriers, and it is possible that once swine are infected they remain carriers for life. Conditions that may lead to shedding by such carriers are ill defined. Other reservoirs of PRV have not been identified, but feral animals as well as dogs and cats have been suspected of transmitting the virus from one premise to another. Although only a single virus serotype has been recognized, the technique of restriction endonuclease analysis of viral deoxyribonucleic acid (commonly referred to as finger-printing) holds promise for strain differentiation.

There is no evidence that subclinical infection of pregnant swine with PRV will result in reproductive failure. In fact, under controlled experimental conditions, even severe maternal illness often has no detectable effect on reproductive performance. Nevertheless, assuming all other factors are constant, the likelihood of abortion or transplacental infection or both is probably directly related to the severity of maternal signs. Abortion may be coincident with other clinical signs, or it may follow apparent recovery if fetuses have been infected transplacentally. Stillbirth and neonatal death are common if fetuses are infected late in gestation. Developmental anomalies have not been reported. Mummified fetuses are not a suitable sample to submit to a diagnostic laboratory for testing because PRV is relatively unstable and quickly inactivated in such tissues. However, virus can be isolated from aborted fetuses and stillborn pigs if samples are kept cold to minimize decomposition before testing. Internal organs, such as spleen and liver, may have lesions of focal necrosis that are evident macroscop-ically as well as microscopically, and viral antigen can be detected around the periphery of such lesions by immunofluorescence microscopy. Pseudorabies virus produces cytopathic changes in a variety of cell cultures.

Prevention requires either isolation of susceptible stock during gestation or vaccination. Vaccines are available and are used extensively in some areas, but they do not appear to contribute much to elimination of PRV. The present consensus in the United States is that all additions to a PRV-free herd should be free of antibody for PRV. The reason is that the presence of antibody indicates past exposure to PRV and the possibility that the animal is an immune carrier of the virus.

Hog Cholera Virus. Hog cholera virus[2] is distributed worldwide but is notably absent from countries such as the United States, England and Canada following eradication programs. There is a single serotype; however, antigenic variants have been reported. The virus is maintained by chronically affected swine and also has been disseminated by the use of modified-live-virus vaccines. Viremia is a feature of both clinical and subclinical hog cholera, thus providing ample opportunity for transplacental infection.

Abortion is a common sequela of severe maternal illness, whereas embryonic resorption, fetal mummification, developmental anomalies, stillbirth and weak pigs result from transplacental infection during mild or subclinical maternal illness. Virus and viral antigen can be detected in tissues of stillborn and weak pigs and sometimes in tissues of fetuses that die near term. Since HCV is not cytopathogenic, its identification in cell culture is usually made by immunofluorescence microscopy. Both inactivated and modified-live-virus vaccines are effective for immunization.

SUMMARY

Selected features of maternal reproductive failure associated with each of the viruses previously discussed are summarized in Table 1. If involvement of a virus in a particular epizootic is probable, then thorough evaluation of such features and consideration of the geographic distribution of each virus should provide sufficient evidence for a tentative diagnosis. Note, for example, that although each of these viruses can cause fetal death and mummification in utero, only PRV and HCV are likely to cause obvious maternal illness, only PRV and HCV are likely to cause abortion and only JEV and HCV are likely to cause macroscopically obvious developmental anomalies. The seasonal nature of JEV is an additional discriminating factor. Reproductive failures caused by PPV and PEV may be clinically indistinguishable, but examination of tissues from a few mummified fetuses, if available, by immuno-fluorescence microscopy will definitively establish whether PPV is involved. Always keep in mind, however, that reproductive problems in swine are common and a significant proportion of these—

Table 1. Selected Features of Porcine Reproductive Failures Associated with Viral Infection

Feature	Porcine Parvovirus	Porcine Enterovirus	Japanese Encephalitis B Virus	Pseudorabies Virus	Hog Cholera Virus
Transmission by copulation	Yes, but relatively uncommon	Yes, but relatively uncommon	No	Possible, but unlikely	Possible, but unlikely
Illness of dam	Usually subclinical	Usually subclinical	Subclinical to mild	Mild to severe*	Subclinical to severe
Maternal viremia and transplacental infection necessary for reproductive failure	Yes	Yes	Yes	No, but transplacental infection is common	No, but viremia and transplacental infection are characteristic
Most susceptible stage of gestation	Primarily first half	Primarily first half	Throughout, but most susceptible first half	Throughout	Throughout, but most susceptible first half
Incidence of abortion	Low or nil	Low or nil	Low or nil	High	Variable, depends on severity of maternal illness
Embryonic and fetal death	Yes	Yes	Yes	Yes	Yes
Developmental anomalies	Not reported	Yes, but uncommon and microscopic	Yes, common	Not reported	Yes, common
Demonstrable antibody in serum of neonate before nursing	Yes, common	Yes	Not reported	No	No
Likelihood of demonstrating virus and/or viral antigen at farrowing in:					
Dead fetus	Excellent	Poor	Poor	Fair	Poor
Live pig	Good, but difficult if pig also has homologous serum antibody	Fair	Fair	Fair	Excellent

*Although subclinical infections with pseudorabies virus are common, there is no evidence that such an infection results in reproductive failure.

especially repeat breeders and what appears to be early embryonic death—are probably manifestations of a variety of non-infectious causes.

References

1. Huang J, Gentry RF, Zarkower A: Experimental infection of pregnant sows with porcine enteroviruses. Am J Vet Res 41:469, 1980.
2. Johnson KP, Ferguson LC, Byington DP, Redman DR: Multiple fetal malformations due to persistent viral infection. I. Abortion, intrauterine death, and gross abnormalities in fetal swine infected with hog cholera virus. Lab Invest 30:608, 1974.
3. Kluge JP, Mare CJ: Swine pseudorabies: Abortion, clinical disease, and lesions in pregnant gilts infected with pseudorabies virus (Aujeszky's disease). Am J Vet Res 35:911, 1974.
4. Mengeling WL, Paul PS, Brown TT: Transplacental infection and embryonic death following maternal exposure to porcine parvovirus near the time of conception. Arch Virol 65:55, 1980.
5. Shimizu T, Kawakami Y, Fukuhara S, Matumoto M: Experimental stillbirth in pregnant swine infected with Japanese encephalitis virus. Jap J Exp Med 24:363, 1954.

Bacterial Endometritis

Michael J. Meredith, B.Sc., B.Vet.Med.,
Ph.D., M.R.C.V.S.
University of Cambridge, England

The most common inflammatory disorder of the porcine uterus is endometritis, i.e., an inflammatory process that primarily involves the tunica mucosa (endometrium). On rare occasions this progresses to the more severe condition of metritis, in which all layers of the uterine wall are acutely inflamed.

Noninfectious endometritis is rarely encountered, but can result, for example, from uterine lavage with irritant drugs or antiseptics. Most cases of endometritis are associated with the presence of bacteria. Large numbers of these bacteria can be found in the uterine lumen and less commonly in the uterine wall.

Only direct bacterial infections of the uterus will be considered in this article, but there is a wide range of extragenital infections that are capable of affecting reproductive processes indirectly as a consequence of their pyrexic, toxemic, metabolic or nutritional effects.

On the basis of bacteriologic surveys of uteri from abattoirs it has been suggested that intrauterine bacteria may be responsible for impaired fertility (particularly the death of embryos) in the absence of endometritis. Further evidence is needed to confirm this, but it is our experience that bacterial contamination of uteri can easily arise during commercial abattoir procedures and during transportation to the laboratory.

ETIOLOGIC AGENTS

The bacterial species that have been isolated in our laboratory from the uterus of spontaneous cases of endometritis are listed in Table 1. It can be seen that a wide range of organisms is involved and that the organisms belong to species that are commonly found at various sites in healthy pigs.

Another bacterium that is widely associated with endometritis is *Brucella suis*. This is a zoonotic agent, and in many countries it is a disease that must be reported. Biotypes 1, 2 and 3 are pathogenic for pigs.

Leptospirae are not known to cause endometritis in pigs, although they can result in other reproductive disorders, including neonatal mortality, still-birth, mummification of fetuses and abortion. In addition, hepatic or renal damage from leptospirosis can debilitate sows with adverse consequences for ovarian function and embryo survival.

EPIDEMIOLOGY

Sporadic cases of bacterial endometritis occur in all herds of breeding pigs, but the disease can also attain epidemic or endemic proportions.

It is scarcely surprising that the peak occurrence of endometritis is in the puerperal period, at a time when the uterus is most likely to experience a combination of trauma and bacterial contamination. The major part of uterine involution and repair occurs in the first week after farrowing, and new cases rarely arise during the remainder of lactation. Endometritis is rarely seen in the postweaning period, before puberty or in anestrous pigs. However, it can be a significant problem in cyclic gilts and sows. This is probably a reflection of predisposing factors associated with mating and insemination (e.g., venereal transmission, genital trauma, contamination), predisposing physiological features of the estrous cycle, dilation of the vaginal ostium and cervical canal during estrus,[4] and a diminution of nonspecific uterine resistance mechanisms (motility and leucotaxis) during the luteal phase.

Bacterial endometritis is present in some cases of abortion and in many cases of fetal maceration, although in many of these instances it may well be secondary to a primarily fetal problem.

Brucella suis is not ubiquitous as are the other bacteria associated with endometritis. The distribution of the organism is worldwide, but many countries remain free of it. Even in those countries that have the disease, it is rarely present in herds in which good management and precautions against disease introduction are followed. Infection usually enters a herd by means of carrier pigs, but infection

Table 1. Bacteria Isolated from Cases of Endometritis

Bacteroides melaninogenicus
*Clostridium perfringens**
*Corynebacterium pyogenes**
Corynebacterium sp. (unclassified)
*Escherichia coli**
*Klebsiella pneumoniae (Aerobacter aerogenes)**
Pasteurella multocida
*Proteus mirabilis**
Pseudomonas aeruginosa
*Staphylococcus aureus**
Staphylococcus epidermidis
Streptococcus (group C)*
Streptococcus (group L)*

*Primary pathogenicity has been demonstrated experimentally.

from wildlife (feral pigs or European hares), semen, ova or contaminated feedstuffs is also possible. Venereal and oral routes of transmission are the usual means of spread within herds.

PATHOGENESIS

The normal bacterial flora of the uterus is a subject of great controversy. There have been a number of reports that bacteria are normally present in the uterus of a substantial proportion of pigs, even during pregnancy. In our laboratory we have rarely isolated bacteria from normal uteri obtained under controlled conditions except in the first few days after parturition or in the first 24 hours after mating. Experimental introduction of bacteria into the uterus post partum or during estrus has resulted in their rapid elimination. However, the inoculation of field strains of bacteria (Table 1) into the uteri of animals in the luteal phase or in pregnancy has induced endometritis. These findings indicate that the uterus does not have a significant resident population of bacteria and that endometritis can ensue from an abnormal persistence and proliferation of bacteria that have entered, as is usual, during the puerperium or estrus period. Bacterial persistence could be a consequence of uterine trauma or delayed involution (dystocia), uterine debris (placental or fetal), foreign bodies, intrauterine hemorrhage, overwhelming bacterial contamination or a particularly pathogenic bacterium (e.g. B. suis).

An additional type of pathogenesis arises when bacteria gain access to the uterus at an unusual time, i.e., in the luteal phase or during pregnancy. At these times, uterine resistance to bacterial infection is very low. This can occur by hematogenous spread of an extragenital infection, by ascending infection from the vagina and cervix or by mating or artificially inseminating sows when they are not in estrus.

Extragenital infection with B. suis is followed by a period of intracellular multiplication in local lymph nodes, which may progress to bacteremia 1 to 7 weeks after exposure, followed by localization at various sites, including the genital tract.[1]

CLINICAL MANIFESTATIONS

Endometritis can exhibit a wide spectrum of presentations, but in many cases clinical signs are not obvious. Vulval discharge is the most common feature of this condition, but in many cases the discharge is very intermittent. The disease is rarely fatal, but in severe cases there may be inappetence, lethargy or pyrexia. Postpartum endometritis is not consistently associated with either agalactia or mastitis.[2]

In gilts and dry sows endometritis can result in fertilization failure, embryo death or, more rarely, abortion. In a recent survey of pigs culled because of repeated returns to service, endometritis was diagnosed in 24 per cent of the gilts and in 25.8 per cent of the sows.[3] When endometritis occurs after breeding, there can be a regular or a delayed return to estrus. Delayed returns to estrus are easily missed and may therefore appear as a "not in pig" problem some months after breeding.

B. suis infection can result in abortion at any stage of gestation but usually occurs quite early and is apparent as delayed returns to estrus. Orchitis and locomotor problems resulting from arthritis may also occur.

CLINICAL DIAGNOSIS

Diagnosis is undoubtedly problematic. Vulval discharge occurs at some time or other in most, if not all, affected pigs. However, discharges are easily missed. On the other hand, some of the vulvar discharges that are seen (Table 2) lead to an erroneous diagnosis of endometritis, particularly when the veterinarian has to rely on stockmen's observations.

In cases in which endometritis is suspected, evidence and samples of discharge may be obtained from the undersurface of the tail where it contacts the vulva or, even better, by use of a vaginal speculum (a human sigmoidoscope is particularly suitable). The stage of reproduction at which a discharge occurs, its gross appearance, odor and microscopic appearance can help to pinpoint its probable origin and significance. Urolithiasis is very common in sows and is frequently misdiagnosed as vaginitis or endometritis. These chemical sediments sometimes appear remarkably like purulent exudate and may linger on the vulva, floors or pen fittings after the urine has disappeared. A simple microscopic examination for the presence of crystals, amorphous material or leukocytes will quickly differentiate between urolithiasis and inflammatory discharges.

Rectal examination of the genital tract can be an invaluable diagnostic aid in detecting delayed uterine involution, thickening of the uterine horns, pyometra, retained fetuses or presence of a normal pregnancy. A vaginal speculum can be helpful in ascertaining the site of origin of a discharge.

Bacteriologic examination of discharge or of swabs taken of the genital tract is of very limited diagnostic value except in the rare cases in which a definite pathogen such as B. suis is isolated. Unfortunately, most cases of endometritis involve bacterial species that can also be isolated from the lower genital tract of healthy pigs. Long-sheathed swabs of the cervical lumen can occasionally be diagnostic when large numbers of a potentially pathogenic species are isolated. However, negative results are unreliable.

Serologic tests of the herd are the most convenient method of detecting B. suis infection. However, both positive and negative results can be unreliable in individual pigs.

Table 2. Differential Diagnosis of Vulval Discharge

Type of Discharge	Quantity	Consistency	Color	Malodorous
Normal				
1. Proestrous/estrous	Small	Watery, slightly tacky	Clear, cloudy or white (depending on cell content)	No
2. Seminal (during/shortly after mating or AI)	Varied	Mainly semen components, some fluid and cells from female	Clear, cloudy or white	No
3. Postmating (8 to 48 hours after service or AI)	Small	Thick, tenacious	White, gray or yellow	No
4. Pregnancy (probably mainly from cervix)	Small	Thick, tenacious	White, gray or yellow	No
5. Postpartum lochia (up to 5 days post partum)	Up to about 15 ml present at one time Decreasing by third day	Usually thick	Varied	Slightly
Abnormal				
1. Vaginitis/cervicitis	Small	Thick, tenacious	White to yellow	Not usually
2. Endometritis (in gilts or dry sows)	Varied	Varied	Varied	Sometimes
3. Endometritis (puerperal)	Often > 15 ml present at one time	Usually thin, may be lumps present	Varied	Usually
4. Urolithiasis (oxalates, phosphates)	Varied	Often slightly gritty when rubbed between fingers	Cloudy, white or yellow	No
5. Cystitis/pyelonephritis	Varied	Varied	Varied	Sometimes

POST-MORTEM DIAGNOSIS

The most important feature to look for is the presence of uterine exudate, which is present in the majority of unequivocal cases of bacterial endometritis. Histologic diagnosis of endometritis requires considerable experience of the normal uterine histology of the pig under a wide range of reproductive states because the classical features of inflammation are normally present at certain stages of breeding. There is no doubt that endometritis will be over-diagnosed by histopathologists who are unfamiliar with this fact. Reliable interpretation of uterine histology can only be achieved if information about the functional condition of the ovaries at the time of slaughter and a full breeding history are available. The sensitivity and specificity of post-mortem diagnosis is greatly improved if pigs are not killed during proestrus, estrus, metestrus or in the first few days after farrowing.

Bacteriologic isolations from porcine uteri should be interpreted with caution, particularly if unsupported by gross or histopathologic lesions. Urine can pass from the bladder to the uterus unless carcasses and excised genital tracts are handled with great care. This urine reflux can introduce bacteria into the uterus from the urinary system or lower genital tract.

TREATMENT AND CONTROL

Parenteral and in-feed antibiotics are widely used to treat confirmed or suspected problems of endometritis. A subsequent improvement in reproductive performance does not necessarily confirm that endometritis was present or that it has been resolved.

When using antibiotics, it is advisable to choose broad-spectrum agents in view of the variety of gram-positive and gram-negative bacteria that can be involved. Mild cases of endometritis tend to resolve spontaneously during lactation, proestrus and estrus. In cases of severe endometritis antibiotics have an important role in reducing sow and piglet mortality, shortening the period of illness and inappetence and preserving lactation. However, we believe that retention of such pigs for future breeding should be avoided whenever possible because permanent uterine damage and low fertility may occur.

Intrauterine installation of antibiotics or antiseptic chemicals has been shown to be beneficial in the treatment of puerperal endometritis. However, intrauterine therapy is time consuming, requires some training and experience and introduces additional microorganisms from the lower genital tract. The cervical lumen remains dilated for a few days after

Table 3. Prevention of Bacterial Endometritis

General Principles	Gilts/Dry Sows	Periparturient Sows
1. Minimize contamination of genital tract by microorganisms and foreign material.	Pen hygiene: cleanliness, good drainage, accommodation divided into subunits to allow all-in, all-out stocking with thorough cleansing, disinfection and drying between batches. Avoid systems in which sows have to lie or to sit (when rising) in dung and urine. Wash perineum of sows that get dirty. Avoid periods of prolonged recumbency by prompt attention to flooring problems, locomotor problems and cases of illness.	
	Supervise and assist mating to minimize contamination of penis (e.g., by rectal intromission).	Minimize time spent in (dirtying) farrowing pen before parturition (e.g., delay moving, induce farrowing).
	Take hygienic precautions during AI.	Take hygienic precautions when assisting parturition.
2. Avoid trauma to genital tract.	Supervise/assist mating.	Maintain prompt detection of and skilled attention to dystocia problems (control of farrowing time with prostaglandins can help). Avoid overdosage and unnecessary use of ecbolics (risk of uterine spasm/hypoxia/trauma from obstructed fetus).
3. Avoid impairment of innate resistance to infection.	Control genital virus infections (e.g., parvovirus and pseudorabies). Avoid chilling effects of drafts and damp, particularly in pigs whose movement is severely restricted. Do not restrict water intake (flushing effect of urine).	

farrowing. At most other times intrauterine administration is very difficult and likely to result in traumatic damage. Fluids can be introduced into the uterus easily during estrus by means of a catheter, which locks into the swollen cervical prominences. However, the indications for therapy at this time, let alone the efficacy of it, are dubious.

Oxytocic drugs can be useful in the treatment of post partum endometritis because they induce expulsion of debris and exudate and hasten uterine involution. Oxytocin is particularly safe and effective for this purpose, although recommended doses are often unnecessarily large. The uterus remains highly sensitive to oxytocin for several days after farrowing, therefore it is unnecessary to give more than 5 units intramuscularly. Unfortunately, the effect of oxytocin is short lived (30 minutes or less), so repeated administration is desirable. In sows that are suckled regularly, endogenous oxytocin is highly effective in stimulating uterine motility and involution. The benefit of giving exogenous oxytocin in these circumstances is very questionable. It is also doubtful if oxytocin is of any benefit for the treatment of endometritis in gilts or dry sows.

Estrogens and prostaglandins are sometimes used to treat endometritis. Estrogens are contraindicated, except in puerperal endometritis, because they can have a luteotrophic effect in pigs. In puerperal endometritis the benefit of estrogens is dubious because endogenous levels are already high. Prostaglandins are useful for preventive purposes, but their therapeutic role is not yet clear. In cyclic pigs their luteolytic effect is insignificant. Theoretically, they could be useful if persistent

corpora lutea are present, but this seems to be uncommon in pigs except for cases of total litter mummification.

Antibiotics and vaccines can reduce the clinical severity of *B. suis* endometritis, but effective control of herd infection requires slaughter and restocking.

PREVENTION

Unfortunately, there has been very little controlled assessment of preventive measures, so the recommendations outlined in Table 3 rely rather heavily on clinical impressions and deductions from what is known of the pathogenesis of uterine infections in pigs and other species. Some practitioners believe that boars play an important role in spreading nonspecific endometritis and undertake lavage of the prepuce with antibiotics or antiseptics, prescribe oral or parenteral courses of antibiotics or even excise the preputial diverticulum. Use of vasectomized boars to "vaccinate" gilts prior to breeding has also been suggested.

References

1. Deyoe BL: Brucellosis. In Diseases of Swine. 5th ed., Ames, Iowa State University Press, 1981.
2. Jones JET: Bacterial mastitis and endometritis in sows. Proc Int Pig Vet Soc, Ames, E.6, 1976.
3. Karlberg K, Rein KA, Nordstoga K: Histological and bacteriological examination of the uterus from the repeat breeder gilt and sow. Nord Vet Med 33:359, 1981.
4. Meredith MJ: Clinical techniques for the examination of infertile sows. Proc Pig Vet Soc 8:49, 1981.

Diagnosis of Reproductive Failure in Sows Manifested as Abortion, Mummified Fetuses, Stillbirths and Weak Neonates

Ross Cutler, B.V.Sc., Ph.D.

Department of Agriculture and Rural Affairs, Bendigo, Victoria, Australia

MECHANISMS INVOLVED IN REPRODUCTIVE FAILURE

The dam and her litter in utero respond to infectious and environmental insults in different ways, depending on the nature of the insult, the effect it has on the dam and the stage of gestation.

The environmental factors that may affect the outcome of pregnancy include temperature (both high and low), atmospheric carbon monoxide levels in the farrowing house and toxic chemicals. Many infectious diseases cause reproductive failure through their effect on the dam or the fetuses. Abortion is the most commonly recognized sequela to systemic maternal disease during pregnancy, but other outcomes are equally possible.

OUTCOME OF INFECTIOUS DISEASES

Abortion occurs when the sow is no longer able to maintain pregnancy. Through a series of events, which may include a febrile clinical illness with viremia or toxemia, the corpora lutea (CL) cease to function. Progesterone levels plummet and premature farrowing commences. It has been suggested that prostaglandins, by-products of the inflammation associated with maternal disease, cause destruction of the CL. Endocrine events are undoubtedly associated with some noninfectious abortions, but the mechanisms are unknown.

In many animals with or without clinical disease infectious microorganisms cross the placenta. Sometimes, as is the case with leptospirosis or brucellosis, placentitis occurs and abortion results. The abortion follows destruction of the CL through the action of inflammatory by-products or through an interruption to the uterine signal to maintain pregnancy.

With some viral infections, placentitis is mild, and the pregnancy continues, but in other infections the placentitis is severe enough to terminate the pregnancy.

Some pathogens are spread during coitus. Brucellosis and streptococcal infections are venereal diseases. After service from an infected boar, the sow suffers a low-grade endometritis, which ultimately progresses to a placentitis and abortion at a later stage. Abortion follows venereal *Brucella suis* infection as early as 17 days after breeding. Although vaginal discharges are uncommon in sows infected with *Brucella suis* (except just before and after abortion), they are common with venereal staphylococcal and streptococcal infection.

Following an infectious disease early in pregnancy (before day 30), the whole litter may be killed and the fetuses resorbed by the uterus. The sow returns to estrus after a period outside the normal 18 to 24 days—a delayed return to estrus.

In other cases the infection may result in abortion, which, because the fetuses are very small, goes undetected. The sow returns to estrus about 5 days after the abortion.

If the fetuses die after day 30 or, if following an earlier infection, some fetuses survive beyond days 30 to 35, they will not be resorbed by the uterus. Such fetuses, because of the development and calcification of their skeletal systems, remain in utero and appear at farrowing as shrivelled, small, dark, mummified fetuses.

Infections occurring late in gestation, depending on the virulence of the pathogen, may result in the appearance of stillborn pigs or weak neonates— often with clinical signs indicative of central nervous system disease. This is a reflection of the rapid development of central nervous system (CNS) tissues, particularly cerebellum, late in gestation and the predilection viruses have for rapidly growing tissues. Mummified fetuses sometimes accompany these pigs. The size of the mummified fetuses is a useful guide to the stage of pregnancy when the sow was first infected. Thirty-day fetuses are about 2.0 cm long, 50-day fetuses, 10 cm long, and by 90 days fetuses are about 20 cm long. At term fetuses are about 23 to 29 cm long.

Effect of Environment

In heat chamber experiments extremely high temperatures cause sows to abort. Such experimental results are supported by observations of abortions in sows kept outside during temperatures in excess of 40°C in summer.

The effect of season is less obvious, but an increase in the incidence of abortion (as distinct from delayed returns to service) during fall has been observed in a number of studies. These abortions occur at every stage of gestation.

Field observations associate abortions in sows held in stalls with the onset of very cold weather. Such sows are huddled, visibly chilled but display no signs of clinical illness. The aborted fetuses appear normal. Pathogens have not been demonstrated. The field observations of abortions associated with cold weather need to be validated by experimental evidence.

Delayed returns to estrus are characteristic of seasonal breeding failure in sows mated during late summer. Based on the estrone sulfate assay, which is a very reliable indicator of pregnancy, bred sows with delayed returns were once, in fact, pregnant and had suffered either an abortion or embryo resorption.

Elevated farrowing house temperatures during summer are responsible for an increase in the stillbirth rate. The piglets die during farrowing, and these deaths are most likely associated with an increase in the duration of parturition of heat-exhausted sows.

Litters of stillborn pigs and autolyzed full-term fetuses have been observed in sows farrowing in poorly ventilated barns heated with malfunctioning propane gas burners. The propane is incompletely burned, and carbon monoxide is produced instead of carbon dioxide. Fetal methoxyhemoglobin takes up carbon monoxide in preference to oxygen. The sows are unaffected but the fetuses die in utero or at term.

The fetus is also extremely sensitive to some toxic chemicals. Treatment with organophosphate before farrowing causes fetuses to tremble and shake at birth. Also, procaine penicillin has been implicated as the cause of early embryonic deaths and abortions later in gestation.

Establishing a Diagnosis

History. When abortions, stillbirths and mummified fetuses occur and are observed, diagnostic procedures are straightforward. It remains only to establish the extent of the problems from farm records so that the costs of a potentially extensive investigation can be balanced against the cost of the problem. Establishing the severity of the problem helps in determining control strategies and also helps to pinpoint the most likely infectious agents.

Pseudorabies, porcine parvovirus (PPV), leptospirosis, brucellosis and streptococcal infections usually affect a group of animals and commonly cause disease in replacement females or young sows when the disease is enzootic in a herd. Most of the other infectious agents cause sporadic abortion involving only isolated sows. Abortions following live erysipelas vaccinations have been reported.

When requesting diagnostic assistance with herd abortion problems, many farmers may not have actually observed sows aborting but merely assumed that their sows failed to farrow because they had aborted. In these cases it is most important to define that pregnancy was actually established. Failure to detect estrus, conception failure, failure to mate and inaccurate pregnancy diagnosis are all possible and just as likely, if not more likely, causes of sows failing to farrow, than abortions.

Small litters of pigs born alive may be part of a herd infection with PPV and perhaps other infectious diseases. However, it is unusual for these syndromes to occur without at least some mummified fetuses. Documentation of mummified fetuses by farrowing house attendants is commonly neglected. Also, mummies are often not differentiated from stillbirths. Thorough questioning will usually elucidate these details.

In normal herds it is expected that about 2 per cent of sows abort, 6 to 8 per cent of piglets are born dead and about 0.5 per cent of pigs are born mummified. During reproductive crises, for any group of farrowings, abortions may exceed 5 to 10 per cent of the group, 10 to 14 per cent of pigs are stillborn and 10 per cent of sows may have three or more mummified fetuses in their litters. In addition, 10 per cent of the group may have litters with fewer than six pigs born alive. Data such as these provide a basis for thorough investigation. In these cases there is ample material available to enable a diagnosis to be reached.

Tissues for Submission to a Laboratory. The submission of fetal tissues to a diagnostic laboratory is an essential component of diagnosis. Maternal blood samples for serology are useful when combined with fetal tissues but useless on their own. At best they indicate exposure to a pathogen or a degree of age group or herd susceptibility. While blood samples may identify some of the potential pathogens involved in a reproductive crisis, they do nothing to confirm a specific diagnosis. If blood sampling is pursued, 10 samples from a group is a minimum sample size.

Entire litters, together with placenta, are best submitted fresh (within 12 hours) to a diagnostic laboratory, but when this is not possible, appropriate samples need to be selected. Weak or shaking neonates should be submitted alive if possible. Mummified fetuses are always useful specimens.

Liver, kidney, heart, lung, spleen, brain and placenta from at least two fetuses from each aborted litter should always be collected for routine histopathology. These samples are particularly important from weak or shaking neonates. Swabs from fetal lung, liver, stomach and placenta can be transported in media. Samples of liver, lung, brain and kidney should be forwarded frozen and fresh to the laboratory for viral and/or bacterial isolation. Individual, isolated, stillborn pigs add little to diagnostic efforts. Stillborn pigs, from a litter of stillbirths or from a litter of three or more stillborn pigs, are preferred. Serum samples from both the sow and the aborted or stillborn fetuses are useful. Presuckling serum samples from weak or trembling neonates may also indicate in utero exposure to a specific pathogen.

Thoracic fluids examined under dark-field mi-

Table 1. Bacteria Causing Reproductive Failure

Bacteria	Principal Clinical Signs	State of Pregnancy when Infection Causes Disease	Transmission	Pathogenesis	Essential Tissues for Diagnosis	Other Comments
Leptospira interrogans	Abortion, stillbirths, mummified fetuses, weak neonates	Second half	From infected urine or aerosol infection-carriers	Subclinical maternal bacteremia and placentitis	Fetal kidney to demonstrate leptospires in silver-stained sections; thoracic fluids to demonstrate leptospires by dark-field examination; liver or kidney for culture	Vaccination does not eliminate carriers but does prevent abortion and fetal infection
serovars: *pomona Icterohemorrhagiae grypotyphosa, tarassovi, hardjo*						
Brucella suis	Abortion, stillbirths, large mummified fetuses, weak neonates, delayed returns to service	Throughout	Venereal or ingestion	Endometritis or subclinical maternal bacteremia, suppurative placentitis	Fetal stomach contents for culture, uterus to demonstrate characteristic miliary abscessation	Infection in wild pigs common. These animals easily gain entry into most piggeries and transmit infection venereally
Staphylococcus aureus & *Streptococcus* spp	Abortion, vaginal discharge	Early	Venereal	Local endometritis and placentitis	Fetal stomach for culture	Infection may occur during mating but sow may not abort until midterm
Erysipelothrix rhusiopathiae	Abortion	Throughout	Fecal or urinary spread	Acute febrile septicemia in sows	Fetal stomach for culture	Abortion has been reported following vaccination of sows with live erysipelas vaccine. Some pigs in the herd will likely have characteristic skin lesions or erysipelas

Other bacteria, which following infection commonly cause a maternal septicemia and abortion, include: *Bacillus anthracis, Rhodococcus equi* (formerly called *Corynebacterium equi), C. pyogenes, Pseudomonas* spp., *Pasteurella multocida, Escherichia coli* (including live *E. coli* vaccines), *Salmonella* spp., *Actinobacillus* spp., *Mycobacterium avium, Chlamydia* spp., *Mycoplasma hyorhinis, Listeria monocytogenes*.

Other micro-organisms include: *Aspergillus fumigatus*, which is occasionally demonstrated in aborted fetuses and placenta. Routine tissues together with placenta and fetal stomach contents are needed for laboratory diagnosis. Toxoplasmosis as a cause of stillbirths has been diagnosed histologically.

Table 2. Viruses Causing Reproductive Failure

Virus	Principal Clinical Signs	Stage of Pregnancy when Infection Causes Disease	Transmission	Pathogenesis	Essential Tissues for Diagnosis	Other Comments
Porcine parvovirus (PPV)	Mummified fetuses; failure to farrow	First Half	Fecal contact; semen possible	Subclinical maternal viremia and transplacental infection	Mummified fetal lung or liver for FA* or HA†; thoracic fluids from stillborn pigs in litter for serology	Mummified fetuses in aborted litters are observed; litters with fewer than 6 born alive are common
Porcine enterovirus (PEV)	Mummified fetuses; abortion	First half	Fecal contact; semen possible	Subclinical maternal viremia with transplacental infection	Thoracic fluids from stillborn pigs for serology; fetal lung or liver for virus isolation	PEV is a common isolate from aborted litters
Japanese B encephalitis virus	Mummified fetuses; stillbirths; weak neonates with nervous signs	Throughout	Mosquito borne	Subclinical maternal viremia with transplacental infection; fetuses develop a nonsuppurative encephalitis	Brain for histology and virus isolation; fetal sera for serology	Disease restricted to Asia; it is a zoonosis
Pseudorabies virus (PRV)	Abortion, mummified fetuses, stillbirths, weak piglets with nervous signs, high mortality	Throughout	Fecal or aerosol contact	Clinical, febrile, maternal disease; transplacental infection possible	Fetal tonsil or brain stem for FA* or culture	
Hog-cholera virus (HCV)	Abortion, mummification, stillbirths, weak piglets with nervous signs	Throughout	Fecal contact, "attenuated" vaccines, mechanical vectors possible	Clinical or subclinical viremia with transplacental infection	Fetal tonsil for FA*; brain for histology	Subclinical maternal HCV infections are associated with low virulence field strains of HCV or "attenuated" virus vaccines

Other viruses causing reproductive failure are African swine fever, foot and mouth disease virus and swine vesicular disease virus. Abortion usually follows a period of acute febrile disease. Infectious bovine rhinotracheitis virus and bovine virus diarrhea virus also infect pigs subclinically and have been associated with reproductive failure. Encephalomyocarditis virus disease, which causes acute mortalities in pigs of all ages, has been linked to late abortion and stillbirths without clinical infection in sows.

*FA = Fluorescent antibody

Table 3. Environmental Causes of Reproductive Failure

Cause	Clinical Signs	Pathogenesis	Diagnostic Approach	Other Comments
High temperature	Abortion, stillbirths	Heat stress; prolonged farrowing in exhausted sows	Routine tissues to eliminate common pathogens	Sows may die around farrowing time during periods of high temperature
Season	Abortion, delayed returns to estrus, conception failure, postweaning anestrus	Unknown, evolutionary trend, pigs are seasonal breeders	Routine tissues to eliminate common pathogens	Seasonal breeding patterns are most apparent in late summer
Low temperature	Abortion	Cold, thin sows innately unable to sustain pregnancy	Routine tissues to eliminate common pathogens	Low temperature abortions occur during the first cold weather snaps in under-fed, cold sows. Observations need experimental substantiation
Carbon monoxide	Stillbirths, autolyzed fetuses	Fetuses take up CO in preference to O_2. Propane gas heaters malfunction in poorly ventilated barns	Blood from fetuses is very red; routine tissues to eliminate common pathogens; environmental CO testing	Disease observed in new "air-tight" barns
Organophosphate (OP) poisoning	Weak, shaking neonates	Toxic effect of OP on developing fetal cerebellum	Clinical signs, history	Follows oral and skin treatment of sows with organophosphates 30 to 35 days before term

croscopy may permit a diagnosis of leptospirosis, but cultures are essential to identify the precise leptospira serotype involved. Histopathology is of value if dark-field microscopic examination leads to uncertain results because of excessive autolysis or fibrin accumulation in thoracic fluids. Fetal serology (microscopic agglutination test) is of little value in the diagnosis of leptospirosis.

Slaughterhouse samples from sows that have aborted rarely yield useful diagnostic materials.

Interpretation of laboratory results is usually conclusive if *plenty* of diagnostic submissions are made. Diagnosis and field action may be confused if they depend on isolated or individual submissions. Insufficient and inappropriate tissues selected for diagnosis may also complicate an otherwise simple diagnosis. Nevertheless, it is important to recognize that successful diagnostic conclusions are reached only in 30 per cent of cases submitted to a laboratory. Hence, correct tissue collection, a thorough

history and astute observation of clinical signs are of paramount importance in reaching a diagnosis.

In Tables 1 to 3 the clinical signs, transmission, pathogenesis and most appropriate diagnostic tissues for diagnosis of the common reproductive pathogens and environmental causes are summarized.

Suggested Readings

1. Cutler RS, Hurtgen JP, Leman AD: Reproduction. In Leman AD (ed): Diseases of Swine. Ames, Iowa State Press, 1981.
2. Holter JA, Andrews JJ: Evaluation of current diagnostic methods for causes of abortions. Am Assoc Vet Lab Diag 22nd Ann Proc pp. 85–96, 1979.
3. Kirkbride CA, McAdaraugh JP: Infectious agents associated with fetal and early neonatal death and abortion in swine. JAVMA 172:480, 1978.
4. Mengeling WE: Porcine parvo virus. In Leman AD (ed): Diseases of Swine. Ames, Iowa State Press, 1981.

Noninfectious Infertility in Swine

John P. Hurtgen, D.V.M., Ph.D.
New Freedom, Pennsylvania

Swine are usually considered highly fertile in relation to other domestic animal species. However, the results of two large surveys that included more than 50,000 hand-mated sows and gilts indicated that the farrowing rate was about 72 per cent per estrus. Noninfectious forms of infertility may be manifested as anestrus, conception failure, early embryonic death, abortion, failure to farrow and reduced litter size. The outward signs of infectious and noninfectious causes of infertility are strikingly similar. In fact, both forms of infertility may occur at the same time within a given herd. This article will present some of the major causes of noninfectious infertility.

DELAYED PUBERTY

Gilts normally reach puberty at 6 to 8 months of age. Much of the variation in age at onset of puberty within and among herds is related to breed of female, access to boar stimulation, season of the year and selection and management factors.

Breed. Landrace and Large White gilts reach puberty at least 4 to 6 weeks earlier, on the average, than gilts of the Duroc, Hampshire and Yorkshire breeds. In general, crossbred females reach puberty at a younger age than purebred gilts. It is becoming increasingly apparent that the average age at onset of puberty can be decreased within a herd or breed through selection for this trait.

Boar Exposure. Once the genetic composition of the gilt has been established, the single most important factor in determining the age at onset of puberty is exposure of the prepubertal gilt to sexually mature boars. It is recommended that gilts be exposed to boars by direct or fence-line contact when gilts are 160 to 180 days of age. This practice will hasten the onset of puberty by approximately 30 days. Use of boars less than 8 months of age is less stimulatory than boars over 12 months of age. Research suggests that 1 to 2 hours of boar contact is as beneficial as continuous stimulation. The use of different boars may be more stimulatory than the same boar. Dependent on breed, some gilts appear to be nonresponsive to the boar stimulus at less than 140 to 150 days of age. In fact, when gilts are exposed to boars at these young ages, they may fail to reach puberty until 7 to 8 months of age.

Season. Gilts expected to reach puberty during summer months are usually 2 to 3 weeks older than gilts expected to reach puberty during winter months.

Confinement. Average age at onset of puberty is somewhat higher for gilts housed in confinement than for gilts housed outside. Gilts held individually in gestation crates or on tethers have a delayed onset of puberty compared with gilts in confinement but placed in pens of four to eight females per pen. Although research studies indicate that the restriction of space does not interfere with onset of puberty, the ability of the boar and herdsman to identify estrous females accurately is markedly reduced, as the number of females per pen increases.

Nutrition. Increased energy intake (flushing) may hasten the onset of puberty in gilts that have been on a restricted plane of nutrition or in undernourished gilts.

Stress Factors. Transportation or movement of gilts nearing pubertal age to a different facility or pen will hasten the onset of puberty. This effect is usually coupled with exposure of gilts to boars, increased space allocation and reduced numbers of females per pen. The mixing of females of different, socially established groups, restriction of feed and water intake and crowding result in restlessness, fighting, reduced feed intake and delay in onset of estrus. These stressful conditions should be minimized in the breeding herd.

Silent Estrus. Occasionally, gilts may initiate normal ovarian activity but fail to demonstrate estrus or standing heat in the presence of boars. This pattern of activity may be called silent estrus or behavioral anestrus. Despite systematic estrous detection practices, certain gilts appear to be behaviorally anestrous during each estrous period. The cause of this condition is unknown. There is presently no treatment for this condition, including hormonal therapy. If mated, such as with artificial insemination, behaviorally anestrous females are fertile. In most cases affected females are culled. However, management aspects of estrous detection must be thoroughly investigated before a presumptive diagnosis of behavioral anestrus is made. The possibility that anestrous females could be pregnant should be eliminated by pregnancy verification using rectal palpation, ultrasonography or serum estrone sulfate determination.

Behavioral anestrus (cyclic ovaries) can be differentiated from delayed puberty or prepubertal ovarian status (absence of corpora lutea) by analysis of plasma or serum for progesterone. It is recommended that two or more blood samples be collected at an interval of 7 to 14 days. Serum progesterone concentration above 2 ng/ml in any one of the samples indicates the presence of corpora lutea on the ovaries.

Treatment of Delayed Puberty. Under practical conditions induction of estrus in gilts does not occur in response to transportation, mixing, restriction of feed or water, increased energy intake and boar exposure once delayed puberty has been established or these stimuli (particularly boar exposure) have previously been applied. Affected gilts may remain prepubertal until 10 to 14 months of age. Owing to the potentially heritable nature of delayed puberty, affected gilts should be culled from the breeding herd.

Prepubertal gilts will respond to hormonal induction of estrus and ovulation with an intramuscular injection of 400 to 600 IU of pregnant mare serum gonadotropin (PMSG). The addition of 200 to 300 IU of a luteinizing hormone such as hCG usually results in estrus and ovulation in 3 to 5 days.

ANESTRUS

Lactating sows and gilts are usually anestrous and have ovaries that are small and lack corpora lutea. Sows are expected to be in estrus 3 to 6 days following the removal of their pigs. However, many factors influence the ability of the weaned sow to reinitiate ovarian cyclicity following weaning.

Parity. On the average, 85 to 90 per cent of multiparous sows are in estrus within 7 days of weaning. However, only 65 to 70 per cent of gilts weaned from their first litter are in estrus the first week after weaning. These parity differences may be because of age, body conditioning, selection or nutritional requirements.

Season. Sows weaned from their pigs during June, July, August and September have a higher incidence of anestrus following weaning than sows weaned at other times of the year. This phenomenon is most pronounced in the first litter gilt. These anestrous females may remain anestrous for as long as 120 days. The cause of this problem is not known. Affected females have ovaries that lack corpora lutea. Therefore, hormone analysis of blood samples usually indicates that serum progesterone concentrations are below 1.5 ng/ml of blood. The influence of season on postweaning estrous activity is evident in sows outside or those in total confinement.

Temperature and Light. Low ambient temperatures do not interfere with postweaning estrous activity of the sow. As ambient temperatures rise above approximately 30°C, ovarian and estrous activities are suppressed. During summer months, evaporative cooling methods may help minimize the severity of postweaning anestrus and infertility. However, under farm conditions various evaporative cooling methods have had minimal value in overcoming seasonal infertility. The role of light in reproductive function of the pig is poorly understood. Limited research suggests that maintaining females in total darkness or in constant light is detrimental. Based on the influence of season on fertility of female swine, it is expected that exposure to more than 12 hours of light per day would have a suppressive effect on estrous activity and fertility.

Group Size. Under most housing conditions, the incidence of anestrus is related to group size. Sows housed in individual crates after weaning have a higher incidence of postweaning estrus than do sows weaned in groups. As group size increases, there is increased bullying, more frequent feet, leg and mammary gland injuries and less control over the nutritional intake of each female within the group. Additionally, as group size increases, the efficiency of boars and farm personnel to identify estrous females decreases. If sows are placed in individual crates or tethers following weaning, it is recommended that the sow be checked for estrus in the direct presence of the boar.

Nutrition. The most common nutritional cause of anestrus appears to be inadequate intake of energy. Body condition of sows during lactation should be closely monitored to minimize weight loss, especially in first litter gilts. Inadequate energy intake during the lactation period is usually complicated by the use of high-fiber diets and reduced feed consumption. Following the first week of lactation, highly productive sows may need to be fed ad libitum. During periods of high environmental temperatures, appetite may be depressed. Therefore, it may be necessary to use low-fiber, high-energy diets, such as the addition of 5 to 8 per cent fat, to maintain adequate energy intake. During very cold weather, it may be necessary to increase feed intake of the females, so they can meet the added energy requirement for maintenance.

It is usually difficult to maintain uniform feed intake by sows housed in groups. The use of feeding stalls may help maintain adequate feed intake by each individual and, therefore, avoid the "thin sow syndrome."

Another management technique that may promote the onset of normal postweaning estrus is to wean two to three of the largest pigs from the thin sows 2 to 3 days prior to weaning the entire litter during the lactation period. This practice may also hasten the onset of postweaning estrus in first litter gilts.

Sows normally reduce feed intake during the immediate postweaning period. However, it is recommended that feed intake not be restricted following weaning, so that stress, fighting among sows and inadequate energy intake are minimized.

Withholding feed and/or water following weaning does not hasten the onset of postweaning estrus.

The ingestion of zearolonone-contaminated feeds may result in an increased incidence of anestrus. Vulvar enlargement and edema may not be present in each female ingesting zearolonone-contaminated feed. Indirectly, other mycotoxins may contribute to infertility problems because of decreased feed consumption. The impact of mycotoxin contaminated feeds on sow herd productivity has not been adequately assessed.

Hormones. Administration of estrogenic compounds or ingestion of zearolonone-contaminated feed by cycling, nonpregnant females may result in persistence of the corpora lutea. Therefore, these females will appear to be anestrous. Estrogenic compounds may contribute to the pseudopregnancy syndrome occasionally observed in bred females. Limited research has suggested that the uteri of affected females are large and edematous, with prominent endometrial folds. On occasion, uteri may also contain clear mucus. These females may not be identified until the expected time of farrowing.

Oral ingestion of progestational compounds, such as allyl trenbolone, or the systemic administration of progesterone will also suppress estrous activity in female swine. Following removal of the progestin, estrous and ovarian activity resume. These compounds are being investigated at the present time as a practical means of controlling the onset of estrus and ovulation in sows and gilts.

Lameness. Lamenesses in sows, gilts and boars frequently result in an increased incidence of anestrus. Commonly observed lamenesses include osteochondrosis, white line disease, pododermatitis and sole bruising or abscessation. These lameness conditions are exaggerated by confinement, rough or wet floor surfaces, narrow gestation crates and sharp edges on concrete slats. There may also be a genetic component to osteochondrosis. Many lameness conditions cause pain and increased stress to the animal. Chronic pain and stressful conditions have a suppressive effect on ovarian function. Additionally, lame sows and gilts are reluctant to rise and move about a pen during estrous detection activities by the boar and personnel. These estrous periods may easily be unobserved. Likewise, lame boars are less physically active and usually have a reduced ability to identify estrous females.

Management Factors. Numerous management factors that contribute to anestrous problems have already been presented. Producers should become very familiar with the signs of proestrus in the female so that their attention and that of the boar can be directed toward these females during the next few days. Signs of proestrus include restlessness, swelling and redness of the vulva, mounting other females, standing near the boar pen, standing while other females are lying down when not disturbed and vocalization. Frequently, untrained personnel are used to conduct heat detection and breeding activities during weekends. Bred females should be tested for estrus 17 to 30 days following breeding. Females failing to return to estrus are tested for pregnancy at 25 to 30 days following service. Due to the high incidence of delayed returns to estrus and early embryonic death in females mated during summer months, estrous detection activities should continue until females are 50 days pregnant and have been retested for pregnancy.

Swine breeding facilities should be designed to allow fenceline or direct contact of young gilts with the boar, beginning when gilts are 160 to 180 days of age. It is probably not necessary for boars to be in direct contact with weaned sows to stimulate onset of postweaning estrus. Gestation crates and pens should be designed to allow the herder to move boars and sows between pens with minimal effort. Sows and boars should always be handled and moved in a calm manner so that their anxieties toward the handler and each other are minimized.

Estrous detection activities of the boar should be complemented by the herder who should "hand pressure test" each female over her loin area. The herder can also direct the boar's interests toward females who have been previously identified as being in proestrus and test-positive to hand pressure, have been weaned 3 to 6 days earlier or have been bred 17 to 24 days previously. It is crucial that estrous detection efforts be conducted in a thorough and systematic fashion on a daily basis.

The herder should also be aware that efficiency of boars to detect estrus in females varies considerably between boars. In general, crossbred boars have greater libido than do purebred boars. Most sexually aggressive boars adapt quickly to the routine of heat detection.

The problem of postweaning and postservice anestrus is usually not detected in herds utilizing pasture or group mating systems. Therefore, anestrus may erroneously appear to be a problem of low conception rates.

Silent Estrus. Silent estrus may be defined as anestrus though in the presence of cyclic ovarian activity. Numerous management and boar and female factors contribute to silent or missed estrous periods. Many of these factors have been presented above. However, there appears to be a behavioral anestrous condition in some females with regular, cyclic ovarian activity and ovulation. This condition appears to be most common in the Yorkshire breed. These silent estrous females have a very low conception rate when constantly housed in groups with boars, presumably due to their unwillingness to stand for mating. The behavioral anestrus is repeated each estrous cycle. If affected females are ovariectomized, they remain nonresponsive to exogenously administered estrogens. The cause of the condition is unknown. These females are fertile if bred by artificial insemination. Because of the possible genetic basis of persistent, behavioral anestrus, affected females should be culled following thorough review of the estrous detection practices in the herd.

Diagnosis of Anestrous Conditions. The possibility that anestrus may be a result of pregnancy should be determined. The most reliable methods for determining pregnancy are ultrasonography, palpation per rectum and serum estrone sulfate determination.

Breeding herd records should be analyzed to determine the incidence of anestrus, age and breed of females affected and seasonal effects.

Estrous detection practices within the herd should

be thoroughly reviewed. Boars used for heat detection should be identified and their degree of sexual aggressiveness should be evaluated.

Serum or plasma from a representative number of anestrous females can be collected and analyzed for progesterone concentration. Two samples collected at 7- to 15-day intervals are preferable to a single sample. If both samples have progesterone concentrations below 1.5 ng/ml, the female probably has inactive ovaries. During diestrus, serum progesterone levels range from 10 to 50 ng/ml.

Evaluation of reproductive organs from a representative number of anestrous females may give meaningful data concerning ovarian, uterine and oviduct pathology.

Treatment and Prevention of Anestrous Conditions. The cause of anestrus must be determined if treatment or prevention efforts are to be successful. The ovarian status of affected females needs to be determined. Many aspects of the treatment and prevention of anestrous conditions have already been outlined. If managerial factors that contribute to anestrus have been corrected, the veterinarian must be concerned with the heritable or genetic nature of the condition within each herd. If it can be determined that heredity is a significant contributor to postweaning anestrus and delayed puberty, efforts should be directed toward culling affected females and selection of replacement females.

LOW CONCEPTION/FARROWING RATE

Pigs are usually considered highly fertile animals. However, numerous studies in the United States indicate that the farrowing rate of sows and gilts is 70 to 78 per cent. Because of the predominance of group mating systems, the actual fertility level within a herd is rarely appreciated. Numerous noninfectious causes of low fertility have been documented.

Age and Parity. The conception and farrowing rate for gilts is approximately 15 to 20 per cent lower than for multiparous sows. The farrowing rate of sows weaned from their first litter is 5 per cent lower than for older sows. It is also expected that the conception rate and litter size would be lower for gilts bred during pubertal estrus compared with subsequent estrous periods.

Season. Season of mating has a striking influence on the farrowing rate of sows and gilts. The farrowing rates for sows and gilts bred during the months of June through September (summer months) average more than 15 per cent lower than for matings during November through March. The decreased fertility during summer months varies considerably between herds and from year to year. This fluctuation may be related to age of females and housing and environmental changes. The influences of season appear to be manifested in confined and nonconfined herds and in herds that utilize evaporative cooling methods during summer months. The litter size of females successfully bred during summer months is similar to that of those bred during other

months of the year. The effects of season on conception and farrowing rates are seen in female swine of all ages and parities.

There is a marked increase in the incidence of delayed returns to estrus (25 or more days after breeding) in females bred during the months of June through September. This suggests that there is a high incidence of early embryonic death but that fertilization rates and boar fertility are minimally altered by seasonal factors. It is common for female swine bred during summer months to be diagnosed as pregnant 20 to 35 days after service but to return to heat in 1 to 8 weeks after pregnancy diagnosis, to abort 1 to 2 months later or to be determined "not in pig" when evaluated at 90 to 115 days of gestation. Aborted materials are rarely observed in females with a delayed return to estrus.

Confinement. There appears to be no detrimental effect of confinement on the fertility of sows and gilts compared with females mated in outside lots. However, as the incidence of lameness increases, fertility decreases.

Group Size. As the number of females per pen increases, the farrowing rate decreases. The effect may be related to the inability to control the nutrition of individual females, increased incidence of injuries and lameness and a greater opportunity for horizontal transmission of disease when females are housed in large groups. The maintenance of sows and gilts in individual crates for 30 days or more following mating resulted in a 10 to 15 per cent increase in the farrowing rate compared with bred females housed in groups during the first 30 days.

Temperature. Ambient temperatures over 30°C have been shown to reduce conception rate and embryonic survival. High ambient temperatures may be partially responsible for the reduced fertility of females mated during hot summer months. However, in one large study the seasonal infertility pattern was not altered in swine housed in confinement, in which temperatures were maintained below 27°C. The use of evaporative cooling methods may be of some benefit during summer in maintaining gilt and sow comfort, improving appetite in hot weather and maintaining boar libido. Systemic fever, such as that following pseudorabies, transmissible gastroenteritis (TGE) or influenza, also reduces conception rate.

Low ambient temperatures (below −25°C) have not been associated with infertility unless gilts are on a restricted plane of nutrition.

Light. The intensity and duration of light does not appear to influence the conception or farrowing rate or litter size of swine.

Breed. Numerous studies have indicated that there are breed differences in conception rate and litter size. Generally, the Landrace, Large White and Chester White breeds are considered more fertile than many of the other breeds. However, large-scale breed comparisons under controlled conditions have not been made. Additionally, it is likely that certain breeds may perform better than others, depending on housing and environmental conditions. Crossbred females are more fertile than pure-breds.

Frequency of Mating. Optimal fertility occurs when sows and gilts are mated 12 hours before ovulation. Ovulation usually occurs 36 to 40 hours after onset of estrus. Gilts are usually in estrus for 2 consecutive days, and sows are in estrus for 3 consecutive days. The conception rate of sows and gilts is 10 to 25 per cent higher for females mated twice using the same boar at an interval of 24 hours compared with females mated only once. The resulting litter size also improves by 0.2 to 0.5 pigs with double mating. When multiple matings are performed using different boars for each service, an additional 3 to 5 per cent improvement in conception rate may be expected. There appears to be little or no advantage to mating sows for 3 consecutive days compared with mating for 2 consecutive days unless boars of low fertility are being used.

Artificial Insemination. The fertility of sows and gilts bred by artificial insemination of fresh semen varies widely from herd to herd but is generally 10 to 15 per cent lower than with natural service. If artificial insemination procedures are less than optimal even lower conception rates occur. Generally, litter size is reduced by about one pig per litter using artificial insemination. The farrowing rate and litter size resulting from the use of frozen semen is about 30 per cent and three pigs lower, respectively, compared with fresh semen.

Diagnostic Efforts in Herds with Low Farrowing Rates. After reviewing the wide range of factors that contribute to reduced farrowing rates, it is obvious that diagnostic efforts need to be directed by the herd history and management system being used. History of the low fertility problem should disclose the onset of infertility, age of females affected, breeds involved, season of year and magnitude of reduced conception. Pregnancy rates at 20 to 35 days after mating should be compared with actual farrowing rates to determine the likelihood of delayed returns to estrus or abortion. Management factors such as group size, mixing of females during gestation and level of feed intake should be determined. The number of females that are double mated should be calculated, if possible. In herds using a group mating system, it may be necessary to determine if low farrowing or conception rates are from failure of females to cycle (anestrus), lack of boar libido or boar infertility. Many infectious causes of low fertility appear clinically similar to noninfectious infertility.

Prevention of Low Fertility. When estrous detection efforts are conducted in a systematic manner, more than 75 per cent of gilts and nearly all sows should be double mated during estrus at an interval of 24 hours. If the same boar is used to mate each female multiply, boars of low fertility can be identified and culled. If group mating is practiced, boars can be rotated in the pen of females at 4- to 12-hour intervals. This practice encourages multiple matings of females, helps prevent boar overuse and allows boars to rest without challenge by sows and gilts. Sows and gilts should be closely monitored for return to estrus 17 to 25 days after breeding. Because of the high incidence of delayed returns to heat during the months of June through October, females should be checked for estrus from 17 to 35 days after service. Females should be tested for pregnancy before 35 days after breeding. Again, during summer and early fall months, females diagnosed as pregnant prior to day 35 should be retested at 45 to 50 days after breeding.

To optimize conception rates, sows and gilts should be placed in individual crates or pens of less than five females per pen following mating. If bred females are to be housed in groups, groups should be established within 3 days of mating and preferably at estrus. Mixing of pregnant females should be avoided, particularly during the first 30 days of gestation. To aid in sow and gilt comfort, the use of evaporative cooling systems during hot weather may be beneficial.

Physical Examination of New Boars Introduced to The Herd

Charles D. Gibson, D.V.M., Ph.D.
Brad J. Thacker, D.V.M., M.S.
Michigan State University,
East Lansing, Michigan

Introducing new boars into the breeding herd is a focal point in disease control, reproductive performance and the future genetic make-up of the herd. Decisions made and actions taken by the herd manager and veterinarian will have a direct impact on the future performance of the breeding herd. The veterinarian and manager must take certain precautions to reduce the potential economic risks associated with introducing boars into the herd. Potential losses can be in the form of disease outbreaks, reduced reproductive performance and undesirable genetic traits.

HISTORY

The disease status, reproductive performance and genetic background of both the boar and the herd of origin are important historical data to consider in the selection of a boar. Many disease organisms can be transmitted by the boar to the breeding herd.[2] The disease status of the herd of origin should be evaluated by analyzing herd health records that include results of post-mortem examinations, slaughter checks and veterinary observations. Documentation of treatments, drugs used and immunization schedules is also useful information in evaluating the disease status of the herd of origin. It is unrealistic to expect seed stock producers to maintain disease-free herds, but health programs to define and to control disease problems correctly should be expected. The herd of origin should be free of diseases such as pseudorabies, brucellosis, tuberculosis and swine dysentery. Clinical experience indicates there is some value in selecting boars from herds having similar facilities and management practices to those of the recipient herd. The general reproductive history should include litter size, pigs weaned per sow and weaning weights from the ancestors of the boar in question as well as averages for the entire breeding herd. The genetic background of the boar should be consistent with his intended use. Breed, terminal versus maternal lines, crossbreeding programs and propagation of breeding stock are all considerations in the selection of the boar. Heritable defects such as scrotal hernias and poor underlines can be avoided by careful analysis of herd health records. Production records that accurately document average daily gain, feed efficiency and back fat thickness of the boar should also be considered when selecting a boar. Those animals having incomplete histories should be viewed as risks to the future disease status, reproductive performance and genetic composition of the recipient herd.

PHYSICAL EXAMINATION

A general physical examination and a thorough reproductive evaluation should be completed during the isolation period. Previous exposure to infectious disease should be evaluated by serologic tests. While blood testing is required for regulated diseases such as pseudorabies and brucellosis, additional blood testing may be desired for evidence of exposure to parvovirus, leptospirosis, *Haemophilus pleuropneumoniae*, transmissible gastroenteritis (TGE), mycoplasma infections and eperythrozoonosis. Intradermal skin tests for avian and bovine *Mycobacterium* species are indicated in areas where tuberculosis is a problem. Immunizations used in the sow herd for parvovirus, erysipelas and other diseases should be administered to the boar during the isolation period. Boars should be evaluated for evidence of both external (mange and lice) and internal parasites, especially if the purchase agreement states that they are not infected. The general physical examination should be carefully performed by a veterinarian. Evaluation of the body condition is important to identify individuals that are too fat or thin and may require special diagnostic or management attention. Conformation of body structure is important in locomotor function and requires special attention. Locomotor function has been shown to be a major reason for culling boars from artificial insemination programs in the United Kingdom.[4] The body conformation examination should include back and leg evaluation (Figs. 1 and 2). Osteomalacia, osteoarthrosis and arthritis resulting in lameness and reluctance to mount or bear weight on the rear legs are serious problems that affect sexual performance.

GENITAL EXAMINATION

The genital examination of the boar includes palpation of testicles, epididymis and scrotum for size, symmetry, consistency and pathologic changes.

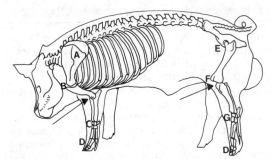

Figure 1. Desirable conformation. Level topline and rump, high tail setting and proper shoulder blade angle (A). Normal shock-absorbing effect of scapulohumerus joint (B). Pressure-absorbing joint (C). Pasterns are sloping and long (60°) to provide cushioning effect (D). The rear leg joints properly angled to provide cushioning effect (E, F, G). (Courtesy of Dr. Howard Miller, Mississippi State University and American Yorkshire Club.)

The penis and prepuce should be examined for abnormalities during the semen collection process.

The testicle is the target of diseases such as brucellosis and is susceptible to mechanical and induced trauma by handlers, other animals and improperly maintained facilities. They should not contain any nodules or soft masses indicative of injury. The initial reaction to trauma or infection of the testicle is swelling, while the long-term result of injury is reduction in size, increased firmness and loss of resiliency. Asymmetry, as a result of unilateral reduction in resiliency and size or swelling, should be considered potentially deleterious to fertility. The resulting semen evaluation may reveal azoospermia or reduced sperm numbers and morphologic changes indicative of testicular damage.

Boars are usually selected for introduction to the breeding herd at 6 to 8 months of age. These boars should be considered to be sexually immature. Spermatogenesis begins by 127 days of age and increases greatly between 5 and 8 months of age. Researchers have shown a great variation between individual boars in onset of puberty and sexual maturity. Boars should be well developed by 8½ months of age, which can be verified by testicle

weight, since both age and testicle weight have been shown to be valid indicators of sexual maturity.[1] Although testicle size is correlated with sperm output, the direct relationship of scrotal measurement to fertility is not known.

The second part of the general examination is observation of libido and mating ability. This is accomplished during semen collection using an estrous female as a mount. Libido may be influenced by psychological, genetic and physical factors. Young boars that lack experience or who have been dominated by older boars or sows may be timid and reluctant to serve. Differences in libido among breeds have also been demonstrated. Selection of a timid, nonaggressive individual over several generations can result in boars with poor libido. Pain and skeletal injury have a strong negative influence on libido. Mating ability is directly affected by penile injuries and anatomic and genetic defects such as persistent frenulum, incomplete erection and diversion of the penis into the diverticulum. These abnormalities are noted during mounting prior to intromission. Abnormal mating behavior, e.g., head mounting or failure to mount, can be detected during observation of the breeding process.

ISOLATION

New boars should be immediately isolated from all other pigs for a minimum of 21 days. They should be housed in a separate building at least 500 feet from the breeding herd and a separate supply of outer clothing and rubber boots should be maintained at this facility. Additionally, these animals should be observed and cared for after the breeding herd on a daily schedule, or preferably, one person should be assigned this duty to avoid inadvertent exposure of the breeding herd to possible infectious organisms. Antibiotics should not be given to the boar during this isolation period, since these drugs may mask or delay the onset of clinical signs of disease. Close attention should be given to clinical signs indicating swine dysentery, transmissible gastroenteritis, mange and pneumonia.

INTRODUCTION TO THE BREEDING HERD

The initial contact with the breeding herd should be limited to nonsexual exposure to facilitate natural immunization. A period of 30 to 45 days of fence contact and close proximity to the breeding herd, especially with gilts, is suggested before the boars are used for breeding. In addition, manure interchange between new boars and gilts is helpful in exposing animals to reproductive diseases caused by enterovirus and parvovirus prior to breeding. Hand-mating should be used for the first breeding experiences of the new male. This allows the handler to assist and to train the boar to mount and enter the female correctly. This is particularly crucial with boars with abnormal mating behavior or

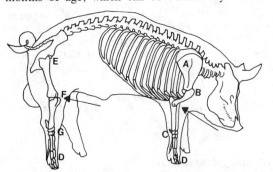

Figure 2. Undesirable conformation. Rump is too steep with tail setting low and back arched. The front limb is too straight with no cushioning effect of the joints (A, B, C, D). The hip, stifle and hock joints lock in a straight line (E, F, G). (Courtesy of Dr. Howard Miller, Mississippi State University and American Yorkshire Club.)

low libido. Overuse and injury are common problems of young boars being introduced into the breeding herd. During the initial 2- to 3-month adjustment period, boars should be handmated to fewer than six females during each 2-week period and a maximum of only once each day. Group or pen mating with several females may result in penile and scrotal injuries and lameness from competitive fighting. Limited exposure to the breeding herd allows the young boar to adjust to the breeding environment with minimal stress, and good breeding habits can be established with proper handling.

Boars should not be expected to reach maximum breeding capacity before 1 year of age.[3]

References

1. Esbenshade KL, Singleton WL, et al.: Effect of housing management on reproductive development and performance of young boars. J Anim Sci 48:246, 1979.
2. Leman AD, Cropper M, Rodeffer HE: Infectious swine reproductive diseases. Theriogenology 2:149, 1974.
3. Leman AD, Rodeffer HE: Boar management. Vet Rec 98:457, 1976.
4. Penny RHC: Locomotor dysfunction causing reproductive failure. In Morrow DA (ed): Current Therapy in Theriogenology. 1st ed. Philadelphia, WB Saunders Co, 1980, pp 1042–1045.

Semen Collection from the Boar

Rolf E. Larsen, D.V.M., Ph.D.
University of Florida,
Gainesville, Florida

Collection of semen from the boar can be accomplished by the use of any of three techniques: the gloved hand method, artificial vagina and electroejaculation. In the majority of cases the most appropriate method will be collection by gloved hand while the boar is mounted on a sow or phantom. The use of an artificial vagina has become somewhat obsolete and is a rather unwieldy technique compared with the gloved hand method. Electroejaculation has a limited but useful place in boar semen collection, typically being used only when circumstances make the use of the gloved hand method impossible.

ADVANTAGES AND DISADVANTAGES OF METHODS

Gloved Hand Method. The gloved hand method of semen collection consists of grasping the coiled portion of the boar's penis during mounting of an estrous female or phantom, so that ejaculation is stimulated. The semen is presumably indistinguishable from that which would be emitted during normal coitus. The use of a glove in this method is not in itself necessary for the collection of an ejaculate. It is, however, considered an important component of hygiene.

The advantages of this method are that very little special equipment is necessary, observation of the penis and seminal fluid throughout the ejaculatory process is possible and a complete ejaculate typical of natural mating can be obtained.

A disadvantage of this method is the necessity for a female in estrus or a restrained sow. If a phantom is used, a training period is usually required for the boar to learn a normal mounting response. In addition, the boar must have both the ability and the inclination to mount the presented sow or phantom under the conditions that prevail for the collection attempt.

Artificial Vagina. Use of the artificial vagina (AV) in other species spurred development of a similar apparatus for the boar. The typical artificial vagina for the boar consists of a hard tubular casing with a rubber liner that is filled with warm water. An air pressure bulb and hose leading through the liner into the water compartment allow the addition of air to increase pressure on the penis during intromission. A container may be attached to the AV, allowing collection of semen directly, without exposure to other environmental factors.

The advantages of this method over the gloved hand technique are few. There may be circumstances in which a boar that objects to direct handling would respond more favorably to the AV. An operator physically unable to perform the gloved hand method may be able to utilize the AV.

Disadvantages include the need for a specialized AV and the inability to observe the penis and its secretions during ejaculation. Use of an AV also shares many of the disadvantages of the gloved hand method.

Electroejaculation. Stimulation for this method is provided by electrical current controlled by one of the several electroejaculators commercially available for use with bulls. The current is applied to pelvic nerves by means of a rectal probe. This is usually done only under general anesthesia.

The circumstances under which use of electroejaculation is indicated are those that make collection by the gloved hand impossible or impractical. Boars unwilling or physically unable to mount a sow or phantom can produce semen adequate for either evaluation or artificial insemination. Boars may be brought to a clinic and, without the presence of a sow or phantom, be collected under circumstances that do not allow for the mount necessary for collection by other methods.

Disadvantages include the need for specialized equipment and provisions for general anesthesia. The probe used in the boar is not one that is standard equipment with commercially available electroejaculators. A long uterine or cervical forceps is usually needed to exteriorize the penis from the prepuce. Anesthesia brings with it the attendant risks of mortality and unpredictable adverse reactions. Since this technique does not involve all of the physical and behavioral reactions used during mating, there is no way to assess the full complement of abilities necessary for reproductive fitness (e.g., physical soundness, libido, ejaculatory reflexes). There is also the risk of poor response to stimulation. Failure to produce a satisfactory sperm-rich aliquot of semen is not absolutely diagnostic for inability to do so. While this is also true for the gloved hand method, it is considerably more difficult to assess and to correct a failure in technique with electroejaculation.

PREPARATION FOR COLLECTION

Regardless of technique used, a collection container capable of holding 300 to 500 cm³ of liquid must be prepared. One suitable readily obtainable container is the wide mouth pint or quart plastic thermos flask. Whatever container is used, it should be insulated and capable of withstanding sterilization procedures. The container should be warmed to 38°C before use. Filtration of gel may be accomplished by fixing two to four layers of gauze over the opening of the container to retain gel outside the collected fluid. Provisions to pour semen through gauze following collection should be made if the gel is not separated at the time of collection.

Gloved Hand Method. While the materials needed for collection by the gloved hand method are simple, it is helpful to consider certain details that will facilitate the procedure. The choice of a glove to be used usually will be limited to latex or vinyl seamless examination gloves. The surface of the vinyl is not as smooth as that of the latex and provides slightly more friction for maintaining a firm grip on the penile surface. Disposable plastic gloves or sleeves of the type used for palpation per rectum are not recommended for this procedure. Paper or cloth towels should be available to wipe the glove dry, in case gel, semen or preputial secretions lubricate the glove too thoroughly to hold the penis during muscular contractions.

When semen collection is performed on the farm, an estrous female should be identified and placed in a breeding pen for use as a mount. If an estrous female cannot be found, a sow held in a stationary position with a hog snare may provide a usable mount. The limitations of this procedure are self-evident, requiring an aggressive boar, a cooperative sow and knowledgeable assistants. Mount of a phantom provides the best conditions for sanitary and safe semen collection. Many boars, however, require training and acclimatization to these conditions.

The use of exogenous hormones to stimulate mounting behavior should be viewed as a potential aid to collection in selected cases, but one that may mask behavioral and physical problems. Prostaglandin $F_{2\alpha}$ can be given immediately prior to collection. A dose of 5 mg administered intramuscularly is usually effective if the animal is capable of responding. Human chorionic gonadotropin (hCG) is sometimes effective when given 24 hours prior to collection. A dose of 2000 IU may be administered either intravenously or intramuscularly.

Artificial Vagina. The short, hard rubber casing used as a boar AV is available from a variety of veterinary supply houses. Rubber liners used for this AV are usually of the smooth latex type, although the roughened rubber sometimes used in bovine AV liners may help in holding the glans penis in a fixed position. A rubber hose should connect the liner to an air bulb, which allows inflation and maintenance of the desired air pressure. A rubber cone attached to one end directs the semen into a collection container. Petrolatum is commonly used as a lubricant. Other preparations for AV collection are similar to those for the gloved hand method.

One variation of AV usage in the boar is a combination of the gloved hand method and an AV. This involves preparation of a short AV with a rubber cone but without the air pressure bulb. The glans penis is allowed to pass completely through the hard casing and into the rubber cone, where it is grasped, as in the gloved hand method.[3] This allows collection of semen through the cone and any connector directly into a container, reducing the possibility of contamination. The rubber cone can, however, be used independently of the hard casing, which is somewhat superfluous if the penis will be secured in the hand of the operator.

Electroejaculation. A variety of electroejaculation devices have successfully been used for collection of semen from the anesthetized boar. They include the Nicholson Transjector, the Standard Precision Electronic and the Lane Pulsator I and Pulsator II.[2] Most attempts at electroejaculation have utilized electroejaculators designed for the bull without modification. The probe required is quite different from the probes available for use in the bull or ram. The type commonly used is constructed of rubber hose 35 cm in length and 3.75 cm in diameter. Six annular electrodes are placed at 5-cm intervals along the length of the probe. A water-based lubricant should be used if lubrication is necessary for placement of the probe in the rectum. Because erection and protrusion of the penis may not occur with electroejaculation, the penis should be removed from the preputial cavity by manual traction. A long uterine or cervical forceps is necessary for atraumatic grasping of the penis. When the penis is exteriorized, gauze can be used to hold it.

General anesthesia is usually necessary for only a short period of time and a single intravenous dose of thiamylal sodium (1gm/115 to 140 kg) is effective, with some boars requiring an additional dose at one half the initial level. Halothane anesthesia alone or after induction with a barbiturate is also effective. The anesthetic agent must be chosen with consideration of the conditions under which the procedure will be performed and the support available in the event of adverse reactions.

TECHNIQUE OF SEMEN COLLECTION

Gloved Hand Method. An understanding of penile reactions during normal coitus in the pig is helpful for successful collection by either the gloved hand method or the artificial vagina. During natural mating the boar will seek the vulva by short thrusts of the penis, with only a small length of the shaft of the penis protruded from the sheath. When the vulva is penetrated, the shaft of the penis is then extended to full protrusion. Both during protrusion and after full extension, the penile muscles are continually contracting, causing a regular partial rotation of the penis in a right-handed direction. After each partial rotation, the penis returns to its original position by a left-handed rotation. The spiral or corkscrew end of the penis has a left-handed thread, so the penis is drawn into the folds of the cervix only during the release of muscular contraction and left-handed rotation. During contraction and right-handed rotation the penis is forced into the cervical folds against the natural corkscrew spiral of the penis by penile extension and thrusting. Release of the contraction then draws the penis into the cervix by rotation with the spiral. When the penis has penetrated the cervix to the extent that muscular contraction cannot rotate the glans penis against the cervical folds, the penis is "fixed," and ejaculation begins.

To collect semen following mount of the sow by the boar, the gloved hand is placed against the vulva so that searching thrusts of the penis strike the palm of the hand, and the penis is deflected toward the operator. As the boar protrudes the penis, the corkscrew end of the penis is grasped firmly with three fingers (Fig. 1). The grip on the penis must be strong enough to prevent rotation within the gloved hand. The shaft of the penis will twist as the boar attempts to force the penis deeper into the hand. If the penis is held fixed, and rotation within the hand is not permitted, the penis will be extended to its fully protruded length and ejaculation will be initiated.

The penis should be grasped only over the spiral. Contact with the shaft proximal to the spiral may cause loss of erection and dismounting. It is not necessary to fit the fingers of the gloved hand into grooves of the spiral. Pressure of the fingers against

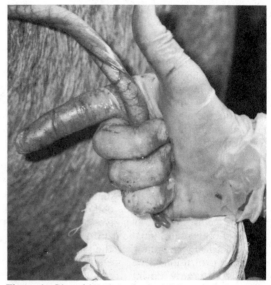

Figure 1. Gloved-hand method of fixing penis for ejaculation during the mount of a sow or phantom. Gel is being filtered through gauze at the opening of the collecting bottle.

the outer curve of the spiral ridges is satisfactory for ejaculation and facilitates holding the penis fixed against the strong contractions.

When ejaculation begins, the urethral opening may not be visible within the hand, and gel may be forced between the penis and glove. Even when this is the case, the grip should not be altered. There should be no detriment to the semen from ejaculation because of contact with the glove; attempting to adjust the grip often results in loss of fixation of the penis. The pattern of secretions should be observed for number and volume of sperm-rich fractions, gel fractions and presence of blood. Depending on potential use of the semen, either the complete ejaculate may be collected or only the sperm-rich fractions. For routine breeding soundness evaluations it is advisable to collect a complete ejaculate.

Ejaculation will usually last 3 to 6 minutes. The erection will be lost and the boar will dismount after secretions cease. Some boars, particularly those collected routinely on a phantom, may remain mounted with penis extended following cessation of ejaculation. In some cases boars will initiate what appears to be a new ejaculatory cycle, and the collection may continue for up to 15 or 20 minutes.

Artificial Vagina. The artificial vagina is filled with hot water, so the final temperature is 40°C. The liner is lubricated with petrolatum. Following mount of the sow or phantom, the AV is placed so that the penis can be deflected from the vulva into the AV. Contact with the lumen of the AV stimulates complete protrusion of the penis as the boar seeks the cervix with the penis. The AV is maintained over the coiled portion of the penis rather than allowing the penis to penetrate completely through. As the penis is extended, the air bulb is pumped to provide sufficient pressure to prevent rotation of the penis within the AV. Ejaculation is stimulated by fixation of the penis.

Electroejaculation. The boar is anesthetized to a light plane, with retention of a mild response to pain. Feces should be removed from the rectum, the anus lubricated and the probe inserted to a depth of 25 to 30 cm. All electrode rings should be within the rectum. Fluid within the preputial diverticulum should be expressed, and the hair around the preputial orifice should be clipped.

Exposure of the penis is often the most difficult aspect of boar electroejaculation. A forceps is passed in a closed position into the preputial cavity to the penis, is opened with slight rotation of the forceps and is closed over the end of the penis, and then the penis is withdrawn. Resistance to extraction may prevent atraumatic exposure of the penis. Mild electrical stimulation via the rectal probe may assist in protrusion. The prepuce may also be pushed posteriorly during traction, reducing the distance of forward movement of the penis necessary for exposure. Once exposed, the end of the penis is grasped with gauze, and the penis is extended. In some animals mild electrical stimulation with manual pressure sliding the prepuce posteriorly will exteriorize the penis adequately to grasp the penis with gauze and extend it without the aid of a forceps.

Electrical stimulations should begin with mild applications of 4 to 5 seconds of stimulation followed by 5 to 10 seconds of rest to allow adequate respiration. The stimulation is increased in a step-wise sequence. Clear fluid, often containing gel, will be emitted after three or four stimulation-rest cycles. As voltage and amplitude are increased, the sperm-rich fraction is ejaculated. Stimulation is continued until the ejaculated fluid begins to clear or no further emissions occur.

Failure of adequate response may be from excessive fecal material surrounding the probe, a prolonged period of stimulations that are too mild to produce the sperm-rich fraction or excessively strong stimulations applied too early in the stepwise sequence of increasing amplitude.

It has been demonstrated that the sperm-rich fraction collected by either electroejaculation or the gloved hand method is equivalent in total numbers of spermatozoa, sperm cell motility and percentage of morphologically normal sperm cells.[1] Regardless of the technique used, the same precautions for temperature maintenance, insulation and protection from cold shock are critical to the success of obtaining a semen sample, which on evaluation, is representative of the boar's potential.

References

1. Basurto-kuba VM, Evans LE: Comparison of sperm-rich fractions of boar semen collected by electroejaculation and the gloved-hand technique. J Am Vet Med Assoc 178:985, 1981.
2. Evans LE: Electroejaculation of the boar. In Morrow DA (ed) Current Therapy in Theriogenology. 1st ed. Philadelphia, WB Saunders Co, 1980, pp 1037–1040.
3. King GJ, MacPherson JW: A comparison of two methods for boar semen collection. J Anim Sci 36:563, 1973.

Evaluation of Boar Semen

Kjell Larsson, D.V.M., Ph.D.

Swedish University of Agricultural Sciences, Uppsala, Sweden

Semen evaluation is an important and critical part of the breeding soundness examination. In many cases boars with lowered fertility have semen abnormalities detectable by routine examination. Although normal semen is needed for normal fertility, not all boars with normal semen have normal fertility. Sperm cell numbers, motility and morphology reflect the function of the seminiferous epithelium and epididymal sperm maturation.

THE NORMAL BOAR EJACULATE

The normal boar ejaculate is voluminous, with a comparatively low sperm cell concentration and a high proportion of progressively motile spermatozoa. During puberty the total sperm numbers increase, and the proportion of abnormal spermatozoa decreases. In sexually mature boars the proportion of any sperm cell abnormality is usually less than 5 per cent, and blood, pus or foreign materials are not present. Table 1 summarizes the characteristics of a normal boar ejaculate.

Data given in Table 1 refer to boars regularly used for breeding or semen collection. Prolonged periods of sexual rest will increase total sperm numbers and, in some cases, decrease progressive motility due to increased numbers of spermatozoa with single-bent tails. Excessive use of the boars will lead to decreased numbers of spermatozoa but will otherwise not alter sperm morphology or motility.

METHODS OF SEMEN EVALUATION

All semen evaluations should have a clinical history, previous fertility status and a complete clinical

Table 1. Some Characteristics of a Normal Boar's Ejaculate

Ejaculate Characteristic	Normal Value	Suggested Limit Value
Ejaculate volume (ml)	100–500	50
Total sperm number ($\times 10^9$)	10–100	10
Progressive motility (%)	70–90	70
Abnormal sperm heads (%)	2–5	10
Proximal cytoplasmic droplets (%)	1–5	5
Acrosome abnormalities (%)	1–2	5
Abnormal midpieces (%)	2–5	5
Single-bent sperm tails (%)	1–5	25

(Compiled from Bane A, et al.: Proc Ann Meet Swedish Vet Assoc, Stockholm, 1977, pp 149–159; Einarsson S, Larsson K: Proc IPVS Congr, Mexico City, 1982, p 215; Gibson C: Comp Cont Ed Pract Vet 5:244, 1983.)

examination, including palpation of testicles and epididymides, as base line data. The procedure of evaluation includes measurement of ejaculate volume, ocular examination of the ejaculate for presence of blood, pus and other foreign materials as well as an estimate of sperm concentration (density) by judgment of semen color. Through microscopy, sperm motility and sperm morphology are evaluated. Accurate estimation of sperm concentration is done by hemocytometric counting or spectrophotometry. All materials and equipment used for semen collection and evaluation should be clean, dry and warm. Semen evaluation should take place as soon as possible after collection, preferably within 15 minutes and not later than 1 hour after semen collection.

Ocular Examination. Ocular examination of the ejaculate is the first step in the evaluation procedure. Ejaculate volume is preferably measured by a glass cylinder. The color of the ejaculate, after removal of the gel fraction, gives a crude estimate of sperm concentration. A gray-watery color indicates a sperm concentration in the range of 50 to 200×10^6 spermatozoa/ml, whereas a milky to creamy color indicates a concentration in the range of 500 to 1000×10^6/ml. Such variations are found among normal ejaculates. The sperm concentration is largely dependent on the volume of postsperm fraction, mainly originating from the seminal vesicles, that has been collected. Neither ejaculate volume nor sperm concentration alone are good quantitative indicators of fertility. The best quantitative measure is the total sperm content in the ejaculate, which is obtained by multiplying ejaculate volume and sperm concentration. A good estimate of sperm concentration is achieved by using hemocytometric counting. A dilution of 1:100 is recommended, and to interrupt sperm motility, water or

formol saline is preferred for dilution. Provided that a proper standard curve is available, spectrophotometry can also be used to estimate sperm concentration. In establishing the standard curve it is important to measure the light uptake by pure seminal plasma. Dilution of samples (sodium citrate or saline) in the range of 1:35 to 1:70 is preferable.

Presence of blood, pus or other foreign materials in the semen should be recorded. If hemospermia occurs, it is important to determine if it is because of trauma during collection or if the blood is actually ejaculated with the semen.

Microscopic Examination. A phase-contrast microscope is preferably used for evaluation of sperm cell motility and morphology in wet preparations, whereas sperm morphology in stained smears should be examined under a light microscope.

Gross motility with a distinct wave-pattern is dependent on the concentration of motile spermatozoa. Thus, in most whole boar ejaculates with a comparatively low sperm cell concentration, distinct wave motion is not apparent. Color of the ejaculate and presence of wave motion might, under field conditions, be used as a rough estimate of sperm concentration.

In the evaluation of sperm motility it is absolutely necessary that warm slides be used. The droplet of semen should be covered with a cover-slip, and motility is preferably estimated at 200 to 400× magnification. If sperm cell concentration is high (presence of wave-motion), dilution of samples in warm saline or sodium citrate will facilitate estimation of motility. Several fields should be judged from two or more droplets of semen. It is important to distinguish progressive motility from passively moving cells and spermatozoa with abnormal movements such as narrow circles. Since motility declines rapidly in the covered preparations, rapid estimates are necessary.

Sperm head morphology should be examined in stained smears. Under field conditions eosin-nigrosin staining can be used; Figure 1 shows spermatozoa stained with this technique. Using this stain, a droplet of semen is added to a drop of stain on a warm slide, mixed and spread to form a thin smear. The smear is allowed to dry immediately, and sperm morphology is evaluated at 1000× magnification using a light microscope. Spermatozoa might be stained or unstained, but a classification of live and dead spermatozoa, as with bull semen, cannot be based on sperm staining. Morphologic characteristics of at least 200 spermatozoa should be recorded.

To obtain more accurate evaluations of sperm morphology, thin smears of raw semen should be prepared on warm slides immediately after collection for subsequent staining with Williams's stain (carbol-fuchsin). This will provide good possibilities for evaluation of shape, size and contour of the spermatozoa. Acrosome morphology, cytoplasmic droplets, midpiece and tail morphology are preferably examined in wet preparations under the phase-contrast microscope at 1000× magnification. An aliquot of semen is fixed in buffered formol saline

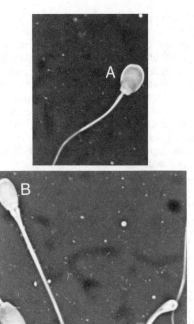

Figure 1. Abnormal boar spermatozoa in eosin-nigrosin stained smears at 1000× magnification in the light microscope. *A,* Short and broad sperm head. *B,* Double midpiece. *C,* Single bent sperm tail with a distal cytoplasmic droplet.

solution.[8] Samples can be stored in a refrigerator for at least 1 month after fixation. Figure 2 is an example of abnormal spermatozoa treated in this way. It is also possible to make smears from the fixed semen for further evaluations. A good estimate of sperm morphology is achieved by evaluation of 500 spermatozoa in smears and 200 spermatozoa in wet preparations.

When thin stained smears are prepared, a proper technique should be used to avoid artifacts caused by damage of spermatozoa. In smears, larger cells

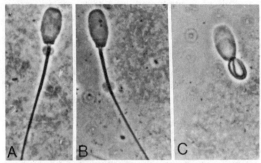

Figure 2. Abnormal boar spermatozoa in formol-saline fixed wet preparations at 1000× magnification in the phase-contrast microscope. *A,* Proximal cytoplasmic droplet. *B,* Distal cytoplasmic droplet. *C,* Coiled sperm tail and missing acrosome.

such as epithelial cells or leukocytes are usually removed. Special smears in which walls of seminal fluid are allowed to dry are preferably prepared for identification of these cells after staining with hematoxylin-eosin.

A spermiogram for boar semen should include sperm head abnormalities (Fig. 1*A*), preferably subclassified into various abnormal forms, presence and position of cytoplasmic droplets (Fig. 2*A, B*), loose or detached sperm heads, acrosome abnormalities (Fig. 2*C*), midpiece abnormalities (Fig. 1*B*) and tail abnormalities. Also, the tail abnormalities should be subdivided into single-bent (Fig. 1*C*) and coiled (Fig. 2*C*) tails and tails coiled around the sperm head.

INTERPRETATION OF RESULTS

Semen examination results should be evaluated against the clinical background. Low-volume ejaculates with no or very few spermatozoa in a watery fluid are often caused by incomplete ejaculation, and in such cases a new collection should be attempted. Total sperm numbers below 10×10^9 are indicative of reduced spermatogenesis, e.g., cases of testicular degeneration or marked overuse of the boar. Also, in pubertal boars sperm numbers are low, and in cases of bilateral total testicular hypoplasia there are no spermatozoa in the ejaculate.

Hemospermia might be caused by trauma of the penis at collection or fistulas from the cavernous tissue, penile lacerations and bleeding from urethral vessels, urethral polyps or the accessory sex glands. Recovery may be possible if bleeding is from trauma of the penis, but otherwise correctional possibilities are limited.

Purulent material in the ejaculate originates from inflammatory processes in the testicles, epididymides, accessory sex glands or the urethra. Efforts should be made, through clinical examination, to localize the site of inflammation, and boars suspected of infection should not be used for breeding.

There is a definite need for more research concerning the relationships between sperm morphology and fertility in boars. The limit values suggested in Table 1 should be considered as guidelines, in the lack of more definite data. In boars with normal fertility the proportion of abnormal spermatozoa is usually below the limits given.

In pubertal boars there is a gradual increase in total sperm numbers together with decreased proportions of abnormal spermatozoa. Proximal cytoplasmic droplets and abnormal sperm heads in proportions above 10 per cent might be used as indicative of delayed puberty in young boars. In such cases a reevaluation within 3 to 4 weeks is preferable before a definite diagnosis is made.

In testicular degeneration experimentally induced by heat stress or local scrotal insulation, there is a rise in all forms of abnormal sperm together with lowered motility and decreased total numbers of spermatozoa in the ejaculate. If regeneration occurs, this will be expressed in normalized morphology, motility and total sperm numbers. In the experimental situation semen alterations occur within 4 weeks. In boars that have suffered from a systemic disease a semen evaluation 4 weeks later has a definite diagnostic value. If abnormalities are found, a reevaluation after another 4 weeks is advisable to detect any possible improvement.

Increased numbers of spermatozoa with distal cytoplasmic droplets have not been related to lowered fertility. Single-bent sperm tails are one of the abnormalities most frequently found. They are caused by epididymal dysfunction,[4,5] and boars with a higher incidence of this abnormality seem to have lowered fertility when used for artificial insemination with liquid semen stored more than 30 hours.[9] However, the definite influence of this defect on fertility in boars used for natural mating remains to be proved.

Acrosome defects—"knobbed spermatozoa"—in a high frequency have been reported in sterile boars.[2] When the abnormality occurred in 35 per cent of the spermatozoa, fertility was severely reduced.[1] Abaxial attachment of the neck-piece to the sperm head does not seem to influence fertility in boars.

References

1. Andersen K: Morphological abnormalities in the acrosome and nucleus of boar spermatozoa. Nord Vet Med 26:215, 1974.
2. Bane A: Acrosomal abnormality associated with sterility in boar. Proc IVth Int Congr Anim Reprod, The Hague, vol IV, p 810, 1961.
3. Bane A, Einarsson S, Larsson K: Fluctuations in sperm morphology and fertility in boars. Proc Ann Meet Swedish Vet Assoc, Stockholm, 1977, pp 149–159.
4. Bonte P, Vandeplassche M, Lagasse A: Functional epididymal disorders in boars. Zuchthyg 13:161, 1978.
5. Einarsson S, Gustafsson B: A case of epididymal dysfunction in a boar. Andrologie 5:273, 1973.
6. Einarsson S, Larsson K: Exposure of boars to elevated ambient temperature: Morphological studies of the ejaculated semen. Proc IPVS Congr, Mexico City, 1982, p 215.
7. Gibson C: Clinical evaluation of the boar for breeding soundness: Physical examination and semen morphology. Comp Cont Ed Pract Vet 5:244, 1983.
8. Hancock JL: The morphology of boar spermatozoa. JR Microscopy Soc 76:84, 1957.
9. Larsson K, Darenius K, Johansson K: Sperm morphology and in vitro viability in diluted semen in relation to fertility of AI boars. Nord Vet Med 32:533, 1980.

Factors Affecting Spermatogenesis and Boar Fertility

Bo G. Crabo, D.V.M., Ph.D.
University of Minnesota, St. Paul, Minnesota

FERTILITY

Documentation of Fertility. Age of puberty, conception rate and litter size are very important components of fertility and strongly influence the economy of pork production. Good records are needed to monitor the fertility level on the farm, but often the recording system is not designed to evaluate the fertility of individual boars.

Influence of the Sow. The normal fertility level on farms can be expected to differ because of the genetic composition of the sow herd and mating system as well as seasonal variations and abnormal conditions. Crossbred sows have a higher conception rate (usually from 80 to over 90 per cent) and farrow larger litters than purebred sows. Higher conception rates are achieved in the first crossing of two purebred breeds than in purebred matings.

Comparisons between some breeds kept in the same facilities have revealed that Landrace sows have significantly higher farrowing rates than Hampshire, Yorkshire and Duroc breeds, in which the farrowing rates are 60 to 70 per cent.[2] Litter size is related to farrowing rate and age of puberty among breeds.

Influence of the Boar. The breed of boar has minimal effect on conception rate and litter size as long as boars with normal semen are used. In this case normal semen denotes not only morphologically but also biochemically normal spermatozoa free from chromosomal defects, since the fertility of boars with morphologically normal semen can vary considerably.[2]

Pubertal boars should be expected to have lower fertility than mature boars. Age of puberty varies considerably and is poorly related to libido. Aged boars often exhibit testicular degeneration to some degree, and their fertility may decrease somewhat. Females mated two or more times during estrus have approximately a 15 per cent higher conception rate.[2] Mating with more than one boar may result in a slightly higher conception rate if boars with normal semen characteristics are used, but a considerably higher rate may result when the boars on the farm have questionable or unknown semen quality.

SEMEN PRODUCTION AND DEVELOPMENT OF THE TESTES

Prepubertal Development. During fetal life primordial germ cells (gonocytes) migrate into the seminiferous tubules of the testicle. Immediately preceding puberty the indifferent cells of the seminiferous tubules mature into Sertoli cells. Differentiation of the gonocytes into dividing spermatogonia signals the onset of puberty. During the first 3 weeks of life the testes undergo a rapid growth phase caused by proliferation of the seminiferous tubules as well as Leydig cells. Endocrine regulation of this development is not fully understood, but it is believed that follicle stimulating hormone (FSH), which peaks at birth in boars but not in gilts, and growth hormone (GH) promotes Sertoli cell proliferation and development and, thus, lays the foundation for sperm production. Testosterone production at the onset of puberty may trigger spermatogonial division directly or via indirect chemical messengers produced by the Sertoli cells. The significance of two testosterone peaks, one during fetal life, which is independent of fetal brain activity, and one neonatal peak, is not understood. LH also peaks during the first week of life. The endocrine pattern of prepubertal pigs is different in several respects from that of other domestic species.[4]

Puberty. Puberty is sometimes defined based on mating behavior or a certain minimal number of spermatozoa in the ejaculate. Based on endocrine data and testicular morphology, puberty can be defined more exactly as the period beginning when spermatogonial divisions are initiated by high testosterone production and ending when sufficient spermatozoa are produced to ensure good fertility. The testes grow considerably during this time because of an approximately threefold increase in diameter of the preformed tubule, caused by lumen formation and spermatogenesis. These events normally start at 80 to 150 days of age, and an ejaculate of 10×10^9 spermatozoa may be produced as early at 5½ to 6 months of age. Large testicular size at a given age during puberty may thus reflect early puberty rather than large mature testicular size. There may be a relation between early puberty and good reproductive performance in mature swine of both sexes.

Semen produced at early stages of puberty is characterized by a high incidence of abnormal spermatozoa, particularly abnormal head shapes and proximal cytoplasmic droplets.

Spermatogenesis. In the boar spermatogenesis is extremely regular and more efficient than in other domestic species. All of the resting spermatogonia in a given cross section of a seminferous tubule of the mature testis divide synchronously every 8.6 days (cycle of the seminiferous epithelium). This initiates spermatogenesis. A number of spermatogonial divisions end in primary spermatocytes undergoing meiosis. These divide into secondary spermatocytes, which last only a few hours before spermatids are formed. The spermatids undergo a metamorphosis into spermatozoa, known as spermiogenesis. The whole of spermatogenesis takes 34.4 days to complete in the boar, and epididymal transit lasts an average of 10 days. Thus, any insult to the testis causing a disturbance of spermatogenesis will take a minimum of 2 weeks to be observed as abnormal sperm in the ejaculate, if the later stages of spermatogenesis are affected, and as long as 44 days when spermatogonial divisions are affected.

Mature boars produce about 24 million spermatozoa per gram of testis per day. Sperm production is thus related to testicular size. There is a positive correlation between daily sperm production and fertility.

Very few abnormal spermatozoa (< 5 per cent) are produced by the testes of a normal adult boar. In older boars foci of testicular degeneration are frequently observed and cause a slightly higher incidence of abnormal spermatozoa in the ejaculate.

Post-testicular Sperm Maturation. Transit from the seminiferous tubule through the rete testis, efferent ductules and the epididymal duct takes 9 to 12 days. During transit the cytoplasmic droplets move from the proximal position at the neck of the spermatozoa to the distal position of the midpiece when the sperm reach a specific region of caput epididymis. It is a membrane related event. Failure of the droplet to move is believed to be of testicular rather than epididymal origin. Spermatozoa further acquire the ability for motility and fertility during passage through the epididymis. The epididymis secretes specific proteins, some of which become part of the sperm membrane. The ionic environment in the epididymis changes along the duct. In the cauda the electrolyte composition of the hypertonic fluid optimizes the stability of the protein conformation. Spermatozoa can be stored in the cauda epididymis for long periods with retained motility and fertilizing ability.

Post-testicular sperm maturation continues in the female tract with capacitation that involves removal of proteins from the sperm membrane. Capacitation can be induced in vitro by diluents used for artificial insemination, and the ionic composition of these influence the extent of protein alteration. It is possible that the incidence of acrosome damage (swollen and lifted acrosomes) as well as sperm elimination by phagocytosis in the female tract is minimized by an intact protein coat.[1]

Ejaculate. The gel-free ejaculate consists of less than 2 per cent cauda epididymal content and approximately 25 per cent seminal vesicle fluid, which supplies most of the proteins and fructose, with the remainder consisting of prostatic secretions high in electrolytes. The osmotic pressure of the ejaculate is lower than that of the epididymis, leading to hydration of the spermatozoa, which in conjunction with a vastly changed ionic environment initiates sperm motility. The distal cytoplasmic droplet is normally lost during ejaculation, but distal droplets per se are not abnormal. Seminal vesicle proteins cause the shedding of the droplet if the spermatozoa are exposed to them before they mix with prostatic fluid. A high incidence of distal droplets is observed at low-serving frequency of the boar under conditions when the spermatozoa are not exposed to seminal vesicle fluid during ejaculation and in conjunction with an increased incidence of proximal droplets.

Normal ejaculates contain 30 to 50 × 10⁹ spermatozoa. At periods of low-serving frequency the number can exceed 100 × 10⁹ and during intensive serving the number can quickly drop to less than 5 × 10⁹ spermatozoa. The seminal volume may vary from 70 to over 500 ml. The sperm concentration is inversely related to the volume. Sperm motility usually exceeds 60 per cent and is often 90 per cent. The sperm-rich fraction of boar semen sometimes exhibits relatively poor motility because of incomplete stimulation by the accessory secretions.

Relation between Fertility and Normal Semen. Morphologically normal sperm do not ensure normal fertility. Chromosomal defects in the form of translocations result in decreased litter size.[3] So-called lethal genes and other genetic deficiencies may possibly result in a similar lowering of fertility.

EFFECT OF ENVIRONMENT AND DISEASE

Light. The effect of light on age of puberty and semen production has recently been studied. Very little or no effect has been observed as a result of supplemental light with the boar.

Environmental Temperature. The temperature regulatory mechanisms of the testis efficiently maintain testicular temperature below body temperature. However, an increased incidence of abnormal spermatozoa has been observed following periods of extremely hot weather. It is possible that the boar may contribute to lowered fertility observed in the seasonal infertility (summer) syndrome. More commonly, boars kept outdoors in the midwestern states of the United States have shown signs of testicular degeneration after exposure to extreme winter temperature. Frost bite may sometimes be seen on the scrotum, but more often there is no physical evidence of injury.

Temperature stress or other conditions leading to elevated corticosteroid levels have not been shown to affect testosterone levels or sperm production in the boar, which is contrary to that of the bull.

Toxic Agents. After ingestion, *heavy metals* accumulate in the testes almost to the same extent as in the liver and kidney. Cadmium, which sometimes is concentrated in sewage sludge, causes classical changes in the testicular vascular bed, with extensive hemorrhages. *Nitrofuran,* sometimes used as an antibacterial feed additive, adversely affects sperm production. A rodenticide, *alpha-chlorohydrin,* is licensed in many countries to control rat populations via male reproduction. Boars become temporarily sterile by ingesting as little as 1 mg/kg body weight, which is one fifth of the effective dose in rats. Semen parameters are unaffected but sperm motility can be lowered at higher doses of the substance. The mycotoxin *zearalenone* has estrogenic actions. However, sows are likely to exhibit anestrus because of retained corpora lutea before semen quality is affected in the boars.

Infections. General infections of bacterial (erysipelas) or viral origin (swine influenza, pseudorabies) causing fever for several days often result in testicular degeneration. Orchitis may be caused by a variety of agents and may have its origin from a general infection such as tuberculosis or brucellosis, or it could be from an ascending genital tract infection. Unilateral orchitis may cause testicular degeneration in the unaffected testis because of local heat. Pseudorabies and porcine parvovirus do not directly alter sperm production, but these viruses have been isolated from semen.

FOREIGN CELLULAR CONTENTS IN SEMEN

Blood, Pus and Microbial Contamination. Leukocyte admixture originates from local infections in the urogenital system and is likely to affect fertility. There is risk for transfer of pathogens to the sow as well. Bacteria of various kinds normally occur in semen and originate in the urethra.[5] Pathogens are uncommon, but blood sometimes occurs in semen. Its origin is usually minor lacerations of the penile surface. Fertility is unaffected by hemospermia, at least by the presence of moderate amounts of blood in the semen. The explanation of this and the fact that venereal transmission of disease via semen is uncommon in swine[5] may lie in a peculiar property of the boar seminal proteins. Boar semen contains basic proteins called hemagglutinins. These coat and agglutinate many foreign proteins and may thus eliminate their harmful effect.

HORMONE TREATMENTS

Attempts to improve sperm production or semen quality with hormonal treatments are generally not advisable and may, in fact, worsen the condition.

In breeding stock hormonal treatments may conceal the genetic ability for reproduction and lead to the selection of inferior replacement animals. *Pregnant mare serum gonadotropin* could, theoretically, increase Sertoli cell numbers and hasten the onset of puberty if given in sufficient quantity at the right time during the prepubertal period. *Human chorionic gonadotropin* may support Leydig cell production of testosterone during or after puberty, but the production of endogenous luteinizing hormone (LH) will be severely decreased by the negative feedback exerted by the excess testosterone produced. Likewise, injections of *testosterone* must lead to blood concentrations many times higher than normal, impairing sperm production because of shutoff of LH release. Testosterone is usually ineffective in improving libido. Injection of *prostaglandin $F_{2\alpha}$* has occasionally proved successful in increasing libido. It is effective within minutes. Its action may be from an increased tonus in the epididymal vas deferens rather than the observed subsequent release of LH followed by a rise in plasma testosterone. Effective release of LH is achieved only by pulsatile administration of *gonadotropic-releasing hormone,* which is difficult to accomplish economically. Spermatogenesis and semen quality in the boar are usually not affected by administration of *estrogens* or *corticosteroids.*

References

1. Crabo BG and Hunter AG. Sperm maturation and epididymal physiology. In Sciarra JJ, Markland C, Speidel JJ (eds): Control of Male Fertility. New York, Harper and Row, 1975, pp 2–23.

2. Crabo BG, Loseth KJ, Henry SC, Kosco MS: Evaluating fertility and evaluating semen. Proc Am Assoc Swine Pract, Cincinnati, 1983, pp 87–97.
3. Gustafsson I, Settergren I, King WA: Occurrence of two different reciprocal translocations in the same litter of domestic pigs. Hereditas 99:257, 1983.
4. Kosco MS, Crabo BG, Bolt DJ, Loseth KJ: Effect of hemicastration on seminiferous tubule development, FSH and GH in prepubertal boars. J Anim Sci 61(Suppl 1):113, 1985.
5. Thacker BJ, Larsen RE, Joo HS, Leman AD: Swine diseases transmissible with artificial insemination. JAVMA 185:511, 1984.

Mating Systems and Boar Management

John P. Hurtgen, D.V.M., Ph.D.
New Freedom, Pennsylvania

Many swine infertility problems are associated with poor boar management. Oftentimes, the particular system of mating used on a farm will predispose the herd or a group of females to a specific etiologic cause of infertility or will frequently mask the etiology. Therefore, it is important that veterinarians and producers understand the mating system and methods of boar management being used.

SEXUAL DEVELOPMENT AND MATING BEHAVIOR

Coordinated sexual behavior and first ejaculation usually occur at 5 to 8 months of age. Age is more important than body weight in determining the onset of puberty. Normal precopulatory behavior between the male and female usually begins as nasonasal or nasogenital manifestations. This behavior may include grunting, grinding of the teeth, excessive salivation, rhythmic urinations, nuzzling of the female's flank area and sniffing of the perineum or head. Mock fighting and biting attempts may also occur.

The estrous female will usually seek out the boar and assume a characteristic immobile stance with arched back and erect ears. Even when the boar cannot be seen, courting grunts and sexual odor are sufficient to attract the estrous female. Therefore, estrous sows and gilts are frequently observed standing along the fence line or gate nearest the boar pen. Boars, however, seem to detect the estrous female more readily by her behavioral activity (immobile stance) than by auditory, olfactory or visual stimuli.

Erection and protrusion of the penis occur after mounting. However, some boars will mount and dismount several times before copulating. After mounting, the boar thrusts until the tip of the penis penetrates the vulva. Following several intravaginal thrusts, the spiral end of the penis becomes fixed in the cervix and ejaculation begins. Muscular, wave-like movements over the perineum and rhythmic contractions of the anal sphincter occur during copulation. The average duration of ejaculation is 3 to 6 minutes.

Fertility gradually increases until boars reach about 12 months of age. Total sperm output and seminal fluid volume increase until the boar reaches 18 months of age, at which time the ejaculate consists of at least 20×10^9 spermatozoa in 150 to 500 ml of semen. The duration of the spermatogenic cycle in the boar is approximately 34 days plus an additional 10 days required for passage of spermatozoa through the epididymis.

BOAR SELECTION

The medical history from the herd of origin is important in selecting new boars. Breeding stock should be purchased from herds free of swine dysentery and transmissible gastroenteritis (TGE) within the past 6 months. The herd should also be free of brucellosis, salmonellosis, pseudorabies and hemophilus pneumonia; individual animals should have negative results on serologic testing for leptospirosis. Swine dysentery, salmonellosis and TGE may be transmitted by recovered carrier animals. The breeder's herd should be observed for signs of lice and mange, lameness, atrophic rhinitis, porcine stress syndrome, campylobacter and chronic pneumonia. Herds with these disease problems should be avoided when purchasing breeding stock. Each group of boars should be purchased from one source in order to reduce disease and fighting among boars. Boars from litters affected by unfavorable genetic traits or traits that increase the degree of inbreeding should not be incorporated into a breeding program. Inbreeding decreases average litter size. Unfavorable genetic traits carried by boars include atresia ani, inguinal and umbilical hernia, myoclonia congenita, reduced libido and delayed puberty.

Conception rate and litter size are influenced by the breed of the dam. Therefore, prolific breeds must be represented in the sow line of a crossbreeding program. Furthermore, individual boars within breeds directly influence conception rate, litter size and piglet viability to weaning. With an increase in conception rate there appears to be a concurrent increase in litter size.

The number of boars required to achieve optimal fertility depends upon the age of the boars, breeding pen size, weaning practices and mating system. Ideally, young boars (< 12 months of age) should not be used more than once daily (maximum of five services per week). Because mating each female two or more times per estrus will improve conception rate and litter size, double mating is recommended. Sows come into a rather synchronous estrus 3 to 6 days after pigs are weaned. Therefore, if sows are weaned from their litters in large groups, the number of boars must be increased.

PRECONDITIONING BOARS

Boars should be purchased at least 6 weeks prior to service to allow a 2-week quarantine and a 4-week preconditioning period. Clinical observations indicate that boars should be at least 8 months old before routine usage. Upon arrival, new boars should be treated for external parasites. They should be observed for signs of swine dysentery, salmonellosis, porcine stress syndrome, and TGE during quarantine. Other diseases carried by the boar are unlikely to be manifested during this time. Boars should be vaccinated with any vaccines and bacterins judged to be necessary for the herd. Treatment for internal parasites and a second treatment for external parasites should also be conducted during quarantine.

Approximately 1 month prior to breeding an immunization program of controlled exposure to viral agents capable of causing reproductive failure should be initiated to establish common immunity among the breeding animals. Porcine enteroviruses and porcine parvovirus are of special concern. Because the epizootiology of these agents is not completely understood, methods by which this common immunity is established are empirical. Clinical evidence suggests that "fence line" contact is insufficient for exposing all breeding animals; therefore, direct contamination may be accomplished by mixing boar fecal material with the feed of nonpregnant females and vice versa or by rotation of animals among pens. Recent experience indicates that new boars should be seropositive for parvovirus for at least 3 weeks prior to mating. If breeding age gilts are vaccinated for erysipelas, porcine parvovirus or leptospirosis, new boars should also be vaccinated. Pregnant sows and gilts should not be exposed to new boars. It is during this preconditioning period that each boar should be evaluated for breeding soundness or should be test-mated to a limited number of females in order to assess potential boar fertility. These females should be closely observed for return to estrus. Serviced females should be checked for pregnancy using an ultrasonic device.

In general, boars are fed 4 to 6 pounds of a balanced ration as outlined in the National Research Council's *Nutrient Requirements of Swine.* Feedstuffs or additives that will uniquely enhance the fertility, libido or longevity of boars have not been identified. Limited research suggests that slightly elevated levels of calcium (0.8 to 1.0 per cent) and phosphorus (0.7 to 0.8 per cent) may reduce the incidence of lameness and the leg weakness syndrome in young growing boars. As with the female, boars should be fed according to body condition and environmental conditions.

Boars housed in pens in confinement should be allotted 80 square feet of space. If boars are housed in individual gestation crates, the crates should be 24 inches wide. Boars should also receive daily exercise. Individually housed boars have a reduced incidence of injuries to the penis. Maintenance of boars in narrow gestation crates may result in traumatic leg injuries, callus formation in the shoulder regions and signs of boredom. Fewer penile injuries also occur in hand-mated boars compared with boars used in pen or pasture mating systems. Because semen production and sperm quality are adversely affected by high environmental or systemic temperatures, attempts should be made to keep boars as comfortable as possible during summer months, and boars with systemic disease or fever should be promptly attended to.

MATING SYSTEMS

Double mating is the servicing of an individual female twice, 12 to 24 hours apart, during the same estrus. This practice significantly increases conception rate and litter size. These benefits are probably a result of breeding nearer the time of ovulation. Maximum conception rates are obtained when females are bred approximately 12 hours prior to ovulation. Heterospermic matings may result in improved fertility. Double mating using different boars masks the effect of a low fertility or a sterile boar and makes the evaluation of the quality of progeny nearly impossible.

Pasture breeding, pen mating, hand mating and artificial insemination are breeding systems in use today. As the result of confinement and intensified production, pasture breeding is being replaced by other practices. The commonly used pen-mating system is a modification of pasture breeding. With these systems a single boar or group of boars is placed in a pasture or pen with females for 23 to 45 (or more) days. It is hoped that estrous animals will be multiple mated, possibly with two or more boars. Various modifications of these practices include the rotation of boars between breeding pens at 8- to 24-hour intervals or removal of boars from breeding pens to assure sexual rest. Disadvantages to these systems are the inability of the manager adequately to identify serviced females, control the number of services per boar, observe mating behavior and libido, identify the sire of offspring and control fighting among strange boars. Some estrous females may fail to be serviced by the boars if pens or groups are large. The effect of social dominance by a boar on fertility and libido of subordinate males has not been investigated. However, observations in beef bulls indicate that one or two bulls may account for all pregnancies in a group of females.

In hand mating, estrous females are selected by the herder, frequently with the aid of a teaser boar, and taken to a breeding pen to be serviced. This practice allows close observation of mating behavior, accurate recording of breeding dates and controlled double mating, insures mating of all identified estrous females and allows control of services per boar per day. This system requires thorough, systematic heat detection and more labor by managers.

Artificial insemination utilizing both frozen and fresh semen is becoming more widely accepted for many reasons: increasing the use of superior, high fertility sires, preventing the introduction of disease from outside sources and spread within a herd, decreasing the number of boars, allowing the pooling of semen from two to four boars to maximize heterospermic mating at each insemination and facilitating the breeding soundness evaluation (including semen evaluation) of each boar at frequent intervals. Boar longevity is greatly enhanced because traumatic foot, leg and penile injuries are less

frequent. Additionally, older boars may be used to service gilts or small females without risk. Demands on time and labor for heat detection, semen collection and insemination are increased, although synchronization of estrus, utilizing group weaning of sows and hormonal therapy, greatly enhances an artificial insemination program. However, artificial insemination is accompanied by a series of factors critical to maintaining high fertility. Quality control must be practiced in the handling, storage and extension of semen. Osmotic pressure, pH and bacterial contamination of the seminal extender should be monitored periodically. Insemination technique must be closely observed. Extended semen should be placed in the uterine body, and a 50 ml minimal volume should be used. It is recommended that sows and gilts be inseminated two to three times during standing estrus, using at least 2 to 5×10^9 spermatozoa per insemination. It is expected that only boars of high fertility be used in an artificial insemination program.

Suggested Readings

1. Signoret JP: Swine behavior in reproduction. In Lucas L, Wagner W (eds): Effect of Disease and Stress on Reproductive Efficiency in Swine. University of Nebraska Cooperative Extension Service, 1970, p 28.
2. Swierstra EE: Duration of spermatogenesis in the boar. J Anim Sci 26:952, 1967.
3. Swierstra EE: Effect of environmental temperature on semen composition and conception rates. In Lucas L, Wagner W (eds): Effect of Disease and Stress on Reproductive Efficiency in Swine. University of Nebraska Cooperative Extension Service, 1970, p 8.

Genetic Influence and Crossbreeding Programs

Charles J. Christians
University of Minnesota, St. Paul, Minnesota

Barbara E. Straw
North Carolina State University, Raleigh, North Carolina

The heritability of a trait is the portion of the average superiority of the selected parents that is passed on to their offspring. Traits such as carcass merit and structural soundness are highly heritable

and respond to individual selection. Production traits associated with growth and feed utilization are moderately heritable and can be improved by individual selection. Since progress is slower for these traits, individual performance records are essential. Reproductive traits such as litter size and birth and weaning weights have relatively low heritabilities and respond very little to individual selection.

In most herds one sire is used for 20 to 25 females; more selection pressure is possible in selection of the sire than of the female. Traits that are highly heritable should be stressed in the sire by individual selection, whereas low heritable traits related to reproduction should be stressed in the gilt by family selection. Fertility, sex drive and mating ability must be evaluated in the boar, and these respond well to individual selection. These selection tools are the primary means available to the seedstock producer.

Commercial producers should use crossbreeding. One can combine desirable characteristics of different breeds and capitalize on heterosis. Heterosis is greatest for traits with low heritabilities.

When a boar of a different breed is mated to

Table 1. Relative Reproductive Performance of Female Breeds*

| | Breed | | | | | | |
Trait	Berkshire	Chester White	Duroc	Hampshire	Landrace	Spotted	Yorkshire
Age at puberty	—	—	94	96	100	99	95
Litter size born alive	87	99	89	84	94	86	100
Litter size weaned	83	95	86	84	89	84	100
Pigs at birth	82	81	94	94	100	92	82
Pig weaning weight	87	87	95	96	100	95	94
21-day litter weight	74	89	84	86	96	84	100
21-day litter weight/female exposed	84	100	78	94	89	91	94

*Composite results from Iowa, Oklahoma, Nebraska, North Carolina and Canada crossbreeding projects. Best breed performance is given a score of 100 and compared with each breed.

Table 2. Relative Reproductive Performance of Crossbred Females*

Breed	Litter Size Born Alive	Litter Size Weaned	21-Day Litter Weight	21-day Litter Weight/Female Exposed
Landrace-Yorkshire	100	100	100	100
Chester-Yorkshire	97	87	86	—
Duroc-Yorkshire	93	85	82	85
Hampshire-Yorkshire	91	87	87	81
Spotted-Yorkshire	91	85	83	93
Berkshire-Yorkshire	90	85	83	93
Hampshire-Landrace	100	95	95	88
Duroc-Landrace	92	93	86	79
Berkshire-Landrace	92	90	87	91
Spotted-Landrace	86	85	85	90
Chester-Landrace	93	83	80	—
Hampshire-Chester	92	81	77	—
Duroc-Chester	83	79	86	—
Hampshire-Chester	86	82	79	76
Berkshire-Duroc	93	82	79	77
Berkshire-Hampshire	81	77	76	74

*Composite results of Iowa, Oklahoma, North Carolina and Canada crossbreeding projects. Best breed performance is given a score of 100 and compared with each breed.

Table 3. Sire Breed Influence on Reproductive Performance*

| | Breed | | | | | |
Trait	Chester White	Duroc	Hampshire	Landrace	Spotted	Yorkshire
Litter size born alive	97	96	98	100	99	100
Litter size weaned	92	96	92	—	—	100
Birth weight	97	100	97	95	98	94
21-day litter weight	84	90	90	—	—	100
21-day litter weight/female exposed	89	91	81	—	—	100
Age at puberty	—	94	98	98	100	95

*Composite results from Iowa, Oklahoma, Nebraska and North Carolina crossbreeding NC-103 project. Best breed performance given a score of 100 and compared with each breed.

Table 4. Average Daily Gain and Feed Efficiency for Boars Tested (to 230 lb) at Central Test Stations*

Breed	Average Daily Gain	Feed Efficiency
Berkshire	96	94
Chester White	92	96
Duroc	100	100
Hampshire	98	98
Landrace	93	90
Poland China	95	95
Spotted	98	96
Yorkshire	98	99

*Summary of 20 Central United States Test Stations. Best breed performance is given a score of 100 and compared with each breed. (From Christians CJ, Johnson RK: Pork Industry Handbook, Extension Folder 361. St. Paul, University of Minnesota, 1979.)

Table 5. Carcass Traits (Adjusted to 230 lb) by Breed for Pigs Tested at Central Test Stations*

Breed	Carcass Length	Back Fat Thickness	Loin-Eye Area
Berkshire	96	87	91
Chester White	95	88	91
Duroc	97	88	88
Hampshire	98	100	98
Landrace	99	78	89
Poland China	94	95	100
Spotted	97	86	95
Yorkshire	100	87	90

*Composite results from National Barrow Show and Minnesota Central Evaluation Station. Best breed performance is given a score of 100 and compared with each breed. (From Christians CJ, Johnson RK: Pork Industry Handbook, Extension Folder 361. St. Paul, University of Minnesota, 1979.)

purebred dams, litter size is not significantly increased. Since the maternal breed in the original cross will influence litter size, breeds that are noted for large litters should be used as foundation females.

Even if litter size at farrowing is not increased, purebred sows will wean about 10 per cent more crossbred than purebred pigs. A greater survival rate results from heterosis responses in the crossbred pigs. A 24 per cent increase in weaning litter size can be expected when a crossbred sow is used. This improvement is a result of an increased number of pigs born alive and greater baby pig survival to 21 days.

Pig survival and growth are the real benefits of a systematic crossbreeding program. When crossbred females are used, about 28 per cent higher 21-day litter weights can be realized per female exposed as compared with purebreds.

Crossbred pigs reach market weight at an earlier age and have a slight improvement in feed efficiency as compared with purebred pigs. Even though traits of intermediate and high heritabilities are not greatly influenced by crossbreeding, overall efficiency can be improved by selecting superior parents. Real breed differences in male and female reproductive efficiency exist; therefore, choice of

breeds appears to be critical in a crossbreeding program.

BREED EVALUATION

Accurately comparing swine breeds for all economically important traits is difficult. Although some crossbreeding experiments are being conducted to evaluate specific breed crosses, all breed combinations have not been adequately compared. Genetic breed composition and frequency of desirable gene combinations do change; therefore, evaluating breeds must be a continuous and endless process.

A comparison of published crossbreeding experiments indicates that Yorkshire females excel in birth and weaning litter size and 21-day litter weight. The Landrace female ranks high in her pigs' birth and weaning weight and 21-day litter weight. The Chester White female excels in 21-day litter weight per female exposed, which is a measure of overall reproductive efficiency (Table 1).

Crossbred sows of Yorkshire and Landrace breeding rank high in reproductive traits evaluated, and the combination of these two breeds is superior to most breed combinations. These results reflect

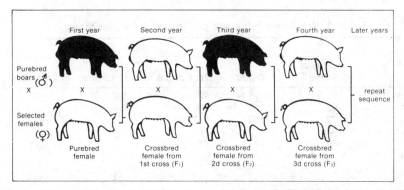

Figure 1. Two-breed rotational cross system. (From Christians CJ, Johnson RK: Pork Industry Handbook. Extension Folder 361, St. Paul, University of Minnesota, 1979.)

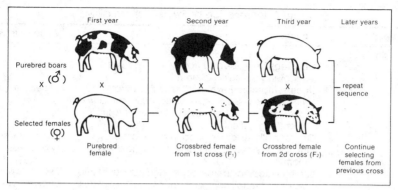

Figure 2. Three-breed rotational cross system. (From Christians CJ, Johnson RK: Pork Industry Handbook. Extension Folder 361, St. Paul, University of Minnesota, 1979.)

the importance of the selection of one of the white breeds in the initial cross and their influence in total reproductive performance. The Hampshire-Landrace combination ranks high in pigs born alive (Table 2).

Because of the increased possibility of disease contamination, most producers should retain their own crossbred females. The influence of sire breed on reproduction, therefore, must be evaluated. Of the breeds evaluated, the Yorkshire sire ranks high, as does the Yorkshire dam, for birth and weaning litter size and 21-day litter weight. In contrast to the female breed evaluation, Yorkshire sires excel Chester White sires for 21-day litter weight per female exposed. Progeny of spotted and Landrace sires reach puberty at a younger age (Table 3).

The Berkshire, as a sire breed, ranks high in 21-day litter weight per female exposed when mated to Yorkshire or Landrace females. The Hampshire sire mated to the Landrace female excels in 21-day litter weight. Duroc sires positively influence pig birth weight and litter size weaned. This advantage in weight is continued throughout the growth phase (Table 4).

CROSSBREEDING SYSTEMS

Crossbreeding provides an opportunity to reap the benefits of many genetic sources. An unplanned crossing program will not be successful. A crossbreeding system must be selected that will capitalize on heterosis, take advantage of breed strengths for carcass traits, and fit the total management program. Colored breeds tend to produce superior carcass merit (Table 5).

Two basic systems may be considered, namely, the rotational cross and the terminal cross. The rotational cross system combines two or more breeds in which a different breed boar is mated to the replacement crossbred females that are produced in the next generation. The two-breed rotational cross (Fig. 1) is a simple program in which two breeds are selected to complement each other. To capitalize on heterosis and other breed strengths, additional breeds can be added. The three-breed

cross is probably the most common (Fig. 2). Using four or more breeds, the percentage of heterosis could be increased; however, management becomes very complicated.

The terminal cross system is well adapted to feeder pig production. A two-breed single or rotational cross female mated to a boar of a third breed producing the terminal market pig fits many of the feeder pig production requirements of reproductive efficiency in the crossbred female and fast growing, efficient pigs that produce superior carcass composition and quality.

The sire breed could be either a purebred or crossbred boar but should be of different breed composition than the crossbred female. Since no replacement gilts are retained from the terminal cross, the sire breed becomes less important; but the individual boar's performance becomes a key criterion of selection. Aggressiveness and breeding ability are important. Testis size and age at puberty will respond to selection and improve breeding efficiency. Since only one breed of boar or terminal sire line is used, females of different ages and groups can be mixed in the breeding groups.

Although limited research information is available on the use of crossbred boars, indications are that crossbred boars are more aggressive breeders, have greater testicular size, reach sexual maturity at a younger age, have less leg soundness problems and improve overall breeding efficiency. A crossbred boar could combine those traits that may not be available in one straightbred breed.

Precaution must be taken in either a terminal or rotational crossing program so that the breed composition of the crossbred boar is different from the crossbred female. If a breed is repeated, an immediate reduction in heterosis will occur and will defeat the purpose of crossbreeding.

ABNORMALITIES AND RESISTANCE TO DISEASE

Plant pathologists have identified and extensively utilized genetic variation in the host species to develop varieties that can tolerate disease. Veterinarians and livestock raisers, on the other hand,

Table 6. Inheritance of Swine Abnormalities

Abnormality/Disease	Comments	Mode of Inheritance
Physical Abnormalities		
Bent legs	Front legs bent, fixed at front knee—causes farrowing difficulty; stillborn	Recessive
Clubfoot	Three symptoms: lower front legs thickened, hooves deformed; eczema on belly, spreads over body; giant alveoli cells in lungs result in breathing difficulty	Recessive
Cryptorchidism	One or both testes retained in body cavity	Recessive, sex-linked
Hairless	Inherited thyroid abnormality; hair follicles not normal	Two recessive
Hernia	Scrotal (intestines come down inguinal canal into scrotum); umbilical ("belly busts"; wall weakness allows intestines to protrude)	Two recessive Undetermined
Hydrocephalus	Brain enlarged and much fluid accumulates in skull cavity (lethal)	Simple recessive
Intersex	Both sex organs present; enlarged clitoris; European Large White and Landrace affected	Recessive, sex-linked
Inverted nipples	Nipples turn into belly wall instead of protruding; nonfunctional	Undetermined
Legless	Pigs born alive without legs and soon die	Simple recessive
Muscle contracture	Lethal condition; front legs born stiff	Simple recessive
Syndactyly (mule foot)	One toe instead of two	Dominant
Thickened front legs	Front legs greatly swollen where connective tissue replaced muscle (lethal)	Simple recessive
Noninfectious Diseases		
Gastric ulcers	Durocs have higher prevalence than Yorkshires; Heritability estimate of 0.50	Undetermined
Goosestep	Pigs lift leg with jerk that often goes as high as the back	One or more recessive
Hemophilia	Pigs normal at birth but bleed to death from induced wounds; full expression of trait occurs at 3 or 4 months of age	Recessive
Leg weakness syndrome	Visual skeletal abnormalities and locomotor patterns lowly heritable in Landrace and Large White pigs; German Landrace heritability estimates 0.50 to 0.60	Undetermined
Melanotic tumors	Moles or skin tumors highly pigmented and containing hair	Recessive
Osteochondrosis	Heritability estimates of 0.14 to 0.30; litter and breed differences in incidence and severity of lesions	Undetermined
Paralysis	Hind legs have muscular tremors, or are paralyzed (lethal)	Recessive
Porcine stress syndrome	Stress, tail and muscle tremors, death; very high prevalence in Pietrain and also in Landrace and Poland China	Recessive
Shaker	25 per cent incidence; a second type found in Landrace, in which only males are blind and shake	Two-pair recessive, sex-linked recessive
Inherited Resistance to Infectious Diseases		
Anthrax	Aerosol or intraperitoneal inoculation of *Bacillus anthracis* failed to induce infection in miniature swine	Undetermined
Atrophic rhinitis	Heritability estimates between 0.10 and 0.60; crossbreds reported to have larger turbinate spaces and be less affected than purebreds; Durocs less affected than Yorkshires; two studies recorded more severe turbinate atrophy in Swedish Landrace than in Yorkshire pigs; Hampshire and Yorkshire pigs had more turbinate atrophy than Landrace pigs	Undetermined
Brucellosis	Certain crossbred Poland China pigs have resisted experimental infection with *Brucella suis* given orally or subcutaneously	Possibly recessive monofactorial, with a penetrance of about 77 per cent

Table continued on opposite page

Table 6. Inheritance of Swine Abnormalities *Continued*

Abnormality/Disease	Comments	Mode of Inheritance
Colibacillosis	K88 positive, enteropathogenic *Escherichia coli* able to establish in the gut and cause disease in "adhesive" pigs	Two alleles at one locus inherited in a simple Mendelian manner; adhesive allele is dominant over the nonadhesive allele
Pneumonia	Two studies recorded higher levels of pneumonia in Yorkshire than in Swedish Landrace; heritability estimated as 0.14; Yorkshire and Hampshire pigs had higher levels of pneumonia than Chester White, Berkshire, Spotted and Poland China pigs	Undetermined
Strongyloides ransomi	Durocs had a low threshold of response to *S. ransomi* exposure and quickly overcame deleterious effects of infestation; Hampshires had a higher threshold and slow rate of compensation; F_1 crossbreds had an intermediate response	Undetermined

have traditionally concentrated all their efforts on eradication of the pathogen or reduction of its levels, and have made little use of genetic differences among animals in ability to live with the organism that cannot be eradicated. Various levels of resistance to infectious disease have been reported between different breeds of pigs or between certain individuals (Table 6). These determinations of variation in breed susceptibility to diseases have required infection with the organisms. Therefore, unless genetic markers can be found that reflect the ability of the pig to resist a disease, selective breeding is not likely to be used in swine as a means of disease control.

In addition to resistance to specific diseases, a general improvement in ability to survive has been seen in the offspring of certain boars. Preweaning mortality rates in the offspring of some boars were found to be twice that of other boars. Genetic influences on postweaning mortality rates have also been recorded. Certain crossbreds have been found to have lower mortality rates than other crossbreds raised in the same facilities. Differential mortality rates were recorded in purebreds. In a 6-year study of purebred pigs raised at two locations, the mortality rate in Yorkshire pigs consistently exceeded the mortality rate in Durocs.

There are reports of heritable chromosome defects in swine. While most chromosome abnormalities are associated with reduced fertility or sterility, their incidence in swine and their impact on productivity is not known.

Castration, Inguinal Hernia Repair and Vasectomy in Boars

H. Neil Becker, D.V.M., M.S.
University of Florida, Gainesville, Florida

PREWEANING CASTRATION

Surgical castration of male pigs will undoubtedly continue to be a procedure that pork producers and veterinarians are required to do. Even though chemical castration is now possible, it will be some time before surgical castration of pigs is abandoned. Surgical castration is most easily done during the time of baby pig processing when iron injections are given, tails are docked, needle teeth are clipped and ears are notched for identification purposes. This is usually between 1 and 4 days of age.

The author prefers the knife blade method, which employs a Bard-Parker No. 3 handle and No. 12 blade. The pig is held by the rear legs, and the first finger is used to push the testicles caudally. After the scrotal skin is tensed, the tip of the hooked blade is pushed through the scrotum with the blade being directed toward the tail. A separate incision is made over and into each testicle. If the incisions are made long enough and deep enough, both testicles will readily be exposed. Each testicle is then grasped separately and pulled upward until the testis and cord are snapped free.

Occasionally, only one testicle will be found because of its failure to descend. It is usually best to identify these pigs in some manner so they may be examined at 6 to 8 weeks of age for descent of the other testicle.

Inguinal hernias are difficult to detect in pigs this young but very few problems of postcastration herniation occur. Tissue swelling, fibrin deposition and blood clotting occur quickly after surgery and almost always prevent intestines from coming through the incisions. In herniated pigs the usual occurrence after castration is for the intestines to fill the inguinal canal and scrotum. This will become visible as a swollen scrotum any time after castration but is usually seen during the first 2 weeks after surgery.

POSTWEANING CASTRATION

Pigs between the ages of 2 and 16 weeks and weighing 5 to 50 kg may be castrated by incisions into the scrotum; however, the incision should be at the most ventral aspect of the scrotum. The pig is restrained by being held by the back legs, with the pig's abdomen toward the operator. The back of the pig is cradled between and squeezed by the legs of the holder. Two incisions are made over and into the testicles that have been forced ventrally by the operator. The testicles will readily drop through the incisions. The testicles are then grasped individually and pulled from the incisions. It is best, but not necessary, to remove the tunic with the testicle. If the spermatic cord does not separate easily, it may be cut or scraped with the knife blade with little resultant bleeding. The incisions should be liberal (6 to 8 cm) to allow for adequate drainage and prevention of seroma formation.

ADULT CASTRATION

Young and adult large boars (50 to 300 kg) may occasionally need to be castrated. Numerous methods of physical and chemical restraint have been described. One common method of chemical restraint is to use 1.0 mg/kg xylazine hydrochloride (Rompun) and 4.0 mg/kg ketamine hydrochloride (Ketaset) admixed and administered intravenously as a preanesthetic. A cannula or butterfly catheter is inserted into a marginal ear vein. Anesthesia is maintained by using 0.5 per cent thiamylal sodium (Bio-Tal) intravenously via the catheter to effect. In all but the largest boars, ½ to 1 gm of thiamylal usually provides adequate time for the surgical castration.

Two incisions are made over each testicle, extending from the dorsal to the ventral aspect of the scrotum about 3 to 4 cm from the lateral margins of the scrotum. The first testicle is removed by dissecting the scrotal skin from the testicular tunic. When the testicle, enclosed within the tunic, has been completely removed from the scrotum, emasculators are applied around the tunic and cord. The spermatic cord is crushed and then severed by the emasculator. The scrotal skin is then incised at the top and bottom in order to join the incision over the second testicle. The second testicle, enclosed in the tunic, is then dissected free and removed as was the first. The remaining scrotal skin is then removed and all loose tissue, including the median raphe, is carefully removed. This procedure leaves a large circular open wound that will drain freely. Anti-

biotic powder is usually applied to the wound and an injectable antibiotic is given intramuscularly for 3 days. Healing is usually complete in 2 to 4 weeks. These boars should be housed individually.

UNILATERAL CASTRATION

Occasionally, an individual testicle may be traumatically injured. The usual result is a large, swollen peritesticular hematoma or seroma. The veterinarian should be certain that the unilateral scrotal enlargement is not an acquired hernia. Anesthesia is induced and the afflicted testicle is removed as previously described. In cases of peritesticular hematoma or seroma, prompt surgery is advised to prevent the contralateral testicle from being damaged by pressure or infectious sequelae.

INGUINAL HERNIA REPAIR

If herniation occurs immediately after castration, replace the prolapsed intestines and suture the external inguinal ring with absorbable suture material and then suture the skin.

Inguinal hernias that are not detected until 1 to 2 weeks after castration may be difficult to repair because of numerous, firm adhesions between the intestines and scrotal tunic. These hernias should be carefully palpated in order to determine if the hernia may be reduced. If adhesions are extensive and the hernia is not reducible, it is best not to attempt surgery. If reducible, the hernia may be repaired as described as follows.

When an inguinal hernia is detected before castration, it is much easier to repair. In the author's experience the majority (> 95 per cent) of inguinal hernias occur in the left inguinal canal. They are also highly heritable.

After anesthesia is induced, the pig is suspended by the rear legs and a 3- to 6-cm incision is made over the external inguinal ring. The tunic is isolated by blunt dissection and freed from surrounding tissues. The intact tunic surrounding the testicle is removed from the scrotum and repeatedly twisted, forcing the intestines back into the abdomen. The twisted tunic is clamped close to the incision, and the stump is ligated with catgut or 6 mm umbilical tape. The tunic and cord are then cut and the external inguinal ring is sutured with absorbable suture material. The wound is sprayed with a mild disinfectant or antibiotic powder. One or two sutures may be placed in the skin.

VASECTOMY

Vasectomized boars may be used advantageously to promote the onset of estrus in young confined gilts or to detect standing heat in gilts or sows, particularly when artificial insemination or very valuable boars are being used for breeding.

Anesthesia is induced, and the boar is placed in dorsoventral recumbency and restrained with leg ties. The surgical area is prepared and is located 2 to 4 cm laterally on either side of the penis and 5 to 10 cm anterior to the base of the scrotum. The initial incision should extend 4 to 6 cm and is made down to the spermatic cord. The cord is freed by blunt dissection and is elevated from the incision. A 1-cm incision is made through the tunic, with care taken not to incise the veins or artery. The vas deferens is a small, firm, white, round band located adjacent to the spermatic artery. A 3- to 4-cm

section of vas deferens is immobilized with clamps or hemostats. The clamped section of vas deferens is ligated and removed. The stumps of the vas deferens may be cauterized. The clamps are removed, and the ends of the vas deferens are replaced in the tunic. The tunic is sutured with absorbable suture material. The procedure is repeated on the opposite vas deferens. The incisions are sprayed with an antibiotic powder. The skin is loosely sutured. Healing should be complete in 2 weeks.

Disease Control Within a Swine Breeding Herd

S. C. Henry, D.V.M.
Abilene Animal Hospital, Abilene, Kansas

M. R. Wilson, D.V.M.
Ontario Veterinary College, Guelph, Ontario, Canada

A. D. Leman, D.V.M.
University of Minnesota, St. Paul, Minnesota

Concepts of "herd health" and "preventive medicine" are embraced by the veterinary profession and livestock industry as innovations of our technologically advanced society. While it is true that modern diagnostic methods enable accuracy unknown in the past and that production systems offer great control over disease, it is not yet possible to ensure freedom from many specific diseases of swine. In considering methods to guard against introduction of disease through breeding stock, a perspective on present practices can be gained from what happened in the past. In 1901 the *Cyclopedia of Livestock* and *Complete Stock Doctor* discussed the philosophy and application of methods to prevent swine disease in terms that are recognizable today.

In the care of swine the prevention of disease is of the utmost importance . . . To prevent disease in swine, the most important thing is so to care for the animals that they shall be kept in general good health. The admission of other swine among the herd should, also, be prohibited until you are well assured that the newcomers are free from disease. The herd should be perfectly isolated during the prevalence of epidemic or contagious diseases, and disinfectants should be freely used.

Little has changed in the current philosophical approach to swine disease prevention, a suggestion that perhaps the foregoing ideas have stood the test of time and are the central concepts of disease prevention in swine herds.

To give our forefathers their due, it must be remembered that another "modern" concept—depopulation, with complete herd replacement—was actually known at the turn of the century. Although it may be suggested today as the panacea for many and varied causes of swine ill health, the 1901 *Complete Stock Doctor* noted

there is only one economical way to treat so-called "hog cholera" which may appear in many forms. . . . When either of these forms of disease attacks swine, the cheapest way to treat it is to send the animals at once to the rendering tanks, and convert them into grease, or kill and bury them at once, and thoroughly disinfect every possible place where contagion may lurk. If a competent veterinarian be near, apply him at once; but beware of quacks who go about doctoring hogs with so-called specifics; they are a delusion and a snare for the unwary.

A veterinarian assumes great responsibility when evaluating the health and soundness of breeding stock. Legal precedent has established that with this responsibility comes liability for omissions or errors in evaluation. Careful physical examination, appropriate laboratory tests and a history of production problems and disease on both the farm of origin and the destination farm are the data base for a professional opinion. Prepurchase discussions among buyers, sellers and veterinarians allow each to emphasize his or her goals and will greatly simplify health and soundness examinations.

KEEPING DISEASE OUT

Physical Examination. Veterinarians have not traditionally been employed by swine producers to examine swine before purchase. Rather, examination is more often requested after pigs arrive at their destination. Communication between the veterinarian who serves the buyer and the veterinarian employed by the seller is an alternative means of collecting information on physical condition before purchase.

Ideally, the herd of origin, not just the animals being purchased, is observed. Evidence of infectious disease is important, but a major goal of such herd observation is to assure physical soundness and to ascertain the physical appropriateness of particular animals to the environment in which they will be housed. Familiarity of the examining veterinarian with production facilities and production goals of the purchaser is imperative if valid, defensible opinions are to be given on subjective conditions such as animal adaptation to new environments.

Herd Production and Disease History. In addition to direct information provided by the seller and his veterinarian, information on medication, immunization, post-mortem and slaughter examinations and production efficiency is helpful. Antibiotics for feed or water medication suggest existing disease conditions. For example, therapeutic antibiotics for swine dysentery fed routinely justifies caution in purchase of animals unless further testing and history show no risk of the disease.

Serologic Screening. The veterinarian, acting as agent for the buyer, must rely on serologic testing in the health evaluation. Serology provides a historic view of a specific disease, indicating whether or not the animals tested have had previous exposure to a particular pathogen. Serology is a simple and economical tool in disease screening. Many serologic tests for specific pathogens are available; few are appropriate in all situations. The following serologic tests are most often used in screening swine herd additions and to gain information about disease in both origin and destination herds.

Brucellosis, now uncommon in U.S. swine, remains a standard test required by law in most interstate movement of breeding swine. Testing is not done when pigs originate from a brucellosis-validated herd.

Leptospira may be carried and shed by vaccinated swine even though immunization has effectively prevented clinical signs of disease. Interpretation of leptospirosis titers is complicated by variations in laboratory methodology and by low titers resulting from vaccination with certain leptospirosis bacterins. Usually, infected animals are found to have serovariant-specific titers severalfold higher than titers induced through vaccination. Many serovariants of *Leptospira interrogans* affect swine, but prepurchase serology screening is most often requested for four serovariants: *L. pomona, L. icterohaemorrhagiae, L. grippotyphosa* and *L. canicola.*

Pseudorabies virus (PRV) serology, now required for certain interstate movements of pigs, is suggested when the destination farm is free of PRV. To decrease the risk of PRV transmission, two serologic samples 30 days apart are recommended. Animals are tested at purchase and again 30 days later to minimize diagnostic error if tested pigs have been infected near the date of purchase; in such cases animals would be virus-infected but seronegative for several days. Pseudorabies virus vaccination results in seroconversion, and vaccination history is important in PRV serology interpretation.

At this time titers induced by field virus and vaccinal virus cannot be distinguished.

Porcine parvovirus (PPV) and *enterovirus* serologic tests are most valuable as disease prevention tools when applied in a comparative fashion. This group of viruses is ubiquitous in U.S. swine, with few herds actually free from serologic evidence of infection. When the serologic status of the destination herd is known, the titers of animals to be added to the herd are useful information. For example, movement of PPV serologically negative gilts into a seropositive herd may result in an unexpectedly high level of fetal mummification in their litters. Comparative serologic testing before purchase serves as a prognostic aid as well as a diagnostic tool. Interpretation of positive serologic titers in an absolute fashion is not valid for ubiquitous diseases; positive titers for such diseases do not infer disease risk but the relative prevalence of pathogen exposure in two groups of pigs.

Haemophilus pleuropneumonia serotesting is especially important in preventing pleuropneumonia spread into seronegative herds. Serotype specific testing is not commonly performed; instead, a pooled antigen complement fixation system is used. Animals from seropositive herds should not enter seronegative herds even if clinical disease has not been noted in the herd of origin. With this particular pathogen, comparative serologic testing may be helpful in judging the risk of disease introduction. Many herds, both origin and destination herds, contain seropostive animals yet there is no history or evidence of clinical disease. When both origin and destination herds contain seropositive animals, some decision must be reached in regard to the relative risks of introduction of separate serotypes versus the merit of new genetic material.

Eperythrozoonosis, transmissible gastroenteritis (TGE) and swine influenza are often included in serologic screening of new herd additions. As all are ubiquitous diseases, results of serology should be compared with the serologic and clinical disease patterns in the destination herd before seropositive animals are rejected as herd replacements.

Serotesting is most valuable as a tool for comparing and contrasting two populations of animals and their history of contact with pathogens. The accuracy of serologic titers as reflections of disease risk is best when adequate sample numbers are compared over a period of time. Such ideal sampling conditions do not occur often under field conditions. While serotesting has been criticized as overstating disease prevalence and risk, it remains one of the few unbiased methods for identification of subclinical disease presence that may pose a risk. Serotesting is a valid tool to apply in preventing disease movement between herds.

Isolation and Quarantine. Following purchase of an animal, an isolation and quarantine period is a valuable practice that serves to safeguard both new animals and the destination herd. It is possible to carry out many diagnostic, therapeutic and immunizing activities during this period. Immunization of new animals should take place with vaccines in use on the destination farm. Adaptation to new diets during this time also acclimates new animals.

The use of sentinel animals from the destination herd may allow detection of subclinical disease not apparent through examination or serology. Enteric diseases are especially difficult to diagnose unless samples are available from clinically ill swine. Commingling new breeding stock with an equal number of age-matched or younger peers from the destination farm encourages expression of disease in both groups. Appropriate diagnostic testing is begun when illness is apparent. Examples of diseases that may be most easily diagnosed through sentinel pig exposure are proliferative ileitis, *Salmonella choleraesuis*, septicemia, swine dysentery, TGE, influenza and pasturellosis. Sophistication of this system to include pre- and postquarantine serologic comparison of sentinels and new stock may be appropriate. Following quarantine, sentinels may be slaughtered and tissues collected, inspected and compared with similar samples from destination farm peers. In addition to the diagnostic benefits from the use of sentinel pigs, new animals have an opportunity to adapt to diseases prevalent at their destination while they are under careful observation.

Isolation and quarantine periods allow for time to administer medication to prevent specific diseases. Administration of bacteriocidal antidysentery compounds may, for example, clear the carrier state of this disease, and such treatment is appropriate during isolation.

Embryo Transfer, Artificial Insemination and Cesarean-derived Pigs. Introduction of genetic material as embryos or semen substantially reduces but does not entirely eliminate risk of disease. Both methods represent recent and potentially practical technologic advances. Cesarean-derived stock has proved very successful in certain areas, as the Specific Pathogen-Free program has demonstrated. At this time for the U.S. swine industry, only a small part of the national genetic base is procurable by these methods. The cost for genetic material is high with these methods, but future refinement should bring extensive use, limiting herd disease risks.

The technologic capability exists to support the veterinarian asked to evaluate prepurchase health and soundness. The depth of concern the owner may have about disease risk and the size of the transaction will influence the effort demanded of a veterinarian in such evaluations. In the past the swine industry has shown slight regard to disease risk and transmission through breeding stock. The centralized shows, sales and test stations all encouraged wide distribution of disease through the swine industry. Closed herd management is becoming an industry standard of operation and, with it, increased demand for assurances of health in breeding stock. The veterinary profession has not developed standards for complete prepurchase examinations,

but application of existing technology can be developed by practitioners to meet the needs of most swine producers on a case-by-case basis.

CONTROLLING DISEASE WITHIN A HERD

The expression of infectious disease is directly proportional to the dose and virulence of the pathogenic microbes and inversely proportional to the animal's resistance. There are many opportunities for veterinarians and pork producers to reduce the dose and increase the resistance.

Reducing Dose of Pathogenic Microbes. Pathogenic microbes are passed from animal to animal through direct animal contact, fecal contact, urine contact and aerosol transmission. Altering these natural routes of disease transmission can effectively reduce the dose of microbes reaching a susceptible animal.

Self-Cleaning Floors. Expanded metal and wire mesh floors offer an excellent opportunity for baby pigs to be born in a manure-free environment. These floors are the only effective treatment for coccidiosis, and they aid in controlling virtually all neonatal enteric diseases. On some farms the cleaning or scraping of the farrowing crate daily or twice daily is a useful diarrhea control procedure.

Fresh Air. There is no better medicine than fresh air. It helps dilute the concentration of microbes and harmful gases and dust. It promotes healthier respiratory tissue, which in turn reduces the dose of microbes that get deep into the lung tissue. The amount of fresh air is a function of the ventilation system, the animal density, the volume of space per animal and the waste management system. There is evidence that pigs with about 4 cubic yards of volume or more have fewer lung lesions at slaughter than pigs with less total air volume.

Current winter ventilation systems in fully slotted barns over a full anaerobic pit do not support optimum performance. Future pork production will feature aerobic waste systems or more air movement than is currently recommended.

Vaccination. Appropriate vaccines will stimulate immunity so the animal will resist the growth and shedding of a pathogenic microbe. Vaccination programs are specifically discussed in the last part of this article.

Early and Effective Therapy. Prompt antibacterial therapy can reduce the multiplication of pathogens and may reduce the number of pathogens shed by the infected animal. Most producers fail to use antibiotics often enough and long enough. A useful rule of thumb is to inject antibiotics at the suggested dose twice daily for 3 consecutive days.

Old Sow Herd. As sows age, they develop specific immunity to many common infections and often clear these pathogens from their bodies. Therefore, old sows will pass a lower dose of pathogens to their offspring.

Disease-Free Dams. Certain diseases, such as internal parasites, mange, atrophic rhinitis and pneumonia are best controlled by eliminating the disease in the dam and thereby reducing the chance of transmission to her offspring. The Specific Pathogen Free (SPF) program has been designed to achieve this status.

Building Design. In addition to floor surface, other factors influence the transmission of pathogens. Solid partitions between pens help reduce nose-to-nose contact and disease transmission. Solid walls help separate groups of pigs and encourage all-in, all-out production.

All-In, All-Out Production. This is an effective, yet underused, method of disease control. It encourages age separation of pigs and facilitates clean-up between groups. All new building and housing systems should be designed with this concept in mind. Existing facilities can often be improved by partitioning pigs into smaller groups.

Selling of Complete Pens of Pigs. Even when facilities do not allow all-in, all-out production, marketing entire pens of pigs will help assure that chronically infected pigs do not remain on the farm.

Age Separation. Divide buildings into rooms and separate pigs according to their ages, to reduce transmission from older to younger pigs.

Clean-Up and Disinfection. This practice helps reduce the dose of infectious organisms in pens and buildings. Fumigation remains the best method of disinfection. In most cases, however, a good cleanup is sufficient.

Farm Security. Every farm should have a well-designed program to keep out potential infections carried mechanically by vehicles, birds, dogs, cats and people. Every farm should have an effective rodent control program. Replacement boars and gilts should come from as few sources as possible. Feeder pigs should come from one farm only.

Sow Health and Longevity. Gestation crates reduce lameness and increase longevity. Wet floors cause hoof damage and lameness. More heat will dry floors and reduce lameness. Cold, underfed sows may abort. Dry, clean floors help reduce bladder and kidney infections.

Increasing Resistance. The pig is a remarkably resilient animal, with a wide range of natural resistance mechanisms. With just a little help from their stewards, they can resist nearly all common diseases.

Elimination of Parasites. Both external and internal parasites are capable of reducing the animal's

Table 1. Vaccination Schedules for Major Infectious Diseases Affecting Swine Reproductive Performance

Disease	Vaccination Schedule*	Comments
1. To protect the sow:		
Erysipelas	First dose to weaned pig; second dose 1 month before first farrowing; repeat at each farrowing	Vaccines and bacterins are effective.
2. To reduce abortion and stillbirth rates:		
Pseudorabies	Live vaccines—3 to 8 weeks of age; repeat every 6 months in breeding stock; dead vaccines—two doses at 14 and 28 days of age, 4 and 2 weeks prior to farrowing	
Leptospirosis	At breeding or weaning	Bacterins are effective but should be used in conjunction with treatment during an outbreak.
Erysipelas	At breeding or weaning	
Embryonic and fetal death associated with parvovirus infection	One dose at time of selection for the breeding herd, a second 2 to 4 weeks before breeding	Vaccination gives assurance against failure of natural immunization through infection.
3. To protect piglets passively from neonatal infections:		
Transmissible gastroenteritis (TGE)	4 and 1 weeks before farrowing and to unweaned piglets	Both intramuscular and oral vaccines give only partial protection.
Pseudorabies	See above	
Enteric colibacillosis	Bacterins at least 1 month and again 1 week prior to farrowing; oral vaccines 10 to 30 days prior to farrowing for 3 consecutive days	Commercially available bacterins or pilus vaccines as well as bacterins and oral vaccines prepared autogenously give good protection.
Bordetella-induced atrophic rhinitis	4 and 2 weeks before farrowing to sows and 1 and 4 weeks of age to piglets	Efficacy varies from herd to herd.
Rotavirus	4 and 1 weeks before farrowing and to unweaned piglets	Independently acquired efficacy data are not available.

*In all cases the manufacturers' directions should be followed when different from those suggested here.

resistance. They can be controlled by currently available chemicals. The technology exists to eliminate sarcoptic mange and the need for deworming in total confinement herds.

Nutrition. Resistance and immunity are directly related to general nutritional status and to several specific nutrients, including zinc and selenium.

Fresh Air. In addition to reducing the dose of irritants and pathogens, an ample supply of fresh air is necessary for healthy respiratory tissue and natural resistance to atrophic rhinitis and pneumonia.

Vaccination. Vaccinations are obviously designed to stimulate specific immunity and resistance to disease.

Animal Comfort. Warm, dry, draft-free conditions allow the animal's defense mechanisms to be fully directed toward fighting disease. When environmental conditions are less than ideal, parts of the animal's feed and energy must be directed toward survival.

Floor Surfaces. Abrasion-free floor surfaces help promote normal hoof development and wear; the chance of damage, infection and lameness is thereby lessened.

Older Sows. Resistance usually increases with age.

CONTROLLING DISEASE BY VACCINATION

Vaccinations during the reproductive period are given for three reasons:

1. To protect the sow.
2. To reduce abortion and increased stillbirth rate.
3. To protect the piglets passively from neonatal infections.

It is important to remember that more than 90 per cent of immunoglobulins in colostrum are obtained from the circulatory system of the sow, whereas more than 70 per cent of the immunoglobulins in milk are produced in the mammary glands. It follows, therefore, that if the objective is to induce protection against a systemic disease of the neonate or the sow, circulating antibodies must be induced in the sow. These are passed into the colostrum and transported to the circulation of the newborn piglets. If protection against an enteric disease in the piglet is desired, for optimal results

stimulation of the immune system in the sow's mammary glands should be attempted. However, reliable and safe methods of effectively achieving this aim have not been documented.

Killed versus Living Biologics. In an article of this length, it is not possible to elaborate upon the merits of killed versus living vaccines. As a generalization, one can say that living porcine viral vaccines are considered by many to be unsafe, whereas killed viral vaccines, although safe, have often given less than desirable protection. Bacterins, however, often give adequate protection and compare favorably with living bacterial vaccines for some conditions.

Finally, there is a form of vaccination that utilizes virulent organisms to attempt to induce immunity at a time when the resultant infection causes no harm to the sow. Such a procedure could be termed "normalizing vaccination." The feeding of feces or dead piglets or both to pregnant animals is of special value when new animals are added to a herd. On some occasions newly added animals will abort because they lack immunity to the resident infections to which the members of the herd are immune. Conversely, on occasion the residents of the herd may abort after introduction of new members; then, the new sows or boars have introduced an infection to which they are immune but to which the residents were not. Feces should therefore be fed from the residents to the newcomers and vice versa.

When tissues or feces are being used, one has no control over what is being fed, as subclinical infection, for example, parvovirus or enteroviruses, could be present. However, the feeding of pure cultures of organisms at a time when there is no danger of inducing abortions or other problems lessens this danger. This procedure is often used with success in enteric colibacillosis and transmissible gastroenteritis. Its disadvantage is that an infection is established in the sow that inevitably results in a considerably increased challenge to piglets if it is a neonatal disease and a carrier state is induced in the infected sow.

Table 1 lists the major infectious diseases affecting the reproductive performance of sows and appropriate schedules for vaccination. It should be noted that in all cases the manufacturer's instructions for vaccination protocol must be followed for optimum results.

Swine Breeding Herd Records

Brad J. Thacker, D.V.M., M.S.
Michigan State University, East Lansing, Michigan

Table 1. Farrowing Data

Sow (#)
Pen or crate (#)
Sire (#)
Parity
Due date
Farrowing date
Total born (#)
Live born (#)
Stillborn (#)
Mummies (#)
Litter birth weight
Transfer in/out date(s)
Date weaned
Weaning weight
Sow and litter treatments
Piglet deaths—date and reason

The recent advances in recording and analyzing breeding herd activities have enhanced our knowledge of swine reproduction and improved diagnostic capabilities to deal with reproductive problems. The high fixed and marginal costs of confinement production mandates the producer and veterinarian to monitor closely, through record analysis, pig flow, inventory, herd reproductive efficiency and individual animal performance. Accurate records of breeding herd activities can then be summarized and analyzed to identify those performance parameters that fall short of intended production levels. Further record analysis is often necessary to define deficiencies accurately before corrective actions can be taken. Finally, the results of recommended remedial actions can be measured by continued monitoring.

Maximum benefits from a record keeping system are obtained with accurate recording, proper collation, careful analysis, willingness to implement remedial actions based on record analysis and continued monitoring to assess remedial actions and identify new problems.

COMPONENTS OF A RECORD SYSTEM

The essential components of a breeding herd recording system include barn records, office records and summary reports.

Barn Records. These should be kept in close proximity to the animals to allow for the immediate recording of events and making day-to-day management decisions. These records should include individual animal data (farrowing crate card or breeding-gestation card) or data from several animals (farrowing or breeding-gestation activity records). Individual animal crate cards are used particularly in the farrowing area, where events are conveniently recorded in conjunction with routine management procedures. In addition to data that are eventually entered into permanent office records, many farrowing crate cards include routine management checklists for castrations, iron injections and needle teeth clipping. A space is also provided for recording sow and litter treatments. The transferral of farrowing data to the office records, and its organization into a form easily summarized by hand calculation, is greatly facilitated by a farrowing activity record. This record lists the same data as the farrowing card but includes information from all animals farrowing in a certain room, time period or group. In the breeding-gestation area most recording occurs near the breeding pens. For this reason, multiple-animal records are often more practical than individual crate cards. They also facilitate data transfer to office records and hand-calculation of summaries. The information contained in a farrowing barn record is listed in Table 1. Breeding-gestation information is listed in Table 2.

Other barn records include breeding herd entry forms and individual boar cards. Entry forms are completed when gilts are selected and placed in the breeding herd. Information recorded onto a separate breeding herd entry form at selection is valuable for monitoring management practices in relation to the onset of puberty in gilts. Gilts can also be entered into the breeding herd records at first mating. Individual boar cards provide for a readily available record for monitoring mating activity.

Office Records. These can be viewed as a file system in which data are stored for future analysis.

Table 2. Breeding-Gestation Data

Sow (#)
Group (#)
Crate or pen (#)
Parity
Date weaned
Wean-to-service interval
Repeat breeder?
Dates serviced
Boars used
Date return to estrus postservice
Interval: regular (18 to 24 days)
delayed (> 24 days)
Pregnancy test—date and result
Due date
Comments—aborted, culled and reason,
not-in-pig and date

They should include permanent sow and boar records and records of farrowing and breeding-gestation events. The permanent sow record should contain a life history, and this is used for culling decisions and the selection of replacement gilts. Many systems include a productivity index to rank sows according to prolificacy and milking ability. The permanent boar record is valuable in detecting the infertile boar and those that sire defective offspring, especially in herds using single-boar matings.

The farrowing and breeding-gestation activity record contains a running account of events in their respective areas. These data provide a framework to generate hand-calculated summary reports with a manual system. The time period of analysis is selected, and the events contained within this period are mathematically summarized. Office records should be updated as necessary to generate summary reports and to provide current information on the permanent sow and boar records, preferably on a weekly basis.

Summary Reports. The key benefit of any record keeping system is the summary report. This information allows the producer and the veterinarian to monitor herd performance, to detect problems and to measure the effectiveness of remedial actions. The absence of detailed information forces the veterinary adviser to base recommendations on intuition rather than fact. Two categories of information are included in the summary report. The first measures the number of activities or events needed to maintain production and pig flow at desired levels, e.g., breedings and farrowings per week, live pigs born per month and death loss per month. The second category measures the efficiency of the herd or the output per activity, e.g., number of live pigs born per litter, farrowing rate and per cent of animals having a positive pregnancy test. Various parameters commonly included in a summary report are listed in Table 3.

RECORD ANALYSIS

The frequency of analysis should be inversely proportional to the herd size. Records from a 100-sow herd would be analyzed monthly or quarterly, whereas a 500-sow herd would be analyzed weekly. Realistically, those parameters effecting management decisions on a weekly basis should be analyzed weekly. For example, the number of breedings per week is managed on a week-to-week basis, and knowledge of the number of breedings in recent weeks is used to target the current week's breedings to maintain proper pig flow. Parameters that monitor efficiencies, such as farrowing rate and liveborn per litter, are used to predict long-term production trends rather than provide weekly information.

The depth of analysis depends on individual herd circumstances. A minimal number of parameters

should be selected to monitor herd performance on a continual basis at either weekly or monthly intervals. Additional parameters can be analyzed less frequently—quarterly or yearly. In-depth analysis

Table 3. Summary Reports

1. **Breeding Herd Inventory Report**
   Sow inventory at end of period
   Average sow inventory
   Average parity
   Number of sows culled
   Number of sows dead
   Boar inventory at end of period
   Net change of sows
   Net change of boars
   Sow-to-boar ratio
2. **Gilt Management**
   Number of gilts entered
   Average age of gilts entering breeding herd
   Days to first service
   Per cent of gilts serviced by 60 days after entrance to breeding herd
   Number of gilts dead
3. **Breeding Management Report**
   Number of services—total, sows, gilts
   Number of first services—total, sows, gilts
   Number of repeat services—total, sows, gilts
   Average weaning-to-estrus interval
   Per cent of sows bred by 10 days postweaning
   Number of regular returns to estrus—total, sows, gilts
   Number of delayed returns to estrus—total, sows, gilts
   Per cent of pregnancy tests positive
   Number and per cent of abortions
   Number and per cent of not-in-pig (NIP)
4. **Farrowing Report**
   Total number of litters farrowed
   Farrowing rate
   Total born—number and average/litter
   Liveborn—number, average/litter, per cent of total born
   Stillborn—number, average, per cent of total born
   Mummies—number, average, per cent of total born
   Average birth weight
   Per cent of litter scatter (< 8 pigs born alive/litter)
5. **Weaning Report**
   Number of litters weaned
   Number of pigs weaned
   Number of pigs weaned/litter
   Average 21-day weaning weight
   Preweaning mortality
     Total number
     Average/litter
     Per cent of liveborn
     Per cent of deaths
       Scours
       Starvation
       Crushing
       Weakness
       Congenital defects
       Miscellaneous
6. **Management Action Lists**
   Sows to be tested for pregnancy
   Sows to be vaccinated
   Sows to be crated
   Sows to be weaned

can be used more clearly to define problems noted in routine performance monitoring. Examination of the parity distribution of an increased number of stillborn piglets would be a classic example. Increased stillborns in older sows may be a normal phenomenon, whereas increased stillborns in gilts may indicate the presence of an infectious disease.

The speed of information recovery is important in persuading the producer to accept record systems. Management action lists, up-to-date permanent sow records and sow productivity index rankings must be available at the time of decision making to be of value.

The manner in which the summary reports are displayed is also of great importance for producer acceptance, usefulness of the information and proper interpretation. Some parameters are best displayed in graphic form; graphs that plot parameters over time are particularly useful to indicate herd trends.

TARGETS AND INTERFERENCE LEVELS

The concepts of using record keeping systems to monitor herd performance and of comparing current production with previously established goals and interference levels have been widely accepted. Interference levels are the minimally acceptable levels of herd performance. When a production parameter drops below the interference level, diagnostic and/or remedial action is undertaken to define and/or to solve the problem. Examples of parameters, goals and interference levels are listed in Table 4.

ANIMAL IDENTIFICATION

Individual animal identification is an essential component of most recording systems. Eartags are commonly used to identify animals. Unfortunately, the loss of a single eartag results in the loss of the animal's identity and ultimately valuable informa-

Table 4. Production Parameters—Target and Interference Levels

Parameter	Target Level	Interference Level
Weaning-to-service interval (days)	7.0	9.0
Returns (per cent)	6.0	12.0
Abortions (per cent)	0.8	2.5
Farrowing rate (per cent)	89.0	80.0
Number alive/litter	10.9	10.0
Per cent born dead	5.0	8.0
Per cent mummified	0.5	1.0
Number weaned/litter	9.6	9.0
Per cent deaths due to weaning	8.0–12.0	12.0–18.0
Litter scatter (per cent)	10.0	18.0
Litters/sow/year	2.2	2.0
Pigs/sow/year	21.0	19.0

tion. Double tagging, one tag in each ear, prevents this loss, providing the missing tag is quickly replaced before the second is lost. Appropriate number changes, if any, are then recorded in the animal's permanent record.

A tattoo placed inside the ear represents a truly permanent form of identification. Gilts and boars are tattooed upon entrance into the breeding herd, and the number is recorded in the animal's permanent record. Dual identification with an eartag, also recorded in the permanent record, is desirable for day-to-day identification, as the reading of tattoos requires handling the ear. When an eartag is lost, the tattoo number is used to locate the animal's permanent record. The animal is then retagged with the same number or a substitute number.

SELECTING A RECORD SYSTEM

Considerations in selecting a record keeping system include the output of information desired, the willingness of the producer to record events accurately and continually, herd size, herd management practices, system cost and labor requirements. For example, summary information that requires breeding dates would be unavailable in herds in which hand mating is not practiced. Emphasis on individual sow productivity would have low priority in herds in which replacement gilts are being purchased. In general, the complexity of a record system should be proportional to herd size. The potential returns of time spent in record keeping and analysis are much greater in large herds. In smaller herds the producer and consulting veterinarian may often have an adequate view of the herd's problem without the use of detailed records.

Computerized record keeping systems greatly enhance analytical capabilities, resulting in more detailed reports. The computer is able to manage the large amounts of data collected on a breeding herd. Summary reports generated from computerized systems have increased the ability to monitor herd performance and have certainly improved diagnostic capabilities in the breeding herd. Once the computer is properly programmed, detailed reports can be generated quickly and easily. Manual, hand-calculated or centralized computer systems are usually recommended for smaller herds (less than 100 sows) when the cost of an on-farm computer cannot be recovered by the expected benefit. Systems using a central computer will cost less than on-farm systems, but the turn around time of analysis may be unacceptable, and the security of herd information is potentially jeopardized.

ROLE OF VETERINARIAN IN RECORD ANALYSIS

The veterinary adviser is in a unique position to assist the swine producer with the interpretation of data. The information generated from a good record

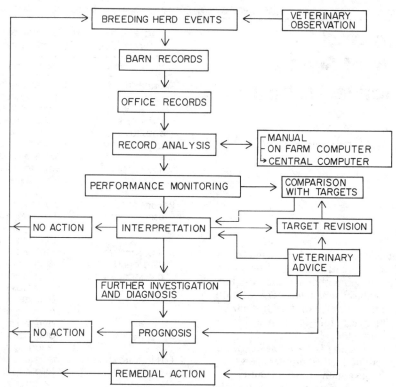

Figure 1. Record analysis in the breeding herd: information flow and veterinary input.

keeping system is extremely valuable, if not essential, for the veterinarian to accurately identify, define and solve the problems of the breeding herd. Currently, many veterinarians include recording systems as an integral part of herd-health programs. The veterinarian needs continually to encourage the producer to maintain good records through the demonstration of its usefulness. If the veterinarian is able to show the producer that record keeping is a successful method for identifying and defining problems and is able to formulate remedial actions and measure their success, the producer will appreciate the benefits. If not, the recording system could fall into disuse, and the value of the veterinarian's advice diminishes. A schematic diagram illustrating the flow of information in monitoring the breeding herd and solving problems is shown in Figure 1.

Occasionally, the veterinarian becomes involved in situations when the recording system does not accurately describe the herd's activities. Periodic physical inventory counts are recommended to crosscheck the figures generated in summary reports. Inaccurate recording of data is occasionally observed because new employees neither understand which information should be recorded nor the meaning of definitions used to describe abnormalities (e.g., stillborns, mummies) and reasons for piglet deaths.

The veterinarian's value as an adviser to swine producers in the future will depend on their willingness and ability to be involved in the various aspects of recording systems. In general, veterinarians need to be more precise in their monitoring and diagnostic activities; records provide the only vehicle for achieving this goal. In addition, the veterinary adviser is in a unique position to guide the producer in the selection of what records are useful for the individual herd situation and continually to demonstrate that record keeping is a cost-beneficial management practice.

References

1. Petter TA, Boyd HW, Rosenberg P: Breeding record analysis in pig herds and its veterinary applications. 1. Development of a program to monitor reproductive efficiency and weaner production. Vet Rec 101:177, 1977.
2. Walton JR, Martin JW, Ward WR: The collection and use of data on a pig farm. Pig Vet Soc Proc 6:23, 1980.
3. Wrathall AE: Investigation and control of reproductive disorders in the breeding herd. In Cole DJA, Foxcroft GR (eds): Control of Pig Reproduction. Boston, Butterworth Scientific, 1982, pp 565–583.

Detection and Diagnosis of Swine Reproductive Failure

Brad J. Thacker, D.V.M., M.S.

Michigan State University, East Lansing, Michigan

Expedient detection and efficient diagnosis of reproductive failure is greatly facilitated by an ongoing herd-health program that includes frequent record analysis, regularly scheduled herd visits by the veterinarian and routine laboratory testing. Diagnosis of reproductive failure is often a difficult task for the following reasons:

1. "Normal" reproduction is a complex series of events. A specific reproductive problem, e.g., repeat breeding, may have many possible causes.

2. Some problems are detected long after the specific failure has occurred. For example, one result of boar over-usage, e.g., decreased liveborn litter size, is detected at farrowing or 114 days after mating.

3. Reproductive problems often have multiple causes. Failure to determine and then to control or to eliminate all of these causes could result in no improvement in reproductive efficiency. Success is often determined by the most limiting factor.

4. Reproductive failure is often from noninfectious causes, especially those related to breeding management and animal care. Traditional diagnostic efforts have dealt primarily with the submission of serum and tissues for the identification of infectious agents. Laboratory methods to support the clinical diagnosis of noninfectious causes are not as well developed or utilized.

5. Detailed record analysis is often necessary to identify when normal physiological events fail. Inadequate record keeping can result in either no diagnosis or an incorrect diagnosis. Records are also essential for estimating the economic importance of a problem, so the costs of remedial actions or additional diagnostic efforts can be compared with the expected benefits.

6. Observation of breeding herd management practices, e.g., heat detection and hand mating, is essential in many instances. Veterinarians and producers are not always willing to make the required investment of time and money to conduct this type of time-consuming investigation.

This article will categorize reproductive failure into general problem areas (primary complaints) that are presented to the veterinarian (Table 1). The detection and diagnosis of reproductive failure through record analysis, observations by breeding

Table 1. Swine Reproductive Problems Presented as Primary Complaints

Primary Complaint	Description
Anestrus in gilts	Caused by delayed puberty or cessation of cyclic activity
Postweaning anestrus in sows	Failure of sows to return to estrus after weaning
Regular returns	Return to estrus 18 to 24 days after mating
Delayed returns	Return to estrus more than 25 days after mating
Returns to estrus—pen mating	Return to estrus at unknown intervals after mating with pen-mating systems
Not pregnant via ultrasound pregnancy test	Negative pregnancy diagnosis at 30 to 40 days after mating indicates a regular or delayed, unnoticed return to estrus. With pen mating, it may also indicate post-weaning anestrus.
Fail-to-farrow; not-in-pig (NIP)	Failure of sows to farrow following a positive pregnancy diagnosis or after appearing pregnant is an indication of fetal death with or without resorption or unobserved abortion.
Abortions	Observed expulsion of fetuses and fetal membranes prior to day 110 of gestation
Mummified fetuses	Dead fetuses that appear discolored (dark green) and shriveled
Stillbirths	Fully developed fetuses that die either before farrowing and are somewhat degenerated (type I) or during farrowing (type II)
Small litters	Liveborn litter size of less than eight pigs per litter without excessive numbers of mummified or stillborn litters
Vaginal discharges	Purulent material observed on, or draining from, the vulva

herd personnel, veterinary inspection and routine laboratory testing is discussed. The specific diagnostic methods and information used for further investigations to identify specific causes with respect to each general problem area are outlined in Table 2. These special diagnostic techniques, which either identify a specific cause or provide additional information for problem definition, are discussed thoroughly in other articles.

RECORD ANALYSIS

Record analysis for monitoring breeding herd performance is discussed in detail in the article Swine Breeding Herd Records. The following factors should be considered when using records to detect reproductive failure:

1. Selection of parameters for monitoring breeding performance and detecting problems is dependent on the complexity of the record system and the breeding management practices. For example, record systems based on individual animal identification and hand mating will generate more detailed reports than those records based on animal groups and pen mating. Selected parameters should indicate reproductive efficiencies (liveborn litter size, farrowing rate), pig flow (breedings per week, farrowings per month) and breeding herd inventory (number of sows, sow-to-boar ratio). Table 3 lists the parameters that provide a fairly complete analysis of breeding herd performance.

2. The frequency of analysis is dependent on the herd size, number of breeding groups and the specific parameters. As herd size increases, so should the frequency of analysis. A breeding system that establishes sow groups on a weekly basis, versus a monthly basis, requires more frequent analysis to ensure that adequate pig flow (especially breedings per week) is maintained. Parameters monitoring reproductive efficiencies are often less subject to dramatic change and require less frequent analysis.

3. The establishment of target and interference levels based on individual herd management practice, genetics, facilities and disease status provide a working guideline to assess herd performance and assist in deciding whether further investigations or control efforts are warranted. Targets and interference levels listed in Table 3 are representative of commercial herds in the United States that feature crossbred females, hand mating, individual gestation stalls, weekly breeding schedules and weaning at 4 weeks.

4. The accuracy of any recording system is based on the ability of the breeding herd personnel to observe breeding herd events and to transcribe this information into a written record. Occasionally, discrepancies between record analysis and visual observation of herd performance are encountered. Conducting a physical inventory of the breeding herd may be necessary to verify records.

5. Records should provide concrete evidence that the recommendations of advisors, e.g., veterinari-

ans, actually result in improved breeding herd performance.

6. When problems are detected, the record system should provide the necessary information to conduct retrospective epidemiological investigations to determine the stage of gestation at which the failure occurred, the group affected (often based on parity) and the expected economic losses. This type of information also provides assistance in the selection of samples to be submitted for laboratory testing.

HERD INSPECTION

Although inspecting the breeding herd usually involves a simple walk through the areas used for breeding, gestation and farrowing, the astute observer can also gain valuable information about current problems and more importantly, point out situations that may eventually contribute to reproductive failure.

The following problems are commonly detected while inspecting the breeding herd:

1. Over- and under-conditioned animals (indicates improper feeding levels).

2. Clinical lameness, defects in foot structure and poor skeletal conformation, particularly in boars.

3. External parasites (mange and lice as evidenced by hair loss, pruritis and sebum and crust formation).

4. Vaginal discharges.

5. Abnormal testicle size and asymmetry.

6. Abnormal development of the external genitalia in gilts (infantile vulvas, hermaphrodites).

7. Physical inventory counts that differ from records.

8. Poor sanitation of facilities, with particular attention to feeders and the back part of gestation crates, boar crates and mating pens.

9. Animals appearing not to be pregnant in groups due to farrow soon (may indicate resorption).

10. Environmental conditions: (A) Effective environmental temperature. In crated gestation barns, room temperature should be more than 18.3°C. If room temperatures exceed 29.4°C during the summer, water sprinklers should be available, especially for sows within 3 weeks of farrowing and for boars. (B) Lighting. Windowless barns should be lighted at least 8 hours and preferably up to 16 hours per day. (C) Ventilation. Air quality and moisture control.

11. Age and body size of breeding gilts.

12. Design of estrous detection facilities is especially important, space allotted and abrasiveness of flooring surface.

Also during each visit, one or more of the following specific areas of breeding herd management should be acutely observed and/or discussed in detail with breeding herd personnel.

1. Weaning-to-breeding management.

2. Postweaning detection of estrus.

Table 2. Investigation of Swine Reproductive Failure: Historical Information, On-farm Observations and Diagnostic Methods

Primary Complaint	Historical Information	On-farm Observations	Special Examinations	Laboratory Tests
Anestrus in gilts	Breeds and breeding program, season, animal movements and mixing, boar exposure and age of boar, housing, stocking density, nutrition	External genitalia (infantile vulvas and hermaphrodites), gilt age, size and condition, light, (space and flooring), estrous detection methods	Slaughter examination to confirm anestrus and to detect developmental defects	Serum progesterone analysis to confirm anestrus
Postweaning anestrus	Parity, season, feed intake during lactation, lactation length, estrous detection routine (especially the interval between weaning and starting estrous checks)	Body condition at weaning and prior to farrowing, estrous detection methods	Slaughter examination to confirm anestrus and to defect pathologic conditions, e.g., metritis, retained fetus	Serum progesterone analysis to confirm anestrus or to assess cyclic activity during lactation
Regular returns	Season (boar infertility during cold winter months), boar usage, percentage of multiple matings, individual boar fertility with single-boar mating systems	Estrous detection routine (after weaning and 18–24 days after breeding), hand-mating technique, quality of coitus, vaginal discharge (hemorrhagic or purulent)	Boar fertility examination, slaughter examination (especially with repeat breeders)	Vaginal cultures, serum progesterone analysis to confirm return to estrus
Delayed returns	Season (especially late summer months), litter size of females that remain pregnant, boar usage, exposure to porcine parvovirus (PPV), parity	Gestational housing, light, vaginal discharges, body condition, effective environmental temperature	Boar fertility and slaughter examination, ultrasonic pregnancy diagnosis (especially Doppler method)	Prebreeding and postbreeding serotests for PPV, serum estrone sulfate analysis to determine if pregnancy was initially established, serum progesterone analysis, vaginal cultures
Return to estrus—pen mating	Season (boar infertility because of cold weather), boar rotation, boar-to-female ratio (factors listed previously under regular and delayed returns)	Daily estrous checks, dominance pattern in boars, postmating bleeding (factors listed previously under regular and delayed returns)	Boar fertility examination with emphasis on detecting penile injuries and libido (factors listed previously under regular and delayed returns)	Tests listed previously under regular and delayed returns
Not pregnant via ultrasound pregnancy test	Factors listed previously under regular returns and delayed returns; with penmating, also include anestrus in gilts and postweaning anestrus; percentage that farrow (false-negatives)	Operator technique, comparison with another instrument, heat detection routine after mating (the number of negative pregnancy tests should not exceed the number of regular returns)	Slaughter examination	Serum estrone sulfate to confirm pregnancy (must be done at 25–30 days after mating)

Table continued on opposite page

Table 2. Investigation of Swine Reproductive Failure: Historical Information, On-farm Observations and Diagnostic Methods *Continued*

Primary Complaint	Historical Information	On-farm Observations	Special Examinations	Laboratory Tests
Failure to farrow (not-in-pig) following positive pregnancy diagnosis	Pregnant or nonpregnant appearance, associated small litters, mummies and stillbirths, new source of virus, parity	Pregnancy diagnosis techniques, heat detection routine during gestation, ability to observe abortions	Slaughter examination especially to detect fetal mummification	Analysis of diet for mycotoxins, estrone sulfate to confirm pregnancy diagnosis, serotests for PPV, pseudorabies, enterovirus
Abortions	Season (autumn and winter), yearly feed intake per sow, vaccination status for leptospirosis and pseudorabies, parity	Light, body condition, effective environmental temperature, ability to observe abortions		Mycotoxin analysis of feed; serotests for leptospirosis, brucellosis, pseudorabies, (eperythrozoonosis) and PPV; examination of placental fetal tissue and fetal fluids for infectious agents or antibody
Mummified fetuses	Parity, exposure to PPV, enterovirus, PRV and mycotoxin-containing feeds; failure to farrow and small litters in contemporary females	Exposure of gilts to the breeding herd prior to mating	Crown-rump length for estimation of fetal age at death (age in days = 21.07 + [3.11 × length in centimeters])	Serotests for PPV, PRV and enterovirus; examination of mummies for presence of virus by fluorescent antibody technique or virus isolation; analysis of feed for mycotoxins
Stillbirths	Parity, age of sows, failure to farrow, mummies or small litters in contemporary females, ambient temperature prior to farrowing	Environmental temperatures, presence of unvented heaters, ventilation, farrowing duration, antepartum (type I) versus intrapartum (type II) stillbirths	Air concentration of carbon monoxide, carbon dioxide and oxygen, post-mortem examination to differentiate between true stillbirth versus found dead (lung expansion with air) and detection of carbon monoxide poisoning, hemoglobin status of sows	Mycotoxin analysis of feed, nutrient analysis of diets (especially calcium and phosphorus levels with relationship to prolonged farrowings); maternal and fetal serotests and fetal tissue examination for leptospirosis, PPV, PRV, enterovirus and eperythrozoonosis
Small litters	Breed, crossbreeding, female heterosis, parity (especially first and second), per cent multiple matings, lactation length, sow-cull rates, boar usage, mummies, stillbirth and failure to farrow in contemporaries	Hand-mating techniques, housing, body condition	Weaning interval versus litter size, ovulation rate via slaughter examination	
Vaginal discharges	Days after mating, association with infertility, association with a certain boar	Sanitation in mating area, boar pens, sow stalls and AI equipment; hand-mating techniques	Speculum examination to determine origin of discharge, necropsy examination of preputial diverticulum	Vaginal culture, semen and preputial diverticulum culture if a certain boar is incriminated

Table 3. Breeding Herd Record Parameters Used to Detect Reproductive Problems

Parameter	Target Level	Interference Level
Sow inventory	Weekly farrowing × 26	—
Gilt inventory	Gilt breedings per week × 1.2 to 1.5 × weeks in gilt pool*	—
Boar inventory	Female inventory ÷ 20	—
Number bred per week	Expected farrowings ÷ farrowing rate	—
Sows	80 to 85% of total breedings	—
Gilts	15 to 20% of total breedings	—
Percentage of sows in estrus by 10 days postweaning	90%	85%
Regular returns	4%	10%
Delayed returns	1%	2.5%
Negative pregnancy diagnosis	4%	Should be less than the per cent of regular returns
Abortion	1%	2.5%
Not-in-pig	1%	2.5%
Farrowing rate	90%	85%
Sows farrowed per week	—	—
Live births/litter	10.5	10.0
Stillbirths	5%	8%
Mummies	0.5%	1%
Litter scatter (< 8 pigs/litter)	10%	15%
Weaned/litter	9.5	9.0
Preweaning mortality	8%	12%
Litters/sow/year	2.2	2.0
Pigs/sow/year	20.0	18.0

*Factor of 1.2 to 1.5 depends on the percentage of selected gilts that are eventually serviced.

3. Hand mating hygiene, quality of coitus, boar libido, postcoital bleeding.

4. Boar handling and usage.

5. Postbreeding management, especially feeding and animal movement.

6. Postbreeding estrous detection.

7. Pregnancy diagnosis (if used).

8. Gilt pool management (especially mixing, movement and boar exposure for estrous stimulation).

9. Observation of abnormal situations, e.g., discharges, abortions, sows not-in-pig.

10. Disease and parasite control.

OBSERVATIONS OF BREEDING HERD PERSONNEL

The ability of breeding herd personnel to observe and to record abnormal situations is the key factor in detecting reproductive failure. Occasionally, confusion occurs over the definitions of terms used to describe and to categorize these observations and events. Terms and definitions that are commonly used to describe abnormal breeding herd events are listed in Table 1. The attending veterinarian should be involved with training new employees to use these terms correctly and to reinforce this initial training with periodic reviews.

ROUTINE LABORATORY MONITORING

Currently, most efforts are directed toward monitoring the infectious disease status of the breeding herd. Future refinements of other diagnostic tests, especially hormone assays, may facilitate pregnancy diagnosis before day 20, litter size determination and prediction of impending reproductive failure. The following program is suggested as a primary monitor of the health and nutritional status of the breeding herd:

1. Incoming animals should be quarantined and serotested for pseudorabies, brucellosis, leptospirosis, eperythrozoonosis, *Haemophilus* pleuropneumonia, transmissible gastroenteritis (TGE) and porcine parvovirus. Interpretation of these tests is discussed in Physical Examination of New Boars Introduced to the Herd.

2. Yearly testing of at least ten breeding-age animals for the previous diseases is advised. Validation of pseudorabies and brucellosis may be advisable in herds that sell breeding stock.

3. Continued serotesting of breeding-age gilts for porcine parvovirus is suggested, especially in unvaccinated herds. The desired situation is the natural seroconversion of gilts prior to breeding.

4. Periodic examination of feces for evidence of internal parasites to assess the efficacy of control programs. It is possible to maintain pigs free of ascarids without using anthelmintics in totally confined herds. Fecal examinations are especially nec-

essary to reconfirm continually this parasite-free status.

5. Routine diet analysis will identify errors in ration formulation, inadequate mixing, malfunctions in delivery systems and poor quality feedstuffs.

SUMMARY

This article has outlined methods for the detection of reproductive problems and the diagnosis of their specific causes. Often, an exact diagnosis is not achieved. In these cases, the adoption of sound reproductive management practices and disease control programs may remedy the situation without actually determining the cause. However, reproductive problems are encountered in well-managed herds in which the latest accepted technologies are utilized. These cases present a diagnostic challenge that requires our best efforts.

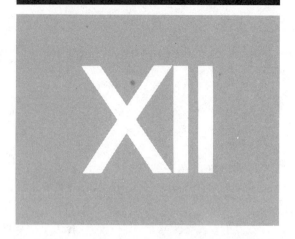

SECTION

XII

LABORATORY ANIMALS

Emerson D. Colby, D.V.M.

Consulting Editor

The Rabbit

Emerson D. Colby, D.V.M., M.S.

Dartmouth Medical School, Hanover, New Hampshire

The rabbit, *Oryctolagus cuniculus,* is of the family Lagomorpha. It is easily kept as a pet and is trainable to some degree. The animals reproduce easily in captivity, with two or more litters per year being the norm. There are many breeds, both large and small, and rabbits are shown by purebred breeders. The larger breeds, New Zealand White, Dutch Belted, Chinchilla and others generally weigh 10 to 15 lb and smaller breeds, most notably the Polish, weigh 5 to 7 lb. The male is a buck, and the female is a doe. The process of parturition is called kindling. Several facts about the rabbit's reproductive life are summarized in Table 1.

ANATOMY

The female reproductive tract is divided into two separate horns, and each has a separate cervix entering the vagina. There is no chance for a crossover of eggs within the uterus. The position of the ovaries is similar to that of either the cat or the dog. Identification of the female is done in a manner common to identifying the sex in other species of animals.

The male has retractable testes, and because of the fur surrounding the scrotal sac, misrepresentation of sex sometimes occurs in the adult animal. The penis in the male may be found to actually overlay the anus in the adult. Male rabbits can be vasectomized or can be orchiectomized by incising the scrotum over each testicle, retracting the organ and surgically excising it and tying off the appropriate structures in the process.

MAMMARY GLANDS

The rabbit has eight pairs of mammary glands. Two glands are located between the front legs. All glands are usually well developed and functional. Does do not normally spend a lot of time nursing and in fact may not nurse more than once per day. The mammary tissue develops rapidly during the last week of pregnancy. Milk letdown may not be apparent until after kindling. The average total daily milk yield may range from 150 to 200 gm/day with the first litter and then increase with subsequent litters. Maximum milk yield usually takes place during the second and third weeks of nursing.

Table 1. Reproductive Characteristics of the Rabbit

Feature	Comments
Sexual maturity	Male: 8 to 9 months; female: 5 to 9 months (seasonal influence)
Estrous cycle	Constant—rhythmic cycling every 4 to 6 days
Ovulation time	10 to 13 hours after mating
Gestation period	31 to 32 days
Mean litter size	Seven to nine, first litter small
Mean litter weight	42 to 55 gm
Weaning age	8 weeks (about 4 lb body weight)
Number of mammary glands	Eight (four pairs)
Body temperature	39.5°C (101°F)
Chromosome number	44
Heart rate	250/bpm resting (increases when handled or disturbed)
Complete blood count	Hb: 9.4 to 13.8 gm/100 ml. Hct: 30 to 42 ml/100 ml. WBC: 2.6 to 11.8/mm³
Food consumption	5 gm/100 gm body weight/day
Coprophagy	Normal; may be observed in young (as early as 3 weeks)
Nutrition	Commercial feed and good quality roughage (hay)
Pseudopregnancy	16 to 19 days
Sperm capacitation time	6 hours
Fertilization time postovulation	1 to 2 hours
Whole blood volume	55 to 57 ml/kg body weight
Number of females/breeding male	8 to 12/1

HOUSING

Rabbits should be housed in a manner that keeps them free of drafts in cold weather and allows for good ventilation during the summer months. Caging should be large enough for mating purposes, so that when the buck mounts the doe there is head room for the encounter. There should also be enough space for the male to get away from the female during a mating encounter, as fighting may occur if the female is not ready (in estrus) or after mating. The cage should be large enough so that the doe may kindle, which will require a small box or other enclosure allowing for privacy. Environmental disturbances will often cause the female to disregard her offspring or to cannabalize them. Body hair is pulled by the female during the nest-making process.

NUTRITION

The average female rabbit will consume 5 gm of feed/100 gm of body weight per day. This amount will increase during gestation and will be two to three times the normal rate during lactation. As most rabbits are fed ad libitum, this is usually not a problem. Fresh water must always be available. Fresh green produce or carrots may be fed, but this is not necessary if commercial rabbit chow is the standard diet. Excessive vitamin A will often cause fetal abnormalities.

PUBERTY

Puberty varies with the breed of the rabbit. The smaller breeds mature earlier and the larger breeds later. Females are sexually competent earlier than the males. The season of the year in which the rabbit is born will also make a difference in the age at puberty. Rabbits born in the fall will generally reach puberty in 5 to 6 months, while rabbits born in the spring attain puberty in 8 to 9 months.

ESTRUS

Domestic rabbits do not show a regular estrous cycle but rather a rhythm. These rhythmic periods, or cycles, do occur at 4- to 6-day intervals and do correlate with periods of peak blood estrogen levels and are indicative of estrus and its associated vaginal cytology. Vaginal smears are not reliable indicators of estrus in the rabbit and, when the procedure is performed, may induce pseudopregnancy; therefore, they are rarely used. Receptivity by the female is usually established by placing her with the male. Breeding will always take place immediately if she is in estrus. This sexual receptivity is not present as long as the mammary glands are active and pups are nursing. Postpartum receptivity varies with the numbers of young born, and nursing will only last

for a very brief period of 1 to 3 days. Congestion of the vulva may be noted during estrus or following mating. This, also, is not a good indicator of the estrous state. Wild rabbits do show a period of true anestrous or estrous inactivity.

MATING

Mating is best accomplished by placing a female in the cage of the male. If the reverse is done, the male may not copulate, as the males are very territorial, and mating efficiency is significantly reduced when the male is placed in unfamiliar surroundings. It is best to observe the mating act, which usually takes place immediately when the female is in estrus and is placed with the male. The females are usually removed immediately after breeding has taken place. A plug is formed following copulation. It is soft, disappears rapidly and is rarely observed. Vulvar congestion does not indicate a fertile mating. Some fluid may be noted in the vulva, but it must be remembered that an initial ejaculate of a male can have a copious amount of seminal fluid.

OVULATION

The rabbit is a postcoital ovulator. Mating causes a rapid increase in the size of the follicles in either ovary, and ovulation usually follows mating by 6 to 10 hours. Ova have a fertilizable life of about 6 hours postcoitus. The mature follicle is about 1.5 mm in diameter and polyovular follicles are not uncommon. Twinning in the rabbit is unknown. Pregnant females have been known to be receptive to the male and allow mating but do not ovulate.

Eosinophilic lipoid inclusions are common in the interstitial cells of the ovary. Among mammals this phenomenon is peculiar to the rabbit.

Ovulation can also be induced by the sight of a sexually active male, a female mounting another female and excessive handling by the owner. Pseudopregnancy will ensue unless the ova are fertilized. Serum luteinizing hormone (LH) peaks about 1 to 2 hours after mating. Purified pituitary luteinizing hormone can be given intravenously at a dose of 2.5 mg/2 to 3 kg body weight to induce ovulation. It is usually not required.

GESTATION

Gestation is generally 31 to 32 days in the average domestic rabbit. A range of 30 to 35 days may be breed dependent. The vagina will enlarge during pregnancy. Pregnancy can be determined by palpation at about 9 days. Radiography may be used for pregnancy diagnosis as early as day 11. Bone structure in the fetus may not be apparent until the last days prior to parturition. The conception rate is higher during the spring breeding season.

There is a period during the normal pregnancy when the uterus enlarges significantly. This appears to be at approximately 22 days of gestation. Stress, in the form of environmental change, drug administration or rough handling may cause the fetuses to either be aborted or resorbed.

The fetuses are fully formed at 17 days of gestation. Litter size is smaller in the small breeds, in which four is the average, with larger breeds averaging many more—eight to ten.

PSEUDOPREGNANCY

This is not an uncommon circumstance in the rabbit. It can be induced by rough handling of the animal, mounting by another female, taking a vaginal smear or using a vasectomized male. The condition produces a persistent corpus luteum for about 2 weeks. At 16 to 19 days of pseudopregnancy the female will begin to behave as though she were about to undergo a normal parturition, with nest building and fur pulling apparent. At this time the female may very well be receptive to the male and if mated, will become pregnant.

KINDLING (PARTURITION)

Parturition usually takes place during the early morning hours. Rabbit pups are presented normally in both the anterior and the breeched positions. Kindling usually requires less than 30 minutes, but occasionally several hours or more will be noted between births. Pups that are retained beyond 35 days will die and if not expelled, will prevent the subsequent pregnancy. There is a definite sequence pertaining to litter size. The largest litters are born to rabbits during their second and third pregnancies, and smallest litters occur with the first pregnancy. Also, there is a definite relationship between ambient temperature and pregnancy and number of offspring. The smallest number of pregnancies and similarly the smallest number of young born are a result of mating during the months of the year with the highest environmental temperature. The reverse is true of mating during the cooler months of the year. This relationship does not appear to be influenced by light.

POSTPARTUM BREEDING

The postpartum pregnancy rate appears to be the inverse of the litter size. The smaller the litter, the greater the chance of the animal's conceiving. Not all does will mate. If the young are removed immediately after delivery, the does will mate and conceive. Rabbits are normally rebred immediately after weaning. A prolonged nursing period causes considerable reduction in the size of the ovaries and, thus, the reduction of numbers in the next wave of follicles to be released.

CESAREAN SECTION

Cesarean sections may be done as in the cat or the dog. A wide variety of anesthetics may be used. Ketamine and xylazine (in combination: 35 and 5 mg/kg body weight, respectively) works well as does premedication with xylazine (3 mg/kg body weight) followed by anesthesia to effect with halothane. Methoxyflurane is not recommended. Rabbits will not vomit when given xylazine and usually do not bother postoperative suture materials. Flank incisions are recommended because of the rapid mammary milk flow, the method of nursing, often only once per day, and hygienic considerations.

ORPHANED RABBITS

A variety of methods have been used to raise orphaned pups. Some have been fostered on other does. This may be best accomplished by removing all of the rabbits of a litter and freely mixing the pups to be fostered with the does' litter and then replacing. It must be kept in mind that there are only eight nipples available for the litter.

The orphaned pups may also be hand reared by feeding them a formula. Puppy formula may be used. Cow's milk may cause uncontrollable diarrhea. The method of administration may be by a stomach tube, usually a No. 5 French catheter, or by using a doll's bottle or a pipette with a rubber bulb on the end. Regardless of the method used, only about 5 ml of formula per day should be given to the neonate. This should be in three to four divided doses throughout the course of the day. This volume may be increased during the second week and so on. Aspiration pneumonia is always a problem that may be encountered. Warm cotton must be used initially to stimulate fecal evacuation and to keep the rabbit clean. The temperature of the diet should be approximately 85°F (29°C) and should be administered very slowly.

Rabbit milk contains 12.3 per cent protein, 13.1 per cent fat, 1.9 per cent lactose and 2.3 per cent minerals. It is richer than cow's milk. Rabbit pups that are about 50 gm in body weight at birth have the greatest potential for survival.

ARTIFICIAL INSEMINATION

Artificial insemination can be done with a high rate of fertilization. This technique has been developed as a result of a need for gnotobiotic rabbits raised for research purposes. Semen from several rabbits are usually pooled prior to insemination.

References

1. Harkness JE, Wagner JE: The Biology and Medicine of Rabbits and Rodents. Philadelphia, Lea & Febiger, 1977, pp 10–13.
2. Cole HH, Cupps PT: Reproduction in Domestic Animals. New York, Academic Press, 1969, pp 484–485.

3. Weisbroth SH, Flatt RE, Kraus AL: The Biology of the Laboratory Rabbit. New York, Academic Press, 1974, pp 24–30.
4. Hafez ESE: Reproduction in Farm Animals. Philadelphia, Lea & Febiger, 1974, p 123.
5. Hamilton CE: Evidences of cyclic reproductive phenomena in the rabbit. Anat. Rec. 110:557, 1951.
6. Doggett VC: Periodicity in the fecundity of male rabbits. Am J Physiol 187:445, 1956.
7. Hamner CE: The semen. In Hafex ESE (ed): Reproduction and Breeding Techniques for Laboratory Animals. Philadelphia, Lea & Febiger, 1970, pp 56–73.
8. Staples RE, Holtkamp DE: Influence of body weight upon corpus luteum formation and maintenance of pregnancy in the rabbit. J Reprod Fert 12:221, 1966.
9. Sanford TD, Colby ED: Effect of xylazine and ketamine on blood pressure, heart rate and respiratory rate in rabbits. Lab Anim Sci 30:519, 1980.

The Hamster

Melvin W. Balk, D.V.M., M.S.
Gilbert M. Slater

Charles River Laboratories, Inc.,
Wilmington, Massachusetts

Hamsters are members of the order Rodentia and are native to temperate regions of Europe and Asia. Although there are over 60 subspecies of the true hamster, the vast majority of those seen as pets or used in medical research are one of the following:

1. The Syrian or Golden hamster (*Mesocricetus auratus*)
2. The Chinese or Gray-Striped hamster (*Cricetus griseus*)
3. The European or Black hamster (*Cricetus cricetus*). This hamster has a black belly and brown dorsum.

The Golden hamster is the most popular animal of these three and can be found frequently as a pet and is widely used in biomedical research. This hamster has been inbred by several investigators, and the color of the animal can range from albino, in some of the inbred strains, to very dark brown and generally has a light gray ventral surface. The majority of the Golden hamsters, however, are the same color as its name (Fig. 1). General husbandry and production information is summarized in Table 1.

PUBERTY

The hamster reaches puberty at a very young age, and although sexual maturity is usually reported in the Golden Syrian hamster as early as 42 days, occasional animals are actually sexually mature and can begin to reproduce as early as 1 month of age (Fig. 2). When litters of hamsters are kept together following weaning, the possibility of inadvertent reproduction is a real possibility. In general, the female Syrian hamster should be 8 to 10 weeks of age and the male hamster 12 weeks of age before reproduction takes place. Sexually mature hamsters can be differentiated from each other based on differences in the external genitalia (Fig. 3).

SEXUAL BEHAVIOR

The female hamster is extremely pugnacious when in the company of the male hamster. In most cases unless the female is sexually receptive, she will not tolerate the presence of the male.

ESTROUS CYCLE

The estrous cycle of the female hamster is very regular and lasts 4 days. There is an obvious external indication of this cycle, which includes the presence of a white, opaque, stringy postestrous discharge on day 2 of the cycle and a waxy secretion that can be found on day 3. In the vagina of the hamster are two lateral pouches that contain cornified epithelial cells. This anatomic finding precludes the use of routine vaginal smears from hamsters to follow the estrous cycle as one would in other female mammals.

MATING OF THE GOLDEN SYRIAN HAMSTER

When the female is exhibiting peak estrus, she will tolerate the male's presence, and lordosis takes place almost immediately once the male is intro-

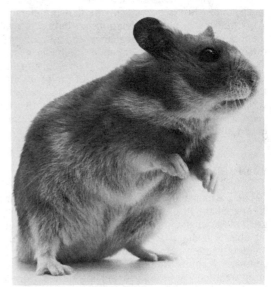

Figure 1. Representative appearance of an adult Golden Syrian hamster with the characteristic posture of a healthy animal.

Table 1. Basic Husbandry and Production Information for the Golden Syrian Hamster

Feature	Comments
Species	Hamster *(Mesocricetus auratus)*
Color	Brown and white
Inbred/outbred	Outbred
Breeding size (male)	100 to 120 gm
Breeding size (female)	80 to 100 gm
Breeding age (male)	12 weeks
Breeding age (female)	8 to 10 weeks
Mating system	Monogamous
Estrous cycle	4 days
Age at onset	6 to 7 weeks
Gestation period	15½ days
Average litter size	10 to 12
Birth weight	1.5 to 2.0 gm
Weaning weight (male)	35 to 40 gm
Weaning weight (female)	35 to 40 gm
Weaning age	21 days
Daily weight gain (male)	3 to 5 gm
Daily weight gain (female)	3 to 5 gm
Breeders retired (male)	12 months
Breeders retired (female)	6 months
Breeders retired (male)	120 to 160 gm
Breeders retired (female)	120 to 160 gm
50 per cent survivability	18 to 24 months
Bedding used	Hardwood chips/5 per cent shavings
Food analysis: Protein	22.4 per cent
Fat	5 per cent
Room temperature	74±2°F
Relative humidity	55±10 per cent
Lighting cycle	On 1:00 AM—off 3:30 PM
Expected weight loss in transit	5 per cent
Average daily food consumption	3 to 5 gm
Average daily water intake	10 ml

Golden Syrian Hamster

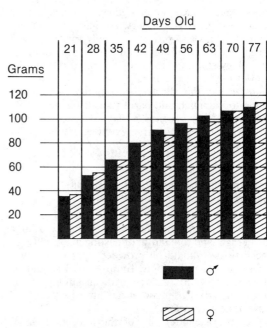

Figure 2. Growth chart of male and female hamsters as a function of age. It should be noted that adult female hamsters are generally larger than males.

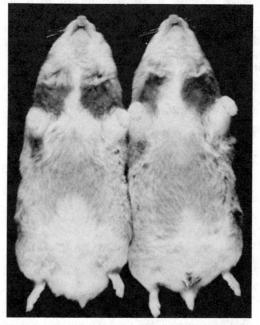

Figure 3. Comparative differences of male and female sexually mature hamsters. The male (left) has testicles that fill the scrotum and partially occlude the tail. The female (right) has an obvious external genital opening that is usually moist following urination.

duced into the cage. Copulation will take place and usually lasts for up to 30 minutes. In most cases, matings are monogamous because of the extremely aggressive behavior of the female hamster.

MATING OF THE CHINESE HAMSTER

The breeding of this particular hamster is much more difficult than that of the Golden hamster because of the disposition of the female Chinese hamster. The male must sometimes be provided protection from the female, and this has been accomplished by providing a safe haven in the form of an 8- to 10-inch section of 1¼ inch pipe in which he can hide. In many cases if a hiding place is not provided, the female will kill the male Chinese hamster.

CONCEPTION, FETAL DEVELOPMENT AND GESTATION

Implantation of the fertilized ova of the hamster takes place on the sixth day after coitus. Hence, care should be exercised in handling hamsters during the sixth day following breeding. Once implantation takes place, embryogenesis proceeds very rapidly for the next 36 hours. At that point organogenesis begins and proceeds rapidly for the next 3 days. The hamster has been used quite often in teratology studies because of the rapid differentiation of the embryo during day 8 of gestation. The hamster has the shortest gestation cycle of any laboratory animal, and parturition takes place 15½ days after coitus (coitus is day 0). The gestation period is *very regular,* varying only ± 2 hours under normal circumstances.

PREPARTURIENT CARE OF THE DAM AND NEONATAL CARE

The gravid female should be transferred to a clean cage, and some form of nesting material (e.g., facial tissue) should be provided approximately 2 days prior to parturition. Enough food should be provided for 7 to 10 days, with an attempt made not to disturb the female or her litter for at least 7 days after parturition.

The average litter size of the hamster is nine, with a range of 4 to 16.

CANNIBALISM

Most first litters are smaller than subsequent litters, and cannibalism can be high in the first litter. It is not, however, restricted to the first litter, and unless care is taken to minimize disturbances it can be a continuing problem. It is extremely important to leave the female undisturbed for the first 7 to 10 days to maximize the chances of survival of the litter.

NEONATAL ANATOMY

The following characteristics are present in newborn hamsters:
1. Teeth are present at birth.
2. They are hairless at birth.
3. Eyes and ears are closed at birth.
4. Ears open first at 4 to 5 days of age.
5. The eyes open at around 14 days of age.
6. They begin to eat solid food at around 7 to 10 days of age.
7. The young animal should not be handled until the female allows the young animals to move around the cage on their own, which is around 18 days of age.

At 10 days of age an extra source of moisture should be provided for young hamsters. A long sipper tube and water bottle that reaches to within ½ inch of the bedding material or some vegetables, an alternative source of water, and nesting material should be provided. If vegetables are provided, care should be taken to remove excess material before it spoils.

WEANING

Hamsters are weaned at approximately 3 weeks of age, and the female is usually remated at this time. Female hamsters will usually mate on the second or third day after weaning.

REPRODUCTIVE LIFE

The reproductive life of the hamster is optimal between 2 and 10 months of age, with a significant depression in reproduction after 1 year of age. During this time the hamster will produce approximately four to six litters of pups.

NUTRITIONAL DEFICIENCIES AND REPRODUCTION

The hamster is particularly susceptible to vitamin E deficiency, which manifests itself in severe muscular degeneration, loss of body weight and reproductive failure and early death. Specifically formulated diets for laboratory rodents should be used as a primary nutritional source for the hamster, and care must be taken to adhere to the proper storage and expiration dates of the laboratory ration.

LIFE SPAN

Hamsters will live for 1 to 3 years, with 18 to 24 months as the norm. Animals over 15 months of age are considered to be senescent, based on histological evidence.

URINALYSIS

The urine of the hamster is normally a milky-white color and has a very high specific gravity. Although urinalysis from a clinical diagnostic viewpoint is not routinely done in the hamster, the appearance of normal hamster urine can cause concern for those individuals not familiar with this information.

HIBERNATION

Hamsters will hibernate when the temperature reaches 48°F or lower and remains constant with respect to temperature and humidity. In fact, the hibernation may be so complete that the hamster may be mistaken for dead. The respiration rate can go as low as 1 to 2 respirations/minute and the heart rate reduced to 6/minute from the normal of 200 to 300/minute.

REPRODUCTIVE RECORDS

Reproductive records and genealogies should be maintained for any well-managed colony. Each breeding female should carry with her a record of matings and the number of offspring weaned from each mating. A future breeder should be selected from a second or later litters with good litter size. Males should also have records of infertile matings, so that poor-producing males can be eliminated.

A good production colony can be expected to produce 1.6 offspring/breeding female/week.

FLANK GLAND

There are sebaceous glands located in the lateral flank areas of the male hamsters, and it is speculated that these are secondary sex glands and/or pheromone producing glands for olfactory identification of territory.

ANTIBIOTIC SENSITIVITY

Hamsters, similar to guinea pigs, develop endotoxemia, which is often fatal, following the administration of a variety of antibiotics. Antibiotics such as erythromycin, tetracycline, penicillin and gentamicin are all contraindicated in the hamster. Following antibiotic administration by usual routes of administration, a significant shift in the microflora of the intestinal tract occurs. This usually results in an enterocolitis, diarrhea and subsequent death. Antibiotics in general are contraindicated for the hamster.

Suggested Reading

1. Hoffman RA, Robinson PF, Magalhaes H: The Golden Hamster, Its Biology and Use in Medical Research. Ames, Iowa State University Press, 1968.

The Gerbil

Donald G. Robinson, Jr., B.S.
Tumblebrook Farm, Inc.,
West Brookfield, Massachusetts

The Mongolian gerbil, or black-clawed jird, *Meriones unguiculatus,* was introduced to the United States as a new experimental animal by Dr. Victor Schwentker of Tumblebrook Farm, Inc., in 1954. Since then, this species has continued to demonstrate a wide range of usefulness in many fields of biomedical research. Its docility, cleanliness and ease of maintenance have also made it popular as a pet. Because it is a relatively new laboratory animal, the practitioner may have to adapt existing procedures or to extrapolate dosages from the literature of other laboratory rodents if the desired data are not available for the gerbil.

PHYSICAL DETERMINATION OF THE MALE AND FEMALE

The functional anatomy of the Mongolian gerbil is similar to that of the laboratory rat (Figs. 1 and 2). In the gerbil, however, the ampullary glands are not as well defined, and the preputial glands are either absent or difficult to locate.

PUBERTY AND SEXUAL AND MATERNAL BEHAVIOR

Data concerning the ages of sexual maturity and other statistics of reproductive behavior are summarized in Table 1.

In the wild, gerbils are polygamous, and most litters are born in the spring and summer. In captivity, they breed throughout the year with little or no seasonal periodicity.

An accurate determination of the gerbil's estrous cycle (4 to 6 days) is difficult, partly because of aggressive behavior when virgin females are repeatedly faced by a strange mate. The vaginal smear has at least three distinct phases: (1) The smear shows almost entirely leukocytes with occasionally a few epithelial and cornified cells; (2) an abundance of epithelial cells is evident and (3) almost entirely cornified cells are present.

Pairing of a male with a female often results in estrus within a few days; estrous behavior may also be induced by sequential treatment with estradiol and progesterone. The male-induced estrus may be a factor that complicates an accurate determination of the estrous cycle.

The majority of matings occur in the late afternoon and at night. The female exhibits lordosis and permits the male to copulate many times; the male's vigorous pursuits are often accompanied by rapid foot-thumping sounds. A small copulation plug is formed, but it lies deep in the vagina and is not easily detected.

The incidence of postpartum matings is about 60 per cent; most of these matings occur within a day following parturition, and the majority (86 per cent) of these are fertile matings.

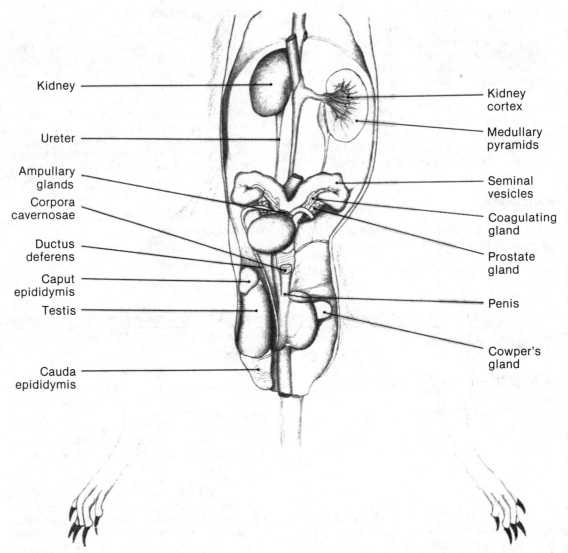

Figure 1. Male reproductive organs. (After Williams WM: The Anatomy of the Mongolian Gerbil [*Meriones unguiculatus*]. West Brookfield, Tumblebrook Farm Inc, 1974, p 107.)

ARTIFICIAL INSEMINATION

Techniques used for artificial insemination in rats or mice can be used with the gerbil, although the success rate to date is only about 50 per cent. Females are given hormone preparations (pregnant mare serum and human chorionic gonadotropin), then they are surgically inseminated with a sperm suspension obtained by flushing one cauda epididymis.

CONCEPTION, FETAL DEVELOPMENT AND PREGNANCY DIAGNOSIS

The corpora lutea of the gerbil are prominent and easy to count under the microscope. Ovulation is generally spontaneous but can be induced by vaginal stimulation. Ovulation occurs 6 to 10 hours after mating. Fertilization is usually effected within 3 hours of ovulation, and the first cleavage division is completed about 24 hours after ovulation. The eggs enter the uterus between 106 and 130 hours, and the embryos are implanted by about 154 hours after ovulation.

A period of pseudopregnancy lasting 13 to 23 days may occur following sterile mating or cervical stimulation; it may also occur spontaneously in paired females. Delayed implantation occurs following postpartum mating if more than two young are being suckled. A large litter may prolong the gestation period (normally 24 to 26 days) and the intervals between parturitions.

Pregnancy can be determined by palpation within a week or more prior to parturition. Within a few days before parturition, the female usually exhibits a general distention of the abdominal area, and often the fetuses will show as one or more external bulges laterally.

EFFECTS OF ENVIRONMENTAL FACTORS ON REPRODUCTION

Limited studies of the gerbil's nutritional needs show that the commercial pelleted feeds for laboratory rodents are adequate for reproductive needs if a protein content of at least 17 per cent is provided; also, a low-fat content (approximately 4 per cent) appears to be desirable.

Factors such as noise and light intensity or light cycle, within limits considered normal by human comfort standards, do not seem of critical importance. The same is true for ambient temperature and humidity, although it is known that reproduction diminishes at the lower temperatures, and a deprivation of drinking water will result in a cessation of reproduction.

EFFECTS OF DISEASES ON REPRODUCTIVE PERFORMANCE

Gerbils are subject to Tyzzer's disease, salmonellosis and nasal (staphylococcal) dermatitis, but the

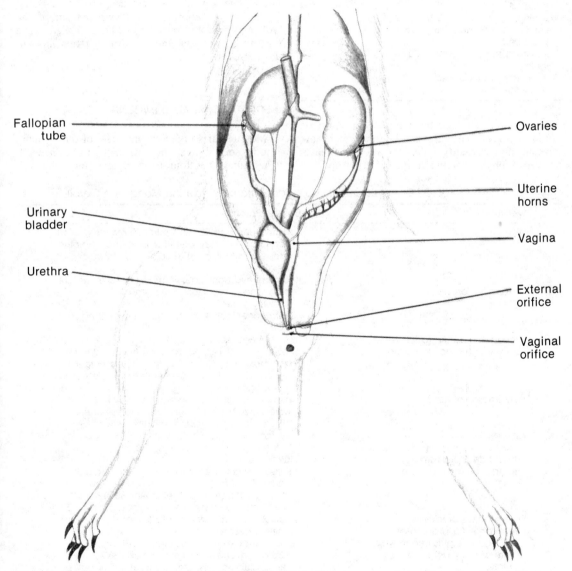

Figure 2. Female reproductive organs. (After Williams WM: The Anatomy of the Mongolian Gerbil [*Meriones unguiculatus*]. West Brookfield, Tumblebrook Farm Inc, 1974, p 107.)

Table 1. Summary of Reproductive Data for the Mongolian Gerbil

Characteristics	Comments
Testes descend	30 to 40 days
Vagina opens	40 to 76 days
Sexual maturity	65 to 85 days
Breeding age	2.5 to 22 months
Estrous cycle	4 to 6 days
Female receptivity	1 to 12 hours after light onset
Duration of female receptivity	5 to 24 hours
Mean ovulation rate	6.6 ova (range 4 to 9)
Gestation period	24 to 26 days
Prenatal mortality	32 per cent
Female weight gain during pregnancy	23 to 36 gm
Mean litter size	4 to 5 (range 1 to 13)
Sex ratio (males to females)	1.03 at birth, 1.00 at weaning
Weaning age	20 to 30 days
Mean number of litters produced	7.6 ± 3.8
Mean number of young	37 ± 20
Age of female at last parturition	462 ± 196 days

effects on reproduction have not been reported. Often these diseases are self-limiting, with low mortality and morbidity, unless the affected animals are very young or debilitated for some reason.

There is some evidence that, as in the rat, continued monogamous breeding may produce reproductive stress in the female that can be detrimental to the animal's health as well as lessening the reproductive performance.

Cystic ovaries in older females can impede reproductive performance significantly. Continued inbreeding can have the same effect and may also be associated with cystic ovaries, so that many inbred strains will die out by about the twelfth generation.

PARTURITION

Parturition usually occurs during the night; about 1 hour is required for delivery of an average-sized litter. The female usually consumes the placental tissues and stillborn fetuses. Cannibalism of the young is rare and may be caused by an excessive disturbance of the female, although this has not been proved.

NEONATAL CARE OF THE YOUNG

Most females take adequate care of their young, and no special precautions or materials are needed. The female has four pairs of teats, and she may

Table 2. Selected Dosages and Physiological Parameters for the Mongolian Gerbil

Feature	Dosage/Parameter
Anesthesia	Sodium pentobarbital: 0.01 ml of 60 mg/ml solution per 10 gm of body weight, with total dose not to exceed 0.10 ml; or 50 to 60 mg/kg of body weight Ketamine hydrochloride: 44 mg/kg of body weight
Antibiotic dosages	Tetracycline hydrochloride: 0.3 gm/100 ml in drinking water Chloramphenicol: 0.083 gm/100 ml in drinking water
Body temperature (adult, rectal)	38.2°C (range of 38.1 to 38.4°C)
Body weights (approximate)	At birth, 2.5 to 3.0 gm; at sexual maturity, 40 to 60 gm; maximum, 140 to 150 gm (male's weight is usually about 10 gm greater than female's at same age)
Chromosomal data	Diploid chromosome number (2n) = 44; 32 autosomes are metacentric or submetacentric, 10 are acrocentric; fundamental number (FN) = 78, including sex chromosomes
Food consumption (approximate)	5 to 8 gm/day/100 gm of body weight
Heart rate (approximate)	360/minute
Hemogram (normal gerbil)	Packed cell volume, 37 to 47 per cent; red cell count, 7 to 8 million/mm³; hemoglobin level, 14 to 16 gm/100 ml; white cell count, 8000 to 11,000/mm³; lymphocyte-to-neutrophil ratio, 3.5:1
Life span (approximate)	Mean, 2 years; maximum, 5 to 6 years
Respiration (approximate)	90/minute (resting)
Sex organ weights (mean weight/100 gm of body weight, adults)	Seminal vesicles and prostate, 946.70 mg; testes, 1.36 gm; ovaries, 98.30 mg; uterus, 233.70 mg
Urinalysis	Proteins, glucose, bilirubin and acetone are all undetectable in normal gerbil urine.
Water consumption (approximate)	4 to 7 ml/day/100 gm of body weight

divide a large litter into two groups for suckling. The male will also often assist in caring for the young.

Some preweaning deaths are common, and occasionally entire litters fail to survive. It is not known whether these deaths are caused by maternal neglect or by lactation failure.

The young may be suckled until about 4 weeks of age. They can eat solid food by about 16 days of age; rolled oats are a good transitional feed, if needed. Weaning should be done by 4 weeks of age to prevent competition from the arrival of a succeeding litter.

BREEDING COLONY MANAGEMENT

A monogamous mating system has proved to be the most effective for breeding gerbils. A solid-bottom cage of at least 144 square inches, with a bedding change at least every 2 weeks, is adequate for a pair and their litter. Pelleted feed and water should be provided ad lib (water need not be provided if adequate amounts of lettuce, carrot or apple are fed).

Breeders are often paired before the age of sexual maturity to minimize aggression. Usually, it is safe to leave the male with the female at all times. Once a mate is lost, the surviving animal may not accept another mate, and even if there is acceptance, there may not be reproduction. Breeders are generally retired at 12 to 15 months of age.

DIAGNOSTIC PROCEDURES AND PHYSIOLOGICAL PARAMETERS

Data concerning anesthesia, antibiotic dosages and normal physiological values for this species are given in Table 2. Blood can be taken from the heart using a ½- or ¾-inch 23- or 24-gauge needle. It may also be obtained from vessels at the medial canthus of the eye, using a capillary tube, or by nicking a lateral tail vein to collect the drops.

Surgical procedures such as castration and ovariectomy are routinely performed using techniques similar to those used for the rat or the mouse.

Selected Readings

1. Allanson M: Gerbils. In Hafez ESE (ed): Reproduction and Breeding Techniques in Laboratory Animals. Philadelphia, Lea & Febiger, 1970, pp 237–243.
2. Arrington LR, Beaty TC, Jr, Kelley KC: Growth, longevity and reproductive life of the Mongolian gerbil. Lab Anim Sci 23:262, 1973.
3. Harkness JE, Wagner JE: The Biology and Medicine of Rabbits and Rodents. 2nd ed. Philadelphia, Lea & Febiger, 1983.
4. Loew FM: The management and diseases of gerbils. In Current Veterinary Therapy III. Philadelphia, WB Saunders Co, 1968, p 426.
5. Marston JH, Chang MC: The breeding, management and reproductive physiology of the Mongolian gerbil, *Meriones unguiculatus*. Lab Anim Care 15:34, 1965.
6. Norris ML, Adams CE: Lifetime reproductive performance of Mongolian gerbils (*Meriones unguiculatus*) with 1 or 2 ovaries. Lab Anim 16:146, 1982.
7. Thiessen D, Yahr P: The Gerbil in Behavioral Investigations. Austin, University of Texas Press, 1977.
8. Williams WM: The Antomy of the Mongolian Gerbil (*Meriones unguiculatus*). West Brookfield, MA, Tumblebrook Farm, Inc., 1974.

The Rat

W. Sheldon Bivin, D.V.M.
Louisiana State University, Baton Rouge, Louisiana

Records indicate that the "Norway rat" or "Norwegian rat" *Rattus norvegicus* was popularized in the early 1800's in France and England for a sport entitled rat-baiting. This sport involved releasing large numbers of rats into an enclosure and recording the length of time required for a trained rat terrier to kill all of the rats. This demand for large numbers of rats soon exceeded local wild-caught supplies and resulted in selected albinos being propagated for show purposes and/or breeding.[39] The first known scientific breeding experiments with rats were performed in Germany in 1877–1885.[40] In 1892, the Wistar Institute in Philadelphia was established, and it was responsible for providing the major contributions on husbandry and reproduction in the rat. Much of what we know today about the rat originated at this institution. Because of the intensive research efforts of the Wistar Institute and many other institutes that have since evolved, the wild rat has been adapted to a laboratory environment. Today, we have in excess of 100 strains and substrains.

At least 35 million rats are used every year in practically every aspect of biologic research. The rat has also gained some popularity as a pet. In either case, the increased usage of this animal by man has placed demands upon the veterinary profession to provide adequate health care. It is the intent of this article to provide essential data and techniques required by the veterinarian to manage the theriogenologic problems of the rat.

PHYSICAL EXAMINATION

Perhaps the most important part of any physical examination is the recording of a thorough medical history. This information must contain complete information on the species, sex, age, genetic background and breeding status; the environment in which the animal is housed, including caging, bedding, sanitation, light cycles, ventilation, room temperature and humidity; and the diet of the animal and any previous medical diseases, treatments, vaccinations or breeding records.

The pet rat is usually tame and will rarely bite unless startled or hurt. Rats should be picked up by placing the hand firmly over the back and rib cage, and the head is controlled by squeezing the thumb and forefinger behind the mandibles. Because the tail skin may easily tear, the tail should be grasped only at the base.

The laboratory rat is characterized by a fusiform body covered by typical mammalian hair except for the nose, lips, ears, palms and soles. Other anatomic characteristics include a dental formula of two (I 1/1 C 0/0, PM 0/0, M 3/3) continuously erupting incisors, an open inguinal canal, a divided stomach, a large cecum, a diffuse pancreas, no gallbladder, masses of brown fat in the cervical and scapular areas and poor eyesight. Male rats exhibit a prolonged period of growth and ossification of the long bones, which is not complete until about 2 years of age. The female is usually smaller and matures within the first few months of life.

The female rat has 12 mammae, three pairs in the thoracic region and three pairs in the abdominal-inguinal area. Female nipples are usually visible when the young are between 8 and 15 days of age. In the adult the ovary appears as a mass of follicles, which lies close to the cranial pole of the kidney. A much convoluted oviduct connects the ovary with a bicornuate uterus (Fig. 1). Although the uterine horns appear to be fused distally, there are two distinct cervical canals opening into the vagina. The vagina is located dorsal to the urethra and is completely separate. The urethra does not enter the vagina or vestibule, as is seen in domestic animals.

Male rats have testicles that are evident at an early age, especially if the rat is held head up allowing the testis to drop into the scrotum. Obviously this means the male rat has retractile testes which can slip back into the abdomen through wide patent inguinal canals.

The epididymis is divided into three portions: the enlarged caput epididymis, a slender corpus epididymis lying on the dorsomedial aspect of the testis and the distal cauda epididymis. The latter gives rise to the ductus deferens, which passes through the inguinal canal and enters the urethra.

Within the pelvis and surrounding the bladder are five pairs of organs (Fig. 2): the glands of the ductus deferens; two pairs of prostate glands, one ventral and one dorsal to the ductus deferens; two large hood-shaped and convoluted seminal vesicles and within the same capsule, the coagulating glands.

The penis lies within a loose prepuce and has a single cartilaginous or bony process, the os penis.

Lying just beneath the skin of the prepuce and opening into its cavity is a pair of slender flattened preputial glands.

Newborn males have a larger genital papilla and a greater anogenital distance than females (5 mm in males and 2.5 mm in females at 7 days).

Other physiological values that are useful in evaluating the reproductive health status of a rat are given in Table 1. The values listed are approximations abstracted from several texts[5, 22, 48] and may not represent the specific range for a given population.

ENDOCRINOLOGY

In both sexes puberty occurs at approximately 50 to 60 days of age. The vagina opens between 35 and 90 days, and the testes descend between 30 and 51 days of age. Usually, rats are first mated between 65 and 120 days, with maximum fertility occurring when they reach 300 days of age.

Ovulatory estrous cycles usually begin at about 77 days. A summary of the changes associated with the estrous cycle of the rat is shown in Table 2. The rat's estrous cycle lasts 4 to 5 days, with an estrous period of about 12 hours. Behavior of the female rat during estrus includes ear quivering when the head and back are stroked, lordosis produced by digital stimulation of the pelvic region and an increased amount of running activity.

The hormonal control of the estrous cycle in the rat is summarized in Figure 3. The arrows show possible causal relationships. A small quantity of luteinizing hormone (LH) is secreted during the late mornings of day 3, which causes estrogen secretion. Luteolysis of the most recent crop of corpora lutea takes place at this time also, probably because of the LH secretion. The estrogen secretion continues until the LH surge, under central nervous system (CNS) control, is released on the day of proestrus. Estrogen is responsible for the uterine and vaginal changes, mating behavior, and luteinizing hormone-follicle stimulating hormone (LH-FSH) release on the following 2 days. The surge of LH necessary for triggering ovulation is released after 14 hours on day 4. This LH release is closely tied to the time of day as defined by the light-dark cycle. There is daily facilitation of this mechanism, but release of LH only occurs on one day of the cycle, which is the day the estrogen level is high. Estrogen levels also promote FSH secretion and possibly prolactin. This LH surge, in addition to causing ovulation, also terminates the ongoing estrogen secretion and starts progesterone secretion by the ovary. The progesterone then acts through the nervous system and helps induce mating behavior. It also causes release of uterine water. As a result of the lowering of estrogen secretion and its negative feedback effect on LH and FSH, the LH and FSH secretion levels are freed to begin increasing, thus initiating the

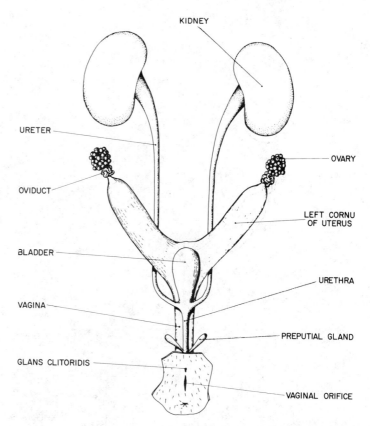

KIDNEY

URETER

OVARY

OVIDUCT

LEFT CORNU OF UTERUS

BLADDER

URETHRA

VAGINA

PREPUTIAL GLAND

GLANS CLITORIDIS

VAGINAL ORIFICE

Figure 1. Female urogenital organs. (From Bivin WS, et al.: In Baker HJ, et al. (eds): Biology of the Rat. New York, Academic Press, 1979, pp 92–93.)

next crop of follicles. The 5-day cycle is similar to the 4-day cycle except that LH and estrogen secretions, luteolysis and uterine changes and the "time of day" signal are all delayed approximately 24 hours.[8]

Synchronization of estrus is a technique that greatly facilitates the production of large numbers of pregnant rats. Although earlier methods involved the placement of medroxyprogesterone soaked sponges in the vagina of 90- to 110-day-old female rats to produce a Whitten effect, which is usually produced by introducing a male to a group of females housed together, newer methods allow us to suppress estrus by administering 40 mg of medroxyprogesterone in 200 ml of ethanol per liter of water. This solution is prepared fresh each day and administered for 6 days, after which estrus is induced by the intramuscular injection of 1 IU of pregnant mare serum, gonadotropin.[4, 8, 33, 34, 42]

BREEDING PROGRAMS

Rats may be monogamously mated for life, as is usually the case with pet rats. However, a more efficient method is to use polygamous mating. One male can be placed with four females and the females are removed as they become pregnant.[32] Pregnant females are placed in a nesting cage and should be left alone as much as possible. If the male and female are not separated before parturition,

cannibalism, litter desertion and agalactia may result. Also, increased handling, especially following parturition, will decrease survivability in the litter. If large numbers are involved, it is best to tatoo the ears to simplify record keeping and to control genetic lines in breeding.[46]

Research laboratories produce large numbers of inbred and random-bred colonies. This is usually accomplished through the use of multistage breeding. Essentially, multistage breeding uses a small colony to provide breeders for a larger colony. This colony is then used to produce breeders for an even larger colony until a colony of sufficient size is established.[4]

PREGNANCY AND REARING

Contrary to popular opinion, vaginal cytology is not the most accurate prediction of pregnancy in rats. However, it has proved to be a useful tool and can be easily accomplished by swabbing the vagina with a small, wet cotton applicator. The cotton swab is then rinsed for 2 seconds in a test tube containing 1.0 ml of physiological saline with two drops of ordinary red fountain pen ink. The cotton swab is then smeared on an albumin-coated slide and covered with a cover glass, and the vaginal cytology is examined under low and high power magnification.[17] A more positive confirmation of conception is the presence of sperm in the vaginal

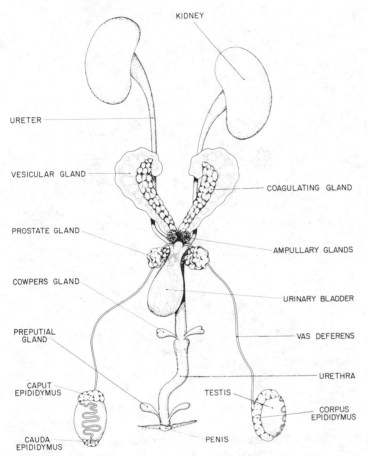

KIDNEY

URETER

VESICULAR GLAND

COAGULATING GLAND

PROSTATE GLAND

AMPULLARY GLANDS

COWPERS GLAND

URINARY BLADDER

PREPUTIAL GLAND

VAS DEFERENS

URETHRA

CAPUT EPIDIDYMUS

TESTIS

CORPUS EPIDIDYMUS

CAUDA EPIDIDYMUS

PENIS

Figure 2. Male urogenital organs. (From Bivin WS et al.: In Baker HJ et al. (eds): Biology of the Rat. New York, Academic Press, 1979, pp 92–93.)

smears.[15] When timed matings are required, a dark paper can be placed under the breeding cage. Newly mated rats will produce a white, waxy copulatory plug in the vagina. After 12 to 24 hours post coitum, the discharged plug will be easily observed on the dark paper. Another accurate estimate of breeding time can be accomplished by placing the male and female together for only 2 hours on the morning of the day of estrus.[6] Further evidence of pregnancy would include palpation, body weights, abdominal enlargement and the development of mammary glands by 14 days of gestation.[15]

Parturition usually occurs 21 to 23 days following conception unless the female is nursing pups, in which case the gestation period may be prolonged for several days. A clear mucoid vaginal discharge appears 1½ to 4 hours prior to delivery, at which time the female is commonly observed licking her perineum. The fact that dystocia in the rat is a rare occurrence can be attributed to selective breeding techniques over many generations and to the adequacy of vitamin A in the diet.[8]

The female will build a nest out of cotton tissue paper, wood shavings and shredded paper. Many people feel that the use of shredded paper greatly improves the ability of the female to suckle her young. Also, the ability to burrow into the paper decreases environmental stresses and increases milk flow, which results in a significant reduction in infant mortality.[36] Be sure the room temperature and bedding are adequate to keep the pups warm. Excessive cooling of the pups, loud noises or handling of the pups may cause the female to abandon or to destroy her litter.

Rat pups are hairless and weigh 5 to 6 gm at birth. Their eyes and ear canals are closed. Litter size is 1 to 20, with an average of about nine. By 12 to 14 days the eyes are open, the pups are fully haired and they have patent ear canals. Young rats are weaned at 21 days, and if the postpartum estrus is not utilized, the female will resume cycling in 2 to 4 days after weaning. Provided that litters are the same age, large litters can be divided or small litters combined with foster mothers.

Hand raising orphaned pups is not easy. A warmed artificial milk formula, Esbilac (Upjohn Veterinary Products), can be fed with a dropper or pipette; however, aspiration of food is a common problem resulting in death. Also, simulated maternal stimulation of defecation and micturition must be provided using a warm, moist cotton applicator.[22]

NUTRITION

Although consumption may vary with the health status, time of day, temperature, humidity, diet or

Table 1. Physiological Values of the Rat

Feature	Value
Life span	2 to 4 years
Adult body weight (male)	400 to 520 gm
Adult body weight (female)	250 to 300 gm
Birth weight	5 to 6 gm
Breeding onset (male)	65 to 110 days
Breeding onset (female)	65 to 110 days
Estrous cycle	4 to 5 days
Gestation period	21 to 23 days
Commerial breeding life	1 year
Postpartum estrus	Fertile
Litter size	6 to 12
Weaning age	21 days
Production of young	4 to 5/month
Milk composition	70 to 74 per cent water, 10 to 15 per cent fat, 7 to 12 per cent protein and 3 to 3.5 per cent sugar
Placentation	discoidal hemochorial
Chromosome number	2n = 42
Body temperature	96.8 to 102.1°F (average 99.2°F)
Blood volume	6 to 7 per cent or 54 to 79 ml/kg
Heart rate	250 to 500/minute
Respiratory rate	70 to 115/minute
Food consumption	10 gm/100 gm of body weight per day
Water consumption	10 to 12 ml/100 gm of body weight per day
Packed cell volume	36 to 48 per cent
Red blood cells	7 to 10 × 10⁶/mm³
White blood cells	6 to 17 × 10³/mm³
Neutrophils	9 to 36 per cent
Lymphocytes	62 to 85 per cent
Eosinophils	0 to 6 per cent
Monocytes	0 to 5 per cent
Basophils	0 to 1.5 per cent
Serum protein	5.6 to 7.5 gm/dl
Urine	Clear, pH 6.0 to 7.5
Activity	Nocturnal

(Compiled from data reported by Williams CSF, 1975; Harkness JE, Wagner JE, 1983; Baker HJ, et al., 1979.)

breeding stage, the average adult will consume 12 to 20 gm of commercial feed each day. The average water consumption is 10 to 12 ml/100 gm of body weight per day. During estrus the food intake may drop as much as 6 gm/day. However, during pregnancy the food intake may increase from a 13 gm/day maintenance level to 19 gm/day by the end of gestation. Lactation is a further burden on the female and will further increase food consumption to about 40 gm/day by the time the pups are weaned. A listing of the minimum nutrient requirements suitable for breeding is given in Table 3.

Most diets of natural ingredients are complete and do not require supplementation. However, many pet store rodent feeds are inadequate in protein and energy and may require supplementation, if used. Purified diets may also have deficient or excessive amounts of certain nutrients.[21] Two other facts of interest are that the rat is coprophagic and that their nocturnal habits result in night feeding and reproduction.

DISEASES OF THE REPRODUCTIVE SYSTEM

Normal genital flora of the female rat include alpha and nonhemolytic streptococcus, *Pasteurella pneumotropica,* diphtheria bacillus, *Staphylococcus epidermidis* and *Proteus mirabilis.*[29]

Because *P. pneumotropica* is a potential pathogen, some researchers feel that this organism should not be considered as part of the normal flora. Casillo and Blackmore[11] reported that 8.2 per cent of their research animals had infected uteri and that *P. pneumotropica* was the predominant organism isolated. They also confirmed[9] that this infection can be easily induced by intravenous, intranasal and intravaginal inoculations. Speculation is that uterine infections are secondary to an upper respiratory infection, and the organisms may enter the uterus during a bacteremic phase or by ascending vaginal infections. It has also been demonstrated that infected male mice will transmit the disease to females by placing their infected noses in close proximity with the female's vulva. It should also be noted that the stage of the estrous cycle has no apparent effect on the susceptibility of the female to uterine infection.

The reproductive problems associated with pasteurellosis include mastitis, infertility and abortion.[22] A definitive diagnosis of *P. pneumotropica* is confirmed by recovery of the organism on blood agar culture. Specific treatments for this condition include 3.5 mg/ml of oxytetracycline in the drinking water for 2 weeks, 9 mg of ampicillin daily for 7 days and/or 0.25 mg/ml of chloramphenicol in the drinking water for 2 weeks. It should be pointed out that treatment rarely eliminates the organism or the infection from the colony.

Another significant disease of the reproductive system is mycoplasmosis. Although *Mycoplasma pulmonis* is usually associated with upper respiratory and middle ear infections, it has been observed to produce an accumulation of a purulent fluid in the uterine horns (pyometra), pus-containing nodules in the uterine mucosa, endometritis, large abscesses at the base of the uterus and a purulent salpingitis.[20] In the ascending genital infections infertility, embryonic resorptions and small litters are common sequelae. Recent studies have demonstrated the infection rate to be as high as 30 to 40 per cent of the females in a given colony and that breeding efficiency may be reduced by 50 per cent.[12] The incidence of this infection in the male genital tract is not known.

Transmission is thought to be by direct contact between the mother and young, respiratory aerosol, sexual transfer, animal carriers and in utero passage. Diagnosis is based on gross and microscopic lesions and by isolation of the organism on a special Hayflick's medium.[23] Other means of diagnosis include

Table 2. Characteristics of the Rat Estrous Cycle

Stage & Duration	Vaginal Fluids	Genitalia	Ovary	Average pH of Vaginal Contents
Proestrus (12 hours)	Small round nucleated cells	Dry vagina	Enlarged follicles	5.4 4.2
Estrus (12 hours)	Cornified cells 25 per cent	Swollen vulva, dry vagina	Large follicles	4.2
Metestrus I (15 hours)	Late cornified stage-pavement cells	Swollen vulva, caseous mass in vagina	Ovulation	—
Metestrus II	Pavement cells and leukocytes	No swelling, moist mucosa	Eggs in oviduct	—
Diestrus	Epithelial cells and leukocytes	No swelling, moist mucosa	Corpora lutea	6.1

(Based on data reported by Baker HJ, et al., 1979; Harkness CSF, Wagner JE, 1983; Nicholas JS, 1949; Asdell SA, 1964; Long JA, Evans HM, 1922; Young WC, et al., 1941; Dewsbury FA, et al., 1977.)

the Giemsa stained touch method of Whittlestone,[47] indirect identification of mycoplasms by immunofluorescence and use of an enzyme-linked immunosorbent assay (ELISA). The latter assay will allow tail blood, nasal washings, genital flushes and oropharyngeal swabs to be used as specimens. Low cost, simplicity, availability and rapidity make this test very useful.

Elimination of mycoplasmosis in a rat colony is impossible at the present time. Tetracycline hydrochloride given in a 2 to 5 mg/ml dose in sweetened drinking water for 5 to 10 days may suppress clinical signs. However, the disease will usually reoccur when treatment is stopped. The fact that this organism may be transferred in utero would suggest that even cesarean derivation is not the answer for

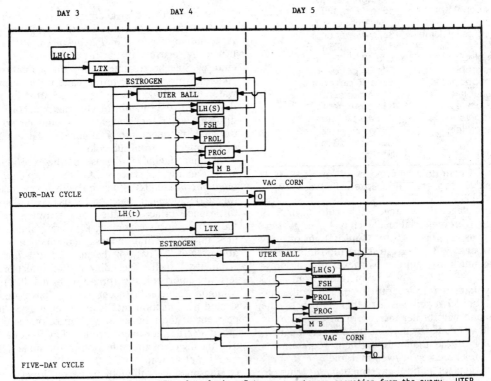

LH (t) = tonic release of LH. LTX = luteolysis. Estrogen = estrogen secretion from the ovary. UTER. BALL. = uterine accumulation of intraluminal fluid. LH(S) = ovulatory surge of LH. FSH = ovulatory surge of FSH. PROL.= prolactin release on day of proestrus. PROG.= progesterone secretion after critical period. M.B. = mating behavior. VAG. CORN. = vaginal cornification. O = ovulation.

Figure 3. Effects of endocrine secretions on estrus. (From Bivin WS, et al.: In Baker HJ et al. (eds): Biology of the Rat. New York, Academic Press, 1979, pp 92–93.)

Table 3. Nutrient Requirements for Optimum Reproduction

Requirements	Amount	
Gross energy	4000	Kcal/kg
Metabolizable energy	3600	Kcal/kg
Crude protein	21.7	per cent
Fat	18	per cent
Net amino acids		
Lysine	1.4	per cent
Arginine	0.75	per cent
Valine	0.70	per cent
Threonine	0.50	per cent
Methionine	1.00	per cent
Phenylalanine	0.90	per cent
Isoleucine	0.50	per cent
Leucine	0.80	per cent
Histidine	0.54	per cent
Tryptophan	0.20	per cent
Nonessential amino acids	4.87	per cent
Essential fatty acids	0.3	per cent
Vitamin B_{12}	23	mg/kg of diet
Vitamin A	400	IU/100 gm
Vitamin D	100	IU/100 gm
Thiamine	0.4	mg/100 gm
Riboflavin	0.4	mg/100 gm
Pyridoxine	0.6	mg/100 gm
Niacin	3.0	mg/100 gm
Tocopherol	3.0	mg/100 gm
Minerals		
Calcium	600	mg/100 gm
Phosphorous	500	mg/100 gm
Sodium	500	mg/100 gm
Potassium	500	mg/100 gm
Chloride	25	mg/100 gm
Magnesium	50	mg/100 gm
Manganese	3.3	mg/100 gm
Iron	2.5	mg/100 gm
Copper	0.5	mg/100 gm
Zinc	0.4	mg/100 gm
Iodine	0.015	mg/100 gm

(Compiled from data reported by Nolan GA, Alexander JC, 1966; Baker DEJ, 1967)

eliminating this disease. Perhaps the development of an effective vaccine may be the only hope for controlling this disease.[13]

Parainfluenza 1 (Sendai) viral infection is common in laboratory rats.[38] The natural disease is usually asymptomatic,[10, 31] but experimental infections have demonstrated that Sendai virus will cause respiratory tract lesions[14, 45] and embryonic resorption.[16] Diagnosis of Sendai virus infection is based upon histopathology, serology and virus isolation. Control of Sendai virus may be accomplished by preventing the introduction of suckling and weaning rats to the colony. Studies in mice have shown that young animals are most susceptible.[7, 37]

Rat parvoviruses (rat virus and H-1 virus) are widespread in laboratory rats.[25, 41] Rat virus infections have been shown commonly to induce intrauterine resorption and teratogenesis and sporadic cerebellar destruction and hepatitis in suckling rats. Adult rats are usually asymptomatic, but a hemorrhagic syndrome can develop in infected immuno-suppressed adults.[19, 26] The clinical disease of enzootic rat virus infection in a production colony may only consist of decreased production because of intrauterine resorption. Diagnosis of infection is best accomplished through serology and virus isolation.[27] Control of rat virus can only be done by purchasing parvovirus-free stock and maintaining the rats behind a laminar flow barrier.[24]

Age will certainly affect the reproductive rate of rats, and the incidence of tumors in reproductive organs is higher in aged rats. In general, breeding efficiency begins to decrease when female rats are between 20 and 30 weeks of age, with menopause beginning at 450 to 540 days of age.[3] The most common age-related lesions involving the reproductive organs of male rats are polyarteritis nodosa of the spermatic arteries, seminiferous tubule degeneration, concretions within the acinar lumens of the prostate and adenitis of the preputial glands.[1] Follicular cysts are common in aged female rats.[28] The most common tumors involving the ovary and testicle are granulosa cell tumor and interstitial cell tumor, respectively.[43]

Other factors that may influence the reproductive rate of adults and the survivibility of their offspring include excessive noise, dirty caging, lack of nesting material or the use of cedar and/or sawdust bedding, agalactia, organophosphate poisoning and nutritional deficiencies.[22]

References

1. Anver MR, Cohen BJ: Lesions associated with aging. In Baker HJ, Lindsey JR, Weisbroth SH (eds): The Laboratory Rat—Biology and Diseases. vol 1. New York, Academic Press, 1979.
2. Asdell SA: Patterns of Mammalian Reproduction. 2nd ed. Ithaca, Cornell University Press, 1964.
3. Baker DEJ: Reproduction and breeding. In Baker HJ, Lindsey JR, Weisbroth JH (eds): The Laboratory Rat—Biology and Diseases. vol 1. New York, Academic Press, 1979.
4. Baker DEJ: Gnotobiotics applied to the standardization of laboratory mice. In Regamey RH, et al. (eds): International Symposium on Laboratory Animals. Karger, Basel, 1967, pp 31–42.
5. Baker HJ, Lindsey JR, Weisbroth SH (eds): The Laboratory Rat—Biology and Diseases; Research Applications. vols 1 and 2. New York, Academic Press, 1979.
6. Bertholet JY: Mating method to produce accurate timed pregnancies in rats. Lab Anim Sci 31:180, 1981.
7. Bhatt PN, Jonas AM: An epizootic of Sendai infection with mortality in a barrier-maintained mouse colony. Am J Epidemiol 100:222, 1974.
8. Bivin WS, Crawford MP, Brewer NR: Morphophysiology. In Baker HJ, Lindsey JR, Weisbroth SH (eds): Biology of the Rat. New York, Academic Press, 1979, pp 92–93.
9. Blackmore DK, Casillo S: Experimental investigation of uterine infections of mice due to *Pasteurella pneumotropica*. J Comp Path 82:471, 1972.
10. Burek JD, Zurchei C, Van Nunen MCJ, Hollander CF: A naturally occurring epizootic caused by Sendai virus in breeding and aging rodent colonies. II. Sendai virus infection in rats. Lab Anim Sci 27:963, 1977.
11. Casillo S, Blackmore DK: Uterine infections caused by bacteria and mycoplasma in mice and rats. J Comp Path 82:477, 1972.
12. Cassell GH, Carter PB, Silvers SH: Genital disease in rats due to *Mycoplasma pulmonis*: Development of an experimental model. Proc Soc Gen Micro 3:150, 1976.

13. Cassell GH, Davis JK: Active immunization of rats against *Mycoplasma pulmonis* respiratory disease. Infect Immun 21:69, 1978.
14. Castleman WL: Respiratory tract lesions in weanling outbred rats infected with Sendai virus. Am J Vet Res 44:1024, 1983.
15. Chow BF, Augustin CE: Induction of premature birth in rats by a methionine antagonist. J Nutr 87:293, 1965.
16. Coid CR, Wardman G: The effect of parainfluenza type 1 (Sendai) virus infection on early pregnancy in the rat. J Reprod Fertil 24:39, 1971.
17. Davis RH, Kramer DL, Sacman JW, Kyriazis G: A simple staining method for vaginal smears using red ink. Lab Anim Sci 24:319, 1975.
18. Dewsbury DA, Estep DQ, Lanier DL: Estrous cycles of nine species of muroid rodents. J Mam 58:89, 1977.
19. El Dadah AN, Nathanson N, Smith KO, et al.: Viral hemorrhagic encephalopathy of rats. Science 156:392, 1967.
20. Graham WR: Recovery of a pleuropneumonia-like organism (P.P.L.O.) from the genitalia of the female albino rat. Lab Anim Care 13:719, 1963.
21. Greenfield H, Briggs GM: Nutritional methodology in metabolic research with rats. Ann Rev Biochem 40:549, 1971.
22. Harkness JE, Wagner JE: The Biology and Medicine of Rabbits and Rodents. 2nd ed. Philadelphia, Lea & Febiger, 1983.
23. Hayflick L: Tissue cultures and mycoplasmas. Tex Rep Biol Med 23:285, 1965.
24. Jacoby RO, Bhatt PN, Jonas AM: Viral diseases. In Baker HJ, Lindsey JR, Weisbroth SH (eds): Biology of the Laboratory Rat. New York, Academic Press, 1979, pp 272–306.
25. Kilham L: Viruses of laboratory and wild rats. Nat Cancer Inst Monogr 20:117, 1966.
26. Kilham L, Margolis G: Spontaneous hepatitis and cerebellar hypoplasia in suckling rats due to congenital infection with rat virus. Am J Pathol 49:457, 1966.
27. Kilham L, Olivier L: A latent virus of rats isolated in tissue culture. Virology 7:428, 1959.
28. King NW: The reproductive tract. In Pathology of Laboratory Animals. New York, Springer-Verlag, 1978.
29. Larsen B, Marovetz AJ, Galask RP: The bacterial flora of the female rat genital tract. Proc Soc Exp Biol Med 151:571, 1979.
30. Long JA, Evans HM: The estrous cycle of the rat and its associated phenomenon. Mem Univ Calif 6:1, 1922.
31. Makino S, Seko S, Nakao H, Midazuki K: An epizootic of Sendai virus infection in a rat colony. Exp Anim 22:275, 1972.
32. Masson P, Comond P: Modalites de production du rat Wistar, A.F. dams uneunite E.O.P.S. Exp Anim 4:73, 1971.
33. May D: Synchronization of estrus in the rat. J Inst Anim Tech 20:155, 1969.
34. May D, Simpson K: An improved method for synchronizing estrus in the rat. J Inst Anim Tech 22:133, 1971.
35. Nicholas JS: Experimental methods and rat embryos. In Farris EJ, Grittith JQ (eds): The Rat in Laboratory Investigation. 2nd ed. New York, Hafner, 1949, p 542.
36. Nolan GA, Alexander JC: Effects of diet and type of nesting material on the reproduction and lactation of the rat. Lab Anim Care 16:327, 1966.
37. Parker JC, Reynolds RK: Natural history of Sendai virus infection in mice. Am J Epidemiol 89:112, 1968.
38. Parker JC, Whiteman MD, Richter CB: Susceptibility of inbred and outbred mouse strains to Sendai virus and prevalence of infection in laboratory rodents. Infect Immun 19:123, 1978.
39. Richter CP: The effects of domestication and selection on the behavior of the Norway rat. J Natl Cancer Inst 15:727, 1954.
40. Richter CP: Rats, man, and the welfare state. Am Psychol 14:18, 1959.
41. Robey RE, Woodman DR, Hetrick FM: Studies on the natural infection of rats with Kilham rat virus. Am J Epidemiol 88:139, 1968.
42. Schwartz NB, Waltz P: Role of ovulation in the regulation of the estrous cycle. In Brown JHG, Gann DS (eds): Engineering Principles in Physiology. vol 1. New York, Academic Press, 1973, p 249.
43. Snell KC: Spontaneous lesions of the rat. In Ribelin WE, McCoy JR (eds): The Pathology of Laboratory Animals. Springfield, Charles C Thomas, 1965, pp 241–302.
44. Szabo KT, Free SM, Birkhead HA, Gay PE: Predictability of pregnancy from various signs of mating in mice and rats. Lab Anim Care 19:822, 1969.
45. Tyrrell DAJ, Coid CR: Sendai virus infection of rats as a convenient model of acute respiratory infection. Vet Rec 86:164, 1970.
46. Van der Waaij D, Van Bekkum DW: Isolation facilities for rat breeding: The efficiency of an isolation unit. Lab Anim Care 17:532, 1967.
47. Whittlestone P: Isolation techniques for mycoplasmas from animal diseases. In Bove JB, Duplan JF (eds): Mycoplasmas of Man, Animals, Plants, and Insects. Paris, INSERM, 1974, pp 143–151.
48. Williams CSF: Practical Guide to Laboratory Animals. St. Louis, CV Mosby, 1976.
49. Young WC, Boling JL, Blandau RJ: In Asdell SA (ed): Patterns of Mammalian Reproduction. 2nd ed. Ithaca, Cornell University Press, 1941, p 333.

The Guinea Pig

John E. Harkness, D.V.M., M.S., M.Ed.

Mississippi State University,
Mississippi State, Mississippi

Guinea pigs or cavies (*Cavia porcellus*) are hystricomorph (hedgehoglike), herbivorous rodents with an absolute requirement for exogenous vitamin C. The English shorthair, Abyssinian (rough hair with whorls), and Peruvian "ragmop" domesticated varieties are related to wild or semidomesticated rodents living in the highlands and grasslands of South America.

Reproductive characteristics of guinea pigs include a relatively long (for rodents) estrous cycle (16 days) and gestation period (68 days); an imperforate vaginal membrane; a fertile postpartum estrus; precocious young; passive nursing and maternal behaviors; spontaneous ovulation within a nonseasonal, continuous, polyestrous pattern and the presence in the blood and placenta of mononuclear, estrogen-stimulated Kurloff cells, whose mucopolysaccharide inclusions may protect fetal antigen. Another distinguishing aspect of guinea pig reproduction is the use of age and weight as determinants for weaning and breeding.

SEXING

Size, conformation and coat color are not reliable indicators of sex, although males are heavier than females of the same strain and age. Both sexes have nipples, but the sow's nipples are longer and overlie

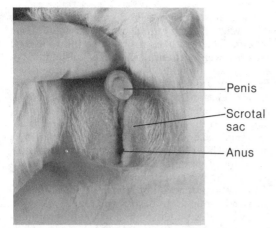

Figure 1. External genitalia of the male guinea pig (penis extruded).

mammary glands. The adult male has bulging scrotal pouches containing testes and lying lateral to the penis. The testes are not descended at birth and can be withdrawn by the adult into the open inguinal canals, but in either case the testes are palpable. On first glance the external genitalia in both sexes appear similar, especially in young animals, but gentle digital pressure applied just anterior to the preputial opening will reveal either the pointed penis (Fig. 1) or the elongated vulva (Fig. 2). The penis may also be palpated under the skin anterior to the preputial opening. The boar has no break in the line from penis to anus, whereas the U-shaped but membrane-covered vaginal opening interrupts the line in sows.

HUSBANDRY AND BREEDING SYSTEMS

Breeding groups of guinea pigs (2 to 11 animals) should be housed in solid-bottomed cages with sides high enough (25 cm or 10 inches) to prevent boars from climbing into other cages. Cages should contain clean, nontoxic, nonedible and nonabrasive wood shaving bedding. Fine beddings, such as saw-

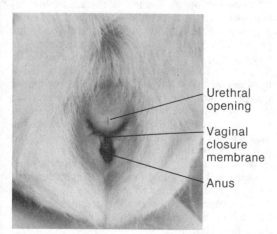

Figure 2. External genitalia of the female guinea pig.

dust, should not be used because the particles cling to the damp genital areas and may interfere with mating. Rectangular rather than square cages should be used to prevent circling and stampeding. Also, animals born onto a solid floor but later placed on wire may develop broken limbs and hair loss and experience decreased weight gains and production.

Each adult (over 350 gm) requires 652 to 950 cm² (101 to 150 inch²) of floor space, and a sow with a litter requires around 1485 cm² (230 inch²). Workable hopper feeders and sipper tube waterers (assuming the guinea pigs are familiar from birth with such devices) should be used and should be accessible to the smallest animals in the cage. The room housing the animals should be well ventilated, draft free, shaded and maintained at a temperature between 18 and 22°C (64 to 72°F). Guinea pigs tolerate cold much better than heat, and they reproduce well in darkened rooms.

Guinea pigs may be bred in monogamous or polygamous systems in which boars and sows are always together (continuous or intensive breeding) or may be separated before parturition and reunited after weaning (discontinuous or nonintensive breeding). In the continuous system, which utilizes the postpartum estrus, a sow will produce around five litters (12 young) per year, whereas annual per sow production in a discontinuous system is around 3.5 litters (nine young). Production, however, also depends on strain, parity, cage density and nutritional status.

In both the monogamous and polygamous systems pregnant sows can be left in the communal pen, or they can be removed to individual or all-female cages. Removal of the sow to an individual cage makes record keeping easier and eliminates problems with paternal aggression and interlitter competition. In harem cages bullying, milk stripping, ear chewing, stampeding and trampling and higher weanling mortality occur. In the polygamous or harem system one boar is housed with 3 to 10 sows.

A system that combines the advantages of isolated parturition and postpartum breeding involves returning the sow to the boar for a 6- to 12-hour period within an hour after parturition. After mating, the sow is returned to her young. In the nonintensive system sows are returned to the male only after weaning.

Litter intervals in guinea pig colonies are around 80 to 96 days, and production ranges from 0.7 to 1.3 young per sow per month. In commercial breeding establishments a breeder's life is around 18 months, but pet guinea pigs remain fertile for 3 years or longer.

MALE REPRODUCTIVE ANATOMY AND PHYSIOLOGY

Boars possess a 45- to 50-mm penis with baculum; 5 to 6 gm testes; elongated (up to 10 cm), clear, smooth seminal vesicles; epididymal fat pads and prostate, coagulating, bulbourethral and rudimentary preputial glands. Seminal and coagulating secretions make up the copulatory or vaginal plug, which blocks the vagina in sows for a few hours after coitus.

At approximately 30 days of age male guinea pigs begin mounting sows, intromission begins around 45 days, and ejaculations begin around 56 days. Boars are first used for breeding when they weigh 600 to 700 gm (3 to 4 months).

FEMALE REPRODUCTIVE ANATOMY AND PHYSIOLOGY

The uterus is bicornate with 30- to 50-mm-long horns. The cervix has two internal ora and one external os, and the vagina is 30- to 40-mm long. Sexual activity in sows is evident around 60 days of age, but they are first bred when they weigh between 350 and 450 gm (2 to 3 months). The average estrous cycle lasts 16.3 days (range 13 to 21) and includes proestrus (1.5 days), estrus (8 to 11 hours), metestrus (3 days) and diestrus (11 to 12 days). Proestrus is indicated by vaginal swelling, vaginal membrane rupture, increased activity and lordosis. At estrus the vulva is swollen and congested, and the vaginal smear contains mucus and a preponderance of cornified epithelial cells. There is no conclusive evidence of cycle synchronization occurring among group-housed sows.

MATING AND PARTURITION

During the receptive period the sow prowls about the cage, runs, mounts other sows, sniffs, vocalizes and assumes lordosis (limbs extended, back arched, perineum up) if mounted or stroked on the rump. The boar mounts, intromits once or twice, then dismounts and scoots about the cage, apparently depositing scent. The sow then resists further mating. Successful mating is indicated by the presence of sperm in the vaginal smear and a copulatory plug either in the vagina or in the bedding. Sixty to 85 per cent of matings, including those occurring during the postpartum estrus, are fertile. The ova remain fertilizable for 30 hours after ovulation, which occurs near the end of the receptive period. The blastocysts implant in 6 or 7 days. The corpora lutea secrete progesterone until around 20 days after coitus when placental gonadotropins and progesterone assume the role of maintaining pregnancy. The corpora lutea can usually be removed at 25 days without terminating pregnancy, and relaxin rather than progesterone apparently regulates myometrial activity in the guinea pig. Pseudopregnancy, if it occurs, does not prolong the estrous cycle. Artificial insemination has been used successfully in guinea pigs, but the technique is of little practical importance to pet or small colony owners. Placentation is hemomonochorionic, with fetal trophoblasts in direct contact with maternal blood.

The uterus, which weighs 2 gm in a nonpregnant sow, weighs 120 gm at midterm and around 300 gm at term. The fetal mass may be one third the total maternal weight at term. Abdominal distention becomes very prominent as pregnancy progresses. Pregnancy is detected by gentle palpation for firm, ovoid bodies in the horns. These swellings are 10 mm in diameter at 25 days and 25 mm at 35 days; after 35 days, parts of bodies can be palpated. Gestation generally lasts 68 days (range of 59 to 72 days), and litter size is usually inversely proportional to length of gestation. Preweaning mortality averages 5 to 15 per cent of implanted embryos.

Placental production of relaxin begins around 30 days and continues to day 63 when the level drops. Relaxin causes the dissolution of the fibrocartilaginous pubic symphysis, and during the last week of gestation the symphysis separates 2 to 3 cm. Impending parturition (within 48 hours) can be detected by palpation for a symphysis separation of two fingers' breadth. In sows bred for the first time at 7 months of age or older symphysis separation may be inadequate to allow for fetal passage.

NEONATAL LIFE AND LACTATION

No nests are built before or after delivery. The vaginal closure membrane again opens, and delivery itself lasts around 30 minutes and occurs at night. The sow squats, delivers, cleans the pups and eat the placentae and membranes. Sows nibble but rarely consume aborted fetuses, or stillborn young. Usually, two to three young are born (range of one to six), and they weigh 45 to 115 gm each; however, young weighing less than 60 gm seldom survive. Neonatal males weigh around 2 gm more than sibling females. The symphysis closes within 24 hours, and a fertile, postpartum estrus lasting around 3.5 hours usually begins within 2 hours (but up to 15 hours) after parturition.

Young are born mobile, haired and with teeth, and eyes and ears are open. The sow cleans and licks the neonates, but otherwise obvious maternal attention is minimal. The neonates learn to discriminate between food and nonfood (other than maternal milk) within a few days of birth, and this prejudicial imprint of taste, odor or texture persists into maturity. Young do poorly if housed alone or deprived of food or water for several hours, and a nursing pup that is off milk for 24 hours or longer may not return to nursing. The young, however, do not feed during the first 24 hours postpartum, and neonatal orphans should not be force fed during this period. Survival of neonates not receiving the sow's milk for the first 3 or 4 days is only around 50 per cent. Fresh pelleted guinea pig chow soaked in cow's milk or diluted evaporated milk, hay and cabbage have been used to feed young guinea pigs. Foster mothers are also readily accepted, and in a harem cage the young will frequently suckle mothers other than their own.

The ovoid, apocrine mammary glands, which

extend ventromedially from the nipples, are very oxytocin sensitive, and the milk contains high levels of saturated, long-chain fatty acids. The milk contains approximately 4 per cent fat, 8 per cent protein and 3 per cent lactose. Milk production, which averages between 45 and 65 ml/kg/day, peaks between days 5 and 8. The supply is not affected by demand, and larger, more aggressive young can strip the milk from harem sows. Agalactia resumes sometime between days 18 and 30, and the young are weaned when they weigh around 180 gm (15 to 28 days) or at 21 days (165 to 240 gm). Males destined for breeding colonies should remain with their siblings and mother to at least 30 days to ensure proper behavioral maturation. The sow resumes cycling during lactation, and a fertile estrus occurs after weaning.

BREEDING DISORDERS

Breeding disorders in guinea pigs include infertility, abortion, stillbirth, dystocia, death of pregnant sows or the neonates, litter desertion or mutilation and mastitis.

Infertility or decreased production of young may be associated with bacterial infection, estrogen contamination of feed, bedding impaction of the genitalia, wire floors, heat stress, immaturity or senescence and various nutritional imbalances and environmental disturbances. Prenatal death in guinea pigs has been attributed to maternal infections with *Bordetella* and *Salmonella* spp. and streptococci, metabolic toxemias, asphyxia at delivery, dystocia and trauma. Small (one to two) or large (over four) litters carried less than 66 days or longer than 72 days, respectively, rarely survive, as is the case for any litter born in less than 62 days or more than 75 days of gestation. Litters of three and four young have the best chance of survival. If a litter of three, for example, is born dead in less than 64 days, abortion has occurred. If the same litter of three is born after 74 days, the young are considered stillborn. Stillbirth is related to litter size, but abortion is not. The major cause of abortion is thought to be a toxemia in the mother, whereas the major cause of death at delivery is probably asphyxia from dystocia or fetal membrane blockage of the nares and mouth.

Dystocia, which is relatively common in obese sows, is manifested clinically by a bloody or green-brown vulvar discharge, exhaustion, depression and death. The impeded delivery, caused by a fetus too large for the pelvic canal, occluding fat pads or an atonic uterus, occurs most often in sows bred for the first time at 7 months of age or older when the pubic symphysis is less likely to separate. Cesarean section and digital manipulation of the fetus may be necessary to save the sow or to effect a delivery. Oxytocin (0.2 to 3.0 units/kg) should be used with care because the pelvic canal is too small for the fetuses. Young guinea pigs are very susceptible to anoxia, and cesarean sections and fetal membrane

removal must be done rapidly. The young should then be dried and kept warm. Death of neonates may be caused by trampling, small size and weakness and maternal agalactia.

Bacterial infections that depress reproduction through general debilitation or metritis include infection with *Bordetella bronchiseptica, Salmonella* spp. and *Streptococcus pneumoniae* or *S. zooepidemicus*. Infection with *Klebsiella* occurs rarely. These bacteria, whose primary foci of infection are in the respiratory or lymphatic system, may cause infertility, stillbirths or abortion, but unfortunately, treatment of these diseases in guinea pigs is in most cases ineffective. Among the antimicrobials only chloramphenicol and the sulfonamides can be used safely in guinea pigs, and even if the bacterium and its sensitivity are known, the guinea pig rarely responds favorably to therapy. A common sequela to bacterial infection is anorexia and either a fatal enteric or metabolic toxemia. Dosages for indicated antibiotics are chloramphenicol palmitate at 30 to 50 mg/kg for 5 days or sulfamethazine at 1 mg/ml in the drinking water for 1 week. A formalin-killed bacterin can be used to prevent infection with *Bordetella,* but the bacterin is not readily available. The *Bordetella* bacterin prepared for use in dogs has not been tested in guinea pigs.

Metabolic toxemias in guinea pigs have been linked to obesity, maturity, large fetal load, anorexia and hypoplasia (or partial blockage) of the arteries supplying the uterus. The condition, which also occurs in boars, is uncommonly seen as a clinical entity in sows, but subclinical cases may be a major cause of fetal loss in breeding colonies. This highly fatal condition occurs in the last trimester of pregnancy or the first week postpartum and more often in winter. Signs include weakness, depression, reluctance to move, obvious pregnancy, incoordination, anorexia, abortion, convulsions and, more often, death. Although many therapeutic regimens have been tried (calcium gluconate, steroids, glucose, antibiotics, propylene glycol), none has been successful in reversing the usually fatal course of the disease. In guinea pigs surviving the metabolic disorder the concomitant stress and anorexia often lead to a fatal enterotoxemia. Prevention of the condition involves feeding an appropriate diet, the avoidance of fasts and stresses, the elimination of affected breeders and the reduction of obesity.

Mastitis is relatively common in guinea pigs, especially in those kept in unsanitary conditions. The causative agents are usually streptococci, coliforms, and *Staphylococcus aureus*. The affected gland and milk become dark red. Either maternal death or a chronic, suppurative condition ensues, but the young are seldom disadvantaged in any case. As with other bacterial infections in guinea pigs, drainage and oral or injected chloramphenicol (30 to 50 mg/kg) are the only possible and practical treatments.

Miscellaneous conditions of the reproductive tract include blockage of the urethra in boars with proteinaceous masses of congealed ejaculum or with uroliths of urinary tract origin. Neoplasia is rare in guinea pigs, but ovarian teratomas, uterine tumors, mammary adenocarcinomas and a single testicular tumor have been reported.

ANESTHESIA AND SURGERY

Guinea pigs should be kept off feed for 6 hours prior to anesthesia and surgery. Atropine (1 to 2 mg/kg) may be used as a preanesthetic. Two satisfactory methods of anesthesia are (1) methoxyflurane administered from a nose cone and (2) ketamine (20 to 40 mg/kg) given intramuscularly with xylazine (5 mg/kg) or acepromazine (2 mg/kg). If neither regimen produces an adequate level or duration of surgical anesthesia, ketamine injection can be followed with methoxyflurane in a nose cone. Ether, halothane and sodium pentobarbital can be used with caution in guinea pigs, but the risk of overdose is great. Halothane causes a profound hypotension in these animals.

In guinea pigs anesthetic concerns include the misleading body weights caused by filled ceca, hypothermia and hypostatic pulmonary congestion occurring during surgery and recovery and the tendency of guinea pigs to move while in the anesthetic surgical plane, giving the false impression that additional anesthetic is needed. Cesarean section may be indicated in dystocia, but no special methods or precautions other than good surgical practice have been described for guinea pigs. Similarly, no specific cautions apply to an ovariohysterectomy in this species.

Castration may be performed to prevent breeding or aggression, but since many aspects of sexual behavior in the boar are extratesticularly determined, undesirable male activities may persist for months following surgery. Live sperm may be found in the ducts 40 days after castration. For the procedure itself, the scrotal pouches are shaved and cleaned. Skin incisions approximately 1.5-cm long are made into each scrotal pouch, followed by a 1-cm cut through the tunica albuginea. The testes are removed, but the epididymis and its nerve and blood supplies remain in the pouch. Because the inguinal canals in rodents remain open for life, the tunic and muscular incisions should be closed to prevent herniation of contents and intestines. Postoperative concerns include hypothermia, hypostatic pulmonary edema and anorexia.

References

1. Cooper MD, Schiller LR: Anatomy of the Guinea Pig. Cambridge, Harvard University Press, 1975, pp 325–357.
2. Kaufman P, Davidoff M: The Guinea Pig Placenta. New York, Springer-Verlag, 1977.
3. Manning PJ, Wagner JE, Harkness JE: Biology and Diseases of Guinea Pigs. In Fox JG, Cohen BJ, Loew FM (eds): Laboratory Animal Medicine. New York, Academic Press, 1984, pp 149–181.
4. Matthews PJ, Jackson J: Pregnancy diagnosis in the guinea pig. Lab Anim Sci 27:248, 1977.
5. Phoenix CH: Guinea pigs. In Hafez ESE (ed): Reproduction and Breeding Techniques for Laboratory Animals. Philadelphia, Lea & Febiger, 1970, pp 244–257.
6. Wagner JE, Manning (eds): The Biology of the Guinea Pig. New York, Academic Press, 1976.

The Laboratory Mouse

Terrie L. Cunliffe-Beamer, D.V.M., M.S.
The Jackson Laboratory, Bar Harbor, Maine

PHYSICAL EXAMINATION OF MALE AND FEMALE REPRODUCTIVE SYSTEM

The distance between the anus and genital orifice is greater in newborn male mice than in newborn female mice. The greater anal-genital distance in the male remains constant throughout life (Fig. 1). By 3 weeks of age, the scrotal sacs of male mice are usually well developed. However, scrotal sac development varies markedly among different strains of mice and thus cannot be used as an indicator of fertility.

The reproductive system of the male mouse (Fig. 2) is similar to that of other rodents. The testicles are paired and may be located in the scrotal sacs or the abdominal cavity. The epididymis and testicle are attached to a large epididymal fat pad, which makes it difficult to palpate the testicle. A single prostate gland divided into ventral and dorsal portions and paired bulbourethral glands surround the urethra. The bulbourethral glands are usually buried in the ischiocavernous muscle. Other accessory sex glands include paired preputial glands, paired coagulating glands, paired vesicular glands (seminal vesicles) and multiple ampullary glands. The preputial glands are located subcutaneously slightly cranial to the prepuce. In some strains of mice normal preputial glands are very obvious and may be misdiagnosed as swollen.

The reproductive system of the female mouse (Fig. 3) consists of paired ovaries, paired oviducts, a Y-shaped uterus with two long horns and a comparatively short body and a single cervix and a short muscular vagina. The urethra opens near the tip of the urogenital papilla—usually exterior to the vaginal orifice.[9]

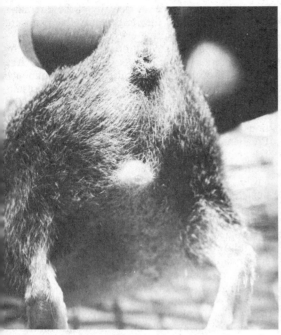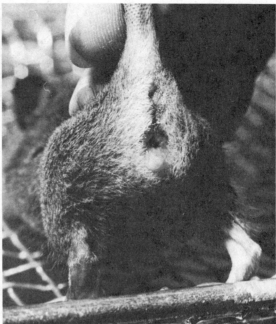

Figure 1. Distance between anus and genital orifice is longer in male mice (left) compared with female mice (right).

PUBERTY AND THE ESTROUS CYCLE

The vaginal orifice is sealed by a thin membrane in the prepubertal female mouse. Vaginal opening and first estrus may occur as early as 24 days of age in some mice. However, complete sexual maturity of female mice usually does not occur until 7 to 9 weeks of age. The mean age of dams at the birth of their first litters ranges from 64 to 92 days of age in sibling breeding pairs that are mated at 3 to 4 weeks of age.[8] Male mice mature approximately 2 weeks later than female mice. Male and female

mice can be expected to reach full adult development between 8 and 10 weeks of age.

The estrous cycle of the female mouse lasts 4 to 5 days or longer and is divided into four stages: proestrus, estrus, metestrus and diestrus. These four stages can be identified by morphologic appearance of the vaginal orifice and by vaginal cytology (Table 1).[1, 3] Housing conditions of female mice influence the length of the estrous cycle. In the absence of a male mouse or male pheromones, individually caged female mice may develop prolonged diestrus. Group-housed female mice become diestrous or

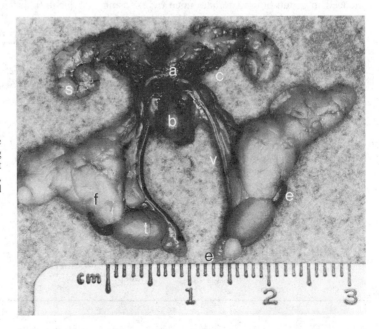

Figure 2. Reproductive system of a male mouse: ampullary glands (a), coagulating gland (c), epididymis (e), epididymal fat pad (f), seminal vesicle (s), testicle (t), vas deferens (v). Prostate gland covered by urinary bladder (b).

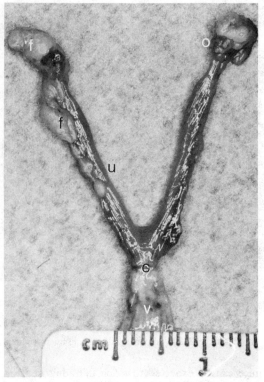

Figure 3. Reproductive system of a female mouse: cervix (c), ovarian and mesometrial fat (f), ovary (o), uterine horn (u), vagina (v).

them to a male mouse. A majority of these females will be in estrus on the third night after exposure to the male (the Whitten effect).[15]

Estrus and supraovulation can be induced by administration of exogenous gonadotropins. Age and strain of the female mouse markedly influence her response to these hormones.[6] For best results the female mice should weigh about 14 gm and should be 18 to 21 days old. Gonadotropin injections are made during the middle of the afternoon. Pregnant mare serum gonadotropin (PMSG 1 to 5 IU in 0.2 ml) is injected intraperitoneally. Forty-eight hours later, human chorionic gonadotropin (hCG, 1 to 5 IU in 0.2 ml) is injected intraperitoneally, and the female mouse is caged with the male. Copulation occurs within hours after hCG administration.

If vaginal smears are to be used to identify estrus, the following technique is recommended. Vaginal smears are obtained using a flat bladed toothpick. A drop of 0.85 per cent NaCl is placed on a glass slide. The end of the toothpick is dipped in the drop of water and then inserted into the vagina. The vaginal walls are gently scraped with the end of the toothpick. Cells adhering to the toothpick are suspended in the drop of saline and examined under 40 to 100 × magnification. The toothpick is used once and discarded. Contact with the cervix or multiple insertions of the toothpick should be avoided in order to prevent pseudopregnancy.

anestrous or mimic pseudopregnancy (the Lee-Boot effect). Pseudopregnancy is also induced by coitus or cervical stimulation during the preparation of vaginal smears. Pseudopregnancy lasts between 10 and 13 days. Pheromones from male mice have an important role in the maintenance of a normal estrous cycle. For example, estrus synchrony can be induced in group-housed female mice by exposing

SEXUAL AND MATERNAL BEHAVIOR

Courtship and mating behavior of mice begins with the male's sniffing the female. This is followed by mounting with multiple intromissions and then ejaculation, after which the male falls on his side and begins postcopulatory grooming. The duration of courtship behavior and the interval between ejaculations vary considerably among inbred strains.

Table 1. Estrous Cycle of the Mouse

Stage in Cycle	Vaginal Orifice	Vaginal Smear	Uterus	Ovary
Proestrus	Red-pink color; moist; dilated orifice; longitudinal folds developing	Nucleated epithelial cells; occasional leukocyte or cornified epithelial cell	Slight distension and hyperemia	Large follicles
Estrus	Lighter color than that of proestrus; longitudinal folds and edema are prominent; dilated orifice	Cornified epithelial cells	Marked distension and hyperemia	Ovulation; distended oviduct
Metestrus	Less edema; dry; pale; white cellular debris may be present	Cornified cells; numerous leukocytes	Collapsed walls; degenerating epithelium; leukocytes in mucosa	Corpora lutea form
Diestrus	Contracted orifice; pale; pink-purple color; moist	Few cells (predominately leukocytes)	Pale; collapsed walls	Follicular growth begins

Courtship lasts between 20 minutes and 1 hour. The interval between ejaculations may be as short as 1 hour or as long as 4 days.[14] A waxy postcopulatory plug (vaginal plug, seminal plug) is found in the vagina after mating. The plug usually is expelled within 12 hours after mating but may persist for 24 to 36 hours.

ARTIFICIAL INSEMINATION AND EMBRYO TRANSPLANT

Artificial insemination can be used to maintain mutant genes that prevent copulation. Sperm are usually obtained by killing the male mouse, excising both epididymides and mincing them in special media. Female mice can be inseminated by transcervical inoculation of sperm or by laparotomy and inoculation of sperm into the uterus. After insemination, the female mouse is mated to a vasectomized male or a vaginal tampon is used to simulate mating.[11]

Embryo transplantation is used to eliminate diseases, to revive cryopreserved strains or to study early embryologic development. Two- to eight-cell embryos are collected by flushing the oviduct between 24 and 72 hours after mating. Morulae or blastocysts are collected by flushing the uterus between 72 and 96 hours after mating. Embryos are transferred to a pseudopregnant foster mother by transcervical inoculation or by laparotomy and intrauterine inoculation.[12]

CONCEPTION, FETAL DEVELOPMENT AND PREGNANCY DIAGNOSIS

The gestation period of the nonlactating female mouse is 19 to 21 days. Lactation can inhibit implantation of fetuses conceived during postpartum estrus and may result in prolongation of gestation by a few days or as many as 16 days. The day that the copulatory plug is observed is counted as day 0 of gestation. By the tenth to twelfth day of gestation, a slight swelling of the abdomen is noticeable in primiparous mice. By the fifteenth day of gestation abdominal enlargment is obvious, and the mouse has a "pear-shaped" appearance. Between the seventh and tenth days of gestation, pregnancy can be diagnosed by palpation. At this time the uterus feels like a piece of string with knots at distinct intervals. Near the fourteenth day of gestation, fetuses are pea sized and can easily be palpated. Between days 15 and 16 of gestation the fetuses begin to elongate, and the uterus feels uniformly enlarged and soft. Between days 17 and 18 fetal heads can be palpated as distinct masses. As parturition approaches, fetal heads become firm, and individual fetuses can be palpated with ease.

Both male and female mice participate in retrieval of newborn. Parturient female mice construct a nest and spend much of their time huddled over the nest. Breeding females should be housed in cages with solid floors and provided with bedding material that permits them to build a nest. Wood shavings (not sawdust), short staple cotton or facial tissues can be used as nesting material. Long staple cotton and other materials with long fibers should not be used because the fibers may become twisted around the neonates' legs and cause pressure necrosis.

EFFECTS OF NUTRITION ON REPRODUCTION

Dietary composition has a marked effect upon reproductive performance of mice. Diets that are formulated to maintain adult rodents (mice, rats and hamsters) will not sustain good reproductive performance in mice, especially inbred mice. Dietary deficiencies can be expected to result in a decrease in the number of offspring per litter, a decrease in the size and vigor of weaned mice, an increase in the mortality of suckling litters or an increase in the number of runts per litter. However, these problems can also be caused by genetic mutations, infectious diseases, improper environmental conditions or rough handling of dam and neonates.

In general, 17 to 19 per cent protein and 5 to 11 per cent fat are recommended as breeding diets for mice.[10] Genetic background and environment also influence dietary requirements. Certain strains of mice seem to require a high fat diet (11 per cent) in order to sustain repeated lactation and pregnancy. Other strains of mice become obese on these high fat diets, and the number of sterile matings increases. Diets for mice that are maintained in germ-free or specific-pathogen–free environments require vitamin fortification because intestinal microflora are limited and pasteurization or sterilization of the diet inactivates some vitamins.

EFFECTS OF INFECTIOUS DISEASES ON REPRODUCTIVE PERFORMANCE

Several viral diseases of mice can affect reproductive performance by increasing morbidity or mortality of suckling litters. Epizootic Sendai virus causes pneumonia and markedly increases mortality of suckling mice, with some increase in mortality of breeding mice.[16] When Sendai virus becomes enzootic within a breeding colony, mortality rates decline, and the infection becomes subclinical. Mouse hepatitis virus (MHV) may cause diarrhea and runting or death of mice between 2 and 3 weeks of age. Some strains of MHV may cause increased mortality among breeders, depending upon the genetic background of the mice and virulence of the virus. However, MHV may also be present as a subclinical enzootic infection. Epizootic diarrhea of infant mice (EDIM) is caused by a rotavirus. EDIM usually presents as a diarrhea with high morbidity, but low mortality, in 10- to 14-day-old mice. EDIM usually does not cause clinical signs in adult mice.

Experimentally induced *Mycoplasma pulmonis* infections have been shown to reduce fertility. However, *M. pulmonis* can be isolated from the vaginas of naturally infected normal mice and is occasionally isolated from uteri that contain viable fetuses. Therefore, the impact of *M. pulmonis* upon reproductive performance is unclear. The role of *Pasteurella pneumotropica* in uterine infections and abortions is also unclear. This bacteria can be isolated from uteri of mice with pyometra or with postabortion suppurative metritis. However, *P. pneumotropica* is also isolated from the vaginas or uteri of normal mice that contain viable fetuses. Infection of mice with *Streptobacillus moniliformis* causes abortions as well as conjunctivitis, polyarthritis and generalized debilitation.[2]

EFFECT OF ENVIRONMENT AND COLONY MANAGEMENT ON REPRODUCTIVE PERFORMANCE

The importance of nesting material and the effects of diet on reproductive performance of mice have been discussed previously. The length of the light and dark cycle also affects reproductive performance. A light-dark cycle of 12 hours light and 12 hours darkness or 14 hours light and 10 hours darkness is recommended. In my experience constant light, resulting from a light timer malfunction, results in a gradual decline in the number of litters born and an increase in the number of infertile matings.

Colony management procedures can also influence reproductive performance. Female mice should be mated by 8 to 10 weeks of age. If mating is delayed until the female is 4 to 5 months of age, an increased number of sterile matings can be expected. The number of females per male also affects reproductive performance. Pair or trio matings (two females per male) are recommended. Harem mating (three or more females per male) of some strains results in a decreased number of offspring because the males do not copulate more than once every 3 or 4 days, or they concentrate their attentions on one female and ignore the others. Group matings (two or more females with two or more males) are not recommended because the male mice will fight. Young mice should be removed from the parents' cage when they are between 3 and 4 weeks of age. If weaning is delayed, young males may be attacked by their sire, young females may be impregnated and survival of subsequent litters is jeopardized because of overcrowded cages.

CONGENITAL AND HEREDITARY CONDITIONS

Three occasionally observed congenital abnormalities of the reproductive tract are vaginal septa, imperforate vagina and hermaphroditism. The incidence of vaginal septa varies from 1 to 38 per cent depending upon the inbred strain. These septa vary in thickness and length and are usually ruptured by coitus or parturition. Reproductive performances of septate and nonseptate female mice are not significantly different.[5] Imperforate vagina is occasionally observed in some inbred strains of mice. These mice are usually asymptomatic until 2 to 4 months of age when a perivaginal swelling that resembles scrotal sacs is noticed. The uterus and vagina are markedly distended by a clear mucoid sterile fluid. No attempts have been made to treat this condition. External genitalia of hermaphroditic mice are usually ambiguous. "Males" have poorly developed scrotal sacs and prepuce and may have mammary glands. "Females" lack mammary glands and have a prominent urogenital papilla.[15]

There are many identified genetic mutations of mice that affect reproductive performance. These mutations result in germ cell deficiencies, hormone imbalances or deficiencies, death of homozygous embryos or inability to copulate. Dr. M. Green's book[7] describes these mutations.

ABORTIONS

Infectious diseases that may cause abortions have been discussed previously. Abortions can also be caused by the stress of shipment from one facility to another. It is recommended that pregnant female mice be shipped between days 10 and 15 of gestation in order to minimize implantation failures or premature parturition. Exposure of the female mouse to a strange male or pheromones from a strange male within 48 to 72 hours of mating prevents implantation (the Bruce effect). This pregnancy block appears to be genetically determined.[15]

PERIPARTURIENT CARE OF THE DAM AND NEONATES

Periparturient female mice can be left with their mates if they are maintained in pair or trio matings and young are weaned by 4 weeks of age. If a harem mating system is used, the female should be removed to a separate cage in order to minimize disruption of her nest and trampling of neonates by other adults in the cage. Male mice are not usually aggressive toward neonates and may retrieve neonates that have wandered out of the nest.

Parturient female mice should be handled gently and quietly. Ideally, the female (and her mate) are transferred to a clean cage 1 to 2 days before the litter is born and not disturbed for 3 to 5 days after the litter is born. If it is necessary to handle a newborn litter, the female should be moved to another cage before her litter is examined. Neonates should be handled with forceps or gloved hand and returned to the nest, not scattered throughout the cage.

SURGICAL PROCEDURES OF THE REPRODUCTIVE SYSTEM

Surgical procedures in the mouse are performed using microsurgery or ophthalmic instruments. Fin pointed sharp/sharp dissecting or corneal scissors are used in place of scalpels. Hair is removed from the incision site by plucking. Scissors or electric dissecters often leave small pieces of hair that tend to migrate into the incision site. Hair can be removed using depilatories; however, the depilatory must be removed quickly in order to prevent chemical burns. Skin is decontaminated by standard techniques using cotton swabs in place of gauze sponges.

Dosages and routes of administration of selected anesthetic agents are listed in Table 2. Most of these anesthetic agents were selected because they are readily available in veterinary hospitals. If large numbers of mice need to be anesthetized, tribromoethanol is an excellent choice. This anesthetic is not available commercially and must be prepared from its basic ingredients, 2,2,2-tribromoethanol and amylene hydrate.[4]

Three surgical procedures that are frequently performed on reproductive tracts of mice are ovariectomy, castration and vasectomy. Ovariectomy can be performed through a ventral midline incision or through two incisions, one in each flank. However, the preferred technique utilizes ventral recumbency and a transverse skin incision that is located midway between the iliac crest and the last rib and is perpendicular to the vertebral column. The skin incision is rotated laterally until the junction of the lumbar muscles and abdominal muscles is visible. A 5- to 8-mm–long incision is made in the abdominal muscles over the ovarian fat pad. The incision should be parallel to segmental blood vessels and nerves and not include lumbar muscles. The ovarian fat pad will be visible at the dorsal end of the incision. Exteriorize the ovarian fat pad and rotate it dorsomedially to expose the ovary. A "crush and tear" technique is used to excise the ovary, oviduct and a portion of the ovarian fat pad. The forceps holding the ovarian pedicle should be held closed

Table 2. Selected Anesthetic Agents for Mice

Drug	Dose	Route of Administration	Comment
Inhalant			
Chloroform		Not recommended	Lethal to males of certain inbred strains.
Ether	To effect	Inhalation	Administer in a covered jar or open drip system. Remove mouse from jar as soon as it is unconscious. Do not use ether for major surgery. Overdose will result if mice come in contact with liquid ether.
Halothane		Not recommended	Margin between anesthetic dose and toxic dose is small.
Methoxyflurane	To effect	Inhalation	Administer using a vaporizer; do not use an open drip system or jar.
Nitrous oxide	To effect	Inhalation	80% NO_2, 15% O_2 for short procedures; or 0.05–1.5% halothane in equal parts NO_2 and O_2 for longer procedures.
Injectable			
Fentanyl and droperidol	0.005 ml/gm of a 10% solution of Innovar-Vet	Intramuscular or subcutaneous	Mice remain responsive to sudden noises.
Ketamine	Not recommended as sole anesthetic agent		Response variable; poor analgesia.
Ketamine and promazine	0.1 mg/gm ketamine given as Ketaset Plus	Intramuscular or subcutaneous	5 to 10 minute induction; 25 to 72 minutes of anesthesia.
Ketamine and xylazine	0.05 mg ketamine/gm 0.05 mg xylazine/gm	Intramuscular or subcutaneous	Final volume should not exceed 0.05 to 0.1 ml.
Pentobarbital	0.05 to 0.08 mg/gm	Intraperitoneal	Dilute in sterile saline so that final dose is 0.01 to 0.02 ml/gm. Length of anesthesia is variable. Keep mouse warm during recovery period.
Tribromoethanol	0.16 mg/gm	Intraperitoneal	See Cunliffe-Beamer TL, 1983 in the References.

for a few seconds in order to be certain that ovarian vessels are crushed. After the pedicle has been returned to the abdominal cavity, a single interrupted or mattress suture is used to close the incision in the abdominal muscles. The skin incision is rotated toward the other side and the contralateral ovary is excised. Then, the skin incision is closed with a small wound clip or everting mattress sutures. The uterus is usually left intact during castration of female mice.

Male mice are usually castrated through two scrotal incisions. The mouse is anesthetized and placed in dorsal recumbency with the head elevated. An incision 5 to 8 mm long and parallel to the median raphe is made in each scrotal sac. Testicles and their associated epididymal fat pads are exteriorized and excised using a "crush and tear" technique. Do not try to dissect the testicle away from the epididymal fat pad. On rare occasions, part of the small intestine herniates through the inguinal canal into the scrotal incision. These hernias can be reduced by adjusting the surgical table so that the mouse's head is lower than his tail. Scrotal incisions are not sutured.

Vasectomy is performed through a ventral midline abdominal incision extending from the pubic symphysis toward the umbilicus. Care must be taken to avoid accidental incision of the preputial glands. Each vas is exteriorized by gentle traction and a 3- to 5-mm portion is excised from the midsection. Testicular vessels or nerves should be left intact.

Postoperative care following these surgical procedures includes trimming toe nails and placing the mouse in a clean warm cage. Anesthetized mice should be placed in lateral or ventral recumbency with the head slightly extended and level. The cage is warmed by placing a 50 or 75 W electric light about 6 inches above the top of the cage in order to prevent hypothermia. "Mouse level" in the cage should feel warm, not hot, to the human hand in order to avoid heat stress.

REPRODUCTIVE RECORDS

Reproductive performance records start with the cage card. The cage card should list breeder identification number, birth dates of litters, number born per litter, weaning dates of litters and number of male mice and female mice weaned per litter. Cage card information is pooled in order to determine average number of mice born per litter, average number of mice weaned per litter, number of sterile matings relative to total matings, interval between birth of consecutive litters and lifetime production of breeding units. These data should be summarized monthly and examined for upward or downward trends of unusual magnitude. Seasonal variation can be expected even in colonies maintained in buildings with sophisticated environmental controls.

DIAGNOSTIC PROCEDURES

In the case of the individual mouse, the clinician relies upon visual examination and palpation in order to make a diagnosis. In the case of a large mouse colony, necropsy, microbiologic cultures and serologic tests are used to obtain information upon which a diagnosis can be made. In either case husbandry practices and the environment should be examined as closely as the mice themselves.

References

1. Bronson FH, Dagg CP, Snell GD: Reproduction. In Green EL (ed): The Biology of the Laboratory Mouse. 2nd ed. New York, Dover Publications, Inc, 1975, pp. 187–204.
2. Casey HW, Irving GW: Bacterial, mycoplasmal, mycotic and immune-mediated diseases of the urogenital system. In Foster HL, Small JD, Fox JG (eds): The Mouse in Biomedical Research. vol 2. New York, Academic Press, 1982, pp 43–54.
3. Champlin AK, Dorr DL, Gates AH: Determining the stage of the estrous cycle in the mouse by the appearance of the vagina. Biol Reprod 8:491, 1973.
4. Cunliffe-Beamer TL: Biomethodology. In Foster HL, Small JD, Fox JG (eds): The Mouse in Biomedical Research. vol 3. New York, Academic Press, 1983, pp 402–438.
5. Cunliffe-Beamer TL, Feldman D: Vaginal septa in mice: Incidence, inheritance and effect on reproductive performance. Lab Anim Sci 26:895, 1976.
6. Gates AH: Maximizing yield and developmental uniformity of eggs. In Daniel JC Jr (ed): Methods in Mammalian Embryology. San Francisco, Freeman. 1971, pp 64–75.
7. Green MC: Genetic Strains and Variants of the Laboratory Mouse. New York, Gustav, Fischer, Verlag, 1981.
8. Heiniger HJ, Dorey JJ: Handbook on Genetically Standardized JAX Mice. Bar Harbor, The Jackson Laboratory, 1980.
9. Hummell KP, Richardson FL, Fekete E: Anatomy. In Green EL (ed): The Biology of the Laboratory Mouse. 2nd ed. New York, Dover Publications, Inc, 1975, pp 247–308.
10. Knappa JJ: Nutrition. In Foster HL, Small JD, Fox JG (eds): The Mouse in Biomedical Research. vol 3. New York, Academic Press, 1983, pp 52–68.
11. Leckie PA, Watson JG, Chaykin S: An improved method for artificial insemination of the mouse (Mus musculus). Biol Reprod 9:420, 1973.
12. Marsk L, Larson KS: A simple method for nonsurgical blastocyst transfer in mice. J Reprod Fertil 37:393, 1974.
13. Whitten WK, Beamer WG, Byskov AC: The morphology of fetal gonads of spontaneous mouse hermaphrodites. J Embryol Exp Morphol 52:63, 1979.
14. Wimer RE, Fuller JL: Patterns of behavior. In Green EL (ed): The Biology of the Laboratory Mouse. 2nd ed. New York, Dover Publications, Inc, 1975, pp 629–654.
15. Whittingham DG, Wood MJ: Reproductive physiology. In Foster HL, Small JD, Fox JG (eds): The Mouse in Biomedical Research. vol 3. New York, Academic Press, 1983, pp 138–165.
16. Zurcker C, Burek JD, van Nunem MCJ, Meihuizen SP: A naturally occurring epizootic caused by Sendai virus in breeding and aging rodent colonies. I. Infection in the mouse. Lab Anim Sci 27:955, 1977.

SECTION

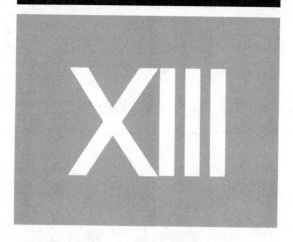

XIII

ZOO ANIMALS

William L. Lasley, Ph.D.

Consulting Editor

Zoo Animals— An Overview

William L. Lasley, Ph.D.
Zoological Society of San Diego, San Diego, California

Until recently, little has been known about the reproductive physiology of nondomesticated species. Hormone profiles reflecting the reproductive processes were traditionally generated through serum evaluations, and the difficulty of collecting blood samples from nontractable species prevented the accumulation of the essential baseline data. This problem has recently been overcome by the development of assay procedures that evaluate hormone metabolites in urine. Urinary hormone profiles reflect both the metabolism of active circulating hormones and, based on the assumption that clearance rate does not change, hormone production.

Urine samples can often be collected on a daily basis without capture and/or restraint of the animal. This aspect of the strategy obviates the worries associated with physical or anesthetic stress and the hormonal perturbations that may be related to these manipulations. Furthermore, urine requires no preparation and can be frozen and stored immediately. The evaluative procedures for urine are, in general, less laborious than hormone assays for serum hormones, thus the entire process can be considered practical.

There are two limitations to this approach that need to be recognized. Since hormone measurements are made on a concentration basis and urine production is not constant, total hormone production can be accurately appraised only through the collection of total urine volumes. This requirement severely detracts from the practicability of the approach and certainly limits breeding or display activities. For this reason, small (5 to 10 ml) daily urine samples are collected and the hormone concentrations are then indexed by the creatinine concentrations in the same samples. The procedure raises some valid questions in regard to the quantitative value of the final measurement, since the excretion rates of both metabolites are assumed to be constant. As a result, it is imperative that urinary hormone profiles be used with an appreciation for daily changes as well as absolute values. These variables underscore the importance of daily samples. The second limitation has to do with the difference in metabolism of the same hormone in different species. Little information exists on this problem and it is difficult to extrapolate from what is known in one species to anything other than another closely related species. Given this limitation, an attempt has been made in this section to describe the urinary hormone profile of representative species. While this sampling approach may convince the reader that most, if not all, species can be monitored, it does little to warn an investigator of instances in which certain evaluations may not be informative.

For some species only a few urine samples are needed to evaluate the reproductive status of the individual and even to diagnose a defect or to stage a pregnancy (as in the gorilla). In most species little or no baseline data exist, preventing the interpretation of results that might be desired at the present time. Such baseline or normative profiles are being accumulated, and those that have been completed are presented in the following sections.

It should be obvious to the reader that for species in which complete urinary profiles have been constructed, previously reported ranges of ovarian cycles and gestations can be narrowed appreciably. Ultimately, once standardized, such measurements will become diagnostic and predictive on an individual animal basis. Currently, this is true for many primate species and a few hoofed species, although little information is available for carnivores.

The following sections represent the first attempt to accumulate data on zoo animals based on the endocrine aspects of reproduction. Companion sections describe recent developments in exotic animal reproductive physiology, including artificial breeding and cryopreservation of germplasm. This rapidly growing field of study is reviewed with emphasis on embryo manipulation and semen collection and storage. Embryo transfer in exotic hoofed stock and carnivores is discussed in detail in the first section. Primate embryo transfer is included in the chapter on embryo transfer in the section on laboratory species. A comprehensive account of current research in semen physiology, collection, analysis and freezing constitutes a second section.

Space, however, does not allow for the complete integration of all aspects of reproduction in zoo animals, and the reader should be aware of the information provided by the authors in the previous edition of this book.

Primates

S. E. Shideler, Ph.D.
N. M. Czekala, B.S.
Zoological Society of San Diego, San Diego, California

APES

Gorilla gorilla

Ovarian Cycle. Data on plasma and urinary hormone levels of the lowland gorilla's menstrual cycle have been available for a number of years, but it is only recently that enough data have been collected, making it possible to begin defining the normal hormone profile of the gorilla ovarian cycle. Based on 22 menstrual cycles of six adult females, Mitchell and colleagues[7] reported the average cycle length of the lowland gorilla to be 32.0 ± 1.0 days (x ± SE), with a range of 25 to 42 days. Total urinary estrogen values (Et) indexed by creatinine (cr) throughout the cycle range from 4.00 to 128.00 ng/mg cr and show a midcycle peak of 76.00 ± 6.00 ng/mg cr as well as a smaller midluteal increase. The follicular phase (defined as the time from the first day of menstruation to the Et peak) is 19.5 ± 1.0 days long (range 11 to 30 days). Urinary pregnanediol-3-glucuronide (Pdg) concentrations range from 0.01 to 2.40 µg/mg cr. Pdg values remain low throughout the follicular phase (0.12 ± 0.01 µg/mg cr), which is followed by a luteal elevation ranging from 0.03 to 2.40 µg/mg cr and averaging 0.44 ± 0.04 µg/mg cr. The luteal phase (defined as beginning the day after the Et peak and continuing until the day before menstruation) is 12.3 ± 0.3 days long (range 10 to 14 days). The observed variation in overall cycle length is accounted for by the variation in follicular phase length within and between females.

Levels of urinary total estrogens and pregnanediol-3-glucuronide (and their duration) established by Mitchell and colleagues[7] for normal gorillas at different phases of their ovarian cycle may be used to identify and to discriminate abnormal, but reproductively functional, cycles from abnormal, dysfunctional cycles. Mitchell and colleagues[8] describe an infertile female gorilla exhibiting an ovarian cycle with an abnormally long follicular phase and normal Et and Pdg levels indicative of ovulation and a luteal phase sufficient to support implantation. An adolescent female gorilla exhibiting Et and Pdg levels indicative of ovulation is also described. The luteal phase of this animal is abbreviated, indicating an insufficient corpus luteum, which is a common luteal phase defect associated with adolescent sterility in humans.[8] Assuming a fertile male is present and compatible with the female, reproductive failure in these cases is a result of determining the optimal time of mating (or artificial insemination) based on the onset of menstruation without regard to follicular phase length in a given individual as well as female infertility. Mitchell and colleagues[8] describe four gorilla cycles monitored before and after artificial insemination attempts were made. These data reveal patterns of hormone excretion incompatible with the success of such clinical manipulations. It is suggested that preovulatory artificial inseminations were suboptimally timed, resulting in decreased steroid production and delayed ovulation. More precise timing of such manipulations coinciding with the occurrence of the ovulatory event appears necessary for successful artificial insemination.

Pregnancy. Czekala and colleagues[2] describe the normal gestation length of *Gorilla gorilla* as 255 days. The total urinary estrogen profile of pregnant gorillas is characterized by a sustained increase in estrogen excretion over that of nonpregnant gorillas, occurring from 9 to 26 weeks of gestation. During this time, estrogen levels increase from 0.15 ± 0.11 to 2.22 ± 0.26 µg/mg cr. Levels reach a plateau during the last 10 weeks of gestation, in which values range from 2.23 ± 0.23 to 3.88 ± 0.91 µg/mg cr. Czekala and colleagues[2] further report that the estrogen profile of pregnant gorillas is qualitatively similar to that of humans but quantitatively dissimilar, since only 10 to 20 per cent of the quantity of estrogen seen during human pregnancy is present in gorilla pregnancy.

Urinary hormone data on normal gorilla pregnancy can be used to establish approximate stages of gestation, which in turn may be used for assessment of fetal well-being during the course of pregnancy. Such data obviate the need for comparisons to human stages of gestation, in which the low estrogens of gorilla pregnancy might be construed as abnormal, resulting in faulty conclusions regarding fetal condition. Czekala and colleagues[2] reported that fetal well-being can be accurately monitored from urinary hormones in the gorilla, citing two pregnancies resulting in fetal death in which a fall in total estrogens precedes abortion and in which the pregnancy associated with placental infarcts and abruptio placentae is characterized by chronically low levels of estrogen. The data support the conclusion that detecting and monitoring gorilla pregnancy through urinary hormones is both more reliable and safer than by any other method.

Chorionic gonadotropin can be used to diagnose pregnancy in *Gorilla gorilla*, and there are a number of test kits, including the Human Pregnancy Test, that effectively measure chorionic gonadotropin.

Tests for gonadotropin, however, are not effective in staging pregnancy, since it is present throughout most, if not all, of gorilla pregnancy.

Pongo pygmaeus abelii

Ovarian Cycle. The ovarian cycle of the orangutan is approximately 30 days. Urinary total estrogen excretion increases from 0.07 μg/mg cr during the follicular phase to 0.10 μg/mg cr at the midcycle preovulatory peak, dropping to less than 0.02 μg/mg cr after ovulation.[6]

Pregnancy. Total urinary estrogen levels increase over nonpregnant levels of 0.02 μg/mg cr to 0.81 μg/mg cr within the first month of orangutan pregnancy, according to Czekala and colleagues.[1] Luteinizing hormone/chorionic gonadotropin bioactivity is detectable in early pregnancy (245.00 μg/mg cr versus 1.50 μg/mg cr in nonpregnant orangutans) and increases to a maximum value greater than 10,000 μg/mg cr within an estimated 6 to 8 weeks after conception. Gonadotropin excretion declines from this maximum but remains above baseline throughout pregnancy. At 8 to 10 weeks of gestation, total estrogen levels begin to increase from 0.2 μg/mg cr to 27.0 μg/mg cr until 15 days prior to parturition, whereupon levels gradually begin to decline. Positive responses to the Nonhuman Primate Pregnancy Test (chorionic gonadotropin) are obtainable until the last 2 months of pregnancy. Gestation lasts 258 days in the orangutan.

Czekala and colleagues[1, 2] report that the orangutan pregnancy closely resembles the human pregnancy qualitatively and quantitatively: both exhibit a steep, sustained estrogen rise from 20 to 30 per cent of gestation until near term, and both reach maximum estrogen levels of approximately 20.00 to 24.00 μg/mg cr during the last one fifth of pregnancy. Because of the overall similarities between human and orangutan pregnancies, orangutan total urinary estrogen levels at different stages of pregnancy (early pregnancy, 0.30 ± 0.05 μg/mg cr; late pregnancy, 16.60 ± 3.78 μg/mg cr) are comparable to those of human pregnancy (early pregnant, 0.46 ± 0.11 μg/mg cr; middle pregnant, 5.80 ± 1.61 μg/mg cr; late pregnant, 23.21 ± 4.44 μg/mg cr) such that it should be possible to stage orangutan pregnancies based on human values.[6]

Pan spp.

Pan troglodytes

Ovarian Cycle. The urinary hormone profile of the common chimpanzee's ovarian cycle is defined by Lasley and colleagues[6] as the interval between the onset of menstruation and 34 days. Total urinary estrogen levels begin to rise approximately 13 days after the onset of menstruation from less than 30.00 ng/mg cr to a maximum of approximately 180.00 ng/mg cr 4 days later. Et levels return to earlier follicular phase levels following ovulation at about day 20. The fall in total urinary estrogens is coincident with a peak in urinary luteinizing hormone (LH) bioactivity (approximately 17.00 μg/mg cr). Sex skin detumescence occurs immediately following the LH peak and menstruation 14 days later. A secondary rise in Et levels (70.00 to 90.00 ng/mg cr) is reported during the luteal phase between days 26 and 32.[3] Taken together, these data suggest a follicular phase of 20 days and a luteal phase of 14 days.

Pregnancy. Lasley and colleagues[6] show that implantation and early pregnancy in the common chimpanzee can be monitored through urinary hormones. Little deviation in hormonal levels is seen during the 10 days following ovulation in fertile versus nonfertile ovarian cycles. Levels of total estrogen and luteinizing hormone/chorionic gonadotropin bioactivity are elevated 2 weeks after ovulation and a fertile mating. Urinary estrogen begins to increase 4 to 5 days earlier from a low of less than 0.05 to 0.20 μg/mg cr 15 to 17 days after conception, falling to between 0.05 to 0.10 μg/mg cr for the next 5 days. Approximately 25 days after fertilization, urinary estrogen levels are above 0.30 μg/mg cr and climbing. Luteinizing hormone/chorionic gonadotropin levels are above 1100 μg/mg cr at this time, having increased from levels below 40.00 μg/mg cr during the first 2 weeks following the fertile mating.

Pan paniscus

Pregnancy. The pregnancy of the pygmy chimpanzee shows a progressive but gradual increase in urinary estrogen excretion throughout gestation.[1] At 20 per cent gestation, estrogen levels are less than 1.0 μg/mg cr and at 85 to 95 per cent gestation are close to 6.00 μg/mg cr (early pregnancy, 0.43 ± 0.05 μg/mg cr; middle pregnancy, 0.59 μg/mg cr; late pregnancy, 5.10 ± 2.5 μg/mg cr).[1, 6] From these data it is apparent that the estrogen excretion of pregnancy in this species is less pronounced than that observed in the human and orangutan and that maximum levels are one third as high and are in fact more similar to gorilla pregnancy values. In general, monitoring and staging chimpanzee pregnancies may be approached in the same way as for the gorilla.

OLD WORLD MONKEYS

Macaca silenus

Ovarian Cycle. Urinary hormone evaluations indicate a 31 ± 0.63 day ovarian cycle for the lion-tailed macaque. The cycle is characterized by a preovulatory increase in estrone conjugates from 126 ± 24.07 ng/mg cr that peak at 471.90 ± 62.95 ng/mg cr, which coincides with a midcycle peak in luteinizing hormone bioactivity.[11] After peaking, estrone levels fall to 62.22 ± 4.85 ng/mg cr and show a secondary rise during the luteal phase, reaching levels of 148.11 ± 13.80 ng/mg cr and then return to early preovulatory levels of less than 90.00 ng/mg cr. Menstruation is observed 17.9 ± 0.38 days after the estrone conjugate peak.

Pregnancy. Instead of returning to preovulatory levels 14 days after ovulation, estrone conjugate values for cycles of fertile lion-tailed macaque increase to over 300.00 ng/mg cr, reaching a level of 515.00 ± 38.00 ng/mg cr 19 days after ovulation then falling to 121.00 ± 36.00 ng/mg cr by the end of the second month of pregnancy.[11] Bioactive luteinizing hormone/chorionic gonadotropin measurements do not show an early pregnancy increase until 18 days, with a peak at approximately 14.00 μg/mg cr 20 days after ovulation. Shideler and colleagues[11] reported that placental sign (as indicated by vaginal bleeding) occurred 24 to 28 days after ovulation in one pregnant female, on day 25 in another and not until 34 to 39 days in a third. It was not observed at all in a fourth female. Gestation length is 172.6 days (n = 4).

The Nonhuman Primate Pregnancy Test may be used to diagnose pregnancy in *Macaca silenus*. Shideler and Lasley[9] reported positive results between 21 and 24 days after ovulation.

Pygathrix nemaeus

Ovarian Cycle. The fertile ovarian cycle of the Douc langur is characterized by a low total urinary estrogen profile (0.05 to 0.10 μg/mg cr) 4 to 12 days preceding the midcycle estrogen peak.[1] Within an additional 3 days a maximum level of 0.20 μg/mg cr of estrogen is reached. This event occurs 1 day prior to the bioactive luteinizing hormone peak of approximately 2.50 μg/mg cr. After peaking at midcycle, estrogen levels drop to early follicular levels 2 days later.

Pregnancy. Following the midcycle fall of estrogen in the Douc langur fertile cycle, estrogen excretion begins to increase 6 days later and shows a sharp early pregnant increase 14 days after the luteinizing hormone peak.[1] Urinary estrogens reach a plateau of more than 1.50 μg/mg cr, where they remain until a second excursion takes place at 20 to 22 weeks of gestation. Bioactive luteinizing hormone/chorionic gonadotropin begins to rise 9 to 10 days after the ovulatory luteinizing hormone peak and reaches levels of approximately 2000 μg/mg cr 10 to 11 days later or 20 to 21 days following presumed ovulation. Gonadotropin values fall, returning to nonpregnant levels at approximately 13 weeks of gestation. After a very steep second increase, estrogen levels oscillate between 4.00 and 9.00 μg/mg cr until 1 week prior to parturition, at which point they begin to fall to approximately 3.00 μg/mg cr. Maximum levels of estrogen excretion are observed at 60 per cent gestation in the Douc langur.

Using urinary estrogen measurements, Czekala and colleagues[1] stage the Doug langur pregnancy as follows: early pregnancy, 1.60 μg/mg cr; middle

pregnancy, 5.20 ± 1.30 μg/mg cr and late pregnancy, 6.48 ± 1.24 μg/mg cr. The Nonhuman Primate Pregnancy Test is also reported as reliable for confirming pregnancy during a 10-day interval 19 to 29 days after the ovulatory luteinizing hormone peak.

NEW WORLD MONKEYS

Ateles fusciceps robustus

Ovarian Cycle. A gradual preovulatory excursion of total urinary estrogens from less than 0.50 to more than 4.50 μg/mg cr is seen in the spider monkey.[4] After the midcycle increase, estrogen excretion declines, returning to early follicular phase levels 6 to 7 days after the total estrogen peak. Bioactive luteinizing hormone peaks on the same day as estrogen, reaching values between 4.00 and 6.00 μg/mg cr. A total cycle length of 20 to 22 days is reported for this species.

Saguinus fuscicollis

Ovarian Cycle. A total cycle length of 18 days, as determined by the interval between successive total urinary estrogen peaks,[4] is reported for the white-lipped tamarin. An abrupt rise in estrogen excretion from less than 50.00 to more than 70.00 μg/mg cr is seen 1 day prior to a luteinizing hormone peak of approximately 3.00 μg/mg cr. Three days after the luteinizing hormone peak, estrogen levels fall to 30.00 to 40.00 μg/mg cr.

Cebus albifrons

Ovarian Cycle. Intervals between successive periods of menstruation and total urinary estrogen or bioactive luteinizing hormone peaks suggest a cycle of 18 to 19 days in the capuchin.[4] During a short follicular phase of 4 to 5 days, estrogen excretion increases from levels below 10.00 μg/mg cr to maximum values ranging between 25.00 and 35.00 μg/mg cr. The luteal phase lasts 13 to 14 days in the capuchin. Urinary estrogens return to earlier follicular phase values 2 days after the midcycle peak and show a secondary increase to approximately 15.00 μg/mg cr 4 to 6 days later. The peak level of bioactive luteinizing hormone (approximately 6.00 to 7.00 μg/mg cr) is coincident with the estrogen peak.[3] Hodges and colleagues[3] also report a successful mating of a socially rejected female, in which the time of ovulation and optimal time of pairing were anticipated through monitoring her urinary estrogen profile. A male was removed from his social group for 3 hours and paired with this female, resulting in the birth of a healthy male offspring 5½ months later.

Pregnancy. Conception in the capuchin is evidenced by a slow sustained increase in total estrogen excretion during the luteal phase of the fertile ovulatory cycle.[1] Eight to eleven days after the ovulatory luteinizing hormone peak, estrogen levels are approximately 20.00 µg/mg cr. An abrupt increase in luteinizing hormone/chorionic gonadotropin bioactivity occurs 20 to 21 days after ovulation, with values higher than 5.00 µg/mg cr. Gonadotropin levels reach their highest levels around 28 to 29 days after conception (approximately 300.00 µg/mg cr) and immediately begin to fall, although they do not return to nonpregnant levels until the last 2 months of pregnancy. Total estrogen concentrations fluctuate around 20.00 µg/mg cr until the last 2 months when a second increase to levels higher than 50.00 µg/mg cr is observed. Estrogens fall sharply at the end of pregnancy, reaching 1.80 µg/mg cr 1 day prior to parturition. Gestation is estimated as 170 days in the capuchin.

Czekala and colleagues[1] stage capuchin pregnancies, based on urinary total estrogen levels, at 23.58 ± 1.14 µg/mg cr for early pregnancy, 14.58 ± 0.75 µg/mg cr for middle pregnancy and 27.00 ± 5.26 µg/mg cr for late pregnancy. In addition, these authors report that the Nonhuman Primate Pregnancy Test gives unambiguous positive results approximately 31 to 61 days after ovulation in the pregnant capuchin.

PROSIMIANS

Lemur variegatus

Ovarian Cycle. Ruffed lemur females (*Lemur variegatus*) are seasonally polyestrous, exhibiting 40- to 44-day intervals between successive cycles. The breeding season begins in mid-December and may continue through March in the northern hemisphere. Females have imperforate vaginas except prior to, during and immediately following estrus (and at parturition). The duration of the onset and termination of genital changes necessary for copulation to occur is 9.85 ± 1.67 days.

The urinary total estrogen profile of *Lemur variegatus* females during their ovarian cycle exhibits a gradual preovulatory estrogen increase over 4 to 6 days, ranging from 7.00 to 12.50 ng/mg cr to 18.00 to 25.00 ng/mg cr. This estrogen increase occurs 30 to 36 days following the previous ovulation or 6 to 8 days prior to ovulation.[13] Serum progesterone measurements by Lasley and colleagues[5] demonstrate that the luteal phase in this species is 28 days, and folliculogenesis, as indicated by increased estrogen production, follows the demise of the previous corpus luteum by 2 to 8 days. In the second or subsequent ovulations following the onset of the breeding season, ruffed lemur females initiate follicular maturation after serum progesterone falls below 2.00 ng/ml. Urinary estrogen progresses to peak levels the day before copulation and assumed ovulation. Copulation is limited to 1 day of the cycle, immediately following estrogen withdrawal and as progesterone levels begin to climb toward peak luteal levels of approximately 30.00 ng/ml.[5, 10, 12, 13]

The occurrence of copulation falls 6 to 7 days after the onset of genital changes, which suggests that these changes are estrogen directed in *L. variegatus* females.

Pregnancy. Gestation is 100.75 ± 1.6 days long in the ruffed lemur.[10] Urinary total estrogen levels are low during the first half of pregnancy, although higher (1.00 µg/mg cr) than those reported for the preovulatory peak (0.018 to 0.025 µg/mg cr) associated with estrus and mating in conceptive cycles.[12] Estrogen concentrations rise steadily during the second half of pregnancy until 10 days prior to parturition, reaching values between 1.50 and 7.20 µg/mg cr. A prepartum drop in total estrogens is observed during the last 10 days of gestation. Luteinizing hormone/chorionic gonadotropin bioactivity remains near the limit of sensitivity of the assay at low levels during the first 18 days of pregnancy and, therefore, is not useful for diagnosing pregnancy in this species.

The broad range in estrogen levels between individual females during the second half of pregnancy is associated with fetal adrenal hyperplasia, but the highest increases among individual dams are strongly related to the number of males in utero and are associated with fetal testicular hyperplasia.

References

1. Czekala NM, Hodges JK, Lasley BL: Pregnancy monitoring in diverse primate species by estrogen and bioactive luteinizing hormone determinations in small volumes of urine. J Med Primatol 10:1, 1981.
2. Czekala NM, Benirschke K, McClure H, Lasley BL: Urinary estrogen excretion during pregnancy in the gorilla (*Gorilla gorilla*), orangutan (*Pongo pygmaeus*) and the human (*Homo sapiens*). Biol Reprod 28:289, 1983.
3. Hodges JK, Czekala NM, Lasley BL: Estrogen and luteinizing hormone secretion in diverse primate species from simplified urinary analysis. J Med Primatol 8:349, 1979.
4. Hodges JK, Gulick BA, Czekala NM, Lasley BL: Comparison of urinary estrogen excretion in South American primates. J Reprod Fert 61:83, 1981.
5. Lasley BL, Bogart MH, Shideler SE: A comparison of lemur ovarian cycles. In Alexander NJ (ed): Animal Models for Research on Contraception and Infertility. New York, Harper & Row, 1978, pp 417–424.
6. Lasley BL, Hodges JK, Czekala NM: Monitoring the female reproductive cycle of the great apes and other primate species by determination of oestrogen and LH in small volumes of urine. J Reprod Fert Suppl 28:121, 1980.
7. Mitchell WR, Presely S, Czekala NM, Lasley BL: Urinary immunoreactive estrogen and pregnanediol-3-glucuronide during the normal menstrual cycle of the female lowland gorilla (*Gorilla gorilla*). Am J Primatol 2:167, 1982.
8. Mitchell WR, Loskutoff NM, Czekala NM, Lasley BL: Abnormal menstrual cycles in the female gorilla (*Gorilla gorilla*). J Zoo Anim Med 13:143, 1982.
9. Shideler SE, Lasley BL: A comparison of primate ovarian cycles. Am J Primatol Suppl 1:171, 1982.
10. Shideler SE, Lindburg DG: Selected aspects of *Lemur variegatus* reproductive biology. Zoo Biol 1:127, 1982.
11. Shideler SE, Czekala NM, Kasman LH, et al.: Monitoring ovulation and implantation in the lion-tailed macaque (*Macaca silenus*) through urinary estrone conjugate evaluations. Biol Reprod 29:905, 1983.
12. Shideler SE, Czekala NM, Benirschke K, Lasley BL: Urinary estrogens during pregnancy of the ruffed lemur (*Lemur variegatus*). Biol Reprod 28:963, 1983.
13. Shideler SE, Lindburg DG, Lasley BL: Estrogen-behavior correlates in the reproductive physiology and behavior of the ruffed lemur (*Lemur variegatus*). Horm Behav 17:249, 1983.

Hoofed Species

N. M. Loskutoff, M.S.
L. H. Kasman
Zoological Society of San Diego, San Diego, California

Evaluating reproductive status and function in exotic hoofed species is difficult because of their size and/or problems with restraining them. For these reasons it is important to utilize all possible methods available in a concerted effort to assess individuals for advanced breeding programs.

Through these methods the following information should be gained:

1. Basic fertility evaluations.
2. Predicting estrus and ovulation.
3. Confirming ovulation and evaluating luteal function.
4. Pregnancy detection and monitoring fetal well-being.
5. Predicting parturition.

This article summarizes the methodology presently available for a number of hoofed species. A great deal of attention has been given to urinary hormone analysis. This has been shown to be a viable method of reproductive evaluation, especially in species that show few if any overt signs of gonadal activity. Additionally, the intractability of many of these species necessitates strategies that limit the need for restraint that could lead to stress or injury.

ARTIODACTYLA

This order is comprised of eight families. The cow, sheep, pig and goat are domestic representatives. Reproductive studies have previously centered around the domestic species for production purposes. The interest in maintaining captive herds of wild species has led to a limited but useful amount of information on their reproductive biology.

Estrous Detection. Until recently, the principal method employed for heat detection has been via behavioral observations. Although this appraisal method can prove to be quite adequate for many hoofed animals, a large number of individuals from diverse artiodactylid species have been known on occasion to fail to exhibit distinct behavioral manifestations of estrus ("silent heat") as well as to tolerate advances of a male merely as an act of submission rather than in response to their estrous cycle. In addition, the various environmental conditions and pressures imposed on captive animals preclude the standardization of objective behavioral data.

Rectal palpation or blood sampling for reproductive hormone concentrations would be impractical because of the restraint methods necessary for their proper administration as well as the lack of sufficient background information necessary for interpreting the findings in exotic ungulates.

Vaginal cytology has been studied in a variety of hoofed species in an attempt to correlate various stages of the estrous cycle with specific cellular characteristics. In the female bongo (*Tragelaphus eurycerus*) a positive correlation was demonstrated between distinct cellular changes in the vaginal vestibule and the sexual behavior patterns of the male.[1] In the okapi (*Okapia johnstoni*) cyclic changes in vaginal cytology were consistent with fluctuations in the concentrations of urinary steroid metabolites (de Groen, personal communication, 1981). In each case the vaginal smears were collected without the need for restraint measures.

The white-tailed deer (*Odocoileus virginianus borealis*) has provided a model for the study of reproductive events associated with seasonal variations as assessed by circulating endocrine evaluations[10] to aid in defining ovarian function in cervid species. The limited data that is presently available on the endocrine systems of cervids results from longitudinal studies requiring serial blood sample collections from surplus animals that either are chemically immobilized or manually restrained. Recent investigations have demonstrated, however, that such restraint measures can significantly alter blood steroid measurements immediately prior to, or during, blood collection[14] because of the adrenal response to the alarm reaction of the animal.[11]

Ovulation—Luteal Function. The development of direct assays for urinary hormone metabolites in their conjugated form has been found to be a practical alternative method for assessing reproductive function in a variety of exotic ungulates. Recent studies have indicated that a principal progesterone metabolite in many artiodactylid species is pregnanediol-3-glucuronide (pdg).[8] Since the limited duration of the follicular phase in most artiodactylid species would not allow sufficient time for estrogen evaluations to time impending ovulations for controlled breeding purposes, the most effective strategy would be to monitor luteal function through pdg evaluations. Luteal regression immediately precedes the next ovulatory event, and behavioral estrus is typically observed at this time. It is assumed that increased estrogen excretion and ovulation

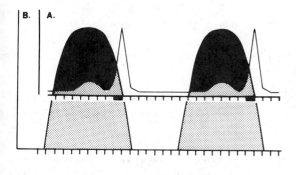

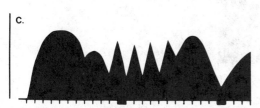

Figure 1. *A,* Typical cyclic ovarian profile of a female okapi as reflected by urinary estrogens (light areas) and pdg (shaded areas). Periods of overt behavioral estrus (dark bars) are indicated. *B,* Typical cyclic ovarian profile of a female giraffe as reflected by urinary PdG levels, shown for comparison with the okapi profile. Urinary estrogens or behavioral data are not available in this example. *C,* Example of a female okapi with reproductive dysfunction in the form of apparent persistent corpora lutea. Periods of overt behavioral estrus (dark bars) are indicated. Urinary estrogen levels were found to remain low throughout this period. (From Loskutoff NM, et al.: J Zoo Anim Med 14:3, 1983.)

occur the day after an estrogen surge, which would be difficult to monitor from urinary analysis.

Pdg has been found to be correlated with circulating progesterone levels in species as diverse as giraffids and bovids. Figure 1*A* illustrates the typical cyclic ovarian profile of a female okapi (a giraffid species) as reflected by urinary estrogens and pdg levels. The luteal phase appears to begin about 6 days after the preovulatory estrogen peak and is characterized by increasing pdg levels, which remain elevated for approximately 7 days.[7] The phase of apparent ovarian inactivity observed from the preovulatory estrogen peak to the subsequent rise in pdg excretion may be from the sensitivity of assay techniques. Baseline pdg levels in the okapi are generally too low to be reliably measured by the current assay system. The urinary pdg profile of a cycling giraffe (*Giraffa camelopardalis*) offers support to this premise (Fig. 1*B*). Because of differences in water intake requirements or habits, the urine of the giraffe studied generally was much more concentrated (by as much as tenfold) than the okapi urine, as determined by creatinine concentrations. Although the typical cycling ovarian profiles of the okapi and the giraffe appear quite similar when the hormonal concentrations are adjusted by

their creatinine content, the increased concentration of mass in the giraffe samples allows for a clearer resolution of the profile through inclusion of points of inflection at the terminal ends of the luteal phase. In reference to their urinary pdg profiles, the total cycle length in the okapi and the giraffe is approximately 15 days.

Urinary estrogens in the giraffid species are found in extremely low concentrations and vary in molecular form at different phases of the cycle. Apparently, urinary estrone and estradiol are found to increase during the luteal phase of the nonfertile cycle and beyond day 50 of gestation.

The scimitar-horned oryx (*Oryx tao*) has a urinary steroid excretion profile typical of most bovids (Fig. 2*A*). The apparent luteal phase begins about 2 days after estrus, and the pdg levels remain elevated for approximately 18 days. The total cycle length in the oryx is about 22 days. As in the giraffids, these species excrete very low levels of estrogens, thus making the routine monitoring of folliculogenesis impractical. In artificial breeding pdg evaluations during hormonal manipulations can confirm the validity of the hormonal regimen by demonstrating appropriate physiologic responses (Fig. 2*B*). On the other hand, pdg evaluations can suggest reasons for protocol failure by revealing aberrations such as an anovulatory cycle, delay of response or luteal insufficiency.

Ovarian dysfunction in the form of apparent persistent corpora lutea can also be identified by the failure of pdg to return to baseline levels but not reaching levels typically observed in pregnancy (Fig. 1*C*). Urinary steroid evaluations not only aid in the diagnosis of a reproductive disorder but also provide additional information during the course of treatment by monitoring the recovery of the animal to a potentially fertile condition.

Pregnancy Diagnosis. In the domestic cow, blood or milk progesterone evaluations have become a routine service available to farmers for pregnancy determinations. A recent study has shown that in the river buffalo (*Bubalus bubalis*), in which returns to estrus are often unobserved because of poor behavioral expression, a single blood evaluation for increased progesterone production 21 days after insemination is an accurate method for detecting pregnancy in that species.[9] In some of the smaller and/or more easily excited hoofed species, however, blood sampling would be inappropriate, owing to the risk involved in harming either the dam or the developing fetus.

In the okapi, pregnancy can be detected 22 days after breeding by an increase in urinary pdg excretion above average luteal phase levels in the nonfertile cycle. Urinary estrogen levels were found to markedly increase 50 days after breeding, apparently as a result of contribution from the developing fetus.

Pregnancy was detected in one of two musk oxen (*Ovibos moschatus*) that was found to excrete high levels of pdg during an otherwise seasonally inactive period as compared with her nonpregnant counter-

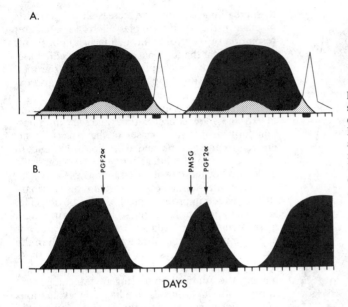

A.

B.

DAYS

Figure 2. *A,* The cyclic ovarian profile of a scimitar-horned oryx as reflected by urinary estrogens (light areas) and pdg (shaded areas). Periods of overt behavioral estrus (dark bars) are indicated. *B,* Example of the physiologic response of an oryx to hormonal manipulation. Urinary estrogen data are not available in this example. (From Loskutoff NM, et al.: J Zoo Animal Med 14:3, 1983.)

part in which only very low, nonfluctuating levels were observed. In the female giraffe, elevated pdg concentrations sharply declined to baseline levels approximately 3 days prior to parturition.

Although limited information is presently available on exotic artiodactyla, preliminary data suggest that predictable hormone changes will allow the early diagnosis of pregnancy, reflect the presence of a viable fetus and predict impending parturition in a variety of these species.

PERISSODACTYLA

The perissodactyla include the families Equidae, Rhinoceroidae and Tapiridae. Except for the domestic horse all are relatively intractable. Presently little data exist concerning the monitoring of reproductive events in most of these species. Again, the domestic horse is the exception and the knowledge of this species should give insight to other Equidae. However, recent endocrine studies of exotic perissodactyla have found differences between the three families and suggest that generalities within this order can be made only with caution.

Estrus Detection. Observation of behavioral changes would provide the simplest and most practical method of detecting follicular maturation. Though teasing methods are a viable method in the domestic mare, they are not feasible in nondomestic species. Of the rhinoceros species, only the Indian (*Rhinoceros unicornis*) shows overt signs of estrus. These include whistling and squirting of urine. This behavior usually lasts from 2 to 4 days, during which time matings often occur.

In the other two major species of rhinoceroses, black (*Diceros bicornis*) and white (*Ceratotherium simum*), behavioral changes are much less pronounced during apparent periods of estrus. Scat-

tered reports of irritability and swelling of the vulva have been observed in cows of these species. The increased aggressiveness of bulls has shown to be a much better indicator of estrus.

Less is known about the tapir species. Apparently, estrus is not associated with any behavioral changes. Physical examination for monitoring follicular maturation is not practical in most members of this order. Rectal palpations not only require restraint measures but are physically impossible in the large rhinos and tapirs. Vaginal cytology is possible in well-trained animals, although no published information exists on its use in these species.

Urinary hormone analysis has been shown to reflect ovarian function in the domestic mare, and its application has recently been applied to other perissodactylids. The report of Kassam and Lasley[6] described the urinary estrogen pattern in the Indian rhinoceros. Cyclic patterns were observed at intervals of approximately 43 days. Behavioral estrus was observed by keepers about ten days after the initial rise of estrogens and lasted approximately 48 hours. Elevated estrogen levels were observed for approximately 15-day intervals in these species. These preliminary studies suggest that ovarian function can be monitored in this species through urinary analysis.

Ovulation—Luteal Function. An important consideration of estrous cycle monitoring is the substantiation of ovulation and competent luteal function. Since ovulatory failure may exist in the face of follicular maturation, the measurement of progesterone in serum or its metabolites in urine is necessary to confirm the completion of ovulation and increased luteal activity. Presently, among the exotic perissodactyla, the Indian rhinoceros is the one species that has been successfully described in this manner. Figure 3*A* represents a typical profile of urinary estrone sulfate (E$_1$S) and pdg in this

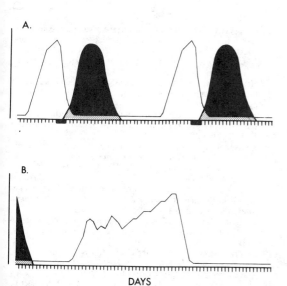

Figure 3. *A*, Cyclic ovarian profile representative of a female Indian rhinoceros as reflected by urinary estrogen (light areas) and pdg (shadowed areas). Periods of overt behavioral estrus (dark bars) are indicated. *B*, Urinary steroid excretion profile of a female rhinoceros with apparent reproductive dysfunction. Behavioral estrus is not clearly detected during the entire collection interval. (From Loskutoff NM, et al.: J Zoo Anim Med 14:3, 1983.)

species. The follicular phase appears to last 15 days, followed by a luteal phase of about 16 days. Ovulation probably occurs just after the E_1S peak when pdg levels are beginning to rise. Behavioral signs of estrus are observed at the E_1S peak and for 2 to 3 days after. When pdg levels decline to baseline values, there are about 12 days of very little ovarian activity. This may in part be caused by the sensitivity of the current assay systems.

Figure 3*B* illustrates the usefulness of these analyses. A female in questionable health produced this profile. No behavioral estrus was observed, and the prolonged elevated E_1S levels were not followed by a luteal phase, as would be indicated by a rise in pdg. Infertility problems as such can only be detected through hormone analysis or physical examination. The urinary analysis offers a noninvasive practical method in exotic species.

Pregnancy Diagnosis. In the mare, the domestic representative of this order, pregnancy determinations include behavioral observation, rectal palpation and serum measurement of estrogens, progesterone and PMSG as well as other less popular methods.[3] In the exotic species some of these methods have been utilized. In those species that show overt behavioral changes according to reproductive state, observations can be useful if good records are kept. Ultrasonography has been attempted in tapirs, but no positive data yet exist.

Physiological monitoring, primarily through hormone analysis, has been successful in diagnosing pregnancy in mares and has shown promise in the exotics. Terqui and Palmer[13] measured plasma levels of estrogens in trotter mares. Levels of total estrogens were significantly higher between days 36 and 45 compared with days 0 and 35.

A recent study measured estrone conjugate in urine of mares, reporting a significant rise between days 37 and 45 after ovulation. Though these findings will probably be valuable for other equine species, preliminary studies in other perissodactyla show different patterns of steroid excretion.

In the Indian rhinoceros urinary estrogens do not appear to be informative in early pregnancy diagnosis. However, by 60 days gestation, levels of pdg and luteal phase levels remain elevated throughout the 6 months proceeding conception. No hormonal evaluations have been completed during early pregnancy in the other species of rhinoceros or in the tapirs. Urine samples from the last 3 months of gestation in the three species of rhinoceros and the Malayan tapir have been obtained and analyzed for steroids.

In the Indian and black rhinoceros species, urinary estrone conjugate (E_1C) levels were uninformative. Pdg levels were elevated and remained so for 1 to 2 weeks after parturition. A late pregnancy in a white rhinoceros showed baseline levels of E_1C 1 month prior to parturition. Pdg levels were found to decline fourfold during the last 2 weeks before delivery.

Some hormonal data have been collected on late pregnancy in the Malayan tapir. Three animals during late pregnancy had elevated levels of both E_1C and pdg compared with nonpregnant levels. Both steroids declined during the last 2 weeks of gestation.

PROBOSCIDEA

Elephants have been the focus of several recent studies in an attempt to define reproductive events in these species. The detailed report of Hess and colleagues[4] described serum levels of estrone (E_1), estradiol (E_2), progesterone (Po) and luteinizing hormone (LH) in Asian elephants (*Elephas maximus*). Estrogen and LH levels showed no apparent pattern. Po levels indicated an estrous cycle with a length of about 16 weeks. Exposure of a bull to female urine elicited a flehmenlike response during late interluteal periods.

Prior to Hess and colleagues' report, the cycle length of this species was thought to be from 18 to 22 days. This was based on behavioral studies,[5] urinary analysis of estrogens[12] and serum measurements of estrogens and LH.[2] Because ovulation was not substantiated in these latter studies, a misunderstanding of actual reproductive events resulted. Apparently, the elephant has waves of follicular maturation before actually ovulating. Additionally, the female appears to be receptive to the male during these waves.

The study by Hess also measured serum levels of Po during pregnancy. Fertile cycles were indicated by a continued rise of Po above luteal phase levels, with a dramatic decline 3 days prior to parturition.

Urinary levels of estrone conjugates (E_1C) have been measured during late pregnancy in both species of elephant. In the African species (*Loxodonta africana*), urine samples have been obtained 1 month prior to parturition. Levels of estrone conjugates were tenfold higher than nonpregnant baseline values. Additionally, there was a substantial decline in the levels of E_1C 2 weeks prior to parturition. In the Asian elephant elevated levels of estrone conjugates have been measured in urine samples from 17 through 23 months of a 24-month gestation compared with nonpregnant levels. No samples have as yet been analyzed through parturition in this species. It should be noted that a quantitative difference of estrone conjugates was found between the two species, with the Asians generally having tenfold higher levels. This must be taken into consideration when applying data from one species to another.

In a species that shows no outward signs of estrus and in which pregnancy is difficult to diagnose until the later stages, a complementary program of management techniques and laboratory methods will become increasingly more important for successful captive breeding of elephants.

References

1. Brownscheidle CM, Dresser BL, Russell PT: The estrous cycle of an African bongo—breeding behavior and cytology of vaginal smears. J Zoo Anim Med 10:41, 1981.

2. Chappel SC, Schmidt M: Cyclic release of luteinizing hormone and the effects of luteinizing hormone–releasing hormone injection in Asiatic elephants. Am J Vet Res 40:451, 1979.
3. Ginther OJ: Reproductive Biology of the Mare. Ann Arbor, McNaughton and Gunn, 1979, pp 248–250.
4. Hess DL, Schmidt AM, Schmidt MJ: Reproductive cycle of the Asian elephant (*Elephas maximus*) in captivity. Biol Reprod 28:767, 1983.
5. Jainudeen MR, Eisenberg JF, Tilakerine N: Oestrous cycle of the Asiatic elephant, *Elephas maximus*, in captivity. J Reprod Fert 27:321, 1971.
6. Kassam AAH, Lasley BL: Estrogen excretory patterns in the Indian rhinoceros (*Rhinoceros unicornis*), determined by simplified urinary analysis. Am J Vet Res 42:251, 1981.
7. Loskutoff NM, Ott JE, Lasley BL: Urinary steroid evaluations to monitor ovarian function in exotic ungulates. I. Pregnanediol-3-glucuronide immunoreactivity in the okapi (*Okapia johnstoni*). Zoo Biol 1:45, 1982.
8. Loskutoff NM, Ott JE, Lasley BL: Strategies for assessing ovarian function in exotic species. J Zoo Anim Med 14:3, 1983.
9. Perera BMAO, Abeywardena SA, Abeygunawardena NA: Early pregnancy diagnosis in buffaloes from plasma progesterone concentration. Vet Rec 106:104, 1980.
10. Plotka ED, Seal US, Schmoller GC, et al.: Reproductive steroids in the white-tailed deer (*Odocoileus virginianus borealis*). I. Seasonal changes in the female. Biol Reprod 16:340, 1977.
11. Plotka ED, Seal US, Verme LJ, Ozoga JJ: The adrenal gland in white-tailed deer: A significant source of progesterone. J Wild Manag 47:38, 1983.
12. Ramsay EC, Lasley BL, Stabenfeldt GH: Monitoring the estrous cycle of the Asian elephant (*Elephas maximus*) using urinary estrogens. Am J Vet Res 42:256, 1981.
13. Terqui M, Palmer E: Oestrogen pattern during early pregnancy in the mare. J Reprod Fert Suppl 27:441, 1979.
14. Wesson JA, Scanlon PF, Kirkpatrick RL, Mosby HS: Influence of chemical immobilization and physical restraint on steroid hormone levels in blood of white-tailed deer. Can J Zool 57:768, 1979.

Carnivore Reproduction

Victor M. Shille, D.V.M., Ph.D.
University of Florida, Gainesville, Florida

Amelia E. Wing, B.S.
Zoological Society of San Diego, San Diego, California

The knowledge of reproductive physiology and related disorders in nondomestic carnivores is primarily anecdotal and has only recently begun to be based on proceptive, systematically collected observational and endocrine data. Practical management of reproduction and infertility is hampered by the lack of appreciation for physiological events on which the zoo clinician could base a logical differential diagnosis. This problem is further compounded by poorly understood environmental and sociobehavioral requirements.

Current developments in this field will be reviewed in this article. For information published before 1978, please refer to the exhaustive review by Seager and Demorest.[24]

MUSTELIDAE

Most mustelidae reach sexual maturity in the spring following their birth, at approximately 1 year of age. A notable exception is the wolverine (*Gulo gulo*), which attains puberty at 3 to 4 years.[30] In ferrets (*Mustela putorius*) exposure to a long-day photoperiod (16 hours of light to 8 hours of darkness) at 15 weeks of age is followed in 2 weeks by increased plasma luteinizing hormone and 17β-estradiol concentrations and sexual activity.[21]

Seasonal sexual behavior of the male badger (*Meles meles*), European marten (*Martes martes*), stone marten (*M. foina*) and polecat (*Mustela putorius*) is reported to occur annually in the spring. Only the badger retains active spermatogenesis throughout the year, while testicular size and spermatozoal numbers in the other species decline between July and March.[2] Female mustelids are seasonally polyestrous, with a breeding period relating to increased daylight.

Cyclic cornification of the vaginal epithelium and vulval edema have been correlated with mating behavior in the ferret, mink (*Mustela vison*) and American marten (*Martes americana*). In the absence of mating, follicular activity continues in the ferret for long intervals (up to 120 days) and the resulting hyperestrinism may lead to aplastic anemia. Unwanted estrus can be terminated in these species with chorionic gonadotropin (1000 IU intramuscularly).[22] Ovulation and termination of estrus are not induced in these species by gonadotropin-releasing hormone (GnRH) treatment.[6] This treatment, however, restricts the duration of coitus in mink to 5 minutes (versus 25 minutes) and reduces fertility.[1]

Gestation length in mustelidae varies according to the need for delayed implantation. Those species with obligatory embryonal diapause generally have longer total gestation intervals (7 to 9 months) than those without. Those without obligatory embryonal diapause have lengths of pregnancy similar to other small carnivores (40 to 65 days). It is reported in mink that the period of embryonal diapause is characterized by low plasma progesterone levels, which gradually increase after implantation, reaching a maximum about 30 days prepartum.[14, 15] Implantation can be advanced and the rise of progesterone hastened by treatment with prolactin.[18]

URSIDAE

The Ursidae are some of the several mammalian species that exhibit an obligatory delay of implantation. In the American black bear (*Ursus americanus*) conception occurs during mid-June, and after rapid development to the blastocyst stage, the embryo remains dormant for about 145 to 164 days. During this period plasma progesterone levels are higher than in nonpregnant bears, but they increase two- to threefold at the approximate time of implantation.[10] These changes may be used to diagnose pregnancy and monitor successful implantation in the bear if baseline progesterone concentrations are known.

The results of a carefully documented, retrospective study of successful birth and rearing of cubs in 11 species of bears has shown that denning arrangements should provide privacy and a sense of security to prevent dystocia caused by interrupted second stage labor and perinatal death through crushing or neglect by the nervous dam.[27]

HYENIDAE

Spotted hyenas (*Crocuta crocuta*) are known to lack sexual dimorphism. The female is actually a completely masculinized individual with a peniform clitoris that contains the urogenital orifice and fused labiae, forming a scrotum. Masculinization takes place during fetal development, probably because of an episode of androgen secretion by the fetal gonad, which affects the external genital primordium but not the wolffian ducts.[13]

Sexing of *Crocuta crocuta* may be done by the buccal smear technique, which although successful, presents the problem of obtaining the necessary scraping without sedation of the animal. Another method for sexing is to use a hair plucked from the animal with its root intact (Olympia test). The hair must be prepared within 15 to 20 minutes of collection for microscopic examination of the external root sheath cells; the sex chromatin in the female appears as a dark body along the inner periphery of the nuclear membrane. No sex chromatin is seen in the male.[31]

Measurement of urinary estrogens has proved to be a successful, noninvasive method for monitoring the estrous cycle of *Hyena brunnea*.[9] Estrus induction with GnRH and follicle-stimulating hormone (FSH) shows that GnRH is a more potent ovarian stimulator in this species.

FELIDAE

Behavioral estrus and patterns of gonadal hormones were studied in the puma (*Felis concolor*),[4] the jaguar (*Panthera onca*)[28] and the lioness (*Panthera leo*).[23] Patterns of ovarian activity suggest that the puma and jaguar are induced ovulators, while the lioness, which shows a repeated spontaneous rise of progesterone related to estrus but not to coitus, may be a spontaneous ovulator. Estrous cycle intervals are 17 to 25 days for the puma, 47 days for the jaguar and 3 to 8 weeks for the lioness; in the latter, progesterone elevation demarcated luteal phases, which lasted 2 to 6 weeks. Vaginal cornification in Felidae is well correlated with estrous behavior but follows the rise of estrogen, so that although estrus could be confirmed by cytology, early phases of the cycle could not be predicted by vaginal smears.

Felidae seem to respond well to efforts for induction of ovarian activity; however, confirmed pregnancies have only been reported in a few cases. A 5-day follicle-stimulating hormone regimen (10 mg/day) was tested in five cheetahs (*Acinonyx jubatus*), five North Chinese leopards (*Panthera pardus japonensis*), four Bengal tigers (*Panthera tigris tigris*), two African lions (*Panthera leo*) and one puma (*Felis concolor*). Folliculogenesis and ovulation, as observed by laparoscopy, were seen in all the treated animals; an injection of a luteinizing-hormone source was not required to induce follicular rupture.[19] A similar regimen for inducing ovulation in cheetahs[29] has proved successful. Bonney and colleagues[4] have reported pregnancies in the puma following treatment with pregnant mare serum gonadotropin and artificial insemination. In the Persian leopard (*Panthera pardus saxicolor*) ovulation was induced during a spontaneous cycle with human chorionic gonadotropin, and pregnancy followed artificial insemination.[7] Other attempts at superovulation and artificial insemination in Bengal tigers, African lions, and Persian leopards have not been successful.[8] Pregnancy also did not result in a trial interspecies embryo transfer from a Bengal tiger to an African lion.[20]

Reproductive diseases reported in felids include ovarian tumors, pyometra/metritis and vaginitis. Management of these conditions is routine, except that in most cases the animals are presented in an advanced state of the disorder.

CANIDAE

Estrogen-induced vaginal cornification has been used to monitor the estrous cycle in the wolf (*Canis lupus*),[25] the blue fox (*Alopex lagopus*),[11] the coyote[12] (*Canis latrans*) and the red fox (*Vulpes vulpes*).[17]

An alternate method for timing fertile periods in canidae is by measurement of electrical resistance in the vaginal mucosa. A probe, connected to an ohm meter and inserted into the vagina of a blue fox, silver fox (*Urocyon cinereoargentes*) and racoonlike dog (*Nyctereutes procyonides*) showed an average rise of resistance from 100 to 700 ohms on the first or second day of sexual receptivity. Since individual variation is high, readings had to be compared with those taken in proestrus on the same animal and not between animals.[16]

Obstetric manipulations, including cesarean section in canids, are similar to the same procedures done in the domestic bitch; however, capture and restraint of the animal presents more of a problem than the actual procedure.

Plasma hormone patterns in the wolf,[25] the red fox[5] and blue fox[15] are remarkably similar to those in the dog. This includes the preovulatory rise of progesterone that correlates with the onset of sexual receptivity and the prolonged luteal function, which is longer in the nonpregnant than the pregnant bitch.

Efforts to induce estrus in blue foxes with gonadotropin hormones have not yielded uniform results. Although most animals come into heat after injection with pregnant mare serum gonadotropin, few conceive.[3] Based on studies in the domestic dog, in which pulses of GnRH were delivered with an attached portable pump, a novel approach to estrus and ovulation induction has been initiated.[26] Small implantable pumps that can be inserted subcutaneously and deliver pulses of GnRH for up to 2 weeks have been tested in a cheetah (*Acinonyx jubatus*), a clouded leopard (*Neofelis nebulosa*), a serval (*Leptailurus serval*) and a golden cat (*Profelis temmincki*); a portable pump has been tested in a wolf (*Canis lupus*). Estrus in the cheetah was monitored using urinary estrogens, plasma progesterone and vaginal cytology. Although still in preliminary stages, these pilot studies may have broad applications throughout the order Carnivora in the future.

References

1. Adams CE, Rietveld AA: Duration of copulation and fertility in mink, *Mustela vison*. Theriogenology 15:449, 1981.
2. Audy MC: Le cycle sexuel saisonnier du male de mustelides europeens. Gen Comp Endocrinol 30:117, 1976.
3. Benjaminsen E, Tomasgard G: Framkalling av brunst hos blarevtispe ved hjelp av hormoner. Nors Vet Tidsskr 86:542, 1974.
4. Bonney RC, Moore HDM, Jones DM: Plasma concentrations of oestradiol-17 beta and progesterone and laparoscopic observations of the ovary in the puma (*Felis concolor*) during oestrus, pseudopregnancy and pregnancy. J Reprod Fert 63:523, 1981.
5. Bonnin M, Mondain-Monval M, Dutourne B: Oestrogen and progesterone concentrations in peripheral blood in pregnant red foxes (*Vulpes vulpes*). J Reprod Fert 54:37, 1978.
6. Donovan BT, ter Haar MB: Effects of luteinizing hormone-releasing hormone on plasma follicle stimulating hormone and luteinizing hormone levels in the ferret. J Endocrinol 73:37, 1977.
7. Dresser BL, Kramer L, Reece B, Russell PT: Induction of ovulation and successful artificial insemination in a Persian leopard (*Panthera pardus saxicolor*). Zoo Biology 1:55, 1983.
8. Dresser B, Kramer L, Russell P, et al.: Superovulation and artificial insemination in Bengal tigers (*Panthera tigris*), African lions (*Panthera leo*), and a Persian leopard (*Panthera pardus saxicolor*). Proc Am Assoc Zool Parks Aquariums, 1981, pp 149–151.
9. Ensley PK, Wing AE, Gosink BB, Lasley BL: Artificial insemination in a brown hyena (*Hyena brunnea*) utilizing urinary estrogens to monitor the estrous cycle. Zoo Biology 1:333, 1983.
10. Foresman KR, Daniel JC: Plasma progesterone concentrations in pregnant and nonpregnant black bears (*Ursus americanus*). J Reprod Fert 68:235, 1983.
11. Jarosz S, Barabasz B: Obraz cytologiczny nablonka pochwy w okresie przedkopulacyjnym i kopulacyjnym u lisow polarnych. Acta Agr Syl Zootech 19:73, 1980.
12. Kennelly JJ, Johns BE: The estrous cycle of coyotes. J Wildl Manage 40:272, 1976.
13. Lindeque M, Skinner JD: Fetal androgens and sexual mimicry in spotted hyenas (*Crocuta crocuta*). J Reprod Fert 65:405, 1982.
14. Møller OM: The progesterone concentrations in the peripheral plasma of mink (*Mustela vison*) during pregnancy. J Endocrinol 56:121, 1973.
15. Møller OM: Progesterone concentrations in the peripheral plasma of the blue fox (*Alopex lagopus*) during pregnancy and the oestrous cycle. J Endocrinol 59:429, 1973.
16. Møller OM: Elektrische Brunstdiagnostik bei Blaufuchsen, Silberfuchsen und Marderhunden—ein neues Hilfsmittel während der Paarungszeit. Deutsch Pelztierzucht 55:17, 1981.
17. Mondain-Monval M, Dutourne B, Bonnin-Lafargue M, et al.: Ovarian activity during the anoestrous and the reproductive season of the red fox (*Vulpes vulpes L*). J Ster Biochem 8:761, 1977.
18. Papke RL, Concannon PW, Travis HF, Hansel W: Control of luteal function and implantation in the mink by prolactin. J Anim Sci 50:1102, 1980.
19. Phillips LG, Simmons LG, Bush M, et al.: Gonadotropin regimen for inducing ovarian activity in captive wild felids. J Am Vet Med Assoc 181:1246, 1982.
20. Reece B, Dresser B, Reed G, et al.: An interspecies embryo transfer from Bengal tiger (*Panthera tigris*) to African lion (*Panthera leo*). Proc Am Assoc Zool Parks Aquariums, 1981, pp 165–167.
21. Ryan DK: Puberty onset in a reflex ovulator: Long-day induced first estrus in the ferret. Biol Reprod Suppl 1:65A, 1981.
22. Ryland LM, Gorham JR: The ferret and its diseases. Am J Vet Med Assoc 173:1154, 1978.
23. Schmidt AM, Nadal LA, Schmidt MJ, Beamer N: Serum concentrations of oestradiol and progesterone during the normal oestrous cycle and early pregnancy in the lion (*Panthera leo*). J Reprod Fert 57:267, 1979.
24. Seager SWJ, Demorest CN: Reproduction of captive wild

carnivores. In Fowler ME (ed): Zoo and Wild Animal Medicine. 2nd ed. WB Saunders Co, 1978, pp 667–706.

25. Seal US, Plotka ED, Packard JM, Mech LD: Endocrine correlates of reproduction in the wolf. 1. Serum progesterone, estradiol and LH during the estrous cycle. Biol Reprod 21:1057, 1979.

26. Vanderlip SL, Wing A, Rivier J, et al.: Induction of ovulation in anestrus bitches using a pulsatile delivery of GnRH. Proc AALAS, San Antonio, Nov 6–11, 1983.

27. van Keulen-Kromhout G: Zoo enclosures for bears, Ursidae: Their influence on captive behavior and reproduction. Int Zoo Yearb, 18:177, 1978.

28. Wildt DE, Platz CC, Chakraborty PK, Seager SWJ: Oestrus and ovarian activity in a female jaguar (*Panthera onca*). J Reprod Fert 56:555, 1979.

29. Wildt DE, Platz CC, Seager SWJ, Bush M: Induction of ovarian activity in the cheetah (*Acinonyx jubatus*). Biol Reprod 24:217, 1981.

30. Wright PL, Rausch R: Reproduction in the wolverine, *Gulo gulo*. J Mammal 36:346, 1955.

31. Yost R: Cytological sex determination in the spotted hyena (*Crocuta crocuta*). Int Zoo Yearb, 17:212, 1978.

Semen Collection, Analysis and Cryopreservation in Nondomestic Mammals

JoGayle Howard, D.V.M.
Mitchell Bush, D.V.M.
David E. Wildt, Ph.D.
Smithsonian Institution, Washington, D.C.

Captive propagation of certain zoologic species could be enhanced by adapting various artificial breeding techniques currently used successfully in domestic animals. Artificial insemination using fresh or frozen-thawed spermatozoa could (1) increase the breeding potential of genetically superior animals, (2) expand gene pools without the risk and expense of maintaining or transporting sires and (3) allow utilization of males unable to mate naturally because of physical or behavioral handicaps. Furthermore, semen evaluation alone has important predictive value in estimating fertility potential. Historically, the production of offspring by natural breeding was the only indication of fertility in nondomestic mammals. Now, reliable techniques are available to retrieve spermatozoa from many of these species and to obtain general estimates of fertility potential. Ongoing studies are in progress at various zoologic parks to improve methods of measuring ejaculate quality and to establish optimal procedures for cryopreserving spermatozoa. Few successful term pregnancies have resulted from artificially inseminating nondomestic species even with fresh spermatozoa. Generally, limited information on reproductive-endocrine function exists for most wildlife species. This lack of baseline knowledge, particularly ovulation time in the female, is the primary reason for the poor efficiency record of artificial insemination. As reproductive norms gradually become established for selected species, artificial breeding will play a more vital role in captive propagation.

TECHNIQUES OF SEMEN COLLECTION

The semen collection method should consistently provide ejaculates of adequate spermatozoal concentration and motility, with minimal stress to the animal. Methods of collection include electroejaculation, manual stimulation, the use of an artificial vagina and post-mortem retrieval. Electroejaculation offers wide application because it can be employed on anesthetized animals and requires no prior training of the animal. Exceptional circumstances allow semen collection by either manual massage or an artificial vagina from unanesthetized nondomestic species. Viable spermatozoa may also be obtained invasively from the caudae epididymides and vasa deferentia of animals shortly after death.

Electroejaculation

Electroejaculation has been used extensively as a method of semen collection in species as diverse as the mouse and elephant. Ejaculates from over 90 different species of nondomestic mammals have been collected in our laboratory. Most species respond to this procedure by producing seminal fluid containing spermatozoa, yet few published reports exist on what constitutes a normal ejaculate; exceptions include the Dorcas gazelle,[3] cheetah,[15] elephant[4] and various species of nonhuman primates.[13]

Most electrical stimulators manufactured for the collection of domestic animal semen can be adapted for use to zoologic specimens. Unfortunately, comparative evaluations of stimulator requirements are often confounded because most studies have not standardized the basic traits of stimulation current, frequency, voltage and waveform. Various designs of ejaculators delivering either alternating current (AC) or direct current (DC) are effective.[7] Our laboratory uses a commercially available AC, 60 Hz electroejaculator requiring 110- to 120-volt current

(Fig. 1). For field studies a DC electroejaculator with a 12-volt rechargeable battery pack is used (Fig. 2). Both electrostimulators are equipped with gauges, permitting the monitoring of voltage and amperage.

When anesthesia is used in conjunction with electroejaculation, food is withheld for 12 to 24 hours in monogastric species and up to 72 hours in ruminants. Certain sedatives relax the musculature surrounding the urethra, which can cause urine contamination of the semen during electroejaculation. These drugs include xylazine (Rompun), diazepam (Valium) or phenothiazine derivatives such as acetylpromazine (acepromazine). This procedural problem appears more prevalent in nondomestic carnivores. Certain species, particularly exotic ungulates, can tolerate a low sedative dosage in combination with a general anesthetic agent to smooth anesthesia without compromising ejaculate quality.

Traditionally, two types of electroejaculation techniques have been adapted to nondomestic species. A penile electrode procedure has been used in various nonhuman primates.[13] In this approach the unanesthetized male is restrained and an ejaculatory response induced by direct electrical stimulus of the penis. Although effective in monkeys, this technique is neither practical nor humane when considered for zoologic specimens.

A viable alternative is rectal probe electroejaculation, which is performed when the animal is in a surgical plane of anesthesia. A probe containing copper or stainless steel electrodes is used to deliver the stimulus. The probe is generally fabricated of plastic or Teflon, and the electrodes are mounted on the probe surface in either a circular or longitudinal configuration (Fig. 3). Recently, there appears to be an increase in the use of longitudinal electrodes, primarily because this type produces only moderate somatic stimulation. The diameter of the rectal probe required generally conforms to the size of a normal, excreted stool and should permit adequate contact between electrodes and the adjacent rectal mucosa.

The anesthetized male is placed in lateral recumbency or in a position that facilitates access to both the anus and penis. Feces are removed manually from the rectum, and the probe is lubricated and inserted. The depth of insertion varies with the species and is such that the electrodes are positioned over the expected orientation of the male accessory organs. Usually, longitudinal electrodes are mounted on only a portion of the probe circumference, allowing the electrodes to be positioned ventrally (against the accessory organs) during electroejaculation. A standardized electroejaculation regimen, in which males of a particular species receive the same number of electrical stimuli at the same voltage increments, is beneficial for comparison of males and ejaculate traits.[3] Our laboratory uses a regimen consisting of sets of 10 stimulations applied at increasing increments of voltage and amperage. Generally, the total sequence is divided into three series of 30 to 40 stimuli/series. Stimuli are given in a 3-second on and 3-second off pattern, with a continuous rise in voltage from 0 volts to the desired peak, then a return to 0 volts. Initial selected voltage is based on the animal's limb response during stimulation. A moderately rigid extension of the hind legs is indicative of an adequate electrical stimulus. Leg extension also can be used as an index of proper probe positioning; for example, a lack of extension could indicate improper dorsal-directed stimulation. Initial voltages used for the majority of

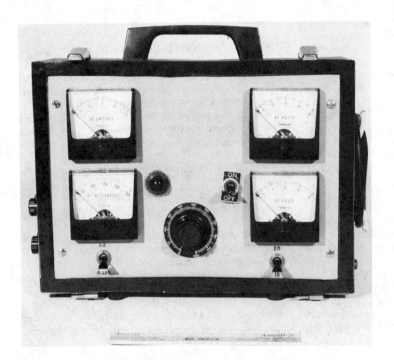

Figure 1. AC electroejaculator.

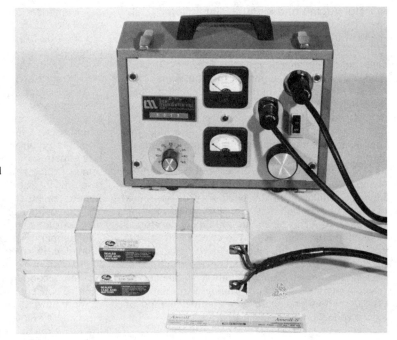

Figure 2. DC electroejaculator and 12-volt rechargeable battery pack.

nondomestic species range from 2 to 5 volts and at the end of collection rarely exceed 10 volts.

Most nondomestic mammals respond to electroejaculation by producing a spermic ejaculate that is collected into a prewarmed plastic vial, which prevents temperature shock to the spermatozoa. Erection may or may not accompany ejaculation. Unexplicably, ease of collection and semen quality often vary among even closely related species. For example, high quality semen has been obtained more easily from certain equids such as the Mongolian wild ass and Przewalskii's horse than in the zebra or domestic horse. Similarly, although electroejaculates have been obtained in various nondomestic canids (timber wolf, fox),[1] this collection method is not routinely effective in the domestic dog. When used correctly, rectal probe electroejaculation is safe. Unfortunately, there is little specific information on libido or breeding ability of nondomestic species subjected to such treatment. Recent results demonstrate that electroejaculation elicits a stress response (increased serum cortisol) in certain exotic Felidae.[14] However, the response is acute, with cortisol concentrations declining coincident with the termination of the semen collection procedure.

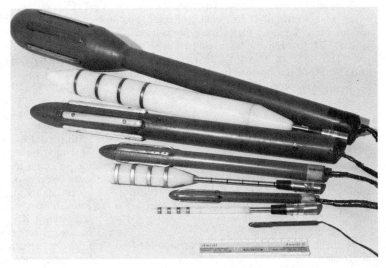

Figure 3. Rectal probes with ring or longitudinal electrode configuration used for electroejaculation.

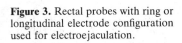

Artificial Vagina and Manual Stimulation

The artificial vagina (AV) is commonly used in farm species (horses, cattle, sheep, goats) for semen collection. The animal mounts either a "teaser" female or fabricated dummy, and the penis is directed into an AV containing a collection vial. Although the AV is a "natural approach," the animal training required and the potential danger of a conscious animal to personnel preclude the routine use of this method in most nondomestic species. However, semen has been collected with an AV from the camel, reindeer, red deer, alpaca, chimpanzee, Eld's deer and Pere David deer.[11, 12] Manual stimulation of the penis to produce reflex erection and ejaculation also has been used in certain canids. This technique, originally developed in the domestic dog, has proved effective in collecting semen from both blue and silver-black foxes and timber wolves, with pregnancies resulting in each case after artificial insemination.[11] Animal type (canids), temperament and training again limit the efficacy of this procedure as a routine method of semen collection.

Post-Mortem Spermatozoal Recovery

Recovery of mature spermatozoa post-mortem involves flushing the vasa deferentia and caudae epididymides with air or warmed saline. Because tissue degeneration is rapid, the reproductive tract requires flushing immediately after death. Epididymal spermatozoa frequently have negligible motility upon recovery, which can often be stimulated by dilution and incubation at 37°C. For example, spermatozoa of wild African elephants collected by flushing the excurrent testicular duct with air within 15 minutes after death develop motility immediately after dilution with phosphate-buffered saline solution. The percentage of motile spermatozoa of this species increases after the addition of potassium and fructose to the saline medium and incubation for 3 hours.[5] These spermatozoa are presumed fertile, as epididymal sperm cells collected postmortem from domestic cattle have been used for artificial insemination and have resulted in pregnancies.[11] The cause of animal death requires investigation to avoid the possibility of disease transmission at artificial breeding.

SEMEN ANALYSIS

Semen is evaluated immediately after collection for ejaculate volume and pH. Aliquots are assessed microscopically at 37°C for per cent spermatozoal motility and status (speed of forward progression). Spermatozoal status is a subjective evaluation based on a scale of 0 to 5 as follows:

0 = no motility or movement

1 = slight side-to-side movement with no forward progression

2 = moderate side-to-side movement with occasional slow forward progression

3 = side-to-side movement with slow forward progression

4 = steady forward progression

5 = rapid, steady forward progression.

At least four separate fields at 400 × are examined, and an average motility and status rating are calculated. Spermatozoal concentration is determined using a hemacytometer and a commercially available erythrocyte determination kit. The capillary pipette of the latter is filled with 10 μl of semen, which is mixed with the reservoir solution, resulting in a 1:200 dilution ratio. Both hemacytometer chambers are filled with the diluted semen, and the number of spermatozoa in the four large (1 mm²) corner squares of each chamber are counted. The number of sperm cells counted in each chamber is divided by two to obtain a spermatozoal count in millions/ml of ejaculate. The procedure is repeated for the second hemacytometer chamber, and an average concentration is calculated.

Spermatozoal morphology is evaluated by fixing ejaculate aliquots in 1 per cent glutaraldehyde followed by microscopic examination of 100 or more spermatozoa at 1000 × magnification. The classification system for spermatozoal morphology categorizes cells as either being normal or having primary or secondary abnormalities. Primary abnormalities include abnormal head shapes, tightly coiled tails or bicephalic or biflagellate features. Secondary abnormalities include bent midpieces, bent tails or protoplasmic droplets. Primary abnormalities originate in the testes during spermatogenesis and are considered to be more detrimental than secondary abnormalities that occur in the excurrent duct system.

Often, a wide range in ejaculate values is reported for a given species. Much of this variation can be attributed to differences among laboratory[1] techniques and subjective criteria.[7] However, it is not unusual for ejaculate volume, sperm count and per cent sperm motility to vary considerably within a species or even among ejaculates from a single individual. Therefore, when assessing male fertility it is important to accumulate semen data on each male over a period of time. Males suspected of reproductive dysfunction should be electroejaculated at least three times at 3- to 4-week intervals before final judgment of fertility status. The influence of season on seminal quality should also be considered.

No single seminal trait should be used to assess fertility status. Per cent spermatozoal motility is probably the most important criterion in establishing potential fertility. However, in the past insufficient emphasis has been placed on progressive sperm status and morphologic forms of spermatozoa. The per cent motility factor is of questionable importance if sperm cells are showing circular or backward movement or no advanced progression. Likewise, spermatozoa could show forward motion but experience a high incidence of pleiomorphic defects. As the percentage of abnormal cells increases, the semen quality decreases, and consequently, its potential fertilizing capacity is reduced. Aberrant spermatozoal morphology is often observed in the ejaculates of nondomestic species and is particularly prevalent in the gorilla[10] and certain exotic felids.[15] The cause of this finding is unknown but could be related to the stresses of captivity or the genetic consequences of inbreeding.[15]

Because the primary focus on spermatozoal evaluation concerns the gamete's ability to move through the female reproductive tract and fertilize the ovum, functional assessment tests have also been developed. These techniques involve the (1) sperm migration media assay to determine gamete migration distance through a synthetic polyacrylamide gel simulating cervical mucus[6] and (2) ova penetration assay to ascertain the ability of heterologous capacitated spermatozoa to fertilize hamster ova in vitro.[16] Originally, these procedures were developed for the study of fertility potential in humans, and both may have eventual application to nondomestic species. However, these assays have been tested using domestic mammalian spermatozoa, and although they may be useful in formulating a multitrait evaluation system for ejaculate quality, both are labor intensive. The ova penetration assay is also expensive to maintain and requires sophisticated laboratory procedures and a knowledge of capacitation requirements for spermatozoa.

SEMEN HANDLING

Little is known about the maintenance of nondomestic animal semen to optimize viability before artificial insemination or freezing. The semen of primates, rodents and macropod marsupials coagulates immediately after ejaculation, posing difficulties in handling and evaluation. The ejaculatory plug can be deposited in the recipient female for artificial breeding; however, a coagulum-free suspension is required for spermatozoal freezing. Coagulum digestion can be accomplished in some species by incubating the ejaculate in normal saline at 37°C or by adding low concentrations (1 to 2 per cent) of the enzymes trypsin or pronase.[13]

Spermatozoal motility is rapidly depressed if the semen sample is contaminated with urine. Although urine contamination can usually be detected macroscopically because of its yellow coloration, pH evaluation more accurately detects subtle urine volumes. In many mammals spermatozoal motility is severely compromised by constituents within the seminal fluid. Undiluted, raw spermatozoa from exotic felids in particular generally maintain in vitro motility for 5 hours or less. Motility of fresh spermatozoa from these and other species can be markedly improved by dilution with a tissue culture media or by removing seminal fluid following low-speed centrifugation.[3]

SEMEN CRYOPRESERVATION

The concept of semen banking of nondomestic animals is of considerable interest to the zoologic community. Technical advances in cryopreservation of domestic animal spermatozoa offer methods that may be applicable to wildlife species. However, it should be realized that basic research to determine optimal spermatozoal requirements for each species is needed prior to extensive storage of nondomestic animal spermatozoa. No cryopreservation protocol is universally appropriate for all species. The effects of various cryoprotective diluents on spermatozoal survivability require investigation. Additionally, further studies are needed to compare different freezing techniques and to examine functional and structural alterations of spermatozoa after freeze-thawing.

Published reports on optimal semen diluents, cryoprotectants and freezing methods for nondomestic mammals are extremely limited. Most previous studies have involved examining only one freezing method with a single cryoprotective diluent.[1] Although semen diluents used successfully in domestic species have application to zoologic species, a wide range in success rates can be expected. Comparative studies have demonstrated marked variations in spermatozoal post-thaw motility and structural integrity following freezing of wild ungulate spermatozoa in various cryoprotective diluents.[2] Therefore, it would appear that a prerequisite to the massive banking of spermatozoa from any one species is a comparative analysis of seminal fluid constituents, spermatozoal requirements and cryoprotective diluents that will provide optimal post-thaw recoveries.

Various cryopreservation techniques available for investigation include semen storage in straws, ampules or pellets. Each requires prefreezing equilibration of diluted semen at 5°C prior to processing for storage in liquid nitrogen. For the straw or ampule approach, cooled semen is deposited into the respective container and vapor frozen by suspending the samples 4 to 5 cm above liquid nitrogen. The pelleting technique involves pipetting single drops of equilibrated semen into 3-mm diameter indentations made in a block of dry ice (Fig. 4A).[8] After a 3-minute interval, the block is inverted, plunging the pellets into liquid nitrogen (Fig. 4B). The pellets are then transferred into labeled vials for storage in liquid nitrogen (Fig. 4C and D). Methods of thawing frozen semen vary widely. In general, straws are thawed rapidly in a 35°C water bath.[9] Usually, ampules are allowed to thaw slowly in an ice-water bath for 10 minutes before the semen is transferred to the insemination catheter.[9] Pellets are rapidly thawed by plunging them into a 0.9 per cent saline solution warmed to 37°C. For most zoologic species the pelleting and straw approaches have been studied more intensely than the ampule technique. Results from our laboratory indicate that the pelleting method is particularly effective in

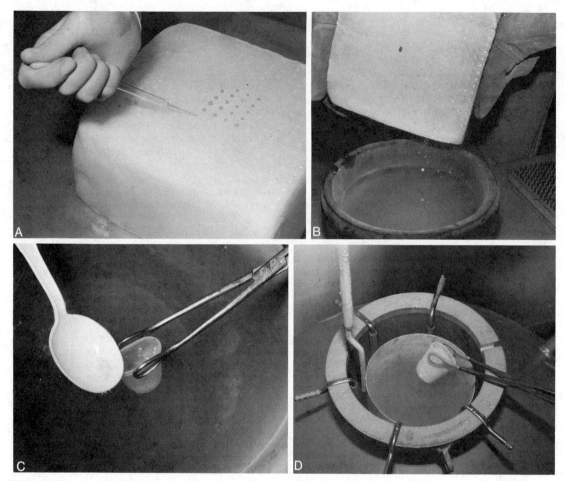

Figure 4. Procedure for freezing semen by pellet method. *A*, Pipetting single drops of diluted semen into indentations made in a block of dry ice. *B*, Inverting block of dry ice and plunging pellets into liquid nitrogen. *C*, Transferring pellets into labeled vials. *D*, Storing vial containing pelleted semen in liquid nitrogen tank.

freeze-preserving nondomestic carnivore and ungulate spermatozoa.

Methods for evaluating spermatozoal damage during freezing assist in determining the cryoprotective abilities of various methods and diluents. Post-thaw per cent motility and status of spermatozoa are frequently used criteria. However, acceptable spermatozoal motility has been observed in thawed semen of certain species in which detailed morphologic evaluations reveal high percentages of spermatozoa with damaged or disintegrating acrosomes.[2] Because the acrosome is critical to the fertilization process, the fertilizing capacity of these damaged spermatozoa must be questioned. Consequently, ultrastructural examination is a necessary adjunct to assessing the effects of spermatozoal freezing. Acrosomal integrity is assessed using phase-contrast microscopy (2500 ×) and is categorized into four morphologic classes: (1) normal apical ridge, with the acrosome possessing a smooth, crescentic apical ridge; (2) damaged apical ridge, with the acrosome possessing an irregular-shaped apical ridge; (3) missing apical ridge, with the apical

ridge absent, but the acrosomal cap firmly adhered to the nucleus and (4) loose acrosomal cap, with the acrosomal cap loosened and vesiculated. The feasibility of acrosomal morphology assessments in nondomestic species appears to be species specific. The apical ridge of spermatozoa of certain wild ungulate species (blesbok and gazelle) extends anteriorly, well beyond the nucleus, similar to that observed in the domestic bull and boar. This type of structural configuration allows easy evaluation of acrosomal integrity at high magnification.[2] In contrast, the acrosome does not protrude anteriorly and is relatively small and thin in certain nondomestic species, particularly in exotic felid spermatozoa.[15] Therefore, definitive examinations of structural integrity in these species require electron microscopic evaluations.

References

1. Graham EF, Schmehl MKL, Evenson BK, Nelson DS: Semen preservation in non-domestic mammals. Symp Zool Soc London 43:153, 1978.

2. Howard JG, Pursel VG, Wildt DE, Bush M: Comparison of various extenders for freeze-preservation of semen from selected captive wild ungulates. J Am Vet Med Assoc 179:1157, 1981.

3. Howard JG, Wildt DE, Chakraborty PK, Bush M: Reproductive traits including seasonal observations on semen quality and serum hormone concentrations in the Dorcas gazelle. Theriogenology 20:221, 1983.

4. Howard JG, Bush M, de Vos V, Wildt DE: Electroejaculation and semen characteristics of free-ranging African elephants (*Loxodonta africana*). J Reprod Fert 72:187, 1984.

5. Jones RC: Collection, motility and storage of spermatozoa from the African elephant, *Loxodonta africana*. Nature 243:38, 1973.

6. Lorton SP, Kummerfeld HL, Foote RH: Polyacrylamide as a substitute for cervical mucus in sperm migration test. Fert Ster 35:222, 1981.

7. Martin ICA: The principles and practice of electroejaculation of mammals. Symp Zool Soc London 43:127, 1978.

8. Nagase H, Niwa T: Deep freezing bull semen in concentrated pellet form. In Proc 5th Int Cong Anim Reprod Artif Insem, Trento, Italy, IV:410, 1964.

9. Pickett BW, Berndston WE: Procedures for handling frozen bovine semen in the felid. In Morrow DA (ed): Current Therapy in Theriogenology. 1st ed. Philadelphia, WB Saunders Co, 1980, p 354.

10. Platz CC, Wildt DE, Bridges CH, et al.: Electroejaculation and semen analysis in a male lowland gorilla, *Gorilla gorilla*. Primates 21:130, 1980.

11. Watson PF: A review of techniques of semen collection in mammals. Symp Zool Soc London 43:97, 1978.

12. Wemmer C: Unpublished data.

13. Wildt DE: Reproductive techniques of potential use in the artificial propagation of nonhuman primates. In Heltne PG (ed): The Lion-Tailed Macque: Status and Conservation. New York, Alan R. Liss Inc, 1985, p 161.

14. Wildt DE, Chakraborty PK, Meltzer D, Bush M: Adrenal-testicular-pituitary relationships in the cheetah subjected to anesthesia/electroejaculation. Biol Reprod 30:665, 1984.

15. Wildt DE, Bush M, Howard JG, et al.: Unique seminal quality in the South African cheetah and a comparative evaluation in the domestic cat. Biol Reprod. 29:1019, 1983.

16. Yanagimachi R: Penetration of guinea pig spermatozoa into hamster eggs in vitro. J Reprod Fert 28:477, 1972.

Embryo Manipulations

Barbara S. Durrant, Ph.D.
Zoological Society of San Diego, San Diego, California

It is imperative that reproductive physiologists begin to employ the most sophisticated techniques of embryo manipulation to aid in the propagation of captive animal species. As populations of wild animals continue to dwindle, it becomes increasingly important to manage captive groups of exotic species as efficiently as commercial livestock. Selection of sires and dams of the next generation based on genetic value will replace random mating. Artificial aids to reproduction will enhance the breeding potential of superior animals. Embryo transfer and freezing are techniques now employed by a small number of zoo researchers. In vitro fertilization and micromanipulation of embryos, although not presently used in zoos, have the potential to become powerful tools in the management of exotic species.

EMBRYO TRANSFER AND FREEZING

The technique of embryo transfer provides the means for maximizing the number of offspring a valuable female is capable of producing during (and after) her lifetime. It also allows for genetic input from females unable to sustain a pregnancy because of deformities or infirmities known not to be heritable. Aging females no longer ovulating spontaneously can be hormonally induced to ovulate, and their gametes can be transferred to younger animals capable of carrying a fetus to term. Embryo transfer may become an increasingly important method of introducing exotic species into the United States as import regulations become more restrictive.

Unlike cattle, whose vast numbers allow selection of only superior females as embryo donors, there are species (e.g., Arabian oryx, Przewalskii's horse) of such limited numbers that "cull" females are not available to be used as recipients. One solution to this problem is the use of interspecies embryo transfer. With this technique closely related but less rare exotics or domestic species can be used for the rapid propagation of a rare species or for the introduction of a species to an area or zoo where no same-species recipients are available. It is interspecies embryo transfer that has received the most attention from zoo workers.

Donor-recipient pairs are most likely to be compatible for embryo transfer if they can hybridize, e.g., mouflon with domestic sheep, gaur and banteng with domestic cattle. But an understanding of the structure and endocrine function of the reproductive tracts and placentae of each species as well as the nature of the estrous cycle must be achieved before interspecific or intergeneric embryo transfers can be expected to be routinely successful.

Differences in hormone production by the placenta is a likely cause of early embryonic death in interspecies embryo transfers. For example, mares carrying mule fetuses characteristically have very low titers of pregnant mare serum gonadotropin (PMSG) compared with mares carrying horse fetuses.[3] Allen and Rowson[1] in their studies of mule and hinny embryo transfers into donkeys and mares suggest that hybrid fetuses are intermediate in placental hormone production while the maternal-fetal differences in full cross-species transfers are much greater and lead to a high percentage of early embryonic death.

Understanding the structure and function of the fetal-maternal attachment is essential for matching donors to recipients with a high rate of embryo acceptance. Although epitheliochorial placentation is common to all bovids, the number, size, arrangement and function of the cotyledons differ among species. Placentae examined at the Zoological Society of San Diego have exhibited as many as 185 small (30 × 20 mm) cotyledons on a term placenta of a sable antelope and as few as 30 large (70 × 50 mm) ones in the placenta of the Congo buffalo. Vast differences in fetal-maternal attachment would certainly preclude successful embryo transfer.

Another largely ignored factor that should be considered when transferring embryos between distantly related species is the behavioral consequences of the offspring either being raised by a foreign species or hand raised. Particularly in highly intelligent and social animals such as primates, an improper social environment during early development often leaves an animal unable or unwilling to interact with its own species and to mate or to raise its own offspring normally. If interspecies embryo transfer is to be used as a tool to enhance the propagation of exotic species, care must be taken to avoid producing individuals that will never breed naturally.

Artiodactyla

The first interspecies embryo transfers involving exotic animals were performed by Bunch and colleagues[2] between mouflon (*Ovis musimon*) and domestic sheep (*O. aries*). Estrus synchronization was achieved with subcutaneous progesterone implants for 14 days. PMSG (1000 IU), given at the time of implant removal, was sufficient to superovulate the mouflons. Higher doses resulted in greater ovulatory response but complete loss of fertility. It was suggested that horse anterior pituitary extracts (HAP) might be the best gonadotropin for superovulating ewes. Two mouflon were carried to term in domestic ewe uteri. The authors concluded that embryos in this interspecies cross must reach the 16- to 32-cell stage, and the donor and recipient must be estrus-synchronized to within 4 hours for the transfer to be successful.

The estrous cycles of Cretan goats (*Capra aegagrus cretica*) were synchronized with African pygmy goats (*C. a. hircus*) at the Zoological Society of San Diego using subcutaneous progesterone implants (Sil-estrus) for 14 days. Estrus occurred 24 to 48 hours after implant removal in the pygmy goats but was not detectable in the Cretan goats. To further synchronize the two species prior to embryo transfer, 125 μg of prostaglandin $F_{2\alpha}$ (PGF$_{2\alpha}$) (Cloprostenol) was administered on day 12 of the new cycle, followed 8 days later with PMSG and another PGF$_{2\alpha}$ injection 2 days after gonadotropin administration. PMSG (500 IU; Gestyl) resulted in superovulation (10 embryos) in Cretan goats. Further work with pygmy goats has resulted in the superovulation (up to 26 ova) with 1000 IU of PMSG. Elevated blood progesterone levels of the recipients to day 40

indicated survival of Cretan goat 8-celled embryos transferred to pygmy goats. Maintenance of corpora lutea to this stage indicates that the transferred embryos were of sufficient age to establish pregnancy and that the synchronization of donor and recipient animals was adequate. The failure of the pregnancy after the beginning of placental attachment (25 to 30 days) suggests the absence of a placental luteotropin, which in normal goat pregnancy may stimulate the increase in size of luteal cells over the period of 40 to 110 days gestation, concomitant with an increase in peripheral plasma progesterone concentration. All females responded to this treatment in November during the natural breeding season of the Cretan goat. However, attempts to stimulate ovulation in this exotic goat during anestrus with the same hormone regimen failed to elicit an ovarian response.

The Bronx Zoo, in cooperation with the Pennsylvania Embryo Transfer Service, synchronized Holstein and gaur (*Bos gaurus*) cows with two PGF$_{2\alpha}$ injections 10 days apart. Superovulation of the gaur donor with 2000 IU of PMSG on the seventh day after the first PGF$_{2\alpha}$ treatment resulted in the nonsurgical collection of five embryos. Of four gaur embryos surgically transferred to the domestic cows, one resulted in a live term birth.

The Cincinnati Wildlife Research Federation researchers synchronized African eland (*Taurotragus oryx*) cows with two 25-mg injections of prostaglandin (PG) (Lutalyse) 11 days apart. Twelve days after the second prostaglandin treatment, the eland were superovulated with 1800 IU of PMSG. The next day (recipients) or 2 days later (donors) a third PG injection was given. The eland exhibited behavioral estrus 48 hours after the last PG treatment. Eight embryos were nonsurgically collected from the two eland donors. One was transferred to the recipient eland, and five were transferred to Holstein cows naturally synchronized or synchronized with one PG injection. No pregnancies resulted. Later work by this group has produced one successful eland to eland nonsurgical embryo transfer calf.

Embryo transfer projects at the Zoological Society of San Diego have involved the attempted superovulation of three species of oryx: Arabian (*Oryx leucoryx*), scimitar-horned (*O. dammah*) and fringe-eared (*O. callotis*). One Arabian oryx was mildly superovulated (three ova) in response to an injection of 1200 IU of PMSG 8 days after behavioral estrus. A second Arabian oryx, whose cycle was unknown, was treated with two 125 μg injections of PGF$_{2\alpha}$ (Cloprostenol) 14 days apart. Twelve days after the first PG injection, she was treated with 2500 IU of PMSG. Surgical flushing of the uterus resulted in the recovery of one normal morula, which was frozen, using the methods established for cattle embryos, and later surgically transferred to a naturally synchronized scimitar-horned oryx. No pregnancy resulted. One hatched blastocyst was recovered nonsurgically from a fringe-eared oryx after treatment on day 10 with 1800 IU of* PMSG followed 2 days later with 125 μg of PG. One scimitar-horned oryx was induced to ovulate only one ovum in response to a 4-day treatment with follicle-stimulating hormone (FSH-P). Although these studies lack the numbers of animals to be significant, they indicate that oryx species may be more difficult to superovulate than domestic cattle. Perhaps the day of gonadotropin treatment is more critical in these antelope, as a day 8 treatment resulted in mild superovulation, but day 10 treatments failed to hyperstimulate the ovaries of several animals.

The Munich Zoo has recently successfully transferred banteng (*Bos javanicus*) embryos into domestic cattle using a hormone regimen similar to that described for the eland using PG and PMSG for synchronization and superovulation.

Embryos have been successfully transferred nonsurgically between water buffalo (*Bubalus bubalis*) using methods and techniques established for domestic cattle. Two cattle morulae were transferred to two water buffalo recipients, and one pregnancy was established. Although the recipient aborted the intergeneric pregnancy after 78 days gestation, these experiments by the University of Florida Department of Reproduction indicate that embryo transfers of this kind may soon be successful.

Several significant findings can be distilled from the experiments described in the preceding section: First, prostaglandins are efficacious in synchronizing estrus in all hoofstock described. The hormone has been successful in inducing estrous behavior leading to natural breeding in each species. Second, the gonadotropins PMSG and FSH, while not yielding the high numbers of ova seen in cattle, have been proved satisfactory in the induction of ovulation and mild superovulation in exotic species. In addition, ovulation has occurred without the use of exogenous luteinizing hormone (LH), and none of the stimulated animals had large numbers of unovulated follicles following treatment.

Carnivora

Cincinnati Zoo researchers have attempted embryo transfer from the Bengal tiger (*Panthera tigris*) to the African lion (*Panthera leo*). The donor tigresses were treated with FSH for 5 consecutive days; 10 mg the first day, followed by 5 mg daily for 4 days. Human chorionic gonadotropin (hCG; 2000 IU) was administered the day after the last dose of FSH. The same hormone regimen was used to synchronize the recipient lionesses except the treatment began 2 days later and consisted of only four 5-mg injections of FSH. All females exhibited estrous behavior 4 days after their first FSH injection. Superovulation was successful in both tigresses (35 and 25 ova), but only two normal morula could be recovered from one animal. The embryos were surgically transferred to one lioness, but a pregnancy did not result.

Wildt and co-workers have reported the success of the hormonal induction of ovulation in wild felids.[5] Prior to hormone treatment for ovulation or prior to artificial insemination or embryo transfer, it is necessary to determine if the animal is an induced or spontaneous ovulator. Of the wild felids studied to date, the cheetah, clouded leopard and tiger have been observed laparoscopically to ovulate spontaneously. The jaguar must receive hCG or gonadotropin-releasing hormone (GnRH) for ovulation to occur. PMSG administered to lionesses results in variable ovulation rates (from 3 to 34), with many unruptured follicles in the superovulated female, although hCG had been given. FSH-P treatment resulted in more uniform ovarian stimulation in cheetahs and tigers when 10 mg was administered for 5 consecutive days. hCG (500 IU; Pregnyl) was used in the cheetah and the tiger to rupture hormonally stimulated follicles. GnRH (100 μg) was similarly effective in causing ovulation in both the cheetah and the tiger.

Ensley and co-workers[4] have recently reported that induction of ovulation and estrus in the brown hyena (*Hyena brunnea*) may be more effectively stimulated with GnRH than with FSH.

Although very few embryo transfers have been attempted in exotic animals and even fewer have been successful, progress is being made in the understanding of the reproductive processes of zoo animals.

Estrus synchronization and superovulation prior to embryo transfer in exotics have been similar to those used for domestic animals. Superovulation has been successful in a variety of species using FSH or PMSG, sometimes in conjunction with hCG or GnRH. Estrus synchronization has been achieved in hoofed stock with $PGF_{2\alpha}$ with or without prior progesterone treatment.

FUTURE TECHNIQUES

The mechanics of advanced techniques in embryo manipulation are described in another section of this book. The importance of these techniques in the study of reproduction in exotic animals will be discussed here.

In vitro fertilization can be a useful method of utilizing valuable genetic material from females unable to transport ova or sperm through the reproductive tract. Natural fertilization may be precluded because of the stenosis of the oviduct as the result of infection or adhesions. Ovaries taken from necropsied females shortly after death can be a source of viable oocytes to be used for in vitro fertilization.

Determining the sex of an embryo prior to embryo transfer can be a valuable tool in the management of exotic species. Space and economic limitations in zoos dictate the number of animals that can be maintained for exhibition and breeding. The ability to select the sex of the embryo will allow the production of more female offspring and, hence, a greater reproductive potential of a group of captive animals. Valuable male embryos may be frozen for use when and where their genetic input is needed. Discarding male embryos is preferable to selective abortion or neonatal euthanasia as a means of changing the sex ratio of a population.

Microsurgical splitting of embryos to form identical twins or quadruplets may become a valuable method of duplicating genetic material while selectively increasing a population size.

Another microsurgical technique that has the potential to become an aid to interspecific or intergeneric embryo transfer is the transposition of inner cell masses. As discussed earlier in this article, proper fetal-maternal attachment is critical for the maintenance of a pregnancy. If a native placenta in its earliest form, the trophoblast layer of a preimplantation embryo, can be "grafted" to the isolated inner cell mass of a foreign embryo, much greater success can be expected after embryo transfer. This may allow the transfer of embryos between very distantly related animals and will be of greatest

value to those species that do not have an easily manipulated nonendangered or domestic species counterpart, e.g., okapi (*Okapi johnsoni*), gorilla (*Gorilla gorilla*), koala (*Phascolarctos cinerius adustus*), cheetah (*Acinonyx jubatus*) and giant panda (*Ailuridae melanoleuca*).

References

1. Allen WR, Rowson LEA: Transfer of ova between horses and donkeys. VII Int Cong Anim Reprod Artif Insemin, Munich 1:484, 1972.
2. Bunch TD, Foote WC, Whitaker B: Interspecies ovum transfer to propagate wild sheep. J Wildl Manage 41:726, 1977.
3. Clegg MT, Cole HH, Howard CB, Pigon H: The influence of foetal genotype on equine gonadotrophin secretion. J Endocrinol 25:245, 1962.
4. Ensley PK, Wing AE, Gosink BB, et al.: Application of noninvasive techniques to monitor reproductive function in a brown hyena (*Hyena brunnea*). Zoo Biol 1:333, 1982.
5. Wildt DE, Platz CC, Seager SWJ, Bush M: Use of gonadotropic hormones to induce ovarian activity in domestic and wild felids. Am Assoc Zoo Vet Ann Proc, pp 44–47, 1980.

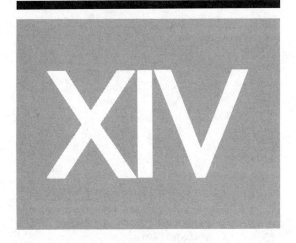

SECTION XIV

COMPUTERS IN REPRODUCTIVE HEALTH PROGRAMS

Edward Mather, D.V.M.

Consulting Editor

Use of Computers in Bovine Theriogenology

Paul C. Bartlett, D.V.M., M.P.H.
Michigan State University, East Lansing, Michigan

The rapid proliferation of relatively inexpensive microcomputers in the 1980's has had a major impact on many different businesses and industries in our society. As hardware prices have dropped, it has become increasingly cost effective for veterinary offices, dairy farms, cow-calf operations and feedlots to computerize various aspects of their operation. This article will discuss the application of this new computer technology to the practice of bovine theriogenology.

BASIC ASPECTS OF COMPUTER USE

Computer Systems

The first generation of computerized herd health systems primarily used large central "mainframe" computers. The 1972 British Melbread system, adapted from a system developed at the University of Melbourne in Australia, was one of the pioneers of this type of program. Data were collected from the farms and then transported to the location of the mainframe computer for keypunching. Reports were then distributed to the participating farmers at monthly intervals. In the United States, the various Dairy Herd Improvement Associations (DHIA) have used a similar centralized mechanism for over 70 years. One difficulty with such centralized systems has been that the users (farmers, veterinarians, bankers) have limited access to their computer records. Also, the output has usually been produced at monthly intervals, which is too infrequent to provide heat predictions, action lists and information regarding reproductive disorders. More recently, some mainframe record systems have been adapted for operation from on-farm terminals. The DHIA processing center in Provo, Utah, was one of the first mainframe systems to develop this capability. In a similar effort, the DHIA system in Raleigh, North Carolina, has instituted DART (Direct Access to Records by Telephone). Terminal access solves many of the communication problems inherent to the mainframe computer but is plagued by the ever increasing cost of long-distance telephone charges. Regardless of whether on-farm terminals are used, mainframe systems can offer tremendous computing power for relatively little expense. They are able to produce output that compares each farmer's performance to that of his peers and can also establish a valuable data base that may be used for educational and research purposes.

As the cost of microcomputers dropped throughout the 1980's, the use of on-farm microcomputers expanded. On-farm systems have the advantage of offering immediate access to records, adaptability to one's individual needs and independence from a central processing center. In the United States, many different dairy management and herd health systems have been written for a wide variety of computer equipment. Some are designed to replace the need for DHIA. Others are designed to supplement DHIA or to interact with DHIA records. One disadvantage of on-farm microcomputers is that they require more skill in computer operation than some farmers are willing to develop. Also, because stand-alone, on-farm microcomputers are isolated from other users, there is no mechanism for comparing one's performance with that of one's peers. In addition, calculation of the more sophisticated herd health diagnostic indices stresses the computational limits of some smaller machines.

Several DHIA organizations and universities are developing computerized herd health networks that use microcomputers on farms or in veterinarians' offices that are linked to a central mainframe system. The networking of the microcomputer and the mainframe computer may offer both the independence and the convenience of the on-farm microcomputer as well as the inexpensive computing power and interherd comparative capabilities of the mainframe systems. In networked systems, output is available from the more convenient microcomputer for timely and immediate functions, while output from the mainframe computer can be produced less frequently to address more long-term functions relating to disease surveillance, reproductive performance and economic impact. In addition, resulting central data bases can be used as educational and research resources, which will also help defray the cost of the system.

Animal Identification

The need for unique animal identification can be a perplexing problem for the operation of any computerized herd health system. Cattle may be identified by any of several identifiers such as DHIA control number, barn name, stall number, registration number, electronic transducer number or brucellosis ear tag number. This may cause a problem for the developers of microcomputer software because they may be asked to provide a cross-referenced index of these different numbering systems and be prepared to enter and retrieve data by any one of them. It may also cause a problem for the data entry person who must continually decide which numbering system the dairyman is using when he records data. For example, if the herdsman writes down that he dried off number 29, is he referring to DHIA control number 29, barn number 29, stall number 29, or transducer number 29?

Confusion may result if a herdsman insists on using a nonunique animal identifier. An example of a nonunique animal numbering system would be neck chain numbers or barn names that are commonly reused when a cow is culled from the milking herd and replaced by a new heifer. Most dairymen do not want to delete a cow's record when she is culled. Also, persons interested in using this data for research or genetic testing will be interested in maintaining inactive records. However, if the old cow's record is not deleted, some mechanism must be provided to prevent data from being mistakenly entered in the wrong cow's record.

Frequently a cow will be assigned a different barn number when she enters the milking herd after each lactation. For example, she may be No. 31 in her first lactation and No. 52 in her second. Also, the number most often used by the dairyman may change depending upon the cow's status or place in the herd. For example, the brucellosis ear tag may be used to identify the calves, the registration number may be used for the pregnant heifers and the barn name used for the lactating cows. It takes heroic measures on the part of the programmers and the users to operate with numbering systems like these. Such complicated and nonunique numbering systems wreak havoc with any record system and may create such frequent and perplexing problems as to render the system essentially unusable.

Ideally, any computer system should be adaptable to the farm's pre-existing management and herd health system. The area of animal identifiers, however, may be one issue in which the pre-existing system may need to be changed to fit the needs of the computer. It is strongly recommended that a single unique animal number be assigned to each calf when it is born, and that this number remain with the animal until it dies and not be reused after its death. Cross-referenced lists of different animal identifiers are very helpful and should be encouraged, but there must be a single animal number to which these other animal identifiers refer that uniquely identifies each animal.

Location of the Microcomputer: On-farm vs. Veterinary Office

There are both advantages and disadvantages to locating the microcomputer at the veterinarian's office as opposed to locating it on the farm. Some dairy farms are not large enough to justify the cost of purchasing their own microcomputer. However, several such farms might benefit from the use of a computer at their veterinarian's office. Dairymen may also be reluctant to expend the effort needed to operate their own computer. Presently, most dairymen must perform many of the duties of accountants, veterinarians, mechanics, electricians, and carpenters. Adding "computer programmer"

to this list of required occupational skills is often more than many dairymen care to undertake. Also, dairymen frequently suffer from "fat-finger syndrome," which can be defined as a combination of poor typing skills and a general lack of understanding of the exacting requirements of computer technology. Such dairymen prefer to have others manage their computing needs.

DHIA learned long ago that periodic personal contact from the DHIA technician greatly improves the quality of the data collected from the farm. This same principle can be applied when someone from the veterinary clinic assists the dairyman by managing the herd health program.

On-farm usage should be considered for large farms with above-average management and record-keeping ability. On such farms, the convenience of continual access to the computer record may outweigh the value of outside assistance in managing the herd health program. Under such circumstances, the veterinarian would do best to encourage these clients to purchase their own computer systems and to use the client's computer for producing the information required to operate the herd health program. Perhaps the veterinarian may wish to keep a duplicate copy of a client's data base on his own computer.

Regardless of where support for the computer is located, the availability of hardware and software support is paramount to the smooth operation of any computer system. Hardware support is becoming increasingly convenient as the number of computer stores continues to grow. It is important to choose a computer that can be serviced locally so that "down time" is minimized. Software support should entail initial training in the use of the program, the provision of manuals and other training materials, access to program updates and future versions and telephone support to answer questions regarding the operation of the program.

Veterinary Clinic–Based Systems

When the computer is located in the veterinarian's office, complete and timely data must be transported from the farm at least weekly. A variety of mechanisms have been used, but probably no one method is best for all farms and all veterinary clinics.

The easiest mechanism for transfer of data to the veterinarian's office is to mail or hand-carry the data to the clinic. A form may be used to guide the dairyman in determining what data should be recorded—i.e. calvings, breedings, dryoffs, culls and so on. A carbon copy should be kept and filed on the farm in case the copy sent to the veterinarian's office is lost. The pages should be sequentially numbered so that lost data pages can be easily identified.

In some instances, it is possible to obtain data from the farm over the telephone. This can be expensive if it is routinely attempted for a large herd and if long-distance telephone charges are incurred. This method is useful, however, for smaller herds and on certain occasions when immediate communication is needed.

Electronic communication over the telephone is becoming more popular and reliable. With some systems, farmers with on-farm terminals can telephone the veterinary clinic microcomputer and enter new data. Often, information output can then be printed on the farm. Terminal entry of data can be expensive if long-distance telephone charges are incurred, and it is more complicated for the farmer who must learn how to operate the terminal and to encode the data into the herd health program. Also, this method places more responsibility on the farmer for the successful operation of the program because the veterinary clinic is less involved with the operation of the system. However, the farmer's accessibility to his computer record is greatly improved with the use of an on-farm terminal.

The establishment of a schedule for data submission is very important. Some clinics request that all data be submitted on a particular day of the week so that the data from all the herds using the program can be entered into the computer and reports generated for return to the respective farms on the same day each week. Other clinics receive and enter data whenever it arrives and return the computer output to each farm as soon as possible. Whatever system is used, it is important that herds communicate with the clinic at least every week and that the herdsman be notified over the telephone when data has not been received.

The skill of the herd health system manager is one of the most important factors in determining the success of a computerized herd health system at a veterinary clinic. The system manager might be a veterinary secretary, veterinary technician or other clinic employee. This person encodes and enters the data received from the veterinarian and the dairymen, and, more important, is responsible for detecting data errors, producing and distributing reports on schedule, reminding dairymen and veterinarians to submit their data, teaching and reminding veterinarians and dairymen to record the needed data, proofreading for evidence of possible erroneous or missing data and coordinating the activities of the dairymen and the veterinarian. It is important that this employee be able to communicate effectively with clients. Considerable tact is often required to compete effectively, in a nonoffensive manner, for the time of the veterinarian and dairyman. System managers must understand that some data may be embarrassing to the dairyman. For example, the system manager may need to ask the dairyman if a record showing a cow to be bred only once and still open at 180 days in milk is, possibly, missing a pregnancy or an insemination report. If the record is accurate, this is an embarrassing situation for the farmer and one to which

he probably does not like attention drawn. Nevertheless, because this record is highly suspicious of being in error, it is necessary for the system manager to question its validity. This must be done as tactfully as possible.

There are a variety of ways in which the system manager can communicate with the herdsman. Some programs allow the system manager to type notes to the dairyman while they are using the data input routine. Handwritten notes accomplish the same purpose with a more personal touch. Notes or telephone calls are frequently needed for the following:

1. Draw attention to records that are suspected of erroneous or missing data.

2. Remind the herdsman as to what data are needed, e.g., sire stud codes are needed with all inseminations.

3. Establish issues of animal identification, e.g., whether control number 313 is named B17 or Delilah.

4. Communicate about the scheduling of the next veterinary herd health visit and what information will be needed for this visit.

DATA COLLECTION

Regardless of the type of computer system or network used, the accuracy and completeness of the available data are of primary importance. The quality of the data is usually the principal limiting factor in the quality of the output. Fancy output formats and complicated statistics can do little to improve the validity of information that is inaccurate or misleading because it was based on incorrect data.

Ideally, the herdsman actually working with the cows should enter his or her observations or management actions directly into the computer. Often it is necessary to record the data on a written record for transport and entry into the computer at another time and place. In general, one should strive for a system that has a relatively direct communication link between the herdsman and the computer.

Computerization may not be beneficial for herdsmen who have difficulty maintaining a traditional written record system such as breeding wheels, cow folders or cow cards. Computers make things run faster but not necessarily better. Chaotic record systems that are computerized will probably result in nothing more than computerized chaos. Records will become confused faster than was ever before possible. Computers cannot supply missing data on inseminations, calvings or culls nor can they know that a cow is pregnant unless they are told. Therefore, as with any record system, the herdsman or veterinarian should not attempt to operate a computer system unless he is willing to diligently record the required data.

An ability and willingness to review the computer output for evidence of missing or incorrectly entered data are also important. Most computer systems have data entry validity routines that check for typographical errors and/or use of proper codes. Some systems also check each entry to see if newly entered data is consistent with the rest of the cow's record. For example, these systems will produce an error message if a cow is called pregnant before she has been inseminated. Although this type of error message is undoubtedly helpful in detecting certain errors, most errors cannot be recognized as definitively incorrect by someone unfamiliar with the management of the herd. Also, complete omission of data is the most frequent data collection problem and the hardest for error-finding subroutines to detect. For example, failure to report a clinical case of mastitis or a second insemination could never be detected by an error-finding routine. In the final analysis, the maintenance of an accurate and current data base depends on the user's ability and willingness to maintain constant vigilance over the computer output for indications of incorrect or missing data. When information that the herdsman suspects is incorrect appears on the computer printout, he must be willing to search the cow's record for the reason for this mistake and provide the necessary correction. Users who do not investigate suspicious output in this manner find that errors and missing data do not self-correct with time but tend to compound until the data base is in disrepair and the information output from the computer has little validity. Like a snowball rolling downhill, the less valuable the information output becomes, the less time the herdsman is going to spend on a computer system that gives "erroneous information." Users must therefore understand that the quality of the information they receive from the computer can be no greater than the quality of the data that is input.

The value of the output is the sole driving force for the human effort required to operate a computerized herd health system. If the value of a particular output section or report is not worth the time spent in data collection and computer operation, then this option should be excluded from the program for this user. For example, the "cost" of having an action list reminder for BVD vaccination is the need to record every vaccination for BVD. If the value of the BVD vaccination action list is not worth this cost, then the herdsman should not use this part of the program.

Confidentiality of records is always a concern whenever on-farm records are contributed to a central data base. Most dairymen who use DHIA are accustomed to allowing their records to leave the farm, but this can be a new experience for most beef producers and one that may cause some initial concern. Herdsmen must be assured that records will be kept confidential and that their data will be seen by others only as part of an average of many herds.

SPECIFIC FUNCTIONS RELEVANT TO THERIOGENOLOGY

Animals Due to Calve

Most good herd health management software can be tailored to notify the user a specified number of days before expected calving. Most systems calculate the time of expected calving by assuming that the last insemination was responsible for conception. Other systems also consider the estimate of gestation length made by a veterinarian at pregnancy examination. Some programs base their calculated date of expected calving on a different length of gestation for each breed of cattle. Dairy managers can usually be notified to change the ration a few weeks before calving and then notified again a few days before calving so that they can move the animal into a maternity stall. Use of this reminder system may increase the utilization of maternity stalls, thereby having an impact on rates of periparturient metritis, retained placenta, dystocia and calf mortality. For beef cattle using natural service, this application has limited value because the exact time of conception is usually less certain.

Many dairy and beef cattle managers need to regulate the size of their herds to maintain a base price for milk or to make maximum use of their physical facilities. For this purpose, a calving calendar can be produced that shows the expected dates of birth of new calves (Table 1).

Animals to Watch for Heat (Table 2)

Heat detection is frequently the most limiting factor in the success of dairy and beef artificial insemination programs. Computers can help by determining which animals are ready to be watched for heat and, when possible, by predicting the day when heat might occur. These predictions can be based on the occurrence of a previous heat or insemination 21 or 42 days ago, observation of postovulation blood 19 days ago, the use of prostaglandin 2 to 5 days ago or the recommendation of a veterinarian after palpation of ovarian structures. Perhaps the most important function of the computer is to prevent any cows from being overlooked for heat detection and being found open long past the date when they should have been pregnant.

Action Lists (Table 3)

Action lists remind the user of certain management actions that should be accomplished on a given day. Perhaps it is not exactly true that the herdsman has many decisions to make each day but rather that he repeats the same decisions many times each day. If so, computers can provide assistance by reminding him of what he has already decided.

Action list reminders should be totally adaptable

Table 1. Calving Calendar Herd #999999, All Groups, 13 Oct, 1983

Number	Name	Sire Name	Stud Code	Anticipated Calving Date
601	421	ERIC	29H3303	19-OCT-83
591	410	ERIC	29H3303	1-NOV-83
680	361	HAKIM	29H3360	14-NOV-83
613	435	ERIC	29H3303	29-NOV-83
612	434	HAKIM	2D9H3360	21-NOV-83
547	367	ERIC	29H3303	1-DEC-83
566	386	ERIC	29H3303	3-DEC-83
597	416	ARTIC	29H3900	7-DEC-83
688	419	ERIC	29H3303	15-DEC-83
679	408	ERIC	29H3303	19-DEC-83
684	373	ERIC	29H3303	19-DEC-83
677	335	DYNAMO	29H3098	3-JAN-84
522	342	ERIC	29H3303	10-JAN-84
602	422	ERIC	29H3303	14-JAN-84
711	437	MAIZ	29H4195	20-JAN-84
530	348	RADAR	29H3845	3-FEB-84
543	363	DYNAMO	29H3098	15-FEB-84
536	357	MAIZ	29H4195	20-FEB-84
689	413	MAIZ	29H4195	20-FEB-84
712	438	MAIZ	29H4195	13-MAR-84
686	442	MAIZ	29H4195	15-MAR-84
705	330	MAIZ	29H4195	15-MAR-84
527	344	ERIC	29H3303	16-MAR-84

Dates of anticipated calvings can be calculated from the date of last breeding or by estimates of length of gestation made at pregnancy examination. This information is used by the farm manager to regulate the size of the milking herd and to remind him of nutritional or housing changes needed as the expected time of calving approaches.

to the producer's individual management goals. For example, a herd health program should allow the farmer to vaccinate for a disease at any age he and his veterinarian choose and to begin watching for estrus at any number of days after calving. Management actions amenable to the use of computer-generated action lists can include vaccinations, weaning, dehorning, worming, hoof trims, dry off, breed registration, moving to another pen, extra teat removal and tuberculosis testing.

Animals for Reproductive Examination (Table 4)

The most useful output for many veterinarians is a list of animals that need a reproductive examination. This list tells the herdsman which animals to have ready to examine when the veterinarian arrives for a regularly scheduled herd health visit. It also gives the veterinarian an explanation of why each animal has been selected for examination. Cows may be selected for reproductive examination on the basis of many different adjustable criteria discussed below. When initiating a new herd on such a program, it is important that the veterinarian and the dairy client discuss exactly what criteria should be used by the computer for selecting the cows to be examined at the reproductive visits.

Pregnancy Examination. Most programs now available provide reminder systems for pregnancy examinations at an adjustable number of days after the last breeding. On many of the less sophisticated software, pregnancy examination may be the only available criteria for selecting a cow for a reproductive examination.

Prebreeding Checks. Herdsmen and veterinarians can select to examine heifers at a specified number of days of age. Cows can be selected for prebreeding examinations following calving or at a specified number of days prior to anticipated insemination.

Anestrus. Heifers over a specified number of days of age and cows that have calved more than a specified number of days ago may be identified as being in anestrus when estrus has not recently been reported. These animals can then be examined by the veterinarian to determine the cause, if any, for failure to show estrus.

Abnormal Cycle. Cows with too many estrous periods reported during a specified time period can be examined by the veterinarian for the possibility of follicular cysts or other causes of irregular cycling.

Problem Cows. Cows with reported problems such as cystic follicles, metritis, retained placenta and milk fever can be selected for an examination.

Repeat Breeders. Cows that have been inseminated more than a specified number of times without becoming pregnant can be selected for examination.

Suspect Abortion. Cows that have a heat, insemination or nonpregnant reproductive examination when they are thought to be pregnant should be selected for a pregnancy recheck.

Table 2. Cows to Observe for Heat Herd #999999 All Groups, 17 Jan, 1983

Criteria

Open cows fresh over 30 days ago
Heat predicted 19 to 23 days following previous heat (Heat)
Heat predicted 17 to 21 days following post-ovulation blood (Blood)
Heat predicted 19 to 23 and 40 to 44 days following breeding (Bred)
Heat predicted by veterinarian (Vet)
Heat predicted 2 to 5 days after prostaglandin (induced)

Number	Name	Comments	Prediction
560	380	Open 75 days, LN 5, bred 3X Last service sire MAIZ, 29H4195	16-JAN to 20-JAN (Bred)
569	389	Open 57 days, LN 4, bred 0X	20-JAN to 24-JAN (Heat)
596	415	Open 52 days, LN 5, bred 0X	24-JAN to 28-JAN (Heat)
604	425	Open 89 days, LN 2, bred 1X Last service sire, 29H3360	20-JAN to 24-JAN (Bred)
606	427	Open 75 days, LN 2, bred 1X Last service sire RADAR, 29H3845	18-JAN to 22-JAN (Bred)
613	435	Open 43 days, LN 2, bred 0X	
680	361	Open 60 days, LN 1, bred 0X	
684	373	Open 51 days, LN 1, bred 0X	
688	419	Open 50 days, LN 1, bred 0X	
692	352	Open 50 days, LN 1, bred 0X	
707	424	Open 71 days, LN 1, bred 1X Last service sire, 29H4195	24-JAN to 28-JAN (Bred)
713	440	Open 113 days, LN 1, bred 4X Last service sire ERIC, 29H3303	24-JAN to 28-JAN (Bred)

Six different criteria can be used to predict when cows or heifers should be watched especially closely for standing heat. Other optional information such as lactation number (LN), times bred (X) and last service sire can also be included to assist the inseminator.

Pregnancy Rechecking. Some veterinarians like to confirm every pregnancy diagnosis at least once. Also, it is sometimes necessary to be able to request explicitly a follow-up examination on an animal after a specified number of days have elapsed.

Failure to Calve. Animals that fail to calve after their calculated gestation period should be checked immediately to identify those that have aborted and to diagnose possible problem pregnancies.

History. Some computer programs produce a reproductive worksheet that gives a short history of the animal that is scheduled to be examined.

Ration Analysis

Nutritional anestrus, fat cow syndrome, and specific vitamin and mineral deficiencies are just some of the nutritional problems that may interfere with the normal reproductive cycle. There are many computer programs now available that analyze a ration for minimal nutritional requirements, and some that calculate a ration on the basis of the least cost required to meet these nutritional requirements.

Table 3. Cows Due to Dry Before Aug. 20, 1982

Cow #	Str #	Breeding Date	Date to Dry	Date to Calve	Trtmt/Cndtn	Action Date Dried
0289	2	12/26/81	08/07/82	10/06/82	Good-6/15	....
0271	2	01/01/82	08/13/82	10/12/82	100CC RM-12/1	....

Total number of cows due to dry = 2

Farmplan Demo: Aug 10, 1982
Numerous action lists are possible to remind farm managers of needed actions such as vaccinations, dry-off, calving date predictions and disease preventive procedures. Reminders should be adjustable to all possible days of age, days before calving or days after calving.

Table 4. Cows to Have Up for Reproductive Exam Herd #999999 All Groups, 17 Jan, 1983

Number	Name	Reason	Comments
457	277	Repeat breeder	Bred 3X. Open 135 days
499	319	Recheck	Requested on 3-JAN-83
517	332	Recheck	Requested on 3-JAN-83
520	340	Cyst, 30 mm	Diagnosed on 10-NOV-82. Open 109 days
547	367	Post partum	Open 26 days
560	380	Repeat breeder	Bred 3X. Open 125 days
566	386	Ret placenta	Diagnosed on 1-JAN-83. Open 18 days
604	425	Preg check	Bred 11-DEC-82. Bred 1X. Open 89 days
607	428	Post partum	Open 26 days
667	3086	Anestrus	478 days old, no heat reported
668	3096	Anestrus	478 days old, no heat reported
669	3084	Anestrus	461 days old, no heat reported
670	3092	Anestrus	478 days old, no heat reported
671	3087	Anestrus	467 days old, no heat reported
687	286	Preg check	Bred 18-DEC-82. Bred 1X. Open 91 days
689	413	Post partum	Open 26 days
690	372	Post partum	Open 25 days
691	CH321	Preg check	Bred 21-NOV-82. Bred 1X.
		Anestrus	476 days old, no heat for last 57 days
703	302	Preg check	Bred 2-DEC-82. Bred 3X. Open 152 days
		Repeat breeder	Bred 3X. Open 152 days
706	337	Recheck	Requested on 3-JAN-83
713	440	Preg check	Bred 15-DEC-82. Bred 4X. Open 313 days
		Susp abort	Open repro exam at 153 days gest
745	301	Preg check	Bred 25-NOV-82. Bred 1X
		Anestrus	456 days old, no heat for last 53 days

Veterinarians and their dairy clients can adjust the computer program to select cows for reproductive examinations on the basis of several criteria.

Individual Cow Records

Computers can also be used as electronic filing cabinets to store and retrieve animal histories to be used for individual animal clinical medicine. Most systems produce a cow page that gives summary information regarding genetic lineage, health history, pregnancy status and calving history (Fig. 1).

Semen Inventory

Some computer systems provide a frozen semen inventory to help the herdsman keep track of what frozen semen is available for use. In addition to helping to ensure that the right semen is available, a semen inventory can help to reduce the use of outmoded genes, which tend to collect in some artificial insemination freezers (Fig. 2).

Reproductive Diagnostic Indices

Herd health is the practice of veterinary medicine in which the herd is the basic unit of involvement. The practice of herd health is dependent on the availability of various diagnostic indices of herd performance. These diagnostic indices are used to identify and delineate herd problems and to monitor the effect of attempted disease control and preventive strategies. In this way, computerized herd health and management programs are the tools used by veterinarians to obtain the information needed to practice herd health. Most diagnostic indices were developed long before the impact of computer technology. However, computers calculate these indices much faster and more economically, enabling a herd health approach to be feasible for a greater number of herds.

Some of the more common reproductive diagnostic indices are shown in Table 5. There are many different ways to calculate each index, depending on how heifers and culled cows are processed and whether maximum and/or minimum values are set to prevent extreme values from having a large influence on the mean. The method of calculation should be made known to everyone who is using the program.

By using diagnostic indices to monitor reproductive efficiency, problem areas can be more quickly identified. Once problems are identified, the effectiveness of implemented solutions can be ascertained by monitoring these same diagnostic indices. In the future, this trial and error approach may be replaced by more sophisticated computer-simulated models.

It is almost impossible to practice dairy herd health medicine with a high degree of success without a means for routinely obtaining information on total herd performance. Attempting to practice herd health medicine without reliable epidemiologic information is as difficult as attempting to practice

```
MATTERHORN FARMS                        *** ANIMAL PROFILE ***                    Herd No: 99  Date: 10/01/84
--------------------------------------------------------------------------------------------------------------
----------------------------------------------- IDENTIFICATION AND PEDIGREE -----------------------------------

Ear Tag   : B70        Name      : Coquette Bradley T A 19    Sire       : Proton Bradley T A      Reg # 8081795
Regist No : 8698249    Group     : 5 - Brood Cow             Sire's Sire: Astro Bradley T A 50     Reg # 7214482
Tattoo(L) : B245       Birthdate : 11/08/75                  Sire's Dam : Carman 5 of Blau Velt    Reg # 7005555
Tattoo(R) : B245       Birth Wt  : 65
Location  : 3B         Origin    : Pasture exposure          Dam        : Coquette Bradley T A 13   Reg # 7399623
Dam's Tag : B69        Breed     : Angus                     Dam's Sire : Astronaut Bradley T A 2   Reg # 6900451
Dam's DOB : 04/21/71   Reg Class : B - Breeding Stock, Registered  Dam's Dam : Coquette Bradley T A 4  Reg # 7222222
--------------------------------------------------------------------------------------------------------------
------------- Weanling --------------|-------------- Yearling -----------------|--------- Acquisition & Sale ----------
Date  : 06/15/76  Weight Ratio: 108  |Date  : 11/15/76      Weight Ratio: 108  |Acquired: BIRTH       Date: 11/08/75
At Age: 220       B V R  Ratio: 105  |At Age: 373                 Ratio:       |For Sale? NO         Sale Price $ 0.00
Treat : 1         Shldr  Meas: 42.5  |Treat :            Shldr  Meas: 47.25     |---------------------------------------
Weight: 475       Hip    Meas: 43.75 |Weight: 1050       Hip    Meas: 49        |--------------- Disposition -----------------
Adj Wt: 454       Dam/Wt Meas: 1220  |Adj Wt: 1036       Scr/Pl Meas: 0         |Code: H- MY HERD  Date: 00/00/00   $ 0.00
A-D-G : 1.8636    Scurs  Meas: 0     |A-D-6 : 2.6407            Meas: 0         |                  :
Wt/DOA: 2.159            Meas:       |Wt/DOA: 2.815      Show?  Meas: Yes       |Comment           :
Comment: Has exceptionally good frame.| Possible embryo donor.                 |                  :
--------------------------------------------------------------------------------------------------------------
--------------------------------------------- HEALTH ACTION HISTORY (MONTH/YEAR) ------------------------------
   H/A #  1.  Clostridia 7Way:  05/79
          2.  I B R          :  05/79
          3.  Leptospirosis   :  10/81  10/80
          4.  PI-3            :  10/80
          5.  Deworm          :  10/82  04/82  10/81  04/81  10/80  04/80  11/79  05/79
          6.  B V D           :
          7.  Vibriosis       :  10/81
          8.  Degrub          :  04/82  04/81  04/80  05/79
          9.  Brucellosis     :  01/76
--------------------------------------------------------------------------------------------------------------
--PREG/CHECK------------------------------------ CURRENT INSEMINATION STATUS ----------------------------------

Date: 05/08/82   Date: 01/11/82 A-I  Gen-DamR# 8698249   Edc: 10/20/32   Date: 02/15/82 P-E  Gen-DamR# 8698249  Edc: 11/24/82
Stat: Positive   Bull       : 6749031   COLUMBUS ADVENTURE 310              Bull       : 8910080   LANSBURY OF WYE
Est Days? 60     Bull's Sire: 6700000   COLUMBUS OF WYE                     Bull's Sire: 4020204   CYRUS OF WYE
Born: 3  Lost: 0 Bull's Dam : 6600000   PRIM LASSIE 21                      Bull's Dam : 4792463   LILMA OF WYE
--------------------------------------------------------------------------------------------------------------
------------------------------------------------ CALVING HISTORY INFORMATION ----------------------------------
  Date     Calf
 Calved    Ear-Tag    Calf Name             Sex  Wt E Wt  B V R  Orig Dam's Reg#  Sire's Reg#  Sire's Name

03/15/79    913    M F BLACKCAP GRANDEUR 913   M   75 1 101  112   P-E  8698249   7500000   HAPPYVALE BLACK GRANDEUR 046H
05/06/80    017    M F COPYRIGHT PROTON 017    M   75 1 112  101   P-E  8698249   9120000   DOUBLE FOUR COPYRIGHT 84 H
08/19/81    133    MATTERHORN LASSIE 133       F   68 1 098  096   A-I  8698249   9210000   MATTERHORN SAMSON 485

Matterhorn Systems, Inc., a subsidiary of Matterhorn Farms
```

Figure 1. Animal profile.

clinical medicine without such information as history, clinical signs and laboratory results.

Veterinary Consultation

For computerized record systems to be successfully used in a herd health program by the practicing veterinarian, the system must provide information gained from analyses of the data collected from the producer, veterinarian and other sources. The analyzed information must be presented by the veterinarian to the producer so that the interpretation is very clear and understandable. The information should be compared with predetermined goals established early in the consultation. Comparison with performance of peer groups may also be helpful. All the data should be utilized to at least some extent to stimulate the producer to collect and input the data accurately. Failure to use some of the data in a meaningful way will cause the producer to wonder why he must collect it at all. Whenever possible, the information should be used to monitor progress of the preventive program in terms of improved conditions and economic benefits to the producer. Feedback to the producer must be given at regular intervals and in a personal manner.

Merely mailing the farmer the computer printouts without further comment may eventually cause lack of interest owing to the producer's failure to understand the resulting analyses. Regular opportunities to talk about the progress of the program, both its positive and negative aspects, should be scheduled. These times should not be hurried or squeezed into a busy work load of service on the farm. They should take place where the records are kept on the farm and not out in the alleyway or on the hood of a truck. These times are of utmost importance to the program and should be treated as such.

If at all possible, the veterinarian should be involved in most of the decision-making processes in the farm enterprise. To bring this about, the veterinarian must demonstrate competence in the areas of individual cow diagnosis and therapy, dairy husbandry and housing principles, management, nutrition and economics. His input into the decisions on the farm will ensure that the objectives of the herd health program will be considered when an important decision is made. Without this input the program might be needlessly weakened.

Prior to starting on the program, the method of charging fees for the computer service must be frankly discussed with the producer. Data collection must be undertaken primarily by the farmer. If dat

SEMEN INENTORY REPORT

DATE: 10/01/84   HERD NO: 99   MATTERHORN FARMS   PAGE: 1

Tank No: 1 BIG BARN IN STOREROOM

| Tank | Cpt | Bull's Reg # | Bull's Name | | ----------Bull's Parents---------- | | | ON HAND | |
					Reg. No.	Names	Amps	Straw	Total
1	1	9189920	DOUBLE FOUR COPYRIGHT 84 H	Bull's Sire:	7111111	MASSIVE OF KAHARAU	0	150	150
				Bull's Dam:	72222222	PAULA GR 31D			
1	2	8974207	PS POWERPLAY	Bull's Sire:	71222222	EARLY SUNSET EMULOUS 60E	0	28	28
				Bull's Dam:	72333333	PS MONTEITH BLANCHE 205			
1	3	9189920	DOUBLE FOUR COPYRIGHT 84 H	Bull's Sire:	7111111	MASSIVE OF KAHARAU	0	150	150
				Bull's Dam:	72222222	PAULA GR 31D			
1	4	9064530	BRIARHILL BARTMAN	Bull's Sire:	7252525	BAR HEART WINTONS IMAGE	0	59	59
				Bull's Dam:	7262626	BRIARHILL BLACK LADY 2553			
1	5	6749031	COLUMBUS ADVENTURE 310	Bull's Sire:	6252525	COLUMBUS OF WYE	0	8	8
				Bull's Dam:	6333333	PRIM LASSIE 21			
1	6	8989216	KEN CARYL MR ANGUS 8017	Bull's Sire:	7000000	NRTHRN PROSPECTOR 1125	0	124	124
				Bull's Dam:	8000000	BLKBRD OF KEN CARYL 2744			

Matterhorn Systems, Inc. A subsidiary of Matterhorn Farms

                                                              *** Tank Totals   0   519   519

                                                                  Report Totals 0   519   519

Figure 2. Semen inventory report.

input into the system is provided by the veterinarian, a fee should be charged. Likewise, a fee (perhaps on a per cow per year basis) should be charged for managing the computer system. The interpretation of the analyzed data should be an additional charge at a rate equal to the hourly rate for on-farm veterinary services. The charges should not be hidden within another fee but should be properly identified as a fee for consultation.

Table 5. Diagnostic Indices

Abortion incidence
Services per pregnancy
Pregnancy rate from first inseminations
Pregnancy rate from all inseminations
Percent of open cows bred 3 or more times
Percent of open cows over 150 days in milk
Percent of milking herd culled for reproductive
  problems
Interval to first heat
Interval to first service
Heat detection efficiency
Days open
Calving interval
Calf mortality (1 wk, 6 wk, 1 yr)
Cull rate
Reproductive cull rate
Incidence of metritis
Incidence of cystic ovaries
Incidence of retained placenta
Incidence of dystocia

Measures of herd reproductive efficiency and disease incidence can be used by the veterinary practitioner to identify herd reproductive problems and to evaluate the apparent effect of herd disease control and management techniques.

SUMMARY

Utilization of computer technology by the food animal industry will undoubtedly continue to grow in future years. In most instances, the information needs specific to the theriogenologist will be integrated with other areas of interest such as nutrition, management, disease control, production and economics. Theriogenologists must establish themselves as active users and consumers of agricultural computer technology if theriogenology is to benefit effectively from the data processing revolution now under way. Theriogenologists will need to participate actively in the design of such integrated systems to ensure that their information needs are met.

References

1. Agpros Livestock Source Book. Agpros Micro Systems, Lubbock, Texas, 1982.
2. Agricultural Computing Source Book. Doane Wester Inc., St. Louis, 1983.

3. Blood DC, Morris RS, Williamson NB, et al.: A health program for commercial dairy herds. Aust Vet J 54(5):207, 1978.
4. Elmore RG, Bierschwal CJ: A microcomputerized dairy herd reproduction program. In Symposium on Computer Applications in Veterinary Medicine. Starkville, Mississippi, 1982.
5. North Central Dairy Health Management Database Workshop, March 1984. Madison, Wisconsin, NCCI, pp 51–58.
6. Bartlett PC, Kirk JH, Mather EC, et al.: FAHRMX—A computerized dairy herd health management network. Comp Cont Ed Pract Vet 7:S124, 1985.

Swine Reproductive Performance: Data Collection, Analysis, and Interpretation

Thomas E. Stein, D.V.M., M.S., Ph.D.
University of Minnesota, St. Paul, Minnesota

Many swine producers have maintained individual sow records for years by manually recording information on sow cards, and have stacked the completed cards on a shelf in the barn office. Few producers or veterinarians attempted to analyze herd performance using these records. However, individual initiative, microcomputers and the value of information have changed the attitude of swine producers and veterinarians so that they are no longer passive record keepers.

In late 1983, the National Pork Producers Council (NPPC) formed an ad hoc committee to formulate standard definitions and calculations for the swine industry. In March, 1984, the Council released its final report, which includes over 300 definitions and over 70 formulas. Many commercial software developers agreed to standardize their calculations based on the NPPC report. The report, Generally Accepted Terms and Formulas for the Pork Industry, is available for $2.50 from the NPPC, Des Moines, Iowa.

In the last two years, many specialized veterinary practices have either designed their own computer record system using electronic spreadsheets or contracted with a service bureau to provide a record system for their clients in the swine industry.

Swine production and swine veterinary practice are becoming information-oriented. The major trends are toward more active data collection from more farms, and toward a service orientation in which the service rests not with a computer program and record-keeping service but with the analysis and interpretation of performance and diagnostic profiles of herd records.

RECORD-KEEPING SYSTEMS FOR SWINE BREEDING HERDS

A reliable, flexible, well-documented and clearly structured system should include the following parts:

1. An individual sow base; that is, all data should be entered into a sow record, from which a computer program will derive all measures and calculate all indices.

2. An internal structure that ensures data integrity so that reports contain useable information—informative, believable and interpretable.

3. A report program that compiles and summarizes sow data in a concise format.

4. Various report levels so that the data stored for each sow can be used to show trends, view performance over time, provide diagnostic profiles and monitor population changes.

DATA COLLECTION

Although it might appear that an individual sow system would increase the record-keeping burden, one of its major advantages is that it keeps record-keeping to a minimum.

Data collection can be divided into six categories: (1) animals entering the herd; (2) animals leaving the herd, i.e., deaths, culls or transfers; (3) breeding information; (4) farrowing information; (5) weaning information; and (6) other information such as sow diseases.

However, only four types of data (at a minimum) are essential for each sow on file. It should be at the producer's option to add more information to a system, such as birth weights and weaning weights. The events and data collected for each event are as follows:

1. *Farrowing data:* date, sow number or name, numbers alive, stillborn and mummified, and piglets fostered on or off.

2. *Weaning data:* date, sow and number weaned.

3. *Removal information:* sow, type of removal (cull or death), date and reason for removal.

4. *Service data:* sow number or name, date and boar identification.

5. *Entry data:* gilt or sow number, date, birthdate, sire, dam, origin and breed.

Although service data are listed as a minimum requirement, *breeding information is not essential for a system to function.* That is, individual sow record-keeping systems can be used successfully on farms that are pen-mating, although some of the capability to identify problems is lost if breeding dates and full boar details are not available.

Another useful option that permits development of a more complete breeding record is the capacity to store entry dates of gilts to the breeding herd separately from a first-service date. This in turn allows the producer to monitor the state of the gilt pool.

Other events that can be recorded include pregnancy examination results, abortions, sow weights, information about sow disease incidents and treatments and general comments.

CONCEPTS USED TO DESIGN A COMPUTER PROGRAM FOR INDIVIDUAL SOW RECORDS

File Structure

Record-keeping programs are of two types, classified by their file structure: they store sow data in either a fixed length format or a flexible, variable-length format.

In a fixed format system, there are limited number of spaces for each sow, and all information for each sow's cycle must fit into these "boxes." If more than, say, 30 things happen in one farrowing-to-farrowing cycle, the extra information cannot be added to the record without removing some of the previous information. If spaces are given for services during one cycle, and a sow has four services, then the fourth service cannot be added without removing one of the previous services. Further, if after having used the system, one wanted to keep track of new information such as sow condition score, a computer programmer would have to change the entire structure of the original program.

The most adaptable programs use a variable-length record so that the size of each sow record reflects the amount of data stored for that sow and expands like an accordion: sows with few events have short records, but as more events occur, a sow's record expands to make room for the new events and cycles. There should be no limit to the number of events that any sow can have in her record. If it is desired to begin recording sow condition score, sow weight at farrowing, and sow weight at weaning, a variable-length format can accommodate these new, previously undefined or unspecified events without major programming changes.

Data Integrity and Error Detection

Since data collection is error-prone, a computer program must have ways of ensuring that the herd data base is as credible as possible, especially when the data will be used by people other than the farmer—e.g., veterinarians, bankers, nutritionists and management consultants. Missing dates, inconsistent information (farrowing a dead sow), and duplicate identification (two or more sows with the same number) are the most common problems that may lead to an inaccurate and potentially misleading data base. Any recording system must have ways of maintaining data quality that are built into the internal structure of the program.

Farm data is never perfect. Sows may farrow but the event may not be written down; sows may die or be culled and be forgotten. Even on well-managed farms this often happens. An effective computerized record system will have multiple levels of error detection to ensure that a herd data base contains credible, high-quality information.

Data should be checked for its logical consistency, for missing dates, for dates in correct sequence and for valid ranges.

The stages during the sow's parity can be described and used to maintain logical consistency. Sows may be lactating, removed, served (gestating), entered, served before weaning or pregnancy terminated, and each of these would be referred to as a sow's *current status*. During data entry a sow's current status can be checked against the information being entered for her. If the data do not fit (weaning a sow before she has farrowed), the program may comment "inconsistent with current sow status." For more serious consistency problems (farrowing a sow that has been dead for 3 years) the program should not accept the entry unless the original sow record is first changed. Table 1 lists sows by current status. In the example, sows are listed by parity, current status and average and current sow productivity indices. Reports of this type can be used to quickly discover the status of all animals in the herd, including past farrowing and weaning performance.

Missing dates, a common problem, are detected by a logical consistency check because if a date is missing, an expected event will also be missing in an event-oriented system. If the system (like many current systems) were of the "pigeon-hole" type, using a fixed format into which each item of data must fit, then missing dates (e.g., farrowing dates, weaning dates) would be difficult to detect unless one could view the entire sow record during data entry. An "event-oriented" computer system, in which the structure of the record is determined by what actually happens to each sow, not what the programmer says should happen to every sow, is a superior approach to design.

Dates not in the correct sequence (farrowing a sow in 1985, then weaning her in 1984) must also be detected. Again, an event-oriented system ensures that events are entered in correct sequence.

In a fixed-format system the only way to detect incorrect dates is with a range check on the interval between two dates. For example, sows should farrow no earlier than 110 days and no later than 120

Table 1. List of Sows by Current Status

Sow ID	Parity	Status	Last Event		Productivity Index Average	Current
275	1	Presumed Pregnant	Served	30 Jul 84	198	198
276	1	Presumed Pregnant	Served	25 Jul 84	186	186
277	1	Presumed Pregnant	Served	21 Sep 84	212	212
279	1	Presumed Pregnant	Served	4 Sep 84	218	216
280	1	Presumed Pregnant	Served	6 Sep 84	216	216
281	1	Weaned	Weaned	27 Sep 84		
283	1	Lactating	Farrowed	18 Sep 84		
284	1	Lactating	Farrowed	20 Sep 84		
285	1	Lactating	Farrowed	12 Sep 84		
287	1	Lactating	Farrowed	6 Sep 84		
288	1	Lactating	Farrowed	23 Sep 84		
289	0	Presumed Pregnant	Served	24 Aug 84		
306	2	Presumed Pregnant	Served	22 Sep 84	190	
3079	7	Presumed Pregnant	Served	20 Aug 84	225	
3084	7	Presumed Pregnant	Served	20 Aug 84	222	233
309	2	Weaned	Weaned	10 Sep 84	184	182
3097	7	Presumed Pregnant	Served	6 Aug 84	199	
3102	7	Presumed Pregnant	Served	6 Sep 84	194	179
3113	7	Presumed Pregnant	Served	2 Sep 84	205	184
3116	7	Lactating	Farrowed	30 Aug 84	213	
312	2	Lactating	Farrowed	6 Sep 84	196	
32	5	Presumed Pregnant	Served	14 Sep 84	197	225
321	2	Lactating	Farrowed	13 Sep 84		
322	2	Presumed Pregnant	Served	22 Sep 84	196	
35	4	Presumed Pregnant	Served	13 Jul 84	187	196
356	2	Lactating	Farrowed	30 Aug 84	190	
36	4	Presumed Pregnant	Served	17 Jul 84	209	169
360	2	Lactating	Farrowed	5 Sep 84	217	
37	4	Presumed Pregnant	Served	14 Jul 84	198	184
3736	10	Presumed Pregnant	Served	4 Jul 84	216	217
3928	11	Weaned	Weaned	27 Sep 84	212	
3S	0	Presumed Pregnant	Served	22 Aug 84		
400	0	Presumed Pregnant	Served	9 Sep 84		
401	0	Presumed Pregnant	Served	1 Sep 84		
402	0	Presumed Pregnant	Served	6 Sep 84		
403	0	Presumed Pregnant	Served	7 Sep 84		
404	0	Presumed Pregnant	Served	8 Sep 84		
405	0	Presumed Pregnant	Served	9 Sep 84		
406	0	Presumed Pregnant	Served	11 Sep 84		
4481	9	Lactating	Farrowed	30 Aug 84	204	
4487	9	Lactating	Farrowed	30 Aug 84	206	
509	4	Presumed Pregnant	Served	21 Aug 84	191	216
509A	1	Presumed Pregnant	Served	24 Jul 84	196	196
511	4	Presumed Pregnant	Served	7 Sep 84	221	228
511A	1	Presumed Pregnant	Served	13 Jul 84	232	232
512A	1	Presumed Pregnant	Served	21 Aug 84	250	250
514	1	Presumed Pregnant	Served	3 Jul 84	187	187
516	1	Presumed Pregnant	Served	16 Jul 84		
52	5	Weaned	Weaned	27 Sep 84	184	
534	1	Presumed Pregnant	Served	13 Aug 84	226	226
538	1	Presumed Pregnant	Served	24 Jul 84	233	233

Each sow is listed by ID number, parity (number of times farrowed), status, last significant event (farrowed, weaned, served, culled or entered) and sow productivity index.

days after breeding. However, a range check on the gestation length can be done only if producers record service dates.

Other types of data should be checked to see that they are valid or make sense. The number of pigs born per litter should fall between 0 and 25, the litter weight between 0 and 50 pounds. Valid range checks are used primarily for trapping data entry errors and cannot ensure logical consistency.

Definition and Description of Events

The most flexible computer systems are event-oriented and based on some sow cycle, such as breeding-to-breeding or farrowing-to-farrowing (a parity model). For clarity and simplicity each parity should begin with a farrowing and end with the next farrowing or removal. Many things may happen as sows move through a cycle, and each thing can be defined as an event. A sow may enter the herd, farrow, foster some pigs on or off, wean, be served or be removed from the herd (death, cull, or some other sale or transfer). Other events occur less frequently, such as pregnancy exam, abortion, sow weight, sow condition score and so on. A group of these events is included in one sow parity.

For example, sows 200 and 201 (Table 2) have moved through the herd together from the time they entered in February, 1983. Each is parity three, having farrowed three times since entering the sow herd. During each parity each sow farrowed, fostered some pigs on or off, was weaned, then served. Notice that sow 201 was served twice in her first parity, in July and again in August.

The records of these sows also illustrate another advantage of an event-oriented computer program: sows with few events have short records, and as more events are added to a sow's record, the record expands to make room for the new events and cycles, as an accordion would expand. There should be no limit to the number of events that any sow can have in her record, in contrast to a typical fixed-format record system.

Definitions of Variables and Implementation of Formulas

A record system should be based on a set of concise, well-defined indices and terms and should provide examples of the way each index, rate or average is calculated. These explanations are critical to the accurate interpretation of the numbers that the program generates. A simple example should suffice: are mummified pigs included in the number born dead, or are they exclusive so that the total pigs born is a sum of live, dead and mummified? Without explicit definitions and formulas the reports become impossible to interpret.

Consider the difference between definitions and concrete expressions of calculations. The definition of conception rate is straightforward: the number of animals that conceive out of a group of animals that were served in a specified time period or group. But notice the distinction between definition and calculation: when writing a computer program, the programmer needs to know how to implement the calculation. Conception measured by what, as of when? Is it a 24-day, a 28-day, or a 30-day conception rate? Is it a nonreturn rate? Is it a 38-day pregnancy rate determined as the proportion pregnant by ultrasound pregnancy detector?

Even more critical are the calculations for overall indices such as pigs born per sow per year, litters per sow per year or pigs weaned per sow per year. Which animals should be included in the denominator, and when should newly entered gilts be added

Table 2. Individual Sow Records, Complete History of All Events Since Entry into a Breeding Herd

Sow: 200 Birth date:	Parity: 3 Sire:	Status: Served Dam: Breed:	
Parity	Date	Event	Event Data
0	16 Feb 83	Enter	Comment:
	14 Mar 83	Service	Boar: 20B
1	6 Jul 83	Farrow	Alive: 8 Stillborn: 0 Mummies: 0 Weight:
	7 Jul 83	Foster	1 pig on
	28 Jul 83	Wean	Pigs weaned: 8 Litter weight: 93.0
	1 Aug 83	Service	Boar: 3542
2	22 Nov 83	Farrow	Alive: 6 Stillborn: 0 Mummies: 0 Weight:
	23 Nov 83	Foster	4 pigs on
	12 Jan 84	Wean	Pigs weaned: 8 Litter weight: 174.0
	16 Jan 84	Service	Boar: 44B
3	12 May 84	Farrow	Alive: 13 Stillborn: 2 Mummies: 0 Weight:
	12 May 84	Foster	2 pigs off
	14 Jun 84	Wean	Pigs weaned: 11 Litter weight: 215.0
	18 Jun 84	Service	Boar: 187
	19 Jun 84	Service	Boar: 187

Sow: 201 Birth date:	Parity: 3 Sire:	Status: Served Dam: Breed:	
Parity	Date	Event	Event Data
0	16 Feb 83	Enter	Comment:
	9 Mar 83	Service	Boar: 4012
1	2 Jul 83	Farrow	Alive: 12 Stillborn: 0 Mummies: 0 Weight:
	21 Jul 83	Wean	Pigs weaned: 10 Litter weight: 94.0
	26 Jul 83	Service	Boar: 4012
	22 Aug 83	Service	Boar: 4012
2	15 Dec 83	Farrow	Alive: 12 Stillborn: 1 Mummies: 1 Weight:
	16 Dec 83	Foster	2 pigs off
	12 Jan 84	Wean	Pigs weaned: 10 Litter weight: 129.0
	16 Jan 84	Service	Boar: 4012
3	12 May 84	Farrow	Alive: 14 Stillborn: 0 Mummies: 0 Weight:
	12 May 84	Foster	3 pigs off
	14 Jun 84	Wean	Pigs weaned: 10 Litter weight: 169.0
	18 Jun 84	Service	Boar: 4012
	19 Jun 84	Service	Boar: 17

to the denominator? The NPPC report provides some needed standardization; it recommends using mated females (any sow or gilt that has had at least one service) as the denominator. Indices that use mated females monitor the biology of reproduction in a population because they include only those sows that would have the opportunity to farrow. Indices that include all females in the population (total females, served and unserved) monitor both the efficiency and biology of herd reproduction but become difficult to interpret.

Data Transfer and Telecommunication

Since no record-keeping program and no brand of microcomputer are standard, the ability to communicate (transfer data electronically) between computers or computer programs is essential. In this way, veterinarians may access on-farm computers and abstract the breeding herd data to run through their own reproductive analysis program. With the introduction of integrated electronic spreadsheet/data base programs, electronic transfer provides even greater flexibility so that data stored in a dedicated breeding herd computer program can be sent to a spreadsheet for special analyses or for graphic reports.

Thus, programs should have the ability to read and write text files using ASCII (American Standard Code for Information Transfer) characters. ASCII files are generic text or data files (sequential access). To reduce the size of data files, most computer programs store data in binary format, so that a printout of the file looks like a lot of 1's and 0's. An ASCII file is a data file stored in characters people can understand when they see it on a computer screen or printout. For example, a sow record in ASCII format might look like this: Y120, 3, 130284, 10, 02. The commas separate (delimit) data, so sow Y120, parity 3, farrowed on February 13, 1984, with 10 pigs born live and 2 born dead. ASCII files are essential for those who wish to transfer data between computers or computer programs.

ANALYSIS AND INTERPRETATION OF REPRODUCTIVE PERFORMANCE AND HEALTH REPORTS THAT MONITOR CURRENT PRODUCTION AND HEALTH

Performance Monitor

The actual production or performance of a breeding herd over time must be monitored closely. A performance report should reflect current performance (number of sows farrowed last week, pigs weaned per sow this week, and so on) and should be able to generate a retrospective picture or "profile" of past performance (Table 3). As such, electronic spreadsheets can work well for this type of report but unfortunately cannot be used to produce diagnostic profiles.

Four major areas of breeding herd production should be monitored continuously:

Breeding performance (sows bred, repeat services, weaning to first service interval, percent of sows bred by 7 days after weaning); *Farrowing performance* (sows farrowed, pigs born alive, farrowing rate, litters per mated female per year); *Weaning performance* (sows weaned, pigs weaned per sow, pre-weaning mortality, pigs weaned per mated female per year); and *Population* (total inventory, average parity of the herd, replacement rate, sows removed, net change in herd inventory).

Monitoring Trends

The practice of monitoring trends provides a broad perspective with which to judge the performance of a herd over time and to remove the considerable effect of short-term biologic variation inherent in herd production. Thirteen-week, 21-week, monthly, or yearly rolling averages can be used to plot trends. It is much easier to see trends and changes when data is presented as a continuous graph. Rolling average calculations are especially suited to electronic spreadsheets but changes in rolling averages become difficult to interpret if the data cannot be explored in more detail.

REPORTS USED PRIMARILY FOR DAILY HERD MANAGEMENT

Action Lists

On some farms, action lists make it easier to manage the herd. Farmers can keep track of sows that may have otherwise been "lost" in the system, due either to a vital piece of information being mistakenly omitted from the system or to the event never taking place for a specific sow. Common examples include a sow that has not been served for some weeks following weaning or a gilt that has not been bred since she entered the herd many weeks before.

Two of the most important action lists are for *sows due to farrow* and *sows weaned but not served*, which tend to include most of the "lost" sows in a herd. These and other action lists can be used for scheduling treatments, such as prostaglandin treatment for sows that have reached 15 days postweaning without showing estrus, or for scheduling an activity, such as the 21-day heat check or the 35-day pregnancy check.

Action lists also help maintain data integrity. The five action lists in Table 4 function by checking for a specific event in each sow's record. For example, for gilts that have entered the herd, all entered gilts without subsequent service dates would be included on the list of gilts entered but not yet served. Their inclusion means that neither a service date nor a culling date had been recorded. Their presence acts

Table 3. Performance Monitor

	Jul 83 Sep 83	Oct 83 Dec 83	Jan 84 Mar 84	Apr 84 Jun 84	Jul 83 Jun 84
Breeding Performance					
Total females served	34	52	68	72	222
Females served 1st service	34	49	66	69	215
Females served repeat service	0	3	2	3	7
Per cent repeat services	0.0	5.8	2.9	4.2	3.2
Weaning—1st service interval	5.9	6.3	4.8	5.3	5.5
Per cent sows bred by 7 days	84.8	87.2	95.8	93.1	91.0
Entry—1st service interval			35.6	78.8	55.0
Farrowing Performance					
Total sows farrowed	40	38	51	66	195
Average parity of farrowed sows	4.0	4.6	3.8	4.0	4.1
Total pigs born alive	372	301	415	604	1692
Average total pigs per litter	9.8	8.8	8.8	9.8	9.3
Average pigs born alive/litter	9.3	7.9	8.1	9.2	8.7
Average pigs born dead/litter	0.5	0.9	0.7	0.6	0.7
Per cent born dead	5.6	10.1	7.6	6.4	7.2
Per cent mummies	0.0	0.0	1.8	1.7	1.0
Litters less than 7 born live	4	11	14	8	37
Per cent < 7 born live	10.0	28.9	27.5	12.1	19.0
Average birth weight	3.4	4.0	4.0	3.7	3.8
Farrowing rate					
Farrowing interval	155.5	142.0	148.1	140.0	145.4
Litters/mated female/year					
Weaning Performance					
Number of sows weaned	34	39	48	64	185
Total pigs weaned	266	274	342	505	1387
Average pigs weaned per litter	7.8	7.0	7.1	7.9	7.5
Preweaning mortality	20.6	15.4	16.0	14.4	16.2
Average weaning weight	11.1	11.7	11.1	11.0	11.2
Average age at weaning	19.3	19.0	18.7	19.8	19.3
Average Sow Productivity Index	168	164	159	163	163
Pigs weaned/mated female/year					
Population					
Total ending inventory	56	74	120	137	137
Average parity	3.9	3.5	2.6	2.7	2.7
Average inventory	48.7	62.6	99.0	134.1	85.9
Gilts entered	12	18	46	19	95
Replacement rate	24.7	28.8	46.5	14.2	110.6
Sows and gilts culled	0	0	0	2	2
Culling rate	0.0	0.0	0.0	1.5	2.3
Average parity of culled sows				1.5	1.5
Sow and gilt deaths	0	0	0	0	0
Death rate	0.0	0.0	0.0	0.0	0.0

An example of a performance monitor that measures herd performance over time for the four keys areas of a breeding herd. Columns one through four are quarterly figures, the last column is a summary for the year. Notice the low averages for total pigs born per litter and pigs born alive per litter.

as a flag or prompt to either breed or cull the gilts on the list or update their records.

History

Record systems should have the ability to produce an individual sow lifetime history (Table 2) containing all recorded events for the duration of the sow's existence in the herd (a sow card). In fact, a computer program should mimic the manual process of posting daily activity (farrowings, weanings, breedings, deaths, culls) to a paper sow card.

DIAGNOSTIC REPORTS

These are reports that can help in finding the causes of problems that are identified by continuous monitoring of performance. They provide diagnostic profiles for the herd to refine the summarized information in the performance profile.

Parity Distribution

Each item monitored on the performance profile should also be grouped by individual parity (Table 5). For example, to define a problem of generally poor reproductive performance may require analysis of returns to service by parity, pigs born alive and dead by parity, pigs weaned by parity, or the number of litters with less than seven pigs born alive by parity.

Table 4. Action Lists

1. Gilts Entered But Not Served

Sow ID	Entered	Days Open
1302	6 Sep 84	69

1 sow listed

2. Sows Served Requiring Heat Checks/Pregnancy Tests

Sow ID	Served	21 Days	35 Days

0 sows listed

3. Sows Due to Farrow

Sow ID	Served	Due Date	Overdue
542	24 Jul 84	16 Nov 84	
276	25 Jul 84	17 Nov 84	
608	26 Jul 84	18 Nov 84	
6617	29 Jul 84	21 Nov 84	
247	30 Jul 84	22 Nov 84	
275	30 Jul 84	22 Nov 84	
6606	30 Jul 84	22 Nov 84	
6609	30 Jul 84	22 Nov 84	
249	6 Aug 84	29 Nov 84	
250	6 Aug 84	29 Nov 84	
3097	6 Aug 84	29 Nov 84	
6622	6 Aug 84	29 Nov 84	
255S	7 Aug 84	30 Nov 84	
602	10 Aug 84	3 Dec 84	
606	12 Aug 84	5 Dec 84	
534	13 Aug 84	6 Dec 84	
6926	13 Aug 84	6 Dec 84	
18	20 Aug 84	13 Dec 84	
231	20 Aug 84	13 Dec 84	
3079	20 Aug 84	13 Dec 84	
3084	20 Aug 84	13 Dec 84	

4. Sows Farrowed But Not Weaned

Sow ID	Farrowed	Days Lactating
3116	30 Aug 84	76
356	30 Aug 84	76
4481	30 Aug 84	76
4487	30 Aug 84	76
6786	30 Aug 84	76
195	5 Sep 84	70
360	5 Sep 84	70
239	6 Sep 84	69
240	6 Sep 84	69
287	6 Sep 84	69
312	6 Sep 84	69
285	12 Sep 84	63
184	13 Sep 84	62
321	13 Sep 84	62
6927	13 Sep 84	62
6931	13 Sep 84	62
6932	13 Sep 84	62
954A	13 Sep 84	62
283	18 Sep 84	57
132	20 Sep 84	55
134	20 Sep 84	55
175	20 Sep 84	55
284	20 Sep 84	55
951A	20 Sep 84	55
288	23 Sep 84	52
1338	27 Sep 84	48
177	27 Sep 84	48
214	27 Sep 84	48
6831	27 Sep 84	48

29 sows listed

5. Sows Weaned But Not Served

Sow ID	Weaned	Days Open
309	10 Sep 84	65
281	27 Sep 84	48
3928	27 Sep 84	48
52	27 Sep 84	48
6824	27 Sep 84	48
731	27 Sep 84	48

6 sows listed

Examples of five action lists that can be used to check for missing information or for management action.

Removal Analysis

The ability to analyze all culls, deaths, or other removals by reason and by parity (Table 6) is a powerful tool, especially when exploring demographic patterns and the effect of culling on herd age distribution.

Farrowing Rate Analysis

A farrowing rate measures success—i.e., sows farrowed divided by sows bred. However, if the farrowing rate declines then it is also important to measure the failures, the nonpregnant females, by examining the components of the nonfarrowing rate. Nonfarrowing animals can be grouped as returns-to-service, diagnosed not pregnant, failures-to-farrow, abortions, or other reasons (cull or death). Failure-to-farrow animals are presumed to be pregnant (pregnancy test positive) that do not farrow.

A farrowing rate analysis (Table 7) is a useful management and diagnostic aid because by examining the reasons that animals "drop-out" of their breeding group, patterns can be recognized that may be consistent with infectious or non-infectious causes of reproductive failure (parvovirus or seasonal infertility, for example).

Table 5. Parity Distribution Report

	Parity					Total
	0	**1**	**2**	**3–6**	**7+**	
Breeding Performance						
Total females served	39	52	40	41	50	222
Females served 1st service	37	50	39	39	50	215
Females served repeat service	2	2	1	2	0	7
Per cent repeat services	5.1	3.8	2.5	4.9	0.0	3.2
Weaning—1st service interval		7.2	5.6	4.5	4.5	5.5
Per cent sows bred by 7 days		75.0	92.5	100.0	98.0	91.0
Farrowing Performance						
Total sows farrowed		55	41	46	53	195
Total pigs born alive		462	322	410	498	1692
Average total pigs per litter		8.9	8.2	9.6	10.5	9.3
Average pigs born alive/litter		8.4	7.9	8.9	9.4	8.7
Average pigs born dead/litter		0.5	0.4	0.7	1.1	0.7
Per cent born dead		5.5	4.5	7.0	10.4	7.2
Per cent mummies		1.8	0.9	0.9	0.5	1.0
Litters less than 7 born alive		9	12	8	8	37
Per cent < 7 born alive		16.4	29.3	17.4	15.1	19.0
Average birth weight		3.4	3.8	4.1	3.8	3.8
Farrowing rate						
Farrowing interval			143.5	153.8	139.6	145.4
Weaning Performance						
Number of sows weaned		51	40	42	52	185
Total pigs weaned		381	288	323	395	1387
Average pigs weaned per litter		7.5	7.2	7.7	7.6	7.5
Preweaning mortality		16.8	12.7	14.3	19.6	16.2
Average weaning weight		10.8	11.3	11.6	11.3	11.2
Average age at weaning		17.9	18.4	20.6	20.2	19.3
Average Sow Productivity Index		170	159	156	165	163
Population						
Total ending inventory	44	25	20	25	23	137
Average inventory	20.8	20.3	13.4	13.7	17.7	85.9
Sows and gilts culled	1	0	0	1	0	2
Sow and gilt deaths	0	0	0	0	0	0

Notice that the format is similar to the performance monitor in Table 3. Parity 0 females are gilts from entry to farrowing, and parity 1 females are gilts that have farrowed once. The last column is a summary for the year.

INTERPRETATION AND ANALYSIS OF REPORTS

Monitoring performance provides a means by which to judge changes in the production or productivity of a swine herd, that is, a baseline.

Certain indices, averages or summary numbers can be monitored, and, if a change occurs, can be investigated more thoroughly. For each index monitored on the herd performance profile there should be a diagnostic profile that can be used to investigate a change or problem more precisely. Below are some examples of the relationship between performance and diagnostic profiles.

Performance Profile
1. Average parity of herd:
   i. Overall population
   ii. Farrowed sows
2. Average litter size
   i. Total born
   ii. Born live
   iii. Born dead
3. Weaning to service interval and
4. Percent of sows mated within 7 days of weaning

Diagnostic Profile
1. Parity distribution: the percent of litters farrowed, by parity

2. Distribution of total, live and dead, by parity
3. and 4. Percent of sows mated within 7 days of weaning, by parity

Attaching significance to a change is the first step toward interpretation. For example, if the stillbirth rate changes from 5 per cent to 10 per cent of total pigs born, some interpretation must be made of its significance. If the change is significant, the next question to ask might be: are all animals experiencing this increase in rate, or can it be traced to a certain subpopulation? By using herd records, one might approach the diagnosis of an increase in stillbirth rate, i.e., above 10 per cent, as follows:

1. Identify the problem by monitoring current reproductive performance. Decide that the change is significant enough to investigate.

2. Define the problem as specifically as possible, using diagnostic profiles of herd records. Do any groups of sows have above average stillbirth rates? Is it a random distribution across all parities? Divide the herd into groups by parity number to calculate parity-specific stillbirth rates and parity-specific litter sizes.

3. Next, consider the parity distribution of the

Table 6. Removal Reasons

Removal Type/Reason	Parity					Total Removed	Per Cent of Total
	0	1	2	3–6	7+		
Cull	47	87	32	105	9	280	98.6
No heat	0	24	4	5	0	33	11.6
Did not conceive	14	4	1	3	0	22	7.7
Not pregnant	12	7	4	2	0	25	8.8
Failed to farrow	15	4	2	5	0	26	9.2
Abortion	1	1	0	0	0	2	0.7
Difficult farrow	0	3	1	0	0	4	1.4
Poor litter	0	1	2	5	0	8	2.8
Mastitis	0	2	0	3	0	5	1.8
Milk problem	0	5	0	5	0	10	3.5
Udder problem	0	1	0	0	0	1	0.4
Farrow performance	0	7	9	27	0	43	15.1
Vaginal prolapse	0	1	0	0	0	1	0.4
Rectal prolapse	1	1	0	0	0	2	0.7
Unsoundness	0	3	2	2	1	8	2.8
Lameness	1	2	0	0	0	3	1.1
Leg injury	0	1	0	1	0	2	0.7
Injury	0	3	0	0	0	3	1.1
Abscess	1	1	0	0	0	2	0.7
Unthrifty	0	3	3	1	1	8	2.8
Old age	0	0	1	40	7	48	16.9
Genitourinary disease	0	0	0	1	0	1	0.4
Central nervous system disease	0	0	1	0	0	1	0.4
Disease, no details	0	0	0	1	0	1	0.4
Behavior problem	0	3	0	0	0	3	1.1
Unknown reason	2	10	2	4	0	18	6.3
Death	3	1	0	0	0	4	1.4
Vaginal prolapse	1	0	0	0	0	1	0.4
Gastro-intestinal disease	1	0	0	0	0	1	0.4
Unknown reason	1	1	0	0	0	2	0.7
Destroyed	0	0	0	0	0	0	0.0
Transfer	0	0	0	0	0	0	0.0
Unknown type	0	0	0	0	0	0	0.0
Total	50	88	32	105	9	284	100.0

An example of a diagnostic analysis of the reasons sows were removed from a herd, including a parity distribution by reason. Notice the many gilts (parity 0) removed for failing to conceive, negative pregnancy diagnosis, or failure to farrow.

Table 7. Farrowing Rate Report

Service Dates	Served	Returns	Negative PRG Test	Abortion	Fail to Farrow	Other Removal	#Preg or Farrowed	% Preg or Farrowed
1 Sep—28 Feb 82	318	22	1	2	24	9	260	81.8
1 Mar—31 Aug 82	333	25	22	3	36	8	239	71.8
1 Sep—28 Feb 83	343	33	7	1	16	7	279	81.3
1 Mar—31 Aug 83	395	50	11	1	21	9	303	76.7
1 Sep—29 Feb 84	365	36	15	3	8	14	289	79.2
1 Mar—31 Aug 84	396	25	7	1	11	7	345	87.1
Total	2150	191	63	11	116	54	1715	79.8

An example of a diagnostic analysis of farrowing rate. Each row begins with the number of served females and their dates of service. The farrowing rate is given in the last column, and the drop-outs for each group are characterized by reason.

Table 8. Example of Problem-Oriented Medicine Population

Process	Example
Performance Profile	
Average litter size:	Problem identified (Table 3)
total born	8.7 pigs born alive per sow
born alive	for sows farrowed from
born dead	July 1, 1983 to June 30, 1984
Diagnostic Profile	
Distribution of pigs born alive, by parity	Problem defined (Table 5) Total born and live-born
Distribution of the breeding herd, by parity	average litter sizes are low across all parity groups, especially parity 1 and 2 females
Diagnostic Investigation	
Specific on-farm investigation, concentrate on the animals contributing the most to the problem	Go to the farm, concentrate primarily on the gilts and parity 2 sows, parvovirus serology, nutritional status, management, age at breeding, and so on

herd: if stillbirth is highest for sows in parity six or older, and the herd is made up of 60 per cent parity six sows or older, then stillbirth rate will not decrease unless the age structure of the herd is changed.

Problem identification using a performance profile, problem definition using diagnostic profiles, and the evaluation of specific treatments or recommendations using either performance or diagnostic profiles is the process of *problem-oriented populaton medicine.*

Both performance and diagnostic profiles can be used to evaluate treatment or management recommendations. Response to treatment (no matter how treatment is defined) is the kind of information veterinarians working with herd populations have not been able to obtain in the past.

Consider what happens on farms. Most problems are multicausal, and the treatment often involves management changes. If there is no feedback or evaluation of the recommended treatment, then little can be added to a veterinarian's armamentarium of experience. By using herd production records to see the effect of their management recommendations or treatments (to decide whether they were successful or not), clinicians can add to their experience. Thus, the ability to evaluate is a critical part of problem-oriented population medicine.

AN APPLICATION OF PROBLEM-ORIENTED POPULATION MEDICINE

Application. We will focus on the identification and diagnosis of an insufficient number of pigs born live per litter farrowed (Table 8).

In this example, a southern Minnesota complete confinement farrow-to-finish hog operation, with Landrace/Large White/Yorkshire and Farmer's Hybrid genetics, had a lower than expected average for pigs born live in 1983. The first step is to recognize that litter size had been smaller than expected, using a performance profile that monitors pigs born live (Table 3).

Once the problem has been recognized and defined as small litter size, a diagnostic profile can be used to further define the problem, in this case a distribution of pigs born live by parity (Table 5). Notice that some animals, parities 3 and greater, had average litter sizes (both total born and live born) above the herd mean, while parities 1 and 2 were below the herd mean.

There are at least two reasons for low litter size in this herd. First, since total and live born averages are low, i.e., less than 11 and 10, respectively, across all parity groups, poor genetic potential must be one of the primary factors ruled out. Second, notice how the demographic structure of the herd causes parity groups 1 and 2 to have such an effect on the herd average.

These two groups farrowed 96 of the 195 litters in the period (about 49 per cent). Thus, when combined, the populations with the smallest litter sizes made up a high percentage of all farrowings relative to the rest of the herd. As long as the parity-specific litter sizes do not change, and as long as the first two parities make up such a high portion of the farrowings, litter size will not improve.

The next step, once the problem has been defined to this level, would be to go to the farm and perform a diagnostic investigation, concentrating on the affected populations, i.e., gilts and parity 2 sows. Serologic profiles for parvovirus may be needed, and gilt management should be assessed carefully (age at breeding, weight at breeding, pen-mating vs. hand-mating, boar exposure, housing after breeding, nutrition, and so on). The advantage of defining the problem as specifically as possible *before* going to the farm is that instead of observing all animals and hoping that a problem will be obvious, one need only investigate selected groups for specific problems of management or disease.

SUMMARY

Management problems, and infectious and non-infectious diseases, can be defined precisely using computerized records for swine breeding herds. Interpretation of records in many cases requires the simultaneous evaluation of two or more complementary measures to fully understand the diagnostic and prognostic implications of the identified problem. Interpretation of problems identified on performance monitors requires swine herd demographic data, specifically the age distribution of the breeding females. A successful computerized system that can be used for problem-oriented population medicine must be based on the collection of data from individual sows.

References

1. Muirhead MR: Constraints on productivity in the pig herd. Vet Rec 102:228, 1978.

2. Pepper TA, Boyd HW, Rosenberg P: Breeding record analysis in pig herds and its veterinary applications—1: Development of a program to monitor reproductive efficiency and weaner production. Vet Rec 101:177, 1977.

3. Wrathall AE: Reproductive failure in the pig: Diagnosis and control. Vet Rec 100:230, 1977.

Computerized Records for Sheep

Marie S. Bulgin, D.V.M., Diplomate, A.C.V.M.
Caldwell Veterinary Teaching Center, Caldwell, Idaho

Anna M. Davis, B.S., M.S.
University of Idaho, Moscow, Idaho

Sheep are more efficient converters of agricultural waste and poor quality forage than most other domesticated food animals. Moreover, they can produce more than one fertile offspring per gestation, have the potential of having two gestations a year, and they produce wool, a second cash crop. For sheep to gain a favorable lead in the face of competition from other livestock species, it will be necessary to fully develop these potentials by using objective selection based on recent research. Research has definitely shown that the desirable traits in sheep (i.e., more lambs per ewe and more pounds of meat per lamb) can be improved through selective breeding. Genetic improvement based on past traditional subjective selection methods have not yet begun to tap the potential of this species to perform; thus, a change in subjective selection of replacement animals to a greater dependency on an objective method is needed.

RECORDS

To improve the efficiency of an operation, objectivity is needed and a record-keeping system becomes crucial. The higher the production goals, the more sophisticated the system must be.

A good record-keeping system can be as simple as a ledger sheet and a pencil and as complicated as a computerized system requiring daily input. A cost-effective system will be affected by the size of the flock, the amount of time that the manager has to devote to record-keeping, the goals of the producer, and the end-product price.

In large commercial flocks where the goal is for a ewe to raise at least one lamb every year, record systems may not be required. In contrast, a producer with goals greater than a 200 per cent annual lamb crop with the lambs gaining over 0.75 pounds per day will require sophisticated written record input. Fortunately, evolution of information-collating systems is perhaps one of the most significant advances of this century. However, these systems are merely a tool that help to make more knowledgeable decisions: The more sophisticated the tool, the more sophisticated the management decision that can be made.

COMPUTERIZED RECORDS

If a flock is adequately culled, using one selection factor such as pounds of meat produced per ewe based on a record system composed of the pencil and ledger sheet, the flock eventually becomes more uniform in production for that factor and selection of replacement animals becomes more difficult. At this point a more sophisticated system is needed that (1) indicates how many pounds of lamb and wool each ewe in the flock has produced, (2) compares the production of a young ewe with that of older ewes, (3) keeps track of health problems or other variables we wish to evaluate and/or eliminate, (4) compares performance of various sires, and (5) ranks lambs on rate of gain, adjusted for sex, type of birth (single, twin etc.), and method of raising (raised as a twin or otherwise) (see Table 1). With this type of information we can more intelligently select replacement animals and thus improve overall flock efficiency.

One such rating has been developed by Dr. Wharton of Ohio State University. Each ewe is given a production score for the year that is a combination of 90-day adjusted weights of lambs raised and the fleece weight of the ewe. A production ratio for the year is calculated for each ewe by dividing her score by the flock average score. In like manner, a probable producing value (PPV) is calculated for each ewe by comparing her lifetime production scores with the average lifetime production scores of the flock. The relative position of each ewe within the flock yields her PPV rank. This rank, combined with the manager's visual appraisal of physical condition and knowledge of possible extenuating factors, provides the basis for accurate culling decisions.

The above record system will also aid greatly in the selection of replacement ewes. A selection score can be calculated for each lamb that combines the

Table 1. Growth Weight Adjustment Factors for 90 Days of Age

	Age of Dam		
	3 to 6 Yr Old	2 Yr or Over 6 Yr	1 Yr Old
Ewe Lamb			
Single	1.00	1.09	1.22
Twin, raised as twin	1.11	1.20	1.33
Twin, raised as single	1.05	1.14	1.28
Triplet, raised as triplet	1.22	1.33	1.46
Triplet, raised as twin	1.17	1.28	1.42
Triplet, raised as single	1.11	1.21	1.36
Wether			
Single	.97	1.06	1.19
Twin, raised as twin	1.08	1.17	1.30
Twin, raised as single	1.02	1.11	1.25
Triplet, raised as triplet	1.19	1.30	1.43
Triplet, raised as twin	1.14	1.25	1.39
Triplet, raised as single	1.08	1.18	1.33
Ram Lamb			
Single	.89	.98	1.11
Twin, raised as twin	1.00	1.09	1.22
Twin, raised as single	.94	1.03	1.17
Triplet, raised as triplet	1.11	1.22	1.35
Triplet, raised as twin	1.06	1.17	1.31
Triplet, raised as single	1.00	1.10	1.25

National Extension Sheep Committee Report, September, 1968, Recommendations for Uniform Sheep Selection Programs, Page 3.

lamb's adjusted 90-day weight and the fleece weight of the dam. The selection score for each ewe lamb is compared to the average selection score of all ewe lambs within the flock to provide a selection score ratio. Producers may also choose to use a weaning index that rates the ewe lamb against all other ewe lambs in terms of a 90-day weight. These numerical scores are always used together with a visual appraisal to prevent selection of ewes with undesirable physical traits.

Ram selection and replacement is a major management decision that is greatly facilitated by the use of good records. Selection of replacement rams should be made not only on physical appearance but also on the basis of the ram's producing value and twinning record, the ram's average daily gain (under test conditions, if possible), birth weight, weaning weight, weaning age, lamb selection ratio and weaning index within the flock.

Good records will also provide the general information about a flock that can make the difference between inefficient and efficient operations. This includes lambing percentage, weaning percentage, pounds of lamb weaned for each ewe in the flock, average lamb birth weight, average ewe age, comparisons of weight gains made by lambs born to ewes of different ages, and death loss.

DATA REQUIRED

The information put into the computer system should be simple and complete. Basic important information would include:

1. Ewe identification, age or date of birth, breed and wool weight.
2. Ram identification and breed.
3. Lamb identification, sex, date of birth, type of birth and rearing, birth weight, weaning weight and date.
4. Type of disposal of ewes culled from the flock.
5. Type of death loss for both ewes and lambs.
6. Date the ram was exposed to the ewes.

In addition, it is advantageous to be able to record some subjective comments. Additional data that may possibly be included in a program are ewe's sire and dam, ewe's wool grade, weight and staple length. It can include lamb fat, muscling and carcass scores or other variables.

INFORMATION GENERATED

General Flock Information. This includes number of ewes, total lambs born and weaned, lambing and weaning percentages, length of lambing season, total wool production and production per ewe, total lamb production and production per ewe, pounds of lamb weaned per ewe in the flock, and averages of lamb birth weight, lamb weaning weight, lamb 90-day adjusted weight, lamb average daily gain and ewe age.

Individual Ewe Information. Information that can be generated for each ewe includes lambing cycle, production score and rank, probable producing value and rank, and lamb production for the current year. In addition, lifetime averages and totals can be generated for wool and lamb production, lambs born and weaned, lamb birth weight, lamb weaning weight and age, lamb 90-day weight and adjusted 90-day weight and lamb index. The poorest individuals as indicated by their PPV values can be so designated.

Individual Ram Information. Information can be generated for each ram to provide number of ewes bred, total lambs born, average lamb birth weight, average lambs born per ewe, estrus cycles per ewe prior to pregnancy, average lamb 90-day weight, adjusted 90-day weight and lamb average daily gain.

Individual Lamb Information. Each individual lamb can be indexed by 90-day weight, given a selection score or replacement value and rank. Weaning age, 90-day weight, adjusted 90-day weight and average daily gain are also usually listed. The top, middle and bottom individuals in the flock as indicated by their selection scores can be designated.

Animal Loss Due to Death or Culling. Summarized ewe culling and lamb death loss, including numbers, ewe age at culling, reason for culling, lamb age at death and cause can be generated.

Economic Information. Economic values for wool and lambs can be assigned and the cost per lamb weaned calculated on an average daily gain basis as well as the maintenance cost for ewes and rams. These values can then be analyzed to provide a profit or loss picture of the operation.

FORMULAS USED IN CALCULATIONS

Since it is sometimes helpful to understand the basis for scores and indices that are used in day-to-day operation, the formulas for calculations are given as follows:

1. Ewe Production Score (PRD SCR)

$$\text{PRD SCR} = \frac{\begin{array}{c} 1.17 \ (\text{90-day adj wt of lambs raised}) \\ + 2 \ (\text{ewe fleece wt}) \end{array}}{\text{No. of lambs raised}}$$

Factor 1.17 is dropped for single lambs. This factor is a bonus given to the ewe based on the repeatability of multiple births.

For 90-day adjusted weight of lambs see Table 1. The factor of 2 is a product of the relative economic importance of wool to lamb combined with the heritability value.

2. Probable Producing Value (PPV) is the ratio of the ewe's production score to the average value of the flock. This takes into account the ewe's production over the entire period of record keeping. The average ewe in the flock has a PPV of 100. The ewe with a PPV of 105 would be expected to produce 5 per cent more pounds of lamb than the flock average for next year. A ewe with a PPV of 95 would be expected to produce 5 per cent less than the flock average.

$$\text{PPV} = 100 + \frac{0.35 \ (N)}{1 + 0.35 \ (N-1)}$$

$$= \frac{\text{Sum (PRD SCR} - \text{Flock Avg PRD} \times \text{SCR)}}{N}$$

$$N = \text{number of years of records}$$

The value of 0.35 is the repeatability factor of the production score.

3. PPV rank. This is an ewe's relative position within the flock based upon her PPV. The ewe with the rank of 1 has the highest PPV in the flock.

4. Lamb 90-day weight. The lamb weaning weight corrected to 90 days of age.

$$\text{90-day Weight} = \frac{\text{90-day weaning wt} - \text{Birth wt}}{\text{Days of age}}$$

5. Lamb 90-day adjusted weight is the lamb's 90-day weight adjusted for ewe age, lamb sex, type of birth and type of rearing (see Table 1).

6. Lamb Selection Score (SS)

$$\text{SS} = (\text{90-day adj wt}) \ (1.1) + 0.4 \ (\text{fleece wt of ewe})$$

1.1 factor is dropped if lamb is raised as a single. This factor is based on the predilection of a lamb to also have multiple births.

7. Lamb selection ratio. Sexes are rated separately. The average lamb within a sex has a ratio of 100.

$$\frac{\text{Selection score of lamb}}{\text{Average selection score of lamb sex}} \times 100$$

8. Lamb index. Sexes are indexed separately. The average lamb within a sex has an index of 100.

$$\frac{\text{Lamb 90-day weight}}{\text{Average 90-day weight for lamb sex}} \times 100$$

HOW TO USE INFORMATION

Individual conformation and eye appeal, the standards by which flocks have been culled in the past, have not appreciably improved productivity over the years. If one is not going to select replacements on the basis of productivity, computerized records have no value. If increased productivity is a major goal, an increase in the following parameters is important:

1. Number of lambs per ewe
2. Average daily gain of lambs
3. Ewe wool weight
4. Feed efficiency

To achieve these goals, the first decision to be made will be that of deciding which ewes should be culled from the flock. The manager must be able to rate each ewe in comparison with others within the flock. (Note: Rating should always be done within a flock rather than between flocks to avoid bias from external factors.)

Apart from the effects of other variables (nutrition, health care, etc.), computerized records can help identify the top producers in a flock by serializing the PPV and SS ratios. There are some limitations in the use of this information, however. For example, a young ewe losing a lamb to predators will have a similar PPV to that of a young ewe losing a lamb due to dystocia. A lamb from superior parentage may lose weight due to illness and thus may be ranked below a lamb that has a genetically based poor rate of gain. Therefore, one should not rely on the computer completely. However, in most cases the bottom 10 per cent of the flock should be culled and replacements should be in the top 25 per cent of the lamb crop and among lambs whose dams rank in the top 25 per cent.

HOW TO COMPUTERIZE RECORDS

The selection of a record-keeping system should depend in large part upon the information that it can generate and the format in which it displays this information. The sheep producer must use care in selecting a system that can be understood easily and that presents information that is important to the producer's specific management system and goals. Thorough investigation of available systems may be time-consuming but is well worth the effort.

Many universities are offering programs and computer services to various livestock producers. One of the first such programs is offered by the Ohio State University Agriculture Experimental Station, Wooster, Ohio 44691. Another is the Idaho Sheep Flock Improvement System available through the Idaho Cooperative Extension Service. Most county extension agents will be helpful in locating available programs in their area. Several private companies also market computer services, such as Sheep Production Services, Shoreham, Vermont 05770, and John Glenn, Ewe-Profit, Dixon, California 95620. Generally, in using one of the above services, the records are kept by the producer as lambs are born and weaned and ewes are sheared. Records are submitted for processing as soon as weaning is completed. The processed information is returned to the producer along with recording forms for the next year that are customized to list each ewe in the flock.

Sheep improvement programs designed for home computers can also be purchased from private companies or through universities and/or cooperative extension studies. These programs are written in specific computer languages. If one is planning to buy a home computer, it may be wise to find the program first, then buy a computer that speaks the same language. Some companies sell the computer and the program together. Such a company is Hometown Computer Services, 2525 South Main Street, Suite 18, Salt Lake City, Utah 84144.

The final alternative is programming one's own computer or hiring someone to make a program utilizing the formulas desired in this chapter and setting forth the specific information desired.

It should be emphasized that a computer does not make record keeping easier. Time needed to gather and enter data will be just as time-consuming as ever, but the computer can synthesize the data and present it in a form that makes it easier to arrive at better decisions. There are many other aspects of efficiency in livestock production besides keeping records and culling. Proper nutrition and health care are important examples. However, records are basic, and any program to upgrade an operation must begin with adequate and accurate records.

If the sheep industry is to survive the challenge of the future, it must fully develop the potential of this versatile species. The objective selection of replacements, based on productivity, particularly by breeders of purebred animals, is absolutely mandatory. Computerized records are essential in this process.

Appendix

Table 1. Unit Equivalents within the Metric System

1 gm (gram)	=	10^3 mg (milligram)	=	10^6 μg (microgram)	=	10^9 ng (nanogram)	=	10^{12} pg (picogram)

Table 2. Metric-English Conversion Factors

Length

Metric to English:
Centimeters (cm) $\times$ 0.394 = inches (in)
Meters (m) $\times$ 39.4 = inches
Meters $\times$ 3.28 = feet (ft)
Meters $\times$ 1.09 = yards (yd)

English to Metric:
Inches $\times$ 2.54 = centimeters
Feet $\times$ 30.5 = centimeters
Feet $\times$ 0.305 = meters
Yards $\times$ 0.914 = meters

Capacity

Metric to English:
Milliliters (ml) $\times$ 0.0338 = fluid ounces (fl oz)
Liters $\times$ 33.8 = fluid ounces
Liters $\times$ 2.11 = pints
Liters $\times$ 1.057 = quarts
Liters $\times$ 0.264 = gallons

English to Metric:
Fluid ounces $\times$ 29.6 = milliliters
Pints $\times$ 473 = milliliters
Quarts $\times$ 946 = milliliters
Quarts $\times$ 0.946 = liters
Gallons $\times$ 3.79 = liters

Weight

Metric to English:
Grams (gm) $\times$ 0.0353 = ounces
Kilograms (kg) $\times$ 35.3 = ounces
Kilograms $\times$ 2.2 = pounds (lb)

English to Metric:
Ounces $\times$ 28.3 = grams
Pounds $\times$ 454 = grams
Pounds $\times$ 0.454 = kilograms

Temperature

Centigrade to Fahrenheit:
($^\circ$C $\times$ 9/5) + 32 = $^\circ$F

Fahrenheit to Centigrade:
($^\circ$F $-$ 32) $\times$ 5/9 = $^\circ$C

Table 3. Convenient Conversion Factors

To Convert:	To:	Do:
gr/lb	mg/lb	Multiply by 65
gr/lb	mg/kg	Multiply by 143
mg/lb	gr/lb	Multiply by 0.015
mg/lb	mg/kg	Multiply by 2.2
mg/kg	mg/lb	Multiply by 0.454
gm/ton	%	Multiply by 0.00011
%	gm/ton	Divide by 11 and multiply by 10^5
%	ppm	Multiply by 10^4
ppm	%	Multiply by 10^{-4}
mg/dl	mEq/L	Multiply by valence times 10 and divide by atomic weight

$$\frac{mg/dl \times valence \times 10}{atomic\ weight} = mEq/L$$

Table 4. Commonly Used Names for Breeding Animals and Their Young

Species	Bovine	Equine	Ovine	Caprine	Porcine	Canine	Feline
Common name	Cattle	Horse	Sheep	Goat	Pig	Dog	Cat
Male	Bull	Stallion	Ram	Buck	Boar	Dog	Tom
Female	Cow	Mare	Ewe	Doe	Sow	Bitch	Queen
Parturition	Calve	Foal	Lamb	Kid	Farrow	Whelp	Queen, kindle
Name of young	Calf	Foal	Lamb	Kid	Pig (litter)	Puppy (litter)	Kitten (litter)
Young male	Bull	Colt	Ram lamb	Buckling	Boar	—	—
Young female	Heifer	Filly	Ewe lamb	Doeling	Gilt	—	—
Castrated male	Steer	Gelding	Wether	Wether	Barrow	—	—

Table 5. Male Reproductive Parameters in Domestic Animals

	Bull	Stallion	Ram	Buck	Boar	Dog	Tom
Age of puberty (months)	10–12	18–24	6–10	3–6	5–6	6–12	6–12
Age of sexual maturity (effective sire)	3–4 yrs	3–4 yrs	18–20 mos	8–12 mos	8–9 mos	12 mos	9–12 mos
Testicle location	Scrotal	Scrotal	Scrotal	Scrotal	Scrotal	Scrotal	Scrotal
Accessory glands†	P, B, VG	P, B, VG	P, B, VG	P, B, VG	P, B, VG	P	P, B
Techniques of semen collection‡	AV, EE	AV	AV, EE	AV, EE	AV	AV	AV, EE
Time required for spermato-genesis (days)	60–70	38–42	59–73	Unknown	50–60	55–70	Unknown
Season	Nonseasonal	Seasonal fluctuation in semen components	Somewhat seasonal; low in summer, highest in fall	Seasonal variation in volume, cell number and quality	Nonseasonal	Nonseasonal	Nonseasonal, depressed somewhat in fall

*Adapted from Mather, E. C. and Rushmer, R. A.: In Alexander, N. J. (ed.): Animal Models for Research on Contraception and Fertility. Hagerstown, Md., Harper & Row, 1979, p. 567.
†P = prostate, B = bulbourethral gland, VG = vesicular gland.
‡AV = artificial vagina, EE = electroejaculation.

Table 6. Averages of Semen Characteristics of Domestic Animals*

	Bull	Stallion	Ram	Buck	Boar	Dog	Tom
Volume (ml)	5	60	1	0.8	225	10	.04
Total sperm/ejaculation ($\times 10^9$)	7	9	3	2.0	45	1.5	.057
Sperm concentration (10^9/ml)	1.2	0.15	3.0	2.4	0.2	0.3	1.7
Motile sperm (%)	70	70	75	80	60	85	78
Normal morphology (%)	80	70	90	90	60	80	90
Ejaculates/week	6–10	3–10	6–24	20	4–10	1–3	2–3

*The editor acknowledges Brian Gerloff, D.V.M., for preparing this table.

Table 7. Number of Females per Male During the Breeding Season in Domestic Animals

Type of Breeding	Bull	Stallion	Ram	Buck	Boar	Dog	Tom
Pasture							
Immature male	10–15	10–15	20–30	20–30	10–20	unk	unk
Mature male	10–25	20–40	40–80	40–60	20–40	unk	unk
Hand (services/week)							
Immature male	2–4	2–5	6–12	6–12	2–4	1–2	3–5
Mature male	4–12	3–12	6–24	6–24	4–10	1–3	7–10

Adapted from Roberts SJ: Veterinary Obstetrics and Genital Diseases. 2nd ed. Ithaca, SJ Roberts, 1971, p 625. Distributed by Edwards Brothers Inc, Ann Arbor, Michigan.

Table 8. Female Reproductive Parameters in Domestic Animals*

	Cow	Mare	Ewe	Doe	Sow	Bitch	Queen
Age of puberty (months)	8–12 (breed differences)	15–24 (seasonal effects)	7–10	6–8	5–8	6–12	5–12
Age of sexual maturity (months)	30	36	10	8 (if born early in year)	10	5–12	6–12
Type uterus	Bipartite	Bipartite	Bipartite	Bipartite	Bicornuate	Bicornuate	Bicornuate
Type placenta, gross	Cotyledonary	Diffuse	Cotyledonary	Cotyledonary	Diffuse	Zonary	Zonary
Type placenta, histologic	Epitheliochorial	Epitheliochorial	Controversial	Controversial	Epitheliochorial	Endotheliochorial	Endotheliochorial
Breeding season	All year	April–Sept., easily maintained all year with lights	Breed variation from autumn to all year	Sept.–Jan. in northern latitudes	All year, slight seasonal influence	All year	Jan.–Oct.
Type estrous cycle	Polyestrous	Seasonally polyestrous	Seasonally polyestrous	Seasonally polyestrous	Polyestrous	Monestrous	Polyestrous
Length estrous cycle	21 days	21 days	17 days (range, 14–19)	21 days	21 days	16–56 weeks	2–3 weeks (if not mated)
Duration of estrus	12–18 hours	4–7 days	36 hours (range, 24–48)	18–36 hours	48–72 hours	9–10 days	3–6 days
Optimal breeding time (hours after onset of estrus)	10–16	48–72	18–24	24–36	12–30	48–96	During estrus
Mechanism of ovulation	Spontaneous	Spontaneous	Spontaneous	Spontaneous	Spontaneous	Spontaneous	Induced
Time of ovulation	4–16 hours after estrus	24–48 hours before end of estrus	24 hours after onset of estrus	12–36 hours after onset of estrus	24–42 hours after beginning of estrus	1–3 days after onset of estrus	25–50 hours after coitus

Table continued on following page

Table 8. Female Reproductive Parameters in Domestic Animals* *Continued*

	Cow	Mare	Ewe	Doe	Sow	Bitch	Queen
Ovulation rate (number of ova)	1	1	1–2	2–3	10–20	6–8	1–12
Transit time of ovum in oviduct (days)	3–4	4	3–4	3–4	2–3	6–8	4–8
Implantation (days)	10–12	25–56	14–18	10–11	11–16	17–21	11–14
Pseudopregnancy	Not reported	Occasionally	Not reported	Frequent	Rare	Common (60 days)	Uncommon (6 weeks)
Gestation length (days)	278–293	330–345	144–151	146–151	112–115	59–68	58–65
Birth numbers	1	1	1–2	1–3	6–12	1–12	1–8
Chromosome number (diploid)	60	64	54	60	38	78	38
Birth weight	18–45 kg	9–40 kg breed variation	4–5 kg	3–5 kg	1–1.5 kg	100–300 gm	~100 gm
Weaning weight	20–180 kg	70–300 kg pony to draft horse variation	10–20 kg	14–16.5 kg	4.5–13 kg	~1400 gm	750–800 gm (8 weeks)
Weaning age	3–205 days (variable management)	4–6 months (variable management)	30–180 days (variable management)	8–10 weeks (variable management)	14–56 days	3–8 weeks	3–8 weeks
Return to cyclic activity postpartum	20–30 days ovulation; conception poor at less than 60 days	4–16 days postpartum estrus; conception slightly lower	Artificially next season unless induction in nonbreeding season	Artificial induction in nonbreeding season	Nonovulatory estrus at 1–3 days; lactational anestrus; estrus 4–9 days postweaning	5–6 months	1–6 weeks
Time to rebreed	45–90 days postpartum	25–30 days postpartum	First estrus	First estrus	First estrus	First estrus	First estrus

*Adapted from Mather, E. C. and Rushmer, R. A.: *In* Alexander, N. J. (ed.): Animal Models for Research on Contraception and Fertility. Hagerstown, Md., Harper & Row, 1979, pp. 568–569.

Table 9. Signs of Estrous Behavior in Domestic Animals*

Species	Signs
Cow	Restlessness, bellowing, mucous discharge and swollen vulva. Stands to be mounted and may mount other cows.
Mare	Association of mare with stallion, elevation of tail to one side when stallion present, squatting or urinating in front of stallion and winking of clitoris. Stands to be mounted by stallion.
Ewe	Restlessness, switching of tail and standing to be mounted. May see cervical mucus and vulvar erythema.
Doe	Rapid side-to-side or up-and-down tail movement is often detected. External genitalia may be swollen, reddened and moist. Restlessness, increased vocalization, increased urination, decreased milk production and decreased appetite may also be observed. Will stand for buck.
Sow	Reduced appetite, restlessness, salivation, frequent grunting and swollen, congested vulvar lips. Sawhorse-like stance to be mounted, which can be induced by boar or pressure of hand on back. Whitish mucous discharge present in late estrus.
Bitch	Follows period of hemorrhagic discharge. Soft vulvar swelling, yellow discharge. Female receptive, "flags" male.
Queen	Crouching, raising and extension of pelvis, treading, lateral deflection of tail, lordosis, crying out and rolling, acceptance of male.

*The editor acknowledges Brian Gerloff, D.V.M., for preparing this table.

Table 10. Characteristics of Gametes within the Female Reproductive Tract in Domestic Animals*

Species	Capacitation Time (hours)	Retention of Sperm Motility (hours)	Retention of Sperm Fertility (hours)	Retention of Ovum Fertility (hours)
Cow	4	15–56	30–48	8–12
Mare	Unknown	70–140	70–140	6–8
Ewe	1.5	48	~24	10–25
Sow	3–6	50	24–48	8–10
Bitch	7†	144–264	150–240	>96
Queen	2–24	48	24–48	26

*The editor acknowledges Brian Gerloff, D.V.M., for preparing this table.
†In vitro.

Table 11. Gestation Length of Domestic Breeds*

Species	Breed	Gestation Length (Days)
Cattle		
(Dairy)	Ayrshire	277–279
	Shorthorn	275–292
	Brown Swiss	288–291
	Holstein	278–282
	Guernsey	282–285
	Jersey	277–280
(Beef)	Angus	273–282
	Brahman	271–310
	Hereford	283–286
	Simmental	285–287
	Charolais	285–287
	Limousin	287–290
Horse	Arabian	335–339
	Morgan	342–346
	Thoroughbred	336–340
	Belgian	333–337
	Clydesdale	334
	Percheron	321–345
Ass		365–375
Hinny	(Stallion × Ass)	348–350
Mule	(Jack × Mare)	355
Sheep	Southdown	143–145
	Dorset	143–145
	Hampshire	144–146
	Shropshire	145–147
	Cornedale	148–150
	Rambouillet	149–151
	Merino	147–155
Goat		146–155
Pig		111–116
Dog		59–68
Cat		56–65
Siamese		63–69

*The editor acknowledges Brian Gerloff, D.V.M., for preparing this table.

Table 12. Characteristics of Milk in Domestic Animals*

	Cow	Mare	Ewe	Doe	Sow	Bitch	Queen
Water (gm/L)	873	890	837	866	788	790	820
Lipid (gm/L)	37	16	53	41	96	85	50
Total protein (gm/L)	33	27	55	33	61	75	70
Calcium (mg/L)	1250	1020	1930	1300	2100	2300	350
Lactose (gm/L)	48	61	46	47	46	37	50
Phosphorus (mg/L)	960	630	1000	1060	1500	1600	700

*The author acknowledges Brian Gerloff, D.V.M., for preparing this table.

Table 13. Male Reproductive Parameters of Representative Nonhuman Primates*

	New World Monkeys		Old World Monkeys				Anthropoid Ape
	MARMOSET	SQUIRREL MONKEY	BABOON	BONNET MACAQUE	CRAB-EATING MACAQUE	RHESUS MACAQUE	CHIMPANZEE
Age puberty (appearance of spermatozoa) (years)	1.2-1.7	3-5	3-4	3-4	4	2.5-3.5	7-8
Age sexual maturity (effective sire) (years)	1.2-1.7	3-5	4-6	3-4	4	4.5	7-8
Testicle location	Scrotal, parapenile	Scrotal	Scrotal	Scrotal	Scrotal	Scrotal	Scrotal
Accessory glands†	SV, P, B	SV, P, B	SV, P, B	SV, P, B	SV, P, B	SV, P, B	SV, P, B
Techniques of semen collection		Electro-ejaculation	Electro-ejaculation	Electro-ejaculation	Electro-ejaculation	Electro-ejaculation	Electro-ejaculation
Volume of ejaculate, ml, mean (range)		0.4(0.2-1.5)	1(0.5-2.0)		1.2(0.6-3.0)	1.1(0.2-4.5)	1.9(0.5-6.2)
Sperm concentration no. × 10^8/ml, mean (range)		2.1(0.8-3.1)	5(3.5-6.5)		4.6(1.6-8.3)	1.1(1.0-3.6)	6.1(2.3-12.7)

*Adapted from Mather, E. C. and Rushmer, R. A.: In Alexander, N. J. (ed.): Animal Models for Research on Contraception and Fertility. Hagerstown, Md., Harper & Row, 1979, p. 562.
†SV = seminal vesicles, P = prostate, B = bulbourethral gland.

Table 14. Female Reproductive Parameters of Representative Nonhuman Primates*

	New World Monkeys		Old World Monkeys				Anthropoid Ape
	Marmoset	Squirrel Monkey	Baboon	Bonnet Macaque	Crab-Eating Macaque	Rhesus Macaque	Chimpanzee
Age puberty (years)	1.5	3	3–4	3–4	4	2–3.5	6–8.5
Age sexual maturity (years)	1.5	3	5–6	3–4	4	3–5	8–11
Type uterus	Bicornuate	Simplex	Simplex	Simplex	Simplex	Simplex	Simplex
Type placenta, gross	Zonary, monodiscoid	Zonary, monodiscoid	Zonary, monodiscoid	Zonary, bidiscoid	Zonary, bidiscoid	Zonary, bidiscoid	Zonary, monodiscoid
Type placenta, histologic	Hemochorial	Hemochorial	Hemochorial	Hemochorial	Hemochorial	Hemochorial	Hemochorial
Breeding season	All year	Restricted, depends on location	All year	All year	All year, decrease in winter	All year cycling, conception fluctuates, max. Jan.–Mar.	All year
Length sexual cycle, days, mean (range)		9	31–32	30(25–36)	28(25–39)	28(23–33)	35(33–38)
Menstrual flow	None	None	3 days	10 days	2–7 days	2–7 days	3 days
Mechanism of ovulation	Spontaneous	Spontaneous?	Spontaneous	Spontaneous	Spontaneous	Spontaneous	Spontaneous
Time of ovulation			2–3 days prior to onset of marked sex skin deturgescence		11–14 days after onset menses	11–14 days after onset menses	22–28 days after onset menses
Ovulation rate (number of ova)	1–3	1	1		1	1	1
Pseudopregnancy	None	None	None	None	None	None	None
Gestation length, days, mean (range)	142–150	155(140–180)	175(164–186)	153–169	160–170	165(156–180)	228(216–260)
Birth numbers	2(1–3)	1	1	1	1	1	1
Birth weight	96 gm		650–800 gm	330–370 gm	230–470 gm	0.5–0.7 kg	1–2 kg
Weaning weight	300–500 gm		2–4 kg			750–900 gm	4–5 kg
Weaning age (months)	6	4	5–7			3–6	12–24
Return to cyclic activity postpartum			4–8 months			3 months or after weaning	After weaning

*Adpted from Mather., E. C. and Rushmer, R. A.: In Alexander, N. J. (ed.): Animal Models for Research on Contraception and Fertility. Hagerstown, Md., Harper & Row, 1979, p. 564.

Table 15. Male Reproductive Parameters of Representative Laboratory Animals*

	Chinchilla	Ferret	Gerbil	Guinea Pig	Hamster	Mouse	Rabbit	Rat
Age puberty (appearance of spermatozoa)	2–3 months			7–8 weeks	4–6 weeks	4–6 weeks	4 months	6 weeks
Age sexual maturity (effective sire)	8 months	9–12 months	10–12 weeks	8–10 weeks	6–7 weeks	6–8 weeks	6–9 months	10–11 weeks
Testicle location	No scrotum; testes inguinal or subcutaneous	Perianal		Perianal	Scrotal	Scrotal	Scrotal	Scrotal
Accessory glands†			VG, P, CG, B, A	VG, P, CG, B	VG, P, CG, B, A	VG, P, CG, B, A	VG, P, CG, B, A	VG, P, CG, B, A
Techniques of semen collection	Manual manipulation, electroejaculation, cauda epididymides maceration		Epididymal maceration	Epididymal maceration, electroejaculation	Epididymal maceration, electroejaculation	Flush female tract, epididymal maceration, electroejaculation	Artificial vagina	Flush female tract, epididymal maceration
Volume ejaculate	0.01–0.02 ml			0.5 ml	0.01–0.02 ml		0.5–1.5 ml	1–2 drops
Sperm/ejaculate	$1–100 \times 10^6$			$2–160 \times 10^6$	$1.8–2.8 \times 10^3$		$10–1000 \times 10^6$	$50–60 \times 10^6$
Season		December–July			Decreased testicular weight Nov.–Jan.		Decreased sperm production in heat	

*Adapted from Mather, E. C. and Rushmer, R. A.: *In* Alexander, N. J. (ed.): Animal Models for Research on Contraception and Fertility. Hagerstown, MD., Harper & Row, 1979, p. 572.

†VG = vesicular gland, P = prostate, CG = coagulating gland, B = bulbourethral gland, A = ampullae.

Table 16. Female Reproductive Parameters of Representative Laboratory Animals*

	Chinchilla	Ferret	Gerbil
Average lifespan (years)	10	5	3
Age puberty	7–12 months	9–12 months (spring)	9 weeks
Age sexual maturity	7–12 months	Bred 1 year from birth	10–12 weeks
Type uterus	2 horns, 2 cervices		
Type placenta, gross		Zonary	
Type placenta, histologic	Hemoendothelial	Endotheliochorial	
Breeding season	Nov.–May	Mar.–Aug.	Slight winter decline
Type estrous cycle	Polyestrous	Seasonally Polyestrous	Polyestrous
Length estrous cycle	41 days (variable)	No regular cycle, in heat until bred	4–6 days
Duration of estrus	2 days	Prolonged	12–18 hours
Mechanism of ovulation	Spontaneous	Induced	Spontaneous
Time of ovulation		30–40 hours postcoitus	
Ovulation rate (number of ova)	4	5–13	7 (4–9)
Pseudopregnancy		41–42 days	13–18 days
Gestation length	111 days (105–118)	41–44 days	24–25 days
Birth numbers	3 (1–5)	8 (5–15)	4 (1–12)
Chromosome number (diploid)	64	40	44
Birth weight (gm)	43 (30–50)	10 (6–12)	3 (4–8)
Weaning weight (gm)		300–450	11–18
Weaning age (weeks)	6–8	6–8	3
Return to cyclic activity postpartum	Estrus 2–48 hours, conception common	After weaning or next season	Postpartum estrus, regular cycles after weaning

Table 16. Female Reproductive Parameters of Representative Laboratory Animals *Continued*

Guinea Pig	Hamster	Mouse	Rabbit	Rat
3–4	2	1–3	13	3
2 months	4–6 weeks	4–6 weeks	5–9 months	50–72 days
3–4 months	6–8 weeks	6–8 weeks	5–9 months	60–100 days
2 horns, single external cervical os	2 horns, 2 cervices, single external os	2 horns, 2 cervices, 2 external ora	2 horns, 2 cervices	2 horns, 2 cervices, 1 external cervical os
Discoidal		Discoidal	Discoidal	Discoidal
Hemochorial		Hemochorial	Hemoendothelial	Hemochorial
All year	All year, some decrease Oct.–Feb.	All year	All year, decrease in late summer	All year
Polyestrous	Polyestrous	Polyestrous	Polyestrous	Polyestrous
16 days 6 hours	4 days	4–6 days	No regular cycle	4–5 days
8 hours	12–20 hours	10–20 hours	Prolonged	10–20 hours
Spontaneous	Spontaneous	Spontaneous	Induced	Spontaneous
10 hours after onset estrus	8–12 hours after onset estrus	2–3 hours after onset estrus	10–13 hours postcoitus	8–11 hours after onset estrus
3–4	10	10	7 (6–10)	10
None	9–10 days	12 days	14–18 days	12 days
63 days (59–72)	16 days	19–21 days	30–32 days	21–23 days
3 (1–6)	7 (5–10)	8 (6–12)	10 (8–12)	9 (7–14)
64	44	40	44	42
90 (60–110)	2	1–3	30–70	5–6
180–240	35–40	10–12	800–1500	40–50
3	3	3	6–8	3
Postpartum estrus, then regular cycles but infertile until weaning	Postpartum infertile estrus, regular cycles after lactation ends	Postpartum estrus, regular cycles after end of lactation	Fertile postpartum and during lactation	Postpartum estrus, regular cycle after end of lactation

*Adapted from Mather, E. C. and Rushmer, R. A.: *In* Alexander, N. J. (ed.): Animal Models for Research on Contraception and Fertility. Hagerstown, Md., Harper & Row, 1979, pp. 573–574.

Table 17. Breeding Data for Felidae*

Species	Age of Puberty	Characteristics of Cyclicity	Duration of Heat	Duration and Frequency of Copulation	Gestation
African lion	Usually 3 years female and 4–6 years male; can be as early as 2 years	Polyestrous all year with peaks in April and Oct. in some areas	4–16 days	21 second avg. duration; 157 times within 55 hours	98–114 days
Tiger	3½–5 years	Polyestrous all year	3–10 days, avg.: 7.1	0.5–3 (avg. 2) minute duration; 3–23 copulations daily for from 3 to 21 days; 100 observed in 6 days	98–110 days
Leopard		Polyestrous all year in most ranges. Peak births occur in April in India. In Manchuria and eastern Siberia mating is seasonal, i.e., Jan. and Feb.	3–14 days, avg.: 6–9		98–105 days
Jaguar	2½–3 years	Polyestrous all year; may be seasonal in some northern ranges (spring)	6–17 days, avg.: 12.9	2–35 second duration; avg.: 9; in excess of 20 times daily	93–110 days
Snow leopard	2–3 years	Seasonal; usually breed during winter months every second year but have been reported breeding as frequently as twice within a single year and as late as May	4–8 days	10–20 pairings/day have been observed	93–105 days
Clouded leopard	About 2–3 years	2 litters born at Frankfurt Zoo and 1 at Dallas Zoo were born in the spring			86–92 days
Cheetah	14–16 months; 9 months possible for 1 female at Whipsnade Zoo	Seasonally polyestrous; Jan.–April appears to be the peak mating period in East Africa	Approx. 10–14 days	1 minute duration; mating usually 1–8 hours apart	Approx. 90–95 days
European wild cat	Females about 1 year, sometimes as early 10 months. Males 9–10 months	Seasonally polyestrous. Males become sexually active in Jan. Occasionally females have more than 1 litter/year. Females usually do not conceive until 2 years but have done so at 1 year	Up to 8 days, 5–6 avg.	Males will continue copulation even when females are pregnant and after parturition	63–69 days
African wild cat or kaffir cat		Polyestrous, with peak litters, 2–3 in summer. Calls a harsh "mwa, mwa" during mating; very vocal	2–3 days		About 56 days
Jungle cat		Probably polyestrous all year. May is the chief mating season in India and Feb.–March in Russian Central Asia			About 66 days

*From Seager, S. W. J. and Demorest, C. N.: Reproduction of captive wild carnivores. *In* Fowler, M. E. (ed.): Zoo and Wild Animal Medicine. Philadelphia, W. B. Saunders Company, 1978, pp. 668–673.

Table 17. Breeding Data for Felidae *Continued*

Litter Size	Weaning Age	Captive Birth Recorded	Young Reared by Mother in Captivity	Second Generation Young Produced in Captivity	Remarks
1–6 mean: 3.04. A litter of 7 has been reported	Approx. 3 months+	Yes	Yes	Yes	Complex social order and reproductive processes interrelated
1–6; avg.: 2–3	3–5 months	Yes	Yes	Yes	Male should have avenue for escape after mating. Complete isolation for mother and kittens
1–5; avg.: 2	6 weeks	Yes	Yes	Yes	Males should be removed after mating. Pairs often not compatible
1–4; usually 1–2		Yes	Yes	Yes	Males should be removed after mating. Pairs often not compatible
1–4	8–12 weeks	Yes	Yes	Yes	Estrous females may not eat about one third of their usual ration
1–4; avg.: 2	5 months	Yes	Yes	Yes	Males notorious for killing females. Females may kill cubs. Young born in tree hollow.
Avg.: about 4 in wild, with high infant mortality. Usually smaller litters in captivity	About 3 months	Yes	Yes	Yes	Large enclosure with view. Live food may stimulate. Various sex ratios are being tried as well as anestral isolation. View of prey species may be helpful. Denning area for female
1–8; avg.: 3 (Prague Zoo), 4 (Berne Zoo)	6–7 weeks	Yes	Yes, but female has been known to kill young	Yes	Young have been raised without removing male, even though in nature these are very solitary cats. Provision of hiding places considered very important for breeding
1–5; avg.: 3		Yes		Yes	
Usually 3–4, up to 5		Yes	Yes		

Table continued on the following page

Table 17. Breeding Data for Felidae *Continued*

Species	Age of Puberty	Characteristics of Cyclicity	Duration of Heat	Duration and Frequency of Copulation	Gestation
Sand cat		Birth recorded in Transcapia from first of April onward			59–63 days
Black-footed cat	21 months (one report of 8 months for first heat)	Mating is in Feb.–March	36 hours, male only accepted by female for 5–10 hours	Males lose interest sooner than domestic toms. Usually no more than 6 couplings with more time between the earlier and later matings	68 days
Serval cat		Polyestrous all year with peaks in Dec. and March. Have produced 2 litters in a single year	Usually 1 day, sometimes 3–4 days		67–77 days; avg.: 74
Leopard cat or Bengal cat	About 2 years	May is chief mating season in India. Have been recorded as producing more than one litter within a year	4–7 days		63–66 days after last copulation
Rusty spotted cat		Young born in spring in India			
Fishing cat		Assumed to be polyestrous all year. Characteristic mating call heard mainly at night			63 days
Iromote cat		Not discovered until 1967; nothing known about reproductive biology			
Flat-headed cat		A young one was found in the wild in Jan.			
Pallas' cat		Mating occurs during April and May in Transbaikalia			
Marbled cat		Scant literature about reproductive biology			
Bay cat		Scant literature about reproductive biology			
Temminck's golden cat		In wild likes to den in hollow trees			
African golden cat		Scant literature about reproductive biology			
Caracal	Less than 2 years	Polyestrous all year with peaks possibly in Feb., March and Aug.		Has been observed to last approx. 10 minutes/copulation	69–78 days
Puma or mountain lion	2–3 years	Polyestrous all year with birth peaks in June–Sept. in the western U.S. Cycle length averages 22.8 days. Most females litter every 2 years	4–9 days		Approx. 3 months·
Pampas cat					

Table 17. Breeding Data for Felidae *Continued*

Litter Size	Weaning Age	Captive Birth Recorded	Young Reared by Mother in Captivity	Second Generation Young Produced in Captivity	Remarks
2–4		Yes			
		Yes	Yes		Smallest member of Felidae, very shy and antisocial; lowered humidity associated with breeding success
1–4; avg.: 2.35		Yes	Yes		Adapt well to captivity. Need a fairly large enclosure
2–3 avg.		Yes	Yes	Yes	Success in rearing has been had with male and female left in enclosure at same time
2–3					
1–4; usually 2	Greater than 6 months	Yes	Yes		Male and female may need to be separated after mating. A quiet denning area is essential for the female
					Very rare
		Yes			Very rare
5–6		Yes	?		Mating call said to resemble a cross between the bark of a small dog and an owl's hoot
		Yes			
1–3		Yes		Yes	Very nervous
		Yes			
1–6; avg.: 2–3		Yes		Yes	Loud calling at mating. Male should be removed after mating. Increased appetite, with anorexia noted the day before parturition
1–5; rarely 6 (usually 2–3)	about 3	Yes	Yes	Yes	Pregnant females should be isolated. Young stay with mother about 1 year in wild
1–3		Yes			

Table continued on the following page

Table 17. Breeding Data for Felidae *Continued*

Species	Age of Puberty	Characteristics of Cyclicity	Duration of Heat	Duration and Frequency of Copulation	Gestation
Mountain cat or Andean highland cat		Nothing known about the reproductive biology			63–70 days
Jaguarundi		Probably polyestrous all year. Peak mating season in Mexico is Nov. and Dec. Solitary at other times. Two litters (March and Aug.) may be produced			63–70 days
Lynx or northern lynx or European lynx	2–3 years	Seasonal: March is primary mating season and May secondary; usually mate at night; females failing to become pregnant probably return to heat in secondary season. Males vocal	7–10 days		63–74 days
Spanish lynx	1 year for females, to 21 months; male, 33 months	Seasonal: Nov.–Feb. Very vocal during mating season	1–4 days		
Bobcat	1–2 years	Seasonal: From Jan.–July depending on locale. Peak is always in March–April. Animals not pregnant from primary mating period may come in heat again in summer and/or early fall. Mating is a series of running encounters	Approx. 1 week	Fewer copulations than most felids	Approx. 63 days
Ocelot	First heat as early as 8 months, usually do not conceive until 2 years	Polyestrous all year with peak mating activity in Dec. and Jan.	7–10 days, can be out if conceives		89 ± 2 days once cat conceives
Brazilian ocelot-cat or tiger ocelot	About 1 year	Mating peak in Dec.–June	Several days		74–76 days
Margay or tree ocelot					83 days
Geoffroy's cat					71–76 days
Kod Kod or Guina					

Table 17. Breeding Data for Felidae *Continued*

Litter Size	Weaning Age	Captive Birth Recorded	Young Reared by Mother in Captivity	Second Generation Young Produced in Captivity	Remarks
2–4					
2–4		Yes			
1–3	12 weeks	Yes	Yes	?	Postpartum aggressiveness and anorexia observed in female. Male may or may not have to be removed. One tom has bred two females in same cage
	About 2 months	Yes			Bear young in a rocky ledge, natural cavity or thicket
1–6; avg.: 3.5		Yes	Yes		Some bobcats may produce 2 litters/year
1–3; avg.: 1–2		Yes			Often mates are not compatible and males have been known to kill females. It is recommended that females in heat not be presented to strange males. Rather poor overall reproductive success, but as many as 3 litters within a year have been reported
1–2		Yes	Yes		Males have been noted to be very aggressive toward females
1–2		Yes	Yes		Estrous females should not be presented to strange males
2–3		Yes			Mate and kitten slaying have been recorded. Rotating males can increase breeding
					Little known of behavior, but some believe this species may be quite social

Table 18. Reproductive Data for Ungulates

Common Name	Breeding Season	Sexual Maturity (months)	Gestation Period (days)	No. of Young	Normal Adult Weight (kg)	Life Expectancy (years)	Herd Size	Comments
Order Perissodactyla:								
Equidae:								
Przevalsky's horse	All year (especially April and May)	36–60	330–360	1	250–300	25–30	Small groups (up to 20)	
Onager	All year	36–48	330	1	200–250	20–25	Singly, small groups or large groups	
African wild ass	All year (especially April and May)	24–60	360	1	250	25–30	10–15	
Grévy zebra	April–Sept.	36–60	350–390	1	400	20–30	10–15 (in large groups during migration)	
Burchell's zebra	April–May	24–48	350–390	1	350	20–30	10–15 (in large groups during migration)	
Mountain zebra	April–Sept.	24–48	300–375	1	350	20–30	Small groups (7–12)	
Tapiridae:								
Brazilian tapir	All year	36–48	390–400	1	225–300	25–30	Alone or in pairs	All tapirs have striped offspring and cycle every 50–80 days with a 2-day heat
Baird's tapir	All year	36–48	390–400	1	225–300	25–30	Alone or in pairs	
Mountain tapir	All year	36–48	390–400	1	225–250	25–30	Alone or in pairs	
Malayan tapir	All year	36–48	390–400	1	225–300	25–30	Alone or in pairs	
Rhinocerotidae:								
Indian rhinoceros	March and April	48–60	510–570	1	2000–4000	50	Solitary	Heat every 46–48 days for 24 hours
Square lipped (white) rhinoceros	July–Sept.	48–60	530–550	1	2000–3000	30	Small groups up to 18	
Black rhinoceros	All year	48–60	530–550	1	1000–1800	30	Singly or in small groups (1–5)	
Order Artiodactyla								
Suidae:								
River hog	Aug. and Sept.	8–10		2–8	75–130	10		Striped offspring
Wild boar	Dec.–Jan. (highest), all year	8–10	115	4–8	150	15		Striped offspring, female cycle every 21 days estrous period 2–3 days
Wart hog	June–July	12	171–175	3	100	15	Small groups	Striped offspring
Forest hog		8–10	125	2–6	200	2	20	Striped offspring
Babirussa		8–10	125–150	2	100	10		
Tayassuidae:								
Collared peccary	All year	10	142–149	2–3	30	20	5–15	
White lipped peccary	All year	10	142–149	2–3	35	13	50–100	

Species								
Hippopotamidae:								
Nile hippopotamus	All year	36	227–240	1	1300–2000	40–45	10	Nurse in water 35-day cycle with 3-day estrous period; wean at 4 months
Pygmy hippopotamus	All year	48	206–210	1	200–250	35	Singly or in pairs	38-day cycle with 1–2 day estrous
Camelidae:								
Dromedary camel	Feb.–March (especially)	24	315–360	1	500	20	Small groups (5–10)	
Bactrian camel	March	30	389–406	1	700	20	6–20	
Llama	All year	6–24	330	1	100	15–20	Small groups	
Guanaco	Nov.–Feb.	24	330	1	100	15–20	Small groups	
Vicuna	Aug.–Sept.	24	300	1	50	15–20	Small groups	
Alpaca		24	330	1	70	15–20	Small groups	
Cervidae:								
Chevrotain	June and July	18	120–180	1–2	2–5	1–2	Singly	Postpartum estrus 1 day after parturition; no antlers-penis has thread-like extension
Musk deer	Jan.	18	160	1–2	7–17	10		
Muntjac	Jan.–Feb.	18	180	1	15–35	16	Singly or in pairs	
Tufted deer	April–May	18	180	1	40–50	7	Singly or in pairs	
Fallow deer	Sept.–Oct.	18	230	1	35–80	20	Small herds (2–3)	
Axis deer	All year	18	210–225	2	75–100	15–20	Small groups (2–3)	
Sanbar deer	All year	18	249–284	1	60–150	10–25		
Barasingha deer	Oct.–Nov.	18	250	1	230–283	20	Small groups (2–3)	
Elk deer	March–May	18	180	1	80–150	20		
Sika deer	Sept.–Oct.	18	222–246	1	25–110	15–20	Small groups	
Red deer	July–Sept.	24	225–262	1	125–350	15–20	Large herds	
American elk	"	"	"	"	"	"	"	
Pere David deer	June–July	30	250–270	1–2	150–200	20	12–15	
White tailed deer	Nov.	7	201	1–2	50–150	10	Singly or in small groups (5)	
Mule deer	Nov.–Dec.	7	210–260	1–2	50–150	10	Singly or in small groups (5)	
Moose	Sept.–Oct.	18	240–250	1–2	80–150	25	Singly or in pairs	Difficult to keep in captivity
Reindeer	Sept.–Oct.	18	240	1–2		15	5–40	
Roe deer	July–Aug.	15		1–3		10	Small groups (2–3)	
Giraffidae:								
Giraffe	All year	42	420–468	1	500–800	25	Singly or in small groups	14-day estrous cycle, 24-hour estrus period, wean 6–9 months
Okapi	June–July	30	426–457	1		15–20	Singly	
Antilocapridae:								
Pronghorn		16	230–240	2	50	7–10	Small to large groups	

Table continued on the following page

Table 18. Reproductive Data for Ungulates *Continued*

Order Artiodactyla (*Continued*)
Bovidae:

Common Name	Breeding Season	Sexual Maturity (months)	Gestation Period (days)	No. of Young	Normal Adult Weight (kg)	Life Expectancy (years)	Herd Size	Comments
Greater kudu	All year	30	210–240	1	200–250	15	6–20 in herd	
Lesser kudu	All year	24	210	1	100	12–15	6 in group	
Sitatunga		24	210–225	1–2	100	17		
Nyala	Jan.–Feb.	30	210	1	100–125	15	Singly or in pairs	
Bushbuck		24	225	1	100	12	Small groups	
Eland	All year	30	255–270	1	1000	25	Singly or in pairs	
Bongo		30	225	1	200	20	Singly or in pairs	
Nilgai	End of March	30		1 first year, 2 thereafter	200	15	Small groups	
Four horned antelope	June–July	24	225–240	1–3	15–25	10	Singly or in pairs	
Anda	All year (especially May)	30	275–315		150–300	28	Singly or in pairs	
Water buffalo	All year	30	300–340	1				
African buffalo	All year	18	300–330	1	1000	20–25	Herds (10–20)	
Gaur	All year	24	270–280	1	300–800	25	Herds (30–60)	Wean 6 months
Banteng	July–Aug.	24	270–280	1	700–1000	25	Groups (8–12)	Wean at 9 months
Kouprey	April–May	24	270	1	500–900	15	Small groups	
Yak	Aug.–Sept.	60	258	1	900	12	Small groups (8–11)	
Bison	May–Sept.	24	270–285	1	1000	25	Large herds 100+	Wean at 12 months
Wisent	Aug.–Sept.	24	260–270	1	1000	20–25	Herds (20–30)	
Duiker			120	1	25	25	Large and small herds	
Hartebeest			240	1	120–215	10	Singly or in pairs	
Sassaby	Dec.–March	24	210–240	1		15	5–30 in group	
Blesbok			225–240	1			Small groups	
White tailed gnu	June	30	240	1	125	15	Small groups (8–10)	
Brindled gnu	June	30	240–270	1	100	15	Small groups (8–10)	
Roan antelope	All year	24	270–280	1	145–270	20	Large herds	
Sable antelope	All year	24	270–281	1	150–300	15	Small groups (3–15)	
Oryx	All year	24	270	1	150–250	15	Small groups (20)	
Addax	March–May (especially), all year	24	300–360	1	100–200	15–20	Small herds, up to 20	
					50–100	18	5–20	

Species	Season		Gestation	Young	Weight		Social grouping	
Waterbuck	All year	24	240–270	1	170–250	15	Up to 30	
Lechwe waterbuck	Oct.–Jan.	24	210	1	60–120	15	Group, up to 50	
Kob	All year	24	240–270	1	50–120	15	Small groups	
Reedbuck	All year	20	180–210	1	25–75	12	Small groups, up to 20	
Dik-dik	All year	6	180	1	2–6	7	Pairs	
Klipspringer		15	210	1	15	15	Singly and pairs	
Steinbok			210		20	12	Singly or pairs	
Gazelles	All year	12	150–180	1–2	15–25	10	5–20, herds	
Blackbuck	All year	12	180	1	25–45	15	6–10, herds	
Impala	Feb.–April	12	190–200	1	40–90	10	6–60	
Gerenuk		15	210	1	35–52	7–8	Pairs or small groups	
Springbok	May	15	180	1	18–45	10	Small to large groups	
Tibetan antelope	Nov.–Dec.		180	1–2	25–35		10–20	
Saiga antelope	Nov.	8	150	1	23–40	4	2–50	
Goral	Sept.–Oct.		180	1	25–35	11	Small groups	
Serow			210–240	1	55–140		Small groups	
Takin			210–240		350		Small herds	
Chamois	Oct.–Jan.	24	80	1	14–62		Small groups, up to 10	
Rocky mountain goat		18	180		150	8	Small groups, up to 10	
Musk ox	July–Aug.	24	255	1	200–300	10	15	
Ibex	Dec.–Jan.	18	150–180	1–3	35–150	15–20	Small herds, up to 20	
Markhor	Nov.–Jan.	18	180		32–40	10		
Wild goat	Nov.–Jan.	18	180	1–3	25–40	10		
Tahr	Dec. (especially), all year	18	150–180	1–3	100	15–20	30–40	
Blue sheep	Oct.–Nov.	18	160	1–3	25–80	15	Small and large herds	
Aoudad (Barbary sheep)	Nov.	18	150–165	1–3	40–140	15	Singly or in small groups	Wean in 6 months
Mouflon	Oct.–Dec.	18	150	1–2	35–50	15–20	Small groups	
Red sheep (Marco Polo)		18	147–188			5–10	Large groups	
Big horn sheep		18	180	1	150		Large groups	

From Boever B: Reproduction of wild ungulates. In Morrow DA (ed): Current Therapy in Theriogenology. 1st ed. Philadelphia, WB Saunders Co. 1980, pp 1120–1123.

Table 19. Criteria For Hand-Raising Ungulates

Name	Weight at Birth (kg)	Type of Nipple	Birth to 2 Weeks		2 Weeks		Formula Recommended
			FEEDINGS/DAY	AMOUNT/FEEDING	FEEDINGS/DAY	AMOUNT/FEEDING	
Zebra	30–50	Albers' calf nipple	4–5	300–500 ml	4–5	500 ml–1 liter	1 part evaporated milk, 1 part distilled water
Tapir	3–10	Lamb or calf nipple	4–5	300–500 ml	4–15	500 ml–1 liter	1 part evaporated milk, 1 part distilled water
Rhinoceros	25–75						1 part evaporated milk, 1 part water
Peccary	0.5–1.0	Albers' calf nipple	4–5	15–60 ml	4–5	30–120 ml	
Nile hippopotamus	30–50						
Pygmy hippopotamus	3–5						
Dromedary camel	30–45	Albers' calf nipple (small cross-cut)	4–6	0.5 liter	4	1.5 liters	3 parts evaporated milk, 3 parts distilled water, 1 part lime water
Llama	7–15	Regular Evenflow nipple (small cross-cut)	4–5	120–240 ml	4	240 ml	1 part evaporated milk, 1 part water
White tailed deer		Evenflow	4–5	60–120 ml	3–5	120–240 ml	Straight evaporated milk
Bison	24–27	Albers' calf nipple	4–6	300 ml–1 liter	4–5	0.5–1 liter	1 part evaporated milk, 1 part distilled water
Eland	31	Albers' calf nipple	3–5	180 ml–1 liter	3–5	240 ml–2 liters	1 part evaporated milk, 1 part water
Springbok	3	Evenflow	4–5	90–150 ml	3–4	150–240 ml	1 part evaporated milk, 1 part water
Impala		Evenflow	2–3	30–180 ml	3	150–240 ml	1 part evaporated milk, 1 part water
Kudu		Lamb or calf nipple	2–6	240–360 ml	4–6	100–240 ml	1 part evaporated milk, 1 part water
Aoudad	2.5–5.0	Evenflow	4–6	60–120 ml	4–5	120–180 ml	1–1.5 parts evaporated milk, 1 part water
Mouflon	2.5–5.0	Preemie large pinhole, small cross-cut	4–6	60–150 ml	4	120–240 ml	1–1.5 parts evaporated milk, 1 part water
Artiodactyla in general			5	Depends on size, approximately 20 ml/kg	5	Depends on size, approximately 20 ml/kg	1 part evaporated milk, 1 part water

From Boever B.: Reproduction of wild ungulates. *In* Morrow DA (ed): Current Therapy of Theriogenology. 1st ed. Philadelphia, WB Saunders Co, 1980, p 1124.

Index

Note: Page numbers in italics indicate illustrations; those followed by (t) indicate tables.